CANCER NURSING
Principles and Practice

The Jones and Bartlett Series in Nursing

Basic Steps in Planning Nursing Research, Third Edition
Brink/Wood

Cancer Chemotherapy: A Nursing Process Approach
Burke et al.

Cancer Nursing: Principles and Practice, Second Edition
Groenwald et al.

Chronic Illness: Impact and Intervention, Second Edition
Lubkin

A Clinical Manual for Nursing Assistants
McClelland/Kaspar

Clinical Nursing Procedures
Belland/Wells

Comprehensive Maternity Nursing, Second Edition
Auvenshine/Enriquez

Cross Cultural Perspectives in Medical Ethics: Readings
Veatch

Drugs and Society, Second Edition
Witters/Venturelli

Emergency Care of Children
Thompson

First Aid and Emergency Care Workbook
Thygerson

Fundamentals of Nursing with Clinical Procedures, Second Edition
Sundberg

1991 Handbook of Intravenous Medications
Nentwich

Health and Wellness, Third Edition
Edlin/Golanty

Health Assessment in Nursing Practice, Second Edition
Grimes/Burns

Human Anatomy and Physiology Coloring Workbook and Study Guide
Anderson

Human Development: A Life-Span Approach, Third Edition
Freiberg

Intravenous Therapy
Nentwich

Introduction to the Health Professions
Stanfield

Introduction to Leadership and Management in Nursing, Second Edition
Holle/Blatchley

Management and Leadership for Nurse Managers
Swansburg

Management of Spinal Cord Injury, Second Edition
Zejdlik

Medical Ethics
Veatch

Medical Terminology: Principles and Practices
Stanfield

The Nation's Health, Third Edition
Lee/Estes

Nursing Assessment: A Multidimensional Approach, Second Edition
Bellack/Bamford

Nursing Diagnosis Care Plans for Diagnosis-Related Groups
Neal/Paquette/Mirch

Nursing Management of Children
Servonsky/Opas

Nursing Research: A Quantitative and Qualitative Approach
Roberts/Burke

Nutrition and Diet Therapy: Self-Instructional Modules
Stanfield

Oncogenes
Cooper

Operating Room Nursing
Fairchild

Psychiatric Mental Health Nursing, Second Edition
Janosik/Davies

Writing a Successful Grant Application, Second Edition
Reif-Lehrer

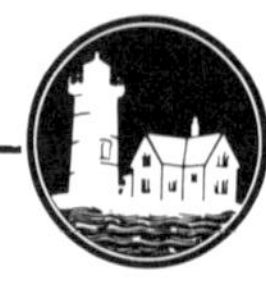

CANCER NURSING
Principles and Practice

Second Edition

EDITED BY:

Susan L. Groenwald, RN, MS
Assistant Professor of Nursing—Complemental
Department of Medical Nursing
Rush University College of Nursing

Rush-Presbyterian-St. Luke's Medical Center
Chicago, Illinois

Margaret Hansen Frogge, RN, MS
Senior Vice President, Clinical Services
Coordinator, Community Cancer Program

Riverside Medical Center
Kankakee, Illinois

Michelle Goodman, RN, MS
Assistant Professor of Nursing
Rush University College of Nursing
Teacher/Practitioner, Department of Surgical Nursing
Section of Medical Oncology

Rush-Presbyterian-St. Luke's Medical Center
Chicago, Illinois

Connie Henke Yarbro, RN, BSN
Editor, *Seminars in Oncology Nursing*
Clinical Associate Professor
Department of Medicine
Division of Hematology/Oncology

University of Missouri—Columbia
Columbia, Missouri

JONES AND BARTLETT PUBLISHERS
Boston

"Any one cell, embodying as it does the record of a billion years of evolution, represents more an historical than a physical event. You cannot expect to explain such a wise old bird in a few simple words."

MAX DELBRUCHT
California Institute of Technology

DEDICATION

To our colleagues in cancer nursing . . .
Who strive to meet the challenges imposed by the manifestations of wayward cells, and . . .
Who care for the complex human beings who live with those manifestations.

SLG, MHF, MG, CHY

Editorial, Sales, and Customer Service Offices

Jones and Bartlett Publishers
20 Park Plaza
Boston, MA 02116

Printed in the United States of America
10 9 8 7 6 5 4 3 2 1

Library of Congress Cataloging-in-Publication Data

Cancer nursing: principles and practice/edited by Susan L.
Groenwald . . . [et al.].—2nd ed.
p. cm.
Includes bibliographical references.
ISBN 0-86720-435-4
1. Cancer—Nursing. I. Groenwald, Susan L.
[DNLM: 1. Neoplasms—nursing. WY 156 C2197]
RC266.C356 1990
610.73'698—dc20
DNLM/DLC
for Library of Congress 89-71658
CIP

ISBN: 0-86720-435-4

The selection and dosage of drugs presented in this book are in accord with standards accepted at the time of publication. The authors and publisher have made every effort to provide accurate information. However, research, clinical practice, and government regulations often change the accepted standard in this field. Before administering any drug, the reader is advised to check the manufacturer's product information sheet for the most up-to-date recommendations on dosage, precautions, and contraindications. This is especially important in the case of drugs that are new or seldom used.

Production: CRACOM Corporation
Production Services Coordinator: Judy Salvucci
Cover Design: Rafael Millán

CONTRIBUTORS

Katherine T. Alkire, RN, MN
Oncology Clinical Nurse Specialist
St. Luke's Regional Medical Center
Boise, ID

Barbara D. Blumberg, ScM
Director of Education
Komen Alliance Clinical Breast Center
Charles A. Sammons Cancer Center
Baylor University Medical Center
Dallas, TX

Joy H. Boarini, RN, MSN, CETN
Professional Education Manager
Hollister Incorporated
Libertyville, IL

Ann Rohman Booth, RN, BSN
Clinical Research Nurse
Hematology and Oncology
University of Arizona Cancer Center
Tucson, AZ

Jean K. Brown, RN, MS, PhD Cand.
University of Rochester
School of Nursing
Rochester, NY

Patricia Corcoran Buchsel, RN, BSN
Director, Outpatient Nursing
Fred Hutchinson Cancer Research Center
Seattle, WA

Candace Carter-Childs, RN, MS
AIDS Project Case Manager
Hospice of Marin
Marin County, CA
Assistant Clinical Professor
University of California
San Francisco, CA

Jane C. Clark, RN, MN, OCN
Oncology Clinical Nurse Specialist
Assistant Professor
Emory University
Atlanta, GA

Rebecca F. Cohen, RN, EdD, CPQA
Instructor, Community Health
School of Allied Health Professions
Northern Illinois University
DeKalb, IL

Mary Barton Cook, RN, BSN, OCN
Director of Nursing
Oncology Program Coordinator
CPS Pharmaceutical Services
IV and Nutritional Services Division
Mountain View, CA

Vincent T. DeVita, Jr, MD
Physician-in-Chief
Memorial Sloan-Kettering Cancer Center
New York, NY

Kathy A. Dietz, RN, MA, MS
Nurse Clinician—Hematology
Memorial Sloan-Kettering Cancer Center
Associate
Columbia University School of Nursing
New York, NY

Joanne M. Disch, RN, PhD
Clinical Director
Department of Medical Nursing, Emergency Services and Dialysis
Hospital of the University of Pennsylvania
Assistant Professor of Nursing
University of Pennsylvania School of Nursing
Philadelphia, PA

Michele Girard Donehower, RN, MSN
Student, Nurse Practitioner Program
University of Maryland School of Nursing
Baltimore, MD

Constance T. Donovan, RN, MSN, FAAN
Oncology Clinical Nurse Specialist
Yale New Haven Hospital
Associate Clinical Professor
Yale University School of Nursing
New Haven, CT

Diane Scott Dorsett, RN, PhD, FAAN
Director
Comprehensive Support Services for Persons with Cancer
Associate Clinical Professor
University of California
San Francisco, CA

Susan Dudas, RN, MSN
Associate Professor
College of Nursing
University of Illinois at Chicago
Chicago, IL

Ellen Heid Elpern, RN, MSN
Clinical Nurse Specialist
Section of Pulmonary Medicine
Assistant Professor of Nursing
Rush University
Rush-Presbyterian-St. Luke's Medical Center
Chicago, IL

Dolores Esparza, RN, MS
President
Esparza Oncology Consultants, Inc.
San Antonio, TX

Betty Rolling Ferrell, RN, PhD, FAAN
Research Scientist, Nursing Research
City of Hope National Medical Center
Duarte, CA

Anne Marie Flaherty, RN, MS
Administrative Nurse Clinician
Adult Day Hospital
Memorial Sloan-Kettering Cancer Center
New York, NY

Arlene E. Fleck, RN, MNEd
Clinical Cancer Research Coordinator
Cancer Prevention Center
Kelsey-Seybold Foundation
Houston, TX

Marilyn Frank-Stromborg, RN, EdD, Nurse Practitioner, FAAN
Coordinator
Oncology Clinical Specialist Program
Professor
School of Nursing
Northern Illinois University
DeKalb, IL

Margaret Hansen Frogge, RN, MS
Senior Vice President, Clinical Services
Coordinator, Community Cancer Program
Riverside Medical Center
Kankakee, IL

Gayling Gee, RN, MS
Director, Outpatient Nursing
San Francisco General Hospital
Assistant Clinical Professor
School of Nursing
University of California
San Francisco, CA

Barbara Holmes Gobel, RN, MS
Oncology Clinical Nurse Specialist
Lake Forest Hospital
Faculty, Complemental
Rush University College of Nursing
Chicago, IL

Michelle Goodman, RN, MS
Oncology Clinical Nurse Specialist
Section of Medical Oncology
Assistant Professor of Nursing
Rush University
Rush-Presbyterian-St. Luke's Medical Center
Chicago, IL

Marcia M. Grant, RN, DNSc, OCN
Director of Nursing Research and Education
City of Hope National Medical Center
Duarte, CA

Susan L. Groenwald, RN, MS
Oncology Nurse Consultant
Assistant Professor of Nursing—Complemental
Rush University College of Nursing
Chicago, IL

Shirley M. Gullo, RN, MSN, OCN
Oncology Nurse
The Cleveland Clinic Foundation
Cleveland, OH

Patricia Hakius, RN, MSN
Cancer Care Consultant
Doctoral Student
University of San Diego
San Diego, CA

Nancy E. Harte, RN, MS
Oncology Clinical Nurse Specialist
Section of Medical Oncology
Rush-Presbyterian-St. Luke's Medical Center
Instructor
Rush University College of Nursing
Chicago, IL

Laura J. Hilderley, RN, MS
Oncology Clinical Nurse Specialist
Private Practice of Philip G. Maddock, MD
Radiation Oncology
Warwick, RI

Barbara Hoffman, JD
Private Consultant
Cancer Survivorship and Discrimination
Princeton, NJ

Catherine M. Hogan, RN, MN, OCN
Oncology Clinical Nurse Specialist
Department of Hematology/Oncology
University of Michigan
Ann Arbor, MI

Susan Molloy Hubbard, RN, BA
Director
International Cancer Information Center
National Cancer Institute
Bethesda, MD

Patricia F. Jassak, RN, MS, CS
Oncology Clinical Nurse Specialist
Foster G. McGaw Hospital
Loyola University of Chicago
Chicago, IL

Judith (Judi) L. Bond Johnson, RN, PhD
Nursing Director
North Memorial Medical Center
Minneapolis, MN

Paula R. Klemm, RN, DNSc Cand.
Nursing Instructor II
The Johns Hopkins Oncology Center
Baltimore, MD

Linda U. Krebs, RN, MS, OCN
Oncology Nursing Program Leader
University of Colorado Cancer Center
Denver, CO

Charles E. Kupchella, PhD
Dean
Ogden College of Science, Technology and Health
Western Kentucky University
Bowling Green, KY

Jennifer M. Lang-Kummer, RN, MS
Oncology Clinical Nurse Specialist
Beaumont County Hospital
Washington, NC

Susan Leigh, RN, BSN
Cancer Survivorship Consultant
Tucson, AZ

Julena M. Lind, RN, MN
Executive Director
Center for Health Information, Education and Research
California Medical Center
Adjunct Assistant Professor of Nursing
University of Southern California
Los Angeles, CA

Ada M. Lindsey, RN, PhD
Dean and Professor
School of Nursing
University of California
Los Angeles, CA

Lois J. Loescher, RN, MS
Research Specialist
Program Coordinator
Cancer Prevention and Control
University of Arizona Cancer Center
Tucson, AZ

Alice J. Longman, RN, EdD
Associate Professor
College of Nursing
University of Arizona
Tucson, AZ

Jean McNicholas Lydon, RN, MS
Oncology Clinical Nurse Specialist
Department of Therapeutic Radiology
Rush-Presbyterian-St. Luke's Medical Center
Chicago, IL

Mary B. Maxwell, RN, C, PhD
Oncology Clinical Nurse Specialist
Nurse Practitioner
Veterans' Administration Medical Center
Portland, OR

Mary Dee McEvoy, RN, PhD
Robert Wood Johnson Clinical Nurse Scholar
Hematology/Oncology Section
Division of Nursing
Hospital of the University of Pennsylvania
Philadelphia, PA

Rose F. McGee, RN, PhD
Professor
American Cancer Society Professor of Oncology Nursing
Emory University
Atlanta, GA

Deborah B. McGuire, RN, PhD
Assistant Professor
The Johns Hopkins University School of Nursing
Director of Nursing Research
The Johns Hopkins Oncology Center
Baltimore, MD

Joan C. McNally, RN, MSN
Executive Director
Michigan Cancer Foundation Services, Inc.
Detroit, MI

Nancy Miller, RN, MS
Assistant Director of Testing Services
National Council of State Boards of Nursing, Inc.
Chicago, IL

Ida Marie (Ki) Moore, RN, DNS
Assistant Professor
College of Nursing
University of Arizona
Tucson, AZ

Theresa A. Moran, RN, MS
Oncology/AIDS Clinical Nurse Specialist
Oncology/AIDS Clinic
San Francisco General Hospital
Assistant Clinical Professor
School of Nursing
University of California
San Francisco, CA

Marian E. Morra, MA
Assistant Director
Yale University Comprehensive Cancer Center
New Haven, CT

Lillian M. Nail, RN, PhD
Assistant Professor
University of Rochester School of Nursing
Clinician II
University of Rochester Cancer Center
Rochester, NY

Susie Lee Nakao, RN, MN
Nurse Manager
Clinical Research Center
Los Angeles County
University of Southern California
Los Angeles, CA

Denise Oleske, RN, DPH
Research Associate
Department of Health Systems Management
Department of Preventive Medicine
Rush-Presbyterian-St. Luke's Medical Center
Assistant Professor
College of Health Systems Management
Rush University
Chicago, IL

Sharon Saldin O'Mary, RN, MN
Home Care Coordinator
Stevens Cancer Center
Scripps Memorial Hospital
LaJolla, CA

Edith O'Neil-Page, RN, BSN
Nursing Supervisor
The Kenneth Norris Jr. Hospital and Research Institute
Los Angeles, CA

Diane M. Otte, RN, MS, ET
Administrative Director—Cancer Program
St. Luke's Hospital Cancer Center
Davenport, IA

Geraldine V. Padilla, PhD
Associate Professor
Associate Dean for Research
School of Nursing
University of California
Los Angeles, CA

Mary Pazdur, RN, MS, OCN
Head Nurse
Discharge Planning
The University of Texas
M.D. Anderson Cancer Center
Houston, TX

Patricia A. Piasecki, RN, MS
Joint Practice
Section of Orthopedic Oncology
Rush-Presbyterian-St. Luke's Medical Center
Chicago, IL

Sandra Purl, RN, MS, OCN
Oncology Clinical Nurse Specialist
Section of Medical Oncology
Rush-Presbyterian-St. Luke's Medical Center
Instructor
Rush University College of Nursing
Chicago, IL

Kathy Ruccione, RN, MPH
Division of Hematology Oncology
Children's Hospital of Los Angeles
Los Angeles, CA

Beth Savela, RN, BSN
Graduate Student
Oncology Clinical Specialist Program
School of Nursing
Northern Illinois University
DeKalb, IL

Vivian R. Sheidler, RN, MS
Clinical Nurse Specialist in Neuro-Oncology
The Johns Hopkins Oncology Center
Baltimore, MD

Joy Stair, RN, MS
Education Specialist
Department of Nursing Education, Quality and Research
Catherine McAuley Health Center
Ann Arbor, MI

Debra K. Sullivan, RD, MS
Research Specialist in Nutrition
Center for Handicapped Children
University of Illinois Hospital
Chicago, IL

Debra J. Szeluga, RD, PhD
Assistant Professor of Clinical Nutrition
Assistant Professor of Medicine
Section of Medical Oncology
Co-Director
Nutrition Consultation Service
Rush University
Rush-Presbyterian-St. Luke's Medical Center
Chicago, IL

Mary Taverna, RN
Executive Director
Hospice of Marin
Marin County, CA

Claudette G. Varricchio, RN, DSN, OCN
Associate Professor
Medical-Surgical Nursing
Niehoff School of Nursing
Loyola University of Chicago
Chicago, IL

JoAnn Wegmann, RN, PhD
Assistant Administrator
Director of Nursing Services
Poway Community Hospital
Poway, CA

Deborah Welch-McCaffrey, RN, MSN, OCN
Oncology Clinical Nurse Specialist
Good Samaritan Cancer Center
Phoenix, AZ

Debra Wujcik, RN, MSN, OCN
Oncology Clinical Nurse Specialist
Oncology/Hematology
Vanderbilt University Medical Center
Adjunct Instructor of Nursing
Vanderbilt University School of Nursing
Nashville, TN

Connie Henke Yarbro, RN, BSN
Clinical Associate Professor
Department of Medicine
University of Missouri-Columbia
Editor, *Seminars in Oncology Nursing*
Columbia, MO

J. W. Yarbro, MD, PhD
Professor of Medicine
Director of Hematology and Medical Oncology
University of Missouri-Columbia
Columbia, MO

FOREWORD

The pace of development in the cancer field and the gratifying assumption of a greater role for nurses in the delivery of cancer care dictates the need for freshness in a modern nursing text on cancer. The second edition of this text provides the opportunity to maintain that freshness. It also provides the opportunity to reflect on where we have been and where we are going. Much of the progress taking place can be described as occurring in two overlapping waves; a breathtaking wave of new technology, developed as a consequence of the biologic revolution, lapping at a wave of significant improvements in technology in existence before 1971. Nineteen seventy-one is a good benchmark year; the key event that year was the passage of the National Cancer Act. The vision of the architects of that Act was prescient. The resources supplied by the US Congress fueled the biologic revolution that is now affecting all of medicine. Before then we had little appreciation of the mechanism of uncontrolled growth we call cancer and how the cell machinery was damaged in the process of carcinogenesis. We knew early diagnosis was useful but not why, and while we had refined methods to control primary tumors with surgery and radiotherapy, more than 65% of the patients died of their disease as a result of micrometastases already present at the time of diagnosis, not included in surgical or radiation treatment fields. To overcome this problem, surgery and radiotherapy had become radicalized, and often mutilating, in an attempt to widen their impact on the illusive cancer cell, which was envisioned as spreading by contiguous involvement of adjacent tissue before entering the blood stream. The use of systemic therapy, concomitant with local treatment, was controversial and of unproven value. Attempts at prevention were almost nonexistent.

In other words, cancer was like a black box. We could remove it or destroy it, when we could identify it; we could examine it, we could measure it, we could weigh it, but we could not out-think it because we could not effectively look inside the cell itself. The biologic revolution wrought by the Cancer Act provided the tools of molecular biology that changed all that.

Now the cancer cell is like a blue print; not only is the machinery of the cancer process exposed for examination and manipulation, but also in this exposure we have uncovered important information in developmental biology—the essence of life itself. We now know that cell growth is controlled by a series of growth regulating genes that operate in a biologic cascade from recessive suppressor genes to dominant genes we know as proto-oncogenes in normal tissue and as oncogenes in cancer tissue, of which there are now more than 40 identified. These genes code for growth factors, their receptors, membrane signal transducing proteins, protein kinases, and DNA binding proteins, all important in signal transmission, which in turn is the way multicellular organisms maintain order in their community of cells. While these genes are involved in normal growth and development, mother nature has wisely provided a means for suppressing their expression in mature organisms since their continued operation would be dangerous. Similarly, the metastatic process is no longer thought to be a random phenomenon tied only to tumor growth but has been found to be an aberration of the process of cell migration in normal development and, like the growth controlling function of oncogenes, subject to manipulation by molecular methods. Cancer can result from damage to any of several of the steps in this genetic cascade. Inherited loss or damage of an allele of a recessive suppressor gene appears to lead to a release of the cascade of oncogenes and uncontrolled expression. Damage to a dominant oncogene can lead to escape from control by suppressor genes. Overproduction of a normal or abnormal protein product of an oncogene can occur due to failure of the cell to respond to "off" signals. The startling advances in molecular technology make it possible to isolate and manipulate the products of these genes with ease and use them as diagnostic and therapeutic targets. This was the promise of the cancer program and this is the payoff.

This new wave is, however, just now reaching the level of practical use. For example, in diagnosis, molecular probes and the extraordinarily sensitive polymerase chain reaction can be used to diagnose gene rearrangements to determine cell lineage in malignancies of lymphoid origin, and specific sequences at break points of nonrandom chromosome translocations can be used to diagnose solid tumors. The polymerase chain reaction can be used as a tool to monitor the effects of treatment by detecting one residual malignant cell out of a million normal cells. A molecular approach to treatment also is surfacing in the form of antisense message compounds, chemically stabilized pieces of DNA complementary for, and inhibitory to, the message strand of the DNA of an operational gene or the message of specific target genes such as oncogenes. An extension of this approach will be the use of analogs of the recently identified products of suppressor genes to attempt to bring the oncogene cascade under control. A crest of this new wave of technology in treatment has reached the clinic in the practical application of the colony-stimulating factors produced through DNA recombinant technology, which is already influencing the use of chemotherapy, and the recombinant-produced interleukins and interferons, which have already produced useful antitumor effects by themselves.

Perhaps the most important and often overlooked implication of the biologic revolution is in its potential to allow meaningful approaches to cancer prevention. One of the main roadblocks to testing new ways to prevent cancer has been the identification of groups of high-risk populations small enough to allow prospective prevention trials to proceed at reasonable costs and with a reasonable prospect of answering important questions in the lifetime of the involved investigators. Genetic analysis of common tumors such as colon, breast, and lung cancers following on the heels of the first work on the identification of deletion of suppressor genes in the rare tumor retinoblastoma indicates that deletions of suppressor genes are common and likely to be tumor specific. These new approaches, when applied to the population at large, should allow us to identify individuals at high risk for getting common cancers. Then and only then can we accurately determine if the many interesting leads in prevention identified in the vast number of epidemiologic studies supported by the cancer program over the last two decades can truly be exploited to prevent common cancers.

This then is the new wave. A simultaneous wave of advancement in existing technology of a more practical nature has occurred in cancer management. The emergence of high-speed computers converted roentgenographic diagnosis and staging from plain film and linear tomography to computerized tomography and made magnetic resonance imaging an indispensable tool. Older, less precise, more morbid methods of diagnosis and staging have slowly, and appropriately, fallen into disuse. In 1971, we had just become aware that drugs could cure some types of advanced cancer, and the exploration of adjuvant chemotherapy had just begun. Now adjuvant drug treatments have proven beneficial in breast, colon, rectal, ovarian, head and neck, bladder, and pediatric tumors and in some kinds of lung cancer and bone and soft tissue sarcoma. Chemotherapy has quietly become the primary treatment for all stages of some types of lymphomas and for some stages of some types of head and neck cancers and bladder cancers. We also have developed a greater appreciation of the reason for treatment failure. A form of multiple drug resistance has been described in common tumors, derived from tissue exposed to the environment, that affects drugs derived from natural sources like some of our best antitumor antibiotics. We are just now beginning to design protocols to circumvent multidrug resistance. The use of bone marrow transplantation to support high doses of chemotherapy has made us acutely aware of past treatment failures due to inadequate dosing that can now be overcome with concomitant use of colony-stimulating factors to promote more rapid recovery of bone marrows. New radiotherapy equipment, coupled with computerized tomography treatment planning, has made radiotherapy less morbid and more acceptable as an alternative to radical surgery.

As a consequence of all this, combined modality treatment is no longer what it was in the early 1970s. It no longer means doing the standard radical surgical procedures, adding the standard extensive and toxic radiation therapy fields, and later the standard drug combination, but instead initial treatment is being offered with a precise design based on the capability of each modality in controlling local tumor and metastases while minimizing toxicity. In other words, cancer management has become a complex medical jigsaw puzzle administered by dedicated professionals, many of whom are nurse practitioners, and almost unnoticed, has become far less morbid. Since cancer treatment is still far too morbid, this latter change has been difficult for many to appreciate. However, those of us who have seen both ends of the spectrum over the past two decades have a greater appreciation of the change in morbidity of treatment than a newcomer. Nowhere is this change more evident than in breast cancer where 15 years ago a radical mastectomy followed by postoperative radiation cured a handful of patients, while leaving the few survivors with the morbid effects of a denuded chest wall and a swollen nonfunctional arm. Now survival is improved with specifically tailored local and systemic treatment with fewer side effects and excellent cosmetic results. Fifteen years ago nausea and vomiting, pain, and marrow suppression were largely uncontrollable side effects, and now all can be managed to a great degree.

Unlike the new wave of advances in molecular biology, which remains to be widely implemented before it will have an impact on cancer mortality, the improvement in current technology has already had an impact on national statistics. In 1971, the relative survival rate for all cancers combined was barely 36%; it has increased to 49% in the last available data ending in 1985. Declines in national mortality, formerly only noted in children under the age of 15, are now apparent in all age groups up to age 65, and if one excludes lung cancer, a largely preventable disease, a decline in national mortality is noted all the way up to age 85.

The challenge before us is to smooth the transition of these successive waves of progress into medical practice. It has never been easy because one must recognize them as they exist, separate and distinct bodies of knowledge, each affecting medical practice in different ways, but waves that will eventually summate. Their combined impact gives us the means to effect a significant reduction in cancer mortality by the year 2000. Successful reduction in cancer mortality, however, depends on a cooperative partnership between the medical profession and the public to use modern information to prevent cancer and to implement newly developed treatment rapidly and effectively nationwide. Aside from lagging support for cancer research, which threatens the momentum of change, the machinery in place to do all this is hampered by outdated regulations, unimaginative reimbursement policies, medical territoriality, and unwarranted pessimism about the prospects for controlling cancer in our lifetime. The prospects have never been better but, as the framers of the National Cancer Act knew, nonscientific reasons and failure of all of us to think about controlling cancer on a national scale are major deterrents to success. Nurses reading this text should keep this in mind because they will play an increasingly important role in the next decade in bridging the various medical specialty interests and the delivery of the new cancer care.

VINCENT T. DEVITA, JR, MD

Physician-in-Chief
Memorial Sloan-Kettering Cancer Center
1275 York Avenue
New York, New York 10021

PREFACE TO THE SECOND EDITION

Our goal in the second edition of *Cancer Nursing: Principles and Practice* is to provide the reader with the most comprehensive information about cancer nursing available in the 1990s. Each of the original 44 chapters in the first edition was thoroughly reviewed and updated. Twenty-five new content areas were added, including Relation of the Immune System to Cancer, Cancer Risk and Assessment, Biotherapy, Bone Marrow Transplantation, AIDS-Related Malignancies, Late Effects of Cancer Treatment, Psychosocial Dimensions: Issues in Survivorship, Sexual and Reproductive Dysfunction, Oncologic Emergencies, Delivery Systems of Cancer Care, Economics of Cancer, Teaching Strategies: The Public, and Teaching Strategies: The Patient. This edition contains 60 comprehensive chapters representing the contributions of over 75 recognized oncology nursing experts.

The exponential increase in information about oncogenes resulting from a massive research effort has provided a greater understanding of the nature of carcinogenesis. This improved understanding is reflected in this second edition and will continue to have a significant impact on the nature of clinical care. Even with this research effort and greater understanding of the nature of carcinogenesis, however, it is unlikely that a magic cure or vaccine for cancer will be available in the near future. There will continue to emerge new approaches to early diagnosis of cancer, new techniques to treat cancer, new measures to ameliorate distressing manifestations of cancer and its treatment, and new approaches to improve the quality of life for cancer survivors. Cancer nurses are integral to these developments. It is to these nurses that this text is dedicated.

The editors wish to gratefully acknowledge the tremendous effort of the contributors who enthusiastically shared their knowledge and expertise and gave their time and energy to this endeavor. We wish to especially acknowledge our husbands Keith, Jim, Larry, and John for their assistance, support, and patience during this mammouth project.

The editors have developed this text to be a comprehensive resource for nurses who provide or manage care for patients in the home, hospital, or community, who teach patients and nurses, and who conduct research to find better approaches to patient care—all of whom contribute to our steady gains in providing quality care to individuals with cancer.

Susan L. Groenwald
Margaret Hansen Frogge
Michelle Goodman
Connie Henke Yarbro

PREFACE TO THE FIRST EDITION

This text is one I always wished to have. As a graduate student of oncology nursing, and later as an oncology clinical nurse specialist and educator at Rush-Presbyterian St. Luke's Medical Center, I became frustrated by the dearth of texts written at the level of the oncology graduate student or oncology nurse specialist. Oncology nursing texts lack the depth and breadth of scientific information that I believe is an essential element in the armamentarium of the professional nurse; medical literature, while it contains the necessary scientific information, lacks application of scientific principles to the nursing care arena.

In this text, the contributors and I committed ourselves to presenting the reader with the most comprehensive information about oncology nursing available, including relevant science and clinical practice content that addresses both the whys and hows of oncology nursing practice. All chapters cite original published research as the scientific foundation for the application of these findings to clinical practice. All students of oncology nursing—beginning or advanced—will find this book valuable as a text and as a reference for clinical practice.

The disease of cancer in the adult is approached from many angles to address the complex learning needs of the oncology nurse specialist. Part I includes cancer epidemiology and deals with individual and societal attitudes toward cancer and the impact of attitudes on health behaviors. Part II provides the foundation of scientific information about the malignant cell on which all subsequent chapters are built. Concepts such as carcinogenesis, oncogenesis, metastasis, invasion, and contact inhibition are included in Part II, and thorough attention is given to changes that occur in a normal cell and its behavior as it transforms to a malignant cell.

In Part III, the psychosocial dimensions of cancer are approached according to critical phases through which patients, families, and caregivers may pass as they cope with the stressors induced by cancer. Part IV presents a conceptual approach to the most common manifestations of cancer and their effects on the individual with cancer. Each chapter includes pathophysiology, assessment, and medical and nursing therapies. Part V describes each of the major cancer treatment methods, their uses, adverse effects, and nursing care considerations for individuals receiving cancer therapy. Included in this part is a chapter on unproven methods of treatment. Part VI is a comprehensive review of most of the major cancers by body system and the problems experienced by people who live with cancer. (Information pertaining to pediatric malignancies and nursing care of the child with cancer has been omitted. Although pediatric oncology is a critical area of interest for many nurses, it could not be covered in sufficient depth within this text.) Part VII presents continuing-care options for the individual living with the problems imposed by cancer. Part VIII analyzes several issues relevant to the oncology nurse: consumerism, ethics, cancer nursing education, and cancer nursing research. Part IX, which lists oncology resources of many types, is a handy reference tool.

Some of the information presented in this text is out of date even as it is written because of ever-expanding knowledge about cancer and its treatment. As Dr. Vincent DeVita remarked at his swearing-in as Director of the National Cancer Institute (*The Cancer Letter,* 1980:4), "What we now know of the cancerous process and what we do to prevent, diagnose, and treat it will be outmoded and radically different by the end of the 80s." This book is our best effort to put down in writing the science and art of cancer nursing in the 1980s.

SUSAN L. GROENWALD

CONTENTS

PART V
MANIFESTATIONS OF CANCER AND CANCER TREATMENT

PART I

THE CANCER PROBLEM

Chapter 1

Epidemiology of Cancer

Denise Oleske, RN, PhD

Susan L. Groenwald, RN, MS

INTRODUCTION

Although there are methods and processes specific to epidemiology, epidemiologists, like nurses, share the philosophy that health problems are complex and multifactorial. Using techniques from statistics, demography, and the natural and social sciences, epidemiology studies the distribution and determinants of diseases and health problems in human populations with the ultimate goal of controlling or preventing the health problem.

In the past, epidemiology has been equated with the study of infectious disease. Although mortality from communicable diseases has declined significantly, health care practitioners are faced with a concomitant increase in chronic health problems. Interest in epidemiology as a tool for understanding the genesis and control of chronic health problems has been gaining momentum since the 1940s, when these trends became apparent. Neoplasms of all sites began to constitute a major proportion of chronic health problems among all ages and races and for both sexes. Cancer is the second leading cause of death, being responsible for 25% of all deaths in the United States in 1987.[1] Unlike diseases attributable to a specific biologic agent, no single causative factor has been identified for cancer. Even some of the classic epidemiologic studies of lung cancer indicated that not all cigarette smokers developed neoplasms and that even when adjustments were made for smoking habits, risk varied with place of residence (urban vs rural), sex, and race.

Epidemiology can be divided into two major areas: descriptive and analytic. *Descriptive epidemiology* describes the characteristics of the disease or health problem in terms of who is affected, where the areas of concern are, and when the problem occurs. Data from descriptive studies are used to generate hypotheses for further study. *Analytic epidemiology* seeks to establish causation, direct or indirect, by testing hypotheses derived from descriptive studies and examining how various factors contribute to the manifestations of the disease or health problem being studied. Thus, analytic epidemiology searches for reasons why certain patterns emerge in specific groups.

The first half of this chapter focuses on how the cancer problem is viewed using descriptive and analytic epidemiologic methods. In the remainder of the chapter, the techniques that epidemiologists use in their efforts to unravel the effects of various factors and their relative contribution to the promotion of cancer and impact on its course are presented.

Oncology nurses should be familiar with epidemiologic techniques and findings. An understanding of epidemiologic methods can enhance the nurse's assessment skills. The knowledge gained from epidemiologic findings gives greater insight on the magnitude of risk for cancer or its complications that are inherent within the individual or community being served. Recognition of the factors that affect the preservation of health or quality of life is necessary to plan and evaluate nursing strategies employed, whether for primary (prevention), secondary (detection), or tertiary (therapeutic) cancer intervention.

CHARACTERISTICS OF THE HOST

The nature and magnitude of the health problems a nurse must face when dealing with a particular individual can be predicted best if the nurse understands the characteristics of the population being served or studied. Individuals can be described according to an infinite number of variables. The variables that have been most often evaluated in cancer epidemiologic studies are:

- Age
- Sex
- Ethnic group or race
- Marital status
- Genetic predisposition
- Psychologic factors
- Previous disease

Age

Age is the most important descriptive determinant. The vulnerability of the host changes throughout each phase of the life cycle, varying because of the intrinsic physiologic states and the life experiences in which the individual is exposed to different social, cultural, and environmental conditions. Table 1-1 illustrates the impact of age on cancer incidence.[2] There is generally a sharp and steady increase in cancer incidence from childhood to old age. Diseases such as colon and prostate cancer are generally diseases of old age, whereas acute lymphocytic leukemia and Wilms' tumor are almost exclusively childhood cancers (Table 1-2). Even within a site-specific category, variations in incidence among age groups may be discernible. For example, Silverman found that Hodgkin's disease peaks between 25 and 34 years of age and again after 55 years of age.[3]

Sex

There is a wide divergence between the sexes with respect to the incidence of cancers not thought to be sex-linked (breast and prostate) (see Table 1-1[2]). Women have an overall lower rate of cancer development and also have higher survival rates for most types of cancer.[4] If these non–sex-linked cancers are environmentally related, the rates for women should become more similar to those of men because of increasing comparable exposure to certain habits and occupations. The effects of the environment can be seen in the increased rate of lung cancer in women, which is attributed to the increased proportion of women smokers. As more women take on life-styles and occupations traditionally held by men, other similarities in the incidence of non–sex-linked cancers are likely to occur.

Ethnicity and Race

A number of ethnic and racial groups have been studied regarding their risk of cancer. Many unique patterns have been found. It has been found that cervical cancer is rare among Jewish and Mormon women; the incidence of gallbladder, cervical, pancreatic, and stomach cancer is excessive among Indians; the mortality rates for Japanese-Americans with stomach cancer are significantly higher than for the white American population, but the breast cancer rates are significantly lower for the former group; and Mexican-Americans are at higher risk for stomach, liver, and cervical cancers but at lower risk for bladder, lung, breast, colon, and rectal cancer than are Anglo-Americans.[5-9]

Before 1950, the mortality rate for cancer among blacks was lower than that among whites. Today, both the incidence and mortality rates for cancer among black Americans are higher than for white Americans. Lung, cervical, colon, pancreatic, esophageal, and bladder cancers are increasing faster among black Americans than white Americans, with a concomitant steep increase in mortality rates. For blacks, cancer incidence has increased 27% since 1960, and cancer mortality has increased by 34%. Among whites, cancer incidence has increased 12%, and cancer mortality has increased 9%.[4,9]

Although some genetic or hormonal factors may prevent or promote cancer development in individuals of a certain sex or among various ethnic or racial groups, strong epidemiologic evidence suggests that culture and other environmental factors, such as economic and social variables, play an important role in determining host susceptibility to cancer.

Marital Status and Childbearing Patterns

Marital status is probably important only as it affects the likelihood of pregnancy and the nature of sexual activity. The incidence of breast cancer is lower in women who were pregnant before 20 years of age and higher in single women than in married women.[10] Conversely, delayed childbearing is linked to an increased incidence of breast cancer.[11] Ovarian cancer has been associated with low fertility.[12] Women who were sexually active at an early age and have multiple sexual partners are at increased risk for cervical cancer, since these practices increase the likelihood of acquiring human papillomavirus, recently implicated as an important etiologic agent for cervical cancer.[13]

Genetic Predisposition

The data regarding the genetic basis of cancer have been derived from a number of sources. A large body of information was derived from the investigation of chromosome instability syndromes, congenital abnormal karyotypes, familial patterns, and cytogenetics of induced chromosomal change.

Individuals with instability syndromes (Bloom's syndrome, Fanconi's anemia, ataxia-telangiectasis, and xeroderma pigmentosum) have a significantly higher risk of cancer than the general population. Although the mechanism by which neoplastic growth emerges from these conditions is not fully understood, it is thought that faulty DNA synthesis or incorrect repair of chromosome breakage may be fundamental to the transformation.[14]

Persons with congenital abnormal karyotypes also are at increased risk of cancer. Turner's syndrome (XO) is associated with increased neural crest and brain and pituitary tumors; Klinefelter's syndrome (XXY), with breast cancer; and Down syndrome, with leukemia. In Turner's and Klinefelter's syndromes, information from the X chromosome is thought to play a role in malignant growths, whereas in Down syndrome, a link has been identified with the G chromosome group.[15]

Heredity has been found to influence the development of breast cancer in some families and the development of some types of colon cancer.[10,16]

Familial patterns have been studied in an attempt to elicit features of transmission of neoplastic tendency. Some forms of retinoblastoma, most bilateral, are inherited. The mechanism of inheritance has not been established. Dysplastic nevi, which are precursors of cutaneous malignant melanoma, are inherited in an autosomal dominant fashion.

Through studies of families with an increased tendency toward cancer, it has been found that heritable malignancies are characterized by earlier onset, commonality in organ site, increased tendency toward cancer in multiple organ sites and paired organs, and limited range of histologic expression. Caution must be exercised in the conduct and interpretation of family studies because the probability of identifying a cancer family increases with the number of affected individuals, which, in turn, is influenced by the actual size of the family. Familial aggregates of cancer also may represent differential attentiveness to the disease because of a previously identified case within the family. In addition, common exposure to an environmental carcinogen or carcinogens may play a significant role in the development of cancer in a "cancer family" but be overlooked because of the mistaken assumption that the disease was precipitated solely by genetic factors.

Cytogenetics has not only helped to clarify the relationships described but has also shed light on the manner in which the host is made vulnerable to neoplastic transformation through induced chromosomal changes, particularly changes caused by viruses, chemicals and ionizing radiation.

The major dilemma facing epidemiologists is filtering out the relative contributions of genetics and the environment, raising the question of what came first, the genetic tendency or the environmental exposure to modify the genetic message.

Psychologic Factors

The effect of the individual's psychologic makeup on the development of cancer is difficult to ascertain. Stress has been related to a variety of illness states. The hormonal imbalances caused by stress could alter the immune sys-

TABLE 1-1(a) Age-Specific Cancer Incidence Rate per 100,000 for Males, by Site*

Age (Yr)	Buccal Cavity	Pharynx + Larynx	Lung: Small Cell	Lung: Non-small Cell	Esophagus	Stomach	Pancreas	Colon	Rectum
<5	0.00	0.12	0.00	0.00	0.00	0.00	0.00	0.00	0.00
5–9	0.00	0.00	0.00	0.03	0.00	0.00	0.03	0.00	0.00
10–14	0.14	0.17	0.00	0.03	0.00	0.00	0.03	0.06	0.00
15–19	0.20	0.15	0.00	0.13	0.00	0.05	0.05	0.15	0.05
20–24	0.32	0.17	0.02	0.12	0.02	0.12	0.15	0.32	0.07
25–29	0.60	0.36	0.05	0.36	0.00	0.29	0.05	1.04	0.47
30–34	1.30	0.89	0.17	1.38	0.17	0.75	0.20	2.13	0.46
35–39	2.90	1.87	0.81	7.23	0.51	1.65	0.84	3.89	1.69
40–44	7.23	6.55	3.39	19.05	1.60	3.75	3.39	9.02	4.58
45–49	12.98	13.96	8.41	48.19	5.06	9.19	6.76	17.75	10.21
50–54	20.75	27.48	20.80	97.72	9.01	14.11	12.44	34.17	22.00
55–59	30.25	41.54	33.01	153.16	13.82	22.58	20.53	59.88	37.97
60–64	40.78	51.27	46.37	229.90	20.36	35.82	33.97	96.38	58.89
65–69	44.80	63.73	62.04	313.87	24.17	51.87	46.57	144.56	80.31
70–74	46.50	54.81	64.15	378.67	27.72	66.95	61.35	209.47	107.75
75–79	49.39	48.27	53.37	395.40	29.47	92.40	70.89	263.82	121.23
80–84	60.15	39.35	44.98	371.89	25.86	110.75	71.40	330.57	139.98
85+	56.37	36.38	20.79	281.06	24.79	125.14	83.96	371.42	145.93

*Source of data is the SEER Program, 1984.

†"Childhood" sites were analyzed with rates for ages under 15 years only. Adult ALL + AML was analyzed with rates for ages 15 and over only. *ALL*, adult lymphocytic leukemia; *AML*, adult myelogenous leukemia.

Source: Greenwald P, Sondik EJ: Appendix A: Use of models to project cancer mortality in the year 2000, in Cancer control objectives for the nation: 1985–2000. NCI monograph no. 2. Washington DC, US Government Printing Office, 1986.

TABLE 1-1(b) Age-Specific Cancer Incidence Rate per 100,000 for Females, by Site*

Age (Yr)	Buccal Cavity	Pharynx + Larynx	Lung: Small Cell	Lung: Non-small Cell	Esophagus	Stomach	Pancreas	Colon	Rectum
<5	0.03	0.03	0.00	0.00	0.00	0.00	0.00	0.00	0.00
5–9	0.03	0.06	0.00	0.00	0.00	0.00	0.00	0.03	0.00
10–14	0.15	0.03	0.00	0.00	0.00	0.00	0.03	0.21	0.00
15–19	0.16	0.21	0.00	0.08	0.00	0.03	0.03	0.16	0.08
20–24	0.32	0.12	0.00	0.10	0.00	0.10	0.15	0.32	0.17
25–29	0.70	0.36	0.03	0.49	0.03	0.13	0.16	1.06	0.28
30–34	0.94	0.51	0.06	1.39	0.00	0.54	0.37	2.24	0.88
35–39	1.31	0.62	0.51	4.61	0.22	1.60	0.69	4.46	1.16
40–44	2.40	2.18	2.00	13.31	0.62	2.54	1.83	8.55	3.38
45–49	4.93	5.45	5.12	24.99	1.35	3.44	3.82	18.48	7.21
50–54	7.95	7.78	10.53	41.82	3.02	5.77	8.22	31.73	16.13
55–59	11.59	11.59	15.54	58.44	4.92	9.31	14.27	48.70	22.48
60–64	15.04	12.05	19.88	82.37	5.46	12.83	19.73	77.84	34.98
65–69	16.17	12.25	22.27	91.00	7.24	18.28	31.92	113.39	43.09
70–74	17.62	9.30	21.81	91.90	7.09	28.52	38.36	163.97	58.57
75–79	18.44	10.12	13.33	83.77	8.52	39.18	47.69	212.32	74.45
80–84	19.86	6.86	8.47	71.86	10.81	55.94	61.05	275.75	82.52
85+	20.50	4.86	4.34	59.59	8.86	69.15	70.71	298.32	91.56

*Source of data is the SEER Program, 1984.

†"Childhood" sites were analyzed with rates for ages under 15 years only. Adult ALL + AML was analyzed with rates for ages 15 and over only. *ALL*, adult lymphocytic leukemia; *AML*, adult myelogenous leukemia.

Source: Greenwald P, Sondik EJ: Appendix A: Use of models to project cancer mortality in the year 2000, in Cancer control objectives for the nation: 1985–2000. NCI monograph no. 2. Washington DC, US Government Printing Office, 1986.

Bladder	Melanoma	Childhood Brain	Childhood ALL	Childhood AML	Adult ALL + AML	DHL	Prostate	Testis, Nonseminoma	All Other Sites
0.09	0.03	2.53	5.03	0.44	†	0.09	0.00	0.47	8.85
0.00	0.06	2.75	2.38	0.37		0.12	0.03	0.12	4.74
0.03	0.11	2.35	1.70	0.59		0.08	0.00	0.03	6.48
0.20	0.93		†		2.29	0.38	0.10	2.44	12.56
0.57	2.41				1.45	0.49	0.00	6.00	16.37
0.70	4.76				1.56	0.55	0.05	5.90	22.74
1.88	7.70				1.44	0.52	0.03	4.36	30.59
3.34	9.99				1.65	1.03	0.11	2.39	38.96
6.96	12.04				1.88	1.47	1.47	1.19	68.26
13.18	15.22				2.43	1.60	5.83	1.02	115.83
25.30	14.34				3.57	3.06	23.40	0.65	184.76
42.83	19.10				4.38	4.48	71.89	0.43	270.66
68.87	21.22				5.65	5.13	172.86	0.35	377.03
101.38	20.41				10.54	7.22	323.75	0.22	478.09
144.39	23.46				14.01	10.69	516.93	0.31	583.69
181.93	26.13				18.64	13.70	726.77	0.48	686.14
211.10	20.24				21.64	16.02	890.79	0.28	754.45
221.49	25.19				22.39	11.19	951.54	0.40	833.60

Bladder	Melanoma	Childhood Brain	Childhood ALL	Childhood AML	Adult ALL + AML	DHL	Breast	Ovary	Cervix	Corpus Uteri	All Other Sites
0.03	0.10	2.39	5.17	0.62	†	0.07	0.00	0.00	0.00	0.00	10.06
0.00	0.13	1.97	2.65	0.36		0.10	0.00	0.16	0.03	0.00	3.90
0.00	0.21	1.77	1.00	0.44		0.09	0.00	0.47	0.09	0.03	4.95
0.05	1.40		†		0.91	0.34	0.16	1.19	7.97	0.10	12.19
0.15	4.07				0.91	0.37	1.26	2.24	63.49	0.20	15.94
0.21	7.31				0.67	0.54	8.26	3.16	120.28	0.83	21.41
0.51	9.67				1.25	0.45	25.45	4.31	122.67	2.81	25.55
1.34	11.18				1.52	0.51	59.28	5.99	95.54	6.10	31.08
2.36	12.29				1.38	0.58	105.52	12.02	74.40	12.29	46.62
4.51	13.17				2.00	1.30	155.32	17.69	49.01	25.32	67.73
6.60	14.90				2.23	2.40	177.65	27.18	35.18	52.09	100.52
10.49	12.08				2.99	2.28	199.31	31.44	32.14	75.13	142.59
18.55	13.50				4.02	4.89	234.29	38.79	34.31	109.26	189.22
24.86	12.85				5.07	6.28	258.89	41.16	34.16	101.99	254.71
33.02	12.96				6.86	8.31	278.06	40.65	31.27	91.29	315.89
42.18	11.52				8.92	10.52	296.39	48.80	29.66	81.86	398.60
50.97	13.88				15.48	13.14	291.09	41.19	27.90	66.02	474.53
69.85	18.94				12.86	9.21	320.73	36.31	26.06	50.21	521.06

TABLE 1-2(a) Mortality for the Five Leading Cancer Sites for Males by Age Group, United States—1985

All Ages	Under 15	15–34	35–54	55–74	75+
All Cancer 246,914	**All Cancer 1,042**	**All Cancer 4,029**	**All Cancer 25,733**	**All Cancer 136,869**	**All Cancer 79,220**
Lung 83,854	Leukemia 418	Leukemia 679	Lung 8926	Lung 53,756	Lung 20,996
Colon and rectum 27,612	Brain and CNS 230	Skin 469	Colon and rectum 2247	Colon and rectum 14,749	Prostate 15,132
Prostate 25,943	Non-Hodgkin's lymphomas 66	Brain and CNS 444	Brain and CNS 1272	Prostate 10,488	Colon and rectum 10,422
Pancreas 11,542	Connective tissue 50	Non-Hodgkin's lymphomas 438	Non-Hodgkin's lymphomas 1214	Pancreas 6652	Pancreas 3672
Leukemia 9422	Bone 33	Hodgkin's disease 301	Skin 1208	Stomach 4485	Bladder 3380

Source: Data from Vital Statistics of the United States, 1985.

TABLE 1-2(b) Mortality for the Five Leading Cancer Sites for Females by Age Group, United States—1985

All Ages	Under 15	15–34	35–54	55–74	75+
All Cancer 214,649	**All Cancer 798**	**All Cancer 3,608**	**All Cancer 27,001**	**All Cancer 106,299**	**All Cancer 76,921**
Breast 40,383	Leukemia 296	Breast 649	Breast 8297	Lung 24,322	Colon and rectum 14,542
Lung 38,839	Brain and CNS 192	Leukemia 347	Lung 4960	Breast 20,301	Breast 11,131
Colon and rectum 28,839	Bone 41	Uterus 347	Colon and rectum 1911	Colon and rectum 12,200	Lung 9279
Pancreas 11,560	Bladder 36	Brain and CNS 321	Uterus 1778	Ovary 6380	Pancreas 5211
Ovary 11,531	Non-Hodgkin's lymphomas 36	Non-Hodgkin's lymphomas 202	Ovary 1666	Pancreas 5542	Ovary 3346

Source: Data from Vital Statistics of the United States, 1985.

tem, which in turn may lead to cancer. When the individual is under stress, however, coping mechanisms may involve heavy smoking, drinking, drug abuse, and alterations in sleeping and eating habits. These mechanisms may increase the risk of cancer.

There are conflicting findings on the relationship of personality to cancer development.[17-24] Two main groups of psychologic factors have been implicated in an increased risk of cancer[24]: (1) loss of or lack of a close relationship to an important person (often a parent) early in life and (2) inability to express hostile feelings. The major drawback of studies conducted on the relationship of psychologic factors to cancer development is that they are likely to be retrospective, meaning that the personality differences may be attributed to the individual's knowledge of the cancer diagnosis.

A few prospective studies have been conducted. One study examined the ability of a number of selected psychosocial risk factors (childhood instability, job instability, marital instability, lack of future plans, recent significant loss) to be predictors of lung cancer morbidity.[25] The composite scale accurately predicted the diagnosis in 80% of persons with benign disease and 61% of persons with lung cancer. Thomas et al conducted a prospective study by studying a cohort of 1337 Johns Hopkins medical students who graduated between 1948 and 1964.[23] In medical school the students were administered a variety of physiologic, psychologic, and metabolic examinations. By 1979, more than 95% of the study participants were between 40 and 59 years of age. The 55 men who had developed cancer perceived themselves to be significantly less close to their parents than did their healthy counterparts. In a prospective study, Fox et al found that individuals classified as having type A personality were more likely to die of cancer than those who were type B personality. The mechanism for cancer development is hypothesized to be through repeated episodes of suppression and recovery of the immune system, increasing the probability of the growth of transformed cells.[26] These findings seem to add support to the hypothesis that certain personality traits may predispose individuals to cancer. More prospective studies must be undertaken before firm conclusions can be made; however, the data are provocative and suggest areas for further research.

Previous Host Disease

Some preexisting pathologic conditions may place an individual at increased risk of cancer, including colon-rectal polyps, some forms of benign breast disease, some infectious diseases (type B hepatitis, schistosomiasis, malaria), leukoplakia, cervical dysplasia, previous malignancy, skin keratosis, gallstones, kidney or bladder stones, cirrhosis, ulcerative colitis, Crohn's disease, adenomatous polyps, pancreatitis, hydatidiform mole, pernicious anemia, obesity in women, and Paget's disease of bone. Thorough, regular follow-up is recommended for individuals at increased risk because of these conditions.

ENVIRONMENT

The influences of factors outside the host on the manifestations of disease must be considered. The analysis of external factors ordinarily begins with descriptive techniques that evaluate the extent of occurrence of cancer types and seek to identify any emerging patterns. A particular feature is investigated further using analytic methods.

Place

The descriptive approach to analyzing the environment focuses on place. Place is used to evaluate the spatial orientation of the phenomenon being studied. Place influences a number of population variables and contains features (smog, humidity, soil composition, water supply, and so on) that may contribute to the type and magnitude of health problems in the population. In addition, individuals with many similar characteristics tend to congregate in a circumscribed area, facilitating the study of the effect of urbanization, culture, latitude, physical environment, and socioeconomic conditions on cancer incidence, prevalence, and mortality.

The most common spatial units used in cancer epidemiology are those created by political boundaries. In these analyses, mortality rates are the predominant data type because they are often the only reliable source of population-based data available. Worldwide cancer mortality rates or country versus country comparisons are the major sources of cross-cultural information on cancer. Conclusions based on worldwide mortality data must be drawn with particular caution. Biases originating from lack of uniform death reporting, cultural differences in diagnostic methods, differences in access to health care, and receptivity to modern medical services must be evaluated for their impact on the data before any judgments are made about the significance of the differences in data among countries.

The county as a geograhic unit is particularly valuable because it is frequently homogeneous with respect to demographic and environmental characteristics. A classic example of this can be found in the *Atlas of US Cancer Mortality Among Whites: 1950–1980*.[27] In this source, death rates for 35 site-specific cancers are mapped by color, revealing some unique patterns in disease distribution among the predominant white population of the United States. For example, breast cancer in postmenopausal women is most common in the north-central and northeast regions of the United States, whereas the mortality distribution among premenopausal women is quite uniform throughout the country. The rates for colon and rectal cancer for both sexes are above average in the northeast and urban areas along the Great Lakes. The similar distribution suggests that the two diseases may share a common etiologic factor. An atlas of site-specific cancer mortality in nonwhites was published in 1976.[28]

By definition, environment is a set of extrinsic factors that influence the appearance of cancer in an individual. Thus a consideration of environment should include nutrition, workplace, habits (especially tobacco and alcohol use), iatrogenic sources, social influences, and the physical, chemical, and biologic environment.

Nutrition

The relationship of what individuals eat and drink to cancer is receiving growing attention. Worldwide patterns of food consumption, when compared with cancer mortality and incidence rates of various countries, have been the initial clue regarding the influence of nutrition on cancer.

Armstrong and Doll[29] examined international cancer incidence data in relation to patterns of gross food product consumption in an attempt to develop hypotheses regarding the role of nutrition in cancer. They found a strong correlation between dietary variables and some cancer types, notably cancer of the colon and meat consumption, and breast and uterine cancer and fat consumption.

There are a number of methodologic difficulties with conducting such nutritional epidemiologic studies. Error may exist because of differences in diagnosis of causes of mortality, lack of uniform death reporting, and inaccuracies in assessing what people in a specific country eat. Most of the studies conducted rely on the individual subjects' recall of their diet over a period of time. Because it is impossible for individuals to remember exactly what they ate at previous times, this method is not entirely accurate. Nevertheless, many of the dietary studies that have been conducted have used the interview-recall method, and much valuable information has been obtained that, when combined with other data derived from other sources, may produce significant findings about the relationships of food intake to the development of cancer.

Most of the work on nutrition and cancer has been based on data from laboratory studies. The applicability of these data to human populations is still controversial. For example, the saccharin controversy arose when high doses of this compound (8 kg of sodium saccarin per kilogram of weight, representing 5% of the diet) were administered to animals and the animals subsequently developed tumors. Based on several studies showing an increased incidence of bladder cancer in rats who were exposed to high doses of saccharin, the Food and Drug Administration (FDA) banned saccharin in 1977. Except for one study that showed increased use of saccharin to be associated with bladder cancer in men but not in women, human epidemiologic studies show no relationship between bladder cancer and the ingestion of saccharin.[30] Thus the epidemiologic evidence obtained from the study of human cases is overwhelmingly in disagreement with the animal studies that link the ingestion of saccharin to bladder cancer.

Many hypotheses link specific dietary components to inhibition or causation of cancer. A review of research findings for the more commonly discussed dietary factors is provided in Table 1-3. As is demonstrated by the incongruence among the data, the myriad of interacting factors affecting the relationship between diet and cancer make understanding the role that diet plays in carcinogenesis extremely complicated. Not only are specific food substances involved, but their storage, harvest, cultivation, and preparation for eating also play a role. Many questions are yet to be answered. For example, what effect does dose have on the potential of a dietary factor to inhibit or cause cancer? What dose is optimal? What dose is toxic? At small doses, vitamin A may inhibit carcinogenesis, whereas large doses of vitamin A are known to be toxic (see Table 1-3).

Because scientists do not understand all the nutritional consequences that occur when food is ingested, they cannot yet determine the role that diet plays in carcinogenesis, and a specific diet cannot be recommended for the avoidance of all types of cancer. However, because many laboratory and epidemiologic studies strongly suggest that modifications in diet can reduce cancer risk in humans, the National Cancer Institute (NCI) developed two ongoing programs to research the relationship between diet and cancer, with the goal of reducing cancer mortality.

The first of these programs, the Diet, Nutrition, and Cancer Program, was established in 1975 by the Division of Cancer Prevention and Control of the NCI. The purpose of this program is to study the broad effects of changes in foods or food groups that may lower the incidence of cancer. Large-scale dietary intervention trials are the primary vehicles for researching these relationships.

The second program, the Chemoprevention Program, focuses on micronutrients, introducing vitamins and other defined chemicals into the diet and observing their effect on cancer incidence.[60,106] Both programs combine basic epidemiologic and laboratory data with the hope of applying knowledge gained to clinical practice.

Figure 1-1 on p. 16 illustrates the three components of the Chemoprevention Program: laboratory research, epidemiologic research, and human intervention studies.[105] Each component consists of stages that require decision points that control movement from stage to stage. The laboratory and epidemiologic research run parallel; results are combined and analyzed before advancement is made to human intervention studies.

The same process is followed in the Diet, Nutrition, and Cancer Program, but the nature of factors studied requires that different methods be used to answer questions at each stage. Some of the substances being investigated in the Chemoprevention Program include retinoids (the largest group of studies), vitamin C, selenium (a trace metal), and vitamin E. For the Diet, Nutrition, and Cancer Program, the major issues being investigated are the roles of dietary fat and fiber in the development of human cancer.

The aim of both of these programs is to obtain information that will have a major impact on cancer incidence and mortality. With the amount of research funds being devoted to these programs and the organized manner in which they are being conducted, perhaps some critical answers to the puzzle of diet and cancer will be forthcoming.

TABLE 1-3 Review of Current Research Issues Regarding Diet and Cancer

Food/Agent	Site	Studies	Results of Studies	Clinical Implications
Saccharin	Bladder	*Laboratory studies*		
		Food and Drug Administration, 1973[31]	High-saccharin diets fed to rats over a long period produced bladder tumors in second-generation rats	Saccharin is a weak carcinogen in rats and a tumor promoter; therefore, avoidance in humans is the best policy, especially because there is no apparent health benefit from saccharin in use
		Health and Protection Branch, 1977[32]	Conclusive report linking the ingestion of saccharin to bladder cancer only in male rats	
		Nicholson and Jani, 1988[33]	Saccharin is a tumor promoter	
		Human epidemiologic studies		
		Howe et al, 1977[30]	Increased incidence of bladder cancer in men (but not women) who used artificial sweeteners	
		Burbank and Fraumeni, 1970[34] Armstrong and Doll, 1974[35] Armstrong and Doll, 1978[36] Wynder and Goldsmith, 1977[37] Kessler and Clark, 1978[38] Morrison and Buring, 1980[39] Wynder and Stellman, 1980[40] Hoover and Strasser, 1980[41]	No epidemiologic evidence of an association between artificial sweeteners (including saccharin) and bladder cancer in humans; did not confirm Howe's report of an increased incidence in men	
Alcohol	Oral Cavity Larynx Esophagus Breast Colon	Rothman and Keller, 1972[42] Graham et al, 1977[43]	Ingesting alcoholic beverages increased the incidence of oral cancer; presence of alcohol enhanced the oral carcinogenic effects of tobacco	Alcohol consumed in large quantities acts synergistically with cigarette smoke to increase smoking-related cancer and has other major health implications
		Jensen, 1979[44]	Excessive alcohol ingestion is associated with an increased risk of cancer of the head, neck, and lungs	Even a moderate amount of alcohol ingestion confers a greater risk of cancer of the oral cavity, larynx, esophagus, breast, and colon
		Pottern et al, 1981[45]	The risk of esophageal cancer responds in a dose-response manner, increasing with greater alcohol consumption	
		Vitale et al, 1981[46]	Alcohol does not cause cancer when fed to laboratory animals; no evidence that alcohol is an initiator of cancer, but alcohol may serve as a carrier of carcinogens	
		Wu et al, 1987[47]	Daily alcohol consumption is associated with twofold increased risk of colorectal cancer in men	
		Schatzkin et al, 1987[48]	Moderate alcohol consumption is associated with increased risk of breast cancer and colon cancer	

TABLE 1-3 Review of Current Research Issues Regarding Diet and Cancer (continued)

Food/ Agent	Site	Studies	Results of Studies	Clinical Implications
Coffee	Bladder Pancreas	Hoover and Strasser, 1980[41]	No significant risk of bladder cancer for persons who drink coffee	There is little evidence that coffee drinking causes cancer in humans
		MacMahon et al, 1981[49]	Suggested relationship between coffee consumption and cancer	
		Newel, 1983[50]	Little or no association between coffee consumption and bladder cancer. When present, association is inconsistent, of low strength, and shows no dose-response relationship	
		Wynder et al, 1983[51]	No association between coffee consumption and pancreatic cancer	
Dietary Fats	Colon	Hill, 1975[52] Wynder, 1975[53] Reddy and Wynder, 1977[54]	Increases in dietary fat are accompanied by increases in bile acids and bacteria in feces, which could metabolize fats into carcinogenic substances	All populations consuming a high-fiber, low-fat diet have low rates of colon cancer; all populations consuming low-fiber, high-fat diets have high rates of colon cancer[55]; although the relationship of dietary fat to colon cancer is not entirely understood, in light of the evidence that a high-fat diet contributes to coronary heart disease and other diseases, reducing fat content of the diet is recommended (in conjunction with increasing fiber content)
		Graham et al, 1988[56]	Increased risk of colon cancer is related to the amount of total fats and total calories ingested Total fat and total calorie intake are associated with increased risk of colon cancer in males and females	
Dietary Fats	Breast	Carroll et al, 1968[57]	Positive correlation between breast cancer mortality and per capita intake of fat and calories in 22 countries	Although the precise role of dietary fat in breast cancer has not been determined, the evidence regarding the etiologic role of a high-fat diet is sufficiently strong to justify the recommendation that fat intake in the American diet be reduced by at least 30% of total calories[60]
		Carroll and Khor, 1971[58] Carroll, 1975[59]	Unsaturated fats enhance the risk of mammary cancer in rats	
		Miller et al, 1978[61]	Breast cancer patients are significantly fatter than matched controls	
		Lubin et al, 1985[62]	Body weight is positively correlated with the risk of breast cancer	
		Hems, 1978[63] Carroll, 1981[64]	Breast cancer incidence in 41 countries is positively correlated with estimated per capita fat, animal protein, and total calorie consumption	
		Cohen et al, 1981[65]	Increased incidence of mammary tumors in rats exposed to high-fat diets	

TABLE 1-3 Review of Current Research Issues Regarding Diet and Cancer (continued)

Food/Agent	Site	Studies	Results of Studies	Clinical Implications
Dietary Fiber	Colon Breast Prostate	*Laboratory Studies* Burkitt, 1971[66] Burkitt et al, 1972[67]	Relationship between fiber and decreased incidence of colon cancer; fiber decreases the transit time, thereby decreasing the time carcinogens are in contact with bowel mucosa	Research findings seem to suggest that dietary fiber protects individuals from colon cancer; because foods that contain fiber (fruit, vegetable) also contain important vitamins and nutrients, it is recommended that fiber intake be 20 to 30 g per day[66]
		Fleiszer et al, 1978[68]	Bran diet containing 28% fiber reduced the incidence of colon tumors	
		Reddy et al, 1987[69]	Increased fiber intake in the form of whole wheat and rye bread may reduce the production or secretion of fecal mutagens	
		Human epidemiologic studies Modan et al, 1975[70]	Low risk of colon cancer for Israelis who frequently eat fibrous foods	
		MacLennan and Jensen, 1977[71]	Finns have a low risk of colon cancer and eat more fiber but the same amount of fat as do Danes, whose risk of colon cancer is high	
		Reddy et al, 1978[72]	Compared Finns and New Yorkers; New Yorkers had a higher incidence of colon cancer; they ate similar amounts of fat but less fiber	
		Graham and Mettlin, 1981[73]	High-fiber diet protects against colon cancer	
		Kritchevsky, 1984[74]	Dietary fiber negatively correlated with the incidence of colon cancer	
Cruciferous vegetables (broccoli, cabbage [including sauerkraut and cole slaw], brussel sprouts, kohlrabi, turnip, cauliflower): raw or cooked	Colon	Borchert and Wattenberg, 1976[75] Graham et al, 1978[76]	Chemicals in cruciferous vegetables reduce the number of tumors resulting from carcinogenic challenge in animals	Human studies corroborate animal studies and indicate that cruciferous vegetables seem to protect against colon cancer

TABLE 1-3 Review of Current Research Issues Regarding Diet and Cancer (continued)

Food/ Agent	Site	Studies	Results of Studies	Clinical Implications
Vitamin C (ascorbic acid)	Oral Cavity Esophagus Colon Bladder Lung Stomach Cervix	*Laboratory studies* Mirvish, 1975[77] Raineri and Weisburger, 1975[78] Weisburger, 1977	Ascorbic acid inhibits gastrointestinal cancers by blocking the formation of carcinogenic nitrosamines	In vivo and in vitro studies are inconsistent, but a number of human epidemiologic studies show that vitamin C may protect against cancers of the mouth, larynx, esophagus, stomach and cervix; dose is an important factor because vitamin C has been shown to be toxic and to stimulate tumors at high doses
		Leuchtenberger and Leuchtenberger, 1977[80]	Ascorbic acid inhibits abnormal growth and malignant transformation in hamster lung cells exposed to tobacco smoke	
		Migliozzi, 1977[81]	Guinea pigs given vitamin C in high doses had increased tumors, those given moderate doses had decreased tumors, and those given low doses had inhibition of tumors	
		Galloway and Painter, 1979[82]	High doses of ascorbic acid damage DNA and cause mutations	
		Redding and Hirota, 1979[83]	Ascorbic acid administered in carcinogens inhibits tumor development	
		Park et al, 1980[84]	Ascorbic acid inhibits growth of colonies of human leukemic cells	
		Human epidemiologic studies		
		Marshall et al, 1983[85]	Patients with cancer of the cervix had a previous low intake of foods rich in vitamin C	
		Bussey et al, 1982[86]	Individuals with familial polyposis have reduced polyp area when treated with ascorbic acid	
		Kolonel et al, 1981[87]	Risk of stomach cancer decreases with increases in ascorbic acid ingestion	
		Graham et al, 1981[88]	Increased risk of laryngeal cancer with a decreased intake of vitamin C	
		Mettlin et al, 1981[89]	Increased risk of esophageal and oral cancer with a decreased intake of vitamin C	

Occupation

Investigations into the relationship of occupation to cancer have been prompted largely by the 1970 Occupational Health and Safety Act (P.L. 91-596), which is concerned with worker health and safety. To date, a number of occupations have been found to be associated with particular cancers (Table 1-4).[106]

The major limitations of studies of the workplace in relation to the development of cancer are in calculating exposure. Workers may be exposed to numerous gradients of potential carcinogens acquired from the same or a combination of occupations throughout their lives.

Personal Habits

Certain personal habits have been found to increase the risk of developing certain types of cancer. For example, cigarette smoking is estimated to cause 30% of the cancer mortality in the United States.[107] Cancers of the following anatomic sites have been found to be associated with cigarette smoking: oral cavity, larynx, esophagus, lung, stomach, kidney, pancreas, and uterine cervix.[108,109] Evidence has accumulated to suggest that the incidence of lung cancer increases with the quantity of cigarettes smoked, the duration of smoking, and the amount of tar exposure.[110] The risk of lung cancer has also been found to be attrib-

TABLE 1-3 Review of Current Research Issues Regarding Diet and Cancer (continued)

Food/ Agent	Site	Studies	Results of Studies	Clinical Implications
Vitamin A (retinoids)	Lung Bladder Oral Cavity Larynx Esophagus	*Laboratory studies*		Although there are inconsistencies in data, human studies seem to corroborate laboratory studies suggesting that vitamin A protects against certain types of cancer; until further research offers more definitive answers, the supplemental addition of vitamin A to the diet cannot be recommended
		Chu and Malmgren, 1965[90]	Taken orally, vitamin A reduced uterine cervix tumors	
		Saffiotti et al, 1967[91]	In hamsters, vitamin A reduced squamous cell respiratory tumors	
		Nettesheim and Williams, 1976[92]	Inhibited lung tumors in rats	
		Newberne and Suphakarn, 1977[93] Merriman and Bertram, 1979[94]	Used synthetic retinoids rather than naturally occurring vitamin A; inhibited colon tumors in animals with less toxicity	
		Peto et al, 1981[95]	Animals fed a vitamin A–deficient diet developed metaplastic changes in epithelial cells of a variety of organs and increased susceptibility to carcinogens	
		Verma et al, 1982[96]	Retinoids increase the incidence of tumors in mice	
		Human epidemiologic studies		
		Bjelke, 1975[97]	Vitamin A protected against lung cancer with all levels of cigarette smoking	
		MacLennan et al, 1977[98]	Lower risk of lung cancer in women who had an increased intake of green leafy vegetables	
		Smith and Jick, 1978[99]	Twofold lower risk of cancer in those taking vitamin A in multivitamin tablet form	
		Mettlin and Graham, 1979[100] Graham et al, 1981[88] Mettlin et al, 1981[89]	Increased dietary intake of vitamin A was protective against various cancers (especially lung, bladder, larynx, and prostate)	
		Kark et al, 1981[101]	Prospective study: in blood samples taken at the beginning of the study, people who subsequently developed cancer years later showed lower vitamin A levels at the beginning of the study	
		Kvale et al, 1983[102]	Odds ratio of lung cancer is three times higher in those with the lowest intake of vitamin A, vegetables, and milk	
		Hinds et al, 1984[103]	Total vitamin A intake, vitamin A intake from foods only, and carotene intake were all inversely associated with lung cancer in males but not females	
		Willett et al, 1984[104]	Lung cancer patients had statistically nonsignificant higher levels of serum retinol	

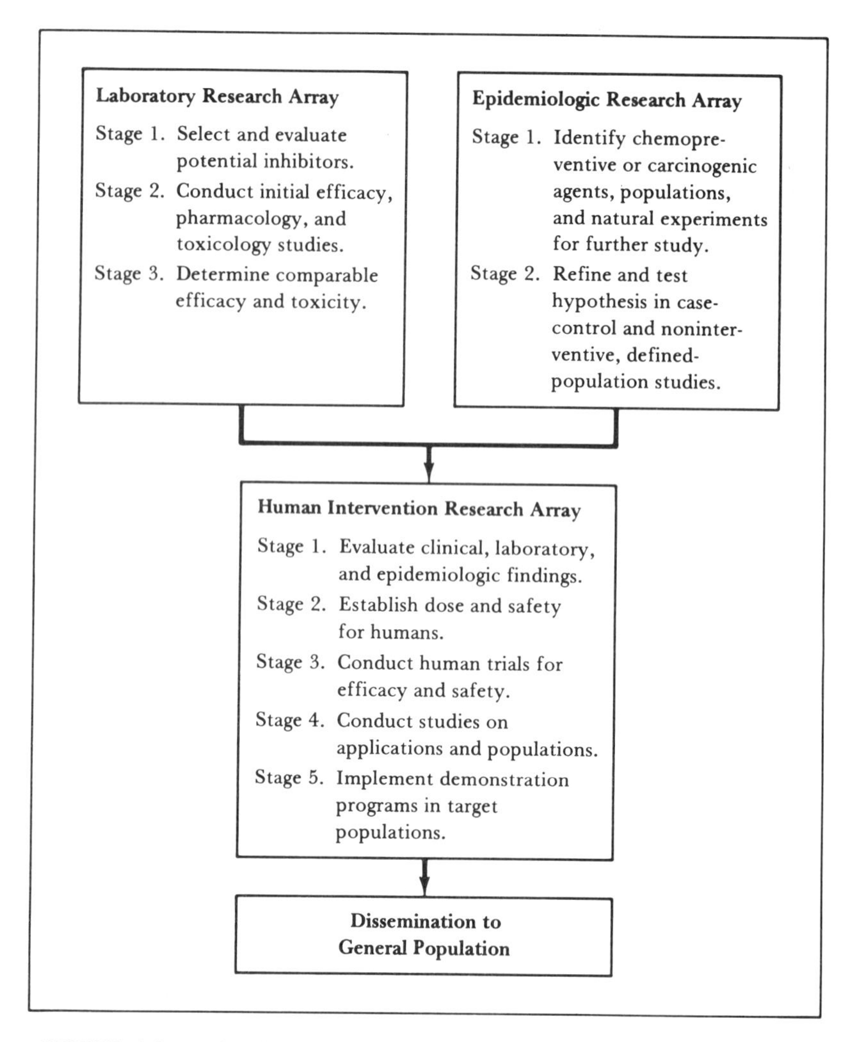

FIGURE 1-1 National Cancer Institute Chemoprevention Program. (Source: From Greenwald P: Manipulation of nutrients to prevent cancer. Hosp Pract 19:120, 1984.

utable to involuntary smoking in a number of studies.[111] The carcinogenic potential of cigarette smoking may also be enhanced when the habit is exercised in certain occupational settings in which other carcinogenic or cocarcinogenic substances, such as asbestos or ionizing radiation, are present.[110]

About 91% of lung cancer in men and about 80% in women is attributable to cigarette smoking. It has only been since 1965 that the percentage of adults who smoke has declined. In 1965, 52% of men over 20 were smokers; 34% of women over 20 were smokers. In 1985, 33% of men and 28% of women were smokers.[112] In addition, cigarettes with less tar are being adopted by smokers.[110] Although the reduction in smoking prevalence may ultimately result in a decline in lung cancer mortality, a less favorable trend is the increase in the percentage of smokers who smoke 25 or more cigarettes a day.[110]

Other personal habits that have been found to increase the risk of developing cancer include tobacco smoking in combination with heavy alcohol consumption (cancer of the head and neck and esophagus) and tobacco chewing (buccal cancer). Risk is generally noted to increase with the frequency and duration of the habit and may persist if the exposure is sufficient despite elimination of the habit. These data provide a strong argument for individual behavior modification to reduce the risk of cancer and continued broad-scale programs for disseminating information about the effects of smoking on health.

Social Environment

Life-style may play a role in an individual's susceptibility to cancer. Life-style is a reflection of social class, and social class dictates the norms and activities to which the individual subscribes. Social class differences in cancer incidence are most pronounced in cervical cancer (affects primarily women of lower socioeconomic status), colon cancer (affects primarily individuals of higher socioeconomic status), and stomach cancer (affects primarily individuals of lower socioeconomic status). Explanations for this phenomenon may include such factors as the "stressful" life-

TABLE 1-4 Occupations/Industries Conveying an Increased Risk of Developing Cancer

Industry/Occupation	Cancer Type *(ICD-9)*	Agent
Vinyl chloride polymerization industry	Hemangiosarcoma of the liver (155)	Vinyl chloride monomer
Vintners Woodworkers, cabinet and furniture makers Boot and shoe industry Radium chemists and processors, dial painters Chromium producers, processors, users Nickel smelting and refining Asbestos industry and users	Malignant neoplasm of nasal cavities (160)	Arsenical pesticides Hardwood dusts Unknown Radium Chromates Nickel Asbestos
Topside coke oven workers	Malignant neoplasm of larynx (161)	Coke over emissions
Asbestos industry and users Uranium and fluorspar miners Chromium producers and processors, users Nickel smelters, processors, users Smelters Mustard gas formulators Ion exchange resin makers, chemists	Malignant neoplasm of trachea, bronchus, and lung (162)	Asbestos Radon daughters Chromates Nickel Arsenic Mustard gas Bis (chloromethyl) ether, chloromethyl methyl, ether
Asbestos industries and utilizers	Mesothelioma, peritoneum (158) or pleura (163)	Asbestos
Dial painters, radium chemists and processors	Malignant neoplasm of bone (170)	Radium
Automatic lathe operators, metalworkers Coke oven workers, petroleum refiners, tar distillers	Malignant neoplasm of scrotum (187.7)	Mineral and cutting oils Soots and tars, tar distillates
Rubber and dye workers	Malignant neoplasm of bladder (188)	Benzidine, alpha and beta naphthylamine, auramine, magenta, aminobiphenyl, 4-nitrophenyl
Coke oven workers	Malignant neoplasm of kidney, other, and unspecified urinary organs (189)	Coke oven emissions
Rubber industry, radiologists	Lymphoid leukemia, acute (204)	Unknown, ionizing radiation
Occupations with exposure to benzene, radiologists	Myeloid leukemia, acute (205)	Benzene, ionizing radiation
Occupations with exposure to benzene	Erythroleukemia (207)	Benzene

Source: Rutstein DD, Mullan RJ, Frazier TM, et al; Sentinnel health events (occupational); a basis for physician recognition and public health surveillance. Am J Public Health 73:1054-1062, 1983.

style of the ghetto, increased exposure to toxic and hazardous substances due to residence or job, inadequate access to adequate health care, differences in dietary patterns, or lack of education about the warning signs of cancer.

Problems in the epidemiologic evaluation of the relationship between cancer and social environment are largely definitional, particularly regarding what constitutes social class and how social and environmental variables contribute to risk.

Iatrogenic Factors

Epidemiologic studies have been used to substantiate clinical impressions of iatrogenic sources of cancer. Radiation for the treatment of an enlarged thymus gland or for tinea capitis has been found to induce thyroid cancers.[113] Women who had radiation treatment for benign gynecologic conditions have been reported to have a higher mortality rate from leukemia and cancers of the pelvic area.[114] Radiation and chemotherapy in the treatment of individuals with cancer have been observed to cause new primary cancers later in life. Individuals receiving immunosuppressive therapy are at increased risk for cancers of the reticuloendothelial system.[115] Radiographic evaluation in utero was found to be associated with increased cancer rates. The sharp decline in endometrial cancer that occurred after information was disseminated on the hazards of estrogen replacement therapy strongly suggests that use of this drug contributed to the development of this form of cancer.[116]

A major concern with these iatrogenic sources is the unresolved question of the risk of cancer among the offspring of those exposed. This issue was raised as a result of the appearance of vaginal adenocarcinoma in the daughters of women who took diethylstilbestrol (DES) to prevent miscarriages.[117]

Physical Environment

Although most cancer-causing substances in the environment are man-made, there also exists a concern over the carcinogenicity of natural substances. The carcinogenicity of ionizing radiation was first discovered by the excess cancer mortality rate among persons in certain occupations, notably radium dial painters (bone sarcomas) and radiologists (leukemia and skin cancer). Further evidence was obtained through observation of the increased incidence of leukemia among atomic bomb survivors and underground miners of uranium, flurospar, and hematite. The widespread addition of fluoride to potable water supplies has been a matter of concern to many people. However, studies to date have found that the rate of cancer is not increased in areas where fluoride has been added to water.[118,119] An association between exposure to sunlight (ultraviolet radiation) and skin cancer (both melanomas and nonmelanomas) has been demonstrated by a number of epidemiologic studies, with the greatest risk related to decreasing latitude.[120,121]

Epidemiologic studies of environmental carcinogens are difficult to perform because of the problems associated with identifying people who have received comparable exposures to a particular agent. The rate of population movement in many areas is quite high; variations in the environment (humidity, wind, temperature, and so on) may affect the degree and nature of the exposure; and, as with occupational studies, the population may have been exposed to a variety of other substances that may not be carcinogenic in themselves but may be cocarcinogens or promoters.

Last, the major controversy involves determining the lowest dose at which exposure to an environmental factor may precipitate a neoplasm. Some authorities feel certain that low levels of environmental carcinogens may be tolerable given the body's tremendous adaptive and detoxifying capabilities and assume that only a minority of the population is highly susceptible. On the other hand, if the clonal theory of cancer is proved (ie, a malignancy need arise from only one cell), the pool of susceptible individuals actually may be growing, particularly in the face of the ever-increasing number of chemicals being introduced into the environment and the burden that this imposes on the human system.

EVALUATING THE INTERACTION BETWEEN HOST AND ENVIRONMENT OVER TIME

Although characteristics of the host and environment each make a unique contribution to a disease entity or health problem, it must be remembered that timing of the interaction ultimately may determine the pattern of observable ill health. Three major epidemiologic techniques are used to examine the effects of these interactions between the host, the environment, and time: *birth-cohort analysis, migrant studies,* and *clustering.*

Birth-Cohort Analysis

A *birth-cohort* is a defined group of persons with similar characteristics or common exposure both in a particular period, usually within 5 years. In this analytic technique, several birth cohorts are compared at the same age to evaluate the extent to which time influenced the emergence of a particular outcome (usually mortality).

Birth-cohort analysis is largely used to determine whether common exposure to a suspected etiologic factor resulted in an increased incidence of disease or to measure how prevention or treatment has altered the course of the disease over time. This method is also particularly useful in identifying those groups at greatest risk, for whom screening and intense follow-up may be a worthwhile investment of resources.

Cohort analysis aids in understanding the impact of changes in the age distribution and other cohort characteristics and medical advances on the dynamics of cancer.

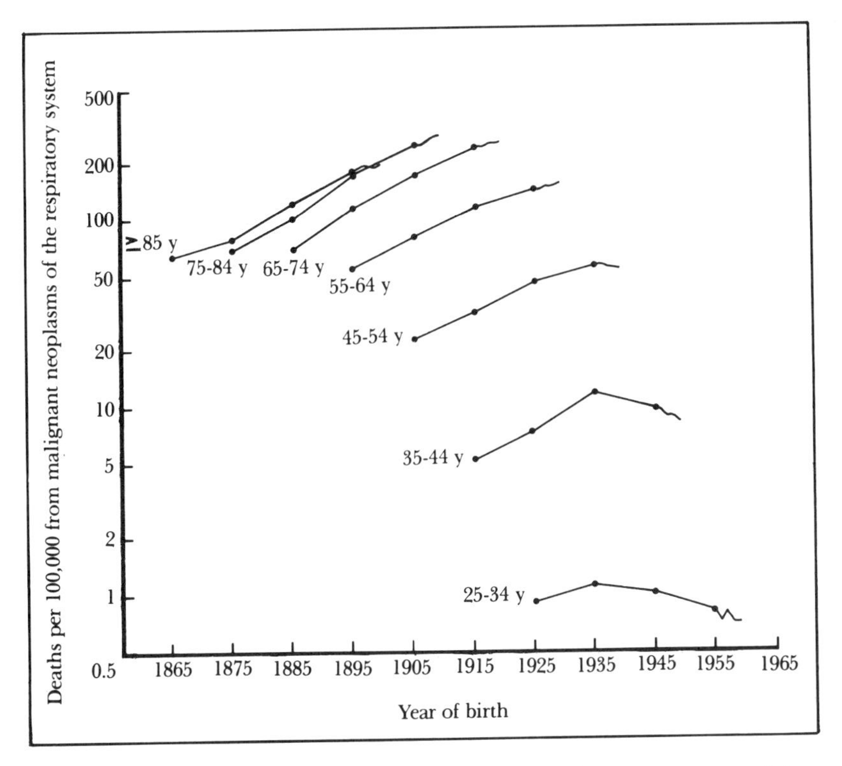

FIGURE 1-2 Cohort age contours for mortality from malignant neoplasms of the respiratory system, 1950 through 1984. Four points plotted within each contour indicate mortality rate for 1950, 1960, 1970, and 1980, respectively. Each contour represents different 10-year age group. (Source: Breslow L, Cumberland WG: Progress and objectives in cancer control. JAMA 259:1690-1694, 1988.)

Figure 1-2 illustrates the cancer mortality patterns between 1950 and 1984 for individuals born between 1865 and 1965. This cohort analysis illustrates that different sets of factors have been operating in the cohort born before 1935 from those individuals born after 1935. In the former cohort, the cancer mortality rates continue to rise. Increased life expectancy and previous high smoking prevalence are likely to explain the increase in lung cancer mortality rates. In the group of individuals born after 1935, earlier diagnosis of cancer, improved cancer treatment, and reduction of smoking may account for the downward trend in respiratory cancer mortality rates.[122]

Migrant Studies

Studies of cancer incidence and mortality trends among populations who migrate afford investigators a unique opportunity to understand the effects of environment and culture on the development of cancer. It is assumed that as populations move from their native land to other areas, some assimilation is made with regard to the new life-style and dietary practices. Migrating individuals also become exposed to the same environmental factors as the host population. In theory, the cancer rates should be intermediate between the rates of the host and native populations, although this is not always the case. Consideration of the age at which migration occurred reveals the length of exposure required for risk to increase or decrease and the critical point at which reversible preneoplastic transformation occurs. Migrant studies as an analytic framework also can reveal if the risk is persistent but delayed with a change in environment. However, migrants may not be representative of their native land (eg, in better or worse health, social outcasts, or more ambitious). Thus, the relatives of migrants may serve as a comparison group.

Although changing patterns of cancer incidence and mortality among immigrants have not been observed for all anatomic sites, some patterns are discernible. Haenszel found that cancer mortality patterns among immigrant populations generally tend to be specific for both site and country of origin.[123] Studies of migrant populations are often based on country-to-country comparisons but can be designed to analyze the effects of other environmental units, such as population movements from rural to urban settings.

Clustering

As described earlier, diseases vary over time and place and exhibit characteristic trends. However, in some circumstances an excessive number of identical cases of a health problem occurs that cannot be explained by natural variation of either time or place or chance alone. Diseases that emerge within a circumscribed place within the same time interval are defined as *clusters*. The presence of clusters raises the question of a common etiologic agent, usually infectious or environmental, but clusters also can be related to genetic or cultural factors. Cluster analysis as applied to cancer involves many methodologic difficulties, especially in determining the size of the geographic place and the time interval required to qualify as a cluster. These variables must be neither too small nor too large.

Epidemiologic methods have been used to evaluate alleged clusters of persons with Hodgkin's disease, for which an infectious etiology is suspected, with equivocal results. Space-time clustering of Burkitt's lymphoma has been demonstrated statistically over a 16-year period in the West Nile district of Uganda. However, it is not known whether an infectious viral agent alone is responsible or whether the virus acts in combination with malaria or some other environmental agent.[124]

The most recent example of astute observations by clinicians of unusual diseases occurring within a similar population was the recognition of acquired immune deficiency syndrome (AIDS), which predisposes the affected individual to infections with opportunistic organisms *(Pneumocystis carinii, Cryptococcus neoformans),* Kaposi's sarcoma, and non-Hodgkin's lymphomas.[125] AIDS was first reported in 1981 by Gottlieb and colleagues, who observed that there was a sudden increase in *P. carinii* pneumonia, other opportunistic infections, and a disseminated form of Kaposi's sarcoma in apparently previously healthy young homosexual men in New York City and San Francisco.[126] This observation drew a great deal of attention, and the Centers for Disease Control (CDC) formed a task force to study this growing disease problem.

Although AIDS was first identified in the homosexual community, it is now found in heterosexual people, in both blacks and whites, and in women and children. AIDS has become a worldwide problem, having been reported in more than 40 countries in five continents.[127] Groups at particularly high risk for AIDS are homosexuals, male bisexuals, intravenous drug abusers, and hemophiliacs.[128] There is increasing evidence that different forms of transmission of AIDS occur among the various risk groups. Among male homosexuals and bisexuals, AIDS infection is acquired through receptive anal intercourse.[129] Among US blacks and Hispanics, contaminated needles used for illicit drugs and perinatal exposure are the primary methods of AIDS transmission.[130] Contaminated blood products, particularly clotting factors, are the primary mode of transmission of AIDS to hemophiliacs.[131] In Africa, frequent contact with different heterosexual partners, especially prostitutes, conveys an increased risk of acquiring AIDS.[132]

AIDS is now known to be caused by human immunodeficiency virus type 1 (HIV-1), which is transmitted through intimate sharing of blood and body fluids; through sexual activity; through medical use of unscreened blood, blood products, and transplanted tissues; and by passage of virus from an infected mother to her unborn child.[127] HIV is a retrovirus that destroys critical immune T cells, producing the syndrome of AIDS.[133] According to the CDC, a total of 72,024 cases of AIDS had been reported in the United States by September 1, 1988.[128] It is projected that by 1992 a cumulative total of 365,000 AIDS cases will have been diagnosed (Figure 1-3).[128]

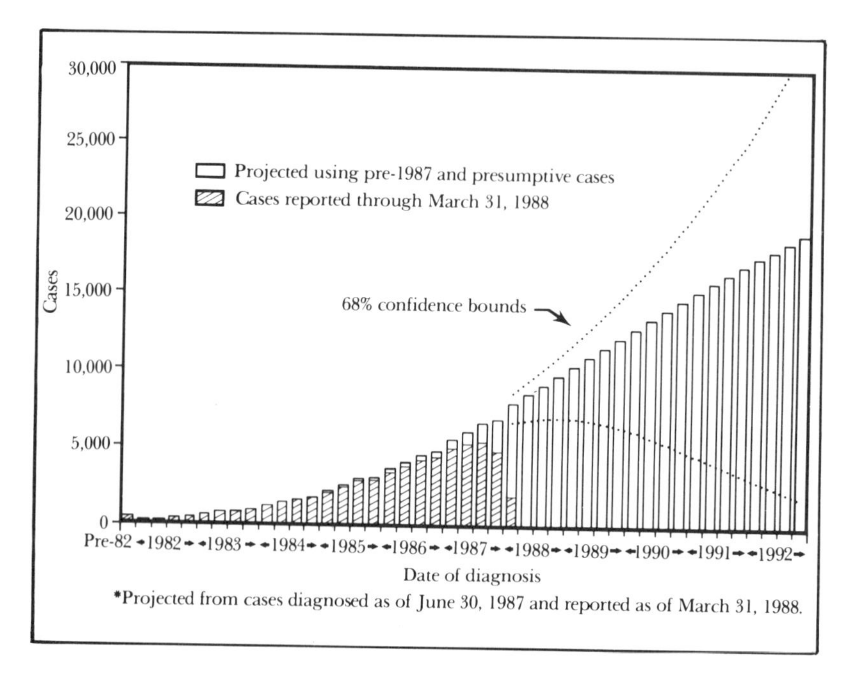

FIGURE 1-3 Incidence of AIDS,* by quarter and year of diagnosis—United States, pre-1982 to 1992. (Source: Centers for Disease Control: Quarterly report of the Domestic Policy Council on the prevalence and rate of spread of HIV and AIDS in the United States. MMWR 37:223-226, 1988.)

AIDS is an excellent example of how knowledge is obtained through observations of clusters of unusual patterns of disease. However, caution is needed before accepting the results of cluster studies. The distribution of cancer cases in space and time may be related to the availability of certain types of diagnostic services, the presence of large families with similar heritages, the movement of a generation of susceptible individuals to a particular area, or to chance. Thus all factors must be examined carefully before decisions about the validity of a cluster phenomenon can be made.

NURSING IMPLICATIONS OF EPIDEMIOLOGIC FINDINGS

The epidemiologic findings cited concerning the etiology of cancer and its consequences as influenced by the host, environment, and their interaction are not meant to be a comprehensive review of the existing literature. They merely illustrate the perspectives to be considered in a comprehensive nursing history of an individual diagnosed with or at risk for cancer, for a community assessment, or for a nursing study.

The categories recommended for assessment are summarized in Figure 1-4. Specific questions to be asked for each category will vary according to the type of individual and population served.

FIGURE 1-4 Nursing history for a cancer patient or potential cancer patient—a categorical outline.

A. Demographic information
   1. Birthdate/birthplace
   2. Sex
   3. Race/ethnicity
   4. Marital status
   5. Longest place of residence
   6. Current place of residence
   7. Socioeconomic status
B. Family history
   1. Family member with diagnosed malignancy
   2. Type of malignancy
   3. Relationship to family member
   4. Consanguinity
C. Habits
   1. Tobacco use (especially cigarettes)
      a. Type; quantity (maximum) per number of year(s); depth of inhalation
   2. Alcohol consumption
      a. Type; quantity per day for how long
   3. Recreational drug usage
      a. Type
      b. Route of administration
      c. Duration of usage
D. Occupational/hobby exposures
   1. Description of job/hobby activities
   2. Nature of carcinogens (insecticides, radiation, and so on)
   3. Route of exposure and type (fumes, particulate matter, and so forth)
   4. Number of years in related positions with common occupational exposures
E. Immunologic status
   1. Cytogenetic abnormalities
   2. Prior therapy affecting the immune system
      a. Drugs (cancer chemotherapy, long-term steroid usage)
      b. Radiotherapy
   3. Primary immune deficiency
F. Diet
   1. Type of foods and nonalcoholic beverages
   2. Eating patterns (considering ethnic preferences)
G. General history
   1. Previous history of cancer
   2. Other diseases or precursor conditions related to malignancy
   3. Stress levels

COMMON EPIDEMIOLOGIC METHODS

Descriptive Methods

Describing the phenomenon observed is the necessary first step in understanding what is occurring. Descriptive methods used in epidemiology are incidence, mortality, and prevalence rates.

Incidence

The *incidence rate* for cancer reflects the number of new cases occurring in a given population at risk during a specified period *(t)*. It is calculated as follows:

$$\text{Incidence rate} = \frac{\text{Number of new cases } (t)}{\text{Population at risk } (t)} \times \text{Factor of } 10$$

The numerator and denominator are multiplied by a convenient factor of 10 or one that is used by convention (eg, cancer incidence rate is expressed as per 100,000 population) to avoid working with fractional units.

This formula can be applied to determine the average annual leukemia rate in Olmstead County, Minnesota, for the years 1965 through 1974, using data from the example opposite:

Total number of leukemia cases, 1965-1974	*Total population Olmstead County, Minn, 1970*
79	83,000

Crude average annual incidence rate = $(79/10 \div 83{,}000) \times 100{,}000$
= 9.5 new cases of leukemia per 100,000 population

Because only a few new cancers of a particular type may occur in a geographic area in any given year, data may be pooled over a 5- or 10-year period and averaged to provide stability to the summary rate calculated. In the above example, the number of cases is "annualized" over a 10-year period.

Incidence data are not readily obtainable for most population areas of the United States because of a lack of legislative requirements for reporting new cases of cancer to the local health authorities. In many developed and some developing countries where health care is subsidized by the government, reporting of cancer is routine. Isolated hospital registries in themselves cannot be used as a source of incidence data because they ordinarily do not draw their cases from a large defined population. Duplication of cases may emerge in individual registries among hospitals sharing cancer treatment facilities or those with overlapping service areas.

To obtain population-based data on site-specific incidence of cancer, mortality, and survival experience, the National Cancer Institute established the Surveillance, Epidemiology, and End Results (SEER) Program in 1973. The SEER Program represents a 12% sample of the US population and includes six large metropolitan areas (San Francisco, Oakland, Detroit, New Orleans, Seattle, and Atlanta), six states (Connecticut, Hawaii, Iowa, New Mexico, Utah, and New Jersey), and the Commonwealth of Puerto Rico.[134] The SEER data provide ongoing information from widely divergent geographic areas and a mixture of ethnic groups.

Before the SEER Program was established, incidence data were derived from three major surveys conducted by the National Cancer Institute (NCI). The first was conducted between 1937 and 1939 and covered ten large metropolitan areas representing approximately 10% of the nation's population. The second survey was conducted between 1947 and 1948 and covered the same ten cities. The Third National Cancer Survey was conducted between 1969 and 1971. The advantage of the SEER Program is that it provides data on an ongoing rather than periodic basis and thus enables identification of emerging patterns in the prevention and treatment of cancer.

The identification of new cancer cases is desirable in many respects. Observation of patterns and trends that emerge may render clues as to how etiology may be related to features of the environment, behavior, or culture. The incidence gives a perspective of the current magnitude of the problem and provides a source for estimating future priorities in cancer control activities. Although these are very important advantages of incidence data, one must always inquire into the reasons for less than expected cancer incidence rates among certain groups of individuals (such as Mormons and Seventh Day Adventists).

Mortality

Another descriptive epidemiologic measure is *mortality rate,* which is the number of deaths that occur in the population at risk in a specific time period. Mortality rate as an epidemiologic measure to describe trends of such chronic conditions as cancer requires that the numbers comprising the numerator and the denominator of the formula be specified by the time period in which they are occurring, and preferably be from the same time period. For example, the crude mortality rate for cancer in 1970 can be calculated as follows:

$$\text{Crude cancer mortality rate in 1970} = \frac{\text{Number of cancer deaths in 1970}}{\text{Total U.S. population in 1970 at mid-year}} \times 100{,}000$$

$$= \frac{330{,}700}{203{,}200{,}000} \times 100{,}000$$

$$= 162.8 \text{ cancer deaths per } 100{,}000 \text{ population per year}$$

Much of the data used in cancer epidemiology are based on mortality rates obtained from death certificates. The entire United States and many countries throughout the world require that causes of death be reported. Because of the wide availability of this information for populations with known demographic characteristics, mortality data are useful in evaluating cancer trends. Where population-based incidence figures are not available, mortality rates can be used to estimate the relative magnitude of cancer in a particular area. The approximation comes close to what can be derived from incidence data, especially for the high and low rates. If the prognosis for a cancer is very limited, the mortality rate tends to parallel incidence for it (eg, lung cancer). On the other hand, if survival of the cancer is long and the likelihood of other factors contributing to death grows, cancer mortality rate may actually decline in the presence of a steady or increasing incidence (eg, thyroid cancer). A certain degree of error is inherent in epidemiologic data gathered from death certificates. Inaccuracies in diagnosis, incompleteness in reporting cancer on a death certificate, and differences in the diagnostic criteria for a neoplastic lesion are the major sources of error.

Prevalence

Prevalence rate is the number of individuals who have a given disease in a given population during a specified period *(t)*. It is a function of both the incidence *(I)* and duration *(D)* of the disease. Prevalence can either be expressed as *point prevalence* or *period prevalence.* The number of cases at one moment in time is called point prevalence. Period prevalence considers the number of cases existing over a period of time, usually 1 year, and is more often used in cancer epidemiology. Prevalence rates include newly diagnosed cases plus individuals with previously diagnosed cancer who are still alive in the period being studied. The formula for prevalence rate is:

$$\text{Prevalence rate} = \frac{\text{Number of cases } (t)}{\text{Number of persons in the population in which cases occurred } (t)} \times \text{Factor of } 10$$

Thus any treatment that prolongs life (duration) would reflect an increased prevalence, even if the incidence is constant. The highest crude cancer prevalence rates found in 1983 to 1985 during the National Health Interview Survey were for female breast, skin, digestive system, and genital system cancers and for prostate malignancies. Of those persons with a malignancy of the lung, 68.2% reported limitation in activity; 48.6% of those with gastrointestinal malignancy reported activity limitation.[135]

Although prevalence is not useful for studying etiology, it can be applied in the planning of facilities and health manpower needs, for diagnostic screening and control programs, and for predicting the long-term economic burden and physical and psychosocial needs of individuals with various types of cancer.

Other rates

The calculations of incidence, mortality, and prevalence previously described do not take into account the relative proportions of age, sex, race, or other variables that might affect the likelihood of cancer in the population at risk. Such calculations of rate are therefore called *crude rates.* It is often necessary to compare groups of individuals or populations with respect to incidence or mortality. To draw appropriate conclusions, measures are taken to ensure comparability of the characteristics of the populations. For example, valid conclusions cannot be drawn about the influence of a suspected environmental carcinogen on cancer incidence on the basis of a comparison of a rural population to a younger inner-city Latino population. Adjustment of rates removes the effect of population characteristics that are particularly influential on the development of or death from cancer. Most often, *age-adjusted rates* are used, although adjustments for other variables such as sex and race may be considered.

Increases in the size of the population and the proportion of aged individuals cause a dramatic increase in the crude death rate from cancer because cancer is largely a disease of old age and because the proportion of elderly people in the United States is increasing. When it is adjusted for age, the increase in the cancer mortality rate between 1970 and 1984 is less than 3%.[122]

Analytic Methods

There are two major analytic designs used in epidemiology: prospective and retrospective studies. The purpose of both is to determine the influence of a cause (or antecedent factor) in relation to an outcome. The major distinction between the two approaches is the time frame used to select the study sample.

Prospective study

In a *prospective study* (also known as a cohort study), individuals are selected with varying degrees of exposure to the suspected factor. These individuals have not experienced the particular outcome thought to be associated with the factor. They are then followed over time and observed to see whether the outcome being investigated occurs. The groups selected for study can be a sample from the general population or a select group of the population such as certain occupational groups. It is also possible to conduct a prospective study by defining a past date for a specific group (eg, HMO enrollees) whose records contain appropriate documentation of the factors under investigation. Follow-up information concerning the outcome is reconstructed, if necessary, through a number of sources, including death certificates, hospital records, and the like. This latter type of study also may be called a historical prospective.

A classic prospective epidemiologic study frequently referred to in the literature was conducted by Doll and Hill.[136] The study, which began in 1951, followed white male British physicians whose smoking habits were surveyed at the onset of the study. Cigarette smoking was related to lung cancer mortality, with dose-response relationships being found. A feature of the Doll and Hill study, like other prospective designs, was that it was able to determine the incidence of the outcome and relate it to the presence of a specific causative factor. It was also able to examine the relationship of smoking to other outcomes and found that although smoking was associated with other diseases, the strength of the association was greatest for lung cancer. These types of conclusions were possible because the denominator of the formula (total population at risk, ie, all British male physicians) was known.

There are several important factors to keep in mind when designing a prospective study: the time the study begins must be clearly defined; individuals must be free of the outcome being studied (this usually requires that members of the study group be evaluated in some way before defining the denominator of the formula); all individuals must be followed in the same manner regardless of exposure level; and every attempt should be made to ensure complete follow-up of all subjects in the cohort.

Retrospective study

In a *retrospective study* (or case-control study), individuals are selected on the basis of a known outcome, and evidence of a factor suspected of being an antecedent to the outcome is sought. The number of instances in which the factor occurs in this group is compared with the number of instances in which it occurs in a control group to determine if there are significant differences between the two groups. The design of a retrospective study can be handled in many ways, depending on the study objectives and certain matters of practicality. Cases (individuals with the known outcome) may either be representative of all the cases or may consist of all possible cases. Controls may consist of the total population when the cases are drawn from a defined geographic population in which the frequency of factors being studied is routinely recorded. Controls also may consist of a sample randomly chosen from a larger population representing all possible controls. Controls also may be selected by a matching schema according to temporal or spatial relation to the cases, for example, a breast cancer case paired with the next noncancer-related diagnosis on an admissions roster living closest to the case, or some effort at matching may be employed. Controls may be matched at the very least on age, sex, and race and on all other major factors except for those being studied to account for confounding variables. The difficulty with this technique is that a match may be difficult to locate, particularly when there are three or more matching variables. Unmatched cases must be discarded from the analysis. Variables that are matched cannot be examined. Alternatives to pairwise matching are possible. With a technique called frequency matching, a random sample of cases is taken and controls are selected in proportion to subgroups reflecting the distribution of the variables used in matching. Last, independent samples of controls and cases may be drawn and statistical analyses may be employed to adjust for any disparities between the controls and cases with respect to potential confounding factors such as age or sex. The decision of whether to match depends on how much is known about the causative factors; matching generally is not employed if little is known about the factors.

A well-done retrospective study is statistically more powerful, more economical, and quicker to do than a prospective study. A retrospective study is usually done when an investigator wishes to conduct a preliminary investigation of a hypothesis. Associations detected or not detected can be used to assess the need for further study. Retrospective studies are often used in studies of cancer etiology where the long latency period and relatively low frequency of a site-specific cancer would make a prospective study extremely expensive and time-consuming.

However, there are many more potential sources of bias in a retrospective study. The medical record from which data for a retrospective study are likely to be obtained may not be complete regarding information needed to define specific parameters. For example, the record may indicate that the individual had an increased temperature, but information needed for the study is documentation of an oral temperature greater than 101° F. Furthermore, because the data are acquired after the disease or health problem is known, the individual's knowledge of the condition might influence the recollection of the factors associated with it. Some individuals with cancer may either have a vague notion of their condition or be completely unaware of their true diagnosis, and criteria for the inclusion or exclusion of this type of individual must be made ahead of time. Knowing which data can be obtained accurately from records or recall can increase the validity of the retrospective study.

A well-done prospective study has the advantage of generalizing the conclusions to the population from which it is drawn. Information derived from a prospective study concerning the rate of occurrence (risk) of the outcome can therefore be calculated directly because the population at risk for the outcome under investigation is well defined. A prospective study also permits a more rigorous and refined definition of the suspect exposure factor, thereby reducing the degree of bias in determining the risk associated with the exposure. Last, other suspect factors can be examined simultaneously in a prospective study.

A decision regarding the type of study design that should be employed depends on the nature of preexisting evidence concerning a particular risk factor. When little is known, a descriptive epidemiologic approach is first employed. Frequency patterns and incidence and mortality rates, when available, are examined in terms of the distribution of the observed outcome, time patterns, and characteristics of the host.

When the outcome is rare or causes are unknown or must be explored further, the retrospective approach is appropriate. The prospective study is conducted when a sufficient body of evidence from retrospective and cross-sectional studies (surveys) is accrued to implicate specific etiologic factors for the disease or health problems under investigation.

Analysis of results

A major end point of prospective and retrospective studies is the determination of *risk*. Risk relates the magnitude of the effect of a particular antecedent (or exposure) factor on the outcome being investigated. The meaning of risk varies depending on how the calculation is made. There are two approaches used to calculate risk: relative and attributable risk.

Relative risk Mathematically, *relative risk* is simply a ratio comparing the rate of the disease among exposed individuals with the rate of the disease among unexposed individuals. Because it is a ratio, it does not reveal the probability that the exposed person will develop the outcome. Rather, the relative risk measures the strength of the association between a factor and the outcome. The higher the relative risk, the greater the evidence for causation. Using the data from Table 1-5, the rate of lung cancer mortality among heavy smokers exposed to low doses of ionizing radiation is 2.7; among nonsmokers the mortality rate is 0.2.[137] The relative risk (2.7/0.2) based on these data is 13.5; that is, the risk of death from lung cancer for smokers is 13.5 times greater than that for nonsmokers given comparable exposure to ionizing radiation.

The disease rates displayed in Table 1-5 were obtained directly because the investigation was based on the experience of a cohort of an occupational group. Disease rates cannot be calculated directly from a study design employing cases and controls; however, the relative risk can still be estimated from such a study.

The odds ratio is a mathematical expression of the odds of having the disease when the factor is present compared with the odds of having the disease when the factor is absent. An odds ratio is an estimate of the relative risk when the disease being investigated is rare. An odds ratio (or estimated relative risk) equal to 1 means that the suspect etiologic factor is as likely to occur among the cases as among the controls. Displayed in Table 1-6 are computations illustrating the concept that the risk of endometrial cancer among users of conjugated estrogens is 7.4 times higher than the risk among nonusers.

The odds ratio is the only means of comparing the results of retrospective and prospective studies. The odds

TABLE 1-5 Mortality from Respiratory Cancer in White Uranium Miners by Smoking Habits and Exposure to Ionizing Radiations

	Annual Death Rate per 1000 Men*		
	Industrial Exposure in Working Level Months		
Smoking Habits	1–359	360–1799	1800 or More
Nonsmokers	0.2(1)	0.9(3)	1.4(2)
Current smokers			
1–19 cigarettes/day	1.6(5)	1.1(3)	8.3(6)
20 cigarettes/day	1.3(9)	3.5(29)	9.4(30)
>20 cigarettes/day	2.7(8)	4.7(17)	13.3(15)

*Five or more years after the start of mining; the number of cases is in parentheses.

Source: From Doll R: Introduction, in Hiatt HH, Watson JD, Winston JA (eds): Origins of Human Cancer, New York, Cold Springs Harbor Laboratory, 1977.

TABLE 1-6(a) Data Layout for a Retrospective (Case-Control) Study

	Exposed	Nonexposed
Cases	*a*	*b*
Controls	*c*	*d*
Odds ratio $= \frac{ad}{bc}$		

TABLE 1-6(b) History of Use of Conjugated Estrogens

	Yes	No
Endometrial cancer	54	40
Controls	29	159
Odds ratio = 7.4		

ratio can be calculated from both retrospective and prospective studies. In this respect it is used to evaluate the consistency of the magnitude of the risk of the outcome in relation to a particular factor across study designs and employed on different populations. A prospective and retrospective study of the same etiologic factor and disease should yield odds ratios or estimated relative risks of the same direction and comparable magnitudes. However, it cannot be overemphasized that even when the odds ratio among studies yields consistent findings, a consistent overestimate or underestimate can occur if individuals are classified improperly regarding their status as eligible cases or controls or if ascertainment of exposure is not adequately evaluated.

Attributable risk Within every time interval, there is an expected or normal number of individuals who are not exposed to the suspect factor but nonetheless experience a particular outcome. The *attributable risk* is the arithmetic difference in the disease rates between the group exposed to the factor and unexposed groups. Using the data from Table 1-5, the mortality rate among the heavy smokers subjected to low doses of ionizing radiation (2.7) minus the mortality rate among nonsmokers at the same dose (0.2) yields an attributable risk of 2.5. This means that an additional 2.5 deaths occurred that were attributable to smoking. Or, to put it another way, these excess deaths would not have occurred if the individuals were not heavy smokers.

The attributable risk can only be calculated directly from a prospective study for the same reasons that were discussed in the section on relative risk. However, the attributable risk in an entire defined population can be estimated from a case-control study if the relative risk and the frequency with which the suspect etiologic factor is found in the population are known. This would reveal that as more individuals in a population are exposed to the suspect factor in the presence of a high relative risk for the factor, a larger number of cases would occur. Thus it would be expected that with the high relative risk associated with heavy smoking among females determined from previous retrospective studies in combination with a greater proportion of females who smoke, a larger number of cases of lung cancer occurring in women could be attributed to smoking. This phenomenon is now being observed.

In summary, the attributable risk is used to calculate the magnitude of change of an outcome (eg, respiratory cancer) with the removal of the suspect antecedent factor (eg, smoking). For more information on calculating relative and attributable risk, the reader is referred to more detailed texts on epidemiologic methods.

OTHER APPLICATIONS OF EPIDEMIOLOGY IN THE FIELD OF CANCER

Survival Analysis

The observation over time of individuals with cancer and the calculation of their probability of dying over several time periods is referred to as *survival analysis*. Survival data for the most common cancer sites are displayed in Figure 1-5.[138] A 5-year relative survival of at least 50% is expected

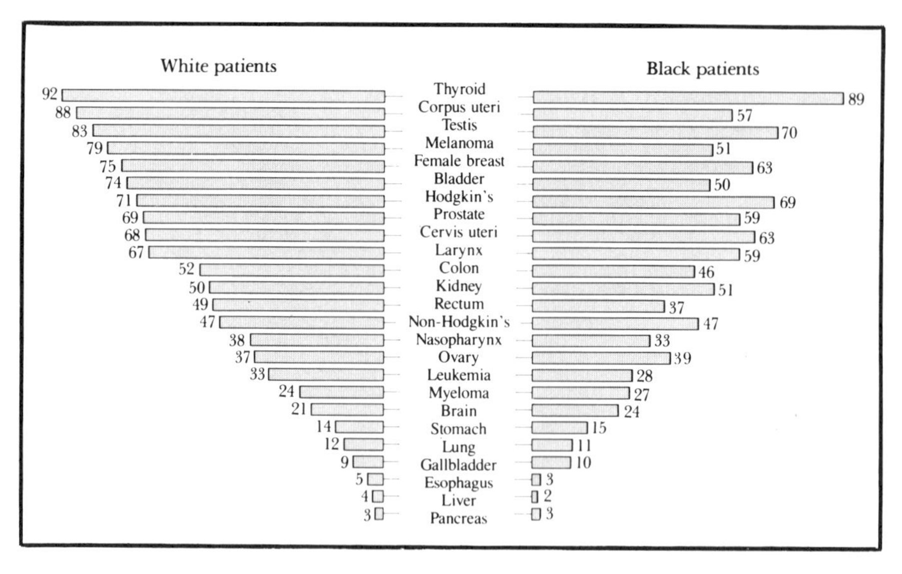

FIGURE 1-5 Five-year relative survival rates (%) for selected cancer sites, white and black patients, SEER Program data, 1973 to 1981. (Source: Greenwald P, Sondik EJ (eds): Cancer control objectives for the nation: 1985-2000. NCI monograph no. 2. Washington DC, US Government Printing Office, 1986, pp 3-14.)

for persons with cancer of the thyroid, corpus uteri, and testis, for persons with melanoma, and for black and white women with breast cancer. The lower survival in blacks for all cancer types is striking and may be because of lower accessibility to health care or lack of knowledge or awareness regarding the importance of seeking diagnosis and treatment for symptoms. Attitudes and knowledge may also be barriers among blacks toward adopting health-promotion behaviors. In addition, blacks may also be assigned or only have employment opportunity in industries or jobs in which the potential exists for higher exposure to carcinogens. These factors may explain some of the black-white survival differences.

Survival analysis has many applications, including evaluating the effectiveness of cancer therapies, determining if the interval between disease onset and commencement of treatment could be modified to reduce cancer morbidity or mortality, and, more recently, as a means of developing hypotheses regarding cancer risk factors.

One interesting pattern recently identified in the 1973 to 1979 SEER data survival analyses was a higher overall survival rate among Japanese vs. Anglos for cancer of the stomach, colon, rectum, prostate, and breast, even when the data are controlled for age and stage of disease. One hypothesis raised from this finding was that different histologies exist in the Japanese, possibly because of different nutritional factors that in turn are associated with higher survival.[139]

An Epidemiologic Perspective of Screening

A major application of epidemiology is the control of disease at a stage where early intervention can significantly improve the quality of life and minimize disability. Although the principles of cancer detection will be discussed at length in Chapter 8, it is worthwhile to mention briefly the applications of epidemiology in this area of cancer control.

Characteristics of the host such as age, sex, race, socioeconomic status, and occupation in relation to the presence of a particular cancer are important because they help identify target populations and assist in decisions regarding what screening strategy must be employed. Equally important are features of the cancer: its incidence, prevalence, distribution, natural history, and the specificity and sensitivity of the screening methods employed.

For an investment in screening methods to prove worthwhile, the cost expended in detection should be more than offset by the number of cancers found. That is, the incidence and severity of a particular disease should be of sufficient magnitude to warrant public health concern, early intervention must have been shown to decrease morbidity and mortality associated with the disease, and the duration of the disease must be such that early intervention would increase longevity.

Critical factors in a screening program are therefore that the screening methods chosen have high specificity and sensitivity in relation to cost, be acceptable and accessible to consumers, and present a minimum of risk. *Sensitivity* is the probability of a positive test response if the individual has the disease. *Specificity* is the probability of a negative test result if the individual is free of the disease.

Few methods for cancer screening exist that possess sufficiently high sensitivity and specificity (over 90%) other than the Papanicolaou test for cervical cancer and mammography for breast cancer. Screening for the most prevalent and lethal cancer, lung cancer, by conventional radiographic means is of little value. By the time this neoplasm is first visible radiographically, it is already 2 cm and is likely to have disseminated. Thus cancer control efforts should be directed toward preventive measures and refinement of knowledge concerning risk factors until early-detection technology improves.

CONCLUSION

Most of the efforts in cancer epidemiology have been directed toward the area of causation. The knowledge derived from work in this area provides a useful basis for assessing risks among individuals, permitting the design and testing of nursing interventions, particularly in the areas of prevention and detection. However, it must be remembered that epidemiologic methods have broader applications for nurses, including the means for assembling data for the planning, implementation, and evaluation of services and the determination of priorities for community or group health programs. Finally, epidemiologic methods are valuable in nursing research. The factors that affect the outcome of cancer subsequent to clinical manifestation and therapy must be investigated. In addition, more studies are needed to determine optimal patterns of cancer detection, treatment, and rehabilitation resource use. Answers to these questions should be of great concern to oncology nurses.

REFERENCES

1. National Center for Health Statistics: Annual summary of births, marriages, divorces, and deaths, United States, 1987. Monthly vital statistics report, vol 36, no. 13. Hyattsville, Md, DHHS pub no. (PHS) 88-1120, 1988.
2. Greenwald P, Sondik EJ: Appendix A: Use of models to project cancer mortality in the year 2000, in Cancer control objectives for the nation: 1985-2000. NCI monograph no. 2. Washington, DC, US Government Printing Office, 1986, pp 59-68.
3. Silverman DT: A comparison of Hodgkin's disease in Alameda County, California, and Connecticut: Histologic subtype and age distribution. Cancer 39:1758-63,1977.
4. Silverberg E, Lubera JA: Cancer statistics. CA 39:3-20, 1989.
5. Gardner JW, Lyon JL: Low incidence of cervical cancer in Utah. Gynecol Oncol 5:68-80, 1977.
6. Rosenwaike I: Cancer mortality among Mexican immigrants in the United States. Public Health Reports 103:195-201, 1988.
7. Creagan ET, Fraumeni JF Jr: Cancer mortality among American Indians, 1950–1967. Natl Cancer Inst 49:959-967, 1972.
8. Haenszel W, Kurihara M: Studies of Japanese migrants. I. Mortality from cancer and other disease in the United States. J Natl Cancer Inst 40:43-68, 1968.
9. Newell GR: Epidemiology of cancer, in De Vita VT, Hellman S, Rosenberg SA (eds): Cancer: Principles and Practice of Oncology (ed 2). Philadelphia, Lippincott, 1985.
10. Kelsey JL, Berkowitz GS: Breast cancer epidemiology. Cancer Res 48:5615-5623, 1988.
11. White E: Projected changes in breast cancer incidence due to the trend toward delayed childbearing. Am J Public Health 77:495-497, 1987.
12. Joly DJ, Lilienfeld AM, Diamond EL, et al: An epidemiologic study of the relationship of reproductive experience to cancer of the ovary. Am J Epidemiol 99:190-207, 1974.
13. Nelson JH, Averetee HE, Richart RM: Cervical intraepithelial neoplasia (dysplasia and carcinoma in situ) and early invasive cervical carcinoma. CA 39:157-178, 1989.
14. Hecht F, McCay-Kaiser B: Chromosome instability syndromes, in Mulvilhill RH, Miller AB, Fraumeni JF Jr (eds): Genetics of Human Cancer. New York, Raven Press, 1977.
15. Rosen N, Isreal MA: Genetic abnormalities as biologic tumor markers. Semin Oncol 2:213-231, 1987.
16. Erbe RW: Current concepts in genetics: Inherited gastrointestinal polyposis syndromes. N Engl J Med 294:1101-1104, 1976.
17. Greene WM: The psychosocial setting of the development of leukemia and lymphoma. Ann NY Acad Sci 125:794-801, 1966.
18. Hagnell O: The premorbid personality of persons who develop cancer in a total population investigated in 1947 and 1957. Ann NY Acad Sci 25:846-855, 1966.
19. Kissen DM: Psychosocial factors, personality, and lung cancer in men aged 55-64. Br J Med Psychol 40:29-43, 1967.
20. Graham S, Snell LM, Graham JB, et al: Social trauma in the epidemiology of cancer of the cervix. J Chron Dis 24:711-725, 1971.
21. Abse DW, Wilkins MM, Kirschner G, et al: Self-frustration, nighttime smoking, and lung cancer. Psychosom Med 34:395-404, 1974.
22. Greer S, Morris T: Psychological attributes of women who develop breast cancer: A controlled study. J Psychosom Res 19:147-153, 1977.
23. Thomas CB, Duszynski KR, Shaffer JW: Family attitudes reported in youth as potential predictors of cancer. Psychosom Med 41:287-302, 1979.
24. Cox T, MacKay C: Psychosocial factors and psychophysiological mechanisms in the aetiology and development of cancers. Social Sci Med 16:381-396, 1982.
25. Horne RL, Picard RS: Psychosocial risk factors for lung cancer. Psychosom Med 41:503-514, 1979.
26. Fox BH, Ragland DR, Brand RJ, et al: Type A behavior and cancer mortality. Theoretical considerations and preliminary data. Ann NY Acad Sci 496:620-7, 1987.
27. Pickle LW, Mason TJ, Howard N, et al: Atlas of U.S. cancer mortality among whites: 1950–1980. DHHS pub. no. (NIH) 87-2900. Washington, DC, US Government Printing Office, 1987.
28. Mason TJ, McKay FW, Hoover R, et al: Atlas of cancer mortality among U.S. non-whites: 1950–1969. DHEW pub. no. (NIH) 76-1204. Washington, DC, US Government Printing Office, 1976.
29. Armstrong B, Doll R: Environmental factors and cancer incidence and mortality in different countries, with special reference to dietary practices. Intl J Cancer 15:617-631, 1975.
30. Howe GR, Burch JD, Miller AB, et al: Artificial sweeteners and human bladder cancer. Lancet 2:578-581, 1977.
31. Food and Drug Administration. Histopathologic evaluation of tissues from rats following continuous dietary intake of sodium saccharin and calcium cyclamate for a maximum period of 2 years: Final report. Project P-169-170. Washington, DC, US Government Printing Office, 1973.
32. Health and Protection Branch, National Health and Welfare Department: Toxicity and carcinogenicity study of ortho-

toluenesulfonamide and saccharin. Project E405/405E. Quebec, Canadian Government Printing Office, 1977.
33. Nicholson LJ, Jani H: Effects of sodium cyclamate and sodium saccharin on focus induction in explant cultures of rat bladder. Intl J Cancer 42:295-8, 1988.
34. Burbank F, Fraumeni JF Jr: Synthetic sweetener consumption and bladder cancer trends in the United States. Nature 227:296-297, 1970.
35. Armstrong B, Doll R: Bladder cancer mortality in England and Wales in relation to cigarette smoking and saccharin consumption. Br J Prevent Soc Med 28:233-40, 1974.
36. Armstrong B, Doll R: Bladder cancer mortality in diabetics in relation to saccharin consumption and smoking habits. Br J Prevent Soc Med 29:73-81, 1978.
37. Wynder EL, Goldsmith R: The epidemiology of bladder cancer: A second look. Cancer 40:1246-1268, 1977.
38. Kessler II, Clark JP: Saccharin, cyclamate, and human bladder cancer. JAMA 240:349-355, 1978.
39. Morrison AS, Buring JE: Artificial sweeteners and cancer of the lower urinary tract. N Engl J Med 302:537-541, 1980.
40. Wynder EL, Stellman SD: Artificial sweetener use and bladder cancer. Science 207:1214-16, 1980.
41. Hoover, RN, Strasser PH: Artificial sweeteners and human bladder cancer. Lancet 1:837-840, 1980.
42. Rothman K, Keller A: The effect of joint exposure to alcohol and tobacco with cancer of the mouth and pharynx. Am J Public Health 55:1578-1585, 1972.
43. Graham S, Dayal H, Rohrer T, et al: Dentition, diet, tobacco, and alcohol in the epidemiology of oral cancer. J Natl Cancer Inst 59:1611-1618, 1977.
44. Jensen OM: Cancer morbidity and causes of death among Danish brewery workers. Intl J Cancer 23:454-463, 1979.
45. Pottern LM, Morris LE, Blot WJ, et al: Esophageal cancer among black men in Washington, DC. I. Alcohol, tobacco, and other cancer risk factors. J Natl Cancer Inst 67:777-783, 1981.
46. Vitale JJ, Broitman SA, Gottlieb LS: Alcohol and cancer, in Newell GR, Ellison NM (eds): Nutrition and Cancer: Etiology and Treatment. New York, Raven Press, 1981.
47. Wu AH, Paginini-Hill A, Ross RK, et al: Alcohol, physical activity and other risk factors for colorectal cancer: A prospective study. Br J Cancer 55:687-94, 1987.
48. Schatzkin A, Jones Y, Hoover RN, et al: Alcohol consumption and breast cancer in the epidemiologic follow-up study of the first national health and nutrition examination survey. N Engl J Med 316:1169-1173, 1987.
49. MacMahon B, Yen S, Trichopoulous D, et al: Coffee and cancer of the pancreas. N Engl J Med 304:630-33, 1981.
50. Newell GR: Food additives and coffee as risk factors, in Mirand EA, Hutchinson WB, Mihich E (eds): Progress in Clinical and Biological Research, vol 132D. New York, Alan R. Liss, 1983.
51. Wynder EL, Hall NEL, Polansky M: Epidemiology of coffee and pancreatic cancer. Cancer Res 43:3900-3906, 1983.
52. Hill MJ: Metabolic epidemiology of dietary factors in large bowel cancer. Cancer Res 35:3398-3402, 1975.
53. Wynder EL: The epidemiology of large bowel cancer. Cancer Res 35:3338-3394, 1975.
54. Reddy BS, Wynder EL: Metabolic epidemiology of colon cancer: Fecal bile acids and neutral sterols in colon cancer patients and patients with adenomatous polyps. Cancer 39:2533-2539, 1977.
55. Burkitt DP: Etiology and prevention of colorectal cancer. Hosp Pract 19:67-77, 1984.
56. Graham S, Marshall J, Haughey B, et al: Dietary epidemiology of the colon in western New York. Am J Epidemiol 128:490-503, 1988.
57. Carroll KK, Gammal EB, Plunkett ER: Dietary fat and mammary cancer. Can Med Assoc J 98:590-594, 1968.
58. Carroll KK, Khor HT: Effects of level and type of dietary fat on incidence of mammary tumors induced in female Sprague-Dawley rats by 7,12-dimethyl benz(a)arthracene. Lipids 6:415-420, 1971.
59. Carroll KK: Experimental evidence of dietary factors and hormone-dependent cancers. Cancer Res 35:3374-83, 1975.
60. Greenwald P, Cullen JW, McKenna JW: Cancer prevention and control: From research through applications. J Natl Cancer Inst 79:389-40, 1987.
61. Miller AB, Kelly A, Choi NW, et al: A study of diet and breast cancer. Am J Epidemiol 107:499-509, 1978.
62. Lubin F, Ruder A, Wax Y, Modan B: Overweight and changes in weight throughout adult life in breast cancer etiology. Am J Epidemiol 122:579-88, 1985.
63. Hems G: The contributions of diet and childbearing to breast cancer rates. Br J Cancer 37:974-982, 1978.
64. Carroll KK: Influence of diet on mammary cancer. Nutrition Cancer 2:232-36, 1981.
65. Cohen LA, Chan PC, Wynder EL: The role of a high-fat diet in enhancing the development of mammary tumors in ovariectomized rats. Cancer 47:66-71, 1981.
66. Burkitt DP: Epidemiology of cancer of the colon and rectum. Cancer 28:3-13, 1971.
67. Burkitt DP, Walker AR, Painter NS: Effects of dietary fibre on stools and transit-times, and its role in causation of diseases. Lancet 2:1408-1412, 1972.
68. Fleiszer D, Murray D, MacFarlane J, et al: Protective effect of dietary fibre against chemically induced bowel tumors in rats. Lancet 1:552-3, 1978.
69. Reddy BS, Sharma C, Simi B, et al: Metabolic epidemiology of colon cancer: Effect of dietary fiber on fecal mutagens and bile acids in healthy subjects. Cancer Res 47:644-8, 1987.
70. Modan B, Barell V, Lubin F, et al: Low-fiber intake as an etiologic factor in cancer of the colon. J Natl Cancer Inst 55:15-18, 1975.
71. MacLennan R, Jensen OM: Dietary fibre, transit-time, faecal bacteria, steroids, and colon cancer in two Scandinavian populations. Lancet 2:207-211, 1977.
72. Reddy BS, Hedges A, Laakso K, et al: Fecal constituents of a high-risk North American and a low-risk Finnish population for the development of large bowel cancer. Cancer Letters 4:217-222, 1978.
73. Graham S, Mettlin C: Fiber and other constituents of vegetables and cancer epidemiology, in Newell GR, Ellison NM (eds): Nutrition and Cancer: Etiology and Treatment. New York, Raven Press, 1981.
74. Kritchevsky D: Dietary fiber and cancer. Nutrition Cancer 6:213-219, 1984.
75. Borchert P, Wattenberg LW: Inhibition of macromolecular binding of benzo(a)pyrene and inhibition of neoplasia by disulfiram in the mouse forestomach. J Natl Cancer Inst 57:173-179, 1976.
76. Graham S, Dayal H, Swanson M, et al: Diet in the epidemiology of cancer of the colon and rectum. J Natl Cancer Inst 61:709-714, 1978.
77. Mirvish SS: Blocking the formation of N-nitroso compounds with ascorbic acid in vitro and in vivo. Ann NY Acad Sci 258:175-180, 1975.
78. Raineri R, Weisburger JH: Reduction of gastric carcinogens with ascorbic acid. Ann NY Acad Sci 258:181-189, 1975.

79. Weisburger JH: Vitamin C and prevention of nitrosamine formation. Lancet 2:607, 1977.
80. Leuchtenberger C, Leuchtenberger R: Protection of hamster lung cultures by L-cysteine or vitamin C against carcinogenic effects of fresh smoke from tobacco or marijuana cigarettes. Br J Exploratory Pathol 58:625-634, 1977.
81. Migliozzi JA: Effect of ascorbic acid on tumor growth. Br J Cancer 35:448-53, 1977.
82. Galloway SM, Painter RB: Vitamin C is positive in the DNA synthesis inhibition and sister-chromatid exchange tests. Mutation Res 60:312-327, 1979.
83. Reddy BB, Hirota N: Effect of dietary ascorbic acid on 1,2-dimethyhydrazine-induced colon cancer in rats. Federation Proceedings, American Society of Experimental Biology 38:714. Abstract 2565, 1979.
84. Park CH, Amare M, Savin MA, et al: Growth suppression of leukemic cells in vitro by L-ascorbic acid. Cancer Res 40:1062-1065, 1980.
85. Marshall J, Graham S, Byers T, et al: Diet and smoking in the epidemiology of cancer of the cervix. J Natl Cancer Inst 70:847-51, 1983.
86. Bussey HJR, DeCosse JJ, Deschner EE, et al: A randomized trial of ascorbic acid in polyposis coli. Cancer 50:1434-1439, 1982.
87. Kolonel LN, Nomura AM, Hirohata T, et al: Association of diet and place of birth with stomach cancer incidence in Hawaiian, Japanese and Caucasions. Am J Clin Nutrition 34:2478-85, 1981.
88. Graham S, Mettlin C, Marshall J, et al: Dietary factors in the epidemiology of cancer of the larynx. Am J Epidemiol 113:675-680, 1981.
89. Mettlin C, Graham S, Priore R, et al: Diet and cancer of the esophagus. Nutrition Cancer 2:143-147, 1981.
90. Chu SW, Malmgren RA: An inhibitory effect of vitamin A on the induction of tumors of the forestomach and cervix in the Syrian hamster by carcinogenic polycyclic hydrocarbons. Cancer Res 25:384-395, 1965.
91. Safiotti U, Montesano R, Sellakumar AR, et al: Experimental cancer of the lung: Inhibition by vitamin A of the induction of tracheobronchial squamous metaplasia and squamous cell tumors. Cancer 20:857-864, 1967.
92. Nettesheim P, Williams ML: The influence of vitamin A on the susceptibility of the rat lung to 3-methylcholanthrene. Intl J Cancer 17:351-357, 1976.
93. Newberne PM, Suphakarn V: Preventive role of vitamin A in colon carcinogenesis in rats. Cancer 40:2553-2556, 1977.
94. Merriman R, Bertram J: Reversible inhibition by retinoids of 3-methylcholanthrene-induced neoplastic transformation in C31/10T 1/2 2/8 cells. Cancer Res 39:1661-1666, 1979.
95. Peto R, Doll R, Buckley JD, et al: Can dietary beta-carotene materially reduce human cancer rates? Nature 290: 201-208, 1981.
96. Verma AK, Conrad ED, Boutwell RK: Differential effects of retinoic acid and 7,8-benzoflavone on the induction of mouse skin tumors by the complete carcinogenesis process and by the initiation-promotion regimen. Cancer Res 42:3519-25, 1982.
97. Bjelke E: Dietary vitamin A and human lung cancer. Intl J Cancer 15:561-565, 1975.
98. MacLennan R, Da Costa J, Day NE, et al: Risk factors for lung cancer in Singapore Chinese, a population with high female incidence rates. Intl J Cancer 20:854-860, 1977.
99. Smith PG, Jick H: Cancers among users of preparations containing vitamin A. Cancer 42:808-811, 1978.
100. Mettlin C, Graham S: Dietary risk factors in human bladder cancer. Am J Epidemiol 110:255-263, 1979.
101. Kark JD, Smith AH, Switzer BR, et al: Serum vitamin A (retinol) and cancer incidence in Evan's County, Georgia. J Natl Cancer Inst 66:7-16, 1981.
102. Kvale G, Bjelke E, Gart JJ: Dietary habits and lung cancer risk. Intl J Cancer 31:397-405, 1983.
103. Hinds MW, Kolonel LN, Hankin JH, et al: Dietary vitamin A, carotene, vitamin C and risk of lung cancer in Hawaii. Am J Epidemiol 119:227-237, 1984.
104. Willett WC, Polk BF, Underwood BA, et al: Relation of serum vitamins A and E and carotenoids to the risk of cancer. N Engl J Med 310:430-434, 1984.
105. Greenwald P: Manipulation of nutrients to prevent cancer. Hosp Pract 19:119-134, 1984.
106. Rutstein DD, Mullan RJ, Frazier TM, et al: Sentinnel health events (occupational): A basis for physician recognition and public health surveillance. Am J Public Health 73:1054-1062, 1983.
107. Doll R, Peto R: The causes of cancer: Quantitative estimates of avoidable risks of cancer in the U.S. today. J Natl Cancer Inst 66:1191-1308, 1981.
108. US Department of Health and Human Services: The Health Consequences of Smoking. DHHS (PHS) 82-50179. Washington, DC, US Government Printing Office, 1982.
109. Lyon JL, Gardner JW, West DW, et al: Smoking and carcinoma in situ of the uterine cervix. Am J Public Health 73:558-62, 1983.
110. Greenwald P, Sondik EJ, eds: Prevention of cancer, in Cancer control objectives for the nation: 1985-2000. NCI monograph no. 2. Washington DC, US Government Printing Office, 1986, pp 15-32.
111. Fielding JE, Phenow KJ: Health effects of involuntary smoking. N Engl J Med 319:1452-1460, 1988.
112. Shopland DR, Brown C: Toward the 1900 objectives for smoking: Measuring the progress with 1985 NHIS data. Public Health Rep 102:68-74, 1987.
113. Favus MJ: Thyroid cancer occurring as a late consequence of head and neck irradiation. N Engl J Med 294:1019-1025, 1976.
114. Smith PG: Leukemia and other cancers following radiation treatment of pelvic disease. Cancer 39:1901-1905, 1977.
115. Gatti RA, Good RA: Occurrence of malignancy in immunodeficiency disease. Cancer 28:89-90, 1971.
116. Jick H, Walker AM, Rothman K: The epidemic of endometrial cancer: A commentary. Am J Public Health 70:264-267, 1980.
117. Herbst A, Ulfelder H, Poskanzer D: Adenocarcinoma of the vagina: Association of maternal stilbestrol therapy with tumor appearance in young women. N Engl J Med 284:878-881, 1971.
118. Hoover RN, McKay FW, Fraumeni JF Jr: Fluoridated drinking water and the occurrence of cancer. J Natl Cancer Inst 57:757-768, 1976.
119. Traves DR: Fluoridation and cancer mortality, in Hiatt HH, Watson JD, Winston JA (eds): Origins of Human Cancer. New York, Cold Springs Harbor Laboratory, 1977, pp 357-368.
120. Elwood JM, Lee JAH, Walter SD, et al: Relationship of melanoma and other skin cancer mortality to latitude and ultraviolet radiation in the United States and Canada. Intl J Epidemiol 3:325-332, 1974.
121. Scotto J, Fears TR, Gori GB: Measurements of ultraviolet radiation in the U.S. and comparisons with skin cancer data. DHEW pub. no. (NIH) 76-1029, Washington, DC: US Government Printing Office, 1977.

122. Breslow P, Sondik EJ: Progress and objectives in cancer control. JAMA 259:1690-4, 1988.
123. Haenszel W: Cancer mortality among the foreign-born in the United States. J Natl Cancer Inst 26:37-132, 1961.
124. Williams EM, Smith PG, Day NE, et al: Space-time clustering of Burkitt's lymphoma in the West Nile District of Uganda: 1961–1975. Br J Cancer 37:109-119, 1978.
125. Steis RG, Broder S: Acquired immunodeficiency syndrome (AIDS) and Kaposi's sarcoma: Clinical relationship between immune deficiency disease and cancer, in De Vita VT, Hellman S, Rosenberg SA (eds): Important Advances in Oncology. Philadelphia, Lippincott, 1985.
126. Gottlieb MS, Schroff R, Schauker HM, et al: *Pneumocystis carinii* pneumonia and mucosal candidiasis in previously healthy homosexual men. N Engl J Med 305:1425-1431, 1981.
127. Selwyn PA: AIDS: What is now known. Hosp Practice 21:127-164, 1986.
128. Centers for Disease Control: Quarterly report to the Domestic Policy Council on the prevalence and rate of spread of HIV and AIDS in the United States. MMWR 37:223-226, 1988.
129. Winkelstein W Jr, Lyman DM, Padian NS, et al: Sexual practices and risk of infection by the AIDS-associated retrovirus: The San Francisco Men's Health Study. JAMA 257:321-325, 1987.
130. Hopkins DR: AIDS in minority populations in the United States. Public Health Rep 102:677-81, 1987.
131. Stehr-Green JK, Holman RC, Jason JM, et al: Hemophilia-associated AIDS in the United States, 1981 to September 1987. Am J Public Health 78:439-42, 1988.
132. Simonsen JN, Cameron DW, Gakinya MN, et al: Human immunodeficiency virus infection among men with sexually transmitted disease. Experience from a center in Africa. N Engl J Med 319:274-8, 1988.
133. Gallo RC, Saluhuddin SZ, Poporic M, et al: Frequent detection and isolation of cytopathic retroviruses (HTLV-III) from patients with AIDS and at risk for AIDS. Science 224:500-502, 1984.
134. Greenwald P, Sondik EJ, eds: Surveillance, in Cancer control objectives for the nation: 1985–2000. NCI monograph no. 2. Washington DC, US Government Printing Office, 1986, pp 45-52.
135. National Center for Health Statistics: Prevalence of selected chronic conditions, United States, 1983–1985. Advance Data from Vital and Health Statistics, no. 155. DHHS pub. no. (PHS) 88-1250. Hyattsville, Md, Public Health Service, 1988.
136. Doll R, Hill AB: Mortality in relation to smoking: Ten years' observations of British doctors. Br Med J 1:1399-1410, 1460-1467, 1964.
137. Doll R: Introduction, in Hiatt HH, Watson JD, Winston JA (eds): New York, Cold Springs Harbor Laboratory, 1977, pp 357-368.
138. Greenwald P, Sondik EJ, eds: Cancer control objectives, in Cancer control objectives for the nation: 1985–2000. NCI monograph no. 2. Washington DC, US Government Printing Office, 1986, pp 3-14.
139. Pollack ES: Tracking cancer trends: Incidence and survival. Hosp Pract 19:99-116, 1984.

Chapter 2

Carcinogenesis

John W. Yarbro, MD, PhD

INTRODUCTION

Our current understanding of the biology of cancer is that *clonal selection* is the process by which cancer develops and evolves. Stated simply, an initial mutation in the genome of a cell may confer a survival advantage on that cell. If one of the progeny of that cell is hit by a second mutation that also confers a survival advantage, this new clone grows even more vigorously. A sequence of such events leads not only to the selection of a clone with the characteristics of a neoplasm but also allows that clone to progress to ever-greater stages of virulence characterized by invasion, metastatic spread, drug resistance, and other characteristics that ultimately lead to the host's death. This is Darwinian evolutionary natural selection on a clonal basis within a single organism.

Multicellular organisms have evolved an elaborate set of controls regulating cellular growth and repair. There are signals to turn growth on and off as needed. There are complex fail-safe mechanisms to prevent the overgrowth of an unregulated clone while allowing growth and repair to take place when needed. However, cancer escapes this regulation. Step by step, cancer overcomes a complex set of protective growth controls. Indeed, the mutations that lead to cancer are mutations of the very genes that regulate growth. Two types of such genes have been identified. The first set is composed of proto-oncogenes, which are dominant genes that code for growth factors, membrane growth factor receptors, cytoplasmic signal transducers, and nuclear receptors that trigger proliferation; the second set of genes, called anti-oncogenes or cancer-suppressor genes, code for proteins that bind to growth-stimulating proteins to block their action or by other, as yet unknown actions that suppress proliferation and malignant growth.

TARGETS OF CARCINOGENESIS

Proto-oncogenes and anti-oncogenes are the genes that organisms have evolved to regulate growth and repair of tissues. They are the genetic codes for the proteins that function as the "off" and "on" signals that cells send and receive to regulate proliferation. These genes are the targets of carcinogens. Mutation of a proto-oncogene may leave it permanently in the "on" position so that it continually stimulates cell proliferation; mutation of an anti-oncogene may prevent it from exerting the "off" signal at the appropriate time, again leading to uncontrolled cellular proliferation. The multiple mutations leading to most human cancers probably involve both types of genes. Some of these mutations, at least of anti-oncogenes, may be inherited. Oncogenes were first discovered in viruses and later found to be present in the DNA of higher organisms. The term *oncogene* is reserved by some authors for the viral or activated form of the proto-oncogene; other authors use the terms *oncogene* and *proto-oncogene* interchangeably. The term *cancer-suppressor gene* is synonymous with anti-oncogene.

A chromosomal or cellular proto-oncogene is indicated by inserting a "c" before the abbreviation of the gene, that is, *c-ras;* a proto-oncogene captured from a cell by a virus and altered or mutated is designated by a "v" before the abbreviation, that is, *v-ras*. The abbreviation for the gene often relates to the system in which it was first discovered; *ras* was discovered in a rat sarcoma, and *sis* was discovered in a simian sarcoma. In some cases, *sis* for example, the protein product was discovered independently as a growth factor. The protein coded for by *sis* is platelet-derived growth factor (PDGF),[1,2] which is released by blood platelets in a clot to stimulate scar formation. In some sarcomas, the product of *sis* seems to act as a tumor growth factor.

It is becoming increasingly clear that some cancers are related to inheritance of defective anti-oncogenes, that is, cancer-suppressor genes. An inherited defective cancer-suppressor gene is seen in some relatively rare pediatric tumors, for example, retinoblastoma. Anti-oncogenes may be targets for carcinogens in some common adult cancers. The retinoblastoma anti-oncogene has been found to be mutated to an inactive state in a cell line from a bladder carcinoma.[3] The products of proto-oncogenes and anti-oncogenes are only beginning to be elucidated and their actions described. This remains the most difficult part of the story to complete, but it is obviously the most important part, since this research will allow direct intervention in a therapeutic or preventive manner.

STAGES OF CARCINOGENESIS

It is customary to divide carcinogenesis into three stages: initiation, promotion, and progression. These stages can be seen distinctly only in carefully controlled experimental systems, and it is likely that their distinctiveness is lost in the development of most common human cancers. However, for purposes of understanding, it is useful to examine these stages separately. These three terms were coined by Peyton Rous based on a series of experiments in skin carcinogenesis: "initiation," by which was meant some primary change in the target produced by a carcinogen; "promotion," by which was meant some secondary effect of an agent (the promoter) that alone might not be able to induce a malignancy; and "progression," by which Rous intended to designate "the process by which tumors go from bad to worse."[4-6] Foulds[7] codified and expanded this concept of multistage carcinogenesis. Progression to the metastatic phenotype has subsequently been well elucidated by Fidler.[8]

The first stage, *initiation,* is characterized by damage to DNA that is initially reversible and later irreversible. A mutation occurs in a specific gene. The mutation does not lead to malignant growth, but, if not reversed by cell repair mechanisms, it sets the stage for the action of a promoter

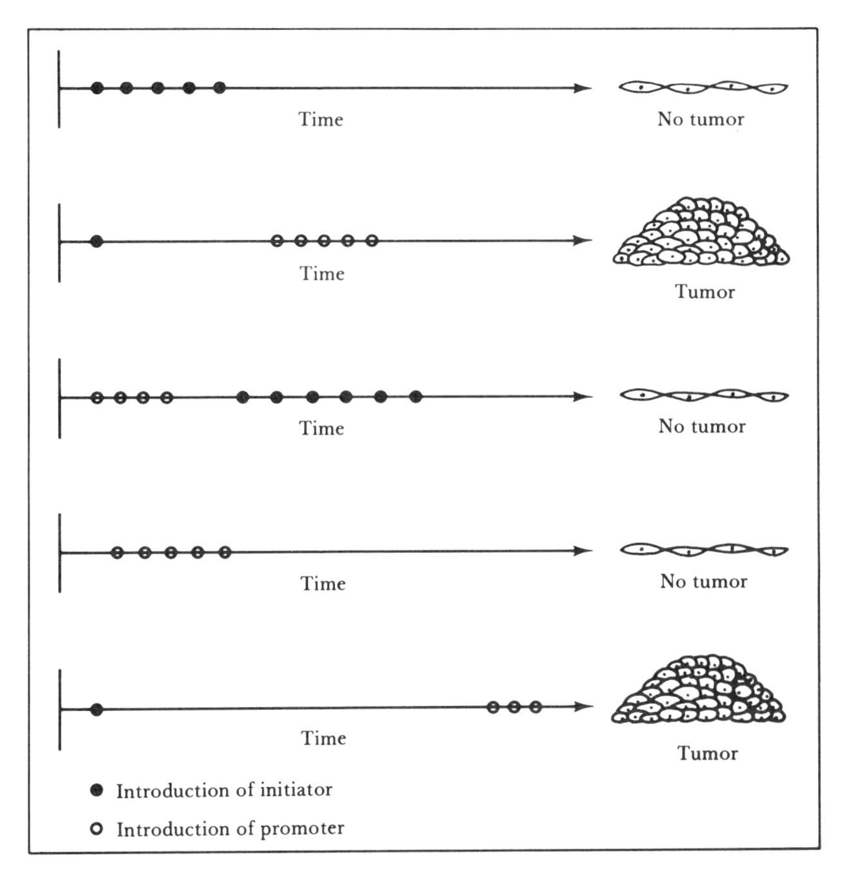

FIGURE 2-1 The interaction of initiation (closed circles) and promotion (open circles) is illustrated. Initiation must precede promotion for a tumor to develop; promotion alone will not produce a tumor. Initiation is permanent, so that there may be a long delay between the initiating and the promoting events.

at a later time. In theory, since the lesion is permanent, application of the promoter can be delayed for long periods, and in experimental animals this is the case.

The second stage, *promotion,* does not involve damage to DNA but usually involves some stimulation of cellular proliferation. Promotion, which is reversible, exhibits a distinct dose-response and measurable threshold. In ways that are poorly understood, perhaps by activating normal cellular genes, continued action of the promoter causes the cell that has undergone initiation to develop an invasive, that is, malignant, behavior. This is often referred to as a maligant phenotype, which means that the cell expresses a genetic change. The relationship between initiation and promotion is shown in Figure 2-1. Promotion alone will not cause cancer. Promotion must follow initiation.

The third stage, *progression,* involves both mutagenic and nonmutagenic events leading to morphologic change and increased grades of malignant behavior, such as invasion, metastasis, and drug resistance. The process is irreversible. The rapidly growing, highly malignant character that the cancer has attained at the time of diagnosis is the result of progression. For example, carcinoma of the cervix can be diagnosed while still in situ, that is, before it has undergone sufficient progression to metastasize. Then it is readily cured by simple excision. Left in place it will progress to extensive invasion and metastasis and become incurable. This is not simply a matter of time; it is a change that the tumor undergoes with time. That change is called progression.

In humans carcinogenesis is much more complex than our well-studied laboratory models. The distinction between the three stages is blurred. More than one type of initiating event is probably common. In some cases it is likely that initiators act as their own promoters; that is, they are complete carcinogens. In other cases an initiator may be a complete carcinogen for one organ and an incomplete carcinogen for another organ. The line between promotion and progression is indistinct. Even when researchers understand a great deal about the carcinogen, it does not seem to fit the laboratory model. For example, in lung cancer, cigarette tars seem to act as both initiators and promoters. Unlike the laboratory model, however, where initiation, once having taken place, becomes irreversible, in humans the smoker who quits returns to the normal low incidence pattern in 10 to 15 years. These complexities are discussed in detail in an excellent review by Pitot.[9]

Obviously much more must be learned before researchers can make reliable predictions in humans, but current knowledge suggests that the process of human carcinogenesis will be found to be much more complex than in animal models. It is also likely that the simple lessons learned from animals will not be simply applied to humans. Some of the notions of identifying a few environmental cancer-causing chemicals and eliminating them may be too simplistic.

Carcinogenesis ordinarily is considered under the headings of chemical, viral, physical, and familial, even though it is likely that human carcinogenesis involves combinations of multiple factors. Carcinogenesis can also be discussed under headings such as occupational, dietary, environmental, life-style, and so forth.

TYPES OF CARCINOGENESIS

Chemical Carcinogenesis

In 1915 cancer was induced in laboratory animals for the first time by the chemical coal tar applied to rabbit skin, at Tokyo University by Yamagiwa and Ichikawa.[10] Perhaps because the English physician Percival Pott had noted in 1775 that soot caused scrotal cancer in chimney sweeps, the chemical carcinogenesis theory became a leading theory. Preceding the often cited observation of Pott, the single most destructive chemical carcinogen yet to be found, tobacco, was identified by an astute clinician, John Hill,[11] only a few decades after it was introduced into common usage in London. From 1761 until 1950, when tobacco was "rediscovered" as a carcinogen,[12-14] the only chemicals discovered to be significant carcinogens in humans were the aniline dyes that caused bladder cancer.[15] The first potent synthetic carcinogen, dibenzanthracene, was discovered in 1930.[16] Subsequently many other chemicals were developed that caused cancer in various animal systems.

The large number of active chemicals discovered raised questions about how they caused cancer, since they seemed to have no common chemical structure. Classic work by the Millers led in 1951 to the understanding that covalent binding within the cell was essential for carcinogenic activity; the active metabolite of the carcinogen was later identified to be an electrophilic reactant that binds to DNA.[17] Carcinogens are converted by a series of metabolic steps into free radicals, that is, compounds with a single unpaired electron. Free radicals are electrophilic, that is, highly reactive with macromolecules that are rich in electrons, such as DNA. Compounds called antioxidants inhibit carcinogenesis because they react with free radicals before the free radicals damage DNA. The role of antioxidants such as vitamin C in the diet is discussed below.

Since different organisms have different metabolic systems, potential carcinogens are metabolized in one way in some organisms and in other ways in other organisms, with the result that some chemicals are carcinogenic for one species but not carcinogenic for another. There may be as yet unidentified metabolic differences that render some people more sensitive than others to certain carcinogens. Ames et al[18] developed a classic assay system to measure carcinogens. The assay employs bacteria and is based on the fact that most carcinogens are mutagens, that is, they damage DNA. The Ames system requires adding liver microsomes to metabolize the chemicals to be tested into active carcinogens. The metabolism of a carcinogen leads to the final active chemical, called the proximate carcinogen, that reacts with the DNA.

In smokers it is possible to identify directly the carcinogen bound to DNA, the so-called hydrocarbon adducts.[19] The proximate carcinogen exerts its effect by binding to DNA and mutating it directly or by causing errors to be made when the host cell tries to repair the damaged DNA. However, many of the lesions produced by carcinogens are repaired. The best evidence for this is the extraordinary incidence of skin cancer in patients with xeroderma pigmentosum, a disease in which patients are unable to repair DNA damage from ultraviolet light.[20]

The specific target proto-oncogenes and anti-oncogenes, the "on" and "off" switches for cell growth, have been identified in some cases. In systems in which known chemical carcinogens and radiation would induce malignant transformation, it was possible to identify mutated cellular proto-oncogenes.[21,22] Further, specific and consistent point mutations were demonstrated in some human malignancies.[23] Movement of a proto-oncogene to a different site on the same or another chromosome that caused activation was also demonstrated.[24] In a few cases the specific structural change in the protein that leads to malfunction has been elucidated, in one case a change that keeps a signal in the "on" condition.[25] However, work has only begun on this complex problem.

Of major importance was the realization that a change in the activity of more than one gene was required to transform a cell to malignant growth and that a long series of genetic changes involving proto-oncogenes and anti-oncogenes leads to tumor progression. Despite the vast array of chemicals discovered to cause cancer in animals, there still remain very few chemicals (other than tobacco) for which there is strong evidence of cancer causation in humans. Occasional industrial chemicals have been documented, such as 2-naphthylamine, vinyl chloride, metals, and benzene, but after extensive study the best estimate is that only 4% of all cancer deaths in America are due to occupational causes.[26] Cancer chemotherapeutic agents are carcinogenic, and cured cancer patients are at risk for leukemia and some other tumors.

Familial Carcinogenesis

Fanconi's anemia, ataxia-telangectasia, xeroderma pigmentosum, retinoblastoma, Wilms' tumor, neurofibromatosis, the dysplastic nevus syndrome, familial polyposis coli (FPC), the cancer family syndrome (CFS), multiple endocrine neoplasia syndromes (MEN I, MEN II, MEN III), and several other heritable cancers all provide ample evidence for a heritable predisposition to cancer.[27] Many inherited cancer syndromes behave as autosomal dominant traits. However, most well-studied syndromes of this sort are rather rare. For the common cancers (lung, colon, and breast), the data are less clear and the syndromes less distinct. There are a variety of estimates, none very reliable, that up to 15% of all human cancers may have a hereditary component. Lynch et al[28] have studied breast cancer and find that 13% have a familial aggregation. When familial, breast cancer seems to segregate as an autosomal dominant trait. Colon cancer, to a lesser degree, provides evidence of a familial pattern.

Familial carcinogenesis of the retinoblastoma type is based in large part on a group of genes that when mutated cause cancer by their absence, that is, they seem to prevent cancer when they are functioning normally. These protective genes have been called anti-oncogenes or cancer-suppressor genes or sometimes emerogenes. The inheritance of a predisposition for cancer had been recognized for many years, the most commonly noted example being breast cancer. But the scientific basis for understanding of one mechanism by which this might occur began in 1971 when Alfred Knudson argued, on the basis of a statistical model, that one of the two mutations required for the development of familial retinoblastoma was inherited and that the second occurred in the retinal cells of the affected eye. In the nonheritable form both mutations occurred in the same cell after birth, with neither mutation being inherited.[29] This model was derived from the observation that acquired retinoblastoma occurred as a single tumor whereas children with hereditary retinoblastoma had multiple primary tumors. This difference indicates that there is an inherited genetic predisposition in all the cells of the retinal tissue. The gene has been identified and named the retinoblastoma gene. The inheritance is dominant, but both copies of the gene must be absent or damaged for a cell to be transformed, so the function of the gene is to prevent malignant growth. When the retinoblastoma gene is introduced into cultured retinoblastoma cells, the malignant growth pattern is suppressed.[30] It was later found that the retinoblastoma gene was present on chromosome 13.

This confirmed in humans the classic laboratory observation that in some tumors, fusing the cancer cell with a normal cell will suppress malignant growth.[31] Analysis of chromosome 13 in hereditary cases of retinoblastoma revealed that the chromosome lost during tumorigenesis was the one from the nonaffected parent, whereas the one retained was from the affected parent,[32] proving dominant inheritance. Final proof of the hypothesis was the suppression of malignant growth by specific gene replacement.[29,30] In one rare tumor, then, the story of carcinogenesis is nearly complete.

Many researchers assumed that the retinoblastoma gene mechanism, although correct for retinoblastoma, was probably not a factor in most human cancers. Slowly, however, the importance of this mechanism in other cancers became evident. A sequence of observations led to the conclusion that a similar mechanism was operative in Wilms' tumor and several associated childhood malignancies. Of greatest interest, loss of the retinoblastoma gene was described in bladder cancer and breast cancer, implying that this gene may be a target for mutagens involved in several common adult cancers. Most recently strong evidence has been presented for a role of the same anti-oncogene associated with familial polyposis as the target for mutagenesis in a large proportion of colon cancer cases. Weinberg[33] has reviewed the implications of the negative regulation exerted on cells by anti-oncogenes such as the retinoblastoma gene and has emphasized the importance of the loss of the normal copy of a gene by the process of mitotic recombination. This is referred to as a reduction to homozygosity because the cell becomes homozygous for the abnormal gene, thus losing its ability to prevent malignant growth. This process may be important in the common adult tumors.

The study of familial carcinogenesis is rapidly expanding. It is becoming increasingly likely that most cancers will be found to result from defects in both oncogenes and anti-oncogenes. It is also likely that some of the defective anti-oncogenes will be found to be inherited. Finally, little evidence exists concerning inherited metabolic pathways that might influence subsequent carcinogenesis.

Physical Carcinogenesis

Physical carcinogens are agents that damage the same proto-oncogenes and anti-oncogenes that chemicals attack, but they exert their action by physical rather than chemical means. In some cases the nature of the reaction is known, as, for example, ionizing radiation that releases sufficient energy to alter DNA. In other cases the mechanism is obscure, as, for example, asbestos, which may act as a promoter by an as-yet-unknown method.

Radiation was recognized as a carcinogen only 4 years after Roentgen's discovery of x-rays.[34] Only a few years later a relationship to leukemia was recognized.[35] Early workers in radiation must have received very large doses to make the association between radiation and cancer so obvious that it would be noticed in such a short time. The excess cancer deaths in the Hiroshima and Nagasaki populations were only about 8%, and leukemia was seen at an incidence of only about 1.5 cases per million people per year per rad of dose.[36] Two forms of radiation can induce cancer: ultraviolet radiation and ionizing radiation.

Ultraviolet radiation

Ultraviolet radiation (UVR) from the sun induces a change in DNA, pyrimidine dimer formation, that if not properly repaired leads to malignant transformation. The very common basal cell and squamous cell carcinomas of the exposed areas of the skin are the result, and these tumors are very common, with nearly a half million cases each year. Melanoma is also linked to ultraviolet exposure, although not as tightly linked as basal and squamous cancers. The most active carcinogenic wavelength of UVR is 280 to 320 nm, which is referred to as UVB.[20]

The most dramatic example of UVB carcinogenesis is seen in patients with xeroderma pigmentosum, an autosomal recessive disease in which DNA repair of UVR damage is defective.[37] These patients are hypersensitive to sunlight and have a very high incidence of skin cancer, including melanoma.

Appropriate preventive techniques include avoidance of direct sunlight and the use of sunblocks that block out UVB radiation. That such measures will be effective is indicated by the protective effect of living in climates with low levels of sunlight, pigmented skin that blocks out UVB, and occupations that minimize sun exposure.

Ionizing radiation

Life evolved in an environment high in radiation, indeed, radiation-induced mutation no doubt accelerated evolution. There are effective mechanisms to repair the damage that results when high-energy radiation interacts with DNA. Ordinarily these mechanisms are very efficient. They are not, however, perfect, and ionizing radiation leads to permanent mutations in DNA. When these mutations involve proto-oncogenes or anti-oncogenes, a cell may transform to malignant growth. As with chemical carcinogenesis, multiple steps are involved. Furthermore, radiation and chemicals interact in a synergistic manner and familial susceptibilities may play a role. There is a hereditary melanoma syndrome that is familial, the familial dysplastic nevus syndrome (FDNS), in which patients have multiple nevi with a strong tendency to evolve into melanoma. Cultured cells from these patients have an increased sensitivity to radiation-induced genetic damage.[38] There are also age and sex variations in sensitivity to radiation-induced cancer.

The average annual exposure of an individual in the United States to radiation from all sources is 360 mrem, 82% of which is from natural sources. The sources of these exposures as reported by the National Council on Radiation Protection Measurements[39] are shown in Table 2-1. Clearly the largest portion of the radiation dose is unavoidable. Recent interest has focused on the radon isotope, for which the home seems to be the major site of exposure. There appear to be substantial geographic variations influencing radon dose. Basements may allow more radon to enter a house, and good insulation may prevent dispersal of radon into the atmosphere.

From the standpoint of prevention, there seems little more to be done than is already being done: minimizing exposure to manmade radiation hazards. Radiation-induced cancer of the lung can best be prevented by stopping smoking, since radon exposure acts synergistically with tobacco smoke. Smokers exposed to radon as miners had ten times the incidence of lung cancer as did nonsmokers because radiation acts synergistically with tobacco smoke.[40]

TABLE 2-1 Sources of Radiation in the Population of the United States According to National Council on Radiation Protection Measurements

Natural Sources (%)		Manufactured Sources (%)	
Radon	55	Medical x-rays	11
Cosmic radiation	8	Medical isotopes	4
Terrestrial radiation	8	Consumer products	3
Internal radiation	11	Occupational	0.3
		Fallout from testing	0.3
		Nuclear power plants	0.1
		All other	0.1
TOTAL	82	TOTAL	18

Values are expressed as a percentage of the total annual dose of 360 mrem.

Asbestos

Asbestos, the major carcinogenic fiber, is thought to be related in the United States to about 2000 cases of mesothelioma annually.[20] Actually it causes more bronchogenic cancers than mesotheliomas, perhaps 6000, because of the synergism between tobacco smoke and asbestos. Lung cancer is rare in asbestos workers who do not smoke. There is characteristically a long latent period between exposure and onset of mesothelioma. Furthermore, the exposure may sometimes be so brief that the patient cannot remember when it occurred unless questioned closely. The mechanism of action of the asbestos fiber is unknown but is thought to be promotion rather than initiation. Presumably the same proto-oncogenes and cancer-suppressor genes are involved as with other forms of carcinogenesis.

Data do not support an association between gastrointestinal cancer and asbestos, an observation of some importance because asbestos-lined cement pipes carry much of the United States' water supply.[41] Physical properties such as crystal type and particle size, of course, play a major role in the physical carcinogenic properties of asbestos. Epidemiologic studies indicate that only certain forms of asbestos increase the risk of mesothelioma.[41] Estimating the risk of exposure to asbestos is much more complicated than estimating risk from a soluble mutagenic carcinogen, and the linear dose-response model probably cannot be applied.

Viral Carcinogenesis

In 1911 Peyton Rous,[42] at the Rockefeller Institute, described a sarcoma in chickens caused by what later became known as the Rous sarcoma virus (RSV). This virus was the source of the first well-characterized oncogene, that is, a gene necessary for a virus to induce transformation rapidly in a target cell.

Heubner and Todaro[43] coined the word "oncogene" in 1969 when they proposed that RNA viruses somehow placed viral genes in the human genome that were then genetically transmitted. These genes were then acted on by chemicals or radiation or aging to cause cancer. Their theory was only partially correct, but the term *oncogene* has persisted. The original concept of viral transmission proposed by Heubner and Todaro has been found to be

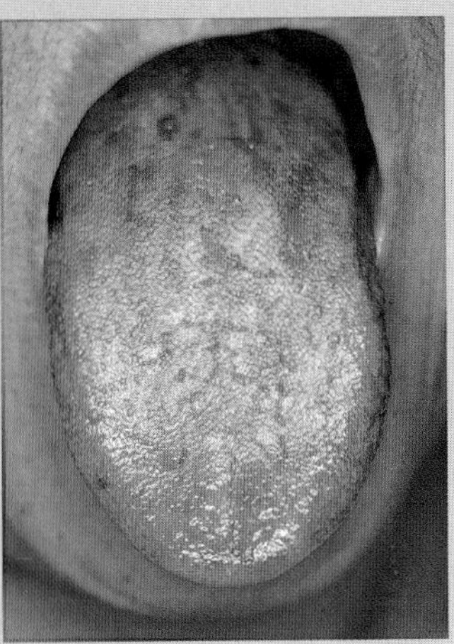

Plate 1: "Black tongue" occurring two weeks following a single doxorubicin injection.

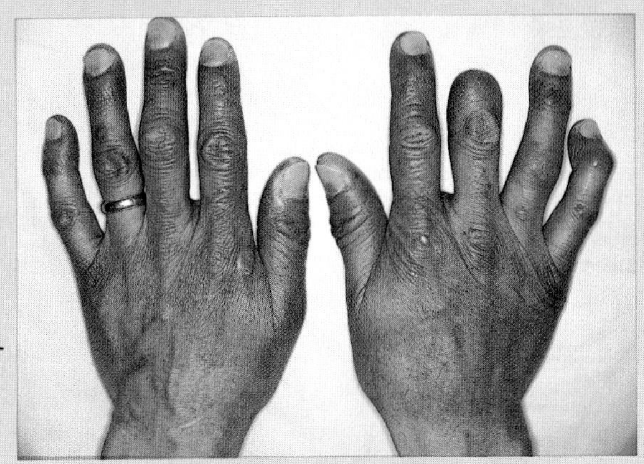

Plate 2: Hyperpigmentation in a white male following long-term 5-FU infusion.

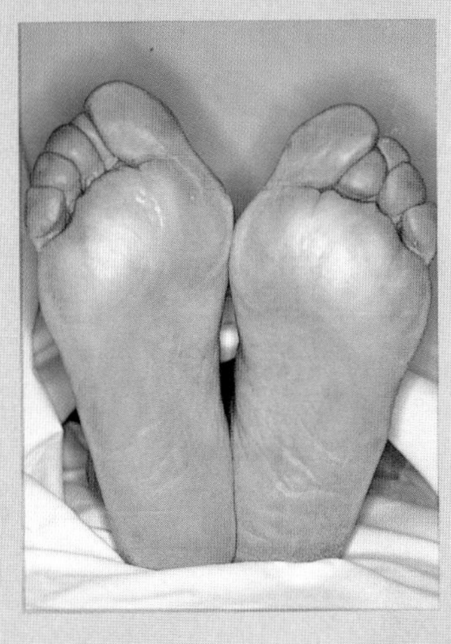

Plate 3: Acral erythema.

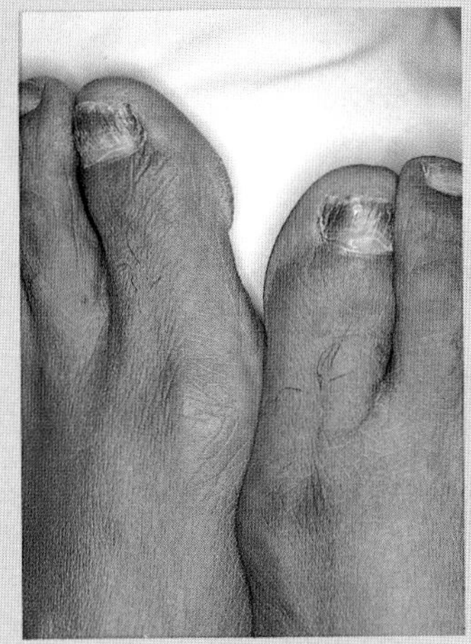

Plate 4: Nail pigmentation following doxorubicin therapy.

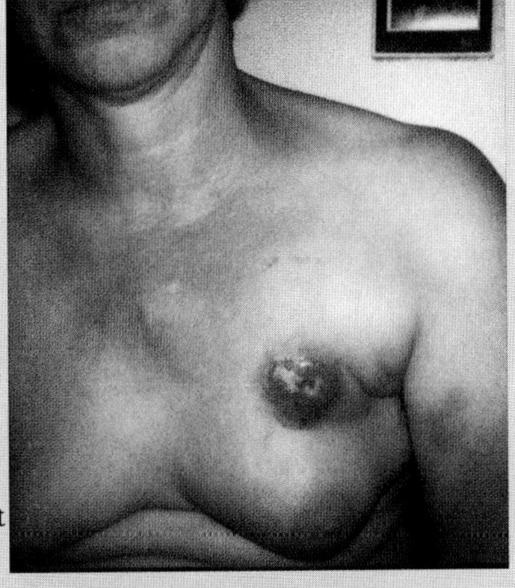

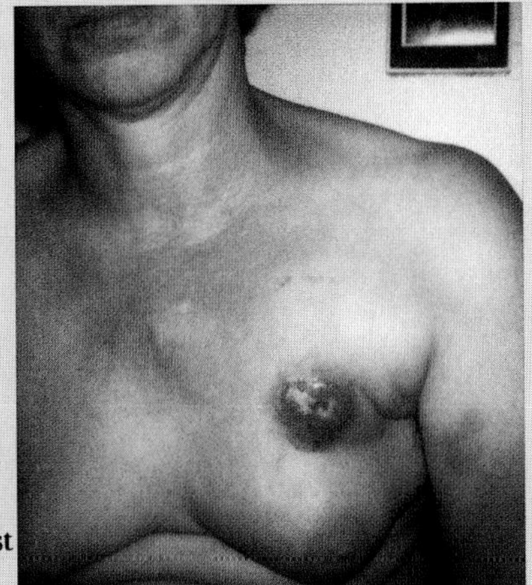

Plate 5: Ulcerating breast cancer.

Plate 6: Metastatic breast cancer invading skin.

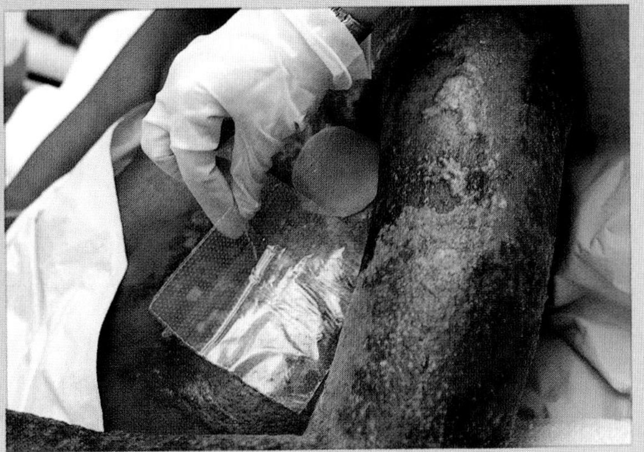

Plate 7: Metastatic breast cancer recurring locally and invading skin of arm. Local therapy includes application of Vigilon dressing.

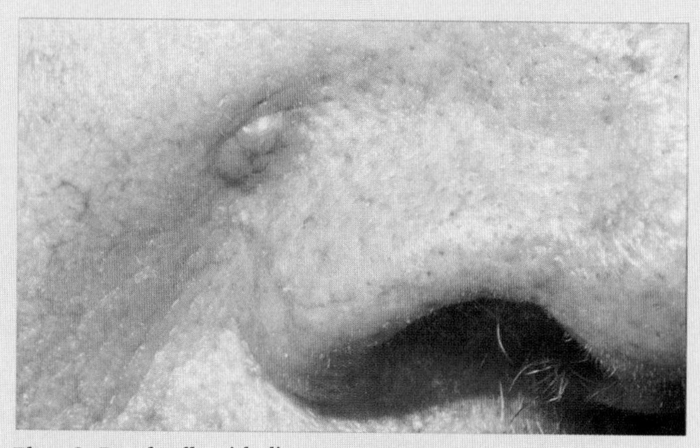

Plate 8: Basal cell epithelioma.

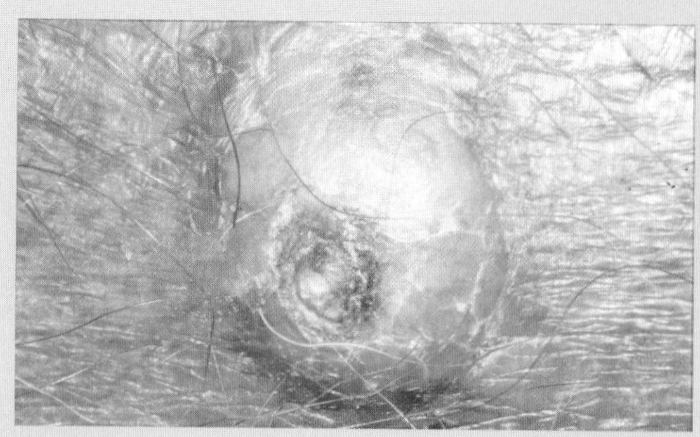

Plate 9: Squamous cell carcinoma.

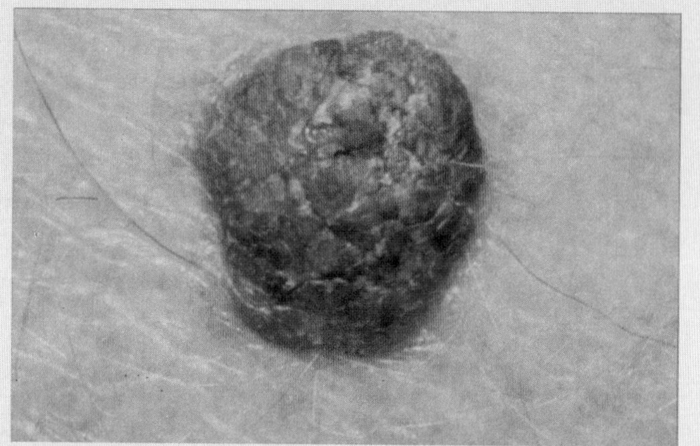

Plate 10: Normal mole.

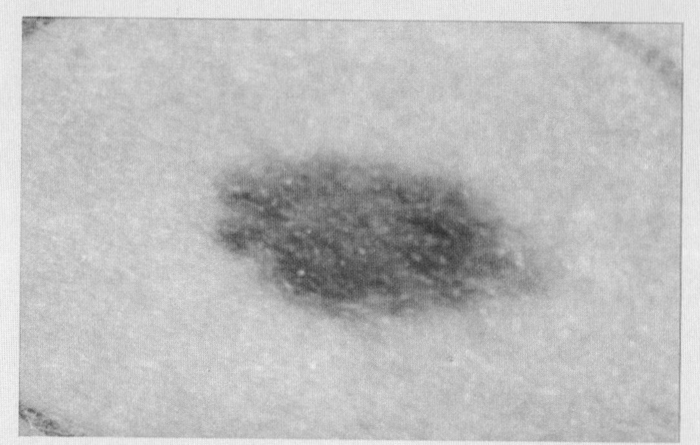

Plate 11: Dysplastic nevus.

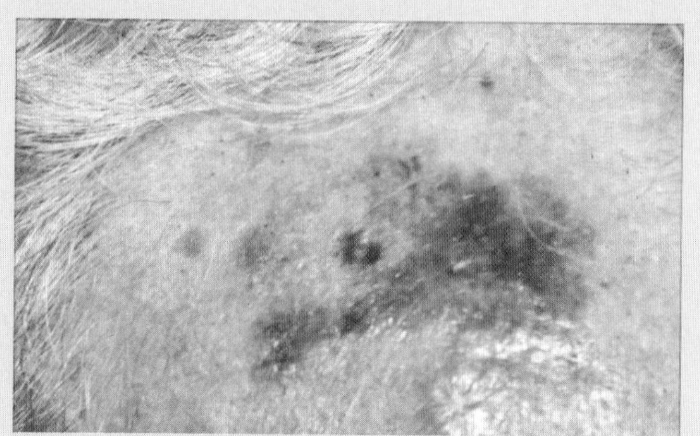

Plate 12: Lentigo maligna melanoma.

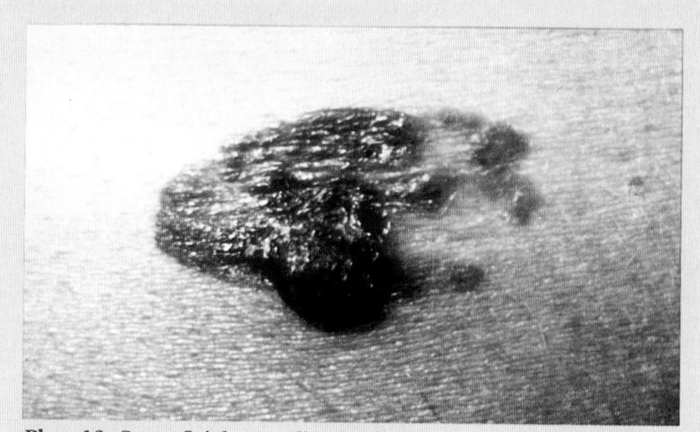

Plate 13: Superficial spreading melanoma.

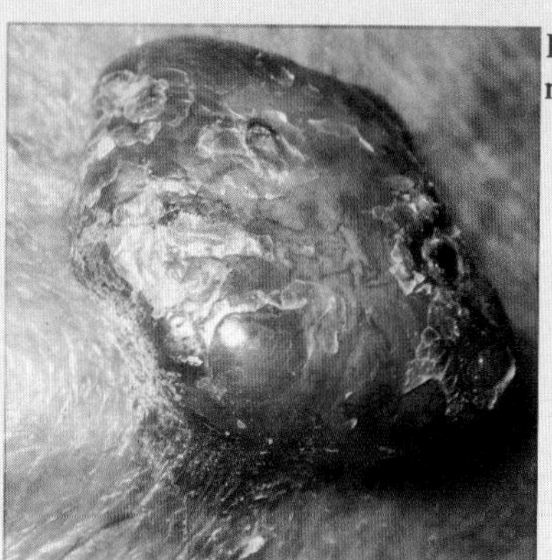

Plate 14: Nodular melanoma.

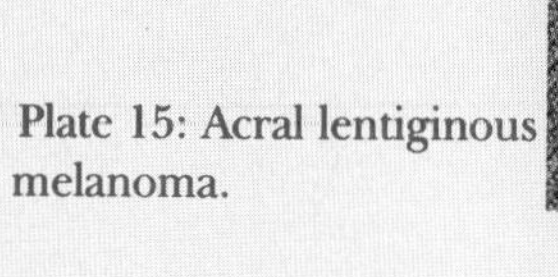

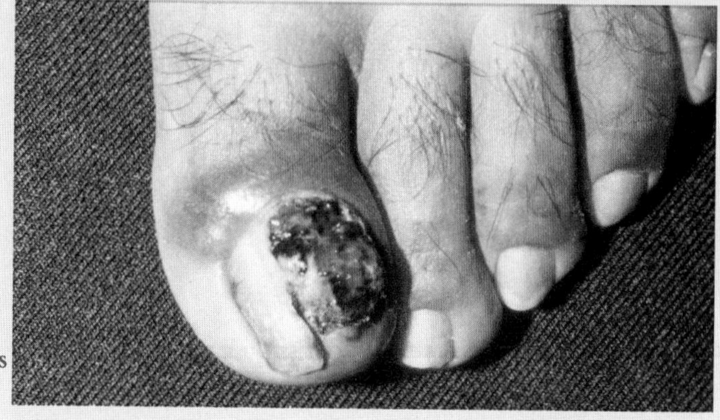

Plate 15: Acral lentiginous melanoma.

very rare. In any case, what were once thought of as viral genes capable of causing human cancer are now thought to be human genes captured by the virus and moved from one cell to another.

In a 1989 review, Henderson[44] presented the evidence for the viral etiology of cancer. The epidemiologic evidence is strongest for a relationship between hepatitis B virus and hepatocellular carcinoma and for human T-cell leukemia/lymphoma virus (HTLV)-I and T-cell lymphoma. Both have a geographic distribution of cancer prevalence and viral infection as well as case-by-case associations. The association between Burkitt's lymphoma and Epstein-Barr virus (EBV) is likewise strong, except that there seems to be a need for an associated immunodeficiency state, perhaps induced by chronic malaria. Similarly, the association between EBV and high-grade lymphoma in Western countries seems to require that an immunodeficiency state be present, either congenital or induced by human immunodeficiency virus (HIV) or by a drug such as cyclosporin. The relationship between EBV and nasopharyngeal carcinoma is less clear, and Henderson interprets the evidence here to suggest that EBV may be a passenger virus, although others see a causative role. Also controversial is the relationship between cervical carcinoma, herpes simplex virus type 2 (HSV-2), and human papillomavirus (HPV), where conflicting data have been reported, although recent biochemical data have strengthened the relationship of HPV to epithelial cancers.[33]

Hepatitis B virus (HBV) is endemic in Asia and Africa, where large numbers of people are chronic carriers, as high as 10% of the population. Epidemiologic studies have established HBV to be etiologic in hepatocellular carcinoma (HCC).[45] In China alone between 500,000 and 1 million cases of HCC occur annually; this is likely to be the most common cancer in the world today. HBV transforms the hepatocyte not because it has an oncogene, but because it integrates copies of itself at random sites into the host DNA. If by chance one of these sites is in the proper relationship to a host DNA proto-oncogene to cause inappropriate activation of that gene, then a clone of malignant cells may be initiated. There is a mean duration of 35 years from the time of HBV infection to the onset of the HCC.[46] There may be other factors that increase risk, although these are not proved. HCC may be induced by a mechanism that does not involve HBV, as, for example, the natural carcinogen aflatoxin, which may be important in the United States, where both chronic HBV infection and HCC are not very common.

Among the human retroviruses, HTLV-1 has clearly been implicated in adult T-cell leukemia (ATL), which is a malignancy of mature T4 lymphocytes endemic in Japan, the Caribbean, parts of Africa, and the southeastern United States.[47] A small proportion of patients with Sézary syndrome and mycosis fungoides also have evidence of HTLV-1. In endemic regions, only a small proportion of infected patients, less than 1%, develop ATL. Transmission of the virus is by sexual contact or through contaminated blood. The latency period between infection and ATL varies from a few years up to 40 years.[45,46] As is the case with HBV, the virus has no oncogene and is randomly incorporated in host DNA. The tumors are monoclonal and vary from one patient to another in the point at which the virus is inserted into the DNA. Presumably, as with HBV, insertion adjacent to a host proto-oncogene may lead to activation of that gene and cell transformation.

Hairy cell leukemia (HCL) is a disease of B lymphocytes for the most part, but a small portion of the cases manifest T lymphocytes. HTLV-2 has been isolated from the T-cell variety of HCL.[45,46]

The Epstein-Barr virus (EBV) causes infectious mononucleosis in the United States and Burkitt's lymphoma in Africa. A double-stranded DNA virus of the herpes family, EBV infects B lymphocytes and stimulates their proliferation. If host immunity is intact, a T-lymphocyte response is generated against an EBV protein expressed on the B-cell membrane, and the proliferating B cells are brought under control. For some reason, in Africa, perhaps because of the effect of chronic malaria on the immune system, a B-cell clone may emerge uncontrolled, which leads to a monoclonal malignancy, Burkitt's lymphoma. The mechanism is associated with an incorporation of the EBV into the host DNA and with visible abnormality of tumor cell chromosomes. Specifically, chromosome 8, which contains the *c-myc* proto-oncogene known to be associated with cell proliferation, exchanges genetic material with chromosome 14, or sometimes chromosome 2 or 22, where genes necessary for antibody synthesis are located. The presumption is that the *c-myc* proto-oncogene is activated when the immune genes are stimulated.

Burkitt's lymphoma is rare in Western countries, and when it is seen, EBV is only occasionally present. An X-linked inherited immune deficiency has been described in which EBV induces a polyclonal lymphoma.[48] Patients with AIDS and patients immunosuppressed for organ transplantation are also at risk for polyclonal lymphomas associated with EBV.[45,46]

The Chinese, no matter where they live, are at increased risk for nasopharyngeal carcinoma. Their tumors are associated with the EBV genome within the tumor cell. There are other causes of this tumor in other races, but the Chinese seem to have a unique association with EBV. The EBV genome is actively transcribed in these tumors in the same way as in latently infected lymphocytes,[49] providing strong evidence for an etiologic role.

Hodgkin's disease has been suspected of being related to EBV, but the data are conflicting. In some cases, the disease may be preceded by an altered antibody pattern against EBV.[50]

The human papillomaviruses (HPV) are double-stranded circular DNA viruses that infect squamous epithelium. There are many strains, some of which cause the common human wart. They are difficult to study because they cannot be grown in the laboratory. Two independent transforming oncogenes have been identified, and the protein product of one of these genes has recently been shown to bind specifically to the protein product of the retinoblastoma gene.[51] This provides strong support for the hypothesis that transformation results when the infecting HPV codes for a protein that blocks the product of a cancer-suppressor gene. It also helps researchers understand how absence of the retinoblastoma genes may lead to malignancy.

HPV causes genital warts. Cervical cancer is associated with promiscuity. DNA from strains HPV-16 or HPV-18 is found in 70% of all cervical carcinomas, and the morphologic changes of cervical dysplasia are linked to HPV infection.[45,46] Thus strong data support a causative role for some strains of HPV in cervical cancer. To a lesser extent there are associations with all genital cancer, including cancer of the penis and prostate.

CONTROVERSIES IN CARCINOGENESIS

Estrogens and Carcinogenesis

One of the most controversial topics in carcinogenesis is the role of estrogens. Animal models have clearly shown that estrogen is involved in the genesis of breast cancer, and a plethora of human studies has demonstrated that estrogen is related to human breast cancer in an as yet poorly defined fashion. That estrogen is in some theoretical way related to breast cancer is not the issue. The central practical issues are two: (1) does postmenopausal estrogen replacement therapy increase breast cancer risk and (2) does oral contraceptive use increase breast cancer risk?

A host of case control studies have provided copious data to support either a yes or no answer to the first question. The only controlled randomized trial, however, showed that after 10 years the placebo group had more breast cancer than the group treated with hormone replacement.[52] In view of the known benefits of postmenopausal estrogen in preventing osteoporosis and reducing cardiovascular risk by up to half,[53] any decision on a contraindication of estrogen based on a hypothetical or poorly documented breast cancer risk must be carefully evaluated. It is likely that replacement therapy has a weak effect, if any, and does not substantially alter breast cancer incidence, although an association with endometrial cancer seems well established.[54]

The role of contraceptives in breast cancer risk, likewise, is controversial and not clearly established, with most of the studies showing no relationship.[53,54] It is possible that long-term use before the first pregnancy may increase risk,[55] and this is obviously an important issue because such a pattern of use is frequent. At present the issue is unresolved, although the preponderant opinion is that contraceptives are safe.

Involuntary (Passive) Smoking

Cullen[56] reviews the evidence for passive or involuntary smoking as causative in lung cancer. There are insufficient data to allow a firm conclusion, but spousal exposure provides some information. Lung cancer mortality may be about one third higher in spouses of smokers than in spouses of nonsmokers. This has served as the basis for estimates that exposure of nonsmokers in proximity to smokers may account for up to 20% of nonsmoker lung cancer deaths each year, or about 2400 deaths. The sex of the spouse would be a factor, since according to a report by the Surgeon General,[57] one-half pack of cigarettes per day increases mortality ratios for women by about 30% to 80% and for men about fourfold to ninefold, indicating that men seem to be more sensitive.

Medical Radiation

The risk of medical radiation exposure has probably been exaggerated, as can be seen in Table 2-1. The large unavoidable radiation doses from our natural environment dwarf the small medical exposure. Still, radiation is carcinogenic, and every attempt should be made to minimize exposure consistent with effective diagnosis and prevention. Of particular public concern is exposure from mammography. This has undoubtedly been exaggerated, and the new techniques provide very low exposures to the breast. Present recommendations of the American Cancer Society for mammography seem reasonable and are likely to save many more lives than those placed at risk by the very low level of radiation.

Radon levels in the home may become a public concern in the future. Presently too little is known to draw firm conclusions or to make useful recommendations concerning prevention.

Environmental Carcinogenesis

Perhaps the most popular subject for the lay press is environmental carcinogenesis. The term *environmental* is subject to a great deal of confusion. Its original use was intended to include all cancers that were not hereditary, that is, all cancers due to viruses, life-style, tobacco, diet, and a host of other causes. Thus it was commonly thought that 85% of cancer was environmental. This was accurate but was misinterpreted in a very limited sense by many people to mean contaminated air, water, and food. And it has been further limited in the media to exclude natural carcinogens in our environment so that the focus has been on man-made chemicals. This has led to the notion that we should identify such cancer-causing chemicals in the air we breathe, the water we drink, and the food we eat and rid our environment of them.

However, such a notion of preventing cancer by eliminating a few chemicals from the environment may be simplistic. Indeed, Ames has suggested just that. A few years ago it was widely believed that we could substantially reduce the incidence of cancer by applying the Ames assay for mutagenic chemicals to identify hazardous wastes, demonstrate the carcinogenicity of each chemical in a laboratory model, and eliminate that chemical from the environment. This is often given a very high priority.

Ames[58] has described what he believes are the mistaken assumptions made by those who argue that environmental

TABLE 2-2 Six Errors Commonly Made Concerning the Role of Environmental Pollutants in the Etiology of Cancer

Error	Argument	Answer
1	Cancer rates are soaring and environmental chemicals are increasing, so there must be a relationship.	Except for lung cancer, age-adjusted cancer death rates are actually falling, and lung cancer is related primarily to smoking, not to environmental pollutants.
2	If we could identify the few carcinogenic chemicals, we could eliminate them from the environment.	Half the synthetic and natural chemicals tested in animals are carcinogenic in high doses, so the world is full of carcinogens and always has been. What is important is not the removal of minute amounts of thousands of theoretically hazardous agents, but giving attention to the high doses of a few agents that clearly cause human cancer.
3	Man made chemical pollutants are present in significant amounts.	Americans ingest 10,000 times more natural pesticides than manufactured pesticides in their diet. Broccoli and cabbage contain a billion times more of a dioxinlike chemical than the Environmental Protection Agency has set as a safe level of dioxin.
4	If a high dose of a chemical will cause a few cancers in rats, a low dose will cause many cancers in a large population.	Present data on radiation and chemical carcinogenesis suggest that a threshold dose exists even for mutagenic agents because of repair of DNA. Furthermore, threshold effects are certainly present for agents acting as promoters, and most agents presently highly publicized are promoters.
5	The Love Canal and other celebrated examples of pollution were associated with increased numbers of cancers.	There are, in fact, no good epidemiologic data proving that the minuscule levels of pollutants detected in most of the celebrated pollution cases led to an increase in cancer rates.
6	Technology is doing us in.	This is true only to the extent that our ability to measure smaller and smaller concentrations of chemicals may be causing us to abandon safe technologies for more dangerous ones and divert our attention from known hazards to theoretical hazards.

Source: Adapted from Ames BN: What are the major carcinogens in the etiology of human cancer? Environmental pollution, natural carcinogens, and the causes of human cancer: Six errors, in DeVita VT, Hellman S, Rosenberg SA (eds): Important Advances in Oncology 1989. Philadelphia, Lippincott, 1989.

pollutants represent our highest priority in cancer prevention. Table 2-2 lists these six commonly made errors, the arguments one hears, and the answers that Ames gives. Ames' views have substantial credibility because he has extensive experience in this area. He points out the dangers of the approach taken today by far too many people. By focusing our attention on trivial or even nonexistent dangers, we divert our attention from significant, very real dangers. There are over half a million deaths each year from tobacco and alcohol, and this number dwarfs the insignificant number of deaths that result from the pollutants we see emphasized so much in the media.

A preferred interpretation of "environmental" would refer to our personal environment or, in usual terminology, our life-style. It is the food we eat, the alcohol we drink, and the tobacco we smoke or otherwise abuse that, more than any other factors, have increased our risk of cancer. The enemy is not the chemical plant down the street, but ourselves. Pitot[9] has emphasized that tobacco is directly related to over 30% of the cancer deaths and that if tobacco-caused cancers are excluded, the cancer death rate is not increasing but is in fact decreasing slightly.

Diet and Carcinogenesis

In Japan cancer of the stomach has long been common and cancers of the colon and the breast uncommon. When Japanese move to the United States, they rapidly develop our pattern of common colon cancer and uncommon stomach cancer. Several generations later they develop our pattern of common breast cancer. Most investigators assume that the explanation for the colon and stomach cancer differences is the change in diet. The reason for the breast cancer difference is less clear. Willett[59] has critically reviewed the data on dietary risk factors for colon and breast cancer. He notes the striking correlation between the amount of fat a nation consumes and the incidence of colon cancer and breast cancer and a similar correlation between meat consumption and colon cancer.

The notion that fat intake may be related to breast cancer has persisted, but there has been an inability to provide individual, compared with national, statistics relating breast cancer to fat intake. This has led to a wide acceptance that the relationship is not to fat but to total calories, and especially to total calories consumed early in life. Willett[59] has interpreted the correlation of height to breast cancer as supporting this hypothesis; in nations where malnutrition is present in some groups, breast cancer incidence is lower in short women; such a relationship is not seen in the United States and Scandinavia. The delay of several generations in Japanese migrants in the development of increased breast cancer rates suggests that the issue is more complex than diet alone.

The role of fat in colon cancer is supported by both the rapid change in incidence with dietary change and the potential relationship of fat consumption to bile acids, which are known to be mutagenic. In Japan since 1945 the improved diet has been associated with an increase in colon cancer but not yet an increase in breast cancer.[59] The well-documented relationship of meat to colon cancer likely reflects animal fat consumption. The role of fiber in colon cancer has repeatedly been postulated to relate to altered transit time, altered bacterial flora in the colon, and altered exposure of the colonic mucosa to potentially carcinogenic bacterially modified bile acids. Epidemiologic studies have suggested an inverse relationship between dietary fiber and colon cancer, and animal studies suggest that the type of fiber consumed may be important.[60] Human studies have shown that wheat bran and cellulose, but not oat bran, are associated with lower stool mutagens by the Ames assay and with reduced secondary bile acids.[61]

Stomach cancer has been suggested to be related to the intake of food that is cured, smoked, pickled, salted, or otherwise preserved but not refrigerated. Some special methods of food preparations have also been incriminated. Long-term use of refrigeration seems particularly important in reducing the incidence of stomach cancer. The records of a group of English hospitals were searched for all cases of gastric cancer diagnosed over a 31-month period starting January 1985. Two controls were selected for each of the 95 cases from a population of patients matched for age, sex, and area of residence. Low intake of fresh vegetables and fruit and high intake of salt were clearly associated with stomach cancer development. No association was found for recent refrigerator use, but risk was cut in half by use of a refrigerator for 29 or more years. Risk was elevated in subjects who as children lived in homes without refrigeration.[62]

The nature of the effect of fruits and vegetables is unclear. There has been speculation that the antioxidant effect of vitamin C might play a role, but this has not been well established. Many food preservatives have an antioxidant effect and may actually antagonize possible carcinogens such as nitrites. Alcohol has been well documented as a risk factor in head and neck cancer and more recently incriminated in breast cancer,[63] although this observation is controversial.

Doll and Peto[64] have suggested that up to 50% of breast cancer and 90% of colon cancer in the United States could be prevented by a change in diet. However, radical changes would be required early in life to effect substantial reductions in incidence. Even reduction in alcohol may not be effective unless it takes place early in life. The potential for substantial reduction in cancer incidence by dietary modification alone seems remote. Nonetheless, a prudent diet rich in fruits, fiber, and cruciferous vegetables and low in animal fat is desirable for many health reasons and may perhaps reduce the risk of cancer.

CONCLUSION

Knowledge of the mechanisms of carcinogenesis has increased greatly in recent years. Researchers have identified many of the targets of carcinogenesis—the proto-oncogenes and anti-oncogenes that are the "on" and "off" switches for cell growth. Specific and consistent point mutations, movement of proto-oncogenes to different chromosomes, and loss of anti-oncogenes have all been demonstrated. In a few cases researchers have found the specific structural changes in growth control proteins leading to malfunction. Still, much remains to be learned.

Despite the vast array of chemicals discovered to cause cancer in animals, there remain very few chemicals (other than tobacco) for which there is strong evidence of cancer causation in humans. Occupational exposures have been examined, but the best estimate is that only 4% of all cancers in America are due to occupational causes. A number of inherited cancer syndromes have been identified, but most are rare, and for the common cancers (lung, colon, and breast), the syndromes are not distinct. It is estimated that up to 15% of all human cancer may have a hereditary component.

Perhaps the most popular subject for the lay press at present is "environmental" carcinogenesis. The term *environmental* is confusing because it leads to the notion that we can prevent cancer by eliminating a few chemicals from the environment. A preferred interpretation would refer to our personal environment, that is, our life-style. It is the food we eat, the alcohol we drink, and the tobacco we smoke or otherwise abuse that, more than any other factors, increase our risk of cancer. The enemy is not the chemical plant down the street, but ourselves. Tobacco is directly related to a third of all cancer deaths, and if tobacco-caused cancers are excluded, the cancer death rate is in fact decreasing. The paradox of carcinogenesis is simply this: Lung cancer is the most common, the most deadly, and the most preventable of all cancers in the United States.

REFERENCES

1. Waterfield MD, Scrace GT, Whittle N, et al: Platelet derived growth factor is structurally related to the putative transforming protein p28-sis of simian sarcoma virus. Nature 304:35-39, 1983.
2. Doolittle RF, Hunkapiller MW, Hood LE, et al: Simian sarcoma virus onc gene v-sis is derived from the gene (or genes) encoding a platelet derived growth factor. Science 221:275-276, 1983.

3. Horowitz JM, Yandell DW, Park SH, et al: Point mutational inactivation of the retinoblastoma antioncogene. Science 243:937-940, 1989.
4. Rous P, Beard JW: The progression to carcinoma of virus induced rabbit papillomas (Shope). J Exp Med 62:523-548, 1935.
5. Rous P, Kidd JG. Conditional neoplasms and subthreshold neoplastic states. J Exp Med 73:365-389, 1941.
6. Friedewald WF, Rous P: The initiating and promoting elements in tumor production. An analysis of the effects of tar, benzpyrene, and methylcholanthrene in rabbit skin. J Exp Med 80:101-126, 1944.
7. Foulds L: The experimental study of tumor progression. A review. Cancer Res 14:327-339, 1954.
8. Fidler IJ: The evolution of biological heterogeneity in metastatic neoplasms, in Nicolson GL, Milas L (eds): Cancer Invasion and Metastasis: Biologic and Therapeutic Aspects. New York, Raven Press, 1984.
9. Pitot HC: Principles of carcinogenesis: chemical, in DeVita VT Jr, Hellman S, Rosenberg SA (eds): Cancer: Principles and Practice of Oncology. Philadelphia, Lippincott, 1989.
10. Yamagiwa K, Ichikawa K: Experimentelle Studie uber die Pathogenese der Epitheliageschwulste. Mitteilungen Med Facultat Kaiserl Univ Tokyo 15:295, 1915.
11. Redmond DE Jr: Hill cautions against snuff in 1761. N Engl J Med 282:18-23, 1970.
12. Wynder EL, Graham EA: Tobacco smoking as a possible etiologic factor in bronchiogenic carcinoma: A study of 684 proved cases. JAMA 143:329-336, 1950.
13. Doll R, Hill AB: Smoking and carcinoma of the lung: Preliminary report. Br Med J 2:739-748, 1950.
14. Levin ML, Goldstein H, Gerhardt PR: Cancer and tobacco smoking: A preliminary report. JAMA 143:336-338, 1950.
15. Rehn L: Blasengeschwulste bei Fuchsin-Arbeitern. Arch Klin Chir 50:588, 1895.
16. Kennaway EL, Hieger I: Carcinogenic substances and their fluorescence spectra. Br J Med 1:1044, 1930.
17. Miller EC: Some current perspectives on chemical carcinogenesis in humans and experimental animals: Presidential Address. Cancer Res 38:1479-1496, 1978.
18. Ames BN, Durston WE, Yamasaki E, et al: Carcinogens are mutagens: A simple test system combining liver homogenates for activation and bacteria for detection. Proc Natl Acad Sci USA 70:2281, 1973.
19. Perera FP, Weinstein IB: Molecular epidemiology and carcinogen-DNA adduct detection: New approaches to studies of human cancer causation. J Chronic Dis 35:581-600, 1982.
20. Fry RJM: Principles of carcinogenesis: Physical, in DeVita VT Jr, Hellman S, Rosenberg SA (eds): Cancer: Principles and Practice of Oncology. Philadelphia, Lippincott, 1989.
21. Sukumar S, Pulciani S, Doniger J, et al: A transforming ras gene in tumorigenic guinea pig cell lines initiated by diverse chemical carcinogens. Science 223:1197-1199, 1984.
22. Guerrero I, Villasante A, Corces V, et al: Activation of a c-K-ras oncogene by somatic mutation in mouse lymphomas induced by gamma radiation. Science 225:1159-1162, 1984.
23. Bos JL, Toksoz D, Marshall CJ, et al: Amino acid substitutions at codon 13 of the N-ras oncogene in human acute myeloid leukaemia. Nature 315:726-730, 1985.
24. Dalla-Favera R, Martinotti S, Gallo RC, et al: Translocation and rearrangements of the c-myc oncogene locus in human undifferentiated B-cell lymphoma. Science 219:963-967, 1983.
25. Tong L, de Vos AM, Milburn MV, et al: Structural differences between a *ras* oncogene protein and the normal protein. Nature 337:90-93, 1989.
26. Doll R, Peto R: The Causes of Cancer. New York, Oxford University Press, 1981.
27. Levine EG, King RA, Bloomfield CD: The role of heredity in cancer. J Clin Oncol 7:527-540, 1989.
28. Lynch HT, Albano WA, Heieck JJ: Genetics biomarkers and the control of breast cancer. Cancer Genet Cytogenet 13:43-92, 1984.
29. Knudson A: Mutation and cancer: statistical study of retinoblastoma. Proc Natl Acad Sci USA 68:820, 1971.
30. Huang HJS, Yee JK, Shew JY, et al: Suppression of the neoplastic phenotype by replacement of the RB gene in human cancer cells. Science 242:1563-1566, 1988.
31. Pereira-Smith OM, Smith JR. Evidence for the recessive nature of cellular immortality. Science 221:964-966, 1983.
32. Cavenee WK, Hansen MF, Nordenskold M, et al: Genetic origin of mutations predisposing to retinoblastoma. Science 228:501-503, 1985.
33. Weinberg RA: The Rb gene and the negative regulation of cell growth. Blood 74:529-532, 1989.
34. Frieben A: Demonstration lines cancroids des rechten Handruckens, das sich nach langdauernder Einwirkung von Roentgenstrahlen entwichelt hatte. Fortschr Geb Roentgenstr 6:106, 1902.
35. von Jagic N, Scwarz G, von Siebenrock L: Blutbefunde bei Roentgenologon. Berl Klin Wochenschr 48:1220-1222, 1911.
36. Preston DL, Kato H, Kopecky KJ, et al: Studies on the mortality of A-bomb survivors. VIII. Cancer mortality, 1950–1982. Radiat Res 111:151-178, 1987.
37. Cleaver JE: Defective repair replication of DNA in xeroderma pigmentosum. Nature 218:652-656, 1968.
38. Standford KK, Parshad R, Green MH, et al: Hypersensitivity to G_2 chromatid radiation damage in familial dysplastic nevus syndrome. Lancet 2:1111-1116, 1987.
39. National Council on Radiation Protection Measurements (NRCP): Ionizing radiation exposure of the population of the United States. NCRP Report No 93. Bethesda, MD, The Council, 1987.
40. Nicholson WJ, Perbep G, Selikoff IJ: Occupational exposure to asbestos: Population at risk and projected mortality. Am J Ind Med 3:258-311, 1987.
41. Mossman BT, Gee JBL: Asbestos related diseases. N Engl J Med 320:1721-1730, 1989.
42. Rous P: Transmission of a malignant new growth by means of a cell free filtrate. JAMA 56:198, 1911.
43. Heubner RJ, Todaro GJ. Oncogenes of RNA tumor viruses as determinants of cancer. Proc Natl Acad Sci USA 64:1087-1094, 1969.
44. Henderson BE: Establishment of an association between a virus and a human cancer. JNCI 81:320-321, 1989.
45. Beasly RP, Linn CC, Hwang L, et al: Hepatocellular carcinoma and hepatitis B virus: A prospective study of 22,707 men in Taiwan. Lancet 2:1129-1133, 1981.
46. Howley PM: Principles of carcinogenesis: Viral, in DeVita VT Jr, Hellman S, Rosenberg SA (eds): Cancer: Principles and Practice of Oncology. Philadelphia, Lippincott, 1989.
47. Poiesz BJ, Ruscetti FW, Gazdar AF, et al: Detection and isolation of type C retrovirus particles from fresh and cultured lymphocytes of a patient with cutaneous T-cell lymphoma. Proc Natl Acad Sci USA 77:7415-7419, 1980.
48. Purtilo DT, Sakamoto K, Barnabai V, et al: Epstein-Barr virus induced diseases in boys with the X-linked lymphoproliferative syndrome (XLP): Updates on studies of the registry. Am J Med 73:49-56, 1982.
49. Pagano JS: Epstein-Barr virus transcription in nasopharyngeal carcinoma. J Virol 48:580-590, 1983.
50. Mueller N, Evans A, Harris NL, et al: Hodgkin's disease and

Epstein-Barr virus: altered antibody pattern before diagnosis. N Engl J Med 320:689-695, 1989.
51. Dyson N, Howley PM, Munger K, et al: The human papilloma virus-16 E7 oncoprotein is able to bind to the retinoblastoma gene product. Science 243:934-936, 1989.
52. Nachtigall LE, Nachtigall RD, Beckman EM: Estrogen replacement therapy. II. A prospective trial on the relationship of breast cancer and cardiovascular and metabolic problems. Obstet Gynecol 54:74-79, 1979.
53. Barrett-Connor E: Postmenopausal estrogen replacement and breast cancer. N Engl J Med 321:319-320, 1989.
54. Thomas DB: Do hormones cause breast cancer? Cancer 53:595-604, 1984.
55. Pike MC, Henderson BE, Casagrande JT, et al: Oral contraceptive use and early abortion as risk factors for breast cancer in young women. Br J Cancer 43:72-76, 1981.
56. Cullen JW: Principles of cancer prevention: Tobacco, in DeVita VT Jr, Hellman S, Rosenberg SA (eds): Cancer: Principles and Practice of Oncology. Philadelphia, Lippincott, 1989.
57. US Department of Health and Human Services, Office of Smoking and Health: The Health Consequences of Smoking: Cancer. A Report of the Surgeon General, DHHS pub. no. (PHS) 82-50179, 1982, p 38.
58. Ames BN: What are the major carcinogens in the etiology of human cancer? Environmental pollution, natural carcinogens, and the causes of human cancer: Six errors, in DeVita VT Jr, Hellman S, Rosenberg SA (eds): Important Advances in Oncology 1989. Philadelphia, Lippincott, 1989.
59. Willett W: The search for the causes of breast and colon cancer. Nature 338:389-394, 1989.
60. Wynder EL, Reddy BS: Dietary fat and fiber and colon cancer. Semin Oncol 10:264-272, 1983.
61. Reddy B, Engle A, Katsifis S, et al: Biochemical epidemiology of colon cancer: Effect of types of dietary fiber on fecal mutagens, acid, and neutral sterols in healthy subjects. Cancer Res 49:4629-4635, 1989.
62. Caggon D, Barker DJP, Cole RB, et al: Stomach cancer and food storage. J Natl Cancer Inst 81:1178-1182, 1989.
63. Willett WC, Stampfer MJ, Colditz GA, et al: Moderate alcohol consumption and the risk of breast cancer. N Engl J Med 314:1174-1180, 1987.
64. Doll R, Peto R: The causes of cancer: Quantitative estimates of avoidable risks of cancer in the United States today. J Natl Cancer Inst 66:1191-1308, 1981.

Chapter 3

Cellular Biology of Cancer

Charles E. Kupchella, PhD

INTRODUCTION

The two deceptively simple-sounding *basic* aims of cancer research are (1) find out how cancer is *caused* and then use this information to *prevent* cancer and (2) find out how cancer cells are *different* and use this information to *detect, control,* or *cure* cancer.

The two aims are actually related to one another—through genes. Cancer is caused by things that alter genes or disturb genetic control. The products of the affected genes express themselves as the features of cancer cells. Put another way, the second objective can be expressed as a series of questions: "What do these genes do? What protein products do they speed up, slow down, establish, or fail to complete? What are the ultimate consequences in terms of cell structure and function, and what pathways connect them to the gene(s)?" If clinicians could answer these questions, they would have ways to "get at" cancer even if they never did establish its *genetic* essence. Even if they could not get at the responsible genes, they *might* be able to get at the gene products or at products of the products, or both. Obviously, all those concerned want the answers.

Maybe, in seeking the answers, researchers will find that one or a few gene products are the primary or principal expressions of malignancy; maybe few key gene products cause every other feature of cancer cells through some kind of "domino effect." If a way could be found to block or influence such a key product, the cancer problem would be a long way toward being solved.

As the remainder of this chapter will show, there are many differences between cancer cells and noncancer cells. Some of the differences are the same as those between dividing and nondividing normal cells. When we try to exploit these differences, normal dividing cells get "hit" along with cancer cells. Cancer patients lose their hair and have problems with their intestines because drugs designed to kill dividing cancer cells also kill dividing hair-producing cells and intestinal epithelial cells.

Researchers obviously must find more fundamentally distinctive features of cancer cells. It should be noted that this chapter is written in general terms. There are approximately 100 different kinds of cancer, and even individual tumors contain many different kinds of cells in terms of their production of marker substances, susceptibility to elements of the immune system, and ability to metastasize. Such overtly functional differences are undoubtedly due to structural-organizational differences. Simply put, cancer cells are far from all alike.

Because of this heterogeneity, it is difficult to determine the nature of cancer cells. Despite their many differences, however, all cancer cells are manifestations of cells gone wrong in terms of cell division and social relationships. The following pages describe what is known about what goes wrong and the differences between cancer cells and normal cells.

TRANSFORMED CELLS AND OTHER MODELS

Background

One problem that complicates the search for key differences between cancer and normal cells is that there is no sure way of identifying the normal counterpart of a human cancer cell.

For most, if not all, human cancer, the normal precursors are unknown. All normal tissue from which tumors arise is made up of a variety of types of cells and cells in different stages of becoming what they will be. By the time human tumors are looked at, many have undergone considerable evolution. The historical connection to the original tissue may be far from obvious.

Liver tumors have been, are being, and no doubt will continue to be compared with normal liver tissue. Although clinicians can learn from such comparison, comparing normal human tissue from which cancer arises with cancer tissue itself may not be the same as comparing a cancer cell with the normal cell from which it came.

Because of this limitation, tumor biologists have tended to rely on cell culture models. They use stable cell lines derived from a variety of animal species as "normal" cells, and for "cancer" cells they use normal cell lines "transformed" by chemical carcinogens, radiation, or viruses. This approach solves the problem of not having a definitive "before" and "after," but problems still arise when we try to apply what we have learned to human cancer.

The unannounced shifts from "real" tumor cells to "transformed" cells in the following pages will imply that the two are one and the same. They are in fact *not* the same. We simply assume that transformed cells and *actual* cancer cells share many identical features and that things found out about transformed cells may well be applicable to "real" cancer. This presumption may *or may not* be confirmed by future experimentation.

Transformed Cell Lines

Transformed cells are cells derived from "normal" cell lines. Cell lines are cells that grow out of small pieces of normal tissue or embryonic tissue put into a cell culture flask under the right conditions. Such cells become permanent or continuous cell lines when they acquire the ability to be propagated indefinitely in tissue culture (see Figure 3-1).

Normal cells can go through only about 50 divisions in cell culture before they die out. Sometimes arising spontaneously from such normal cell cultures are variants that do not die out but go right on dividing as long as they are fed, subcultured, and maintained properly. With qualification, they serve very nicely as models of normal cells. Except for their "immortality," which disqualifies them from *absolute* "normalcy," the cells of cell lines behave nor-

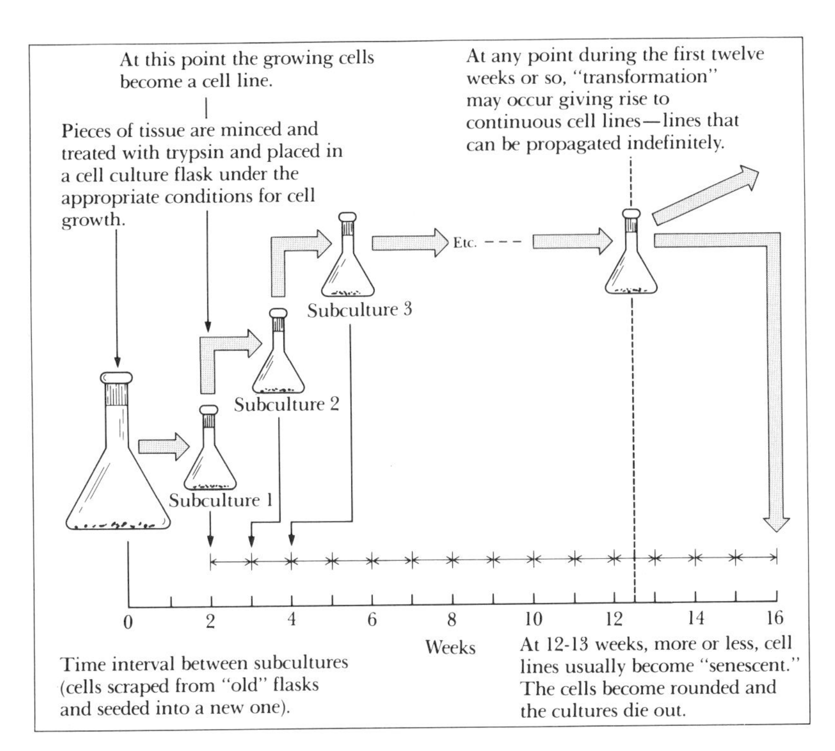

FIGURE 3-1 How cell lines and continuous cell lines are derived. Continuous cell lines arise from normal cells by some kind of spontaneous change or "transformation." Except for their immortality, continuous cell lines behave like normal cells in culture. They are referred to throughout this chapter as if they *were* normal. The term *transformed cell* means cell lines derived from continuous cell lines (by exposure to radiation, chemical carcinogens, or oncogenic viruses) that behave like cancer cells. (Source: Kupchella CE: Dimensions of Cancer. Belmont, Calif, Wadsworth, 1987. © 1987 by Wadsworth, Inc. Used by permission of publisher.)

mally. The cells of cell lines can be transformed—converted to cells that behave like tumor cells in culture.

Although the ultimate test of a transformed cell line is its ability to develop into a malignant neoplasm when implanted into an appropriate host species, transformed cells can be recognized by other characteristics. Pitot[1] and Ruddon[2] list the most important criteria of "transformedness." These include altered antigenicity, diminished contact inhibition, reduced requirements for certain nutrients, and the ability to grow in suspension or otherwise unattached to a solid substratum. Not all transformed cell lines exhibit *all* the characteristics *generally* found in transformed cells.

Cell lines are transformed by the same kinds of agents that cause tumors to arise in animal tissue, namely, viruses, chemical carcinogens, and radiation.

The beauty of cell line or transformed cell systems is that they provide "pure" untransformed cells and "pure" transformed counterparts that can then be compared. Particularly useful have been the "temperature-sensitive mutants" discovered along the way. Temperature-sensitive mutants are cell lines that express transformedness only at certain temperatures. At other temperatures, they revert to the *un*transformed phenotype. By providing a means by which to turn transformation on or off quickly, these mutants make it possible to evaluate the *tightness* of connections between chemical changes and other features of the transformed state.

We will move on now to describe how *actual* cancer cells look under the microscope.

CANCER CELLS LOOK DIFFERENT

Characteristics

A pathologist looking at cancer tissue under the microscope sees tissue that lacks the high level of structural organization seen in normal tissue. The degree of deviation from normal varies from one type of tumor to another.

"Fixed," static sections of tumor tissue stained with hematoxylin and eosin (a mixture of dyes that colors the cytoplasm of a cell red and the nucleus blue) often give the impression of motion or disarray. Some of the disarray is caused by the presence of variable amounts of dead cells, connective tissue, and infiltrating white cells. Actual cancer cells are often clearly recognizable, mostly because of their hyperchromatism—more strongly stained chromatin and

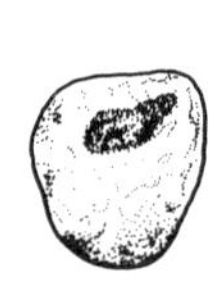

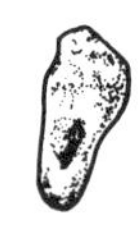

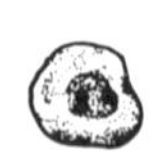

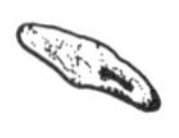

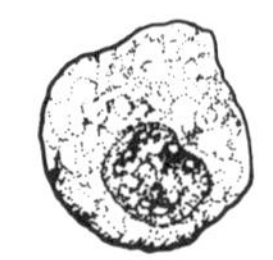

(a) Pleomorphism
Normal
(b) Hyperchromatism
Cancer
Normal
(c) Increased nuclear to cytoplasmic ratio
Normal
Unequal segregation
Tricentric
Tetracentric
(d) Abnormal mitoses
Normal. Highly differentiated columnar ciliated epithelium
Dysplasia. Deranged cell growth leading to tissue made up of cells of variable size, shape, and appearance
Anaplasia. Primitive-looking, undifferentiated cells
(e) Anaplasia

FIGURE 3-2 General features of cancer cells.

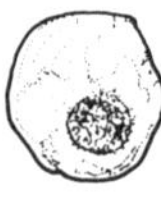

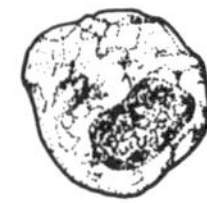

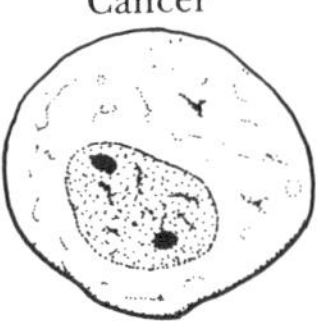

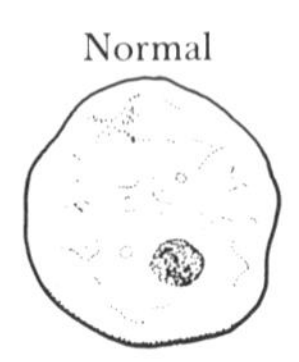

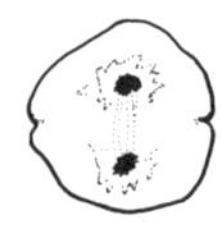

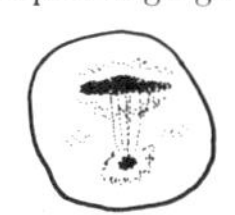

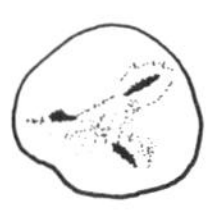

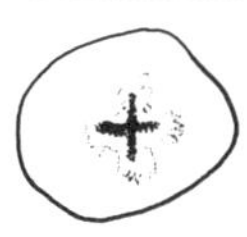

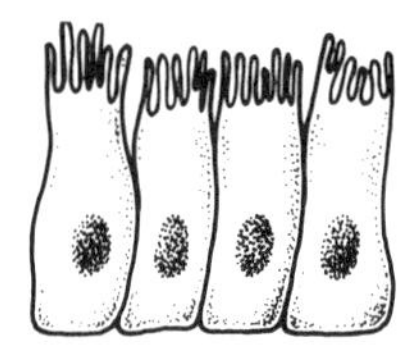

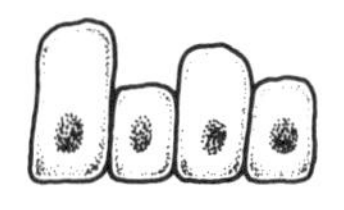

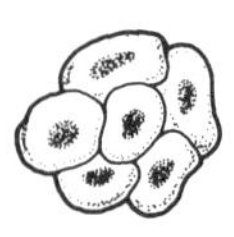

larger nuclei (Figure 3-2b). When a pathologist is evaluating a tumor, blue is bad!

There are other important features of cancer cells. Cancer cells tend to be pleomorphic—they have variable sizes and shapes (Figure 3-2a). Cancer cells have a high nucleus-to-cytoplasm ratio; their nuclei are disproportionately large (Figure 3-2c). In a group of cancer cells, there will tend to be more cells undergoing mitosis than in normal tissue, and often there is a large number of *abnormal* mitotic figures (Figure 3-2d).Cancer cells have unusually prominent nucleoli. Finally, cancer cells tend to be anaplastic; they tend to be less well differentiated than the cells of surrounding normal tissue (Figure 3-2e). For example, liver tumor cells do not look like normal liver cells. Some cancer cells are so poorly differentiated that it can be difficult to identify the tissue origin.

Cancer Cells and Differentiation

As a fertilized human egg divides and divides again, the individual cells in the expanding mass become different from one another. Ultimately, some results of this process look like "fully differentiated" liver, kidney, skin, and muscle cells.

For a long time it was thought that all cancer cells emerged from fully differentiated normal cells that had "*de*differentiated" due to transformation. It was thought that cells that had reached their mature appearance reverted—in the direction of embryologic forms—when "hit" by a carcinogen. Later it was more generally believed that cancer cells all come from the small number of undifferentiated cells already present in normal tissue (Figure 3-3).

Today, researchers know that genes (oncogenes) previously turned off during differentiation can be reactivated by carcinogenic agents. We also know that it is possible to cause the cells at one level of differentiation to become transformed into less well-differentiated cells by exposing them to carcinogenic agents. There are also other indications that the differentiated state is quite plastic. Blau et al[3] showed, for example, that when muscle cells are fused with various *differentiated* nonmuscle cells from different species, muscle gene expression is activated in the nonmuscle cells.

Although it is still not entirely clear, it may be that human cancer can arise by the transformation of either partially differentiated cells or at least some kinds of more fully differentiated cells. It may simply be easier (require fewer changes) to transform undifferentiated cells.

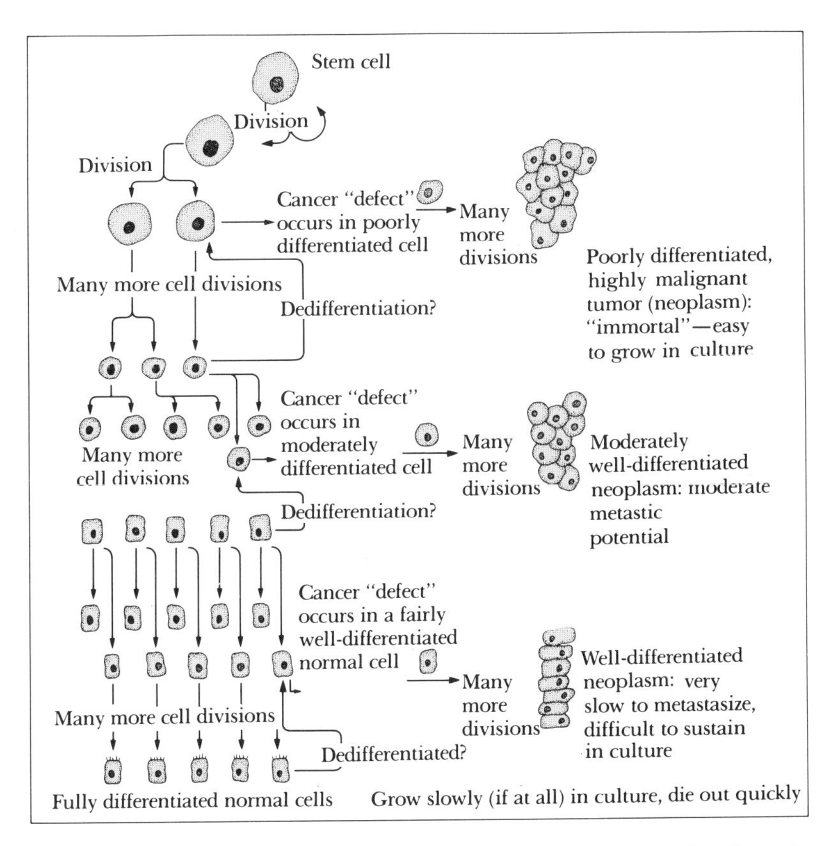

FIGURE 3-3 The normal differentiation of cells (left) and the origin of poorly differentiated, moderately well differentiated, and well-differentiated neoplasms. The relationship between differentiation and metastatic behavior is far from precise; poorly differentiated cancers tend to be highly metastatic, however. (Source: Kupchella CE: Dimensions of Cancer. Belmont, Calif, Wadsworth, 1987. © 1987 by Wadsworth, Inc. Used by permission of publisher.)

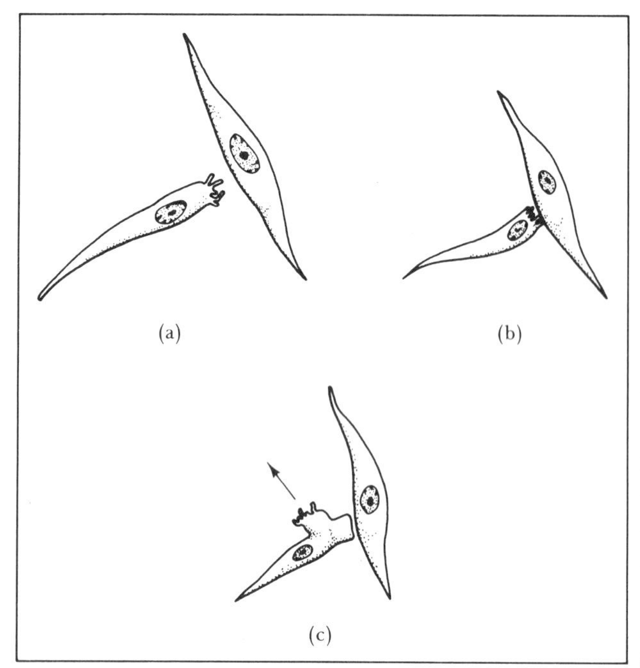

FIGURE 3-4 Contact inhibition of movement.

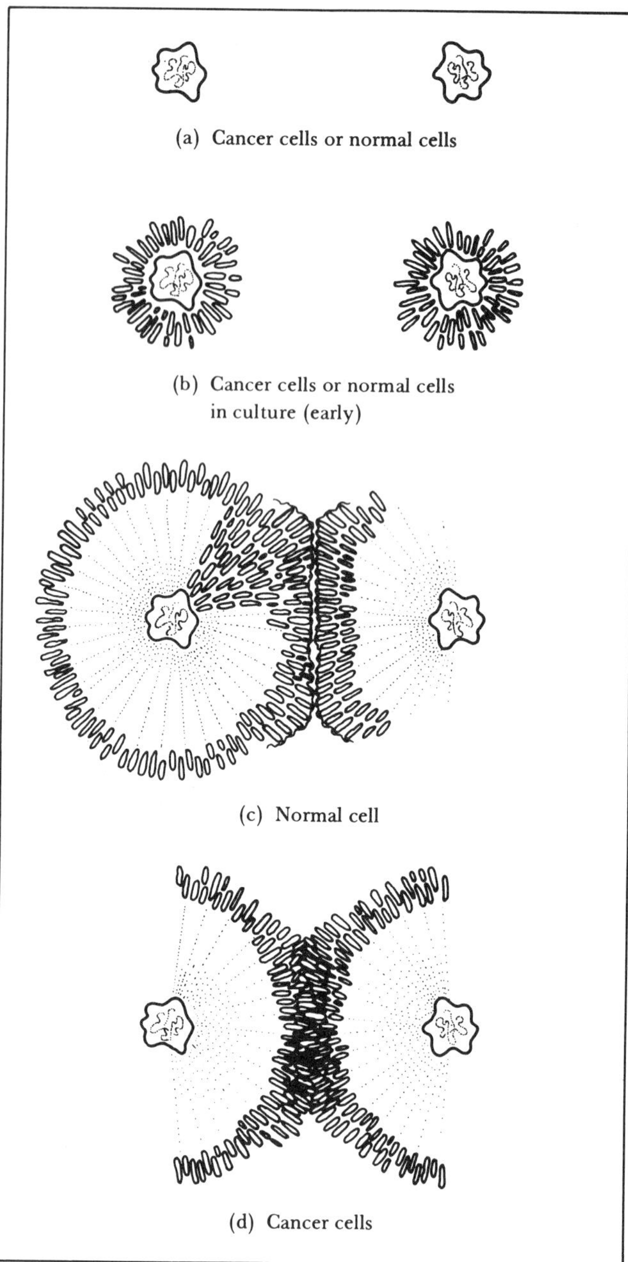

FIGURE 3-5 Impaired contact inhibition of cancer cells.

CANCER CELLS BEHAVE DIFFERENTLY

The spread of cancer from a primary tumor to regional lymph nodes and to other organs was noted by early physicians, and they must have deduced that cancer cells *behaved* abnormally. After it became possible to grow cancer cells and transformed cells in culture, a number of characteristic behavioral features of these cells were documented:

1. Altered contact inhibition of movement
2. Altered contact inhibition of cell division
3. Altered ability to recognize other cells
4. Altered intercellular adhesion

As we consider each feature in turn, note that they all have *something to do with the cell surface.*

Diminished Contact Inhibition of Movement

If a small clump of normal cells is placed in fresh medium in a tissue culture flask, the cells will slowly migrate along the glass or plastic surface outward. Ambercrombie[4] showed that this migration resulted from cell-contact regulation of movement. Through time-lapse photography, he showed that, as a migrating cell made contact with another cell, forward motion stopped; after a short time, the cell began moving off in another direction (Figure 3-4). In experiments in which colonies of normal and then transformed cell lines were placed in a flask and allowed to migrate toward one another, cells of normal colonies stopped when they encountered the advancing edge of the other colony. Under the same circumstances, colonies of transformed cells climbed over and past one another (Figure 3-5). The normal phenomenon has come to be called *contact inhibition of movement.* This feature appears to be lost or at least diminished in malignant cells.

Diminished Contact Inhibition of Cell Division

If normal cells are placed in a tissue culture flask under the appropriate conditions, the cells begin to divide, moving outward, until the flask is covered with a single layer of cells that looks like a flagstone patio. At this point cell division ceases. If a few of the cells are scraped off, cells in that region begin dividing again until the blank space is filled in.

Such experiments indicate that normal cells quit dividing at "saturation density," not because they run out of nutrients, not because of accumulated waste, but because of "full contact" with other cells. When they are surrounded, they simply quit dividing. This kind of contact inhibition is sometimes called *contact inhibition of growth*.

Cancer cells generally lack or exhibit diminished contact inhibition of growth. Cancer cells continue to divide even after the bottom of a culture flask is covered. Apparently oblivious of other cells, cancer cells go right on dividing; they even pile up. They look less like a flagstone patio and more like a pile of flagstones dumped off the back of a truck.

The General Defect in Cell-to-Cell Recognition

It makes sense that normal cells *are* growth- and movement-inhibited by contact with other cells. This pattern helps explain how liver and skin cells stay where they belong and why the liver and kidneys only get so big.

The fact that cancer cells are defective in these traits helps explain (1) the invasion of normal tissue by tumor cells, (2) the spread of cancer, and (3) the fact that cancer manifests itself as lumps. The basis of these contact-mediated properties of normal cells and their alteration in the cancer cell must certainly involve both the cell surface and some kind of intercellular chemical interaction or recognition. Quite a number of studies have clearly indicated that normal cells can "recognize" and interact with one another chemically.

If a sponge is disassociated into individual cells and then mixed with cells of other strains of sponge, the cells from the same strain "find" one another and form multicellular clumps. Similarly, if rat cells and mouse cells are mixed, rat cells sort themselves out, forming aggregates with other rat cells, and mouse cells aggregate with other mouse cells. Moscona[5] showed that if kidney and liver cells from the same species were mixed, preexisting individual liver cells formed tiny liver "organoids," and kidney cells did likewise (Figure 3-6). Liver cells did not bind to kidney. All such examples of selective adhesion suggest the presence of very highly specific cell surface recognition systems normally serving to segregate and then stabilize cells into differentiated tissues. Cancer cells tend not to adhere to other cancer cells very well, and so naturally there is a great deal of interest in the chemical basis of cell-cell recognition and adhesion.

So far, among the chemicals known to be involved in cell-cell recognition are certain divalent cations, notably calcium and magnesium, and sugar-containing macromolecules that can be stripped off the surface by trypsin (indicating that they are glycoproteins). Whatever macromolecules are interacting from cell to cell, it is most likely the *distribution* of arrays of the molecules—a kind of molecular Braille—that accounts for the specificity. One compelling reason for such an explanation is that if liver had a different code from kidney—even in the same animal, as indicated by Moscona's experiments—there are too few different kinds of sugars on the surface to account for the number of different codes that would be required by the many kinds of tissue present in every animal. Just a few different kinds of glycoproteins could, however, be arranged in a large number of different patterns.

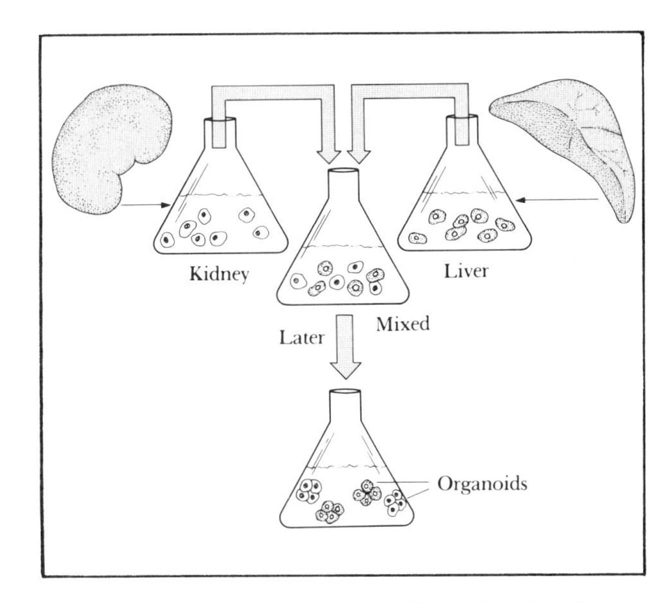

FIGURE 3-6 Moscona's experiment illustrating the adhesive specificity of cells of different organs in the same species. (Source: Kupchella CE: Dimensions of Cancer. Belmont, Calif, Wadsworth, 1987. © 1987 by Wadsworth, Inc. Used by permission of publisher.)

It has been suggested that enzymes may be involved in the initial stages of cell-cell adhesion. Glycosyl transferases, for example, are enzymes able to attach sugar residues to the carbohydrate portion of glycoprotein molecules. They put the finishing touches on protein-sugar complexes. It may be that such enzymes on *one* cell bind to the residues of their substrates on the *other*, accounting for the specific initial attachment of one cell to another. If not enzymes and substrates, then something very much like this process must account for the apparently very specific association of like cells.

We should be prepared to find out that many kinds of cell surface changes might all lead to the same end—the effective failure of the cell to know when it meets up with another cell. A recognition code could be disturbed by *additions* and *changes* as well as outright *deletions* of the molecules directly and indirectly involved.

It is not hard to imagine some kind of molecular hand-and-glove interaction between adjacent cells serving to appraise each cell of the existence of the other. If the glove does not fit very well because of some change in either the hand or the glove, the cells act as if they were alone. Molecular hands and gloves are probably made of glycolipids and glycoproteins (see below).

Growth

Above all else, cancer cells are different in the way they divide. The very fact that neoplasms express themselves as lumps indicates that cancer cells increase in number faster than do the cells of surrounding normal tissue. Actual measurements of many different kinds of human tumors indicate that the average human neoplasm doubles every 2 months. Since the cell cycle time of cancer cells is generally not much different from that of normal cells, this rate means that only a fraction of the cells in a tumor are dividing at any one time. The fact that neoplasms become lumps indicates that, whatever the fraction is, it is enough to keep cell division ahead of cell death or loss. This imbalance contrasts with the case in mature normal tissues capable of growth, where cell division matches cell loss. What keeps too high a fraction of cancer cells in the so-called growth fraction? This is one of the burning questions in cancer research—and, indeed, in all of cell biology.

A CATALOG OF CHANGES IN THE CANCER CELL SURFACE

Often sited as the first clear demonstration that there are surface differences between normal and cancer cells was the work of Coman[6] in the 1940s. He showed that tumor cells could be pulled apart more easily than their normal counterparts.

Driven by interest in basic cell biology, the basic biology of tumor cells, and in finding ways to control and cure cancer, there has since been, and continues to be, an enormous research effort directed at the cancer cell surface. The result to date has been the cataloging of a long list of things that are true about the cell surface. These, along with some cytoplasmic and nuclear changes, are summarized in Figure 3-7[7] (see also [8-16]).

Nearly all the known changes in the cell surface are still under active investigation. We still need to know if, and just how, these changes influence overt behavior features of cancer cells, and indeed, just how *general* these changes are.

The next few pages will describe what is known so far about the nature and possible significance of the most profound and important of these changes. We'll begin with glycoproteins and glycolipids.

Among the generalized changes in cell surface glycoproteins and glycolipids found in cancer cells are the following:

1. New glycoprotein molecules appear on the surface.
2. Some of the same glycolipid and glycoprotein molecules found on normal cell surfaces appear to be changed on transformed cell surfaces; some of these appear to be incompletely processed.
3. Certain high-molecular-weight glycolipids and glycoproteins are missing.
4. Another family of protein-carbohydrate complexes called *proteoglycans* are represented on the cell surface and in the intercellular matrix. These, too, appear to change in association with malignancy. Because these are large, negatively charged molecules in a position to interfere with the chemistry of the cell surface, it is important that the synthesis of certain of them increases in cancer cells. (Few clear generalizations about the relationship between proteoglycans and cancer have emerged thus far; we mention them only in passing.)

All this could be summarized by saying that some new molecules appear, some of the regular molecules are lost, and some of the regular molecules are changed.

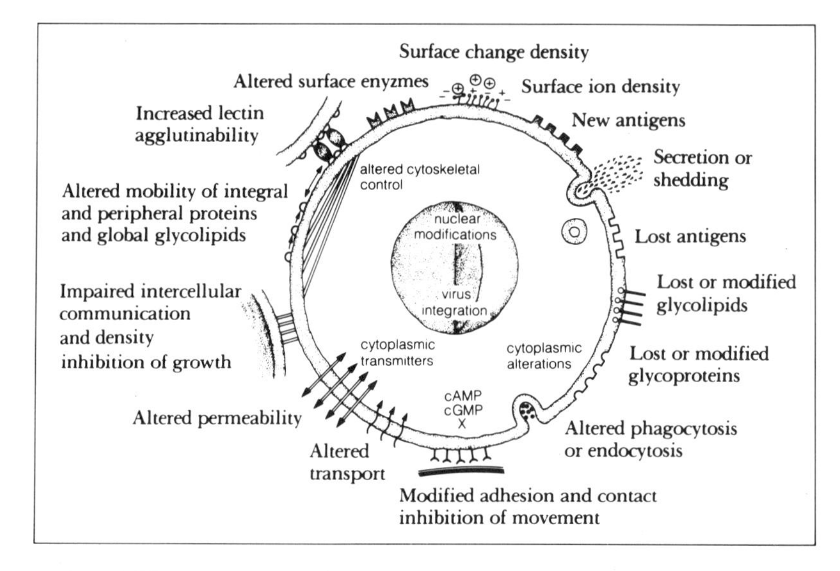

FIGURE 3-7 Summary of the cell surface and cell surface–related alterations generally seen in cancer cells. (Source: Adapted from Nicolson GL: Trans-membrane control of the receptors on normal and tumor cells. II. Surface changes associated with transformation and malignancy. Biochim Biophys Acta 458:16, 1976.)

Glycoprotein Changes

Transformation is almost invariably associated with alterations in cell-surface glycoproteins.[8] Although in some instances the complexity of malignant cell glycoproteins is increased,[17] the trend, by far, is toward a lower protein content of the transformed cell surface. Many of the glycoproteins that *are* present are altered, mostly by being simpler. Much evidence shows that transformed cells have deranged mechanisms by which polysaccharides are made and attached to proteins.

Fibronectin

Among the most profound or overt cell surface changes associated with transformation is the *loss* of a large glycoprotein, at first unimaginatively called *L*arge *E*xternal *T*ransformation-*S*ensitive protein, or LETS. LETS was found by Yamada and by others[13] to have something to do with adhesion. When investigators added LETS to red blood cells, it caused them to clump. LETS also caused the aggregation of previously disaggregated, transformed kidney cells and isolated cells derived from chicken embryos. It has also been observed that LETS levels are greatest in normal cells at rest and that they decline to near zero during cell division, suggesting the possibility of a basic role in controlling cell division.

As interest in LETS gathered steam, it was discovered that LETS was really a glycoprotein known by another name, *fibronectin.* Fibronectin is a large-molecular-weight glycoprotein found in soluble form in the blood of vertebrates and on normal cell surfaces. It is a component of the matrix or stroma in which cells are imbedded. Fibronectin is an anchoring molecule. Together with various proteoglycans, collagen, and elastin, fibronectin forms a fibrillar network that holds cells in place in tissue. It is also believed to serve as an organizing grid for the integral proteins of the cell surface. It acts like an exoskeleton; in other words, it holds receptor molecules in particular arrays. Fibronectin also influences organization inside the cell. Fibronectin molecules apparently interact specifically with actin filaments within the cytoplasm, probably through proteins that span the cell membrane.[13] Perhaps it is through this interaction that fibronectin also has something to do with the shapes of cells. When fibronectin is removed from fibroblasts, they lose their spindle shape, round up, and develop numerous microvilli, making them look much like transformed cells. All this suggests that fibronectin may lie close to a "primary defect" in cancer cells.

Hynes[13] suggests that the simplest explanation for why cancer cells have low levels of fibronectin associated with their surfaces is that cancer cells stop making fibronectin. Although there is some evidence for this, there is also evidence that cancer cells may make a defective form of fibronectin—a form they cannot hold on to. Cancer cells may also make a defective transmembrane fibronectin-binding protein, and there is some evidence that cancer cells may break down fibronectin as soon as they make it (see following discussion). In any case, it seems to be more than coincidental that cancer cells are deficient in fibronectin and that this substance plays important roles in cellular organization, cell-to-cell adhesion, cellular migration, and normal cytoskeletal structure.

Protease

Plasma fibronectin levels rise in the blood of cancer patients, and fibronectin is shed into the medium in which transformed cells are growing. It could be that all this is a direct consequence of a rise in protease (the general name for enzymes that break up protein molecules) secretion by cancer cells. The proteases may simply clip the fibronectin connections to the surface, allowing it to float away.

Transformed cells secrete "plasminogen-activating factor," which activates plasminogen. It actually converts plasminogen, an inactive protease, into plasmin, the active form. The secretion of plasmin and other proteases may be part of a general mechanism by which cells lose fibronectin.

The possibility that protease secretion or activation may be a "first cause" in the expression of the malignant phenotype is suggested by experiments in which it has been shown that when normal cells are treated with exogenous proteases, they begin to behave like transformed cells. Additional support for this possibility comes from experiments in which it was shown that abnormal behavior of transformed cells can be reversed or at least modulated by protease inhibitors. Other contributing evidence comes from the observation that certain normally masked features of the *normal* cell surface appear to be uncovered or exposed in the transformed cell.

Glycolipid Changes

In vitro experiments with fibroblast cell lines and their virus-induced transformants indicate that cell-surface glycolipid changes may be another general attribute of transformation. In general, the glycolipid content of transformed cell membranes is *reduced;* also, the complexity of membrane glycolipids is reduced—terminal sugar groups are often missing. Experimental evidence indicates that these changes are attributable to reduced synthesis and incomplete processing. Perhaps the fact that transformed cells are continually dividing simply does not leave the glycolipid synthesizing and processing machinery enough time to finish its work.

Changes in glycosphingolipids in particular have been linked to a number of important features of the transformed state.[18] Although glycosphingolipids are sometimes identified as blood group antigens, they are found in all animal cells and in some plant cells as well. The expression of glycosphingolipids on the surface of cells changes as normal cells divide and differentiate. Of interest is that the composition and metabolism of certain glycosphingolipids have been shown to change when normal cells are transformed. It has been suggested that by interacting with receptor proteins on the surface of normal cells, glycosphingolipids may inhibit cell responsiveness to growth factors in some general way. Changes or decreases in the amounts of glycosphingolipids associated with cell surfaces may thus move cells toward increasing responsiveness to growth factors. The experimental addition of certain glycosphingolipids to proliferating cells has been shown to inhibit them. The addition of another glycosphingolipid was shown to induce differentiation.[18]

Another cancer connection is that glycosphingolipids have been shown to serve as components of surface markers involved in cell-cell recognition.[18] How might all the cell surface changes described thus far be connected in their relationship to cancer cells?

THE FUNCTIONAL SIGNIFICANCE OF CELL SURFACE CHANGES IN CANCER

Glycoprotein as well as glycolipid changes may mean changes in receptor configurations on cell surfaces and a resultant disability to respond to other cells and to chemical signals from other parts of the organism. Glycoprotein and glycolipid changes may likewise be important to immune defense against cancer because they are a means (as antigens) by which the cells that bear them might be recognized by the immune system.

Alterations in the Cell Membrane as a Control Panel

The cell membrane plays an important role in all cells in the signaling that goes on between cells and the organism at large. The reader may recall that the enzyme, adenyl cyclase, which is bound to the inside of the cell membrane, is influenced by extracellular hormones that bind to receptors on the outside. Adenyl cyclase converts intracellular adenosine triphosphate (ATP) to the "second messenger," cyclic adenosine monophosphate (cAMP), which is an important regulator of the things that go on inside the cell.

Work by Pastan[19] and Levitzki[20] has shown that cAMP levels fluctuate with the state of cellular activity. Levels are generally high in resting normal cells and are low in dividing cells, including cancer cells. Another important regulatory molecule, cyclic guanosine monophosphate (cGMP), has been found to vary in a way opposite that of cAMP. Cell division is usually associated with *low* cAMP levels and *high* cGMP levels. Cyclic GMP has been found to stimulate RNA synthesis in some cells, and tumor promotors have been found to influence cAMP levels.

Although these changes may simply be part of a long list of secondary characteristics generally true of "turned-on" cells, the key regulatory position of cAMP makes it especially interesting to cancer researchers. Conceivably, the decreased cAMP level seen in transformed cells is a major primary stimulus or key to autonomous growth. If membrane changes turn out to be among the key initial expressions of malignancy, the very next change in the cascade of events leading to the full expression of malignancy could well be suppression of adenyl cyclase and a drop in cAMP levels. Especially intriguing is the observation that transformation traits such as roundedness and diminished adhesiveness can be restored to normal when transformed cells are prevented from degrading cAMP, causing its levels to rise toward normal.

Tumor-Associated Antigens

Our immune systems are designed to deal with foreign proteins and other foreign "antigenic" substances. We could just as easily have used the word *new* in place of *foreign*. Human immune systems conduct a survey early in neonatal life and declare all proteins there at that time to be "self." Proteins that show up after that survey are dealt with by the immune system as if they were parts of hostile, foreign organisms. As might be expected from the fact that *new* proteins and protein complexes appear on the surfaces of cancer cells, cancer cells are often immunologically distinguishable from their assumed or actual normal counterparts (see Chapter 5).

Some such antigenic differences can be recognized only by *other* species, the so-called heterologous antigens. Some can be recognized by other members of the same species, the alloantigens. Alloantigens are the kinds of antigens—such as histocompatibility antigens and blood-type antigens—that make it difficult to achieve successful organ and tissue transplants and that make it necessary to cross-match blood before giving transfusions.

Sometimes tumor cells bear isoantigens, tumor-associated antigens that the tumor-bearing animal recognizes as new or foreign. Some of these are antigens of tumor-inducing viruses; others are simply *neo*antigens associated with the transformed state. Some, if not all, tumor-specific antigens may be altered histocompatibility antigens, that is, a "normal" histocompatibility antigen of the host, modified beyond recognition as far as the immune system is concerned. Some antigens found on cancer cells are immunologically identical to fetal antigens—antigens found in that tissue normally but only in the fetal state. Such antigens are apparently expressed as a result of the reactivation of genes turned off at the end of fetal development. Unfortunately, although the existence of tumor-specific antigens has been demonstrated in many cell-culture and animal-tumor models, the evidence for tumor-*specific* antigens in human tumors is very weak. Most human tumors do, however, exhibit tumor-*associated* antigens, antigens that normally appear only during embryologic development or that appear in lesser amounts in normal cells.

The fact that cell surface protein changes are detectable immunologically has tremendous practical significance, even though we may not have the slightest idea what the antigenic substance actually *does* on the cell surface. Examples of the uses of immunologic properties of tumors in detection, diagnosis, and treatment of cancer are discussed at length in other chapters.

Altered Permeability and Membrane Transport

Materials are transported at generally higher rates across the membranes of transformed cells. Materials that show enhanced uptake include glucose, other sugars, and certain amino acids. It has been shown that the basis of increased transport of glucose is a rapid increase in the production of a glucose transporter protein following transformation.[21,22] Enhanced transport is consistent with the greater metabolic demand for certain raw materials characteristic of cancer cells and parallels a similar change seen in normal cells undergoing cell division. Increased transport of sugars and amino acids is probably not a *primary* change *responsible* for the malignant state; it is more likely that whatever triggers malignant behavior ultimately also increases transport. Still, the fact that cancer cells are different with respect to transport is important. Perhaps ways could be developed to retard selectively transport across cancer cell membranes and thereby help control the expression of malignancy.

Altered Secretion: Export

Another dimension of transport is *export*. Export is abnormal in cancer cells. Although this fact may reflect changes or problems with many aspects of the cell, including the integrity of the membrane, it most often is the result of (1) the excess production of *normal* secretions or (2) the "inappropriate" secretion that results from the "inappropriate" activation of normally turned-off genes. See Chapter 26 for a discussion of abnormal secretions from the viewpoint of their *general* effects on the host. Of direct relevance to the present discussion is the fact that "proteases" are among the things abnormally exported.

Altered Cell-to-Cell Junctions

Cells make connections with one another that are far more elaborate than simple contact. Among the discrete types of junctions (anatomically distinct kinds of points of contact) between cells are (1) tight junctions, junctions that appear to function as seals between cells and that appear to be derived from the fusing of parts of the plasma membranes belonging to adjacent epithelial cells; (2) desmosomes, junctions that appear to function as structural anchoring points possibly serving in tissue organization; and (3) gap junctions, which are actually channels between adjacent cells, through which cells may exchange chemical substances.

Junctions appear to be deranged in at least some cancer cells. Decreases in the number of desmosomes have been reported in cervical carcinoma as well as in tumors of breast, skin, and liver. If failure to form organizational and communicative junctions proves to be generally true of cancer cells, this may be part of the general reason why cancer cells characteristically do not communicate or otherwise relate to one another very well.

Changes in Surface Charge

If transformed cells are placed in an electric field, they tend to be drawn toward the positive pole. Although this is also true of normal cells, transformed cells move faster (Figure 3-8), indicating that cancer cells are more negatively charged than their normal counterparts. This enhanced negative-charge density has been linked to phospholipid and nucleic acid changes but mostly to glycoprotein changes. Negative charges associated with transformation are nearly all reduced if the cell is treated with the enzyme neuraminidase, an enzyme that removes sialic acid residues from glycoprotein molecules.

Cell Membrane Summary

A number of changes in the cell membrane have been found to be associated with the transformed state. Changing cyclic nucleotide levels, membrane fluidity, surface receptors, protease activity, and the like are *all* good candidates as primary changes from which the rest of the malignant state may unfold. Yet it is not known how, or even *if*, all these changes are related to one another or to other features of the transformed cell in terms of cause and effect. In other words, we do not have a unifying concept that describes just how the cell membrane fits in

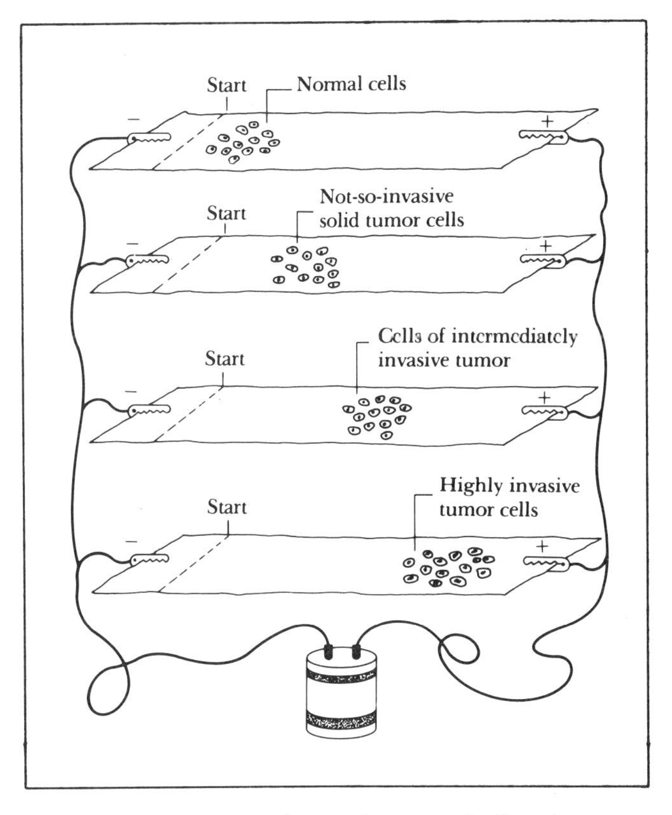

FIGURE 3-8 In one experiment, when normal cells and cancer cells were placed on an appropriate support strip in an electrical field, the more malignant cells moved most toward the positive pole, indicating greater electronegativity. (Source: Kupchella CE: Dimensions of Cancer. Belmont, Calif, Wadsworth, 1987. © 1987 by Wadsworth, Inc. Used by permission of publisher.)

the overall scheme of transformation and tumor cell behavior. The relationships among "oncogenes," cell membrane changes, and transformation (see Chapter 2) will continue to be a major focus of cancer research.

CYTOSKELETON ALTERATIONS IN CANCER CELLS

In cancer cells, microfilaments and microtubules are not well organized. They exist in pieces rather than in finished form. As indicated earlier, microfilaments and microtubules are important in maintaining the shapes of cells and in "setting" the character of the cell surface. Microfilaments and microtubules are also deranged in normal cells during division, and it is not known if this fact has any specific significance with respect to cancer.

CHANGES IN THE NUCLEUS AND IN THE REGULATION OF GENETIC MACHINERY

Among the changes often seen in cancer-cell machinery by which genetic plans are "translated and transcribed" into protein are the following:

1. Transfer RNA is different; it may have too many or too few methyl groups (CH_3) attached.

2. Some differences appear in proteins that regulate genes.

3. Differences appear in the enzymes involved in nucleic acid synthesis.

4. As previously pointed out, cancer cells often exhibit abnormal mitoses, and they have large nuclei with prominent nucleoli.

5. Almost all cancer cells seem to have unusual numbers of chromosomes but very few such abnormalities—such as the Philadelphia chromosome associated with leukemia (see Chapter 42)—appear to have any *consistent* relationship to cancer.

All these differences are potential influences of the expression of malignant state, but their actual significance is unknown.

It now appears that the most likely primary defects in malignant transformations involve normally quiescent, normal host-cell oncogenes activated in different ways by viruses and other carcinogenic agents. Some oncogenes prescribe products that activate certain enzymes—some of the same enzymes that are activated when cell-surface receptors bind to growth factors. Other oncogene products apparently mimic activated cell surface receptors, and others mimic growth factors; the products of still other oncogenes regulate the expression of other genes in the nucleus. What we know of oncogenes thus far seems to suggest that they all have something to do with one or more parts of a complex chain of molecular interactions involved in the control of cell division and suggests that transformation is something that can be induced in more than one way. Oncogenes and their products are considered fully in Chapter 2. In this chapter, let us consider some of the general things that have been discovered about regulator substances in cancer cells and some other possibilities that have been proposed.

Growth and Differentiation Inducers

Various gene-control factors have been described that *induce* transformation; other factors have been described that reverse or *inhibit* the expression of "transformedness." Perhaps such factors are balanced in normal cells, unbalanced in cancer.[23,24] Perhaps some cancer cells are unable to respond to growth-suppressor factors; perhaps others are chronically stimulated. It seems likely, in any case, that interrelated, on-off gene-regulating switches control both cell division *and* differentiation and that some *correct sequence of switching* brings the division of embryonic cells and other stem cells to a controlled end point. Anything that interferes with the normal cascade of gene–gene-product interaction leads to cancer—abnormal growth and differentiation.

Positive and negative regulatory elements that work only in certain types of cells have now been identified.[25] Transforming growth factor (TGF) beta, inhibits the growth of most cells but stimulates the growth of fibroblasts. In most cells it inhibits by shutting off genes. One group of researchers found that it somehow leads to the shutting off of the *myc* gene (which is known to be turned on by a variety of stimulatory factors); in fibroblasts, TGF beta somehow turns on the *sis* gene, a gene that encodes for a growth factor.[24] Other growth inhibiting agents include interferons and tumor necrosis factor.

Sachs[26] and others, using normal and leukemic blood cells (all of which are derived from the same multipotent stem cell in the bone marrow), have isolated and characterized both growth inducers *and* differentiation inducers and have found, among other things, that:

1. Growth inducers and differentiation inducers are different proteins; growth inducers cannot cause stem cell derivatives to mature; if anything, differentiation inducers *inhibit* growth.

2. The actions of growth inducers and differentiation inducers are coupled. *Different* growth inducers stimulate cells at different stages of differentiation to produce *different* inducers of differentiation at different times. The result? Variable *numbers* of different *types* of differentiated cells derived from the same stem cell type. Since terminally differentiated cells usually no longer divide, differentiation must ultimately neutralize *growth* inducers.

If growth inducers induce the production of differentiation inducers that bring an end to growth, this would amount to an orderly way of reaching a final, quiet, configuration of differentiated cells. Sachs[26] suggests that whereas normal cells depend on other cells for growth inducer, cancer cells either need little or no growth inducer, or they make their own. Cancer cells have also been found to have a defective coupling of growth and differentiation. Not only do the cancer cells not need growth inducer, but even when it is supplied artificially, growth inducer fails to stimulate the production of differentiation inducer. The result? Steadily dividing cells that are not differentiated. Instead of a quiet configuration—cancer.

As stated earlier, all this suggests that the normal processes of cell division and differentiation are driven and guided by a highly synchronized sequence of gene activation and gene suppression. Although the work of Sachs[26] and others suggests that sequences involved may be complex and will thus take some time to unravel, the potential payoff in terms of possible breakthroughs in cancer therapy is enormous. Imagine, for example, how exciting it would be to find differentiation inducers that cause cancer cells to differentiate and stop dividing.

Agents able to stimulate cancer cells to differentiate and to stop dividing have been identified and are now being tested clinically.[27] Some are chemotherapeutic agents that apparently have both cell-killing and differentiation-enhancing effects. Agents with differentiation effects on cancer cells include cytosine arabinoside (Ara C) (low doses), 6-thioguanine (low doses), hexamethylene bisacetamide (HMBA), and various hematopoietic growth factors.

Trigger Protein

There is a so-called restriction point, R, in the first (G-1) phase of the cycle. Once the restriction point is passed, the cell is irreversibly committed to another division. The cell will either divide or literally die trying. Although it is not known what determines whether a cell will go beyond this point—what triggers cell division, in other words—cancer researchers would clearly like to know because in cancer cells, something keeps the trigger pulled. Rossow et al[28] have hypothesized that cells must accumulate a certain amount of an unstable "trigger" protein (also called "U," for unstable, protein) to reach and pass the restriction point. Any condition or thing that would tend to reduce the rate of protein synthesis by cells—say, crowding or starvation—would tend to lengthen G-1 because it would take longer for "U" protein to accumulate. Unless protein synthesis proceeds faster than "U" protein breaks down, a cell could *never* reach R. Such a model would explain many experimental observations about cell division and its control. It has been suggested that if indeed there is a "trigger protein" operative in normal cells, perhaps cancer cells make it faster or make a more stable variety. Since we do not yet know if there is such a protein, we obviously do not know how it might trigger DNA synthesis, how it might be related to growth inducers, or how it otherwise sets the cell division cycle into motion.

Chalones

Skin, liver, kidney, and other tissues contain specific chemical substances able to arrest or retard the growth of cells in those specific tissues. These substances, called *chalones,* are believed to help account for the fact that organs such as the liver get just "so big" and then stop growing. Each normal liver cell theoretically produces some liver chalone. When the right number of liver cells is present, enough chalone is produced, collectively, to halt further growth of liver. If part of the liver is removed, the chalone level drops and liver cells start dividing and continue until the right number is present once again.

Could it be that cancer cells are deficient in their ability to make chalones or to respond to them? Maybe. Some cancer cells have in fact been found to contain greatly reduced chalone levels. It is not known how chalones might be related to the regulatory molecules described above.

ALTERED METABOLISM

Biochemists and biologists have long been intrigued by the possibility that some key metabolic differences could account for all the overt differences between cancer cells and normal cells. Maybe some metabolic pathway is speeded up. Maybe some metabolic regulator fails to regulate. Such possibilities have been explored since about 1920, and many biochemical-metabolic differences have been catalogued.

In 1930 Otto Warburg published a book on the metabolism of tumors in which he suggested that neoplasms may originate from normal cells because of a defect in their respiratory pathways for which they compensate by increased glycolysis. Normally, glycolysis is greatly suppressed in the presence of oxygen. This phenomenon is called the *Pasteur effect.* Warburg found that cancer cells engage in anaerobic glycolysis and in a concomitant, rapid use of glucose even in the presence of oxygen. Although it does seem to be generally true that cancer cells burn up sugar faster than their supposed normal counterparts, the "Warburg theory" has little standing today. For one thing, any rapidly growing tissue needs more glucose; increased glycolysis is most likely a *secondary* consequence of increased rates of cell division. Also, many kinds of neoplasms have since been found to have normal glycolytic rates, and many normal tissues have been found to have glycolytic rates that *exceed* those of tumors. Cancer cells apparently do *not* have a universal defect in their ability to "respire."

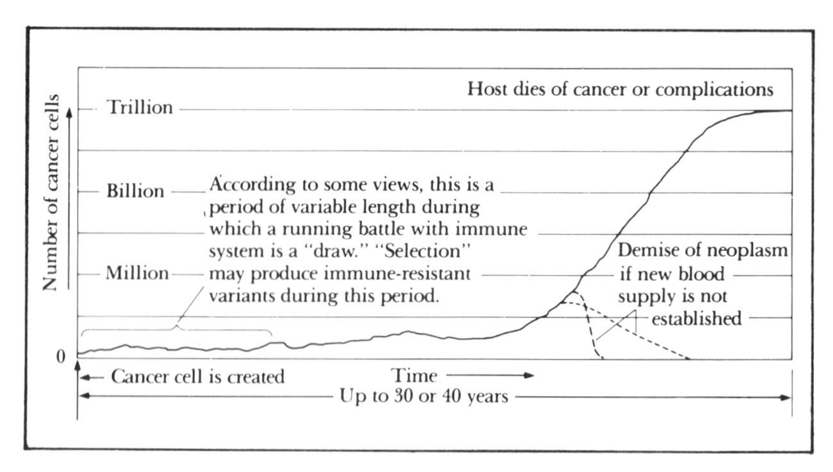

FIGURE 3-9 The generalized natural history of a neoplasm. (Source: Kupchella CE: Dimensions of Cancer. Belmont, Calif, Wadsworth, 1987. © 1987 by Wadsworth, Inc. Used by permission of publisher.)

Twenty-five years ago, Jesse Greenstein published *The Biochemistry of Cancer,* in which he proposed that all tumors seemed to share certain common enzymatic patterns—including some that had to do with respiration. This proposal also fell by the wayside as exceptions were catalogued.

Other attempts have been made to formulate similar "unifying" descriptions of cancer biochemistry, but none have stood up. When Harold Morris developed his series of transplantable liver tumor lines*—all derived from rat liver—it quickly became clear that tumor cells have widely different biochemical characteristics, even when the tumors come from the same organ of the same species.

Over the last few decades, Weber et al[29,30] took advantage of the fact that the Morris hepatomas spanned a wide range of growth rates and degrees of differentiation to see if there were any correlations between enzyme patterns and growth rate or differentiation. Although correlations have been found, certain pathways are enhanced and others diminished with increasing growth rate, and so forth, it is most likely that these are all *secondary* effects.[31] They happen because cells *are* dividing and are not likely the *cause* of uncontrolled division.

The bottom line? Cancer cells do generally have certain metabolic features in common—features they share with other rapidly dividing cells such as those found in embryos and fetuses. There is no evidence for any key metabolic change that accounts for the difference between normal cells and cancer cells.

*Morris ultimately developed dozens of transplantable hepatoma lines that came to be known as the *Morris hepatomas.* All the lines were induced by feeding rats carcinogens and then transplanting the resulting tumors from rat to rat over many transplant generations. Morris made the lines available worldwide to investigators interested in them because they exhibited a spectrum of growth rates ranging from fast to slow and a spectrum of degrees of differentiation. They enabled scientists to study the ramifications of metabolic and other features of malignancy in cells that otherwise came from the same organ of the same species.

TUMORIGENESIS

The term *tumorigenesis* refers to the development of a neoplasm after the initial carcinogenic event—after a cancer cell first appears. It is far more than simple cell division that carries the initial cancer to the large mass stage, where it may contain billions or even trillions of cancer cells.

The natural history of a typical tumor is depicted in Figure 3-9. It would be impossible for a few cancer cells to graduate to a large mass without lots of help. Cancer cells must be nourished and oxygenated just like any other living cells. If they simply divided, they would quickly outgrow their blood supply, and they would then wither and die. They flourish—temporarily, at least, because they are somehow able to induce the development of blood vessels and they somehow induce the development of supporting structures—connective tissue and intercellular cement.

As it grows, a neoplasm may wage a running war with the host's immune system, with the survivors possibly becoming increasingly resistant to the immune system. A neoplasm evolves—its more slowly dividing cells fall by the wayside, and the fast-growing cells "take over." In a "malignant progression," the tumor becomes increasingly hostile. In some cases, selective progression is actually accelerated by therapy. The most susceptible cancer cells are killed by initial treatment, leaving the more resistant cells to survive. At some point in the process of tumorigenesis, cells begin to invade adjacent tissues and ultimately break away to metastasize (see Chapter 4).

CONCLUSION

Many things happen to cells as they become cancer cells. Although a few of these changes may be the keys to all the others, no particular feature of malignant cells has yet been found to have such fundamental importance. Among the possible key expressions of "oncogenes" still under active consideration are protease secretion, decreased cAMP and increased cGMP, and altered cytoskeleton, altered glycoprotein, and altered glycolipids on the cell surface.

The quest continues. It is driven both by the desire to understand fully the basic biology of tumors and to identify differences that can be exploited in detection, diagnosis, and treatment of cancer—even before the biology is fully understood.

• • •

This chapter is an adaptation of Chapter 4 in the author's book *Dimensions of Cancer* published by Wadsworth, Belmont, Calif., 1987.

REFERENCES

1. Pitot HC: Fundamentals of Oncology. New York, Dekker, 1978.
2. Ruddon RW: Cancer Biology. New York, Oxford University Press, 1981.
3. Blau HM, Pavlath GK, Hardeman EC, et al: Plasticity of the differentiated state. Science 230:758-766, 1985.
4. Abercrombie M: The contact behavior of invading cells. In Cellular Membranes and Tumor-Cell Behavior. Baltimore, Williams & Wilkins, 1975, pp 21-37.
5. Moscona AA: Development of heterotypic combinations of dissociated embryonic chick cells. Proc Soc Expl Biol Med 92:410-416, 1956.
6. Coman DR: Decreased mutual adhesiveness, a property of cells from squamous cell carcinomas. Cancer Res 4:625-629, 1944.
7. Nicolson GL: Transmembrane control of the receptors in normal and tumor cells. II. Surface changes associated with transformation and malignancy. Biochim Biophys Acta 458:1-72, 1976.
8. Smets LA, Van Beek WP: Carbohydrates of the tumor cell surface. Biochim Biophys Acta 738:237-249, 1984.
9. Burger MM: Surface properties of neoplastic cells, in Weissman G, Claiborne R (eds): Cell Membranes. New York, Hospital Practice, 1975, pp 215-222.
10. Chen LB, Gallimore PH, and McDougall JK: Correlation between tumor induction and the large external transformation sensitive protein on the cell surface. Proc Natl Acad Sci 73:3570-3574, 1976 (abstr).
11. Curtis A, Pitts J (eds): Cell Adhesion and Motility. New York, Cambridge University Press, 1980.
12. Hynes RO: Surfaces of Normal and Malignant Cells. New York, Wiley, 1979.
13. Hynes RO: Fibronectins. Sci Am 254:42-51, 1986.
14. Nicolson GL, Poste G: The cancer cell: Dynamic aspects and modification in cell surface organization. N Engl J Med 295:197-203, 1976.
15. Nicolson GL, Poste G: The cancer cell: Dynamic aspects and modification in cell surface organization. II. N Engl J Med 295:253-257, 1976.
16. Pollack RE, Hough PVC: The cell surface and malignant transformation. Ann Rev Med 25:431-446, 1974.
17. Dennis JW, Laferte S, Waghorne C, et al: Beta 1-6 branching of Asn-linked oligosaccharides is directly associated with metastasis, Science 236:582-585, 1987.
18. Hakomori S: Glycosphingolipids. Sci Am 254:44-53, 1986.
19. Pastan IH, Johnson GS, Anderson WB: Role of cyclic nucleotides in growth control. Ann Rev Biochem 44:491-522, 1975.
20. Levitzki A: From epinepherine to cyclic AMP. Science 241:800-806, 1988.
21. Birnbaum MJ, Haspel HC, Rosen OM: Transformation of rat fibroblasts by FSV rapidly increases glucose transporter gene transcription. Science 235:1495-1497, 1987.
22. Flier JS, Mueckler MM, Usher P, et al: Elevated levels of glucose transport and transporter messenger RNA are induced by ras and src oncogenes. Science 235:1492-1495, 1987.
23. Marx JL: The yin and yang of cell growth control. Science 232:1093-1095, 1986.
24. Marx J: Cell growth control takes balance. Science 239:975-976, 1988.
25. Maniatis T, Goodbourn S, Fischer JA: Regulation of inducible and tissue-specific gene expression. Science 236:1237-1244, 1987.
26. Sachs L: Growth differentiation and the reversal of malignancy. Sci Am 254:40-47, 1986.
27. Marx J: Human trials of new cancer therapy begin. Science 236:778-779, 1987.
28. Rossow PW, Riddle VG, Pardee AB: Synthesis of labile, serum-dependent protein in early G_1 controls animal growth. Proc Natl Acad Sci USA 76:4446-4450, 1979.
29. Weber G: Molecular correlation concept: Ordered pattern of gene expression in neoplasia. GANN Monograph Cancer Res 13:47-77, 1972.
30. Weber G: Enzymology of cancer cells. I. N Engl J Med 296:486-492, 1977.
31. Weinhouse S: Metabolism and isozyme alterations in experimental hepatomas. Fed Proc 32:2162-2167, 1973.

Chapter 4

The Spread of Cancer: Invasion and Metastasis

Charles E. Kupchella, PhD

INTRODUCTION

In his book *Recherches du Cancer*, published in 1820, the French physician Joseph Claude Anselme Recamier (1774 to 1852) introduced the term *metastasis* to describe the *secondary* growth of cancer in the brain of a patient with breast cancer. This description carried the understanding of cancer a step beyond the earlier recognition of local invasion and the spread of cancer to regional lymph nodes. Medicine quickly came to recognize metastasis as the crux of the cancer problem.[1]

Were it not for metastasis, curing cancer would be a simple matter because surgery would almost always achieve cure. But metastasis spreads destruction to critical organs throughout the body, which makes cancer impossible to excise. Metastasis is clearly the worst feature of a disease that is sometimes simplistically described as "the uncontrolled division of cells." Thus one key to finding a cure is a better understanding of those factors that influence the detachment of cells from the primary tumor, their movement into the circulation, and their implantation in other locations. Researchers have some idea what these factors are,[2-12] but they are a long way from a complete understanding.

CANCER CELLS AND CELLS THAT ARE SIMILAR

Some normal cells of the human body can move about. In their role as scavengers and defenders, white blood cells (leukocytes) can leave blood vessels and "invade" tissue in response to infection, trauma, and other stimuli. Leukocytes thus share some key behavioral features with cancer cells, but there are some important differences. An especially important difference is that blood cells normally lose their ability to divide when they enter the general circulation. Cancer cells do *not* surrender this option.

Invasion and metastasis also resemble the behavior of the cells of normal embryos. Embryonic cells migrate, they invade, and they establish new growth where they come to rest. But embryonic cells differ from cancer cells in that *embryonic cells follow a genetic program that has a nonchaotic end point*—namely, the limited development of tissue having a functional interrelationship with all other tissues.

Still other examples of noncancer cells express metastatic behavior. Cells from the chorion (one of the membranes of the placenta) can be found in the lungs of pregnant women. Such cells nearly always die shortly after the birth of the fetus when the hormone environment changes—but then, certain types of cancer respond to hormonal changes in a similar fashion. Viable bone-marrow fat cells sometimes spread to distant sites after fractures. Another example is the spread of endometrial cells to various locations in the abdomen (endometriosis).

All the foregoing examples suggest that there may be something to learn about metastasis by studying normal cells. Perhaps all cells capable of exhibiting invasive or metastatic properties share some key chemical or surface structural features.

METASTATIC SEQUENCE

The metastatic sequence is illustrated in Figure 4-1.[13] Metastasis begins with *local invasion* and ends with secondary tumors at remote sites. Between these points are a number of discrete steps that include (1) *continuous extension* of the tumor along paths of least resistance, (2) *detachment* of cells or clumps of cells, (3) *dissemination* of cancer cells through lymphatics and blood vessels, (4) *arrest* of tumor cells at distant sites, and (5) *reinvasion* by the tumor cells, this time out of the circulation into tissues where the tumor cells secrete various factors that help create an environment conducive to the growth of the secondary tumor *(angiogenesis)*.

Local Invasion

Except for the amoeboid movement that enables lymphocytes and other cells of the immune system to move in and out of tissue spaces, the tissues of the human body are normally *not* freely permeable to the migration of cells. This leads to the question, what is it about the cancer cell and its cell surface that enables it to invade?

Research has revealed at least five factors possibly important in enabling invasiveness: (1) pressure buildup resulting from the expanding mass (producing mechanical forces that figuratively "inject" cancer cells into tissue), (2) production of toxins or enzymes that, respectively, damage and digest adjacent tissues, allowing cancer to extend, (3) phagocytic properties (cancer cells may eat their way out), (4) cell motility (cancer cell motility is relatively uninhibited by contact), and (5) loss of cellular adhesiveness (changes in cell properties such as adhesiveness could make cancer cells "slippery"). It may be that all these factors are important in invasion by cancer cells.

Pressure and fracture lines

Perhaps the first thing that the crablike extension of cancer into normal tissue suggests is that the extension is a result of the buildup of pressure. Uncontrolled division would certainly produce rather densely packed, expanding masses of cells that must certainly exert pressure on adjacent tissues. Indeed, tumors do seem to extend into normal tissue along "natural fracture lines"—into spaces that could be expected by an architect to "part" in response to pressure.[7]

Further support for this concept is that expanding tumors often seem to be stopped by "capsules"; that is, by architectural barriers to fracture. Kidney capsules, for ex-

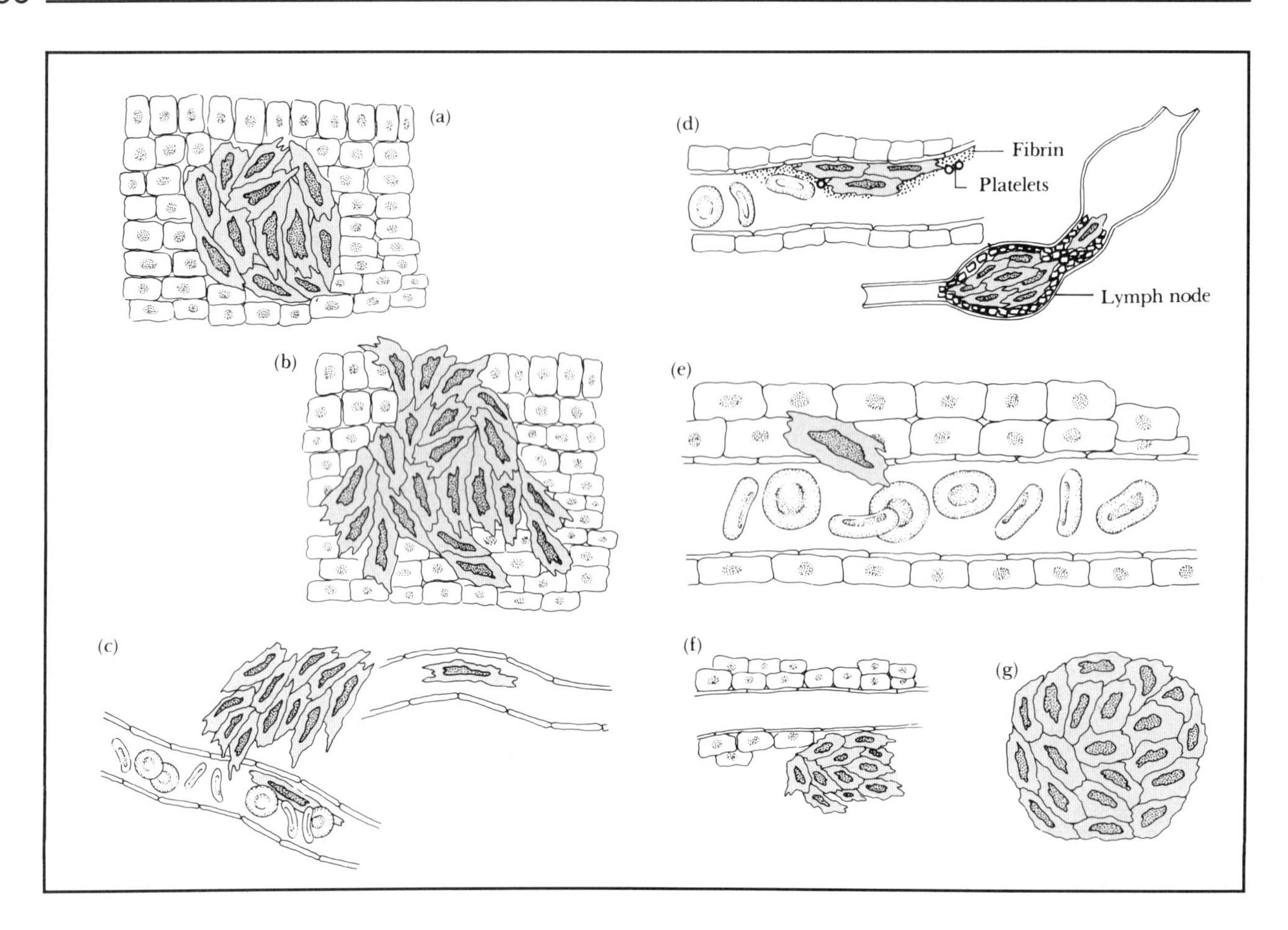

FIGURE 4-1 The metastatic sequence. The metastatic cascade occurs in a series of stages. The entire sequence is shown here, including (a) the establishment and growth of the primary tumor, (b) the invasion of adjacent tissue and body cavities, (c) continuous extension into vascular and lymphatic channels and dissemination through the bloodstream or the lymphatics, (d) the arrest of tumor cells and clumps of cells in lymph nodes or on the vascular epithelium, (e) the penetration of vascular walls (extravasation) by the tumor cells (reinvasion), (f) early proliferation of metastatic cells and the establishment of a blood supply (angiogenesis), and (g) the growth of the secondary tumor into a discernible mass. Cells can also escape from the secondary mass, and the entire process can be repeated, giving rise to tertiary neoplasms. (Source: Kupchella CE: Dimensions of Cancer. Belmont, Calif, Wadsworth, 1987. © 1987 by Wadsworth, Inc. Used by permission of publisher.)

ample, seem to be able to contain tumors and to limit or at least redirect their extension.

Pressure spreading is an attractive hypothesis. However, apparently it does not tell the whole story. Cancers in experimental systems in which pressure is *known* to be *non*existent still exhibit invasiveness, clearly indicating that pressure is not the *only* factor involved.

Enzymes and spreading factors

Do cancer cells digest their way through normal tissues by secreting enzymes? At one time it was a popular notion that certain kinds of bacteria had the ability to secrete hyaluronidase, an enyzme that digests intercellular "cement." Hyaluronidase came to be called "spreading factor" and was believed to play a role in the invasion of normal tissues by bacterial cells. In time, this concept fell out of favor. Very little positive correlation was found between invasiveness and whether a particular bacterial species could synthesize and secrete hyaluronidase. All this research nevertheless suggested the possibility that tumor invasion may be aided by enzyme secretion.[13]

Many types of malignant neoplasms have been found to shed enzymes capable of altering ground substance. Nakajima et al[15] reported that the more highly invasive and metastatic sublines of a spectrum of B16 melanoma lines had more of the enzymes that are able to digest the glycosaminoglycans of the extracellular matrix, suggesting that cancer cells may slip into and out of the circulation by digesting the cement between cells.

The picture is still not clear. Some highly invasive tumors have negligible degradative enzyme capacities, while some relatively noninvasive tumors have been found to have *high* degradative enzyme activities. Recent evidence does show, however, that there is a fairly good correlation between invasiveness and the secretion of plasminogen activator (a protease activator). The strongest statement that can be made in summary is that enzymes probably facilitate invasion in some if not all neoplasms.[6]

Do cancer cells kill their way out?

Another possible mechanism of invasion is that cancer cells kill their way through adjacent normal tissue. Cancer cells *do* have the ability to kill normal cells; however, this effect is thought to be a result of competition for nutrients or disruption of blood supplies. There has been no definitive demonstration that cancer cells produce poisons that serve as a principal mechanism of invasion.

Migration as a factor

As described in the preceding chapter, experiments have shown that cancer cells do *not* exhibit the same degree of contact inhibition of migration seen in normal cells. This suggests, of course, that cancer cells may actually move under their own power into adjacent tissues. The migration of transformed animal cells grown in tissue cultures *into* and over other cells further suggests that such a mechanism would be operative even in the absence of "pressure buildup."

A number of investigators have suggested that there may actually be chemical stimulants to invasive migration. It has been proposed, for example, that tumor cells tend to move according to acid-base gradients; that is, they move from high or low acidity to zones of relative neutrality. Easty and Easty[7] describe a possible "chemotactic" influence (based on data presented by Koono et al[16]) suggesting that cancer cells may secrete a substance that causes cells and tissues in remote locations to secrete a *second* chemical that serves as a "beacon" for the migrating cancer cell. Liotta et al[6] claim to have isolated an autocrine motility factor—a factor secreted by tumor cells that binds to surface receptors, causing more than a 100-fold increase in cell movement.

Slippery cells

Many of the changes that take place in cancer cell surfaces could well contribute to invasion. Cancer cells do not adhere to one another or to various substrates as well as normal cells. Perhaps this trait helps them "slip" between normal cells in the process of invasion.

• • •

In summary, a number of factors contribute to invasiveness in cancer. Research to date, rather than having provided definitive answers, seems simply to have identified a number of possibilities, all of which still seem viable to some degree.

Continuous Extension

The first consequence of invasion could be called "continuous extension." The primary and anatomic *routes* of local extension of cancer are (1) tissue spaces, (2) lymph vessels, (3) blood vessels, (4) coelomic cavities, (5) cerebrospinal spaces, and (6) epithelial cavities. Neoplasms may extend into any one of these areas, without loss of overall continuity; that is, without breaking away from the parent mass. Willis stressed that *venous channels* appear to be involved in at least *half of all fatal cancers.*[17]

Detachment

Once the extension of a tumor carries it into a body cavity or a blood or lymphatic vessel, cells break away from the main mass rather regularly. Although single cells can break away from tumor masses, cancer cells are much more likely to break away as emboli or *clusters* of cells. Experimental observation has indicated that for every gram of adenocarcinoma in a rat, as many as a million cells or cell clumps were released into the blood in a 24-hour period.[18] Most of these cells perish, but it does not take many survivors to cause problems.

Metastasis by contact?

It has been suggested that cancer might be transplanted by contact between a neoplasm and an "opposite" area; for example, from one lip to another. Metastasis by contact implantation appears that it might occur in tumors of the urinary tract and perhaps the lung. However, what *appears* to be spread by contact may actually be the simultaneous development of independent tumors spread through blood or lymph channels.

Gravitational dissemination within body cavities

Neoplasms frequently extend into and invade body cavities such as nasal and pharyngeal cavities, the uterus, the bladder, and the bronchi of the lung until the cavities are literally filled up with cancer. During the spread of cancer over the serous membranes of larger body cavities such as the pleural and peritoneal cavities, cancer cells sometimes break away and gravitate to the lower reaches of such cavities. Gravity, therefore, can be a casual factor in metastasis.

Dissemination: The Transport of Cancer Cells to Distant Sites

Transport through lymphatic vessels

For many types of cancer, the very first evidence of disseminated disease presents itself as a mass in the lymph nodes that drain the area or region of the body carrying the primary tumor. Usually these secondary tumors come from emboli carried to the lymph nodes by the *down*stream flow of lymph. Occasionally, upstream lymph nodes become infiltrated by metastatic cancer. This exception is thought to be a result of blockage or the reversal of lymphatic flow, allowing cancer cells to migrate upstream.

Involvement of lymph nodes can be very rapid or very slow, depending on the neoplasm. In some animal tumor models, regional lymph node metastasis can be demonstrated a few days after implantation of a transplantable tumor. *In humans, lymph node involvement is found in about half of all fatal cancers.* The readiness with which cancer spreads to lymph nodes varies considerably from one human cancer to another.

The variability of lymph node involvement in cancer

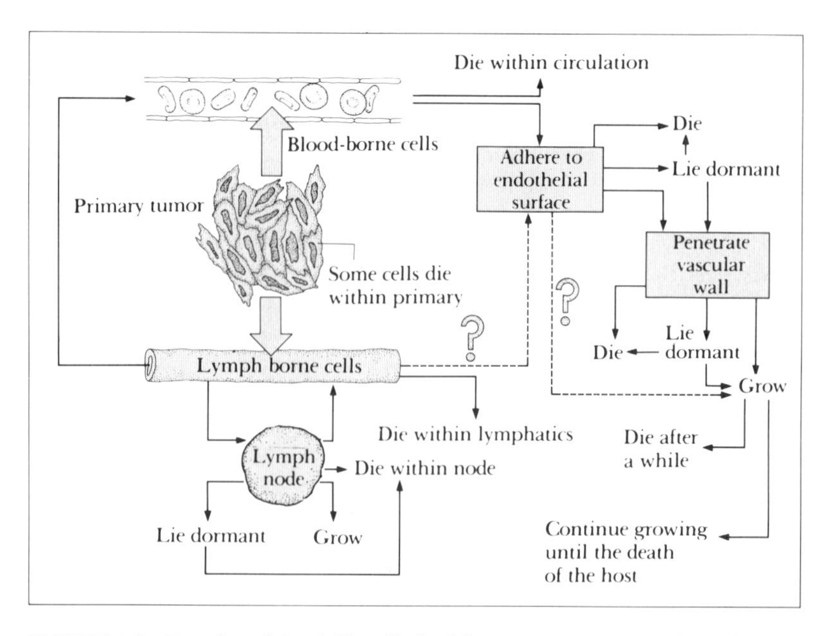

FIGURE 4-2 Very few of the viable cells shed from a tumor mass survive to become established as a metastasis. Illustrated here are some of the many possible fates of shed tumor cells. (Source: Kupchella CE: Dimensions of Cancer. Belmont, Calif, Wadsworth, 1987. © 1987 by Wadsworth, Inc. Used by permission of publisher.)

is at least partly a result of the fact that many things can happen to the cancer cells that become lodged in lymph nodes. They may die as a result of a local inflammatory reaction; they may die because of lack of the proper environment; they can grow into a discernible lump; or they can remain dormant for reasons unknown (Figure 4-2).

It was once thought that the filtering action of the lymph nodes was responsible for nodal metastasis, but experimental investigation has revealed that filtration is a relatively minor factor, and perhaps some part of the physiochemical cell surface and lymph node interaction is also important in whether cancer cells become lodged in lymph nodes.

An important feature of the lymphatic system is that the main lymphatic trunk enters the venous system just before the veins enter the heart. Thus, the lymphatic and blood vessel systems of the body are interconnected, and cancer cells that reach the lymphatics are able to get into the blood stream as well. Lymphatic drainage channels appear to be a common route by which tumors spread locally and regionally, perhaps reflecting a favorable environment for the survival of cancer cells in the lymphatic vessels.

Transport through the bloodstream

Although some cancer cells that get into blood are believed to get there through the lymphatics, it is generally believed that the more aggressive cancer cells that reach the bloodstream get there through direct invasion of capillaries and veins. Although the local spread of cancer may well occur predominantly through the lymphatic vessels, metastatic spread to remote organs and tissues is almost invariably the result of cells being transmitted through the bloodstream.[17]

The mechanism by which cancer cells enter the bloodstream is not known. Apparently, arteries are only rarely invaded by cancer cells. It has been suggested that this resistance to invasion may be a result of high pressures, enzyme inhibitors (such as collagenase inhibitors) found in arterial walls, or the relative impermeability of the artery vessel wall. However, cancer cells do enter capillaries and veins.

What happens to cancer cells once they get into the bloodstream? In the blood, aggregates of cancer cells interact with one another, with platelets, with various soluble substances in the bloodstream, and with elements of the immune system. This interaction gives metastatic cells additional complex characteristics, some of which are possibly important in the eventual arrest and establishment of metastatic tumor masses.

Because only a very small fraction of the cancer cells that "leave home" through the bloodstream—or in any other way—become successful colonists of distant places, the mere presence of cancer cells in the bloodstream does not in itself constitute a metastasis. The circulatory system is really a very hostile environment. We tend to think of it as being otherwise because of the system's role in nurturing the cells of our tissues. But although it is good to have the circulation pass nearby, to be inside the circulatory system is a different matter.

Arrest of Tumor Cells

If a metastatic cancer cell or a cluster of cells adrift in the circulatory system is to become established as a metastatic tumor, it must first come to rest. This fact raises some important questions: Why would a cell having invaded its way out of tissue, and having become detached from the parent tumor, stop somewhere and "crawl back into" normal tissue? What could possibly stop a cell that obviously has a tendency to "slip away"? Such a cell might be expected to spend the remainder of its life as an aimless drifter in the bloodstream.

A number of factors have been found in identifying those qualities of cells and hosts that determine when and how cancer cells arrest and attach to surfaces of blood vessels to develop a metastasis. The four main factors involved are (1) *blood flow mechanics*, (2) *blood coagulation factors*, (3) *immune system factors*, and (4) unknown features of host tissue and of the cancer cells themselves.

Hemodynamic and mechanical factors

One popular notion about tumor cells is that they become lodged in places where large total cross-sectional area capillary beds (lung, brain, etc.) cause them to stall or slow down or where they become lodged because they are too large to pass through. Morphologic aspects of the arrest and attachment of tumor cells leading to the establishment of metastasis were reviewed by Chew et al.[19] Although the mechanical trapping of tumor cells is both a simple and appealing idea, it does not seem to tell the whole story. Tarin[20] cited a number of studies indicating that tumor fragments *do not necessarily* come to rest in the *first* capillary bed they enter. It has also been shown that cancer cells can "squeeze" through capillaries that "look" too small.

The major evidence against a simple trapping concept is that metastatic cancers simply do *not* faithfully exhibit distributions that support it.

Blood-clotting factors

Chew et al[19] present a picture of cancer cells, having once entered the bloodstream, becoming associated with both cellular and humoral constituents of blood. Platelets and fibrin may be the most important of these constituents. In studies with the Walker 256 rat tumor model, Chew et al found the following: (1) *platelets* were seen in almost every case in association with tumor cells attached to the vascular epithelium, (2) fibrin was present in the complex of platelets and tumor cells at the site of arrest, (3) as the fibrin-platelet complex disintegrated, the tumor cells remained attached to the blood vessel wall and then passed through the vascular wall by *destroying* cells of the vascular epithelium (rather than passing between cells).

Another observation in support of a role for platelets and fibrin in tumor cell arrest is that anticoagulants have been shown to *reduce* the frequency of metastasis.[21] Heparin has been implicated as an antimetastatic agent. Tsubura et al[22] also presented data illustrating that xylan sulfate, a sulfated polysaccharide, was able to inhibit metastasis. They postulated that this compound worked by inhibiting some step in the coagulation cascade. Unfortunately, some conflicting results have been found,[21,22] and the overall effects of anticoagulants on tumor cell arrest are unclear. The consensus in the literature seems to be that too little is known at the moment to even begin considering manipulating anticoagulation-coagulation forces to treat or control metastatic cancer.

The laminin connection

Laminin, a basement membrane glycoprotein, may be involved at several points in the metastatic cascade but particularly at the point of arrest. Interaction between tumor cells and the extracellular matrices of metastatic target organs is obviously important in the metastatic cascade. Forms of interaction would include both initial attachment and degradation of the target organ extracellular matrix. Since these interactions are obvious target points for possible interference with metastasis, it is not surprising that a fair amount of work is being done to try to understand the interactions better. Laminin has been shown to increase both invasive and metastatic activity, and a pentapeptide portion of one of the laminin chains was shown to reduce lung colony formation, possibly by competing with would-be metastatic cells for laminin-binding sites.[23] Another possible connection is that the specificity of metastasis to particular organs (see below) could be related at least in part to relationships between particular tumor cells and particular extracellular matrices.[4,24] In some experimental systems, fibronectin appears to be able to block interaction between laminin receptors on metastatic cells and laminin.[4,6,24]

• • •

In summary, *arrest* of tumor cells—as with all other aspects of metastatic dissemination—is a result of interaction between (1) the properties inherent in the cancer cells themselves and (2) factors and modifiers present in each host.

Why do metastatic deposits occur where they occur?

Experience with human tumors clearly indicates that particular kinds of tumors tend to metastasize to particular places. Breast tumors tend to metastasize to the brain and to the lungs, lung tumors tend to metastasize to the brain, and prostatic cancer tends to spread to bone. The tendency for certain types of cancers to metastasize to certain sites, particularly the lymph nodes, bones, lung, and liver, is documented in Table 4-1.[25] These data and others suggest that metastatic dissemination of cancer is far from random, raising the question "Why do these patterns exist?"

There are related intriguing questions. Why is it, for instance, that metastasis rarely occurs in the spleen? Or in the thymus? Why is it common for carcinomas to metastasize to lymph nodes, while sarcomas rarely do? Why are metastases only rarely seen in skeletal muscle or skin? Are vascular pressures and blood flow rates too high in muscle and skin to allow cancer cells to come to rest there? Or are other factors at work? And why do some patients show completely nontypical distributions of metastatic disease?[20]

Answers offered for these kinds of questions over the years have all revolved around mechanical factors: (1) tumors cannot become established in certain places because flow rates are too high and tumor cells cannot stop long enough to become attached and (2) cancer cells become lodged in capillary beds because blood flow rates are slow in capillaries and the passageways are small enough to trap

TABLE 4-1 Patterns of Metastases. Sites of Metastasis in 1000 Consecutive Autopsied Cases and in More than 100 Cases Each of Breast, Lung, and Colon Cancer

Site of Metastatic Involvement	In 1000 Consecutive Autopsies (%)	In 167 Cases of Primary Breast Cancer (%)	In 160 Cases of Primary Lung Cancer (%)	In 118 Cases of Primary Colon Cancer (%)
Abdominal nodes	50	44	29	59
Liver	49	61	40	65
Lungs	47	77	47	37
Mediastinal nodes	42	67	83	14
Pleura	28	65	28	14
Bone	27	73	33	9
Adrenal	27	54	36	14
Gastrointestinal tract	27	15	11	27
Diaphragm	20	25	16	11
Brain (cerebral)	18	9	43	—

Source: Bodansky O: Biochemical criteria of metastatic growth in human cancer, in Day SB, Meyers WPL, Stansley P, et al. (eds): Cancer Invasion and Metastasis: Biochemical Mechanisms and Therapy, New York, Raven Press, 1977, p 201.

cancer cells. But there are apparently some other possibilities. First, a "seed and soil" hypothesis suggests that certain tissues and organs have special characteristics that enable cancer cells to flourish. A corollary is that cells that travel to other sites and become lodged there never appear as metastases. A second hypothesis involves the receptors or recognition signals on the surface of cancer cells, causing them to associate with cells of particular organs and tissues (Figure 4-3).[26] A more recent hypothesis is that only in certain locations can metastatic cancer cells elicit the production (by surrounding cells) of growth factor(s) needed to support cancer cell-division.

Nicolson[27] has shown that metastatic patterns do not really correlate all that well with patterns of blood flow and the locations of capillary beds. Fidler and Nicolson[28] found that even after injecting B16 melanoma cells into the *left* ventricle of the mouse heart, in effect requiring that the cells pass through capillary beds *other than those in the lung first*, there was *still* preferential metastasis to lung. Similarly, Sugarbaker[29] showed (using another model system) that cells injected into the left side of the heart did not develop metastasis in all peripheral organs. Clearly, capillaries do not *necessarily* stop all cancer cells.

Kinsey[30] showed that if portions of normal lung were transplanted to various nonlung locations in an animal body, lung-seeking melanoma cells established metastasis in association with lung *and* the transplanted piece of lung but not anywhere else in the body. Control grafts using other organs ruled out the possibility that surgical disturbance itself had anything to do with metastatic deposits. And, since a transplanted piece of lung would be physiologically quite different in many ways from the normal lung, this experiment suggests that something about particular cancer cells causes them to bind to certain types of tissue. In other words, this finding seems to favor the "adhesive-specificity" explanation as opposed to patterns of blood flow or the "congeniality of soil."

Several experiments[28,31] have demonstrated that neoplasms are not homogeneous with respect to metastatic potential. By isolating single cells from a B16 mouse melanoma line, allowing these to grow, and then characterizing them by their metastatic potential, Fidler[31] found that the isolates had different tendencies to metastasize and that the tendencies were genetically faithful.

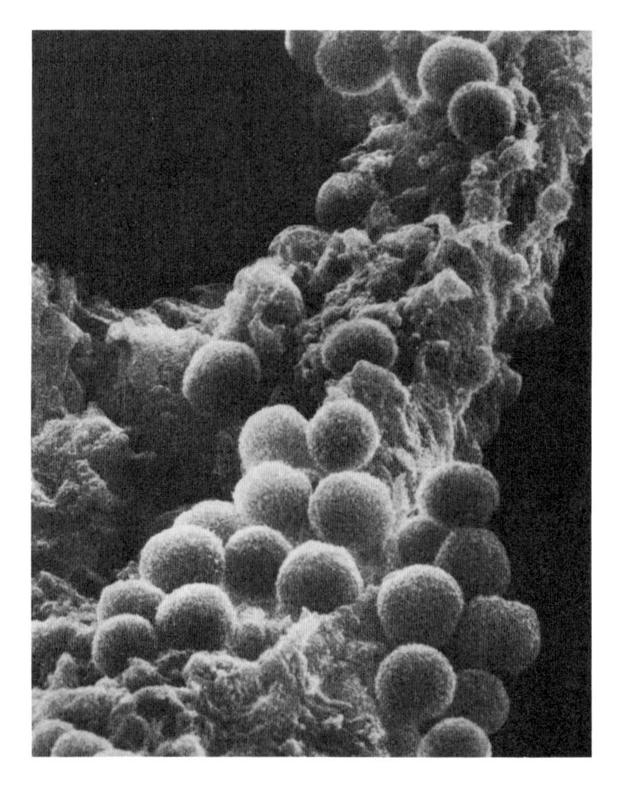

FIGURE 4-3 Scanning electron micrograph of mouse B16-F10 melanoma cells binding to mouse lung tissue (×8800). Even outside of mice, these metastatic tumor cells adhere preferentially to the tissue they colonize in a living mouse (see Netland and Zetter[26]). (Source: Netland PA, Zetter BR: Organ-specific adhesion of metastatic cells in vitro. Science 224:1113-1114, 1984. Copyright 1984 by the AAAS.)

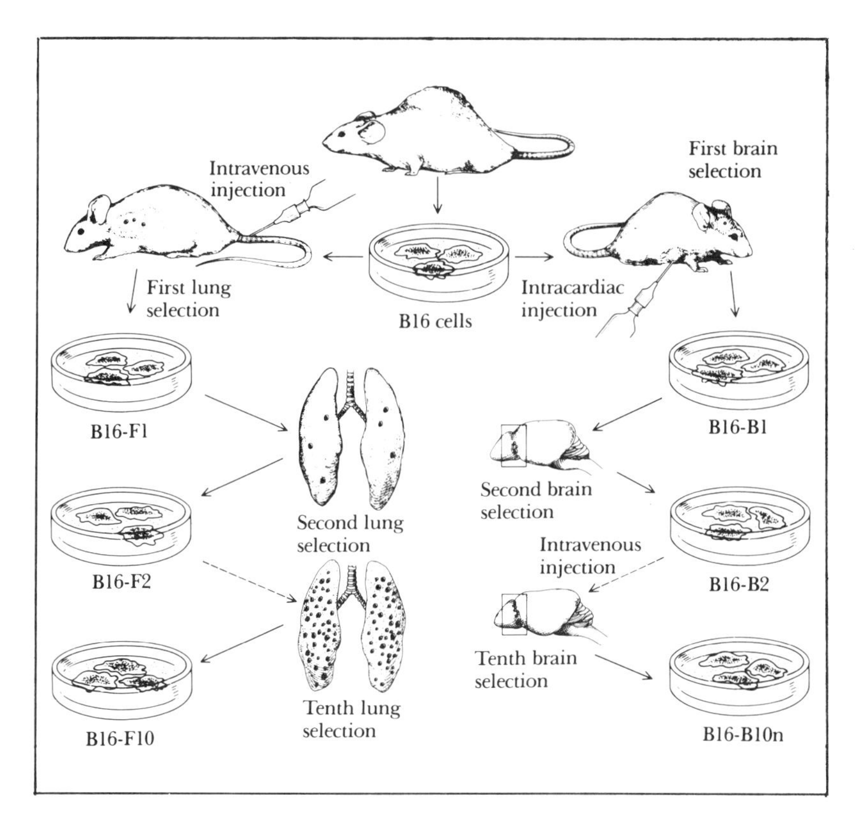

FIGURE 4-4 Selection of melanoma cell lines with enhanced ability to metastasize to lung (left) and to a particular part of the brain (right). The selections were accomplished by repeatedly isolating tumor cells from the target organ, culturing them, and then injecting them into the tail veins of other mice. Highly lung–selective B16-F10 cells were produced by ten such cycles. Similarly, ten "selections" resulted in a B16-B10n cell line highly selective of rhinal fissure of the brain. (Source: Adapted from Nicolson GL: Cancer metastasis. Sci Am 240:66, 1979, p 71. Used by permission of WH Freeman and Company.)

Fidler and Nicolson[28] were able to select sublines of B16 melanoma cells that preferred lung almost exclusively, and thus they concluded that metastatic localization is *genetically* determined. A primary tumor is an aggregation of genetically *dis*similar cells having phenotypic shades of variation, including different metastatic preference.* The metastatic potential of individual cells in a primary tumor is apparently quite variable, and genetic selection can establish lines from an individual tumor with high degrees of selectivity and efficiency of metastasis to particular organs (Figure 4-4).[33]

Lung-seeking lines do not become lung-seeking lines because they become adapted to lung by spending a lot of time there. If a line is grown in lung (or brain), excised, and then reimplanted in the same organ ten times, the tendency to colonize that organ (when injected into the circulation) does not change. Apparently cells with particular metastatic preferences are present from the first.

The experiments just described notwithstanding, it seems likely that the "congeniality of soil" is also an important factor in metastatic distribution. In one experiment, Fidler and Nicolson[27] radioactively labeled lung-preferring B16 melanoma cells and then injected these in different sites in mice. After a few hours, the B16 melanoma cells were found in *many* types of organs and tissues but mostly in the lung (Table 4-2). After 2 weeks, however, viable labeled cells were found only in the lung.[34]

The implication of all these findings is that the distribution of metastatic cancers is governed to some degree by factors other than circulation. The data also clearly suggest that the "congeniality of soil" hypothesis has some validity and that the adhesive-specificity hypothesis also has something to it. The data in Table 4-2 suggest that these factors may even somehow be related—that cancer cells may preferentially stop where they are more likely to survive.

There appear, experimentally at least, to be multiple bases for the specificity of metastases. These include (1) differential tumor cell adhesion to the microvessel endothelial cells of particular organs or to the organ's parenchymal cells,[26] (2) specificity of invasion of basement membranes and organ tissues, and (3) differential responses to organ-derived growth-stimulatory and inhibitory factors.[35] Nicolson[35] suggests that each tumor-host system may "achieve" organ specificity through these multiple properties and through the suitability of the "soil" offered by a particular organ. It should be noted that as a general rule, as malignancy progresses, relative organ

*Fidler and Hart[32] say that this diversity may arise either by virtue of the multicellular origin of the primary tumor *or* by the "evolution" of diversity as a neoplasm develops from a single cell.

TABLE 4-2 Distribution of 200,000 Viable Radioactively Labeled B16 Melanoma Cells Injected Intravenously into Normal C57B1/6 Mice

Time of Death After Injection	Number of Viable Tumor Cells			
	Lung	Liver	Blood†	Urine‡
1 minute	136,000	2,200	3,750	—
5 minutes	105,700	7,600	2,200	—
10 minutes	130,500	9,350	2,600	100
1 hour	108,000	3,500	3,800	10,000
12 hours	5,500	700	1,050	10,500
1 day	1,700	600	580	1,700
3 days	450	200	40	0
14 days	400	0	0	0

*These data suggest that metastatic deposition may have a considerably dynamic nature in the early stages. The data also illustrate the "harshness" of the various environments into which metastatic cells travel.

†Per 1.0 ml blood.

‡Urinary bladder and contained urine.

Source: Fidler IJ: Patterns of tumor cell arrest and development, in Weiss L (ed): Fundamental Aspects of Metastasis. New York, American Elsevier, 1976, p 278.

specificity gives rise to more of a multisite tendency, probably because of increasing heterogeneity.

Reinvasion

The next critical phase in the metastatic cascade is the phase between the point at which the cancer cell becomes attached to the wall of the vessel and the point at which it becomes established as a secondary tumor on the other side of the blood vessel wall.

Although some metastatic deposits may originate from cells that block a capillary, shut off blood flow, and begin to proliferate in place (and after a while, changes induced in and around the growing deposit may erase all evidence that the deposit originated in a capillary), the weight of experimental observation indicates that tumor cells most commonly must migrate out (Figure 4-5) of the vasculature before they can establish a thriving "colony."

Of the cancer cells that merely come to rest and attach to blood vessel surfaces, *most never become clinically manifest metastatic deposits.* Perhaps some are unable to get through the blood vessels, and perhaps many of these that do are unable to establish a blood supply fast enough and die because of the lack of oxygen or the buildup of toxic byproducts of metabolism. The trick, then, is to get through the blood vessel and establish supply lines quickly. The mechanism by which cancer cells move off the vascular highway back into the tissues is unknown. It seems likely that some form of *diapedesis*—the mode of invasion of white blood cells—is involved.[33] The ability to slip through capillary vessel linings into tissue would require that cancer cells be highly deformable, and we have already mentioned they are sufficiently deformable to pass through capillaries smaller than they are.

Sato and Suzuki[36] have studied various strains of transplantable ascites tumors in the rat and have developed a way to measure deformability of tumor cells by recording the pressure required to "suck" a hemispheric bulge in cells (using a micropipette). They have compared metastatic potential and deformability and concluded that deformability of tumor cells is a "potentially important" factor in metastasis.

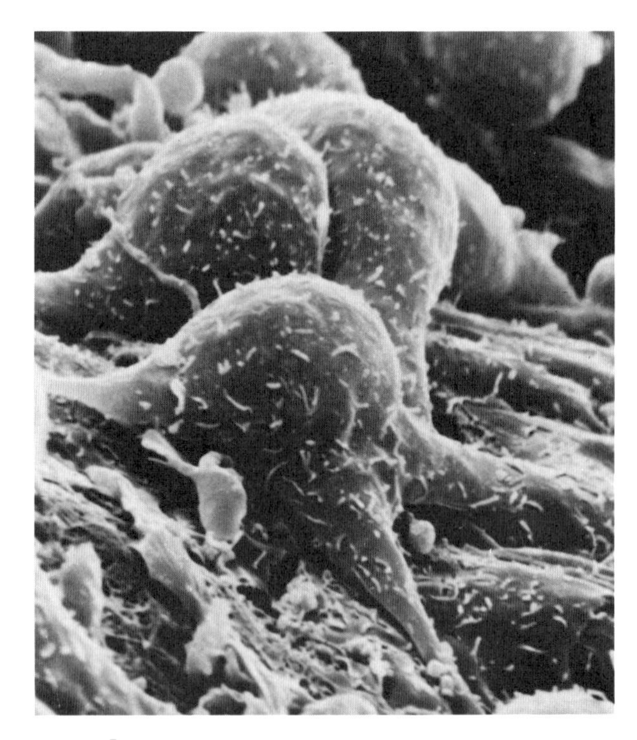

FIGURE 4-5 Scanning electron micrograph of metastatic melanoma cells invading the wall of a blood vessel (×2200). (Photograph courtesy Dr. Garth L. Nicolson, University of Texas, M.D. Anderson Hospital and Tumor Institute at Houston.)

Another possibility is that cancer cells destroy the cells that form capillary walls. Chew et al[19] observed that in the Walker 256 rat tumor line, tumor cells passed through the vascular wall after attachment, by destroying cells of the vascular epithelium.

Establishing a Beachhead: Angiogenesis

A cancer cell leaving the bloodstream and invading local tissue is not unlike an advancing army outdistancing its supply lines. Such a military maneuver can be accomplished only by developing ways to live off the territory being invaded. Apparently, metastatic cancer cells come equipped to do just that. Or perhaps it would be more accurate to say that cells that come so equipped are the ones able to develop full-blown metastatic tumors.

Once cancer cells reinvade remote tissue, a number of things can happen. They may die, they may lie dormant for many years and then grow to a large size even well after the primary tumor has been removed, or they may immediately begin to grow to a larger size.

According to Folkman and Tyler,[37] metastatic tumors cannot grow more than a few millimeters in diameter or achieve population densities of more than a million cells or so without having new blood vessels established to sustain them.

A number of studies have revealed that malignant tumors do not form their own blood vessels; they cause the host to make blood vessels for them[37-39] through a chemical substance called *angiogenesis factor* or *tumor angiogenesis factor* (TAF).[40-44]

Folkman and Tyler[37] have presented some dramatic and interesting evidence that tumors are able to induce the formation of blood vessels and that this ability is more highly developed in cancer cells than in embryologic cells. Their experiments were based on inducing blood vessel growth into the cornea of rabbit eyes (Figure 4-6).

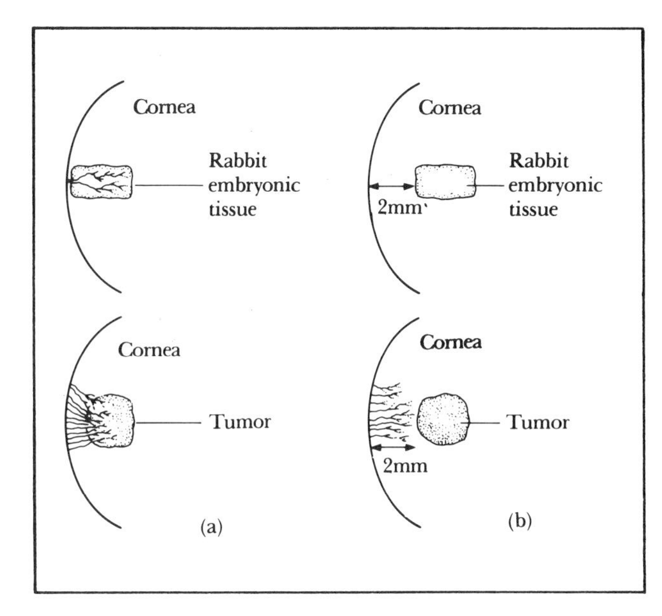

FIGURE 4-6 Angiogenesis. Illustrated here are the experiments of Folkman and Tyler.[37] Tumors are apparently able to release a diffusable chemical substance that stimulates nearby normal blood vessels to send out new capillaries that grow toward and eventually "nourish" the tumor. This substance is also apparently released by embryonic tissue but to a lesser degree. **A,** Vascularization of embryonic tissue implanted in the rabbit cornea compared with tumor implanted in the cornea when both grafts are placed adjacent to the vessels at the edge of the cornea. **B,** Comparison of corneal implants of embryonic tissue and tumor tissue when the grafts are placed at a distance from the vessels at the edge of the cornea. In this situation, the embryonic tissue is *un*able to attract new vessels, whereas the tumor graft *does* attract new vessels and becomes vascularized. (Source: Adapted from Folkman J, Tyler K: Tumor angiogenesis: Its possible role in metastasis and invasion, in Day SB, Meyers WPL, Stansley P et al (eds): Cancer Invasion and Metastasis: Biological Mechanisms and Therapy. New York, Raven Press, 1977, p 96.)

The cornea does not normally have blood vessels. Implantation of embryologic tissue and tumor tissue in the cornea at variable distances from its edge induces vessels to grow out from the edge of the cornea to the implant. Normal tissues do *not* induce vascularization, but embryonic tissue will cause blood vessels to grow out only if implanted relatively close to the edge of the cornea.[37] As illustrated in Figure 4-6, tumor implants induced the outgrowth of vasculature over a greater distance.

Another difference between embryologic and tumor tissue illuminated in this experimental model is that the intact blood vessels of *embryonic tissue* grafts lined up and became spliced to the vessels growing out from the edge of the cornea. In contrast, the original vessels within the *tumor* implant disintegrate, and new host vessels induced by the tumor and originating in the surrounding stroma take their place.

TAF has been isolated from human cancer cells by researchers at Harvard in collaboration with scientists at the University of Washington; they characterized the protein and named it *angiogenin.*[39] This achievement was a major breakthrough, not only because it should now be easier to find ways to block angiogenin and thus keep blood vessels from developing in tumors, but also because angiogenin may be useful in other areas of medicine. For example, it may be used to speed up the development of blood vessels in burns and other wounds or to encourage the growth of new blood vessels in the heart after a heart attack.

In recent years, a number of angiogenic factors have been purified. Among these are the polypeptides, fibroblast growth factor (both acidic and basic forms), and transforming growth factors alpha and beta, as well as angiogenin. Nicotinamide has been reported to have angiogenic properties.[42] Other less-well-characterized angiogenic factors, including some lipids, have also been described.[43] Some of the angiogenic factors act directly on vascular endothelial cells; others appear to act indirectly through other cells, for instance, macrophages, causing them to release vascular endothelial growth factors. Still other factors, such as some steroids, have been found to inhibit angiogenesis.[44]

HOST AND TREATMENT FACTORS IN METASTASIS

In some model systems, metastatic efficiency is related to hormone levels. Hormones may influence delay in the development of metastases, and they have also been implicated in the arrest of tumor cells.

Age may be another factor. Willis[17] cited studies carried out in the 1930s concluding that older rats were less susceptible to metastases than young rats.

The host may influence metastatic development in other ways, as suggested by the observation that metastatic efficiency is influenced by the site of experimental implantation of tumor cells. Certain strongly metastatic animal tumors (eg, the Lewis lung carcinoma) were found to become nonmetastatic when implanted in certain body cavities.[45]

According to Nicolson,[27] protection against metastatic disease through immunization has been achieved in a number of experimental animal systems. Another important experimental observation suggesting that the immune system can defend against metastasis is that certain normally nonmetastasizing cells *will* metastasize in animals whose immune systems have been suppressed. It has long been known that human tumors found on histologic examination to be surrounded or infiltrated by cellular elements of the immune system have a more favorable prognosis.

One key research question in tumor immunology has been "Why doesn't the host mount an immunologic response against neoplastic cells if they do indeed have antigens not found in normal tissues?" Research has made it clear that the immune system may even be guilty of treason. Tumor cells that are mildly immunogenic apparently can cause certain immunoglobulins to attach to their surfaces, making them "invisible" to the macrophages and other elements of the cell-mediated immune system. This interaction may also help cancer cells invade adjacent normal tissue and even increase the likelihood that cancer cells will metastasize.

Lymphocytes may actually promote metastasis by clumping cancer cells, making them more likely to become trapped in capillary beds.[33] It has been shown that in animals without mature T cells the metastatic efficiency of B16 melanoma cells was *lower* than in normal animals.[27] Apparently tumor immunity can markedly modify tumor metastasis in both positive and negative ways. This fact led Fidler et al[46] to suggest that immunologically sensitized experimental animals are really more appropriate animal models for studying the mechanisms of metastasis than "normal" animals. Obviously, metastasis and the immune system do not have a simple relationship.

METASTASIS AS A CLINICAL PROBLEM

The Recognition of Metastatic Potential

The patient diagnosed as having cancer but who shows no metastases presents a special problem to the clinician. Because treatment plans are based on whether disease has been disseminated, the diagnostician must try to determine through x-ray studies, scans, and other means if disease has spread. The clinician is often faced with tentative evidence of metastatic disease. In the absence of histopathologic confirmation of metastases, this problem is especially acute because of significant rates of false-positive and false-negative results using other methods.

It would obviously be helpful if a primary tumor could somehow be evaluated and the probability of dissemination at a certain point in its tumorigenesis established. Unfortunately, clinicians cannot yet make accurate estimates. It is nearly impossible to assess the efficiency of metastatic spread of cancer in human beings or to determine exactly when metastatic spread begins in the natural history of a tumor. The problems are multiple. One notable difficulty is that simple measurements of a neoplasm cannot distinguish between cells lost because of cell death and those lost through metastatic dissemination.

Certain general types of tumors grow faster and are more likely to metastasize than other types of tumors. So far no morphologic or histochemical attribute of cancer cells has been identified that consistently parallels metastatic behavior.

Among the types of tumors that will rarely metastasize, regardless of degree of differentiation, are basal cell carcinomas of the skin. Some thyroid tumors metastasize frequently even though they are well differentiated, so that overall, although morphologic characterization and tumor grade are good indicators of likely metastasis, other factors must also be operating that are not expressed morphologically or that cannot yet be identified.

The Latent Primary Tumor

It is not uncommon for metastatic disease to reveal itself even before the primary tumor has given any indication of its presence. In some situations, patients come in with broken bones and are later found to have a primary carcinoma of the thyroid with a metastasis to bone. It is not unusual in head and neck cancer to find a secondary mass in the neck that results from an unsuspected primary tumor in some area of the head, neck, or even lung. Skin metastases may be the very first symptom of latent gastric cancer.

The Dormant Secondary Tumor

It is also not unheard of for malignant growth to appear in cancer patients many years after they were thought to be cured. In breast cancer, for example, metastases can appear in the vertebrae 30 years later. There has been enough documentation of this phenomenon to lead to the notion that metastatic tumor cells can actually remain *dormant.* It is not known, however, what causes metastatic tumor cells to go into and remain in a dormant state or what causes them to eventually reemerge.

A number of clinically important questions are related to the dormancy of metastatic cancer, such as, How do tumor cells become dormant? How do they avoid destruction by the immune system while dormant? Are dormant metastases more common in some types of tumors than others? Does dormancy occur after a period of rapid cellular division, or does it reflect the body's successful effort to control the tumor? What treatments will be available to combat dormant tumor cells?

Apparently, a number of factors can influence the rate of division of metastatic cancer, that is, can increase the division of metastatic cancer cells abruptly and possibly stimulate dormant metastatic cells to emerge from dormancy. Simpson-Herren et al[47] cited evidence that surgical removal of primary tumors or even sham surgical operations in experimental models stimulate the growth rate of metastatic lung tumors. This concept has received support in a number of studies and suggests that a primary tumor is able to repress or hold in some intermediate state of dormancy the metastatic cells present in the same body. Experiments in which sham surgery produced a similar effect suggest that the reason may be a little more complicated, possibly involving suppression of the immune system.

The observation that taking out the primary tumor results in a spurt of growth in metastatic tumors suggests that drugs toxic to rapidly dividing cells might be used to special advantage immediately following surgery. Indeed, such strategies have been employed with success.

The Detection of Metastasis

The following are methods used to assess the presence of metastases.

Chemical methods

Among the differences between normal cells and cancer cells discussed are abnormal hormone secretions, abnormal secretions of certain enzymes, and the release of cell surface components into extracellular fluid, blood, urine, and cerebrospinal fluid. A number of strategies have been devised based on the persistence of abnormal secretions after the primary tumor has been resected. Alkaline phosphatase was one of the very first biochemical markers used to monitor the presence of metastases, and human chorionic gonadotropin (HCG) has been one of the most useful of the peptide hormones. Of more recent vintage is the use of carcinoembryonic antigen assays in blood to find indications of tumors persisting after surgical excision. A number of other biochemical parameters have also proved useful in following the growth or progression of metastatic disease. These will all be considered in more detail in Chapters 5 and 9.

Radiographic and radiologic methods

Radiographic techniques are also useful in the detection of metastatic deposits. In the lungs, the differential contrast between normal lung tissue and densely packed metastatic masses can be seen on x-ray film. X-ray studies are also able to detect defects in bone produced by calcium resorption and other abnormalities of calcium deposition caused by the presence of metastatic disease. These methods are far from perfect. In recent years, routine radiographic analysis of the long bones has been found to be rather insensitive in the detection of disseminated disease, and the use of scans and imaging agents has become more popular (see Chapter 9). Radiopaque materials put into the circulation reveal areas of the liver where the contrast medium is retained an extra length of time, that is, leaves a lingering "blush." This method takes advantage of the hemorrhagic character or abnormal vasculature within metastatic tumor masses. Other approaches to imaging metastatic lesions include use of radiolabeled monoclonal antibody to tumor-associated-antigens. The radioactive antibody label reveals the presence of tumor through the interaction between the tumor antigens and the tagged antibody.

Unfortunately, a number of things can cause false-negative findings in searches for metastases. Preoperative and postoperative workups miss metastatic disease later confirmed at autopsy.

False-*positive* findings are obviously also a considerable clinical problem. Among the factors responsible for false-positive findings are gall bladder artifacts, cirrhosis of the liver, abscesses, and other types of benign diseases. All these errors show that additional research must be aimed at improving the methods of detecting and evaluating metastatic cancer.

CONCLUSION

Metastasis is clearly the most significant feature of cancer. Contrary to what was once thought to be the case, the development of metastases involves much more than random survival of a very small proportion of the clumps of cells that break away from primary masses to become trapped in capillary beds. Rather, metastasis appears to result from a complicated interplay between host factors and a small subpopulation of cancer cells (in the primary mass) with the ability to invade adjacent tissue, enter the circulation, leave the bloodstream by passing through capillary walls, induce the development of a blood supply, and continue to proliferate. Difficulty in accurately assessing metastatic spread remains one of the biggest problems in clinical cancer treatment.

Cancer cells differ in many respects from normal cells. Although many of these differences are subtle, they offer a considerable array of potentially exploitable differences and suggest numerous points of attack on cancer. The metastatic sequence—from invasion through the establishment of a vascular blood supply for a secondary tumor—offers some especially strategic points of attack on cancer. Some very significant work has gone on in recent years, but the stimulus for additional work remains; improved understanding of metastasis is fundamental to any prospect for significant improvements in how cancer is treated.

• • •

This chapter is an adaptation of Chapter 6 in the author's book *Dimensions of Cancer* published by Wadsworth, Belmont, Calif., 1987.© 1987 Wadsworth, Inc. Used by permission of publisher.

REFERENCES

1. Paget S: The Distribution of Secondary Growths of Cancer of the Breast. Lancet 1:571-573, 1889.
2. Fidler IJ, Balch CM: The biology of cancer metastasis and implications for therapy. Curr Probl Surg 24:129-209, 1987.
3. Eisenbach L, Kushtai G, Plaskin D, et al: MHC genes and oncogenes controlling the metastatic phenotype of tumor cells. Cancer Rev 5:1-18, 1986.
4. Terranova VP, Hic S, Diflorio RM, et al: Tumor cell metastasis, CRC Crit Rev Oncol Hematol, 5:87-114, 1986.
5. Hagmar B, Ryd W, Erkell LJ: Why do tumors metastasize? An overview of current research. Tumor Biol 5:141-149, 1984.
6. Liotta LA, Wewer U, Rao NC, et al: Biochemical mechanisms of tumor invasion and metastases. Progr Clin Biol Res 256:3-16, 1988.
7. Easty GC, Easty DM: Mechanisms of Tumor Invasion, in Symington T, Carter RL (eds): Scientific Foundations of Oncology. Chicago, Heinemann Medical Books/Yearbook Medical Publishers, 1976, pp 167-172.
8. Nicolson GL, Milas L: Cancer Invasion and Metastasis: Biologic and Therapeutic Aspects. New York, Raven Press, 1984.
9. Feldman M, Eisenbach L: What makes a tumor cell metastatic? Sci Am 259:60-85, 1988.
10. Schirrmacher V: Cancer metastasis: Experimental approaches, theoretical concepts, and impacts for treatment strategies. Adv Cancer Res 43:1-73, 1985.
11. Welch DR, Bhuyan BK, Liotta LA (eds): Cancer Metastasis: Experimental and Clinical Strategies. New York, Alan R. Liss, 1986.
12. Talmadge JE, Wolman SR, Fidler IJ: Evidence for the clonal origin of spontaneous metastases. Science 217:361-362, 1982.
13. Kupchella CE: Dimensions of Cancer. Belmont, Calif, Wadsworth, 1987, pp 50-69, 79-101.
14. Sylven B, Bois I: Protein content and enzymatic assays of interstitial fluid from some normal tissues and transplanted mouse tumors. Cancer Res 20:831-836, 1960.
15. Nakajima M, Inmura T, DeFerrante D, et al: Heparin sulfate degradation: relation to tumor invasive and metastatic properties of mouse B-16 melanoma sublines. Science 220:611-613, 1983.
16. Koono M, Ushijima K, Hayashi H: Studies of the mechanisms of invasion in cancer. III. Purification of a neutral protease of rat ascites hepatoma cells associated with the production of a chemotactic factor for cancer cells. Int J Cancer 13:105-115, 1974.
17. Willis RA: The Spread of Tumors in the Human Body (ed 3). London, Butterworth, 1973.
18. Glaves D, Weiss L: Initial arrest patterns of circulating cancer cells: Effect of host sensitization and anticoagulation, in Weiss L (ed): Fundamental Aspects of Metastasis. New York, American Elsevier, 1976, pp 263-273.
19. Chew EC, Josephson RL, Wallace AC: Morphological aspects of arrest of circulating cancer cells, in Weiss L (ed): Fundamental Aspects of Metastasis. New York, American Elsevier, 1976, pp 121-150.
20. Tarin D: Cellular interactions in neoplasia. In Weiss L (ed): Fundamental Aspects of Metastasis. New York, American Elsevier, 1976, pp 151-190.
21. Carter RL: Metastasis, in Symington T, Carter RL (eds): Scientific Foundations of Oncology. Chicago, Heinemann Medical Books/Yearbook Medical Publishers, 1976, pp 172-178.
22. Tsubura E, Yamashita T, Higuchi Y: An inhibitory mechanism of blood-borne metastasis by sulfated polysaccharides, in Day SB, Meyers WPL, Stansley P, et al, (eds): Cancer Invasion and Metastasis: Biological Mechanisms and Therapy. New York, Raven Press, 1977, pp 367-381.
23. Iwamoto Y, Robey FA, Graf J, et al: YIGSR, a synthetic laminin pentapeptide, inhibits experimental metastasis formation. Science 238:1132-1134, 1987.
24. Terranova VP, Williams JE, Liotta LA, et al: Modulation of the metastatic activity of melanoma cells by laminin and fibronectin. Science 226:982-984, 1984.
25. Bodansky O: Biochemical criteria of metastatic growth in human cancer, in Day SB, Meyers WPL, Stansley P (eds): Cancer Invasion and Metastasis: Biochemical Mechanisms and Therapy. New York, Raven Press, 1977, pp 199-211.
26. Netland PA, Zetter BR: Organ-specific adhesion of metastatic cells in vitro. Science 224:1113-1114, 1984.
27. Nicolson GL: Experimental tumor metastasis: Characteristics and organ specificity. Bioscience 28:441-447, 1978.
28. Fidler IJ, Nicolson GL: Organ selectivity for implantation, survival, and growth of B16 melanoma variant tumor lines. J Natl Cancer Inst 57:1199-1202, 1976.
29. Sugarbaker ED: The organ selectivity of experimentally induced metastases in rats. Cancer 5:606-612, 1952.
30. Kinsey DL: An experimental study of preferential metastasis. Cancer 12:674-676, 1960.
31. Fidler IJ: Review: biologic heterogeneity of cancer metastases. Breast Cancer Res Treatment 9:17-26, 1987.
32. Fidler IJ, Hart IR: Biological diversity in metastatic neoplasms: origins and implications. 'Science 217:998-1003, 1982.
33. Nicolson GL: Cancer metastasis. Sci Am 240:66-76, 1979.
34. Fidler IJ: Patterns of tumor cell arrest and development, in Weiss L (ed): Fundamental Aspects of Metastasis. New York, American Elsevier, 1976, pp 275-289.
35. Nicolson G: Organ specificity of tumor metastasis: role of preferential adhesion, invasion and growth of malignant cells at specific secondary sites. Cancer Metastasis Rev 7:143-188, 1988.

36. Sato H, Suzuki M: Deformability and viability of tumor cells by transcapillary passage, with references to organ affinity to metastasis in cancer, in Weiss L (ed): Fundamental Aspects of Metastasis. New York, American Elsevier, 1976, pp 311-317.
37. Folkman J, Tyler K: Tumor angiogenesis: Its possible role in metastasis and invasion, in Day SB, Meyers WPL, Stansley P, et al (eds): Cancer Invasion and Metastasis: Biological Mechanisms and Therapy. New York, Raven Press, 1977, pp 95-103.
38. Knighton DR, Hunt TK, Scheuenstuhl H, et al: Oxygen tension regulates the expression of angiogenesis factor by macrophages. Science 221:1283-1285, 1983.
39. Fett JW, Strydom DJ, Lobb RR, et al: Isolation and characterization of angiogenin, an angiogenic protein from human carcinoma cells. Biochemistry 24:5480-5486, 1985.
40. Salahuddin SZ, Nakamura S, Biberfeld P, et al: Angiogenic properties of Kaposi's sarcoma-derived cells after long-term culture in vitro. Science 242:430-433, 1988.
41. Marx J: Angiogenesis research comes of age. Science 237:23-24, 1987.
42. Kull FC, Brent DA, Parikh I, et al: Chemical identification of a tumor-derived angiogenic factor. Science 236:843-845, 1987.
43. Folkman J, Klagsbrun M: Angiogenic factors. Science 235:442-447, 1987.
44. Crum R, Szabo S, Folkman J: A new class of steroids inhibits angiogenesis in the presence of heparin or a heparin fragment. Science 230: 1375-1378, 1985.
45. Garattini S: Concluding remarks on cancer dissemination and metastases, in Day SB, Meyers WPL, Stansley P, et al (eds): Cancer Invasion and Metastasis: Biological Mechanisms and Therapy. New York, Raven Press, 1977, pp 501-505.
46. Fidler IJ, Gersten DM, Riggs CW: Quantitative analysis of tumor: Host interaction and the outcome of experimental metastasis, in Day SB, Meyers WPL, Stansley P, et al (eds): Cancer Invasion and Metastasis: Biological Mechanisms and Therapy. New York, Raven Press, 1977, pp 277-303.
47. Simpson-Herren L, Springer TA, Sanford AH, et al: Kinetics of metastasic experimental tumors. In Day SB, Meyers WPL, Stansley P, et al (eds): Cancer Invasion and Metastasis: Biological Mechanisms and Therapy. New York, Raven Press, 1977, 117-133.

Chapter 5

Relation of the Immune System to Cancer

Katherine Alkire, RN, MN

Susan L. Groenwald, RN, MS

INTRODUCTION

The relation of the immune system to cancer is complex and only partially understood. During the last two decades, as research has begun to sort out the components and interactions of the immune system, theories about the immune system's impact on disease have surfaced. The origin of most cancers remains a mystery. However, through epidemiologic and immunologic study, theories about causation, detection, and treatment of cancer have included some aspect of the immune system with increasing frequency. Failure of the immune system has been cited as a possible reason for the appearance of some tumors. Research into tumor-associated antigens has provided clinical indicators of cancer growth from a sample of blood. Administration of immune products has shown moderate success in the treatment of certain types of tumor. It is obvious that cancer care now demands a thorough understanding of immune system function and its relation to cancer.

OVERVIEW OF THE IMMUNE SYSTEM

Function

The classic function of the immune system is to protect the body against injury from foreign substances (antigens), distinguishing self from nonself and destroying nonself substances. There are four elements to the process of differentiating self from nonself. The first is recognition—the ability of the body to recognize something as nonself. Degree of recognition correlates with the immune system's previous exposure to the invader. The second is activation, in which components of the immune system become activated against the invader. Third is actual destruction, and fourth is clearance or removal of the nonself target from the body. The immune system is relatively specific in its ability to recognize, destroy, and clear nonself targets.

A second function of the immune system is that of homeostasis. Immune cells are responsible for preserving the body's internal environment by degradation and removal of damaged or dead cells from the body.

A third function is surveillance—prevention of the growth and development of aberrant cells that might otherwise develop into neoplasms. It is estimated that mutant cells arise at a rate of 100 to 1000 per day.[1] The immune system effectively eliminates most of these aberrant cells.

Each of these functions is distinct; yet all are provided by the same system.

Components

There are both specific and nonspecific components of the immune system. Specific components are those that recognize and attack only one type of nonself invader or antigen. Nonspecific components are those that can respond to a variety of nonself targets.

TABLE 5-1 Humoral Versus Cellular Immunity

Type of Immunity	Specific Components*	Nonspecific components†
Humoral (noncellular)	Immunoglobulin (Ig)	Complement (C)
Cell-mediated (cellular)	T lymphocytes	Mononuclear phagocytes Polymorphonuclear (PMN) leukocytes Natural killer (NK) cells

*Attack only one nonself target.
†Attack different targets.

An antigen is any cell that is capable of eliciting an immune response. A target cell is any cell against which the destructive forces of the immune system are directed, self or nonself.

There are two main subsystems of the immune system that work together to recognize and remove nonself invaders. These two subsystems, shown in Table 5-1, represent humoral immunity and cell-mediated immunity. The humoral immunity subsystem comprises two types of noncellular serum protein: (1) Immunoglobulins (Ig) or antibody molecules are produced by B lymphocytes and provide the body with the ability to specifically attack nonself invaders. (2) Complement is a group of nonspecific, noncellular proteins in the blood that work together in a cascade of events initiated by an antigen-antibody reaction, culminating in the lysing ("poking holes in") of target cells to which complement is directed.

The cell-mediated immunity subsystem also has both specific and nonspecific components. The system is mediated by T lymphocytes, of which there are several types. Each type is specific in its action; that is, it recognizes only one type of nonself invader and will not respond to others.

The cells of the immune system are distributed throughout the body but are concentrated primarily in the lymphoid system, which comprises bone marrow, liver, lungs, thymus gland, spleen, lymph nodes, and lymphatic vessels and fluid. Cells of the immune system travel from one part of the immune system to another by way of lymphatic vessels and blood vessels and mount an immune response to any nonself invaders that are discovered.

The cells of the immune system are derived from a common bone marrow stem cell through the process of differentiation. Figure 5-1[2] depicts the development of each type of cell. White blood cells can be divided into two groups: (1) The polymorphonuclear (PMN) leukocytes are neutrophils, basophils, and eosinophils. PMN cells help defend the body nonspecifically against bacterial invasion. (2) The mononuclear leukocytes (MNLs) comprise two groups of cells—(a) mononuclear phagocytes, which are

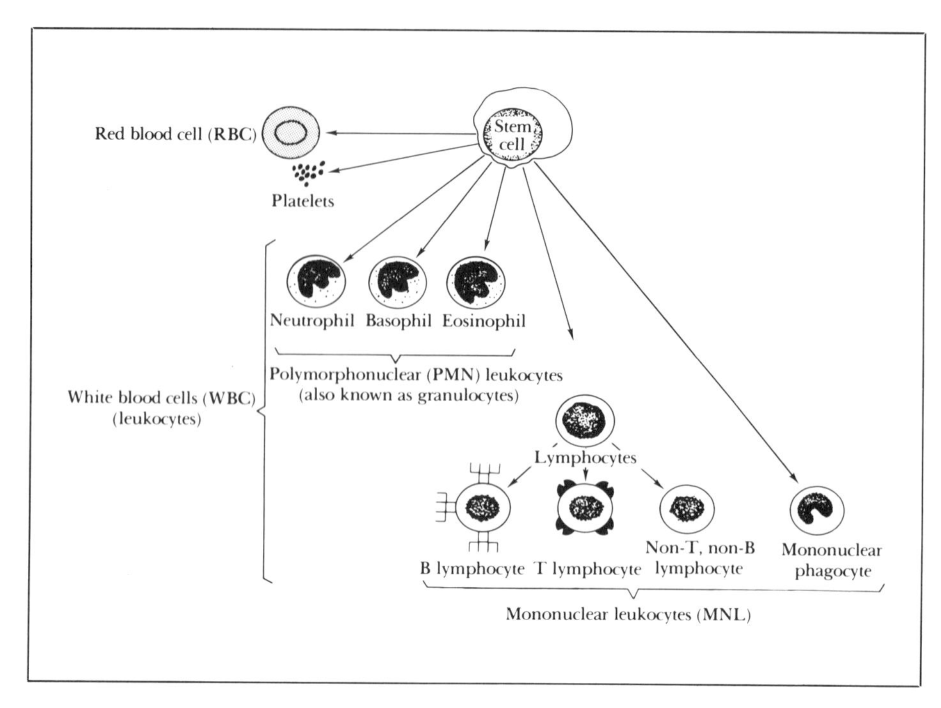

FIGURE 5-1 Differentiation of leukocytes from common stem cell. (Source: Huffner TL, Kanapa DJ, Stevenson GW: Introduction to Immunology. Boston, Jones and Bartlett, 1986, p 78.)

responsible for nonspecific action against nonself invaders, (b) lymphocytes, which are subdivided into B lymphocytes, T lymphocytes—and a third group that is neither T nor B, called large granular lymphocytes or natural killer (NK) cells.

T lymphocytes

T lymphocytes account for approximately 80% of all circulating lymphocytes and may be identified by the special receptors for antigen found on their surfaces. The T lymphocyte differentiates into a mature cell in the thymus gland and then migrates to lymphoid tissues.

T lymphocytes are responsible for specific cell-mediated immune responses. They enhance the actions of other immune components; direct or participate in destruction of antigen, specifically viruses, fungi, and parasites; and are responsible for immunosurveillance and graft rejection.

For purposes of this chapter, there are four main subsets of T lymphocytes: (1) helper T lymphocytes, (2) suppressor T lymphocytes, (3) killer T lymphocytes (cytotoxic), and (4) memory T lymphocytes.[3]

Helper T lymphocytes produce lymphokines that enhance the activity and efficacy of other lymphocytes and phagocytes. Helper T lymphocytes also trigger B-lymphocyte proliferation and maturation and immunoglobulin production.

Suppressor T lymphocytes decrease activity in lymphocytes and phagocytes, keeping the immune system from a state of overreaction. A delicate balance between helper and suppressor cell activity is needed for normal immune function. An example of imbalance between helper and suppressor cells occurs in acquired immune deficiency syndrome (AIDS), in which the helper T lymphocytes function at a normal level while the activity of suppressor T lymphocytes is increased, leading to overall suppression of immune system function.

Killer cytotoxic T lymphocytes can directly kill target cells bearing a specific antigen.

Memory T lymphocytes are antigen-specific T lymphocytes that have memory of antigens previously recognized by the body. T memory and B memory cells act together to enhance response time on each subsequent occasion the antigen is introduced.

The products of lymphocytes are cytokines called lymphokines. Table 5-2[4] summarizes lymphokines and their functions.

B lymphocytes

B lymphocytes account for 12% to 15% of circulating lymphocytes. They are responsible for humoral immunity, including production of immunoglobulins. They may be identified by the antigen-specific immunoglobulins found on their cell surfaces. They also have on their surfaces

TABLE 5-2 Types and Functions of Lymphokines

Function	Lymphokine
Enhanced phagocytosis	
Stimulates macrophage activity	Macrophage activation factor (MAF)
Prevents migration of macrophage from site of antigen	Macrophage inhibition factor (MIF)
Recruits macrophages to site of antigen	Macrophage chemotactic factor (MCF)
Enhanced T-cell function	
Increases clonal proliferation of T cell	Interleukin-2 (IL-2)
Enhanced B-cell function	
Stimulates activated B lymphocyte clonal proliferation	B-cell growth factor (BCGF)
Causes activated B cells to differentiate into antibody-secreting plasma cells	B-cell differentiation factor (BCDF)
Enhanced cytoxicity	
Stimulates cytotoxicity of NK cells	Gamma interferon (γ-IFN) Interleukin-2 (IL-2)
Enhanced destruction of tumor cells	
Secreted by killer T lymphocytes	Tumor necrosis factor (TNF)

Source: Adapted from Grady C: Host defense mechanisms: An overview, Semin Oncol Nurs 4:86-94, 1988.

receptors for C3b (a complement split product) and the Fc portion of immunoglobulin.

When B lymphocytes are stimulated by helper T lymphocytes and an encounter with a foreign antigen, they mature and divide into plasma cells that secrete antigen-specific immunoglobulins. Some of the resultant progeny of stimulated B lymphocytes become B memory cells, which enhance the ability of the immune system to deal with that particular antigen each time it is encountered.

Antibody

Antibody is an antigen-specific immunoglobulin that is synthesized and secreted by a mature plasma cell, the final cell of B lymphocyte differentiation. Each plasma cell produces only one type of antibody, and each antibody is specific for only one type of antigen. There are five classes of immunoglobulins: IgG, IgA, IgM, IgD, and IgE (Table 5-3).[4]

One end of the immunoglobulin molecule is called Fab (antigen-binding fragment). The sequence of amino acids on the Fab section is highly variable, depending on the type of antigen for which the immunoglobulin was produced. The other end of the molecule, the Fc or constant fragment, has a constant sequence of amino acids that is consistent within a class of antibody.

Complement

Complement is a group of circulating proteins that amplify immune response and destroy antigens. Complement consists of nine serum proteins numbered C1 through C9. They are synthesized primarily by mononuclear phagocytes. C1 through C4 are primarily regulatory components; C5 through C9 are the effector cells responsible for destruction of the antigen.

The ultimate goal of complement activation is lysis of the target cell; however, the split products of complement activation—chemotoxins, opsonins, and anaphylatoxins—augment the immune system by enhancing phagocytosis.[5]

Phagocytic cells

Mononuclear phagocytes, polymorphonuclear (PMN) leukocytes, and natural killer (NK) lymphocytes are the nonspecific effector cells of the cell-mediated immune response (see Table 5-1). They are nonspecific because, although they are able to recognize nonself, they cannot distinguish one antigen from another. These effector cells are targeted to antigens by specific signals received by other immune system components.

TABLE 5-3 Human Immunoglobulins

Immunogobulin	Serum Concentration and Location	Activity	Other
IgG	75% in serum; Intravascular, Extravascular	Opsonization Neutralization Complement fixation	Crosses placenta Secondary response ab
IgA	17% in serum; Also found in mucous membranes and secretions	Neutralization Prevention of surface attachment	Found in breast milk
IgM	7% in serum; Intravascular	Agglutination Complement fixation	Primary antibody, natural blood group AB
IgE	0.1% in serum; bound to cells (mast cells and basophils)	Release of histamine and other mediators from mast cells "reaginic antibody"	Involved in type I hypersensitivity reactions
IgD	Nondetectable in serum Surface of B cells	Unknown	May function as a receptor on the B-cell surface

Source: Grady C: Host defense mechanisms: An overview. Semin Oncol Nurs 4:86-94, 1988.

Mononuclear phagocytes Mononuclear phagocytes exist in three forms in the body: promonocytes, monocytes, and macrophages. Promonocytes represent the earliest form in the differentiation process from the common stem cell (see Figure 5-1) and exist only in the bone marrow. When promonocytes differentiate into monocytes (cells with a characteristic horseshoe-shaped nucleus), they are dispersed into the circulation and within 48 hours become lodged in lymphoid tissues of the lymphoreticular system (liver, spleen, and lymph nodes). They differentiate into macrophages (literally "large eater" cells). Mononuclear phagocytes are responsible for antigen processing and the removal of dead or damaged self or nonself cells. Like the lymphokines secreted by T lymphocytes, monocytes release a number of important cytokines called *monokines*. Monokines include the following:

1. Alpha interferon (IFNα). Enhances NK cell killing. Increases phagocytic action of macrophages.
2. Interleukin 1 (IL-1). Stimulates T lymphocyte proliferation and mobilizes monocytes and macrophages to a site of injury.
3. Colony-stimulating factor (CSF) causes proliferation of mononuclear phagocytes and PMN leukocytes in the bone marrow.
4. Tumor necrosis factor (TNF) causes death of tumor cells.

PMN granulocytes Polymorphonuclear granulocytes are short-lived mobile phagocytic cells (they live only 2 days in the bloodstream) that attack invading bacteria and fungi. Granulocytes comprise 60% to 70% of the total leukocyte population. There are three categories of PMN cells: (1) neutrophils (60% of the granulocyte population); (2) eosinophils (2% to 4%); and (3) basophils (0.02% to 0.5%). Neutrophils are the primary PMN cells involved in phagocytosis.

NK cells

The natural killer lymphocyte is a large non-T, non-B lymphocyte with prominent granules in its cytoplasm (called large granular lymphocyte [LGL]).[6] NK cells exist throughout the reticuloendothelial system and are abundant in the bloodstream. NK cells are antigen-nonspecific effector cells that are thought to kill aberrant cells in the body, thus preventing the development of tumors.[7]

THE IMMUNE RESPONSE

Recognition

Before T lymphocytes and B lymphocytes can respond to the presence of an antigen, the antigen must be processed by mononuclear phagocytes and other nonspecific effector cells of the cell-mediated immune system. It is the role of the mononuclear phagocytes to localize the antigen and to ingest it, destroying, inactivating, or processing it for presentation to lymphocytes. Processing involves enzymatic modifications of the antigen and the reexpression of the processed antigen on the phagocyte's surface along

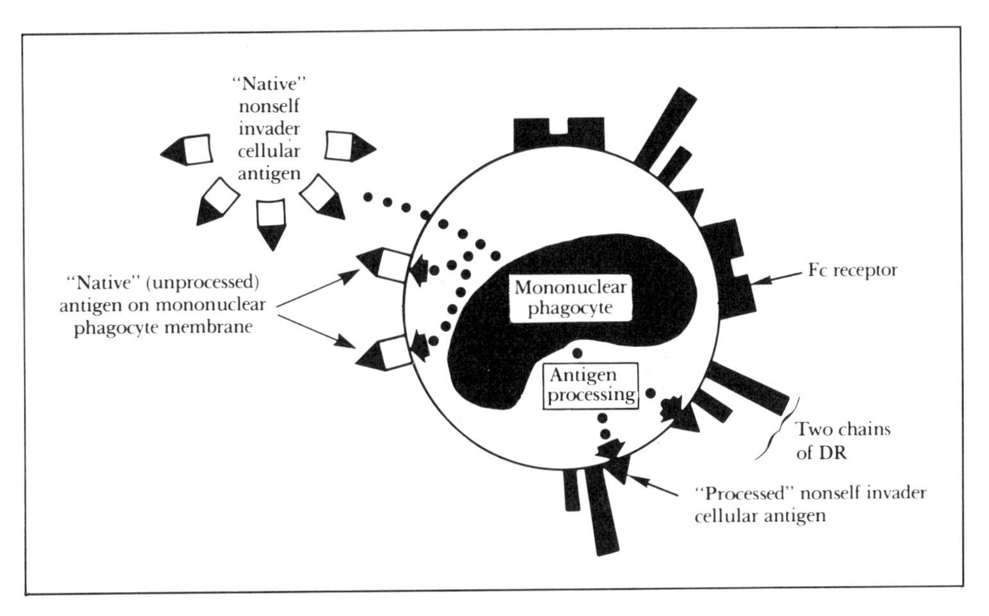

FIGURE 5-2 Details of antigen processing. (Source: Huffner TL, Kanapa DJ, Stevenson GW: Introduction to Immunology. Boston, Jones and Bartlett, 1986, p 99.)

with the set of membrane proteins known as "DR" (Figure 5-2).[2] DR is a Class II gene located on the sixth chromosome that is part of the major histocompatibility complex known as human leukocyte antigen (HLA) genes.[8] Class I HLA genes code for the classic histocompatibility antigens found on all cell surfaces. Class II HLA genes code for HLA-D and HLA-DR antigens that are found on the surfaces of macrophages and B lymphocytes. The DR gene is known as the immune response gene and provides the capability for an individual's immune system to respond to an antigen.[5]

Processed antigen must be presented on the surface of a mononuclear phagocyte in association with the DR proteins. The complex of DR and processed antigen activates lymphocytes.

Activation and Destruction

T lymphocyte activation

The T lymphocyte requires at least two signals for activation to occur. In addition to binding antigen to the T lymphocyte's surface antigen receptor, the T lymphocyte must also bind to the Class II DR molecule that is expressed on the surface of the mononuclear phagocyte for which the T lymphocyte has receptors. Both signals must be present simultaneously. If receptors on the surface of the mononuclear phagocyte do not match receptors on the T lymphocyte, activation does not occur[2] (Figure 5-3).

Macrophages, in addition to their role in processing the antigen, also release a cytokine IL-1 to stimulate T lymphocytes to proliferate and mobilize other macrophages.[9] Once activated, T lymphocytes begin clonal expansion to produce many similar cells and emit lymphokines that send powerful signals to enhance the activities of other immune system components.

Within a few days of invasion by an antigen (bacteria, fungus, virus, or tumor cell), T lymphocytes of an immunized individual will surround the antigen and arrange for its direct destruction by the T lymphocytes and its indirect destruction by the nonspecific PMN leukocytes, mononuclear phagocytes, and NK cells. The process is assisted by the release by the T lymphocytes of a variety of lymphokines.

B lymphocyte activation

The B lymphocyte becomes activated by recognizing and binding to the partially exposed antigen on the surface of the macrophage that is already bound to the T lymphocyte. Simultaneously, receptors on the T lymphocyte bind to the DR molecules on the B lymphocyte surface. This tricellular complex causes the B lymphocyte to become activated and generate receptors for the lymphokine, B-cell growth factor (BCGF), which causes the B lymphocyte to proliferate into two different cell types.[10] Some of the resultant progeny of the clonal proliferation develop receptors for another lymphokine, B-cell differentiation factor, which causes a B lymphocyte to differentiate into plasma cells that have lost their surface immunoglobulin and instead secrete large amounts of immunoglobulin. The immunoglobulins are released into the blood to seek and bind with antigen (Figure 5-4).[2]

The second type of cell resulting from B lymphocyte proliferation is the memory B lymphocyte that is responsible for the recall component of the system.

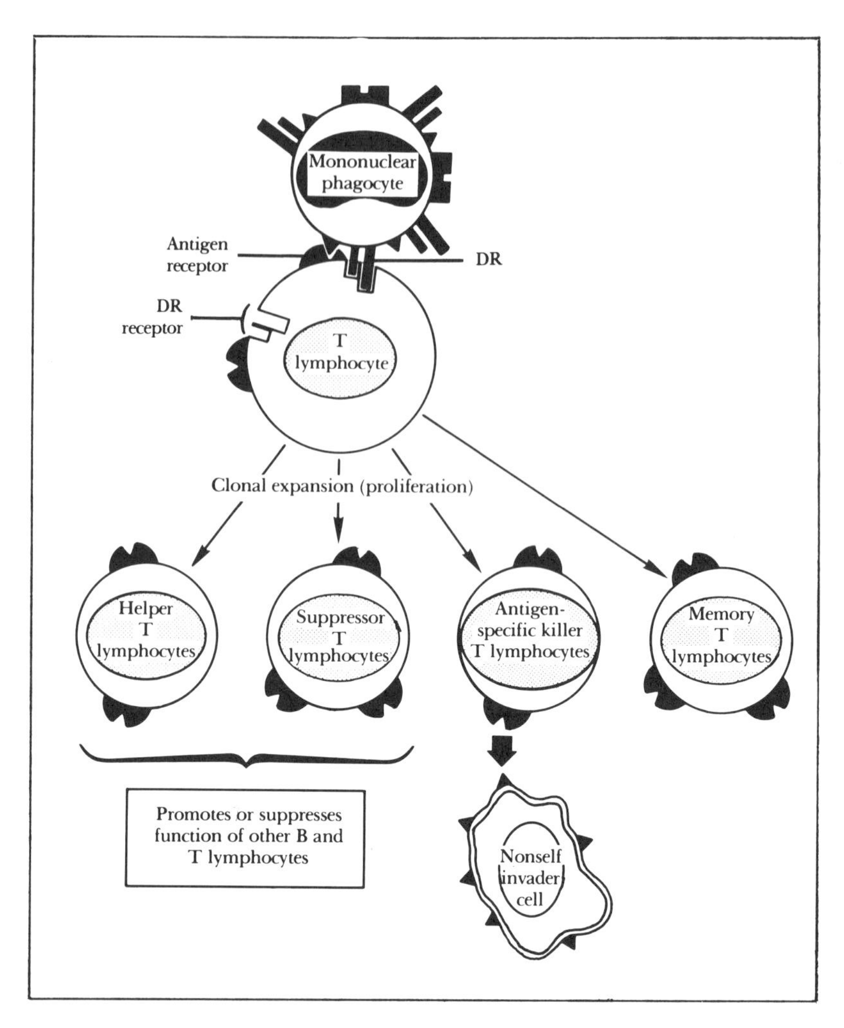

FIGURE 5-3 Details of T-lymphocyte activation. (Source: Huffner TL, Kanapa DJ, Stevenson GW: Introduction to Immunology. Boston, Jones and Bartlett, 1986, p 101.)

Antibody reactions

Antigen-specific antibody binds with antigen for which it was made by combining at the variable (Fab) portion of the immunoglobulin molecule. The resulting bond of antigen-antibody is called an immune complex.

On initial exposure to an antigen, there is a delay during which little or no antibody can be detected in the serum. It is during this delay that the antigen is recognized by the B lymphocyte; this causes the B lymphocyte to divide and differentiate into a plasma cell and to form antibody. The primary antibody response usually is evident 4 to 10 days after the initial exposure to the antigen.

The first antibody produced is of the IgM type. As the immune response progresses, it matures, with resultant production of IgG antibody. The same cell produces both types of antibody, converting from one type of production to another.[5]

The antibody usually does not reach a high level or persist unless a second encounter with the antigen occurs. At that time, a secondary antibody response ensues. In the secondary response, antibody is produced within 1 to 2 days and the titer of antibody produced may be up to 50 times greater than that in the primary response. This secondary response is maintained at high levels and falls slowly over a period of months. The secondary response is faster, stronger, and more persistent and is boosted to even higher levels with each subsequent exposure to the same antigen. B-lymphocyte memory cells retain a memory of the antigen, even months or years after exposure of the individual.

Antigen-antibody reactions against antigen can involve (1) precipitation, when insoluble antibody combines with a soluble antigen, resulting in antigen-antibody complex precipitates; (2) agglutination, when antigen is attached to particulate matter such as red blood cells and the antigen-antibody reaction results in agglutinated aggregates (eg, blood transfusion reaction); (3) neutralization, when the antibody neutralizes toxins released by bacteria or renders the antigen harmless by interfering with its ability to attach to cells; (4) opsonization, when the antibody coats the surface of the antigen to facilitate phagocytosis.

Some immune complexes are eliminated by cytotox-

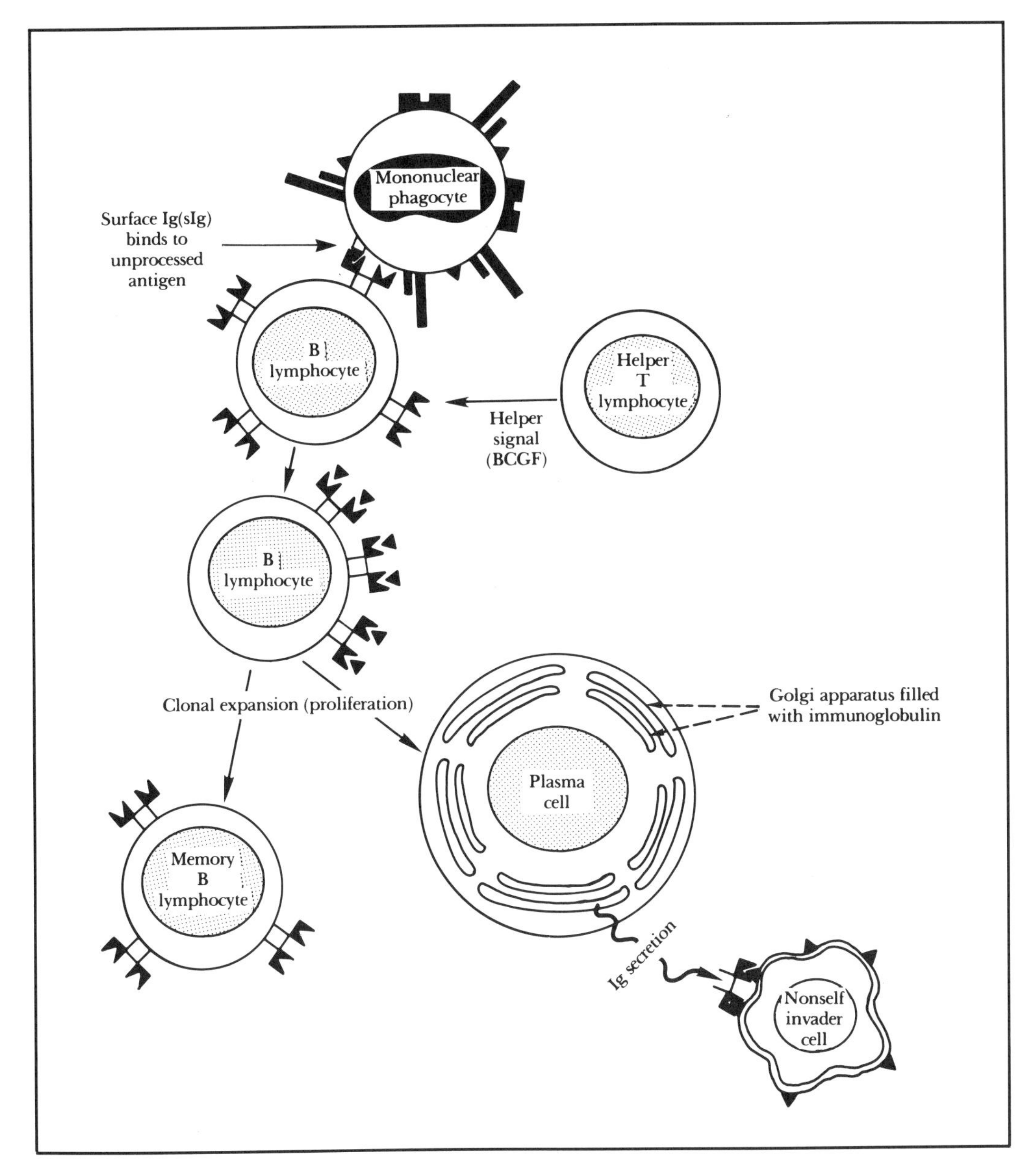

FIGURE 5-4 Details of B-lymphocyte activation. (Source: Huffner TL, Kanapa DJ, Stevenson GW: Introduction to Immunology. Boston, Jones and Bartlett, 1986, p 106.)

ic cells with receptors for Fc. Mononuclear phagocytes, PMN leukocytes, and NK cells bear Fc receptors in great abundance and are highly efficient at killing target cells by this mechanism. The cells with Fc receptors bind to the Fc portion of an immunoglobulin that is bound to an antigen. The cytotoxic cell is capable of destroying the antigen and eliminating the immune complex.[10] This process is called antibody-dependent cellular cytotoxicity (ADCC). ADCC is indirectly dependent on T lymphocytes, as T lymphocytes are required to activate B lymphocytes to proliferate into antibody-secreting plasma cells. ADCC or complement-mediated lysis must occur in order for the antibody-coated target cell to be killed. Antibody alone will not harm a target cell. ADCC is diagrammed in Figure 5-5.[2]

Complement activation

One of the most powerful results of antigen-antibody binding is activation of complement. Complement is considered an amplifier of the humoral immune system. Complement proteins activate one another in a stepwise action to cause a cascading of events. Each C component is completely inactive until activated by the C enzyme above it in the cascade. To initiate the cascade, C1 must be activated by an antigen-antibody reaction that usually involves IgG or IgM; IgE or IgA in large amounts also may activate the complement system.[11] When C5 through C9 are activated, they come together to form a needlelike tube configuration that attacks any cell (self or nonself) in the vicinity by poking a hole in its cell membrane (lysing); this allows the intracellular contents to leak out, thus killing the cell.

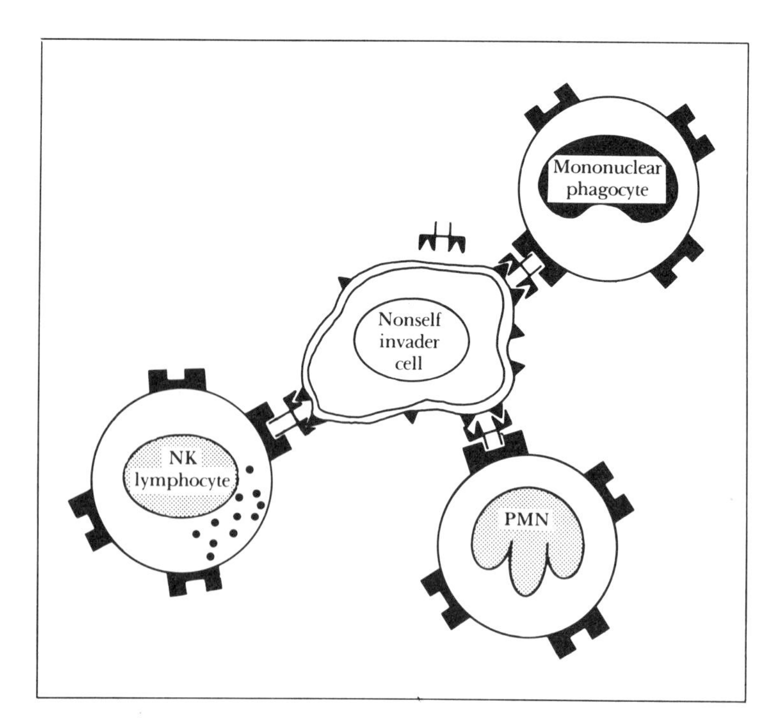

FIGURE 5-5 Details of antibody-dependent cellular cytotoxicity (ADCC). (Source: Huffner TL, Kanapa DJ, Stevenson GW: Introduction to Immunology. Boston, Jones and Bartlett, 1986, p 109.)

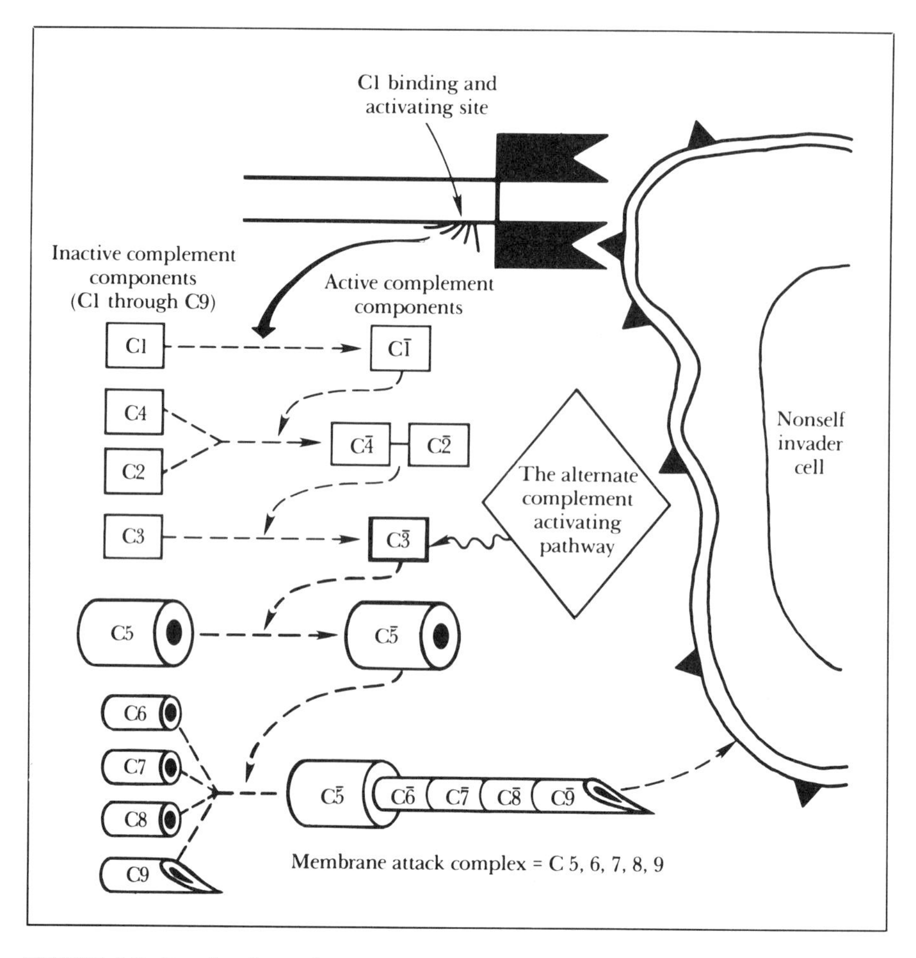

FIGURE 5-6 Details of complement components. (Source: Huffner TL, Kanapa DJ, Stevenson GW: Introduction to Immunology. Boston, Jones and Bartlett, 1986, p 111.)

Figure 5-6 diagrams the cascade of events in complement activation.

Natural cytotoxicity

Target cell killing can be accomplished by two mechanisms: (1) with immunoglobulin, and (2) without immunoglobulin or natural cytotoxicity. NK lymphocytes kill a wide range of tumor and virally infected cells without antibody. The function of NK cells in natural killing can be boosted if NK lymphocytes are exposed to alpha interferon (IFNα), a monokine, at the time of their encounter with a target cell.[6]

PMN leukocytes can also kill nonself target cells efficiently without antibody. PMN cells are a first line of defense against bacterial and fungal infection. They kill by ingesting the target cell.

Finally, mononuclear phagocytes are also capable of natural cytotoxicity and are especially useful in ridding the body of bacteria, fungi, tumor cells, and dead cells. The cytotoxicity of mononuclear phagocytes can be enhanced by gamma interferon, a lymphokine.

Immune Response as a System

Components of the immune system act in concert to maintain immune function (Figure 5-7).[12] When a foreign substance enters the body, macrophages distinguish it as "nonself," process the antigen, and present it to both humoral and cellular immune components. B-lymphocyte activa-

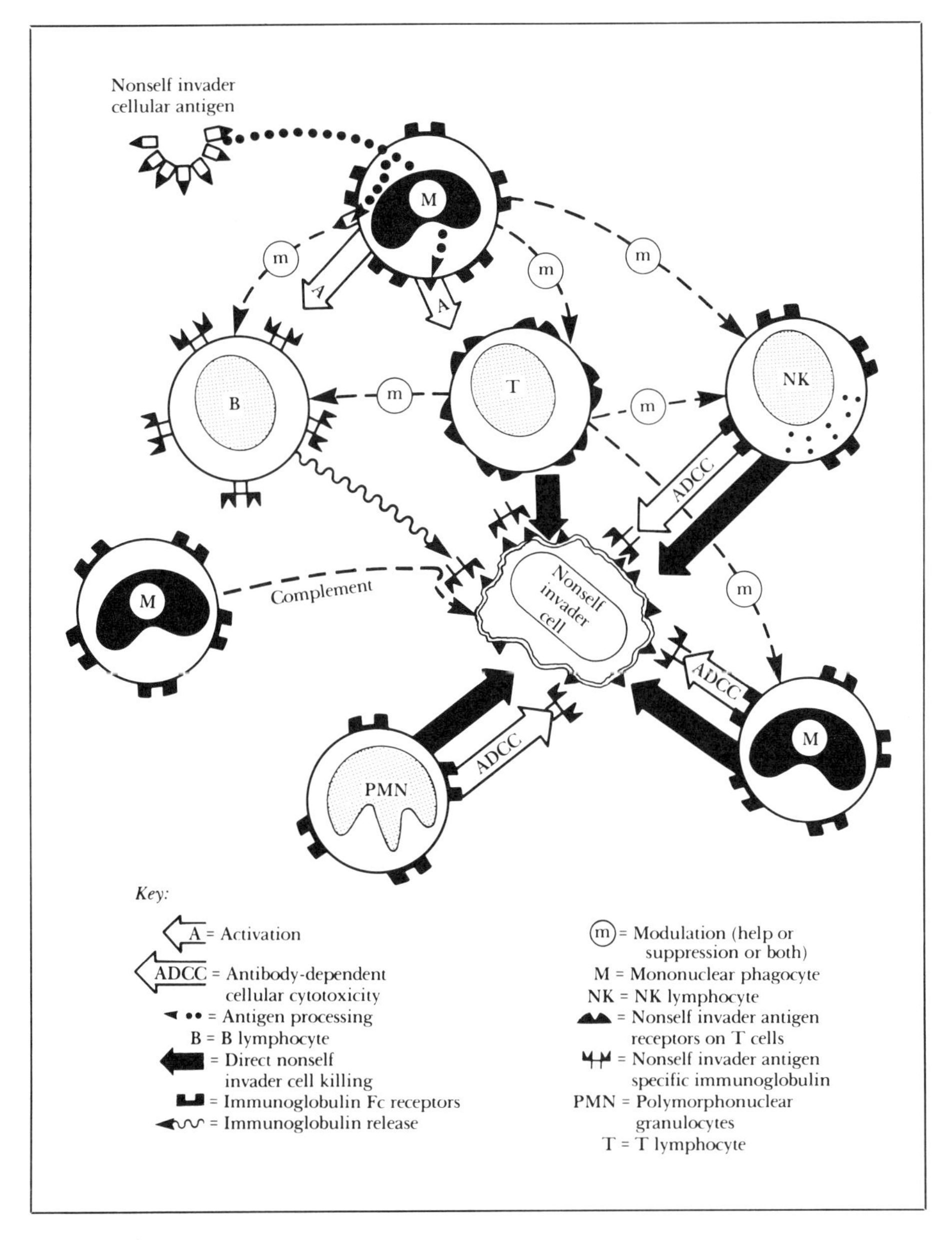

FIGURE 5-7 Simplified drawing showing major relationships between and among lymphocytes and lymphokines of immune system. A description of the relationships is given in the text. (Source: Huffner TL, Kanapa DJ, Stevenson GW: Introduction to Immunology. Boston, Jones and Bartlett, 1986, p 119.)

tion occurs as B lymphocytes recognize the antigen. Once activated, B lymphocytes mature into plasma cells and release immunoglobulins specific to the invading antigens. Immunoglobulins, with the help of complement, kill the antigen. Memory B lymphocytes produced in this process retain information about the invader and store that information to later call into action a faster immune response to a subsequent invasion by the same antigen.

T-lymphocyte activation occurs when the mature T lymphocyte is confronted by "processed" antigen and proliferates into helper, suppressor, specific killer, and memory T lymphocytes. Helper T lymphocytes release lymphokines to aid in immune response. Memory T lymphocytes serve as enhancers of cell-mediated immunity when an antigen subsequently enters the system. T lymphocytes also augment B lymphocyte activity.

Killer T lymphocytes destroy antigen as well as attract phagocytes into the area to aid in cleanup of the casualties of the battle. Complement and phagocytes destroy antigens by damaging cell membranes and consuming internal components. Various cytokines regulate this activity, allowing immune components to work on foreign invaders but halting overproduction of immune system components. As the function of the immune system becomes better understood, methods of using immune system components and actions to treat disease states will increase.

TUMOR IMMUNOLOGY

There has been a long-standing interest in the relationship between tumor growth and the immunologic response of the host. At the turn of the century, physicians intermittently observed unexpected extended survival of individuals with cancer who developed secondary infections. Such unusual occurrences stimulated curiosity among the medical community regarding a possible correlation between tumor growth and immune stimulation. After the development, in the 1930s, of inbred animal strains, the science of transplantation genetics was developed. The knowledge thus gained enabled investigators to eliminate issues of a person's response to foreign tissues and to more clearly address questions involving host reactions to malignancy. More recently, the discovery of tumor antigens on the surfaces of malignant cells supplied the necessary foundation for more intense and advanced research in the field of tumor immunology.

Tumor Antigens

Definition

All cells have on their surfaces normal antigens, called transplantation antigens, that reflect individual specificity and induce rejection of allogeneic transplanted tissue. When a cell becomes malignant it undergoes biochemical changes that result in the production of new cellular antigens. The most basic concept of tumor immunology is that these alterations in the surface antigens are sufficiently aberrant that they are recognized by the host as foreign and an immune response is initiated.

In animals

This concept of the immunogenicity of tumor cell antigens was first confirmed by animal research in 1953. Foley[13] injected methylcholanthrene, a polycyclic hydrocarbon, into inbred mice. Soft tissue sarcomas developed and, if left untreated, resulted in death of the mice. In those mice from which the tumor was removed, subsequent rechallenge with the same tumor resulted in an immunologic resistance. In 1957 Prehn and Main[14] confirmed and extended the observation by demonstrating that since there was no decrease in tolerance to skin grafts from other mice of the same strain, the normal histocompatibility antigens of these tumor cells must not be involved in the response. The antigens involved were at that time thought to be unique to the tumor tissue and not shared by normal tissue, and they were referred to as tumor-specific transplantation antigens (TSTAs). Today it is known that they are not unique to the tumor but are preferentially expressed on tumor tissue and are thus called tumor-associated transplantation antigens (TATAs or TAAs).[15,16] The degree of antigenicity depends on the cause of the tumor, the stage of tumor growth, and a variety of host factors.

A variety of antigens has been identified on the surface of neoplastic cells, including normal histocompatibility antigens, differentiation antigens, virus- or chemical-induced antigens, oncofetal antigens, and viral structural antigens. Studies suggest that all chemically induced and virally induced TAAs are related.[17] Such cross-reactivity of tumor antigens has beneficial implications when new strategies for cancer treatment are being considered. Immunization specifically directed at TAAs of a particular type of malignancy would destroy tumor cells and yet have no harmful effect on the host since the antigenic determinant would be found only preferentially on tumor cells.

In humans

Evidence of tumor antigenicity in human neoplasms has been presented for several types of malignant lesions: melanomas, sarcomas, gastrointestinal cancers, testicular cancers, hepatomas, leukemias, and lymphomas.[15] As yet, no antigens have been identified that are specific for a type of malignancy.[18] Following are tumor antigens that have been identified in humans.

Oncofetal antigens Fetal TAAs have been identified successfully on human tumor cells in colon, rectal, pancreatic, and breast cancers as well as neuroblastoma. There is evidence that these antigens are associated with tumor growth.

Carcinoembryonic antigen (CEA) was first described in 1965, when Gold and his associates[19] inoculated rabbits with extracts of colon carcinoma and obtained antibody directed against the tumor antigen, even after exhaustive absorption by normal colon tissue. The antigen detected was found on cells from colon carcinoma and normal fetal guts in the first two trimesters of pregnancy; hence the name *carcinoembryonic* antigen. CEA is shed from cell surfaces and is released into the circulation, making it possible to follow CEA antigen levels through radioimmunoassay. CEA determinations have been used in screening for cancer in persons without symptoms, diagnosing cancer, determining prognosis at diagnosis, and monitoring treatment efficacy.[20]

However, CEA lacks specificity. CEA levels may be elevated in individuals with nonmalignant conditions such as bronchitis, cirrhosis, emphysema, gastrointestinal inflammatory diseases, and uremia. Males have higher levels of CEA than females, and smokers have higher levels than nonsmokers. Although CEA may be used as a monitor for predicting the clinical course of individuals whose tumors yield elevated CEA levels, the lack of specificity limits its clinical usefulness.

Alpha-fetoprotein antigen The second tumor-associated antigen of the fetal class is alpha-fetoprotein (AFP), identified in hepatomas by Abelev and coworkers[21] in 1963. This protein factor was described in the serum of the human fetus. It is synthesized by the fetal liver, yolk sac, and gastrointestinal tract. It is the major serum protein of the human fetus. Although AFP is not detectable in normal adults except by radioimmunoassay, it is present in the majority of persons with primary hepatoma or testicular cancer. AFP has also been identified in some ovarian, pancreatic, and lung cancers. A quantitative relationship has been shown to exist between circulating AFP levels and the extent of malignant disease.[22]

Differentiation antigens are found on cells in normal differentiating tissue as well as tumor cells. These antigens generally are associated with T or B lymphocytes or their precursors. T-lymphocyte differentiation antigens are found in approximately 20% to 25% of all cases of acute lymphoblastic leukemia.[22] They also appear in chronic lymphoblastic leukemia (predominantly of the B-lymphocyte type) and lymphoblastic lymphoma.[16]

Lineage-associated determination antigens are being studied in solid tumors. One example, CA-125, appears in the serum of patients with ovarian cancer. Generally, CA-125 levels are used to assess responsiveness to treatment every 2 or 3 months; level fluctuations have been shown to be closely associated with tumor burden, indicating disease response to chemotherapy.[22]

Viral antigens represent another class of tumor-associated antigens. In Burkitt's lymphoma, EBV-infected cells shed T-lymphocyte antigens. Viral T-lymphocyte antigens are also present in T-cell leukemia. Antibodies to these virally induced antigens may be useful as a treatment option.[18]

Tumor-associated antigens are not perfect predictors of cancer occurrence or response. These antigens lack specificity for tumor; they may also lack correlation to true tumor burden when used as a measurement of treatment success. Tumor-associated antigen levels also may be falsely increased or decreased in individuals who do not have cancer.

Therapy options using TAAs remain open. Antigen-specific monoclonal antibodies may be used to identify and attack specific cancer cells. Whether antigens will be used as treatment markers or as diagnostic indicators, nurses will need to understand the importance of antigen use and ensure that sampling times and methods are accurate.[23] Explanations to patients regarding tumor-associated antigens used to determine tumor response to treatment and to detect early recurrence will be necessary. Although these antigens are a source of information to the clinician, they may also be a source of anxiety to patients.

Immune Surveillance Concept

The demonstration of a cell-mediated immune reaction to the presence of tumor antigens led Thomas[24] and later Burnet[25] to postulate the "immune surveillance" theory of the lymphoid system. They suggested that many cells undergo neoplastic transformation in the body but that the T cells of the lymphoid system continually seek out and destroy these malignant cells through recognition of tumor-associated antigens. If a tumor cell manages to escape this surveillance and supposed destruction, a clinically evident tumor will eventually develop. Any compromise in the immune system itself would, therefore, interfere with this surveillance capacity.

Evidence

Many clinical laboratory observations offer supportive evidence of this surveillance theory. The first observation is the increased incidence of cancer existing in the elderly. The body tends to lose its ability to differentiate self from nonself in the later years; autoimmune connective tissue disorders begin to appear. The surveillance mechanism becomes impaired and the ability to respond to the challenge of foreign antigens decreases. Abnormal cells may be allowed to proliferate unnoticed and cancer sometimes results.

Additional evidence in support of this theory lies in the fact that genetically thymectomized mice will accept tumor transplants, whereas such transplants are rejected by mice with normal thymic function. These same thymectomized animals were shown to have an increased incidence of cancer growth when exposed to oncogenic DNA viruses.[26] The presence of thymus-dependent T lymphocytes, therefore, seems to have an essential role in the recognition or destruction of foreign invaders.

Reports of spontaneous tumor regressions, although usually anecdotal in nature, add enthusiasm to the support of immune surveillance. These cases involve the shrinkage or total regression of tumors without the benefit of present-day systemic therapy. Regressions have been reported most frequently in persons with non-Hodgkin's lymphoma, renal cell carcinoma, breast and ovarian carcinoma, and malignant melanoma.[27,28] The concept that the immunogenicity of these clinically evident tumors has initiated recognition and launched a spontaneous immune reaction offers an attractive explanation for these otherwise unexplained phenomena.

The widely differing courses of some types of tumors in different persons is an unexplained phenomenon in oncology. Some tumors progress very slowly while others of the same type advance rapidly and unsparingly. After therapy for some malignancies patients often appear to have no evidence of disease; yet they will frequently have a recurrence long after the initial treatment. The answer to such mysteries may lie in the natural defenses of the host. Individual levels of immunocompetence may result in variability in the course of the disease.

The significance of tumor lymphocyte infiltration also offers strong evidence of the feasibility of the concept of immunosurveillance. The histologic picture of tumors infiltrated with lymphocytes, plasma cells, and macrophages is commonly seen during the rejection of antigenic tumors in animals.[29] A similar histologic picture is seen in normal tissue grafts of both animals and humans during the process of rejection. This reaction, an apparent hallmark of tissue rejection, has not only been carefully observed in some individuals with breast cancer, but the presence of such cellular infiltrates could be correlated with more favorable prognoses than in persons whose tumors did not appear to be infiltrated. This reaction suggests that the host immune cells were capable of reducing the rate of growth and metastasis of primary tumors.[30]

Observations regarding the immunosuppressed or immunodeficient individual offer further credence to the existence of immunosurveillance. Persons receiving long-term immunosuppressive therapy after renal or cardiac transplantation have an approximately 300-fold increased incidence of cancer compared with a normal population.[15] Individuals with congenital immunodeficiency diseases were reported to have a 10,000 times greater likelihood of developing cancer than a normal, age-matched control population.[31] Although such findings seem to point to the necessity of an intact immune system in the protection against cancer, a flaw in this argument must be considered. In both patient populations mentioned, the cancers reported were not representative of the types one would expect to see. In 80% of the immunodeficient persons tumors tended to develop in the lymphoreticular tissues—the site of their primary pathogenic disturbance. Perhaps the increased incidence of malignancy in this population is a direct result of some pathogenic abnormality, genetic or acquired, in the lymphoid tissue rather than being due to an actual decrease in immunity. The immunosuppressed persons also showed an unusual pattern of neoplasms, with a high incidence of lymphoid malignancies. This deviation may be a result of overstimulation of the lymphoid system in an attempt to reject the transplanted organ. The increased incidence of malignancy could also be a carcinogenic effect of the immunosuppressive drugs rather than an actual immune suppression reaction.

This theory has been similarly applied to persons who, having been cured by chemotherapy of their original neoplasms, are being seen with second malignancies. Scientists are considering the carcinogenic effect of chemotherapeutic agents; however, studies suggest persons with malignancy may have inherent immune-response abnormalities. Forty-seven long-term survivors of Hodgkin's disease who had undergone methotrexate-oncovin-prednisone-phenylalamine (MOPP) chemotherapy[32] demonstrated persistent immunologic abnormalities that could not be attributed to chemotherapy alone, since such abnormalities were not noted in a control group of survivors of diffuse histiocytic lymphoma who had received similar chemotherapeutic regimens.

Although some researchers remain skeptical of immunosurveillance as the specific mechanism whereby the body destroys naturally occurring tumors, the theory remains attractive for analyzing observations of the occurrence of cancer. Mitchell and Bertram[15] suggest that the theory, as proposed by Burnet in 1967, may need some modification. They suggest that non-T cells may be more important in immunosurveillance than T cells and that the target of the surveillance may be the etiologic agent rather than the cell itself. Further testing of the hypothesis will continue to shed light on the controversy.

Mechanisms of Tumor Destruction

Tumor cell destruction is accomplished by the coordination of a number of immune system components:

Lymphocyte

The lymphocyte response to tumor burden involves two lymphocyte populations. Helper T lymphocytes mediate the secretion of lymphokines, which activate macrophages or NK cells to nonspecifically destroy tumor cells. Lymphokines released by helper T lymphocytes also activate killer (cytotoxic) T lymphocytes that are capable of directly lysing tumor cells. Helper T lymphocytes also stimulate immunity by interacting with antigen presented by macrophages and subsequently with B lymphocytes in the production of antibody.

Macrophage

Macrophages initiate virtually every immune response by attaching antigenic material on their cell membrane and presenting it to T lymphocytes. This event stimulates the release of lymphokines such as interleukin-1, leading to the activation and clonal proliferation of T-lymphocyte subsets. In turn, macrophages are nonspecifically activated by the lymphokines to kill tumor cells and are major effector cells for this process.

Effector macrophages participate in killing tumor cells

directly, primarily by inhibiting their growth and, less important, by cytolysis.[1,18,19]

Natural killer cells

The hypothesis that NK cells can prevent the growth of a tumor is based on laboratory research demonstrating that "nude" mice that are genetically deficient in T lymphocytes but in which NK cells are particularly active are not susceptible to tumor development. In contrast, "beige" mice, which lack NK-cell activity, are susceptible to tumor development.[33]

NK cells are antigen-nonspecific effector cells that are capable of lysing tumor cells in vitro and are thought to inhibit tumor cell metastasis.[6] NK cells are thought to provide the host with a "natural immunity," for they are capable of effecting an immune response without prior sensitization to the agent.

B lymphocytes

Research has suggested that antibody responses occur to tumor antigens shed from human tumors.[10] Antibodies may mediate tumor lysis by binding to tumor cell and activating complement or by antibody-dependent cell-mediated cytotoxicity (ADCC), in which IgG antibodies bridge tumor cell receptors with macrophage or granulocyte receptors, causing lysis of tumor cells.

Escape of Tumor Cells from Antitumor Immunity

In the face of apparently effective antitumor immune mechanisms, how do antigen-bearing tumors proliferate seemingly undetected by the body's immune system? Ironically, the same mechanisms designed to prevent tumor cell proliferation are altered by the tumor in such a way that tumor proliferation is allowed or enhanced. A number of "escape" mechanisms are described below.

Suppressor cells

Suppressor cells participate normally in the body's immune response but are also an important factor in escape of tumors from antitumor immune mechanisms. Tumor cells release antigens that exaggerate immune regulation leading to excessive activity of suppressor T lymphocytes and subsequently to diminished antitumor immunity.[3] Some investigators have demonstrated that certain types of antitumor chemotherapeutic agents (cyclophosphamide, busulfan, 6-mercaptopurine, and mitomycin-C) have eliminated suppressor T-cell activity in vivo.[34,35]

Blocking factors

The presence of "blocking factors" was first documented by Hellstrom and Hellstrom[36] when it was thought that tumor antibodies coated the surfaces of tumor cells, preventing recognition and destruction of tumor antigen by sensitized T lymphocytes. It is now established that specific antigen-antibody complexes are responsible for the blocking of antitumor mechanisms, probably through stimulation of suppressor T-cell activity.[37] Circulating immune complexes have been noted in melanoma, neuroblastoma, breast and ovarian carcinomas, and Hodgkin's disease.[16]

Antigenic modulation

Antibody is thought to be capable of suppressing antigen synthesis, thus permitting altered cells to proliferate undetected in a highly immunized host; this process is called antigenic modulation.[38] Antibody may stimulate movement or shedding of antigens, which affects the immunogenicity of the cell.

Tumor antigen heterogeneity

A tumor may have many different antigens on its cell surface. These antigens may be expressed by the tumor at different times. Thus the body would need to mount an immune response to many different antigens on one tumor. Individual immune systems may not be able to respond to all expressed antigens, or the immune system may miss them in their sporadic presentation.[39]

Others

All other factors that are known to decrease the immune response, such as aging, genetic defects, infection, stress, chemotherapy, surgery, infection, or malnutrition, must be considered as obstacles to human immune surveillance.

RATIONALE FOR IMMUNOTHERAPY

Since there is evidence supporting theories that the immune system has an impact on the formation of cancer, it is reasonable to examine the immune system as a possible modality for the treatment of cancer. If the immune system can be stimulated to overcome tumor growth, a fourth treatment modality exists, to be used alone or in combination for the treatment of cancer. Questions remain as to which cellular components of the immune system should be enhanced, or whether certain steps of the immune process should be targeted. Barriers to immune destruction of tumor exist when host immunocompetence is compromised, tumor burden is large, and immunogenicity of neoplasms changes or is difficult to identify. As we gain a better understanding of the immune system and of a person's biologic response to malignancy, we will learn techniques to manipulate that response in a beneficial way.

IMMUNOCOMPETENCE AND CANCER

How Immunocompetence Affects Malignancy

Cancers, specifically lymphomas and leukemias, appear when the immune system is compromised. Aberrations in B cells yield chronic lymphocytic leukemia and multiple myeloma; aberrations in T cells yield Hodgkin's disease and squamous cell cancer of the head and neck.[40] The reasons these diseases become manifest in immunocompromised patients are unknown. Decreased T- or B-cell competence may be the precursor of cancer formation, but altered immunoregulatory function, such as decreased phagocytic activity, may also be important. Recent research has focused on regional immune function and its reaction to malignancy. Research into the immunology of the skin has shown that carcinogens and/or radiation make functional alterations in epidermal Langerhans cells, which are antigen-presenting (phagocytic) cells of the skin. As a result, outside antigens fail to elicit a normal immune response and, instead, have shown to increase suppressor T-cell activity. The hypothesis is that carcinogens may affect local immune cells, causing suppressive immune responses and allowing malignancy to develop.[41] Similar response of suppressive T-cell activity is noted in individuals with acquired immune deficiency disease in whom Kaposi's sarcoma develops. Thus it is clear that the immune system needs to be considered as a factor in the development of malignancy.

How Malignancy Affects Immunocompetence

Changes in immunocompetence may occur as a result of cancer. Cancer produces immune system depression, progressing to a state of immune unresponsiveness (anergy). Several changes are noted in persons with tumors. Granulocyte abnormalities are found in patients with acute lymphoblastic leukemia, acute and chronic myelogenous leukemia, and multiple myeloma.[42] Research indicates that patients with a variety of cancers have a defect in monocyte chemotactic response. One model proposes that certain proteins may be responsible for suppressing lymphocyte and natural killer cell and macrophage and monocyte activity in the person with cancer.[43]

Bone marrow tumors eliminate normal immune cellular growth within the marrow, predisposing patients to low white blood cell counts and subsequent infection. Lymph organs, such as nodes or spleen, may become necrotic because of a compromised blood supply or may be directly invaded by tumor, with interruption of lymphogenous flow. Tumors may cause organ or tissue breakdown through direct growth and extension, increasing the likelihood of infection. Decline in nutritional status from cancer anorexia or cachexia leads to further immunocompromise.[42]

How Cancer Treatment Affects Immunocompetence

The effect of cancer treatment on immunocompetence is great in an already compromised host. Each type of treatment brings unique problems to the immune system. (See Part III, Treatment Modalities.)

Surgery

Surgery affects immunocompetence by eliciting the stress response, including glucocorticoid release from the adrenal glands. Surgery increases cortisol release in patients both with and without cancer. The action of cortisol has to be examined if its effect on the immune system is to be understood. Cortisol affects metabolism, immunity, and blood volume.

Normal amounts of cortisol regulate production of inflammatory mediators (namely, interleukin, histamine, and bradykinins) released in response to injury. When large amounts of cortisol are released, many immunologic functions are inhibited. Glucocorticoids also inhibit macrophage and neutrophil chemotaxis, suppress natural killer cell activity, and decrease the action of complement. Thus when cortisol is released during surgery, the patient's immune function is potentially compromised.[44]

Surgical removal of lymph tissue (such as axillary lymph node dissection in modified radical mastectomy) impairs the transport of lymph from the affected area, predisposing patients to swelling, lymphadenopathy, and infection. Decreased immune function caused by the tumor also increases susceptibility to postsurgical infection. Removal of other organs of the immune system, for example, the spleen alters immune function and predisposes the patient to infection.

Chemotherapy

The action of chemotherapy at therapeutic dose levels decreases immunoresponsiveness anytime within 1 to 3 weeks of therapy. The immune suppression is understood to be a consequence of general inhibition of cell proliferation and specifically of bone marrow stem cells. Higher doses, in frequent-interval dosing schedules, increase immunosuppressive effects. Subtherapeutic small doses have been shown to potentiate the immune responses in certain chemotherapeutic agents. Mastrangelo et al.[45] explains that in vitro cytoxan augments immunity by selective toxicity for suppressor T lymphocytes and their precursors, allowing helper T lymphocytes greater activity.

Glucocorticoids administered in conjunction with chemotherapeutic agents further inhibit immune function and cell proliferation but are used to enhance the cell-killing capacity of chemotherapy.[44]

The immunosuppressive effects of chemotherapeutic agents depend on the type of drug administered and at what point in cell division an agent attacks the cell. Alkylating agents, for example, kill both proliferating and nonproliferating cells, but antimetabolites work more effectively on actively dividing cells. Thus the amount of damage to bone marrow immunologic stem cells depends on combinations of chemotherapy used, the dosages, and the timing of therapy. Frequently, in patients receiving high-dose chemotherapy, immune system dysfunction will limit further doses and may require increased intervals between treatment cycles to avoid total collapse of the immune response.[46,47]

Despite the decreased immune function in patients undergoing chemotherapy, anaphylaxis remains possible with the administration of several chemotherapeutic agents. Anaphylaxis-inducing chemotherapeutic agents include L-asparaginase, cisplatin, cyclophosphamide, cytarabine, bleomycin, doxorubicin, methotrexate, and dacarbazine. Since anaphylaxis is largely an immunoglobulin-driven process that is not affected by cytotoxic drugs, patients with immune compromise from previous therapy can still mount an anaphylactic response to chemotherapy and blood products. In certain situations, test doses should be given before the first dose of the drug. Anaphylaxis can occur in response to subsequent drug doses as well.

Chemotherapy further contributes to compromised immune function by often necessitating the use of multiple intravenous sites that disturb the skin barrier and by compromised nutritional status resulting from drug treatment–induced anorexia.

Radiotherapy

Radiotherapy to the bone marrow destroys stem cells, thereby affecting the population of lymphocytes available to effect an immune response. While lymphocytes are most readily affected by radiation, macrophages and plasma cells remain relatively radioresistant.[40] In adults, when the sternum or pelvis is included in the radiation field, immune function must be monitored by observation of white blood cell levels. In children, marrow cells of long bones produce stem cells and thus, when included in the field, predispose the patient to a decreased immune response. Total nodal radiation used in lymphoma therapy produces prolonged T-cell depression. Radiation effects on bone marrow occur when any significant body area is irradiated, with the exception of the head and neck.

Fractionated radiation therapy, which is used most frequently today, diminishes damage to marrow stem cells; thus decreases in white blood cell function are small and often transitory. Radiation in preparation for bone marrow transplantation produces massive suppression of the immune system, since it is designed to eliminate functioning bone marrow.

CONCLUSION

Research into the response of the immune system continues to provide information that aids in tumor detection, monitoring, and treatment. A thorough understanding of the immune system is now an essential part of oncology nursing.

REFERENCES

1. Roitt I, Broff J, Male D: Immunology. St Louis, CV Mosby Co, 1985.
2. Huffner TL, Kanapa DJ, Stevenson GW: Introduction to Immunology. Boston, Jones and Bartlett, 1986.
3. Barrett J: Textbook of Immunology. St Louis, CV Mosby Co, 1983.
4. Grady C: Host defense mechanisms: An overview. Semin Oncol Nurs 4:86-94, 1988.
5. Bellanti J: Immunology Basic Processes. Philadelphia, WB Saunders, 1985.
6. Lotzova E: Immunobiology of Natural Killer Cells. Boca Raton, Fla, CRC Press, 1986.
7. Herberman R, Ortaldo J: Natural killer cells: Their role in defenses against disease. Science 214:24-30, 1981.
8. Miller WU, Rodey G: HLA without tears. Chicago, American Society of Clinical Pathologists, 1981.
9. Kluger MJ, Oppenheim JJ, Powanda MC (eds): The Physiologic, Metabolic and Immunologic Actions of Interleukin-1. New York, Alan R. Liss, 1985.
10. Stites D, Stobo J, Funderberg H, et al: Basic and Clinical Immunology (ed 6). Los Altos, Calif, Lange, 1987.
11. Hood LE, Weissman IL, Wood NB, et al: Immunology. Menlo Park, Calif, Benjamin Cummings, 1984.
12. Kupchella CE: The immune system and cancer, in Dimensions of Cancer. Belmont, Calif, Wadsworth Publishing, 1987, pp 240-246.
13. Foley EJ: Antigenic properties of methylcholanthrene-induced tumors in mice of strain of origin. Cancer Res 13:835-837, 1953.
14. Prehn RT, Main JM: Immunity to methylcholanthrene-induced sarcomas. J Natl Cancer Institute 18:769-778, 1957.
15. Mitchell MS, Bertram JH: Immunology and biomodulation of cancer, in Calabresi P, Schein PS, Rosenberg SA (eds): Medical Oncology. New York, Macmillan, 1985, pp 363-391.
16. Turk JL, Hosokawa M: Regulation of the immune response, in Mihich E, Sakurai Y (eds): Biologic Responses to Cancer. vol 3. New York, Plenum Press, 1985, pp 29-46.
17. Lennox ES, Howe AB, and Evan G: Specific antigens on methylcholanthrene-induced tumors of mice. Transplantation Proceedings 13:1759-1761, 1981.
18. Virji M, Mercer D, Herberman R: Tumor markers in cancer: Diagnosis and prognosis. CA-A Cancer Journal for Clinicians 38:104-126, 1988.
19. Gold P, Freedman SO: Demonstration of tumor-specific antigens in human colonic carcinomata by immunological tolerance and absorption techniques. J Exp Med 121:439-462, 1965.
20. Fletcher RH: Carcinoembryonic antigen. Ann Intern Med 104:66-73, 1986.
21. Abelev GI, et al: Production of embryonal alpha globulin by transplanting mouse hepatomas. Transplantation 1:174-180, 1963.
22. Sulitzeanu D: Human cancer associated antigens: Present status and implications for immunodiagnosis. Adv Cancer Res 44:1-33, 1985.
23. Lovejoy N, Thomas M, Hallisburton P, et al: Tumor markers: Relevance to clinical practice. Oncol Nurs Forum 14:5, 75-82, 1987.
24. Thomas L: Discussion, in Lawrence HW (ed): Cellular and humoral aspects of the hypersensitive states. New York, Harper and Row, 1959.

25. Burnet FM: Immunologic aspects of malignant disease. Lancet 1:1171-1174, 1967.
26. Allison AC, Taylor RB: Observations on thymectomy and carcinogenesis. Cancer Res 27:703-707, 1967.
27. Drobyski WR, Qzai R: Spontaneous regression in non-Hodgkin's lymphoma: Clinical and pathogenic considerations. Am J Hematol 31:2, 138-141, 1989.
28. Pitot HC: Fundamentals of Oncology. New York: Marcell Dekker, 1986.
29. Herberman RB: Immune defense mechanisms in tumor immunity, in Bellanti JA, et al (eds): Immunology III. Philadelphia, WB Saunders, 1985, pp 330-345.
30. Berman LD: Immune parameters in the host response to neoplasia: Morphological considerations, in Reif AE (ed): Immunity and Cancer in Man. New York, Marcel Dekker, 1975, pp 121-129.
31. Good RA, Finstad J: Essential relationship between the lymphoid system, immunity, and malignancy. National Cancer Inst. Monograph 31:41-58, 1969.
32. Fisher RI, et al: Persistent immunologic abnormalities in long term survivors of advanced Hodgkin's disease. Ann Intern Med 92:595-599, 1980.
33. Riesenfeld I, Morgan AC, Bumol TF, et al: Positive correlation between in vitro NK activity and in vitro resistance to AKR lymphoma cells. Int J Cancer 25:399-403, 1980.
34. Ray PK, Raychaudhuri S: Low dose cyclophosphamide inhibition of transplantable fibrosarcoma growth by augmentation of the host immune response. J Natl Cancer Inst 67:1341-1345, 1981.
35. Kataoka T: Effect of antineoplastic agents on the induction of suppressor macrophages by concanavalin A-bound tumor vaccine. Cancer Res 41:5151-5157, 1981.
36. Hellstrom I, Hellstrom RE: Immunologic enhancement of tumor growth, in Green I, Cohen S, McClaskey RT (eds): Mechanisms of Tumor Immunity. New York, Wiley, 1977, pp 98-116.
37. Mitchell MS, Rao VS: The interrelationship of immune complexes and suppressor T cells in the suppression of macrophages, in Saunders JP, Daniels JC, Serrau B, et al (eds): Fundamental Mechanisms of Human Cancer Immunology. New York, Elsevier—North Holland, 1981, pp 279-291.
38. Kirkpatrick CH, Fahey J: Tumor immunology: clinical aspects. JAMA 248:20, 2722-2726, 1982.
39. US Department of Health, Education, and Welfare. "Immunology—Its Role in Disease and Health," Summary Report of Task Force on Immunology and Disease. NIH 75-940.
40. Bast RC: Principles of cancer biology: Tumor immunology, in DeVita V, Hellman S, Rosenberg S (eds): Principles and Practice of Oncology. Philadelphia, JB Lippincott, 1985, pp 125-150.
41. Kripke L: Immunoregulation of carcinogens: Past, present, and future. J Natl Cancer Inst 80:10, 722-727, 1988.
42. Gallucci B: The immune system and cancer. Oncol Nurs Forum 14:6, 1987, (suppl 3-10).
43. Cianciolo GJ, Synderman R: Effects of tumor growth on host defenses. Cancer Metast Rev 5:15-27, 1981.
44. Schwartz SI, Shires GT, Spencer FC: Principles of Surgery (ed 5). New York, McGraw-Hill, 1989, pp 1563-1564.
45. Mastrangelo M, Berd D, Magoine H: The immunoaugmenting effects of cancer chemotherapeutic agents. Semin Oncol 13:2, 186-194, 1986.
46. Carter SK, Glafstein E, Livingston RB: Principles of Cancer Treatment. New York, McGraw-Hill, 1982, p 85.
47. DeVita VT: Principles of chemotherapy, in Devita VT, Hellman S, Rosenberg SA (eds): Cancer: Principles and Practice of Oncology (ed 4). Philadelphia, JB Lippincott, 1989, pp 276-296.

PART II

PREVENTION, DETECTION, AND DIAGNOSIS

Chapter 6

Factors Affecting Health Behavior

Joanne Disch, RN, PhD

Mary Dee McEvoy, RN, PhD

INTRODUCTION

Social scientists and health care professionals have long sought to ascribe some method, some predictability to health behavior. More important, once a pattern was formed, the goal was to modify the behavior and effect healthful practices—in other words, to promote compliance with health care regimens.

Of particular relevance to this text is health and illness behavior as it relates to cancer. Although much of the general data available on health and illness behavior apply to this more specific subgroup, some factors are either specific to or heightened by the diagnosis of cancer. Also of particular importance to the practitioner for whom this book is written are suggestions for interventions to foster a positive health orientation and to facilitate the incorporation of healthful behaviors into an individual's lifestyle.

This chapter presents information on some of the different forms of health and illness behavior, particularly as they occur in individuals with cancer. Two models (the health belief model and models of helping and coping) are described briefly and are used as frameworks within which to identify factors that influence health behavior related to cancer. Several of these predominant factors are presented, and strategies for assisting individuals who have cancer to cope with their disease are offered.

HEALTH BEHAVIOR

Health behavior consists of a set of activities in which a person engages to maximize wellness and avoid illness. These activities include measures that are initiated and controlled by the individual, as well as those that occur in a more structured setting, such as preventive health programs or screening or diagnostic opportunities.

A person can exhibit positive health behaviors in relation to cancer in various ways:

- By performing a monthly self-examination of breasts or testes
- By undergoing regular Papanicolaou (Pap) smear testing
- By giving up smoking or never starting to smoke
- By decreasing fat intake and increasing amount of fiber in daily diet
- By avoiding excessive exposure to known carcinogens

A person can therefore maximize wellness by actively doing something to promote health or by avoiding something that would endanger health. Health behavior, then, can represent acts of commission or of omission with regard to health matters.

ILLNESS BEHAVIOR

The person in whom a particular disease has been diagnosed or is suspected engages in illness behavior. Illness behavior has been defined as "any activity undertaken by a person who feels ill, to define the state of his health and to discover a suitable remedy."[1] Activities involved in this endeavor include perceiving a symptom, complaining of it, and seeking and undergoing treatment. Illness behavior pertaining to cancer might involve a return visit to the physician because a Papanicolaou smear report indicated atypical cells. It might involve undergoing chemotherapy or radiotherapy, or it might involve ceasing to smoke in response to the development of persistent hoarseness.

The distinction between health behavior and illness behavior for an individual is understandably blurred and in some instances nonexistent. What is done to maintain health in some situations may overlap with what is done to decrease the effects of a particular illness in others. Furthermore, blurring occurs because health-related activities engaged in by a person who has been found to have a disease depend not only on the fact that a diagnosis has been made but also on that person's perception of the disease. For example, is the person with no apparent symptoms engaging in health behavior or illness behavior with relation to cancer when visiting the physician for a checkup? Is a person considered to be ill or to be a patient when the diagnosis is made or when feeling ill? The distinctions are subtle and are considered unimportant by some health professionals, but they influence how individuals respond to persons with cancer, particularly if there is dissonance between perceptions.

MALADAPTIVE BEHAVIOR

As there are positive health and illness behaviors, there are also negative or maladaptive behaviors, which can adversely affect a person's health. Examples of negative or maladaptive behaviors include continuing to smoke after various suggestive signs have appeared; failing to have periodic Pap smears; forgetting to do or choosing not to do monthly breast self-examinations; failing to report a change in the appearance of a mole; and deciding that the hoarseness that has persisted for 6 months is a result of encroaching old age.

Noncompliance

One form of behavior that has often been labeled as maladaptive is noncompliance. Compliance exists when an individual carries out orders with regard to a health-related regimen. Individuals who fail to adhere to recommendations are termed noncompliers or defaulters, and health care researchers have extensively scrutinized the characteristics of these persons. Factors related to compliance include individual characteristics (age, sex, education, and race), perceptions of the disease, disease and treatment factors (stage of the disease and complexity and duration of the treatment), and social support.[2] Noncompliance has been further examined in relation to the concept of barriers. Barriers can be defined as the general costs associated with taking a particular health action and include system barriers, time, distance, cost, availability, and discrimination.[3]

Failure to participate in available preventive health programs or to adhere to indicated health care programs can present many problems. Possible benefits of treatment may be interrupted or decreased and, at the very least, are usually difficult to measure. Treatable disease may progress unnecessarily to untreatable states. Compliance is seen as a major, if not *the* major, determinant of efficacy in regard to some medications. If the expected benefits of a drug are not evident, additional diagnostic tests or treatments may be required, thus increasing costs. Additional time must be spent in counseling and in the administration and interpretation of tests.

Persons who diverge from expected health behavior are labeled noncompliant, deviant, unreliable, disobedient, and uncooperative. The relationship between the patient and the health caregiver is usually affected. The physician or nurse becomes frustrated, and the patient becomes dissatisfied with either the lack of improvement or the relationship. Dissatisfaction with the health care system ensues. More important, the patient's health can deteriorate unnecessarily and perhaps irreversibly.

In recent years there has been a trend away from compliance as a goal and toward the concept of adherence. Whereas to some compliance implies passive obedience, adherence connotes a greater degree of active participation. The patient adheres to a regimen because it seems, for one reason or another, to be consistent with his or her estimation of the situation.

Delay in Seeking Care

One form of maladaptive behavior—delay in seeking health services—has been seen especially often in the person who is seeking health care for the diagnosis or treatment of cancer. Delay can occur in several ways. There can be delay in reporting symptoms or in following up with an indicated regimen. Occasionally, however, an individual may not intend, consciously or unconsciously, to put off diagnosis or treatment. That person may truly not appreciate the importance of the symptoms or events. If the symptoms are subclinical, the individual may not even be aware of them.

Unavoidable delay occurs when no signs or symptoms are readily apparent to an individual or can be overlooked easily or ascribed to a benign cause (for example, a persistent cough after influenza). What also may be considered as unavoidable delay is the situation in which an individual is aware of a symptom but cannot see a physician for some time. In addition, legitimate turnaround time between the presentation of the individual for evaluation and the reporting of results and the initiation of treatment can contribute to unavoidable delay.

Avoidable delay, the focus of most of the articles on delay in the literature, is usually considered to occur when there is some earlier stimulus for action that could or should have moved the person to seek health care. In this type of situation, lack of knowledge or the vagueness of a symptom may have contributed to the person's hesitation to seek help. The person who was more knowledgeable or vigilant in matters related to health might have sought help earlier. Recently attention has been given to ways to encourage patient response to positive screening results. For example, Lauver[4] has studied how the manner of presentation of the results of a Papanicolaou smear in a positive or a negative way affects a woman's delay in coming for colposcopy. She found that there was no relationship between how information is presented and follow-up care.

THEORETICAL FRAMEWORKS

Health Belief Model

Much research has been devoted to development of theories that attempt to explain human behavior as it relates to health. Probably one of the better known theories that attempt to explain the vagaries of health behavior is the Health Belief Model.[5,6] Devised by Leventhal and colleagues in the early 1950s, it is a model often used in oncology, particularly to study breast self-examination practices.[7,8] It originated in the theories of Kurt Lewin, who postulated that the individual is the prime determinant of action in a given situation. The environment is important only as it is perceived by the individual. Certain areas in life are viewed positively, whereas others are negative. Fear of cancer, for example, could be considered as a positive force because it motivates the individual to perform a particular action, such as monthly breast self-examination. However, if performing the examination brings the individual into an area of negativity (for example, finding a lump means chemotherapy or possibly loss of a breast), that person may consciously or subconsciously "forget" to do the breast self-examination. Therefore, life may be viewed as a series of positive and negative forces influencing a person's daily activities.

In this framework, then, beliefs are important and are thought to be supremely influential in a person's decision about a particular action. The major determinant influencing a particular action is the perceived threat of a specific disease. This perception of threat arises from two factors: perceived susceptibility to or possibility of contracting a particular disease and the perceived severity of the disease.

Another important determinant influencing the chosen course of action is the individual's belief concerning the usefulness of the various courses of action available. The person must believe that one or more courses of action could decrease the likelihood of getting the disease or improve the prognosis if the disease is already present and that the action or actions would not entail a greater cost (in the form of pain, time, money, and so on). To participate in preventive actions, the individual must believe that prevention is available and know where and how to obtain the required service. To participate in screening or diagnostic procedures, the individual must believe, at least to some extent:

- That it is possible to have the disease and not have symptoms
- That techniques currently available can detect the presence of both symptomatic and asymptomatic disease
- That symptoms may indicate a specific disease
- That early detection improves the prognosis
- That the facilities and personnel available can perform the test competently

To adhere to a treatment regimen, the patient must believe that the potential benefits of therapy outweigh the negative aspects.

A final crucial determinant is the importance the individual places on health and health matters. The person who values health is more likely to take steps to ensure its maintenance. The person who gives little thought or emphasis to health and illness may place a low priority on health-related activities.

Beliefs arise from various origins, including personal experience, tradition, and introduction by others. They gain strength by (1) concurrence in the belief by family and significant others, (2) successful testing of the belief over time, (3) compatibility of the belief with other beliefs or known facts, and (4) reinforcement of the belief by valued sources.

Foremost in the decision to seek health care is belief in the efficacy of care. Does the person perceive the course of action to be available, effective, and relatively "cost" free? Opinions vary widely in regard to cancer screening programs and available treatment methods. Hence, an almost fatalistic perception in this area could modify and possibly counteract a strong belief concerning severity or susceptibility to cancer.

One confounding aspect in the application of the Health Belief Model is that persons who are more inclined to initiate preventive health measures do not show a greater tendency to participate in diagnostic programs or increased compliance with a specific treatment regimen. In fact, studies show that adherence to one component of a regimen is not necessarily a valid predictor of whether a person will adhere to other components.[1,5] This is true partly because the stimulus that may direct a person to seek treatment is often the presence of a symptom (eg, persistent hoarseness), whereas the motivation to participate in preventive or diagnostic procedures when symptoms are absent may be unknown or a complex interplay of contributing variables. Kasl[5] has found that compliance in one role is correlated only modestly with compliance in another role. There seems to be no general health orientation to behavior, but there may be medical care habits or clinic habits by which patients get into more routine patterns of behavior and therefore use health care services as a general rule and not in response to specific diseases.

Models of Helping and Coping

Because the Health Belief Model alone does not completely explain behavior in a number of instances, the use of additional models in conjunction with the Health Belief Model offers an interesting perspective. These are the models of Helping and Coping.[9,10] The four models within the set differentiate between attribution of responsibility for a problem (who is to blame for a problem occurring) and attribution of responsibility for the solution (who is to deal with the situation). Thus the theory addresses the behavior of both helpers and recipients of help (helpees). Consequently, the framework is called the model of Helping and Coping, depending on the perspective.

The four models are summarized in Table 6-1. Individuals operating under the *moral model* view themselves as being responsible for creating the problem, as well as for solving it. A problem persists because the individual is lazy or has not exerted the necessary effort to deal with it. Professionals or friends are not expected to help; nor are they really able to help, except for perhaps encouraging the individual to change and improve. The problem is the individual's own doing, and he or she needs to correct it. The philosophy of the *est* movement exemplifies the moral model.

With the *compensatory model,* individuals are not responsible for the existence of their problems. These may be due to a failure of the environment to provide adequate resources or services, or they may be due to an act of God. The individual, however, is responsible for correcting the problem, using whatever is necessary: creativity, special effort, or collaboration with others. Professionals can help by identifying and providing opportunities through which the patient can compensate for the deficit.

The moral and compensatory models are similar in that individuals are seen as responsible for resolving their own problems. Moreover, the decision as to what is or is not helpful rests with the helpees, not with the helpers. Brickman and colleagues[9] hypothesized that this would result in increased competence in the individual. In contrast, the other models have been hypothesized to increase dependence. The *medical model,* exemplified by the practice of modern medicine, assumes that individuals cannot solve their problems without expert help. In this way individuals cannot be blamed for their problems or given credit for solving them. Decisions as to the helpfulness of interventions rest with the professionals.

The *enlightenment model* also requires the efforts of others to solve a person's problems. However, this model places responsibility for the existence of the problem with the individual, thus inducing guilt and dependency. The model is so labeled because the individual has been enlightened and has seen the error of his or her ways, but control of the solution rests in the hands of others. Al-

TABLE 6-1 Consequences of Attribution of Responsibility in Four Models of Helping and Coping

Attribution to Self of Responsibility for Problem	Attribution to Self of Responsibility for Solution	
	High	Low
High	*Moral model*	*Enlightenment model*
Perception of self	Lazy	Guilty
Actions expected of self	Striving	Submission
Others beside self who must act	Peers	Authorities
Actions expected of others	Exhortation	Discipline
Implicit view of human nature	Strong	Bad
Potential pathology	Loneliness	Fanaticism
Low	*Compensatory model*	*Medical model*
Perception of self	Deprived	Ill
Actions expected of self	Assertion	Acceptance
Others beside self who must act	Subordinates	Experts
Actions expected of others	Mobilization	Treatment
Implicit view of human nature	Good	Weak
Potential pathology	Alienation	Dependency

Source: From Brickman P, et al: Models of helping and coping. Am Psychol 37:370, 1982. Copyright © 1982 by the American Psychologist Association. Reprinted by permission of the author.

coholics Anonymous is an example of a therapy based on this model.

Implications arising from the use of the models of Helping and Coping focus on the roles of helpers and helpees. Cronenwett[11] has raised a number of questions that may influence an individual's health behavior:

- Who is considered responsible for defining the patient's problems?
- Is the patient blamed for the problems?
- Is the patient expected to take responsibility for deciding on the appropriate solutions to the problems?
- Who judges the success or failure of the solutions?
- Are different helping models advocated in different situations, or is one model suggested for all nurse-patient relationships?

Understanding of the individual's attributions for responsibility is important, in that people may reject certain forms of therapy if the therapy is not congruent with the individual's perception of the cause of the disease. In addition, some may needlessly assume guilt when they accept the idea that their life-style or deficiencies have caused or influenced the course of their illness.

Application of the models of helping and coping to the person in whom cancer has been diagnosed suggests that no one model is sufficient for all situations. Although the medical model, historically used more frequently than the others, might be appropriate in some situations, it would be inappropriate in others. For example, a person who develops colorectal cancer of unknown origin and who has the involved area excised by an expert surgeon would not be held responsible for the problem or the solution. In another situation, however, when sustained management of a chronic form of cancer is indicated, use of the compensatory model may be more appropriate so that the patient can assume responsibility for carrying out the prescribed regimen.

An interesting application of this theory can be seen in the current debate on the relationship between psychosocial factors and cancer. Matje[12] has reviewed a number of studies that reported a relationship between these factors and the cause or course of malignant disease. In many instances it has been postulated that patients not only exert a positive influence on the course of their disease but may even be responsible for its existence. This would suggest assumptions compatible with the moral or compensatory models. Research by Cassileth and colleagues,[13] however, suggests that the psychosocial factors are not useful clinical predictors for certain patient populations and that the individual has perhaps less responsibility for influencing the course of his or her disease than had previously been thought. In a longitudinal study, Cassileth and colleagues[14] reported on psychosocial factors related to survival in two groups of patients, one with advanced disease and a poor prognosis and a group with an intermediate prognosis. The psychosocial factors studied included social ties, marital history, job satisfaction, life satisfaction, subjective view of health, and hopelessness. No psychosocial factor was found to relate to survival or remission.

Application of this theory also may shed light on why the use of the Health Belief Model alone as the theoretical framework is insufficient in some situations to predict a person's health behavior. It is conceivable that an individual could hold certain beliefs very strongly and yet not engage in health behavior if there were dissonance between the individual and the health professional as to each person's role in attributing responsibility for the cause of the problem, identifying the appropriate course of treatment, or evaluating the outcomes.

The Health Belief Model and the models of Helping and Coping suggest that a number of factors influence the health behavior of persons with a diagnosis of cancer. Among these are the individual's perception of the illness and the course of therapy, the character of the cancer, and the individual's sense of role identity and acceptance of role expectations in relation to cancer.

FACTORS AFFECTING HEALTH BEHAVIOR RELATED TO CANCER

Nature of the Disease

A major factor affecting health behavior in relation to cancer is the fact that cancer is the disease involved.[15,16] Although any disease is undesirable and connotes certain images, cancer seems to evoke special feelings, impressions, and reactions. This, in turn, affects the individual's behavior. In the provocative book entitled *Illness as Metaphor,* Sontag[17] speaks of the concept of punishment in relation to cancer:

> Punitive notions of disease have a long history, and such notions are particularly active with cancer. There is the fight or crusade against cancer; cancer is the "killer" disease; people who have cancer are "cancer victims." Ostensibly, the illness is the culprit. But it is also the cancer patient who is made culpable. Widely believed psychological theories of disease assign to the luckless ill the ultimate responsibility both for falling ill and for getting well. And conventions of treating cancer as no mere disease but a demonic enemy make cancer not just a lethal disease but a shameful one.

Cancer may force many individuals into a dependent role. Unlike other chronic diseases, cancer is often pictured as an invasion, a foreign substance that takes over certain body parts or functions. Individuals with cancer often see themselves as "victims," and this feeling may be accentuated by the fact that there are, for some forms of cancer, no guaranteed preventive measures to "ward off" the invader.

As an alternative point of view, Frank-Stromborg and colleagues[15] point out that the universal reaction to the diagnosis of cancer has not been supported through research but has emerged as a result of observations and anecdotes about individual reactions to the diagnosis of cancer. Of a total of 484 responses in a survey of ambulatory cancer patients, 27% reflected a positive attitude when the patients were asked their feelings on receiving the diagnosis of cancer. Comments such as "It came as such a relief because I was expecting the worst" or "I decided to beat/conquer the cancer" suggest that not everyone goes through predictable stages in reacting to the diagnosis of cancer.

Beliefs About the Disease

Studies have shown that people view cancer as being serious and likely to occur. A study in 1978 by the American Cancer Society[18] found that approximately one in three persons agreed with the following statements: "Getting cancer is the worst thing that could happen to a person" (37%) and "Getting cancer is a death sentence for most people" (36%). Moreover, almost half of the 1553 respondents agreed that "the word 'cancer' itself scares me." Regarding the public's perception of the incidence of cancer, only 24% correctly indicated that one out of four persons will get cancer; the incidence was underestimated by 63% of the respondents. Most people also underestimate the survival rate. In answer to the question, "How many people who get cancer will survive?" 65% of the respondents incorrectly chose the category "fewer than one out of three." More recent research indicates that negative attitudes continue to exist in spite of an effort toward public education. In a survey of black residents of northern California, it was found that, although knowledge of cancer was high, belief in the efficacy of treatment was low.[19] Although 89% of the sample believed that "someday a cure would be found," 65% of the women continued to believe that cancer was a "death sentence" and 75% believed that surgery caused it to spread through the air.

Yet research has also demonstrated that those with cancer often exhibit a positive frame of mind. For example, in a study of 33 women with breast cancer, Brandt[20] found that all but two subjects reported feelings of hopefulness. Further, in a study by Herth,[21] hopefulness was found to be positively correlated with coping.

Attitudes about cancer have been shown to influence whether and how soon a person seeks health care. An increasing belief in the curability of cancer has led to a decrease in delay, whereas the feeling that cancer is shameful has been shown to increase delay.[22] The individual who believes that one can have a disease without visible symptoms is more likely to seek help.[23] The person who perceives the symptoms as mild is less likely to seek help.[24] In a study requesting subjects to respond to a vignette describing a woman discovering a lump in her breast, Timko[25] found that delay in seeking care was related to attitudes toward delay and social pressure. Specifically, delay related to the perception of control over one's health and life as well as the belief that the symptom was not serious. It is logical, then, to expect that a person's beliefs (about health and illness, cancer, treatment, and health care) will have some impact on decisions related to health and illness behavior. These beliefs need to be recognized and incorporated in the formulation of a profile of the factors that influence a person's decision about health behavior.

Knowledge About the Disease

Exposure to facts about cancer is, in itself, inadequate to change behavior, because there may be other factors that are either unresponsive to education or are not always under the complete control of the individual. These factors include the nature of the health care system that is available; the social, economic, and political climate in which the individual and the health care system exist; and the individual's social and physical environment or lifestyle. Education alone cannot remove every obstacle to adherence to a therapeutic regimen. The more informed individual is not necessarily more compliant.

Education can, however, facilitate adherence. In a study of the health beliefs and knowledge about testicular cancer in a group of college men, Reno[26] reported that only 12 of 126 subjects practiced testicular self-examination. There was a significant difference in the amount of knowledge related to testicular cancer and testicular self-examination between those who practiced the screening examination and those who did not. However, the data on the practice of breast self-examination demonstrates conflicting results. Although 96% of women have knowledge of breast self-examination,[27] studies[28-30] indicate that it is practiced by only 14% to 40%. Lauver[31] studied the relationship between the practice of breast self-examination and the method of instruction. No difference was found between the groups receiving different types of instruction and the frequency of the practice of breast self-examination. However, regardless of type of instruction, the frequency of breast self-examination increased after teaching.

Knowledge may be necessary but not sufficient for actions relating to health. Knowledge of the seven danger signals can alert an individual as to what to watch for and report if an individual is so inclined and is able to do so; information as to where screening centers are located can direct an individual; facts about risks from cigarette smoking can frighten an individual. Education about cancer (the risk factors, warning signs, and diagnosis and treatment opportunities) is important. Knowledge about cancer will not, of itself, move a person to act. Therefore, it cannot be the only component in programs of cancer prevention and control if successful screening and treatment are to be accomplished.

The mass media have a tremendous influence on education of the public about health, illness, cancer, and so on. In addition, the mass media frequently direct persons toward the appropriate facilities. With the increased incorporation of messages about cancer into news articles, programs, television, movies, talk shows, and the like, people have become more willing to participate in screening programs, seek treatment, and share their experiences for the benefit of others. The visibility associated with former President and Mrs. Reagan's cancer experiences, for example, stimulated many people to undergo screening for cancer and made it more acceptable for those with cancer to share their experiences with others.

Modifying Factors

Several demographic factors combine to influence health behavior, including education level, socioeconomic status (SES), age, and sex. Each factor alone probably does not exert a direct influence on behavior but perhaps places an individual in a particular group that supports or encourages general activities that are congruent with health-seeking behaviors. For example, if persons with a higher SES participate more often in certain health-related activities, it cannot be said that the more money one has, the more likely one is to comply with a health regimen. Rather, preventive health behavior may involve certain activities commonly found in the social structure seen in formal organizations, of which those in higher SES groups are commonly members. Along this line, cost of therapy, originally considered to be a major hindrance to the poor in their participation in health programs, is not as great a factor as was once thought. When programs have been heavily subsidized and offered at minimal expense, participation has not risen accordingly.[32] Therefore, ability to pay for services, which is often associated with SES, does not necessarily correlate with participation in health care practices.

Membership in a particular ethnic group also can affect a person's involvement in health care activities. Sugarek and colleagues[33] studied the beliefs and attitudes about cancer screening in three groups of women: Mexican-American, black, and white. They found that the Mexican-American population was significantly less educated than the other two groups, valued early diagnosis the least, and were the most fatalistic in outlook.

Age is of particular importance as a factor that influences health behavior. Although considerable attention has been given to children and cancer, little attention is given to the elderly in relation to cancer. This is particularly troublesome, given the tendency of some cancers to be diagnosed at a more advanced stage with increasing age. Gray[34] identified fears relating to death, institutionalization, dementia, fatalism, and feelings of worthlessness as factors that inhibit screening practices in the elderly.

Gender also plays an important role in determining participation in health practices. Women are more active health care consumers and usually set or at least influence the tone in a family with respect to health care matters. Moreover, women are exposed more on a daily basis to sources promoting health practices, such as women's magazines, television, and women's clubs.

The extent to which a person's personality can serve as a modifying factor in the progression of cancer is a subject that has received much attention. The concept of a cancer personality goes back as far as Galen (AD 200), who postulated a relationship between the existence of melancholy in women and breast cancer. More recently, Cassileth and colleagues[35] studied the psychologic attributes of five groups of physically ill persons (with arthritis, diabetes, cancer, renal disease, and dermatologic disorders) and found that they did not differ significantly from one another or from the general public. However, persons whose diseases had been diagnosed recently in all the groups had poorer mental health scores than did persons whose illness had been diagnosed more than 4 months previously. In another study,[36] the same researchers found that the psychosocial factors that were studied (social ties, marital history, job satisfaction, general life satisfaction, subjective view of adult health, and degree of hopelessness/helplessness) were unrelated to the specific diagnosis, extent of disease, or therapy.

Influence of the Family and Significant Others

The importance of the patient's family and significant others as a factor in health behavior has been well documented.[37-41] The family is responsible for introducing certain beliefs or practices to its members. The family exerts tremendous influence on an individual's definitions of health and illness, the value placed on health care, and the perception of how trustworthy a particular health care system or agent is. Norms are established within the family, so that certain health-related activities are either supported or impeded, overtly or covertly. It is certainly true that a health professional must direct attention to both the family and the person in whom cancer has been diagnosed if successful outcomes are sought. For example, it is crucial that the patient accept chemotherapy, but if her husband considers it useless and makes disparaging remarks, the full benefits of therapy probably will not be realized. In short, the family's reaction to illness is determined by several factors, and the feelings generated by these factors, in turn, determine how supportive the family will be.

In addition, the family's concerns and perceptions must be addressed. Just as the family influences the person with cancer, so too does the existence of cancer influence the family and significant others. For example, Cassileth and colleagues[36] found that the psychologic status of patients and relatives was closely correlated. Wright and Dyck[42] discovered that the needs of family members differed at different times throughout the course of the disease. Cooper[43] found that more spouses than patients reported feelings of stress and loneliness. These studies and those cited earlier reflect the reality that the family and significant others have extensive needs during this period, and the nurse plays an important role in identifying these concerns and addressing them.

Influence of Health Care Professionals and Indicated Regimens

The type of treatment regimen that is indicated for a particular disease significantly affects an individual's decision and ability to adhere. Strauss[44] listed a number of characteristics that make it difficult, undesirable, and sometimes impossible for a person (and family) to carry out any regimen. A person may have difficulty with a regimen if

- It is difficult to learn and/or carry out.
- It takes too much time.
- It causes dangerous side effects.
- It causes too much discomfort or pain.
- It requires much energy or effort to carry out.
- It is visible to others.
- It is obvious (thus stigmatizes).
- It does not seem efficient.
- It is expensive.
- It leads to increased social isolation.

With a majority of cancer treatments, characteristics of these regimens make adherence and cooperation difficult. The literature is replete with examples and accounts of negative side effects or potential toxic effects, high cost, possible disfigurement, lengthy treatments, and recurrent pain. Richardson and colleagues[45] examined side effects of treatments and compliance and found that neither the occurrence of side effects nor the difficulty of dealing with them were related to compliance with oral treatment. However, difficulty in tolerating an effect and the degree of interference with activities were correlated with decreased keeping of appointments. Missing from this same literature is the assurance that these treatments will help. Statistics support the likelihood that certain treatments work well against certain cancers. At this stage in cancer control, however, the patient's usual option is to follow a regimen with a hope that it will be helpful.

A number of studies have explored the attitudes of nurses toward cancer and cancer therapy.[46-49] Newlin and Wellisch[47] found that many health care professionals had common reactions to caring for persons with cancer. These included the following:

- The feeling that the whole world has cancer
- Cancer phobia
- Mourning each patient's diagnosis
- Identification with patients and families
- Frustration at inability to completely eradicate patient's physical pain
- Frustration at the inability to alleviate the patient's and family's emotional pain
- Conflict over involvement in experimental therapy or therapy that causes unpleasant side effects
- Conflict caused by time required for providing physical care and emotional support
- Depression and mourning related to progression of disease or death

In a more recent study by Fanslow,[48] it was found that nurses perceived cancer as hopeless and leading to death. Wilson and Williams[49] surveyed 937 oncology nurses and found that there was a positive relationship between attitudes of the cancer patient's sexuality and nursing care practices related to sexuality. Lack of knowledge was a commonly given reason for not dealing with sexuality issues.

The physician or health care professional who prescribes and supervises a plan of care exerts an impact on the health care behavior of patients.[50,51] Depending on the relationship that has been established, the patient may implicitly follow the recommendations, adhere to some and disregard others, or ignore all of them. The patient can become discouraged if he or she and the professional set mutual goals but only the professional decides how these goals are to be achieved.

Thorne[52] found significant differences between helpful and unhelpful communication from nurses or physicians in four areas: perceived intent of and concerns expressed by the caregiver; the expected outcome of the course; and the context of the interaction. For example, doctors more often communicated about the decision and the treatment, while nurses communicated about the treatment and illness experience. Physicians more often gave information, whereas nurses were perceived as giving advice (interpreted as an unhelpful action generally). This is consistent with findings from Frank-Stromborg and Wright[53] who found that ambulatory cancer patients were more satisfied with their interactions with doctors.

The health care worker can be a source of confusion if a patient goes away from an appointment not completely understanding the prescribed regimen. What may appear to be noncompliance may actually be a lack of comprehension and, depending on the health care worker's response, the patient can be made to feel guilty, stupid, or uncooperative. The health care worker has a responsibility to make sure that the patient completely understands the plan of care.

Health care workers and patients need to be partners in the program of care. The professional contributes experience and expertise with certain diseases, and the patient contributes information that individualizes the particular situation. A partnership is especially important for a person with cancer because:

1. This disease frequently causes dependency or a feeling of helplessness. The opportunity to actively participate as a partner can relieve some of these feelings.
2. Treatment is often complex, prolonged, and unpleasant, so the patient with cancer and the health care professional have to pull together to ensure that communication is maintained and cooperation is maximized.
3. The person with cancer needs the support, close contact, and hopeful outlook that a trusted professional can provide in dealing with such possible outcomes as pain and death.

Persons with cancer sometimes switch their allegiances among various health professionals at different stages in their diseases. The health care professional may see this as a lack of faith in his or her ability when it may really represent a search for the impossible cure. This is not maladaptive behavior if the person is merely seeking a second opinion before coming to a decision about therapy, for example. It does become a problem if the patient seeks opinion after opinion, all the while ignoring the recommendations or information given. The tone set by the oncology clinician greatly influences a person's decisions regarding health and illness behavior.

To effectively assist the patient and family during this critical period, the practitioner needs to follow several guidelines. The clinician primarily needs to obtain a comprehensive data base regarding the patient's beliefs and attitudes about health and illness. The process begins during the earliest of diagnostic tests. The following questions would provide some baseline information on the person's perceptions of health, illness, and normal coping mechanisms:

1. How would you rate your health generally?
2. For what kinds of things have you seen a physician in the past year? In the past 5 years?
3. What supports are available to you?
4. How do you normally handle stress?
5. What kinds of things are stressful to you?
6. What do you think is the problem?

Additional questions could be asked to elicit the person's attitudes about cancer and treatment methods. The answers could then direct educational and supportive interventions, as well as give some sense of the patient's motivation to act. Questions could include the following:

1. Have you had experience with cancer before? Were you yourself involved, or another family member or friend? What was the outcome of the experience?
2. How successful do you consider cancer therapy to be?
3. What do you think causes cancer? What can be done to prevent it? What kinds of things have you done to reduce the risk for yourself?
4. How has cancer interfered with your life? Your family's life?
5. What would you like to see accomplished during this hospitalization (visit)?

Obviously, questions of this kind do not lend themselves to a checklist style of interviewing. They can be introduced through discussion and development of the nurse-patient relationship.

An assumption frequently made is that persons develop a certain coping style and will rely on this to handle problems. A woman who is self-directed and who has taken active responsibility for her own health is likely to want an active role in decision making.[51] Research by Pierce[54] suggests that this may not be the case. Her findings in a study of decision making after the diagnosis of breast cancer but before therapy indicated that women who held what would be considered to be strong, responsible positions were not necessarily more likely to participate actively in decisions regarding therapy and that women who in some situations had actively participated in certain decisions related to their health did not necessarily wish to participate actively in decisions related to cancer therapy.

In a major study by Degner and Beaton[55] decision making was studied in a qualitative fashion. They sought to answer the question of how treatment decisions are made for patients with life-threatening illnesses within the context of modern health care. Four major patterns of control over treatment-decision making were identified: provider-controlled, patient-controlled, family-controlled, and jointly controlled. The selection of treatment options is determined by whoever maintains control. Degner and

Beaton found that provider control was the dominant pattern in the health care system.

Further analysis of the decision-making process identified several calculations that are made, including risk-benefit calculations, getting better–getting worse, cost-benefit calculations, and quality-of-life calculations. The importance of this work lies in making explicit the way decisions are made so that patients as well as health professionals understand treatment options. This understanding should assist patients in gaining more control over their decisions.

That major work was followed by a study of the preferences for control over treatment decisions of 60 adults with cancer.[56] Results indicated that most patients preferred to have joint control of treatment decisions with the physician and that patients were willing to give control over to physicians rather than to family members.

The implication from the work on decision making is that, in addition to gathering information from the patient about general health beliefs and beliefs about cancer, it is important to gather information about this particular experience or situation and not to form expectations based on previous situations until data support doing so. Degner and Beaton[55] suggest a series of questions to evaluate decisions made in health care. Examples include:

1. Is someone designated as having final responsibility for decisions?
2. Are life-style information and the experiential knowledge base of the patient/family considered?
3. Is the patient/family allowed to express a preference for the degree of control they desire over treatment decisions?
4. Is the type of decision process used clearly specified?
5. Does the decision process demonstrate sensitivity to quality-of-life factors?

A second data base that must be compiled relates to the clinician. Research has shown that nurses themselves may have misperceptions about cancer and the possible outcomes of care, which can affect their approach.[57,58] The clinician needs to examine his or her own feelings about cancer and the efficacy of certain treatments, as well as the reactions to the patient's feelings. A health professional may be comfortable with his or her own feelings about cancer and therapy but have difficulty in accepting, for example, the patient's feelings or rejection of a plan of care. Or the clinician may accept the concept of death with dignity and therefore have difficulty with the person who seeks every possible treatment, option, or recommendation. Feelings of both patient and professional must be recognized, accepted, and dealt with.

By incorporating these two assessments, the clinician has several options for changing an individual's health patterns. For every patient it is helpful to do the following:

1. Identify beliefs and perceptions the individual has regarding health, the cancer, advantages and disadvantages of therapy, and so on.

2. Support the positive aspects of the patient's decision to seek or follow the indicated regimen.

3. Educate the patient about health maintenance practices, such as testicular and breast self-examinations.

4. Enlist the support of family and/or significant others in the care of the individual with cancer.

5. Obtain information from the patient and family regarding their expectations of treatment, support realistic goals, and explore the impetus behind unrealistic hopes.

6. Use follow-up letters or telephone calls before appointments to remind patients of their scheduled times.

7. Provide time during appointments or sessions to answer questions and ascertain perceptions of progress.

8. Validate that the patient understands clearly what is expected of him or her. Provide written instructions where possible and go over them with the patient. Have the patient repeat the instructions. Ask the patient whether he or she anticipates any problems in following a particular regimen. Incorporate any modifications so that the total plan fits the patient's life-style.

9. If a person holds beliefs that are contradictory to certain aspects of the regimen, do not give up. It may be possible to motivate the person to follow the regimen through some other mechanism and then, once the behavior is established, work to modify the belief. For example, a person may be skeptical about screening tests and refuse to participate in them. Should they be offered in the work setting, however, and be an expectation of the person's position, he or she may engage in them until they have become a routine part of life.

10. Encourage the patient to be as active a partner as possible in defining the desired level of wellness, as well as in planning and carrying out the health program. The person's patterns, to a large extent, have already been established, but the practitioner can benefit from the person's self-knowledge and perspective.

Given and Given[40] identified problem-solving strategies for use with the person with cancer:

- Assist the patient as he or she overcomes barriers that could interfere with the therapeutic regimen.
- Test solutions to find those that best fit the patient's life-style and preferences.
- Show those patients who wish more control how they can participate more fully in their therapy.
- Help patients secure ongoing social support.

CONCLUSION

The individual with cancer offers a complex and unique challenge to the oncology nurse. Although there have been a number of studies on patient perceptions of the disease, their reactions to therapy, and strategies for care, the only consistent and valid strategy that can be applied to all patients universally is to begin from their perspective—with their words, perceptions, and objectives.

REFERENCES

1. Kasl SV, Cobb S: Health behavior, illness behavior and sick role behavior. Arch Environ Health 12:246-266, 1966.
2. Given BA, Given CW: Compliance among patients with cancer. Oncol Nurs Forum 16:97-103, 1989.
3. Melnyk K: Barriers: A critical review of recent literature. Nurs Res 37:196-212, 1988.
4. Lauver D: Personal communication.
5. Kasl SV: The health belief model and behavior related to chronic illness. Health Educ Monogr 2:433-454, 1974.
6. Janz N, Becker M: The health belief model: A decade later. Health Educ Q 11:1-47, 1984.
7. Rutledge DN, Davis GT: Breast self-examination compliance and the Health Belief Model. Oncol Nurs Forum 15:175-179, 1988.
8. Williams RD: Factors affecting the practice of breast self-examination in older women. Oncol Nurs Forum 15:611-616, 1988.
9. Brickman P, et al: Models of helping and coping. Am Psychol 37:368-384, 1982.
10. Cronenwett L, Brickman P: Models of helping and coping in childbirth. Nurs Res 32:84-88, 1982.
11. Cronenwett L: Helping and nursing models. Nurs Res 32:342-346, 1982.
12. Matje DM: Stress and cancer: A review of the literature. Cancer Nurs 7:399-404, 1984.
13. Cassileth B, Lusk EJ, Miller DS, et al: Psychosocial correlates of survival in advanced malignant disease. N Engl J Med 312:1551-1555, 1985.
14. Cassileth B, Walsh W, Lusk E: Psychosocial correlates of cancer: A subsequent report 3 to 8 years after cancer diagnosis. J Clin Oncol 6:1753-1759, 1988.
15. Frank-Stromborg M, Wright PS, Segella M, et al: Psychological impact of the cancer diagnosis. Oncol Nurs Forum 11(3):16-22, 1984.
16. Welch-McCaffrey D: Cancer anxiety and quality of life. Cancer Nurs 8:151-158, 1985.
17. Sontag S: Illness as metaphor. New York, Vintage Books, 1978, p 57.
18. American Cancer Society: Public Attitudes Toward Cancer and Cancer Tests. New York, American Cancer Society, 1978.
19. Bloom J, Hayes W, Saunders F, et al: Cancer awareness and secondary prevention practices in black Americans: Implications for intervention. Family Commun Health 10:19-30, 1987.
20. Brandt B: The relationship between hopelessness and selected variables in women receiving chemotherapy for breast cancer. Oncol Nurs Forum 14:35-39, 1987.
21. Herth KA: The relationship between level of hope and level of coping response and other variables in patients with cancer. Oncol Nurs Forum 16:67-72, 1989.
22. Eardley A: Triggers to action: A study of what makes women seek advice for breast conditions. Int J Health Educ 17:256-265, 1974.
23. Antonovsky A, Hartman H: Delay in the detection of cancer: A review of the literature. Health Educ Monogr 2:98-128, 1974.
24. Green LW, Roberts BJ: The research literature on why women delay in seeking medical care for breast symptoms. Health Educ Monogr 2:129-177, 1974.
25. Timko C: Seeking medical care for a breast cancer symptom: Determinants of intentions to engage in prompt or delay behavior. Health Psychol 6:305-328, 1987.
26. Reno D: Knowledge and health beliefs about testicular cancer and testicular self-exam. Cancer Nurs 11:112-117, 1988.
27. Howe H: Social factors associated with breast self-examination among high-risk women. Am J Pub Health 71:251-255, 1981.
28. Morra ME: Breast self-examination today: An overview of its uses and its values. Semin Oncol Nurs 1:170-175, 1985.
29. Nettles-Carlson B, Field M, Friedman B, et al: Effectiveness of teaching breast self-examination. Res Nurs Health 11:41-50, 1988.
30. Rutledge DN: Factors related to women's practice of breast self-examination. Nurs Res 36:117-121, 1987.
31. Lauver D: Instructional information and breast self-examination practice. Res Nursing Health 12:11-19, 1989.
32. Battistella RM: Factors associated with delay in the initiation of physician's care among late adulthood persons. Am J Pub Health 61:1348-1362, 1971.
33. Sugarek NJ, Deyo RA, Holmes BC: Locus of control and beliefs about cancer in a multi-ethnic clinic population. Oncol Nurs Forum 15:481-486, 1988.
34. Gray J: Education for health in old age, in Gray J: Prevention of Disease in the Elderly. London, Churchill Livingstone, 1985, pp 200-220.
35. Cassileth BR, Lusk EJ, Strouse TB, et al: Psychosocial status in chronic illness, N Engl J Med 311:506-511, 1984.
36. Cassileth BR, Lusk EJ, Strouse TB, et al: A psychological analysis of cancer patients and their next-of-kin. Cancer 55:72-76, 1985.
37. Welch D: Planning nursing interventions for family members of cancer patients. Cancer Nurs 4:365-370, 1981.
38. Northouse L: Mastectomy patients and the fear of recurrence. Cancer Nurs 4:213-220, 1981.
39. Welch-McCaffrey D: When it comes to cancer—think family. Nursing 83 12(12):32-35, 1983.
40. Given BA, Given CW: Creating a climate for compliance. Cancer Nurs 7:139-147, 1984.
41. Valentine AS, Sheldon T: Health behaviors of family members of cancer and cardiac patients. Oncol Nurs Forum 11(5):49-52, 1984.
42. Wright K, Dyck S: Expressed concerns of adult cancer patients' family members. Cancer Nurs 7:371-374, 1984.
43. Cooper ET: A pilot study on the effects of the diagnosis of lung cancer on family relationships. Cancer Nurs 7:301-307, 1984.
44. Strauss AL: Management of regimens, in Chronic Illness and the Quality of Life. St Louis, CV Mosby Co, 1975.

45. Richardson J, Marks G, Levine A: The influence of symptoms of disease and side effects of treatment on compliance with cancer therapy. J Clin Oncol 6:1746-1752, 1988.
46. Whelan J: Oncology nurses' attitudes toward cancer treatment and survival. Cancer Nurs 7:375-384, 1984.
47. Newlin NJ, Wellisch DK: The oncology nurse: Life on an emotional roller coaster. Cancer Nurs 1:447-449, 1978.
48. Fanslow J: Attitudes of nurses toward cancer and cancer therapies. Oncol Nurs Forum 12:43-47, 1985.
49. Wilson ME, Williams HA: Oncology nurses' attitudes and behaviors related to sexuality of patients with cancer. Oncol Nurs Forum 15:49-53, 1988.
50. Hackett TP, Cassem NH, Raker JW: Patient delay in cancer. N Engl J Med 289:14-20, 1973.
51. Valanis BG, Rumpler CH: Helping women to choose breast cancer treatment alternatives. Cancer Nurs 8:167-176, 1985.
52. Thorne SE: Helpful and unhelpful communication in cancer care: The patient's perception. Oncol Nurs Forum 15:167-172, 1988.
53. Frank-Stromborg M, Wright P: Ambulatory cancer patient's perception of the physical and psychosocial changes in their lives since the diagnosis of cancer. Cancer Nurs 7:117-130, 1984.
54. Pierce P: Decision-making by women recently diagnosed as having breast cancer. Doctoral dissertation, University of Michigan, 1985.
55. Degner L, Beaton J: Life-death decisions in health care. Washington, Hemisphere Pub Co, 1987.
56. Degner L, Russell C: Preferences for treatment control among adults with cancer. Res Nurs Health 11:367-374, 1988.
57. Craytor JK, Brown JK, Morrow GR: Assessing learning needs of nurses who care for patients with cancer. Cancer Nurs 1:211-220, 1978.
58. Craytor JK, Fass M: Changing nurses' perceptions of cancer and cancer care. Cancer Nurs 5:43-50, 1982.

Chapter 7

Cancer Risk and Assessment

Rebecca F. Cohen, RN, EdD, CPQA

Marilyn Frank-Stromborg, RN, EdD, NP, FAAN

INTRODUCTION

Health risk appraisal has been credited to Dr. Lewis C. Robbins, who worked extensively on the prevention of cervical cancer and heart disease during the 1940s. He developed a "health hazard chart" to give the medical examination a more prospective orientation toward preventive efforts. By the end of the 1960s life insurance actuarial principles were being applied to risk assessment, and risk multipliers were quantified for patient characteristics that affect mortality risk. The presence of these necessary elements thus led the way to quantitative risk appraisal. In 1970 Robbins and Hall[1] published a manual entitled *How to Practice Prospective Medicine*, which provided a complete health risk assessment (HRA) package, including questionnaire, risk computations, and feedback strategy.

When HRAs were first presented for use, the medical profession generally ignored their presence. However, the potential for computerization of the risk-estimation procedure, commercial interest, and the involvement of government agencies led to a proliferation of HRA programs. As of 1985, there were approximately 52 HRAs identified by the Office of Disease Prevention and Health Promotion in the US Department of Health and Human Services. While questions have been raised concerning the validity of the data bases and procedures used in HRA risk estimation, few empirical evaluations of the adequacy of the HRA procedures have been reported.[2]

Precise prediction of disease or mortality by any means is currently an unattainable goal because of incomplete knowledge of the total set of risk factors, their time-dose levels, and the true functional form of their contribution to risk. Similar risk models are successful in differentiating high-, medium-, and low-risk persons and in estimating relative risk but are much less successful in estimating absolute risk in individuals or across populations. In contrast, measurements applied to individuals should attain higher levels of accuracy than measurements used only in correlational studies, where there is opportunity for random errors to offset one another.[2]

HRA as a vehicle for what might be termed "prospective health assessment" potentially has a number of very desirable qualities for clinicians and health educators: preventive orientation, systematic approach, ability to emphasize modifiable factors, and a scientific knowledge base. However, a major concern is the value of quantitative estimates of absolute risk. Would the use of relative risk, risk scores, health scores, and other less quantitative measures, given the limitations in scientific knowledge and risk-estimation methods, be more helpful than the dependence on absolute risk assessment? Schoenbach[2] suggests that while HRAs may have valuable purposes, sophistication and precision in risk estimation are not necessarily the measure of their quality.

DEFINITIONS OF RISK

Risk is the potential realization of unwanted consequences of an event. Both a probability of occurrence of an event and the magnitude of its consequences are involved.[3,4] According to Rowe,[5] *hazard* implies the existence of some threat, whereas *risk* implies both the existence of a threat and its potential for occurrence. Since a risk can occur only if a potential pathway for exposure exists, a hazard may exist without implying risk. For example, there are toxic chemicals that are hazardous, but until the chemical actually exists in some form with a potential pathway to man or the environment there is no risk. A risk estimate in this case involves both potency of the substance and exposure to a population in terms of the number of persons who might receive specified dose levels. This definition of risk does, however, imply that risk is always negative. A more general definition of risk, which would not be in conflict with other definitions, is that risk "is the downside of a gamble."[5] This definition implies that (1) living itself involves gambles, (2) some gambles are involuntary, (3) tradeoffs are often required between quality and quantity of life, and (4) there is no such thing as zero risk, only involuntary and voluntary gambles for which minimum risk for acceptable gain is one criterion for decision making.[5]

A person's "cancer risk" would generally mean a factual estimate of the likelihood and severity of adverse effect, or the odds of incurring cancer. The estimation of health risks is an empiric problem filled with many uncertainties. After risks are estimated, decisions must be made about whether to bear the risks or to reduce them by reducing their source or taking protective actions. These decisions, often referred to as risk evaluation, are based on personal and social value judgments.[3,4] As Rowe[5] has stressed, the issue is really whether a particular risk is "acceptable" or is similar to risks already accepted or to the risks of alternatives.

Two approaches that can be used to calculate risk are relative and attributable risk. *Relative risk* is a ratio that compares the rate of the disease among exposed persons with the rate of the disease among unexposed persons. Although relative risk does not reveal the probability that the exposed person will have the disease, it does measure the strength of the association between a factor and the outcome.[6] The *attributable risk* is the difference in the disease rates between the group exposed to the factor and unexposed groups. Attributable risk is used to calculate the magnitude of change when a particular factor is added or subtracted.[6]

CANCER RISK FACTORS

Cancer risk factors are specific risk factors or individual characteristics that are associated with an increased cancer risk: personal behavior, genetic makeup or familial traits, and exposure to a known cancer-causing agent.[3-9] Breslow[8] divides the factors that cause cancer into two groups: those under a person's control (personal habits, such as cigarette smoking) and those outside a person's control (age, bodily characteristics such as familial polyposis). Risk factors have also been divided according to whether they are unique to an individual or shared by a group of persons. Individual risk factors include the individual's life-style, nutritional habits, medical conditions, and exposure to radiation or drugs. Group risk factors are those shared by persons from the same geographic residence or the same occupation.[9] Eventually the role of such factors may be describable in terms of chemical or metabolic mechanisms that might relate to multistage or cocarcinogenesis in humans.[3]

In general, the predominant carcinogenic risk factors believed to be responsible for 70% to 90% of cancers in humans in Western industrial societies can be put into the following categories:

A. Environmental:
  1. Nonoccupational
    a. Habits
      i. Smoking
      ii. Alcohol consumption
      iii. Sunbathing
      iv. Dietary factors
    b. Customs (eg, noncircumcision)
    c. Air and water pollution
  2. Occupational
    a. Chemical (eg, asbestos)
    b. Physical (eg, radiation)
B. Sex differences (eg, hormonal)
C. Virus
D. Racial differences
E. Habitat: urban versus rural environmental
F. Genetic factors
G. Marital status
H. Socioeconomic class
I. Psychologic
  1. Personality profile theory
  2. Stressful life events
J. Medical therapy–related cancers

It is important to categorize risk factors because this provides a data base from which to develop an individual's cancer-risk profile, make recommendations about risk factors, and plan specific interventions for risk reduction.[9] In addition, categorization emphasizes the many causative factors and the complex etiology of cancer. For example, some cancers, such as skin cancer, appear to have one factor that is especially important (ie, ultraviolet radiation). For most types of cancer, however, it appears that an interaction of multiple factors is probably necessary.[3,10-14] Risk factors for specific cancers are discussed below and summarized in Table 7-1.

Bladder Cancer

The strongest risk factors for bladder cancer involve occupational exposures and life-style practices. In developing countries, bladder infection with the parasite *Schistisoma haematobium* has been linked to the development of bladder cancer.[15] In the United States, however, risk factors for bladder cancer primarily involve occupational ex-

TABLE 7-1 Risk Factors for Selected Cancers

BLADDER CANCER	
Personal risk factors	Male White Infection with schistosomiasis
Life-style	Cigarette smoking Coffee drinking? Drinking liquids with artificial sweeteners?
Occupation	Occupations working with benzidine, aniline dye, and 2-naphthylamine—apparel, textile and leather workers, workers in dye industry, rubber workers, metal workers, painters
Drugs	Cyclophosphamide (alkylating drug).
BREAST CANCER	
Personal risk factor	History of benign breast disease Being Jewish Being single Some researchers believe that all women should be treated as being at risk
Life-style	Alcohol consumption Higher socioeconomic status Diet high in fat
Reproductive history	Early menarche Nulliparity Late menopause Late age at birth of first child
Family history	Family history of breast cancer
CERVICAL CANCER	
Personal risk factors	Black women Dysplasia Infection with herpes genitalis and condyloma accuminatum (HPV)
Reproductive history	Early age at first marriage or coitus Multiple marriages or sexual partners Use of nonbarrier contraceptives

TABLE 7-1 Risk Factors for Selected Cancers (continued)

COLORECTAL CANCER

Personal risk factors	Increasing age Disease with hereditary predisposition—Gardner's syndrome, Turcot syndrome, Peutz-Jeghers syndrome, familial polyposis of colon Ulcerative colitis Crohn's disease History of colon cancer, female genital cancer, bladder cancer, breast cancer Sporadic colorectal adenomas
Life-style	A diet high in fat, low in fiber, and low in fruits and vegetables containing vitamins A and C Obesity Sedentary life-style
Geographic location	Living in highly developed countries

LUNG CANCER

Personal risk factors	Cigarette smoking Family history of lung cancer
Life-style	Exposure to smokers over a period of time Exposure to high levels of indoor radon
Occupation	Working with iron oxide, nickel, arsenic, chromium, asbestos, petroleum-related products, mustard gas, chloromethyl methyl, ether; occupations involved: iron ore miners, nickel smelters, miners, chromium producers, millers, textile workers, insulation workers, shipyard workers, mustard gas workers, chemical workers, diesel jet testers, iron foundry workers, oil refiners, vintners
Geographic location	Living in an urban area or coastal community

ORAL CANCER

Personal risk factors	Tobacco use Heavy alcohol use Nutritional deficiencies Poor dentition and oral hygiene Plummer-Vinson syndrome
Occupation	Long-term exposure to the sun (lip cancer)

OVARIAN CANCER

Personal risk factors	White upper income groups in the Western Hemisphere Cancer of the breast
Reproductive history	Delayed age at first pregnancy Nulliparity
Medical treatments	Radiation to the pelvic area
Occupations	Occupations involving asbestos

PROSTATE CANCER

Personal risk factors	Increasing age Black males—highest incidence in the world
Life-style	Diet high in fats, oils, sugar, eggs, milk, animal protein (under investigation) Sexual activity? History of venereal disease?
Occupation	Occupations related to use of cadmium.

SKIN CANCER

Personal risk factors	Light-skinned, fair-haired, freckles, burns easily History of severe sunburn under the age of 20 Increasing age Presence of congenital moles Personal history of dysplastic nevi, cutaneous melanoma History of excessive sunbathing Xeroderma pigmentosum (a progressive sun-sensitive disease that develops in early childhood) Albinism Epidermodysplasia verruciformis (multiple virus-induced warty lesions that develop in early childhood) History of tropical ulcers, burns, and scars related to squamous cell carcinoma and increased incidence
Family history	History of melanoma in children, siblings, and parents
Occupation	Outdoor work—farming, ranching Uranium miners, radiologists
Drugs	Treatment for psoriasis known as PUVA
Precursor lesions	Solar (actinic) keratosis Bowen's disease
Chemicals	Polycyclic aromatic hydrocarbons
Immunologic factors	Organ transplant recipients

TESTICULAR CANCER

Personal risk factors	White males Family history Younger men (ages 20 to 40) Cryptorchidism Higher socioeconomic status[2]

ENDOMETRIAL (UTERINE CORPUS) CANCER

Personal risk factors	Obesity Hypertension Diabetes mellitus
Life-style	Higher socioeconomic class
Reproductive history	History of menstrual irregularities Nulliparity Infertility through anovulation
Drugs	Long-term use of conjugated estrogens

VAGINAL CANCER

Personal risk factors	Mother's use of DES during pregnancy Radiation of cervix for cancer Elderly

posure and tobacco use. Workers exposed to aromatic amines (B-naphthylamine, benzidine) have a fourfold greater risk of bladder cancer.[16,17] Persons in high-risk occupations include apparel, textile, and leather workers, workers in the dyestuffs industry, rubber workers, metal workers, and painters.

Cigarette smoking is the most important known risk factor for bladder cancer. Smokers develop bladder cancer two to three times more often than nonsmokers.[18] Drug use has also been found to increase the risk of bladder cancer. Cyclophosphamide can cause bladder cancer.[20] In addition, long-term use of analgesics containing phenacetin may contribute to the development of transitional cell carcinoma of the renal pelvis, ureter, or bladder.[18] It has been reported that there is a latency period of as much as 18 years before bladder tumors develop after exposure to carcinogens.[19]

There is conflicting information concerning the role of coffee drinking and the use of artificial sweeteners and the risk of bladder cancer. Further research is needed to determine the association between these two substances and the incidence of bladder cancer.[18,21]

Breast Cancer

The primary risk factors for breast cancer are a family history of breast cancer, history of benign breast disease, late age at first live birth, nulliparity, early age at menarche, late age at menopause, higher socioeconomic status, being Jewish, and being single. However, several authors[22,23] stress that all women 35 or older should be treated as being at risk for breast cancer.

There are conflicting data on the relationship between consumption of alcohol and risk of breast cancer. One study[24] reported that moderate alcohol consumption is associated with an elevation in the risk of breast cancer of 50% to 100%. Several other reports[25,26] found no association between alcohol and breast cancer. The same type of debate has revolved around the use of birth control pills and increased risk of breast cancer.[27] A study by the Centers for Disease Control and the National Institute of Child Health and Human Development[28] found that use of birth control pills did not increase the risk of breast cancer in women. However, use of oral contraceptives around menopause and onset of puberty may increase the risk of breast cancer.[29]

There is considerable debate about the influence of diet on the development of breast cancer. Since the worldwide distribution of breast cancer is very similar to that of colorectal cancer, it is believed by many researchers that a high fat intake is a causative factor in breast cancer, especially in older women.[30,31] Additional evidence of this association comes from clinical and laboratory animal studies.[32] How much reduction in fat intake is necessary to lower the risk of cancer is also unknown at this time. Willett et al.[33] reported from their study of 85,538 US nurses that a moderate reduction in fat intake by women is unlikely to result in a substantial reduction in the incidence of breast cancer.

Cervical Cancer

Race, personal factors, and venereal disease are the major risk factors associated with cervical cancer. Personal risk factors include early age at first coitus, multiple marriages or sexual partners, and use of nonbarrier contraceptives.[34,35] Venereal infections associated with increased risk are herpes genitalis and condyloma accuminatum caused by human papillomaviruses (HPV).[36,37] Black women in the United States have a twofold greater risk than white women. Certain religious groups in the United States have been noted to have low incidence rates of cervical cancer; these groups are Jews, Mormons, and Seventh-Day Adventists.[38]

Colorectal Cancer

High rates of colorectal cancer are found in highly developed countries (eg, North America, northern and western Europe, New Zealand) and low rates are found in Asia, Africa, and most countries of Latin America.[39] There is substantial evidence that differences between nations in the incidence of colorectal cancer are due at least in part to environmental factors, such as diet. Obesity, high fat intake, low fiber content, and a dearth of fruits and vegetables containing vitamins A and C have been identified as risk factors. A sedentary life-style has also been implicated as a risk factor for colorectal cancer.[40-45]

Age is considered a significant risk factor for colorectal cancer. Risk begins to increase at age 40, increases rapidly above age 55, and roughly doubles with each successive decade, reaching a peak at age 75.[46]

Familial and hereditary factors are another significant risk factor, believed to account for at least 20% of colorectal cancers. The specific diseases with a hereditary predisposition are Gardner's syndrome, Turcot syndrome, Peutz-Jeghers syndrome, and familial polyposis of the colon.

Having ulcerative colitis is another significant risk factor for colorectal cancer. The risk of carcinoma of the large intestine is 20 times greater than in the general population among individuals with extensive ulcerative colitis for 10 years or more.[39,47,48] Crohn's disease also places individuals at higher risk of colorectal cancer.[46] Persons with a past history of colon cancer and adenomatous intestinal polyps are also at increased risk.[48]

Lung Cancer

The major risk factors for lung cancer are geographic location, social class, occupation, and tobacco use. Cigarette smoking increases the risk of lung cancer to a greater degree than any other risk factor. It is estimated that in the United States cigarette smoking may contribute to at least 80% of all lung cancer in males and 40% in females.[49,50] Studies have also found an elevated risk of lung cancer among individuals who have never smoked but are living with a spouse who smokes cigarettes.[51] There is a wide body of evidence that points to the likelihood that the involuntary inhalation of tobacco smoke has a causal effect on the risk of lung cancer in nonsmokers. It is estimated that in the United States between 2500 and 8400 of the approximately 12,200 annual deaths from lung cancer that are not due to smoking may be attributable to environmental tobacco smoke.[52]

Another environmental risk factor for lung cancer is indoor radon exposure. It is estimated that indoor radon exposure causes about 13,000 lung cancer deaths a year.[53] However, almost all of the increased risk seems to occur in smokers. There has been some suggestion that radon acts synergistically with cigarette smoking to enhance the risk of lung cancer.

High-risk occupations are those in which persons work with asbestos, polycyclic hydrocarbons, chromium, mustard gas, chloromethyl ethers, radon, nickel, and inorganic arsenic. Included in this group are welders, gas workers, roofers, uranium miners, workers in the chrome pigment industry, nickel refinery workers, copper smelter workers, vineyard workers, and insulation workers.

International studies of geographic variation have shown that lung cancer is most common in urban and coastal communities.

Oral Cancer

Tobacco is a major risk factor for this cancer. The habits of chewing tobacco and smoking cigarettes have long been associated with oral cancer.[54,55] In other countries different tobacco-chewing habits place users at increased risk of oral cancer. In India betel nut or "pan" is chewed, in Bombay "bidi" is chewed, "keeyo" is chewed in Thailand, and "nass" is chewed in Soviet Central Asia. These mixtures of tobacco with other products increase the risk of oral cancer. Another significant risk factor for oral cancer is excessive alcohol intake. The risk of oral cancer among heavy drinkers and smokers is approximately seven times greater than it is in nonsmokers and nondrinkers.[54] Alcohol appears to act chiefly by augmenting the effects of tobacco.

Other risk factors are nutritional deficiencies and poor dentition. Plummer-Vinson syndrome has a positive association with oral cancer. However, other nutritional deficiencies linked with an increased risk of oral cancer may be related to heavy use of alcohol, which influences dietary intake.[56]

Occupations related to long-term exposure to the sun have been associated with cancer of the lip.

Ovarian Cancer

The risk factors for ovarian cancer are less well known than those of the other major gynecologic cancers.[57] Ovarian cancer tends to be more common among white upper income groups in highly industrialized countries.[58] The risk of ovarian cancer is associated with delayed age at first pregnancy and with a smaller number of pregnancies. These risk factors suggest an abnormality of endocrine secretion as an important component of ovarian carcinogenesis.[59] Present information suggests that oral contraceptive use might protect against ovarian cancer.[60,61] Other risk factors are radiation to the pelvic area, cancer of the breast, and occupations involving asbestos.

Prostate Cancer

Age and race are significant risk factors for prostate cancer. Black Americans have the highest prostate cancer incidence rate in the world.[62,63] Prostate cancer affects the elderly more than the young to a greater extent than any other cancer.[65]

Other risk factors for prostate cancer are tentative at this time and require more research. A positive relationship has been found between the consumption of fats, oils, sugar, animal protein, eggs, and milk ("overnutrition") and mortality rates among men with prostate cancers.[30,65] There may be a familial tendency toward the development of prostate cancer. However, whether it is due to environmental or genetic factors has not been determined. An increased risk of prostate cancer in association with an increasing number of sexual partners, prior history of venereal disease, frequency of sexual intercourse, and an early onset of sexual activity has been suggested.[63] Occupations that have been linked to increased risk of prostate cancer are those in which workers are exposed to cadmium (eg, welding, electroplating, alkaline battery production). However, other studies have linked the development of prostate cancer with a multitude of other occupations that have no common carcinogenic exposure. At this time the evidence relating occupation and increased risk of prostate cancer is weak and needs further study.

Skin Cancer

The chief risk factor for the development of basal cell and squamous cell carcinomas of the skin is exposure to ultraviolet radiation. Melanoma is also related to ultraviolet radiation, but there are several other influential risk factors: familial predisposition, hormonal factors, and dysplastic nevus syndrome. Overall, those at greatest risk of skin cancer are fair-skinned white persons, particularly those with reddish or blond hair, blue or light eyes, those with a tendency to freckle or burn easily, and individuals who have spent considerable time in the sun. Table 7-1 lists other risk factors for skin cancer related to occupation, personal risk factors, family history, drugs, precursor lesions, chemicals, and immunologic factors.[66-70]

Testicular Cancer

A significant risk factor for testicular cancer involves race and age. This cancer occurs about 4.5 times more frequently in whites than in blacks and in men between the ages of 20 and 40 years. Another significant risk factor is undescended testicles, especially in men who have a testicle that descended after the age of 6 or a testicle that never descended (cryptorchidism).[71] Other possible risk factors are a familial tendency, trauma, hormonal drugs, and socioeconomic status.

Endometrial (Uterine Corpus) Cancer

The risk factors for cancer of the uterus are well known. Obesity, hypertension, and diabetes mellitus have been correlated with the development of endometrial cancer.[72] Women who have a history of menstrual irregularities and infertility through anovulation are also at increased risk.[73] Long-term use of conjugated estrogens is an iatrogenic risk factor for this cancer.[74] On the other hand, the use of oral contraceptives (containing both estrogen and progesterone in each pill) for at least 1 year has a protective effect against endometrial cancer.[75] In addition, women of high socioeconomic status are at increased risk.

Vaginal Cancer

A risk factor for vaginal cancer that has received much attention is diethylstilbestrol (DES). Adenosis of the vagina has been identified in the offspring of women who received DES during pregnancy. This agent is no longer given to women to prevent threatened miscarriages. Another risk factor is radiation of the cervix for cancer of this organ. Postradiation carcinoma in situ of the vagina is of the epidermoid type and may occur 1 or more years after apparently successful treatment of cancer of the cervix.[76]

CANCER RISK ASSESSMENT

The purposes of a cancer risk assessment include (1) providing an individual with information about his or her health-related behavior that may increase cancer risk, (2) serving as an effective aid for educating patients about the relationship between risk factors and the likelihood of cancer, and (3) stimulating a person to participate in activities aimed at changing life-style and improving health.[9,77,78] In addition, analysis of cancer risk may help patients identify their options so that they can make realistic decisions about their health care. Physicians have also found that risk analyses help in the development of health regimens that are tailored to each individual's risk and tolerance for living with that risk.[77]

Before information is provided about an individual's specific risks, however, it is important that there be an understanding of the risk to an average person in the population.[77] This average risk serves as a baseline against which individuals can measure the magnitude of their increased risk, if any. Also, tables that show risks to various ages are useful because they indicate that cancer risk in the general population usually increases with certain activities (ie, smoking) and with age.

One of the problems that exists in assessment of cancer risks is that some persons are unwilling to seriously consider what their risks might be. If a relative has had cancer, they may assume that their risk is "high" but fear that an examination of this assumption might in some way further increase their risk. They may also be dealing with various emotions such as low self-esteem, denial, fear, anger, guilt, embarrassment, and insecurity, which are often seen in persons who come from families with a history of cancer. These emotions act as barriers to effective communication and can result in an inability to face a risk analysis. Other individuals may believe that as long as they suffer by worrying about their high risk, their worry will act as a shield and they will be spared the suffering of cancer itself. Finally, there often is the belief that if one worries about risks, one is engaging in "negative thinking that can cause cancer." Through the process of learning to understand one's fears, learning that such ideas are perfectly normal, and taking positive action to reduce the risks, an individual can be helped to understand the importance of risk assessment. Those who have received information about risk are more likely to schedule regular checkups and undergo necessary diagnostic procedures than are those who hold unrealistic health beliefs.[77]

It is also extremely important that a clear definition of the meaning of risk be provided when a health risk analysis is conducted. Many believe that when one's cancer risk is considered to be "high," it means that their risk of dying is high. This, of course, is inaccurate because risk implies occurrence of disease and complications, not just mortality rate. Therefore, health professionals need to make sure that the health care consumer understands such concepts as "carcinogen," "risk," "cancer risk," "carcinogenic risk factors," and "cancer risk assessment" in order that they will know exactly what the assessment can and cannot do for them and how to use the data obtained.

When a cancer risk assessment is done, the carcinogenic risk of exposure of individuals or populations to a particular risk factor is quantified.[79] However, assessment is only one aspect of a complete risk analysis. A comprehensive risk analysis should include: (a) the identification of risks and the estimation of the likelihood and magnitude of risk occurring and (b) an evaluation that measures risk acceptance (the acceptable levels of societal risk) and risk management (the control of risks, including methods of reducing and avoiding risk).[5]

Constanza et al[80] point out that risk assessment is not only a part of cancer prevention but must also be included in detection procedures to maximize the chance that one can discover cancer at its smallest or earliest possible stage.

Evaluation

The assessment of every patient should start with the history. The history format should include information on the following factors[4]:

A. Demographic data
B. Current past medical problems
C. Family medical history
D. Surgical and (if appropriate) obstetric history
E. Childhood illnesses
F. Allergies
G. Current medications
H. Psychologic status
I. Social history
J. Environmental background
K. Review of systems

In most cases, this information, excluding the review of systems, can be supplied by the patient on one of the many questionnaire forms available (see Table 7-2). It is important to remember that there is an element of fear of the diagnostic implications of admitting to certain symptoms that can create problems in cancer prevention/detection. The history, therefore, is helpful not only in detecting early, vague symptoms but also in identifying signs and symptoms that the patient might deny if asked outright. In addition, the history helps to identify factors, such as a family history of genetic susceptibility, that

TABLE 7-2 Health Risk Assessment Instruments

Instrument	Description	Source
	COMPUTER-SCORED HRAs	
COSTPREDICT AND HEALTHPREDICT	It calculates costs and savings related to 51 health-related conditions and 44 risk factors. Reports give predicted costs and savings related to risks, absenteeism, and hospitalization. (200-item questionnaire re: habits, stress, medical history, and women's health.)	CompuHealth Associates (also available for IBM-PC)
HEALTH AND LIFESTYLE QUESTIONNAIRE	It emphasizes current quality of life over long-term risks. Report assigns scores ranging from "excellent" to "immediate attention" and discusses the individual's risks. (54-item questionnaire re: health habits, psychological and job attitudes, and social relationships.)	Health Enhancement Systems
HEALTH HAZARD APPRAISAL	Computer analysis provides a 4- to 5-page report that is a combination of bar graph, narrative, and tabulated data, including summaries of health age, projected health cost, and stress. (80-item questionnaire re: medical history, family history, lifestyle, stress, and women's health.)	Prospective Medicine Center
HEALTHLINE	A 4-page report discusses leading probable causes of death and alterable risk factors. A 15-page report shows specific risks such as frustrations, satisfactions, and stresses. (44-item questionnaire re: medical history, life-style, women's health, stress, social and psychological factors, exercise, and nutrition.)	Health Logics
HEALTHLOGIC	20-page report focuses on impact of life-style changes on health, fitness, and risk of chronic disease. (17-page booklet has questions on health history, men's and women's health, stress, and motor vehicle safety.)	HMC Software Inc.
HEALTHPATH	14-page report scores participants in 11 health habit areas. (72-item questionnaire covers 13 risk/life-style areas. Physical measurements and laboratory data are optional.) Helps to serve cost-containment objectives of a corporation.	Control Data Corp.
HEALTH WRAP	Both a standard risk profile and a "wellness index" are provided. (93-item questionnaire.)	Lifestyle and Health Promotion
LIFE	Report lists 20 major risk indicators (mostly physical measurements), patient's values for these, and recommended values. Also lists 20 leading causes of death for patient's age and sex, making recommendations to reduce risks where appropriate. A nutrition profile, stress profile and appraisal, and achievable ages are included. (16-page questionnaire re: personal and family medical histories, habits, and life-style, attitudes about health, physical measurements, diet, exercise, and other health habits.)	Wellsource
LIFESCORE PLUS	Report projects lifespan and identifies risks. (62-item questionnaire: biomedical measurements, life-style habits, health history.) Booklet suggests guidelines to reduce or eliminate health risks.	Center for Corporate Health Promotion

TABLE 7-2 Health Risk Assessment Instruments (continued)

Instrument	Description	Source
	COMPUTER-SCORED HRAs—cont'd	
LIFESTYLE ASSESSMENT QUESTIONNAIRE (LAQ)	Printout suggests specific resources on topics selected and compares level of wellness with average of others who have taken the LAQ. The top 10 risk factors are listed, as well as ways to reduce them. (270-item questionnaire re: "Wellness inventory" section with six dimensions of wellness and "Personal Growth" section to identify preferred topics for further information.)	National Wellness Institute
LIFESTYLE DIRECTIONS	Short 30-question instrument, which covers diet, exercise, and health. Report presents graphic information on risks for five major diseases.	Lifestyle Directions, Inc.
PERSONAL STRESS PROFILE	12-page booklet aimed at employees in a workplace environment contains explanations on stress and specific recommendations for behavior change. (167-item questionnaire re: personal and family medical history, life-style behaviors, socioeconomic status, and stress.)	General Health, Inc.
HEALTHPLAN AND HEALTHPLAN PLUS	12-page booklet provides narrative and graphic information on 8 health areas, current risk as compared to average and achievable risk, and specific recommendations for behavior change. Individual's 5 leading health problems in order of importance are included. HealthPlan Plus has a longer and more detailed profile. (111-item questionnaire re: personal and family medical history, behavior habits, socioeconomic status, and women's health.)	General Health, Inc.
HEALTH RISK APPRAISAL	4-page report tabulates risks for 5 leading causes of death, recommends ways to reduce risks, and gives a 20-year future projection. (50-item questionnaire re: health habits and medical status.) A wider-ranging Lifestyle Development Questionnaire is available.	University of Michigan (also available for IBM-PC)
HEALTH RISK APPRAISAL QUESTIONNAIRE	2-page report explains patient's risk factors for the 12 leading causes of death as percentages by which he or she deviates from the average; appraisal and achievable ages are given as behavioral changes that could reduce risks. (39-item questionnaire re: personal and family medical history, health habits, and women's health.)	St. Louis County Health Dept.
HEALTH RISK ASSESSMENT	Report recommends ways to reduce risks and compares the client's risk factors with those of others of the same age, sex, and race. (85-item questionnaire re: personal and family medical history, alcohol, smoking, and driving habits, women's health.)	University of California
HEALTH RISK ASSESSMENT QUESTIONNAIRE	3-page report describes risks and gives information on health age, achievable age, and top 10 mortality causes and risk factors sorted into 4 categories: ideal, average, risky, and nonmodifiable. (96-item questionnaire re: medical history, physical examination, family history, women's health, personal health habits.)	Wisconsin Center for Health Risk Research
HEALTH RISK QUESTIONNAIRE	Report discusses risk factors for 15 major diseases with an emphasis on cancer.* (39-item questionnaire re: lifestyle, medical history, physical and laboratory measurements.)	Health Enhancement Systems (also available for IBM-PC)

TABLE 7-2 Health Risk Assessment Instruments (continued)

Instrument	Description	Source
	COMPUTER-SCORED HRAs—cont'd	
RHRC HEALTH RISK APPRAISAL	In addition to assessing individual risks, this instrument estimates the impact of workplace wellness programs. 5-page report includes 10-year mortality estimates for the 12 leading causes of death, estimated annual hospital days, and advice on reducing risks. A group profile includes the estimated reduction in work force mortality and hospitalization achievable through specific wellness programs. (39-item questionnaire re: lifestyle, medical history, frequency of medical screening, optional laboratory data, and women's health. An additional "General Well-Being Questionnaire" measures stress.)	Regional Health Resource Center (also available for IBM-PC)
WELL AWARE HEALTH RISK APPRAISAL	Emphasis is on quality of life and current risks. 16-page report includes mortality predictions and stresses practical measures to improve health. (Questionnaire includes health habits, life-style, health knowledge, stress, women's health, diet, motor vehicle safety, alcohol use, sociability, physical and laboratory data.)	Well Aware About Health
	MICRO-COMPUTER–BASED HRAs	
AVIVA	Provides an overall risk score adjusted for age and sex, the contribution of each risk factor to the score, and suggestions for modifying risks. This instrument assesses hospitalization risks, but concerns only those risks which an individual can modify. (5- 10-minute or 15- to 20-minute versions available. Screens users to ensure that the interview is appropriate; questions cover alcohol use, driving habits, weight, blood pressure, cholesterol levels, depression, and smoking. User can ask why certain information is requested and receive explanations.)	Center for Research in Medical Education and Health Care, Jefferson Medical College
HEALTH AWARENESS GAMES	This is a set of 5 microcomputer programs that draw on statistics about life-style and health as they relate to life expectancy. Appropriate for junior high school through college and is suitable for home use. (5 programs include Coronary Risk, Why Do You Smoke? Exercise and Weight, Life Expectancy, and Life-Style.)	Queue Inc.
HEALTH RISK APPRAISAL	Profile displays the user's risks for 10 leading causes of death and provides a 1-page summary printout. (40-item questionnaire re: life-style and physiologic indicators. For Apple II, II+, IIe, and IBM-PC.)	University of Minnesota Media Distribution
LIFESCAN	Each individual receives a printout listing his or her top 10 risk factors and suggested methods to reduce those risks. Special feature is a listing of the individual's positive life-style behaviors. (40-item questionnaire re: physical activity, drug usage, driving habits, cholesterol level, medical history, and women's health issues. For IBM-PC.)	National Wellness Institute
PERSONAL HEALTH APPRAISAL	There are two versions: The personal version is interactive and the professional version can be used in either an interactive or batch-processing mode and can store and update profiles. The user's life expectancy is calculated at the end and it includes an analysis of the user's "Cancer Early Warning Signs" and preventive health practices. (84-item questionnaire re: medical history, occupational health information, life-style, women's health. For IBM-PC.)	MedMicro
SPHERE	The 25-item questionaire covers medical and life-style characteristics. Reports explain each user's risks and appraisal and achievable ages. Available in English and French. (For IBM-PC.)	University of British Columbia

TABLE 7-2 Health Risk Assessment Instruments (continued)

Instrument	Description	Source
	SELF-SCORED QUESTIONNAIRES	
HOW DO YOU RATE AS A HEALTH RISK?	Booklet includes 40 questions on smoking, alcohol and other drugs, nutrition, weight control, exercise, stress, and safety. Provides suggestions to improve the individual's present condition.	Channing L. Bete Co., Inc.
HOPE HEALTH APPRAISAL	A complete health kit designed to help an individual manage his/her health risk and improve life-style.	International Health Awareness Center
HEALTHSTYLE: A SELF-TEST	2-page, 24-item questionnaire published by US Public Health Service. Gives specific suggestions for reducing risks. Topics covered include nutrition, alcohol and drug use, smoking, fitness, stress, and safety.	ODPHP National Health Information Center
LIFESCORE-C	Designed for employee health programs. Results yield an individual score and can be batch-processed to yield a group profile. Questions cover life-style, environmental factors, family medical history, and utilization of health care. Scores are given for general health and life expectancy.	Center for Corporate Health Promotion (also available as LIFESCORE-M FOR IBM-PC)
	OTHER INSTRUMENTS	
INCREASED RISK ASSESSMENT	Check-off list related to carcinogenic exposure, genetic predisposition, personal history of cancer, and certain associated diseases. Next to each item is the associated cancer for which the person is at increased risk.	Costanza, Li, Green, and Patterson. Cancer prevention and detection: strategies for practice, in Cancer Manual, ed 7, American Cancer Society, Boston, 1986.
C.A.R.E.S. (CANCER AWARENESS RISK EDUCATION SERVICE)	C.A.R.E.S. was designed to assist health educators in providing cancer risk reduction information to the general public. It is used on a Compaq 386 with 1024K of memory and an EGA board. User responds to questions about personal health history, family history, personal habits related to skin, lung, colorectal, breast, gynecologic, prostate, testicular, stomach, head and neck, and esophageal cancers. A comprehensive component on dietary habits, stress, and exercise is also included. The user receives a printed analysis of his/her personal risk for developing the cancers listed.	H. Lee Moffitt Cancer Center and Research Institute, Inc. P.O. Box 280179, Tampa, Florida 33682-0179
CANCER RISK ASSESSMENT	Check-off questions for men and women related to cancer risks. Specific areas include skin, head and neck, lung, breast, colon-rectum, cervix, endometrium, vulva, vagina, prostate, testes.	White, L.N. Cancer risk assessment. Semin Oncol Nurs 2: 184-190, 1986
RISK APPRAISAL FORM	A Risk Appraisal Form that is practical and useful for office or clinic setting was developed. Questions are presented related to risk for cardiovascular disease, malignant diseases, auto accidents, suicide, diabetes. Scores are summarized to provide total number of risk factors for which the patient is in the highest risk level and this is then converted to a percentage. Form indicates factors that provide low, medium, and high risk for patient.	Pender, N. Health Promotion in Nursing Practice. New York, Appleton-Century Crofts, 1982

TABLE 7-2 Health Risk Assessment Instruments (continued)

Instrument	Description	Source

RESOURCES FOR HEALTH RISK ASSESSMENT INSTRUMENTS

Center for Corporate Health Promotion
1850 Centennial Park Dr.
Suite 520
Reston, VA 22091

Center for Research in Medical Education and Health Care
Jefferson Medical College
Philadelphia, PA 19107

Channing L. Bete Co., Inc.
200 State Rd.
South Deerfield, MA 01373

Compu Health Associates
13795 Rider Trail
Earth City, MO 63045

Control Data Corp.
StayWell/EAR Division
901 East 78th St.
Minneapolis, MN 55420

General Health, Inc.
3299 K. St., NW
Washington, DC 20007

Health Enhancement Systems
9 Mercer St.
Princeton, NJ 08540

Health Logics
111 Deerwood Pl
San Ramon, CA 94583

HMC Software Inc.
4200 North MacArthur Blvd.
Irving, TX 75038

International Health Awareness Center
157 South Kalamazoo Mall
Suite 482
Kalamazoo, MI 49007-4895

Lifestyle and Health Promotion
59 Monterrey Ave.
Kenner, LA 70065

Lifestyle Directions, Inc.
300 Ninth St.
Conway, PA 15027-1696

MedMicro
6701 Seybold Rd.
Suite 220A
Madison, WI 53719

National Wellness Institute
University of Wisconsin-Stevens Point
South Hall
Stevens Point, WI 54481

ODPHP National Health Information Center*
P.O. Box 1133
Washington, DC 20013

Prospective Medicine Center
Suite 219
3901 North Meridian
Indianapolis, IN 46208

Queue Inc.
562 Boston Ave.
Bridgeport, CT 06610

Regional Health Resource Center
Medical Information Laboratory
1408 West University Ave.
Urbana, IL 61801

St. Louis County Health Department
1001 East First St.
Duluth, MN 55805

University of British Columbia
Health Care and Epidemiology
5804 Fairview Crescent
Mather Building
Vancouver, BC V6T W5
Canada

University of California
Epidemiology and International Health
1699 HSW
San Francisco, CA 94143

University of Michigan
Fitness Research Center
401 Washtenaw Ave.
Ann Arbor, MI 48109-2214

University of Minnesota
Media Distribution
Box 734, Mayo Building
420 Delaware St., SE
Minneapolis, MN 55455

Well Aware About Health
P.O. Box 43338
Tucson, AZ 85733

Wellsource
15431 Southeast 82nd Dr.
Suite E
P.O. Box 569
Clackamas, OR 97015

Wisconsin Center for Health Risk Research
University of Wisconsin Center for Health Sciences
600 Highland Ave., Room J5/224
Madison, WI 53792

*Source for Health Risk Assessment Instruments (excluding "other instruments") and Resources: ODPHP National Health Information Center. *Healthfinder: health risk appraisals.* Public Health Service, US Department of Health and Human Services, Washington, DC, November, 1988. The *Healthfinder* includes other HRAs and can be ordered for $1.

may increase an individual's risk of specific cancers. In such situations, the physician may order special tests that are not included in the guidelines for the public in general.[80] A complete physical examination should follow the health history to provide objective data that can complement and verify the health history's subjective data.

For patients identified as having a high risk of cancer, advice should be given about avoiding additional exposure to carcinogens, and rigorous intervention may be indicated (eg, excision of the colon in a patient with chronic ulcerative colitis before the appearance of cancer or removal of a dysplastic nevus to prevent progression to melanoma). In high-risk patients, screening might also be carried out more frequently and in greater detail than in low-risk patients. Women at high risk of breast cancer may need to have mammography and periodic physical examinations performed more frequently and started at an earlier age than women who are at low risk. The recommended schedule of prevention and detection procedures for the general population, as suggested by the American Cancer Society[81,82] is as follows:

A. WOMEN

1. Physical Examination:
Age 20 to 40: Pelvic examination every year. Examination of the mouth, thyroid, breasts, rectum, ovaries, skin, and lymph nodes every 3 years.
Age 40 and over: Every year to include examination of the above.

2. Health Teaching:
To teach proper diet, exercise, health habits, breast self-examination (should be done every month), and how to stop smoking.

3. Mammography:
Age 20 to 40: Between the ages of 35 and 40, an initial mammography to profile later changes should be done.
Age 40 and over: Between 40 and 49, a mammography should be done every year or two. Over the age of 50, it should be done every year.

4. Pap test for the cervix:
Should be done annually for all women who are sexually active or who are 18 years of age and older. After three or more consecutive normal annual examinations, it should be done as often as the doctor advises, regardless of age.

5. Tissue sample for endometrium:
Should be done for high-risk women at menopause. High risk includes obesity, abnormal uterine bleeding, estrogen therapy, history of infertility, and failure to ovulate.

6. Stool blood test for cancer of the colon and rectum:
Age 20 to 40: Should be done as often as the physician advises if a woman is at higher risk, which includes personal or family history of colon or rectal cancer, personal or family history of polyps in the colon or rectum, and ulcerative colitis.
Age 40 and over: Between 40 and 50, a stool blood test for cancer of the colon and rectum should be done as often as the physician advises if the patient is at high risk. After age 50 it should be done every year.

7. Protologic examination for cancer of the colon and rectum:
Age 20 to 40: Should be done as often as physician advises if a woman is at high risk. (High risk includes personal or family history of colon or rectal cancer, personal or family history of polyps in colon or rectum, ulcerative colitis.)
Age 40 and over: At age 50+, a protologic examination should be done annually for 2 years, then every 3 to 5 years as the physician advises.

B. MEN

1. Physical Examination:
Age 20 to 40: An examination should be done at least every 3 years to include mouth, thyroid, breasts, testes, prostate, rectum, skin, and lymph nodes.
Age 40 and over: An examination should be done every year and should include the above.

2. Stool blood test for cancer of the colon and rectum:
Age 20 to 40: Should be done as often as the physician advises if the patient is at higher risk which includes personal or family history of colon or rectal cancer, personal or family history of polyps in colon or rectum, and ulcerative colitis.
Age 40 and over: Between 40 and 50, a stool blood test should be done as often as the physician advises if one is at higher risk. After age 50 it should be done every year.

3. Proctologic examination for cancer of the colon and rectum:
Age 20 to 40: The proctologic examination should be done as often as the physician advises if the patient is at higher risk (as stated above for stool blood test).
Age 40 and over: At age 50+, a proctologic examination should be done annually for 2 years, then every 3 to 5 years as the physician advises.

4. Health Teaching:
Instruction in proper diet, exercise, health habits, testicular self-examination, and how to stop smoking.

EDUCATION

Education of persons at high risk of cancer cannot be treated as something separate and distinct from general education of the public about cancer, although it has certain features. The aims of public education are

1. To inform and educate about treatable forms of cancer and to reassure people that treatment is advantageous;
2. To persuade people, particularly those at special risk, to undertake preventive action, to undergo tests so that cancer can be detected at an earlier stage, or to seek medical advice quickly when recognizable signs of ill health occur.[83]

Consequently, organized cancer education attempts to maintain positive health behavior or to interrupt a behavior pattern that is linked to increased risks of cancer. The behavior usually is that of the persons whose health is in question, but it often includes the behavior of others who control resources or rewards for behavior, such as community leaders, parents, employers, peers, teachers, and health professionals. Whether it is at the primary, secondary, or tertiary stage of prevention, a cancer education program is an intervention to prevent disability, illness, or death or to enhance quality of life through voluntary change of cancer-related behavior.[84]

Areas that should be covered in educational programs include tobacco, alcohol, occupations and cancer, environmental pollutants, sexual activity, radiation, infective and genetic factors, and diet.[56] Each of these areas should be discussed in terms of the risks they impose for certain types of cancer, actions to reduce risks, signs and symptoms of specific cancers, screening and detection methods, and personal responsibility in prevention. To reduce fears that may prevent compliance, reassurance must be given that some forms of cancer respond well to treatment. These deep-seated fears influence behavior and often create situations in which the person knows what ought to be done but does not do it.

CONCLUSION

From experience to date, we know that more than 80% of the causes of cancer are theoretically avoidable. This tells us that cancer is not inevitable and that cancer prevention is feasible and practical. As LeMaistre[14] points out, "If we are willing to use the knowledge we now have about how to prevent cancer as effectively as we do the knowledge about how to cure cancer, then and only then will we be on the road to eliminating cancer." The concept of prevention is sound, but successful application will require that we move forward aggressively in two directions: (1) basic research in cancer prevention and (2) understanding more about motivating human behavior change. A first step in refocusing our cancer-prevention efforts occurred when a consensus was achieved that cancers are caused by specific risk factors in our environment and in our lifestyle. However, efforts at developing effective cancer-prevention strategies have been hampered by the fact that the knowledge base and understanding of each risk factor varies. We must, therefore, acquire additional knowledge about each individual risk factor and determine how it affects the body. This information, combined with strong public education, will prove to be the cornerstone of cancer prevention.

REFERENCES

1. Robbins LC, Hall JH: How to Practice Prospective Medicine. Indianapolis, Methodist Hospital of Indiana, 1970.
2. Schoenbach V: Appraising health risk appraisal. Am J Pub Health 77:409-411, 1987.
3. Higginson J: Existing risks for cancer, in Deisler P (ed): Reducing the Carcinogenic Risks in Industry. New York, Marcel Dekker, 1984, pp 1-19.
4. Bodnar B, Pedersen S: The nursing process, in Edelman C, Mandle C (eds): Health Promotion Throughout the Lifespan. St. Louis, CV Mosby Co, 1986, pp 44-71.
5. Rowe W: Identification of risk, in Risk and Reasons: Risk Assessment in Relation to Environmental Mutagens and Carcinogens. New York, Alan R Liss, Inc, 1986, pp 3-22.
6. Oleske D, Groenwald S: Epidemiology of cancer, in Groenwald S (ed): Cancer Nursing: Principles and Practice. Boston, Jones and Bartlett, 1987, pp 3-28.
7. Groer M: Risk factors and theories of carcinogenesis, in Groenwald S (ed): Cancer Nursing: Principles and Practices. Boston, Jones and Bartlett, 1987, pp 47-63.
8. Breslow L: Review and future perspectives of cancer screening programs, in Nieburgs H (ed): Prevention and Detection of Cancer. Part II. Detection. New York, Marcel Dekker, 1978, pp 1177-1212.
9. White L: Cancer risk assessment. Semin Oncol Nurs, 2:184-190, 1986.
10. Hammond E: Epidemiologic basis for cancer prevention. Cancer 33:1728-1731, 1974.
11. Hammond E: The epidemiological approach to the etiology of cancer, in Kruse L, Reese J, Hart L (eds): Cancer: Pathophysiology, Etiology and Management. St. Louis, CV Mosby Co, 1979, 44-46.
12. Lin R, Kessler I: A multifactorial model for pancreative cancer in man. JAMA 245:147-152, 1981.
13. Woods N, Woods J: Epidemiology and the study of cancer, in Marino L (ed): Cancer Nursing. St. Louis, CV Mosby Co, 1981, pp 139-175.
14. LeMaistre C: Reflections on disease prevention. Cancer, 62:1673-1675, 1988 (suppl).
15. Gray N: Cancer risks and cancer prevention in the third world, in Vessey M, Gray M (eds): Cancer Risks and Prevention. Oxford, Oxford University, 1985, pp 269-299.
16. Schulte P, Ringen K, Hemstreet G, et al: Risk assessment of a cohort exposed to aromatic amines. J Occup Med 27:115-121, 1985.
17. Schulte P, Ringen K, Hemstreet G, et al: Risk factors for bladder cancer in a cohort exposed to aromatic amines. Cancer 58:2156-2162, 1986.
18. Morrison A, Cole P: Urinary tract, in Schottenfeld D, Fraumeni J (eds): Cancer Epidemiology and Prevention. Philadelphia, WB Saunders, 1982, pp 925-937.
19. Wakefield J: Education of the public, in Fraumeni J (ed): Persons at High Risk of Cancer: An Approach to Cancer Etiology and Control. New York, Academic Press, 1975, pp 415-434.
20. Skegg D: Other drugs, in Vessey M, Gray M (eds): Cancer Risks and Prevention. Oxford, Oxford University, 1985, pp 211-230.
21. Whitmore W: Bladder cancer: An overview. CA 38:213-221, 1988.
22. Seidman H, Stellman S, Hushinski M: A different perspective on breast cancer risk factors: Some implications of the non-attributable risk. CA 32:301-313, 1982.
23. Berg J: Clinical implications of risk factors for breast cancer. Cancer 53:589-591, 1984.
24. Schatzkin A, Jones Y, Hoover R, et al: Alcohol consumption and breast cancer in the epidemiologic follow-up study of the first national health and nutrition examination survey. N Engl J Med 316:1169-1173, 1987.
25. Harris R, Wynder E: Breast cancer and alcohol consumption: A study of weak associations. JAMA 259:2867-2871, 1988.
26. Good news for women who booze—CDC finds no breast cancer increase. Cancer Lett 14:6-7, April 8, 1988.
27. Petrakis N, Ernster V, King M: Breast, in Schottenfeld D, Fraumeni J (eds): Cancer Epidemiology and Prevention. Philadelphia, WB Saunders, 1982, pp 855-870.
28. The Cancer and Steroid Hormone Study of the Centers for Disease Control and the National Institute of Child Health and Human Development: Oral contraceptive use and the risk of breast cancer. N Engl J Med 315:405-411, 1986.
29. Henderson B, Ross R, Bernstein L: Estrogens as a cause of human cancer: The Richard and Hinda Rosenthal Foundation Award Lecture. Cancer Res 48:246-253, 1988.
30. Kerr G: Nutritional counseling for cancer prevention, in Newell G (ed): Cancer Prevention in Clinical Medicine. New York, Raven Press, 1983, pp 165-189.
31. Wynder E, Rose D: Diet and breast cancer. Hosp Pract 19:73-88, 1984.

32. Wynder E, Rose D, Cohen L: Diet and breast cancer in causation and therapy. Cancer 58:1804-1813, 1986.
33. Willett W, Stampfer M, Colditz G, et al: Dietary fat and the risk of breast cancer. N Engl J Med 316:22-28, 1987.
34. Cramer D: Uterine cervix, in Schottenfeld D, Fraumeni J (eds): Cancer Epidemiology and Prevention. Philadelphia, WB Saunders, 1982, pp 881-908.
35. Lovejoy N: Precancerous lesions of the cervix: Personal risk factors. Cancer Nurs 10:2-14, 1987.
36. Bender M: A clinician's guide to genital papillomavirus infection. Curr Concepts Skin Disorders Fall:11-16, 1988.
37. McCauley K, Ol R: Evaluating the papanicolaou smear: Part I. Consultant 28:31-40, 1988.
38. Hendershot G: Coitus-related cervical cancer risk factors: Trends and differentials in racial and religious groups. Am J Pub Health 73:299-301, 1983.
39. Schottenfeld D, Winawer S: Large intestine, in Schottenfeld D, Fraumeni J (eds): Cancer Epidemiology and Prevention. Philadelphia, WB Saunders, 1982, pp 703-727.
40. Carrott K, Braden L, Bell J, et al: Fat and cancer. Cancer 58:1818-1825, 1986.
41. Hennekens C, Mayrent S, Willett W: Vitamin A, carotenoids, and retinoids. Cancer 58:1837-1841, 1986.
42. Kritchevsky D: Diet, nutrition, and cancer: The role of fiber. Cancer 58:1830-1836, 1986.
43. McDonough B: Sedentary lifestyle invites colon cancer. Oncol Biotechnol News, August 1988, p 19.
44. Weinhouse S: The role of diet and nutrition in cancer. Cancer 58:1791-1794, 1986.
45. Tornberg S, Holm L, Carstensen J, et al: Risks of cancer of the colon and rectum in relation to serum cholesterol and beta-lipoprotein. N Engl J Med 315:1629-1633, 1986.
46. Stroehlein J, Newell G: Detecting colon cancer early: Suggestions for the primary care physician. Your Patient & Cancer 3:87-90, 1983.
47. Fleischer D, Goldberg S, Browning T, et al: Detection and surveillance of colorectal cancer. JAMA 261:580-585, 1989.
48. Winawer S: Screening for colorectal cancer: An overview. Cancer 45:1093-1098, 1980.
49. Fraumeni J, Blot W: Lung and pleura, in Schottenfeld D, Fraumeni J (eds): Cancer Epidemiology and Prevention. Philadelphia, WB Saunders, 1982, pp 564-582.
50. Hammond EC: Tobacco, in Fraumeni J (ed): Persons at High Risk of Cancer: An Approach to Cancer Etiology and Control. New York, Academic Press, 1975, pp 131-138.
51. Humble C, Samet J, Pathak D: Marriage to a smoker and lung cancer risk. Am J Public Health 77:598-602, 1987.
52. Fiedling J, Phenow K: Health effects of involuntary smoking. N Engl J Med 319:1452-1460, 1988.
53. NAS says radon causes 13,000 lung cancer deaths yearly. Med World News, Feb 8, 1988, p 97.
54. Mahboubi E, Sayed G: Oral cavity and pharynx, in Schottenfeld D, Fraumeni J (eds): Cancer Epidemiology and Prevention. Philadelphia, WB Saunders, 1982, pp 583-595.
55. Holmstrup P, Pindborg J: Oral mucosal lesions in smokeless tobacco users. CA 38:230-235,1988.
56. Peto R: The preventability of cancer, in Vessey M, Gray M (eds): Cancer Risks and Prevention. Oxford, Oxford University, 1985, pp 1-14.
57. Weiss N: Ovary, in Schottenfeld D, Fraumeni J (eds): Cancer Epidemiology and Prevention. Philadelphia, WB Saunders, 1982, pp 871-880.
58. White L: The nurse's role in cancer prevention, in Newell G (ed): Cancer Prevention in Clinical Medicine. New York, Raven Press, 1983, pp 91-112.
59. Henderson B, Gerkins V, Pike M: Sexual factors and pregnancy, in Fraumeni J (ed): Persons at High Risk of Cancer: An Approach to Cancer Etiology and Control. New York, Academic Press, 1975, pp 267-284.
60. Vessey M: Exogenous hormones, in Vessey M, Gray M (eds): Cancer Risks and Prevention. Oxford, Oxford University, 1985, pp 166-194.
61. The Cancer and Steroid Hormone Study of the Centers for Disease Control and the National Institute of Child Health and Human Development: The reduction in risk of ovarian cancer associated with oral-contraceptive use. N Engl J Med 316:650-655, 1987.
62. Cutler S, Young J: Demographic patterns of cancer incidence in the United States, in Fraumeni J (ed): Persons at High Risk of Cancer: An Approach to Cancer Etiology and Control. New York, Academic Press, 1975, pp 307-360.
63. Greenwald P: Prostate, in Schottenfeld D, Fraumeni J (eds): Cancer Epidemiology and Prevention. Philadelphia, WB Saunders, 1982, pp 938-967.
64. Doll R, Peto R: The Causes of Cancer: Quantitative Estimates of Avoidable Risks of Cancer in the United States Today. New York, Oxford University Press, 1981.
65. Rose D, Boyar A, Wynder E: International comparisons of mortality rates for cancer of the breast, ovary, prostate, and colon, and per capita food consumption. Cancer 58:2363-2371, 1986.
66. Fitzpatrick T, Rhodes A, Sober A: Prevention of melanoma by recognition of its precursors: Reply to letter. N Engl J Med 312:1388, 1985.
67. Rhodes A, Weinstock M, Fitzpatrick T, et al: Risk factors for cutaneous melanoma: A practical method of recognizing predisposed individuals. JAMA 258:3146-3154, 1987.
68. Finley C: Malignant melanoma: A primary care perspective. Nurse Pract 11(4):18-38, 1986.
69. Kinlen L: Infections and immune impairment, in Vessey M, Gray M (eds): Cancer Risks and Prevention. Oxford, Oxford University, 1985, pp 149-165.
70. Friedman R, Rigel D, Kopf A: Early detection of malignant melanoma: The role of physician examination and self-examination of the skin. CA 35:130-151, 1985.
71. Schottenfeld D, Warshauer M: Testis, in Schottenfeld D, Fraumeni J (eds): Cancer Epidemiology and Prevention. Philadelphia, WB Saunders, 1982, pp 947-957.
72. de Waard F: Uterine corpus, in Schottenfeld D, Fraumeni J (eds): Cancer Epidemiology and Prevention. Philadelphia, WB Saunders, 1982, pp 901-908.
73. Gusberg S: Detection and prevention of uterine cancer. Cancer 62:1784-1786, 1988.
74. Shapiro S, Kelly J, Rosenberg L, et al: Risk of localized and widespread endometrial cancer in relation to recent and discontinued use of conjugated estrogens. N Engl J Med 313:969-972, 1985.
75. Mishell D: Contraception. N Engl J Med 320:777-787, 1989.
76. Koss L: Precancerous lesions, in Fraumeni J (ed): Persons at High Risk of Cancer: An Approach to Cancer Etiology and Control. New York, Academic Press, 1975, pp 85-102.
77. Kelly P: Counseling persons who have family histories of cancer, in Newell G (ed): Cancer Prevention in Clinical Medicine. New York, Raven Press, 1983, pp 147-164.
78. Cohen J, Jaffe D: Holistic health—the future, in Edelman C, Mandle C (eds): Health Promotion Throughout the Lifespan. St. Louis, CV Mosby Co., 1986, pp 643-666.
79. Baeck M, Eisenberg M: Carcinogenic risk assessment: Concepts and issues. Md Med J 34:672-674, 1985.

80. Constanza M, Li F, Green H, et al: Cancer prevention and detection: Strategies for practice, in American Cancer Society: Cancer Manual (ed 7). New York, American Cancer Society, Massachusetts Division, Inc, 1986, pp 14-35.
81. American Cancer Society: Cancer-related checkups. ACS Publication 2070-LE. New York, American Cancer Society, Inc., 1987.
82. American Cancer Society: Recommendations for the early detection of cancer in asymptomatic persons. ACS Publication 3409-PE. New York, American Cancer Society, 1988.
83. Wakefield J: Education of the public, in Fraumeni J (ed): Persons at High Risk of Cancer. New York, Academic Press, 1975, pp 415-434.
84. Green L, Rimer B, Elwood T: Public education, in Schottenfeld D, Fraumeni J (eds): Cancer Epidemiology and Prevention. Philadelphia, WB Saunders, 1982, pp 1100-1110.

Chapter 8

Assessment and Interventions for Cancer Prevention and Detection

Marilyn Frank-Stromborg, RN, EdD, NP, FAAN

Rebecca Cohen, RN, EdD, CPQA

INTRODUCTION

Despite the long history of cancer, it became a relatively important health problem only during the twentieth century. It was among the first chronic diseases recognized as potentially "controllable," that is, amenable to public health strategies consistent with its magnitude and social impact. In 1937 the Congress of the United States took its first significant action on the problem of cancer by passing the National Cancer Institute Act. This law established the National Cancer Institute for purposes of conducting research relating to the cause, diagnosis, and treatment of cancer and the application of research results with a view to the development and prompt widespread use of the most effective methods of prevention, diagnosis, and treatment of cancer.[1] Congressional intent toward the cancer problem was reaffirmed by the passage of the National Cancer Act of 1971. The Act expanded activities "to develop, through research and development efforts, the means to significantly reduce the morbidity and mortality from cancer by: preventing as many cancers as possible, curing patients who develop cancer, providing maximum palliation to patients not cured, rehabilitating treated patients to as nearly normal a state as possible."[2]

Although a clear expression of congressional intent existed regarding cancer control, results of the 1971 legislation tended to be in the direction of research. It had been hoped that the legislation would result in cancer control efforts (1) to improve identification of techniques or methods with a potential for combating the disease, (2) to improve community testing of these technologic methods for safety and efficacy, (3) to provide for evaluation of the results of the testing, and (4) to enhance promotion of the appropriate general use of technologic techniques in the community through professional and public education. Obstacles existed, however, that made it much more difficult to initiate cancer control efforts than it had been to control other communicable diseases. One of the obstacles included the fact that physicians generally did not view cancer as epidemic in nature. It was believed that governmental action to establish public services for cancer diagnosis or treatment was an intrusion into physicians' freedom to practice. In addition, economic resistance to control measures, for example, by the tobacco industry, was assisted by the fact that the long latency period of cancer helped to make etiologic factors less identifiable. Finally, cancer's multiple etiology engendered an extensive research effort when an additional attack on the disease was mounted. Money for research and training of personnel was held onto tightly by special interest groups that resisted public expenditures for cancer control as a threat to their own existence.[3,4]

Thus organized cancer control in the United States has had three strong adversaries: the private medical world, the private industrial world, and the biomedical research establishment that emerged after the passage of the National Cancer Institute Act of 1937 and the subsequent creation of the National Institutes of Health in 1948. In some situations these forces, feeling threatened by cancer control, have developed strong lobbies against cancer control.

Can We Prevent Cancer?

The arguments that cancer can be prevented are familiar to almost everyone. Different populations throughout the world suffer from different kinds of cancer, but those who migrate tend to acquire the pattern of cancers characteristic of their new home. It is therefore concluded by scientists that the incidence of most kinds of cancers is determined by environment.[5,6] Research indicates that Americans could cut their incidence of cancer to little more than half the national average simply by adopting the lifestyle of the Seventh-Day Adventists and moving to the Rocky Mountain states or becoming Mormons and migrating to Utah.[7]

Evidence clearly illustrates that trying to change life-styles may create some resistance.[8-12] Such attitudes as "there is not much a person can do to prevent cancer" or "scientists say everything causes cancer" create further resistance to the prevention of cancer.[13] Everyone knows about the link between cigarettes and lung cancer, and people expect to be exposed to lectures about the dangers of smoking. However, it has become customary to brush this aside and concentrate attention on modern industry as the supposed cause of most of our ills. It is attractive to distrust science and technology because they lay the blame on the imagined avarice of others rather than on one's own self-indulgence.[7]

In fact, some scientists[7,12] believe that there is really no evidence that any of the products of modern technology (except cigarettes) contribute to the common cancers. Thus most of the major cancers, except lung cancer, are not any more common today than they were 50 years ago.[7,12] It is suggested, however, that new industrial products be monitored for mutagenicity and carcinogenicity and that industries are deterred from adding hazardous ingredients or waste to our environment. However, cancer cannot be conquered simply by the surveillance and control of industry. To effectively conquer the common cancers, preventive measures must reach the individual and seek to modify personal habits and life-styles.[7,12] For example, cancer of the lung is due to a highly addictive habit; cancer of the head and neck is associated with tobacco and excessive alcohol use; cancer of the large intestine and breast are most common in affluent countries and are thought to be related to diet; cancer of the skin is linked to ultraviolet rays and for some individuals it is connected with increased leisure time.[10,12] The preventive strategies for these cancers may conflict with the immediate desires of some.[11] Apart from giving up smoking, sunbathing, and alcohol, the most recent change that we have been asked to make is in diet—the consumption of less fat, less cholesterol, and more fruits, vegetables, and cereals.[14-20]

Whether people will be willing to give up certain immediate desires for health and prolonged life remains to be seen. However, the National Cancer Institute has established as its "Year 2000 Cancer Control Objective" a 50% reduction in the cancer mortality rate.[10] It is the belief of the National Cancer Institute that through the application of current knowledge about cancer prevention, screening, and detection; access to the latest treatment; and continuing advances in cancer treatment, the 1980 mortality rate can be reduced by 25% to 50%.

LEVELS OF PREVENTION

How, then, can we approach the problem of cancer prevention? According to Edelman and Milio[21] we must begin by broadening our definition of prevention. Prevention, in a narrow sense, means averting the development of disease. In a broad sense, however, it consists of all measures, including definitive therapy, that limit the progression of disease at any point of its course. This concept is important because it implies that prevention can take place anywhere along the continuum of health. By adopting this definition, one could employ preventive strategies while healthy, during the phase of determining whether one has the disease, and during the phase of dealing with a disease already contracted. It has therefore been suggested that there are three levels of prevention: primary, secondary, and tertiary.[22,23] Each level of prevention occurs at a distinct point in the development of the disease process and requires specific interventions.

Primary Prevention

Primary prevention is true prevention; it precedes disease or dysfunction and is applied to a population generally considered both physically and emotionally healthy. Primary prevention is not therapeutic, does not use therapeutic treatments, and does not involve symptom identification. The purpose of primary prevention is to decrease the vulnerability of the individual or the population to illness or dysfunction through health-promoting strategies, as well as to provide specific protection.[21]

Contrary to the popular belief that preventive medicine will decrease medical expenditures, it actually may increase the nation's steadily rising medical bills. Preventive activities must be assessed in terms of health and not just cost. This is necessary because there are certain preventive measures that will create enormous benefits in terms of health but actually will increase medical expenditures. Society must decide whether better health is worth the higher cost, and individuals must determine what best meets their own personal needs. The final choice depends on the value that one places upon health benefits, risks, and costs.[24,25]

Health promotion

Edelman and Milio[21] point out that health promotion efforts focus on maintaining or improving the general health of individuals, families, and communities. These activities are carried on at both the public level, such as government programs that promote adequate housing, and the personal level. There are two strategies of health promotion, passive and active. Passive strategies involve the individual as a passive participant or recipient. Examples of passive strategies may include maintaining clean water and sanitary sewage systems or enforcing governmental regulations within industries to make sure that employees are protected from industrial agents/chemicals, lights, and injuries.[21] On the other hand, active strategies depend on the individual adopting a proposed program of health promotion. Examples include changes in eating or exercise habits or enrollment in a stress management class.

Nursing interventions are directed toward developing the resources of persons to maintain or enhance their well-being. Health promotion activities related to cancer include[26]:

1. Identifying risk factors in individuals or groups
2. Educating and counseling people for risk factor reduction
3. Identifying existing primary cancer prevention activities (eg, stop-smoking programs)
4. Planning and implementing new cancer prevention programs, such as (a) nutrition education, (b) hazards of cigarette smoking, alcohol consumption, and poor diet, and (c) programs for children, the elderly, and disadvantaged that are aimed at their particular health needs
5. Genetic screening
6. Periodic selective examinations
7. Conducting epidemiologic research

Although health promotion is a desirable concept, the health care system in the United States responds to the most pressing matter at the moment. Health promotion lacks the demanding element of immediacy and thus tends to be regulated to lower levels of importance. The federal government policy advocates health promotion, as evidenced by the establishment of the Office of Health Information and Health Promotion and the publication of *Healthy People* in 1982, but it has yet to show a major commitment to the allocation of more funds for research and demonstration projects in this field.[21]

Personal health promotion most commonly is provided by health education. However, because health education is concerned principally with creating changes in human behavior, it must involve more than the provision of health information and must be considered an important function of nurses, physicians, parents, and allied health professionals. The goal is to assist individuals to develop a sense of responsibility for their own health and a shared sense of responsibility for avoiding injury to the health of others. Health education encourages health-promoting habits, values, and attitudes that must be learned through practice. These, in turn, must be reinforced through systematic instruction in hygiene, bodily function, physical fitness, and use of leisure time. Another important goal of health education is to help the individual understand how to appropriately use health services.[21]

Specific protection

Specific protection focuses on protecting persons from disease by providing immunization and reducing exposure to occupational hazards, carcinogens, and other environmental health risks. Primary prevention is considered health protection because it emphasizes shielding or defending the body from injury.

Specific protection strategies include[21]:

- Attention to personal hygiene
- Use of environmental sanitation
- Protection against occupational hazards
- Protection from accidents
- Use of specific nutrients
- Protection from carcinogens
- Avoidance of allergens

Secondary Prevention

Secondary prevention activities include defining and identifying high-risk groups and groups with precursor stages of disease. It is important to acknowledge that there is no sharp break between primary and secondary prevention or between precursors and "early" stages of a disease.[23]

Secondary prevention ranges from early diagnosis/detection, screening, and treating early stages of disease to limiting disability by averting or delaying the consequences of advanced disease.

Early diagnosis and prompt treatment

Early detection is the identification of a precancerous lesion or the diagnosis of a cancer when it is still localized, curable, or manageable. Screening has been defined as the presumptive identification of unrecognized disease or defect by the application of tests, examinations, or other procedures that can be applied rapidly. Although the two terms often are used interchangeably, there is a difference between them. Early detection is the early identification of disease in an individual, who may or may not have symptoms, through the use of tests, examinations, and observations. On the other hand, screening is an organized effort to find cancer in its early stages in a defined population.[26]

Activities carried out to ensure early diagnosis and prompt treatment include[21,26]:

1. Case-finding measures both on an individual basis and for the community as a whole
2. Screening procedures based on identified risk factors
3. Monthly breast self-examinations
4. Periodic Papanicoulaou (Pap) smears
5. Attending a cancer detection clinic
6. Seeking medical attention for one of cancer's seven warning signals
7. Prevention of complications and sequelae

Limiting disability

Providing adequate treatment to arrest a disease process and to prevent further complications and sequelae, as well as providing facilities to limit disability and prevent death, are important functions in this category. Delayed recognition because of incomplete knowledge of some disease process in early secondary prevention results in the need to limit future disability in the late stage of secondary prevention. Certain economic environmental changes may aid in preventing sequelae, but the preventive measures primarily are therapeutic to arrest the disease and prevent further complications.[21]

Tertiary Prevention

Tertiary prevention takes place when a disability is permanent and irreversible. It involves minimizing the effects of disease and disability by surveillance and maintenance aimed at preventing complications and deterioration. This level of prevention focuses on rehabilitation to help persons attain and retain an optimal level of functioning regardless of their disabling condition.

ROLE OF THE NURSE IN PRIMARY AND SECONDARY CANCER PREVENTION

Activities undertaken by the nurse in promoting primary and secondary cancer prevention include assessment, counseling, teaching, screening, planning, and acting as an advocate. In addition, increasing knowledge and skills to carry out the preventive strategies in an effective manner is important. This requires that the nurse have knowledge of and be able to teach the individual about risk factors associated with the development of cancer and factors that affect health behaviors. It also requires that the nurse be competent in carrying out cancer screening and detection methods and making recommendations for their use.[12,14,26-29]

The nurse begins any intervention by assessing the needs of the individual or target group. Intervention then can consist of one-on-one teaching or counseling; participating in planning, conducting, and evaluating new primary and secondary cancer prevention programs; serving as an information resource; or encouraging participation in existing cancer prevention and detection programs.[26-28]

Advocacy is an important aspect of cancer prevention. The nurse should act as an advocate to help promote and maintain healthier lives for people. Nurses must also encourage, or participate in, research that will investigate cancer prevention and learning methods on how to motivate human behavior change.[26-28]

DETECTION OF MAJOR CANCER SITES

In the last 10 years, physical assessment has become a vital part of the nursing role regardless of the nurse's setting. The use of physical assessment techniques is not limited to nurses who have completed a nurse practictioner program. Rather it is now routinely taught in all undergraduate nursing programs, and the expectation is that nursing students will incorporate the four cardinal techniques (inspection, palpation, percussion, and auscultation) into their daily clinical practice. Physical assessment techniques enable the nurse to assume an active role in the early detection of cancer.

Cancers of the lung, breast, cervix, colon/rectum, and prostate are among the cancers that result in the highest morbidity and mortality rates in the United States.[30] The nursing interventions for these five cancers and for skin, testicular, head and neck, and other gynocologic cancers will be discussed. Each section presents the nursing role in terms of obtaining the health history, conducting the physical examination, using screening tests for asymptomatic persons, and initiating patient education for primary and secondary prevention of the cancer.

Lung Cancer

It is estimated that in 1989, 155,000 Americans will be diagnosed with lung cancer.[31] It is the leading cause of death from cancer in men and women over 35 years old. Once considered a male disease, within the last 5 years it has replaced breast cancer as the chief cause of cancer deaths among women. Of all the known risk factors for lung cancer, the most important environmental carcinogen related to the increased incidence of lung cancer is cigarette smoking. Cigarette smoking is the largest single preventable cause of premature death and disability and the major single cause of cancer mortality.[32]

History assessment

When obtaining the history, the nurse should inquire into smoking habits, including marijuana use, occupational history, and the general respiratory environment in both the workplace and home. Persons at high risk for lung cancer are those exposed to high levels of respiratory carcinogens in their workplace, in their general environment, and in their homes. Because of the risks of passive smoking, a detailed history should be taken of the number of smokers in the home and the length of time the individual has been exposed to the smoke environment.[33,34]

Although the process of obtaining a detailed, lifetime occupational history is time-consuming, it is strongly recommended for anyone who has worked in shipyards or who is believed to have been exposed to asbestos; significant exposures may have been as brief as 1 month and may have occurred many years ago, even during World War II. Because the World War II work force was composed of women as well as men, the female patient should not be overlooked. The same type of detailed, lifetime occupational history should be obtained if exposure to other known carcinogenic respiratory agents, such as those found in the following occupations, is suspected: clothing and textile workers, laundry workers, meat wrappers and cutters, hairdressers, agricultural workers, chemical workers, electrical machinery manufacturers, and health care workers.[35] In the assessment of elderly persons, prior employment in settings unregulated by the National Institute of Occupational Safety and Health, the Occupational Safety and Health Act of 1970, or the Toxic Substances Control Act of 1976 must be considered because of possible exposure to toxic chemical or carcinogens that are no longer manufactured or permitted in unsupervised occupational settings.

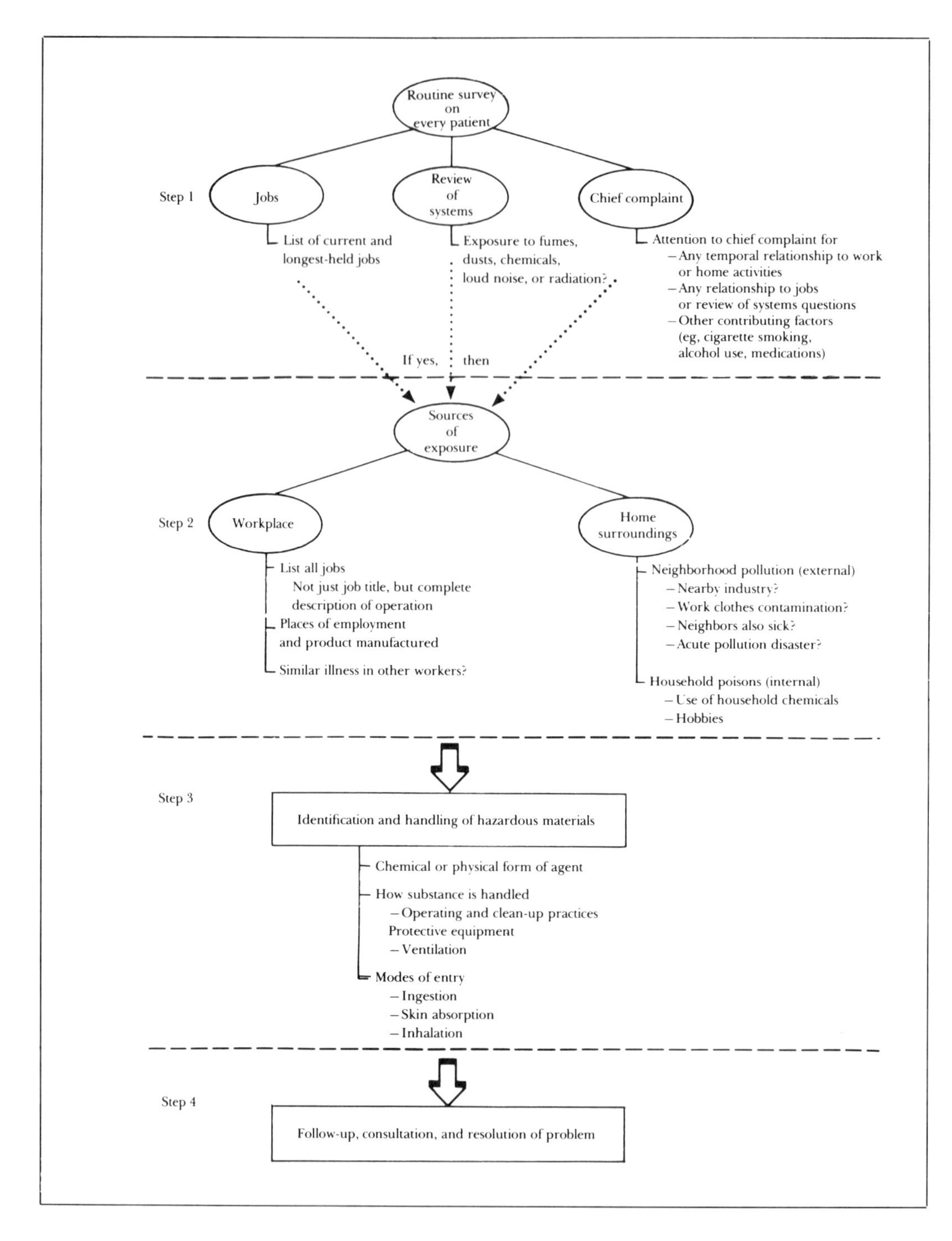

FIGURE 8-1 Systematic approach to the occupational and environmental health history. (Source: Goldman R, Peters J: The occupational and environmental health history. JAMA 246:2832-2836, 1981.)

An occupational history includes dates of employment, a list of current and longest-held jobs, average hours worked per week, exposure to potential hazards in the workplace, common illness in coworkers, and personal protective equipment worn on the job. Figure 8-1 presents a systematic approach to the occupational and environmental health history.[36]

Questions that should be included in the history and review of systems for lung cancer consist of the following items:

1. When was your last chest x-ray?
2. When was your last tuberculin skin test? If positive, what was the treatment?
3. Do you presently smoke? How many packs a day and for how many years? (Pack years equal packs per day

times years of smoking.) What do you smoke? Are they filtered? What's your style of smoking? Have you ever tried to stop smoking? What happened? Do you have a "smoker's" cough? Who else in the home smokes, and how much do they tend to smoke a day?

4. Do you have bronchitis or asthma?
5. Have you ever had pneumonia?
6. Do you get short of breath with walking? climbing stairs? while resting? exercise?
7. Have you ever been told you have emphysema?
8. How many pillows do you sleep on? What happens if you don't?
9. Do you ever spit or cough up blood?
10. Smokers: What color is the sputum you cough up? Does it have a smell? How much is routinely coughed up in the morning?
11. What occupations have you had?
12. Chronic obstructive pulmonary disease: How often do you get flu shots? Have you been taught ways to drain the secretions from your lungs?
13. Have you ever had a pulmonary function test? What were the results?
14. Do you ever wheeze?
15. Do you cough a lot?
16. Do you have any skeletal deformities? Or were you born with any skeletal conditions?
17. Have you had any broken ribs?
18. Do you have to purse your lips to breathe?
19. Are you aware of any sounds when you breathe?
20. Have you noticed any color changes of your lips or nails?
21. Do you now (or have you been some time in the past) exposed to fumes, chemicals, dust, or radiation?

The majority of patients have no profound early symptoms, but most have some combination of cough, chest pain, weight loss, dyspnea, fever, fatigue, or transient hemoptysis. Because these symptoms are general in nature, they usually cause no alarm and delay diagnosis. The most frequently reported symptom of lung cancer is a cough that is productive and often associated with hemoptysis or chest pain. Cough may be the primary or only complaint in such varied diseases as congestive heart failure, asthma, upper respiratory infection, pneumonia, or bronchitis. The irritative cough may occur at night accompanied by mucoid expectoration. However, if the lung cancer is centrally located or if only the main carina is involved, the cough is non-productive.

Later symptoms are increased frequency of early symptoms and some combination of wheezes, pleuritic pain, hoarseness, nerve disorders from local invasion, edema of head, neck, or arms, or dysphagia. There is a high index of suspicion in anyone with a history of smoking or exposure to carcinogenic agents who complains of pneumonitis that persists longer than 2 weeks despite antibiotic therapy. Unfortunately, the first symptoms of lung cancer are usually not alarming and therefore tend to be considered lightly by health professionals. Because elderly persons experience changes in respiratory structure and function, their initial vague respiratory complaints go unnoticed or are attributed to the aging process or chronic illnesses (eg, congestive heart failure).

Physical examination

Inspection On inspection there may be many systemic, as well as localized, signs that will alert the practictioner to the possibility of lung cancer.

Finger clubbing This may be either an early or a late sign of thoracic disease, and it may be absent even in the presence of advanced disease. Clinically 5% to 12% of the patients with carcinoma of the lung will have clubbing of the fingers. It also may be seen in other diseases such as industrial lung disease (eg, asbestosis).[37] It is important to closely inspect the nails and to palpate them for sponginess. With clubbing, the nail bed becomes thickened and boggy, which is first observed by palpating the nail bed to elicit fluctuation. Clubbing usually occurs first in the thumb and index finger and then spreads to the other fingers.

The changes associated with clubbing usually occur gradually over many weeks, months, and years. However, they have been noted to appear within a week of the onset of lung cancer. Clubbing is best assessed by viewing the finger from the side. A normal finger viewed from this direction has an angle of about 160 degrees between the base of the nail and the skin next to the cuticle (Figure 8-2). In clubbing, this base angle is obliterated and becomes 180 degrees or more.[38]

Barrel chest This is characterized by prominence of the sternum and a barrel-shaped configuration of the chest that appears to be held in a state of full inspiration.[39] This finding is associated with pulmonary emphysema or normal aging. Emphysema can be inherited, but the vast majority of persons with this disease have acquired it from a lifetime of smoking. Those with emphysema are at high risk for lung cancer. Typical physical findings of emphysema are pursed lips during breathing, retraction of the intercostal spaces during inspiration, use of accessory muscles during quiet respirations, and audible wheezes.

Abnormal breathing With obstructive types of pulmonary disease, expiration is prolonged and inspiration is gasping and may require the use of the accessory muscles of respiration in the neck and about the shoulder girdle.[40] Figure 8-3 shows the stance taken by individuals with pulmonary obstruction. This stance is called the professorial attitude because is resembles a professor lecturing.

Bulges on the thorax With the use of indirect lighting, the practitioner may observe a bulge on the chest. Neoplasm of the ribs may protrude and will be visible on inspection.

Breathlessness During the history-taking process the patient's breathlessness may indicate obstruction of the lungs.

Superior vena cava obstruction Obstruction of the superior vena cava is a common complication of lung cancer; approximately 80% of these cases are caused by undif-

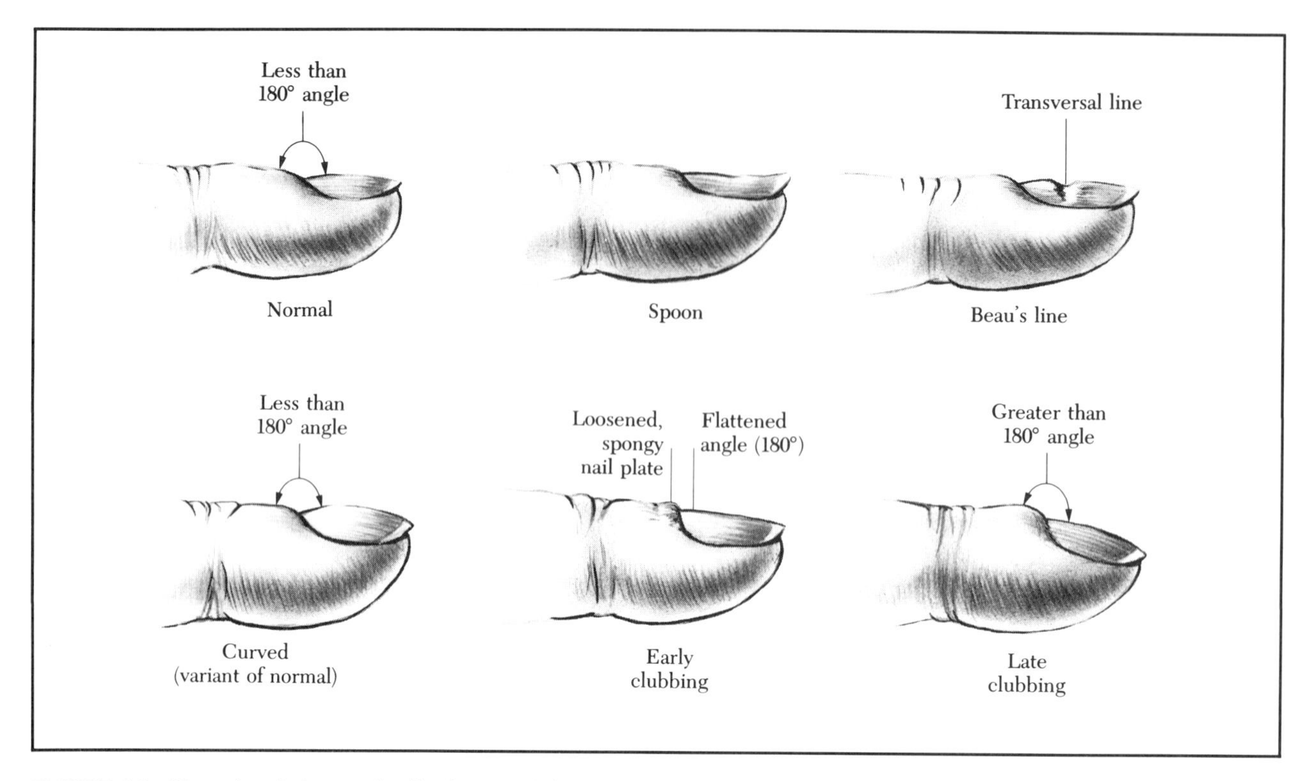

FIGURE 8-2 Normal and abnormal nails. (Source: Grimes J, Burns E (eds): Health Assessment in Nursing Practice (ed 2). Boston, Jones and Bartlett, 1987.)

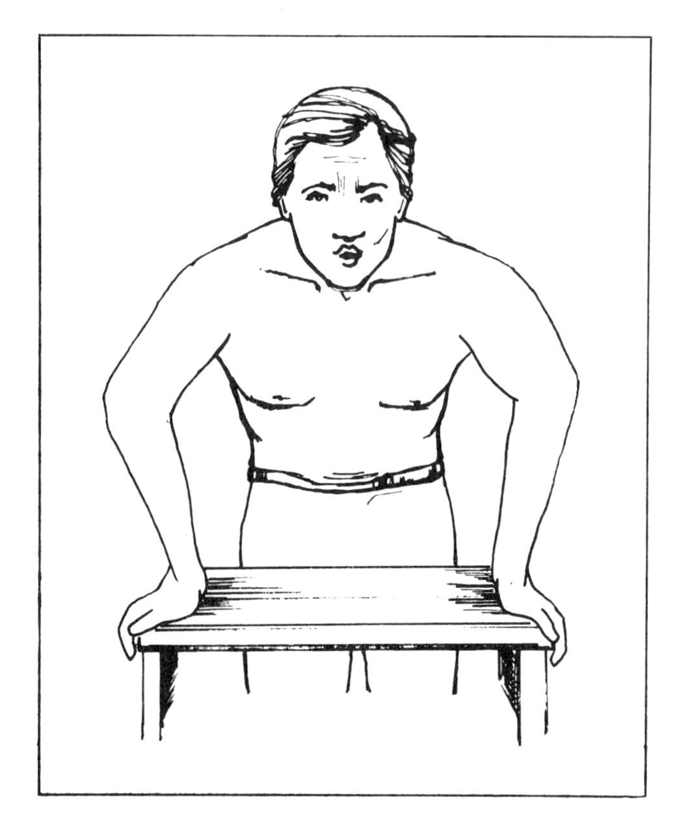

FIGURE 8-3 Patient fixes the arms and leans forward to use pectoral muscles as accessory inspiratory muscles for obstructed breathing. (Source: Buckingham W: A Primer of Clinical Diagnosis (ed 2). New York, Harper & Row, 1979.)

ferentiated neoplasms arising in proximal right bronchi.[41] The clinical picture is described by Buckingham:

> . . . Edema of both eyelids, arms, and hands develops and will "pit" on pressure; . . . the face is a dusky blue color, the lips are deeply cyanotic; and the swollen, blue head sits on a thick "bull neck" which is distended by many large, tense collateral views. The shoulders, chest, and upper abdomen are covered with a lacy collateral venous pattern.[40]

Palpation Palpation of the thorax includes testing for vocal fremitus, respiratory excursion, and compression and ascertaining the position and movability of the trachea. The following discussion presents physical signs of palpation that may indicate lung cancer.

Deviation and fixed trachea Normally the trachea is located in the midline and is freely movable. Localized disease may produce tracheal shift, or the trachea may be fixed by disease in the surrounding structures. Carcinoma of the lung rarely causes displacement except by producing atelectasis.[42]

Thoracic wall Palpation of the thoracic wall reveals masses.

Vocal fremitus Decreased or absent vocal fremitus indicates local bronchial obstruction from bronchial carcinomas, adenomas, or foreign bodies. Sound transmission through the bronchus is interrupted, causing the change in fremitus. Absent vocal fremitus also may indicate pleural effusions. Lung tumors immediately adjacent to the visceral pleura often cause early, insidious formation of pleural effusion that is responsible for the initial complaint of dyspnea.[41]

Percussion and auscultation These may provide the final clues to assessment of the individual who is at high risk for lung cancer. Auscultation is best done with the diaphragm of the stethoscope in a slow methodical sequence of upper, middle, and lower zones and front, sides, and back. Physical signs that would require referral are discussed here.

Dullness Dullness on percussion indicates either pleural effusion or a consolidated lung. The normal sound percussed over the lung is resonance. Lung cancer is the most common cause of hemorrhagic pleural effusion in middle-aged and elderly male smokers. The early production of pleural fluid by most tumors produces the classic signs of pleural effusion: flatness, absence of fremitus, and breath sounds.[42] An excellent technique for assessing dullness in the thorax is the auscultatory-percussion technique. This technique is accomplished by having the examiner lightly percuss the patient's manubrium while listening with the diaphragm piece on the posterior chest wall (Figure 8-4[43]).

In the normal chest the sound on auscultatory percussion is resonant. If any pathologic condition exists between the sound source (manubrium) and the reception point (stethoscope), the sound produced is a duller tone than normal. This technique enables the examiner to detect small, deep areas of pathologic disease.

Decreased or absent breath sounds Breath sounds are decreased or absent when air flow is decreased or when fluid or tissue separates the air passages from the stethoscope.

Unilateral wheezing and the bagpipe sign Tumors in the main bronchus may cause a localized expiratory and/or inspiratory wheeze, or "honk," which sometimes is reproduced only when the individual lies on the affected side. When a continuous wheeze is heard at the end of expiration as air continues to whistle out past a partial obstruction, this is known as the *bagpipe sign.*[41]

Presence of whispered pectoriloquy, bronchophony, and egophony When the lungs are normal, whispered test words are faint and their syllables are not distinct when the examiner listens with a stethoscope over the lungs. When a lung is consolidated or compressed by a pleural effusion, transmission of voice sounds is altered. The sounds are louder, clearer than usual, and sometimes changed in quality. On the basis of these three criteria, the following changes are noted:

1. *Whispered pectoriloquy.* The patient whispers numerals (eg, one, two, and three). Normally these sounds are muffled; in consolidation they are clearly transmitted.[44]

2. *Bronchophony.* When the patient says a number (eg, 99), the sound normally is muffled. When the sound transmitted is a clear sound of the vocalized numerals, it is created by mucous- or fluid-filled alveoli or by cellular mass replacing alveolar tissue.[45]

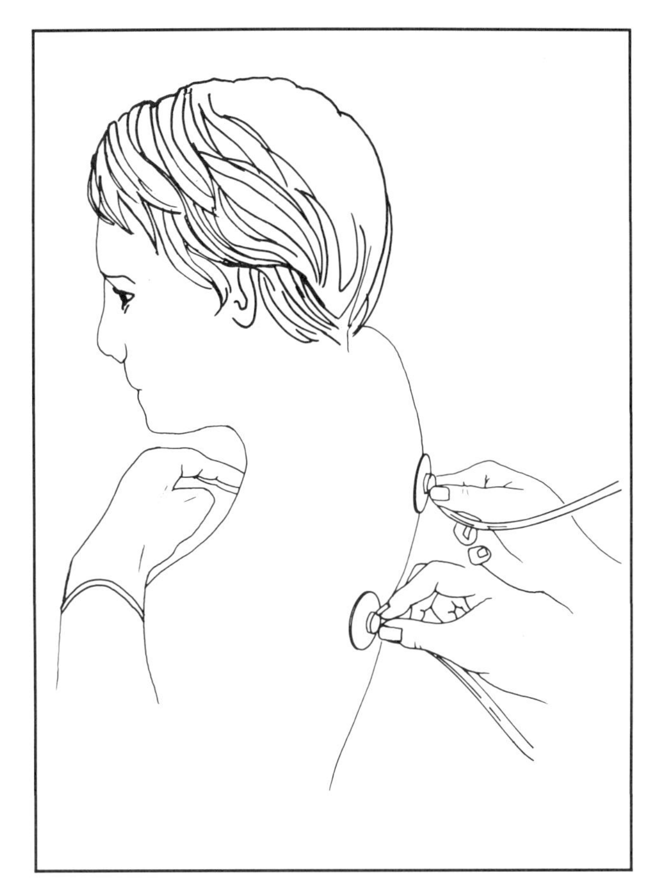

FIGURE 8-4 Auscultatory-percussion technique. (Source: Guarino J: Auscultatory-percussion, a technique for detecting unsuspected lung disease. Diagnosis, January: 20-26, 1981.)

3. *Egophony.* The patient says "e," which normally results in a muffled, indistinct sound. In pleural effusion the "e" sound is heard as a nasal-sounding "a."

In conclusion, there are no physical signs or symptoms in the early stage of lung cancer. The majority of physical signs the practitioner would discover during physical assessment are the result of late and far-advanced carcinoma of the lung. Figure 8-5 presents a synopsis of the physical findings commonly seen with tumors of different anatomic sites in the lungs. The majority of physical signs discussed previously are found in late or advanced lung cancer. The *only early* physical finding that most strongly suggests lung cancer is wheezing localized to a single lobe of the lung in an elderly person with a long history of smoking.

Screening tests for asymptomatic individuals

There are no recommended screening programs or tests for lung cancer because studies have not shown any evidence of a significant reduction in mortality from these programs. The American Cancer Society focuses on primary prevention: helping smokers to stop and keeping nonsmokers from starting.[46]

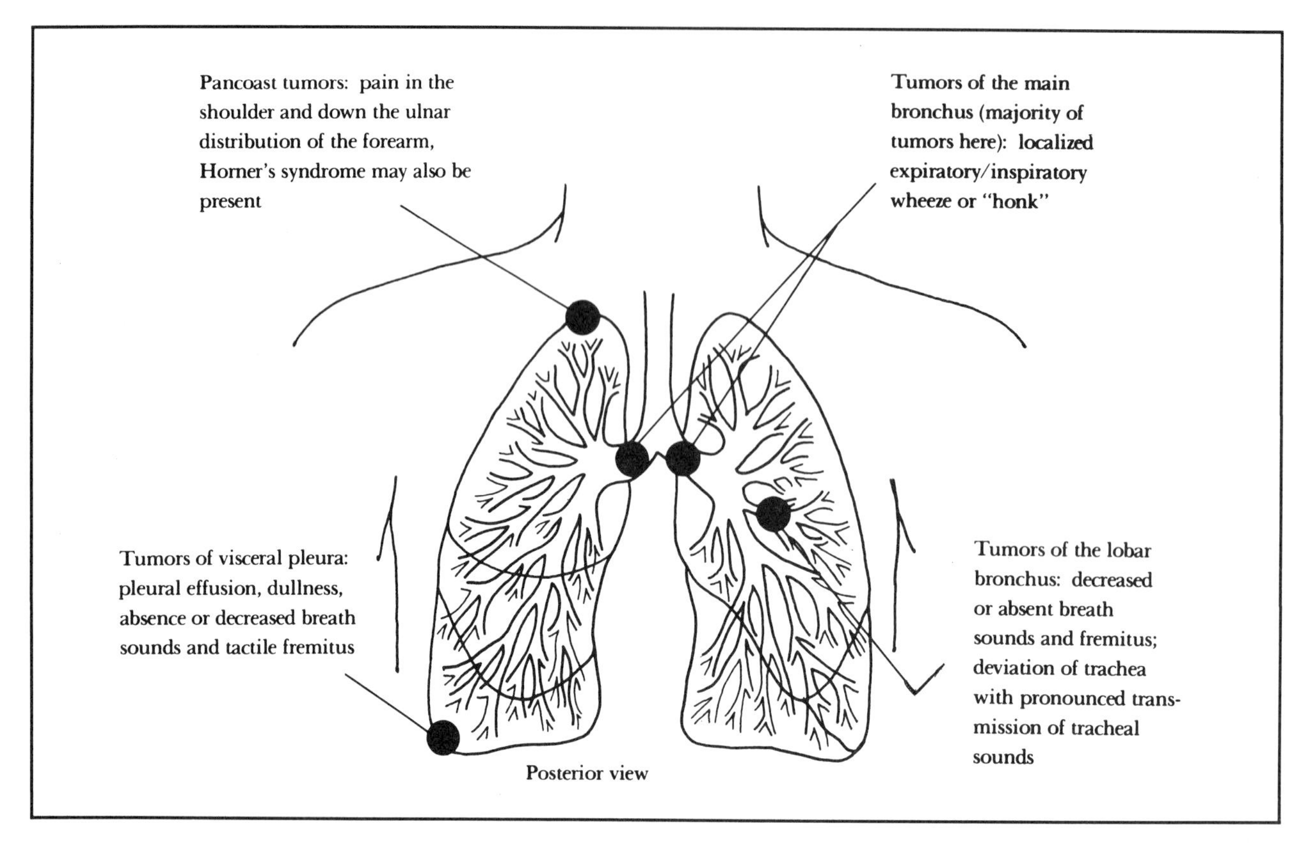

FIGURE 8-5 Synopsis of physical findings of lung cancer.

Smoking cessation

The greatest reduction in mortality can be achieved by cessation of smoking. Between 80% to 85% of deaths from lung cancer are directly attributable to smoking, thus making smoking the leading cause of cancer mortality in the United States.[47] Smoking in the United States is on the decline. Per capita cigarette consumption among adults fell from 4141 in 1974 to 3196 in 1987, and this is the lowest per capita consumption since 1944.[48] In general, smoking prevalence is decreasing across all race-gender groups, although at a slower rate for women than men.[49] However, there are distinct groups of Americans who start or who continue to smoke. In general, blue collar workers, high school graduates, and men with lower incomes are more likely to smoke than men with college educations, white collar occupations, and high-level incomes.[47] In contrast, women who work are more likely to smoke than housewives and women in households with low family incomes. The latest data collected by the National Health Interview Surveys indicate that educational level is the major demographic predictor of whether an individual will smoke cigarettes. Regardless of gender, a person who does not attend college is more than twice as likely to start smoking than the person who does. In addition, smoking cessation occurs more frequently in groups with higher levels of education than in groups with less education, and the gap is widening over time.[50]

Several cigarette advertising campaigns have been directed to groups that tend to smoke (women, minorities, and blue-collar workers) in order to recruit new smokers or increase cigarette consumption among smokers.[51] Knowing the groups that tend to smoke and that are being targeted by the tobacco industry should assist health professionals in identifying and predicting patterns of cigarette use and in developing health-promotion materials specifically designed for these high-risk groups.[52] The Yellow Pages at the back of this text list smoking cessation materials specifically written for blue-collar workers, minorities, and women.

Obviously, the nurse wants to monitor most aggressively those who smoke, who have had a history of heavy smoking, or who were employed in high-risk occupations. These individuals should have (1) a complete baseline respiratory assessment, (2) a thorough assessment of respiratory symptoms, and (3) physical assessment of their respiratory system at periodic intervals. Deviations from normal merit referral for chest x-ray studies and/or sputum cytologic findings. In this high-risk population a cold that lingers or "smoker's cough" that is accompanied by fatigue and weight loss should not be ignored.

One fallacy commonly heard about individuals who smoke is that because they have smoked for years, "what harm is there in letting them continue?" Nothing could be further from the truth or more detrimental to their health. Continual smoking damages not only their already compromised respiratory system but their cardiovascular system as well. Research clearly documents that smoking cessation results in improved sensory, respiratory, and cardiovascular status.[53] Fielding,[47] in a review on the health effects of smoking, noted that a British physican study reported that ex-smokers who had not smoked for 5 years had a lung-cancer mortality rate approximately 40% that of a current smoker. After 15 years without smoking the mortality rate of ex-smokers was only slightly greater than that of nonsmokers. No one is ever too old nor has smoked too long to *stop* smoking.

The nurse should take a nonjudgmental approach with those who refuse or are unable to stop smoking. The 1988 surgeon general's report stated that "an extensive body of research has shown that nicotine is the drug in tobacco that causes addiction. However, the processes that determine tobacco addiction are similar to those that determine addiction to drugs such as heroin and cocaine."[54] Because of the addicting qualities of nicotine, many ex-smokers are not able to give up the habit on the first attempt but must try three or more times before finally succeeding.[49] In the hope of reducing the adverse health consequences of smoking, health professionals frequently advise individuals who cannot quit to smoke fewer cigarettes, to smoke cigarettes with less than 10 mg of tar, to smoke filtered cigarettes, and to smoke only half of each cigarette. However, habitual smokers may compensate for the reduced number of cigarettes by taking in more smoke per cigarette ("oversmoking").[55]

The nurse needs to be aware and share with the smoking public that the introduction of smokeless cigarettes by tobacco companies (eg, RJ Reynolds) will expose smokers to the same levels of carbon monoxide and nicotine as conventional cigarettes.[56] Many authorities view the new smokeless cigarette as a novel device for nicotine delivery.

It is the nurse's responsibility to actively and assertively disseminate information on the disease potential of smoking whenever possible. Every assistance should be afforded to help those who want to stop smoking. Nurses who smoke are less likely to discuss health-promoting behaviors with patients, that is, the need to stop smoking or the various smoking cessation methods that can be employed to stop successfully.[57,58] It is essential that nurses act as role models by not smoking and by actively working at creating nonsmoking environments in both their employment and home settings.

Nurses have frequent opportunities to advise smokers to quit either in health care settings or in the community. The importance of counseling smokers to quit is underscored by the research of Anda et al.[59] In their study of 5875 Michigan adults who smoked, of those who had seen a physician in the previous year, only 44% reported being told to quit smoking by a physician. In general, most smokers did not perceive physicians to be even minimally involved in their efforts to quit. In fairness to physicians, there may be a tendency for smokers to hear only what they want to hear.[60] For this reason, the US Preventive Services Task Force recommends that smokers should be exposed to a variety of intervention techniques on multiple occasions delivered by *both* physicians and nonphysicians to improve smoking cessation rates.[61] Kottke et al[62] also found that the best results for helping smokers quit was using a team of physicians and nonphysicians that used multiple intervention modalities to deliver individualized advice on multiple occasions. The multiple smoking cessation interventions suggested by all authorities include the following:

1. Direct, face-to-face advice and suggestions on smoking cessation
2. Smoking cessation self-help materials that are culturally and educationally relevant for the individual person
3. Referral to community smoking cessation programs
4. Drug therapy when appropriate (eg, nicotine gum)
5. Scheduled reinforcement with the smoker

Table 8-1 lists the process the nurse should follow to successfully assist the smoker in quitting, and Table 8-2 lists the factors associated with successful smoking cessation.[63] When individuals are referred to smoking cessation programs, it is advised that cost effectiveness be considered in the selection. Altman et al[64] found that although self-help programs had the lowest total cost and lowest time requirement for participants, their quit rate percentage was the lowest. In contrast, smoking cessation classes were expensive but had the most success in getting individuals to stop smoking.

Significant changes in the social and work-related environments have occurred in this country that have resulted in less tolerance for smoking and that have made smokers more receptive to the antismoking messages of health professionals. In 1987 the Bureau of National Affairs surveyed 623 large corporations and found that 54% had adopted some type of plan to restrict employee smoking. This was a 36% increase from a similar survey the previous year.[65] In the health care field more than 90% of hospitals have a smoking policy; 8% of those have banned smoking completely.[66] In addition, 43 states have passed laws that place limitations on smoking.[48] These antismoking policies appear to have a dramatic effect on the nation's smoking habits. Theoretically, they will encourage people to quit smoking by increasing the social pressure against it and by restricting the time available for it.

Gastrointestinal Cancer

Colorectal cancer incidence and mortality in the United States are second only to lung cancer. It is estimated that in 1989, 151,000 new colorectal cases will be diagnosed and 61,300 people will die of this cancer. In both men and women 35 years of age and older, colorectal cancer is one of the leading causes of deaths from cancer.[31]

History assessment

Several conditions and health practices must be questioned to obtain a realistic picture of the patient's gastrointestinal system. For example, after the age of 50 years

TABLE 8-1 Smoking Cessation Intervention Process

1. Initiate discussion of patient's smoking behavior
   - Review smoking history
   - Provide risk-benefit information, personalizing when possible
   - Assess health beliefs about smoking
2. Assess interest in smoking cessation
   - Determine patient's readiness to quit in terms of motivation, intention, and self-efficacy
3. Set the target quit-date
   - Pick a realistic calendar quit-date
   - Stop smoking "cold turkey"
4. Suggest smoking-cessation strategies
   - Provide materials and referral sources
   - Describe preparatory techniques
     - List reasons for quitting
     - Become aware of smoking-related situations
     - Seek social support
     - Reduce number of cigarettes and/or amount of nicotine
     - Replace cigarettes with gum or food (preferably low-fat, low-calorie)
     - Eliminate environmental cues
     - Avoid, distract, delay
   - Discuss withdrawal symptoms
   - Review cognitive and behavioral strategies to use in high-risk situations—social, relaxation, work, and upsetting situations
5. Follow-up
   - Encourage the maintenance of successful abstinence and discuss "slips"
   - Review relapse—motivate patient to resume cessation

Source: From Gritz E: Cigarette smoking: The need for action by health professionals. Reprinted by permission from Ca-A Cancer Journal for Clinicians in (CA 38:194-212, 1988). Copyright 1988 American Cancer Society. Preparation of this article was supported by the National Cancer Institute of the National Institutes of Health (Grants CA36409 & CA43461).

TABLE 8-2 Factors Associated with Successful Smoking Cessation

Motivational Factors
Desire to overcome minor smoking-related symptoms (coughing, wheezing, shortness of breath)
Expectation of improved future health
Sense of personal vulnerability to risk
Desire to increase self-mastery and self-esteem
Expectation of many quitting benefits—health, freedom, social, and economic
Expectation of success
Expectation that benefits will outweigh difficulties
Support and encouragement from family (especially spouse), friends, work associates

Effective Quitting Skills
Quitting abruptly instead of tapering off
Using a variety of coping methods for withdrawal symptoms, such as deep breathing, positive thinking, and specific cigarette substitutes
Using a variety of methods to remain off cigarettes, such as avoiding temptations to smoke, finding alternative ways to relax and cope with stress (such as hobbies or exercise), using substitute self-rewards to counteract sense of loss and prevent relapse
Taking a long-range, problem-solving approach

Social Supports/Psychosocial Assets
Personalized and medical quit-smoking advice and support
Encouragement, inspiration, and advice from ex-smokers
Good psychosocial resources (such as education and income)

Smoking Habit Factors
Lower smoking rate and nicotine intake/dependence
Less reliance on cigarettes for regulation of negative effect
Past success in quitting for 6 months or more
Good stress management skills

Source: From Orleans CT: Understanding and promoting smoking cessation: Overview of guidelines for physician intervention. Annu Rev Med 36:51-61, 1985.

approximately 25% of the population has demonstrable diverticulosis, and by age 80 years the proportion is 70%.[67] Slight rectal bleeding commonly is found with this disorder. Another condition that causes symptoms that mimic gastrointestinal cancer is depression. Depression is more common in the elderly than in the young because of increasing losses and limitations that accompany the aging process.[67] Some of the cardinal manifestations of depression are anorexia, constipation, and somatic pains. In addition, weight loss in the elderly may be due to nutritional disturbances rather than a malignancy. Loss of income, depression, decreased sensation of taste, loss of teeth, and difficulty swallowing all contribute to decreased food intake. Another important part of the nursing assessment is a thorough history of drug intake. The elderly tend to use aspirin frequently for the pain of arthritis and to abuse laxatives. Laxative abuse is the most common cause of diarrhea in this age-group, especially among women.[68] Considering these factors, the history and review of systems should include the following questions:

1. Do you have a history of cancer of the bowel or ulcerative colitis?
2. Have you ever been told you have polyps of the bowel? Gardner's syndrome? Have you had any polyps removed?
3. Do any of your relatives have (or have any had) bowel cancer?
4. Would you characterize your diet as consisting of more red meat than fish, veal, and poultry? Has your

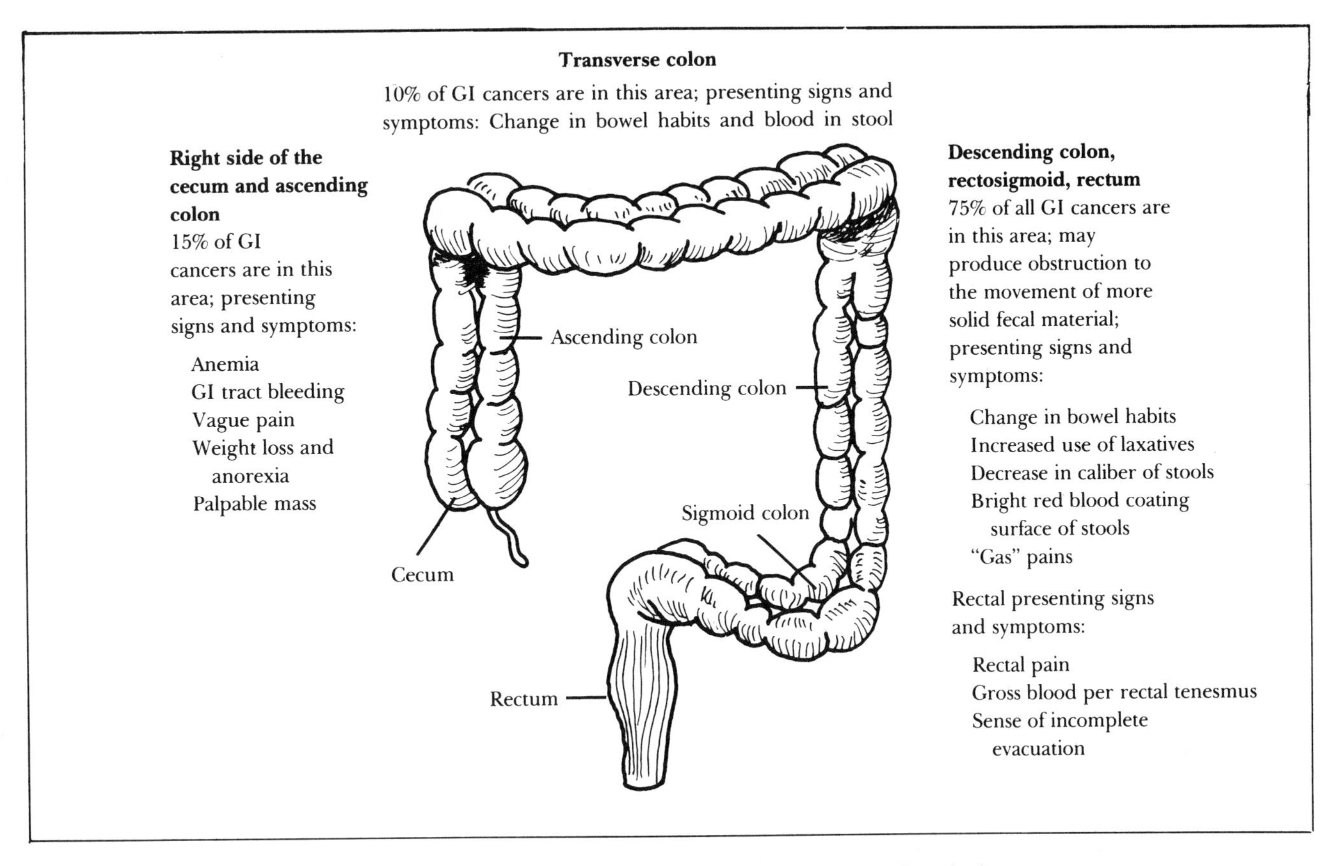

FIGURE 8-6 Presenting signs and symptoms of colorectal cancers based on location in the intestinal tract.

diet usually consisted of more starches and sweets than vegetables and fruits? Would you characterize your diet as being high in fats?

5. Do you take laxatives? If so, what kind, how often, what amount? How long have you taken laxatives?
6. Have you noticed a difference in your bowel habits? Do you have more constipation, more diarrhea? Do these two conditions seem to alternate?
7. What is your usual bowel habit? Has this changed in the last few years? Has the shape of your bowel movements changed recently?
8. Have you ever been told you have diverticulosis? Ulcers? Nervous stomach?
9. Have you had gastrointestinal x-ray studies within the last 2 to 3 years? Have you had a barium enema, proctoscope, or related procedure to examine your rectum and colon in the last 2 to 3 years? If you did, why was the test done and what were the results?
10. Do you take aspirin? How often and how much? What other medications (antacids, stool softeners, antispasmodics) are you now taking?
11. Are you familiar with at-home stool guaiac testing? Have you ever used this?
12. Do you have hemorrhoids or anal fissures?
13. Have you noticed any change in appetite? Are you experiencing nausea or vomiting?
14. Have you experienced any weight loss recently?
15. Do you have excessive gas? Feelings of being bloated? Abdominal pain?
16. Do you have the feeling after you have a bowel movement that you still have to go to the bathroom and expel more stool? Do you experience pain before, with, or after defecation?

The signs and symptoms of cancers of the colon and rectum often are related to the portion of intestine involved. Figure 8-6 identifies the most frequent presenting signs and symptoms of each area of the intestinal tract affected by cancer.

Physical examination

Inspection The assessment of the gastrointestinal system begins with inspection. The findings that may suggest cancer of the system include the following:

1. Nodular umbilicus. Abdominal carcinoma, especially gastric, may metastasize to the navel. This is called Sister Joseph's nodule.

2. Masses that distort the abdominal profile and indicate organomegaly.

3. Subcutaneous nodules under the skin that are visible with tangential lighting.

4. Distention. The abdominal profile should be inspected because neoplasms can distort the profile. The examiner

may see distention of the lower half, lower third, or upper half of the abdomen.

5. Venous distention caused by blockage of the inferior vena cava, which can occur from spread of cancer. In this condition there is edema of the eyelids, a bluish face and lips, prominent neck veins, and pitting edema of the arms and large veins over the upper portions of the chest and shoulders.

6. Visible peristaltic waves, which may appear in normal persons with thin abdomens and may be accentuated in patients with obstruction to the forward passage of gastrointestinal contents. Small bowel obstruction gives rise to a condition resembling a "bag of worms" or a "step ladder." Numerous segments of small bowel contract and relax in an irregular manner, and the peristalsis has no recognizable pattern.[39]

7. Bulging of the flanks may signal intra-abdominal fluid.

Auscultation After a thorough inspection of the abdomen is performed with the use of tangential lighting, the abdomen should be auscultated. Bowel sounds that are heard without the use of a stethoscope are called *Borborygmi.* Bowel sounds heard with the stethoscope bell range from absent to frequent. The significance of the different types of bowel sounds includes the following:

1. High-pitched, long, intense peristaltic rushes occur with any hypermotile state such as partial obstruction.
2. High-pitched, "tingling" sounds indicate a more complete mechanical intestinal obstruction.
3. Extremely weak or infrequent sounds may also indicate bowel immobility.
4. Absent bowel sounds, determined by listening to the bowel for at least *5 minutes,* may indicate advanced intestinal obstruction.

Another sound that may signal obstruction of the small intestines is a *Succussion splash.* Succussion splash is produced by a combination of air and fluid in the gut when the examiner "tingles" the stomach or vigorously moves the abdomen. The sound resembles very loud splashes.

Some abdominal circulatory sounds also signal cancer (Figure 8-7). A bruit heard over the liver with the bell of the stethoscope when the patient takes a deep breath may indicate a hepatoma with arteriovenous shunting. In addition, a hepatic friction rub heard with the bell of the stethoscope may also indicate a hepatoma. A bruit heard over the pancreas may indicate pancreatic carcinoma. A murmur over the left hypochondrium is one of the rare physical signs that suggests an early carcinoma of the body of the pancreas. Thus auscultation of the abdomen may indicate a bowel obstruction, a hepatoma, or pancreatic carcinoma.

Palpation and percussion The information obtained from inspection and auscultation should alert the examiner to expected findings during palpation and percussion of the abdomen. It is important to remember that on palpation of the abdomen the organs that are normally palpated are the abdominal aorta, the edge of the liver, the lower pole of the right kidney, the descending colon and the sigmoid, and the ascending colon. The following findings on palpation and percussion merit further attention and many signal colorectal cancer.

Hepatomegaly Total liver span is the best estimate of liver size because liver height cannot be determined by feeling only the edge. Palpation alone detects the inferior portion as it descends below the costal margin. A normal liver at the midclavicular line is 10 to 12 cm in span. Nodules on the liver or an irregular edge suggests malignancy.

Splenomegaly Because the normal spleen is rarely palpable, a spleen that descends below the left costal margin on deep inspiration is enlarged. Cancer conditions that enlarge the spleen are leukemias and lymphomas.

Enlargement of the colon Carcinoma of the colon may produce a palpable mass anywhere along the course of the colon.

Fluid Several tests can be used to determine if there is free fluid in the abdomen. The presence of intraperitoneal fluid is suspected when there is abdominal distention with bulging flanks and possibly an everted umbilicus. *Shifting dullness* and *fluid wave* are two tests frequently used to detect fluid in the abdomen. The *puddle sign* has the advantage of detecting small amounts of intra-abdominal fluid. After the patient has been on hands and knees for several minutes, the examiner percusses the periumbilical area to detect a line between fluid and air, as in the determination of shifting dullness. As little as several hundred milliliters of ascitic fluid can be detected by this method.[42]

Rectal examination Half the cancers that occur in the rectum and colon are within reach of the examining finger. Lesions high in the rectum are sometimes felt more readily when the patient bears down as if having a bowel movement. On palpation the examiner may feel a *rectal shelf* that is a stony hard mass above the prostate on the anterior rectal wall. In women it is felt as a stony hard mass in the cul-de-sac. The shelf indicates a carcinoma that has metastasized to the pelvic floor and therefore is a sign of advanced malignancy. Carcinoma of the rectum causes plateaulike, nodular, annular, and cauliflower masses in the rectum.[40]

• • •

Several physical findings in other parts of the body, which are not revealed in the abdominal examination, are typical in abdominal carcinoma. For instance, enlargement of a single node, usually in the left supraclavicular group, is the site of carcinomatous metastasis from a primary lesion in the upper portion of the abdomen. This node is called *Virchow's node* and is frequently behind the clavicular head of the left supraclavicular group. The Valsalva maneuver causes the node to rise and enables the nurse to palpate Virchow's node.

Another physical finding that indicates abdominal carcinoma is *acanthosis nigricans,* a skin lesion. Acanthosis nigricans is probably the most well-known cutaneous marker

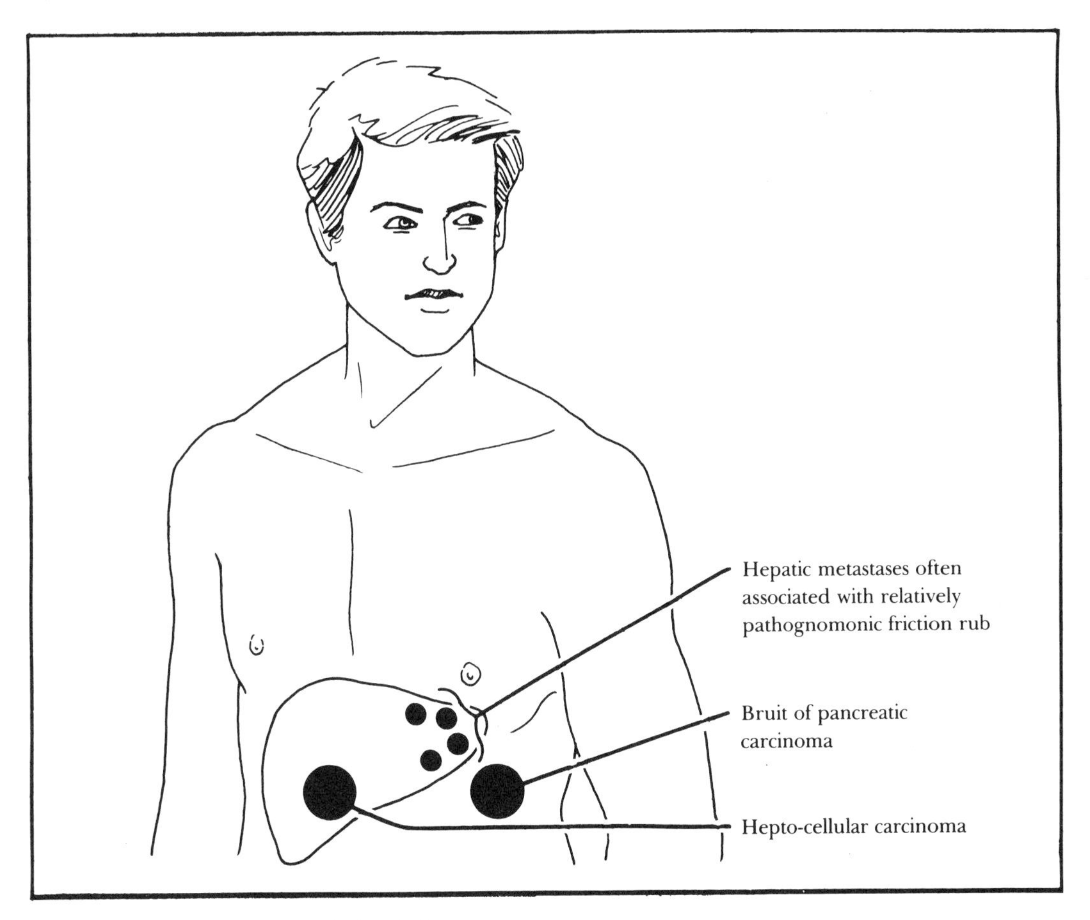

FIGURE 8-7 Abdominal sounds that indicate cancer.

of internal malignancy. It is a velvety, brownish skin eruption that strongly suggests an intestinal malignancy when it occurs in patients older than 40 years of age.[39,69]

Another systemic finding that is connected with pathologic findings of the gastrointestinal system is jaundice. Jaundice and accompanying steady pain may indicate hepatic or pancreatic lesions. Although painless obstructive jaundice is said to be a feature of carcinoma of the head of the pancreas, about 70% of patients with pancreatic cancer have some degree of anterior abdominal or back pain.[39] By means of daylight or fluorescent light the sclerae, the undersurface of the tongue, and the frenulum of the tongue should be examined for jaundice.

In conclusion, although there are many physical findings that suggest cancer of the gastrointestinal system, the findings that *most strongly* suggest cancer of the colorectal area are (1) a mass palpated in the rectum, (2) a palpable mass in the abdomen, and (3) evidence of blood in the feces. Nurses who work with the elderly or high-risk individuals in nursing homes, residential settings, acute-care institutions, and physician's offices are encouraged to take the time to thoroughly assess an individual's gastrointestinal complaints. Often the elderly will share their complaints with the nurse rather than the physician because they hesitate to bother the doctor with "trivial" problems.

Screening tests for asymptomatic individuals

Presently the two most important screening tests for asymptomatic persons are examination of the feces for occult blood and the digital rectal examination.[70] There is professional debate about the use of fecal occult blood tests as a mass screening tool. The results from the only true randomized controlled study in this country that assessed the effect of occult blood screening on colorectal cancer mortality has thus far failed to show any reduction in mortality.[71] The University of Minnesota School of Public Health has been amassing data on colorectal cancer detection since 1975. More than 46,000 people between the ages of 50 and 80 years have participated in the study. They were randomly assigned to three groups. One group was given an annual fecal occult blood test, another group was screened with the test every second year, and a control group was not offered the test. Only 2.3% of those with a positive slide result have been found to have colorectal cancer.[72] It is argued that although the test itself is inexpensive, the recommended follow-up diagnostic procedure is expensive. For instance, if 1 million people were screened, about 100,000 of them (10%) would show positive findings and the costs of the follow-up tests would be $50 million for the detection of 2300 colorectal cancers.[72]

Another problem with occult blood tests is the number of false-positive results that necessitate additional tests. It is recommended by the manufacturer that fecal occult test slides be rehydrated with a drop of water before development. This increases the sensitivity but decreases the specificity of the test.[73] The increased sensitivity after rehydration means that the number of false-positive test results increases as the specificity decreases. A Swedish study[73] documented that rehydration of Hemoccult II slides is necessary because significantly more carcinomas were found in the rehydrated group compared with the unrehydrated group of slides. Table 8-3 presents the causes of false-positive and false-negative test results in the use of Hemoccult slides.[74]

The American Gastroenterological Association and the American Society for Gastrointestinal Endoscopy recommend the following screening techniques for identification of colorectal adenomas and early detection of cancer. For the asymptomatic average-risk population a digital rectal examination should be performed in persons 40 years of age and older, and fecal occult blood testing and flexible sigmoidoscopic examination in those 50 years of age and older.[75] In contrast, the US Preventive Services Task Force states that there is "insufficient evidence to make a recommendation either for or against fecal occult blood screening for individuals aged 45 years and older. Screening of individuals younger than age 45 years is not recommended. Based on the higher expected prevalence in individuals aged 45 years and older with a family history of colorectal cancer in a first-order relative, a stronger a priori argument can be made for screening in this group."[76]

Although it is acknowledged that the role of fecal occult blood tests in the early detection of colorectal cancer is still being evaluated, the nurse should be aware of specific recommendations that will increase the accuracy of the test.

TABLE 8-3 Causes of False-Positive and False-Negative Tests Using the Hemoccult Method

False-Positive Tests	False-Negative Tests
Meat in diet	Failure to employ high-residue diet
Medications: antibiotics, aspirin, anti-inflammatories, oral iron compounds	Vitamin C in diet
Diverticulosis	Time lag between specimen collection and specimen examination
Minor anorectal problems	Failure to prepare slides properly or complete all six slides
Hemorrhoids	Follow-up examinations which failed to detect lesion
Fissures	Lesion not bleeding at the time of stool collection
Proctitis	Outdated Hemoccult slides or reagent
Peroxidases in skins of vegetables and fruits (tomatoes and cherries)	
Upper gastrointestinal pathology	
Gastritis from ASA ingestion	
Ulcer disease	
Hiatus hernia	
Gastric malignancy	

Source: Sugarbaker P, Gunderson L, Wittes R: Colorectal cancer, in DeVita V, Hellman S, Rosenberg S (eds): Cancer: Principles and Practice of Oncology (ed 2). Philadelphia, JB Lippincott, 1986, pp 795-884.

1. Duplicate samples should be taken from different parts of the feces each day for three consecutive days while the patient follows a meat-free diet.[77] It is important for the nurse to encourage the patient to collect stool for three consecutive days because not all bowel cancers bleed nor is occult blood always uniformly distributed in feces. Increasing the numbers of tests may therefore address these two causes of false-negative tests.[78] Presently no scientific validation exists for a high-residue diet during the 3 days of stool specimen collection.[78]

2. During the 3 days of stool collection, patients should avoid:

- **a.** Aspirin-containing compounds (cause false-positive reaction)
- **b.** Antibiotics (cause false-positive reaction)
- **c.** Anti-inflammatory drugs (cause false-positive reaction)
- **d.** Ascorbic acid (cause false-negative reaction)
- **e.** Foods high in peroxidase—broccoli, cabbage, potatoes, cantaloupe, turnips, apricots, apples, pears horseradish (cause false-positive reaction)
- **f.** Oral iron compounds (cause false-positive reactions)[79]

3. The stool specimens should be read within 6 days of collection because delay contributes to false-negative reactions.

Because of the false-positive and false-negative results frequently obtained with the present tests for occult stool by means of guaiac-impregnated cards, alternate methods to detect colorectal cancer are being sought. Several researchers have published preliminary data on immunochemical tests that do not rely on blood loss to detect gastrointestinal changes caused by cancer.[76,80,81] Clinical studies to validate the usefulness of these tests are being conducted. HemoQuant (Smith-Kline Diagnostics, Sunnyvale, Calif) is a quantitative assay based on the conversion of heme to fluorescent porphyrins. It appears to be unaffected by dietary factors, specimen storage and hydration, and medication and seems to be as effective as the Hemoccult slide test. HemoQuant also distinguishes between heme that has been converted chemically during gut transmit and heme that has not, thus giving information about the level of bleeding in the gastrointestinal system. However, it costs several times as much as Hemoccult.[75,76]

In general, compliance with the collection of fecal occult blood tests tends to be poor, with rates of 22% to 30% reported.[78] Those who are most likely to be helped by screening (eg, the elderly) are less likely to cooperate.

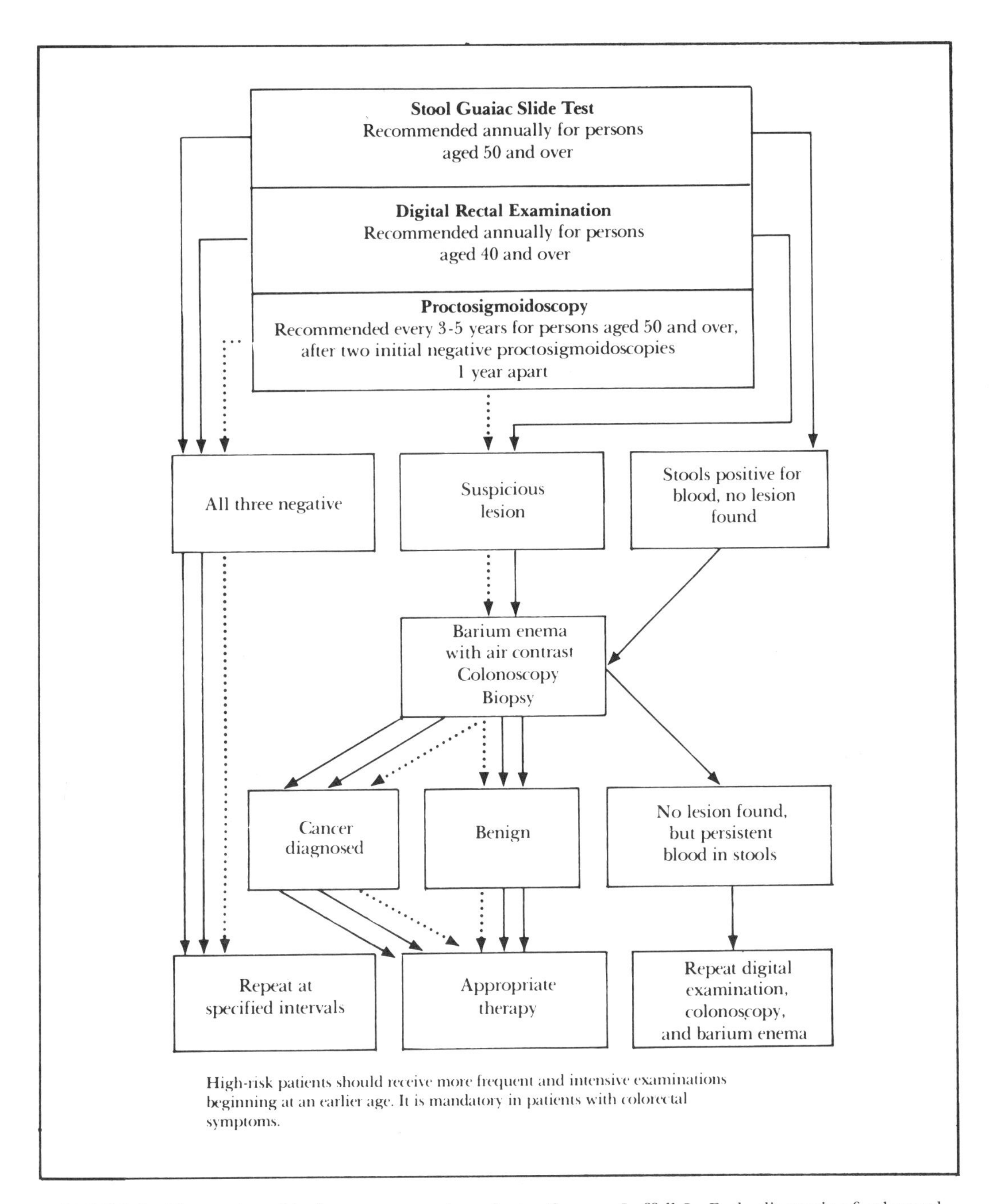

FIGURE 8-8 Diagnostic guide for asymptomatic patients. (Source: Leffall L: Early diagnosis of colorectal cancer. New York, American Cancer Society [Professional Educational Publication 81-50M-No 3311-PE], 1981.)

Those studies that report good compliance usually deal with a highly motivated or selected group of volunteers.

The carcinoembryonic antigen (CEA) assay is not conclusive for the initial proven diagnosis of colorectal cancer.[70] A normal level does not rule out colon cancer, and elevated levels have been found in cancer of the pancreas as well as in nonmalignant diseases of the colon, lung, and liver. Because it is nonspecific, it is not considered a good screening test for colorectal cancer.

The American Cancer Society recommendations for screening asymptomatic patients for colorectal cancer are shown in Figure 8-8.

Additional nursing interventions

Nurses have a variety of roles in colorectal cancer detection. Not only are they practitioners; they also are educators, coordinators, counselors, and researchers. One of the most important roles the nurse assumes is that of educator. Two surveys conducted by the Gallup Organization for the American Cancer Society have found that only a small percentage of the public has taken the necessary steps to detect colorectal cancer at its earliest stages.[82] The surveys also revealed that very few people were asking their physicians for the tests during regular physical examinations. There was also little knowledge about this type of cancer, and attitudes toward its early detection were pessimistic. A little more than one third of Americans in the 40-plus age-group knew that colorectal cancer was one of the most common forms of cancer. More than 40% believed that surgery for colorectal cancer would result in a permanent colostomy, and more than 50% had little faith that anything could be done to cure colorectal cancer. In addition, there were general misconceptions about the recommended early detection tests. Twenty-five percent believed that if no blood is found in a stool blood test, then the digital rectal and proctoscopic examinations would not be needed.

As educators, nurses can play an important role in colorectal cancer detection by (1) informing the general public about colon and rectum cancer, as well as by making a special effort to inform the elderly and other high-risk groups, and (2) encouraging the participation of the general public and high-risk groups in early detection of the disease through the use of a stool guaiac slide test, digital rectal examination, and, after 50 years of age, proctosigmoidoscopic examination. The most effective public education approach to general screening for colorectal cancer ("the cancer nobody talks about") is (1) to emphasize the effectiveness of the stool guaiac test, (2) to stress that it is painless and convenient (it can be administered in the privacy of one's home), and (3) to indicate the value of early detection of colorectal cancer (eg, President Reagan's successful bout with a malignant tumor of the colon).[83]

Nurses who work in community organizations, clinics, nursing homes, retirement centers, geriatric day-care centers, and hospitals are in ideal settings to provide education and plan and participate in colorectal screening programs. These screening programs could be conducted by community organizations such as the American Cancer Society, local service groups, or community religious groups, with the nurse coordinating the efforts.

Another role as educator relates to the following dietary recommendations of the American Cancer Society and the National Cancer Institutes to lower overall cancer risk including colorectal cancer:

1. Avoid obesity.

2. Decrease total fat intake. It is recommended that fat be only 30% of total calories. The year 2000 cancer control objective is to reduce average consumption of fat from 40% to 25% or less of total calories.[84] There are many simple methods to reduce dietary fat in the diet: (1) use low-fat cottage cheese instead of sour cream for dips, (2) use baked potatoes instead of French fries, (3) use nonstick pans or a spray for grilling sandwiches instead of grilling them in oil, and (4) select bagels or whole wheat bread for breakfast instead of doughnuts, rolls, or croissants.

3. Consume more high-fiber foods, such as whole grain cereals, fruits, and vegetables. The year 2000 cancer control objectives are to increase the average consumption of fiber from 8 to 12 g/day to 20 to 30 g/day.

4. Include foods rich in vitamins A and C in the daily diet. Foods rich in carotene, a form of vitamin A, are carrots, tomatoes, spinach, apricots, peaches, cantaloupes. In general, dark green and deep yellow vegetables are rich in vitamin A.

5. Be moderate in the consumption of alcoholic beverages.

6. Be moderate in the consumption of salt-cured, smoked, and nitrite-cured foods.

7. Include cruciferous vegetables in the diet, such as cabbage, broccoli, brussels sprouts, kohlrabi, and cauliflower.[85-87]

Research supports the assumption that Americans will change their diet in an effort to be healthier. A survey in Illinois, conducted in 1982 and in 1986, found that 42% of the 46,830 subjects reported a major change in their diet since the first survey. Subjects reported eating less meat and pork and more fish and chicken, and there was a shift toward whole grains from refined grains and an increase in the number of times per week that subjects eat cruciferous vegetables.[88]

In the role of researcher, it is extremely important that nurses be knowledgeable about the emerging information on the relationship between diet and colorectal cancer. Future research may establish definitive relationships, as well as additional relationships not presently known. Nurses also should be able to evaluate research findings. Those reports that are based on sound, ethical research principles may be judged appropriate for inclusion in patient education. Because of debate about the use of stool guaiac tests in screening programs in terms of lowering mortality from colorectal cancer, nurses need to remain alert to new research that either supports or refutes the use of this early detection test. Nurses also can plan or participate in the wide range of research projects related to colorectal cancer such as health behaviors, dietary habits, motives that facilitate early detection and dietary changes, and effective educational approaches for changing dietary patterns. Results certainly would benefit existing nursing practice as it relates to the prevention and early detection of colorectal cancer.

As practitioners, nurses are urged to use their physical assessment skills when they deal with individuals who have gastrointestinal complaints. Geriatric patients often share their symptoms first with a sympathetic nurse. Thus the nurse is in the ideal position to detect colorectal cancer in its *initial stages*. Physical assessment of the abdomen may reveal subtle clues of a pathologic condition that merits referral, one that otherwise might be overlooked by an elderly patient. Hospital-based nurses are cautioned not to assume that elderly patients must have had a thorough physical examination because they are in the hospital. If the complaints are not related to the gastrointestinal system, that system may not have been thoroughly assessed.

Prostate Cancer

Prostate cancer is currently the second most common cancer in American men. In men older than 75 years of age, it is estimated that the prevalence of prostate cancer is 500/100,000. The American Cancer Society estimates that in 1989 there will be 103,000 new prostate cases and 28,500 deaths caused by this cancer.[31] A large percentage of men have advanced disease at the time of diagnosis; approximately 35% have metastases to the bones or lymph nodes, and another 40% have extracapsular invasion.[89] Black American men have the highest incidence of prostate cancer in the world. Between 1937 and 1985 the incidence of prostate cancer increased 53.3% among white men and more than 100% in black men.[90] Prostate cancer increases in incidence with age more rapidly than any other cancer.

History assessment

There are *no* real symptoms of early, probably curable, disease. Most symptoms are related to late complications of stage C or D prostate cancer. Because many of the initial symptoms may be related to carcinomatous obstruction of the prostatic urethra, the inquiries made during the history should be about nonspecific urinary symptoms. The following questions are recommended:

1. Do you have to wait for your stream to begin?
2. Does your stream stop while you still have the urge to void?
3. Do you have to strain to urinate?
4. Does your stream seem very weak to you?
5. Do you have the urge to urinate but find you can't?
6. Have you noticed blood in your urine? Has your urine changed in color or smell at all?
7. Does the blood seem to come at the beginning or end of your stream?
8. Do you dribble after urinating?
9. Do you find you have to urinate more than you used to?
10. Do you have pain on urination?
11. Do you ever wet your pants?
12. How often do you urinate during the day? Do you get up at night to urinate? How often?
13. When was your last rectal examination? Why was this done? What was found?

Symptoms that suggest prostatic cancer are urinary difficulty manifested by a decrease in urinary stream and a frequency and urgency to urinate, often associated with pain. These symptoms also are found with prostatic enlargement (benign prostatic hypertrophy) that is extremely common in older men. The most frequent initial symptoms of prostate cancer are, in order of frequency, frequency of urination, difficult or painful urination, pain, complete urinary retention, and hematuria.[91]

Physical examination

An early diagnosis of prostate cancer can be done only by rectal palpation of the prostate (Figure 8-9). It is rec-

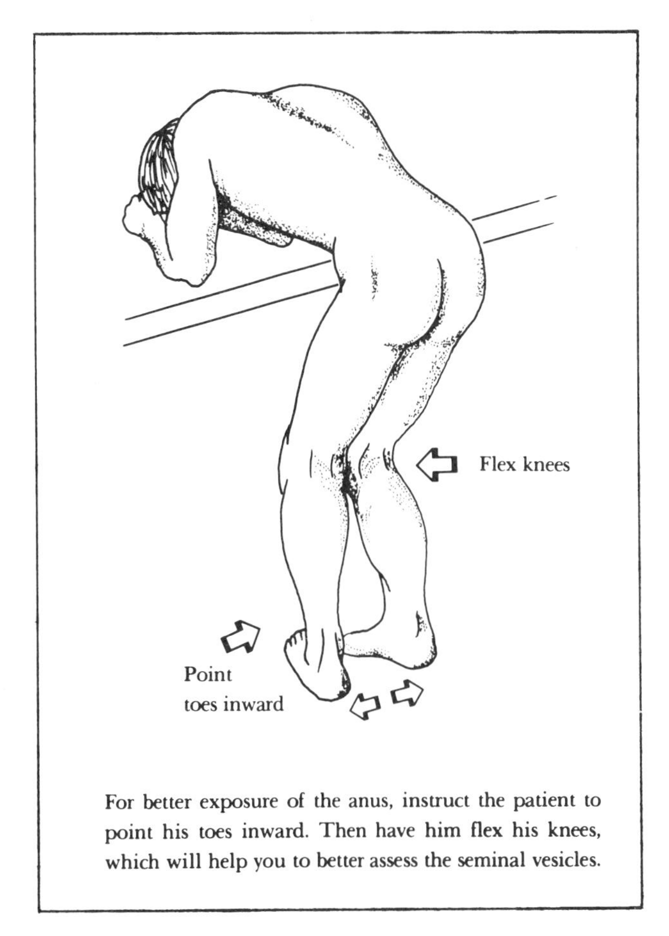

FIGURE 8-9 Recommended position for digital rectal examination. (Source: Adapted from Guinan P, Sharifi R, Bush I: Prostate cancer: Tips toward earlier detection. Your Patient & Cancer 4:37-42, 1984.)

ommended that the examiner flex the distal finger joint 2 to 3 mm into the gland substance rather than keep the finger straight (Figure 8-10). The Valsalva maneuver during the rectal examination will bring the prostate gland closer to the examining finger. Early prostatic carcinoma is a nodule *within*, not *on*, the gland. Simply rubbing the gland is not effective for early detection of prostate cancer.[92]

The normal prostate on palpation is usually a rounded structure about 4 cm in diameter, feels firm rather than boggy, soft, or rock hard, and usually is not tender. Some examiners describe the consistency of the normal prostate as that of a pencil eraser. Cancer of the prostate typically appears as a stony-hard nodule.[91] On the other hand, benign prostatic hypertrophy usually results in a diffuse enlargement of the prostate without masses.

It is extremely common to find in older men a diffusely enlarged prostate gland without masses (benign prostatic hypertrophy). Carcinoma of the prostate is manifested by a palpable hard nodule near the posterior surface of the prostate. As the carcinoma grows, the entire gland may become stony hard, or there may be several hard nodules.[42]

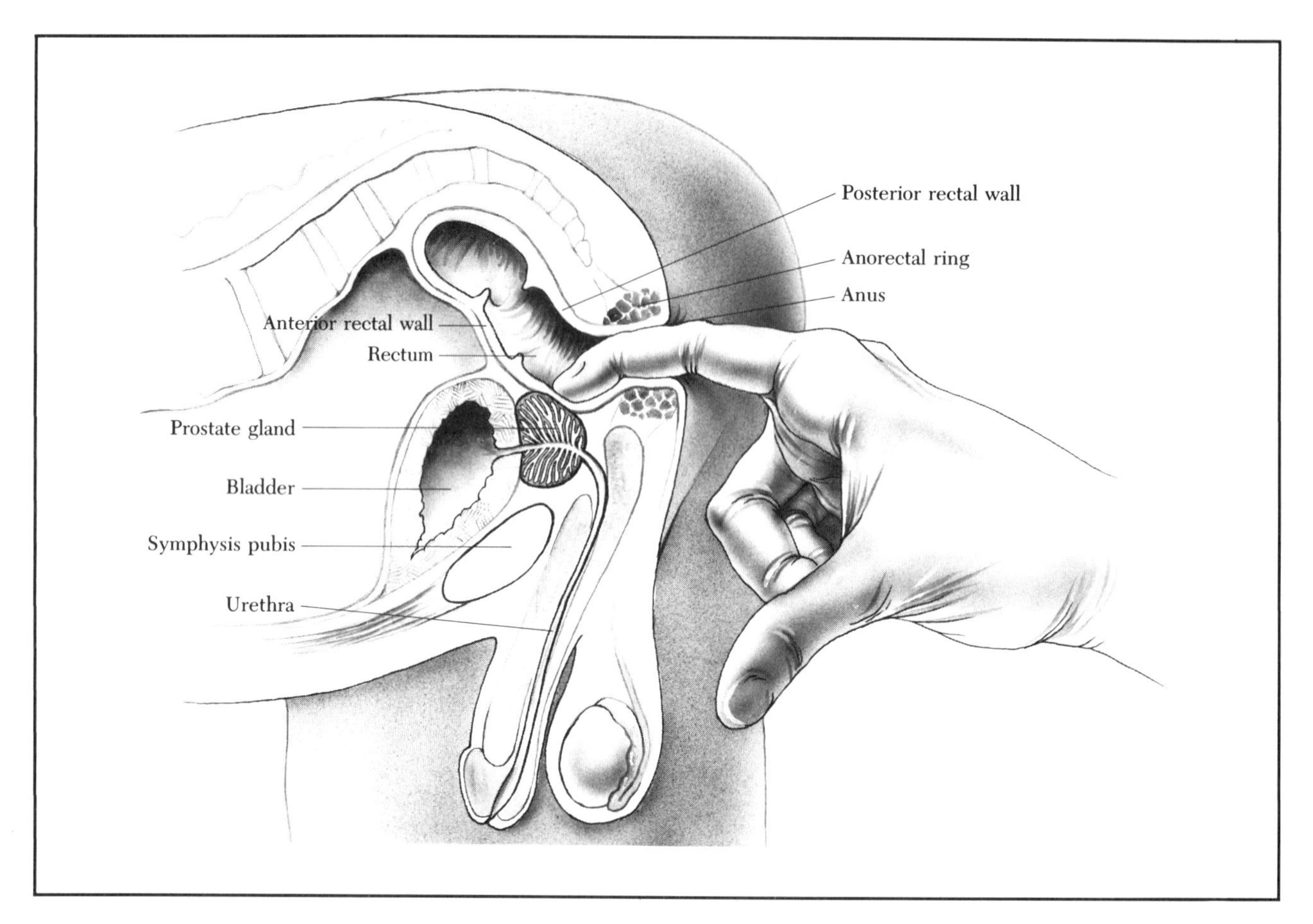

FIGURE 8-10 Technique for palpation of the prostate gland. (Source: Grimes J, Burns E (eds): Health Assessment in Nursing Practice (ed 2). Boston, Jones and Bartlett, 1987.)

Screening tests for asymptomatic individuals

The most sensitive method of diagnosis of early prostate cancer is the digital rectal examination. Guinan et al[93] compared the digital rectal examination with nine other laboratory tests designed to detect prostate cancer. Their data on 300 men suggest that the digital rectal examination is the most efficient test for the diagnosis of prostate cancer.

Research is being conducted to determine whether transrectal ultrasound has greater accuracy in the early detection of prostate cancer than the digital rectal examination.[94-96] The transrectal sonography, commonly used in Japan, involves a machine that is a large chair with a square hole through which an ultrasound probe protrudes. The probe is inserted into the rectum, and ultrasound images of the prostate are recorded on film. It is considered by most men to be less uncomfortable than a digital examination. Lee and colleagues[97-99] report that ultrasound is superior to the digital examination in a screening and detection program for prostate cancer in men older than 60 years of age. In their study of 784 men in this age-group, findings of transrectal ultrasound examination alone resulted in biopsy recommendation for 83% of the biopsies performed, whereas digital examination resulted in biopsy recommendation for only 38%. A total of 22 cancers were found at biopsy, giving an overall detection rate of 2.8% and 1.3% for transrectal ultrasound and digital examination, respectively. Transrectal ultrasound demonstrated 100% (17/17) of tumors with the most favorable prognosis compared with 41% (7/17) for digital examination.[99]

A tumor marker is a biochemical indicator for the presence of a tumor. In clinical use the term refers to a molecule that can be detected in plasma or other body fluids.[100] Two tumor markers, prostate-specific antigen and prostatic acid phosphatase, are useful in monitoring therapy and disease progression of prostate cancer, but they have not as yet been shown to be specific or sensitive enough to use in the early detection of prostate cancer.

In the detection of early prostate cancer, one of the most important roles the nurse can assume is that of educator. All men older than 40 years of age, especially black American men, should be informed of the importance and rationale for yearly or biannual rectal examinations. Men with strong family histories of prostate cancer should be urged to *request and expect* rectal examinations at their annual physical inasmuch as early detection can result in cure and rectal examination is presently the most effective means of detecting early prostate cancer.

In some communities it may be necessary for the nurse to conduct the physical examination that includes the rectal examination for prostate as well as colorectal cancer. Female nurses who conduct physical examinations but omit the rectal assessment because of their embarrassment or the patient's discomfort must request a male physician or nurse practitioner to complete this portion of the examination rather than omitting it. In other settings it may be possible to develop a once-a-year volunteer transportation program that will enable infirm or geographically isolated elderly patients to have the recommended yearly examination. The development of a prostate screening program for each isolated, poor, or infirm elderly man is a problem all nurses should attempt to solve. At the very least the nurse should question all hospitalized elderly men about their last rectal examination and contact the physician about those men who have not had one within the last year (or who have "deferred" written on their chart next to "rectal examination").

Breast Cancer

Breast cancer is the most common cancer in women in the Western World.[101] It is the leading cause of cancer deaths in women 15 to 54 years of age and the second cause of cancer deaths in women older than 55 years of age.[31] It is estimated that in 1989, 142,900 women will be diagnosed with invasive breast cancer and 43,300 will die of the disease.[31] In women 40 years of age breast cancer develops each year in approximately 1/1000; by 60 years of age this rate rises to 2/1000 per year.[102] In the last 20 years the probability of breast cancer developing in a woman's lifetime changed from 1/20 to 1/11.[101,103]

History assessment

Questions that may be asked during the history include the following:

1. Do you practice breast self-examination (BSE)?
   a. "Yes" response. How often do you do BSE? Where did you learn to do this? Do you feel comfortable doing BSE, or would you like me to go over it with you?
   b. "No" response. Have you ever been shown BSE? Would you be interested in learning BSE? Some women don't examine their breasts because they feel unsure, embarrassed, or frightened about doing it. Do you feel this way about BSE?
2. Have you ever been advised to have a mammogram? If you have had a mammogram, what were the results?
3. Do you experience sore breasts?
4. Have you ever been told you had "lumpy" or "cystic breasts"?
5. Have you noticed any color or temperature change on your breasts? Do you have trouble with scaly, itching nipples?
6. Have you ever had breast infections?
7. Have you ever had breast surgery or cosmetic surgery of your breasts? Tell me about the surgery that was done.
8. Do you have any sores or open wounds on your breasts?
9. Have you noticed any "dimpling" of your breasts?
10. Have you noticed any change in your nipples or discharge?
11. Have you ever been told that you had cancer of the breast?
12. Do you have or have you discovered any breast lumps?
13. Is there anyone in your family—grandparents, siblings, cousins, parents, aunts and uncles—who have or had cancer? Breast cancer? Can you remember how old your ______________ was when she first was diagnosed as having breast cancer?
14. At what age (or grade in school) did you start menstruating? At what age did you stop menstruating?

The *most common* presenting complaint of women with breast cancer is a painless lump or mass in the breast. It is estimated that 90% of all palpable breast tumors are discovered by women themselves either accidently or through planned self-examination.[103]

Physical examination

Inspection The physical examination begins with inspection of the breast with the woman sitting with her arms at her side, sitting with her arms elevated, sitting with pectoral contraction, and sitting bending forward (Figure 8-11a-d). Visible signs of cancer of the breast include the following:

1. *Dimpling of the breast* results from a shortening of Cooper's ligaments as the tumor spreads in the breast.
2. *Unilateral flattening of the nipple* is caused by fibrosis and contraction of this fibrotic tissue, thus producing retraction signs, including flattening or deviation of the nipple.[44]
3. *Abnormal contours or flattening* becomes apparent as the woman changes positions. It is important to compare one breast with the other. An excellent position for observing this is when the woman leans forward.
4. *Peau d'orange,* orange peel skin, is caused by interference with the lymphatic drainage of the skin (Figure 8-12).
5. *Increased venous prominence* usually is unilateral. Carcinomas demand an increased blood flow; thus the dilated venous channels will be obvious on inspection.[104]
6. *Scaling or eczematoid lesions* of the nipple indicate Paget's disease, a slow-growing intraductal carcinoma.

It is essential that the woman be examined with good lighting (eg, the use of a gooseneck lamp) so that subtle contours will be detected by the examiner. Also, the initial inspection *must* include all positions previously mentioned

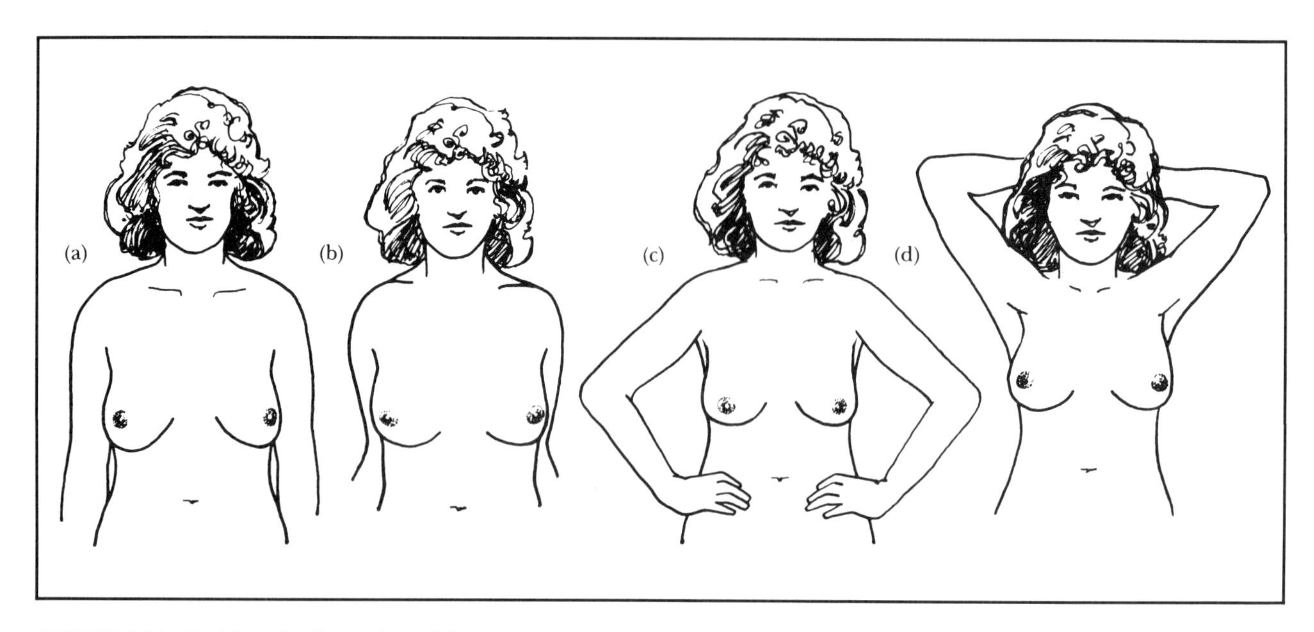

FIGURE 8-11 Positions for inspection of the breast. (a) Arms at side with woman relaxed; (b) arms at side pressed against body; (c) hands on waist pressed against body; (d) arms over head. (Source: Adapted from Olsen S: Examinations for detecting breast cancer. Cancer Prevention Program, Wisconsin Clinical Cancer Center, 1300 University Ave-7C, Medical Science Center, Madison, WI 53706.)

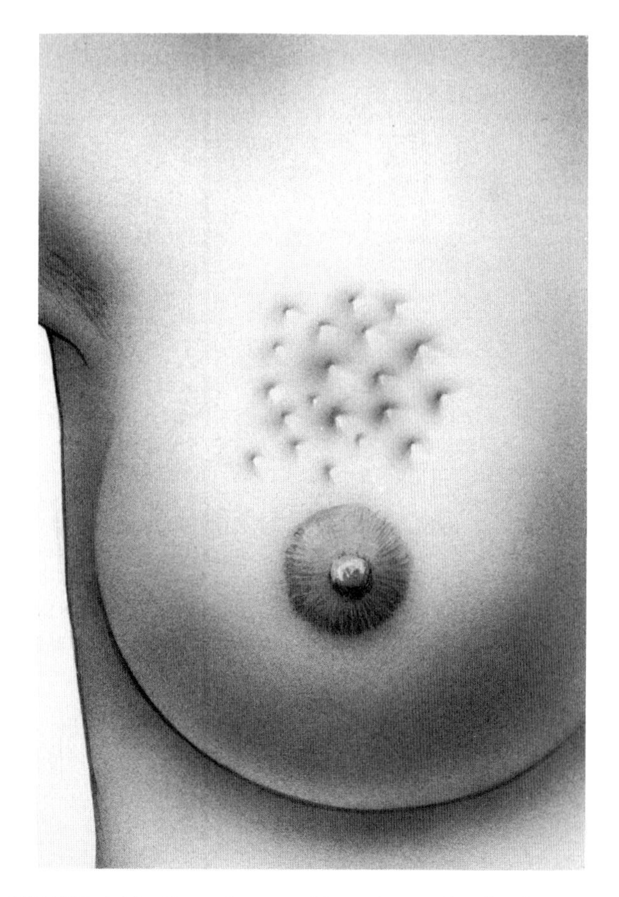

FIGURE 8-12 Peau d'orange. Note the rough, pitted appearance. (Source: Grimes J, Burns E (eds): Health Assessment in Nursing Practice (ed 2). Boston, Jones and Bartlett, 1987.)

and shown in Figure 8-11; omitting a position may cause the nurse to miss important pathologic findings. The photographs in Figures 8-13 and 8-14 show the differences when the woman has her hands at her sides and when she raises her arms.

Palpation After inspection, the entire breast should be lightly palpated for thickening. This is accomplished by using the pads of your fingers. Palpation for thickening is done very lightly and slowly toward the nipple and enables the nurse to detect subtle differences in consistency in the breasts. This technique has evolved from 15 years of clinical practice as a nurse practitioner (MF-S). It should be viewed as a "scouting expedition" before palpation for masses is begun. If the woman complains of a lump, she should find it for the examiner. It is best to first palpate the normal breast. Cancer occurs as a hard, poorly circumscribed nodule, fixed to the skin or underlying tissue.

If cancer is suspected, the breast should be gently moved or compressed and observed for dimpling. A malignant lump that may be attached to the deep fascia will limit the mobility of the breast on the chest wall. The examiner checks for such a lump by having the patient place her hands on her hip; then the examiner moves the breast medially and laterally with the muscles relaxed and then with the muscles under tension by forced adduction.

The breasts need to be thoroughly palpated while the woman is supine with her arms above her head. One of us (MF-S) uses powder on the breasts to establish a frictionless surface. Palpation should be done with the flat part of the tips of three fingers. Using a spiral motion, rotate the fingers in small circles. It is recommended that the nurse start at the areolar margin and examine the

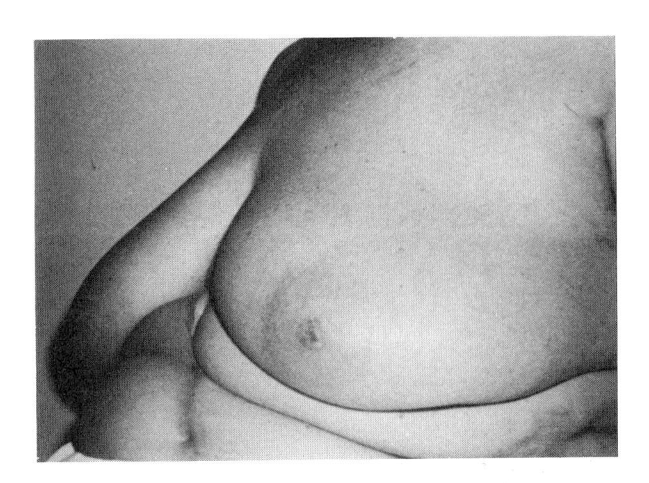

FIGURE 8-13 Woman sitting. Note that breasts appear normal. (Source: Rosemond G, Maier W: Breast Cancer. New York, Famous Teachings in Modern Medicine, Medcom, 1974.)

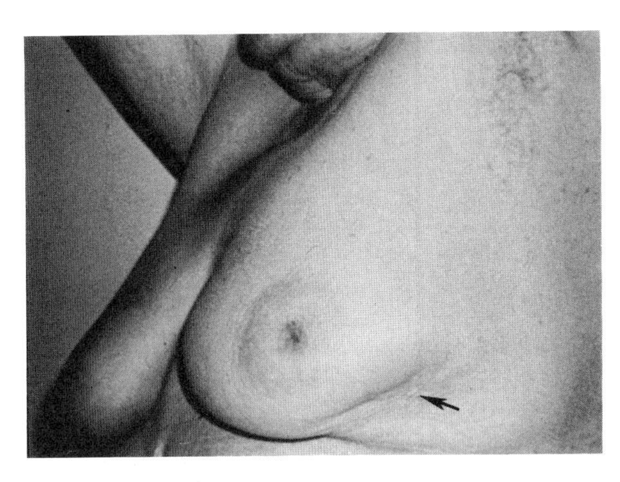

FIGURE 8-14 Woman raising her hands during breast inspection. Note dimpling, which becomes evident with this maneuver. (Source: Rosemond G, Maier W: Breast Cancer. New York, Famous Teachings in Modern Medicine, Medcom, 1974.)

breast by palpation in ever-widening concentric circles. Any mass that is felt should be charted as to its location, size, shape, consistency, discreteness, mobility, tenderness, erythema, and dimpling over the mass. Location of a nodule should be charted in terms of the quadrant, that is, right upper, left outer, and so forth. Special attention should be paid to the breast tissue along the inframammary crease. In its early stage cancer in this area may be hidden under the overlying breast tissue, and the normal induration of the inframammary crease can be confusing.[105]

Heymann[106] recommends that physical examination of a woman's breasts include right and left semilateral decubitus positions (Figure 8-15). The rationale for this is as follows: Lesions deep within the medial aspects, upper outer quadrants, or axillary tail, especially in large breasts, may be hidden within dense parenchyma or a thick layer of fat or may sink between ribs onto intercostal muscles when they are examined in the usual erect and supine positions (Figure 8-15a). By means of the right and left semilateral decubitus positions with both of the patient's arms elevated (Figure 8-15b), both breasts will fall dependently, thereby thinning the lateral aspects, upper outer quadrant, and axillary tail of the upper portion of the breasts and the medial aspect of the lower portion of the breast[106] (Figure 8-15c).

Next, the examiner needs to check for nipple discharge. Because the ducts are spoke wheel–like, a discharge from the 10 o'clock position indicates trouble in the upper inner quadrant, and so forth. The nipple should be gently compressed in *all* directions for the presence of discharge. Smears should be taken for cytologic examination of any suspicious discharge.

Because carcinoma of the breast may metastasize to regional lymph nodes, a careful palpation of the axillae and the supraclavicular regions is necessary. Most clinicians believe that the axilla is best palpated with the patient sitting erect and at a higher level than the examiner. Hard, fixed nodes palpated in the axillae or the supraclavicular region raise the suspicion of cancer. Normally, lymph nodes are felt as soft, movable structures.

When the clinician examines the breasts of the older woman, it should be kept in mind that the physiologic changes which normally occur with aging may simulate cancer of the breast. As a woman ages, there is atrophy of glandular elements that accentuates anatomic landmarks and reduces the amount of palpable tissue. Shrinkage and fibrotic changes of the breast may cause retraction of the nipple, and the terminal ducts are more visible. Both these changes may cause the examiner to suspect cancer. Because of the high incidence of breast cancer in elderly women, it is best to refer all suspicious findings rather than assume they are due to aging.

In conclusion, the physical signs that most *strongly* suggest cancer of the breast are dimpling, peau d'orange, abnormal contours of the breast, flattening of the nipple, palpable hard, poorly circumscribed nodules that are fixed to the skin or underlying tissue, and palpable hard, fixed nodes in the axillae or supraclavicular region.

Screening tests for asymptomatic individuals

Three methods frequently are used in screening for breast cancer: physical examination of the breast by the health professional, teaching the woman BSE and mammography.

The American Cancer Society's revised recommendations for screening for breast cancer are as follows:

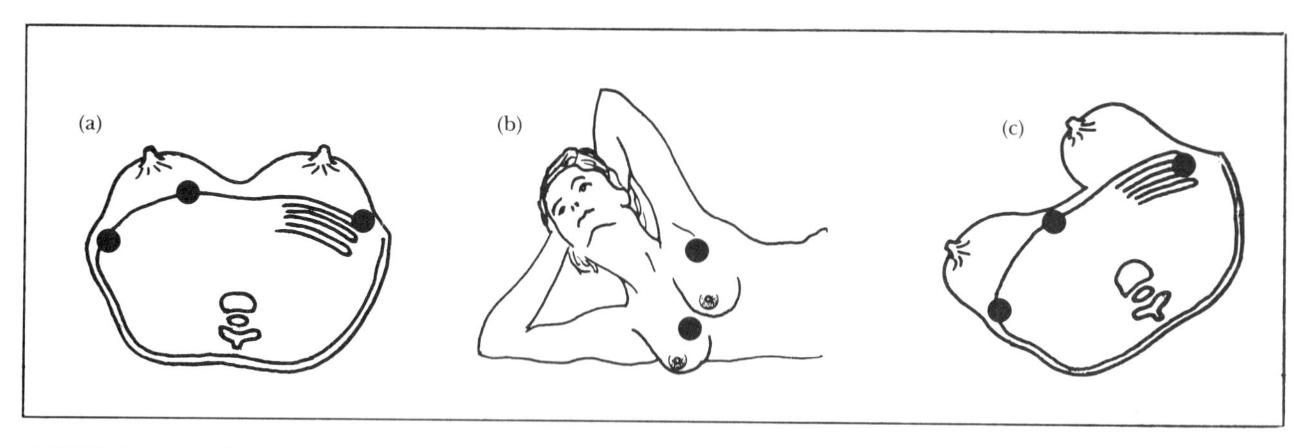

FIGURE 8-15 Semilateral decubitus breast examination. (a) Small masses obscured by breast parenchyma or ribs when breast is examined in upright or supine position; (b) Semilateral decubitus position; (c) Thinning of parenchyma with clarification of obscured masses when patient is in semilateral decubitus position. (Source: Adapted from Heymann A: Semilateral decubitus breast examination. JAMA 243:1713, 1980.)

1. All women from age 20 years should perform BSE monthly.
2. Women 20 to 40 years of age should have a breast physical examination every 3 years, and women older than 40 years should have a breast physical examination every year.
3. Women should have a baseline mammogram between the ages of 35 and 40 years; women 40 to 49 years of age should have a mammogram every 1 to 2 years; and women older than 50 years of age should have a mammogram every year.[107,108]

The National Cancer Institute's cancer control objectives for the year 2000 are to increase the percentage of women from age 50 to 70 years who have an annual breast examination and mammogram from 45% to 80%.[109] The mortality rate of carcinoma of the breast can be reduced by a combination of physical examinations and mammography, as shown by a study conducted by the Health Insurance Plan of New York (HIP)[110]:

> About one third of the cancers were detected on mammography alone, and were negative on initial clinical examination. At the same time, two fifths of the cancers were found on clinical examination alone, and were negative on mammography. About one fifth of the cancers were detected on both modalities. It was concluded that both modalities were needed for proper yield in screening.[101 (p 666)]

The Breast Cancer Detection Demonstration Project (BCDDP) showed that mammography alone was responsible for the detection of 41.6% of 3557 cancers diagnosed in 280,000 women. In women 40 to 49 years of age, mammography alone detected 35.4% of 762 cancers. These percentages are better than the mass screening study of 160,000 women developed by HIP a decade earlier, which showed that mammography alone detected 33.3% of all cancers and 19.4% of the cancers in women 40 to 49 years of age. At 10 years, mortality is reduced 30% in women older than 50 years of age who are screened for breast cancer by mammography and physical examination. A study in Sweden duplicates the 30% mortality reduction found in the HIP study.[111] The BCDDP study also showed results consistent with the reduction in mortality from breast cancer found in the HIP and the Swedish study.[109] In all the studies, there is unequivocal benefit for those older than 50 years of age. However, the benefits for those 40 to 50 years of age have been widely debated in the literature.[110] In the HIP study women in the 40 to 49 age-group exhibited only a 5% decrease in mortality.

A new analysis of the HIP data has found significant reductions in breast cancer mortality for women younger than 50 years of age, which may help settle the under-50 screening debate. The investigators attribute the new finding to longer follow-up and more efficient statistical methods. At the same time, recent analysis of the BCDDP data supports the new HIP findings that mammographic screening lowers mortality for the 40 to 49 age-group. The National Cancer Institute, the American Cancer Society, and the American College of Radiology now recommend that women between 40 and 49 years of age have a mammogram every 1 to 2 years.[108,112,113]

Breast self-examination The importance of BSE is based on the fact that approximately 95% of breast cancers are self-discovered either accidentally or through planned examination. Because approximately 10% of cancers termed *interim cancers* will become apparent within a year of an examination with negative results, reliance has been placed on BSE to find these lesions. In the last few years there has been considerable debate about the value of BSE in reducing mortality and increasing survival rates.[114-117] The problem is that to date there have been no prospective randomized studies testing the benefits of BSE. The World Health Organization is sponsoring a prospective trial of BSE in Russia, and there is also a British randomized trial of breast cancer screening under way, but any data from these trials are several years away.[115] Because BSE has not been studied in a prospective, controlled trial with mor-

TABLE 8-4 Educational Efforts to Help Women Detect Breast Cancer Early

1. *Increase competence of women in doing BSE*
   a. Cognitive component—educate women about importance of becoming familiar with their breasts in order to identify changes if they occur.
   b. Tactile-skill competence—women are shown BSE and then *return* the demonstration. Women should be seen 6 months later to again demonstrate their technique and findings.
2. *Increase frequency and retain persistence of BSE*
   a. Habit component of BSE—provide calendar or other stimulus memory aid noting date on which BSE should be performed.
   b. Memory component of BSE—provide woman with a record form to be filled out each month; form should enable woman to chart findings.
   c. Reinforcement component of BSE—offer praise whenever possible either verbally or through tangible rewards (ie, buttons, stickers)
3. *Reduce delay in reporting findings and increase access to physicians*
   a. Share the fact that BSE is not enough if something different is discovered. Need to have suspicious findings followed up by mammography and biopsy if necessary.
   b. Educate women about the favorable outcome of breast cancer that is found at stage I and the substantial risk in delay.
   c. Encourage woman to have physician who will welcome her if she finds differences in any monthly findings. Women should change physicians if their present physician is not supportive of her early detection efforts.

Source: From Kegeles S: Education for breast self-examination: Why, who, what and how? Prev Med 14:702-720, 1985.

tality as an outcome, the US Preventive Services Task Force does not make a recommendation about the inclusion or exclusion of teaching BSE during the periodic health examination.[116] In addition, the World Health Organization does not recommend BSE screening programs as public health policy, although there is insufficient evidence to change them where they already exist.[116]

Although there probably is not sufficient evidence to justify BSE as a large-scale, community-based intervention, many authorities believe it should be encouraged as part of a woman's regular medical care.[115,118] A study by Huguley et al[119] of 2093 women with breast cancer found that self-examiners tended to seek medical care more rapidly and to have earlier stages of disease at diagnosis than non-self-examiners. Five years after diagnosis the cumulative observed survival rates in breast cancer were 76.7% among self-examiners and 60.9% among nonexaminers ($p < 0.0001$). The researchers acknowledge that the observed survival advantage may be due to characteristics of the self-examiners other than BSE per se; however, they encourage BSE as an adjunctive technique for the early detection of breast cancer.[119]

In any discussion of BSE it must be remembered that the majority of American women do not practice monthly BSE. Although nearly all women (90% to 99%) are aware of this early detection practice, only 15% to 40% perform BSE monthly.[117] Bennett et al[120] interviewed 616 women and found that women who were more likely to practice BSE on a frequent basis were living with their sexual partner, had a maternal history of breast disease, had been shown how to perform BSE, and were confident in their examination technique. They found no association between monthly BSE practice and formal education. Studies consistently have shown that lack of knowledge and low confidence are related to low rates of practice or no practice at all. In a review article on BSE, Kegeles[121] noted that knowledge of how it should be done and confidence in one's ability were the characteristics that consistently differentiated frequent from less-frequent practitioners of BSE.[121] Table 8-4 provides several educational approaches to help women detect breast cancer early.

Many researchers, including those of the Gallup poll, found that personal instruction results in more frequent BSE than do films, pamphlets, or lectures. It also has been shown that individual contact is successful in bringing both low users of health services and women at high risk for cancer into cancer screening programs.[121] Self-instruction includes teaching a woman to do BSE by *using her own hand on her breast under the direct guidance of a professional.* Because women can be taught to detect lesions of 1 cm or less in their own breasts, those who practice regular BSE will detect tumors within a size range that will maximize chances for survival and minimize chances for axillary node involvement.[122] When teaching BSE, the nurse should also review the American Cancer Society guidelines, stressing the importance of a yearly physical examination by a health professional and mammographic examination at intervals determined by the woman's age.

Because a high percentage of cancerous lesions are potentially palpable, it is important for nurses to include one-on-one instruction in BSE techniques whenever possible. Research documents the effectiveness of personal instruction in self-examination techniques by registered nurses as part of a cancer education program through their place of employment.[103,123,124] In the BSE program reported by Styrd,[125] more than 60% of the eligible female employees participated in the program and 1 year later 80% reported performing BSE some time during the 3 months before being surveyed. In addition, the proportion of employees who indicated that they had performed BSE on a monthly basis increased significantly after the program ($p < 0.001$).

Primary nursing, as well as public health and occupational health nursing, afford the nurse excellent opportunities for BSE education. To date, there is some empirical evidence that supports nurses' ability to promote the practice of BSE in the acute care setting. Shamian and Edgar[126] studied the knowledge and the frequency pattern of 223 women who were taught BSE by nurse clinicians. They concluded that nurses influence positively the factual and proficiency knowledge base and the frequency of BSE practice. To reinforce personal instruction in BSE there could be posters, multimedia events such as slide-tape and films, and educational panels portraying the techniques of BSE. These methods, however, should reinforce, *not* replace, personal instruction.

Testicular Cancer

Although testicular cancer is relatively rare (1% of all cancers), it is the most common solid tumor in young men between 20 and 35 years of age.[127] A lesser peak occurs in early childhood. Testicular cancer, which is uncommon after 40 years of age, affects white men more than black. It is estimated that in 1989, 5700 men will be diagnosed with this cancer and 350 will die from testicular cancer.

History assessment

When obtaining the health history, the nurse should inquire about the following:

1. Do you have a history of undescended testicles? Was this surgically corrected? At what age?
2. Is there a history of mumps, orchitis, or testicular cancer in the family? History of inguinal hernia?
3. Did your mother take any type of hormones while she was pregnant with you?
4. Are you aware of any lumps in your scrotum?
5. Were there signs of early puberty as a child?
6. Have you noticed any changes in your genital organs or interest in sex?
7. Are you aware of any scrotal heaviness or heavy discomfort in the scrotum or lower portion of the abdomen and groin?
8. Are you aware of any breast swelling or nipple tenderness?
9. Do you practice testicular self-examination (TSE)? If not, have you ever been shown?
10. Are you aware of any recent trauma to the genital organs?

Although there is no direct proof that trauma causes testicular cancer, many men link swelling or a lump to a recent trauma. The most common presenting complaint is a painless enlargement of the testis, or "heaviness," which is noticed by about two third of men.[128] Nodules in the testes are typically small, hard, and usually painless, and they are slightly more common in the right testis (52.3%) than in the left (47.7%).[129]

The major obstacle to early detection of testicular cancer is the delay that commonly occurs between initial detection of the lesion in the testis to the time of treatment. Approximately 6 months will elapse before treatment is either sought by the patient or begun by the physician.[128] The uninformed young man may ignore the unilateral enlargement for quite some time for the following reasons: (1) the man may hope that the testis will spontaneously revert to normal; (2) he may feel a certain pride in his enlarging sexual organ; (3) he may perceive the tumor as punishment for past sexual sins; (4) he may perceive the lack of pain as an indication that the lump is innocent; and (5) he may fear it is cancer.[128,130]

In 1978 Conklin and coworkers[131] explored the need for and the interest in a health education program about TSE at the University of Vermont. Although 58% of the 90 students interviewed had taken a health-related course in the previous 2 years, 75% had never heard of testicular cancer. None knew how to examine their testes correctly, and only one knew what to palpate for. In 1986 Blesch[132] surveyed a random sample of 233 professional men about their knowledge and perceptions of testicular cancer and TSE and found the same lack of knowledge about TSE as Conklin and colleagues. Of 129 responses, only 31.1% of the sample subjects were aware of TSE and only 9.5% practiced TSE. Although more than half the sample (61.2%) were aware of testicular cancer, 4/9 men with a personal history of undescended testis (a significant risk factor) had not heard of testicular cancer.[132] Because the effectiveness of TSE in lowering mortality has not been documented, there is debate about recommending this practice for men in screening programs.[109]

Physical examination

The examination begins with inspection of the scrotum. Cancer of the testes may be manifested by asymmetry of the scrotum. In most men the left side of the scrotal sac descends lower than the right because of the greater length of the left spermatic cord.[133] Another clue to the presence of a tumor in the scrotum is scrotal skin that appears stretched and thin over the tumor.

Palpation of the scrotal contents can be done with the man standing or in a recumbent position; however, the examination should be thorough and gentle because the testes are exquisitely tender to physical pressure.[134] The examiner must conduct the palpation as gently as possible to avoid eliciting the cremasteric reflex. Stimulation of the scrotum or inner thigh may elicit this reflex and cause the testes to be retracted into the inguinal canal (migratory testis). Several procedures are recommended for palpating the testes. Some authors advocate that the examiner palpate the scrotal contents with both hands to help differentiate the testicles from the other scrotal structures—epididymis, vas deferens, and spermatic cord. Palpating bimanually also improves the chances of detecting any weight differential between the testicles, an important clue to malignancy.[135] The bimanual procedure of using index and middle fingers to separate testes and scrotum so that the right testis and epididymis can be examined with left

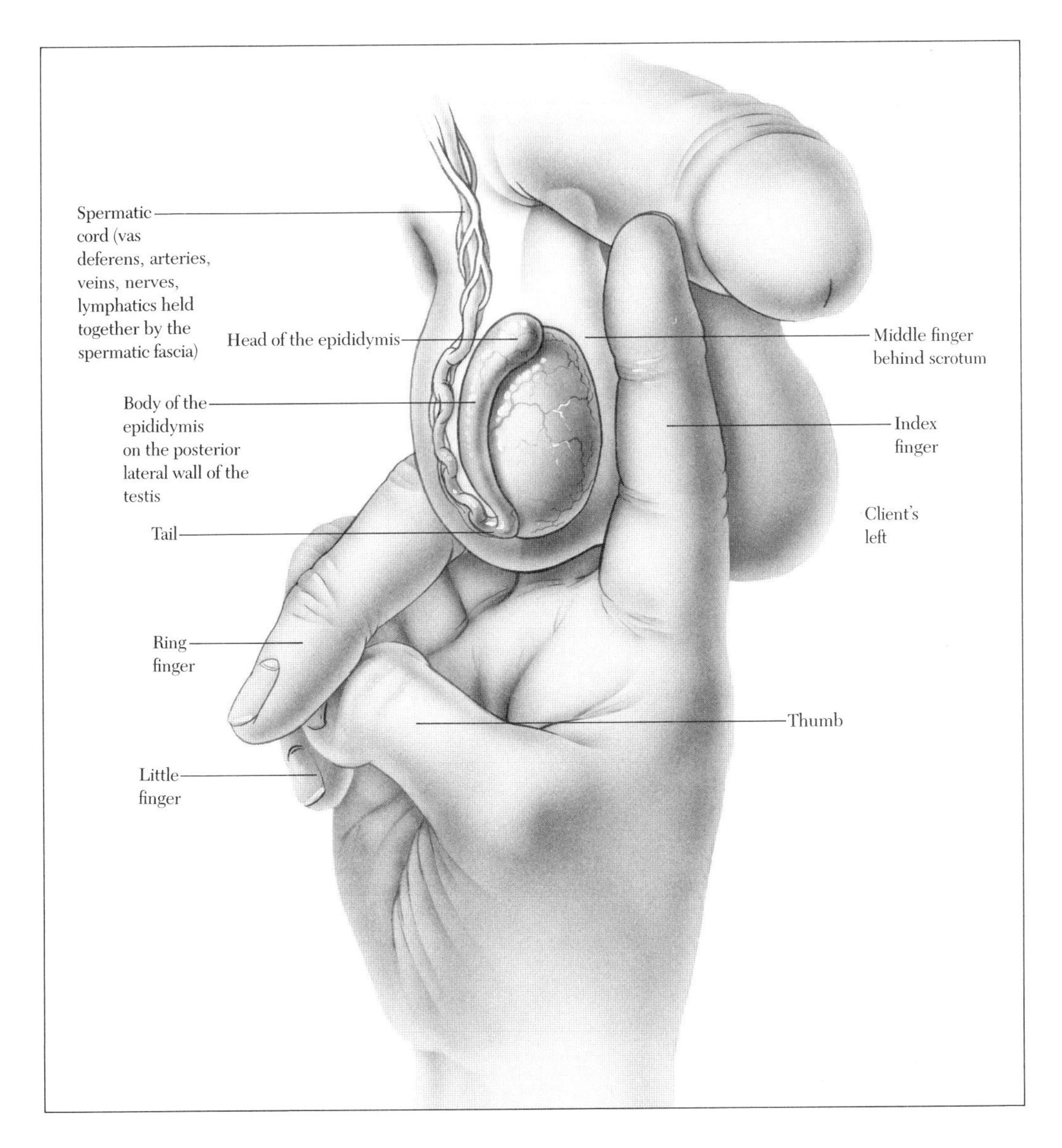

FIGURE 8-16 Palpation of the scrotum. (Source: Grimes J, Burns E (eds): Health Assessment in Nursing Practice (ed 2). Boston, Jones and Bartlett, 1987.)

hand and vice versa is illustrated in Figure 8-16. DeGowin and DeGowin[42] recommend comparing both testes simultaneously by grasping one with each hand, using the thumb and forefinger. As is true with breast lesions, if the man has symptoms, the uninvolved testis should be examined first to provide a baseline comparison.[136]

A normal testicle has a somewhat rubbery, spongy consistency, and the consistency is uniform throughout with a surface free of lumps or indurations. Diffuse induration of the testis in the absence of discrete nodularity also may be the initial abnormality.[137] The most common sites for tumors are on the testicular anterior and lateral surfaces.[138] In the young male, the testis is apt to feel firm and smooth whereas in the elderly male it may be very soft, almost mushy.[133] Even though the testes feel normal, they each should be transilluminated. One may be atrophied and the normal size attained by a hydrocele.[42] Transillumination is helpful in distinguishing cystic from solid masses. Transillumination can be accomplished by aiming a small flashlight behind or on the side of the scrotum in a darkened room. It should be remembered that hydroceles may develop as a result of a tumor.[139] Typically, a testicular tumor occurs as a painless scrotal mass that does not transilluminate. The size may range from less than 1 cm to 10 cm in diameter.[127] The examiner needs to be aware that the scrotal skin overlying the tumor is rarely attached, although attachment may exist in lymphomatous involvement of the testis.[133]

Other areas should be checked to ascertain if there has been metastases, for example, a mass in the epigastrium or an enlarged left supraclavicular node (Virchow's node) may be palpable.[127] The examiner also should palpate the abdomen for retroperitoneal lymph node involvement. To feel any metastatic nodes the examiner will have to palpate the abdomen fairly deeply. Metastatic nodes usually lie at the level of, or slightly caudal to, the umbilicus. Ultrasonographic examination is often useful in further defining an abnormality of the testicular parenchyma.[137]

Education: testicular self-examination

There is a need for nurses to educate themselves, their colleagues, and their patients about testicular cancer and TSE. The major deterrent to early detection and treatment is young men's lack of knowledge of the great danger of testicular cancer and the lack of awareness of the need for regular self-examination.[132] Because the prognosis is good when the tumor is treated early, there is a vital need to educate the public about early detection and treatment. The majority of men discover the changes in the testes while bathing or showering, or it is found by their sexual partners. Only 4% of tumors are detected by clinicians doing a work-up for infertility.[129]

Pediatric hospital and office-based nurses, pediatric nurse practitioners, and school nurses must instruct the parents of high-risk boys and adolescents, ie, those who have or have had undescended testis, how to correctly palpate the scrotum and what physical findings are significant. These same children should be instructed in TSE as they mature. TSE techniques should be included in health education classes just as breast self-examinations are now routinely included in these classes. Education should emphasize the importance of reporting abnormal findings immediately because delay in reporting testicular lesions is common. Table 8-5 summarizes what should be taught during TSE.[140]

Nurses who work in the military, in occupational health settings, in physicians' offices, and in educational settings are in ideal clinical settings for teaching TSE and providing education that will dispel the myths that contribute to delay once a testicular lump is found. Teaching TSE should be incorporated into routine physical examinations by the examining health professional. A nursing assessment of any male younger than 40 years of age should include a health history to elicit any subjective symptoms and established risk factors for testicular cancer. A man who complains of vague scrotal symptoms should be referred for a careful genital examination, and those men identified as being at high risk for testicular cancer should be instructed in TSE.

The following methods to disseminate information about testicular cancer and TSE have been proposed by Carlin[129]:

1. Teaching male clients in sexually transmitted disease clinics
2. Publishing articles on TSE and early detection in local papers, radio, and television
3. Including discussions of TSE in all health education classes at the junior high and high school levels
4. Distributing TSE pamphlets to physicians' offices (especially offices of urologists), hospitals, pediatric clinics, clinics for women, infants, and children, immunization clinics, and other health care settings
5. Teaching personnel in public health departments the importance of including discussions of testicular cancer and how to perform TSE when they work with parents of young boys and with men who attend the health clinic
6. Publishing articles in college newspapers and offering health programs at the university infirmary on the early detection of testicular cancer
7. Discussing testicular cancer and TSE in all health-related programs for new military recruits
8. Providing classes and written materials to male employees in occupational settings, particularly young men in the "high-tech" occupations

In summary, the best defense against testicular cancer is a well-educated male population that practices TSE and understands the importance of seeking medical attention when a "lump" is discovered. Much progress has been made in the last 10 years in discussing and promoting breast self-examination among women. The time has come for nurses to address the issue of testicular cancer in the same forthright open manner that breast cancer has been discussed so that men will incorporate this health practice into their lives.[141]

TABLE 8-5 Summary Chart: Testicular Self-Examination (TSE)

Perform monthly while bathing or showering. Lather hands with soap to increase the fingers' sensitivity.
Hold the scrotum in the palm of the hands and compare each half of the sac for equal heaviness.
Examine the side of the scrotal sac individually. Place index and middle fingers on the underside of the testis and the thumb on top. Palpate the ovoid-shaped testis for lumps. Locate the epididymis and palpate. It is a comma-shaped structure on top of and extending down behind the testicle. It is usually soft and slightly tender. Position the thumb and fingers into the deep groove between the anterior oval testis and the posterior epididymis. The testis is firmer than the epididymis.
Identify the spermatic cord or vas deferens that ascends from the epididymis. It is a smooth, firm, moveable, tubular structure.
During TSE, apply gentle pressure. If there is pain, too much pressure is being applied.
Examination of the testis should be done with a slow, gentle, rolling action. Check for any small lump, slight enlargement, or change in consistency.
Repeat the same procedure for the opposite testicle.
Report any changes found to a physician for immediate evaluation.

Source: From White L: The nurse's role in cancer prevention, in Newell G (ed): Cancer Prevention in Clinical Medicine. New York, Raven Press, 1983, pp 91-112.

Skin Cancer

Cancers of the skin are the most common cancers in humans. In the United States it is estimated that in 1989, 27,000 people will be diagnosed with melanoma and 8200 will die of skin cancer (6000 of melanoma and 2200 of other skin cancers[31]). Annually new cancers of the skin will develop in more than 500,000 people in the United States.[142] Thus approximately one in three newly diagnosed cancers is a malignancy of the skin.

Malignant melanoma accounts for about 74% of all deaths that result from cutaneous cancers.[143] The mortality rate from malignant melanoma is increasing faster than that of any other cancer except lung cancer. Since 1930 the lifetime incidence of malignant melanoma has increased from 1/1500 people to 1/150—a tenfold increase.[144] Today the majority of persons with malignant melanoma are relatively young: the median age at diagnosis is 45 years.[145]

History assessment

When obtaining the health history, the nurse should inquire about the following:

1. Have you noticed any changes in any of your moles in terms of color, size, surface characteristics, sensation, areas around the mole, and elevation of the mole?
2. Are you aware of any skin lesions on your body that are new or don't seem to "go away"?
3. Are you aware of the development of any new moles?
4. Have you ever been told you should have a mole removed? Why were you told this?
5. Have you (or any members of your family) ever been told you have dysplastic nevi? Have you (or any members of your family) ever had skin cancer? Melanoma? If yes, where was the cancer?
6. Do you feel you have a lot of moles? Where are the majority of these moles?
7. Do you sunbathe? How often? Do you use sunscreen?
8. Do you go to a tanning salon or use a tanning bed? How often?
9. Does your skin generally burn when in the sun or tan?
10. What is your occupation? Have you ever worked in a position in which you were outside for long periods of time? How long did you hold that job?
11. Have you ever worked in occupations in which you were exposed to tar and pitch, oils, paraffins, arsenic, x rays, and radium?
12. Were you ever burned, or do you have scarring from corrosive or thermal damage?
13. Do you have any outdoor recreational habits or hobbies that you consistently engage in?

When obtaining a health history, the nurse must inquire whether any of the aforementioned changes in moles have occurred. A history of change, often extending over a period of weeks or months, in a preexisting mole or the development of a new mole in an adult is of great importance and requires inspection. The nurse needs to be aware that almost half the melanomas arise in moles or pigmented areas; thus there should be a high index of suspicion in any mole that is changing or enlarging.[146]

Physical examination

It is essential that the entire integument be inspected during the examination of a patient. Skin assessment includes inspection of the inner lip mucosa, the axillae, the nail beds, the external genitalia, the webs between the toes, the soles of the feet, and the areas in skin folds.[147] This is best accomplished in a setting with good lighting (eg, a gooseneck lamp) that enables the nurse to project the light obliquely across the body surface. A pen light can be used instead of a gooseneck lamp. A magnifying glass also allows closer inspection of minute details.[148]

All areas that are chronically exposed to the sun should be meticulously assessed, including the neck, ears, shoulders, face, scalp, arms, and hands. Areas that have been chronically exposed to sunlight are common sites for basal cell and squamous cell carcinomas. However, melanoma are found on head, neck, and trunk, which may or may not be exposed to sun, and on the legs in women; occurrence of malignant melanoma is infrequent in rarely exposed or unexposed areas (breasts and bathing suit area of women and bathing-trunk area of men).[149] The surface distribution of melanomas in black persons differs from that in white persons; the relatively depigmented palms, soles, nail beds, and mucous membranes are primary sites in almost all black patients.[150]

It is recommended that the entire posterior and anterior aspect of the body be viewed and the location of moles be mapped to serve as baseline data for future skin assessments. If a skin lesion is detected, the nurse has three responsibilities: accurate documentation (size, location, description of the lesion), referral of the patient to a physician for diagnosis, and follow-up for recurrent disease.[147]

There are three types of skin cancer: basal cell carcinoma, squamous cell carcinoma, and melanoma. The nurse should be aware of the following precancerous skin lesions: leukoplakia (found in the oral mucosa), senile and actinic keratoses, and dysplastic nevi. Table 8-6[143,151-153] lists the incidence, clinical characteristics, and common sites of actinic keratoses and basal cell and squamous cell skin cancer. Table 8-7 compares the clinical features of a normal mole, dysplastic mole, and malignant melanoma.

Education

Of all the known risk factors, ultraviolet radiation from the sun is the leading cause of skin cancer. Fortunately, the most carcinogenic of the ultraviolet wavelengths can be blocked by sunscreening agents. Sunscreens are rated according to *sun protection factor* (SPF), on a scale currently ranging from 2 to 23. An SPF of 2 in a sunscreen means that proper application allows users to stay in the sun twice

TABLE 8-6 Incidence, Clinical Characteristics, and Common Sites of Premalignant Skin Cancers and Skin Cancer

Skin Carcinoma	Incidence	Clinical Characteristics	Common Sites
Actinic keratoses (senile keratoses, solar keratoses)	Most common premalignant keratoses; develop in persons with fair complexions as result of excessive exposure to light; located on sun exposed areas	Appear as circumscribed dry patches with adherent scales on slightly red inflamed skin	Most commonly on the face and the backs of hands. In 20% of cases lead to squamous cell carcinoma
Basal cell carcinoma	Most common form of skin cancer; it occurs primarily in persons exposed to intense sunlight, especially fair complexioned white persons with light eyes and hair	Nodular basal cell carcinoma: elevated papule to lesions with an ulcerated center, raised margin, and waxy or "pearly" border; firm. Superficial basal cell carcinoma: plaque, usually with a crusted and erythematous center, flat, and defined margins	Commonly found on the nose, eyelids, cheeks, and neck Commonly found on trunk and extremities
Squamous cell carcinoma	Less common than basal cell carcinoma, it occurs primarily on areas exposed to actinic or ultraviolet (UV) radiation	Appearance varies from an elevated nodular mass to a punched-out ulcerated lesion or a large fungating mass. Unlike basal cell carcinoma, squamous cell tumors are opaque and aggressive	Commonly found on head and hands

Source: Adapted from Friedman et al[143]; Helm and Helm[151]; Epstein[152]; Gumport et al.[153]

as long as they could without any protection at all.[144] Sunbathing should be avoided during the 2-hour period around noon because two thirds of the day's ultraviolet light comes through during that time. Skin types are similarly rated from 1 to 6 according to intensity of sunburn in the first 30 to 45 minutes of unprotected exposure to the sun after a period of no exposure. Skin type 1 burns easily and never tans whereas skin types 5 and 6 rarely burn and tan well.

The following information about decreasing or eliminating skin cancer risks should be discussed with each patient:

1. Ultraviolet rays can penetrate thin clothing like cotton T-shirts; thus those who desire protective clothing should select hats, long-sleeved shirts, and beach robes rather than rely on T-shirts.
2. Persons with skin types 1 and 2 should avoid sunbathing.
3. Persons who live or vacation in areas of higher altitudes need to be aware that there is less atmosphere to filter out the ultraviolet rays so that the sun's effects are more intense.
4. Persons need to be informed that the sun's rays are reflected off snow, sand, and water and that significant sun exposure can result from activities on these surfaces.
5. As the ozone layer of the earth changes, persons need to be aware that this significantly changes the amount of ultraviolet radiation that reaches the Earth.

Routine self-examination of the skin is the best defense against skin cancer, especially malignant melanoma. It is inexpensive, noninvasive, and totally free of danger. Periodic self-examination for melanoma and examination by others may result in improved survival.[154] It is recommended that persons older than 30 years of age who have fair skin and are subject to heavy sun exposures be taught skin self-assessment. Those with dysplastic nevus syndrome or a history of melanoma in a first-degree relative also should have regular medical examinations that include measurement and charting of location of unusual pigmented lesions.[143] It also is recommended that patients be given copies of blank body charts so that they can chart lesions found during self-skin assessment. Figure 8-17 illustrates the correct procedure for self-assessment of skin.

TABLE 8-7 Comparison of Common Nevi, Dysplastic Nevi, and Malignant Melanoma

Characteristic	Common Nevi	Dysplastic Nevi	Malignant Melanoma
Color	Uniformly tan or brown	Variable mixtures of tan, brown, black, or red/pink within a single nevus; nevi may look very different from each other	Variegated colors ranging from various hues of tan and brown to black and sometimes intermingled with red and white
Shape	Round; sharp, clear-cut borders between the nevus and the surrounding skin; may be flat or elevated	Irregular borders; pigment may fade off into surrounding skin; always have a flat portion level with the skin, which often occurs at the edge of the nevus	Borders of early malignant melanomas usually irregular, notched or angular
Size	Usually <6 mL in diameter like this:	Usually >6 mL; may be >10 mL; occasionally <6 mm	Diameters of macular malignant melanomas often >5 mm (it is not unusual to see 1.0 to 1.5 cm); 98.5% had a diameter ≥5 mm
Number	In a typical adult: 10 to 40 are scattered over the body	Often very many (>100), but some people may not have an unusual number of nevi	
Location	Generally on the sun-exposed surfaces of the skin above the waist; the scalp, breasts, and buttocks rarely are involved	Sun-exposed areas: the back is the most common site but also may be seen on the scalp, breasts, and buttocks	Relatively uncommon body areas that are always covered, especially the breast and pelvic area in women; sharp increase in incidence in the head, neck, trunk of men, and arms and lower legs of women

Source: Adapted from Friedman R, Rigel D, Koff A: Early detection of malignant melanoma: The role of physician, examination and self-examination of the skin. CA 35:130-151, 1985.

Along with self-assessment of the skin, patients should be instructed about the changes in moles that merit immediate medical attention: size, color, elevation, surface characteristics, and sensation. Melanoma is more likely to develop in individuals and families with a history of dysplastic nevus syndrome (DNS) than it is in most people. The initial diagnosis is based on a physical examination and confirmed by the removal and biopsy of several moles. Individuals with familial DNS should visit their clinician or dermatologist twice a year for assessment and follow-up. They also should conduct self-assessments of the skin on a monthly basis. Assistance usually is necessary because many of the nevi are present in areas such as the scalp or back that are difficult for the individual to inspect.

The elderly constitute the highest-risk group for skin cancer because of the number of years of exposure to the sun. It is estimated that 40% to 50% of all those who live to be 65 years of age will have at least one skin cancer during their lifetime.[155] Changes normally occur in the skin with age, which increase the risk of skin cancer. Keratoses, lentigines, and pigmented alterations develop with aging and in areas of chronic solar exposure. Elderly persons should be taught skin self-assessment and the importance of having a health professional examine any new lesions or changing lesions. Any setting where older adults congregate offers the nurse an excellent opportunity to provide an educational program on skin self-examination and early detection for skin cancer. Again, any areas that have been chronically exposed to the sun should be meticulously screened.

Oral Cancer

In 1989 it is estimated that there will be 30,600 new cases of oral cancer in the United States. The majority of these cancers (11,700) will be cancers of the mouth. There will be 8650 deaths from oral cancer.[31] These figures indicate that oral cancer incidence is not in decline nationally and that success in treatment has not made significant headway during the last decade.[156] Approximately 95% of all oral malignancies begin in the surface mucosa. Although the

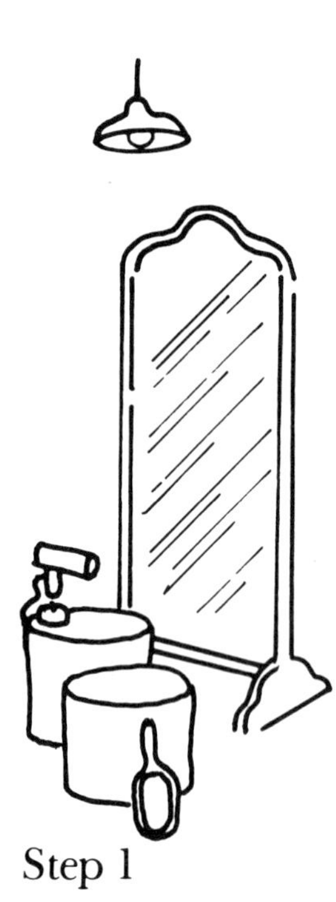

Step 1

Make sure the room is well-lighted and that you have nearby a full-length mirror, a hand-held dryer, and two chairs or stools. Undress completely.

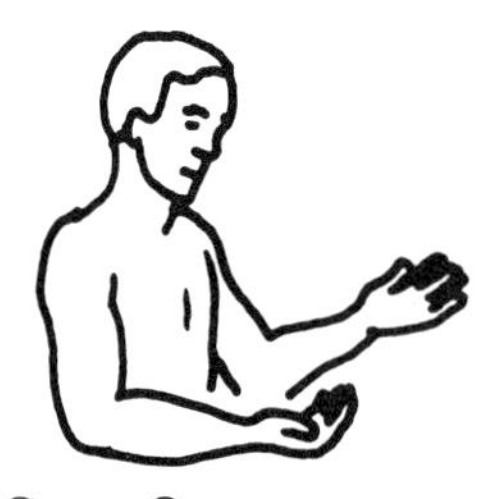

Step 2

Hold your hands with the palms face up, as shown in the drawing. Look at your palms, fingers, spaces between the fingers, and forearms. Then turn your hands over and examine the backs of your hands, fingers, spaces between the fingers, fingernails, and forearms.

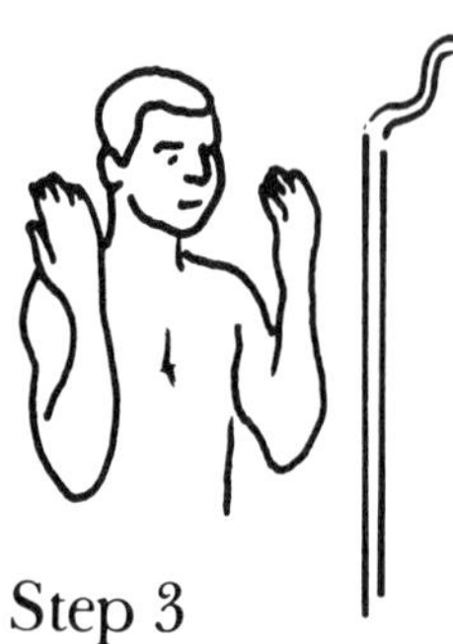

Step 3

Now position yourself in front of the full-length mirror. Hold up your arms, bent at the elbows, with your palms facing you. In the mirror, look at the backs of your forearms and elbows.

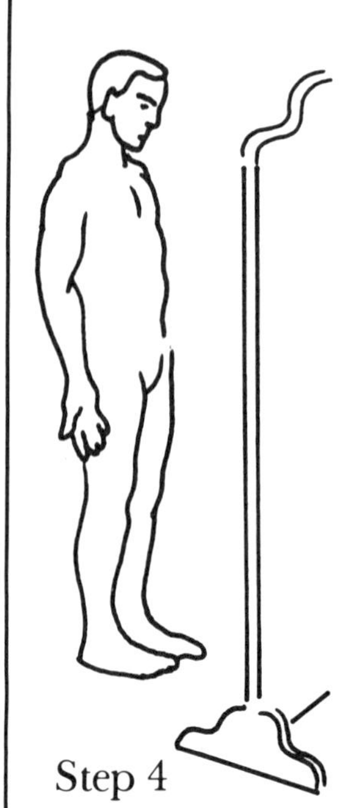

Step 4

Again using the full-length mirror, observe the entire front of your body. In turn, look at your face, neck, and arms. Turn your palms to face the mirror and look at your upper arms. Then look at your chest and abdomen, pubic area, thighs and lower legs.

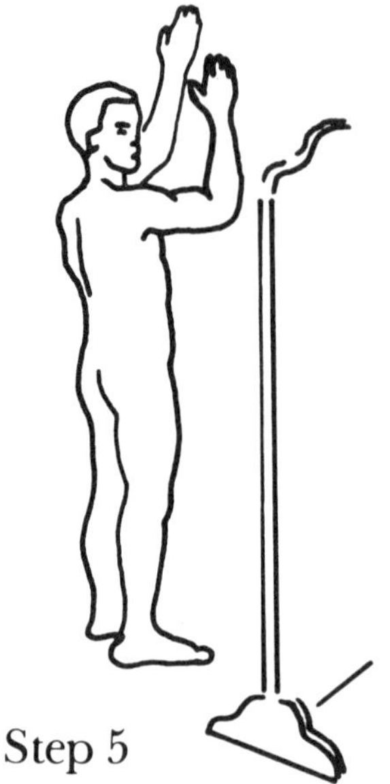

Step 5

Still standing in front of the mirror, lift your arms over your head with the palms facing each other. Turn so that your right side is facing the mirror and look at the entire side of your body—your hands and arms, underarms, sides of your trunk, thighs, and lower legs. Then turn, and repeat the process with your left side.

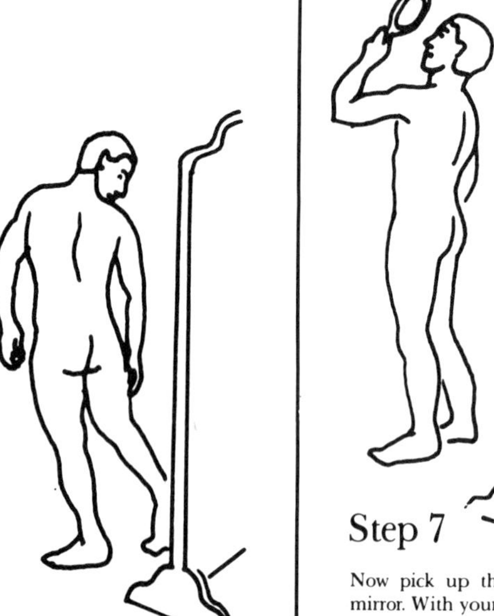

Step 6

With your back toward the full-length mirror, look at your buttocks and the backs of your thighs and lower legs.

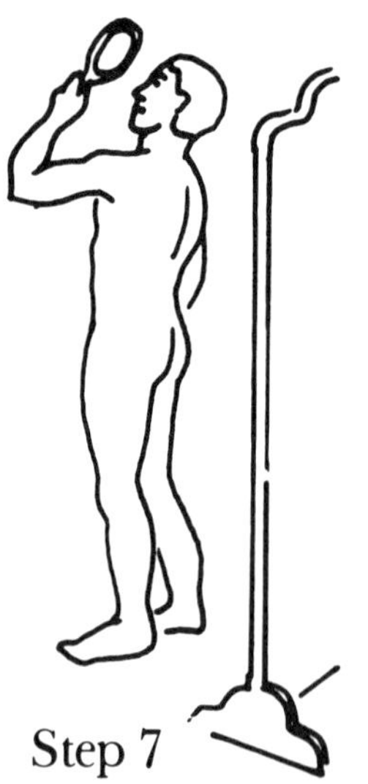

Step 7

Now pick up the hand-held mirror. With your back still to the full-length mirror, examine the back of your neck, and your back and buttocks. Also examine the backs of your arms in this way. Some areas are hard to see, and you may find it helpful to ask your spouse or a friend to assist you.

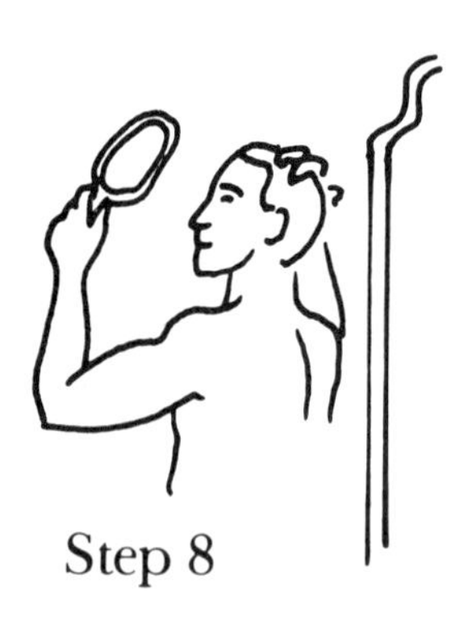

Step 8

Use the hand-held mirror and the full-length mirror to look at your scalp. Because the scalp is difficult to examine, we suggest you also use a hand-held blow dryer turned to a cool setting to lift the hair from the scalp. While some people find it easy to hold the mirror in one hand and the dryer in the other, while looking in the full-length mirror, many do not. For the scalp examination in particular, then, you might ask your spouse or a friend to assist you.

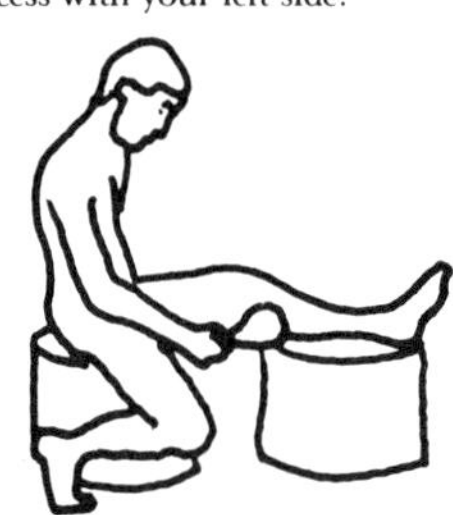

Step 9

Sit down and prop up one leg on a chair or stool in front of you as shown. Using the hand-held mirror, examine the inside of the propped-up leg, beginning at the groin area and moving the mirror down the leg to your foot. Repeat the procedure for your other leg.

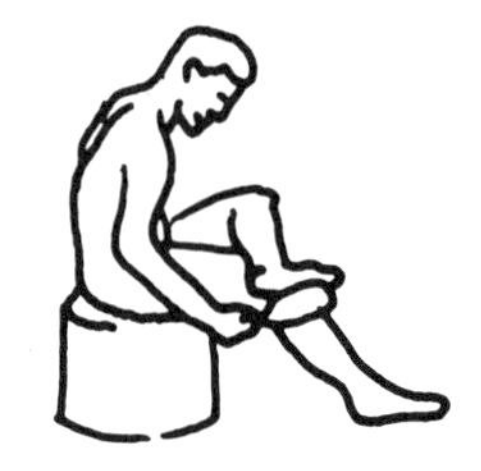

Step 10

Still sitting, cross one leg over the other. Use the hand-held mirror to examine the top of your foot, the toes, toenails, and spaces between the toes. Then look at the sole or bottom of your foot. Repeat the procedure for the other foot.

FIGURE 8-17 Self-examination of the skin. (Source: Friedman R, Rigel D, Kapf A: Early detection of malignant melanoma: The role of physician examination and self-examination of the skin. CA 35:130-151, 1985.)

surface of the oral mucosa is easily inspected and palpated, by the time of diagnosis more than 60% of oral cancers have spread to the lymph nodes.[156]

History assessment

When the nurse obtains the health history, it is important to ask the following questions:

1. Do you smoke? How much do you smoke, and how many years have you smoked (pack years)?
2. Do you chew tobacco or dip snuff? How long have you done this? How much tobacco do you use in a day? Can you describe where you place the tobacco in your mouth?
3. Do you smoke a pipe? How long have you smoked a pipe? Do you smoke a cigar?
4. Do you drink alcohol? Approximately how much alcohol do you drink in a day? What type of alcohol do you consume?
5. For the patient from Southeast Asia or Central Asia—do you chew *betel quid?* Do you use betel quid with any form of tobacco (chewing or smoking)?[157]
6. Do you wear dentures? Do you have any sore spots in your mouth from your dentures? Do you inspect under your dentures at least weekly?
7. When was your last dental examination?
8. How often do you brush your teeth? Floss your teeth?
9. Have you ever been in an occupation in which you spent a lot of time outside? Do you have any hobbies or sports interests that involve spending a great deal of time outdoors? Do you wear lip balm when outdoors to protect your lips?
10. Have you noticed any white or red sores in your mouth for longer than a month? Any lumps, swelling, or rough spots?
11. Have you been aware of any limitation of tongue or jaw movement?
12. Have you noticed taste changes, dry mouth, speech changes, hoarseness, or chronic cough?
13. Are you aware of any sores or crusts on your lips?
14. Are you aware of any lumps or growing "bumps" in your neck or face?
15. Do you have problems with persistent halitosis that does not seem to respond to any home remedies?

Physical examination

The majority of oral cancers cause no symptoms in their early stages. Most individuals who notice a white or bright red spot, "sore," or a swelling in their mouth attribute it to their teeth or dentures and thus seek the consultation of a dentist.

Physical examination of the mouth includes inspection, digital palpation, and olfaction of the oral cavity. The following maneuvers should be performed during the oral examination:

1. Have the patient extend the tongue and move it from side to side. The patient also should be asked to move the jaw from side to side and up and down. Limitation of normal movement could indicate that a tumor is interfering with muscle action.

2. Palpate the tongue with a gloved hand. Palpation may reveal a lesion not otherwise visible. Palpation of a hard lesion should be referred for biopsy to establish the diagnosis.[158]

3. Inspect the anterior two thirds of the tongue by grasping the tip of the tongue with a piece of gauze and gently pulling the tongue forward and to each side. Lesions of the base of the tongue are most often overlooked and must be both inspected and palpated. The nurse should be aware that most tongue cancers appear on the lateral surfaces.

4. The floor of the mouth should be inspected by having the patient place the tongue on the hard palate. Squamous cell carcinomas frequently are found on the floor of the mouth. The floor of the mouth should be palpated bimanually, with the fingers of one hand in the floor of the mouth and the fingers on the other hand placed on the skin under the right side of the jaw.

5. Inspection of the mouth may reveal snuff keratosis from the use of snuff in one spot in the mouth and nicotine stomatitis from cigar or pipe smoking. Nicotine stomatitis is a diffuse white condition that contains numerous red dots. This lesion usually covers the entire hard palate and is almost always associated with pipe smoking and has minimal or no malignant potential. Complete resolution should occur with cessation of smoking.

Individuals who use smokeless tobacco may develop leukoplakias in the exact region where they hold the quid. The leukoplakia may vary from just a very mild whiteness, which may be difficult to see, to a very obvious white lesion.[159,160] When a white oral lesion is found, the area should be rubbed to see if it can be removed. White lesions that adhere to the surface are classified as keratotic and have a greater probability of malignancy. Leukoplakia occurs in men more commonly than in women, and the vast majority are seen in individuals older than 40 years of age.

In erythroplakia, also considered premalignant, a red plaque or well-defined red patches have a velvety consistency and often have tiny areas of ulceration. Erythroplakia (red) lesions usually have a more malignant histologic component than does leukoplakia.[158] Erythroplakia patches are characteristically painless and occur with about equal frequency in men and women who usually are older than 50 years of age.

6. While inspecting the lips, they should be observed for any skin changes, such as keratosis of the lips from excessive sun exposure and pipe smoking. Solar keratoses occur on sun-exposed surfaces and are flat, reddish-to-tan plaques that are usually scaly. In the earliest stages a cancerous lesion may appear as a small swelling or induration that may be difficult to see but that can be palpated. An area of roughness, induration, or granularity often is the best clue to the diagnosis of early carcinoma. The upper lip should be grasped between the index finger and the thumb and bidigitally palpated along its complete length to discover masses that may be located deep to the surface.[158]

7. Olfaction of the breath. An odor of sourness may indicate obstruction and fermentation, whereas fetid and foul odors may signal necrotic neoplasms indicative of advanced disease. All large, fungating oral cancers produce a marked halitosis; however, small oral cancers are not particularly associated with mouth odor.[159] Referral to a dentist may be necessary if the breath odors indicate advanced dental decay and poor oral hygiene.

8. Palpate the parotid, submandibular, and submental areas and the cervical lymph nodes.

Screening

Because alcoholics who smoke constitute the largest risk group for oral cancers, screening programs should be geared to this population. Any screening programs would have to be conducted in settings in which alcoholics could be approached as a group such as in reform organizations, Salvation Army facilities for this population, shelters for the homeless, or alcoholic rehabilitation units. Although primary prevention by limiting alcohol intake and cessation of smoking is a more desirable goal, many alcoholics cannot be reached by these types of programs. Thus the more realistic approach with this group is to encourage periodic oral examinations so that cancer can be detected in the early stages.

It is important for the nurse to explain to individuals 40 years of age and older that it is necessary to have a complete oral and dental examination on a periodic basis to detect serious lesions. Individuals with complete dentures frequently believe that they no longer require periodic oral examinations because of their loss of natural teeth.[161]

The use of smokeless tobacco (eg, snuff and chewing tobacco) has risen dramatically in the last 10 years. The increase in the sales of smokeless tobacco, predominantly snuff, since the early 1970s has been estimated at 11% per year, representing an estimated 7 to 12 million users.[162] In the early 1970s a majority of users were men 50 years of age and older; now most are young men between 16 and 29 years of age. Nurses need to stress that smokeless tobacco is *not* a safe substitute for smoking. Long-term use of smokeless tobacco increases the risk of gingival and buccal carcinomas nearly 50-fold.[159] Many young people are not aware that smokeless tobacco is as addicting as cigarette smoking.[163] Information about the health hazards of smokeless tobacco should be shared with young people. Because so many users are very young children, it is advocated that education on the dangers of smokeless tobacco should begin with children as young as 6 and 7 years of age.[164] School nurses and nurses who work in settings with young people need to actively initiate educational programs on this subject or make sure that whenever smoking is discussed in health and science classes that the issue of smokeless tobacco also is addressed. In addition, parents, teachers, and athletic coaches should not neglect the powerful influence they can have as positive role models. Youngsters perceive the use of smokeless tobacco as "macho," and athletic coaches can have a tremendous influence in dispelling this myth. The Yellow Pages section lists sources for obtaining patient education materials on smokeless tobacco.

In summary, education first begins with the identification of persons at high risk for oral cancer. Depending on the risk factors identified, the individual could be referred to a physician or a dentist or taught oral self-examination for the early signs of cancer, or the nurse could conduct the oral examination at predetermined intervals. Grabau[165] found that about half those taught self-examinations for early signs of cancer continued these examinations at regular intervals. It is advocated that oral self-examination techniques need to be popularized in the same manner as breast self-examination techniques.

Gynecologic Cancer

In 1989 it is estimated that 34,000 cases of endometrial cancers and 13,000 cases of cervical cancers will occur. However, the anticipated mortality rate reverses the prevalence because 7000 deaths from cervical cancer, but only 3000 deaths from endometrial cancer, are expected in this same period.[31] The risk of endometrial cancer is age-related; the disease usually occurs in women 50 to 60 years old.

In stark contrast are the incidence and mortality rates for ovarian cancer. It is estimated that in 1989, 20,000 women will be diagnosed with this cancer and 12,000 will die of the disease. Ovarian cancer accounts for about 26% of all gynecologic cancer and about 52% of all genital cancer deaths. The greatest number of cases of ovarian cancer are found in the age-group comprised of 55- to 59-year-old women.

History assessment

The health history should include questions that will elicit an accurate menstrual, obstetric, gynecologic, and sexual history. The majority of women at risk for cancer of the reproductive organs can be identified only after a thorough and complete gynecologic history has been obtained. The following questions will help identify high-risk women:

1. When was your last Pap smear? Do you remember the results? Was any follow-up done or recommended?
2. Have you ever been told that you have herpes? genital warts? Were the genital warts treated? What type of treatment was done for the genital warts? Have you been treated for pelvic inflammatory disease or any other sexually transmitted diseases?
3. Do you have any vaginal bleeding or discharge not connected with menses?

4. Do you have spotting between menstrual periods?
5. Do you have bleeding or spotting although you no longer have menstrual periods?
6. Do you have bleeding after intercourse or douching?
7. At what age did you start sexual activity?
8. Have you had a consistent sexual partner since beginning sexual activity, or have you had different partners?
9. What is the approximate number of sexual partners you have had?
10. What age did you start menstruation?
11. What age did you start menopause? When was your last period?
12. How many pregnancies have you had? How many live births? miscarriages? elective abortions?
13. Have you ever taken birth control pills? How long did you take birth control pills? Do you remember the name of the pill that you took?
14. Have you ever taken estrogens? How long did you take these? What was the dose that you were given? What follow-up tests were recommended for you while taking estrogens?
15. Have you ever had infertility problems? Have you ever had endometriosis? polycystic ovaries? Stein-Leventhal syndrome? uterine fibroids?
16. Are you aware of abdominal distention or vague abdominal discomfort?
17. Are you aware if your mother received diethylstilbestrol (DES) when she was pregnant with you?
18. Have you had any gynecologic surgery—hysterectomy, tubal pregnancy, sterilization, ovarian cysts, cancer?
19. Have you ever had office procedures for a gynecologic problem, such as cervical cautery and colposcopic examination?
20. Has your present sexual partner ever had a sexual partner who had cervical cancer?

Physical examination

The early signs and symptoms of gynecologic cancer are as follows. Ovarian cancer usually has no early manifestations. There may be vague abdominal discomfort, dyspepsia, indigestion, gas with constant distention, flatulence, eructation, a feeling of fullness after a light meal, or slight loss of appetite.[166] The majority of patients with endometrial cancer have unexplained bleeding. In postmenopausal women, abnormal bleeding takes the form of intermittent spotting or bleeding that the patient describes as a "very light period." A malodorous watery discharge may be noticed as an early sign. The symptoms of cervical cancer typically are abnormal vaginal discharge, irregular bleeding, elongation of menstrual period, or bleeding that may occur after douching or intercourse.[167]

The gynecologic examination includes *inspection* and *palpation*. The nurse should be aware of the following maneuvers performed during the gynecologic examination and related signs that indicate cancer.

Abdomen The abdomen must be thoroughly and slowly palpated to detect any masses, areas of tenderness, or inguinal adenopathy. A mass in the upper portion of the abdomen may suggest the presence of omental cake, the solid mass formed when the omentum is infiltrated with cancer, which is a sign of advanced ovarian disease. It may be palpated or detected by ballottement during the abdominal examination. Other signs of advanced ovarian cancer are abdominal distention and ascites.[166]

Vulva The vulva should be inspected and palpated for signs of cancer of the vulva: excoriation of skin because of pruritis, ulcers, lumps, leukoplakia, bleeding, atrophy of the labia, and narrowing of the introitus.[168]

Infection with human papillomavirus (HPV) may produce the typically raised exophytic tumors (warts) that can be seen with simple inspection of the vulva. There is, however, a variety of anogenital warts known as "flat" or "noncondylomatous" warts that may be invisible before the application of acetic acid. Several gauze pads (4-in diameter) that are soaked in 3% to 5% acetic acid should be compressed on the vulva and left in place for 10 minutes. After the compress is removed, the area should be inspected with a high-quality magnification lens for the *acetowhite reaction*. Acetic acid will cause the surface of both flat and exophytic warts to turn white.[169] Colposcopic examination also can be used to inspect lesions after acetic acid application. Further, carcinoma in situ also may appear as a hyperpigmented lesion. In addition, HPV can infect the entire lower female genital tract—the vagina and cervix. Patients with vulvar HPV lesions should have a thorough examination of the vagina, cervix, and perirectal epithelium with the use of an acetic acid compress application and a colposcopic examination.[169] In 1989 it is estimated that a minimum of 10% of the population, and probably much higher, are infected with HPV.[170] About half the individuals infected with HPV are carriers of the high-risk types of HPV virus.[16,18,31,33]

Vagina The vagina should be inspected and palpated for cancer—masses, vaginal bands, texture changes, ulcers, erosions, leukoplakia, pink blush, induration, telangiectasis, and erythematosus. Induration and nodulation may indicate submucosal vaginal lesions. Most squamous cell carcinomas are found in the posterior vaginal wall, but 25% involve the anterior wall and at least 15% arise from the lateral walls.[171] The majority of lesions occur in the upper third of the vagina.

The nurse may elect to do a Schiller's test on any suspicious area of the vagina or cervix. The mucosa is painted with an iodine solution (Lugol's solution), and the normal mucosa becomes brown whereas areas of abnormal epithelium remain uncolored. This test is merely an adjunctive aid to colposcopic examination or used when colposcopy is not available. It indicates a glycogen-free area and delineates biopsy sites.[168]

Cervix The cervix should be inspected and palpated, and a Pap smear should be taken for cytologic examination. To avoid contamination of the cell sample with foreign material vaginal jelly should not be used before Pap smears are obtained. The cervical sample should contain cells from the squamous epithelium of the vaginal portion of the cervix, from the squamocolumnar junction (also known as the transformation zone), and from the endocervical epithelium.[170,172] With aging the transformation zone becomes increasingly invisible as it moves into the endocervical canal. In women during and after menopause, a sample of the vaginal pool cells is obtained, in addition to the cervical smear, to identify cancer cells from the endometrium, tubes, and ovaries.

The nurse should inspect and palpate the cervix for position, shape, consistency, regularity, mobility, friability, and tenderness. The cervix is freely movable, firm, and smooth, and if it has been invaded by cancer, it becomes hard and immobile. In addition to rendering the cervix much harder than normal, malignancy produces a rough, granular surface and is likened to both the feel and appearance of a cauliflower.[133] However, the nurse needs to be cognizant of the fact that early carcinoma has an appearance that cannot be well differentiated visually from erosion. Cancer arising within the cervical canal may cause no abnormal appearance of the cervix.

Several physical changes may be apparent in the cervix that indicate possible patient exposure to DES in utero. Cervical ectropion, or cervical bumps or ridges ("cockscombs," "hoods," or "collars"), and other nonneoplastic changes are immediate clues to DES exposure. These physical signs merit referral to a physician.

The conventional Pap smear, taken in the usual manner for cervix cancer screening, is inaccurate for a diagnosis of endometrial lesions.[173] For this reason an annual suction curettage is recommended for menopausal women and women who have taken estrogen without progestational modification for a prolonged period after menopause. Suction curettage can provide an excellent sample and in most cases can be done in the office without need for anesthesia. Monitoring of women who have received long-term estrogen therapy will detect those whose endometrium is overstimulated (adenomatous hyperplasia), and appropriate referrals can be made.

Uterus and adnexa A bimanual examination of the uterus and adnexa should be done. The nurse should note the size, shape, mobility, position, tenderness, and consistency of the uterus. Uterine tenderness, immobility, or enlargement merits further investigation and appropriate referrals. An enlarged boggy uterus is an indication of advanced disease.

Ovaries Palpation of the ovaries in prepubertal girls or postmenopausal women also merits investigation because (1) the normal ovary and tube are usually not palpable, (2) ovaries in these two groups of women are smaller than the usual ovarian size of 4 cm in its largest dimension, and (3) 3 to 5 years after menopause the ovaries usually have atrophied and are no longer palpable. In actively menstruating women, any ovarian enlargement that persists or increases more than 5 or 6 cm requires prompt referral.[166] In general the findings on the pelvic examination that can alert the nurse to a possible ovarian cancer are adnexal enlargement, fixation or immobility, bilateral irregularity or nodulation and masses, relative insensitivity of the mass, and bilaterality of the mass.

Rectovaginal palpation *Rectovaginal* palpation, as well as rectal palpation, should be done. It is extremely important that the anterior rectal wall in the region of the peritoneal rectovaginal pouch, or Douglas's cul-de-sac, be palpated. Thickening of this area occurs from spread of cervical carcinoma, whereas spread from ovarian cancer may be felt as a shelf, nodule, or handful-of-knuckles on rectal palpation.

Screening of asymptomatic individuals

The American Cancer Society recommends that all women who are, or who have been, sexually active or have reached 18 years of age, have an annual Pap test and pelvic examination. After a woman has had three or more consecutive satisfactory normal annual examinations, the Pap test may be performed less frequently at the discretion of her physician.[174] Numerous other professional health organizations also have approved a similar or identical recommendation.

Cervical smears Because of the Pap test, the death rate from invasive cervical cancer has decreased by at least 70% over the last 40 years.[84] However, 15% to 20% of American women do not have regular Pap testing.[174] The majority of women in whom cervical cancer develops have not had the test on a regular basis.

The importance of regular Pap smears was documented by Stenkvist and colleagues.[175] They studied 207,455 women for 10 years and found that when women were screened at least once, the incidence of cervical cancer dropped from 32/100,000 to 10/100,000 (a 75% decrease in invasive cervical cancer incidence among women who had smears taken at least once during the 10-year period). Among women with at least one normal smear, the incidence drops still lower, to 7/100,000. Because elderly women will constitute 17.3% of the adult population by the year 2020, screening programs for older, high-risk women will be needed.

Mandelblatt and Fahs[176] conducted a study of the cost effectiveness of a cervical cancer screening program for infrequently screened elderly women. The results of the Pap smears were abnormal in 11/816 women screened. This early detection of cervical neoplasia saved $5907 and 3.7 years of life per 100 Pap tests. The average medical costs per year of life extended by screening were included, and the program cost $2874 per year of life saved. The researchers concluded that the benefits from cervical cancer screening for elderly women can offset the costs of these programs.

Several factors contribute to false-negative results from Pap smears and other errors:

1. Patient error. Patient error consists of women failing to have follow-up annual examinations, delay in seeing a physician while symptoms are present, and refusal to undergo diagnostic measures.

2. Physician error. Physician error consists of failure to act on reports of abnormal cytologic findings, failure to perform a pelvic examination with a Pap smear, reading of Pap smears by untrained physicians, and diagnosis of "dysplasia," which is considered inconsequential by uninformed physicians.

3. Laboratory error. Koss[170] reports in his excellent review article that studies have found a false-negative laboratory rate for invasive cancer of approximately 50%. The rate of screening errors for precancerous lesions was at least 28%.

Although nurses generally do not have control over laboratory errors, they can play a significant role in decreasing patient and physician error (1) by educating women about the early symptoms of gynecologic cancer and the necessity of seeking medical advice with these early symptoms; (2) by educating women about the recommended intervals for Pap smears; (3) by educating women, particularly older women, to the necessity of asking for a Pap smear when they have a physical examination; (4) by educating women to request information about the mechanism used by the health care setting to inform them about the results of their Pap smears: women with a history of abnormal or questionable Pap smear results should be encouraged to personally call about their results rather than rely on the health professional to alert them; (5) by educating women about the importance of receiving additional medical care with an abnormal or a questionable Pap smear finding; and (6) by performing Pap smears only after they are thoroughly versed in the proper procedures for obtaining a smear. Improperly done smears probably contribute to at least half of the 10% to 35% false-negative rate generally reported for Pap smears.[177] Errors made by cytotechnologists may be minimized in the future by new experimental technologic techniques that measure the DNA content of standard Pap smears. Several groups of researchers are investigating the feasibility of automating the procedure of reading Pap smears on the basis of optical density of the specimens or DNA content of cell nuclei.[178,179] Studies are being conducted to determine the feasibility of these approaches.

Two classification methods are used to identify abnormal changes in the Pap smear. One method is the classification system accepted by the World Health Organization. This system identifies two types of lesions, dysplasia and carcinoma in situ. The dysplasias are subdivided into very mild, mild, moderate, and severe grades, depending on the extent of involvement of the epithelium.[180] Another classification method is the cervical intraepithelial neoplasia (CIN) nomenclature. CIN is a continuum of change and generally begins as a well-differentiated lesion (CIN 1 or mild dysplasia), passes through a less well-differentiated phase (CIN 2 or moderate dysplasia), and leads to an undifferentiated intraepithelial lesion (CIN 3).[172] CIN 3 is the severe dysplasia/carcinoma in situ in the World Health Organization system. Table 8-8 compares the commonly used Papanicolaou terminology and relationship to the CIN classification method, and Figure 8-18 is a schematic representation of precancerous cervical lesions.[181]

TABLE 8-8 Classification and Comparative Nomenclature of Cervical Smears

Class I
Normal smear
No abnormal cells
Class II
Atypical cells present below the level of cervical neoplasia
Class III
Smear contains abnormal cells consistent with dysplasia
Mild dysplasia = CIN 1
Moderate dysplasia = CIN 2
Class IV
Smear contains abnormal cells consistent with carcinoma in situ
Severe dysplasia and carcinoma in situ = CIN 3
Class V
Smear contains abnormal cells consistent with invasive carcinoma of squamous cell origin

CIN, Cervical intraepithelial neoplasia.
Source: From Nelson J, Averette H, Richart R: Dysplasia, carcinoma in situ, and early invasive cervical carcinoma. CA 34:307, 1984. Courtesy of James H. Nelson Jr.

Colposcopic examination is an accurate and reliable method for evaluating the cervix and vagina of a woman with an abnormality revealed by Pap smear. This modality (a well-illuminated binocular microscope) not only provides visualization of the cervical transformation zone but also allows directed biopsy of specific areas of the epithelium, removing only small amounts of tissue.

Additional nursing interventions

Reaching those women who are at high risk for gynecologic cancer is one of the most challenging roles for nurses. Patient acceptance and increasing the availability of screening are areas that will require major effort on the part of nurses if the entire population at greatest risk is to be reached. Because cytologic screening is closely tied to obstetric care and contraceptive services, a higher proportion of women are screened among the groups that require such attention than among those that do not. This is effective for screening for cervical and vaginal cancer in the reproductive years but does not reach the postmenopausal women who are at risk for ovarian and endometrial malignancies. Nurses who work in retirement centers, extended care facilities, physicians' offices, factories, public health agencies, and ambulatory care settings are urged to provide health education programs that include the early signs and symptoms of ovarian, cervical, and endometrial cancer and to stress the need for gynecologic examinations after menopause as well as during

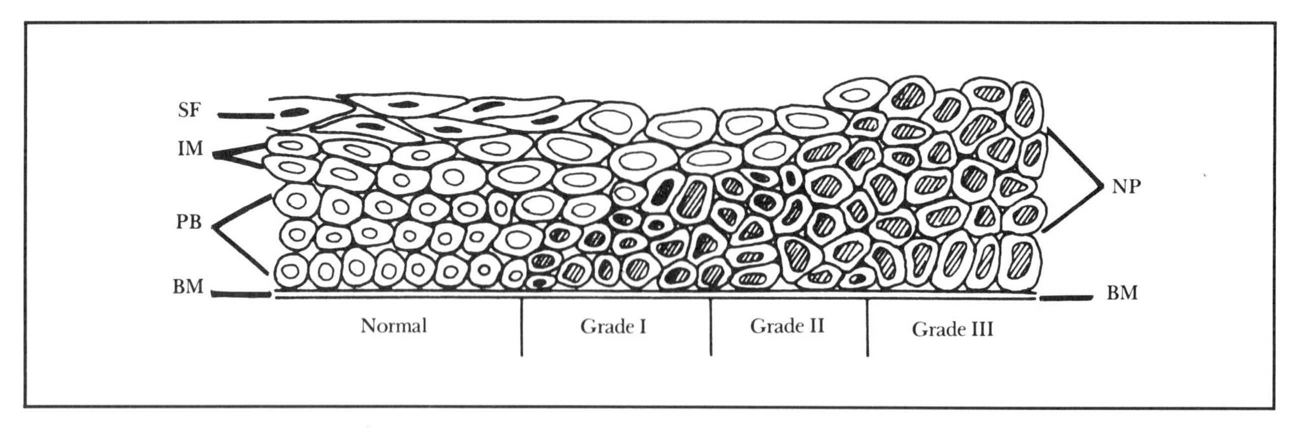

FIGURE 8-18 Cervical intraepithelial neoplasia *(CIN)*, shown infiltrating normal epithelium. CIN is dysplasia that occurs in the transformation zone. When CIN is suspected from abnormalities seen on a Pap smear of cervical secretions, a colposcopic examination should be done. (*SF* = superficial cells; *IM* = intermediate cells; *PB* = parabasal cells; *BM* = basement membrane; *NP* = neoplastic cells. *Grades* refer to degree of epithelium involved by dysplasia. *Grade I* = ¼ in thickness; *grade II* = ¼ to ¾ thickness; and *grade III* = ¾ to full thickness of epithelium. (Source: From McCauley K, Oi R: Evaluating the Papanicolaou smear: Part I. Consultant 28(12):31-40, 1988.)

the reproductive years. Female patients being followed routinely for chronic problems (such as hypertension, diabetes, heart condition, or chronic lung disease) should be asked when they had their last pelvic examination.

When appropriate, nurses should discuss the myths about menopause with women who are in their late 30s and early 40s. There are several significant barriers to early detection of gynecologic cancer in older women. Many women have the mistaken belief that once they are past childbearing years and/or are sexually inactive, they no longer need pelvic examinations. There are also physical changes that occur that make the gynecologic examination difficult for older women. There is decreased mobility of the femoropelvic structure, which leads to pain when they are put in the lithotomy position for a gynecologic examination. Nurses need to be aware of this physical barrier and suggest the use of the left lateral Sims' position instead of the traditional lithotomy position. Because the vaginal orifice may have narrowed with age, the insertion of the traditional speculum may cause discomfort or admit only the passage of one finger.

Nurses need to conduct educational programs in community settings that dispel these myths that surround menopause and aging and provide factual information on the early signs and symptoms of the common gynecologic cancers in older women, as well as discuss methods to make the gynecologic examination more comfortable for the woman. Women taking estrogens should be advised that they need to be routinely monitored by their physician in terms of an examination to detect endometrial cancer.[182,183]

Nurses need to be aware that older women are at high risk for endometrial, vulvar, vaginal, and ovarian cancer. Several premalignant conditions commonly found in elderly women predispose them to gynecologic cancers. These premalignant conditions are leukoplakic vulvitis, which precedes epidermoid carcinoma; lichen sclerosus et atrophicus, which precedes epidermoid carcinoma; and endometrial adenoma, which precedes hyperplastic lesions. Normal changes that occur with aging frequently obscure the early symptoms of cancer. The vaginal mucosa thins with aging, and there is a decrease in vaginal/cervical lubrication. Bleeding that results from endometrial or vaginal cancer is shrugged off as normal "postmenopausal bleeding" or attributed by health professionals to atrophic vaginitis and often is not followed up.[173]

Young women who have had venereal disease (syphilis, gonorrhea, genital herpes, or HPV infection) must be alert to the necessity of having regular Pap smears. Women with vulvar condyloma acuminatum should be referred for a thorough examination of the vagina, cervix, and perirectal epithelium with the use of acetic acid compress application, a colposcopic examination, and a Pap smear. It also is recommended that these women (and infected male partners) have frequent follow-up examinations to detect precancerous conditions caused by a latent virus in clinically and histologically normal tissue.[169] Infection of the genital tract by HPV is a common disease and often encountered in clinics for family planning, prenatal care, and sexually transmitted diseases. Women whose Pap smears indicate the presence of warty infections such as koilocytotic cells or who show cells consistent with squamous papilloma or warty atypia also should be referred to a physician for further evaluation.[184]

Nurses are urged to acquire physical assessment skills that will enable them to perform pelvic examinations. It has been documented that nurses who perform pelvic examinations can detect gynecologic malignancies, that patient acceptance and satisfaction are high, and that pelvic examinations done by nurses are cost effective.[173,185] Nurses trained to conduct gynecologic examinations are in an ideal position to reach those women who are at highest risk for the development of various types of gynecologic cancers but who are least likely to use conventional screening programs or have routine health examinations, such as older women in residential settings or older poor women in the community. Nurses actively involved in conducting pelvic examinations also would increase the availability of screening programs and thus reach more women.[185]

REFERENCES

1. The National Cancer Institute Act, Aug 5, 1937. PL 244, 75th Congress, 1st Session. Chapter 565 (S. 2067).
2. The National Cancer Act of 1971. JNCI 48:577-584, 1972.
3. Schottenfeld D, Fraumeni JF: Cancer Epidemiology and Prevention. Philadelphia, WB Saunders, 1982.
4. Vessey MP, Gray M: Cancer Risks and Prevention. Oxford, Oxford University Press, 1985.
5. Enstrom J, Austin D: Interpreting cancer survival rates, in Kruse L, Reese J, Hart L (eds): Cancer: Pathophysiology, Etiology and Management. St Louis, CV Mosby, 1979, pp 28-37.
6. Bailar JC, Smith EM: Progress against cancer. N Engl J Med 314:1226-1232, 1986.
7. Hamburg D: Healthy people: The surgeon general's report on health promotion and disease prevention, background papers. Washington DC, DHEW pub no. (PHS) 79-55071A, 1979, p 162.
8. Schottenfeld D: Cancer Epidemiology and Prevention: Current Concepts. Springfield, Ill, CC Thomas, 1975.
9. Pollner F: Debate over cancer survival rates is heating up. Medical World News 72: Apr 25, 1988.
10. Sondik E: Cancer control objectives for the year 2000. Oncology 1:27-34, 1987.
11. Fisher S: Cancer: Prevention, screening and early diagnosis. Aust Fam Physician 6:269-277, 1977.
12. Van Parifs LG, Eckhardt S: Public education in primary and secondary cancer prevention. Hygiene 111:16-28, 1984.
13. Slenker S, Spreitzer EA: Public perceptions and behaviors regarding cancer control. J Cancer Educ 3:171-180, 1988.
14. Kennedy BJ: Principles of cancer prevention. Oncology Time 6:2, 1984.
15. Blonston G: Cancer, the new synthesis: Prevention. Science 28:36-39, 1984.
16. Breslow L: A positive strategy for the nation's health. JAMA 242:2093-2095, 1979.
17. Whelan E: The politics of cancer. Policy Review 33:46, 1979.
18. Woods N, Woods J: Epidemiology and the study of cancer, in Marino L (ed): Cancer Nursing. St Louis, CV Mosby, 1981, pp 139-175.
19. Becker CE, Coye MJ: Cancer Prevention: Strategies in the Workplace. Washington, Hemisphere Publishing, 1986.
20. American Cancer Society: Cancer Facts and Figures: 1988. New York, American Cancer Society, 1988.
21. Edelman C, Milio N: Health defined: Promotion and specific protection, in Edelman C, Mandle CL (eds): Health Promotion Throughout the Lifespan. St Louis, CV Mosby, 1986, pp 2-18.
22. Leavell H, Clark AE: Preventive Medicine for Doctors in the Community. New York, McGraw-Hill, 1965.
23. Fraumeni J: Persons at High Risk of Cancer: An Approach to Cancer Etiology and Control. New York, Academic Press, 1975.
24. Russel LB: Prevention often costs more. Medical World News, Jan 27:76, 1986.
25. Eddy DM: The economics of cancer prevention and detection: Getting more for less. Cancer 47:1200-1209, 1981.
26. Glasel M: Cancer prevention: The role of the nurse in primary and secondary cancer prevention. Cancer Nurs 8:5-8, 1985 (suppl 1).
27. Gianella A: Teaching cancer prevention and detection. Cancer Nurs 8:9-12, 1985 (suppl 1).
28. White L, Taylor D: Cancer Prevention and Detection in Nursing Practice. Houston, The University of Texas System Cancer Center, MD, Anderson Hospital and Tumor Institute (no date), pp 12-20.
29. LeMaistre C: Reflections on disease prevention. Cancer 62:1673-1675, 1988 (suppl).
30. Hospital discharge rates for four major cancers—United States, 1970-1986. JAMA 260:3412-3416, 1988.
31. Silverberg E, Lubera J: Cancer statistics, 1989. CA 39:3-20, 1989.
32. Gritz E: Cigarette smoking: The need for action by health professionals. CA 38:194-212, 1988.
33. Fielding J, Phenow J: Health effects of involuntary smoking. N Engl J Med 319:1452-1460, 1988.
34. Humble C, Samet J, Pathak D: Marriage to a smoker and lung cancer risk. Am J Public Health 77:598-560, 1987.
35. Stellman J, Stellman S: Occupational lung disease and cancer risk in women. Occup Health Nurs 31:40-46, 1983.
36. Goldman R, Peters J: The occupational and environmental health history. JAMA 246:2832-2836, 1981.
37. Asbestos exposure. Washington DC, National Cancer Institute, 1978; DHEW pub no. 78-1622.
38. Grimes J, Burns E (eds): Health Assessment in Nursing Practice (ed 2). Boston, Jones and Bartlett, 1987.
39. Bouchier I, Morris J: Clinical Skills. A System of Clinical Examination. London, WB Saunders, 1976.
40. Buckingham W: A Primer of Clinical Diagnosis (ed 2). New York, Harper and Row, 1979.
41. Rohwedder J: Neoplastic disease, in Guenter C, Welch M (eds): Pulmonary Medicine. Philadelphia, JB Lippincott, 1977, pp 300-320.
42. DeGowin E, DeGowin R: Bedside Diagnostic Examination (ed 5). New York, Macmillan, 1987.
43. Guarino J: Auscultatory-percussion, a technique for detecting unsuspected lung disease. Diagnosis, January: 20-26, 1981.
44. Bates B: A Guide to Physical Examination (ed 3). Philadelphia, JB Lippincott, 1983.
45. Burns K, Johnson P: Health Assessment in Clinical Practice (ed 2). Englewood Cliffs, NJ, Prentice-Hall, 1980.
46. Ca screening: Auditing the payoff. Medical World News 26:42-55, 1985.
47. Fielding J: Smoking: Health effects and control. N Engl J Med 313:491-498, 1985.
48. Fiore M, Novotny T, Pierce J, et al: Trends in cigarette smoking in the United States. The changing influence of gender and race. JAMA 261:49-55, 1989.
49. American Cancer Society: General Facts on Smoking and Health. Press release from the ACS, New York, Nov 17, 1988.
50. Pierce J, Fiore M, Novotny T, et al: Trends in cigarette smoking in the United States. Educational differences are increasing. JAMA 261:56-60, 1989.
51. Davis R: Current trends in cigarette advertising and marketing. N Engl J Med 316:725-732, 1987.
52. Ernster V: Trends in smoking, cancer risk, and cigarette

promotion: Current priorities for reducing tobacco exposure. Cancer 62:1702-1712, 1988.
53. Hermanson B, Omenn G, Kronmal R, et al: Participants in the Coronary Artery Surgery Study: Beneficial six-year outcome of smoking cessation in older men and women with coronary artery disease. N Engl J Med 319:1365-1369, 1988.
54. Koop report equates nicotine with narcotic addiction. Oncology & Biotechnology News 2(6):3, 1988.
55. Benowitz N, Jacob P, Kozlowski L, et al: Influence of smoking fewer cigarettes on exposure to tar, nicotine, and carbon monoxide. N Engl J Med 315:1310-1313, 1986.
56. Cigarette chokes health experts. Medical World News 28:30, 1987.
57. Nurses' smoking habits and attitudes influence patients. Cancer Lett 1(12):4-5, 1987.
58. Johnson J: Nurses: The challenge to action in anti-smoking efforts. New York, American Cancer Society [Professional Education Publication No 80-50M-No 3340-PE], 1980.
59. Anda R, Remington P, Sienko D, et al: Are physicians advising smokers to quit? The patient's perspective. JAMA 257:1916-1919, 1987.
60. Smith J: Letter to the editor. JAMA 258:472, 1987.
61. US Preventive Services Task Force: Recommendations for smoking cessation counseling. JAMA 259:2882, 1988.
62. Kottke T, Battista R, Defriese G, et al: Attributes of successful smoking cessation interventions in medical practice. A meta-analysis of 39 controlled trials. JAMA 259:2883-2889, 1988.
63. Orleans CT: Understanding and promoting smoking cessation: Overview and guidelines for physician intervention. Annu Rev Med 36:51-61, 1985.
64. Altman D, Flora J, Fortmann S, et al: The cost-effectiveness of three smoking cessation programs. Am J Public Health 77:162-165, 1987.
65. New rules extinguish "smoking lamp" in growing number of public places. JAMA 259:2809, 1988.
66. More "no smoking" signs seen in hospitals. JAMA 259:2814, 1988.
67. Schuster M: Disorders of the aging GI system, in Reichel W (ed): The Geriatric Patient. New York, HP Publishers, 1978, pp 73-81.
68. Evans J: Cancer of the colon and rectum, in Murphy G (ed): Cancer Signals and Safeguards. Littleton, Mass, PSG Publishing 1981, pp 155-160.
69. Braverman I: Skin signs of systemic disease. Philadelphia, WB Saunders, 1970.
70. Leffall L: Early diagnosis of colorectal cancer. New York, American Cancer Society [Professional Education Publication 81-50M-No 3311-PE], 1981.
71. Collins J: Colon cancer screens unproven. Medical World News 29:77-78, 1988.
72. Minnesota study aimed at finding final answer on Hemoccult screening. Cancer Lett 13(30):4-6, 1987.
73. Kewenter J, Bjork S, Haglind E, et al: Screening and rescreening for colorectal cancer. Cancer 62:645-651, 1988.
74. Sugarbaker P, Gunderson L, Wittes R: Colorectal cancer, in DeVita V, Hellman S, Rosenberg S (eds): Cancer: Principles and Practice of Oncology (ed 2), Philadelphia, JB Lippincott, 1986, pp 795-884.
75. Fleischer D, Goldberg S, Browning T, et al: Detection and surveillance of colorectal cancer. JAMA 261:580-585, 1989.
76. Knight K, Fielding J, Battista R: Occult blood screening for colorectal cancer. JAMA 261:587-593, 1989.
77. Rakel R: A clinician's guide: Tips on fecal occult blood testing. Your Patient & Cancer 3:33-38, 1983.
78. Simon J: Occult blood screening for colorectal carcinoma. A critical review. Gastroenterology 88:820-837, 1985.
79. Winawer S: Introduction to position papers from the Third International Symposium on Colorectal Cancer. CA 34:130-133, 1984.
80. Dorozynski A: Test for early detection of colorectal cancer under development. Oncology & Biotechnology News 1(2):3, 1987.
81. Colorectal ca found earlier with new quick office tests. Oncology News/Update 2(2):1-7, 1987.
82. Poll finds public misconceptions re colorectal cancer detection. Oncology Times, September:9, 25, 1986.
83. Callahan L: Colo-rectal cancer: Clinical trial/community outreach. Proceedings of the Fourth National Cancer Communications Conference. Washington, DC, National Institutes of Health, 1977, DHEW publication no (PHS) 78-1463.
84. Greenwald P, Sondik E, Lynch B: Diet and chemoprevention in NCI's research strategy to achieve national cancer control objectives. Annu Rev Public Health 7:267-291, 1986.
85. American Cancer Society Special Report: Nutrition and cancer: Cause and prevention. New York: American Cancer Society [Professional Education Publication 84-50M-No 3389-PE], 1984.
86. Palmer S: Dietary considerations for risk reduction. Cancer 58:1949-1953, 1986.
87. Carroll K, Braden L, Bell J, et al: Fat and cancer. Cancer 58:1818-1825, 1986.
88. The changing diet: Illinois 1982-1986. American Cancer Society Cancer Prevention Study II Newsletter 5(2):3, Fall 1987.
89. Chodak G, Schoenberg H: Early detection of prostate cancer by routine screening. JAMA 252:3261-3264, 1984.
90. National Cancer Institute: Cancer among blacks and other minorities: Statistical profiles, Washington, DC, NIH publication no 86-2785, March 1986.
91. Sagalowsky A, Wilson J: Carcinoma of the prostate, in Petersdorf R, Adams R, Braunwald E, et al (eds): Harrison's Principles of Internal Medicine (ed 10). New York, McGraw-Hill, 1983, pp 795-798.
92. Guinan P, Sharifi R, Bush I: Prostate cancer: Tips toward earlier detection. Your Patient & Cancer 4:37-42, 1984.
93. Guinan P, Gilham N, Nagubadi S, et al: What is the best test to detect prostate cancer? CA 31:141-145, 1981.
94. Diggs A: A case for the rectal exam. Medical World News, Feb 25:82, 1985.
95. New prostate cancer detection group to study potential of ultrasound. Cancer Lett 13(10):4-5, 1987.
96. Murphy G: Urologic cancer. Cancer 62:1800-1807, 1988.
97. Lee F, Gray J, McLeary R, et al: Transrectal ultrasound in the diagnosis of prostate cancer: Location, echogenicity, histopathology and staging. Prostate 7:117-129, 1985.
98. Lee F, Gray J, McLeary R, et al: Prostatic evaluation by transrectal sonography: Criteria for diagnosis of early carcinoma. Radiology 158:91-95, 1986.
99. Lee F, Littrup P, Torp-Pedersen S, et al: Prostate cancer: Comparison of US and digital rectal examination for screening. Radiology 168:389-394, 1988.
100. Virji M, Mercer D, Herberman R: Tumor markers in cancer diagnosis and prognosis. CA 38:104-126, 1988.
101. Strax P: Mass screening for control of breast cancer. Cancer 53:665-670, 1984.
102. Olsen S: Examinations for detecting breast cancer. Cancer Prevention Program, Wisconsin Clinical Cancer Center, 1300 University Ave-7C, Medical Science Center, Madison, WI 53706.

103. Wilkes B: The development of a two-tier BSE educational program, in Progress in Cancer Control III: A Regional Approach. New York, Alan R Liss, 1983, pp 127-131.
104. Burnside J: Adams' Physical Diagnosis (ed 15). Baltimore, Williams and Wilkins, 1977.
105. Scanlon E: A photo checklist for a better breast palpation. Primary Care & Cancer 7:13-20, 1987.
106. Heymann A: Semilateral decubitus breast examination. JAMA 243:1713, 1980.
107. Feig S: Mammography screening: Published guidelines and actual practice. Recent Results Cancer Res 105:78-88, 1987.
108. Mammography screening advised for both younger and older women. Oncology News/Update 2(6):2, 13, 1987.
109. Greenwald P, Sondik E: Cancer control objectives for the nation: 1985-2000. Washington, DC, National Institutes of Health, 1986. NIH pub no. 86-2880, no. 8.
110. Dodd G: Screening for the early detection of breast cancer. Cancer 62:1781-1783, 1988.
111. Tabar L, Fagerberg C, Gad A, et al: Reduction in mortality from breast cancer after mass screening with mammography. Lancet 1:829-832, 1984.
112. New analysis of HIP study supports mammographic screening age 40-49. Cancer Lett 14(37):4-6, 1988.
113. Status of breast cancer research updated in overview compiled by NCI. Cancer Lett 14(32):3-5, 1988.
114. Frank J, Mai V: Breast self-examination in young women: More harm than good? Lancet 2:654-657, 1985.
115. Foster R, Costanza M, Worden J: The current status of research in breast self-examination. NY State J Med 85:480-482, 1985.
116. US Preventive Services Task Force: Recommendations for breast cancer screening. JAMA 257:2196, 1987.
117. O'Malley M, Fletcher S: Screening for breast cancer with breast self-examination. A critical review. JAMA 257:2197-2203, 1987.
118. Feldman J: Breast self-examination—a practice whose time has come? NY State J Med 85:482-483, 1985.
119. Huguley C, Brown R, Greenberg R, et al: Breast self-examination and survival from breast cancer. Cancer 62:1389-1396, 1988.
120. Bennett S, Lawrence R, Fleischmann K, et al: Profile of women practicing breast self-examination. JAMA 249:488-491, 1983.
121. Kegeles S: Education for breast self-examination: Why, who, what, and how? Prev Med 14:702-720, 1985.
122. Study shows survival advantage for women who examine their breasts. Medical World News 25:31, 1984.
123. Boyle M, Michalek A, Bersani G, et al: Effectiveness of a community program to promote early breast cancer detection. J Surg Oncol 18:183-188, 1981.
124. Diem G, Rose D: Has breast self-examination had a fair trial? NY State J Med 85:479-480, 1985.
125. Styrd A: A breast self-examination program in an occupational health setting. Occup Health Nurs 30:33-35, 1982.
126. Shamian J, Edgar L: Nurses as agents for change in teaching breast self-examination. Public Health Nurs 4:29-34, 1987.
127. Garnick M, Scully R, Weber E, et al: Cancer of the testis, in Cady B (ed): Cancer Manual (ed 7): New York, American Cancer Society, Massachusetts Division, 1986, pp 268-277.
128. Swanson D: Why you should conscientiously promote self-examination. Consultant 27(4):142-147, 1987.
129. Carlin P: Testicular self-examination: A public awareness program. Public Health Rep 101(1):98-102, 1986.
130. Borski A: Diagnosis, staging and natural history of testicular tumors. Proceedings of the National Conference on Urologic Cancer. New York, American Cancer Society, 1973 [Professional Education Publication no. 3080-PE].
131. Conklin M, Klint K, Morway A, et al: Should health teaching include self-examination of the testis? Am J Nurs 78:2073-2074, 1978.
132. Blesch K: Health beliefs about testicular cancer and self-examination among professional men. Oncol Nurs Forum 13(1):29-33, 1986.
133. Smith J, Hollenbeck Z: Genitalia, in Prior J, Silberstein J, Stang J (eds), Physical Diagnosis. The History and Examination of the Patient. St Louis, CV Mosby, 1981, pp 330-364.
134. Delp M, Manning R: Major's Physical Diagnosis. An Introduction to the Clinical Process (ed 9). Philadelphia, WB Saunders, 1981, pp 381-383.
135. Office urology: When your patient fears testicular cancer. Patient Care 9:102, 1975.
136. Frank-Stromborg M: The role of the nurse in cancer detection and screening. Semin Oncol Nurs 2:191-199, 1986.
137. Garnick M: Urologic cancer, in Rubenstein E, Federman D (eds): Oncology, vol 9. New York, Scientific American Medicine, 1988, pp 1-17.
138. Murray B, Wilcox L: Testicular self-examination. Am J Nurs 78:2074-2075, 1978.
139. Malasanos L, Barkauskas V, Moss M, et al: Health Assessment. St Louis, CV Mosby, 1986, pp 401-414.
140. White L: The nurse's role in cancer prevention, in Newell G (ed): Cancer Prevention in Clinical Medicine. New York, Raven Press, 1983, pp 91-112.
141. Frank-Stromborg M: Nursing's contribution to case finding and the early detection of cancer, in Marino L (ed): Cancer Nursing, St Louis, CV Mosby, 1981, pp 176-233.
142. Kopf A: Prevention and early detection of skin cancer/melanoma. Cancer 62:1791-1795, 1988.
143. Friedman R, Rigel D, Kopf A: Early detection of malignant melanoma: The role of physician examination and self-examination of the skin. CA 35:130-151, 1985.
144. Adler J, Gosnell M, Springen K, et al: The dark side of the sun. Newsweek, June 9:60-64, 1986.
145. Legha S: Malignant melanoma. Pitfalls and controversies in diagnosis and treatment. Consultant 28(6):111-124, 1988.
146. Schleper J: Cancer prevention and detection: Skin cancer. Cancer Nurs 7:67-84, 1984.
147. White L, Patterson J, Cornelius J, et al: Cancer Screening and Detection Manual for Nurses. New York, McGraw-Hill, 1979, pp 9-16.
148. Finley C: Malignant melanoma: A primary care perspective. Nurse Practitioner 11(4):18-38, 1986.
149. Fitzpatrick T, Rhodes A, Sober A: Prevention of melanoma by recognition of its precursors. N Engl J Med 312:115-116, 1985.
150. Smith T, Mihm M, Sober A: Malignant melanoma, in Cancer Manual (ed 7). New York, American Cancer Society, Massachusetts Division, 1986, pp 106-113.
151. Helm F, Helm J: On guard against skin cancer, in Murphy G (ed): Cancer. Signals and Safeguards. Littleton, Mass, PSG Publishing, 1981, pp 67-80.
152. Epstein E: Common skin disorders. A manual for physicians and patients. Oradell, NJ, Medical Economics, 1979.
153. Gumport S, Harris M, Kopf A: Diagnosis and management of common skin cancers. New York, American Cancer Society, 1974 [Professional Education Publication No 3373-PE].
154. Rhodes A, Weinstock M, Fitzpatrick T, et al: Risk factors for cutaneous melanoma. A practical method of recognizing predisposed individuals. JAMA 258:3146-3154, 1987.

155. Diekmann J: Cancer in the elderly: Systems overview. Semin Oncol Nurs 4:169-177, 1988.
156. Wood N: Oral cancer: An overview. Ill Dental J 57:323, 1988.
157. Winn D: Smokeless tobacco and cancer: The epidemiologic evidence. CA 38:236-243, 1988.
158. Sawyer D, Wood N, Lehnert J: Examination, detection, diagnosis and referral. Ill Dental J 57:326-329, 1988.
159. Silverman S: Early diagnosis of oral cancer. Cancer 62:1796-1799, 1988.
160. Holmstrup P, Pindborg J: Oral mucosal lesions in smokeless tobacco users. CA 38:230-235, 1988.
161. Kabot T, Heffez L, Bergschneider J: Prevention, detection and referral. Responsibility of the dental team: Prevention and patient education. Ill Dental J 57:324-325, 1988.
162. Squier C: The nature of smokeless tobacco and patterns of use. CA 38:226-229, 1988.
163. Benowitz N: Nicotine and smokeless tobacco. CA 38:244-247, 1988.
164. Schroeder K, Iaderosa G, Chen M, et al: Bimodal initiation of smokeless tobacco usage: Implications for cancer education. Cancer Education 2:15-21, 1987.
165. Grabau J: Oral/facial self-examination, in Nieburgs H (ed): Prevention and detection of cancer. Part I (vol 2), Prevention. New York, Marcel Dekker, 1978, pp 2263-2274.
166. Williams T: Ovarian cancer. Fewest signs, greatest challenge. Diagnosis 3(5):53-60, 1981.
167. White L: Cancer prevention and detection: Cervical cancer. Cancer Nurs 7:335-345, 1984.
168. Beecham J, Helmkamp BF, Rubin P: Tumors of the female genital tract, in Rubin P (ed): Clinical oncology for medical students and physicians (ed 6). New York, American Cancer Society, 1983, pp 428-481.
169. Bender M: A clinician's guide to genital papillomavirus infection. Curr Concepts Skin Disorders, Fall: 11-16, 1988.
170. Koss L: The Papanicolaou test for cervical cancer detection. A triumph and a tragedy. JAMA 261:737-743, 1989.
171. Jones H: Vaginal cancer. Common signs, uncommon cause. Diagnosis 3(5):71-85, 1981.
172. Nelson J, Averette H, Richart R: Dysplasia, carcinoma in situ, and early invasive cervical carcinoma. CA 34:306-327, 1984.
173. Gusberg SB: Detection and prevention of uterine cancer. Cancer 62:1784-1786, 1988.
174. Fink D: Change in American Cancer Society checkup guidelines for detection of cervical cancer. CA 38:127-128, 1988.
175. Stenkvist B, Bergstrom R, Eklund G, et al: Papanicolaou smear screening and cervical cancer. What can you expect? JAMA 252:1423-1426, 1984.
176. Mandelblatt J, Fahs M: The cost-effectiveness of cervical cancer screening for low-income elderly women. JAMA 259:2409-2413, 1988.
177. Guintoli R, Mikuta J: Cervical cancer. Regular office exams can stamp it out. Diagnosis 3(5):25-36, 1981.
178. Diagnosing cervical cancer by measuring DNA content. Primary Care & Cancer 8:13, 1988.
179. Jones G: Densitometric screening found accurate for detecting cervical cancer. Oncology & Biotechnology News 2(2):3, 1988.
180. Lovejoy N: Precancerous lesions of the cervix. Personal risk factors. Cancer Nurs 10:2-14, 1987.
181. McCauley K, Oi R: Evaluating the Papanicolaou smear: Part I. Consultant 28(12):31-40, 1988.
182. Braunstein G: The benefits of estrogen to the menopausal woman outweigh the risks of developing endometrial cancer [Opinion: Pro]. CA 34:210-219, 1984.
183. Morrow C: The benefits of estrogen to the menopausal woman outweigh the risks of developing endometrial cancer [Opinion: Con]. CA 34:220-231, 1984.
184. Jones W, Saigo P: The "atypical" Papanicolaou smear. CA 36:237-242, 1986.
185. Stromborg M, Nord S: A cancer detection clinic: Patient motivation and satisfaction. Nurse Pract 4:10-14, 1979.

Chapter 9

Diagnostic Evaluation, Classification, and Staging

Sharon Saldin O'Mary, RN, MN

DIAGNOSTIC EVALUATION

Factors That Affect the Diagnostic Approach

Early detection is the key to survival for patients with cancer. Early diagnosis of a precancerous lesion or a malignant neoplasm affords the best opportunity for cure, extended survival, and less extensive treatment. For example, the breast mass found on a screening mammogram or the isolated tumor found incidentally on a chest film holds the best chance for a diagnosis of localized disease amenable to treatment. More typically, the tumor goes undetected until specific signs or symptoms become apparent and the patient consults a physician. Frequently, these symptoms include the complaints of weight loss, persistent pain, unexplained fever, fatigue, or one of cancer's seven warning signals (Table 9-1).[1] The worst prognosis can be expected in those patients who delay seeking medical evaluation at the onset of their symptoms, in those cancers for which technologic methods are unavailable to make an early diagnosis, and in patients with an unknown primary lesion. Altering health care behaviors and developing detection programs that are accessible, affordable, and ethnically relevant are areas in which nurses can intervene.

The major goals of the diagnostic evaluation for suspected cancer are to determine the tissue type of the malignancy, the primary site of the malignancy, and the extent of disease within the body. This information is the critical first step in determining the therapeutic management. Ideally there would be uniformity in cancer staging and classification to facilitate comparison of clinical data on appropriate treatment, the natural history of the disease, and prognosis. Although an international system of staging solid tumors is now available,[2] fundamental differences in tumor biology have necessitated diverse approaches to classification.

An effective clinical evaluation of the patient with a suspected malignancy includes a comprehensive history with the identification of known risk factors, a thorough physical examination, laboratory and imaging tests, and the histologic verification of the malignancy. Known biologic characteristics of the suspected malignancy and the typical routes of regional and distant metastases will direct the approach of further diagnostic and staging procedures. In some situations extensive laboratory and imaging examinations precede tissue biopsy in the attempt to locate the primary or an accessible tumor. In other patients results of a biopsy specimen that confirm the presence of malignancy precedes further testing that will be done to accurately stage the extent of disease. Obtaining tissue for histologic examination or cells for cytologic analysis is paramount in the diagnosis of malignancy and precedes any decision for treatment.

Many diagnostic tools are available and the modern armamentarium is elaborate. Rapidly changing technology will only improve the imaging modalities and biochemical tests that affect the field of diagnostic medicine. Those tests that are the least taxing to the patient and family, that are cost effective, and that yield the information necessary for treatment planning are considered. The diagnostic approach depends on the following factors: the patient's presenting signs and symptoms, the biologic characteristics of the suspected malignancy, the patient's clinical status and ability to tolerate invasive procedures, the diagnostic equipment available in the patient's community, and the anticipated goal of treatment when the diagnosis is made.

TABLE 9-1 Seven Warning Signals for Cancer That Alert People to the Need for Medical Attention

1. Change in bowel or bladder habits
2. A sore that does not heal
3. Unusual bleeding or discharge
4. Thickening or lump in breast or elsewhere
5. Indigestion or difficulty in swallowing
6. Obvious change in wart or mole
7. Nagging cough or hoarseness

If you have a warning signal, see your doctor.

Source: Cancer Facts and Figures. American Cancer Society, New York, 1988, p 28.

In the present era of cost containment in health care the judicious selection and sequencing of diagnostic studies are stressed. The proper test is one that yields information on the suspicious site of malignancy and complements rather than merely confirms known information. The relative benefits of competing imaging technologies such as computed tomography and magnetic resonance imaging currently are being evaluated for several organ sites by the National Cancer Institute.[3] The increased availability of sophisticated equipment, the fear of litigation, and pressure from patients and families are all factors that influence the physician to overinvestigate. At least one study has indicated that patients believed extensive test ordering correlated with physician quality.[4] It is apparent that third party payers and health maintenance organizations also will play an important role as financial gatekeepers in the diagnostic evaluation.

Nursing Implications in Diagnostic Evaluation

The diagnostic evaluation can evoke fear and anxiety in patients and families. Oncology nurses play a key role in providing information and support. An accurate assessment of the patient's and family's desire to know, in addition to their ability to understand, is the first step in providing this much needed support. Educational preparation for an examination should include an explanation of the procedure to be followed, as well as a description of any physical sensations that might be expected, such as pain, discomfort, or facial flushing. The purpose of the examination, when the results can be expected, and from whom to expect them should be identified. Nurses also must be cognizant of any potential complications that may occur after a procedure. More specific nursing interventions depend on identified nursing diagnoses. These include the following: (1) knowledge deficits related to lack of exposure to or misconceptions about cancer, (2) anticipatory grieving related to the stigma of cancer or probable prognosis, (3) ineffective coping related to the meaning of the diagnosis, financial stress, inadequate support, and the demands of decision making, (4) spiritual deficit related to challenged belief because of diagnosis, (5) fear of death, treatment, and body-image changes related to inability to control events and knowledge deficit, and (6) self-care deficit related to effects of the malignancy.[5]

Laboratory Techniques

Laboratory studies are performed to help formulate a clinical diagnosis and to monitor the patient's response to a specific therapy. The data provide information on the functioning of specific organs and metabolic processes that may be altered by disease or a malignant process.

Biochemical analysis of blood, serum, urine, and other body fluids identifies chemical values outside the narrow, homeostatic range. Specific malignancies characteristically alter chemical composition of the blood, but no single value is diagnostic for a malignancy.

Malignancy may alter the hematologic status of the patient. For example, distinct changes such as immature blast cells may be seen in some leukemic processes. Nonspecific changes such as anemia, leukocytosis or leukopenia, and thrombocytosis or thrombocytopenia also may be significant in the diagnostic evaluation.

The value of a particular laboratory study or imaging technique often is reported in terms of sensitivity or specificity. Sensitivity establishes the percentage of patients with cancer who will have positive (abnormal) test results, known as true positive results. Test results of patients with cancer that are negative (normal) are false negative findings. Specificity establishes the percentage of patients without cancer who will have negative (normal) test results, known as true negative results. Patients who are free of disease and show positive (abnormal) results are considered to have false positive results. A clinically useful test will detect a malignant abnormality early in its development (sensitivity) and exclude nonmalignant sources for the abnormality (specificity). In reality many tests are highly sensitive but not very specific, whereas the opposite is true for other tests.

Tumor markers are proteins, antigens, genes, ectopically produced hormones, and enzymes that are released from the tumor into the blood or produced by normal tissue in response to the tumor. Ideally, a tumor marker would be produced exclusively by the tumor cell and not in other conditions (highly specific) and would be present and detectable in early, occult disease (highly sensitive). The only marker that approaches this ideal is human chorionic gonadotropin in gestational trophoblastic tumors.[6] Several other markers are clinically useful in monitoring tumor activity during treatment and in detecting recurrent cancer even though they lack specificity and are poor screening tools. The assay for carcinoembryonic antigen is highly sensitive and correlates well with tumor burden and prognosis in gastrointestinal neoplasms.[7,8] It lacks specificity, however, because the antigen is expressed by normal as well as malignant cells.[9]

Radioimmunoassay, an important technique in the measurement of tumor markers, determines the amount of tumor antigen in a serum sample. A known amount of radiolabeled antigen combined with antibody is added to a serum sample. The patient's unlabeled antigen displaces the radiolabeled antigen, which permits quantification.

All laboratory studies must be evaluated in conjunction with the results of other clinical data. Table 9-2 identifies several laboratory values and their clinical significance in the diagnosis and monitoring of cancer.[10,11] Reference ranges for normal values vary, depending on the specific method of testing and on institutional values.

Tumor Imaging

Many diagnostic procedures are available to ascertain the presence of a tumor mass, localize the mass for biopsy, provide tissue characterization, and further assess or stage the anatomic extent of disease. Although diagnostic imaging has benefited from the technology that produced computerized tomography and magnetic resonance imaging, an important role remains for the conventional diagnostic procedures. Examinations are selected that are efficient in detecting suspicious lesions and that also result in the least risk, discomfort, and expense for the patient. Table 9-3 identifies preferred imaging procedures for tumor definition and staging in several organ sites. Table 9-4 elaborates on the patient preparation and education for select examinations.[12,13] The following section discusses imaging techniques available for diagnosis and staging.

Radiographic techniques

Radiographic studies, or x-ray films, allow visualization of internal structures of the body. Distinction is made between normal and abnormal structure and function. X rays or gamma rays are passed through the body, absorbed variably by tissues of differing densities, and react on specially sensitized film or fluoroscopic screens. Radiographs may be site specific, such as the standard chest film or mammogram, or they may view the dynamic function of an entire organ system. For example, in a gastrointestinal series a continuous flow of x rays passes through the digestive tract to assess the action of peristalsis, to detect displacement of structures, and to visualize mucosal abnormalities.

Mammographic examination now is performed primarily in x-ray units dedicated solely to this procedure. These units are distinguished by the incorporation of a tissue compression device or cone that improves the quality of the image and reduces the amount of primary and scatter radiation. Imaging is done by either the screen-film mammography or the xeromammography process.

TABLE 9-2 Select Laboratory Values from Blood Samples and Their Clinical Significance in the Diagnosis and Monitoring of Malignant Disease

Laboratory Test	Normal Reference Range	Oncologic Clinical Significance
	BIOCHEMICAL TESTS	
Acid phosphatase	M: 2.5-11.7 U/L F: 0.3-9.2 U/L	↑ Acute leukemia, multiple myeloma, metastatic prostate and breast cancer (bone)
Alkaline phosphatase	30-150 IU/L	↑ Cancer of bone, liver, leukemia, lymphoma, tumors causing extrahepatic biliary obstruction
Calcium	8.5-10.5 mg/dL	↑ Leukemia, lymphoma, multiple myeloma, bone metastasis, cancer of lung (squamous), kidney, esophagus, pancreas, bladder, liver, parathyroid
Immunoglobulins		
IgG	650-1600 mg/dL	↑ IgG myeloma
IgA	50-400 mg/dL	↑ IgA myeloma
IgM	18-280 mg/dL	↑ Waldenström's macroglobulinemia
IgD	0.5-3.0 mg/dL	↑ IgD myeloma
IgE	0.1-0.04 mg/dL	↑ IgE myeloma ↓ Advanced neoplasms
Lactic dehydrogenase (LDH)	70-250 IU/L	↑ Lymphoma, liver cancer, acute leukemia, metastatic carcinoma
Lysozyme	4.0-13.0 mg/L	↑ Acute leukemia (monocytic or myelomonocytic), chronic myeloid leukemia
Parathyroid hormone	430-1860 ng/L (C-terminal fragment) 230-630 ng/L (N-terminal fragment)	↑ Ectopic hyperparathyroidism from cancer of the kidney, lung (squamous), pancreas, ovary
Progesterone	M: 0.12-0.3 ng/mL F: 0.02-30 ng/mL	↑ Luteinizing tumors, adrenocortical tumors
Serum alanine aminotransferase (SGPT)	6-24 U/mL	↑ Metastatic liver cancer
Serum aspartate aminotransferase (SGOT)	10-30 U/mL	↑ Metastatic liver cancer
Serum gamma glutamyl transferase (SGGT)	1-70 U/mL	↑ Metastatic liver cancer, pancreas cancer
Testosterone	M: 300-1200 ng/dL F: 10-100 ng/dL	↑ Cancer of adrenals, ovary, extragonadal tumors producing ectopic gonadotropin
Uric acid	M: 4.0-8.0 mg/dL F: 2.5-7.5 mg/dL	↑ Leukemia, multiple myeloma, disseminated cancer ↓ Hodgkin's disease, multiple myeloma, lung cancer
	TUMOR MARKERS	
Alpha-fetoprotein (AFP)	0-30 ng/mL	↑ Nonseminomatous germ cell testicular cancer, choriocarcinoma, gonadal teratoblastoma in children, cancer of the pancreas, colon, lung, stomach, biliary system
Carcinoembryonic antigen (CEA)	Nonsmokers: 0-2.5 ng/mL Smokers: 0-3 ng/mL	↑ Cancer of the colon, rectum, stomach, pancreas, prostate, lungs, breast
Human chorionic gonadotropin, beta subunit (HCG_{β})	0-5 IU/L	↑ Choriocarcinoma, germ cell testicular cancer, ectopic production in cancer of stomach, pancreas, lung, colon, liver
Prostate acid phosphatase	<4.0 ng/mL	↑ Metastatic cancer of prostate
Calcitonin	<100 pg/mL	↑ Cancer of thyroid (medullary), lung (small cell), breast, carcinoid
CA-125	<35 U/mL	↑ Cancer of ovary (epithelial)
Prostatic specific antigen (PSA)	0-4 ng/mL	↑ Prostate cancer

M, adult male; *F*, adult female; ↑, elevated; ↓, decreased.

TABLE 9-2 Select Laboratory Value from Blood Samples and Their Clinical Significance in the Diagnosis and Monitoring of Malignant Disease (continued)

Laboratory Test	Normal Reference Range	Oncologic Clinical Significance
	HEMATOLOGY	
Hematocrit	M: 41-53% F: 36-46%	↓ Anemia, nonspecific
Hemoglobin	M: 13.5-17.5 g/dL F: 12.0-16.0 g/dL	↓ Anemia, nonspecific
Leukocyte count (WBC)	M: 3.9-10.6/mm^3 F: 3.5-11.0/mm^3	↑ Leukemia, lymphomas, tumors involving peripheral blood marrow ↓ Leukemia, ↓ metastatic disease to bone
Leukocyte differential (%)		
Neutrophils	54-75	↑ Acute myeloblastic leukemia, chronic myelocytic leukemia, lymphoma ↓ Carcinoma, leukemia, sarcoma, myeloma
Lymphocytes	29-40	↑ Leukosarcoma, lymphocytic leukemia, multiple myeloma, lymphoma, carcinoma ↓ Hodgkin's disease, leukemias, (chronic, granulocytic, monocytic) lymphosarcoma, terminal carcinoma
Monocytes	2-8	↑ Hodgkin's disease, lymphoma, monocytic leukemia, chronic myelogenous leukemia, multiple myeloma ↓ Hairy cell leukemia
Eosinophils	1-4	↓ Chronic myelogenous leukemia, Hodgkin's disease, metastatic carcinoma, eosinophilic leukemia
Basophils	0-1	↑ Chronic myelogenous leukemia, Hodgkin's disease
Platelet count	150,000-400,000/mm^3	↑ Myeloproliferative disorders, chronic myelogenous leukemia, carcinoma, Hodgkin's disease, lymphoma ↓ Acute leukemia, myelogenous or lymphocytic, monocytic leukemia, multiple myeloma

TABLE 9-3 Preferred Imaging Procedures for Tumor Definition and Staging

Sites	Tumor Definition and Staging	Comments
Brain	MRI superior	MRI for cord tumors In most CNS applications, MRI is more accurate and justifies the 25% increased cost over CT MRI with skull base or intracranial extension
Head and neck	CT adequate in most instances	Contrast-enhanced CT best for tumor definition, staging, and follow-up
Lung	CT adequate for parenchyma, mediastinal nodes; ? MRI advantages: chest wall, vascular invasion	No role identified to support MRI over CT CT used to identify abnormal nodes for biopsy and to avoid unnecessary surgery
Esophagus	CT preferred for T and N staging; contrast esophagram best for tumor measurement	Contrast esophagography better to measure lesion length; CT best for penetration; ? role for endoscopic ultrasound
Stomach	Contrast studies better at defining tumor	CT of limited staging value (nodes too small) MRI not shown to have advantage over CT
Colon	Double-contrast barium enema acceptable for tumor definition; CT not accurate for staging	CT has role in evaluation of liver for metastasis and in follow-up of abdominoperineal resection patient but not for general colon cancer staging; ? role for MRI (high-signal intensity for recurrent tumors)
Liver	CT (with contrast); ? MRI role (ferric and gadolinium contrast)	CT-dynamic scan (? role of delayed 4-hr scan); controversy over MRI role
Kidney	CT preferred study for T and N definition (with and without contrast)	CT preferred for staging and follow-up
Musculoskeletal	After detection with plain films and radionuclide bone scan, MRI is preferred for staging	MRI has overtaken CT in most bone and soft tissue primary tumors for staging and follow-up

Source: Adapted from Bragg DG: State-of-the-art assessment: diagnostic oncologic imaging. Cancer 64:262, 1989 (suppl).

TABLE 9-4 Several Tumor Imaging Techniques with Instructions for Preparing the Patient

Tumor Imaging Examination	Patient Instruction
Barium studies	Restriction of diet, smoking, most medication before examination Laxatives and enemas to cleanse bowel before colon examination Will lie on tilting x-ray table, secured Barium will taste chalky, milkshake consistency Barium enema will feel cool, may cause cramping Time: 30-60 min
Computerized tomogram	Diet restrictions before examination Will lie still on adjustable table; x-ray tube rotates around patient to take many pictures Machinery noisy Test painless May receive intravenous contrast dye; may feel burning sensation as injected May report feelings of nausea, vomiting, flushing, itching, bitter taste Time: 30-90 min
Angiogram	Diet restriction before examination May receive sedative just before examination Will lie still on x-ray table Skin over selected artery site cleansed and anesthetized Cannula passed into artery or vein Contrast die rapidly injected; may feel burning sensation as injected Several x-ray films taken May report feelings of nausea, vomiting, flushing, itching, bitter or salty taste Cannula removed after examination; pressure applied, limb immobilized Time: 1-3 hr
Lymphangiogram	No diet restrictions Blue dye injected into interdigital webs of feet; some discomfort May discolor urine, stool, skin for 48 hr Skin over lymphatic vessel on foot anesthetized Small incision made on each foot and cannula inserted
Lymphangiogram, continued	Contrast dye infused for 1-2 hr May be uncomfortable during beginnning of infusion but must lie still X-ray films taken after dye infused Time: 2-3 hr Must return following day for more x-ray studies (Time: 30 min)
Magnetic resonance imaging	No diet restriction Remove anything affected by a magnet Lie still on table, secured with Velcro straps Table will move into narrow magnetic opening Knocking or beating sound in machinery is normal Painless May recieve intravenous contrast die May report nausea, vomiting, itching if given contrast die Time: 45-60 min
Ultrasonogram	Diet restriction before examination Full bladder for pelvic ultrasound Will lie on examination table Ultrasound gel applied over skin of area to be examined Transducer passes over skin May feel presure; no pain Time: 30 min
Nuclear medicine imaging	No diet restriction Radioisotope injected before examination (15 min-2 hr) Will lie on scanner table; may have to vary positions Scanner moves back and forth, taking several pictures Procedure painless Radiosotope harmless Time: 30-60 min
Endoscopy	Diet restriction before examination Mild sedation before procedure, but patient remains conscious Intravenous infusion for medications and hydration *Oral:* Local anesthetic sprayed in mouth

TABLE 9-4 Several Tumor Imaging Techniques with Instructions for Preparing the Patient (continued)

Tumor Imaging Examination	Patient Instruction
Endoscopy (continued)	Flexible tube passed through mouth to level to be examined Tongue and throat feel swollen; difficult to swallow May feel pressure and fullness if scope in stomach *Rectal:* Prepared for examination with laxatives, enemas Lubricated endoscope inserted anally Feels cold; urge to defecate May need to change positions during examination as scope is advanced Time: 30-60 min
Mammogram	Breast is compressed between two plates on x-ray cassette Compression may feel tight but not painful Two views taken of each breast: one view is from head to foot (craniocaudal), the other lateral Radiation exposure is minimal and safe Time: 15 min

The xeromammographic process penetrates deeper into the tissue and is able to better image the retromammary space. For this reason it may be preferred for diagnostic imaging. Thermography, which images variations in radiant heat produced by blood flow through the breast, now is considered to be an ineffective modality for breast cancer screening.[14]

Tomography provides a radiographic image of a selected layer or plane of the body that would otherwise be obscured by shadows of other structures. Tomograms are particularly helpful in evaluating small calcified or cavitated lesions in the chest, hilar adenopathy, and mediastinal abnormalities.

Computerized axial tomography (CT or CAT) also provides sectional (axial, coronal, or sagittal) views of structures in the body. After serial x-ray exposures are taken through different angles of the body, a computer analyzes the information and provides a three-dimensional, reconstructed picture of the area studied. Computerized tomography is one of the most useful, informative, and available tests in the diagnosis and staging of malignancies. It is able to detect minor differences between tissue densities in any area of the body. Its major drawback is its production of artifact in areas of cortical bone content. Tissues surrounded by bone, such as the posterior fossa, the base of the skull, and the spine are most affected.[15] CT may be completed with or without contrast agents. Intravenous radioiodinated contrast enhances the projected image by highlighting the blood vessels. CT frequently is used to direct a needle to a tumor site for percutaneous biopsy.

Several radiographic examinations rely on contrast materials to enhance or outline the structures to be visualized. Angiography, venography, cholangiography, and urography, in addition to computerized tomography, all rely on the intravascular administration of iodinated contrast agents for optimal visualization of body structure and function. An example is the excretory radiograph, also known as the intravenous pyelogram, which is used in the initial diagnostic evaluation of renal masses.

Approximately 5% of the patients who undergo examinations with iodinated contrast material experience an adverse reaction to the contrast medium.[16] Most commonly this reaction includes nausea, localized pain at the injection site, a metallic or bitter taste, and a sensation of warmth and flushing, lasting from 1 to 3 minutes. These symptoms do not require treatment and will not progress to life-threatening reactions. The incidence of a severe reaction such as cardiopulmonary arrest is extremely uncommon, occurring in only 0.1% of patients.[16] There is not a good predictor for severe reactions; however, patients with any history of allergic response should be closely monitored. Patients who are considered to be at risk for reaction may receive a test dose of the contrast agent and be given premedication with diphenhydramine, adrenocorticotropic hormone, or epinephrine.

An oily iodinated contrast material is employed in lymphangiography. The lymphatic vessels in each foot, or less commonly, each hand, are injected to allow visualization of the lymphatic vessels and nodes. This is indicated in the diagnosis and staging of Hodgkin's and non-Hodgkin's lymphomas and in some pelvic cancers. In addition to the risk of a reaction to the iodine in the contrast medium, as described previously, it is important to be aware of the potential reaction of pulmonary microembolization. This is of greatest concern if the lymph channels of the upper portion of the body are imaged. The thoracic duct empties into the lungs, and a degree of embolization is likely to occur. Patients with compromised pulmonary reserve are at highest risk. Symptoms to be observed for are shortness of breath, chest pain, hypotension, and cyanosis. Nursing actions after lymphangiogram include instruction in deep breathing and coughing to keep the lungs expanded.

Intrathecal contrast agents are used in myelography and in computerized tomography. Radiographs of the subarachnoid space are taken after the injection of either an oily or a water-soluble contrast agent. The contrast agent will flow only to the point of obstruction, and more than one injection may be required. This is one reason why magnetic resonance imaging has become the superior examination for detection of spinal cord compression as well as for skeletal metastatic deposits. A water-soluble myelographic contrast agent often is used with computerized tomography if a single disease site within the spinal canal is suspected.[12]

Barium sulfate is a nonabsorbable, radiopaque contrast

agent used in the examination of the gastrointestinal tract. Studies that use barium include esophagography, upper gastrointestinal series, small bowel series, barium enema, and hypotonic duodenography. Barium is ingested or introduced into the gastrointestinal tract and allowed to coat the intraluminal surfaces. Radiographs are taken that can detect primary malignancies of the gastrointestinal organs or extrinsic compression from other tumor sites. By combining barium and air, a double contrast study is performed that is more sensitive than barium alone in detecting primary gastrointestinal tumors.[17] There are seldom complications to this examination unless there is an obstruction or a perforation of the digestive tract. Retention of the barium may cause fecal impaction and discomfort in some patients. The administration of a laxative or enema may be necessary to assist with bowel evacuation.

Nuclear medicine techniques

Nuclear medicine imaging involves the intravenous injection or the ingestion of radioisotope compounds (technetium-99m methylene diphosphate, technetium-99m diethylenetriaminepentaacetic acid, technetium-99 sulfur colloid, iodine-123/131, or gallium-67 citrate), followed by the sensitive camera imaging of those organs or tissues that have concentrated the radioisotopes. Scans of the bones, liver and spleen, brain, thyroid, and kidneys are used in the detection of malignancy. Nuclear medicine studies are very sensitive and often will detect sites of abnormal metabolism or early malignancy several months before changes are seen on a radiograph. Gallium scans are particularly sensitive in detecting bronchogenic carcinomas and lymphomas. However, the increased use and the sensitivity of computerized tomography have replaced many radioisotope examinations.

Positron emission tomography is an imaging modality that provides information based on the biochemical and metabolic activity of tissue. Infused biochemical compounds such as glucose are tagged with radioactive particles that emit positrons. The image is detected by gamma camera tomography. The best clinical application has been in brain imaging. Practical limitations of this modality are its expense (estimated at $1000 in 1989) and the need for a cyclotron to produce the isotopes.[18] Single photon emission computed tomography uses commercially available radioisotopes and has much broader application.

Nuclear imaging with radiolabeled monoclonal antibodies is employed, thus far investigationally, to visualize microscopic sites of metastasis or suspected malignancy. This technique requires that a monoclonal antibody targeted against a specific tumor antigen be combined with tracer amounts of radioactivity, usually iodine-131 or iodine-123. After intravenous injection, the antibody binds to antigen on the tumor. These tumor sites then "light-up" with imaging scanners. Sensitivity and specificity at levels of 90% have been achieved in some tumor types, occult lesions missed by other imaging modalities have been found, and the antibody has been administered without serious side effect.[19] In clinical trials, imaging has been successful in several disease sites, including the colon,[20] the breast[21] and ovaries,[21] and in melanoma[22] and T-cell lymphomas.[23]

Ultrasonography

Ultrasonography is a nonradiographic and noninvasive technique of imaging deep structures within the body. The reflecting echoes of high-frequency sound waves directed into specific tissues are recorded on an imaging screen. The echoes are variable, depending on the tissue density, and can be used to discriminate masses. Ultrasonography is most applicable in detecting tumors within the pelvis, retroperitoneum, and the peritoneum of patients with cancer.[12] Masses greater than 2 cm in diameter can be detected and localized for possible percutaneous biopsy.

Magnetic resonance imaging

Magnetic resonance imaging (MRI) creates sectional images of the body, similar to computerized tomography, but does not expose the patient to ionizing radiation. Images are created by placing the patient within a powerful magnetic field that aligns the body's hydrogen nuclei in one direction. Radiofrequency pulses are used to excite the magnetized nuclei and change their alignment. Between radiofrequency pulses the nuclei return to a state of relaxation, and variable signals are transmitted on the basis of tissue characteristics. These signals are analyzed by the computer, and multiplaner (sagittal, coronal, and axial) images are produced with exquisite clarity. Magnetic resonance imaging can be enhanced with the intravenous paramagnetic contrast agent, gadolinium diethylenetriaminepentaacetic acid (DTPA). This agent, the first of its kind to receive Food and Drug Administration approval (in 1988), works by reducing tissue relaxation time, thus increasing signal intensity and image production. Adverse reactions to gadolinium DTPA, which are rare, include nausea, pain localized to the injection site, and headache that occurs several hours after the examination.

Magnetic resonance imaging is most applicable in the detection, localization, and staging of malignant disease in the central nervous system, spine, head and neck, and musculoskeletal system. Contrast-enhanced MRI is the superior imaging modality in brain tumors (Figure 9-1).[24] MRI imaging of the spinal cord essentially has eliminated the use of myelography in patients with cancer.[3]

Significant limitations do exist in the use of MRI. Patients with aneurysm clips, pacemakers, or any ferromagnetic metallic implant cannot undergo MRI examination. The magnetic pull of the MRI is easily capable of removing the object from the patient's body. Acutely ill patients with life support or monitoring devices are excluded. Claustrophobic patients require sedation if they are able to undergo the test at all. The cost and somewhat limited availability of this relatively new diagnostic tool are additional disadvantages of the MRI at this time.

(a)

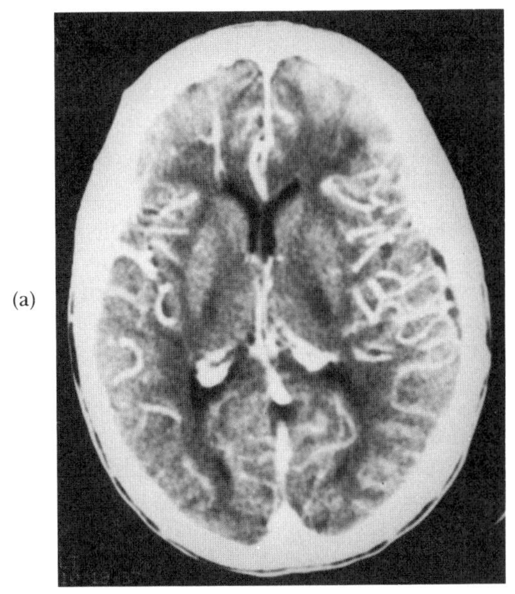

(b)

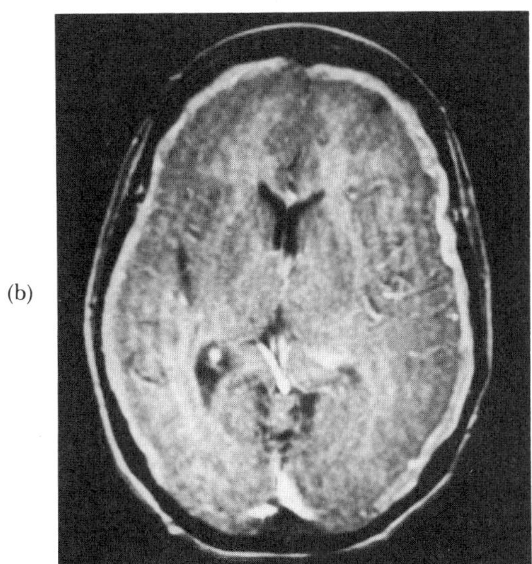

FIGURE 9-1 Contrast enhanced CT (a), and contrast enhanced MRI (b) of metastatic intracranial tumor. MRI shows "rind" of metastatic deposit around brain that was invisible on CT due to bone artifact.

Invasive Diagnostic Techniques

Endoscopy

Endoscopy is a method of directly visualizing the interior of a hollow viscus by the insertion of an endoscope into a body cavity or opening. The endoscope contains fiberoptic glass bundles that transmit light and then return an image to the optical head of the endoscope. The instrument may be rigid or flexible. Visual inspection, tissue biopsy, cytologic aspiration, staging the extent of disease, and the excision of pathologic processes are possible through the endoscope. Endoscopic examinations can visualize directly the larynx, the upper airway passages and the bronchial tree, the esophagus, the stomach, and the upper duodenum by the passage of a flexible scope through the mouth. Endoscopic retrograde cholangiopancreatography combines the diagnostic procedures of endoscopy and contrast-enhanced radiography to evaluate biliary tract obstruction and pancreatic masses. Visualization of the distal sigmoid colon, the rectum, and the anal canal is performed by means of a rigid scope. The entire large intestine can be viewed with a flexible colonoscope that is inserted anally. The cervix and vagina are visualized with the use of the magnification lens of the colposcope. Peritoneoscopy or laparoscopy permits assessment of surfaces within the peritoneal cavity by the insertion of a peritoneoscope through a small incision below the umbilicus. Thoracoscopy allows visualization of the visceral and parietal pleura, the mediastinum, and the diaphragm by means of a thoracoscope passed through an incision in the midaxillary line of the sixth to eighth intercostal space.[25] The direct visualization of the tissues and organs of the mediastinum is performed under general anesthesia. The endoscope is introduced into the mediastinum through a small incision above the manubrium.

Biopsy

The importance of obtaining histologic or cytologic proof of malignancy cannot be overstated. Treatment decisions for cancers arising within the same organ differ on the basis of the histopathology report. An example is the very different treatment regimens for small cell cancer of the lung and adenocarcinoma of the lung.

Exactly what tissue is to be biopsied depends on several factors: the clinical status of the patient, the patient's willingness to undergo invasive procedures, the size and location of the identified tumor, and the amount of tissue needed by the pathologist for analysis.[26]

The cytologic examination of aspirated fluid, secretions, scrapings, or washings of body cavities may reveal malignant cells that have exfoliated from a primary or metastatic tumor. Tissue will not be obtained by this method, and the pathologist's ability to establish the primary site of the malignancy may be limited. Cancer of the cervix often is detected by the cytologic examination of cells acquired from a Papanicolaou smear.

A biopsy provides tissue for histologic examination. The following are commonly recognized techniques for obtaining a biopsy: needle biopsy, incisional biopsy, excisional biopsy, and bone marrow aspiration. These procedures and their nursing implications are discussed in Chapter 11. For a definitive diagnosis of malignancy it is imperative that the pathologist receive an adequate, representative, and well-preserved tissue specimen. A cytologic or histologic report that is negative for malignancy may signify only a specimen that is inadequate for diagnostic evaluation, thus requiring repeat biopsy. An equivocal biopsy report should be sent to an outside source for a second evaluation.

CLASSIFICATION AND NOMENCLATURE

Basic Terminology

The terms *cancer* and *tumor* often are used interchangeably and inappropriately and can be misleading for patients, families, and professional colleagues. Tumor is a swelling or mass of tissue that may be benign or malignant. Cancer, synonymous with malignant neoplasm, is an uncontrolled "new growth" capable of metastasis and invasion that threatens host survival. The use of the term *tumor* in place of cancer because of its safer emotional connotation is misleading.

The term *primary* site is used to describe the original histologic site of tumorigenesis. A *secondary* or metastatic tumor resembles the primary tumor histologically but sometimes may be so anaplastic as to obscure the cell of origin. A *second primary* lesion refers to an additional, histologically separate malignant neoplasm in the same patient. Although this is a relatively unusual occurrence, it must be excluded at the time of an apparent recurrence.

Benign and Malignant Tumor Characteristics

Certain biologic, histologic, and cytologic characteristics distinguish a benign tumor from a malignant tumor. However, with the exception of the properties of invasion and metastasis, which are found only in cancer, the differences between a benign process and a malignant process are relative. In some circumstances a definitive diagnosis of benign tumor versus malignant tumor cannot be made.[27] For example, a well-differentiated follicular carcinoma of the thyroid may be solitary and encapsulated and may mimic a benign adenoma of the thyroid. Occasionally a benign tumor will transform into a malignant tumor over time. An adenomatous polyp of the colon is an example of a relatively benign process that can transform into cancer of the colon if left untreated.

In general, the following features distinguish benign tumors from those that are malignant. The benign tumor is relatively slow-growing. Tumor stasis or regression may occur. Growth occurs as the tumor expands locally within a capsule of fibrous tissue. Benign tumors do not invade adjacent tissues, destroy normal tissue, or metastasize elsewhere in the body. Symptoms result from pressure on adjacent tissue or from ectopic hormone production. Cytologic examination reveals uniform, well-differentiated cells that resemble those of the adult tissue of origin and demonstrate little or no anaplasia and rare mitoses. In contrast, the malignant tumor is characterized by its generally high mitotic rate, rapid growth, and disregard for normal growth limitations. Malignant tumors are almost never encapsulated. The malignant cells invade surrounding tissue, lymphatic vessels, and blood vessels and metastasize to distant sites. Tumor cells are anaplastic, vary in morphologic characteristics within the same tumor, are poorly differentiated, and have abnormal and inconstant numbers of chromosomes.

Tumor Classification System

The most relevant classification systems will universally communicate clinical and prognostic information. Tumors may be classified not only by their biologic behavior (benign versus malignant) but also by their tissue of origin.

To understand the nomenclature of tumors it is useful to review normal cell differentiation in the embryonic state. An early occurrence in the life of the embryo is the development of three primary germ layers: the ectoderm, the mesoderm, and the endoderm. The cells within these layers divide, specialize, and give rise to all cells, tissues, and organs within the body. The ectoderm differentiates into the skin and nervous system. The mesoderm differentiates into several organs and connective tissue: bones, blood, cartilage, fat, fibrous tissue, muscle, blood and lymph vessels. The endoderm differentiates into the lining of the digestive and respiratory tracts, bladder, and urethra.

Virtually every cell type in the body is capable of transforming into a malignant cell. Chapter 3 provides a complete discussion of carcinogenic transformation. It is fairly well accepted that the malignant cell derives from a postembryonic cell that is arrested in the process of differentiation.

Most tumors will retain sufficient characteristics of the normal, differentiated cell to allow recognition of the type of tissue from which they were derived, which is the basis of distinguishing tumors in the histogenetic classification system (Table 9-5).[28,29] Specific nomenclature provides information on characteristics of the neoplasm. A suffix is added to the name of the tissue or cell type under pathologic study to designate its benign or malignant nature. Benign tumors usually end in the suffix *oma,* the Greek root for tumor. Lipomas are benign tumors of fat tissue. Most malignant tumors end in either the suffix *sarcoma* or *carcinoma,* depending on the tissues from which they arise. Sarcoma specifies a malignant tumor of the connective tissues, that is, those tissues originating from the mesodermal embryonic layer. Liposarcoma is a malignancy of fat tissue. Carcinoma specifies a malignant tumor arising from epithelial tissues. Epithelium is the tissue that covers or lines surfaces in the body and arises from the ectodermal, mesodermal, or endodermal embryonic layers.

Carcinomas are further delineated by the prefixes *adeno,* for tumors that arise from glandular epithelial tissue, and *squamous,* for tumors that originate from squamous epithelial tissues. Descriptive terms such as cystic, follicular, papillary, medullary, exophytic, and polypoid are added to further define histologic characteristics.

Blastoma is the suffix that refers to malignant tumors that resemble the primitive blastula phase in embryonic development. Examples are neuroblastoma and retinoblastoma.

TABLE 9-5 Selected Benign and Malignant Neoplasms Listed by Histogenetic Classification

Tissue of Origin	Benign	Malignant
Epithelial (endodermal)		
Squamous	Squamous cell papilloma	Squamous cell or epidermoid carcinoma
Glandular	Adenoma	Adenocarcinoma
	Papilloma	Papillary carcinoma
	Cystadenoma	Cystadenocarcinoma
Respiratory tract	—	Bronchogenic carcinoma
Renal epithelium	Renal tubular adenoma	Renal cell carcinoma (hypernephroma)
Urinary tract	Transitional cell papilloma	Transitional cell carcinoma
Placental epithelium	Hydatidiform mole	Choriocarcinoma
Testicular epithelium	—	Seminoma, embryonal carcinoma
Liver	Liver cell adenoma	Hepatocellular carcinoma (hepatoma)
Biliary tree	Cholangioma	Cholangiocarcinoma
Stomach	Gastric polyp	Gastric carcinoma
Colon	Colonic polyp	Carcinoma of the colon
Mesenchymal (mesodermal)		
Connective		
Fibrous	Fibroma	Fibrosarcoma
Adipose	Lipoma	Liposarcoma
Cartilage	Chondroma	Chondrosarcoma
Bone	Osteoma	Osteosarcoma
Smooth muscle	Leiomyoma	Leiomyosarcoma
Striated muscle	Rhabdomyoma	Rhabdomyosarcoma
Blood vessels	Hemangioma	Hemangiosarcoma
Lymphatic vessels	Lymphangioma	Lymphangiosarcoma
Hematopoietic and lymphoreticular		
Hematopoietic cells	—	Leukemias
Lymphoid tissue	—	Lymphomas, plasmacytoma (multiple myeloma), Hodgkin's disease
Neuro-ectodermal		
Meninges	Meningioma	Meningeal sarcoma
Glia	Astrocytoma	Glioblastoma multiforme
Nerve cells	Ganglioneuroma	Neuroblastoma, medulloblastoma
Melanocytes	Nevus	Malignant melanoma
Mixed tissues		
Kidney	—	Wilms' tumor
Salivary gland	Mixed tumor of salivary gland (pleomorphic adenoma)	Malignant mixed tumor of salivary gland

Mixed tumors, such as adenosquamous carcinoma of the bronchi, represent tumors with mixed squamous and glandular elements, but they arise from the same germ layer and tissue. Some tumors, although rare and highly malignant, have such primitive differentiation that characteristics of a carcinoma and sarcoma may be evident.[28,30]

Teratoma and its malignant counterpart, teratocarcinoma, arise from tissue of all three germ layers and have no relationship to the site of origin.[28]

Several exceptions exist to the classification system described. Lymphoma, melanoma, and hepatoma are malignant tumors with the *oma* suffix. Additionally, some malignancies are named after the person who characterized them. Hodgkin's disease, Ewing's sarcoma, and Wilms' tumor are examples. The hematopoietic malignancies are classified separately by predominant cell type and their acute or chronic nature.

Tumors of Unknown Origin

A significant number of patients have metastatic cancer of an unknown primary site. Most frequently the histologic classification will be adenocarcinoma, but the site of origin may never be determined, even on autopsy. The goal of proceeding with a diagnostic investigation in this situation is to identify those malignancies that are potentially curable or effectively palliated with systemic treatment, even if they are disseminated. For example, lymphomas, germ cell tumors, acute leukemia, ovarian cancer, and pediatric sarcomas are potentially curable.[31] Effective palliation with hormonal therapy can be achieved in breast, prostate, and endometrial malignancy.

STAGING AND GRADING CLASSIFICATIONS

Staging the Extent of the Disease

The staging process is a method of classifying a malignancy by the extent of its spread within the body. It is a clinical and histologic determination that depends on the natural course of each particular type of cancer. Staging is based on the premise that cancers of similar histologic features and site of origin will extend and metastasize in a predictable manner. Although most staging classifications are based on the anatomic extent of disease, not all malignancies can be categorized by this criterion.

The objectives of solid tumor staging are multiple: to aid in treatment planning, to give prognostic information, to assist in treatment evaluation, and to facilitate the exchange of information and comparative statistics between treatment centers.[2]

With the goal of developing an internationally consistent system of staging solid tumor malignancy, the TNM committee of the International Union Against Cancer and the American Joint Committee on Cancer (AJCC) have agreed on the TNM staging system.

The TNM staging system classifies solid tumors by the anatomic extent of disease, as determined clinically and histologically. Three categories are quantified. The extent of the primary tumor (T) is evaluated on the basis of depth of invasion, surface spread, and tumor size. T0 signifies no evidence of primary tumor, and Tis signifies carcinoma in situ. The gradations of T1, T2, T3, and T4 indicate progressive tumor size or extent. The absence or presence and extent of regional lymph node (N) metastasis are considered, with attention to the size and location of the nodes. N0 signifies no regional involvement. N1, N2, and N3 signify increasing involvement of regional lymph nodes. The absence or presence of distant metastasis (M) is assessed as the third category. M0 signifies no evidence of metastasis. M1, M2, and M3 indicate distant metastasis, single versus multiple sites, and degree of organ involvement. A subscript may also specify the site of metastasis. For example, M1PUL denotes pulmonary metastasis.

The TNM classification is based on clinical and pathologic analyses. The clinical classification (cTNM or TNM) takes into account the information obtained from the physical examination, laboratory and imaging studies, biopsy, and surgical exploration. Clinical staging refers to all information obtained before the initiation of definitive treatment. The pathologic classification (pTNM) includes all information from the clinical TNM staging plus information from the pathologic examination of a resected specimen. This includes resected tumor (pT), lymph nodes (pN), and distant metastasis (pM) if they are evident on clinical staging.

For reporting purposes the TNM stage classification remains constant throughout the disease process. Progression of disease will not change the initial stage of disease. Two other TNM classifications are seen less frequently. Retreatment TNM (rTNM) is used after a disease-free interval or at the time of a second-look surgery. The extent or absence of disease recurrence is documented before retreatment planning is begun. Autopsy TNM (aTNM) is a postmortem classification that requires pathologic confirmation of TNM involvement. This method of staging helps to define the natural history of a tumor type relative to the treatment: response to treatment, recurrence patterns, and extent of disease at the time of death.

After numerical values are assigned to the T, N, and M categories, they are clustered into one of four stages (I through IV), or stage 0 for carcinoma in situ. All tumor sites are grouped differently on the basis of characteristics of the disease. A typical TNM grouping is depicted in Table 9-6.

Not all malignant tumors fit precisely into the TNM categories. Several other established and accepted staging systems for particular malignancies exist. Melanomas are staged histologically by the level of invasion of the primary lesion, inasmuch as this is the major determinant of prognosis. The Clark levels of invasion are widely accepted. The TNM stages for melanoma incorporate Clark's classification into primary tumor (T) assessment. The Duke's staging system for colorectal cancer, with its many subsequent modifications, classifies colorectal tumors by their

TABLE 9-6 A Typical Stage Grouping Based on TNM Classification

- *Stage 1, T1, N0, M0:* Clinical examination reveals a mass limited to the organ of origin. The lesion is operable and resectable with only local involvement, and there is no nodal and vascular spread. This stage affords the best chance for survival (from 70% to 90%).
- *Stage II, T2, N1, M0:* Clinical examination shows evidence of local spread into surrounding tissue and first-station lymph nodes. The lesion is operable and resectable, but because of greater local extent, there is uncertainty as to completeness of removal. The specimen shows evidence of microinvasion into capsule and lymphatics. This stage affords a good chance of survival (50% ± 5%).
- *Stage III, T3, N2, M0:* Clinical examination reveals an extensive primary tumor with fixation to a deeper structure, bone invasion, and lymph nodes of a similar nature. The lesion is operable but not resectable, and gross disease is left behind. This stage affords some chance of survival (20% ± 5%).
- *Stage IV, T4, N3, M+ :* There is evidence of distant metastases beyond the site of origin. The lesion is inoperable. There is little to no chance of survival (<5%).

Source: From Rubin P: Statement of the clinical oncologic problem, in Rubin P (ed): Clinical Oncology for Medical Students and Physicians: A Multidisciplinary Approach (ed 6). New York: American Cancer Society, 1983, p 10.

depth of invasion and presence of nodal metastasis. The International Federation of Gynecology and Obstetrics has an accepted staging system for cervical and endometrial cancers. Hodgkin's disease and non-Hodgkin's lymphoma are standardly described by the Ann Arbor classification, which recognizes disease distribution and symptoms. Cancers of the brain are not entirely suited to the TNM system because there are no lymphatic structures to categorize nodal (N) involvement.

The nonsolid tumors do not conform to solid tumor staging principles because of their disseminated nature. Leukemias are best classified according to their predominant cell types (ie, lymphocytic or nonlymphocytic), cell maturation, and acute or chronic nature. Clinical and morphologic factors such as age, platelet and blast counts, and periodic acid-Schiff stain reaction are indicators of favorable or unfavorable prognostic categories in acute lymphoblastic leukemia. The French-American-British classification has some clinical significance in acute myeloblastic leukemia but is not a staging system. In chronic lymphocytic leukemia two staging systems exist: the Rai classification and a relatively new system prepared by the International Workshop on chronic lymphocytic leukemia.[32] For patients with myeloma there is a staging classification that correlates M proteins with myeloma cell mass to provide prognostic information.[33]

Patient Performance Classification

A patient's physical performance status at the time of diagnosis and staging often will influence the type of treatment selected and provide prognostic information.[34] Patients who are bedridden are much less likely to respond to any treatment than those who are asymptomatic and able to maintain the activities of daily living. Performance scales are used frequently in the eligibility criteria for cooperative group clinical trials and also periodically to evaluate the effects of treatment and disease. The most prevalent performance scales are the Karnofsky Performance Status scale and the Eastern Cooperative Oncology Group scale. In an attempt to standardize this classification the American Joint Committee on Cancer (AJCC) has developed a simplified performance scale (Table 9-7).[35]

TABLE 9-7 Patient Physical Performance Scale Developed by the American Joint Committee on Cancer

Host Performance Scale	
H	The physical state (performance scale) of the patient, considering all cofactors determined at the time of stage classification and subsequent follow-up examinations
H0	Normal activity
H1	Symptomatic and ambulatory; cares for self
H2	Ambulatory more than 50% of time; occasionally needs assistance
H3	Ambulatory 50% or less of time; nursing care needed
H4	Bedridden; may need hospitalization

Source: From Beahrs OH, Henson DE, Hutter RVP, et al: American Joint Committee on Cancer: Manual for Staging of Cancer (ed 3), Philadelphia, JB Lippincott, 1988, p 9.

Grading

Grading a malignant neoplasm is a method of classification based on histopathologic characteristics of the tissue. It assesses the aggressiveness or degree of malignancy of tumor cells by comparing the cellular anaplasia, differentiation, and mitotic activity with normal counterparts. Specific characteristics vary with each type of cancer.

In grading a tumor the pathologist's objective is to quantify information to assist with treatment planning and prognostic determinations. For selected tumors such as soft tissue sarcomas, astrocytomas, and cancer of the prostate, the grade of the tumor is considered more significant than staging in terms of prognostic value. For other tumors, such as melanoma and renal cell carcinoma, grading has little prognostic value.

Two grading systems are commonly seen. One descriptively identifies the tumor as well differentiated, ie, retaining most characteristics of the normal cell of the tissue of origin, moderately well differentiated, poorly differentiated, or undifferentiated. The other system numerically grades from 1 to 3 or 4, with 1 being the most differentiated and 3 and 4 being the least well differentiated. The AJCC recommends the following grading classification[2]: GX, Grade cannot be assessed; G1, Well differentiated; G2, Moderately well differentiated; G3, Poorly differentiated; G4, Undifferentiated.

Certain problems exist with grading classifications. A tumor's level of differentiation may vary with time. Also, several grades of malignancy may exist within one tumor, and there must be certainty that a representative biopsy specimen has been obtained.

CONCLUSION

The diagnostic phase of a cancer illness is a time of adjustment, learning, anxiety, and uncertainty for the patient and family. During this time nurses will interact with the patient in several health care settings, eg, primary clinics, inpatient and outpatient units, and extended care units, as well as in the community. With adequate knowledge of the diagnostic evaluation nurses can help prepare patients for their tests, thereby easing the anxiety associated with the unknown. Awareness of the significance of a malignant tumor's grade and stage will permit the nurse to respond realistically to questions about treatment and prognosis.

REFERENCES

1. Cancer Facts and Figures. New York, American Cancer Society, 1988.
2. Beahrs OH, Henson DE, Hutter RVP, et al: American Joint Committee on Cancer: Manual for Staging of Cancer (ed 3). Philadelphia, JB Lippincott, 1988.
3. Bragg DG: State-of-the-art assessment: Diagnostic oncologic imaging. Cancer 64:261-265, 1989 (suppl).
4. Marton KI, Sox HC, Alexander J, et al: Attitudes of patients toward diagnostic tests: The case of the upper gastrointestinal series roentgenogram, Medical Decision Making 2:439-448, 1982.
5. Herberth L, Gosnell DJ: Nursing diagnosis for oncology nursing practice. Cancer Nurs 10:41-51, 1987.
6. Braunstein GD, Vaitukaitis JL, Carbone PP, et al: Ectopic production of human chorionic gonadotropin by neoplasm. Ann Intern Med 78:39-45, 1973.
7. Wolmark N, Fisher B, Wieand HS, et al: The prognostic significance of preoperative carcinoembryonic antigen levels in colorectal cancer. Results from NSABP clinical trials. Ann Surg 199:375-381, 1984.
8. Zamcheck N: The present status of carcinoembryonic antigen (CEA) in diagnosis, detection of recurrence, prognosis and evaluation of therapy of colonic and pancreatic cancer. Clin Gastroenterol 5:625-638, 1976.
9. Bates SE, Longo DL: Use of serum markers in cancer diagnosis and management. Semin Oncol 14:102-138, 1987.
10. Tietz NW: Clinical Guide to Laboratory Tests. Philadelphia, WB Saunders, 1983.
11. Byrne CJ, Saxton DF, Pelikan PK: Laboratory Tests: Implications for Nursing Care (ed 2). Menlo Park, Calif, Addison-Wesley, 1986.
12. Borg SA, Rosenthal S: Handbook of Cancer Diagnosis and Staging: A Clinical Atlas. New York, John Wiley & Sons, 1984.
13. Diagnostics: The Nurse's Reference Library. Nursing 81 Books. Springhouse, Penn, Intermed Communications, 1981.
14. Paulus DD: Imaging in breast cancer. CA 37:133-150, 1987.
15. Bragg DG, Harnsberger HR: Specialized techniques of diagnosis: New radiologic techniques, in DeVita VT, Hellman S, Rosenberg SA (eds): Cancer Principles and Practice of Oncology (ed 2). Philadelphia, JB Lippincott, 1985, pp 388-405.
16. Ehrlich RA, McCloskey ED: Patient Care in Radiography. St Louis, CV Mosby, 1989, pp 139-167.
17. Thompson WM: Imaging strategies for tumors of the gastrointestinal system. CA 37:165-185, 1987.
18. Treseler KM: Clinical Laboratory and Diagnostic Tests: Significance and Nursing Implications (ed 2). Norwalk, Conn, Appleton & Lange, 1988, pp 556-559.
19. Goldenberg DM: Targeting of cancer with radiolabeled antibodies. Arch Pathol Lab Med 112:580-587, 1988.
20. Goldenberg DM, Kim EE, Bennett S, et al: CEA radioimmunodetection in the evaluation of colorectal cancers and in the detection of occult neoplasms. Gastroenterology 84:524-532, 1983.
21. Epenetos A, Britton KE, Mather S, et al: Targeting of I-123 tumor associated antibodies to ovarian, breast, and gastrointestinal tumors. Lancet 2:999-1005, 1982.
22. Siccardi AG, Buraggi GL, Callegaro L, et al: Multicenter study of immunoscintiragraphy with radiolabeled monoclonal antibodies in patients with melanoma. Cancer Res 46:4817-4822, 1986.
23. Carrasquillo JA, Bunn PA, Keenan AM, et al: Radioimmunodetection of cutaneous T-cell lymphoma with ^{111}In-labeled T101 monoclonal antibody. N Engl J Med 315:673-680, 1986.
24. Stack JP, Antoun NM, Jenkins JPR, et al: Gadolinium-DPTA as a contrast agent in magnetic resonance imaging of the brain. Neuroradiology 30:145-154, 1988.
25. Sugarbaker PH, Roth JA: Specialized techniques of diagnosis: Endoscopy, in DeVita VT, Hellman S, Rosenberg SA (eds): Cancer Principles and Practice of Oncology (ed 2). Philadelphia, JB Lippincott, 1985, pp 353-374.
26. Neiman RS, Smith TJ: Biopsy principles, pathologic evaluation of specimens and staging of cases, in Cancer Manual (ed 7). Boston, American Cancer Society, 1986, pp 36-44.
27. Bonfiglio TA, Terry R: The pathology of cancer, in Rubin P (ed): Clinical Oncology for Medical Students and Physicians: A Multidisciplinary Approach (ed 6). New York: American Cancer Society, 1983, pp 20-29.
28. Pitot HC: Fundamentals of Oncology (ed 3). New York, Marcel Dekker, 1986, pp 21-33.
29. Robbins SL, Cotran RS: Neoplasia, in Pathologic Basis of Disease (ed 2). Philadelphia, WB Saunders, 1979, pp 141-187.
30. Sirica AE: Classification of neoplasms, in Sirica AE (ed): The Pathobiology of Neoplasia, New York, Plenum Press, 1989, pp 25-39.
31. Robert NJ, Garnick MB, Frei E: Undifferentiated neoplasms and cancers of unknown primary: a clinicopathological perspective, in Fer MF, Greco FA, Oldham RK (eds): Poorly Differentiated Neoplasms and Tumors of Unknown Origin, Orlando, Fla, Grune & Stratton, 1986, pp 541-555.
32. Santoro A: Chronic leukemias, in Bonadonna G, Robustelli della Cuna G (eds): Handbook of Medical Oncology, Milano, Italy, Masson, 1988, pp 756-777.
33. Durie BGM, Salmon SE: A clinical staging system for multiple myeloma. Cancer 36:842-854, 1975.
34. Stanley KE: Prognostic factors for survival in patients with inoperable lung cancer. J Nat Cancer Institute 65:25-32, 1980.
35. Rubin P: Statement of the clinical oncologic problem, in Rubin P (ed): Clinical Oncology for Medical Students and Physicians: A Multidisciplinary Approach (ed 6). New York: American Cancer Society, 1983, pp 2-19.

PART III

TREATMENT MODALITIES

Chapter 10

General Principles of Therapy

Mary Maxwell, RN, PhD

INTRODUCTION

Because "cancer" includes more than 101 different disease presentations involving virtually every organ system in the body, understanding the basis for choosing among the therapeutic alternatives in attempting to eradicate or control the disease is a tremendously complex task. Fundamentally, therapeutic decisions in oncology are based on the location, cell type, and extent of the malignancy, with established modes of therapy directed toward the particular disease presentation. The aim of treatment is to cure or to palliate, causing minimal structural or functional impairment of the individual. The sequence and intellectual constructions in treatment planning are the same as in any problem-solving activity: gathering information, planning, executing the plan, and evaluating. In this chapter the factors involved in this kind of problem-solving are examined in detail. The material is organized temporally, following the usual sequence in planning treatment for a patient. A brief historical look at treatment will set the context for understanding the philosophy of past and contemporary therapy, from which projections can be made for the future.

Much of the material covered in this chapter is of necessity purely scientific. However, it should always be kept in mind that cancer is a disease that occurs in human beings. By seeking medical help, the person with cancer asks to participate in the extraordinary experiment that constitutes modern health care. The patient wants to be rid of bothersome symptoms or to obtain relief that will allow a return to work and a normal life. From the clinician who performs the experiment, the patient requests the drugs, operations, communication, and compassion that will achieve these ends. The diagnostic names employed by the clinician and his or her concepts of etiology and pathogenesis are interesting and useful, but the nomenclature and mechanistic explanations of the disease are of secondary importance to a sick person; they are but the means to the primary goal, which is treatment. The recipient of treatment is a unique human being, and every aspect of the design and evaluation of therapeutic activities must take this into consideration. A therapeutic plan that seems indicated by abstract scientific analysis may have to be modified or changed by many human events in the real world. Care and treatment should be an "art," a humanistic application of established modes of therapy to the person with cancer.[1]

HISTORICAL PERSPECTIVES ON CANCER TREATMENT

From the earliest times, the treatment of cancer has been based on the prevalent ideas about the disease in that particular era. In the haste to find better ways to treat the disease, new therapeutic methods were and are constantly being devised. However, treatment assumptions that can seem so logical are often not borne out with time or by the application of rigorous scientific research methods. Five hundred years from now, the treatments in use today may seem as bizarre to future clinicians as those used by ancient healers seem to us. Because understanding cancer involves unraveling the mysteries of the basis of life itself, therapeutic interventions have always been and will continue to be subject to change as new knowledge accumulates.

The Egyptians used arsenical ointment in 1500 BC to attack cancer's external manifestations, which were probably believed to be the most important.[2] Hippocrates cauterized cancer in the neck in the fourth century BC. Celsus (30 BC–38 AD) excised breast cancer, leaving the pectoral muscles intact. Cato administered charcoal, and many therapists employed metallic salts, particularly copper and lead, treatments that persisted for centuries. Galen (131–203 AD) advocated vegetable diets and purging, cautioning against eating walnuts. He classified tumors and considered cancer a systemic disease related to an excess of black bile, being thereby beyond the cure of operation. His ideas predominated until the eighteenth century, so for the intervening time the objective of cancer therapy was purely palliation. In 1704 Valsalva advanced the theory that cancer was first a local lesion capable of cure by surgery, which then spread through the lymphatics to regional nodes, consequently tending to recur as secondary lesions.[3] The principles on which modern cancer surgery are based were formulated on this theory. In keeping with the understanding of the disease at the time, an "anatomic" basis for cancer surgery arose about 100 years ago. "En bloc" dissections, where the primary tumor as well as adjacent lymphatics and lymph nodes were removed in one continuous section, was deemed the "proper" cancer operation. Radical cancer surgery based on these considerations has persisted, with the desired goal being surgical removal of every single cancer cell. Bigger and better operations were devised. However, the superradical surgical procedures of the 1960s, such as forequarter and hindquarter amputations and hemicorpectomy, are no longer being performed regularly because it was shown that they do not increase patient survival time.

As a consequence of conceptual changes arising from new information about tumor biology, a new biologic basis for cancer surgery is emerging. Because it is now generally accepted that even the smallest solid tumor that can be diagnosed with contemporary methods (usually 1 cm) is already systemic at presentation, the primary aim of oncologic surgery is moving toward an attempt to reduce the tumor burden of the individual to a number of viable cells that can be destroyed by host immunologic factors, systemic chemotherapy or immunotherapy, local irradiation, or a combination of these methods. The combination of various therapies in this way is known as adjuvant therapy. When surgery is used alone, the "en bloc" excision may still be appropriate; when combined with other methods, a more conservative procedure may be in order. The objective, to eradicate each malignant cell, remains the same, but the method for its accomplishment has been modified.

The discovery of x rays, radioactivity, and radium before the turn of the century was soon followed by the therapeutic application of the new agents. By 1899, a basal call carcinoma had been cured by radiation.[4] It was thought that a miraculous new cure for cancer had been discovered because of the dramatic initial responses seen in the treatment of skin and superficial lesions. Then followed a period of disillusionment and pessimism as recurrence and serious injuries to normal tissues developed. These first 25 years were the "dark ages" of the new discipline, radiotherapy. The physical nature and biologic effects of the new agents were not understood, and equipment was primitive. There was no reliable way to measure dose. Many scientists lost their lives through their work with radiation during this time. Because most of the earliest practitioners were surgeons, they adopted treatment methods involving single, massive exposures aimed at eradicating a tumor in a single treatment. As might be expected, those individuals who lived through the immediate postirradiation period, although they had impressive initial regressions of their lesions, usually developed serious complications as well as early recurrences. Starting in 1919, clinical research tempered these early developments. Slowly, the technique of successive fractionated daily doses of radiotherapy evolved. Impressive results began to emerge in the treatment of head and neck and cervical lesions. Advances in the technologic and physical aspects of the new discipline emerged and are ongoing. In the early 1950s, the emergence of megavoltage equipment, such as the betatron and linear accelerator, greatly improved delivery. Where previously radiation was used only for palliation, it began to be used for cure in some instances.

Only during the past 30 years has chemotherapy abandoned empiricism and become a rational therapy of present value and future promise. In the 1940s, the laborious task of ascertaining which of some 200,000 known chemicals possessed cancericidal properties was begun.[2] By grouping chemicals with similar structural formulas and observing their effects on transplanted tumors in animals, on cancer tissue cultures, and on inoculated tumor growths in egg embryos, scientists were able to move from "chemotherapy by trial-and-error" to a system of rational choice. The majority of chemical and biologic agents recommended in earlier years, such as colloidal lead and Coley's toxin, were abandoned. Effective chemotherapeutic agents were produced by the synthesis of toxic radicals with chemical substances required by the malignant cell for metabolism and division (such as nucleic acid); when the cancer cell ingests or absorbs these compounds, it is damaged or destroyed. Where at first single agents were given continuously over a period of time, the application of systemic chemotherapy to cancer during the ensuing years has included such advances as combined drug therapy, pulse dosing (high doses given intermittently), infusions and perfusions of body segments, and the use of chemotherapeutic agents as adjuvant to other therapies.

During the first 50 years of the twentieth century, survival rates for cancer improved tremendously, and morbidity associated with treatment fell dramatically. However, by the 1950s, cancer survival had plateaued, primarily because cancers believed to be localized were shown to have occult micrometastases at diagnosis. Because surgery, radiotherapy, and chemotherapy are not competitive, treatment aimed at covering all bases by using more than one therapeutic approach began to emerge.

Traditionally, surgeons had managed the treatment of most people with cancer. During the 1960s, medical oncology became a specialty in its own right as an offshoot of internal medicine. Radiotherapy is a consultative discipline, and radiation oncologists see patients only on referral by other physicians. Where up to 20 years ago the primary qualifications sought in an oncology nurse were a kind heart and the ability to improvise, the recent expansion of treatment and care possibilities calls for a new breed of professional. Advanced formal education and clinical sophistication are mandatory as nursing roles expand and increased responsibility for all aspects of patient management is sought.

The modern care of people diagnosed with cancer is increasingly a team effort involving the expertise of specialists from several disciplines. The consultative assistance of qualified oncologic specialists is freely available to all physicians and their patients throughout the United States through the consultative tumor boards that exist in all hospitals with accredited cancer programs. With this assistance, patients can often be treated in their communities, avoiding the necessity of long periods away from home and family. The care provided by the major cancer centers is becoming increasingly palliative and research-oriented as more patients receive their primary treatment in their own communities from the growing number of qualified surgical and medical oncologists and oncology nurses. The recent surge of interest in the possibilities for improving care of individuals with cancer who are living and undergoing treatment longer has led to the establishment of special oncology units and cancer rehabilitation programs in local hospitals and hospice development in local communities.

But the care of the person with cancer has not always been so enlightened. The first cancer hospital opened in Rheims in 1740 under the supervision of the Hotel Dieu (the oldest hospital in Europe).[2] In 1770, because of the superstition that cancer was contagious, the hospital was moved outside the city. The first establishment of a cancer service in a general hospital occurred in England, at the Middlesex Hospital. It consisted of 12 beds for patients who were permitted to remain until they improved or succumbed to their disease. In the United States, the present Memorial Center in New York was finally established in 1884 by J. Marion Sims, who was ridiculed and threatened for his efforts to treat cancer.

As people with cancer are living longer because primary therapy has improved and as combined methods offer a wider variety of interventions to manage the disease after recurrence, a new objective has emerged to take its place with "cure" and "palliation"—that of "control." Control indicates that by the serial use of various combinations of surgery, radiation, chemotherapy, and immu-

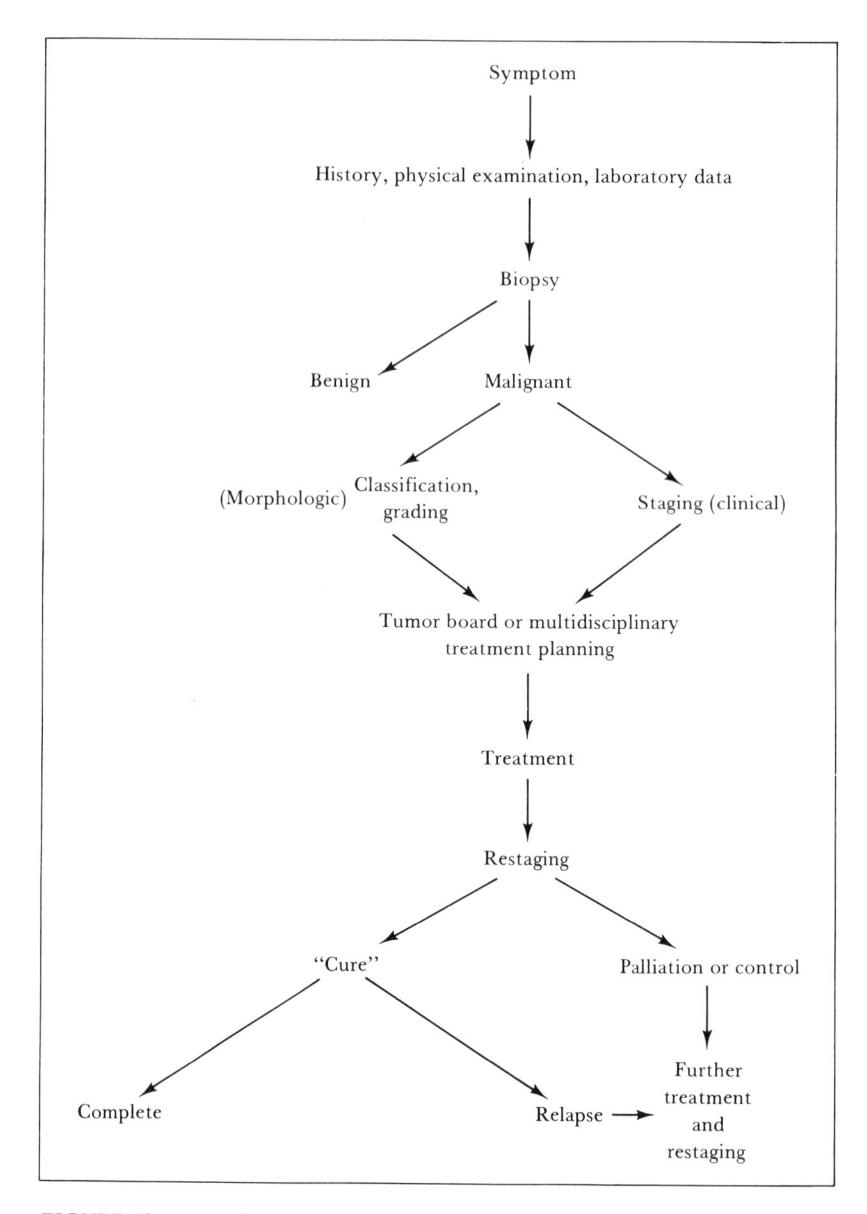

FIGURE 10-1 Usual sequence of events in planning cancer treatment.

notherapy, cancer can be kept within bounds for increasingly longer periods. This often means many therapeutic planning sessions and visits to the tumor board as new problems arise. Figure 10-1 charts the usual sequence of events that occur in planning cancer treatment.

FACTORS INVOLVED IN TREATMENT PLANNING

The Patient Presents

Any person who seeks medical care with a complaint may have cancer. Any complaints of weight loss, unexplained pain, unexplained loss of energy, irregularities of the alimentary, respiratory, genital, urinary, or neurologic system, or complaints of lumps or bumps should alert the primary clinician to the possiblity of cancer.

A Diagnostic Workup Is Begun

When a neoplastic disease is suspected, a detailed history, physical examination, and hematologic, biochemical, and radiologic studies must be performed to establish the likelihood of cancer as the diagnosis and the necessity for obtaining histologic proof. When the clinical evidence points to the presence of a primary malignancy, the next step is to establish by biopsy the nature of the neoplasm.

A Biopsy Is Done

Histologic proof of malignancy is an essential prerequisite to planned treatment. This allows full investigation of the person and prevents hasty local treatment measures that might jeopardize later plans. It can be a useful guide to prognosis, and it fosters the economical, orderly, and planned use of all available resources. Chapter 11 describes the methods of performing biopsies.

Any biopsy report that is equivocal or inconsistent with the clinical findings should be reviewed by an outside source (such as the Armed Forces Institute of Pathology) or a new biopsy obtained. Recurrent or metastatic disease requires the same critical diagnosis as the primary lesion.

The Biopsy Establishes the Diagnosis

The pathologist's report is crucial in oncology because it conveys the special significance of a given neoplasm. The information given to the clinician is expressed in a kind of shorthand, condensing abundant information into a few terms.

The shorthand used in communicating information about cancer is critical. The language used must be understood by all involved, it must be simple enough to be practical for use in the clinical setting, and it should be standardized so that cross-comparisons of different cancers in different persons in different geographic locations can be made.

National and international committees are working to standardize the language of malignant disease. The two major agencies involved are the International Union Against Cancer (UICC) and the American Joint Committee for Cancer Staging and End Results Reporting (AJCCS). Not only does a common language assist the individual clinician in planning treatment and determining the person's prognosis, but it will assist clinicians around the world to share the results of their evaluation of treatment regimens. Research efforts will be improved as the population of people that can be studied increases. The potential end result may be improvement in the treatment of malignant disease.

Classifying the tumor

One type of nomenclature used by the pathologist in communicating the diagnosis to the clinician is tumor classification. The current and best classification system is a combination of two approaches: histogenesis (tissue of origin) and anticipated biologic behavior. Knowing the organ of origin does not provide much information because tumors arising from different tissues in the same organ behave quite differently. Conversely, tumors of the same tissue from different organs behave in a similar fashion. For example, adenocarcinoma of the lung and adenocarcinoma of the rectum behave similarly, whereas adenocarcinoma of the lung and squamous cell carcinoma of the lung have different natural histories. Consequently, the general region of the tumor is primarily descriptive, as, for example, a testicular carcinoma or a rectal carcinoma. The tissue of origin determines the behavior of a tumor, and the cell type of a tumor can be relied on not to change.

The second method of tumor classification concerns biologic behavior. Tumors can be divided into benign or malignant groups. Usually, a benign tumor is well circumscribed or encapsulated: microscopically, it appears orderly and is made up of cells similar to those of its parent tissue. A typical malignant tumor, on the other hand, invades the organs from which it originated and eventually the surrounding tissues; it is made up of cells that vary greatly in size and shape and contains large, hyperchromic nuclei and prominent nucleoli. There are many mitotic figures, some of which are atypical, and lymph and blood vessels are often permeated by tumor cells.[5]

Various suffixes are used to complete the nomenclature of tumors. "Oma" implies simply tumor, and benign tumors are usually named by adding this suffix to the name of the cell type of tissue (such as fibroma or lipoma). Malignant tumors arising in epithelial tissues are known as *carcinomas. Sarcoma* refers to malignant tumors involving mesenchymal tissues. Because epithelial tissue contains three germ layers, neoplasms of the squamous epithelium are called *squamous cell carcinomas*, neoplasms of the transitional epithelium are called *transitional cell carcinomas*, and those involving glandular epithelium are called *adenocarcinomas*.

Grading establishes the degree of malignancy

The pathologist also uses the language of grading in describing tumors. Grading refers to the appearance of tumor cells, specifically to their degree of anaplasia or differentiation. Grading can be done numerically from I to IV. Grade I indicates that the cells are so well differentiated that they closely resemble the normal parent cells. Grade IV tumor cells are so anaplastic that it is often difficult for the pathologist to determine their cell of origin. Grade II and III are intermediate designations. Grading also can be expressed by the terms well differentiated (grade I), moderately differentiated (grade II), poorly differentiated (grade III), or undifferentiated (grade IV).

The prognostic value of grading varies with different types of tumors. In some tumors, such as bladder cancers, the grade of the tumor is directly related to the ultimate prognosis for the person, with the prognosis deteriorating as the cells become less differentiated. For other tumors, however, such as melanoma, grading has little or no prognostic value.

Years of accumulated experience have shown that a tumor with a particular appearance of cells, with a certain level of differentiation, arranged in a certain way, and originating in a particular organ will behave in a predictable way. This knowledge permits the medical team to plan therapy based on information about what happened to numerous individuals with the same tumors in the past.

For instance, a pathologic report revealing a "seminoma" carcinoma of the testes means that metastasis to the nearby lymph nodes is likely. This type of tumor has a fairly good prognosis because the primary lesion is usually resectable and lymph node metastasis is radiosensitive. High cure rates are expected, with only a 10% mortality rate. On the other hand, a report of an embryonal cell carcinoma of the testes is ominous. This type of tumor tends to metastasize early to the lung, liver, bone marrow, and brain. It is radioresistant, with a 50% mortality rate. From the knowledge gained by the pathologist's report, treatment can be planned.

The Staging Reveals the Clinical Extent of the Disease

Once the diagnosis is established, further definitive testing is needed to assess the anatomic extent of the disease as meticulously as possible. A knowledge of the natural history and patterns of spread of the neoplasm can be expected to focus and expedite the staging workup of each person. Depending on the tumor type, whole-lung tomography, metastic surveys, bone, brain, or liver scans, abdominal ultrasound, xerograms, or more routine procedures such as cystoscopy and proctoscopy serve to focus on areas of possible hidden metastasis. In Hodgkin's disease, lymphangiography is valuable in detecting occult disease in the retroperitoneal and pelvic nodes, and arteriography is often helpful in evaluating lesions in the kidney. A surgical procedure may be indicated, such as the diagnostic exploration of the abdomen (staging laparotomy) used in Hodgkin's disease. This often reveals occult involvement of the liver and spleen.

When all the essential information is at hand, the disease can be clinically staged. The UICC has standardized the clinical staging of many tumors by the use of the TNM system (Table 10-1). Using the TNM system, the extent of disease is evaluated separately with respect to the primary tumor site (T), the regional lymph nodes (N), and the presence or absence of metastasis (M). The basic TNM model is expanded by using subcategories to describe how far the disease has progressed and the extent of metastasis, if any. Tis indicates tumor in situ, or tumor with all the histologic characteristics of malignancy except invasion. T with possible numbers 1, 2, 3, and 4 denotes increasing primary tumor extension. Increments of progressive lymph node involvement are indicated by N0, N1, N2, and N3. In like manner, M0, M1, M2, and M3 mean an advancing metastatic involvement and degree of organ impairment.

On the basis of information derived about each of the compartments, "T," "N," and "M," a stage designation can be assigned. Stage designations differ among primary tumor types. The American Joint Committee on Cancer Staging and End Results Reporting (AJC) describes a typical stage grouping:

- *Stage I, T1, N0, M0:* Clinical examination reveals a mass limited to the organ of origin. The lesion is operable and resectable with only local involvement, and there is no nodal and vascular spread. This stage affords the best chance for survival (from 70% to 90%).
- *Stage II, T2, N1, M0:* Clinical examination shows evidence of local spread into surrounding tissue and lymph nodes. The lesion is operable and resectable, but because of greater local extent, there is uncertainty concerning completeness of removal. The specimen shows evidence of microinvasion into capsule and lymphatics. This stage affords a good chance of survival (50% ± 5%).
- *Stage III, T3, N2, M0:* Clinical examination reveals an extensive primary tumor with fixation to deeper structure, bone invasion, and lymph nodes of a similar nature. The lesion is operable but not resectable, and gross disease is left behind. This stage affords some chance of survival (20% ± 5%).
- *Stage IV, T4, N3, M+:* There is evidence of distant metastases beyond the site of origin. The lesion is inoperable. There is little to no chance of survival (<5%).

TABLE 10-1 TNM Staging System

Tumor	
T0	No evidence of primary tumor
Tis	Carcinoma in situ
T1, T2, T3, T4	Progressive increase in tumor size and involvement
Nodes	
N0	Regional lymph nodes not demonstrably abnormal
N1, N2, N3	Increasing degrees of regional lymph node disease
Metastasis	
M0	No evidence of distant metastasis
M1, M2, M3	Progressive distant metastasis

TNM classifications differ at each anatomic site depending on the knowledge of spread and clinical evaluation of the specific cancer. TNM classifications for cancers of many primary sites have now been adopted and are available to all interested clinicians.

Nevertheless, the TNM system is not perfect. Confusion and controversy over it exist in the medical community. Except for a few sites (eg, head and neck cancer), it is not widely used by practicing physicians. Some authorities think it is unnecessarily complex, whereas others criticize it for being too simplistic to include all important prognostic factors.[6] Cox et al have pointed out the problems with the TNM system and conceptualized an approach that emphasizes these individual clinical features and constitutes a better description of the person with a given type of cancer.

For some cancers, especially the inaccessible ones, the TNM system cannot be used. In brain tumors, for

TABLE 10-2 Karnofsky Performance Status Scale

Condition	Percentage	Comments
Able to carry on normal activity and to work. No special care is needed	100	Normal; no complaints; no evidence of disease
	90	Able to carry on normal activity; minor signs or symptoms of disease
	80	Normal activity with effort; some signs or symptoms of disease
Unable to work. Able to live at home, care for most personal needs. A varying degree of assistance is needed	70	Cares for self; unable to carry on normal activity or to do active work
	60	Requires occasional assistance but is able to care for most needs
	50	Requires considerable assistance and frequent medical care
Unable to care for self. Requires equivalent of institutional or hospital care. Disease may be progressing rapidly	40	Disabled; requires special care and assistance
	30	Severely disabled; hospitalization is indicated, although death is not imminent
	20	Hospitalization is necessary; very sick; active supportive treatment necessary
	10	Moribund; fatal processes progressing rapidly
	0	Dead

Source: Karnofsky DA, Burchenal JH: The clinical evaluation of chemotherapeutic agents in cancer, in MacLeod CM (ed): Evaluation of Chemotherapeutic Agents. New York, Columbia University Press, 1949.

instance, where metastasis does not occur and no lymph nodes are involved, the "T," "N," and "M" are irrelevant. Tumors that metastasize primarily by vascular routes, such as bone sarcoma and renal and hepatic carcinomas, do not lend themselves well to the TNM system, primarily because there is no lymph node involvement. For these tumors, other systems have been devised. In Hodgkin's disease and the lymphomas, where the primary site is usually a lymph node and where there can be no clear distinction between the "T" and "N" components, other staging schemes have been adopted. The Ann Arbor classification is the system currently most widely used for lymphomas (see Chapter 44). Duke's staging of rectal and colonic cancer is another type of staging system.

These clinical staging classifications play a very important dual role. They estimate the chances of survival in the individual, and they assist physicians in selecting appropriate treatments. They facilitate the valid comparison of the results of different treatment regimens from a variety of institutions.

The major weakness of the classification systems is that they often cannot use any histologic criteria, such as loss of cellular differentiation, blood vessel invasion, invasion into lymphatic vessels, and growth into connective or adipose tissue, to describe the grade, or degree of malignancy, of the tumor. This may be important in understanding why some tumors of apparently similar type and stage do not all respond to the same treatment.

During this time of staging, additional factors that might further influence the treatment plan must be considered. It is important to evaluate the person's general clinical condition in terms of such factors as age, general debility, previous treatment for the same or other cancers, the presence of preexisting cardiovascular, hepatic, renal, or other major illnesses, and presence of a second primary neoplasm. The person's performance status can be determined, giving a quantitative measure of the activity of which the person is capable at the moment. The person's performance status can then be measured periodically throughout the treatment regimen. Although first devised by Karnofsky[7] (Table 10-2), who used increments of ten, ranging from 100 (fully active) to 0 (dead), other similar types of performance rating scales can be used. The measurement of activity for statistical purposes in this way is widely used by the cooperative research groups, who are interested in comparing not only objective tumor response but also the total effect of tumor and treatment on the person's ability to carry on his daily activities. The Veterans Administration Lung Group, which used the original Karnofsky Scale, excluded people from participating in their cooperative studies if their performance status measured less than 40. It was anticipated that at that level of functioning, the person would not live long enough to provide meaningful data. The Veterans Administration Lung Group used the performance status for stratifying individuals entering research studies because a person with a higher initial Karnofsky rating may live longer than one who begins at a lower level, regardless of the treatment approach or tumor cell type.

DECIDING ON THE TREATMENT METHOD

When the clinical stage of the disease has been established, a series of crucial decisions concerning management must be made. Careful integration of the extent of disease and the individual's condition with a large body of knowledge relating to prognosis, anticipated response to various forms of treatment, anticipated complication rates, and other relevant clinical considerations is required.

Should Treatment Be Aimed at Cure?

This is the vital question. In general, the oncologist tends to think of tumors with 5-year survival probabilities in the range of 1% to 5% as having no or only a minimal chance for cure. The oncologist will therefore ask whether any method can offer the person even such a small chance for cure. The risks involved must then be related to the person's age and general condition, any previous treatment that might modify or limit tissue tolerance, and other pertinent considerations. An intensive treatment program that offers a small chance for permanent cure may be justified for a young, vigorous adult but inappropriate for a frail, elderly person, even though their cancers may be of the same type and extent. A correct decision on whether to treat for cure is one of the most important decisions that the oncologist must make, and it calls on the full extent of background and prior experience. Overly aggressive attempts can expose individuals who are incurable to needless morbidity, prolonged and expensive treatment, and distressing complications. On the other hand, therapeutic decisions that are too pessimistic deprive the person who has a small but significant chance for cure of the chance to live out the rest of life.

A person's feelings and values are crucial to the decision. Some people, even knowing that they have only a slight chance for cure, will strongly prefer an aggressive plan of action. Others will make it clear that they have lived a long and fruitful life and prefer to be allowed to die in peace.

Although in many instances the therapeutic decision is straightforward and clearly follows an established treatment pattern, there is often a fine line to be balanced regarding what would be best for a given person.

Which Method Should Be Used?

After it has been decided that the person is best treated with a curative attempt, the next decision involves choosing the best method or combination of methods. Again, a broad body of knowledge about all aspects of clinical oncology must be used, including a familiarity with the anticipated results of surgery, chemotherapy, and radiotherapy used either alone or in combination with other procedures. Surgery and radiotherapy alone may be curative if the disease is truly localized. On the other hand, chemotherapy may be curative when widespread disease is present. Each major technique has its advantages and shortcomings. When used by themselves, surgery and radiotherapy may leave behind viable malignant cells. Chemotherapy may eliminate micrometastasis but leave behind viable cancer cells if a bulky tumor mass is present. Modern treatment programs are designed to allow the greatest curative potential of each method by using each to exploit the different biologic characteristics of a variety of cancers.

When choosing the treatment for a given person, the best approach is for an interdisciplinary group to share in the decision-making process. The surgeon specifies the therapeutic potential and operability of the person's tumor. The radiotherapist tells the expectation of curability by primary radiotherapy or the augmentation effect that radiotherapy might have before or following surgery or chemotherapy. The chemotherapist specifies the contribution that chemotherapy can make to cure the particular tumor and the potential for chemotherapeutic or hormonal palliation should surgical or radiotherapeutic cure be impossible. The pathologist's role involves explaining the details of the biopsy and microscopic appearance of the tumor. The radiologist reviews the various radiographs and scans. As cancer treatment planning becomes more of a team effort, nurses may have one or a number of roles; a nurse practitioner who is the primary care provider may present the person's case to the board. An enterostomy nurse may have contributions to make regarding postoperative care feasibility and rehabilitation. A research assistant nurse may explain details of a chemotherapy protocol under consideration. A primary nurse for a person who is hospitalized may have contributions to make based on his or her knowledge of the person, including such pertinent details as pain, vocational incapacitation, familial problems, emotional reactions, financial burdens, geographic location, or other aspects of the panorama of human life. The nurse can be very helpful in providing a broader perspective on the person's overall situation and care. Although the ultimate decision regarding treatment of the tumor legally rests with the physicians, as oncology nurses become increasingly clinically and professionally sophisticated, they undoubtedly will have a greater role to play.

Cancer treatment is by necessity radical because extraordinary measures are needed to control this aggressive disease. Because the basic principle is to cure the person with the least functional and structural impairment, interdisciplinary planning provides consideration on how radical a treatment should be based on the following factors: the aggressiveness of the cancer, the predictability of its spread, the morbidity and mortality that can be expected in the individual from the therapeutic procedure being considered, the cure rate that could be expected from it, and the patient's desires. These can be hard decisions, and the choice is often relative. What percentage of survival is acceptable for a debilitating surgical, radiotherapeutic, or chemotherapeutic maneuver? Is the tendency to be more radical justified as the chance for cure diminishes? Will a more conservative approach only lead to recurrence? There is no magic formula other than personal opinion based on clinical experience and the experiences of others that have been published in the literature. For this reason, it is in the patient's best interest to have a multidisciplinary approach. The therapeutic aggressiveness of one member of the team is often tempered by the more conservative bent of a colleague, and each member present brings a fresh approach to the question at hand. Although in the majority of instances the indications for one discipline or the other are clear-cut and noncompetitive, the decisions made by an interdisciplinary team are never easy. Each patient thus benefits from the highly individualized prescription that a tumor board consultation affords.

The construction of a treatment plan for the overall care of the individual takes into consideration not only the nature and extent of the disease and therapeutic potentials of each method, but also the facilities available for treatment, the experience of the consultant or family physician, and the ability of the patient and family to accept the recommended therapy. The treatment plan should provide for both immediate management and anticipated future developments.

Clinical Trials

The choice of treatment is difficult and tends to become quite arbitrary in some situations. Clinicians, realizing the limitations of their own experience and of haphazard observations in general, turn for guidance to organized clinical trials. At present and for the future, these constitute the only sure foundation for therapeutic progress.

The scientific method associated with clinical trials involves objectivity, control, rigor, and the use of empirical data in a systematic manner. A clinical trial can be defined as a carefully and ethically designed experiment with the aim of answering a precisely framed question.[8] An absolute necessity is a valid protocol that covers all foreseeable eventualities and ambiguities. Clinical trials for chemotherapy drug testing proceed through phases that are described in Chapter 13. The publication of the results of clinical trials allows clinicians around the world to build on treatment successes. Replication of the experiments at other institutions ensures that treatment outcomes are not serendipitous.

A well-conducted clinical trial can achieve a number of objectives:

1. It can demonstrate the effectiveness or ineffectiveness of a particular form of treatment and can make direct comparisons between two or more treatment regimens.
2. It can assess the toxicities of the treatment.
3. It can identify prognostic features within the group of patients as a whole.
4. It can identify subgroups responding in a particular way to any of the treatment schedules.
5. The organization of a trial may facilitate the collection of data relating to the disease irrespective of prognosis or treatment.
6. Analysis of the results may reveal variations in clinical practice that influence the course of the disease or response to treatment.
7. Following a protocol ensures a certain standard of investigation, care, and treatment.

Incidental advantages include the freedom from having to make individual choices of treatment for each patient, and the actual conduct of the trial can provide opportunities for a valuable exchange of ideas among the physicians involved. Clinical trials are not perfect. No trial can absolutely determine the best treatment for an individual. Also, it is hard to control the confounding variables that are possible with a human subject. Any type of therapy or combination thereof for any form of malignant disease can be made the objective of a clinical trial.

The epitome of the multidisciplinary approach to cancer treatment is the cooperative clinical study groups. Rubin[9] defines such cooperation as:

> multidisciplinary undertakings at the local level, and they involve multiple universities and medical centers at the national level and even the international level. Although the hope for rapidly achieving good data lies in cooperative national protocols, this ideal will be difficult to achieve. It assumes that clinicians and pathologists at different institutions can agree on classifications, and that treatment selection can be unbiased.

Despite the problems inherent in such cooperative efforts, several groups are actively engaged in cooperative clinical studies. Examples of such groups include the Southwest Oncology Group (SWOG), the Eastern Cooperative Oncology Group (ECOG), Radiation Therapy Oncology Group (RTOG), Gynecology Oncology Group (GOG), the Northern California Leukemia Group (NCLG), and the National Surgical Adjuvant Breast Project (NSABP). Such cooperative groups achieve the goal of obtaining adequate numbers of study patients so that meaningful answers can be derived to improve therapeutic regimens for specific categories of malignant disease.

How Treatment Plans Are Recommended

The optimal treatment situation from the physician's point of view would be for a patient to be entered into an existing clinical trial. However, this is not always possible. The facility where the patient is being treated may not participate in a cooperative study group. There may not be a protocol available that fits the patient's stage of disease. If a protocol exists, the patient might be ineligible. The patient may refuse to be in a study for one reason or another.

An alternative approach is to use a "conventional" treatment program. Conventional or standard regimens are those that have been studied extensively, used for a long time, and are widely accepted for common cancers. For instance, MOPP (nitrogen mustard, oncovin, procarbizine, prednisone) is a standard treatment choice for stage III and IV Hodgkin's disease. CMF (cyclophosphamide, methotrexate, 5-fluorouracil) is a commonly used treatment for metastatic breast cancer, and weekly 5-fluorouracil is common for colon cancer. Conventional treatment programs involve drugs that are commercially available; clinical trials often test recently developed drugs that are only available to patients entered into the studies. These newest drugs may provide a breakthrough not available with commercial drugs, another reason why a clinical trial treatment program could offer the patient an advantage.

If a patient is not eligible for an existing clinical trial and there is not a conventional treatment program pertinent to the case, the physician usually tries to find a study in the literature that documents a successful treatment program for the situation. Publications in journals usually involve larger numbers of patients and a longer period for evaluating the effectiveness of the therapy. More details are provided in a journal article about side effects and dose reduction. If a journal article is not available, an abstract publication could be used. Abstracts are published overviews of oral presentations at national meetings. Abstracts offer few protocol details but often provide information about the latest drug combinations and doses.

Finally, if no existing treatment programs are available, the physician puts together a protocol specific to the situation. Agents that are active against the tumor are specified for a regimen unique to that patient, the disease state, and the coexisting medical problems.

A treatment plan may involve a single modality or multiple modalities. *Primary therapy* indicates the best, most definitive treatment aimed at cure for a given cancer. Primary therapy could be surgery, chemotherapy, or radiotherapy. *Adjuvant therapy* refers to a situation where other modalities are used after the primary treatment (usually surgery).[10] Adjuvant means "assisting or aiding." Thus chemotherapy, radiation therapy, immunotherapy, or some combination thereof follows surgery in an attempt to eradicate any tumor cells that may have been left behind. *Neoadjuvant* therapy, a newer concept, uses the aforementioned modalities to treat micrometastatic disease before the primary, definitive treatment. It is not particularly concerned with the primary tumor itself, although the primary tumor often shrinks, facilitating surgical removal.

With chemotherapy, *first-line* drugs are used during initial treatment. First-line drugs are those known to be most effective against the tumor, thus most likely to lead to "cure" or remission. If the tumor recurs, *second-line* drugs are in order. At that point, the first-line drugs would be considered failures, since the disease returned despite their use (probably due to resistance). Second-line drugs are those with less activity against the tumor, but a response or a second remission may be possible. In some cases, third- and fourth-line drugs may be available.

ASSESSING THE RESPONSE TO TREATMENT

Responses may be classified as objective or subjective. Objective responses are described as follows[11]:

Complete Response	Complete disappearance of signs and symptoms of cancer, lasting at least 1 month
Partial Response	A 50% or more reduction in the sum of the products of the greater and lesser diameters of all measured lesions, lasting at least one month, without the development of any new lesions during therapy
Progression	A 25% or more increase in the sum of the products of the greater and lesser diameters of all measured lesions, or the emergence of new lesions

Objective parameters are measured before initiating therapy to give a baseline for evaluation. Frequently used parameters include pulmonary lesions, as seen on radiographs; liver involvement, as measured on a liver scan or by liver function tests; and enlarged lymph nodes, which can be palpated and compared with the initial measurements. In acute leukemia a complete response (or remission) indicates the disappearance of all clinical evidence of disease and normal bone marrow.

With some tumors, the response to treatment is assessed by restaging. Restaging involves reestablishing the clinical extent of disease at the completion of a prescribed course of therapy or at the time of relapse. For instance, individuals with Hodgkin's disease who have received a course of 6 to 8 cycles of combination chemotherapy are subsequently restaged to confirm remission or assess the extent of residual disease. Physical examination and radiography and laboratory examinations, such as scans and bone marrow aspiration and biopsy, are repeated. Particular attention is paid to studies that were positive at diagnosis to search out any remaining evidence that treatment should continue. Restaging does not imply that a person who goes into remission reverts to a lesser stage. The stage at the time of diagnosis is the one that characterizes the illness throughout, even if there is no clinical evidence of disease after treatment.

When there is no objective evidence of decrease in the tumor burden but the person feels better, gains weight, and becomes more active, this is termed a *subjective* response. It represents improvement from the patient's point of view.

In the face of a lack of objective or subjective response, no progression of the disease can be a worthy goal. The criteria for improvement then include (1) to achieve and maintain complete remission of the tumor, (2) to achieve partial remission for varying periods, (3) to keep the disease from progressing, and (4) to help the person feel better. Accurate assessment of the response to treatment is very important.

EVALUATING THE EFFECTIVENESS OF TREATMENT

In oncology it is often difficult to evaluate the comparative efficacy of therapeutic interventions. If a person succumbs after being treated, therapy has clearly failed. On the other hand, normal recovery, with the return of health, weight gain, and the resumption of normal activity, is not conclusive evidence that therapy has been curative. The nature of cancer is such that after an interval of apparently perfect health, the disease may reappear and the person die.

If at autopsy there is no evidence of tumor, a cancer can be said to have been cured. This is the only precise definition of "cure." For obvious reasons, this criterion is not of much practical value. Therefore, most clinicians accept freedom from clinical evidence of recurrent metastatic disease during the person's lifetime as a reasonably reliable estimate.

Cure is also assessed by survival statistics. A time interval is selected that must elapse without evidence of recurrence. The time at which survival can be called cure varies according to how soon after the primary treatment residual disease becomes evident. It is best understood as the time after treatment at which the annual death rate of the treated person is no longer greater than that of the normal population. Because this does not occur for 15 to 20 years after primary treatment in many tumors, 5-year survival rates, which are customary to report the results of treatment, are important only in the more aggressive tumors.

To compare various clinical sites of disease, it must be clear whether "5-year cure" means survival with evidence of tumor or without. Survival times also must be corrected for age by comparison with healthy groups of comparable age distribution.

Follow-up of patients is extremely important for the compilation of conclusive data. An integral part of most hospitals' cancer program is a tumor registry, where data are compiled over time on each person diagnosed with cancer at that institution. These data not only aid in systematic follow-up of individuals with cancer but facilitate the hospital's evaluation of therapy. In addition, many states or regions have cancer data programs in which the information from each individual tumor registry is fed into a larger program. Such a regional cancer database is helpful in examining trends in cancer therapy and patient survival. The widely used standardized methods of reporting the results of therapy go a long way to making such evaluation possible.

WHEN CURE IS NOT ACHIEVED

Should the attempt to "cure" fail and disease recur, there may be a fairly long period during which treatment is aimed at "control." For this reason, cancer is viewed as a chronic disease. In general, the principles of treatment of advanced disease take into consideration the specific diagnosis and the site or sites of the disease, the status of the bone marrow, the status of liver and renal function, the presence of complications due to the tumor, the immunologic status, and the person's general condition.

With some tumors, such as myeloma, cure is not yet an option, and therapy is aimed at control from the onset. In these instances survival can be prolonged and improved with proper treatment. Here, comparison can be made with such chronic illnesses as diabetes or heart disease, where cure is impossible and control is the objective.

If a person is deemed an inappropriate candidate for treatment for cure or control, the next question that must be entertained is: Does the person present symptoms that require palliation? Radiation or even chemotherapy may be quite effective in relieving pain, bleeding, compression, or obstruction of vital organs. A palliative surgical procedure may provide relief from a bulky tumor mass that is impinging on other organs. Palliative treatment should always be used with discretion and based on sound clinical indications because injudicious measures could increase the discomfort of a dying person, be unnecessarily expensive, or deprive the person of precious remaining days or weeks at home. Again, these are often hard decisions to make. Palliative measures may need to be used for people who are asymptomatic in whom the impending development of a catastrophic problem can be predicted, such as obstruction of the superior vena cava or a major bronchus or a collapsing vertebral body due to metastatic disease. Individuals with advanced illness may need palliative treatment aimed more at their emotional well-being than at inducing a remission of the disease. For instance, individuals receiving chemotherapy may insist on continuing their treatments even in the face of obvious disease progression. To these people, hope is maintained through active therapy, even though there may be no physical benefits to the therapy. Although this may conflict with the values and philosophy of the clinician, it can be a crucial factor in doing what is best for an individual.

Aside from these exceptions, palliative treatment of the person who is asymptomatic and incurable is usually deferred until the appearance of specific problems. If these cannot be relieved with simple medication, more aggressive palliative measures can be considered. These individuals should be followed closely to offer emotional support and should be reassured frequently that appropriate palliative therapy will be initiated should the need arise.

CANCER THERAPY IN THE FUTURE

Most clinicians who treat individuals with cancer in their daily practice realize that the present therapeutic methods do not hold the complete answer to the disease. We have already seen how the different methods of treatment have evolved and changed and how they have been integrated into programs of current use. None of these methods is really adequate for this most difficult of diseases. However, until clinicians have more answers from basic science research, there are no alternatives but to proceed with what has been proved to be most effective up to this time.

As the primary therapeutic measure, oncologic surgery may have reached its limit.[12] It is difficult to imagine how more elaborate operations could improve the results presently attainable, except for reconstructive surgery. It is hoped that the experiments with radiotagged antibodies to allow for detection of tumors at earlier stages will make more cures by surgical removal possible in the future. Less extensive surgery may be seen, such as the present tendency to do less extensive mastectomies for breast cancer. Laser surgery and microsurgery bring greater precision to oncologic surgery.

Because any area of the body can only tolerate a certain amount of irradiation, advances in radiotherapy, when used alone, will probably depend on technologic innovations, such as beam-modifying devices. Radiation sensitizers and radioprotectors are being evaluated to enhance the tumoricidal effect of radiation therapy.[13] Intraoperative radiation therapy enables large doses of radiation to be given to less accessible sites. The best hope for the future probably lies in the combined use of surgery, chemotherapy, and radiation therapy in the prophylactic treatment of minimal residual disease.

Refinements in chemotherapy and immunotherapy theoretically also hold promise for the future. In the case of chemotherapy, however, certain major problems must first be solved. Agents are needed that can exploit biologic differences between normal and malignant cells, destroying only those that are harmful. Until this is possible, chemotherapy will be used more and more in combination with other forms of treatment, such as occurs in bone marrow transplantation. The present forms of immunotherapy and other biologic agents in use are still primarily experimental. Clinical trials are currently evaluating the use of immunomodulators. Monoclonal antibodies, the interferons, interleukin 2 and 3, tumor necrosis factor, and granulocyte-macrophage colony-stimulating factors as single agents or in combination hold future promise as therapeutic modalities.[14,15] See Chapter 14 for an in-depth discussion of immunologic therapies.

There is one further dimension of treatment that should be mentioned, that is, the idea of "hope." It is hard to measure objectively the hope that is generated in the individual and family as therapy proceeds. Although not always the case, the observation that treatment enhances hope for the individual can be made again and again in clinical practice. During illness, a person badly needs hope and the feeling that all possible is being done. If the person is participating in a clinical trial, the knowledge that he or she might be helping others may be comforting. Even if the drug or treatment fails to meet expectations, its psychologic value to the person may be inestimable. As a final therapeutic principle, the transmission of an attitude of optimism vis à vis therapy on the clinician's part will greatly benefit the patient, who is usually quite sensitive to the attitudes of caregivers.

REFERENCES

1. Feinstein AR: Clinical Judgement. Baltimore, Williams & Wilkins, 1967.
2. Pack GT, Ariel IM: The history of cancer therapy, in Cancer Management, A special post graduate course on cancer sponsored by the American Cancer Society. Philadelphia, JB Lippincott, 1968.
3. Veronesi U: Principles of cancer surgery, in Holland JF, Frei E (eds): Cancer Medicine. Philadelphia, Lea & Febinger, 1982, pp 555-570.
4. Ahiya RK, Milligan AJ, Dobelbower RR: Radiation therapy in cancer management: principles and complications, in Moossa AR, Martin C, Schimpff SC (eds): Comprehensive Textbook of Oncology. Baltimore, Williams & Wilkins, 1986, pp 257-268.
5. Rosai J, Ackerman LV: The pathology of tumors. III. Ca—A Cancer Journal for Clinicians 29:56-77, 1979.
6. Cox EB, Laszlo J, Freiman A: Classification of cancer patients: beyond TNM. JAMA 242:2691-2695, 1979.
7. Karnofsky DA, Burchenal JH: The clinical evaluation of chemotherapeutic agents in cancer, in MacLeod CM (ed): Evaluation of Chemotherapeutic Agents. New York, Columbia University Press, 1949.
8. Knobf MD, Fischer DS, Welch-McCaffrey D: Cancer Chemotherapy: Treatment and Care. Boston, GK Hall, 1984, pp 15-22.
9. Rubin P: Statement of the clinical oncologic problem, in Rubin P (ed): Clinical Oncology for Medical Students and Physicians (ed 5). New York, American Cancer Society, 1983, pp 2-19.
10. Klastersky J: Adjuvant chemotherapy, in Moossa AR, Martin C, Schimpff SC (eds): Comprehensive Textbook of Oncology. Baltimore, Williams & Wilkins, 1986, pp 239-243.
11. Haskell CM: Principles of cancer chemotherapy, in Haskell CM (ed): Cancer Treatment (ed 2). Philadelphia, WB Saunders, 1985, p 37.
12. Cole JW: Principles and complications of surgical therapy, in Moossa AR, Martin C, Schimpff SC (eds): Comprehensive Textbook of Oncology. Baltimore, Williams & Wilkins, 1986, pp 269-271.
13. Phillips TL: Radiation sensitizers and protectors, in DeVita VT, Hellman S, Rosenberg SA (eds): Cancer: Principles and Practices (ed 2). Philadelphia, JB Lippincott, 1985, pp 2256-2271.
14. Baird S (ed): The biotherapy of cancer. Oncol Nurs Forum 15:2-40, 1988 (suppl).
15. Oldham RK, Smalley RV: Newer methods of cancer treatment, in DeVita VT, Hellman S, Rosenberg SA (eds): Cancer: Principles and Practices (ed 2). Philadelphia, JB Lippincott, 1985, pp 2223-2234.

Chapter 11

Surgical Therapy

Margaret Hansen Frogge, RN, MS

Michelle Goodman, RN, MS

INTRODUCTION

The natural history of cancer is such that the initial treatment plan, whether single approach or multimodal therapy, is the critical opportunity to cure a person with cancer. Once disease recurs, cure is unlikely. Surgery is the treatment of choice for many tumors, but current understanding of tumor biology and advances in interdisciplinary cancer management have changed the reliance on surgery as the only form of curative therapy for cancer and precipitated a change in the magnitude of surgical resections. Approximately 55% of all individuals with cancer are treated with surgical intervention. Of the 40% that are treated by surgery alone, one third are cured.[1] By using combinations of surgery, chemotherapy, radiotherapy, or immunotherapy, disease-free intervals have been significantly lengthened. Surgery can be used for prevention, diagnosis, definitive treatment, rehabilitation, or palliation.

Recent advances in surgical oncology have been greatest in preoperative assessment, intraoperative management, and postoperative care.[2] Major improvements in surgical techniques include use of lasers and surgical stapling devices.[3-6]

FACTORS INFLUENCING THE SELECTION OF SURGERY FOR THE TREATMENT OF CANCER

Tumor Cell Kinetics

An understanding of the biology and natural history of individual tumors is fundamental to the surgical treatment of cancer. Tumor cell characteristics such as growth rate, differentiation, metastatic potential, and metastatic pattern affect the teatment decision. It was once thought that cancer was essentially a mass of uncontrolled, rapidly proliferating cells that extended into surrounding tissues and lymph nodes and inevitably reached the circulatory system. With this in mind, surgeons felt that time was of the essence in curing cancer and that the lymph nodes had to be included in any resection because metastatic extensions would rest there. With these ideas guiding surgeons to extend the surgical margin and resect more tissue, extensive radical procedures such as hemicorporectomies and radical mastectomies were performed with better but still disappointing results. Such radical procedures have failed to significantly increase cure rates.[1,7-10]

In the past 20 years, an explosion of knowledge in the field of tumor biology has led clinicians to recognize that interdisciplinary collaboration and treatment planning is necessary to select the most effective treatment method for cancer. Oncology practitioners must have an understanding of the potential of surgery, chemotherapy, radiation, and immunotherapy to select the most effective course of therapy intelligently.[11] The factors that affect the decision of whether an individual with cancer should be treated by surgery will be discussed in the following sections.

Growth rate

The rate of growth of a tumor is expressed in terms of volume-doubling time. The time it takes for a tumor mass to double in size depends on the cell cycle activity of proliferating cells comprising the tumor; the growth fraction, or number of cells that are proliferating in the tumor; and the rate of cell loss from the tumor. In general, tumors that are slow growing and consist of cells with prolonged cell cycles lend themelves best to surgical treatment because these types of tumors are more likely to be confined locally.

Invasiveness

Any cancer cell remaining after treatment constitutes a potential risk for recurrence or metastasis if that cell is capable of proliferating. Therefore, a surgical procedure that is intended to be curative must involve resection of the entire tumor mass and normal tissue surrounding the tumor to ensure a margin of safety for removal of all cancer cells. Some cancers (eg, melanomas) invade deeply into adjacent tissues, thus requiring extensive surgical procedures to remove the tumor mass or making surgery an impractical treatment option. Other tumors, such as basal cell carcinoma or chondrosarcomas, are highly coherent and are more amenable to complete surgical excision. Local, less radical procedures are performed for particular tumors where research has demonstrated an equally effective result compared with radical surgery.[10,12-15]

Metastatic potential

The initial operation performed for removal of a cancer has a better chance for success than a subsequent operation performed for a recurrence; thus, knowledge of metastatic patterns of individual tumors is crucial for planning the most effective therapy.

Some tumors metastasize late or not at all and, even if advanced, may be cured by aggressive therapy. Other tumors predictably metastasize to local or regional sites, and cure may be achieved by a procedure that involves removal of the primary tumor-bearing organ and the involved adjacent tumor sites or lymph nodes. Some tumors are known to metastasize early. In such cases surgery may not be warranted (eg, lung cancer), or surgery may be used to remove all visible tumor in preparation for adjuvant system therapy or after a number of courses of chemotherapy to resect remaining disease (eg, testicular cancer).[12-14,16,17]

Subclinical metastasis or occult disease is responsible for most recurrences when surgery is the only treatment used. It is now believed that micrometastases are present in 50% of individuals by the time a tumor is large enough to be detected clinically.[18] Interdisciplinary planning and selection of the most appropriate treatment methods are important to improve survival and to lower an individual's risk of systemic metastasis.[19]

Tumor Location

Once the location and extent of the tumor are determined through diagnostic and staging procedures, the clinician can assess the structural and functional changes that can be expected as a result of the surgical procedure. This assessment will assist the clinician and patient and family in weighing the benefits and risks involved in treatment. In some cases the decision to treat an individual's cancer with surgery may rest solely on whether the tumor involves vital structures. Superficial and encapsulated tumors are more easily resected than those that are embedded in inaccessible or delicate tissues or those that have invaded tissues in multiple directions.

Physical Status

Careful preoperative assessment is critical for evaluating the significant factors that would potentially increase the risk of surgical morbidity and mortality. In-depth evaluation of respiratory, cardiovascular, nutritional, immunologic, renal, hydration, and central nervous system (CNS) status are important. The severity of the underlying illness and comorbid conditions are considered in the decision regarding surgical therapy. The health care team assesses the patient's rehabilitation potential, particularly if the intended surgery will significantly alter normal physiologic function. In some cases the intended surgical procedure may produce physiologic alterations that are beyond that particular person's capabilities. The elderly often experience effects of aging that limit their dexterity and ability to manage difficult surgical deficits.[20] Since cancer incidence is much greater in elderly patients, age can be a factor to weigh in the treatment decision. In general, elderly patients have a higher surgical risk than younger patients. However, the elderly patient should also be treated as aggressively as possible but may require additional preoperative support (eg, hyperalimentation, blood products). Elderly patients with cancer do not appear to have a higher risk or complication rate than their age-related cohorts.[2]

Quality of Life

The goal of therapy for the person with cancer varies according to the stage of disease. Selection of the treatment approach includes consideration of the quality of the individual's life when treatment is complete. Research has shown that some radical surgical procedures are not warranted either because they do not improve the end result or because they interfere unduly with the person's functional or psychological well-being. Multidisciplinary planning that includes the individual with cancer and family will facilitate the selection of a treatment plan tailored to that individual's unique needs and desires.

SURGERY IN THE PREVENTION OF CANCER

Certain conditions, genetic or congenital traits, and diseases are known to be associated with a higher risk of developing cancer. In some instances, surgical removal of a nonvital benign tissue or organ that is responsible for predisposing the individual to higher risk can lower incidence and possibly prevent occurrence of cancer. Polyposis is an excellent example of a condition that increases the individual's risk for developing colon cancer. Surgical excision of colon polyps is a relatively simple preventive procedure to reduce the person's risk for colon cancer. Another more complex situation is that of women who have a high risk for breast cancer. After careful review and thorough explanation, some women may benefit from prophylactic mastectomy to lower significantly the risk of breast cancer. The role of surgery in cancer prevention is somewhat limited at this time; however, future epidemiologic and etiologic findings may indicate a more extensive role for surgery.

SURGERY IN THE DIAGNOSIS OF CANCER

Each type of cancer responds differently to therapy; therefore, a histologic diagnosis is crucial to selecting effective treatment. Surgical techniques such as endoscopy, needle aspiration, incisional biopsy, excisional biopsy, or needle biopsy are frequently used to obtain tissue specimens for histologic examination.

An adequate biopsy requires careful planning by the physician. The biopsy specimen should contain normal cells and tumor cells for comparison; it should be intact and not crushed or contaminated; and it should be labeled and preserved properly for complete evaluation. An important principle to note in the diagnosis of cancer is that only positive biopsy findings are definitive. A negative biopsy finding can mean no cancer, but it can also mean that the biopsy specimen was not representative of the tumor. If a high index of suspicion for cancer exists, another biopsy technique may be in order.

Before selecting the most appropriate biopsy technique, the surgeon will consider the possible treatment regimens that will be used if cancer is diagnosed. Because tumor cells can contaminate the biopsy site, tracts, or new tissue planes, either the biopsy site should be placed so that it will be removed at surgery or the biopsy itself should contain the tumor in toto.[20] If multiple biopsies are to be taken, instruments that may have contacted the tumor should not be used for other sites. Aesthetic results are also considered during biopsy so that incision lines and subsequent incisions will be located in cosmetically acceptable areas or folds if possible.

Use of incisional, excisional, aspiration, or needle biopsy depends on tumor size, location, and growth characteristics. Possible complications following any biopsy are bleeding, hematoma, infection, dehiscence, or tumor cell seeding. Individuals should be instructed about biopsy site care and recognition of complications.

Incisional Biopsy

Incisional biopsy is a careful and delicate procedure performed to secure a wedge of tumor tissue. Incisional biopsies are generally selected to diagnose large tumors that will require major surgery for complete removal. The biopsy is usually performed at the tumor margin so that the sample contains both normal and abnormal tissue. Incisional biopsies are often small incisions placed in a position to be completely excised by subsequent definitive surgical procedures.

Excisional Biopsy

Excisional biopsy is performed on small, accessible tumors to remove the entire mass and little or no margin of surrounding normal tissue. In some cases, such as tumors of the lip, nose, ear, or breast, excisional biopsy alone will be definitive therapy. The pathologist and surgeon will determine whether the extent of the excisional biopsy is sufficient to eliminate the possibility of residual disease or whether more extensive surgery is indicated.

Aspiration Biopsy

Aspiration biopsy is a method using a carefully guided needle to aspirate cells or tissue from a suspicious lesion. If the aspiration biopsy yields a tentative diagnosis of malignancy, further definitive biopsy is usually performed before aggressive therapy is initiated. Needle aspiration specimens can be erroneously interpreted more frequently than other types of biopsies.

Needle Biopsy

Needle biopsy is performed during surgery or with the percutaneous technique, which does not require open surgery. Needle biopsy is done with local or topical anesthesia. A needle is inserted through the skin into the tumor site, where a core of tissue is obtained. An unfortunate limitation of needle biopsy is the possibility that the tumor will be missed; therefore, only a positive finding of malignancy is diagnostically significant.[21] Various types of biopsy needles are used. Some have carrier needles that shield and guide the actual biopsy needle, cup, or punch used to obtain the specimen. The purpose of the carrier is to reduce the possibility of contaminating the needle tract with tumor cells from the specimen as the needle is withdrawn.

Endoscopy

Endoscopy is a surgical technique that is used for diagnosis of tumors in accessible lumen. Tumors of the gastrointestinal, genitourinary, or pulmonary system can be diagnosed by inserting an optical instrument into the lumen to examine the area and secure a biopsy or secretions. Flexible instruments have made endoscopy more tolerable for the patient and more functional for the clinician.

SURGERY IN THE STAGING OF CANCER

Surgical procedures have a significant role in the diagnosis of cancer and in defining the extent of tumor involvement. For example, staging laparotomy is an important diagnostic measure for lymphomas. At laparotomy, liver and lymph nodes are biopsied and a splenectomy is performed. Clips are sometimes placed to define the tumor and mark specific areas for radiotherapy and evaluation of treatment response.

Exploratory surgical procedures can be done to diagnose most intracavitary tumors or to define the extent of tumor growth, size, nodal involvement, implants, or multiorgan involvement.

The Amerian Joint Committee for Cancer Staging and End Results Reporting has developed a system for staging many cancers by site. The TNM classification defines the extent of solid tumors based on size and local extension (T), the presence or absence of nodal involvement (N), and the presence or absence of distant metastasis (M) and degree of organ dysfunction. This classification can be used to classify the disease before, during, and following therapy (see Chapter 9 for more details on the TNM system).

Clinical diagnostic staging (cTNM) is accomplished by physical examination, laboratory studies, radiographic studies, cytologic examination, and other select diagnostic procedures. With these data, the clinician is able to determine the stage and classification of a tumor before initiating therapy or definitive treatment. Easily accessible tumors, such as those of the cervix or larynx, are often evaluated in this manner.

Surgical evaluative staging (sTNM) is reserved for tumors that are inaccessible, difficult to evaluate, or inadequately staged by any other means. For example, surgical evaluation staging is useful in evaluating tumors of the stomach, ovary, lung, and pancreas.

Postsurgical-pathologic staging (pTNM) is used to define the tumor following therapeutic surgical resection and pathologic examination. If residual tumor is suspected or confirmed, it will be noted.

This histopathologic analysis and grade of the tumor are other important determinants in tumor classification. Descriptions of staging and classification of each tumor are included throughout this text.

Before definitive diagnosis, or staging, the person with cancer will probably experience profound anxiety, which can be alleviated or reduced to some extent by astute nursing care. It is important to assess the possible factors that could contribute to anxiety, such as previous hospitalizations, experience with other persons with cancer, influence of the mass media, and formal and informal sources of information.[22] The nurse should consider the person's understanding of the diagnostic procedures and the significance of the findings. Does the person have a general understanding of the procedures, what to expect, and how he or she will feel afterward?

Although information-seeking is considered a healthy coping mechanism, only the patient can cue the nurse on how much information is adequate. Assessing the individual's learning needs will allow the nurse to teach the patient what he or she should know about the diagnostic procedure. Visual aids, pamphlets, slide tapes, and group sessions are all supplementary teaching techniques that have met with good results.

SURGERY IN THE TREATMENT OF CANCER

After diagnosis, staging, and classification of the tumor, the interdisciplinary oncology team will choose the most appropriate plan and sequence of therapy. The goal of therapy will be based on a collation of the patient's desires, general condition, and tumor stage and classification. The sequence and methods used will be guided by the most effective treatment protocols presently available for that particular tumor type. Surgical intervention may be the definitive treatment or may be part of a sequence of multimodal therapy. Preoperative chemotherapy or radiotherapy are used for some tumors, such as head and neck cancers.

Preoperative considerations include a thorough patient and family history and physical examination. Assessments are made of life-style, habits, concomitant disease, general physical condition, nutritional status, hematologic status, and pulmonary status. Measures to improve the patient's overall status are initiated before surgery whenever possible.[23] In addition, an assessment of the patient's understanding of the surgery and rehabilitation should be completed. Involving the patient's family in preoperative teaching will often facilitate understanding and reduce anxiety.

Surgery Aimed at Cure

Advances in understanding of cancer biology have changed the surgical approach from the "more is better" concept to an approach that considers tissue and functional preservation and relies more on effective use of radiotherapy, chemotherapy, or immunotherapy. Tumors that are solid, accessible, and have relatively well-defined margins can generally be surgically excised. Several cardinal surgical principles guide the surgical oncologist[16]:

1. Surgery should not be done if the end result or potential impairment is unsuitable to and for the individual.
2. The patient understands and agrees that the surgeon will do as much surgery as necessary to eradicate the tumor and as little surgery as possible within that premise.
3. Maximum exposure of the tumor facilitates adequate accessibility and margins for resection without leaving residual tumor. A bloodless surgical field is important for gross observation of the tumor at all times.
4. Human tissue is friable and is handled delicately, especially if the area has been previously irradiated. The "no-touch" technique minimizes seeding, contamination of new tissue planes, and local recurrence.
5. Free tumor cells in the operative site can be a source of recurrent or metastatic disease. Careful surgical techniques such as glove changes, instrument cleaning, and extensive wound irrigation with cytotoxic agents (eg, 5% formaldehyde, hypotonic saline) will help reduce the risk of local recurrence.
6. Successful surgical resection for cure depends on the ability to resect the tumor en bloc with an adequate tumor-free border. This ensures a margin of safety of normal tissue. Surgical skill and patience in defining the entire tumor boundaries are requisite.
7. Reconstruction and rehabilitation are essential components of quality cancer therapy.

Excision of primary tumors

The type of surgical procedure selected for curative treatment of primary tumors depends on the specific tumor cell characteristics and site of involvement. In the preoperative period, the surgeon is challenged to identify those patients who will be treated best by local or extensive surgery and to select the surgery and adjuvant therapies that will control local and distant disease.[20]

Local excision is used to resect small lesions where the entire tumor and a margin of safety can be encompassed. Tumors of the ear, skin, or lip are typical areas where local excision can provide definitive therapy. Hemostasis and infection are the major postoperative concerns. Aseptic measures and prophylactic antibiotics provide control.

The magnitude of the surgical approach for many tumors has been greatly modified in recent years. A better understanding of the biology and natural history of specific cancers combined with advances in adjuvant treatment modalities have led to less radical surgeries for some cancers. Breast cancer is probably the best example of a tumor that is approached much differently now, especially from the surgical perspective.[10]

Major surgical resections are performed when the tumor is surgically accessible, and there is hope that the tumor can be resected en bloc along with the necessary local or regional tissues and lymphatics. All the surgical principles outlined previously apply. Before recommending a surgical resection of the tumor for cure, the physician will undertake a search for evidence of distant metastasis. This metastatic workup is important for accurate staging of disease. Such a time can be difficult for the patient because the chance for cure is debated during this time. Surgical resections can greatly alter the person's body image as well as the structure and function of the person's body. Extensive surgery may be needed if the disease is to be eradicated and the person given the chance to live a normal life span. There are obvious tradeoffs and concessions that the person with cancer must acknowledge. Striking a balance between length of life and quality of life is a major challenge in surgical oncology.

During the preoperative period, the nurse instructs the individual on what to expect in the postoperative period so that the person is aware of and can contribute to expected outcomes. Discussion of nursing management and rehabilitation of the person following various surgical procedures are included in Part VI on the management of specific malignancies.

Excision of metastatic lesions

Surgery also may be done to resect a metastatic lesion if the primary tumor is believed to be eradicated, if the metastatic site is solitary, and if the patient can undergo surgery without major morbidity. Resection of the metastatic lesion is not indicated if there is evidence of additional metastatic disease or if the metastatic lesion is particularly aggressive or inaccessible. A solitary pulmonary lesion, liver lesion, or a cerebral mass are examples of metastatic sites that may be amenable to resection with a curative intent.[20]

Metastasis from primary tumors of unknown origin are another example of how surgery may be employed for optimal tumor control. It is not uncommon for a primary tumor to remain undetected for many years. When the only identifiable site of the disease is the metastasis, it is reasonable to manage the person's disease in an aggressive manner, particularly if the metastatic disease is life threatening. The decision to treat the metastasis in an aggressive manner is made only after a thorough search is conducted for the primary tumor. These particular circumstances create uncertainty and anxiety for the patient and family.

Surgery and adjuvant therapies

Surgery is local treatment and is therefore limited in what can be accomplished. Surgery was once the sole therapy for many solid tumors such as carcinoma of the breast, colon, and head and neck. Survival rates for these cancers and others have not been satisfactory with surgery alone. For this reason, combination or adjuvant therapies are being used to improve the rates of cure and disease-free survival. Adjuvant therapy can be given preoperatively, intraoperatively, or postoperatively. Surgery may be combined with radiotherapy for local tumor control. Chemotherapy is given to provide systemic control of micrometastases and distant metastases. In some situations, surgery is used to debulk or reduce the tumor mass to a size where radiation or chemotherapy can be most effective.[16] Ovarian cancer is often approached in this manner, since it is usually spread throughout the peritoneum at diagnosis and debulking procedures improve therapeutic results. The individual may undergo definitive therapy for months or even years. This adjuvant approach to the treatment of the person with cancer requires a multidisciplinary team effort.

Surgery Aimed at Palliation

Many surgical procedures are performed for the palliation of the debilitating manifestations of cancer. These procedures are aimed at controlling the cancer and improving the quality of life for the person with cancer, even when all the cancer cannot be removed. If the quality of the person's life cannot be improved as a result of the surgery, then the surgery is not warranted. If the surgery carries an unnecessary risk of morbidity or mortality, it is also not indicated. Issues such as biologic pace of the disease, the person's life expectancy, and expected outcome of the palliative procedure all require careful consideration if the person is to benefit from the procedure. Open communication between the patient, family, and physician is of paramount importance. The patient must know the goals of the procedure and have a realistic understanding of the expected outcome. If the person's hope is unrealistic, the potential disappointment experienced postoperatively can be devastating. For instance, consider the person experiencing chronic pain who is offered a surgical procedure that can possibly alleviate suffering. It is more compassionate to ensure that the person understands and accepts that the pain may be relieved only temporarily rather than indefinitely. The person who lives with cancer knows well the meaning of palliation. Clinicians should always respect the courage and will of the individual with uncontrolled cancer and promote his or her active participation in the plan of care.

The goal of palliative surgery is to relieve suffering and minimize the symptoms of the disease. For example, palliative surgery may involve removal of a tumor that has become ulcerative and a likely source of infection or the amputation of a nonfunctioning, painful limb with sarcoma. Some tumors are slow growing, and although metastatic sites are evident and the person is technically incurable, resection of the primary tumor is warranted to prevent future complications such as bleeding or obstruction. Several surgical techniques are used for palliation of cancer: fulgeration, electrocoagulation, lasers, photodynamic therapy, shunts, and bone stabilization procedures.[2,24]

Palliative procedures are not undertaken unless the clinician is reasonably confident that the wound will heal. For example, surgery is contraindicated for the person who has a local recurrence and lung metastasis following radiotherapy to an oropharyngeal lesion. In this case a surgical wound would probably not heal without extensive skin flap reconstruction, which would not be warranted in view of the distant metastasis.

Alleviation of obstruction

Palliative surgery is particularly useful in relieving suffering caused by an obstructive process. Obstruction occurs in the respiratory, gastrointestinal, or urinary system. For example, a tumor of the hypopharynx can obstruct the upper aerodigestive tract, resulting in respiratory compromise, malnutrition, and weight loss. Surgical interventions such as a tracheostomy will restore airway patency, and a gastrostomy tube will facilitate adequate nutrition. Through palliative procedures, the individual can be maintained nutritionally while therapy is initiated to control the primary disease.

Decompression of vital structures

Tumors also may compress vital structures. A large portion of a brain tumor that is causing neurologic deficits may be resected and the residual primary tumor controlled with radiation, chemotherapy, and steroids. A decompression laminectomy to relieve spinal cord compression caused by a metastatic tumor is another example of surgical palliation. The goal is to prevent paraplegia, decrease morbidity, and increase the quality of life.[25]

Control of pain

Palliative surgery is useful for pain control. Solid tumors can cause pain when they grow large enough to displace other organs or tissues. Palliative surgical debulking can temporarily alleviate such debilitating pain.

The surgical interruption of nerve pathways to control pain may be instituted to provide maximum comfort. Neurosurgical approaches to pain control are generally not undertaken unless the person's pain cannot be controlled by noninvasive measures and the source of the person's pain is in an area that is amenable to surgical interruption of nerve pathways. These procedures may be performed at the level of a peripheral nerve (nerve block), a dorsal nerve root (rhizotomy), spinothalamic tract (cordotomy), or by a direct approach to the thalamus. See Chapter 20 for detailed discussion of surgical procedures for pain control.

Surgery for Rehabilitation

Although surgical procedures have long been used to treat cancer, their use in rehabilitation of individuals with cancer is fairly recent. Today great emphasis is being placed on the quality of life for the person with cancer. With this emphasis has come an effort to develop techniques to restore an individual to as near a normal life as possible following surgery for cancer. Cosmetic or functional success has been achieved through breast reconstruction following mastectomy, facial reconstruction after head and neck surgery, and skin grafting following major resections for melanoma, to name a few.

Rehabilitation potential is considered before initiation of primary therapy. Careful interdisciplinary planning will assist the clinician to prepare the person emotionally and physically for both the primary treatment and subsequent rehabilitation. In preparing an indivdiual for rehabilitation, the clinician strikes a fine balance between optimism and realism. Rehabilitative teaching and counseling generally are begun before primary surgical therapy is initiated. Some people fear that their desire for rehabilitative surgical procedures will be interpreted as valuing their physical appearance or function as more important than the length of their life. Nurses can assist the patient to see that rehabilitation is desirable and sometimes necessary for achieving the highest possible level of functioning.

Rehabilitative success is measured not only by cosmetic improvement but also by improvements in function and self-esteem. As rehabilitative techniques improve, more people with cancer will select and enjoy the benefits of surgical rehabilitation.

NURSING CARE OF THE INDIVIDUAL UNDERGOING SURGERY FOR THE TREATMENT OF CANCER

Nursing care of the person with cancer undergoing surgery is much the same as that for an individual undergoing non-cancer-related major surgery. Nurses should be acutely aware of problems that can occur as a result of the cancer disease process itself, as well as possible postoperative complications. The person with cancer is cared for with a keen eye to the following complications, which are common to this disease.

Nutrition

The nutritionally debilitated person with cancer is a poor surgical risk and often cannot undergo major surgery without preoperative correction of the underlying nutritional deficit. Because of the nutritional deficit, the individual also might not be a candidate for adjuvant therapy either.

When subjected to a major stress such as surgical trauma or infection, the undernourished person is often unable to adapt with preservation of lean body mass and will develop a negative nitrogen balance. As a result, the individual is at risk for poor wound healing, infection, pneumonia, and increased morbidity.[26,27] An important principle in the management of the malnourished surgical cancer patient is that the nutritional management should be first aimed at reversing protein calorie malnutrition and preventing weight loss. Once this is accomplished, the nutrition plan should be as aggressive as the anticancer plan. It is generally agreed that people who are nutritionally compromised should receive preoperative enteral or parenteral nutritional support, since studies have shown reductions in postoperative complications and surgical mortality from nutritional support of individuals preoperatively.[28] Specific nursing measures to improve nutritional status of patients are discussed in Chapter 24.

Hemostasis

Another common manifestation of cancer that can significantly increase the risk of postoperative complications is altered hemostasis, especially hypercoagulability and thrombosis.[29] Elevated clotting factors and shortened partial thromboplastin and prothrombin times have been noted to occur in individuals with cancer.

The person with cancer therefore is highly susceptible to minor changes in the hemostatic process. A person with cancer is more likely to develop postoperative thrombophlebitis than is a person witihout cancer. Other malignancies most commonly associated with recurrent deep vein thrombosis are pancreas, brain, lung, and stomach cancer and mucinous adenocarcinomas.

The nursing managment of the individual with cancer undergoing surgery is based on accurate assessment of hemodynamic parameters and an understanding of the implications of abnormalities in clotting factors, which can result in bleeding tendencies and hemorrhage.

The importance of early postoperative ambulation cannot be overemphasized. Because these individuals are at high risk for deep vein thrombosis, the nurse observes the patient for signs and symptoms of this disorder. Bleeding abnormalities in individuals with cancer are discussed in more detail in Chapter 22.

Complications of Multimodal Therapy

The multimodal treatment of cancer has introduced a new set of challenges for health care providers in surgical oncology. Chemotherapy, radiation therapy, and immunotherapy are now being given for certain tumors in various sequences: preoperative, intraoperative, and postoperative. The interactive and compounding effect of these therapies produces sometimes difficult problems and side effects to manage.

Preoperative chemotherapy or radiotherapy, alone or in combination, is being used more frequently with particular tumors that have better response rates when multimodal therapy is sequenced in this manner, especially tumors of the head and neck.[13,14] The timing and extent of surgery may require modification following radiation or chemotherapy depending on the individual's response to therapy and the side effects experienced. Sometimes, surgical procedures become necessary during active radiation or chemotherapy, such as inserting vascular access devices, relieving obstructions, or repairing perforations.

Intraoperative radiotherapy and intraoperative chemotherapy are being researched for their potential to decrease recurrence. Intraoperative radiotherapy and chemotherapy is a method used to deliver a single, high dose directly to the surgically exposed tumor or tumor bed. Intraoperative therapy requires extensive multidisciplinary collaboration. Patient and staff safety are carefully considered. Potential side effects of intraoperative therapy are not yet fully known but appear to be similar to traditional delivery methods. Intraoperative treatments, used predominantly in major cancer centers, are administered for locally advanced abdominal and pelvic malignancies. Gastric, pancreatic, ovarian, bladder, and colorectal are a few of the tumor types being investigated.[30]

A major challenge in multimodal therapy is the problem of postoperative wound healing in the person who has previously received radiation to the surgical site. Radiation may cause long-term damage to the underlying tissues such as fibrosis and obliteration of lymphatic and vascular channels.[31] Once the integrity of the tissue is damaged by radiation, additional traumas are not tolerated well. Postoperative wound dehiscence, infection, and tissue and bone necrosis are potential complications that can occur when surgery is performed on previously irradiated tissue.

In some cases, it becomes necessary or highly desirable to initiate chemotherapy early in the immediate postoperative period. There are questions regarding the appropriate timing and effects of specific chemotherapeutic agents on wound healing. Methotrexate, 5-fluorouracil (5-FU) doxorubicin, and corticosteroids have been shown to modify the process of wound healing at specific times during the postoperative period.[27,32] Bleomycin administered intraoperatively causes a decrease in fascial wound-bursting strength up to 7 days postoperatively but has no detrimental effect when given after the seventh postoperative day.[27,32] Supratherapeutic doses of doxorubicin diminish fascial wound-bursting strength if administered before wound healing occurs.[27] Increased morbidity due to abnormal wound healing can occur if 5-FU is given before the 14th postoperative day. Corticosteroids administered in the perioperative period lead to decreased granulation tissue and epithelialization and delayed wound contracture. Perioperative corticosteroid administration reduces the wound inflammatory response, delays fibroplasia, and results in increased local wound complications.

Given the trend toward more aggressive chemotherapy and radiotherapy, wound healing may become a significant problem in the future, since wound strength and integrity can be affected by certain antineoplastic agents and radiation doses. Such information points to the need for further research to determine the optimal doses and timing sequence for multimodal therapy.

The nurse should be aware of the overall plan for therapy, particularly the type and extent of treatment before surgery. This will enable the nurse to anticipate and take measures to minimize the predictable postoperative complications that can occur as a result of multimodal therapy.

Certain chemotherapeutic agents are toxic to specific organ systems, resulting in long-term side effects that can increase the individual's risk of surgical complications. For example, bleomycin therapy given before surgery may predispose the person to postoperative development of an acute adult respiratory distress syndrome. Bleomycin can cause interstitial fibrosis and thus increase intraoperative and postoperative pulmonary complications. Preoperatively, individuals previously treated with bleomycin should undergo pulmonary function tests to determine functional lung capacity and to define the potential risk for anesthesia and the appropriate anesthesia and oxygen concentration to be used during surgery. In most cases, fluid restriction, diuretics, and aggressive pulmonary hygiene can prevent interstitial pulmonary edema associated with prior bleomycin therapy. Methotrexate and busulfan are two other drugs that can produce a diffuse interstitial and alveolar pneumonitis. Cis-platinum (cisplatin), streptozocin, and methotrexate can result in a persistent decrease in glomerular filtration rate (GFR) due to renal tubular damage. The patient is at risk for further impairment of renal function at surgery if the GFR is not maintained. The anesthesiologist and surgeon will take special precautions during and following surgery to ensure adequate kidney function. Nephrotoxic anesthetics are avoided in these individuals. During and after surgery, mannitol may be infused to provide an adequate GFR and diuresis. Intravascular fluid volume is monitored with central venous pressure readings. In the postoperative period, the nurse pays particular attention to the individual's fluid balance to ensure adequate kidney perfusion and output. A rise in blood urea nitrogen (BUN) and creatinine levels coupled with decreased urinary creatinine clearance can signal deterioration of kidney function.

Other drugs used commonly in the treatment of a variety of neoplasms are the anthracyclines, doxorubicin, and daunorubicin (daunomycin). A cumulative dose of 500 mg/m^2 or more of either of these drugs increases the risk of intraoperative and postoperative congestive heart failure and pulmonary edema. Before surgery, the person undergoes testing of left ventricular function to assess the level of cardiac function. During surgery, the individual's fluid balance is managed carefully. A preoperative dose of digitalis may be given to strengthen ventricular contractility. A Swan-Ganz catheter may be needed to monitor physiologic parameters intraoperatively and postoperatively. If the individual has had prior mediastinal irradiation as well as an anthracycline, the risk of cardiomyopathy is greater.

These are but a few examples of the types of complications that can occur in the individual with cancer undergoing surgery as a result of prior therapy. The nurse must be alert to the need for a thorough history of drug therapy and possess knowledge of the implications of such therapy.

CONCLUSION

Surgery for cancer is the oldest form of cancer therapy still in use; however, there have been advances and changes in the scope and reliance on surgical therapy. Surgery continues to be the mainstay of effective cancer treatment for many tumors. Current knowledge of cancer biology and the natural history and progression of certain tumors has caused the role of surgery to be questioned and modified in many instances. Radical surgery is still a reasonable and valid approach for several tumor types. It is not a reasonable approach for others, however. Breast cancer is the most profound example of modified surgical approaches.[8]

Surgery is now frequently combined with multimodal therapy including chemotherapy, radiation therapy, or immunotherapy. Adjuvant therapy can lengthen survival and disease-free intervals and improve the quality of life. There are three potential sequences for introduction of adjuvant therapy: preoperative, intraoperative, and postoperative. The potential side effects and complications of surgery and adjuvant therapy present new challenges to health care practitioners.

Prospective clinical research that includes active participation of surgical practitioners is sorely needed.[8,12,34-37] Effective surgical cancer therapy depends on a solid integration of the biologic and clinical sciences of cancer. In addition to important strides in the understanding of the biology of cancer, clinicians have learned a great deal about the educational, psychological, social, and rehabilitative needs of individuals undergoing surgical procedures for cancer therapy.[37,38]

REFERENCES

1. Morton DL, Sparks FC, Haskel CM: Oncology, in Swartz SI (ed): Principles of Surgery (ed 4). New York, McGraw-Hill, 1984.
2. Patterson WB: Surgical issues in geriatric oncology. Semin Oncol 16:57-65, 1989.
3. Burke TW, Weiser EB, Hoskins WJ, et al: End colostomy using the end-to-end anastomosis instrument. Obstet Gynecol 69:156-159, 1987.
4. Penalver M, Averette H, Sevin BU, et al: Gastrointestinal surgery in gynecologic oncology: evaluation of surgical techniques. Gynecol Oncol 28:74-82, 1987.
5. Aronoff BL: State of the art of lasers in oncologic surgery. Semin Surg Oncol 5:3-5, 1989.
6. Bandiermonte G, Chiesa F, Lupi M, et al: The use of laser in microsurgical oncology. Microsurgery 7:95-101, 1986.
7. Eilber FR: Principles of cancer surgery, in Haskell CM (ed): Cancer treatment (ed 2). Philadelphia, WB Saunders, 1985.
8. Herfarth C: Advances in surgical oncology—introduction. World J Surg 11:405, 1987.
9. Jeekel J: Can radical surgery improve survival in colorectal cancer? World J Surg 11:412-417, 1987.
10. Veronisi U: Rationale and indications for limited surgery in breast cancer. World J Surg 11:493-498, 1987.
11. Hutchinson WB: The surgeon's future role in the conquest of cancer. J Surg Oncol 34:73-75, 1987.
12. Douglass HO: Adjuvant treatment in colorectal cancer: an update. World J Surg 11:478-492, 1987.
13. Schuller DE, Laramore G, Al-Sarraf M, et al: Combined therapy for resectable head and neck cancer. Arch Otolaryngol Head Neck Surg 115:364-368, 1989.
14. Shepard FA, Ginsberg RJ, Patterson GA, et al: A prospective study of adjuvant surgical resection after chemotherapy for

limited small cell lung cancer. J Thorac Cardiovasc Surg 97:177-186, 1989.
15. Schwartz GF, D'Ugo DM, Rosenberg AL: Extent of axillary dissection preceding irradiation for carcinoma of the breast. Arch Surg 121:1395-1398, 1986.
16. Silberman AW: Surgical debulking of tumors. Surg Gynecol Obstet 155:577-585, 1982.
17. Hereber G, Denecke H, Demmel N, et al: Local procedures in the management of rectal cancer. World J Surg 11:499-503, 1987.
18. Liotta LA: Mechanisms of cancer invasion and metastasis, in DeVita VT, Hellman S, Rosenberg SA (eds): Important Advances in Oncology. Philadelphia: JB Lippincott, 1985.
19. Enker WE, Heilwell M, Janoy AJ, et al: Improved survival in epidermoid carcinoma of the anus in association with preoperative multidisciplinary therapy. Arch Surg 121:1386-1390, 1986.
20. Rosenberg SA: Principles of surgical oncology, in DeVita VT, Hellman S, Rosenberg SA (eds): Cancer: Principles and Practice of Oncology (ed 3). Philadelphia, JB Lippincott, 1989, pp 236-246.
21. McDonald TW, Shepard JH, Morley GW, et al: Role of needle biopsy in the investigation of gynecologic malignancy. J Reproduct Med 32:287-292, 1987.
22. Martocchio BC: Family coping: helping families help themselves. Semin Oncol Nurs 1:294-295, 1985.
23. Wilson RE: Surgical oncology. Cancer 54:2595-2598, 1984.
24. Russin DJ, Kaplan SR, Goldberg RI, et al: Neodymium-YAG laser. Arch Surg 121:1399-1403, 1986.
25. Klein PW: Neurologic emergencies in oncology. Semin Oncol Nurs 1:278-284, 1985.
26. Shiplacoff TA: Concepts in surgical oncology, in Vredevoe DL (ed): Concepts of Oncology Nursing. Englewood Cliffs, NJ, Prentice-Hall, 1981.
27. Falcone RE, Nappi JF: Chemotherapy and wound healing. Surg Clin North Am 64:779-794, 1984.
28. Mueller JM, Dienst C, Brenner U, et al: Preoperative intravenous feeding in patients with gastrointestinal carcinoma. Lancet 1:68, 1982.
29. Kempin S, Gould-Rossbach P, Houland WS: Disorders of hemostasis in the critically ill cancer patient, in Howland WS, Carlon GC (eds): Critical Care of the Cancer Patient. Chicago, Year Book, 1985.
30. Yasko J: Care of the Client Receiving External Radiation. Reston, V: Reston, 1982.
31. Haibeck SV: Intraoperative radiation therapy. Oncol Nurs Forum 15:143-147, 1988.
32. Smith RW, Sampson MK, Lucas CE: Effects of vinblastine, etoposide, cisplatin and bleomycin in rodent wound healing. Surg Gynecol Obstet 161:323-327, 1985.
33. Langer B: Presidential address, 1988. Surgical research: Its importance in the evolution of the specialty of general surgery. Can J Surg 32:154-158, 1989.
34. McKenna RJ: The privileges and the responsibilities of a surgical oncologist. Cancer 55:1159-1162, 1985.
35. Avis FP, Ellenberg S, Friedman MA: Surgical oncology research. Ann Surg 207:262-266, 1988.
36. Jacobs JR, Pajak TF, Snow JB, et al: Surgical quality control in head and neck cancer. Arch Otolaryngol Head Neck Surg 115:489-493, 1989.
37. Thorne SE: Helpful and unhelpful communications in cancer care: the patient perspective. Oncol Nurs Forum 15:167-172, 1988.
38. Morra ME: Choices: Who's going to tell the patients what they need to know. Oncol Nurs Forum 15:421-425, 1988.

Chapter 12

Radiotherapy

Laura J. Hilderley, RN, MS

THE CURRENT APPLICATION OF RADIOTHERAPY IN THE MANAGEMENT OF THE PERSON DIAGNOSED WITH CANCER

Radiotherapy is often combined with surgery or chemotherapy and immunotherapy, as well as being the sole treatment for cancer in some instances. For example, stage IIB adenocarcinoma of the endometrium is treated with preoperative radiation followed by hysterectomy, whereas Stage IIB squamous cell carcinoma of the cervix is treated with radiation alone.

The aim or intent of radiotherapy may be curative, as in skin cancer, carcinoma of the cervix, Hodgkin's disease, or seminoma. Treatment is vigorous and often lengthy, but the prognosis and probability of long-term survival make such an attempt worthwhile.

For certain other lesions, cure or eradication is not possible, and control of the cancer for periods ranging from months to years may be the aim. Recurrent breast cancer, some soft tissue sarcomas, and lung cancer are examples of cancers controlled by radiotherapy in combination with surgery or chemotherapy.

Palliation may be another goal of radiotherapy. Relief of pain, prevention of pathologic fractures, and return of mobility can be achieved with radiation to metastatic bone lesions from breast, lung, and prostate tumors. Pain relief is often dramatic, and it is not uncommon for one individual to receive multiple palliative courses to different bony structures over the course of several years. Between such metastatic episodes the person can sometimes carry on a near-normal life. Palliative radiotherapy is also given for the relief of central nervous system (CNS) symptoms caused by brain metastasis or spinal cord compression. Hemorrhage, ulceration, and fungating lesions can be effectively reduced and in some instances eliminated by palliative radiotherapy.

"Anticipatory" palliation is a useful application of radiotherapy in treating potentially symptomatic lesions before they become a problem. Examples of anticipatory palliation include treatment of a mediastinal mass that threatens to produce a superior vena caval syndrome and treatment to a vertebral lesion when spiral cord compression is impending.

Although treatment techniques and equipment may vary, the fundamental principles of radiobiology and radiation physics form the basis on which a course of treatment is selected and designed for each patient. Understanding these principles will enable the oncology nurse to support and care for the person diagnosed with cancer receiving radiotherapy, meeting the emotional as well as physical needs that result from the disease and therapy.

APPLIED RADIATION PHYSICS

The use of ionizing radiation in the treatment of cancer is based on the ability of radiation to interact with the atoms and molecules of the tumor cells to produce specific harmful biologic effects. Ionization affects either the molecules of the cell or the cell environment.

An understanding of atomic structure is basic to understanding the ionizing effects of radiation. The atom, the basic unit of molecular structure, consists of two parts: the nucleus, containing positively charged protons and neutrons that have mass but no charge; and the shells (orbits), containing electrons (equivalent to the number of protons) that each have a negative charge. Each shell can accommodate only a certain number of electrons, and if this number is exceeded, a second or third shell is established more distant from the nucleus (Figure 12-1). The negatively charged electrons orbit the nucleus, held in place by the attractive force of the positive protons in the nucleus, thus maintaining a stable state. Certain atoms are known to be unstable, however, and it is in this process of decay or breakdown into a more stable state that alpha, beta, or gamma rays may be emitted. Radium, radon, and uranium are examples of unstable atoms that produce radiation.

Stable atoms also may be made to produce ionizing radiation through excitation, ionization, and nuclear disintegration. Radiation produced by these processes can be classified into two groups: *electromagnetic radiation* and *particulate radiation*. The electromagnetic spectrum can be further divided into five levels of decreasing wavelength:

1. Radiowaves
2. Infrared radiation
3. Visible light
4. Ultraviolet radiation
5. Ionizing radiation

Ionizing radiation has the shortest wavelength and greatest energy of the electromagnetic spectrum and is therefore the form of energy used in radiotherapy. A classification system for ionizing radiations is shown in Figure 12-2.

As seen in Figure 12-2, the terms *x ray* and *gamma ray* both describe ionizing electromagnetic radiation and dif-

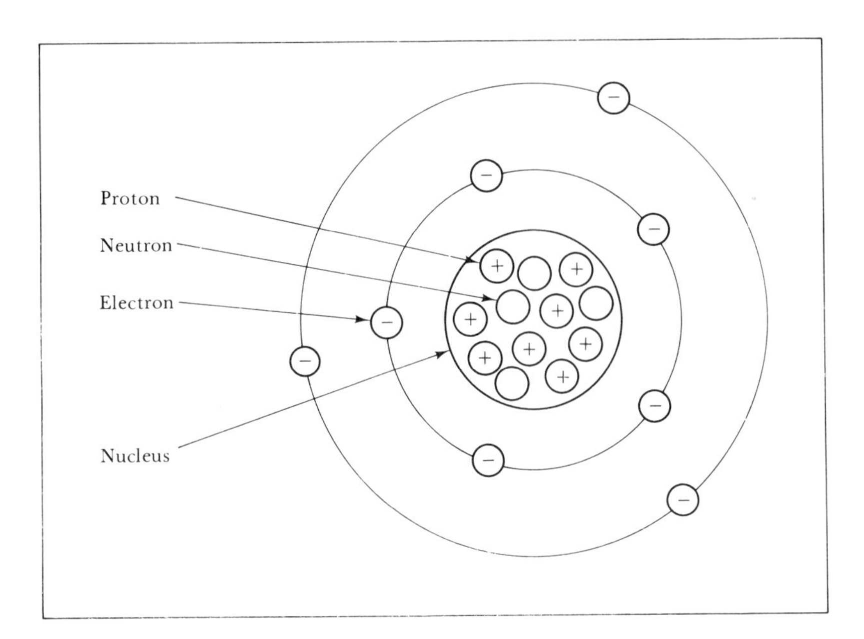

FIGURE 12-1 Basic structure of an atom. Protons, which are positively charged, and neutrons, which have no electrical charge, are the major components of the nucleus of an atom. The number of protons is equal to the number of negatively charged electrons orbiting the nucleus. Atoms of any given element may have different numbers of neutrons in the nucleus, thus giving atoms of the same element different atomic weights. An atom of a given element that differs only in its atomic weight is called an isotope.

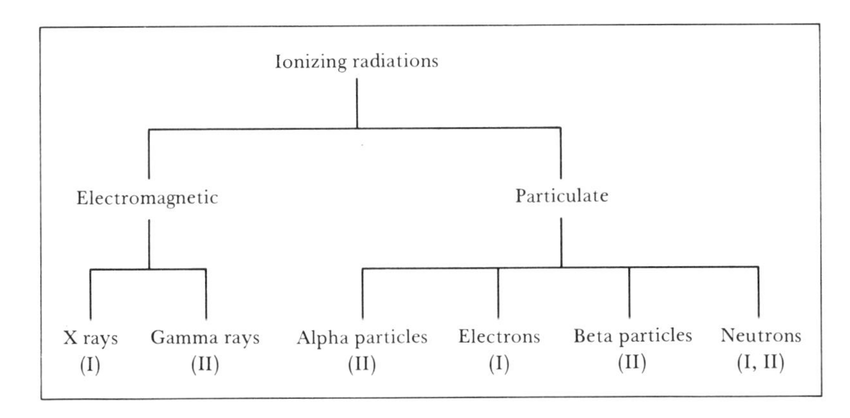

FIGURE 12-2 Classification system for ionizing radiations.

fer only in their means of production. That is, x rays are produced by specially designed equipment, and gamma rays are emitted by radioactive materials such as ^{60}Co undergoing nuclear transition. Both x and gamma rays have no mass but rather are packets of available energy ready to be released on collision with a substance. Because they have no mass, x and gamma rays can penetrate much deeper into tissue before releasing their energy.

Particulate radiation, on the other hand, is composed of alpha and beta particles, as well as electrons and neutrons, which have a mass. The relatively large size of alpha particles allows them to penetrate only a short distance into tissue before collision and energy release take place; beta particles, which are smaller than alpha particles, will penetrate deeper but, because of their mass, do not have the ability to reach as deeply into tissues as do x and gamma rays. The significance of these variations in ability to penetrate tissue will be obvious when treatment beams and equipment are discussed.

X rays are produced when a stream of fast-moving electrons, accelerated by the application of high voltage (between the filament and the target), strikes the target, and the electrons give up their energy. This radiation loss occurs because the electron is attracted to and slowed down by the nucleus of the tungsten (target) atom. Figure 12-3 illustrates the basic structure of an x-ray tube.

In addition to x rays, some treatment machines (betatron, linear accelerators) are equipped to produce par-

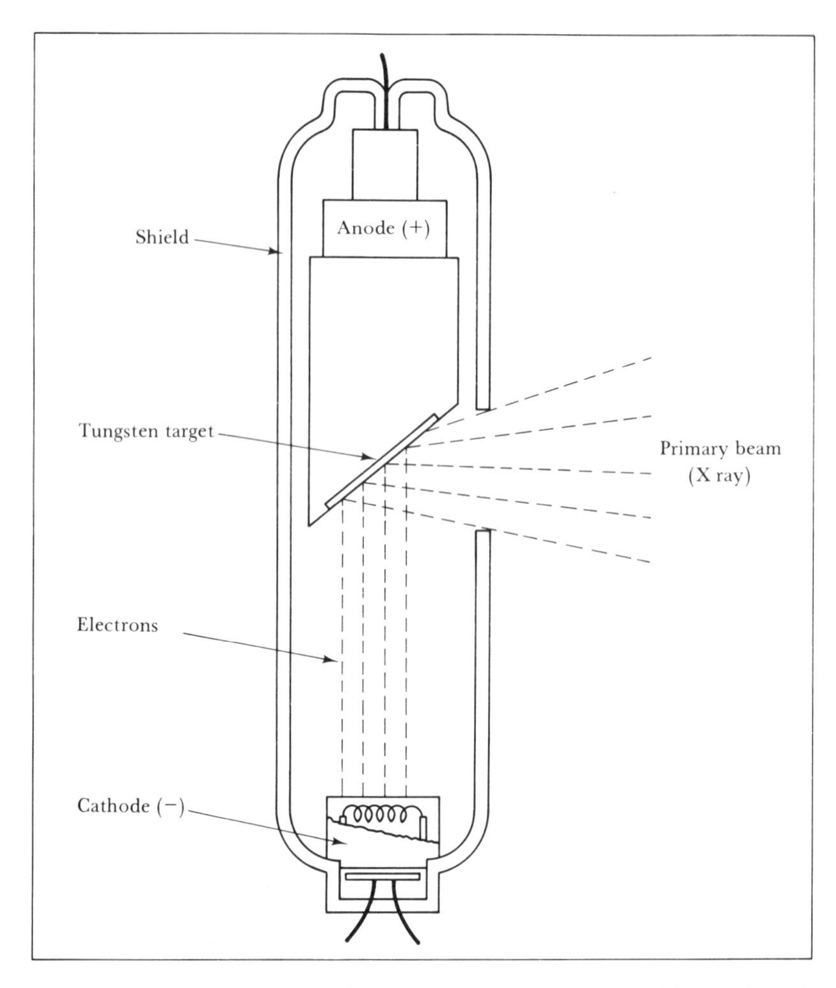

FIGURE 12-3 Basic structure of an x-ray tube. Electrons emitted from a heated tungsten filament are accelerated across a high-voltage source. These high-speed electrons then strike a positively charged tungsten target, producing x rays. The primary beam of radiation thus produced penetrates tissues. The greater the voltage, the greater the penetrating power of the beam.

ticle irradiation in the form of electrons. Electron energy is produced in an x-ray tube by bypassing one of the steps used to produce x rays (see Figure 12-3). Electrons from the heated tungsten filament are injected into the vacuum tube, accelerated at a high velocity, and emerge from a window in the vacuum tube, thus bypassing the tungsten target and emerging as electron particles suitable for treating surface lesions and those located a few centimeters below the skin.

Electromagnetic and particulate radiations are also produced through the process of decay of radioactive elements and radioactive isotopes. This process, which produces radiation in the form of alpha, beta, or gamma rays, is illustrated as follows:

$$\text{Atom X} \xrightarrow{\text{radioactive decay}} \text{Atom Y and radiation}$$

The time required for half the radioactive atoms present at any time to decay is known as the *half-life* of that radioactive element or isotope.

Because most radioisotopes are produced by neutron bombardment of stable elements (^{60}Co, ^{32}P, ^{182}Ta, ^{198}Au) or nuclear fission of uranium in a nuclear reactor (^{90}Sr, ^{137}Cs), they are referred to as *artificial isotopes* to distinguish them from naturally occurring radioisotopes such as ^{226}Ra and ^{222}Rn. Radioisotopes are listed in Table 12-1.

EQUIPMENT AND BEAMS USED IN RADIOTHERAPY

The types of equipment and beams used in radiotherapy are numerous and vary considerably in their application to clinical practice. A large radiotherapy center will have available a selection suitable for the treatment of almost any malignancy in any part of the body. On the other hand, the equipment available in a private office or small general hospital may be limited to that which is easiest to use and maintain.

Equipment can be classified according to use: external radiation, or *teletherapy* (radiation from a source at a dis-

TABLE 12-1 Radioactive Isotopes Used in Radiotherapy

Isotope	Symbol	Half-Life	Emissions		
			Alpha	Beta	Gamma
Cesium	^{137}Cs	30 years			X
Cobalt	^{60}Co	5.3 years		X	X
Gold	^{198}Au	2.69 days		X	X
Iodine	^{131}I	8.0 days		X	X
Iridium	^{192}Ir	74.5 days		X	X
Phosphorus	^{32}P	14.3 days		X	
Radium	^{226}Ra	1622 years	X	X	X
Radon	^{222}Rn	3.83 days	X	X	X
Strontium	^{90}Sr	28 years		X	
Tantalum	^{182}Ta	118 days		X	X

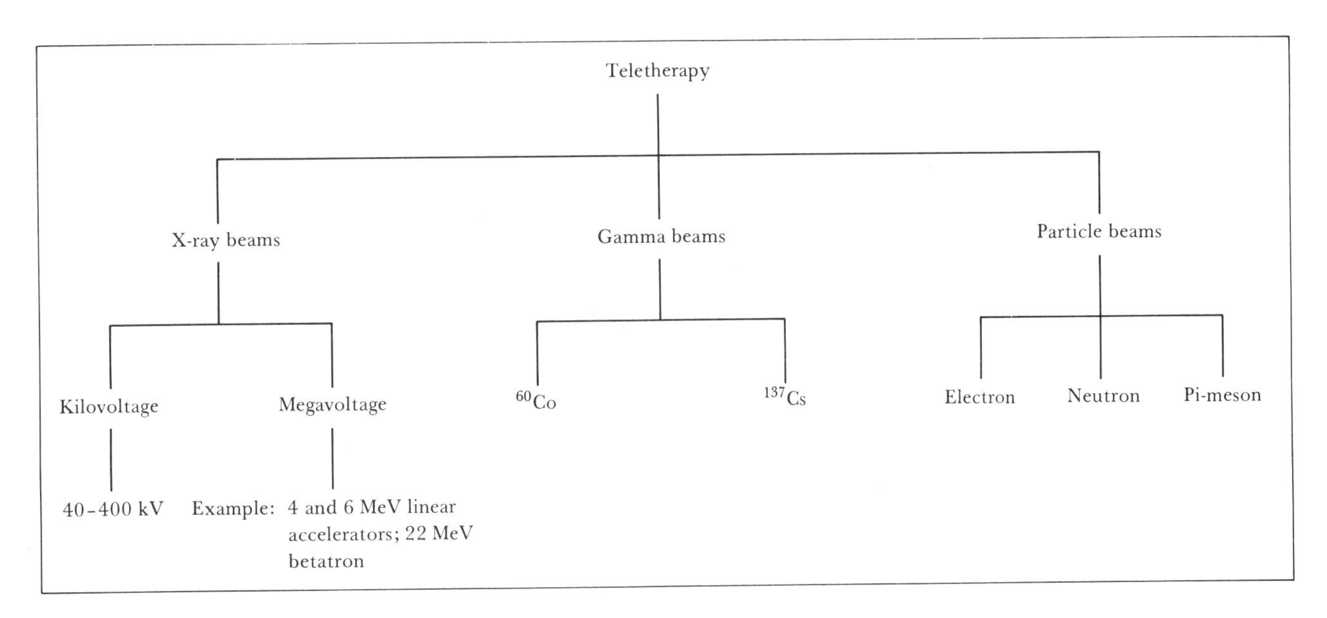

FIGURE 12-4 Classification system of teletherapy.

tance from the body), or internal application, or *brachytherapy* (radiation from a source placed within the body or a body cavity).

A useful classification system of various beams, equipment, and radioactive materials is given in Figures 12-4 and 12-5. In addition to teletherapy and brachytherapy, radiotherapy may be administered systemically using radioisotopes. *Contact therapy* using ^{90}Sr isotopes for conjunctival lesions and *surface (mould) therapy* for superficial skin lesions are additional applications of brachytherapy.

Teletherapy Equipment

Conventional or orthovoltage equipment

Conventional or orthovoltage equipment produces x rays of varying energies depending on the voltage used. The higher the voltage, the greater the depth of penetration of the x-ray beam. In selecting the proper beam for treatment of a particular lesion, the percentage depth dose of the beam must be known, as well as the depth within the body of the lesion. *Percentage depth dose* is defined as the percentage of the intensity of any given beam at a

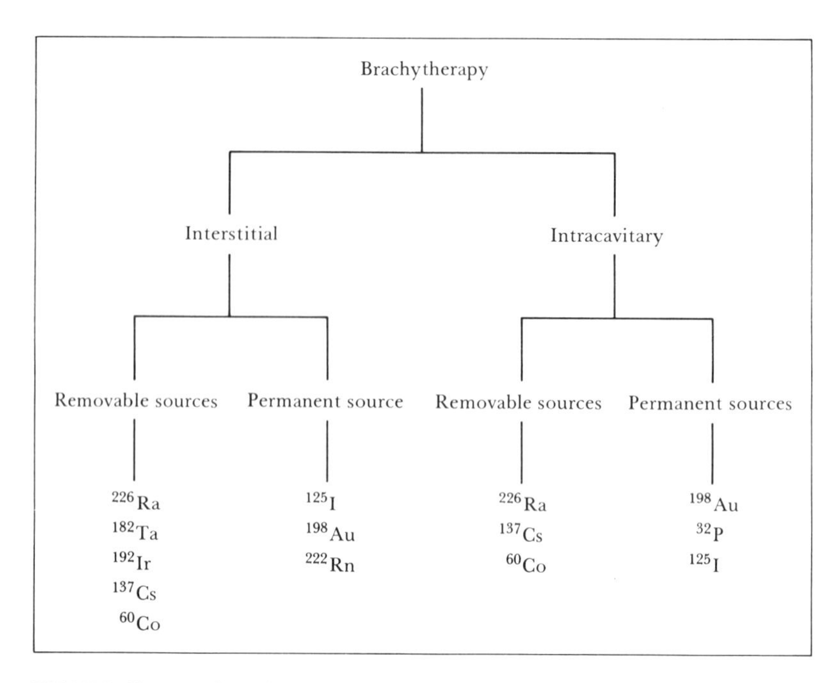

FIGURE 12-5 Radioactive sources used in brachytherapy.

given depth in tissue compared with the presumed 100% dose level. The maximum, or 100%, level occurs at varying depths depending mainly on the energy of the radiation being produced. Equipment in the range of 40-120 kV (1kV = 1000 V) is suitable only for superficial skin lesions and those no deeper than 1 cm. Beams in the 250 to 400 kV range (orthovoltage) have greater penetration and have been in use for many years. There are, however, a number of disadvantages to orthovoltage beams in addition to the poor depth of penetration. Most important are the severe skin reactions, due to the fact that most of the dose is at skin level, and bone necrosis, which may result from the fact that bone absorbs more orthovoltage radiation than does soft tissue. As a result of bone absorption, tumor located distal to bone in the treatment field receives less than the desired dose of radiation.

Megavoltage equipment

Megavoltage equipment operating at from 2 to 40 MeV (million electron volts) has distinct advantages over orthovoltage beams. The primary advantages of megavoltage therapy are (1) deeper beam penetration, (2) more homogeneous absorption of radiation (minimizing the excessive absorption by bone that occurs with orthovoltage treatment), and (3) greater skin sparing. Equipment used in megavoltage therapy includes the Van de Graaff generator, cobalt and cesium units, the betatron, and linear accelerators. Largely experimental units such as those producing heavy ions, neutron beams, and negative pi-meson particle beams will be briefly mentioned.

The Van de Graaff generator, operating at 2 million volts, was one of the forerunners in megavoltage equipment. Its use today is relegated primarily to the experimental laboratory, having been replaced in cancer therapy by more sophisticated equipment.

Cobalt-60 radiotherapy units were once the most common megavoltage equipment used. The cobalt machine is easy to operate and maintain, having no complicated electronics, as do linear accelerators. Because the radiation source is a radioactive isotope of cobalt, it is undergoing constant decay, at the rate of about a 10% per year decrease in output. Cobalt sources are measured in curies, and 3000 to 9000 Ci are typically needed in a teletherapy unit. Gamma rays are emitted as the ^{60}Co atoms decay, and with a half-life of 5.3 years, this means that the source would need to be replaced every 5 to 6 years to avoid lengthy treatment times. Cobalt units are also characterized by lower dose rates and a lower percentage depth dose compared with a linear accelerator of 10 MeV.

Cesium in the form of ^{137}Cs is also used in teletherapy units, primarily those used outside of the United States. Because of the low specific activity of a ^{137}Cs source, the source must be placed about 35 cm from the skin. This short source-to-skin distance (SSD) adds to surface skin dose by electron contamination, producing greater skin reactions. In comparison, ^{60}Co is usually placed at 80 cm SSD.

Linear accelerators, although more complex in terms of operation and maintenance than cobalt units, are widely used in most hospital-based radiotherapy departments as well as in the private practice setting. Linear accelerators have distinct treatment advantages, including the speed with which treatments can be given. Not only is this an advantage in terms of efficient use of time, but more important, it means that the person being treated spends less time in awkward and sometimes uncomfortable positions. In addition, a sharply defined field of irradiation can be obtained, thus treating only the desired tissue volume.

Linear accelerators are so named because of the method of x-ray production, which involves accelerating electrons along a radiofrequency electromagnetic wave, achieving energies equivalent to those that could only be obtained in a conventional x-ray tube at excessively high voltage. Some linear accelerators are also equipped to allow use of the electron beam (particulate radiation) itself. Electron beam therapy is useful in relatively superficial lesions such as chest wall recurrence of breast cancer, skin cancers, and superficial nodes and may be used to provide a booster dose to a limited site following treatment with megavoltage therapy. Electron particles are the equivalent of beta particles, differing only in their origin (beta particles are produced by radioactive decay), and, because of their mass, they have limited penetration into tissue. This is a distinct advantage over x or gamma radiation in that almost all the electron energy is expended at a particular tissue depth, sparing whatever structures lie beyond the tumor site.

The betatron is a therapy machine that predates the development of the linear accelerator for electron therapy. Electrons produced from a heated tungsten filament are injected into a doughnut-shaped porcelain envelope and accelerated by a changing magnetic field. These high-velocity electrons range in energy from 10 to 30 MeV and are useful for deep-seated lesions. X rays (18 to 40 MeV) also may be produced by the betatron when the electron beam is directed at a tungsten target.

High-energy radiation

There are two basic forms of radiation used in radiotherapy, those classified as low LET (linear energy transfer) radiation, such as x rays, gamma rays, and electrons, and high LET radiation, such as neutron beams, heavy ions, and negative pi-mesons (pions). Basically, the difference between low and high LET radiation is in the deposition of energy in the tissue molecule. (See Figure 12-13 in the section entitled Radiobiology.) Low LET radiation could conceivably pass through a molecule without damaging it. In contrast, the number of ionizing events produced in molecules by high LET radiation is much greater.

High-energy radiation facilities are limited in distribution in the United States and elsewhere. Years of experimentation have shown that there are distinct advantages to this form of therapy, yet the cost of such facilities and the technologic sophistication needed to operate them has meant that they must remain as referral centers for very carefully selected individuals with cancer. According to Orton,[1] high LET radiation has several advantages over low LET radiation:

1. More biologically effective (greater relative biologic effectiveness [RBE])
2. Reduced relative radioresistance of hypoxic cells in tumors (low oxygen enhancement ratio [OER])
3. Less intertreatment recovery of tumor cells in fractionated dosage

Neutron beam therapy Fast neutrons are produced by a cyclotron in which high-energy deuterons are used to bombard targets of either beryllium or tritium. Neutron therapy is less expensive than other high LET energy producers; however, technologic problems and the low dose rate (5 to 6 cGy/min) are some of the disadvantages to this form of therapy.

Heavy ion therapy Heavy ions such as protons, helium, and nitrogen are useful mainly for small tumors because the dose distribution is best when treating a small volume. As the treatment volume increases, the oxygen enhancement ratio (OER) will also increase.

Negative pi-meson therapy Negative pi-mesons (pions) are small, negatively charged particles found in the nuclei of atoms that "cement" protons and neutrons together. Pions are produced when protons are accelerated at approximately 131,000 miles/sec before striking a carbon target. The pions are then collected by a system of magnets, and the beam of high LET energy is directed at the target tissue. The first application of this form of treatment for human subjects took place at the Los Alamos Meson Physics Facility in Los Alamos, New Mexico, in 1974. The advantage of pion therapy, like other forms of high LET radiation, is that the beam can be shaped to fit the tumor precisely, thus minimizing the amount of radiation to surrounding normal structures. Pions can be aimed and stopped at a specific target site by adjusting the momentum of the particles.

Brachytherapy Equipment

Brachytherapy, the use of sealed sources of radioactive material placed within or near a tumor, is the treatment of choice in a variety of lesions. Brachytherapy is frequently combined with teletherapy and also may be used preoperatively and postoperatively.

Radioactive isotopes for brachytherapy application are contained in a variety of forms such as wires (^{182}Ta), ribbons or tubes (^{192}Ir), needles (^{137}Cs, ^{226}Ra), grains or seeds (^{198}Au, ^{222}Rn), and capsules (^{137}Cs,^{226}Ra). The source is selected by the radiotherapist according to the site to be treated, the size of the lesion, and whether the implant is to be temporary or permanent.[2]

Needles, wires, and ribbons (either preloaded or afterloaded) are particularly useful in treating head and neck lesions. Intra-abdominal and intrathoracic lesions may be implanted with gold or iodine seeds introduced either through hollow needles or tubes or through a "seed gun" that injects the radioactive sources into the tumor bed. Isotopes implanted in this manner are usually permanent, and radiation precautions may be needed after the person is discharged.

Intracavitary radiotherapy is most often employed in the treatment of gynecologic lesions. A variety of techniques and types of equipment have been designed (Figure 12-6) to provide a desired dosage to the tissues around the radiation source.[3] Most gynecologic applicators are based on the "Manchester method."[4] According to this method, the radioactive source is contained in two vaginal ovoids separated by a spacer, and a central uterine tandem is added when both the corpus and cervix are to be treated. Many of these applicators are the afterloading type that can be positioned in the operating room and loaded with the radioactive source at a later time after the proper position has been checked by radiograph and the patient returned to her room. The afterloading method is most desirable because it prevents unnecessary radiation exposure to personnel.

Surface (mould) therapy is often classified as a type of brachytherapy because it involves close contact of the source with the lesion. Radon, a chemically inert gas that is the product of radium decay, is well suited for this type of therapy. Techniques vary, but in most instances the ^{222}Rn seeds are embedded in a plastic mould especially built to the individual's contours, or the seeds are placed on a piece of adhesive plaster and then taped in place on the person's skin.

Mould therapy is suitable for small surface lesions in irregularly contoured areas such as the face. Because this type of plaster or device may be worn by the person at home, it is ideally suited for elderly or otherwise infirm individuals who would find daily treatment in the radiotherapy department difficult. Cosmetic results are excellent.

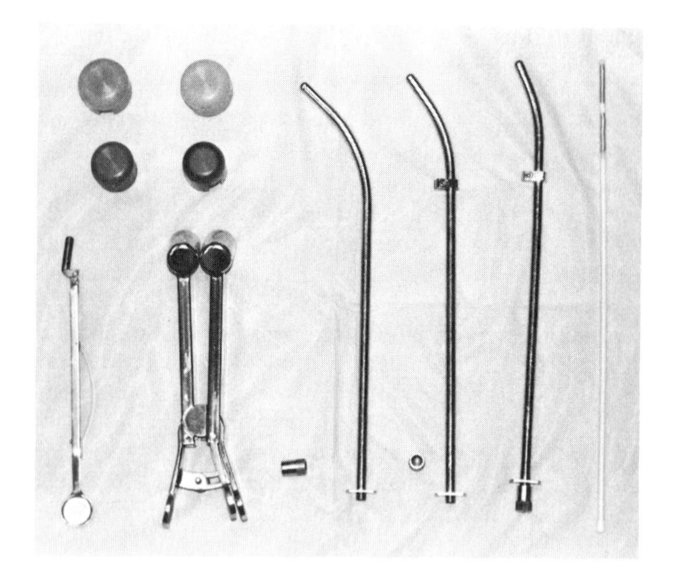

FIGURE 12-6 Examples of gynecologic applicators. Left to right: carrier for radioactive source to be inserted in colpostat: afterloading vaginal colpostats with plastic caps used to increase the size; afterloading uterine tandems; plastic tube containing radioactive sources to be inserted into tandem.

SIMULATION AND TREATMENT PLANNING

The decision to employ radiotherapy is made after consideration of a number of factors. Histologic confirmation of the diagnosis and staging of the disease by appropriate clinical, surgical, and laboratory procedures are necessary before a treatment decision can be made. In addition, such factors as the person's age and general condition, site of tumor, radioresponsiveness of the tumor, risk versus benefit, patient consent, and availability of treatment facilities must all be considered when selecting a plan of therapy.

When the decision has been made to treat a person with radiotherapy, the radiation oncologist devises the treatment plan, often utilizing an array of sophisticated equipment and involving a team of personnel.

One of the first steps in planning is localizing the tumor and defining the volume to be treated. Although some lesions are visible and their dimensions can be determined clinically, it is often necessary to employ a simulator to determine treatment volume accurately. A simulator may have several component parts (Figure 12-7). It contains a diagnostic x-ray unit for visualizing the proposed treatment site. Fluoroscopic examination may also be done. From radiographs taken on the simulator, the physician can determine the field of treatment and draw in the proposed field outline on the radiograph. The radiotherapy technologist then duplicates these markings on the patient's skin using anatomic points and outlines projected onto the patient's skin by the simulator. Treatment portals may be identified by several small tattoos placed at the corners of the field. Tattooing is a simple process in which a drop of India ink is placed on the skin and a needle is used to introduce the ink into the skin, leaving a tiny permanent black dot. This procedure, which produces only momentary discomfort, can be distressing to the person if it is not explained carefully beforehand. For individuals receiving head and neck irradiation, where the field markings are particularly visible, tattoos may be substituted for lines once the reproducibility of the field has been ensured. In many instances, however, tattoos are not placed until the end of the treatment course because a field may shrink or change as surface contours change and tumor volume shrinks. Tattoos are a useful means of identifying a previously treated area if a person returns for further therapy. Injection moulding equipment has recently been employed to form masks or head holders of clear plastic. Field markings may be placed on these masks rather than on the skin, avoiding conspicuous facial marks.

Some simulators are also capable of transverse axial tomography. Tomography is a radiographic technique for showing detailed images of body structures at any given plane in the body. This technique allows a three-dimensional view of the tumor and surrounding structures to be obtained, allowing greater precision in planning and delivering treatment. Computerized tomography (CT scan) provides the radiotherapist with even finer detail for treatment planning.

Some simulators are also equipped with an ultrasound device that produces an image of internal structures. This technique employs ultrasound (inaudible sound with fre-

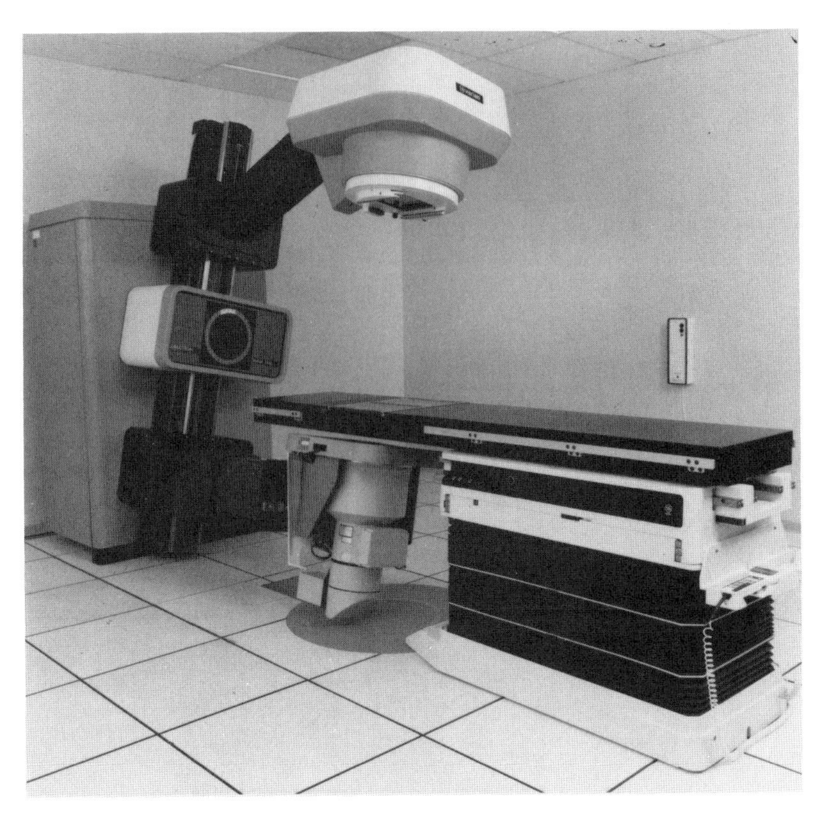

FIGURE 12-7 A Varian Ximatron™ C-Series radiation therapy simulator. (Photo courtesy of Varian Associates, Inc., Palo Alto, CA.)

quencies ranging from 16,000 to 10,000,000,000 cycles per second [cps]) that is reflected back as an echo from the varying tissues it strikes. Differences in density and elasticity of tissues and organs produce differences in the echo, which are recorded as an image of the target structures. Ultrasound is another means of defining tumor volume and relationship to nearby vital structures.

Various restraining or positioning devices may be designed at the time of simulation to aid in immobilizing the person. Lying still in exactly the same position each day is sometimes difficult but is necessary to deliver the prescribed treatment to the prescribed volume. For children, especially, a custom-made body cast is sometimes used to ensure immobility. The adult also may be more accurately positioned by means of various headrests, armboards, handgrips, and the like.

An important part of simulation and treatment planning is shaping the field and determining what structures are to be blocked and protected from radiation. The therapy machine produces a rectangular field, which can, within limits, be made larger or smaller. However, that rectangular field must then be trimmed and shaped with portions eliminated in varying patterns to meet individual requirements. Blocks to protect vital body organs and tissues are secured to a plastic tray that is then placed on the head of the treatment machine between the beam and the person being treated. *Portal films* (sometimes called *beam films*) are radiographs taken through the treatment machine to confirm the treatment field and placement of blocks in the desired position.

During simulation, contours of the person's body may be obtained and then traced onto paper. Information from the tracings is fed into a computer, which then produces an isodose plot to guide the radiotherapist and physicist in designing the best field arrangement possible. Some examples of various field arrangements for treating tumors in different locations are shown in Figures 12-8 and 12-9.

The physicist plays an important role in simulation and treatment planning. Working together, the physicist and radiotherapist design the field arrangement, determine the dose calculations, monitor tumor response, and ensure accuracy of technical aspects. Physicists are also often involved in the maintenance and calibration of treatment machines.

For the person with cancer, the process of simulation and treatment planning is usually the first introduction to the machinery of a radiotherapy department. Thorough and careful explanation about the purpose of this preliminary phase of treatment is important to allay fears, not only of the procedures themselves, but also anxiety about the delay in getting treatment started. If the person can be helped to understand the importance of careful planning, the necessary steps will be accepted or at least tolerated better.

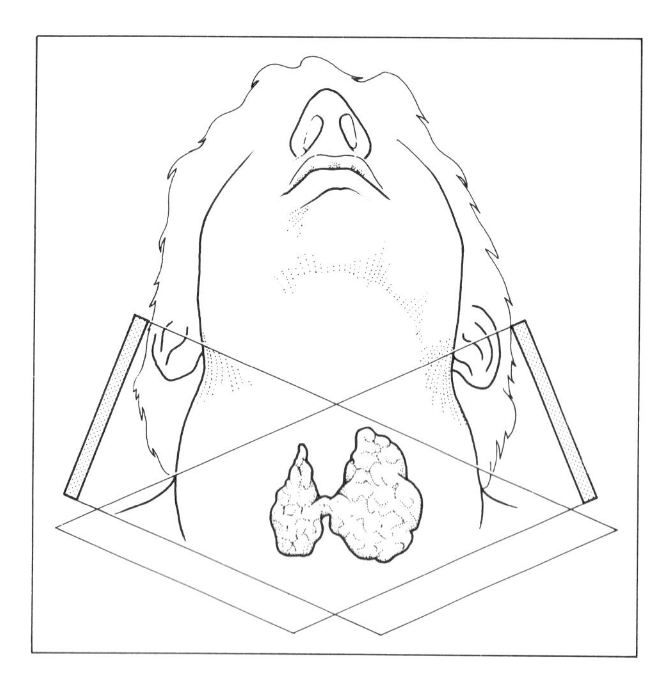

FIGURE 12-8 Two vertically wedged field arrangements for the treatment of thyroid carcinoma.

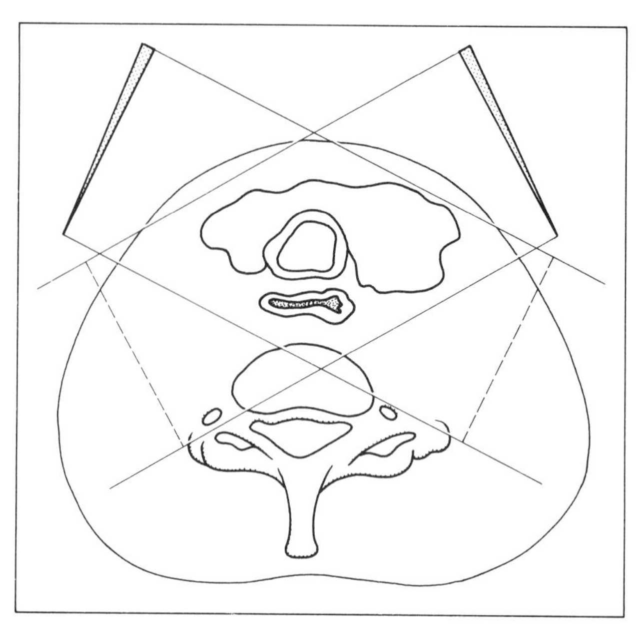

FIGURE 12-9 Cross-section of the neck showing the zone of high-dose irradiation to a thyroid tumor; the dose to the spinal cord is low, although the skin dose is high.

RADIOBIOLOGY

The biologic effects of radiation on humans are the result of a sequence of events that follows the absorption of energy from ionizing radiation and the organism's attempts to compensate for this assault. Radiation effect takes place at the cellular level, with consequences in tissues, organs, and the entire body. Factors contributing to radiation response will be presented, and the reader is referred to Chapter 3 on cell biology for background.

Cellular Response to Radiation

Radiation effect at the cellular level may be either direct or indirect. According to the target theory,[4,5] a *direct* hit occurs when any of the key molecules within the cell, such as DNA or RNA, are damaged. Among the types of damage observed after high-dose radiation of DNA molecules in vitro are (1) change or loss of a base (thymine, adenine, guanine, or cytosine), (2) breakage of the hydrogen bond between the two chains of the DNA molecule, (3) breaks in one or both chains of the DNA molecule, and (4) cross-linking of the chains after breakage. Such unrepaired breaks or alterations in the base lead to mutations, which bring about impaired cellular function or cell death.

An *indirect* hit, according to target theory, occurs when ionization takes place in the medium (mostly water) surrounding the molecular structures within the cell. Radiation absorbed by the water molecules results in a free radical when an electron is literally knocked out of orbit surrounding the ion. The resulting free radical is then available to join with the others, and this high degree of reactivity in itself can damage the macromolecules of the cell. Such free radicals may trigger a variety of chemical reactions, producing new compounds that are toxic to the cell. Figure 12-10 illustrates the ionizing effect of radiation on the water contained within a cell.

It is generally agreed that a direct hit (ie, DNA damage and chromosomal aberrations) accounts for the most effective and lethal injury produced by ionizing radiation.[6] However, because of the relative proportions of water to DNA in a single cell, the probability of indirect damage through ionization of cellular water is much greater.

In addition to the damage produced by a direct or indirect hit, experimental evidence shows that radiation can cause damage to proteins, carbohydrates, and enzymes within the cell. Damage to these molecules, as well as alterations in the permeability of the cell membrane, also may be implicated in the ultimate effect of radiation at the cellular level.

Cell cycle and radiosensitivity

According to Richter et al,[7] radiosensitivity appears to be maximum during the M and G_2 phases of the cell cycle (Figure 12-11). Thus the maximum effect from radiation should occur just before and during actual cell division. Bergonie and Tribondeau[8] in early research formulated their law, which says that the sensitivity of cells to irradiation is in direct proportion to their reproductive activity and inversely proportional to their degree of differentiation. A differentiated cell is one that is morphologically or functionally specialized (such as the erythrocyte) and

The final products of the ionization of water molecules (HOH) by radiation are an ion pair (H^+, OH^-) and free radicals ($H^\cdot$, $OH^\cdot$), which are capable of damaging the cell. The ionization of water is shown in the following steps:

$$HOH \xrightarrow{\text{Radiation}} HOH^+ + e^-$$

The free electron (e^-) is then captured by another available water molecule and, as shown in the next step, forms the second ion:

$$HOH + e^- \longrightarrow HOH^-$$

Because the two ions (HOH^+, HOH^-) produced by these reactions are unstable, rapid breakdown occurs (in the presence of other normal water molecules), forming yet another ion and a free radical as follows:

$$HOH^+ \longrightarrow H^+ + OH^\cdot$$

$$HOH^- \longrightarrow OH^- + H^\cdot$$

Although the resulting ion pair (H^+, OH^-) have some potential for cellular damage through chemical reactions, they are more likely to recombine and form water (HOH). The free radicals ($H^\cdot$, $OH^\cdot$) are extremely reactive, and they too may simply recombine to form water. However, free radicals appear to be more likely to undergo chemical interactions with other free radicals, forming cytotoxic agents, as shown in this reaction:

$$OH^\cdot + OH^\cdot \longrightarrow H_2O_2 \text{ (hydrogen peroxide)}$$

Free radicals that result from the interaction of radiation with water are capable of triggering a variety of chemical reactions within the cell and are therefore believed to be a major factor in the production of damage in the cell.

FIGURE 12-10 The effect of ionizing radiation on water molecules.

does not undergo mitosis. An undifferentiated cell (such as the red blood cell stem cell or erythroblast) has few specialized morphologic or functional characteristics, and its primary purpose is to divide and provide new cells to maintain its own population. Because the effect of radiation is known to be greatest during mitosis, undifferentiated cell populations are generally most sensitive to radiation. In contrast, well-differentiated cells are relatively radioresistant.

Changes in mitotic activity due to radiation can be classified as *delayed onset* or *complete inhibition.* Delay in the onset of mitosis indicates that although damage occurred at some point during prophase, repair was accomplished and division takes place. *Complete inhibition* of mitosis, or cell sterilization, renders the cell incapable of division, although it may continue to live in a nonreproducing state.

Cell death

There are three types of cell death: mitotic (or genetic) death, interphase death, and instant death. *Mitotic death*

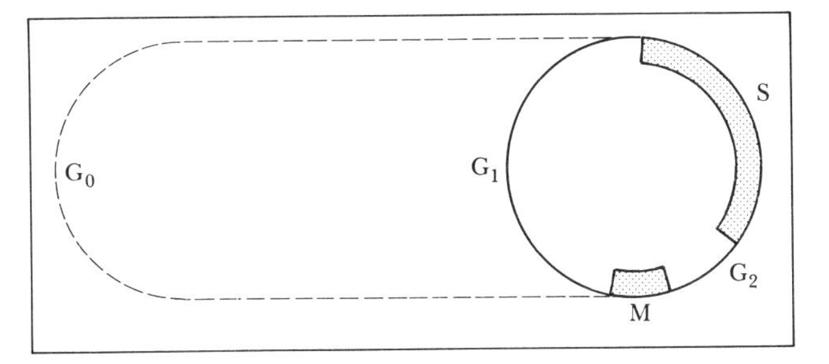

FIGURE 12-11 Stages in cell replication cycle:
S, DNA synthesis
G_2, the gap between DNA synthesis and mitosis
M, mitosis
G_1, the gap between the end of mitosis and the start of DNA synthesis

occurs after one or more divisions and usually with much smaller radiation doses than those required to produce interphase death. *Interphase death* takes place many hours after irradiation and before the cell begins the mitotic process. *Instant death* occurs following extremely high doses of radiation and would take place only in the experimental laboratory or in the event of a nuclear accident.

Other factors

A number of additional factors directly affect the biologic response to radiation and ultimately the treatment outcome. Among these are the oxygen effect, linear energy transfer (LET), relative biologic effectiveness (RBE), dose rate, radiosensitivity, and fractionation.

Oxygen effect Well-oxygenated tumors show a much greater response to radiation, that is, are more radiosensitive than poorly oxygenated tumors. Extensive laboratory and clinical research[6,9] has shown that the existence of oxygen tension between 20 and 40 mm Hg at radiation greatly enhances the radiosensitivity of the cells. Theoretically, the mechanism of the oxygen effect is related to the ability of oxygen to combine with the free radicals formed during ionization, producing new and toxic combinations. A second theory states that the presence of oxygen at irradiation prevents the reversal (and thus the repair) of some of the chemical changes that occur as the result of ionization. The clinical significance of the oxygen effect is that oxygen modifies the dose of radiation needed to produce a given degree of biologic damage. The magnitude of the oxygen effect is expressed as the *oxygen enhancement ratio* (OER). The OER is the ratio of radiation dose in the absence of oxygen (or hypoxia) to the radiation dose in the presence of oxygen required for the same biologic effect.

Linear energy transfer Linear energy transfer (LET) describes the rate at which energy is lost from different types of radiations while traveling through matter. Its usefulness is seen in designating the quality of radiation emitted from various radiations such as x rays, neutrons, and alpha particles. Low LET radiations (x and gamma rays)

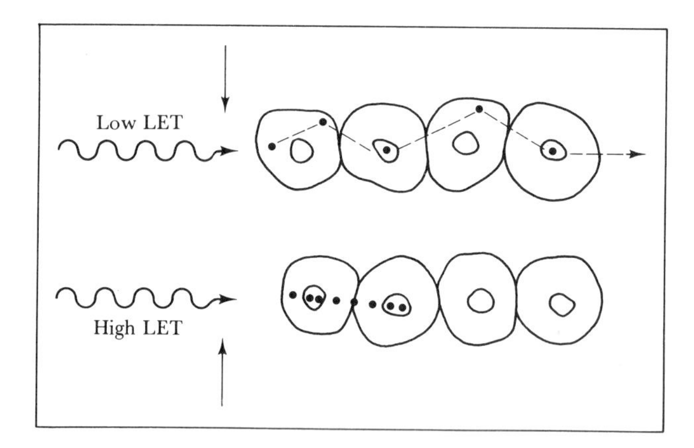

FIGURE 12-12 Comparison of the effects of low and high LET radiations on a population of cells. Note the irregular path of the low LET radiation, interacting with four cells, compared with the relatively straight path of the high LET radiation, which is interacting with only two cells. However, the low LET radiation produces only *one* hit in two nuclei, whereas the high LET radiation produces *two* hits in two nuclei. (Source: Travis EL: Primer of Medical Radiobiology. Chicago, Year Book Medical Publishers, 1975, p 71. © 1975 Year Book Medical Publishers. Reproduced with permission.)

are sparsely ionizing, having a random pathway that results in few direct hits within the cell nucleus. Radiation of higher LET (alpha particles, neutrons, and negative pimesons) has a greater probability of interacting with matter and producing more direct hits (Figure 12-12).[5]

Relative biologic effectiveness Because different radiations have varying rates of energy loss, the biologic response will be different. Therefore, the term *relative biological effectiveness* (RBE) is used to compare a dose of test radiation with a dose of standard radiation that produces the same biologic response. The following formula is used to express RBE:

$$\text{RBE} = \frac{\text{Dose of reference radiation to produce a given biologic effect}}{\text{Dose of test radiation to produce the same biologic effect}}$$

Dose rate *Dose rate* refers to the rate at which a given dose is delivered by a treatment machine. Studies have shown low dose rates to be much less effective in producing lethal cell damage than high dose rates, primarily because low dose rates permit cell repair to occur before the lethal dose has been reached.

Radiosensitivity According to Bergonie and Tribondeau's law, ionizing radiation is most effective on cells that are undifferentiated and undergoing active mitosis.[8] Laboratory and clinical experience has shown this to be true in most tissues.

Fractionation Fractionation, or the dividing of a total dose of radiation into a number of equal fractions, is based on four important factors: *repair, redistribution, repopulation,* and *reoxygenation,*[5,6,10] commonly referred to as the four Rs of radiobiology.[11]

Repair of intracellular sublethal damage by normal cells between daily dose fractions is one benefit of fractionation. The goal of fractionation is to deliver a dose sufficient to prevent tumor cells from being repaired while allowing normal cells to recover before the next dose is given. Although some tumor cells may be repaired between daily doses, they also may reoxygenate, rendering them more radiosensitive when the next dose is given. Thus although some degree of repair of tumor cells is possible between fractionated doses, repeated daily doses would ultimately lead to tumor control.

Redistribution of cell age (within the cell cycle) as a result of daily radiation is advantageous because more tumor cells are made radiosensitive. Theoretically, with succeeding daily doses of radiation, more and more tumor cells would be delayed in cycle and reach the mitotic phase as the next dose is given, thus increasing the cell kill. Certain chemotherapeutic agents, such as methotrexate and hydroxyurea, are being used in combination with radiation to take advantage of this synchronization in the cell cycle.

Repopulation of normal tissues takes place through the process of cell division at some time during a multifraction treatment course. Fractionation of dose allows this repopulation in normal tissues, sparing them from some of the late consequences that might occur if repopulation (new growth) was inhibited. On the other hand, those tumor cells that do succeed in dividing while undergoing a fractionated course of radiotherapy are usually incapable of surviving because of the radiation effect. Thus fractionation favors normal tissue while still eradicating tumor.

Reoxygenation is the fourth consideration favoring fractionation of the radiation dose. Whereas normal tissues are usually well oxygenated, tumors characteristically range from normal to hypoxic to anoxic. As discussed earlier, radiosensitivity is closely related to oxygen tension in the tumor cell; hypoxic or anoxic cells are generally radioresistant, whereas oxygenated cells are radiosensitive. Fractionating the dose allows time between treatments for the tumor to reoxygenate.

Tissue and organ response to radiation can now be understood on the basis of sensitivity of cellular components. It is important to note that tissues and organs are composed of more than one cell category, each cell category having different degrees of radiosensitivity. A second factor in determining tissue response is related to the parenchymal versus stromal substance found in that tissue. The parenchyma is composed of cells characteristic of the tissue or organ, and if those cells are radiosensitive (eg, the testis), ionizing radiation has its greatest impact on the parenchyma. However, if parenchymal tissue is relatively radioresistant (eg, the spinal cord), radiation response in that organ is due to the indirect effects on the stromal components (epsecially the vasculature) that support the parenchyma.

Table 12-2 lists various organs according to their degree of radiosensitivity as measured by parenchymal hypoplasia.

TABLE 12-2 Degree of Radiosensitivity of Various Organs Based on Parenchymal Hypoplasia

Organ	Radiosensitivity
Lymphoid organs, bone marrow, blood, testes, ovaries, intestines	High
Skin, cornea, oral cavity, esophagus, rectum, bladder, vagina, cervix, ureters	Fairly high
Optic lens, stomach, growing cartilage, fine vasculature, growing bone	Medium
Mature cartilage or bone, salivary glands, respiratory organs, kidneys, liver, pancreas, thyroid, adrenals, pituitary gland	Fairly low
Muscle, brain, spinal cord	Low

CHEMICAL AND THERMAL MODIFIERS OF RADIATION

Radiosensitizers and Radioprotectors

The goal of radiotherapy is to achieve maximum tumor cell kill while minimizing injury to normal tissues (therapeutic ratio). Efforts to improve the therapeutic ratio have resulted in the development of certain compounds that act to increase the radiosensitivity of tumor cells or to protect normal cells from radiation effect. Combined modality therapy with both radiation and certain cytotoxic agents also takes advantage of enhanced tumor cell kill. Drugs such as doxorubicin, actinomycin-D, cyclophosphamide, bleomycin, and cisplatin are often used along with radiation to achieve greater cell kill than either therapy could achieve if used independently. When used alone, chemical modifiers of radiation therapy (radiosensitizers), however, are generally not cytotoxic like the chemotherapeutic agents.

Phillips[12] proposed several definitions useful in describing the various interactions of radiation with other agents. *Enhancement* or *potentiation* describes any radiation effect that is greater in the presence of the chemical than in its absence. If the effect is less than that caused by the most active agent in the combination, then this is known as *interference*. *Antagonism* is the term used to describe an outcome less than that of the least effective agent in a given combination. In clinical radiotherapy, enhancement by noncytotoxic sensitizers is called *radiosensitization*. Antagonism by protective compounds is called *radioprotection*.

Radiosensitizers are compounds that apparently promote fixation of the free radicals produced by radiation damage at the molecular level. The mechanism of this action is similar to the oxygen effect described earlier, in which biochemical reactions in the damaged molecules prevent repair of the cellular radiation damage. Free radicals (such as OH•) are captured by the electron-affinic radiosensitizers, rendering the molecules incapable of repair.

The two most biologically active radiosensitizing compounds first tested in phase II and III studies were metronidazole (Flagyl) and misonidazole (RO-07-0582). Major side effects are neurotoxicity, including peripheral neuropathies and CNS symptoms of somnolence, confusion, and transient coma. Nausea and vomiting are also fairly frequent side effects that seem to be dose-related. Early clinical trials using misonidazole as a radiosensitizer indicated some degree of effectiveness in treatment of squamous carcinoma of the head and neck and of the uterine cervix. Overall results were disappointing, however, due to severe toxicity and only marginal improvement in tumor control. Brown[13] concludes that a new hypoxic cell radiosensitizer is needed. Misonidazole is the only such substance to have undergone extensive clinical trial evaluation, and most studies have failed to demonstrate a significant effect with the addition of misonidazole.

The compound SR-2508 (etanidazole) has been tested with promising results in phase I trials.[14] This member of the nitroimidazole group of compounds appears to be less toxic to the CNS tissue than misonidazole. It is currently being used in a number of phase II and III trials.

Early studies[15] with nitroimidazoles used *invitro* showed that these radiosensitizers are also capable of cytotoxic activity in hypoxic cells after periods of long exposure. The high doses required to achieve actual cell kill *invitro* have, however, prohibited their use *invivo* for this purpose.

Misonidazole also has been shown to increase the cytotoxicity of alkylating agents, nitrosoureas, 5-fluorouracil (5-FU), cyclophosphamide, and melphalan.[16] However, the side effects commonly experienced with these agents are also apparently enhanced by the addition of misonidazole. This nonselective enhancement detracts from the potential benefits to be gained.

Radioprotectors are compounds that can protect aerated (nontumor) cells while having a limited effect on hypoxic (tumor) cells. This selective action thus serves to increase the therapeutic ratio by promoting the repair of irradiated normal tissues. Repair or return to a nondamaged state takes place through the chemical process of reduction. Free electrons are captured by the radioprotective substance and are thus unavailable to participate in further chemical reactions that lead to cellular damage. This process can be viewed as the opposite of what occurs when radiosensitizers are used.

The sulfhydryl groups contained in the nonprotein fraction of most cells aid in the reduction process following radiation damage. Thiophosphate compounds (such as cysteine and cysteamine), containing sulfhydryl and aminopropyl groups, were among the earliest radioprotectors synthesized. The compound that appears to be most useful at present is designated WR-2721.[17]

The study of radiosensitizers and radioprotectors has

extended to phase II and III clinical trials in the continued effort to achieve better results in cancer treatment with radiotherapy. With combined therapy, toxicity can be increased and patient comfort may be compromised. Clinical trials are no longer confined to major cancer centers. Thus the nurse in a community hospital setting may be involved in caring for the person receiving radiosensitizers or radioprotectors.

Some nursing responsibilities in the use of radiosensitizers and radioprotectors would include:

1. Providing patient and family education
2. Participating in obtaining informed consent
3. Administering investigational agents
4. Timing and coordinating drug administration with radiotherapy treatment
5. Observing and documenting expected and previously unreported effects and side effects
6. Managing side effects, including developing interventions for those newly observed

A thorough discussion of the nursing implications for patients receiving chemical modifiers of radiation can be found in Noll.[18]

Pretreatment evaluation phase

1. Assess suitability for treatment
2. Assess ability to tolerate treatment
3. Assess cardiac and neurologic status
4. Assess for presence of metal objects
5. Provide thorough patient and family education

Treatment phase

1. Vital signs, gastrointestinal preparation, sedation
2. Assist during surgical placement of thermometry probes
3. Position for comfort and access to applicator probes
4. Monitor patient throughout treatment
5. Provide physical and emotional support

Posttreatment phase

1. Clean and dress cannula sites
2. Observe and document thermal changes at treatment site
3. Provide discharge instructions
4. Manage subsequent local reactions

FIGURE 12-13 Potential Nursing Responsibilities in Hyperthermia Treatment

Hyperthermia

The use of hyperthermia to achieve a synergistic effect with radiotherapy has been studied and applied in clinical situations with considerable enthusiasm. Although it is technically arguable whether hyperthermia actually sensitizes tumor cells to radiation effect or simply combines to produce a greater effect than either modality can achieve on its own, researchers agree that this combined technique is warranted.[19-22]

The biologic basis for combining hyperthermia with radiation is based on several factors. Heat is cytotoxic to cancer cells but is also destructive to healthy tissue if applied in excess of tolerable ranges. Controlled hyperthermia combined with radiation achieves tumor cell kill without excess toxicity.

Tumor cells are *least* radiosensitive during S-phase. Hyperthermia is *most* effective during S-phase; therefore, the combined effect on a tumor produces greater cell kill than does either alone. Similarly, hypoxic cells, which are generally radioresistant, have been found to be quite thermosensitive. Heat is also known to inhibit the repair of radiation damage, thus increasing the therapeutic ratio.

Valdagni et al[23] reviewed the important parameters that may influence tumor response to combined hyperthermia and radiation therapy. Pretreatment parameters include tumor size, histologic findings, and disease site. Treatment parameters include total dose of radiation and dose per fraction, thermal dose, total and weekly number of hyperthermia sessions, and, finally, the sequencing of hyperthermia and radiation.

Hyperthermia is achieved in various ways, including immersion of the local area in a heated bath, ultrasound, microwaves, interstitial implants, and perfusion techniques. The choice of technique depends on whether local, regional, or whole-body hyperthermia is desired.[24-29]

Side effects of combined hyperthermia and radiation include local skin reaction, pain, fever, gastrointestinal effects, and cardiac arrhythmias. Late effects such as necrosis and ulceration can occur but do not seem to be significant enough to preclude continued use of this combined modality. Wojtas[30] details the nursing care of persons receiving hyperthermia treatments as well as the role nurses might take in administering the actual treatment. Figure 12-13 provides an overview of the nursing care.

TISSUE AND ORGAN RESPONSE TO RADIATION

When discussing the effect of radiation on tissues, one must consider both the acute, or immediate, effects, seen within the first 6 months following treatment, and the late effects, seen after 6 months. In general, acute effects are due to cell damage in which mitotic activity is altered in some way. If early effects are not reversible, late or permanent tissue changes occur. These late effects can be attributed to the organism's attempt to heal or repair the damage inflicted by ionizing radiation.

The unit of radiation dose is called a *gray* (Gy). This term was officially adopted in 1985, replacing the term *rad* (an acronym for *r*adiation *a*bsorbed *d*ose). One gray equals 100 rad. One cGy equals 1 rad.

In the following sections, radiation changes in normal tissues are presented according to body systems. It is important to remember that treatment volume, *dose rate* (number of cGy in a given unit of time), and *dose-time* factor (total number of cGy in a total number of days), as well as beam quality, may alter the tissue reaction. Except for those systemic effects described, radiation response is seen only in the tissues and organs that are within or immediately adjacent to the treatment field. Thus, an individual being treated to an abdominal field will not lose scalp hair from radiation, nor will the person being treated to the mediastinum develop radiation-induced diarrhea. Similarly, those persons undergoing brachytherapy will develop site-specific reactions to treatment, which vary with the site, dose, volume, and energy of the source. For example, cesium needle implants to the tongue will produce intraoral mucositis but usually no skin reaction. Application of a radioactive source intravaginally produces vaginal mucositis and often results in diarrhea due to the effect of radiation on the adjacent rectal mucosa. The important point to remember is that side effects from radiation are specific, and therefore preparation, teaching, and care must be planned for each individual.

Integumentary system

The outer layer of skin (epidermis) is composed of several layers of cells, with mature nondividing cells at the surface and immature dividing cells at the base. Normal mature cells are constantly being shed from the skin surface and replaced by new cells from the basal layer. This continuous state of reproductive activity accounts for the high radiosensitivity of skin. Although the skin may be the primary site of radiation (as in skin cancer), it is also irradiated when any other site within the body is treated because radiation must pass through whatever tissues it encounters before reaching the target site. Depending on the equipment used and the beam quality, skin of the exit portal also may be affected. Erythema may be the only manifestation, or the skin reaction may progress to dry and then moist desquamation. Healing may be slow but is usually complete and leaves minimal evidence of the acute damage except for changes in pigmentation. Fibrosis and atrophy may occur after high doses, as may ulceration, necrosis, and skin cancer. Such changes are uncommon with modern equipment and techniques. It is important to note that skin in certain areas, such as the groin, gluteal fold, axilla, and under the breasts, usually exhibits a greater and often earlier reaction to radiation due to the natural warmth and moistness in these areas and to friction caused by apposition of skin surfaces.

Use of the term *burn* or *radiation burn* to describe skin reactions is no longer appropriate. The severe skin reactions of the past are uncommon because of the skin-sparing effect of modern equipment. *Burn* implies accidental or unexpected damage, neither of which should take place in a controlled therapeutic setting. There are specific instances in which the person being treated will experience a severe reaction, especially when receiving electron beam therapy in the range of 5500 to 6000 cGy.

Skin reactions of this nature progress from a brisk erythema to a florid state, followed by a moist desquamation and loss of the epidermis. This, however, is an *expected* reaction because of the particular beam quality (see the section entitled Equipment and Beams Used in Radiotherapy), and despite the severity of the acute reaction, the involved skin usually heals well.

Hair follicles and glands (sweat and sebaceous) are also radiosensitive. The radiosensitivity of the hair follicle is due to the relatively high rate of growth (mitotic activity) taking place; thus, these follicles are more susceptible to radiation damage. Under normal circumstances, hair grows and new hair is formed at a rate that keeps pace with the regular loss or shedding of the mature hair, with the net result being no obvious change in the amount of hair on the head. However, when the scalp is irradiated, the resulting inhibition of growth of new hair coupled with the accelerated hair loss due to damage to the follicle produces a net loss of hair, or *alopecia*. Epilation occurs in doses as low as a single dose of 500 cGy but is usually temporary. Regrowth may not begin for several months following the end of treatment, and the new hair may have a different quality or color. Higher doses (4500 cGy or greater) may produce permanent alopecia or delay regrowth for a year or more. Sebaceous and sweat glands will usually experience a decrease in activity during treatment and may cease functioning altogether at high doses (over 6000 to 7000 cGy). Return of function is proportional to the dose received.

Hematopoietic system

Red bone marrow is responsible for producing mature functional cells for the circulating blood. The stem cells are highly radiosensitive, and when large areas of red bone marrow (in the adult) are irradiated, including ilia, vertebrae, ribs, metaphyses of the long bones, skull, and sternum, the amount of circulating mature cells decreases because production is suppressed. More erythroblasts (red blood cell precursors) are damaged by moderate doses than myeloblasts but recover rapidly, and thus anemia is not a prominent or early feature. Myeloblasts (white blood cell precursors) are suppressed at the same rate as erythroblasts, but the rate of recovery is much slower. Megakaryocytes (platelet precursors) are affected 1 to 2 weeks after exposure and take the longest time to recover (2 to 6 weeks).

Mature, nondividing blood cells in the circulating blood have a limited life span and are relatively insensitive to radiation. Peripheral blood does, however, reflect marrow activity. Thus, the person receiving radiotherapy may have depressed blood counts if sufficient radiation was given to active red bone marrow, especially if prior or concomitant chemotherapy has been given. The usual pattern seen in individuals whose marrow has been affected is a drop first in lymphocytes, then in neutrophils, and then in platelets and red blood cells. It is sometimes necessary to interrupt a course of radiotherapy for varying periods to allow the bone marrow to recover.

Radiation to the spleen alters its physiologic functions of hemolysis, red blood cell and iron storage, and antibody production, as well as causing shrinkage of the spleen itself.

Lymph nodes, like the spleen, are highly radiosensitive, whereas lymphatic vessels appear to be relatively radioresistant. Interference with lymphatic vessel function is thought to be caused by fibrotic changes and obstruction.

Gastrointestinal system

The gastrointestinal tract, from mouth to rectum, is lined with mucous membrane that contains layers of cells. A large proportion of these cells are undifferentiated and mitotic and are thus extremely radiosensitive. In addition, glandular tissue, ranging from large distinct bodies such as the parotids to multiple small mucous glands, is embedded in much of the mucous membrane. The effect of radiation on glandular tissue can be summarized as follows:

1. Initial swelling and edema of the epithelial lining of the ducts results in partial obstruction.
2. Secretion is inhibited by damage to the acini.
3. Atrophy and fibrosis occur as healing takes place, with permanent reduction in secretion, the amount depending on the dose received and volume of mucous tissue irradiated.

Oral mucous membrane may develop a confluent mucositis, especially on the soft palate and floor of the mouth, during the third and fourth weeks of therapy at the usual dose rate. Salivary function is altered as damage to the serous and mucous acini occurs, and saliva becomes viscous after moderate doses. Higher doses lead to atrophy of the salivary glands, with greatly diminished saliva and increased acidity. Such changes in saliva production and acidity are often permanent and are a factor in the development of radiation caries and infection. Alterations in the sense of taste occur early in treatment but are rarely permanent, depending on the dose of radiation received.

The esophagus and stomach also develop dose-dependent reactions. Changes in the glandular tissues of the stomach brought about by radiation are even more complex than those that occur in the glands of the oral mucous membranes. Gastric secretions, in addition to mucus, include pepsin and hydrochloric acid. When 1600 cGy are delivered in approximately 10 days to the stomach, all three secretions will be reduced; this may be accompanied by nausea, dyspepsia, and pyloric spasm. Inflammation of the mucosa (esophagitis and gastritis) occurs with moderate to high doses and produces dysphagia, anorexia, and sometimes nausea and vomiting. Late changes may include atrophy, ulcerations, and fibrosis.

The most sensitive area of the entire gastrointestinal tract is thought to be the small intestine. When one considers the length of the small intestine and also the fact that its loops overlap and fill a large portion of the abdomen, even a small radiation field of 5 × 8 cm on the abdomen will contain a large surface area of intestinal mucosa. Crypt cells (rapidly dividing, undifferentiated stem cells) arise from the base of the villi on a continuous basis to replace mature cells of the villi that are lost as part of the normal sloughing process. The high degree of radiosensitivity of these crypt cells and resultant changes in the intestinal villi account for the sometimes severe reactions that occur when abdominal or pelvic radiation is given.

Radiation reaction in the small intestine is characterized by shortening of the villi and loss of absorptive surface. Temporary reactions can usually be tolerated with minimal nutritional consequences. However, if reactions are prolonged and severe, as in some individuals receiving 5000 to 6000 cGy to the abdomen or pelvis, the nutritional consequences can be major. Shortening of the villi and denuding of the intestinal mucosa prevent adequate absorption of the end products of digestion, namely, amino acids (protein), simple sugars (carbohydrates), and glycerol and fatty acids (fats). Late changes following high doses of radiation include fibrosis, ulcerations, necrosis, and hemorrhage. Intestinal obstruction, although not common, can occur in a person receiving abdominal or pelvic irradiation. This is more likely to happen postoperatively, when the trauma of surgical manipulation combined with the previously discussed effects of radiation can result in paralytic ileus.

Such a reaction depends on many factors, including total dose, fractionation, volume, site, and so on. Most individuals receiving pelvic irradiation experience only some degree of anorexia, nausea, diarrhea, or cramping, which can be managed readily with appropriate medication and diet.

The effect of radiation on the colon and rectum is similar to that seen in the small intestine, with the addition of the distressing symptom of tenesmus, which sometimes occurs when the anal sphincter is irradiated.

Liver

The liver is considered an accessory digestive organ and has been shown to be moderately radiosensitive. Although the parenchymal cells do have a regenerative capacity and are therefore vulnerable, the greatest damage produced by radiation to the liver is due to vascular injury. Early changes may be detectable only by liver function tests. However, radiation hepatitis is a possible consequence of doses over 2500 cGy, and the severity will depend on the volume irradiated.

Respiratory system

Mucous membrane lines the pharynx, trachea, and bronchi, and reactions that occur are due to the response of that sensitive tissue to irradiation. Hoarseness due to laryngeal mucous membrane congestion sometimes occurs. More significant in terms of radiation is the response of the bronchial tree and alveoli. Radiation pneumonitis, usually a transient response to moderate doses, is the result of changes in the alveolar wall plus the accumulation of exudate in the air sac, similar to pneumonia. Late changes are manifested by fibrosis in the lung tissue itself plus some thickening of the pleura. Such changes will compromise respiratory function in the area treated, but the degree of disability is related to the amount and condition of remaining untreated lung tissue.

Reproductive system

The cervix and uterine body are quite radioresistant and usually present no problem for the person being irradiated. However, vaginal mucous membrane responds to radiation much the same as the oral mucous membrane with mucositis and inflammation. Following brachytherapy, vaginal stenosis due to permanent fibrotic changes is a potential problem. Radiation to the ovaries produces either temporary or permanent sterility, depending on the age of the person being treated and the dose of radiation. Permanent sterilization will occur at doses of 600 to 1200 cGy, and older women are sterilized at lower doses than younger women.

Maturation of graafian follicles and release of ova are essential for fertility. Radiation is most damaging to the intermediate follicle, thus preventing its development into a mature form. Small follicles are most radioresistant, and fertility may return if these small follicles are able to undergo repair and release ova. Mature graafian follicles are only moderately radiosensitive, and an ovum can be released, which accounts for the period of fertility that sometimes occurs after moderate doses of radiation.

In addition to sterility, hormonal changes (especially loss of estrogen production) and early menopause may occur. Perhaps most significant in terms of late or long-term consequences of radiation to the gonads in both the male and female is the potential for genetic damage. Chromosomal aberrations are a possibility that must be considered, especially at low doses. (For further reading on the genetic effects of radiation, the reader is referred to Travis,[5] BEIR III[31] and Lushbaugh and Casarett.[32])

Radiation to the male testes damages and prevents maturation of the immature spermatogonia. Sterility can be permanent even after a dose of 500 to 600 cGy, and temporary sterility is usually seen following doses as low as 250 cGy.

Urinary system

Radiation-induced cystitis and urethritis are early and transient effects on the urinary tract that usually respond well to symptomatic treatment. Of major significance when considering the effect of radiation on the urinary system is damage to the kidneys in the form of nephritis. Early changes brought about by high doses of radiation lead to permanent fibrosis and atrophy, largely due to sclerosis of the vasculature. Renal failure and death can result. Protection of the kidneys is essential when the abdomen is irradiated.

Cardiovascular system

Damage to the vasculature of an organ or tissue (ie, to stroma) can be the primary reason for the radioresponsiveness of that organ or tissue. Blood vessels (lined with epithelium) may become occluded when excessive cell production takes place during repair and regeneration in response to radiation injury. Thrombosis may be induced by the thickening that occurs during regenerative activity, thus further occluding the vessels. Late changes can be seen in the form of telangiectasia, petechiae, and sclerosis. The heart muscle itself is thought to be relatively radioresistant. However, at doses above 4000 cGy, pericarditis may occur in addition to the damage to the vasculature of the heart muscle.

Nervous system

The brain and spinal cord are considered to be relatively radioresistant, and peripheral nerves are even more so. However, therapeutic doses between 3000 and 6000 cGy have produced transient symptoms in the CNS, usually following a latent period in which no functional damage is seen. Especially noticeable is the response called Lhermitte's syndrome, which may occur following irradiation to the cervical cord. This syndrome is characterized by paresthesia in the form of shocklike sensations that radiate down the back and extremities when the neck is bent forward. Stretching of the cord in this manner compromises circulation, which may partially account for the sensations experienced. Myelopathy is usually transient but at higher doses may lead to paralysis or paresis. When large volumes of the spinal cord (15 cm or more) are irradiated, doses of 4500 to 5000 cGy will produce transverse myelitis. The tissues of the nervous system are composed of a variety of cells, most sensitive of which are the neurons found in olfactory, gustatory, and retinal receptors. Radiation to these neurons can therefore alter or destroy the function of the particular sense organ. Because the nervous system is thought to be relatively radioresistant in itself, damage that does occur following radiation probably relates to vascular insufficiency. As described earlier, the vasculature of the body is radiosensitive. In addition, preexisting disorders such as diabetes, hypertension, and arteriosclerotic changes may enhance the effect of radiation on nervous tissue.

Skeletal system

Mature bone and cartilage are radioresistant and seldom present a problem in planning radiotherapy. However, late avascular necrosis can occur after high doses, causing pain and possible pathologic fracture. This is a relatively rare complication with supervoltage equipment.

Of much greater clinical significance is the effect of radiation on growing bone and cartilage. Children treated for spinal, thoracic, or abdominal tumors are susceptible to deformity as a result of radiation to the vertebrae. Failure to attain normal height due to spinal irradiation has occurred, as has shortening of a limb when the epiphyses are irradiated. Such orthopedic problems, although serious in themselves, may be considered a necessary compromise in terms of tumor eradication.

Systemic Effects of Radiation

Aside from or in addition to the specific local effects of radiation to tissues and organs already presented, the person receiving radiotherapy may experience certain subjective systemic effects, including nausea, anorexia, and malaise. Although the psychologic component of these symptoms cannot be overlooked, these systemic effects can theoretically be linked to the release of toxic waste products into the bloodstream resulting from tumor destruction. The presence of these toxins may account for the nausea and anorexia, whereas the increased metabolic rate required to dispose of the waste products might be partially responsible for the frequent complaint of fatigue. The physical effort needed to make a daily trip to the radiotherapy department for 4 or 5 weeks also may account for the malaise experienced by many individuals.

It is important to note that the response of the whole body (nausea, anorexia, malaise) to radiation of a limited site depends on the volume of the irradiated area, the anatomic site, and the dose. Consequently, not all individuals experience these systemic symptoms, and the degree of disability due to the symptoms will vary from mild to severe. Most individuals receiving radiotherapy tolerate treatment remarkably well and experience only mild systemic symptoms.

Whole body irradiation

Whole body or hemibody irradiation is a relatively infrequent therapeutic application of radiation. The effect on the person being treated varies with the dose, dose rate, and dose-time factor. For example, total body irradiation of 150 cGy is being used in some centers in the treatment of chronic lymphocytic leukemia. This total dose is delivered at the rate of 5 cGy/day for 10 days, followed by a 2-week break and then repeated for two more cycles to reach the total of 150 cGy. When total body irradiation is delivered in this manner, which calls for small daily doses fractionated over a 10-week period, the side effects are negligible.

In contrast, radiotherapy given before bone marrow transplantation involves total body irradiation with 1000 cGy administered over 6 to 8 hours. Although the purpose of treatment in this instance is to suppress the bone marrow totally before transplantation with healthy marrow, this suppression presents a major problem in terms of patient management. With this high dose to the whole body, side effects are much greater and include nausea, vomiting, diarrhea, fever, erythema, alopecia, mucositis, parotitis, and pancreatitis, all of which occur in the immediate posttreatment phase. More severe skin reaction, cataracts, sterility, and major organ damage are delayed side effects.[33]

Chronic low-dose radiation exposure occurs to all persons from background radiation from naturally occurring radioactive substances and cosmic rays.[34,35] Such exposure is largely unavoidable and within the safe limits defined by federal regulations. Radiation workers are exposed to a somewhat higher level of ionizing radiation, but the allowable limit is well below that which will produce ill effects.

Total body radiation syndrome

Total body radiation syndrome refers to the effects of the acute exposure of the organism to doses of radiation received in a matter of minutes rather than hours or days. Acute exposure of human beings has been studied through data obtained from industrial and laboratory accidents, individuals exposed at Hiroshima and Nagasaki, Pacific Testing Grounds fallout exposure, and medical treatment procedures.[36] Doses of 150 to 2000 cGy delivered to the whole body in a short time frame produce life-shortening or lethal damage through effects on the hematopoietic, gastrointestinal, and central nervous systems. The April, 1986, nuclear accident in Chernobyl, USSR, will undoubtedly produce additional significant information about the somatic and genetic effects of exposure to high levels of radioactivity. For greater detail and for information on the effects of radiation exposure to the embryo and fetus, the reader is referred to Travis.[5]

Radiation-induced malignancies in humans

The carcinogenic effects of radiation, often called "late effects," from both chronic low-dose exposure and acute exposure to the whole body are of particular interest and concern to the nurse, especially in providing support to the person who is hesitant about accepting treatment. The key to understanding lies in the fact that acute exposure and chronic low-dose exposure are the exceptions, occurring in radiation accidents, occupational exposure, and the early stages of the development of the science of radiotherapy. The usually prescribed therapeutic doses (in the range of 2500 to 6500 cGy) are believed to be less carcinogenic than lower doses given over a much longer time period. Theoretically, a cell that has survived in a damaged or altered state after low-dose irradiation may undergo carcinogenic mutation in the presence of other conditional factors. On the other hand, a cell that has been sterilized or destroyed by therapeutic doses of radiation should be incapable of malignant changes.

The most common malignancies associated with radiation exposure are skin carcinoma and leukemia, and evidence also implicates radiation in some sarcomas, thyroid carcinoma, and lung cancer.[37-40] Recent reports have suggested the possibility of inducing breast cancer in females by frequent radiographic exposure for screening for tuberculosis, other lung disease, and breast cancer itself.

Radiation carcinogenesis depends on a number of variables. These include a latent period of from 1 to 30 years, radiation dose, concomitant factors in the radiated organism's environment, and the actual fate of the cell as it responds to radiation injury. For a comprehensive review of radiation carcinogenesis, the reader is referred to Bucholtz.[41]

NURSING CARE OF THE PATIENT RECEIVING RADIOTHERAPY

Caring for the person receiving radiotherapy gives nurses an opportunity to put into practice all the theory and science acquired in their education and work experience. The person receiving radiotherapy is first and foremost a person with all the needs and problems generated by the diagnosis of cancer. Care cannot focus solely on the disease site (ie, a "lung" patient, a "cervix" patient, a "Hodgkin's" patient, and so on). Nor can nursing care be based solely on meeting the immediate needs generated by treatment and its side effects without considering the individual's long-term needs. Nursing care must be individualized and holistic, intelligent and thoughtful, scientific and compassionate. All these qualities can be achieved in nursing care of the person receiving radiotherapy. By applying the scientific background material provided in earlier sections of this chapter and using specific nursing care measures detailed in the following pages, the nurse will be able to devise a comprehensive plan of care for each individual receiving radiotherapy.

Assessing the individual's situation is the first step in planning care. A number of questions must be asked and answered:

1. What is the diagnosis? Prognosis?
2. What is the goal of treatment?
3. Does the person know and understand the diagnosis?
4. Does the family (or significant others) know and understand the diagnosis?
5. What is the plan of treatment? Radiotherapy alone? Surgery? Chemotherapy? All three?
6. Will therapy be given on an inpatient or outpatient basis?
7. What does the person know and understand about radiotherapy?
8. Where can the correct information about the individual's treatment plan be obtained?

When the person with cancer is an inpatient, the staff should begin this assessment on admission and build on the care plan as the diagnosis becomes available and treatment plans are formulated by the medical staff. Coping with the diagnosis may be the only crisis a particular person can handle at this early stage; elaborate plans and explanations about treatment may go largely unheard as the person struggles to resolve feelings about the diagnosis of cancer. In contrast, another individual moves quickly past the diagnosis and literally pleads to get treatment under way before a total care plan has been formulated. Each person must be assessed and managed on an individual basis.

In seeking answers to some of the assessment questions posed previously, the hospital nurse can turn to the patient's physician, the patient, and the family. After the person has been referred to a radiotherapist and evaluated, the radiotherapist (and nursing staff from that department, if available) can provide further information that can be useful in devising the care plan.

What are some of the facts about radiotherapy the nurse must understand when caring for the person in the pretreatment phase? How can these facts be incorporated into the nursing care plan? Most individuals newly diagnosed with cancer have a number of misconceptions about treatment stemming from the experiences of other persons. The worst side effects are always the ones that are remembered and are often exaggerated in the retelling. Of course, side effects do occur, but their severity depends on such factors as treatment site, treatment volume, fractionation, total dose, and so on, and especially on the individual being treated. Knowing what side effects can be expected and, most important, knowing that measures are available to alleviate most symptoms can be reassuring to the person. In general, most individuals respond best to a reassuring pretreatment discussion in which side effects specific to their treatment are discussed, stressing that symptomatic relief is available. Knowing what to expect usually helps prevent the person from worrying that a treatment-related side effect represents a worsening or recurrence of disease. At this time the nurse can also mention briefly the reactions that will not occur. Some might argue that this only puts ideas into the anxious person's mind, but most people are reassured to know, for example, that they will not lose their hair or be nauseated if this is the case.

Thus nurses should know the facts about treatment site and potential side effects when they are caring for individuals before and during radiotherapy. Most people experience few or at least manageable side effects in today's modern and well-equipped radiotherapy departments and offices. Many individuals are able to continue working, perhaps with some changes in schedule, or manage a home and family just as they did before diagnosis and treatment. Others are debilitated by the disease or treatment, making it impossible to continue in their former roles.

In planning nursing care for the person receiving radiotherapy, another important consideration is the length of the treatment course. Specifically, it is important to determine the need for transportation following discharge and help the individual and family to obtain this transportation. Although some palliative treatment is given over a period of 7 to 10 days (often while the patient is hospitalized), most individuals receive radiotherapy for an average of 5 weeks, and some may be treated over 7 or 8 weeks. The person with stage III Hodgkins's disease receiving total nodal irradiation will be making trips to the radiotherapy department for approximately 3 months, with several 2-week breaks interspersed. Transportation must be arranged on a daily basis for these lengthy periods.

Some individuals are able and willing to drive themselves, and some have family and friends who can provide this service, but many, especially elderly persons, are without transportation on a steady basis and will need assistance. Sources of transportation vary, but some available services are as follows:

1. Senior citizens transportation (a federal or locally funded service in many parts of the United States)
2. American Red Cross
3. American Cancer Society
4. Religious groups (FISH)
5. Service and civic organizations

In addition to meeting transportation needs, explaining potential side effects, and dispelling misconceptions, the staff nurse or community nurse can provide a great service to the individual undergoing radiotherapy by describing the treatment facilities and equipment. People are sometimes frightened by the size and complexity of the equipment, the perceived impersonal attitude of the staff, and the fact that they must be alone in the room during treatments. Of course, no nurse can be familiar with every radiotherapy facility. However, nurses working in oncology settings or caring for individuals with cancer regularly should make it a part of their own education to visit and familiarize themselves with radiotherapy departments and facilities. Persons being treated and visitors are sometimes disturbed by the fact that a radiotherapy facility is in a basement or underground location. Again, a factual explanation about the necessity for proper shielding will help allay some of these fears.

The well-informed nurse who is familiar with local radiotherapy facilities can provide the support and reassurance needed during the pretreatment phase of a person's illness. The confidence that familiarity brings can significantly increase the nurse's ability to meet some of the pretreatment needs of a person about to begin radiotherapy.

The personnel an individual comes in contact with during radiotherapy can play an important role in alleviating anxiety. The radiotherapist, who prescribes, directs, and evaluates treatment, is primarily responsible for the person's care during treatment and for varying periods afterward. This is often done in conjunction with a family physician, oncologist, or surgeon. Nurses employed by a radiotherapy department can offer much of the supportive care needed to cope with the emotional and physical needs of the person being treated and the family. Symptomatic relief of side effects, nutritional support, and social and financial assistance are all nursing concerns. Coordination of complex treatment schedules and protocols also may be part of the nurse's role. Some departments employ one or more nurses to meet these patient needs, and in others an oncology nurse is shared by both medical and radiation oncology. Realistically, nurses are in short supply in radiotherapy departments, and nursing needs often go unmet. This is why the role of the staff nurse, office nurse, or community nurse is so important.

The person with whom the patient has the most frequent contact and establishes the closest relationship is very often the radiotherapy technologist. The technologist is a highly skilled individual, certified by the American Society of Radiologic Technologists, and is responsible for giving the daily treatments under the direction of the radiotherapist. Although the technologist's primary focus is the physics and mechanics of treatment, attention is also given to the person being treated as a human being with particular wants and needs. Nursing care is sometimes carried out by the technologist in departments where there are no nurses. However, it would be unfair to expect that a radiologic technologist could or would be able to devote as much attention to nursing needs as to the technical responsibilities of the job. In recognition of this need for combined skills, some centers have employed, trained, and prepared nurses for certification as radiotherapy technologists.

Regardless of who will be treating and caring for the person in a radiotherapy department, it is important and comforting for the individual and family to know that caring individuals are available who will try to make the total treatment experience as untraumatic as possible. Most individuals experience few or no treatment-related problems, and those who do can for the most part be managed effectively. The person being treated should be encouraged to ask questions, report symptoms, and regard radiotherapy as part of a total plan for managing the cancer.

Assessment of individual needs and implementation of nursing interventions are ongoing processes in oncology nursing. For individuals receiving radiotherapy, this is especially true because needs change as treatment progresses. Initial nursing concerns focus on diagnosis and the person's acceptance of treatment, preparation (both physical and psychologic) for treatment, transportation arrangements, and so on. As treatment progresses, many of the initial fears and misconceptions disappear, and the person settles into the somewhat routine process of coming for daily treatments. Expected side effects usually occur after 10 to 14 days, depending on dose, volume, and site. Individuals undergoing treatment frequently count the days and keep track of the number of treatments received. Although a plan has been made from the beginning prescribing the number of daily fractions, this plan is subject to change as the radiotherapist deems appropriate. There are a number of reasons for adding to, subtracting from, or changing the plan, and if the person understands this from the beginning, changes will not be interpreted as signs of recurrence or disease progression. Although most individuals want to know how many treatments will be given so that they can adjust their activities accordingly, they should be helped to understand that this number is subject to change.

Apathy or a sense of futility may develop as treatment progresses and the person does not see any obvious changes in his or her disease. Visible lesions frequently can be observed to shrink or disappear with treatment, and this is encouraging. However, when a tumor is not visible or when treatment is an adjunctive measure in cases where no known lesion exists, the person being treated sometimes finds it difficult to continue in the absence of obvious and immediate benefits. This is especially true if side effects produce symptoms that are more troublesome than those created by the disease. Regardless of the setting, the nurse plays a vital role at this point in helping the person to accept and continue treatment for its long-term potential despite the immediate discomforts. A telephone call to the radiotherapist, nurse, or technologist in the department from the nurse caring for the person in another setting can be helpful in such situations.

SPECIFIC NURSING CARE MEASURES FOR PATIENTS RECEIVING RADIOTHERAPY

During a course of radiotherapy, certain treatment-related side effects can be expected to develop, most of which are site specific as well as dependent on volume, dose fractionation, total dose, and individual differences. Many symptoms do not develop until approximately 10 to 14 days into treatment, and some do not subside until 2 or more weeks after treatments have ended.

Nursing care measures and medical management described in the following sections reflect the policy and practices that have proved most effective in one particular institution. It should be noted that alternative means do exist for management and nursing care, any of which may be suitable to the particular setting in which they are practiced.

Fatigue

Fatigue or malaise is common among most individuals during radiotherapy and for varying periods afterward. Extra rest and a reduction in the normal activity level may be necessary during treatment. Individuals receiving radiotherapy should be encouraged to nap, go to bed early, or alter their daily schedule to allow for rest periods rather than to "fight it," as some are prone to do. Some individuals report that taking a nap immediately after returning home from their treatment gives them enough energy for the rest of the day. Others prefer to go to bed earlier than usual at night. The person who is bedridden at home or hospitalized will need provisions for rest and quiet according to individual needs.

Anorexia

Anorexia occurs frequently among individuals receiving radiotherapy regardless of the treatment site. Anorexia, like fatigue, is probably related to the presence in the person's system of the waste products of tissue destruction. Other possible causes for anorexia include anemia, inactivity, medications, alterations in the person's ability to ingest and digest foods, and psychologic factors. The cause often cannot be identified clearly, and therefore the symptom must be treated utilizing all the techniques known to encourage adequate intake. A self-perpetuating cycle of anorexia/weight loss/weakness/inactivity/anorexia can develop if the symptom is untreated.

For detailed information on the management of anorexia and cachexia in the individual with cancer, see Chapter 24.

Mucositis

The reaction produced by radiation to the mucous membranes in any part of the body (gastrointestinal, genitourinary, and respiratory systems) is called mucositis. Mucositis can be described as a patchy, white membrane that becomes confluent and may bleed if disturbed. This reaction is most visible when radiation is given to the mouth and oropharynx, and severe reactions cause considerable discomfort to the person. A number of measures can be employed in treating mucositis in the oral cavity, but it is first important to enlist the patient's cooperation in avoiding irritants such as alcohol, tobacco, spicy or acidic foods, very hot or very cold foods and drinks, and commercial mouthwash products (they are too astringent even when diluted). Although a 1:1 solution of hydrogen peroxide has been used for mouth care for many years, this solution can actually be very damaging to tissues if it is not diluted correctly. Normal saline is an acceptable solution, although it does little to refresh the mouth. One ounce of diphenhydramine hydrochloride (Benadryl) elixir diluted in 1 quart of water provides an ideal agent for mouth care in individuals with mucositis. The diphenhydramine hydrochloride solution provides a soothing, nontoxic, pleasant-tasting means for the person to rinse and gargle as needed. Mouth care should be done as often as every 3 or 4 hours and is especially important before mealtime. One technique is to use an air-powered spray apparatus to deliver a fine mist of the diphenhydramine hydrochloride solution, which can be directed at all surfaces of the mouth and oral cavity. This irrigation technique is effective in loosening retained food particles, breaking up the usually tenacious mucus, and soothing the mucosa. Care should be taken not to dislodge the plaquelike formations of mucositis because dislodgement will cause bleeding and denude the mucosal surface. Outpatients can receive this irrigation treatment daily, as can inpatients when they are brought to the radiotherapy department for their radiation treatment. In addition, inpatients can be given mouth care by a modified technique at their bedside several times daily. A disposable irrigation bag is hung from an intravenous pole, using gravity to deliver a spray of solution to the mouth and oropharynx.

In addition to diphenhydramine hydrochloride mouth care solution, agents that coat and soothe the oral mucosa such as Maalox are sometimes used. Lidocaine hydrochloride 2% viscous solution may provide some relief from discomfort, but the anesthetic effect, especially on the tongue, is objectionable to some individuals. This active approach to mouth care for radiation-induced mucositis enables most individuals to tolerate the effects of radiation better. Occasionally, a break from treatment will have to be given when reactions are excessive, but constant daily nursing support appears to be a factor in promoting tolerance of treatment.

Xerostomia

The dry mouth resulting from radiation to the salivary glands or portions of them is know as xerostomia. Alterations in taste frequently accompany xerostomia. Whether the condition is temporary or permanent depends on the dose received and the percentage of the total salivary tissues irradiated. During the course of radiation, little can be done to relieve this annoying symptom. The sensitivity of the mucous membranes precludes the use of saliva substitutes at this point, and frequent sips of water seem to be the best method of providing moisture. Saliva, although present, is thick and viscous, often causing the person to gag and expectorate with difficulty. Frequent mouth care, especially before meals, will provide some relief. When a course of therapy has ended and any intraoral reaction has subsided, some individuals will benefit from the use of a saliva substitute to provide moisture and lubrication for 2- to 4-hour periods. During the night, xerostomia causes the person to awaken frequently with a dry, almost choking sensation that is relieved only by taking a drink of water. Some individuals find that using the saliva substitute allows them to sleep uninterrupted for several hours. A small container of this mixture can be carried easily in a pocket or purse for use when the person is away from home. The formula for saliva substitute is as follows:

- Cologel 98.2 mL
- Glycerin 110.0 mL
- Saline 1000.0 mL

The solution should be mixed well and refrigerated. It is stable for 3 months. The person with xerostomia should use 1 to 2 teaspoons every 3 or 4 hours. The solution is swished in the mouth and swallowed. Several brands of saliva substitute are available for over-the-counter purchase.

Radiation caries

Although it is a potential late effect of irradiation to the mouth and oropharynx, radiation caries can be greatly reduced or avoided by proper care before, during, and after a course of treatment. Absence or decrease in saliva and the altered pH produced by treatment promote decay. Before the start of therapy, a thorough dental examination and prophylaxis should be carried out. If extensive decay and general poor dentition exist, full mouth extraction is usually the treatment of choice. However, if teeth are in good repair, a vigorous preventive program is begun to protect them from the late effects of radiation. This can include daily diphenhydramine hydrochloride mouth sprays for their cleansing effect, followed by a 5-minute application of fluoride gel. Brushing the teeth with a soft-bristled brush several times daily is also important. Such vigorous efforts to prevent decay in individuals receiving radiotherapy can be initiated by the nurse, and nursing support and encouragement are necessary in helping to ensure continuation of this preventive treatment when radiotherapy is completed.

Esophagitis and dysphagia

When radiation is given to the mediastinum, as, for example, in treating patients with cancer of the lung or breast or Hodgkin's disease, areas of the esophagus may receive a sufficient dose to produce symptoms of esophagitis. This is a transient effect in which the esophageal mucous membrane becomes somewhat edematous, and mucositis can develop. The patient will first notice some difficulty in swallowing solids, which is often described as "a lump in my throat, only deeper." This may then progress to a definite esophagitis, which makes swallowing painful and can be responsible for a decrease in intake of foods and fluids. Newer treatment techniques are available that minimize this effect, and a treatment technique or schedule can be adjusted to allow the reaction to subside. The following mixture provides temporary relief from radiation esophagitis:

Radiotherapy Mixture

Mylanta (Stuart)—450 mL (three 5-oz bottles)

Lidocaine hydrochloride viscous 2%—100 mL

Diphenhydramine hydrochloride elixir—60 mL

Shake well and refrigerate

Dosage: 1 to 2 tablespoons 15 min ac and hs

When esophagitis occurs, ensuring adequate nutrition becomes a major nursing concern. The person receiving treatment should be encouraged to substitute high-calorie, high-protein, high-carbohydrate liquids and soft, bland foods for their regular meals. Eggnogs, milk shakes, "instant" liquid meals, and commercially prepared liquid supplements may all be used between meals as well as substituted for solids. Blenderized foods from the person's regular diet are less expensive than commercial products, and the person with esophagitis should be encouraged to try this method.

The individual and family need continual encouragement and support through this difficult period. Weight loss caused by decreased intake can be interpreted by the person undergoing therapy as treatment failure and lead to a defeatist attitude. The temporary nature of the esophagitis and dysphagia should be emphasized.

Nausea and vomiting

Of the potential side effects from radiotherapy, nausea or vomiting or both are probably the most distressing to the person being treated. Although nausea and vomiting are not common, the fear that they will occur causes great stress in many individuals. As with other side effects, treatment site and volume are the variables to be considered, along with preexisting conditions related to surgery, chemotherapy, and sites of disease. The patient's emotional state and apprehension about the disease and treatment are sometimes responsible for nausea when treatment is unlikely to be the cause.

Generally, the person receiving radiotherapy can be expected to experience some degree of nausea when treatment is directed to any of the following sites: whole abdomen or portions of it, large pelvic fields, hypochondrium, epigastrium, or para-aortic areas.

Some patients report nausea with whole brain irradiation or wide mediastinal fields. However, the majority of patients experience little or no difficulty with this side effect. When nausea does occur, it can usually be controlled by antiemetics administered on a regular schedule and by adjusting the eating pattern so that treatment is given when the stomach is relatively empty. Delaying intake of a full meal until 3 or 4 hours after treatment is also helpful because nausea, if it occurs, will usually appear from 1 to 3 hours after treatment.

Diarrhea

Diarrhea, like nausea and vomiting, is not an expected side effect in most individuals receiving radiotherapy. However, it does occur if areas of the abdomen and pelvis are treated after about 2000 cGy have been given. Some individuals experience only an increase in their usual number of bowel movements, whereas others develop loose, watery stools and intestinal cramping. Occasionally, treatment must be interrupted to allow the bowel to recover from radiation effects, especially in elderly or debilitated individuals. When diarrhea and vomiting both occur, active intervention with intravenous fluids for short-term replacement may be needed, as well as a rest from treatment.

For most individuals with radiation-induced diarrhea, a low-residue diet and prescription of loperamide hydrochloride are usually sufficient. The low-residue diet may be all that is required in some instances. Many individuals are not sufficiently knowledgeable about foods and their composition to manage this on their own, and a low-residue diet sheet has been developed to supplement the teaching done by the nurse (Table 12-3). When reviewing the diet with the person being treated (and with the individual preparing meals at home), it is especially important to emphasize the "Foods Allowed" and to point out that a daily multiple vitamin should be included. Vitamin C is notably lacking from the diet, as well as those vitamins found in leafy green vegetables. A favorite food from the "Foods to Avoid" list may be added now and then, if it does not increase symptoms. Diets such as this one should be individually designed to meet the particular geographic and ethnic food patterns of the population, hence the inclusion of well-washed clams and pasta without sauces on the sample.

Tenesmus, cystitis, and urethritis

Although infrequent, tenesmus, cystitis, and urethritis do occur in some individuals receiving pelvic irradiation. Tenesmus of the anal or urinary sphincter produces a persistant sensation of the need to evacuate the bowel or bladder. Relief can sometimes be obtained from gastrointestinal and urinary antispasmodics and anticholinergic preparations. The problem may persist, however, until after the course of treatment has ended.

Cystitis and urethritis resulting from radiation to the bladder area is distressing to the person being treated and is usually brought to the physician's or nurse's attention soon after it develops. A clean-voided urine specimen for culture and sensitivity testing should be obtained, and appropriate antibiotic therapy instituted if indicated. Usually, no infection is found, and treatment consists of urinary antiseptics and antispasmodics for symptomatic relief. High fluid intake is encouraged. Sitz baths, which are commonly prescribed for tenesmus, cystitis, and urethritis, are contraindicated if the perineal area is being irradiated. The added moisture will only enhance any potential or actual skin reaction.

Alopecia

The loss of hair is traumatic to most people regardless of whether they are prepared for this change in body image. The needless fear of this loss is equally traumatic, and if patients are prepared for radiotherapy that does not include the scalp, they should be reassured that hair loss will not occur as a result of treatment.

During treatment of the whole brain, as in metastatic disease or for primary brain tumor, alopecia will occur and follows a typical pattern. At about 2500 to 3000 cGy fractionated over 2 or 3 weeks, the patient will notice excessive amounts of hair in the brush or comb and a gradual thinning of the hair. This continues for 2 or 3 weeks, and then quite suddenly most of the hair comes out, and the patient awakens to find the remainder of his or her hair on the pillow. The patient who is prepared for this with a wig or attractive scarves or caps will adjust to this change with less emotional trauma than one who is totally unprepared either emotionally or physically.

In some instances hair loss may occur regionally or in patches rather than over the entire scalp. Examples include the patient being treated for a pituitary lesion with a two- or three-field technique involving portals of approximately 6 × 6 cm or the person receiving mantle irradiation for Hodgkin's disease that includes the suboccipital lymph nodes. The latter patient will lose hair at the base of the scalp from the hairline to several centimeters above with a strip remaining in the midline due to a block inserted to protect the spinal cord. Whenever possible, the person being treated with this or similar field arrangements in which patchy hair loss is expected should be advised to grow the hair longer. In some instances the long hair can be combed to cover areas of alopecia.

Care of the hair and scalp while receiving radiation to the scalp includes very gentle brushing or combing and infrequent shampooing. Some radiotherapists request that patients not shampoo at all, whereas others will permit a once-a-week cleaning. Permanent waves and hair coloring are contraindicated because of the potential harm to the irradiated skin of the scalp. Individuals being treated in the neck or facial areas should likewise avoid any pro-

TABLE 12-3 Low Residue Diet for Control of Radiation-Induced Diarrhea

Foods Allowed	Foods to Avoid
Beverages	
Skim or low-fat milk, tea, soda, Gatorade, ice-milk, sherbet, low-fat yogurt (plain, vanilla, lemon), buttermilk	Coffee, beer, liquor, fruit juice, chocolate milk, cocoa, hot chocolate
Breads and cereals	
White bread and rolls, plain muffins, saltines, melba toast, cream of wheat or rice, farina, corn and rice cereals, well-cooked oatmeal	Dark, whole-grain breads, rolls and cereals (eg, whole wheat, cracked wheat, bran, pumpernickel, rye, granola, wheat germ, shredded wheat, bran flakes, cereals with dried fruits and nuts)
Starchy foods	
White potatoes (no skin), plain spaghetti, macaroni, noodles, other pasta (no tomato sauce), white rice	Sweet potatoes, potato skins, brown or wild rice, pizza
Vegetables	
Well-cooked carrots, squash, green beans	All other vegetables (cooked or raw) especially cabbage, broccoli, brussels sprouts, baked beans, kidney beans, peas, radishes, cucumbers, corn
Fruits	
Bananas, apples in any form (baked, raw, applesauce, apple juice)	All other fruits and juices
Meats and meat substitutes	
Chicken (stewed, creamed, broiled, or baked, all without skin), turkey, lean beef, veal, pork, lamb, ham, fish, canned or well-washed clams, cottage cheese, hard cheese, eggs	All fried, tough or spicy meats, hot dogs, sausage, poultry skins, gritty seafood, pork and beans, peanut butter
Miscellaneous	
Broth, bouillion, consomme, creamed soups, salt, sugar, jelly, honey, plain jello, custard, tapioca pudding, other puddings (except chocolate), hard candies	All seasonings, jams, pickles, popcorn, olives, coconut, nuts, dried seeds, chocolate cake and chocolate cookies

Courtesy of Philip G. Maddock, MD, and Laura J. Hilderley, RN, Radiation Oncology, Warwick, RI.

cedures on the hair that involve the use of harsh chemicals because such substances may run down onto treated skin. As in the case of irradiated skin in general, the scalp should be treated with care and caution for several months to a year or more after all healing has taken place. The top of the head, especially in males (who have less of a protective layer of hair), should be protected from sunburn with a cap. The forehead, ears, and neck also may exhibit more sensitivity to the sun than before radiation treatment was given.

Skin reactions

The response of normal skin to radiation treatments varies from mild erythema to moist desquamation that leaves a raw surface similar to a second-degree burn. Because megavoltage and cobalt beams deliver the maximum dose beneath the skin, skin reactions have become less significant. Although an acute response may occur during the course of therapy in which brisk erythema progresses to dry and then moist desquamation, healing and cosmesis are usually satisfactory. Some individuals may exhibit a permanent tanning effect in the treatment area with no change in the texture of the skin and subcutaneous tissues. Other individuals will have fibrosclerotic changes in the subcutaneous structures, and their skin will be smooth, taut, and shiny. Telangiectasia also may be evident.

Acute and chronic changes in irradiated skin depend on many factors that govern the severity and permanence of the radiation effect. As in other treatment-related side effects, total dose, fractionation, and volume are important factors. Quality of the treatment beam and its percentage depth dose (see the section entitled Applied Radiation Physics earlier in the chapter) will determine the amount of skin sparing. Individuals treated with electron beams will exhibit considerable skin reactions when the electron beam is intended for lesions located on the skin or a few centimeters below the surface. Characteristics of the electron beam are such that maximum dose buildup occurs within 1 cm below the skin, especially at energies below 20 MeV. However, even more severe reactions that include areas of moist desquamation and peeling will heal well, leaving some patchy depigmentation and telangiectasis.

Skin in some areas of the body, such as the groin, perineum, buttocks, inframammary folds, and axillas, has a relatively poor tolerance to radiation. This is due to the normal warmth and moisture found in these areas rather than any characteristic of the skin itself. Reactions to radiation in these sites are likely to be more severe than in adjacent areas receiving identical treatment.

Because moisture enhances skin reactions, the person being treated should be advised to keep the skin in the treated area as dry as possible. Bathing or showering is permissible, but long periods of soaking are inadvisable. Treated skin should be bathed gently with tepid water and mild soap. The area should be rinsed thoroughly and gently patted (not rubbed) dry. Lines or markings placed on the skin at simulation should not be removed until the radiation therapy technologist or radiotherapist advises the patient to do so. It may therefore be necessary to take sponge baths rather than tub baths or a shower for some time to avoid washing off the markings.

General guidelines to follow for care of the skin within the treatment site include:

1. Keep the skin dry.
2. Avoid using powders, lotions, creams, alcohol, and deodorants.
3. Wear loose-fitting garments.
4. Do not apply tape to the treatment site when dressings are applied.
5. Shave with an electric razor only. Do not use preshaves or aftershaves.
6. Protect the skin from exposure to direct sunlight, chlorinated swimming pools, and temperature extremes (hot water bottle, heating pad).

Such precautions are necessary throughout the course of treatment and until any skin reaction has disappeared afterward.

Specific measures that are useful in treating skin reactions include the use of a light dusting of cornstarch for pruritus from erythema and dry desquamation. If moist desquamation and denuded areas appear, a thin layer of A and D ointment may be applied, followed by a Telfa (nonstick) dressing to protect the clothing and the skin. The radiotherapist or radiation oncology nurse should always be consulted regarding specific skin care measures appropriate to the individual.

When planning for skin care for the person receiving radiotherapy, it should be remembered that individuals are often treated by parallel opposing portals and only one of these portals may be marked to indicate the field. This means that in addition to the clearly marked portal on the person's abdomen or chest (for example), there may be a corresponding field on the posterior that needs the same careful attention. A telephone call to the radiotherapist or radiotherapy technologist will provide the information needed to identify the treatment portal or portals. Tattoos that indicate the treatment site (as described in the section entitled Simulation and Treatment Planning) also may be present on the person's skin and may be helpful in determining which areas of skin require special care.

Skin care in radiotherapy varies considerably from one treatment center to another. The radiotherapy nurse or physician should always be consulted about skin care if there is any question concerning institutional or office policy. Outpatients should be given explicit directions for managing at home, and written directions are very helpful in addition to the verbal instructions.

One area of skin care about which there is usually some question is the matter of exposure to the sun. Any restrictions on sunbathing apply only to the treated area or areas. No special precautions are needed for sites that are normally covered by clothing when outdoors. (One exception is skin that exhibited a moderate or severe reaction to radiation, which may become sunburned when protected only by a sheer or light fabric covering.) During treatment and for a month or more afterward, treated skin should not be exposed to direct sunlight. Individuals whose treatment site is exposed can usually go from home to car or elsewhere for brief periods without difficulty. However, during seasons when the sun is most intense or in locales where the exposure is more intense, even a brief trip outdoors without protective garments may enhance the reaction on treated skin, depending on the dose of radiation received. Caution and common sense should prevail.

When a course of radiotherapy has ended and after any reaction has subsided and healed, a cautious approach to sunbathing may be resumed. Previously treated areas may be exposed gradually (15 min/day), using a number 15 sunblock. Each person must determine his or her own tolerance to the sun and proceed accordingly.

Because of the skin-sparing effect of today's treatment machines, most individuals are able to enjoy outdoor activities without incident after their treatment course has ended. Again, it is important to emphasize caution and common sense.

Bone marrow depression

When large volumes of active bone marrow are irradiated (especially the pelvis or spine in the adult), the effect on the marrow can be quite significant. Other areas of concern when large fields are treated include the sternum, ribs, metaphyses of the long bones, and skull. During simulation and treatment planning, provision is made for shielding as much of this active marrow as possible without compromising the treatment. Because of careful planning and trimming of fields to include only the necessary volume, the majority of people receiving radiotherapy are able to tolerate a course of treatment without experiencing bone marrow depression. Nonetheless, weekly blood counts should be done on all individuals receiving radiotherapy and two to three times weekly in some instances.

The latter is necessary for individuals receiving concomitant chemotherapy or those who have had extensive chemotherapy before radiation. A notable example would be the person with Hodgkin's disease or non-Hodgkin's lymphoma who has received several cycles of combination chemotherapy. Individuals receiving total body irradiation or splenic irradiation for chronic lymphocytic leukemia will require daily blood counts before treatment to avoid (or at least anticipate) a precipitous drop in the white blood cell and platelet counts.

For the person whose bone marrow is affected by treatment or a combination of factors, a number of support measures can be employed. If available, a laminar flow unit may be used. However, most individuals do not have access to such facilities and can be managed either at home or in the hospital. Transfusions of whole blood, platelets, or other components may be necessary for the patient who has dangerously low counts, and treatment may have to be adjusted or interrupted. Nursing care should include observation of the person for signs and symptoms of bleeding, anemia, and infection. Patients and their families must be taught what to look for and to report to the radiotherapist or nurse whenever symptoms occur.

Radiation side effects: special considerations

As previously stated, most people are less anxious if told ahead of time what specific side effects they may expect from their treatment. Knowing that diarrhea is quite likely to result from pelvic irradiation will help the person prepare for such an event, both in terms of dietary adjustments and in helping to avoid embarrassing accidents. There are, however, a number of side effects that do not occur with any predictability or regularity, and an individual being treated would not necessarily benefit from knowing about them ahead of time. The nurse, who is sometimes the first caregiver to whom a person may report symptoms, should be aware of these less common but possible side effects of radiotherapy to specific sites.

Transient myelitis When lymph nodes in the cervical region are radiated, as in the mantle technique employed when treating patients with stage III Hodgkins's disease, the spinal cord is blocked to protect it from unnecessary radiation. However, a radiation effect on the spinal cord can still occur. Some individuals will experience paresthesia (a shocklike sensation radiating down the back and over the extremities) when flexing the neck. This is known as Lhermitte's syndrome and occurs after a latent period of 2 to 3 weeks after treatment to the site has ended. The symptoms usually improve gradually or spontaneously, leaving no permanent effect. The dose of radiation that can produce a transient myelopathy is well below the dose that results in a permanent injury to the spinal cord. A possible explanation for the symptoms found in Lhermitte's syndrome is the effect of radiation on the vasculature supplying the cervical cord. If the blood vessels are compromised by radiation injury, stretching or bending the neck can cause a temporary occlusion and decrease in blood supply to the cord, resulting in paresthesia. Paresthesias can be frightening to a person. However, the temporary nature of this effect can be stressed and the person reassured that this is a known side effect that sometimes occurs.

Parotitis Parotitis is a painful swelling and inflammation of the parotid glands that sometimes occurs in individuals receiving radiation to the maxillomandibular area. Again, it may occur with mantle irradiation for Hodgkin's disease, as well as with treatment to the area for other forms of cancer. The onset of symptoms is sudden and usually follows the first two or three treatments. Although uncomfortable, the symptoms subside almost as quickly as they arise, and no specific treatment is necessary.

Visual and olfactory disturbances During radiation to the pituitary area, some individuals occasionally experience visual or olfactory disturbances, which can be distressing. Some have reported seeing lights or smelling something burning, among other things, after several treatments. The explanation for this phenomenon lies in the anatomic proximity of the optic and olfactory nerves to the hypophysis and the fact that ionization taking place in or near these structures can cause alterations in the sensations of sight and smell. A multiple-field technique is usually employed when treating patients with pituitary lesions to deliver a high dose to the tumor with a minimal dose to surrounding structures. However, the optic nerves, chiasma, and optic tract lie between the hypophysis and the bulk of the brain, and the oflactory bulb and tract lie superior and anterior to the hypophysis, which means that the olfactory and optic structures are likely to be included in the field arrangement. Again, reassurance and explanation tailored to the person's ability to understand are the best means of handling these disturbing but uncommon side effects.

Radiation recall Although not technically a radiation reaction, *radiation recall* can occur in a previously irradiated site that exhibited mucositis or erythema. Radiation recall occurs in response to the systemic administration of certain chemotherapeutic agents (for example, actinomycin) several months to a year or more after radiation was received. Typically, the person develops intraoral mucositis or a skin reaction in the exact pattern corresponding to the previously treated radiation portal. Treatment is symptomatic, and the drug dosage or choice of agent may be modified if necessary.

NURSING CARE OF THE PATIENT WITH A RADIOACTIVE SOURCE

Nursing care of individuals being treated with implanted radioactive sources is a challenge that goes beyond basic medical-surgical theory and requires an understanding of radiation safety, biology, and physiologic manifestations. Rather than fear, the nurse should develop a healthy respect for all that is implicit in working with radioactive isotopes and proceed to plan and deliver optimum care under the special conditions encountered in each situation.

Radioactive materials for therapeutic usage are listed in Figure 12-2, and specific sources for brachytherapy are outlined in Figure 12-5. In addition to being implanted in tissues or inserted into body cavities, some radioactive isotopes may be administered orally, intravenously, or by installation. These materials are adsorbed or metabolized by the body, and specific safety precautions are required, depending on the particular source and mode of administration. Adsorbed or metabolized isotopes used most commonly include ^{131}I, ^{32}P, and ^{198}Au, all of which are administered as colloids or solutions. Liquid sources such as these present a possibility of contamination of equipment, dressings, and linens, depending on the mode of administration and metabolism. In contrast, sealed sources such as ^{137}Cs and ^{226}Ra for implantation through a mechanical device are not metabolized and are therefore not excreted in body fluids.

The following information is necessary to provide safe and effective nursing care for individuals being treated with brachytherapy (sealed radioactive source placed within a body cavity or tissue) or with metabolized or adsorbed radiation:

1. What is the source being used?
2. What is the half-life of that source?
3. What is the type of emission (alpha, beta, gamma)?
4. How much radioisotope is being used (energy)?
5. What method of administration/application is being used?
6. Is the source metabolized? Adsorbed? Neither?

From this information, the nurse can plan and administer nursing care utilizing the appropriate precautions, including disposal of wastes and care of linens and equipment. This information will also help to determine whether radiation safety precautions are necessary after hospital discharge.

Radiation safety and radiation protection are the concern of every caregiver involved with brachytherapy patients. This includes the radiotherapist, other physicians, nurses, technologists, physicists, and allied health workers who may come in contact with the person being treated. Leading this team is the radiation safety officer employed by the institution to implement radiation safety procedures and monitor all use of radioactive materials. Most institutions will also have a radiation safety committee composed of representatives from among the disciplines listed previously, whose responsibilities are the control and enforcement of the use of radioisotopes in the hospital as required by the Atomic Energy Commission.

Three primary factors in radiation protection should be foremost in the minds of all personnel involved in care of the person being treated: *time, distance,* and *shielding*.

Time

The exposure to radiation that personnel receive is directly proportional to the time spent within a specific distance from the source. Nursing care must be planned and organized so that the nurse spends as little time as possible in close contact with the individual being treated while still providing for his or her needs.

Distance

As radiation is emitted from a point source, the amount of radiation reaching a given area decreases according to the law of inverse square. Figure 12-14 illustrates this principle.

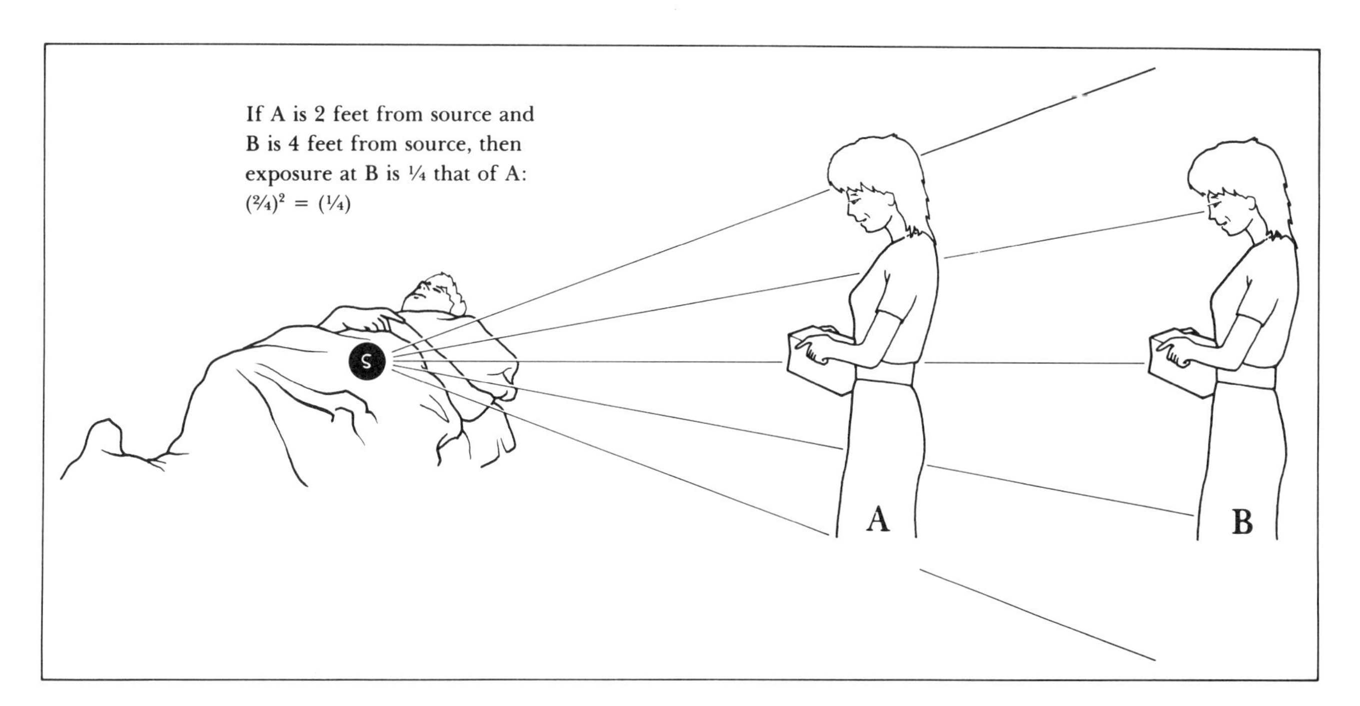

FIGURE 12-14 The inverse square law. As distance from a radiation source increases, exposure decreases by the square of that distance.

Shielding

When a sheet of absorbing material is placed between a radiation source and a detector, the amount of radiation that reaches the detector decreases depending on the energy of the radiation and the nature and thickness of the absorbing material (shield). The thickness of a shielding material that is required to reduce the radiation to half of its original quantity is referred to as the *half-value layer* (HVL). The HVL for ^{137}Cs (a commonly used radioactive source) is approximately 6 mm of lead or 10 cm of concrete. The practical implications of this should be evident.

When planning nursing care for the person with a radioactive source, time and distance are the two variables that can most readily be controlled. Because shielding from gamma radiation requires lead or concrete in the previously specified thicknesses, it is usually impractical to expect that much physical care can be given from behind such a shield. Portable radiation shields (similar in design to a moving blackboard on wheels) are available and do protect the caregiver who places it between himself or herself and the source. However, this is primarily useful in doing tasks within the person's room other than direct care. The so-called lead aprons used in diagnostic radiology are not of sufficient thickness to stop gamma rays and cannot protect the caregiver from exposure when caring for individuals with radium or cesium sources, for example.

Because shielding is not always possible or practical, time and distance are the two factors that nurses must incorporate into the care plan. Some of the ways in which exposure to personnel can be reduced are listed in Figure 12-15.

1. Use appropriate radiation precaution signs, wristbands, and tags.
2. Plan care to avoid delays at the person's bedside.
3. Eliminate the bedbath except what the person can manage alone.
4. Change linens less frequently or only when soiled.
5. Prepare meal trays outside of the person's room instead of at the bedside (cut up meats, open containers, etc.).
6. Work quickly; concentrate on accomplishing the necessary tasks in as short a time as possible.
7. Position the bedside table, call bell, and television controls within easy reach of the person to avoid frequent return trips to the bedside.
8. Use appropriate monitoring devices and heed the information regarding total individual exposure.
9. No nurse should care for more than two individuals with radioactive sources at a time.
10. Keep long-handled forceps and a shielded transport cart in the person's room at all times.
11. Use long-handled forceps to retrieve a radioactive source that has accidentally been dislodged.
12. Arrange the chair so that ambulatory individuals can be seated as far from the bed (and thus the caregiver) as possible while linens are being changed.

FIGURE 12-15 Some ways to reduce exposure to personnel caring for the individual with a radioactive source.

With all the emphasis on haste and elimination of nonessential personal hygiene, it is sometimes easy to eliminate that most important consideration of emotional and social support of the person being treated. Individuals who are isolated for radiation precautions often feel "unclean" or "contaminated." The fact that visitors are allowed only at the doorway and that housekeeping personnel are barred from the room adds to this sense of isolation. Because the nurse also must limit the time spent in giving direct care, the person's sense of rejection is often heightened.

Planning and providing emotional support are major components of nursing care for all individuals, but especially for those with an implant or other form of radioactive material. Preparation for these procedures should include all the following points of information:

1. *Description of the procedure.* For example, although performed in the operating room under anesthesia, insertion of vaginal tandem and ovoids will not involve a surgical incision.

2. *Possible change in appearance.* For example, individuals with needle implants in the facial region often request a mirror and should be prepared for their sometimes grotesque appearance while needles are in place.

3. *Anticipated pain or discomfort and measures available for relief.* For example, the presence of gynecologic applicators (such as in Figure 12-6) combined with bedrest and restricted movement often produces a low backache. Appropriate analgesics are prescribed and should be administered as needed.

4. *Potential short-term and long-term side effects and complications.* An example of a short-term side effect is that needle implants to the tongue usually produce edema, causing the tongue to be noticeably swollen during the procedure and for several days afterward. A long-term complication, such as occurs with vaginal brachytherapy, may result in scarring and the formation of adhesions that cause dyspareunia.

5. *Restrictions on activity while the radioactive sources are in place.* For example, individuals with gynecologic applicators in place are confined to bed for the duration of the treatment, which may be as long as 3 to 4 days.

6. *Visiting restrictions.* For example, policy varies depending on the availability of appropriate shielding devices and the energy of the sources being used. However, visitors are usually restricted from the person's room, and, when allowed, visits must be brief.

7. *Radiation precautions observed by hospital personnel.* For example, individuals should be reassured that their personal care needs will be met but that the nurses' time at the bedside and in the room will be restricted because of the presence of the radioactive sources.

The person also should be helped to prepare for such procedures by planning for suitable activities such as reading, handwork, television, and so on. Boredom and isolation are sometimes the most difficult part of treatment with a radioactive source. The nurse has a primary responsibility to meet those treatment-induced needs, as well as those of a physical nature.

With the proper application of the principles of radiation safety and careful attention to the special emotional needs of individuals being treated with brachytherapy, this challenge for nursing care can be met.

ADVANCES IN RADIOTHERAPY

Radiation oncology in the 1990s will be characterized by continual refinement of treatment techniques and expanded application of multimodal therapy. Numerous cooperative group studies employ radiation as primary or adjuvant therapy. Variations such as hyperfractionation (more than one treatment per day) for particularly resistant tumors are being tested. Whole or hemibody irradiation for widespread metastasis is providing rapid palliation for some individuals.[42]

Use of particle radiation such as fast neutrons, deuterons, helium ion beams, and negative pi-mesons will continue to be tested and refined for use in situations where conventional radiation is of little value. The expense and limited applicability of such treatment methods currently confine their use to a small proportion of cancer patients.

In February 1989, an announcement was made of the first proton beam accelerator built for hospital use. This device will move out of the physics laboratory setting (Fermi Laboratory in Illinois, Harvard University, the University of California at Berkeley, as well as several sites abroad) where limited numbers of patients have been treated since the early 1970s. Loma Linda University Medical Center, Los Angeles, expects to start using the $40 million treatment device in 1990.

Radiolabeled antibody therapy has been the subject of considerable interest and effort through the 1970s and 1980s.[43] This treatment technique is based on the information acquired in recent years regarding immunobiology and the isolation of many tumor-specific monoclonal and polyclonal antibodies. Among the numerous radioactive isotopes that have been used therapeutically, ^{131}I and ^{90}Y, in particular, have been adopted for use in radiolabeled antibody therapy.

The underlying principle of radiolabeled antibody therapy involves attaching a radioactive isotope to the tumor-specific antibody to deliver therapeutic radiation directly to the target tumor. Theoretically, this avoids prolonged radiation exposure to healthy cells while delivering lethal or sublethal doses to the tumor. Among numerous phase I, II, and III clinical trials over the past two decades, some of the more significant results have been achieved in the treatment of hepatoma.[44] Studies involving treatment of intrahepatic biliary carcinoma, nonresectable, non-oat-cell carcinoma, and recurrent Hodgkins's disease are ongoing.[44]

Intraoperative radiotherapy (IOR) was developed in the United States during the late 1970s at Howard University and at Massachusetts General Hospital.[45] Unresectable tumors had been the primary target of IOR before the 1980s. By 1985, however, IOR was used increasingly in a prophylactic approach combined with resection of primary tumors such as locally advanced colorectal carcinoma; pancreatic, gastric, and bladder cancers; and soft tissue sarcomas.

Compared with external beam therapy, intraoperative radiotherapy has the advantage of increasing tumor dose in relation to normal tissue dose. After surgically exposing the target volume, a single, large fraction of radiation is delivered directly to the tumor site by a specially built cone attached to the therapy machine. The surgical procedure is then completed, and a further postoperative course of conventional radiotherapy is given. Some institutions give a preoperative rather than postoperative course of conventional radiotherapy, but rarely is IOR the definitive treatment.

There are a number of differences in the exact IOR procedures at the various institutions in the United States now using IOR.[46,47] Although some have installed radiotherapy equipment in an operating room or built a special room to perform the combined therapy, others have worked out a detailed procedure for transporting the fully anesthetized and surgically opened patient through the hospital corridors to the radiotherapy department. Despite the technical difficulties in performing IOR, it appears to have potential for further development and application in cancer management.

CONCLUSION

Radiotherapy in the treatment of cancer has indeed come a long way from its exciting beginning in the late 1800s. Much has been learned about the beneficial as well as the harmful effects of ionizing radiation. The 1990s continue to hold promise for advances in cancer treatment, with radiotherapy playing a major role in primary treatment as well as in combined modality approaches.

Along with advances in therapy has been increased recognition of the important role of the nurse as educator and care provider for persons receiving radiation treatment and their families. As new radiation centers open and others are restructured, nurses are increasingly being added to the team of caregivers. Previously nurses had been involved somewhat peripherally in care of radiotherapy patients, but they are now taking a major role as collaborative caregivers with the radiotherapist. Advances in nursing science and nursing care parallel advances in radiotherapy as a treatment modality.

REFERENCES

1. Berry RJ: Basic concepts in radiobiology: A review, in Mansfield CM (ed): Therapeutic Radiology: New Directions in Therapy. New Hyde Park, NY, Medical Examination Publishing Company, 1983, pp 1-15.
2. Maddock PG: Brachytherapy sources and applicators. Semin Oncol Nurs 3(1):15-22, 1987.
3. Shell J, Carter J: The gynecological implant patient. Semin Oncol Nurs 3(1):54-66, 1987.
4. Hall EJ, Cox JD: Physical and biologic basis of radiation therapy, in Moss WT, Cox JD (eds): Radiation Oncology: Rationale, Technique, Results. St. Louis, CV Mosby, 1989, pp 1-57.
5. Travis E: Primer of Medical Radiobiology. Chicago, Year Book Medical Publishers, Inc., 1975.
6. Hall EJ: Radiobiology for the Radiologist (ed 2). Hagerstown, Md, Harper & Row, 1978.
7. Richter MP, Share FS, Goodman RL: Principles of radiation therapy, in Calabrese P, Schein PS, Rosenberg SA (eds): Medical Oncology: Basic Principles and Clinical Management of Cancer. New York, MacMillan, 1985, pp 280-291.
8. Bergonie J, Tribondeau L: Interpretation of some results of radiotherapy and an attempt at determining a logical technique of treatment. Radiation Res II: 587, 1959.
9. Gray LH: Radiobiologic basis of oxygen as a modifying factor in radiation therapy. Am J Roentgenol 85:805, 1961.
10. Withers HR, Peters LJ: Biologic aspects of radiotherapy, in Fletcher GH (ed): Textbook of Radiotherapy (ed 3). Philadelphia, Lea & Febiger, 1980, pp 103-180.
11. Withers HR. Biologic basis of radiation therapy, in Perez CA, Brady LW (eds): Principles and Practice of Radiation Oncology. Philadelphia, JB Lippincott, 1987, pp 67-98.
12. Phillips TL: Chemical modification of radiation effects. Cancer 39:987-999, 1977.
13. Brown JM: Hypoxic cell radiosensitizers: Where next? Int J Radiat Oncol Biol Physics 16:987-993, 1989.
14. Coleman CN, Wasserman TH, Urtasun RC, et al: Phase I trial of the hypoxic cell radiosensitizer SR 2508: The results of the five to six week drug schedule. Int J Radiat Oncol Biol Physics 12:1105-1108, 1986.
15. Hall EJ, Miller R, Astor M, et al: The nitroimidazoles as radiosensitizers and cytotoxic agents. Br J Cancer 37:120, 1978 (suppl 3).
16. Phillips TL: Sensitizers and protectors. Semin Oncol 8:65-82, 1981.
17. Fowler JF: Chemical modifiers of radiosensitivity-theory and reality: A review. Int J Radiat Oncol Biol Physics II:665-674, 1985.
18. Noll L: Chemical modifiers of radiation therapy, in Hassey K, Hilderley L (eds): Nursing Perspectives in Radiation Oncology. Albany, NY, Delmar Publishers, 1990.
19. Gonzalez D, van Dijk JDP, Blank LE, et al: Combined treatment with radiation and hyperthermia in metastatic malignant melanoma. Radiother Oncol 6:105-113, 1986.
20. Bicher HI, Wolfstein RS, Lewinsky BS, et al: Microwave hyperthermia as an adjunct to radiation therapy: Summary experience of 256 multifraction treatment cases. Int J Radiat Oncol Biol Physics 12:1667-1671, 1986.
21. Howard GCW, Sathiaseelan V, Freedman L, et al: Hyperthermia and radiation in the treatment of superficial malignancy: An analysis of treatment parameters, response and toxicity. Int J Radiat Oncol Biol Physics 3:1-8, 1987.
22. Valdagni R, Amichetti M, Pani G: Radical radiation alone versus radical radiation plus microwave hyperthermia for N3 (TNM-UICC) neck nodes: A prospective randomized clinical trial. Int J Radiat Oncol Biol Physics 15:13-24, 1988.
23. Valdagni R, Fei-Fei L, Kapp D: Important prognostic factors influencing outcome of combined radiation and hyperthermia. Int J Radiat Oncol Biol Physics 15:959-972, 1988.
24. Hand J, ter Haar G: Heating techniques in hyperthermia. Br J Radiol 56:969-970, 1983.
25. Guy A, Chou CK: Physical aspects of localized heating by radiowaves and microwaves, in Storm F (ed): Hyperthermia in Cancer Therapy. Boston, GK Hall, 1983, pp 279-304.
26. Scott R, Johnson R, Story K, et al: Local hyperthermia in combination with definitive radiotherapy: Increased tumor clearance, reduced recurrence rate in extended followup. Int J Radiat Oncol Biol Physics 10:2119-2123, 1984.
27. Bahman E, Perez C: Interstitial thermoradiotherapy: An overview, Endocuriether/Hypertherm Oncol 1:35-40, 1985.
28. Sapozink M, Gibbs F, Egger M, et al: Abdominal regional hyperthermia with an annular phased array. J Clin Oncol 4:775-783, 1986.
29. Shimm D, Cetas T, Oleson J, et al: Regional hyperthermia for deep-seated malignancies using the BSD annular array. Int J Hypertherm 4:159-170, 1988.
30. Wojtas F: Hyperthermia and radiation therapy, in Hassey K, Hilderley L (eds): Nursing Perspectives in Radiation Oncology. Albany, NY, Delmar Publishers, 1990.
31. BEIR III: The effects on populations of exposure to low levels of ionizing radiation. Report of the Advisory Committee on the Effects of Ionizing Radiation (BEIR III). Washington, DC, National Academy of Sciences, National Research Council, 1980.
32. Lushbaugh CC, Casarett GW: The effects of gonadal irradiation in clinical radiation therapy: A review. Cancer 37:1111-1120, 1976.
33. Schryber S, LaCasse CR, Barton-Burke M: Autologous bone marrow transplantation. Oncol Nurs Forum 14:74-80, 1987.
34. Upton AC: The biological effects of low level ionizing radiation. Sci Am 246:41-49, 1982.
35. Harley N, Physics: Environmental sources of radioactivity levels, and interaction with matter, in Upton AC, Albert RE, Burns FJ, et al (eds): Radiation Carcinogenesis. New York, Elsevier Science, 1986.
36. Kato H, Schull WJ: Studies of the mortality of A-bomb survivors. Mortality, 1950-78. I. Cancer mortality. Radiat Res 90:395-432, 1982.
37. March HC: Leukemia in radiologists in a twenty-year period. Am J Med Sci 220:282, 1950.
38. Pack GT, Davis J: Radiation cancer of the skin. Radiol 84:436, 1965.
39. Conrad RA, Hicking A: Medical findings in Marshallese people exposed to fallout radiation: Results from a ten-year study. JAMA 214:316, 1970.
40. Stewart A: An epidemiologist takes a look at radiation risks. DHEW pub no. 73-8024, Washington DC, US Government Printing Office, 1973.
41. Bucholtz, J: Radiation carcinogenesis, in Hassey K, Hilderley L (eds): Nursing Perspectives in Radiation Oncology. Albany, NY, Delmar Publishers, 1990.
42. Dudjak L: Alterations in fractionation, in Hassey K, Hilderley L (eds): Nursing Perspectives in Radiation Oncology. Albany, NY, Delmar Publishers, 1990.
43. Bucholtz J: Radiolabeled antibody therapy, in Hassey K, Hilderley L (eds): Nursing Perspectives in Radiation Oncology. Albany, NY, Delmar Publishers, 1990.
44. Sitzman JV, Order SE, Klein JL, et al: Conversion by new

treatment modalities of non-resectable hepatocellular cancer, J Clin Oncol 5:1566-1573, 1987.

45. Goldson A: Past, present, and prospects of intraoperative radiotherapy (IOR). Semin Oncol 8:59-64, 1981.
46. Kinsella TJ, Sindelar WF: Newer methods of cancer treatment: Intraoperative radiotherapy, in DeVita VT, Hellman S, Rosenberg SA (eds): Principles and Practice of Oncology (ed 2). Philadelphia, JB Lippincott, 1986, pp 2293-2304.
47. Smith R: Intraoperative radiation therapy, in Hassey K, Hilderley L (eds): Nursing Perspectives in Radiation Oncology. Albany, NY, Delmar Publishers, 1990.

Chapter 13

Chemotherapy

Jean K. Brown, RN, MS

Catherine M. Hogan, RN, MN, OCN

INTRODUCTION

As a systemic mode of treatment, chemotherapy is unique in contrast to older, localized forms of treatment, such as surgery and radiotherapy. This systemic approach is extremely desirable, because it offers hope of effective treatment for many systemic cancers, such as leukemia, lymphoma, and Hodgkin's disease, which cannot be managed effectively with surgery or radiotherapy. It also provides a means of treating early, clinically undetectable metastasis. Thus cancer chemotherapy has become recognized as an essential means of treating cancer by curing some diseases and providing palliation in others, and it is currently one of the three major treatment techniques.

Nurses play an important role in caring for patients who are receiving chemotherapy and their families in both inpatient and outpatient settings. The goal of this nursing care is to ameliorate the impact of treatment on the daily lives of patients and their families. This goal is accomplished in many ways but begins with a thorough assessment of patient and family needs. On the basis of this assessment, the nurse, the person with cancer, and the family develop a plan of care. An essential part of this plan is to provide the patient and the family with information about the specific chemotherapy regimen, side effects that might be experienced, and precautionary and preventive measures that can be taken. In addition, nurses act as coordinators of care, patient advocates, experts on supportive care, and frequently experts responsible for the safe administration of chemotherapeutic drugs. Therefore it is imperative that nurses caring for individuals receiving chemotherapy thoroughly understand this treatment method so that high-quality nursing care may be achieved.

HISTORY

There is evidence of the ineffective use of chemotherapy in the form of metallic salts, such as arsenic, copper, and lead, in early Egyptian and Greek civilizations, and this therapy continued for centuries thereafter.[1] However, effective cancer chemotherapy is a recent medical development. The first effective efforts were developed in the late nineteenth century. Lissauer used potassium arsenite effectively in 1865, and Coley's toxin, a combination of bacterial products, was developed around 1890.[2] Neither of these methods proved reliable and practical enough to be in widespread use.

In the early 1940s, effective, reliable treatment was demonstrated with hormonal therapy for prostate and breast carcinomas.[3,4] This was followed by the identification of cytotoxic substances in World War II research programs in the areas of poisonous gases, nutrition, and antibiotics that provided a basis for postwar chemotherapy research.[5] As a result of poisonous gas research, nitrogen mustard was identified and studied in cancer therapy with excellent temporary responses in chronic leukemia and lymphomas, such as Hodgkin's disease. Nutrition studies focused on folic acids, which led to research by Farber and colleagues[6] on folic acid antagonists (aminopterin) that produced temporary remissions in acute childhood leukemia. With the advent of penicillin, research efforts during World War II focused on large-scale fermentation and isolation of penicillin and other antibiotics. Antitumor activity was reported in crude preparations of penicillin and led ultimately to the isolation of cytotoxic antibiotics, such as the actinomycins. The research on hormones, nitrogen mustard, folic acid antagonists, and antibiotics served as a strong stimulus for chemotherapy research in the following years.

The next three decades witnessed the rapid development of many cancer chemotherapeutic agents. These developments were aided immensely in 1953 when Congress initiated a national program in chemotherapy directed by the National Cancer Institute.[5] A year later the American Cancer Society and the Damon Runyon Memorial Fund for Cancer Research joined the National Cancer Institute, and thereafter grant support was increased. Although the development of new agents has slowed somewhat in recent years, experimental drugs are still being developed and tested. There is a particular emphasis at this time on development of analogues of effective drugs that are less toxic to specific organs and tissues, such as the heart, lungs, kidneys, and nervous tissue.[7]

Along with the development of new drugs over the past four decades, changes have occurred in the treatment regimens for some cancers and in their effectiveness. These have been particularly evident since the United States Congress enacted the National Cancer Act in 1971, which included and expanded the chemotherapy program. This act provided funding for escalating treatment research, and there have been dramatic results. In some instances, chemotherapy can now cure gestational choriocarcinoma, advanced Hodgkin's disease, histiocytic lymphomas, Burkitt's lymphoma, childhood leukemias, and testicular cancers. Increased survival rates also have been reported among persons with many other lymphomas and leukemias.[8] In addition, chemotherapy has contributed significantly to the effective multimodal management of Hodgkin's disease, breast cancer, small-cell lung cancer, Wilms' tumor, Ewing's sarcoma, embryonal rhabdomyosarcoma, and osteogenic sarcoma.[9,10] Many other cancers have been treated with chemotherapy, and the results have given individuals with cancer beneficial palliation and extension of life.

ATTITUDES AND PERCEPTIONS ABOUT CHEMOTHERAPY

Because chemotherapy is a relatively new method of treating cancer, the general public has had limited exposure to it through personal experiences and the mass media. This, coupled with society's great fear of cancer, has led to many negative attitudes and perceptions about cancer drug therapy among both lay people and health care professionals. This can create great anxiety, fear, and avoidance behavior. Patients and their families often display ineffective coping and lack of interpersonal support, leading to frustration among health care professionals. This may result in avoidance and unmet needs. Oncology nurses play an extremely important role in intervening with patients, families, and other health care professionals to provide information and other needed support regarding cancer chemotherapy.

Of all the major cancer treatment techniques, drug therapy is associated most commonly with experimental research. Fears about being a "guinea pig" in the study of experimental drugs are relatively common among individuals and their families. Associated with this is a concern about severe toxic side effects. In addition, individuals with cancer often believe that there is no effective treatment available for their disease and thus no hope of effective management. The strength and scope of these fears and beliefs are altered as the patients and their families progress through the different phases of cancer treatment. Heinrichs and Schmale[11] found that while the initial cancer treatment is anticipated with great anxiety there is hope that no further treatment will be needed and that a cure will result. Information about chemotherapy and possible reactions can be reassuring to these individuals. However, these researchers further found that when faced with treatment for recurrence of the disease, individuals and families inevitably believed that cure was no longer likely. At this stage, skepticism and reluctance were evident, and a great deal of emotional support was needed. All of these attitudes and perceptions have a significant effect on how patients cope with chemotherapy, and it is essential for nurses to consider them as they assess and plan to meet patients' and families' needs.

BIOLOGIC CONCEPTS RELATED TO CHEMOTHERAPY

Cellular kinetics, the study of mechanisms and rates of cellular changes, provides the basis for an understanding of the actions and side effects of anticancer drugs. It is also becoming more and more useful in planning treatment regimens and scheduling drug administration that maximizes therapeutic effectiveness and minimizes toxicity. Because these drugs act primarily on proliferating cells, it is important to examine the cell cycle and the growth of normal and malignant cell populations to understand the rationale for and the effects of drug therapy. Drug specificity, cell kill, and drug resistance are also related directly to the cell cycle and tissue growth.

Cell Cycle

Cycling cells go through four classic phases of G_1, S, G_2, and M to complete a cell growth cycle, as shown in Figure 13-1.[12-15] Some cells move out of the cell cycle after mitosis into G_0, becoming resting and nondividing cells. Other cells enter the first phase, G_1, or the first "gap." This is the period between mitosis and the beginning of DNA synthesis when active RNA and protein synthesis occurs. The G_1 phase is the most variable in time (8 to 48 hours) of all the phases, and its length influences the rate of cell proliferation.[14,15] Cell populations that are growing slowly have many cells in the G_1 phase, whereas populations that are growing rapidly have very few or no cells in the G_1 phase.

As cells emerge from G_1, they enter the S phase, where enzymes necessary for DNA synthesis increase in activity and DNA synthesis occurs. This phase, which is concluded when the cell's DNA content has doubled, takes from 10 to 30 hours. After the S phase, a resting period, called G_2, or the second "gap," occurs. During this phase, the RNA and protein necessary for mitosis are synthesized. This phase extends from the end of DNA synthesis to the beginning of mitosis and takes from 1 to 12 hours. The last

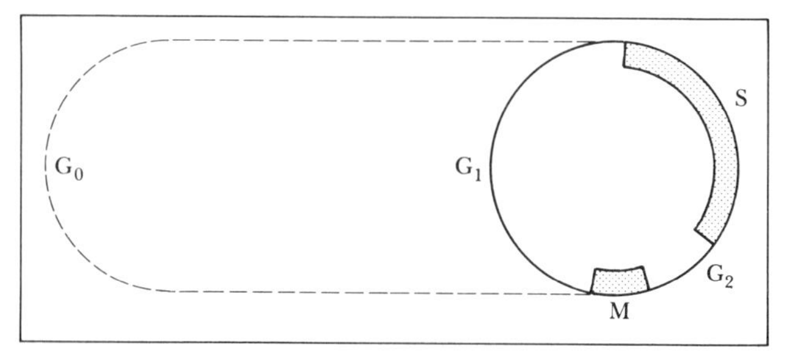

FIGURE 13-1 Stages in the cell replication cycle *S*, DNA synthesis; G_2, the gap between DNA synthesis and mitosis; *M*, mitosis; and G_1, the gap between the end of mitosis and the start of DNA synthesis.

phase of the cell cycle is the M phase, where mitosis takes place. The formation of the spindle, separation of chromosomes, and the division of the cell into two daughter cells occur. The M phase takes about 1 hour. Most investigation to date has focused on mitosis; as more is learned about other phases, however, more information will be available about the action of anticancer drugs.

Normal and Malignant Tissue Growth

In all normal and malignant tissues, three different cell populations affect growth.[14] The first group consists of cells that are dividing continuously and are called cycling cells. The second group consists of cells that divide for a time and then differentiate. These cells complete their life cycle without dividing again and are thus called nondividing cells. The third group is composed of G_0, or resting, cells that leave the cell cycle and remain dormant until conditions stimulate them to reenter the cell cycle and divide. Evidence is being gathered that indicates that cycling cells and G_0, or resting, cells are further divided into stem cells and nonstem cells.[12,16] Stem cells replenish the stem cell pool, which maintains the continued survival and integrity of a specific cell population. Nonstem cells differentiate and enter the maturing groups of cells. As long as G_0 stem cells remain, a damaged cell population can be renewed.

In view of these cell populations or compartments, three things must be considered during assessment of normal or malignant tissue growth: the cell cycle time, the growth fraction, and the rate of cell loss.[14] The *cell cycle time* is the amount of time required for the cell to move from one mitosis to the next. The *growth fraction* is the fraction of cycling cells in the entire cell population, and the *rate of cell loss* is the fraction of cells that die or leave the cell population. Growth depends on the net result of the number of cells produced and the number of cells that die. Rate of growth depends on the cell cycle time, the growth fraction, and the rate of cell loss. In addition, it is believed that the growth of tumors follow the Gompertzian growth curve, which theorizes that as the tissue mass increases in size, the doubling time slows.[17] In tumors, an additional factor that slows the growth rate is the decrease in nutrients available for each cell as the total mass increases and the blood supply is outgrown.[15]

In the past it was believed that tumor cell populations had a shorter cell cycle time and a faster growth rate than normal cells because cancer was characterized by erratic, uncontrolled growth. However, it has been found that some normal cells cycle faster than tumor cells in human beings.[14] For example, the normal crypt cells of the colon and rectum cycle in 39 to 48 hours, whereas cancer cells of the stomach cycle in 72 hours.[18] Also, bone marrow precursor cells cycle in 19 to 40 hours, whereas acute myeloblastic leukemia and chronic myeloid leukemia cells cycle in 50 to 120 hours.[19] Overall, tumor cell cycling times range from 24 to 120 hours, with most ranging from 48 to 72 hours.[15] Because chemotherapy acts on rapidly dividing cells, it will damage some normal cells as well as tumor cells.

As previously stated, the cell cycle times for most tumor cells remain fairly constant at a range of 1 to 5 days, with an average of 2 to 3 days.[15] However, the doubling time of most tumors is substantially longer, ranging from 5 days to 2 years, with a mean of 1 to 3 months.[20] This longer doubling time is due to several factors. First, the growth fraction of human tumors varies widely, from 0% to 100%. Second, many tumor cells die spontaneously. Turbiana, Richard, and Malaise[21] found that 48% of tumor cells may die every day, and their calculations have indicated that at least 5% to 97% of all tumor cells die spontaneously. Spontaneous death results from inadequate nutrition, cumulative genetic damage in tumor cells, and cell differentiation into nondividing cells. Thus a great deal of tumor cell death occurs without any form of treatment.

Drug Specificity

Bruce, Meeker, and Valeriote[22] were one of the first groups to identify successfully the specificity, or selective toxicity, of chemotherapeutic drugs as it relates to cell kinetics. As a result of their findings, chemotherapeutic drugs were classified into three groups according to the sensitivity of cells. Class I nonspecific drugs, such as melphalan, were found to affect both resting and proliferating cells equally. Class II phase-specific drugs, such as vincristine, were toxic to proliferating cells in a specific phase or part of the cell cycle. Resting cells were not affected. Class III cycle-specific drugs, such as doxorubicin, were more toxic to proliferating cells than to resting cells. The results of this research have been verified by clinical experience. At this time, the available drugs are most toxic to proliferating cells. Thus tumors with high rates of cellular proliferation are most amenable to chemotherapy.[23]

Because most chemotherapeutic drugs affect proliferating cells, the cellular kinetic classification method used commonly includes only two classes: phase-specific agents and cycle-specific agents. There has been some confusion in the terms used for these two classes because of the introduction by Skipper[24] of the terms *cell cycle stage–specific* and *cell cycle stage–nonspecific*.[16] The terms *phase-specific* and *cell cycle stage–specific* are comparable and *cycle-specific* and *cell cycle stage–nonspecific* are comparable. Other kinetic classification systems similar to those previously described have been developed. A clear definition of terms is necessary if one is to understand the similarities and differences.

Another factor that affects sensitivity is drug dosage. The dosage affects the action of agents on proliferating cells.[16] High dosages kill the cell at a certain phase or phases in the cell cycle. Low dosages can block or arrest the cell's progression from one phase to the next. In addition, these two effects may not act on the same phases of the cycle. A low dose of a single drug may arrest a cell in a phase that is earlier than the phase in which the drug is lethal.

Tumor Cell Kill

The goal of modern chemotherapy is to destroy all cancer cells; however, many factors can prevent the achievement of this goal. Because most active cytotoxic agents are selectively toxic to rapidly proliferating cells, many G_0 or resting cells remain untouched. As long as resting stem cells remain, the tumor cell population can be regenerated. In addition, as the tumor mass increases in size, the cells cycle at a slower rate, the growth fraction decreases, and the cytotoxic effect of the drug diminishes. Another problem is that these drugs are not only specific to cancer cells but also toxic to normal proliferating cells, particularly those that are rapidly dividing. Normal cells most affected by these drugs include hematopoietic or bone marrow cells, gastrointestinal epithelial cells, hair follicle cells, germinal cells, and embryonal cells.

Two hypotheses have been postulated regarding the ability of chemotherapeutic drugs to kill tumor cells. The first hypothesis evolved from research that has shown that antineoplastic drugs kill tumor cells according to first-order kinetics.[24] This means that a certain drug dose will destroy a constant fraction of tumor cells in the body, rather than a constant number of cells. In addition, these drugs also follow an exponential, or "log-kill," model. Thus cell kill may be expressed as a "log-kill" of two, meaning that the body's tumor burden is decreased from 10^8 to 10^6 cells, from 100,000,000 to 1,000,000 cells, or 99%. The maximum cell kill from a single drug dose has been found to be from two to five logs.[2] Thus treatment must be repeated many times to decrease the number of tumor cells in the body. Because a single dose always kills a fraction of the tumor cells, this hypothesis suggests that chemotherapy can never destroy all the malignant cells in the body.

The second hypothesis has proposed that cell kill caused by antineoplastic drugs is related to the relative growth fraction of the tumor at the time of treatment.[25] Thus the greatest tumor cell kill occurs when the Gompertzian growth fraction is greatest. Only at this time is the log-kill hypothesis valid, whereas at other times a lower fraction of cells are destroyed. The Gompertzian growth fraction is greatest when tumors are of intermediate size and less when they are very small or very large. This hypothesis has not been confirmed clinically but is supported by some observed tumor responses. Further research is needed on both hypotheses.

Drug Resistance

The development of drug resistance by malignant cells is a common problem in cancer therapy. Often the first dose of a drug is very effective, but successive doses have decreasing effectiveness until eventually no effect is seen. Cell resistance to these drugs can be natural or acquired. Natural resistance may result from several factors.[26] The response of normal cells to the drug may be greater than the response of malignant cells. Transport of the drug to the tumor may be inhibited because of the poor vascularity of large, solid tumors. Also, slow-growing tumors may have a very low growth fraction, with dividing cells staying in one phase for long periods of time. Finally, it is theorized that neoplasms mutate spontaneously toward drug resistance, and more resistant mutations are present in large tumors than in small tumors.[27] Accordingly, certain populations of cells within a tumor may be resistant to the drug(s) initially, and this resistance will become evident over time as those cells that are sensitive to treatment diminish. Thus only a certain population of cells receives adequate treatment. This theory is at present the subject of clinical research. All of these naturally occurring phenomena can significantly inhibit the effectiveness of anticancer drug therapy and contribute to recurrence of disease.

Acquired resistance occurs at the cellular level after drug therapy has been given. Although this area still requires substantial investigation, several causes of acquired resistance have been identified.[15,17,28] Alterations in cell membrane permeability occur and inhibit transport of the drug into the cell. Additional alterations can occur in the activity of enzymes that activate or inactivate drugs, and resistant mutagens may develop. There seems to be a similarity between cancer cell resistance to drugs and bacterial resistance to antibiotics.[2] Thus similar approaches, such as large initial doses, combinations of drugs, alternating combinations of drugs, and earliest possible treatment of disease, are used to overcome resistance and eventual tumor recurrence.

All in all, an understanding of the function of chemotherapy at a cellular level is essential. It forms the basis for an understanding of drugs used in treatment, treatment schedules, management of side effects, and research efforts. Further study of the cellular kinetics of cancer holds the key to the successful treatment of malignant disease.

PHARMACOLOGIC CLASSIFICATION OF ANTICANCER DRUGS

The classification of anticancer drugs has developed in two ways. The first was based on the effect of the drugs on cells, as was described previously. The second and most commonly used classification method is based on the pharmacologic properties of the drugs. According to this method, anticancer drugs are classified as alkylating agents, nitrosoureas, antibiotics, antimetabolites, hormones, plant alkaloids, and miscellaneous agents. Table 13-1 compares these two classification methods. A general description of each pharmacologic class follows, and detailed information regarding the specific drugs in each class can be found in Appendix A.

Alkylating Agents

Nitrogen mustard, one of the first effective antineoplastic drugs, is an alkylating agent, and this drug continues to be the prototype of all alkylating agents.[29] Alkylating agents produce highly reactive ions, and alkylation occurs when these ions are covalently bonded to molecules that have nucleophilic centers (reactive protons).[28,30] The most important target molecules are DNA, whereas the effects on other similar molecules, such as protein and RNA, seem to be much less. The No. 7 position of guanine in DNA seems to be most affected by alkylating agents. As a result, DNA cross-linking can occur, leading to the inability of DNA to replicate. DNA strands can also break, and glycolysis, respiration, and synthesis of enzymes and nucleic acid can be inhibited. Most other synthesis at the cellular level continues, causing an imbalance that leads to cell death.[28] Most alkylating agents are cell cycle stage nonspecific, destroying both resting and dividing cells; however, rapidly dividing cells are most sensitive. Commonly used alkylating agents are mechlorethamine (nitrogen mustard, Mustargen), cyclophosphamide (Cytoxan), L-phenylalanine mustard (L-PAM, melphalan), chlorambucil (Leukeran), busulfan (Myleran), and triethylenethiophosphoramide (thiotepa).

The major side effects of these drugs are related to their effect on rapidly dividing normal cells, especially hematopoietic cells, gastrointestinal cells, and reproductive cells. Nausea and vomiting are common, especially with intravenous administration. The effect on hematopoietic cells is primarily leukopenia, which reaches its nadir in 7 to 14 days and recovers in approximately 30 days. Extravasation of nitrogen mustard causes severe necrosis and tissue sloughing. Contact with skin and mucous membranes should be avoided. If accidental contact occurs, the area should be flushed immediately with large volumes of water for 15 minutes, followed by a 2% sodium thiosulfate solution. If eye contact occurs, the eye is irrigated with a 0.9% sodium chloride solution or a balanced salt opthalmic irrigating solution.

Nitrosoureas

The action of the nitrosoureas is similar to that of alkylating agents, causing cross-linking and breaks in DNA strands. These agents may also affect DNA formation by inhibiting several essential enzymatic steps.[28] Because nitrosoureas are lipid-soluble, they cross the blood-brain barrier; this makes them useful in the treatment of central nervous system disease. Nitrosoureas are cell cycle nonspecific, affecting both dividing and resting cells. Commonly used nitrosoureas include carmustine (BCNU), semustine (methyl-CCNU), lomustine (CCNU), and streptozocin.

Side effects of the nitrosoureas include hematopoietic cell suppression and gastrointestinal toxicities. Delayed depression of the hematopoietic cells is a major characteristic of nitrosourea therapy. The nadir is reached at 3 to 5 weeks and can continue for several more weeks. Thrombocytopenia is also common, but anemia occurs less frequently. Severe nausea and vomiting may also occur.

TABLE 13-1 Comparison of Cellular and Pharmacologic Classification Methods of Chemotherapeutic Drugs

Pharmacologic Classification	Cellular Classification
Alkylating agents	Cell cycle phase nonspecific
Antibiotics	Cell cycle phase nonspecific
Antimetabolites	Cell cycle phase specific (S phase)
Plant alkaloids	Cell cycle phase specific (M phase)
Miscellaneous agents	Cell cycle phase specific and cell cycle phase nonspecific

Antibiotics

Antitumor antibiotics have antimicrobial properties, but their cytotoxic properties are most prominent. They are similar in action to alkylating agents. These drugs act by interfering with nucleic acid synthesis through a process called *intercalation* and by blocking DNA-directed RNA and DNA transcription.[28] These drugs are active in all phases of the cell cycle and are thus classified as cell cycle stage nonspecific. Some antibiotics are particularly effective during M and S phases of the cell cycle. Commonly used antitumor antibiotics are dactinomycin (actinomycin D or Cosmegen), mitomycin C (Mutamycin), doxorubicin hydrochloride (Adriamycin), daunorubicin hydrochloride (daunomycin, Cerubidine), bleomycin (Blenoxane), and plicamycin (mithramycin, Mithracin).

The side effects of antibiotics are similar to those of alkylating agents. Bone marrow suppression is common, especially leukopenia and thrombocytopenia, with the nadir at 10 to 14 days and recovery in 21 days.[29] Stomatitis and alopecia result from most of these drugs. In addition, severe tissue necrosis and sloughing occur when all of these drugs except bleomycin and plicamycin are extravasated. A unique side effect of doxorubicin and daunorubicin is dose-related cardiotoxicity, and bleomycin can cause severe pulmonary toxicity.

Antimetabolites

Antimetabolites are structural analogues of natural metabolites essential to cellular functioning. These drugs damage cells by substituting for a natural metabolite in an important molecule, thereby altering the function of the molecule. They compete with an essential natural metabolite for a catalytic site in a key enzyme, and if the natural metabolite is replaced, the catalytic rate of an essential enzyme is altered.[13] Antimetabolites used currently are folate antagonists, purine antagonists, and pyrimidine antagonists. These drugs are most active during the S phase and are thus cell cycle phase specific. Commonly used antimetabolites include methotrexate (MTX, amethopterin), 5-fluorouracil (5-FU), 6-mercaptopurine (6-MP), cytosine arabinoside (ARA-C, Cytosar, cytarabine), and 6-thioguanine (6-TG).

Common side effects of these drugs are bone marrow suppression, which reaches its nadir in 1 to 2 weeks, alopecia, and mucositis. Leukopenia is the most severe, whereas thrombocytopenia and anemia are less severe. Gastrointestinal distress in the form of nausea, vomiting, and diarrhea occurs as a side effect of several of these drugs. Two important side effects occur with specific drugs of this class: methotrexate and the purine antagonists, 6-MP and 6-TG. Methotrexate can be lethal when given in high doses without an antidote. Leucovorin (citrovorum factor) "rescue" provides this antidote. Leucovorin is a reduced form of folic acid that competes with methotrexate for entry into cells and also bypasses the enzymatic block in DNA production that methotrexate induces. It is essential that leucovorin be given 24 to 36 hours after high-dose methotrexate therapy is initiated. The second side effect that is extremely important is the potential for 6-MP and 6-TG to cause liver damage. This can be serious for patients who are undergoing chemotherapy because many of these drugs are excreted through the liver.

Plant Alkaloids

Plant alkaloids are derived from the periwinkle plant *(Vinca rosea)* and are sometimes called the vinca alkaloids. Although several potential drugs have been identified in this group, only two have been used extensively in cancer treatment. These are vinblastine (Velban) and vincristine (Oncovin). These drugs destroy cells by crystallizing the microtubular spindle proteins during metaphase and arresting mitosis at that point.[28] Thus, these drugs are cell cycle phase specific.

Although these drugs act similarly to destroy cells, the side effects of each are different. The major side effect of vinblastine is myelosuppression, with leukopenia being the most prominent symptom. The nadir occurs in 4 to 10 days, and recovery occurs in 10 to 21 days. The major side effect of vincristine, however, is neurotoxicity, evidence by peripheral neuropathy in the form of numbness, weakness, and loss of deep tendon reflexes; cranial nerve palsies; vocal cord paralysis; and autonomic nervous system dysfunction, such as constipation, tachycardia, urinary retention, and paralytic ileus.[28] Both drugs are vesicants that cause tissue necrosis if extravasated.

Hormones

Hormone therapy is not chemotherapy per se because this form of therapy is not cytotoxic and does not always involve the use of drugs. Hormone therapy is effective because many cancers that arise in such tissues as the breast, prostate, and endometrium are dependent on hormones to some degree for cellular proliferation. In some situations the cancer cells do not retain hormone dependency as the tissue of origin and therefore lack the receptor for the hormone. This means that altering the hormonal environment of the cancer cell will have no bearing on the rate of tumor cell division. These patients are therefore spared efforts to manipulate the hormone environment and are given cytotoxic chemotherapy instead. If the tumor tissue demonstrates appropriate receptors or is deemed to be hormone dependent, cancer cell division can be suppressed by pharmacologic or surgical hormone manipulation.

The action of hormones is dependent on the presence of specific receptor proteins inside the cytoplasm of the cell. The binding of the hormone to the receptor proteins facilitates the transport of the hormone into the cell nucleus, where the hormone, once bound to the chromatin, facilitates the synthesis of messenger RNA and ultimately the synthesis of new protein and cell division.[29] Antitumor effects can be achieved by blocking this process or using other hormones that are antagonistic to the process.[28]

Research efforts continue to study the significance of the presence or absence of receptor proteins, such as estrogen and progesterone receptors in breast and endometrial cancer, and the effect that changes in the hormone environment have on tumor response.

Hormones commonly used in cancer treatment include estrogens (diethylstilbestrol, estradiol), androgens (testosterone, Halotestin), progestins (Megace, Provera), and corticosteroids (prednisone, dexamethasone, hydrocortisone). Antiestrogens (tamoxifen), antiandrogens (flutamide), and antiadrenal agents, such as aminoglutethimide (Cytadren, Elipten) are not hormones but significantly alter the hormone environment of those cancer cells that retain hormone dependency. Leuprolide acetate (Lupron) and flutamide are two drugs that are used to treat prostate cancer. They alter the hormonal environment of the cancer cell in different ways and are useful as an adjunct to other cancer treatments. Leuprolide acetate (Lupron) effectively suppresses release of gonadotropin-releasing hormone from the brain, thereby suppressing production of LH and FSH, which normally account for the production of testosterone from the testis. Flutamide, on the other hand, is responsible for preventing formation of the androgen (testosterone)/protein receptor complex with subsequent tumor shrinkage. Hormone therapy is never curative because tumor cell populations are heterogeneous, with some retaining protein receptors and others mutating from this more well-differentiated cell type.

The side effects of hormonal treatment are directly related to the normal action of the hormones. Because dosages of these drugs are higher than the levels that occur normally in the body, the normal hormone action is accentuated. With the sexual hormones, fluid retention, changes in libido, and changes in secondary sexual characteristics (such as deepening of the voice and hirsutism) often occur. Corticosteroids commonly cause appetite stimulation and feelings of euphoria. Long-term use can lead to a cushingoid state, peptic ulcer, hypertension, diabetes, and osteoporosis. Side effects of the antihormonal agents are similar to the natural effects of decreased amounts of their normal hormone counterparts. Antiestrogens cause hot flashes, dizziness, nausea, and vomiting, whereas antiadrenal agents cause adrenal suppression, lethargy, ataxia, and nystagmus. Overall, however, hormonal treatment is generally well tolerated.

Miscellaneous Agents

Several anticancer drugs have been placed in a miscellaneous class, either because their action does not conform to one of the classes described previously or because their action is not fully understood. Drugs used commonly that belong to this group are hydroxyurea (Hydrea), L-asparaginase, procarbazine, hexamethylmelamine, and cisplatin (Platinol). The properties and side effects of each of these drugs are diverse. Hydroxyurea and procarbazine are cell cycle phase specific, whereas the remainder are phase nonspecific. Side effects of these individual drugs are described in Appendix A.

ANTINEOPLASTIC DRUG TREATMENT

Goals of Chemotherapy

The goals of antineoplastic drug treatment are similar to those of other cancer treatment modalities. Curative treatment with chemotherapy is aimed at total eradication of malignant cells, including micrometastasis, whereas the purpose of palliative chemotherapy is to reduce tumor size, extend life, and improve quality of life. Chemotherapy is often combined with other modalities for optimal effectiveness.

Treatment Regimens

Combination chemotherapy

Single-drug therapy was the accepted treatment regimen during the early development of cancer chemotherapy, but it has been replaced almost completely by combination drug therapy. In most cancers, single-drug therapy has proved unsuccessful in achieving long-term remission, has produced tumor drug resistance, and would have created severe or lethal toxicities when given in doses adequate for tumor kill.[31] Combination therapy, however, has demonstrated long-term remissions,[26] more effective prevention of drug resistance, and tolerable side effects with maximal doses.[29]

One of the earliest and most successful drug combinations was MOPP (nitrogen mustard [Mustargen]; vincristine [Oncovin], procarbazine, and prednisone), which was used to treat advanced Hodgkin's disease. DeVita, Serpick, and Carbone[32] reported complete remissions in 80% of the individuals treated, with half of these achieving long-term remissions. Successful results also have been demonstrated with combination therapy for acute lymphoblastic leukemia of childhood.[29]

These improved therapeutic results have occurred as a result of the additive and synergistic effects of the drugs. Most chemotherapy combinations have an additive effect that improves response rates. True synergism occurs rarely, but there are some examples in which antineoplastic drug combinations are more effective than the additive effects of single agents. One example of synergism is the combination of doxorubicin and cyclophosphamide.[28] These individual drugs have a 30% response rate in advanced breast cancer, whereas in combination they have a 70% to 80% response rate.[28] Thus the combination results in a response rate that is greater than the additive effect of each drug. Another example of possible synergism is the combination of 5-fluorouracil (5-FU) and leukovorin in the treatment of colon cancer. The presence of leukovorin enables 5-FU to bind covalently to thymidylate synthetase. This synergism results in an increased intracellular concentration of 5-FU, enhancing cell kill. Not all drugs provide additive or synergistic effects; some combinations are antagonistic, with blocking action occurring at the cellular level. The development of new drug combinations is related directly to cellular kinetics, because the drugs' actions in the cell must be evaluated carefully to determine whether additive, synergistic, or antagonistic actions occur.

Decreased tumor resistance to the drugs is another positive aspect of combination therapy. Drugs are usually chosen from different classes, so there is a wide variety of action at the cellular level. Few cells are resistant to the total effect of all the drugs; therefore few resistant cells survive and continue dividing. This dimension of combination therapy has increased the therapeutic usefulness of the same drug regimen over prolonged periods of time.

Combination therapy has allowed treatment with drug dosages that are adequate for achieving a maximal response without the severe or lethal side effects that would have occurred with maximal doses of single drugs. In the ideal drug combination, each drug has different side effects and different timing or duration of similar side effects.[28] For example, a drug that primarily causes bone marrow suppression might be combined with vincristine, which primarily causes neurologic side effects. Combinations of drugs that cause bone marrow suppression are often scheduled so that the nadir of bone marrow suppression occurs at different times. The goal in all drug combinations is to include drugs with nonoverlapping side effects.

Adjuvant chemotherapy

Despite curative surgery and/or radiotherapy, many individuals experience a recurrence of their malignant disease. It is believed that recurrence is due to clinically undetectable micrometastasis that occurred before the primary tumor was detected. Adjuvant chemotherapy is used in addition to surgery and/or radiotherapy to destroy systemic micrometastases and thus provide a complete cure or a more prolonged period of remission. Several malignant diseases have been noted to recur in a high percentage of individuals, presumably because of micrometastasis. In addition, tumor stage and other clinical indicators related directly to micrometastasis and recurrence have been identified.[29] This knowledge has provided the basis for determining the potential usefulness of adjuvant therapy in specific malignancies. Adjuvant chemotherapy is usually given following definitive therapy (usually surgery) and has proved successful in treatment of Wilms' tumor, osteosarcoma, Ewing's sarcoma, embryonal rhabdomyosarcomas of childhood, nonseminomatous testicular cancer, and breast cancer in premenopausal and postmenopausal women.[2] Prolonged use of adjuvant therapy is needed to evaluate its full impact because disease-free intervals and long-term survival are the only means of evaluating its effectiveness. Because some diseases, such as breast cancer, may not recur for years, it is too early to evaluate the full potential of this approach.

Neoadjuvant chemotherapy, also termed induction or synchronous chemotherapy, is given first, before surgery and/or radiation. The use of induction chemotherapy is particularly appealing in patients with more advanced disease, such as head and neck cancer, sarcomas, and breast cancer. Such treatment is gaining prominence, especially where standard therapy has been ineffective in preventing recurrence. The premise of induction chemotherapy is that it can enhance local/regional control and overall survival by promoting regression of macroscopic disease before surgery or radiation therapy and not only ensures tumor cell sensitivity but also provides the earliest possible treatment of systemic micrometastatic lesions. In addition, with induction chemotherapy, one may select patients who can receive less extensive local treatment without a significant loss in local/regional control.

Scheduling

Evidence from animal studies and clinical observations suggests that designing schedules for chemotherapy on the basis of a cytokinetic and pharmacologic rationale can improve therapeutic results. After a review of this evidence and recognition of the problems of relating animal studies to humans, Hill and Baserga[16] recommend that several principles be followed in the scheduling of drug therapy:

1. Maximal doses should be given in short courses.
2. Courses should be repeated, once hematologic recovery occurs.
3. Repeated low doses should be avoided because of reduced effectiveness and because selective action against malignant cells is reduced since normal stem cells are being induced to cycle.
4. Bone marrow toxicity can be reduced if drugs are not given over more than one to two cell cycle times.
5. Effective combinations include drugs that exert their effects in different phases of the cell cycle.
6. Drugs acting in the same cell cycle phase may not have additive effects.
7. Drugs can be sequenced to have one drug arrest cells in one phase and the following drug kill cells in the phase in which they are arrested.
8. Combinations that are not cross-resistant should be considered and used alternately.

In general, clinicians base the scheduling of chemotherapy on these principles. According to Dorr and Fritz,[28] high-dose intermittent therapy has proved clinically to be the most effective and the least immunosuppressive. The potential tumor doubling time and the recovery time from toxic effects in normal tissue are also important considerations in scheduling. Ideally, chemotherapy should be given before tumor regrowth if cure or tumor regression is to occur. The recovery of normal tissue from toxic effects, however, is most often the major determinant in scheduling. Fortunately, normal tissues generally recover faster than malignant tissues.

The actual drug schedules used vary considerably. Drugs are given in varying sequences and intervals, and treatment courses or cycles are repeated at different intervals, with 4 to 6 weeks being a common interval. One example of treatment scheduling is the MOPP regimen used for Hodgkin's disease (Table 13-2). This regimen is repeated every 28 days.

In hematologic cancers, as well as a few others such as testicular and oat cell lung cancers, a somewhat different scheduling model has been used.[28] Induction therapy is given initially, with large doses to induce remission. Once remission has been achieved, low-dose maintenance therapy is given. If a relapse occurs, reinduction therapy is given with the same induction drugs or different drugs. In some newer treatment regimens, consolidation or early intensification therapy is used during remission to prevent malignant cell growth. Dosages are slightly lower than during induction and are aimed at overcoming tumor regrowth. A few treatment regimens include late intensification therapy given 1 year after remission. The aim of this treatment is to destroy any remaining micrometastases.

Scheduling of chemotherapy needs to be investigated further to determine the best methods. One method dis-

TABLE 13-2 MOPP Treatment Schedule

Drugs and Dosage	Schedule
Nitrogen mustard (Mustargen), (6 mg/m² IV)	Days 1 and 8
Vincristine (Oncovin), (2 mg/m² IV)	Days 1 and 8
Procarbazine (100 mg/m² PO)	Days 1 to 14
Prednisone (40 mg/m² PO)	Days 1 to 14
No treatment	Days 15 to 28

cussed and questioned frequently is the traditional day 1 and 8 treatments, as in the MOPP regimen. Because toxicity causes a hematopoietic nadir for many drugs at 7 to 14 days after treatment, the second dose, given on day 8, is often given at the peak of bone marrow suppression and thus violates one of the recommended principles. The development of new hypotheses for scheduling is ongoing. For example, Norton and Simon[25] hypothesized that drug dosages should increase throughout treatment to destroy the more resistant remaining cells. These researchers proposed that therapy should begin with relatively low doses that are gradually increased in subsequent courses. Such questions and hypotheses are important to the continuing improvement of knowledge related to scheduling of chemotherapy.

Measurement of Tumor Response

Clinical trials have contributed greatly to establishment of uniform terms and definitions for the objective measurement of tumor response. These terms and their definitions are as follows[17,31]:

1. *Complete remission.* The tumor and all signs and symptoms of disease disappear for at least 4 weeks, and normal functional status returns.
2. *Partial remission.* The tumor is reduced by 50% or more, and functional status improves.
3. *Improvement.* The tumor is reduced 25% to 50% and some functional improvement is evident. This is sometimes used to define subjective improvement only.
4. *No response.* The tumor shows no evidence of response, and no significant improvement in functional status is evident.
5. *Progression.* New tumor growth, new metastasis, or reappearance of old lesions occurs.

To identify an individual's response to chemotherapy, measurable tumor markers must be identified. The actual objective measurement is done on the same marker or variable over time. In solid tumors the measurable variables used are clearly defined palpable masses, radiographs of the tumor, and radioisotope scans of the tumor. In some diseases, such as ovarian cancer, "second look" surgery is performed because accurate external objective measurement is not possible. In the hematologic malignancies such as leukemia, blood cell counts and the maturity of blood cells are the variables used to measure response. Other variables used include serum and urinary paraproteins, gonadotropin titers, organ function tests, disappearance of effusions, and tumor-associated antigens.[13] A further description of these variables may be found in Chapter 9, Diagnostic Evaluation, Classification, and Staging.

Instruments that measure physical functional status are also used to determine the person's response to therapy. Two instruments are commonly used. One is the Karnofsky Performance Status Scale (see Chapter 10).[33] This scale ranges from 0 to 100. A score of 0 indicates death, and a score of 100 indicates a normal level of physical functioning. The newer, more simplified Zubrod Performance Scale is used in many clinical trials.[34] This scale ranges from 0 to 4. A score of 0 means that functional level is normal and 4 means the individual is moribund. From a nursing perspective, the Karnofsky Performance Scale is the most useful because it measures several aspects of physical functioning, such as level of activity, symptoms of disease, and amount of assistance needed.

Because both the therapeutic effects and the side effects of cancer chemotherapeutic drugs are so closely related, the presence of side effects is also used as an indicator of response. Obviously, this is a subjective measurement method and can be totally invalid if normal cells respond to the drug and malignant cells do not respond. However, the presence of side effects does provide evidence of the extent of distribution of the drugs in the body.

Clinical Research

Research involving clinical trials investigates the therapeutic effect of various drugs and regimens. This type of research has played an important role in the development of new chemotherapeutic drugs, treatment regimens, and schedules. The majority of this research has been done by national or regional collaborative groups of oncologists (such as the Eastern Cooperative Oncology Group, the Southwest Oncology Group, and the Childhood Cancer Study Group) who have received financial support from the National Cancer Institute, private cancer institutes and foundations, and the Division of Cancer Treatment of the National Cancer Institute. Clinical trials research is an excellent example of an organized research effort that has significantly advanced the body of knowledge concerning cancer therapy in a relatively short period of time. The pooling of data from collaborative efforts has provided for the acquisition of adequate samples much faster than any investigator working alone could.

After new drugs have been developed, have been tested in animal studies, and have demonstrated antitumor activity, they enter clinical trial studies, which are organized into three phases. A decision is made at the end of each phase as to whether a drug warrants continued investigation. Phase I studies determine the effect of the drugs on humans. More specifically, these studies are aimed at identifying and describing the drug toxicities and their reversibility, maximum dose, optimal dose and schedule, and pharmacologic data on metabolism, tissue distribution, and excretion in humans. These studies are performed on consenting patients with advanced cancer who have not responded to other treatment regimens.

Phase II studies are designed to determine the effectiveness of the drug on various common malignant diseases, including leukemia, lymphoma, melanoma, breast cancer, lung cancer, colorectal cancer, ovarian cancer, and brain cancer. Various tumor types are investigated, because a drug may be effective for some tumors and ineffective for others. Patients with advanced cancer also participate in these studies, but measurable disease must be present that can be used to determine objectively the tumor response to the drug.

Drugs that have demonstrated effectiveness in destroying tumor cells and that have tolerable toxicities move into phase III studies. These studies compare the effectiveness of the new drug or drug combination with that of standard forms of treatment. The new drug is evaluated on response rate, speed of response, magnitude of tumor regression, and length of remission. Phase III studies use a large, randomized sample of persons in various stages of disease in which the drug's effectiveness might prove useful. Many individuals entered into phase III studies are those in whom cancer is newly diagnosed. In these studies participants have the opportunity to receive the best new therapy or the best standard therapy. Many new, effective drugs are available only to patients participating in these phase III studies. A large amount of comprehensive data must be obtained before the Food and Drug Administration approves the drugs for commercial distribution. It takes approximately 10 years for new drugs to move through animal and clinical trial studies and to be approved for commercial distribution. Thus it can be beneficial for individuals to participate in phase III clinical trials when new and better drugs have been identified but are still being investigated.

Nurses have been essential participants in clinical trials research. Their role has been primarily twofold: as advocates for individuals with cancer and as data collectors. The role of advocate has focused on the individual's understanding of the treatment and informed consent. Informed consent has become very complex in recent years because of the legal standards that have been established. Although the physician is responsible in most states for informing the person about the proposed treatment, risks involved, and alternatives,[35] the patient and the family often ask the nurse to address their unanswered questions or to interpret the physician's explanation. In addition, physicians often rely heavily on the nurse to reinforce information about side effects and to teach the patient and the family how to manage the side effects. It is the physician's and nurse's shared responsibility to be sure informed consent has been obtained before the patient receives treatment. If the nurse administers treatment and informed consent has not been obtained by the physician, the nurse is potentially liable.[35] It is further the nurse's moral and professional responsibility to serve as the advocate for the individual with cancer in the areas of informed consent and understanding of treatment.

The nurse's role of data collector in clinical trials research requires considerable expertise. The nurse must understand the research and make astute assessments of multiple objective and subjective responses to the treatment. As well as collecting accurate and comprehensive data, the nurse has a responsibility to identify and document nursing interventions that assist individuals to participate in the treatment and minimize its impact on their normal activities. Teaching of patients is a very important intervention used in all of these studies. Other interventions might include development of a method for individuals to take oral medications in the correct sequence and at the correct time or identification of the best timing for initiation of side effect management. In recent years nurses have been taking a much more active role in identifying and developing nursing interventions related to clinical trials research. Nursing research committees have been formed in collaborative oncology groups and at the Clinical Center for the National Cancer Institute in Bethesda, Maryland. Some nursing studies complementing clinical trials have been initiated. (See Chapter 60, Cancer Nursing Research, for a more detailed discussion of nurse participation in clinical trial research.)

Drug Incompatibilities and Adverse Interactions

Antineoplastic drugs are incompatible with many materials, and their safe use requires a great deal of specific knowledge about individual drugs. Incompatibilities and adverse interactions have been demonstrated with other drugs, materials commonly used in preparation and administration of drugs, diet, smoking, alcohol intake, certain temperatures, pH, insecticides, paints, and solvents.[28,36]

There are several general recommendations for avoiding antineoplastic drug incompatibilities and adverse interactions. It is advisable to use only unpreserved diluents in the preparation of parenteral anticancer drugs. Inactivation or increased toxicity of some drugs may occur as a result of preservatives, and prolonged storage of mixed drugs is not advisable.[36] It is also sound practice to physically separate each drug during preparation and intravenous administration. Flushing the intravenous tubing and the proximal vein with 10 mL normal saline solution before initiation of drug administration and between deliveries of individual drugs tests vein patency and eliminates most of one drug before the next is given.[36] The effect of oral medications should be monitored carefully, and dosages should be adjusted if indicated. For example, malabsorption of oral medications, such as digoxin, may occur in persons who are taking cytotoxic drugs that impair the intestinal mucosa.[37]

Since nurses frequently administer or are involved in the administration of antineoplastic drugs, their awareness of incompatibilities and adverse interactions is essential to the safety of individuals receiving chemotherapy. Several common adverse cytotoxic drug interactions are described in Table 13-3. It is cautioned that this list is not exhaustive. The most specific and current information about incompatibilities and adverse interactions can be obtained from drug package inserts and from pharmacists who are knowledgeable about antineoplastic drugs and current references on drug interactions.[38,39]

Chemotherapy Administration

The administration of chemotherapeutic drugs has both similarities and differences when compared with the ad-

TABLE 13-3 Oncology Drug Compatibilities
Part A: Oncology Drug with Oncology Drug

Oncology Drug A	Oncology Drug B	Solution	Concentration of Drugs	Stability and Compatibility Comments
Bleomycin	Cisplatin and Cytarabine	Sodium chloride 0.9%	0.12 units/mL and 0.2 mg/mL and 1.05 mg/mL	Stable for 24 hours at 25°C
	Cytarabine and Cisplatin	Sodium chloride 0.9%	0.12 units/mL and 1.05 mg/mL and 0.2 mg/mL	Stable for 24 hours at 25°C
	Fluorouracil	Sodium chloride 0.9%	0.02-0.03 units/mL and 1 mg/mL	Stable for 7 days at 4°C. May adsorb onto plastic
	Methotrexate	Sodium chloride 0.9%	0.02-0.03 units/mL and 0.25-0.5 mg/mL	Drug decomposes within 7 days at 4°C
	Mitomycin	Sodium chloride 0.9%	0.02-0.03 units/mL and 0.01-0.05 mg/mL	Drug decomposes within 7 days at 4°C
	Vinblastine	Sodium chloride 0.9%	0.02-0.03 units/mL and 0.01-0.1 mg/mL	Stable for 7 days at 4°C. May adsorb onto plastic
	Vincristine	Sodium chloride 0.9%	0.02-0.03 units/mL and 0.05-0.1 mg/mL	Stable for 7 days at 4°C. May adsorb onto plastic
Carmustine	Cisplatin	Manufacturer's package inserts	1.4 mg/mL and 0.86 mg/mL	Both drugs stable for 3 hours at 23°C
Cisplatin	Bleomycin and Cytarabine	Sodium chloride 0.9%	0.2 mg/mL and 0.12 units/mL and 1.05 mg/mL	Stable for 24 hours at 25°C
	Carmustine	Dextrose 5%	0.86 mg/mL and 1.4 mg/mL	Both drugs stable for 3 hours at 23°C
	Carmustine	Sodium chloride 0.9%	0.86 mg/mL and 1.4 mg/mL	Both drugs stable for 3 hours at 23°C
	Cytarabine and Bleomycin	Sodium chloride 0.9%	0.2 mg/mL and 1.05 mg/mL and 0.12 units/mL	Stable for 24 hours at 25°C
	Etoposide	Sodium chloride 0.9%	0.2 mg/mL and 0.2-0.4 mg/mL	Stable for 24 hours at 25°C
	Etoposide	Dextrose 5% and sodium chloride 0.45%	0.2 mg/mL and 0.2-0.4 mg/mL	Stable for 24 hours at 25°C
Cyclophosphamide	Doxorubicin	Sodium chloride 0.9%	0.67 mg and 11.7 mg/mL	Both drugs stable for 7 days at 25°C
Cytarabine	Bleomycin and Cisplatin	Sodium chloride 0.9%	1.05 mg/mL and 0.12 units/mL and 0.2 mg/mL	Stable for 24 hours at 25°C
	Cisplatin and Bleomycin	Sodium chloride 0.9%	1.05 mg/mL and 0.2 mg/mL and 0.12 units/mL	Stable for 24 hours at 25°C
	Daunorubicin and Etoposide	Dextrose 5%	200 mg and 25 mg and 300 mg	All drugs stable for 72 hours at 20°C
	Daunorubicin and Etoposide	Sodium chloride 0.45%	200 mg and 25 mg and 300 mg	All drugs stable for 72 hours at 20°C
	Etoposide and Daunorubicin	Dextrose 5%	200 mg and 300 mg and 25 mg	All drugs stable for 72 hours at 20°C
	Etoposide and Daunorubicin	Sodium chloride 0.45%	200 mg and 300 mg and 25 mg	All drugs stable for 72 hours at 20°C
	Fluorouracil	Dextrose 5%	0.4 mg/mL and 0.25 mg/mL	Both drugs stable for 8 hours at 25°C; no significant UV spectra changes
	Methotrexate	Dextrose 5%	0.4 mg/mL and 0.2 mg/mL	Both drugs stable for 8 hours at 25°C; no significant UV spectra changes
	Methotrexate	Dextrose 5%	30-50 mg/12 mL and 12 mg/12 mL	Hydrocortisone Sodium Succinate 15-25 mg/12 mL; all drugs stable for 24 hours at 25°C
	Methotrexate	Elliot's B solution	30-50 mg/12 mL and 12 mg/12 mL	Hydrocortisone Sodium Succinate 15-25 mg/12 mL; all drugs stable for 10 hours at 25°C

For further information regarding stability and compatibility of oncology drugs, phone (800) CETUS-RX. Please consult complete prescribing information for any drug mentioned.
Source: © 1988 Cetus Corporation. Cetus is pleased to grant reprint privileges for "Stability and Compatibility of Intravenous Oncology Drugs—1988 Reference Guide for Your Practice."

TABLE 13-3 Oncology Drug Compatibilities (continued)
Part A: Oncology Drug with Oncology Drug

Oncology Drug A	Oncology Drug B	Solution	Concentration of Drugs	Stability and Compatibility Comments
Cytarabine—cont'd	Methotrexate	Lactated Ringer's	30-50 mg/12 mL and 12 mg/12 mL	Hydrocortisone Sodium Succinate 15-25 mg/12 mL; all drugs stable for 24 hours at 25°C
	Methotrexate	Sodium chloride 0.9%	30-50 mg/12 mL and 12 mg/12 mL	Hydrocortisone Sodium Succinate 15-25 mg/12 mL; all drugs stable for 24 hours at 25°C
	Vincristine	Dextrose 5%	0.016 mg/mL and 0.004 mg/mL	Both drugs stable for 8 hours at 25°C; no significant UV spectra changes
Daunorubicin	Cytarabine and Etoposide	Dextrose 5%	25 mg and 200 mg and 300 mg	All drugs stable for 72 hours at 20°C
	Cytarabine and Etoposide	Sodium chloride 0.45%	25 mg and 200 mg and 300 mg	All drugs stable for 72 hours at 20°C
	Etoposide and Cytarabine	Dextrose 5%	25 mg and 300 mg and 200 mg	All drugs stable for 72 hours at 20°C
	Etoposide and Cytarabine	Sodium chloride 0.45%	25 mg and 300 mg and 200 mg	All drugs stable for 72 hours at 20°C
Doxorubicin	Cyclophosphamide	Sodium chloride 0.9%	11.7 mg/mL and 0.67 mg/mL	Both drugs stable for 7 days at 25°C
	Fluorouracil	Dextrose 5%	0.01 mg/mL and 0.25 mg/mL	Precipitates; color change
	Vinblastine	Sodium chloride 0.9%	0.5-1.5 mg/mL and 0.075-0.15 mg/mL	May be stable for 10 days at 8 to 32°C, however, HPLC erratic
	Vincristine	Dextrose 2.5% and sodium chloride 0.45%	1.4 mg/mL and 0.033 mg/mL	Both drugs stable for 14 days at 25°C
	Vincristine	Sodium chloride 0.9%	1.4 mg/mL and 0.033 mg/mL	Both drugs stable for 14 days at 25°C
	Vincristine	Sodium chloride 0.45% and Ringer's	1.4 mg/mL and 0.033 mg/mL	Both drugs are stable for 1 and 7 days, respectively, at 25°C
Etoposide	Cisplatin	Dextrose 5% and sodium chloride 0.45%	0.2 mg/mL and 0.2 mg/mL	Stable for 24 hours at 25°C
	Cisplatin	Dextrose 5% and sodium chloride 0.45%	0.4 mg/mL and 0.2 mg/mL	Mannitol 1.875% and Potassium Chloride 0.02 mEq/mL; stable for 24 hours at 25°C
	Cisplatin	Sodium chloride 0.9%	0.2-0.4 mg/mL and 0.2 mg/mL	Stable for 24 hours at 25°C
	Cytarabine and Daunorubicin	Dextrose 5%	300 mg and 200 mg and 25 mg	All drugs stable for 72 hours at 20°C
	Cytarabine and Daunorubicin	Sodium chloride 0.45%	300 mg and 200 mg and 25 mg	All drugs stable for 72 hours at 20°C
	Daunorubicin and Cytarabine	Dextrose 5%	300 mg and 25 mg and 200 mg	All drugs stable for 72 hours at 20°C
	Daunorubicin and Cytarabine	Sodium chloride 0.45%	300 mg and 25 mg and 200 mg	All drugs stable for 72 hours at 20°C
Fluorouracil	Bleomycin	Sodium chloride 0.9%	1 mg/mL and 0.02-0.03 units/mL	Stable for 7 days at 4°C; may adsorb onto plastic
	Cytarabine	Dextrose 5%	0.25 mg/mL and 0.4 mg/mL	Both drugs stable for 8 hours at 25°C; no significant UV spectra changes
	Doxorubicin	Dextrose 5%	0.25 mg/mL and 0.01 mg/mL	Precipitates; color change
	Methotrexate	Dextrose 5%	0.25 mg/mL and 0.2 mg/mL	Both drugs decompose within 1 hour at 25°C; altered UV spectra
	Methotrexate	Fluorouracil (as diluent)	500 mg/10 mL and 50 mg/10 mL	Both drugs stable for 24 hours at 25°C
	Vincristine	Dextrose 5%	0.01 mg/mL and 0.004 mg/mL	Both drugs stable for 8 hours at 25°C; no UV spectra changes

Methotrexate	Bleomycin	Sodium chloride 0.9%	0.25-0.5 mg/mL and 0.02-0.03 units/mL	Drug decomposes within 7 days at 4°C
	Cytarabine	Dextrose 5%	12 mg/12 mL and 30-50 mg/12 mL	Hydrocortisone Sodium Succinate 15-25 mg/12 mL; all drugs stable for 24 hours at 25°C
	Cytarabine	Sodium chloride 0.9%	12 mg/12 mL and 30-50 mg/12 mL	Hydrocortisone Sodium Succinate 15-25 mg/12 mL; all drugs stable for 24 hours at 25°C
	Cytarabine	Lactated Ringer's	12 mg/12 mL and 30-50 mg/12 mL	Hydrocortisone Sodium Succinate 15-25 mg/12 mL; all drugs stable for 24 hours at 25°C
	Cytarabine	Elliot's B solution	12 mg/12 mL and 30-50 mg/12 mL	Hydrocortisone Sodium Succinate 15-25 mg/12 mL; all drugs stable for 10 hours at 25°C
	Cytarabine	Dextrose 5%	0.2 mg/mL and 0.4 mg/mL	Both drugs stable for 8 hours at 25°C; no UV spectra changes
	Fluorouracil	Fluorouracil (as diluent)	50 mg/10 mL and 500 mg/10 mL	Both drugs stable for 24 hours at 25°C
	Fluorouracil	Dextrose 5%	0.2 mg/mL and 0.25 mg/mL	Both drugs decompose within 1 hour at 25°C; altered UV spectra
	Vincristine	Dextrose 5%	0.008-0.1 mg/mL and 0.004-0.01 mg/mL	Both drugs stable for 8 hours at 25°C; no UV spectra changes
Mitomycin	Bleomycin	Sodium chloride 0.9%	0.01-0.05 mg/mL and 0.02-0.03 units/mL	Drug decomposes within 7 days at 4°C
Vinblastine	Bleomycin	Sodium chloride 0.9%	0.01-0.1 mg/mL and 0.02-0.03 units/mL	Stable for 7 days at 4°C; may adsorb onto plastic
	Doxorubicin	Sodium chloride 0.9%	0.075-0.15 mg/mL and 0.5-1.5 mg/mL	May be stable for 10 days at 8 to 32°C, however, HPLC erratic.
Vincristine	Bleomycin	Sodium chloride 0.9%	0.05-0.1 mg/mL and 0.02-0.03 units/mL	Stable for 7 days at 4°C; may adsorb onto plastic
	Cytarabine	Dextrose 5%	0.004 mg/mL and 0.016 mg/mL	Both drugs stable for 8 hours at 25°C; no significant UV spectra changes
	Doxorubicin	Sodium chloride 0.9%	0.033 mg/mL and 1.4 mg/mL	Both drugs stable for 14 hours at 25°C
	Doxorubicin	Dextrose 2.5% and sodium chloride 0.45%	0.033 mg/mL and 1.4 mg/mL	Both drugs stable for 14 hours at 25°C
	Doxorubicin	Sodium chloride 0.45% and Ringer's	0.033 mg/mL and 1.4 mg/mL	Both drugs are stable for 7 and 1 days, respectively, at 25°C
	Fluorouracil	Dextrose 5%	0.004 mg/mL and 0.01 mg/mL	Both drugs stable for 8 hours at 25°C; no UV spectra changes
	Methotrexate	Dextrose 5%	0.004-0.01 mg/mL and 0.008-0.1 mg/mL	Both drugs stable for 8 hours at 25°C; no UV spectra changes

Part B: Oncology Drug with Other Drugs

Bleomycin	Amikacin sulfate	Sodium chloride 0.9%	0.02-0.03 units/mL and 1.25 mg/mL	Stable for 7 days at 4°C
	Aminophylline	Sodium chloride 0.9%	0.02-0.03 units/mL and 0.25 mg/mL	Drug decomposes within 7 days at 4°C
	Ascorbic acid	Sodium chloride 0.9%	0.02-0.03 units/mL and 2.5-5 mg/mL	Drug decomposes within 7 days at 4°C
	Carbenicillin disodium	Sodium chloride 0.9%	0.02-0.03 units/mL and 4-12 mg/mL	Drug decomposes within 7 days at 4°C
	Cefazolin sodium	Sodium chloride 0.9%	0.02-0.03 units/mL and 1 mg/mL	Drug decomposes within 7 days at 4°C
	Cephalothin sodium	Sodium chloride 0.9%	0.02-0.03 units/mL and 2-5 mg/mL	Drug decomposes within 7 days at 4°C
	Cephapirin sodium	Sodium chloride 0.9%	0.02-0.03 units/mL and 3 mg/mL	Stable for 7 days at 4°C; may adsorb onto plastic
	Dexamethasone sodium phosphate	Sodium chloride 0.9%	0.02-0.03 units/mL and 0.05 mg/mL	Stable for 7 days at 4°C; may adsorb onto plastic
	Diazepam	Sodium chloride 0.9%	0.02-0.03 units/mL and 0.05-0.1 mg/mL	Physically incompatible
	Diphenhydramine	Sodium chloride 0.9%	0.02-0.03 units/mL and 0.1 mg/mL	Stable for 7 days at 4°C; may adsorb onto plastic
	Gentamicin sulfate	Sodium chloride 0.9%	0.02-0.03 units/mL and 0.01-0.6 mg/mL	Stable for 7 days at 4°C; may adsorb onto plastic

TABLE 13-3 Oncology Drug Compatibilities (continued)
Part B: Oncology Drug with Other Drugs

Oncology Drug	Other Drug	Solution	Concentration of Drugs	Stability and Compatibility Comments
Bleomycin—cont'd	Heparin sodium	Dextrose 5%	0.02-0.03 units/mL and 10-1,000 units/mL	Stable for 24 hours; may adsorb onto plastic
	Heparin sodium	Sodium chloride 0.9%	0.02-0.03 units/mL and 10-200 units/mL	Stable for 7 days at 4°C; may adsorb onto plastic
	Hydrocortisone sodium phosphate	Sodium chloride 0.9%	0.02-0.03 units/mL and 0.1-2 mg/mL	Stable for 7 days at 4°C; may adsorb onto plastic
	Hydrocortisone sodium succinate	Sodium chloride 0.9%	0.02-0.03 units/mL and 0.3-2.5 mg/mL	Drug decomposes within 7 days at 4°C
	Nafcillin sodium	Sodium chloride 0.9%	0.02-0.03 units/mL and 2.5 mg/mL	Drug decomposes within 7 days at 4°C
	Penicillin G sodium	Sodium chloride 0.9%	0.02-0.03 units/mL and 2,000-5,000 units/mL	Drug decomposes within 7 days at 4°C
	Phenytoin sodium	Sodium chloride 0.9%	0.02-0.03 units/mL and 0.5 mg/mL	Stable for 7 days at 4°C; may adsorb onto plastic
	Streptomycin sulfate	Sodium chloride 0.9%	0.02-0.03 units/mL and 4 mg/mL	Stable for 7 days at 4°C; may adsorb onto plastic
	Terbutaline sulfate	Sodium chloride 0.9%	0.02-0.03 units/mL and 0.0075 mg/mL	Drug decomposes within 7 days at 4°C
	Tobramycin sulfate	Sodium chloride 0.9%	0.02-0.03 units/mL and 0.5 mg/mL	Stable for 7 days at 4°C; may adsorb onto plastic
Carmustine	Sodium bicarbonate	Dextrose 5%	0.1 mg/mL and 0.1 mEq/mL	Drug decomposes within 1 hour at 25°C
	Sodium bicarbonate	Sodium chloride 0.9%	0.1 mg/mL and 0.1 mEq/mL	Drug decomposes within 1 hour at 25°C
Cisplatin	Metoclopramide	Manufacturer's package inserts	173 mg and 10-160 mg	Use immediately
Cyclophosphamide	Metoclopramide	Manufacturer's package inserts	560 mg and 10-160 mg	Physically compatible for 24 hours at 25°C
Cytarabine	Cephalothin sodium	Dextrose 5%	0.8 mg/mL and 1 mg/mL	Both drugs stable for 8 hours at 25°C
	Methylprednisolone sodium succinate	Dextrose 5% and sodium chloride 0.9%	0.36 mg/mL and 0.25 mg/mL	Physically compatible for 24 hours
	Methylprednisolone sodium succinate	Dextrose 10% and sodium chloride 0.9%	0.36 mg/mL and 0.25 mg/mL	Physically compatible for 24 hours
	Methylprednisolone sodium succinate	Sodium chloride 0.9%	0.36 mg/mL and 0.25 mg/mL	Physically compatible for 24 hours
	Methylprednisolone sodium succinate	Ringer's	0.36 mg/mL and 0.25 mg/mL	Physically incompatible
	Methylprednisolone sodium succinate	Sodium lactate 1/6 molar	0.36 mg/mL and 0.25 mg/mL	Physically incompatible
	Metoclopramide	Manufacturer's package inserts	50-500 mg and 10-160 mg	Physically compatible for 48 hours at 25°C
	Prednisolone sodium phosphate	Dextrose 5%	0.4 mg/mL and 0.2 mg/mL	Both drugs stable for 8 hours at 25°C
	Sodium bicarbonate	Dextrose 5%	0.2-1 mg/mL and 0.05 mEq/mL	Stable for 7 days at 8 and 22°C in glass or PVC

	Sodium bicarbonate	Dextrose 5% and sodium chloride 0.225%	0.2-1 mg/mL and 0.05 mEq/mL	Stable for 7 days at 8 and 22°C in glass or PVC
Dacarbazine	Heparin sodium	Sodium chloride 0.9%	10 mg/mL and 100 units/mL	Precipitates in IV line
	Hydrocortisone sodium phosphate	Not specified	Not specified	Physically compatible
	Hydrocortisone sodium succinate	Not specified	Not specified	Precipitates
	Lidocaine hydrochloride	Not specified	Not specified and 1% or 2%	Physically compatible
	Metoclopramide	Manufacturer's package inserts	140 mg and 10-160 mg	Physically compatible for 8 hours at 25°C
Daunorubicin	Dexamethasone sodium phosphate	Not specified	Not specified	Precipitates
	Heparin sodium	Dextrose 5%	0.2 mg/mL and 4 units/mL	Physically incompatible
	Hydrocortisone sodium succinate	Dextrose 5%	0.2 mg/mL and 0.5 mg/mL	Physically compatible
Doxorubicin	Aminophylline	Not specified	Not specified	Color change
	Cephalothin sodium	Not specified	Not specified	Precipitates
	Dexamethasone sodium phosphate	Not specified	Not specified	Precipitates
	Diazepam	Not specified	Not specified	Precipitates
	Furosemide	Manufacturer's package inserts	2 mg/mL and 10 mg/mL	Precipitates
	Heparin sodium	Manufacturer's package inserts	2 mg/mL and 1000 units/mL	Precipitates
	Hydrocortisone sodium succinate	Not specified	Not specified	Precipitates
	Metoclopramide	Manufacturer's package inserts	103.8 mg and 10-160 mg	Physically compatible for 24 hours at 25°C
Etoposide	Metoclopramide	Manufacturer's package inserts	86.5 mg and 10-160 mg	Physically compatible for 48 hours at 25°C
	Morphine sulfate	Not specified	Not specified and 50 mg/mL	Stable for 24 hours
	Potassium chloride	Sodium chloride 0.9%	0.2-0.4 mg/mL and 0.04 mEq/mL	Physically compatible for 8 hours
	Potassium chloride	Dextrose 5%	0.2-0.4 mg/mL and 0.04 mEq/mL	Physically compatible for 8 hours
	Potassium chloride	Lactated Ringer's	0.2-0.4 mg/mL and 0.04 mEq/mL	Physically compatible for 8 hours
	Potassium chloride	Mannitol 10%	0.2-0.4 mg/mL and 0.04 mEq/mL	Physically compatible for 8 hours
Floxuridine	Heparin sodium	Sodium chloride 0.9%	2.5-12 mg/mL and 200 units/mL	Stable for 4 days at 37°C
Fluorouracil	Cephalothin sodium	Dextrose 5%	0.5 mg/mL and 1 mg/mL	Both drugs stable for 8 hours at 25°C; no UV spectra changes
	Diazepam	Not specified	Not specified	Precipitates
	Droperidol	Manufacturer's package inserts	50 mg/mL and 2.5 mg/mL	Precipitates
	Metoclopramide	Manufacturer's package inserts	840 mg and 10-160 mg	Physically incompatible
	Prednisolone sodium phosphate	Dextrose 5%	0.25 mg/mL and 0.2 mg/mL	Both drugs stable for 8 hours at 25°C; no UV spectra changes

TABLE 13-3 Oncology Drug Compatibilities (continued)
Part B: Oncology Drug with Other Drugs

Oncology Drug	Other Drug	Solution	Concentration of Drugs	Stability and Compatibility Comments
Mechlorethamine	Methohexital	Dextrose 5%	0.04 mg/mL and 2 mg/mL	Drug decomposes within 3 hours
	Methohexital	Sodium chloride 0.9%	0.04 mg/mL and 2 mg/mL	Drug decomposes within 3 hours
Methotrexate	Cephalothin sodium	Dextrose 5%	0.4 mg/mL and 1 mg/mL	Both drugs stable for 8 hours at 25°C; no UV spectra changes
	Droperidol	Manufacturer's package inserts	25 mg/mL and 2.5 mg/mL	Precipitates
	Metoclopramide	Manufacturer's package inserts	50-200 mg and 10-160 mg	Use immediately
	Prednisolone sodium phosphate	Dextrose 5%	0.2 mg/mL and 0.2 mg/mL	Both drugs decompose within 1 hour at 25°C; UV spectra changes
	Sodium bicarbonate	Dextrose 5%	0.75 mg/mL and 0.05 mEq/mL	Stable for 7 days at 5°C or for 72 hours at 25°C when exposed to light
Mitomycin	Heparin sodium	Sodium chloride 0.9%	5-15 mg/30 mL and 1000-10,000 units/30 mL	Stable for 48 hours at 25°C
Vinblastine	Furosemide	Manufacturer's package inserts	1 mg/mL and 10 mg/mL	Precipitates
	Heparin sodium	Sodium chloride 0.9%	1 mg/mL and 200 units/mL	Decomposes within 24 hours at 37°C
	Metoclopramide	Manufacturer's package inserts	9.5 mg and 10-160 mg	Physically compatible for 48 hours at 25°C
Vincristine	Furosemide	Manufacturer's package inserts	1 mg/mL and 10 mg/mL	Precipitates
	Metoclopramide	Manufacturer's package inserts	2.4 mg and 10-160 mg	Physically compatible for 48 hours at 25°C

ministration of other drugs. All of the usual care in administering drugs, such as checking the physician's order, preparing the proper dose, using strict aseptic technique, being knowledgeable about the drugs and their side effects, and administering them properly, is essential. However, chemotherapy is administered with the use of a variety of routes and specialized equipment. Special precautions often are required to ensure drug stability related to light exposure and time in solution. Although errors in dosage or administration of other drugs often have minor effects on the individual receiving them, such errors with chemotherapeutic drugs can be lethal or cause severe side effects. Thus administration of cancer chemotherapy should be undertaken only by qualified professional registered nurses and physicians.

The Oncology Nursing Society's *Cancer Chemotherapy Guidelines* include self-learning modules that address the administration of chemotherapy and biologic response modifier agents in a variety of settings.[40] These modules provide a framework for the development of a cancer chemotherapy course, clinical practicum and recommended policies, outcomes and procedures for acute care, and outpatient and home care settings. While this publication was written to guide rather than direct practice, it is important to note that the recommended educational preparation of the nurse administering chemotherapy is specific. Regardless of the practice setting, the nurse is considered qualified to administer chemotherapy only after adequate educational preparation has taken place. Thus oncology nurses at all levels, whether involved in clinical practice, education, or administration, are responsible for developing mechanisms that ensure safe administration of chemotherapy in their practice setting. The ONS *Chemotherapy Guidelines* serve as an excellent resource for the nurse involved in the development of chemotherapy administration courses and policies, in learning chemotherapy administration, and in seeking to upgrade and maintain current skills. Several other excellent nursing resources are available to assist in teaching nurses this skill.[41-43]

Individual and family assessment

Nursing assessment of individuals receiving chemotherapy and their families should focus on the actual and potential impact that cancer and its treatment have on usual physical and psychosocial functioning. Both baseline and ongoing assessments are essential in the designing of interventions to assist the individual and family in optimal functioning. Such an assessment is complementary to that of other health professionals and focuses on those areas within the scope of nursing intervention. Specifically, the nursing assessment should address actual or potential problems related to physical performance, psychosocial functioning, and cognitive status.[40,44-46] Assessment of physical status should include hematopoietic, integumentary, gastrointestinal, respiratory, cardiovascular, genitourinary, and nervous systems. Evaluation of performance status examines the ability to perform normal life activities. The Karnofsky and Zubrod scales (see Chapter 10) are often helpful in quantifying what is often subjective functional data. Psychosocial functioning and cognitive status assessment addresses anxiety level, individual and family coping, knowledge about chemotherapy, social support, and social interaction.

The nurse administering chemotherapy also needs to ascertain other factors relevant to the drugs prescribed before they are administered. Overall physical condition and bone marrow, liver, and renal functions must be within acceptable limits as determined and ordered by the physician or the treatment protocol. In addition, information about previous therapy that may be synergistic with current chemotherapy and severity of side effects should be consistently updated and evaluated. Cumulative doses of drugs with specific organ toxicity (especially cardiac, renal, and pulmonary) should be within safe limits and consistently updated. Any questionable finding should be recorded and concerns should be discussed with the prescribing physician before the drug is administered.

Patient education

Education of the patient and the family is essential in chemotherapy treatment and requires an individualized approach. There are several key components to individualizing patient and family education, as follows[47]:

1. The nurse must identify what patients and their families need and want to know about the disease, treatment, and measures to ameliorate their impact.
2. Mutually agreed-on education goals need to be established with the patient and the family. These should focus on the patient's and family's needs, not on what the nurse intends to teach.
3. Educational methods and resources selected should be consistent with the patient's and family's learning needs and abilities.
4. Implementation of the educational program needs to consider how, when, and by whom the teaching will be done.
5. Evaluation of patient and family learning should be ongoing and focused on the goals established at the outset.
6. All components of the education process should be documented. An organized, systematic approach, such as a form in the medical record, is most efficient and effective.

Chemotherapy-related patient and family education is a multifaceted, ongoing process that emphasizes self-care. Patients and their families must know what specific symptoms require immediate attention as well as how to reach a health care provider 24 hours a day. It is helpful to view patient education within the context of three key areas:

1. What does the patient need to know in order to provide informed consent?
2. What does the patient need to know in order to cope with the immediate side effects of cancer?
3. What does the patient need to know in order to engage in appropriate self-care behaviors?

Numerous studies have indicated that informed consent and patient education should be considered as an ongoing process. Regardless of the level of the patient's and family's sophistication, the uniquely threatening nature of cancer and cancer therapy to the lay public cannot be overemphasized.[48-50] The issue of informed consent with individuals participating in clinical trials is extremely challenging. There are several variables that impede the process of providing these individuals with all the information required to make a truly informed decision. Anxiety, physiologic responses to the disease process, the desire to please the health care team, and the general readability level of the consent document may all adversely affect the individual's right to self-determination. The nurse who provides patient education in an ongoing manner, building on the individual's past experiences, is not only demonstrating patient advocacy but also substantiates the data from which the individual with cancer makes decisions.

Dosages

Dosages of chemotherapeutic drugs are determined by body surface area and expected drug tolerance. Most chemotherapeutic drug dosages are expressed in milligrams per square meter of body surface area (mg/m^2). Accurate measurements of current height and weight are essential in determining body surface area. Although body surface area is the preferred method of calculating the dosage, body weight is sometimes used. This method is expressed as milligrams per kilogram (mg/kg). The body surface area method provides a better method of determining the individual's size than body weight because it minimizes the variation in similar-sized individuals due to weight and provides for dosage differences between adults and children.[51] Debate continues regarding the appropriate mechanism for dosage calculation in the obese individual. Most authorities continue to recommend the use of ideal rather than actual body weight in this population; however, there are conflicting data regarding this issue.[52] The nurse is advised to discuss dosage concerns related to the obese with the prescribing physician on an individual basis.

Another factor that affects the determination of dosages of chemotherapeutic agents is the individual's expected tolerance of the drug.[17] Tolerance is based on such variables as general physical condition, age, and organ function. For example, an elderly person with liver metastasis may be in poor physical condition and unable to degrade drugs. Such an individual may be unable to tolerate the side effects of therapy resulting from optimal dosages, and a lower initial dosage may be required. Side effects of therapy also negatively affect the patient's general physical condition and may cause dosages to be lowered in subsequent courses of therapy. A thorough clinical assessment of the person provides a basis for making judgments about drug tolerance.

Maintenance of chemotherapy dose intensity in spite of untoward side effects is an issue that has received increasing attention.[53] Frequently nurses are in a position to help patients cope with moderately severe side effects while the attempt is made to maintain dose intensity. This challenge occurs in such populations as those with breast cancer and lymphomas, in whom dose intensity has been shown to influence disease-free survival.[53] In these situations, the necessity for the patient and the family to have access to a health care provider 24 hours a day cannot be overemphasized. Severe side effects may become life-threatening within a very short period of time.

The use of conventional chemotherapeutic agents in unconventional doses has gained increasing acceptance. High-dose therapy with such agents as cytosine arabinoside, methotrexate, cyclophosphamide, cisplatin, and carmustine, may be given alone or as part of a bone marrow transplant regimen for either solid tumors or leukemias.[51,54,55] The rationale for such therapy is multidimensional, including the attempt to overcome resistance of cells to conventional doses and to increase the diffusion of the agent across cell membranes. In addition, by using high-dose treatment methods, it is possible to approach therapeutic drug levels in the cerebrospinal fluid by crossing the blood brain barrier. However, the use of high-dose treatments has resulted in the identification of numerous previously unreported toxicities, including renal failure, cerebellar dysfunction, peritonitis, colitis, paralytic ileus, peripheral neuropathies, pulmonary failure, and profound, prolonged bone marrow suppression. Individuals receiving high-dose therapy require ongoing assessment and intensive monitoring.[56,57] Oncology nurses have been in the forefront of describing the toxicities of high-dose regimens as well as developing care plans that address the unique needs of this population.[58]

Routes of administration

Chemotherapy is administered via multiple routes, and the route chosen is an important variable in optimal drug delivery within the body, minimizing side effects and maintaining the person's level of functioning. Bioavailability of the drug is also an important consideration and accounts for the use of some agents such as methotrexate and cyclophosphamide by either the oral or the intravenous route, depending on the disease.[59] The most common routes used are oral and intravenous. The oral route is used for drugs that are well absorbed and nonirritating to the gastrointestinal tract. Obviously, the individual must be able to swallow and have a gastrointestinal tract free of obstruction for this route to be effective.

Compliance with oral cancer therapy is an area that necessitates further research. A study of individuals receiving oral therapy for hematologic cancers indicated that noncompliance with oral therapy was a serious concern in spite of several different types of patient education programs.[60] Of greatest concern in this study is the fact that according to serum samples, self-reported compliance was overestimated by a factor of two. The nurse who is caring for the ambulatory oncology patient must consider the possibility of noncompliance in a person who has verbalized fear of the disease process and is responsible for their own chemotherapy administration. Further, individuals with poor social support structures and individuals who are receiving oral regimens that may cause nausea, such as cyclophosphamide or procarbazine, are more likely to be noncompliant.[61]

The intravenous route is the most common route of chemotherapy administration because it has several advantages. First, the intravenous route achieves a therapeutic blood level quickly. Second, most chemotherapeutic agents are not absorbed in the gastrointestinal tract.

Routes used commonly for other drugs, including the subcutaneous and intramuscular route, have limited use in administration of chemotherapy because the chemotherapeutic drugs are irritating to the tissues. Continuous or intermittent subcutaneous infusion of chemotherapy agents that are not irritating to the tissues, such as cytosine arabinoside or bleomycin, may be accomplished through the use of ambulatory infusion pumps.[62-64]

Other less common methods of drug administration that are used in anticancer drug therapy seek to cross the blood-brain barrier, localize the drugs in a selected area of the body, minimize systemic side effects or maximize therapeutic effectiveness. Some drugs do not cross the blood-brain barrier. When it is desirable for the drug to reach the central nervous system, intrathecal administration is used. This route allows the drug to be given directly into the cerebral spinal fluid. Methotrexate and cytosine arabinoside are the drugs most commonly given by this route in treating central nervous system leukemia or carcinomatosis meningitis. Intracavitary drug administration instills the drugs directly into body cavities, such as the bladder, peritoneum, pleura, or pericardium. This technique is used most frequently to control malignant effusions, but it is also used for well-localized malignancies.

The intraperitoneal administration of chemotherapy is being used more frequently, especially in the treatment of ovarian carcinoma where metastatic seeding of the peritoneum is common. Intraperitoneal administration allows for a high concentration of drug to reach the affected area. Chemotherapeutic agents, including cisplatin, cytosine arabinoside, doxorubicin, and 5-fluorouracil, have all been administered in this fashion.[65] For the intraperitoneal technique to be effective, the patient must have limited intra-abdominal adhesions, as adhesions interfere with the flow of chemotherapy to the site of disease. Hoff[66] has described three major problems related to intraperitoneal therapy, including fluid imbalance related to inadequate drainage of intraperitoneal fluid, pain due to fluid infusion, and the potential for peritonitis due to catheter-related infection. Education of the patient concerning intraperitoneal chemotherapy is complex and will depend on the type of catheter being used. An excellent patient education resource has been developed for use with this population by Eriksson and Swenson.[67]

Intra-arterial infusion is used when large amounts of localized disease are present, such as primary or metastatic liver cancer, primary head and neck tumors, primary brain tumors, and widespread metastatic disease in the pelvis.[68,69] In this method large concentrations of the drug are given through the artery supplying the area. The rationale for this approach is that it maximizes the concentration of drug that is effective for a specific tumor.[70]

The isolation-perfusion method has been used to deliver high drug dosages to extremities while limiting their absorption into the rest of the system.[71] Tourniquets are used to isolate the extremity, and then the extremity's major artery and vein are cannulated and connected to a reservoir and pump. This allows the drugs to be perfused in a closed system. Isolation perfusion is used to treat sarcomas or malignant melanoma in an extremity after surgical excision. The incidence of complications, including tissue necrosis, resulting from this method of administration is high. Thus patients receiving chemotherapy by this route must be monitored closely.

Antineoplastic drugs also can be applied topically or injected directly into the tumor. These methods have had limited usefulness and are therefore employed infrequently.

Equipment

Cerebrospinal fluid reservoirs Many kinds of specialized equipment have been and continue to be developed to administer chemotherapy with increased precision, safety, and comfort. One of the earliest was the subcutaneous cerebrospinal fluid reservoir, or the Ommaya reservoir. An Ommaya type of reservoir is a silicone rubber device that is implanted surgically under the scalp and provides access to the cerebrospinal fluid through a burr hole in the skull,[72] as shown in Figure 13-2. Drugs are injected into the reservoir with a hypodermic syringe, and then the domed reservoir is depressed manually to

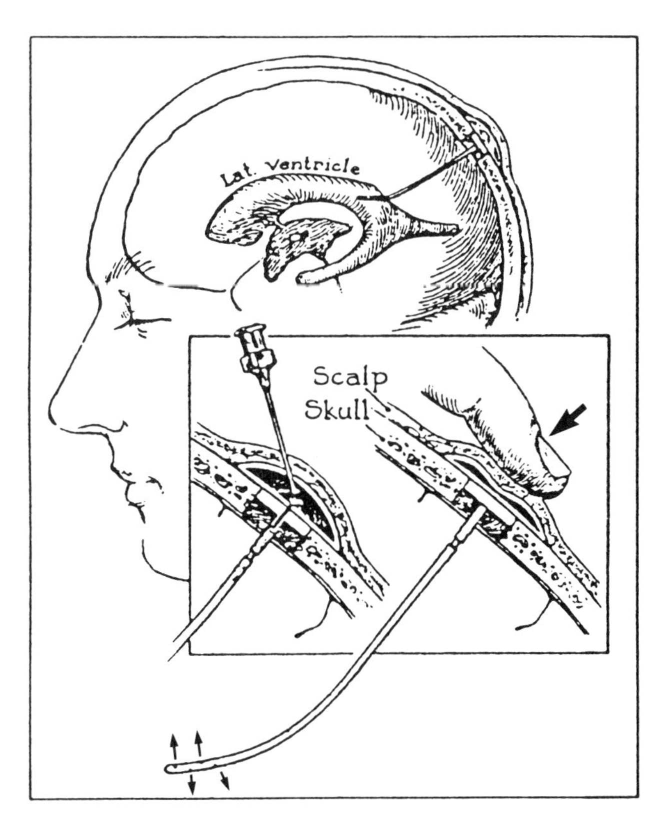

FIGURE 13-2 Cerebrospinal fluid reservoir and mode of use. (Source: Ratcheson RA, Ommaya AK: Experience with the subcutaneous cerebrospinal fluid reservoir. N Engl J Med 229:1025-1031, 1968. Copyright © 1968 by the New England Journal of Medicine. Reprinted by permission.)

mix the drug with the cerebrospinal fluid. The use of this reservoir has been extremely effective for intrathecal chemotherapy and continues to be well tolerated. The patient's comfort is increased because the need for multiple lumbar puncture is eliminated. The reservoir has several other uses, such as draining tumors or ventricles, obtaining cerebrospinal fluid for diagnostic studies, giving antibiotic therapy, and administering intravenous therapy.[73]

The primary focus of nursing care for patients with cerebrospinal fluid reservoirs must be on teaching of patient and family and assessment of mental status and potential infection.[74,75] Assessment of mental status is often complicated by cognitive and other neurologic impairments of individuals with central nervous system metastasis who are receiving therapy by this method. Nursing assessment is also focused on drug toxicities and malfunctions of the reservoir, such as leakage of cerebrospinal fluid, bleeding, or clogging of the catheter tip. When chemotherapy is administered by this route, a strict aseptic technique must be used. Any medication or diluent used to prepare medication administered by the intrathecal route must be free of preservatives to avoid neurotoxicity.[76] Because individuals often receive chemotherapy with a reservoir for an extended period of time, effective patient and family teaching and ongoing assessment for complications are essential.

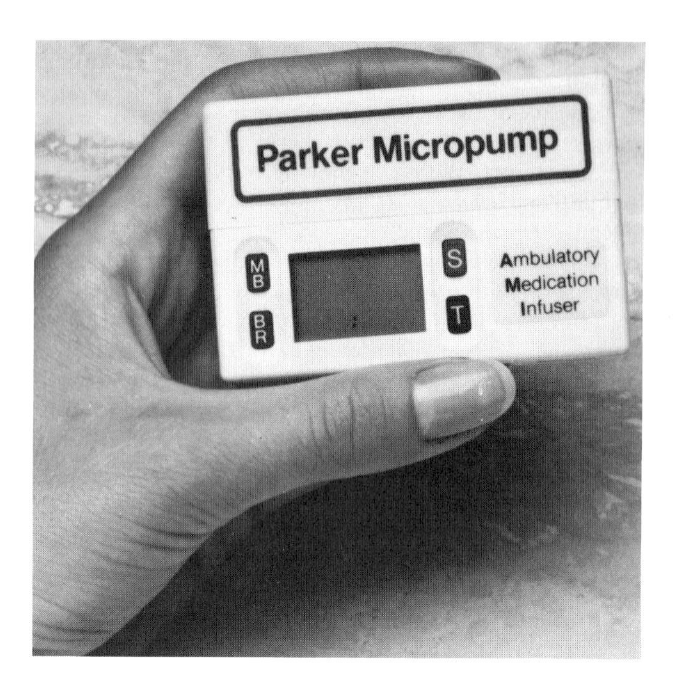

FIGURE 13-3 Portable infusion pump. (Courtesy of Parker Hannifin Corporation, Biomedical Products Division, Irvine, CA.)

Infusion pumps Infusion pumps have been widely used in chemotherapy administration to provide continuous and intermittent drug delivery with precision. They are essential in intra-arterial administration, where the drug must be given against arterial pressure. These pumps administer fluids by controlling the gravity flow or by peristaltic action, exerting positive pressure on the intravenous tubing.[77,78] Pumps that control the gravity flow are useful in intravenous therapy, and pumps that exert positive pressure are useful for both intravenous and intra-arterial therapy. All of these pumps can be set for the rate of fluid administration desired. Many have alarm devices that go off if the pump cannot maintain the set rate of fluid administration for any reason, such as infiltration, an empty bottle, air in the intravenous line, or occlusion of the intravenous tubing.

Pumps are available in two sizes and may be nonportable and portable. Nonportable pumps are usually designed to clamp onto an intravenous pole, are quite bulky, and run on AC current or a battery. Therefore, they are used primarily in the hospital or for intermittent infusions in the home. Compact, battery-operated portable pumps have enabled individuals to receive continuous chemotherapy on an outpatient or home care basis,[79,80] and they allow greater mobility for hospitalized patients. The pumps can be attached to a belt or carried in a shoulder bag. Microcomputer technology has greatly increased the number and types of pumps available. Drug delivery may be accomplished through a variety of mechanisms, including battery-powered pulsatile pumps, such as the Auto Syringe, or battery-powered peristaltic pumps, such as the Cormed, the Pancreatec Infuser, and the Parker Micropump.[63] Many of the pumps offer the option of pulse bolus administration during continuous infusion. This flexibility greatly enhances drug delivery options. An illustration of a portable pump is shown in Figure 13-3.

Several factors must be considered when one is choosing an ambulatory infusion pump. The insurance coverage for ambulatory infusion therapy varies considerably among insurance carriers. Determination of coverage may be a service provided by pump manufacturers or by medical equipment companies. Individuals using ambulatory pumps and their families must have access to a health care provider on a 24-hour basis in the event of pump failure or occlusion. Ambulatory pumps vary in the degree of manual dexterity needed to change tubing, cartridges, and cassettes. Therefore, the choice of pump should be consistent with the individual's manual dexterity, learning ability, and anxiety level. For the individual who has difficulty mastering such equipment, the Travenol Infuser may provide an alternative if a fixed drug infusion rate is appropriate and bolus infusion is not required.[63]

The advantages of ambulatory chemotherapy are obvious in terms of both comfort and economic feasibility. Individuals with appropriate support are able to maintain increased control of their life-style, including both work and leisure activities. Nurses provide critical education in terms of the early detection of complications, including thrombosis, pump occlusion, and extravasation.[81] The economic savings in minimizing hospitalization seem obvious but are mitigated by the wide variety of insurance coverage, often in policies by the same company.

The totally implanted infusion pump, shown in Figure 13-4, offers another option for chemotherapy administration in the ambulatory population.[82-85] The advantages of the implanted pump include the ability to provide con-

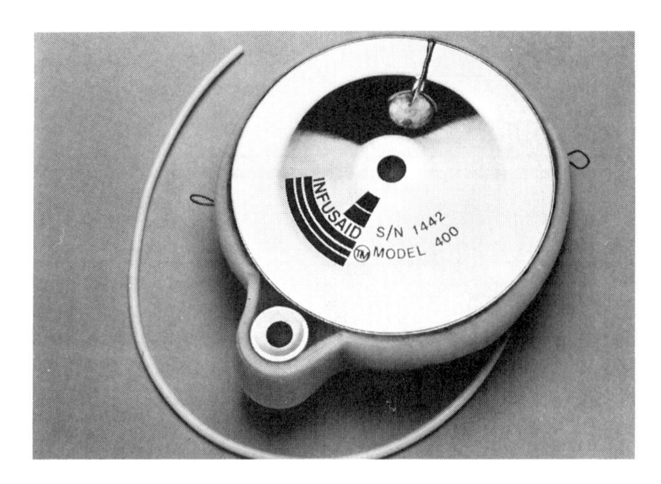

FIGURE 13-4 Implantable infusion pump and inner mechanism. (Source: From Infusaid Corporation. Reprinted by permission.)

tinuous or intermittent infusions on a systemic or regional basis to primary or metastatic tumors of the head and neck, brain, liver, and thorax. The pump is implanted in a subcutaneous pocket that is usually formed in the left lower quadrant of the abdomen or the upper chest. The septum of the pump is then easily palpated for filling. Placement of the catheter is determined by the goal of the infusion.

Regional infusions require ligation of arteries that supply the area. Systemic therapy usually necessitates the use of the cephalic vein with the tip resting in the superior vena cava.[84] Although the Infusaid pump is the most widely used, other models, including the Medtronic pump, have been developed for use on an experimental basis.[86] The technology of these pumps continues to develop; for example, the flow rate of the pump can now be recalculated by means of a noninvasive programmer.[85] In the Infusaid pump, flow rate is determined primarily by the manufacturer but is influenced by changes in temperature, drug viscosity, and atmospheric pressure.[84]

Because the pump is not visible, minimal limitations in normal activities are experienced, and the individual needs to return to health care providers only for refills. Dressler and colleagues[87] described key aspects of patient education for the individual with an implanted pump. The patients should avoid situations that raise body temperature, including saunas, electric blankets, heat-producing ointments, and hot tubs, showers, or tub baths that last longer than 30 minutes. In addition, individuals should seek medical attention before they travel by air because cabin pressure may affect the flow rate of the drug. Individuals who are being treated with an implanted pump also need to avoid engaging in contact sports or recreational activities that involve a change in atmospheric pressure.

The implantable pump system is reliable and has been acceptable to individuals receiving treatment in this manner. However, as experience with these systems has increased, untoward reactions, including extravasation of vesicants, have been reported.[88] Throughout the period the patient is treated with an implanted pump, patient education strategies should reinforce the need to notify the health care provider of the presence of fever, signs of infection at the incision site, pain, and fluid leakage at the incision site.[87]

The use of all infusion pumps for chemotherapy administration requires ongoing nursing assessment. Pumps are tools that are used to administer drugs and fluids accurately, and therefore the nurse must monitor administration just as carefully as when a pump is not used. Areas to be assessed include (1) the site of venipuncture or incision for signs of infiltration, infection, leakage, hemorrhage, or phlebitis; (2) rate of flow; (3) total volume intake; and (4) condition of the intravenous tubing and fluid. Strict asepsis must be maintained, air in the tubing should be avoided and any intravenous fluids that may be contaminated or contain precipitate should be discarded.

Patient education is also essential for the successful use of infusion pumps. Patients and their families should know the purpose of the pump in administering their therapy, any actions needed to maintain its proper functioning and side effects of the drugs received. For hospitalized individuals who are using nonportable pumps, the knowledge needed is limited and includes information about any restrictions in movement required to maintain fluid flow; signs of infiltration, leakage, hemorrhage, and infection; and the alarm device on the pump. Implanted pump systems also require a limited amount of patient and family teaching, which should include restrictions in activities; signs of fluid leakage, hemorrhage, and infection; preoperative and postoperative care; and instructions regarding appointments for refilling.[83] External, portable pumps require extensive patient education. In addition to the knowledge needed for other pumps, teaching must include care of the venipuncture site, maintenance of the pump, drug administration procedures, sterile technique, and the management of problems.[89,90] Manufacturers of portable pumps have developed patient education materials specific to their products that are useful.

Vascular access devices Vascular access devices have revolutionized the care of individuals who receive chemotherapy. Individuals who have poor venous access, either as a primary problem or as a result of chemotherapy, or who demonstrate a fear of needles experience a dramatic increase in comfort as a result of vascular access devices. In addition, vascular access devices have made safe administration of chemotherapy feasible in the home.[80] These devices allow for blood sampling as well as administration of blood components, chemotherapy, and analgesics without the anxiety or discomfort associated with multiple attempts at venipuncture.

There are numerous types of vascular access devices available for use in the oncology population. These include indwelling silicone rubber (Silastic) right atrial catheters, peripherally inserted central venous catheters, and vascular access ports. These devices vary in terms of design, construction, and number of lumens. Vascular access ports are also available in arterial and intraperitoneal varieties.

TABLE 13-4 Characteristics of Selected Silicone Silastic Atrial Catheters*

Right Atrial Catheters (Manufacturers)	Features/Internal Diameter	Uses	Maintenance Outpatient Routine Care
Hickman (Davol)	Single/double/triple lumens: 1.6 mm, 1.3 mm Pediatric: 0.7 mm	Blood drawing/administration Total parenteral nutrition Fluids, antibiotics Chemotherapy Double lumen when vascular access is needed frequently for multiple infusates Leukemic Bone marrow recipient Outpatient infusion of chemotherapy and total parenteral nutrition	Irrigation QOD with 3 mL of heparin/saline solution (10-100 units of heparin/mL) Brisk irrigations may help prevent outflow obstruction Routine clamping is not recommended Clamp over protective covering when clamping catheter Dressing changes every other day up until 2-3 weeks after insertion, then dressing is not necessary; apply Band-Aid to exit site Prevent undue tension on the catheter Catheter is taped to the person at all times Change cap(s) every 7 days Showering/bathing is permitted
Broviac (Davol)	Single lumen: 1.0 mm Pediatric: 0.7 mm, 0.5 mm	Broviac is used more for total parenteral nutrition than for blood drawing	Same as above
Chemocath Silastic (HDC)	1.0 mm, 1.6 mm Pediatric: 0.8 mm Single/double lumen		Same as above
Hemed Silicone (Gish)	0.6 mm, 1.0 mm, 1.6 mm Single/double lumen		Same as above
Quinton Silastic	1.5 mm, 1.0 mm, 0.75 mm		Same as above
Raaf catheter (Quinton)	1.1 or 1.5 each Single/double/triple lumen		Same as above
Groshong (catheter) technology	1.33, 1.1 mm Single/double/triple lumen		• Never clamp the catheter • Requires no heparinization • Pressure-sensitive valve remains closed when not in use • Irrigate briskly with 5 mL of normal saline solution once every 7 days or after use • Irrigate with 20 mL saline solution following blood aspiration or transfusion of blood component • Do not use needle through injection cap

*Catheters are radiopaque or contain a radiopaque strip to visualize on x-ray. All have repair kit and patient-teaching material available.

Source: Adapted from Goodman MS, Wickham R: Venous access devices. Oncol Nurs Forum 11(6):25-30, 1984.

The advantages and disadvantages of each type of device have been reviewed by numerous authors.[85,91-94] Tables 13-4, 13-5, and 13-6 describe the features of three types of vascular access devices and give suggestions for their maintenance.[92,95] The particular brand of access device used is often determined by the physician's experience and preference.[96]

Several factors should be considered when one is recommending a particular type of vascular access device. If possible, individual preference should be the primary factor considered in decision making. The decision may also be influenced by the cost, frequency, and method of dressing changes associated with atrial catheters. Recommendations vary considerably regarding the frequency and extent of dressing changes as well as the permissibility of swimming or tub baths.[97,98] The decision may also be uncomfortable with the visibility of right atrial catheters. Conversely, while implanted ports require no dressing changes and swimming is generally allowed, a needle "stick" is required to access the port. The person who experiences needle phobia may find an implanted port unacceptable. Also, frequent blood sampling may be more difficult with an implanted port.

Individuals with hematologic malignancies or those receiving aggressive multiple drug treatment by continuous infusion will often benefit from the early placement of vascular access devices.[93] However, the choice of vascular access devices in hematologic malignancies is controversial

TABLE 13-5 Characteristics of Selected Small-Gauge Silastic Silicone Central Venous Catheters for Percutaneous Use

Catheter	Features*	Indications	Maintenance
Per-Q-Cath (Gesco International)	Peripherally placed central venous catheter placed in the antecubital 20 gauge ID 18 gauge ID 16 gauge ID 58 cm long Made of Silastic Not sutured in place Available in single and double lumen	Single, intermittent chemotherapy injections Outpatient infusion of chemotherapy Short-term treatment (30-60 days). Catheter may remain in place indefinitely Blood drawing is discouraged in small-diameter catheters; permissible in larger-diameter catheters	Irrigate catheter with heparin 10-100 μ/mL, 5-10 mL 1 or 2 times daily Change injection cap every 2 weeks Sterile dressing change every other day or once a week. Transparent dressing (ie, Op-site or Tegaderm) Do not clamp catheter Microgauge tubing is available to attach to connector hub of catheter for clamping
Cook Percutaneous (Cook, Inc)	Single lumen: 16 gauge, 5 french Double lumen: 7 french, 16 gauge, 21 gauge Pediatric: Single lumen: 18 gauge, 4 french Double lumen: 4 french, 20 gauge, 23 gauge Polyurethane catheter Phalanges are sutured in place Also available in triple lumen	Same as above	Same as above
Hickman (Davol)	Lumen: 1.6 mm, 9.6 french Single/double/triple lumen available Sold without cuff for percutaneous placement	Same as above	Same as above
Broviac (Davol)	Lumen: 1 mm, 6.6 french Pediatric: 0.7 mm, 4.2 french Single/double/triple lumen available Sold without cuff for percutaneous placement		

*All catheters are radiopaque and distributed with introducer kits.

Source: Adapted from Goodman MS, Wickham R: Venous access devices. Oncol Nurs Forum 11(6):25-30, 1984.

TABLE 13-6 Characteristics of Selected Implanted Infusion Ports

Implanted Infusion Ports	Reservoir Body	Septum	Catheter	Maintenance
Groshong Port (Catheter Technology)	Titanium body	Silicone rubber	3-position groshong valve *Does not* need heparin to maintain patency	Puncture with Huber point needle only Irrigate every 4 weeks with heparin/saline solution, 3-5 mL (100 units of heparin/mL) Normal saline flush following blood drawing (20 mL) For arterial ports, irrigate once a week with 3-5 mL (100 units heparin/mL) Flush catheter after each use No restrictions for patient because the port is entirely implanted
Chemoport (HDC)	Titanium or stainless steel Height 0.61 in. Diameter 0.795 in. Base 1.25 in.	Silicone rubber	Arterial and venous	Same as above
Hickman SQ Port (Davol)	Stainless steel, titanium or implantable grade plastic	Silicone rubber	Arterial (0.5 mm) Venous (1.6 mm)	Same as above
Infuse-A-Port, Infusaid Microport (Shiley Infusaid)	Polysulfone plastic Contoured body No metal Height 15.8 mm Base diameter 48 mm Weight 12.1 g	Silicone rubber Septum diameter 7 mm Septum depth 3 mm 2000 punctures (22-gauge needle)	ID 0.6 mm OD 2.3 mm ID 1.0 mm (arterial) OD 2.5 mm (venous)	Same as above
Port-a-Cath (Pharmacia Nutech)	Titanium Height 13.5 mm Base diameter 25.4 mm Weight 28 g	Silicone rubber Septum diameter 11.4 mm Septum depth 11.5 mm 2000 punctures (22-gauge needle) 1000 punctures (19-gauge needle)	ID 0.5 mm (arterial) OD 2.0 mm ID 1.02 (venous) OD 2.8 mm Radiopaque	Same as above
Life Port, single and double lumen (Strato Medical)	Titanium Diameter 1.25 in.	Silicone rubber Target area of 0.625 in.		Sames as above
S.E.A. Port, side entrance port (Harbor Medical)	Titanium Height 12 mm Base 33 × 40 mm	2 Silicone rubber septa on sides of port	Polyurethane	Same as above Needle lies flat against skin
Norport SP (Norport Medical)	Polysulfone Dacton base Height 15 mm Base 38 × 38 mm	Silicone rubber		Same as above Needle lies flat against skin Puncture with butterfly non-coring needle

Source: Adapted from Goodman MS, Wickham R: Venous access devices. Oncol Nurs Forum 11(6):25-30, 1984.

and influenced by the frequent need for at least two lumens to facilitate the administration of blood components, chemotherapy, and nutritional support.[91,92] While two lumen-implantable ports are available, these devices have had limited use in patients with acute hematologic problems.[85,92]

As experience with vascular access devices has grown, a wide variety of untoward effects have been described. Occlusion, spontaneous rupture of the catheter, thrombosis, extravasation and catheter migration have been reported by several authors.[96,99,100] Although these complications are relatively rare, they underscore the necessity of applying the same previously described principles of safe administration of chemotherapy in this group of patients. Nurses have been instrumental in developing procedures that address the technical aspects of access device care, including specimen collection, catheter occlusion procedures, and catheter repair.[93,101] Nurses have also been instrumental in the development of excellent patient education materials that address patient preference and home management of vascular access devices.[97,102,103]

Educational programs in chemotherapy administration

Many educational programs have been developed to teach nurses how to administer chemotherapy. Such programs have provided a comprehensive, practical approach to learning to administer cancer chemotherapy as well as testing to determine competency. Information commonly included in these educational programs is the pharmacology of anticancer drugs, principles of cancer chemotherapy, preparation, handling, and administration of these drugs; nursing assessment and management; and documentation. Both didactic course content and a clinical practicum are recommended. An excellent outline of content to be covered in a cancer chemotherapy course is included in *Cancer Chemotherapy Guidelines* developed by the Oncology Nursing Society.[40] The successful development and evaluation of a course based on these guidelines has been reported by Welch-McCaffery.[104] Additional information on development of continuing education programs may be helpful in the development of cancer chemotherapy courses designed to meet the unique needs of individual agencies.[105-109] Chemotherapy competency courses are essential to the safe practice of nurses who administer and monitor chemotherapy in hospitals, ambulatory clinics, physicians' offices, and home health care agencies.[104,110]

Legal implications for nurses

Many nurses have become experts in administration of cancer chemotherapy and are relied on by physicians to administer treatments. As a result, independent nurse decision making is often increased. In these circumstances an awareness of the legal statutes governing nursing practice is essential if one is to keep within the boundaries of the law. The laws related to nursing practice vary from state to state, and nurses should be familiar with the statutes of their own states.[111]

There are several general areas to be considered when one is examining the statutes of a particular state and the resulting implications for nurses. These include informed consent, responsibility and supervision, documentation, dispensing of drugs, and liability insurance.[35] The nurse is not responsible for obtaining informed consent. Most states consider this a physician's responsibility. However, the nurse should not administer treatment without proof of the patient's consent. Treatment without consent is battery, and the nurse can be held liable.[35] The nurse also has an obligation to help the patient and the family understand the treatment regimen and its side effects and to communicate openly with the physician. In the state of Ohio, nurses are responsible and accountable for providing information to patients about their medications. "Therefore, assuring that consent is informed is solely a nursing responsibility."[112]

In the area of supervision, an institution or physician employing nurses can be held liable for their actions under the doctrine of "respondent superior," which means "let the master answer."[35,113] This does not dismiss nurses' liability for their own actions, however. It is therefore beneficial for nurses to have a clear, written description of their responsibilities, including the identification of their supervisor. Nurses are responsible for acquiring the skills necessary to do their jobs and to perform their duties in a manner that could be expected of a qualified, prudent nurse.[35]

The dispensing of drugs by nurses is not permitted in most states. "Dispensing means preparing, delivering, distributing, disposing of, or giving away a drug, medicine, or prescription."[35] Nurses involved with investigational chemotherapy, especially oral agents, should use care in this area. The pharmacist or physician should prepare the correct dosage and label according to the physician's written orders, and the nurse can then administer it. The dispensing of drugs is the responsibility of the physician or the pharmacist.

Thorough documentation of nursing care is essential because it provides a record of the nurse's actions. In the event of legal proceedings, the medical record is critical evidence. Schulmeister[113] reviewed 12 cases of litigation involving oncology nurses and found that documentation was incomplete or inconsistent in all cases. Vital elements of documentation include significant events or action, the care given to the person receiving treatment, the condition and response to care, and the physician's involvement.[35] All care, including telephone follow-up and problem solving, needs to be documented. In addition to the legal necessity of nursing documentation, the Joint Commission for the Accreditation of Healthcare Organizations requires documentation of the nursing process. This includes a nursing assessment, care plan, interventions, and evaluation of the person's response. Documentation of nursing care is a critical professional responsibility for quality care as well as for fulfilling legal requirements.

Nurses who administer cancer chemotherapy should investigate their need for professional liability insurance. Some hospitals carry liability insurance for their professional employees, but the amount and scope of coverage vary. According to one source, only about 10% of the hospitals in the United States provide professional liability coverage.[114] Even if a hospital does provide liability coverage for nurses, the insurance company may seek reimbursement from the nurse if damages are paid. Physician employers may or may not carry liability insurance for the nurses they employ. Another consideration is that nurses who supervise or teach nurses or nursing students are accountable for them under the "respondent superior" doctrine. The decision to purchase professional liability insurance is ultimately the nurse's after thorough investigation of potential risk of liability and existing insurance coverage. Personal liability insurance for the professional nurse can provide increased security and is available at low cost through the Oncology Nursing Society or the American Nurses' Association.

Safe handling and disposal

Several studies have reported findings that suggest that antineoplastic drugs may pose a significant hazard to those who handle them routinely. Scientists in Finland and Norway identified an increased frequency of mutagens in the urine, chromosome gaps, and a slight increase of frequency in sister chromatid exchange among nurses handling cytostatic drugs.[115,116] The frequency of chromosomal changes was related directly to the total period of time nurses had been exposed to the drugs.[116] All nurses claimed to have worn gloves and masks while handling these agents. Another study, however, showed no urine mutagenicity in nurses who wore no protective clothing.[117] Knowles and Virden[118] described absorption of these drugs through inhalation and skin contact, even when certain kinds of rubber and synthetic gloves were used. They also described these agents as having the potential to irritate the skin, eyes, mucous membranes, and other tissues. One study has reported that polyvinylchloride gloves prevented nitrogen mustard penetration.[119] In a well-controlled, longitudinal study of pharmacy personnel by Nguyen, Theiss, and Matney,[120] a twofold increase in mutagenic activity in the urine over 8 days was reported when study subjects mixed antineoplastic drugs in open-faced, horizontal laminar flow hoods. However, when drugs were mixed in a closed-faced, vertical laminar flow hood, no increase in urine mutagenic activity was found. Increased urinary mutagenicity has also been reported in oncology nurses working in a bone marrow transplant unit despite controlling for dietary mutagens, use of latex gloves, and use of premixed drugs.[121]

As a result of these and other findings, the National Study Commission on Cytotoxic Exposure and the Occupational Safety and Health Administration of the US Department of Labor developed recommendations for the safe handling of cancer chemotherapeutic drugs.[122,123] These recommendations are aimed at minimizing absorption through direct skin contact and inhalation. In the preparation of injectable antineoplastic drugs, all procedures should be carried out under a class II laminar flow biologic safety cabinet (type B3 preferred) with filtered exhaust to the outdoors. The work surface should be covered with plastic-backed absorbent paper to reduce the dispersion of spills. Persons who prepare the drugs should wear surgical latex gloves and closed-front surgical gowns with knit or elastic cuffs. These should be changed whenever overt spillage occurs and when preparation of the drugs is completed. Polyvinylchloride gloves should not be used, because they are permeable to many drugs. Aseptic technique should be used at all times, and measures are taken to avoid spray when one is reconstituting vials or breaking ampules. Placement of alcohol-soaked cotton or gauze around the neck of the ampule or venting vials with a hydrophobic filter is recommended to minimize spray. After preparation is complete, surfaces of intravenous bottles and cabinets should be wiped clean, gown and gloves removed, hands washed thoroughly with soap and water, and needles, syringes, vials, gloves, unused drugs, and other equipment disposed of in accordance with federal, state, and local codes (usually incineration or in landfills) regarding toxic chemical wastes. No eating, drinking, smoking, gum chewing, or application of cosmetics should occur in the preparation area.

During administration of injectable antineoplastic drugs, similar precautions should be taken. A protective gown with knit or elastic cuffs and surgical latex gloves should be worn. Sterile, alcohol-soaked gauze should be placed over the tips of needles or intravenous tubing when air bubbles are removed. All drug-contaminated products should be disposed of as toxic chemical wastes. Needles should not be clipped to avoid drug spray; nor should they be capped to avoid accidental puncture. Hands should be washed after drug administration, or immediately in case of skin contact. Protective clothing with double gloving should be used for clean-up in the event of a small spill. If a large spill occurs, a respirator should also be worn.

The effect of handling excreta of persons who are receiving antineoplastic drugs has not been determined, but it has been suggested that this may pose a hazard. Most antineoplastic drugs are excreted in the urine and feces.[124] Detailed information on drug excretion can be obtained from the drug package inserts. Persons who handle excreta and body wastes should avoid contact of the materials with the skin, wear surgical latex gloves and a gown, and wash hands thoroughly after disposing of excreta.[125-127]

The preparation, administration, and disposal of equipment, excreta, and body fluids in the physician's office or in the home should follow the same recommended procedures. Office nurses were found to handle more drugs and use fewer precautions than nurses in other settings.[128] Nurses in physicians' offices often mix and administer drugs. Although precautionary measures may be costly or inconvenient, the acquisition of such equipment as a vertical laminar flow hood is very important to occupational safety.[129] Safety precautions in the home present unique problems. If possible, drugs should be prepared at a hospital or pharmacy and transported to the home in a leak-proof container. All equipment and leftover drugs should be returned to the hospital or agency for disposal. Handling of excreta and body fluids should be done cautiously with the use of gloves and protective clothing. Dilution in sewer systems is believed to be adequate to decrease risk of exposure to the family and the environment. Soiled clothing and bedding should be washed twice and kept separate from the other family laundry.[127,130]

COMMON SIDE EFFECTS OF CHEMOTHERAPEUTIC DRUGS AND THEIR MANAGEMENT

Most side effects of antineoplastic agents are related to the fact that these drugs have a nonspecific effect on all rapidly dividing cells. Many side effects result from the drugs' actions on normal rapidly dividing cells, including hematopoietic or bone marrow, gastrointestinal, hair follicle, and germinal cells. Other side effects unrelated to normal cell proliferation, including organ toxicities, local tissue irritation, allergic reactions, and long-term effects, also can occur. The side effects an individual experiences are related directly to the drugs received. In some situations the side effects are an indication that an effective drug level has been achieved, as was discussed earlier in relation to tumor response. Thus strategies for the management of side effects must not compromise the desired therapeutic intent.

In managing these side effects, the nurse's comprehensive, astute assessment and appropriate intervention are critical. Nursing interventions are focused on minimizing the effect of chemotherapy on the ongoing, daily functioning of the patient and the family. Information giving, support, and competence in chemotherapy-related procedures are key nursing interventions. Nursing research has made significant contributions in the area of management of side effects and continues to do so.

Bone Marrow Suppression

The most important dose-limiting factor in chemotherapy is bone marrow suppression or myelosuppression. It is also an important means of ensuring that effective drug levels have been given because chemotherapy acts on all rapidly dividing cells. The bone marrow cells most affected are the white blood cells (leukocytes) and platelets (thrombocytes). The red blood cells (erythrocytes) are also affected, but this is rarely critical except in cisplatin therapy, where hemolysis may occur after prolonged treatments.[59,131] Individuals with anemias from other causes or thrombocytopenia may be at some risk and require red blood cell transfusions. The primary concerns in myelosuppression are leukopenia and thrombocytopenia, which are expected side effects of most anticancer drugs.

Leukopenia is the most serious form of myelosuppression. Decreased lymphocytes and granulocytes lead to suppression of humoral and cellular immunity, and the risk of serious infection is heightened. The leukocytes generally are divided into two classifications: nongranulocytes and granulocytes. The granulocytes also are referred to as polymorphonuclear leukocytes or "polys" or "PMNs." Normally the majority, or about 60%, of granulocytes are neutrophils (as opposed to basophils and eosinophils) and are responsible for fighting infection. It is a decrease in the number of neutrophils that places the individual at risk of infections. In addition to the total white blood cell count, the granulocyte count, particularly neutrophils and maturing "bands" and "segs," are assessed most frequently to evaluate the patient's ability to fight infection and whether an adjustment in chemotherapy dosage is indicated. To evaluate a person's ability to mount a response to infection, the absolute granulocyte count (AGC) is determined. The white blood cell count (WBC) is multiplied by the sum of segmented neutrophils and band cells. A value greater than 1200 cells/m^3 indicates an adequate and recovering bone marrow, whereas a value less than 1000/m^3 indicates risk of infection. When the AGC is 500/mm^3 and below, the patient is at severe risk of an infection in which endogenous opportunistic organisms can flourish, possibly resulting in life-threatening sepsis.

The majority of chemotherapy drugs cause an expected nadir in 7 to 14 days, with complete recovery in 14 to 28 days. The nitrosoureas, however, cause a delayed myelosuppression with a nadir of 4 to 6 weeks and recovery at 6 to 8 weeks.

In an attempt to minimize the risk of infection as well as foster greater dose intensity, numerous studies are investigating the use of the various growth factors (see Chapter 14, Biotherapy) in conjunction with chemotherapy. Preliminary study reports indicate that normal neutrophil production and development are stimulated by growth factors. The use of growth factors is an exciting development in the quest to minimize the complications of myelosuppression, including oral toxicities.[132,133] Considerable effort will be needed in ongoing studies to address the most effective use of these agents in terms of dose, timing, and expected side effects of the growth factors themselves. The medical management of leukopenia may include prophylactic antibodies and antiviral agents. Granulocyte transfusions are rarely used because of limited effect and multiple side effects.[134]

Thrombocytopenia can also cause severe consequences and can occur at the same time as leukopenia. Symptoms of thrombocytopenia include bruising, petechiae, and hemorrhaging. Platelet counts of more than 100,000 to 120,000/mm^3 [51] indicate that patients can be given a 100% dose at their next drug treatment. Lower platelet counts indicate the need for a dose adjustment, withholding of drugs, and/or transfusion of platelets.

Myelosuppression has been graded by toxicity level. This is useful both in clinical practice and in clinical trials research. The grades of myelosuppression are listed in Table 13-7.

Nursing assessment in relation to myelosuppression is extremely important, because nurses generally have the greatest contact with individuals undergoing chemotherapy. The assessment of fever patterns in the individual who is taking steroids or the individual who is neutropenic is extremely important, as these patients may not be able to manifest the usual signs of infection, including those of

TABLE 13-7 Grades of Myelosuppression

Toxicity Grade	White Blood Cell Count/mm³	Granulocyte Count/mm³	Platelet Count/mm³
Normal	5000–10,000	2000–7000	150,000–350,000
0	≥4000	≥1500	≥100,000
1	3000–3999	1000–1499	75,000–99,999
2	2000–2999	500–999	50,000–74,999
3	1000–1999	250–499	25,000–49,999
4	<1000	<250	<25,000

Source: Haskell CM (ed): Cancer Treatment (ed 2). Philadelphia, WB Saunders, 1985.

high fever, redness, or pain.[135,136] For persons with thrombocytopenia, it is important to assess for bruising and signs of bleeding tendencies, such as bleeding mucous membranes, petechiae, ecchymosis, tarry stools, bloody urine, coffee-ground emesis, and hypermenorrhea. The assessment of the individual at risk of anemia requires careful attention to the patterns of problems experienced. Shortness of breath and fatigue are difficult symptoms to assess objectively, since they are subjective in nature. Therefore such symptoms may cause the patient greater distress than those that are apparent objectively. The problem of fatigue in the cancer patient is the subject of increased nursing research efforts aimed at defining the phenomenon and development of effective nursing interventions. Several excellent articles have addressed the problem of fatigue. The reader is referred to the work of Nail and King,[137] Aistairs,[138] and Piper, Lindsey, and Dodd[139] and to Chapter 23 of this text for excellent discussions related to the incidence and management of fatigue in individuals with cancer.

The most important nursing intervention in both the hospital and the ambulatory clinic is teaching patients and their family members what symptoms to report to their health care team as well as how to minimize the risk of both infection and bleeding.[135,136] Specific self-care strategies should be taught, as well as the necessity of contacting a member of the health care team immediately if symptoms occur. Patient education materials, such as *Chemotherapy and You,*[140,141] address the symptoms related to infection, bleeding, and anemia in a manner that is understood by lay persons. The challenge to the nurse who provides patient education about chemotherapy is in teaching patients and their families about the very real risk of life-threatening infections and bleeding problems without overwhelming them to the point that they are paralyzed with fear.

The use of nursing protocols[142] that are based on institutional policy helps to specifically tailor patient education efforts. Information related to fever, the prevention of infection by avoiding contact with individuals who have viral or bacterial illnesses, and self-care strategies that minimize trauma to the skin and mucous membranes should be given to the patient and the family, both verbally and in writing. Additional general self-care instructions related to maintenance of adequate nutrition and fluid intake and minimizing of fatigue, with attention to activity and rest patterns, are provided on an ongoing basis.

To minimize the risk of bleeding in the individual with thrombocytopenia, the need to avoid trauma is emphasized. Surgery and dental work are performed only after consultation with the oncology health care team. In addition, patient education includes the rationale for avoiding all over-the-counter drugs, such as aspirin-containing compounds that disrupt platelet function, and the importance of avoiding constipation, subsequent straining, and the use of rectal suppositories and enemas. Self-care measures emphasize the use of electric razors and soft toothbrushes. Patients are taught to report excessive gingival bleeding, unusual rectal bleeding, coffee-ground emesis, and the onset of petechiae or nontraumatic bruising, hematemesis, or hematuria. Menstruating patients are taught to report changes in their menstrual cycle, including excessive bleeding and between-cycle spotting. Postmenopausal women are taught to report vaginal bleeding immediately. Patient education related to sexual intercourse in the presence of thrombocytopenia or leukopenia emphasizes the avoidance of rectal intercourse and the importance of good hygiene and adequate lubrication to avoid trauma to mucous membranes.[45,143-145]

There are additional threats for the myelosuppressed individual who is hospitalized. The risk of nosocomial infection is great. Careful handwashing by hospital personnel before contact with the myelosuppressed patient is critical and has been found to be the most effective way of preventing nosocomial infection. Personnel with infections should not have contact with the patient. The nurse also uses care in relation to equipment and supplies. Keeping equipment in the patient's room rather than moving it from room to room, as well as adequate cleaning to prevent bacterial growth, is important in minimizing the risk of infection. Intravenous tubing, fluids, and dressings should be changed as recommended by the manufacturer and in compliance with the hospital's infectious disease policies (usually every 24 to 48 hours). Procedures or equipment that may break the integrity of the mucous membranes or skin, such as rectal temperatures, enemas, stiff toothbrushes, blood drawing, or unnecessary injections, should be avoided. Attention is focused on all avenues of potential spread of infection, and every effort is made to minimize this potential. Various nursing care protocols that theoretically decrease the risk of infection in the neutropenic patient have been described.[135,146] Controversy remains, however, about such recommendations as reverse isolation and cooked food diets. At least once during each shift the nurse systematically assesses the myelosuppressed patient for physical findings that indicate an increased possibility of infection.

The hospitalized individual with thrombocytopenia is also at greater risk. Injections and drawing of blood should be minimized or avoided. If these procedures are necessary, pressure is applied to the site until bleeding has stopped (usually about 15 minutes). Care is taken in oral hygiene and temperature taking to avoid breaking the mucous membranes. Often soft toothbrushes or commercially available swabs are recommended for oral care, and oral temperatures are advisable. As with the individual who has leukopenia, attention must focus on avoidance of all possible trauma that might initiate hemorrhage.

Gastrointestinal Side Effects

The most common gastrointestinal side effects of cancer chemotherapy are nausea and vomiting; however, it must be stressed that these do not occur with all drugs. Other gastrointestinal side effects that may occur are stomatitis, pharyngitis, esophagitis, anorexia, alterations in taste, diarrhea, and constipation. These symptoms result from irritation or destruction of the gastrointestinal epithelial cells.

Nausea and vomiting

While tremendous strides have been made in the management of chemotherapy-induced nausea and vomiting, this symptom remains a very distressing side effect for up to 30% of the individuals who undergo chemotherapy.[147] Study findings suggest that most chemotherapy-induced vomiting ends within 48 hours after treatment, while nausea may persist for 72 hours or more.[148] Uncontrolled nausea, vomiting, and retching may cause the development of fluid and electrolyte imbalances as well as esophageal tears and severe psychologic distress.[149,150] Therefore, every effort should be made to minimize this side effect. Patients and their families are taught that nausea and vomiting are not inevitable side effects and that the patient does not have to experience nausea and vomiting in order to achieve a response from chemotherapy.

Chemotherapy-induced nausea and vomiting are complex phenomena with both physiologic and psychologic components. Borison and McCarthy[151] described much of the physiology of the emetic center. The vomiting center is located in the floor of the medulla and consists of two components: the chemoreceptor trigger zone and the true vomiting center. The chemoreceptor trigger zone does not initiate vomiting on its own but, rather, provides afferent stimulation of the true vomiting center as a result of changing chemical levels in the brain and cerebral spinal fluid. Afferent pathways from numerous other sources also stimulate the true vomiting center. These pathways include (1) vagal visceral afferents that arise from inflammation, edema, and irritation of the gastrointestinal tract, (2) sympathetic visceral afferents stimulated by obstruction or ischemia of hollow visceral organs, (3) the cerebral cortex and limbic system stimulated by pain and previous experiences, and (4) the vestibulocerebellar afferent. The vestibulocerebellar afferents are responsible for the vomiting associated with motion sickness and are believed to have little involvement in pharmacologically induced nausea and vomiting. Physiologic stimulation of the vomiting center is thought to be mediated by a variety of neurotransmitters, including serotonin, histamine, glutamine, acetylcholine, dopamine, and norepinephrine.

A psychologic component of chemotherapy-induced nausea and vomiting has been suggested in several studies.[152,153] Several subjects in these studies had nausea and vomiting before chemotherapy; this suggests a conditioned response. Anticipatory nausea and vomiting usually begin the day before actual drug administration and may be elicited by a variety of stimuli, including sights, sounds, smells, and activities associated with drug administration. Morrow[154] reported that one in four persons will begin to experience anticipatory nausea and vomiting by the fourth cycle of treatment. A variety of factors, such as susceptibility to motion sickness, age of 50 or less, and posttreatment responses to chemotherapy (feeling warm or hot, cold or clammy, nauseated or vomiting) have been reported to be associated with the development of anticipatory nausea and vomiting.[154-158]

The most common treatment of nausea and vomiting is with antiemetics. Combinations of antiemetic drugs attempt to block as many of the neurotransmitter sites as possible, thus minimizing stimulation of both the chemoreceptor trigger zone and the true vomiting center. The phenothiazines, substituted benzamides, and butyrophenones are groups of drugs used primarily to suppress activity near the chemoreceptor trigger zone. The benzodiazepines depress the central nervous system and also cause temporary amnesia, which is theoretically advantageous in minimizing the nausea and vomiting conditioning of individuals undergoing cancer chemotherapy.[159] The side effects of substituted benzamides range from restlessness and diffuse anxiety to dystonia. The combination of steroids and diphenhydramine may mitigate some of these side effects.[160] Antihistamines minimize some of the untoward side effects of phenathiazines and substituted benzamides.[149] The experimental use of serotonin inhibitors has indicated extremely promising antiemetic activity with minimal toxicity.[161,162]

Nurses play a vital role in determining which regimen is most efficacious for an individual patient. Rhodes and colleagues[163] have systematically investigated patterns of nausea, vomiting, and distress in individuals receiving a variety of cancer chemotherapy protocols. Their work provides a framework for selection of antiemetic agents and patient education. Determination of the most appropriate antiemetic regimen should be based on the individual's previous experience with emetogenic chemotherapy, the emetogenicity of the current regimen, and the tolerance of side effects experienced. Instructions regarding antiemetic administration, dietary counseling, sleep, and rest are extremely important nursing interventions, not only on the day chemotherapy is administered but on posttherapy days as well.[164] A prophylactic approach for antiemetic regimens is recommended; the antiemetics are administered about 30 to 60 minutes before chemotherapy in order to block neurotransmitter sites and minimize stimulation of the chemoreceptor trigger zone and the true vomiting center.[28] The problems of delayed-onset nausea

(a)

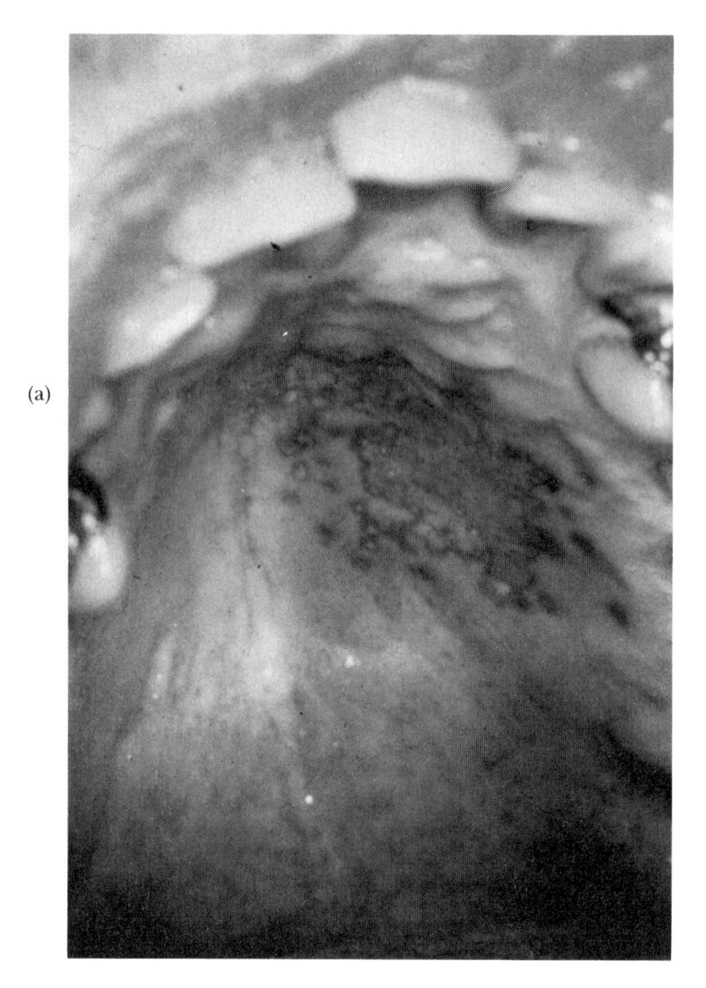

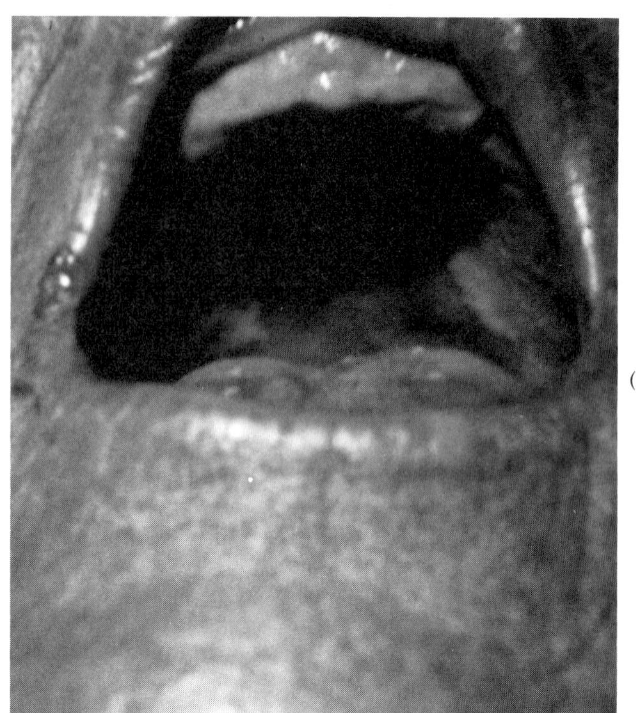

(b)

FIGURE 13-5 Chemotherapy-induced stomatitis. (a) Early-stage stomatitis illustrating reddened, irritated mucosa. (b) Severe mucosal ulceration. (Source: Reprinted by permission of Reidun Daeffler, RN, MSN.)

and vomiting induced by the highly emetogenic cisplatin as well as effective antiemetic interventions have been described by Kris and colleagues.[165]

The problem of anticipatory nausea is very distressing and may actually result in delays in administration of therapy as well as other avoidance behaviors.[149] Assessment of individuals with symptoms of anticipatory nausea and vomiting needs to be done in a manner that reassures them that they are not mentally ill and that such sensations are a result of learned behavior and classic conditioning. Burish and Lyles,[166] Cotanch and Strum,[167] and Redd et al[168] have indicated that a variety of behavioral interventions may be quite effective in controlling this phenomenon. Nurses have increasingly integrated techniques, such as progressive muscle relaxation and hypnosis, into their daily practice in an effort to minimize anticipatory nausea and vomiting and improve the quality of the individual's life with subsequent chemotherapy treatment.

Many other interventions have been used by nurses to alleviate nausea and vomiting, with varying success. These techniques have focused on patient education and support, adjustments in food intake, relaxation, and distraction techniques, alterations in the environment, and position of the individual during treatment.[169] However, there is considerable empirical evidence in support of patient education interventions which aid individual coping. The research of Johnson and colleagues[170,171] has indicated that individuals can be helped to cope if they are given information about the sensations they will encounter, the time sequence of events, and coping behaviors that may be helpful. These investigators also reported that telling individuals that they may experience a noxious side effect such as vomiting does not necessarily lead to their exhibiting the side effect.

Stomatitis

Chemotherapy-induced stomatitis, illustrated in Figure 13-5, occurs with the use of selected antimetabolites and antibiotics, including methotrexate, 5-fluorouracil, dactinomycin, daunorubicin, bleomycin, and doxorubicin. Stomatitis is caused by chemical tissue injury, infection, or both. Chemical tissue injury damages the basal layers of the oral mucosa and inhibits replacement of the superficial cell layers, resulting in ulcerations that occur 5 to 7 days after chemotherapy. Infection can occur as a result of immunosuppression and oral tissue breakdown and is caused by a wide variety of organisms such as *Staphylococcus, Candida,* and herpes simplex virus. A definitive review of the pathology, assessment, and interventions related to chemotherapy-induced stomatitis has been described by Sonis.[172]

Stomatitis is a distressing side effect for many individuals. Pain and irritation have a negative effect on nutritional and emotional status. Nursing care focuses on the management of oral care hydration and pain control. Patients and their families require education related to the cleansing regimen and the use of topical agents.

Although some nursing research has been done concerning assessment and interventions for stomatitis, more is needed. The impact of a systematic oral care protocol was studied by Beck,[173] who found that it improved oral status and reduced infection. The protocol included an assessment done twice a day, mouth care before and after meals and at bedtime, and treatment guidelines for mild and severe stomatitis. The assessment was begun before chemotherapy was initiated to establish a baseline and included systematic inspection of the lips; tongue; mucous membranes of the palate, tonsillar fossa, and gingiva for moisture, color, texture, and debris; teeth; amount of saliva; and changes in taste, voice, or comfort. Mouth care included brushing the teeth with a soft toothbrush and toothpaste, rinsing the mouth with Cepacol mouthwash, and putting petroleum jelly on the lips to prevent dryness. If stomatitis occurred, an oral culture, a complete blood cell count, and a differential leukocyte count were obtained; the patient was placed on a bland diet; oral hygiene procedures were carried out every 1 to 2 hours with a soft toothbrush or soaked gauze and equal parts of Cepacol, hydrogen peroxide, and water; and anesthetics, antibiotics, and analgesics were used as needed.

A second study done by Daeffler[174] surveyed cancer hospitals in the United States to determine the management of oral care. A wide variety of agents, equipment, and methods were used. The most widely used agents were hydrogen peroxide and water in combination with various other products, such as analgesics or lubricants. The use of hydrogen peroxide in cleansing the oral cavity is controversial because it may cause irritation, breakdown of granulation sites in the mouth, and aspiration brought about by the foaming action. It is useful, however, for loosening crusts and debris.

As a result of Daeffler's survey, a nursing procedure for oral care was delineated and many research questions were identified.[175] This procedure includes daily assessment of the oral mucosa, oral care before and after meals and at bedtime, and keeping the lips soft and intact. If stomatitis occurs, cleansing is increased to every 2 hours during the day and every 6 hours at night, and measures to alleviate pain and discomfort are taken. Cleansing is done with 0.9% sodium chloride, saline solution (1 teaspoon of salt to 1 pint of water), or Cepacol or another mild mouthwash diluted 1:5 with water. If the individual is unable to rinse all parts of the mouth effectively, a Water Pik or other irrigation device, a foam stick, or gauze is used to apply the mouthwash to all oral surfaces. Sodium bicarbonate (1 teaspoon to 1 pint of water) followed by a water or saline rinse can be used for thick mucus, and hydrogen peroxide 3% and water (1:4) or Amosam in water (1:2) followed by a saline solution or water rinse can be used for hardened debris, as well as Gly-Oxide alternating with saline solution every 2 hours. A soft toothbrush and dental floss should be used every 24 hours to clean the teeth if tolerated. If such cleaning is not tolerated, a disposable foam swab can be used. Dentures and bridges should be removed and cleaned. After cleansing, a water-soluble jelly is used to moisten the lips. Pain and discomfort are relieved by a bland diet and local anesthetics or analgesics, such as Dyclone 0.5%, lidocaine 2% Vicous or Benadryl elixir with Kaopectate. Although these procedures are complex, they are very effective means of reducing and minimizing oral ulceration and infection.

Eilers, Berger, and Petersen[176] have reported the use of an oral assessment instrument to increase interrater reliability. This instrument, which involves eight categories (voice, swallow, lips, saliva, mucous membrane, gingiva, teeth, or dentures) rated on a three-point ordinal scale, significantly refines those used previously. The study also reported valuable information related to stomatitis in a bone marrow transplant population.

The patient who has stomatitis related to myelosuppression is at an increased risk of esophagitis as well as systemic infections. Because up to 80% of the individuals with lymphoma and leukemia may test seropositive for herpes simplex virus[177] and there is a very high incidence of fungal infection[179] in individuals with leukemia and those who are receiving prednisone, it is important to culture oral lesions that are not healing in spite of a recovering bone marrow. Topical medications, such as chlortrimazole or mycostatin, may be needed. There have been anecdotal reports of the use of multiple topical agents, either for cleansing the oral cavity or in the treatment of pain. While controversy continues regarding the efficacy of such cleansing agents as hydrogen peroxide, saline solution, and sodium bicarbonate, the importance of frequent cleansing cannot be overemphasized. Anecdotal evidence regarding the use of such agents as sucralfate suspension, a combination of antacids, antihistamines, and lidocaine is frequently reported. More nursing research can be extremely helpful in delineating oral care further.

Anorexia

A common and frustrating side effect of cancer treatment and of the disease itself is anorexia. There are many well-documented side effects of specific cancer chemotherapeutic drugs that have the potential for decreasing food intake. These side effects include nausea and vomiting, mucositis, stomatitis, diarrhea, changes in taste acuity, and learned food aversions. In addition, some chemotherapeutic drugs, such as cyclophosphamide, give individuals an unpleasant, often metallic taste during administration. Several authors[179-183] have hypothesized that these effects have a negative impact on caloric intake. Bernstein and Bernstein[184] clearly demonstrated the development of learned food aversions in individuals undergoing gastrointestinal toxic chemotherapy and postulated that this decreased food intake. There is currently little or no empirical evidence to support these hypotheses, and they need to be investigated.

Studies that examined nutritional status and weight loss in individuals undergoing chemotherapy have been few and sample sizes were small.[181,185,186] Findings indicated that weight loss and changes in nutritional status were minimal. Unfortunately, none of the studies distinguished between the effects of the cancer and those of the chemotherapy or indicated whether the negative changes were due to decreased intake or increased energy expenditure. More study of the effect of chemotherapy on nutritional intake is needed.

Nursing interventions designed to relieve chemotherapy-induced anorexia aim to prevent or alleviate the cause, give support to patients and their families, and provide nutritional teaching that emphasizes making the most of the nutrients and calories the person eats. For example, to reduce the smells of cooking, food can be prepared in advance and frozen. Because neither prevention nor alleviation may be possible, provision of support and nutritional counseling regarding methods of increasing caloric and protein intake is essential.

Diarrhea

Diarrhea and abdominal cramping most often result from antimetabolites.[187] If assessment determines that the cause is related to chemotherapy rather than to laxatives or an impaction, therapy may have to be stopped temporarily until the intestinal mucosa has regenerated. A low-residue (see Chapter 12, Radiotherapy) or liquid diet usually is advised until the diarrhea stops. Electrolytes and fluid intake and output should be monitored carefully to assess for fluid and electrolyte imbalances.

Alopecia

The hair follicles are another group of rapidly dividing normal cells that are affected by the nonspecific action of some chemotherapeutic drugs. The most commonly used drugs that cause alopecia are doxorubicin, cyclophosphamide, vincristine, and methotrexate. Chemotherapy-induced hair loss is reported to occur by two mechanisms, depending on the drug and dosage received.[188] If the insult is great enough, marked atrophy of the hair bulb occurs, and the hair falls out spontaneously or in response to a mechanical action such as combing. If the insult is of a lesser nature, a marked constriction of the hair shaft occurs, and the hair breaks off. Hair loss from chemotherapy is not permanent, and regrowth is clinically evident in 4 to 6 weeks. Texture and color of the hair often change with regrowth.[189,190] Nurses should be sensitive to the fact that alopecia may not be limited to the scalp but may include all body hair. Patient teaching also should address the loss of body hair in addition to scalp hair.

Several nursing interventions are useful in helping individuals deal with hair loss. Giving the person information about hair loss and presenting different methods for dealing with it before it occurs are primary interventions. Both men and women need this information, because hair loss can be devastating to the body image of both sexes.[192] Information about hair and scalp care, when and to what extent hair loss can be expected, obtaining a wig, and protecting the scalp from sun and cold are important considerations. Some cancer hospitals have hairdressers who specialize in caring for hair damaged by chemotherapy in a manner that minimizes hair loss. Gentle care of the hair and scalp is essential, and wigs or hairpieces should have a soft "cap."

Two additional methods that claim to prevent hair loss are in use: the scalp tourniquet and the ice turban. However, research findings are in conflict.[192,193] Both methods operate on the principle of decreasing the blood supply to the hair follicles, which decreases the amount of chemotherapeutic agent reaching the hair and thus prevents hair loss. The scalp tourniquet consists of rubber bands, soft rubber tubing, or inflatable cuffs that are placed around the head and tightened for 20 minutes. Research has indicated no statistically significant difference between a control group of individuals receiving cyclophosphamide (40 mg/kg), vincristine (2 mg), methotrexate (0.6 mg/kg), and actinomycin D (2 mg) at 2-week intervals only and an experimental group receiving the same chemotherapy along with use of a scalp tourniquet.[194] Although patients in the latter group did not experience dizziness, headache, or syncope, the head did feel constricted and the scalp soon became numb. However, other investigators in less well-documented studies claim that this approach is effective in minimizing or delaying alopecia.

The second and more popular method of trying to prevent alopecia is use of the ice turban, which decreases the blood supply to the scalp by cooling. In one study ice packs were applied to the scalp 5 minutes before and 30 minutes after doxorubicin treatment for a total of 35 to 40 minutes.[195] Excellent to good protection from hair loss was provided for 70% of the individuals. However, there was a difference between individuals receiving doses of 40 to 50 mg and those receiving more than 60 mg in that those who received the lower doses had significantly more protection. Parker[196] reported the use of a hypothermia cap with good results in individuals receiving intravenous cyclophosphamide, methotrexate, and 5-fluorouracil for breast cancer. None of the patients in the small sample required a wig.

Since both of these methods have been described in the mass media, individuals undergoing chemotherapy often request these treatments. However, many physicians and nurses are concerned that micrometastasis to the scalp may not be exposed to proper doses of chemotherapy and potentially curative treatment is thereby prevented. In malignant diseases in which skin metastasis is documented, such as leukemias, lymphomas, sarcomas, and multicentric solid tumors, these methods are not used in curative therapy. Keller and Blausey[197] and Lindsay[193] have provided an excellent overview of the complexity of this problem as well as the need for nurses and individuals undergoing anticancer therapy to approach with caution measures that prevent alopecia.

Germinal Tissue Effects

The effect of cancer chemotherapy on sexual function and reproduction is an area in which there has been increased research activity because of the emphasis on long-term survival and quality of life. Chapman[198] provides an excellent overview of the physiologic effects of cytotoxic therapy on sexual and gonadal function. General effects of chemotherapy, such as fatigue, anxiety, and change in body image, may contribute to the decreased libido.

Men may experience impotence as a result of the neurologic toxicity associated with the vinca alkaloids and cisplatin. Sperm counts and morphology may be temporarily or permanently depressed. Alkylating agents cause a particularly high incidence of infertility in the male, with aspermia seen as early as the third cycle of nitrogen mustard therapy for Hodgkin's disease.[199] The diagnosis of lymphoma or testicular cancer has been associated with impaired sperm counts before therapy.[200] Counseling related to sperm banking should be viewed from the perspective of positive results in the management of idiopathic male infertility[201] as well as from the individual's religious and moral beliefs regarding masturbation and artificial insemination.

Women frequently report irregular menses, vaginal dryness, and amenorrhea. Reproductive dysfunction is related directly to the woman's age at the time chemotherapy is initiated. Efforts to protect ovarian function with the use of oral contraceptives in women who do not have hormonally dependent tumors have been reported by Chapman.[202] A study of pregnancy outcome in cancer patients reported that 8 of 10 infants who were exposed to chemotherapy during the first trimester were normal.[203] Of pregnancies occurring after cancer therapy, 40% had abnormal outcomes, which were due mainly to low birth weight and premature terminations of pregnancy. Most abnormalities were concentrated in the first year after treatment. Women receiving chemotherapy need to be informed of effects related to reproduction and counseled appropriately.[204]

It is strongly recommended that individuals do not become parents during or immediately after their course of treatment; therefore counseling regarding birth control and mutagenic and teratogenic effects is needed. Tarpy[205] has developed an excellent patient education booklet regarding birth control during cancer therapy. If cured cancer patients have children, long-term follow-up of the children is critical to increasing knowledge about germinal tissue effects and maximizing the child's health.

Lamb and Woods[206] have identified six ways in which nurses can promote sexual health:

1. Foster open communication with the individual. This usually means that the nurse must initiate any discussion related to sexuality.
2. Provide anticipatory guidance. Information is given regarding the sexual changes that can be expected.
3. Validate the normality of the individual's sexual behavior.
4. Explore values and attitudes, as well as information about changes in the patient's physical functioning or appearance.
5. Provide counseling about alternate methods of sexual expression. This includes suggestions for optimal sexual functioning, as well as alternatives to genital intercourse.
6. Educate fellow health professionals through consultation and continuing education.

Nursing knowledge related to individuals who are experiencing sexual and reproductive dysfunction as a result of cancer treatment has increased in the last decade. Research efforts need to be continued in this area that is so crucial to the quality of life of long-term cancer survivors. (For more in-depth discussion, see Chapter 28, Sexual and Reproductive Dysfunction, and Chapter 29, Altered Body Image and Sexuality.)

Local Tissue Irritation

Local tissue irritation resulting from chemotherapy occurs infrequently and usually results from extravasation. The reactions that are seen range from mild to severe and include hyperpigmentation, burning, erythema, inflammation, ulceration, and necrosis. The severity of the reaction depends on the particular drug involved, the amount that leaked into the tissues, and the length of exposure.[207] Delayed local tissue irritation associated with mitomycin C (Mutamycin) that is unrelated to extravasation has been reported by Wood and Ellerhorst-Ryan.[208] Reactions of hyperpigmentation, venous thrombosis and fibrosis, ulceration, and tissue necrosis have occurred up to 6 months after administration of mitomycin C at sites both proximal and distal to the infusion site.

Drugs that commonly are associated with severe necrosis when extravasated are known as vesicants, whereas those associated with less severe reactions of burning or inflammation are known as irritants. Known vesicants and irritants are listed in Table 13-8. The extent of vesicant extravasation reactions depends on the drug and the amount extravasated. The degree of tissue damage often is obvious within 7 to 10 days after most extravasations. Reactions to vesicant drug extravasations may last for several months. Reactions to irritant drugs occur during administration as burning or several days after administration as inflammation and phlebitis and are of much shorter duration.

Extravasations and the severity of reactions can be due to several physiologic factors, as well as poor venipuncture technique.[207] In elderly, debilitated patients vessels may be fragile, small in diameter, and have less blood flow, all of which increase the risk of extravasation. Individuals with elevated venous pressure, such as occurs in superior vena caval syndrome or obstructed venous drainage and edema of an extremity after axillary surgery, are at risk of severe reactions if extravasation occurs. This is a result of venous pooling due to poor circulation, which delays drug absorption. Local reactions also may be more severe as a result of extravasation into a previously irradiated site. Radiation is potentiated by the action of some drugs, such as doxorubicin; thus previous reactions to radiation can be reactivated, even in distant sites. These conditions should be avoided whenever possible when chemotherapy is administered. If the condition cannot be avoided, a highly skilled professional will be most successful in avoiding extravasation.

TABLE 13-8 Vesicant and Irritant Antineoplastic Drugs

Vesicant Drugs	Irritant Drugs
Amsacrine (M-AMSA)	Carmustine (BCNU)
Bisantrene	Dacarbazine (DTIC)
Dactinomycin (Actinomycin D)	Etoposide (VP-16-213 Vepesid)
Daunomycin (Cerubidine)	Mitoguazone (Methyl-GAG)
Daunorubicin hydrochloride (Adriamycin)	Plicamycin (Mithracin)
Estramustine phosphate (Estracyte)	Streptozotocin (Zanosar)
	Teniposide (VM-26)
Maytansine	
Mechlorethamine (nitrogen mustard)	
Mitomycin C (Mutamycin)	
Pyrazofurin (Pyrazomycin)	
Vinblastine sulfate (Velban)	
Vincristine (Oncovin)	
Vindesine (Eldisine)	

Source: Oncology Nursing Society. Cancer chemotherapy: Guidelines, Modules I-V. Pittsburgh, Oncology Nursing Society, 1988. See Module V, p 7.

Several aspects of venipuncture technique can aid in preventing extravasation or minimizing its effect. Any area in which sloughing would expose critical nerves and tendons, such as the antecubital fossa, wrist, and hand, should be avoided as injection sites.[207] Extravasation in these areas can lead to permanent dysfunction. In addition, extravasations in the antecubital fossa are difficult to detect. The optimal site of injection is the forearm, where there is sufficient tissue protecting nerves and tendons.

Another aspect of venipuncture technique that should be avoided is the use of multiple puncture sites in the same vein. This can result in leakage into surrounding tissues, once an intravenous line is established. If multiple puncture sites are necessary, a different vein should be chosen when possible. If this is not possible, a proximal (closer to the heart) point on the same vein should be used, because leakage could occur from a previous more distal puncture site.

Extravasation can occur in spite of preventive measures. When it occurs, prompt treatment frequently can minimize the severity of the reaction. Definitive management of doxorubicin, mechlorethamine, and vinca alkaloid extravasations has been identified. Treatment of doxorubicin extravasation has received the most study, but a definitive pharmacologic antidote has not been identified. Although local injection of steroids, sodium bicarbonate, and topical application of DMSO was reported to be effective in anecdotal reports and some studies, these findings have been negated.[209] It is now clear that the positive effect of these agents can be explained by the clinical finding that 89% of all extravasations never progress beyond mild local irritation, even in the absence of any local pharmacologic therapy.[210] Animal studies indicate that the current best treatment for doxorubicin extravasation is immediate removal of the intravenous line and application of ice to the site for 30 minutes to 10 hours after the extravasation and intermittently for up to 7 days thereafter.[211,212] These findings have been confirmed in humans by Larsen[210] with a program of intermittent ice application for 3 days. Since ulceration usually occurs 3 to 4 weeks after the extravasation, close observation of the wound should continue during this time.[210] An example of untreated doxorubicin extravasation is shown in Figure 13-6.

An effective pharmacologic antidote for mechlorethamine (HN_2, nitrogen mustard) has been clearly demonstrated. "Sodium thiosulfate 1/6 M, given immediately following HN_2 extravasation, significantly reduced HN_2-induced skin ulceration."[209] The 1/6 M isotonic solution of sodium thiosulfate should be injected at the extravasation site in a dose of at least 20-fold molar excess of the amount of HN_2 extravasated. Delayed treatment is ineffective.

Dorr and colleagues[209] also identified an effective antidote for the extravasation of the vinca alkaloids, vincristine, vinblastine, and vindesine. Hyaluronidase dissolved in saline solution should be injected liberally into the extravasation site immediately after removal of the intravenous tubing. Heat is applied to activate the hyaluronidase. Cold application or steroids should

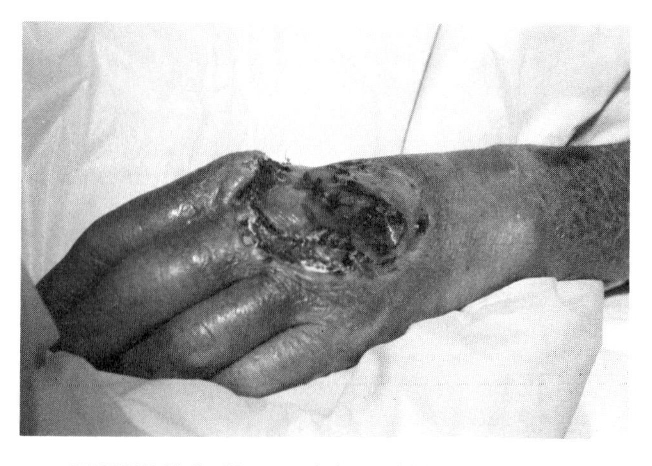

FIGURE 13-6 Untreated doxorubicin extravasation.

not be used, because they increase the skin toxicity of vinca alkaloids.

Unfortunately, effective antidotes for other vesicants, such as mitomycin C, are not known. It is clear, however, that early recognition of extravasation and termination of the vesicant infusion are very important in reducing skin irritation and toxicity.

Although nurses do not order treatment for extravasations, they may be the first to recognize that an extravasation has occurred and to administer treatment. To provide prompt treatment, a previously approved treatment protocol is recommended. It should be included in the administration orders of any vesicant drug for each individual patient. In areas in which chemotherapy is administered frequently, an extravasation tray can expedite treatment. Astute observation by nurses and prompt treatment can prevent severe necrosis in doxorubicin, mechlorethamine, and vinca alkaloid extravasations.

If extravasation occurs and severe necrosis results, surgical consultation may be needed for debridement and repair. Recovery can be a very long process that includes physical rehabilitation.

Allergic Reactions

Allergic reactions to chemotherapeutic drugs have received little attention in the literature. These reactions do occur, however, and can be uncomfortable and even life-threatening.[213,214] Allergic or hypersensitivity reactions result from overstimulation of the immune system. Type I sensitivity reactions are most frequently seen in chemotherapy. In type I reactions, hypersensitivity occurs by exposure to a foreign substance or antigen, resulting in the development of IgE antibodies. After sensitization has occurred, subsequent exposures to the antigen result in allergic reactions, with such symptoms as agitation, urticaria, facial edema, rhinitis, dyspnea, and anaphylaxis. Allergic symptoms usually become worse with each additional exposure to the antigen.

The antineoplastic drug that most often causes allergic reactions is L-asparaginase, with hypersensitivity reactions occurring in 6% to 43% of the individuals studied.[214] The highest incidence of reactions has been when L-asparaginase was administered intravenously as a single agent at doses greater than 6000 IU/m^2 and given three or more times per week. Sensitization usually occurs after 2 weeks of daily treatment, but occasionally it occurs after one dose. The most common symptom is urticaria; other symptoms are agitation, dyspnea, hypotension, facial edema, abdominal cramps, laryngospasm and stridor, rash, pruritus of the hands and feet, and loss of consciousness. Most individuals recover after treatment is stopped and epinephrine and glucocorticoids are given. However, some deaths have occurred.

The second most common drug associated with hypersensitivity is cisplatin, with reactions occurring in 1% to 20% of the individuals studied.[214] Reactions are most common when cisplatin is used in combination with other drugs and have occurred after a wide variety of dosages. Symptoms have included anxiety, flushing, burning and tingling sensations, pruritus, cough, dyspnea, diaphoresis, periorbital edema, bronchospasm, vomiting, erythema and urticaria, maculopapular rash, and hypotension. Most individuals have recovered after treatment with glucocorticoids, antihistamines, and epinephrine. Some individuals have been able to tolerate further treatment with cisplatin when premedicated with glucocorticoids and antihistamines.

Other drugs that have been associated with hypersensitivity reactions are bleomycin, cyclophosphamide, daunorubicin, doxorubicin, intravenous melphalan, nitrogen mustard, methotrexate, teniposide (investigational), and zinostatin (investigational). The incidence of hypersensitivity to these drugs is low. Symptoms vary widely and range from mild to severe. One fairly common local hypersensitivity reaction may be seen by nurses who administer doxorubicin. A "flair," or localized urticaria, develops along the course of the vein at the injection site.[214] Patchy or diffuse erythema, urticarial wheals, and pruritus may occur. This reaction may occur with the first dose but not with subsequent doses. If it continues, premedication with antihistamines or further dilution of the drug may be helpful in preventing the problem.

Because nurses often administer chemotherapy, their assessment and interventions are extremely important in the effective management of allergic reactions. A nursing care plan designed to deal with hypersensitivity reactions includes interventions before drug administration as well as after a reaction occurs.[213] Before each treatment, a nursing history is taken; this includes previous allergic responses, especially to antineoplastic and other drugs, and a baseline recording of pulse, respirations, blood pressure, and mental status. The nurse makes sure that emergency drugs and equipment are available and knows their location. In addition, the patient is taught to report any symptoms of an allergic reaction and is reminded of this each time chemotherapy is given. When chemotherapy is administered, the full course of the vein is exposed to the nurse's view. In administration of bleomycin, test dosing has been advocated to determine individual sensitivity.[215]

If an allergic reaction occurs, the flow of drug is stopped immediately, but the intravenous line is kept open. The nurse then makes a careful but rapid assessment of symptoms. If an anaphylactic response is suspected, the nurse requests medical and emergency services, maintains an airway, places the individual in a Trendelenburg position (unless that is contraindicated by respiratory distress), monitors vital signs, reassures the patient, and institutes cardiopulmonary resuscitation if necessary. If anaphylaxis does not occur, the patient is carefully observed until the threat of an anaphylactic reaction has passed. These nursing actions can be lifesaving, and therefore a nursing protocol that includes them should be used for all individuals receiving chemotherapeutic drugs.

Organ Toxicities

Cardiotoxicity

Both acute and chronic cardiac toxicity can occur as a result of cancer chemotherapy.[216] Several agents are associated with transient electrocardiogram changes evidenced by sinus tachycardias, ST and T-wave changes, and premature beats. These changes occur immediately, usually resolve quickly, and are rarely life-threatening. The exception is ventricular fibrillation associated with amascarine (m-AMSA), especially in the presence of hypokalemia.[51] Kaszyk[217] provides an excellent overview of the chemotherapy agents associated with cardiac toxicity.

Cumulative cardiomyopathy syndrome is a chronic form of cardiotoxicity that results from the anthracyclines, doxorubicin and daunomycin. Cardiomyopathy is irreversible. Clinical characteristics are classic congestive heart failure with low-voltage QRS complexes and other physical symptoms of heart failure. Traditionally, it has been recommended that cumulative doses of doxorubicin in adults with normal cardiac function not exceed 550 mg/m^2 and that total doses of daunorubicin not exceed 550 to 600 mg/m^2. Previous or concurrent cardiac irradiation is synergistic with doxorubicin, and these individuals receive a total cumulative dose no greater than 450 mg/m^2. Individuals with hypertension or heart disease do not receive cumulative doses exceeding 450 mg/m^2, and those with a history of heart failure probably should not receive the drug at all.

Dosages greater than those recommended may be possible in responsive individuals. This is determined on an individual basis through the use of endomyocardial biopsy to assess cardiac myocyte damage.[218] In addition, continuous infusions or low weekly doses of doxorubicin may decrease the risk of cardiomyopathy.[216,219] Newer generations of less toxic anthracyclines are also promising.

Nurses should keep an accurate record of total cumulative dosages of doxorubicin and daunorubicin, do a baseline and subsequent electrocardiograms before each treatment, assess the patient for symptoms of heart failure, and teach the patient and family to assess and report symptoms of heart failure immediately. Nursing measures for the individual in whom cardiomyopathy develops include patient teaching on conservation of energy, managing fluid retention, and minimizing sodium in the diet.[217]

Hepatotoxicity

Liver dysfunction may result from many antineoplastic drugs and is usually diagnosed by transient elevations of the hepatic enzymes during treatment.[220] Some drugs, however, can cause fibrosis, cirrhosis, and acute hepatotoxicity that may be dose-limiting. Long-term administration of methotrexate, mercaptopurine, and azathioprine (metabolized to 6-MP) has produced significant hepatic fibrosis and cirrhosis. L-asparaginase and plicamycin often cause decreased albumin and clotting factor synthesis, impaired lipid metabolism, elevated lactic dehydrogenase (LDH), and azotemia. Previous liver impairment as a result of hepatitis increases the likelihood of liver dysfunction.

Dosages producing acute toxicity are variable, and symptoms occur immediately or very early in treatment. Assessment of baseline hepatic enzyme levels is essential before therapy with these drugs. Liver function tests should be assessed periodically throughout the course of treatment. When hepatotoxicity occurs, the toxicity of drugs such as doxorubicin or the vinca alkaloids will increase markedly because of impaired liver metabolism and excretion.[221] In these situations, dosage reduction of 50% to 75% may be necessary.

Neurotoxicity

Drugs that commonly produce neurotoxicity include vincristine, vinblastine, and L-asparaginase. High doses (>2 mg) and cumulative doses of vincristine commonly produce dose-limiting toxicities. Symptoms include paresthesias of the hands or feet, constipation, loss of deep tendon reflexes, weakness, and frequently impotence. Ongoing assessment of neurologic function is required. Preventive stool softeners or laxatives are needed, as well as education of the patient and family concerning safety precautions related to sensorimotor impairment.

High-dose (2 gm/m^2) cytosine arabinoside has been associated with severe neurologic toxicity.[222,223] The combination of daunorubicin and L-asparaginase with these agents increases the potential for neurologic toxicity.[224] The symptoms may include cerebellar toxicities, such as tremor, loss of balance, and fine motor movement; severe peripheral neuropathies; confusion; and somnolence. Conrad[225] describes nursing assessment of patients receiving higher doses (2 gm/m^2) of cytosine arabinoside.

Peripheral neuropathies also have been reported with the use of cisplatin therapy, especially in higher doses.[226] Symptoms include loss of feeling in the extremities, auditory and visual impairment, and inability to determine placement of extremities.[227] These symptoms result in impairment of motor function, ability to provide self-care, and ability to perform occupational and recreational activities. Holden and Felde[227] describe an excellent and extensive nursing care plan for individuals experiencing cisplatin-related neurologic toxicity. The essential components are thorough ongoing nursing assessment, patient and family education, and supportive nursing care.

Pulmonary toxicity

A high risk of pulmonary toxicity is associated with bleomycin, busulfan, and carmustine.[228] Bleomycin has the highest risk of pulmonary toxicity, which occurs in 10% to 40% of patients in the form of severe pneumonitis and interstitial fibrosis. These dose-related and dose-limiting toxic effects occur with greater frequency with cumulative doses greater than 200 to 250 U/m^2 without chest irradiation and 120 to 150 U/m^2 with chest irradiation. However, toxicity has been seen in total doses as low as 40 U/m^2. The risk and incidence increase greatly in individuals over 70 years of age, those with previous chest irradiation, and those with preexisting pulmonary disease. Simultaneous administration of another drug, such as mitomycin, with some risk of pulmonary toxicity may be synergistic.

Clinical symptoms include dry cough, fever, exertional dyspnea, basilar fine rales, and occasionally tachypnea. Treatment includes discontinuation of the drug and administration of corticosteroids, which may be beneficial in relieving symptoms. The onset of toxicity is usually slow, taking place over several months; therefore ongoing assessment of pulmonary function and total cumulative dose is needed. The lifetime cumulative dose of bleomycin is 400 U.

Busulfan produces clinically evident pulmonary toxicity in 2% to 10% of individuals. Pulmonary problems associated with this drug occur at any time from 10 months to 10 years and are associated with the total duration of treatment, rather than the total dose. Chest irradiation and treatment with other pulmonary toxic drugs are synergistic.

The incidence of lung toxicity with carmustine (BCNU) is 20% to 30% and is associated with the total cumulative dose given. Toxicity has occurred with total doses ranging from 240 mg/m^2 to 2400 mg/m^2. However, a cumulative dose of 1200 to 1400 mg/m^2 has been correlated with a significant rise in lung injury and death, so this is usually the dosage at which therapy is discontinued. Unlike bleomycin, age does not appear to be correlated with risk of toxicity. Once pulmonary toxicity produced by carmustine occurs, it is irreversible and usually fatal. Therefore prevention through careful assessment for symptoms of respiratory problems, records of total cumulative dose, and discontinuation of the drug is the only recourse.

Several other drugs have lower risks of pulmonary toxicity. Medium- to low-risk drugs include chlorambucil, cyclophosphamide, cytarabine, melphalan, methotrexate, and mitomycin. Very low risk is associated with azathioprine, 6-mercaptopurine, procarbazine, semustine, teniposide, uracil mustard, and zinostatin. Wickham[229] provides an excellent review of the mechanism of chemotherapy-induced pulmonary damage.

Nephrotoxicity

Nephrotoxicity usually is not dose-limiting, but it is important in the renal clearance of drugs. Other side effects, such as myelosuppression, can be enhanced even by mild nephrotoxicity. Renal toxicity can occur in the urinary bladder as a result of cyclophosphamide or in the renal tubules as a result of cisplatin, methotrexate, streptozocin, mitomycin (rare), and the nitrosoureas (rare). Lydon[230] provides a thorough review of the nephrotoxicity associated with cancer therapy.

Cyclophosphamide can produce acute hemorrhagic cystitis with doses of 1 to 2 g/m^2, but this is at least partially preventable with large volumes of fluid each day. Symptoms include dysuria, frequency, urgency, or hematuria occurring from 24 hours to several weeks after treatment. Symptoms generally subside when the drug is discontinued. The most important nursing intervention is provision of adequate hydration.

Cisplatin may cause acute tubular necrosis with cumulative doses greater than 50 mg/m^2 and repeated doses of 0.25 mg/kg for 5 days. The toxicity occurs rapidly within 1 week and is diagnosed on the basis of elevations in blood urea nitrogen, creatinine, or uric acid. Prophylactic therapy consisting of hydration and diuresis with mannitol may reduce the incidence and severity of toxic effects. Administration of adequate fluids to a well-hydrated individual minimizes nephrotoxicity. Adequate hydration of at least 3 L per day should be maintained for 3 days after treatment to maximize excretion of cisplatin and preserve renal function.[221]

Streptozocin commonly causes dose-limiting nephrotoxicity because 10% to 20% of the active drug is excreted via the kidneys within 2 hours. Early symptoms of toxicity include proteinuria, hypophosphatemia, and aminoaciduria. If the drug is discontinued at this time, toxic effects are reversed in 2 to 4 weeks. However, if therapy is continued or if large doses are given (>1.5 g/m^2 per week or >500 mg/m^2 per day for 5 days), severe renal failure and death may occur. Prophylactic hydration may reduce the incidence of complications or prevent severe toxicities, and careful ongoing assessment is essential.

Methotrexate can produce acute renal tubular necrosis when given in high doses (>1 g/m^2) or to individuals with renal disease, because a large amount of this drug is excreted by the kidneys. This occurs rapidly within 48 hours and is detected by serial serum creatinine levels. Toxicity results from the precipitation of the drug in the tubules, causing dilatation and damage. Alkalinization of the urine to a pH of 7 prevents precipitation. This is done by administering 3 g of sodium bicarbonate orally every 3 hours for four doses before, during, and after treatment. Hydration greater than 3 L/day is also recommended. Patients are taught to avoid taking vitamin C because it acidifies the urine and can cause methotrexate retention.[221]

Long-Term Effects

In addition to short-term side effects, individuals undergoing chemotherapy are at risk of long-term effects of these drugs. The three potential problems that have been identified are second malignant diseases, sterility or impaired gonadal functioning, and genetic defects in offspring.[231] In addition, psychosocial sequelae may have a long-term impact. Although research is limited or nonexistent, especially on psychosocial problems, more will be learned as individuals survive longer and are cured. (See Chapter 19, Psychosocial Dimensions: The Survivor.)

The development of second malignant diseases after cancer treatment contributes only a small percentage to the mortality of cancer survivors.[229] The majority of chemotherapy-related malignancies are acute nonlymphocytic leukemia associated with alkylating agent therapy. The mechanism by which chemotherapy induces second malignancies is not known, but it is believed to be associated with the ability of these drugs to alter DNA.[29] Second malignancies may develop up to 20 years after treatment.

Sterility and impaired gonadal functioning may also be long-term effects of chemotherapy. As discussed previously, both ovarian and testicular functioning often are affected by chemotherapy, and function can be impaired for several years. Some individuals have impaired gonadal functioning for long periods of time, whereas others recover.[29,228] There are several reports of individuals who have received chemotherapy and became parents of healthy infants.[203] Genetic defects resulting from chemotherapy are also suspected as a possible long-term effect, but there is no supporting evidence to date.

Much more research is needed regarding the long-term effects of chemotherapy, and this will be possible as more individuals survive for long periods of time. Until more is known, individuals should be taught methods to identify second malignancies early. They also should be encouraged to remain in follow-up with their physicians indefinitely. If they have children, they should be encouraged to monitor their children's health carefully. Cancer nurses, as well as nurses in other specialties, should be alert to the long-term problems associated with cancer chemotherapy. (See Chapter 32, Late Effects of Cancer Treatment.)

CONCLUSION

Cancer chemotherapy is a treatment modality in which nursing participation is essential. Nursing skill and expertise is needed both in the administration of these drugs as well as in the management of side effects. The nurse's competence, patient teaching, and support is fundamental to assisting patients and families with the successful integration of chemotherapy into their lives.

Nursing research related to chemotherapy-induced problems is critical. There is a need to document systematically the characteristics of such problems as hair loss, infections, and impact on daily living, both cross-sectionally and longitudinally, and to study nursing interventions with experimental methods to determine effectiveness. Some valuable nursing research has been done but more is needed to enhance patients' and their families' adaptation to this treatment.

REFERENCES

1. Pack GT, Ariel JM: The history of cancer therapy, in American Cancer Society (ed): Cancer management: A Special Graduate Course on Cancer. Philadelphia, Lippincott, 1968, pp 2-27.
2. Cline MJ, Haskell CH: Cancer Chemotherapy (ed 3). Philadelphia, Saunders, 1980.
3. Haddow A, Watkinson JM, Paterson E: Influence of synthetic estrogens upon advanced malignant disease. Br Med J 2:393-398, 1944.
4. Huggins C, Hodges CV: Studies on prostatic cancer. I. The effect of castrations, of estrogen and of androgen injection on serum phosphatases in metastatic carcinoma of the prostate. Cancer Res 1:293-297, 1941.
5. Saunders JF, Carter SK (eds): U.S.A.-U.S.S.R. monograph: Methods of development of new anticancer drugs. National Cancer Institute Monograph 45 (DHEW publication no. 76-1037), 1977.
6. Farber S, Diamond LK, Mercer RD, et al. Temporary remissions in acute leukemia in children produced by folic acid antagonists, 4-aminopteroyl-glutamic acid (aminopterin). N Eng J Med 238:787-793, 1948.
7. Krakoff LH: Cancer chemotherapeutic agents. CA 31:130-140, 1981.
8. Stonehill EH: Impact of cancer therapy on survival. Cancer 42:1008-1014, 1978.
9. Burchenal JH: The historical development of cancer chemotherapy. Semin Oncol 4:135-146, 1977.
10. Lane M: Chemotherapy of cancer, in del Regato JA, Spjut HJ, Cox JD (eds): Ackerman and del Regato's Cancer: Diagnosis, Treatment and Prognosis (ed 6). St. Louis, Mosby, 1985, pp 93-118.
11. Heinrichs MH, Schmale AH: Principles of psychosocial oncology, in Rubin P (ed): Clinical Oncology for Medical Students and Physicians: A Multidisciplinary Approach (ed 6). Rochester, NY, American Cancer Society, 1983, pp 482-488.
12. Hill BT: Cancer chemotherapy: The relevance of certain concepts of cell cycle kinetics. Biochem Biophys Acta 516:389-417, 1978.
13. Haskell CM (ed): Cancer Treatment (ed 2). Philadelphia, Saunders, 1985.
14. Baserga R: The cell cycle. N Engl J Med 301:454-459, 1981.
15. Henshaw EC: Introduction, in Rosenthal SN, Bennett JM (eds): Practical Cancer Chemotherapy. Garden City, NY, Medical Examination Publishing Co, 1981, pp 1-13.
16. Hill BT, Baserga R: The cell cycle and its significance for cancer treatment. Cancer Treat Rev 2:159-175, 1975.
17. Carter S, Bakowski M, Hellman K: Chemotherapy of Cancer (ed 3). New York, Wiley, 1987.
18. Baserga R: Multiplication and Division in Mammalian Cells. New York, Marcel Dekker, 1976.
19. Killman SA: Acute leukemia: The kinetics of leukemic blast cells in man; an analytical review. Series Haematologia 1:38-102, 1968.
20. Turbiana M, Malaise E: Comparison of cell proliferation kinetics in human and experimental tumors: Response to irradiation. Cancer Treat Rep 60:1887-1895, 1976.
21. Turbiana M, Richard JM, Malaise E: Kinetics of tumor growth and of cell proliferation in U.R.D.T. cancers: Therapeutic implications. Laryngoscope 85:1039-1052, 1975.
22. Bruce WR, Meeker BE, Valeriote FA: Comparison of the sensitivity of normal hematopoietic and transplanted lymphoma colony-forming cells to chemotherapeutic agents administered *in vivo*. J Nat Cancer Inst 37:233-245, 1966.
23. Valeriote FA, Edelstein MB: The role of cell kinetics in cancer chemotherapy. Semin Oncol 4:217-226, 1977.
24. Skipper HE: Combination therapy: Some concepts and results. Cancer Chemother Rep 4(Part 2):137, 1974.
25. Norton L, Simon A: Tumor size, sensitivity to therapy, and design of treatment schedules. Cancer Treat Rep 61:1307-1317, 1977.
26. Krakoff IH: Systemic cancer treatment: Cancer chemotherapy, in Horton J, Hill GJ (eds): Clinical Oncology. Philadelphia, Saunders 1977, pp 157-182.

27. Goldie JH, Coldman AJ: A mathematical model for relating the drug sensitivity of tumors to their spontaneous mutation rate. Cancer Treat Rep 63:1727-1733, 1979.
28. Dorr R, Fritz W: Cancer Chemotherapy Handbook. New York, Elsevier, 1980.
29. Murinson DS: Clinical pharmacology, in Rosenthal SN, Bennett JM (eds): Practical Cancer Chemotherapy. Garden City, NY, Medical Examination Co, 1981, pp 14-74.
30. del Regato JA, Spjut HJ, Cox JD: Ackerman and del Regato's Cancer: Diagnosis, Treatment and Prognosis (ed 6). St. Louis, Mosby, 1985.
31. Hubbard SM: Chemotherapy and the nurse, in Marino LB (ed): Cancer Nursing. St. Louis, Mosby, 1981, pp 287-343.
32. DeVita VT, Serpick A, Carbone P: Combination chemotherapy in the treatment of advanced Hodgkin's disease. Ann Intern Med 73:881-895, 1970.
33. Karnofsky DA, Burchenal JH: The clinical evaluation of chemotherapeutic agents in cancer, in McLeod CM (ed): Evaluation of Chemotherapeutic Agents. New York, Columbia University Press, 1949, pp 191-205.
34. Zubrod CC, Schneiderman M, Frei E, et al: Appraisal of methods for the study of chemotherapy of cancer in man: Comparative therapeutic trial of nitrogen mustard and triethylenethiophoramide. J Chron Dis 11:7-33, 1960.
35. Miller SA: Legal implications for the nurse involved in cancer chemotherapy, in Dorr RT, Fritz WL (eds): Cancer Chemotherapy Handbook, New York, Elsevier, 1980, pp 743-754.
36. Dorr RT: Incompatibilities with parenteral anticancer drugs. Am J Intravenous Ther 6(2):42-52, 1979.
37. Hansten PD: Drug Interactions: Clinical Significance of Drug-Drug Interactions (ed 5). Philadelphia, Lea and Febiger, 1985.
38. Stockley IH: Drug Interactions: A Source Book of Adverse Interactions, Their Mechanisms, Clinical Importance and Management. Oxford, Blackwell Scientific Publications, 1981.
39. Griffin JP, D'Arcy PF, Speirs CJ: A Manual of Adverse Drug Interactions (ed 4). London, Wright, 1988.
40. Oncology Nursing Society: Cancer Chemotherapy Guidelines, Modules I-V, Pittsburgh, Oncology Nursing Society, 1988.
41. Spross J, Cullen ML, Frogge MH (eds): Update on Nursing Issues: Issues in chemotherapy administration. Oncol Nurs Forum 9:50-54, 1982.
42. Lauffer BE, Yasko JM: Care of the Client Receiving Chemotherapy: A Self-learning Module for the Nurse Caring for the Client With Cancer. Reston, Va, Reston, 1984.
43. Fischer DS, Knobf MT: The Chemotherapy Handbook (ed 3). Chicago, Yearbook Medical Publishers, 1989.
44. Engelking CH, Steele NE: A model for pretreatment nursing assessment of patients receiving cancer chemotherapy. Cancer Nurs 7:203-212, 1984.
45. McNally JC, Stair JC, Somerville ET: Guidelines for Cancer Nursing Practice. New York, Grune & Stratton, 1985.
46. American Nurses' Association, Oncology Nursing Society: Standards of Oncology Nursing Practice. Kansas City, American Nurses' Society, 1987.
47. Oncology Nursing Society: Outcome Standards for Cancer Patient Education. Pittsburgh, Oncology Nursing Society, 1982.
48. Gross J: Clinical research in cancer chemotherapy. Oncol Nurs Forum 13:59-65, 1986.
49. Morrow GM: How readable are subject consent forms? JAMA 244:56-58, 1985.
50. Chammaro T, Applebaum J: Informed consent: Nursing issues and ethical dilemmas. Oncol Nurs Forum. 15:803-808, 1988.
51. DeVita VT: Principles of chemotherapy, in DeVita VT, Hellman S, Rosenberg SA (eds): Cancer: Principles and Practice of Oncology (ed 3). Philadelphia, Lippincott, 1989, pp 276-300.
52. Gelman RS, Tormey DC, Belensky R, et al: Actual vs. ideal weight in the calculation of body surface area: Effects on the dose of 11 chemotherapy agents. Cancer Treat Rep 71:907-910, 1987.
53. DeVita VT: Principles of chemotherapy, in DeVita VT, Hellman S, Rosenberg SA (eds): Cancer: Principles and Practice of Oncology (ed 3). Philadelphia, Lippincott, 1989, pp 276-300.
54. Duffy TP: How much is too much high dose cytosine arabinoside. J Clin Oncol 3:601-602, 1985.
55. Goorin AM, Perez-Atayde A, Gebhardt M: Weekly high dose methotrexate and doxorubicin for osteosarcoma: The Dana-Farber Children's Hospital study. III, J Clin Oncol 5:1178-1184, 1987.
56. Ford R et al: High dose etoposide (Vepesid or VP16), in Brown MH, Kiss, ME, Outlaw E: Standards of Oncology Nursing Practice. New York, Wiley, 1986.
57. Conrad K: Cerebellar toxicities associated with cytosine arabinoside: A nursing perspective. Oncol Nurs Forum 13(5):57-59, 1986.
58. Holden S, Feld E: Nursing care of patients experiencing cisplatin related neuropathy. Oncol Nurs Forum 14:13-19, 1987.
59. Chabner B, Myers C: Clinical pharmacology of cancer chemotherapy, in DeVita VT, Hellman S, Rosenberg SA (eds): Cancer: Principles and Practice of Oncology (ed 3), Philadelphia, Lippincott, 1989, pp 349-388.
60. Levine AM, Richardson JL, Marks G, et al: Compliance with oral drug therapy in patients with hematological malignancy. J Clin Oncol 5:1469-1476, 1987.
61. Barofsky I: Therapeutic compliance and the cancer patient. Health Educ 10:43-56, 1984.
62. Sticklin LA, Dubbelde K, Larson E: Nursing care of the patient receiving subcutaneous low-dose ARA-C therapy. Oncol Nurs Forum. 16:365-369, 1989.
63. Mioduszewski J, Zarbo A: Ambulatory infusion pump: A practical view of an alternative approach. Semin Oncol Nursing. 3:106-111, 1987.
64. Harvey VJ, Slevin ML, Aherne GW, et al: Subcutaneous infusion of bleomycin: A practical approach to intravenous infusion. J Clin Oncol 5:648-650, 1987.
65. Markman M, Howell SB, Lucas WE, et al: Combination intraperitoneal chemotherapy with cisplatin, cytarbine and doxorubicin for refractory ovarian carcinoma and other malignancies principally confined to the peritoneal cavity. J Clin Oncol. 2:1321-1326, 1984.
66. Hoff S: Concepts in intraperitoneal chemotherapy. Semin Oncol Nurs 3:112-117, 1987.
67. Eriksson JH, Swenson KK: Your guide to intraperitoneal chemotherapy. Oncol Nurs Forum 13(5):77-81, 1986.
68. Levin V, Sheline G, Gutin P: Neoplasms of the central nervous system, in DeVita VT, Hellman S, Rosenberg SA (eds): Cancer: Principles and Practice of Oncology (ed 3). Philadelphia, Lippincott, 1989, pp 1557-1611.
69. Sugarbaker PH, Gianda FJ, Speyer J, et al: Prospective randomized trial of intravenous use intraperitoneal 5-FU in patients with advanced primary colon or rectal cancer. Semin Oncol 12:101-111, 1985.

70. Collins J: Pharmacologic rationale for regional drug delivery. J Clin Oncol 2:498-504, 1984.
71. Ghussen F, Nagle K, Grouh W, et al: A prospective randomized study of regional extremity profusion in patients with malignant melanoma. Ann Surg 200:764-769, 1984.
72. Racheson RA, Ommaya AK: Experience with the subcutaneous cerebrospinal-fluid reservoir. N Engl J Med 279:1025-1031, 1968.
73. Esparza D, Weyland J: Nursing care for the patient with an ommaya reservoir. Oncol Nurs Forum 9(4):17-20, 1982.
74. Wujcik D: Meningeal carcinomatosis: Diagnosis, treatment, and nursing care. Oncol Nurs Forum 10(2):35-40, 1983.
75. Speery R: Ommaya resevoir, in Brown MH, Kiss M, Outlaw E, et al: Standards of Oncology Nursing Practice, New York, Wiley, 1986, pp 606-610.
76. Fisher DS, Knobf MT: The Cancer Chemotherapy Handbook (3 ed). Chicago, Year Book Medical Publishers, 1989, p 142.
77. Beland IL, Passos JY: Clinical Nursing: Pathophysiological and Psychosocial Approaches (ed 3). New York, MacMillan, 1975.
78. Ostrowski MJ: Continuous intravenous infusion of cytotoxic agents. Nurs Times 75:919-920, 1979.
79. Bishop C: Home parenteral chemotherapy. Top Hosp Pharm Management 11:35-42, 1984.
80. Garvey EC: Current and future nursing issues in the home administration of chemotherapy. Semin Oncol Nurs 3:142-147, 1987.
81. Nieweg R, Greidanus J, de Vries E: An outpatient education program for a continuous infusion regimen on an outpatient basis. Cancer Nurs 10(4):177-182, 1987.
82. Gullatte M, Foltz A: Hepatic chemotherapy via an implantable pump. Am J Nurs 83:1674-1676, 1983.
83. Cozzi E, Hagle M, McGregor ML, et al: Nursing management of patients receiving hepatic arterial chemotherapy through an implanted infusion pump. Cancer Nurs 7:229-234, 1984.
84. Von Roemling R, MacDonald M, Langevin T: Chemotherapy via implanted infusion pump: New perspectives for delivery of long term continuous treatment. Oncol Nurs Forum 13(2):17-24, 1986.
85. Hagle M: Implantable devices for chemotherapy: Access and delivery. Semin Oncol Nurs 3:96-105, 1987.
86. Vogelzang N, Ruane M, DeMeesler T: Phase I trail of an implanted battery powered programmable drug system for continuous doxorubicin administration. J Clin Oncol 3:407-414, 1985.
87. Dressler S, Lanon F, Galowitz H, et al: Administration of floxuridine (FUDR) via implanted pump, in Brown MH, Kiss M, Viamontes C (eds): Standards of Oncology Nursing Practice. New York, Wiley, 1986, pp 602-605.
88. Steele C: A complication of hepatic chemotherapy via implantable port: A case report. Oncol Nurs Forum 13:25-29, 1986.
89. Garvey E, Kramer R: Improving cancer patients' adjustment to infusion chemotherapy: Evaluation of a patient education program. Cancer Nurs 6:373-378, 1983.
90. Teich CJ, Raia K: Teaching strategies for an ambulatory chemotherapy program. Oncol Nurs Forum, 11(5):24-28, 1984.
91. Goodman MS, Wickham R: Venous access devices: An overview. Oncol Nurs Forum, 11(5):16-23, 1984.
92. Moore C, Erikson K, Yanes L, et al: Nursing care and management of venous access ports. Oncol Nurs Forum 13(3):35-39, 1986.
93. Simon R: Small gauge central venous catheters and right arterial catheters. Semin Oncol Nursing 3(2):87-95, 1987.
94. Camp L: Care of the groshong catheter. Oncol Nurs Forum 15:745-748, 1988.
95. Winters V: Implantable vascular access devices. Oncol Nurs Forum 11(6):25-30, 1984.
96. Lokich J, Bothe A, Benotti P, et al: Complications and management of implanted venous access catheters. Clin Oncol 3:710-717, 1985.
97. Howser D, Meade C: Hickman catheter care developing organized teaching strategies. Cancer Nurs 10(2):70-76, 1987.
98. Petrosino B, Becker H, Christian B: Infection rates in central venous catheter dressings. Oncol Nurs Forum 15:709-717, 1988.
99. Fraschini G, Jadya J, Lawson M, et al: Local infusion of urokinase for the lysis of thrombosis associated with permanent central venous catheters in cancer patients. J Clin Oncol 5:672-678, 1987.
100. Noyen J, Hoorntje J, deLangen Z, et al: Spontaneous fracture of a catheter of a totally implantable venous access port: A case report of a rare complication. J Clin Oncol 5:1295-1299, 1987.
101. Almadrones L, Goldbold J, Raaf J, et al: Accuracy of activated partial thromboplastin time drawn through central venous catheters. Oncol Nurs Forum 14(2):15-18, 1987.
102. Wainstock JM: Making a choice: The vein access method you prefer (a patient education booklet). Oncol Nurs Forum 14(1):79-82, 1987.
103. Goodman M: External venous catheters: Home management. Oncol Nurs Forum 15:357-360, 1989.
104. Welch-McCaffery D: Rationale, development, and evaluation of a chemotherapy certification course for nurses. Cancer Nur 8:255-262, 1985.
105. Fernsler J: Developing continuing education programs in cancer nursing: An overview. Oncol Nurs Forum 14:59-60, 1987.
106. Volker DL: Developing continuing education programs in cancer nursing: Learning needs assessment. Oncol Nurs Forum 14:60-62, 1987.
107. Itano J: Developing continuing education programs in cancer nursing: Developing educational objectives. Oncol Nurs Forum 14:62-65, 1987.
108. Belcher AE: Developing continuing education programs in cancer nursing: Defining content and methods. Oncol Nurs Forum 14:65-67, 1987.
109. McMillan SC: Developing continuing education programs in cancer nursing: Program evaluation. Oncol Nurs Forum 14:67-70, 1987.
110. Hubbard SM, Seipp CA: Administration of cancer treatments: Practical guide for physicians and oncology nurses, in DeVita VT, Hellman S, Rosenberg SA (eds): Cancer: Principles and Practice of Oncology. Philadelphia, Lippincott, 1985, pp 2189-2222.
111. Plumer AL: Principles and Practice of Intravenous Therapy (ed 3). Boston, Little, Brown & Co, 1982.
112. Krohner K: Patient education tool serves as consent. Oncol Nurs Forum 14:91-92, 1987.
113. Schulmeister L: Litigation involving oncology nurses. Oncol Nurs Forum 14:25-28, 1987.
114. Fiesta J: The Law and Liability: A Guide for Nurses. New York, Wiley, 1983.
115. Falck K, Grohn P, Sorsa M, et al: Mutagenicity in urine of nurses handling cytostatic agents. Lancet 1:1250-1251, 1979.
116. Waksvik H, Klepp H, Brogger A: Chromosome analysis of nurses handling cytostatic agents. Cancer Treat Rep 65:607-610, 1981.
117. Cloak MM, Conner TH, Stevens KR, et al: Occupational

exposure of nursing personnel to antineoplastic agents. Oncol Nurs Forum 12(5):33-39, 1985.
118. Knowles RS, Virden JE: Handling of injectable antineoplastic agents. Br Med J 281:589-591, 1980.
119. Thomson K, Mikkelsen HI: Protective capacity of gloves used for handling of nitrogen mustard. Contact Dermatitis 1:268-269, 1975.
120. Nguyen TV, Theiss JC, Matney TS: Exposure of pharmacy personnel to mutagenic antineoplastic drugs. Cancer Res 42:4792-4796, 1982.
121. Caudell KA, Vredevoe DL, Dietrich MF, et al: Quantification of urinary mutagens in nurses during potential antineoplastic agent exposure. Cancer Nurs 11:41-50, 1988.
122. National Study Commission on Cytotoxic Exposure: Recommendations for Handling Cytotoxic Agents, Providence, Rhode Island Hospital, 1984.
123. US Department of Labor, Office of Occupational Medicine, Occupational Safety and Health Administration: Work Practice Guidelines for Personnel Dealing With Cytotoxic (Antineoplastic) Drugs, publ no. 8-1.1, 1986.
124. Barry LK, Booher RB: Promoting the responsible handling of antineoplastic agents in the community. Oncol Nurs Forum 12(5):41-46, 1985.
125. Zimmerman PF, Larsen RK, Barkley EW, et al: Recommendations for safe handling of injectable antineoplastic drug products. Am J Hosp Pharm 38:1695-1697, 1981.
126. Miller SA: Issues in cytotoxic drug handling safety. Semin Oncol Nurs 3:133-141, 1987.
127. Gullo SM: Safe handling of antineoplastic drugs: Transplanting the recommendations into practice. Oncol Nurs Forum 15:595-601, 1988.
128. Vlanis B, Shortridge L: Self-protective practices of nurses handling antineoplastic drugs. Oncol Nurs Forum 14:23-27, 1987.
129. Barhamand BA: Difficulties encountered in implementing guidelines for handling antineoplastics in the physician's office. Cancer Nursing 9:138-143, 1986.
130. Stevens KR: Safe handling of cytotoxic drugs in home chemotherapy. Semin Oncol Nurs 5:15-20, 1989.
131. Maxwell MB: When the cancer patient becomes anemic. Cancer Nurs 7:321-326, 1984.
132. Gabrilove JL, Jacubowski A, Sher H, et al: Effect of granulocyte colony stimulating factor on neutropenia and associated morbidity due to chemotherapy for transitional cell carcinoma of the urothelium. N Engl J Med 318:1414-1422, 1988.
133. Mortsyn G, Campbell L, Souza LM, et al: Effect of granulocyte colony stimulating factor on neutropenia induced by cytotoxic chemotherapy. Lancet 1:667-671, 1988.
134. Deisseroth A, Wallerstein R: Use of blood and blood products, in DeVita VT: Cancer: Principles and Practice of Oncology (ed 3). Philadelphia, Lippincott, 1989, pp 2043-2059.
135. Brandt B: A nursing protocol for the client with neutropenia. Oncol Nurs Forum 11:24-28, 1984.
136. Henschel L: Fever patterns in the neutropenia patient. Cancer Nurs 8:301-305, 1985.
137. Nail LM, King KB: Fatigue. Semin Nurs Oncol 3:257-262, 1987.
138. Aistairs J: Fatigue in the cancer patient: A conceptual approach to a clinical problem. Oncol Nurs Forum 14(6):25-30, 1987.
139. Piper BF, Lindsey AM, Dodd MJ: Fatigue mechanisms in cancer patients: Developing nursing theory. Oncol Nurs 14:17-22, 1987.
140. Office of Cancer Communication: Chemotherapy and You. Bethesda, Md, National Cancer Institute, 1986.
141. Myers J, Davidson J, Hutt P, et al: Standardized teaching plans for the management of chemotherapy and radiation therapy side effects. Oncol Nurs Forum 14(5):95-99, 1987.
142. Medvec BR: Nursing protocols in outpatient chemotherapy. Outpatient Chemother 1(4):7, 1987.
143. Chernecky C, Ramsey P: Critical Nursing Care of the Client With Cancer. Norwalk: Appleton-Century Crofts, 1984, pp 61-66.
144. Kelly JO: Neutropenia and thrombocytopenia, in Brown MH, Kiss ME, Outlaw EM, et al: Standards of Oncology Nursing Practice. New York, Wiley, 1986, pp 78-86.
145. Sanford AC: Injury, potential for, related to thrombocytopenia, in McNally JC, Stair JC, Sommerville ET: Guidelines for Cancer Nursing Practice. New York, Grune & Stratton, 1985, pp 147-151.
146. Chernecky CC, Ramsey PW: Critical Nursing Care of the Client With Cancer. Norwalk, Appleton-Century-Crofts, 1984, pp 147-157.
147. Craig JB, Powell BL: Review: The management of nausea and vomiting in clinical oncology. Am J Med Sci 293:34-44, 1987.
148. Rhodes VA, Watson PM, Johnson MH: Patterns of nausea and vomiting in chemotherapy patterns: A preliminary study. Oncol Nurs Forum 12(2):42-48, 1985.
149. Laszlo J: Antiemetics and Cancer Chemotherapy. Baltimore, Williams & Wilkins, 1983.
150. Ingle R, Burish T, Wallston K: Conditionability of cancer chemotherapy agents. Oncol Nurs Forum 11(4):97-102, 1984.
151. Borison HL, McCarthy LE: Neuropharmacology of chemotherapy induced emesis. Drugs 25:(Suppl 1) 8-17, 1983.
152. Scogna DM, Smalley RV: Chemotherapy-induced nausea and vomiting. Am J Nurs 79:1562-1564, 1979.
153. Pratt A, Lazar RM, Penman D, et al: Psychological parameters of chemotherapy-induced conditioned nausea and vomiting: A review. Cancer Nurs 7:483-490, 1984.
154. Morrow GR: Clinical characteristics associated with the development of anticipatory nausea and vomiting in cancer patient undergoing chemotherapy treatment. J Clin Oncol 2:1170-1176, 1984.
155. Rhodes V, Watson P, Johnson M: Association of chemotherapy related nausea and vomiting with pretreatment and post treatment anxiety. Oncol Nurs Forum 13(1):41-47, 1986.
156. Coons H, Leventhal H, Nerenz D, et al: Anticipatory nausea and emotional distress in patients receiving cisplatin-based chemotherapy. Oncol Nurs Forum 14(3):31-35, 1987.
157. Headly J: The influence of administration time on chemotherapy-induced nausea and vomiting. Oncol Nurs Forum 14(6):43-47, 1987.
158. Nerenz DR, Leventhal H, Easterling D, et al: Anxiety and drug taste as predictors of anticipatory nausea in cancer chemotherapy. J Clin Oncol 4:224-233, 1986.
159. Gagen M, Gonchour D, Young D, et al: A randomized trial of metoclopramide and a combination of dexamethasone and lorazepam for prevention of chemotherapy induced nausea and vomiting. J Clin Oncol 2:696-701, 1984.
160. Kris MG, Tyson LB, Gralla RJ, et al: Extrapyramidal reactions with high dose metoclopramide. N Engl J Med 309:433-437, 1983.
161. Kris MG, Gralla RJ, Clark RA, et al: Dose ranging evaluation of the serotonin antagonist GRC 507-75 (GR 38032F) when used as an antiemetic in patients receiving cancer chemotherapy. J Clin Oncol 6:659-662, 1988.
162. Hesketh PJ, Murphy WK, Lester EP, et al: GR 38032C (GC507/75): A novel compound effective in the prevention of acute cis-platinum-induced emesis. J Clin Oncol 7:700-705, 1989.

163. Rhodes VA, Watson PM, Johnson MH, et al: Patterns of nausea vomiting and distress in patients receiving antineoplastic drug protocols. Oncol Nurs Forum 14(4):35-44, 1987.
164. Goodman M: Cisplatin: Outpatient and office hydration regimens. Semin Oncol Nurs 3(Suppl-February):36-45, 1987.
165. Kris MG, Gralla RJ, Clark RA, et al: Incidence course and severity of delayed nausea and vomiting following the administration of high dose cisplatin. J Clin Oncol 3:1379-1384, 1985.
166. Burish TS, Lyles JN: Effectiveness of relaxation training in reducing adverse reactions to chemotherapy. J Behav Med 4:65-78, 1981.
167. Cotanch P, Strum S: Progressive muscle relaxation as antiemetic therapy for cancer patients. Oncol Nurs Forum 14(1):33-37, 1987.
168. Redd W, Anderson G, Minagawa R: Hypnotic control of anticipatory emesis in patients receiving chemotherapy. J Counseling Clin Psychol 50(3):14-19, 1982.
169. Grant MM: Environmental influences on the occurrence of chemotherapy-associated nausea and vomiting. Oncol Nurs Forum 9(1):50-51, 1982.
170. Johnson JE, Fuller S, Endress MP, et al: Altering patients' responses to surgery: An extension and replication. Res Nurs Health 1:111-121, 1978.
171. McHugh NC, Christman NJ, Johnson JE: Preparatory information: What helps and why. Am J Nurs 82:780-782, 1982.
172. Sonis ST: Epidemiology, frequency, distribution, mechanisms, and histopathology, in Paterson D, Sonis S (eds): Oral Complications of Cancer Chemotherapy. New York, Nijhoff, 1983, pp, 1-20.
173. Beck S: Impact of a systematic oral care protocol on stomatitis after chemotherapy. Cancer Nurs 2:185-199, 1979.
174. Daeffler R: Oral hygiene measures for patients with cancer. II. Cancer Nurs 3:27-432, 1980.
175. Daeffler R: Oral hygiene measures for patients with cancer. III. Cancer Nurs 4:29-35, 1981.
176. Eliers J, Berger A, Peterson M: Development, testing, and application of the oral assessment guide. Oncol Nurs Forum 15:325-330, 1988.
177. Greenberg MS, Friedman H, Cohen S, et al: A comparison study of herpes infections in renal transplant and leukemic patients. J Infect Dis 156:280-286, 1987.
178. Driezen S, McCredie KB, Kealing MJ, et al: Chemotherapy associated oral infections in adults with acute leukemia. Postgrad Med 7:133-146, 1982.
179. Carter SK: Nutritional problems associated with cancer chemotherapy, in Newell GR, Ellison NM (eds): Nutrition and Cancer: Etiology and Treatment. New York, Raven Press, 1981.
180. Costa G, Donaldson S: The nutritional effects of cancer and its therapy. Nutr Cancer 2:22-29, 1980.
181. Donaldson SS, Lenon RA: Alterations of nutritional status: Impact of chemotherapy and radiation therapy. Cancer 43:2036-2052, 1979.
182. Ohnuma T, Holland JF: Nutritional consequences of cancer chemotherapy and immunotherapy. Cancer Res 37:2395-2406, 1977.
183. Kokal WA: The impact of antitumor therapy on nutrition. Cancer 55:273-278, 1985.
184. Bernstein IL, Bernstein ID: Learned food aversions and cancer anorexia. Cancer Treat Rep 65(suppl 5):43-47, 1981.
185. Black ML, Gallucci BB, Katakkar SB: The nutritional assessment of patients receiving cancer chemotherapy. Oncol Nurs Forum 10:53-58, 1983.
186. de Graaf SSN, Meeuwsen-Van Der Roest, WP, Koops HS, et al: Dissociation of body weight and lean body mass during cancer chemotherapy. Eur J Cancer Clin Oncol 23:731-737, 1987.
187. Lane CG: Nursing management—cancer chemotherapy. J Nurs Care 13:7-11, 1980.
188. Crounse RG, VanScott EJ: Changes in scalp hair roots as a measure of toxicity from cancer chemotherapeutic drugs. J Invest Dermatol 35:83-90, 1960.
189. Gauci L: Letter: Changes in hair pigmentation associated with cancer chemotherapy. Cancer Treat Rep 64:193, 1980.
190. Welch D, Lewis K: Alopecia and chemotherapy. Am J Nurs 80:903-905, 1980.
191. Baxley KO, Erdman LK, Henry EB, et al: Alopecia: Effect on cancer patients' body image. Cancer Nurs 7:499-503, 1984.
192. Cline BW: Prevention of chemotherapy-induced alopecia: A review of the literature. Cancer Nurs 7:221-228, 1984.
193. Lindsay AM: Building a knowledge base for practice. Part II. Alopecia, breast self-exam and other human responses. Oncol Nurs Forum 12:27-34, 1985.
194. Maxwell MB: Scalp tourniquets for chemotherapy-induced alopecia. Am J Nurs 80:900-903, 1980.
195. Dean JC, Salomon SE, Griffith HA: Prevention of doxorubicin-induced hair loss with scalp hypothermia. N Engl J Med 301:1427-1429, 1979.
196. Parker R: The effectiveness of scalp hypothermia in preventing cyclophosphamide induced alopecia. Oncol Nurs Forum 14(6):49-53, 1987.
197. Keller J, Blausey L: Nursing issues and management in chemotherapy induced alopecia. Oncol Nurs Forum 15:603-607, 1988.
198. Chapman R: Effect of cytotoxic therapy on sexuality and gonadal function. Sem Oncol 9:84-94, 1982.
199. Redman J, Bajournas D, Goldstein M, et al: Semen cryopreservation and artificial insemination in Hodgkin's disease. J Clin Oncol 5:233-238, 1987.
200. Thachil JV, Jewett MS, Reider WD: The effects of cancer and cancer therapy on male fertility. J Urol 126:14-144, 1981.
201. Cohen J, Edwards J, Fehilly C, et al: *In vitro* fertilization: A treatment for male infertility. Steril 43:422-432, 1985.
202. Chapman RM, Sutcliff SB: Protection of ovarian function by oral contraceptives in women receiving chemotherapy for Hodgkin's disease. Blood 58:849-851, 1981.
203. Mulvihill JJ, McKeen EA: Pregnancy outcome in cancer patients: Experience in a large cooperative trial. Cancer 60:1143-1150, 1987.
204. Kaempfer S, Wiley F, Hoffman D: Fertility considerations and procreative alternatives in cancer care. Semin Oncol Nurs 1(1):25-34, 1985.
205. Tarpy CC: Birth control considerations during chemotherapy. Oncol Nurs Forum 12(2):75-78, 1985.
206. Lamb MA, Woods NF: Sexuality and the cancer patient. Cancer Nurs 4:137-144, 1981.
207. Ignoffo RJ, Friedman MA: Therapy of local toxicities caused by extravasation of cancer chemotherapeutic drugs. Cancer Treat Rev 7:17-27, 1980.
208. Wood HA, Ellerhorst-Ryan JM: Delayed adverse skin reactions associated with mitomycin-C administered. Oncol Nurs Forum 11:14-18, 1984.

209. Dorr RT: Discussion: What is the appropriate management of tissue extravasation by antitumor agents? Plast Reconstr Surg 75:403-405, 1985.
210. Larsen DL: What is the appropriate management of tissue extravasation by antitumor agents? Plast Reconstr Surg 75:397-402, 1985.
211. Harwood KV, Bachur NR: Evaluation of dimethyl sulfoxide and local cooling as antidotes for doxorubicin extravasation in a pig model. Oncol Nurs Forum 14:39-44, 1987.
212. Oncology Nursing Society: Cancer chemotherapy guidelines, module A revised. Oncol Nurs Forum 16:275, 1989.
213. Kreamer KM: Anaphylaxis resulting from chemotherapy. Oncol Nurs Forum, 8:13-16, 1981.
214. Weiss RB, Bruno S: Hypersensitivity reactions to cancer chemotherapeutic agents. Ann Intern Med 94:66-72, 1981.
215. Schulmeister L: Developing guidelines for bleomycin test dosing. Oncol Nurs Forum 16:205-207, 1989.
216. Von Hoff D, Rozencweig M, Piccart M: The cardiotoxicity of anticancer agents. Semin Oncol 9(1):23-33, 1982.
217. Kaszyk L: Cardiac toxicity associated with cancer therapy. Oncol Nurs Forum 13(4):81-86, 1986.
218. Druck M, Gulenchyn K, Evans W, et al: Radionuclide angiography and endomyocardial biopsy in the assessment of doxorubicin toxicity. Cancer 53:1667-1674, 1984.
219. Torti F, Bristow M, Howes A, et al: Reduced cardiotoxicity of doxorubicin delivered on a weekly schedule. Ann Intern Med 99:745-749, 1983.
220. Perry M: Hepatoxicity of chemotherapeutic agents. Semin Oncol 9(1):65-74, 1982.
221. Goodman M: Managing the side effects of chemotherapy. Semin Oncol Nurs 5(Suppl 1):29-52, 1989.
222. Herzig R, Hines J, Herzig G, et al: Cerebellar toxicity with high dose cytosine arabinoside. J Clin Oncol 5:927-932, 1985.
223. Dworkin L, Goldman L, Fuchs PC: Cerebellar toxicity with high dose cytosine arabinoside. J Clin Oncol 3:613-616, 1985.
224. Powell B, Capizzi R, Lyerly S, et al: Peripheral neuropathy after high dose cytosine arabinoside, daunorubicin and asparaginase consolidation for acute nonlymphocytic leukemia. J Clin Oncol 4:95-97, 1969.
225. Conrad KJ: Cerebellar toxicities associated with cytosine arabinoside: A nursing perspective. Oncol Nurs Forum 13(5):57-59, 1986.
226. Legha S, Dimery I: High-dose cisplatin administration without hypertonic saline: Observation of disabling neurotoxicity. J Clin Oncol 3:1373-1378, 1985.
227. Holden S, Felde G: Nursing care of patients experiencing cisplatin-related peripheral neuropathy. Oncol Nurs Forum 14:13-19, 1987.
228. Weiss RB, Trush DM: A review of pulmonary toxicity of cancer chemotherapeutic agents. Oncol Nurs Forum 9(1):16-21, 1982.
229. Wickham R: Pulmonary toxicity secondary to cancer treatment. Oncol Nurs Forum 13(5):69-76, 1986.
230. Lydon J: Nephrotoxicity of cancer treatment. Oncol Nurs Forum 13(2):68-77, 1986.
231. D'Angio GJ: Complications of treatment encountered in lymphoma-leukemia long term survivors. Cancer 42:1015-1025, 1978.
232. Fraser MC, Tucker MA: Late effect of cancer therapy: Chemotherapy-related malignancies. Oncol Nurs Forum 15:67-77, 1988.

APPENDIX A Chemotherapeutic Drugs

Name	Classification	Adult Dosage	Major Side Effects	Nursing Implications
Amascarine (M-AMSA)	Miscellaneous	30-120 mg/m² IV in 1 hour infusion for 21-28 days; frequency of dosing is dependent on marrow recovery	Leukopenia, thrombocytopenia, and stomatitis are dose-limiting toxicities; thrombocytopenia may be severe in patients who have been irradiated previously to bone-marrow–producing sites. Nausea and vomiting are dose dependent; elevated liver function tests have been reported; ventricular fibrillation has been reported in the presence of decreased serum potassium; vesicant properties; pruritus and rash have been reported; neurologic toxicities in the form of peripheral neuropathy, headache, and seizures; discoloration of skin and urine	Assess serum potassium level before drug administration; assess liver function status. Patients with poor liver function may not be considered to be appropriate candidates for this agent; provide appropriate antiemetic support; monitor cardiac status; do not dilute in saline solution as precipitates may occur; assess for neurologic toxicity
Aminoglutethimide (Cytadren)	Miscellaneous: hormone suppressant	500-1500 mg/day/PO with 2000 mg/day the upper dose limit	Rash, which disappears in 5-8 days; lethargy, ataxia, dizziness and nystagmus; decreased aldosterone and cortisol secretion; elevated thyroid-stimulating hormone levels	Teach the individual and family to observe and report symptoms of somnolence; teach the person the importance of cortisone replacement if needed
L-Asparaginase (Elspar)	Miscellaneous: enzyme	Variable, many schedules; 10,000 IU/m² IM weekly for two to three doses possible	Acute liver dysfuntion; nausea and vomiting are common and may be severe; mild anorexia; hypersensitivity reactions in 20%-35% of individuals; usually mild with urticarial eruptions but can be life threatening; transient fever; depression, lethargy, and drowsiness in 30%-60% of individuals	Assess hepatic enzyme levels, liver impairment, and alcohol ingestion; observe for possible anaphylaxis for at least 20 minutes after administering the drug. Have the physician and appropriate medications and resuscitation equipment available; observe the person's level of consciousness and neurologic signs, especially the first day after treatment; solution is unstable, discard after use; test dosing recommended according to individual institution protocol.
5-Azacytidine (5-AZA-C)	Antimetabolite	150-300 mg/m² IV daily × 3-5 days	Bone marrow depression, especially leukopenia, with a nadir of about 25 days; leukopenia is occasionally prolonged; nausea and vomiting are common and occur about 1½-3 hours after IV injection; diarrhea occurs in about 50% of individuals; neurologic toxicity including lethargy and coma has been reported	Premedicate the person with antiemetics; two daily divided doses can lessen gastrointestinal toxicities; very unstable after reconstitution; use within 3 hours; Ringer's lactate provides optimal stability and pH; observe the person's level of consciousness and neurologic signs
Bleomycin (Blenoxane)	Antibiotic	10-20 U/m² IM, IV, or SC one to two times per week; continuous infusions of 15 mg/m² over 24 hours for 4 days; maximum cumulative lifetime dose is 400 U	Pulmonary toxicity is the most serious side effect; dose, age and lung disease increase the risk; most common in individuals over 70 years of age; also synergistic with chest irradiation; hypersensitivity reactions include fever, chills, and occasionally anaphylaxis; skin reactions are common, including pruritic erythema, rash, striae, hyperpigmentation, edema, and vesiculation; reversible alopecia with regrowth occurring several months later; related to dose and occurs 3 weeks after therapy is initiated; mucositis, stomatitis, and mild nausea and vomiting; combination with radiation can be devastating	Assess for pulmonary problems; a record of cumulative dose should be kept; anaphylaxis precautions should be taken; teach the person regarding possible alopecia and fever; premedicate with Tylenol; special mouth care as needed; test dose prior to first dose is recommended as per individual institutional protocol; continuous infusion requires glass bottles

Busulfan (Myleran)	Alkylating agent	2-10 mg PO daily to WBC of 10,000/mm^3, then no treatment or reduced doses	Bone marrow depression, particularly leukopenia, with recovery occurring over 24-54 days; menstrual dysfunction, usually amenorrhea; interstitial pulmonary fibrosis as a result of long-term therapy in 2%-10% of individuals; reversible with prompt discontinuation of drug; hyperpigmentation of skin; gynecomastia; nausea, vomiting, and diarrhea	Teach the person about possible changes in sexual characteristics and functioning; observe for pulmonary symptoms and teach the person accordingly; assess for prolonged bone marrow depression; monitor BUN, creatinine, and uric acid; administer allopurinol to relieve hyperurecemia
Carmustine (BCNU)	Alkylating agent	75-200 mg/m^2 IV q 6-8 weeks	Delayed leukopenia 4-5 weeks after administration, with a nadir lasting 1-2 weeks; thrombocytopenia is usually more severe than leukopenia, with a nadir 4-5 weeks after administration and lasting 1-2 weeks; may be prolonged; nausea and vomiting are common, occurring 2-6 hours after administration and lasting 4-24 hours, dose related; painful venous irritation during administration and marked flushing of face; irreversible, dose-related pulmonary fibrosis (20%-30% of individuals) may occur, especially at doses greater than 1200-1400 mg/m^2, often fatal	Cumulative hematopoietic toxicity; infection and bleeding precautions may be necessary; premedicate with antiemetics; drowsiness may occur with doses greater than 100 mg, so the person should not drive immediately after treatment; give via slow IV, and if pain occurs, give the drug more slowly or dilute it more; pain is due to the alcohol diluent; maintain a careful record of the cumulative dose and assess the person for symptoms of pulmonary toxicity
Carboplatin (Paraplatin)	Miscellaneous: Cisplatin analog	240-500 mg/m^2 IV q 4 weeks depending on disease, renal function, and marrow reserves	Bone marrow suppression especially thrombocytopenia is dose limiting; WBC nadir occurs about day 21; recovers in 4-6 weeks; incidence of anemia increases with increased exposure to Paraplatin; patients with creatinine clearance less than 60 mL/min are at increased risk for severe bone marrow suppression; nausea and vomiting, while not as severe as with cisplatin, occurs in about 65% of patients and is severe in about 25% of these patients; patients treated with cisplatin previously are more likely to have severe nausea and vomiting; delayed nausea and vomiting has not been reported with Paraplatin; mild paresthesias have been reported; renal toxicity is uncommon; electrolyte changes occur in about 30% of patients	Monitor blood counts; prepare using nonaluminum needle; mix in sterile water or saline solution; Paraplatin does not require vigorous hydration
Chlorambucil (Leukeran)	Alkylating agent	0.1-0.2 mg/kg PO daily for 3-6 weeks	Bone marrow depression with prolonged use; medium to low risk of pulmonary toxicity; second malignancies have been reported with prolonged use	Well-tolerated drug; administer on empty stomach to reduce nausea
Cisplatin (Platinol)	Miscellaneous alkylating properties	Single doses up to 120 mg/m^2 IV q 3-4 weeks or 10-20 mg/m^2 IV daily for 5 days	Nausea and vomiting are often severe, starting about 1 hour after treatment and lasting 24 hours; anorexia may be cumulative; nephrotoxicity is dose related and cumulative with doses greater than 50 mg/m^2 or 0.25 mg/kg for 5 days; intravenous hydration and/or mannitol diuresis are required; ototoxicity with tinnitus and/or hearing loss, which is dose limiting; moderate leukopenia and thrombocytopenia, with a nadir on day 23 and recovery by day 39; hypersensitivity reactions may occur; neurotoxicity may be dose-limiting; electrolyte disturbances	Keep weight record; monitor renal function closely; hydration and diuresis procedures must be followed according to institutional policy; record the cumulative dose; take anaphylactic precautions, aggressive antiemetic regimen must be followed; dilute the drug in chloride-containing solutions only

APPENDIX A Chemotherapeutic Drugs (continued)

Name	Classification	Adult Dosage	Major Side Effects	Nursing Implications
Cyclophosphamide (CTX, Cytoxan, Endoxan)	Alkylating agent	500-1800 mg/m² IV q 3-4 weeks, 60-120 mg/m² PO daily; bone marrow dose 50 mg/kg/day × 4 days	Leukopenia, with a nadir of 8-14 days and recovery in 18-25 days; acute hemorrhagic cystitis in poorly hydrated individuals at doses of 1-2 g/m²; nausea and vomiting with an onset 4-6 hours after treatment and lasting 8-10 hours; alopecia in about 50% of individuals occurring about 3 weeks after therapy is initiated; medium to low risk of pulmonary toxicity; high risk of amenorrhea and impaired fertility; second malignancies have been reported; hyperpigmentation of skin and nails; cardiac toxicity with high doses	Encourage high fluid intake and frequent urination; monitor output to avoid cystitis; premedication with antiemetics is helpful in minimizing nausea and vomiting; oral doses on an empty stomach and not at bedtime also help decrease nausea and vomiting; teach the person regarding reversible alopecia; hot flashes, lightheadedness, foul taste, and nasal stuffiness often occur during IV administration; slowing the rate of administration helps, and symptoms disappear when the drug is stopped
Cytarabine (ARA-C, Cytosar, cytosine, arabinoside)	Antimetabolite	100-150 mg/m² IV or SC for 5-10 days; 20-30 mg/m² intrathecally; high dose is 3 g/m² q 12 hours for 6 days	Bone marrow depression, including leukopenia and thrombocytopenia, with a nadir in 5-7 days; dose-related nausea and vomiting; medium to low risk of pulmonary toxicity; mild oral ulceration; lethargy, cerebellar toxicity, typhlitis, and keratoconjunctivitis with high doses; acral erythema in higher doses	Premedication with antiemetics is helpful; use preservative-free diluent for intrathecal administration; use Decadron eye drops for conjunctivitis; monitor for typhlitis (inflamation of the cecum) including diarrhea, constipation, and symptoms of bowel obstruction; monitor neurologic toxicity including tremors, loss of balance, nystagmus, and confusion
Dacarbazine (DTIC, DIC)	Alkylating agent	150-250 mg/m² IV daily for 5 days; 650-1450 mg/m² IV q 4-6 weeks	Moderate myelosuppression, including leukopenia and thrombocytopenia, with a nadir at 21-25 days; severe nausea and vomiting are common (90%), ocurring 1-3 hours after injection and lasting up to 12 hours; flulike symptoms with high doses; photosensitivity; local tissue irritant	Inject the drug slowly to prevent local pain at the injection site; avoid extravasation, which may result in tissue damage and severe pain; severe nausea and vomiting may diminish after several treatments, however, aggressive antiemetic management is necessary; restriction of food and fluid prior to therapy may diminish nausea and vomiting
Dactinomycin (Cosmegen, actinomycin D)	Antibiotic	500 μg IV × 5 days q 3-4 weeks; also used for regional perfusion; children: 15 μg/kg/day × 5 days, maximum dose 500 μg	Bone marrow depression occurs in 7-10 days, with a nadir at 3 weeks; leukocytes and platelets are affected primarily; no cumulative toxicity; nausea and vomiting common and can be severe; occurs immediately or a few hours after treatment; lasts 4-20 hours but can be prolonged to 2-3 days; mucositis with ulcerations of the alimentary tract may occur; reversible alopecia may occur; if the person received previous radiotherapy, "recall" skin reactions can occur as acneiform changes, erythema and hyperpigmentation; can be severe; extravasation causes local pain, swelling, and necrosis	Assess blood counts prior to treatment; premedicate with antiemetics; provide aggressive antiemetic support; weigh the person frequently; observe for mucositis, stomatitis, pharyngitis, and dysphagia; assess skin carefully if the person is or was receiving radiotherapy; avoid extravasation

Daunorubicin hydrochloride (daunomycin, Cerubidine)	Antibiotic	30-60 mg/m^2 V × 1-3 days; maximum total lifetime dose of 500-600 mg/m^2	Leukopenia with a nadir in 8-10 days and recovery in 2-3 weeks; thrombocytopenia is less significant, with a nadir at 4-15 days and recovery in 2-3 weeks; nausea and vomiting are moderate to severe; extravasation causes severe pain, necrosis, and fibrosis; cumulative dose is related to acute cardiotoxicity, which is reversible; cardiotoxicity may be aggravated by concurrent radiation therapy or cyclophosphamide; complete alopecia in 3-4 weeks; skin reactions in areas of previous irradiation	Avoid extravasation; the person should be cautioned that urine will be red-colored several days after treatment; maintain an accurate cumulative dose record; prepare the person for reversible hair loss; monitor hepatic status—if bilirubin >1.2, dose reduction is recommended; avoid mixing with $NaHCO_3$ solutions and heparin
Deoxycoformycin (Penostatin)	Miscellaneous antibiotic	2-4 mg/m^2 IV q 2-4 weeks	Profound leukopenia, lymphopenia and thrombocytopenia are dose-limiting toxicities; nausea and vomiting are usually not severe; acute renal failure has been reported at high doses; hepatotoxicity, ocular pain, conjunctivitis, fever, skin rash, lethargy, somnolence and coma have been reported	Monitor blood counts and neurologic status as well as myalgias, skin reactions, and fever patterns
Doxorubicin (Adriamycin PFS, Rubex)	Antibiotic	60-75 mg/m^2 IV q 3-4 weeks; 20 mg/m^2 IV weekly 2-9 mg/m^2 in prolonged infusion; cumulative total lifetime dose of 550 mg/m^2 or 450 mg/m^2 with previous or concurrent heart irradiation	Leukopenia, with a nadir occurring in 10-14 days and recovery by day 19; severe tissue necrosis with extravasation; severe nausea and vomiting in about 50% of individuals may have delayed onset up to 12 hours after therapy; dose-related cardiotoxicity of classic congestive heart failure with electrocardiographic changes; risk of cardiac toxicity may be decreased by prolonged infusions and/or weekly dosing; stomatitis at high doses; "recall" skin reactions at previous sites of irradiation; photosensitivity, skin and nail bed changes; alopecia of all body hair is common in 3-4 weeks but is dose dependent	Avoid extravasation; red discoloration of urine for about 24 hours after therapy; keep an accurate cumulative dose record; assess for previous irradiation, hypertension, and heart disease; obtain baseline electrocardiogram prior to treatments; observe for stomatitis; person is often lethargic and fatigued for 1-2 weeks after therapy; prepare the person for reversible hair loss over the entire body, depending on dose; avoid mixing 5-FU and doxorubicin in same IV line—flush between drugs
Epirubicin hydrochloride (Pharmorubicin)	Antibiotic	60-100 mg/m^2 IV q 3 weeks	Leukopenia is dose-limiting toxicity; nausea and vomiting; mucositis; diarrhea (rare) and acute cardiac arrhythmias have been reported; considered less cardiotoxic than doxorubicin; radiation recall, urticaria, vein streaking, and phlebitis occur; toxicities potentiated by liver dysfunction	Avoid extravasation; administer antiemetics; monitor blood counts and liver function
Etoposide (VePesid, VP16)	Plant alkaloid	50-100 mg/m^2 IV × 5 days; 100-200 mg/m^2 in oral dose days 1-5, q 3-4 weeks; 200 mg/m^2 IV q 3 weeks	Leukopenia is prominent, with a nadir in 12-16 days and recovery by days 20-22; thrombocytopenia also occurs, with a similar nadir; nausea, vomiting, and anorexia in about 33% of individuals, occurring 2-6 hours after therapy; alopecia in 20%-90% of individuals; regrowth occurs after the drug is discontinued; hypotension and bronchospasm occur if the drug is infused too rapidly; oral dose is associated with nausea and vomiting	Premedication with antiemetics may be helpful; advise the person of possible hair loss and measures to deal with it; administer over 30-45 minutes; the drug should be infused in normal saline solution; monitor blood pressure during and after treatment; dose reduction recommended in presence of elevated bilirubin; store capsules in refrigerator

APPENDIX A Chemotherapeutic Drugs (continued)

Name	Classification	Adult Dosage	Major Side Effects	Nursing Implications
Floxuridine (5-FUDR)	Antimetabolite	Intra-arterial dosage is 0.1-0.6 mg/kg daily for 1-6 weeks; highest doses are given by intrahepatic administration of 0.5-1.0 mg/kg/day IV for 6-15 days by continuous infusion	Gastrointestinal toxicities are common, including nausea, vomiting, anorexia, abdominal cramps, and some pain; intra-arterial administration results in fewer side effects but is associated with chemical hepatitis; regional enteritis, duodenitis, and gastritis are common	If administered intra-arterially, symptoms of catheter malfunction, bleeding, and infection must be assessed; monitor liver enzymes; discontinue drug if signs of gastritis or enteritis are evident
5-Fluorouracil (5-FU, Adrucil)	Antimetabolite	12-15 mg/kg IV; larger doses are given for loading, decreased for maintenance; solution or cream is applied topically for basal cell carcinoma; IV infusions weekly with leukovorin	Mild nausea and vomiting in 30%-50% of individuals shortly after administration; granulocytopenia common, with a nadir in 9-14 days; thrombocytopenia is less common, with a nadir in 7-14 days; stomatitis is a sign of impending severe toxicity; diarrhea occurs frequently in a 5-day daily schedule; mild and reversible alopecia occurs in 5%-20% of individuals; dermatitis; hyperpigmentation is common; acral erythema occurs with long-term infusion therapy	Premedication with an antiemetic is helpful in decreasing nausea and vomiting; if precipitate forms because of cold temperatures, heat and shake vigorously until clear; cool to room temperature before administering; oral administration is poorly absorbed; assess for stomatitis; assess palms and soles for erythema and tissue sloughing
Flutamide (Eulexin, Anandron)	Hormone: nonsteroidal antiandrogen	250 mg PO 3× daily	Gynecomastia; impotence; mild elevation of SGOT and LDH have been reported; diarrhea	Generally well-tolerated
Hexamethylmelamine (HMM, HXM)	Alkylating agent or antimetabolite	4-12 mg/kg/day PO in four divided doses for 21-90 days	Anorexia, nausea, and vomiting with occasional abdominal cramps and diarrhea occur in 50%-70% of individuals; mild leukopenia and thrombocytopenia, with nadirs in 3-4 weeks; recovery is rapid; neurotoxicities occur occasionally	Administering the drug after meals and at bedtime helps to minimize nausea and vomiting; premedication with antiemetics is also helpful; observe for neurotoxicities
Hydroxyurea (Hydrea)	Miscellaneous: inhibits DNA synthesis	20-30 mg/kg PO daily	Bone marrow depression is dose related; leukopenia occurs in about 10 days; thrombocytopenia and anemia are less common; mild nausea, vomiting, and diarrhea occur in about 25% of individuals; skin rash; temporary impairment of renal tubular function	Large doses may induce drowsiness; elderly individuals may be more sensitive to effects and require a lowered dosage; large 500 mg capsules can be opened and mixed in juice or water
Ifosfamide (Ifex)	Alkylating agent: cyclophosphamide analog	1.0-2.0 g/m^2 IV per day × 3-4 days q 3 weeks	Mild-moderate bone marrow depression; urinary tract toxicity may be dose-limiting; hematuria, sterile hemorrhagic cystitis; dysuria and acute tubular necrosis have been reported; alopecia is common; lethargy, confusion, psychoses occur occasionally but are increased in individuals with poor renal function. Nausea and vomiting moderate to severe and are dose and schedule related; less myelosuppression but greater urinary tract toxicity than seen with cytoxan	Provide aggressive antiemetic support; aggressively monitor urinary tract toxicity, including hematuria, dysuria, frequency, and urinary output; encourage intake of at least 2 L of water per day orally or intravenously, including 1 day before and 2 days after therapy; bladder toxicity prevented by use of Mesna, a detoxifying agent given by IV bolus injection in dose equal to 20% of Ifex dose at time of Ifex administration and q 4 hours for 2 additional doses; monitor neurologic toxicity; prepare patient for possibility of alopecia

Iproplatin (Chip)	Miscellaneous: Cisplatin analog	180-270 mg/m^2 IV q 4 weeks	Thrombocytopenia is dose-limiting toxicity with nadir reported at 10-21 days; nausea and vomiting are mild-moderate in severity and generally well controlled by antiemetics; rare renal or neurologic toxicity; rash frequently occurs but rarely symptomatic; diarrhea may be severe	Monitor platelet count and gastrointestinal toxicity
Lomustine (CCNU, CeeNU)	Alkylating agent: nitrosourea	100-130 mg/m^2 PO as a single dose q 6 weeks	Delayed and potentially cumulative myelosuppression; thrombocytopenia, with a nadir in 26-34 days, lasting 6-10 days; leukopenia with a nadir in 41-46 days, lasting 9-14 days; nausea and vomiting are common, beginning 2-6 hours after treatment and lasting up to 36 hours; mild anorexia; ovarian, sperm suppression; renal toxicity; hepatotoxicity	Administering the drug at bedtime on an empty stomach is helpful in reducing gastrointestinal side effects; premedication with antiemetics may be helpful; monitor BUN, creatinine, SGOT, SGPT, LDH, bilirubin
Leuprolide (Lupron)	Hormone	1 mg/day subcutaneously; may be continued indefinitely; Depot Form: 7.5 mg/month/IM for prostate cancer	Bone pain flare (similar to tamoxifen) hot flashes in about 50% of patients; gynecomastia and genital atrophy in approximately 3%-7% of patients; rare dizziness, headache, and paresthesias have been reported	Teach and monitor self-injection technique; reassure patient and family that bone pain flare is temporary and not disease related; medicate for pain accordingly
Mechlorethamine (nitrogen mustard, Mustargen, HN_2)	Alkylating agent	0.4 mg/kg IV q 3-4 weeks	Leukopenia and thrombocytopenia within 24 hours, with a nadir at 6-8 days to 3 weeks; severe nausea and vomiting, beginning 1-3 hours after treatment and lasting 8 hours; extravasation or skin contact results in necrosis; amenorrhea and impaired spermatogenesis; tinnitus and skin rash; alopecia; vertigo, ototoxicity	Aggressive premedication with antiemetics is necessary; avoid extravasation and skin contact; local phlebitis may occur with subsequent brown discoloration of veins
Megestrol (Megace)	Hormone	Total dose 40-300 mg PO q day; may be continued indefinitely	Mild nausea and vomiting, stomach cramps; amenorrhea, breakthrough bleeding; fluid retention and weight gain that is not related to fluid retention; alopecia, skin rash and headaches have been reported	Generally well tolerated; weight gain (nonfluid related) may be a beneficial side effect in anorexic patients
Melphalan (Alkeran, L-PAM, phenylalanine mustard)	Alkylating agent	2-15 mg per m^2 PO daily for 5 days q 5-6 weeks	Leukopenia and thrombocytopenia occurring 14-21 days after treatment; onset may be delayed to 5-6 weeks; large doses produce nausea and vomiting; medium to low risk of pulmonary toxicity; maculopapular rash; urticaria; ovarian and sperm suppression; risk for second malignancies	Well-tolerated drug; assess renal function
Mercaptopurine (6-MP, Purinethal, 6-mercaptopurine)	Antimetabolite	1-2.5 mg/kg PO daily	Minimal gastrointestinal toxicity; stomatitis is common with large doses; mild leukopenia and thrombocytopenia, with nadirs at days 16 and 15, respectively; occasionally hepatotoxic with long-term use	Observe for stomatitis and liver dysfunction; decrease doses to one third of normal if allopurinol is given concomitantly

APPENDIX A Chemotherapeutic Drugs (continued)

Name	Classification	Adult Dosage	Major Side Effects	Nursing Implications
Methotrexate (MTX, Amethopterin)	Antimetabolite	10-30 mg IM, PO, or IV in various schedules; 15 mg maximum intrathecally biweekly; high-dose MTX: 2-10 g/m^2 q 3-4 weeks in 6-hour infusion or weekly × 4; *must be followed by leukovorin rescue*	Dose-related leukopenia, with a nadir in 7 days, and thrombocytopenia, with a nadir in 5-12 days; dose-related stomatitis, sore throat, and anal pruritus; diarrhea can be severe; mild nausea; chronic hepatotoxicity with long-term daily use; renal failure in high doses (>1 g/m^2); pneumonitis (medium to low risk); neurologic symptoms resulting from intrathecal administration (eg, headache, back pain, paresis, and confusion)	Assess for stomatitis; assess for adequate renal function and alkaline urinary pH; avoid vitamin C during treatment because the drug precipitates in acidic urine; observe for neurologic symptoms; high-dose MTX is lethal without rescue—therefore, leukovorin rescue *must* be given promptly at prescribed times; avoid aspirin and other compounds that displace MTX from plasma proteins; use preservative-free MTX for intrathecal and high doses
Plicamycin (Mithracin)	Antibiotic	0.025 mg/kg IV push q 3-4 days depending on serum calcium	Anorexia, nausea, and vomiting are common; thrombocytopenia, which may result in hemorrhage, usually rapid onset; headache is common; other neurologic symptoms may occur (eg, irritability, lethargy, and agitation); hepatic and renal function impairment; extravasation causes local irritation and cellulitis; blushing of face with progressive thickening of facial folds	Premedication with antiemetics is helpful; assess carefully for bleeding tendencies; assess hepatic enzyme levels, liver impairment, and alcohol ingestion; avoid extravasation
Mitomycin (Mutamycin, mitomycin-C)	Antibiotic	10-20 mg/m^2 IV as a single dose; 2 mg/m^2 IV daily × 5 days; may be given into the bladder intravesical 20-60 mg weekly	Cumulative myelosuppression, including leukopenia, thrombocytopenia, and anemia, recovery is delayed and takes 2-3 weeks, severity increases with successive courses; occasional nausea, vomiting, and anorexia within 1-2 hours after therapy and persisting for several hours; extravasation causes local irritation, cellulitis, and necrosis; stomatitis and diarrhea may occur; alopecia may occur; occasional nephrotoxicity and possible cardiotoxicity; medium to low risk of pulmonary toxicity	Avoid extravasation; record the cumulative dose; a total dose of greater than 50 mg results in increased toxicity; assess renal function; provide aggressive antiemetic therapy; monitor changes in lifestyle secondary to malaise; monitor for dry cough and dyspnea
Mitotane (Lysoden, Ortho-para-DDD, O'p'-DDD)	Miscellaneous	2-10 g/day PO; maximum tolerated dose is 16 g/day	Nausea, vomiting, and anorexia are common; occasional diarrhea; neurotoxicity in 40%-60% of individuals, resulting in lethargy, somnolence, vertigo, or dizziness; causes atrophy of the adrenal cortex; adrenal insufficiency may occur in doses of more than 3 g/day or stress (eg, shock, infection, or trauma)	Assess for severe nausea and vomiting; advise the person of drowsiness and dizziness and to avoid driving, operating machinery, or using alcohol; mineral and glucocorticoid supplementation needed when the dosage exceeds 3 g/day; assess for increased stress and related adrenal insufficiency
Mitoxantrone (Novantrone)	Miscellaneous: antibiotic	4-12 mg/m^2 IV × 3-5 days or 10-14 mg/m^2 q 3 weeks when used in combination	Neutropenia is the dose-limiting toxicity; mild stomatitis and nausea and vomiting have been reported; mild congestive heart failure has been reported in patients previously treated with anthracyclines; increased cardiotoxicity with cumulative doses >180 mg/m^2	Premedicate with antiemetics; monitor cardiac status; monitor blood counts; avoid extravasation; warn patients that their urine will be green; monitor for stomatitis and treat according to institution's protocol

Procarbazine (Matulane)	Miscellaneous: monamine oxidase inhibitor	50-200 mg/day PO × 14 days	Leukopenia, thrombocytopenia, and anemia are common with a nadir beginning at about 4 weeks and recovery complete in 6 weeks; nausea and vomiting are common in early treatment but then subside; high doses result in neurotoxicities, amenorrhea, and azospermia	Alcohol, antidepressants, central nervous system depressants, and tyramine-rich foods (cheese, wine, bananas, etc) should be avoided because they can result in severe toxicities and hypertensive crises; provide antiemetic therapy and monitor blood count; assess for signs and symptoms of infection
Semustine (MeCCNU, Methyl-CCNU) (Investigational)	Alkylating agent	125-200 mg/m^2 PO q 6 weeks	Delayed and cumulative myelosuppression, with a pronounced platelet nadir at about 4 weeks and white and red blood cell nadirs following at about 6 weeks, recovery occurs in 6-10 weeks; nausea and vomiting are common 4-6 hours after treatment and last 6-8 hours; nephrotoxicity and hepatotoxicity occur infrequently; available for protocol studies only because of increased incidence of secondary leukemia	Administering the drug at bedtime with an antiemetic and on an empty stomach is helpful in diminishing nausea and vomiting; record the cumulative dose; assess renal and liver function
Streptozocin (SZN, Zanosar)	Alkylating agent or nitrosourea	500 mg/m^2 IV daily × 5 days q 4 weeks; 1-1.5 g/m^2 IV q 4 weeks	Moderate to severe nausea and vomiting occurring 1-4 hours after therapy are common; occasional diarrhea; mild, reversible nephrotoxicity if the drug is discontinued with early symptoms; severe renal failure occurs with doses of greater than 1.5 g/m^2/week or greater than 500 mg/m^2/day for 5 days; transient hepatotoxicity with an elevated SGOT 2-3 weeks after treatment; hypoglycemia in some individuals; mild myelosuppression, particularly anemia; burning at the site of infusion	Nausea and vomiting may improve with successive doses; assess for signs of early nephrotoxicity; assess for sudden hypoglycemia; increasing the dilution of the drug and slowing the infusion can decrease perivenous discomfort
Tamoxifen (Nolvadex)	Miscellaneous: antiestrogen	20-80 mg PO daily given in two doses	Minimal myelosuppression; transient hypoglycemia seen in some individuals; nausea in about 20% of individuals; gynecologic problems (eg, vaginal bleeding, menstrual irregularities, hot flashes, pruritus vulvae, and skin rashes); hypercalcemia in individuals with widespread bone metastases, temporary bone pain flare; induces ovulation in premenopausal women; higher doses have caused visual changes	Assess for gynecologic problems; advise premenopausal women to use birth control methods if they are sexually active; prepare patient and family for bone pain flare; medicate for pain accordingly; provide reassurance that bone pain is temporary and does not indicate disease progression
Teniposide (VM 26, Vumon)	Plant alkaloid	100 mg/m^2 IV weekly for 5 weeks; 50 mg/m^2 IV 2× /week	Leukopenia is dose-limiting toxicity; moderate to severe nausea and vomiting; mild peripheral neuropathies and anaphylactic reactions have been reported; fever, hepatotoxicity are mild; hypotension may occur with rapid administration; local tissue damage may occur if extravasated	Phlebitis may occur if medication is not diluted; administer antiemetic; administer over 30-60 minutes; assess for hypersensitivity reaction; assess for numbness and tingling in extremities

APPENDIX A Chemotherapeutic Drugs (continued)

Name	Classification	Adult Dosage	Major Side Effects	Nursing Implications
Thioguanine (6-TG, 6-thioguanine)	Antimetabolite	2 mg/kg PO daily × 4 weeks, then if no serious toxicity or response, the dose can be increased to 3 mg/kg daily	Delayed leukopenia followed by thrombocytopenia and anemia; nausea, vomiting, anorexia, stomatitis, and diarrhea may occur; hepatotoxicity with jaundice occurs infrequently	Administer oral dose on empty stomach because the drug is poorly absorbed; dose reduction is not necessary with allopurinol administration; monitor blood counts and gastrointestinal toxicity
Triethylenethiophosphoramide (thiotepa, TSPA, TESPA)	Alkylating agent	10-30 mg/m² IV q 1-4 weeks; 45-60 mg IM, intracavitary, or into the tumor; 60 mg instilled into the bladder retained 2 hours q 1-4 weeks; 1-10 mg intrathecally one to two times per week	Dose-dependent myelosuppression, with leukopenia and thrombocytopenia nadirs at 14 days and recovery 2-4 weeks after the nadir; anemia also occurs; nausea and vomiting occur infrequently; allergic skin reactions (eg, hives and dermatitis) may occur; irradiation of drug-treated areas may increase toxicity; ovarian and sperm suppression; headache; dizziness	Observe for allergic reactions; mild local pain at the injection site is common; for bladder instillation, encourage patient to change position every 15 minutes; use measures to prevent drug contamination
Vinblastine sulfate (Velban, Velbe, Velsar)	Plant alkaloid	6 mg/m² IV q week or 0.1-0.4 mg/kg q week	Leukopenia, with a nadir in 4-10 days and recovery in 1-2 weeks; serious platelet reduction is uncommon; occasional nausea and vomiting; constipation; stomatitis, which can occasionally be severe; dose-related but not dose-limiting neurotoxicity (eg, mild paresthesias, peripheral neuropathy, depression, headache, dizziness, malaise, jaw pain, and convulsions); dose-related, mild alopecia in 5%-10% of individuals; extravasation results in painful cellulitis and tissue necrosis; phlebitis with vein discoloration is common	Prophylactic stool softeners are helpful in preventing constipation; assess for neurotoxicities; transient lightheaded sensation may follow IV injection; avoid extravasation; teach patient to monitor bowel patterns daily to avoid obstruction

Vincristine (Oncovin, Vincasar)	Plant alkaloid	0.5-2 mg/m^2 IV q week; maximum dose is 2 mg	Reversible but dose-limiting neurotoxicity with constipation and peripheral neuropathy with numbness and weakness; hoarseness, depression, footdrop, abdominal pain, irritability, and convulsions may occur; bone marrow depression is unusual and mild when it occurs; alopecia in 20%-50% of long-term patients; regrowth occurs after drug is stopped; extravasation results in painful inflammatory reaction, leading to cellulitis and phlebitis; severe jaw pain may follow injection in 4-8 hours	Neurotoxicity recovery occurs in 6 weeks to 1 year; teach patient and family safety precautions related to sensory and motor impairments; stool softeners, mild laxatives, or enemas should be used preventatively to avoid constipation; teach patient to monitor bowel patterns daily; avoid extravasation; encourage adequate hydration; observe for signs of neurotoxicity; dizzy sensation may follow IV injection, disappears in a few minutes; aching may occur at the IV site, slower administration may help; repeated doses may cause phlebitis
Vindesine (Eldisine)	Plant alkaloid	2-4 mg/m^2 IV q 7-14 days	Mild to moderate leukopenia is common, with a nadir in 5-10 days; anemia is also common, but thrombocytopenia is infrequent and mild; partial alopecia is common, complete alopecia occurs in about 25% of individuals; neurotoxicity, including general muscle weakness, malaise, paresthesias, myalgias, arthralgia, decreased deep tendon reflexes, muscle spasm, jaw pain, hoarseness, and abdominal cramping; occasional nausea, vomiting, diarrhea, or constipation; mild stomatitis; extravasation results in phlebitis, cellulitis, and tissue necrosis	Assess for signs of neurotoxicity; prophylactic stool softeners may be helpful; avoid extravasation

Sources: Data from Fisher DS, Knobf MT; The cancer chemotherapy handbook (ed 3). Chicago, Yearbook Medical Publishers, 1989. Hubbard SM, Seipp C, Duffey P: Administration of cancer treatments: Practical guide for physicians and oncology nurses. In DeVita VT, Hellman S, Rosenberg SA (eds): Cancer: Principles and Practice of Oncology. Philadelphia, Lippincott, 1989, pp 2369-2402. Tenebaum L: Cancer Chemotherapy: A Reference Guide. Philadelphia, WB Saunders, 1989. McEvoy GK (ed): American Hospital Formulary Service Drug Information. Bethesda, Md, American Society of Hospital Pharmacists, 1989. Physicians' Desk Reference (43 ed). Oradell, NJ, Medical Economics, 1989. Covington TR et al: Drug Facts and Comparisons (1989 ed). St. Louis, JB Lippincott, 1988.

Chapter 14

Biotherapy

Patricia F. Jassak, RN, CS, MS

INTRODUCTION

Although the use of the combined therapeutic modalities of surgery, radiation therapy, and chemotherapy has resulted in increased survival for many persons with cancer, effective treatment measures still are not available for many types and stages of neoplastic disease.

In the search to control or cure cancer the hypothesis that the immune system can be manipulated to restore, augment, or modulate its function has stimulated scientific inquiry since the beginning of this century. Evidence from both animal and human trials clearly indicates that under the proper circumstances, malignant tumors are susceptible to immunologic rejection. And so the search for effective biologic agents continues.

Fortunately, the future is brighter than the past primarily as a result of four major technologic advances that have recently occurred.[1-4] First, scientists have developed an increased understanding of the complex cellular structure of the immune system, which enables them to isolate new cellular components and to accurately measure their function. Second, advances in genetic engineering, specifically the discovery and continued refinement of hybridoma techniques, have made it possible to clone genes and thereby produce large quantities of highly purified agents for analysis and clinical use. Previously, isolation and purification were slow, cumbersome, and costly processes that produced small quantities and impure products. Third, continued advances in molecular biology have allowed scientists to construct and alter molecules synthetically so that they can be investigated or their biologic activities changed. Fourth, technologic advances in laboratory equipment and computer systems have facilitated researchers in their pursuit of the unknown.

Scientists have pursued actively the use of immunologic approaches for cancer therapy for more than three decades. As a result of these technologic advances, biotherapy, the therapeutic use of biologic response modifers (BRMs), previously referred to as immunotherapy, has emerged as the fourth modality of cancer therapy.

The medical community's reaction to the reintroduction of biologic agents into the clinical setting has been varied. Moertel,[5] in a scathing editorial in the Journal of the American Medical Association, condemns his peers for highlighting their limited success with interleukin-2 (IL-2) and lymphokine-activated killer (LAK) cell therapy as a "breakthrough." He points out the extraordinary impact that this claim had on patients, families, and physicians because the prohibitive cost and severe toxicity of this regimen make it unavailable to the general public.

Durant,[6] on the other hand, ponders the possibility that we have reached "the end of the beginning of the search for successful immunotherapy for cancer." He projects that the future of biotherapy will be limited only by how well we use our knowledge base and fit the puzzle pieces together.

Although the majority of agents classified as BRMs are, in fact, agents that modulate the immune system, biotherapy encompasses a broader range of approaches than previously considered under immunotherapy, in particular, those agents responsible for the growth and maturation of cells. A BRM is defined as any soluble substance that is capable of altering (modifying) the immune system with either a stimulatory or a suppressive effect.[7(p 178)] Clark and Longo[8] classify BRMs into three major categories:

- Agents that restore, augment, or modulate the host's immunologic mechanisms
- Agents that have direct antitumor activity
- Agents that have other biologic effects (agents interfering with tumor cells' ability to survive or metastasize; differentiating agents or agents affecting cell transformation)

A wide array of BRMs currently are being investigated, including the interferons (IFNs), interleukins (ILs), colony stimulating growth factors, monoclonal antibodies (MoAbs), and tumor necrosis factor (TNF). The past decade has unveiled a great deal of information about the activities and toxicities of biologic agents. Many of the clinical results are exciting, demonstrating responses in diseases previously unresponsive to our known arsenal of therapy. As we gain a better understanding of the individual's biologic response to malignancy, we will learn techniques to manipulate that response in a beneficial way.

HISTORICAL PERSPECTIVE

Two observations laid the early groundwork in immunology research: first, the observation of a spontaneous regression, in which the tumor becomes smaller and/or disappears without any apparent reason; second, the observation of prolonged survival in which the patient lives longer than clinical experience or statistics would predict. An early pioneer in the field of immunotherapy, Dr. William B. Coley, a surgeon at New York's Memorial Hospital from 1891 until 1936, investigated why some patients with cancer appeared to be cured after surgical resection whereas others quickly relapsed. He identified that many of the patients who remained tumor-free had experienced what we now call *septic episodes* after their surgery. Clinically, Coley used live bacteria and later filtered toxins, referred to as *Coley's toxins,* to induce an infectious response in patients with cancer. These toxins were used clinically until 1975 and provide the background for what is now called TNF.[9] These toxins may have boosted the immune system to identify, detect, and destroy tumor cells from the body.

The application of immunotherapy to cancer therapy gained popularity only since the 1960s when many clinical trials of bacterial agents were initiated, specifically bacille Calmette-Guérin (BCG) and *Corynebacterium parvum.* These early experiments produced positive results in selective laboratory tumor models. In 1969 Mathe et al[10] demonstrated positive therapeutic results in an initial clinical trial using BCG to treat children diagnosed with acute lymphoblastic leukemia. Subsequently, hundreds of clinical trials were undertaken with BCG for the treatment of leukemia and many types of solid tumors with mixed results. Although survival as a result of BCG therapy was shown to increase among individuals with acute myelogenous leukemia, those with solid tumors were shown to derive no therapeutic benefit.[11]

Similarly, no substantial or significant improvement of response or survival rates was documented for individuals with leukemia, carcinoma of the head and neck, colon, breast, cervix, and nonsmall cell carcinoma of the lung and melanoma who received *C parvum*.[1,12] In addition, during this same time period viruses were used to stimulate tumor cells to produce viral oncolysates, again in an attempt to manipulate the immune system to reject tumor cells. Although some of the early clinical trials showed positive results, the majority were discouraging and few if any could replicate the positive responses reported. Therefore, by the late 1970s, most clinicians had developed a negative view of the promise of immunotherapy. Oldham and Smalley[1,2] attribute the early failure of immunotherapy as a discipline to the fact that initially most studies were conducted with the use of impure reagents, which resulted in variability of experimental procedure and lack of generalizable results. Oldham[2] believes that the future of biotherapy lies in the recent technologic advances that have allowed researchers to continue their quest.

As previously cited, four major technologic advances since 1970 have greatly expanded our ability to study BRMs. Genetic engineering has produced a large quantity of purified products, including recombinant IFNs (rIFNs) IL-2, TNF and CSFs, that are available for clinical evaluation and use.

The 1980s saw cumulative positive clinical results in diseases previously deemed unresponsive. In 1986, α-IFN received approval from the Food and Drug Administration (FDA) for use in hairy cell leukemia. Subsequently, in 1989 the FDA also approved α-IFN for clinical use in AIDS-related Kaposi's sarcoma. History was made. BRMs are and do have a therapeutic role in cancer therapy. In the use of BRMs, however, previous failures demand that researchers measure and analyze both the pharmacologic effect of the agent and the biologic response exerted by these approaches. A discussion of a variety of biologic response modifiers under active clinical investigation follows.

SEROTHERAPY (ANTIBODY THERAPY)

The limiting factor in effective cancer therapy is its current lack of specificity. During the 1980s significant strides were made in the field of serotherapy, which promotes specific targeting of cells through an antibody-antigen response. Serotherapy is based on the knowledge that typically all cells (including tumor cells) have antigens present on their surface that are specific to that cell type. Although tumor-associated antigens are found mainly on tumor cells, they also may be present on normal cells in lesser quantities, thus allowing tumor cells to be targeted while sparing normal cells.

Hybridoma Techniques

In 1975, Kohler and Milstein[13] described a technique for the production of monoclonal antibodies. An animal (usually a mouse) is injected with the desired antigen (tumor cells). The mouse's lymphocytes recognize the antigen as foreign and produce antibodies. The immunized lymphocytes are removed from the mouse's spleen and fused with mouse malignant myeloma cells to form a "hybrid" (Figure 14-1[14]). This last step is done to make the lymphocytes immortal and therefore capable of unlimited cell division. The hybrid is then screened for antibody production and the antibody is concentrated and purified. The end result is a highly purified murine (mouse) monoclonal antibody directed against specific human tumor–associated antigens.

All antibodies derived from a single clone are exactly the same, thus the term *monoclonal antibodies* (MoAbs). Thus a hybridoma is the result of a fusion between two cell lines to form a hybrid that shares genetic information. The refinement of the hybridoma technique allowed scientists to obtain a pure antibody to a known antigen and facilitated the development of new therapeutic and diagnostic applications of antibodies in cancer therapy.[15]

Antibody Function

Monoclonal antibodies may be used alone (referred to as *unconjugated*) or in combination *(conjugated)* with radioisotopes, toxins, or chemotherapeutic drugs to stain, destroy, or identify cells with specific antigens on their cell surface. They also are used in vitro to remove tumor cells from bone marrow before autologous transplantation and in conjunction with other biologic response modifiers such as IFN and IL-2. Antibodies can kill tumor cells through a variety of direct or indirect mechanisms.[16]

Direct tumor cell kill

Unconjugated monoclonal antibodies may directly kill tumor cells through several processes. The process of antibody-dependent cell-mediated cytotoxicity (ADCC) occurs when the antibody binding to the target cell acts as a signal to the effector cells to destroy the target cell (see Chapter 5). It is not yet known which cell type is the most important in vivo effector cell of ADCC; however, potential cells include lymphocytes, monocytes, and possibly neutrophils. Antibodies also may bind to the surface of the tumor cell, causing complement-dependent cytotoxicity to be initiated, which results in cell lysis. Opsonization

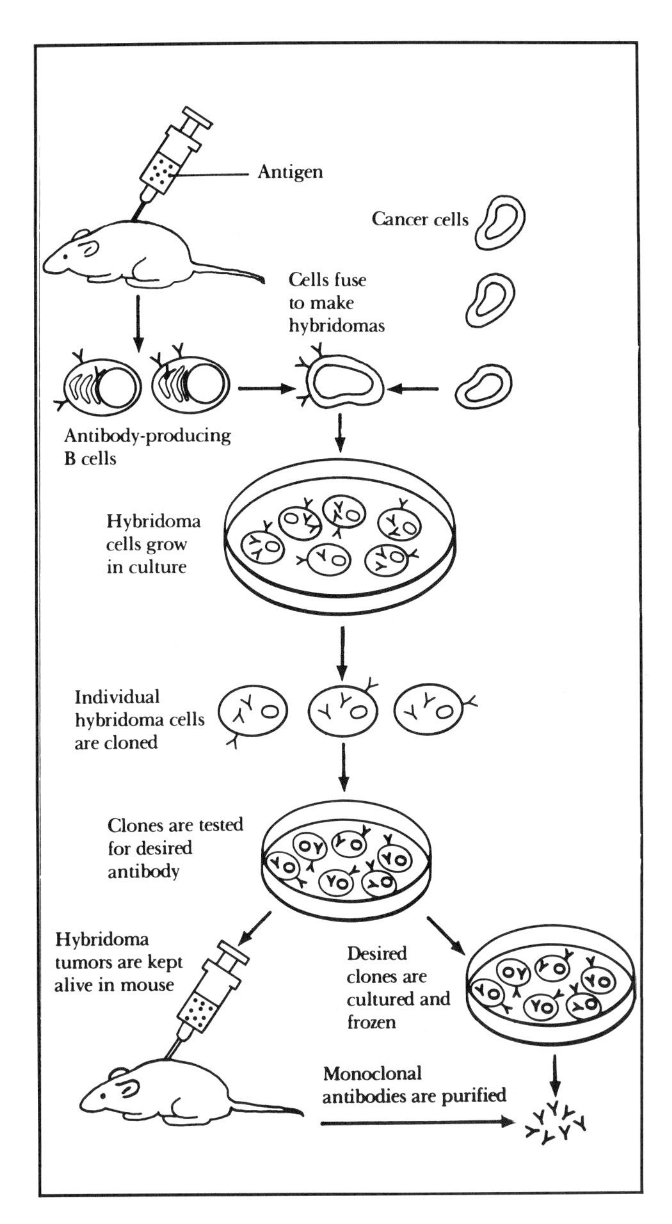

FIGURE 14-1 Use of hybridoma technique to make monoclonal antibodies. (Source: Schindler LW: Understanding the immune system. Bethesda, Md, US Department of Health and Human Services, NIH pub no. 88-529, July, 1988, p 28.)

is the process whereby tumor cells are coated by the antibody to facilitate clearance by the reticuloendothelial system.

Modulation of differentiation/growth

Antibodies also are capable of blocking tumor cell surface growth receptors for growth factors, providing a direct antiproliferative effect. This phenomenon has yet to be demonstrated in vivo, because researchers first need to identify tumor-expressed growth factor receptors and then develop antibodies that are specifically capable of blocking the receptor but that are not active in promoting proliferation.

Regulation of immunity

Antibodies also may be used to regulate immunity. Attempts to develop an effective immunization program to prevent cancer or its recurrence have been impeded by the lack of a reliable supply of immunogenic vaccine of known reactivity.

Anti-idiotype as immunogen

Anti-idiotypic antibodies may be used as surrogate antigen, thus providing a possible solution to the supply and immunogenicity problems of a reliable cancer vaccine. An idiotype is the unique part of an antibody's variable region (Fab) that can in itself act as an antigen to trigger a complementary antibody. Antibodies complementary to idiotopes are termed *anti-idiotypic*. Anti-idiotypic antibodies may be used as a substitute for the original antigen in the preparation of vaccines against infectious microorganisms. Data from clinical trials evaluating the use of anti-idiotypic antibodies as surrogate tumor antigen vaccines are not yet available.

Unconjugated Monoclonal Antibodies

Murine MoAbs have been used in clinical trials since the early 1980s to treat patients with acute lymphocytic leukemia,[17] chronic lymphocytic leukemia,[18-20] B-cell lymphomas,[21-23] and T-cell leukemias and lymphomas.[18,24-27] Transient clinical responses have been reported.

In addition, the effect of murine MoAbs has been studied in patients with gastrointestinal malignancies. Sears et al[28] reported durable remissions, minimal toxicity, and a 17% response rate, which compares favorably with that achieved with 5-fluorouracil.

Most patients, however, did not benefit substantially despite known evidence of an antitumor effect. Attempts to improve response have included the use of in vitro incubation of peripheral blood mononuclear cells with antibody and γ-IFN before administration; however, limited response has been achieved.

Several clinical trials have evaluated murine MoAbs in patients with metastatic melanoma.[29-36] For all studies combined, one complete response and seven partial responses are reported among a total of 54 patients. Although it is clear that MoAbs directed against melanoma antigens are active, data from phase II trials are not yet available; therefore the clinical efficacy cannot be established.

Immunoconjugates

The term *magic bullets* was coined at the turn of the century by Ehrlich who envisioned antibodies as carriers to deliver toxic agents directly to tumor cells. Immunoconjugates are formed when a variety of agents are linked to monoclonal antibodies. These agents include radioisotopes, toxins, chemotherapeutic agents, and biologic agents.

Toxins

A variety of toxins are available for conjugation with antitumor antibodies, including ricin, diphtheria toxin, alpha-toxin, exotoxin, abrin, gelonin, saponin, and pokeweed antiviral protein.[37,38] Toxins are unique in their remarkable potency and are considered to be the most lethal substances known; a single molecule of toxin can kill a cell. Ricin A chain has been conjugated with several antitumor murine antibodies to produce immunotoxins. Clinical trials with ricin A chain immunotoxins currently are under way in the treatment of melanoma, colorectal and breast cancer, and refractory leukemia. Spitler et al[39] report that major toxicities include hypoalbuminemia, with secondary fluid shifts, dependent edema, and intravascular hypovolemia. To date, no major tumor responses have been achieved.

Chemotherapeutic agents

Chemotherapeutic agents conjugated to MoAbs are called *chemoimmunoconjugates*. Agents used include chlorambucil, the anthracyclines, methotrexate, mitomycin C, and cisplatin. Theoretically, through conjugation, the antibody targets the chemotherapeutic agent to the tumor cells, alleviating the expected toxicity to normal cells. Thus higher doses of chemotherapeutic agents can be used with minimal systemic toxicity. Clinical trials are in early stages, with therapeutic efficacy and toxicity still to be determined.

Isotopes

Diagnostic imaging Current diagnostic imaging is limited by the lack of tumor specificity. Radiolabeled MoAbs with the use of iodine (^{131}I), technetium, and indium (^{111}In) allow specific bindings of these agents to tumor cells, thus enhancing the detection of tumor cells.[40-42] In diagnostic imaging these agents demonstrate sensitivity and specificity for tumor detection. In several instances imaging has been compromised because of the reticuloendothelial uptake of these immunoconjugates in the liver and spleen. These issues are under study, and diagnostic use of radiolabeled immunoconjugates is being refined. It is anticipated that the use of radiolabeled MoAbs will allow small tumors clinically undetectable by present technology to be isolated.

Therapeutic radioisotopes Radiolabeled antibody therapy involves conjugation of an antibody active against a specific tumor antigen with a radioactive isotope. This radioimmunoconjugate is administered into the blood stream where the antibody seeks out the tumor and attaches to it, and the radioactive isotope internally irradiates the tumor. Radioimmunoglobulin therapy has been attempted with the use of ^{131}I and ^{90}yttrium. Remissions through the use of radiolabeled polyclonal antiferritin antibodies have been reported in primary hepatomas (48%) and Hodgkin's disease (40%).[43] No acute toxicities have been reported.[44] Problems with nonspecific hepatic uptake, tumor vascularity, and choice and dose rate of the therapeutic isotope remain factors that need continued refinement in the search for effective therapeutic radiolabeled immunoconjugates.

Immunobiologic agents MoAbs may be linked to various lymphokines, cytokines, and hormones. These agents also may be used in conjunction with MoAbs. Possible actions include increasing antigen expression, enhancing the action of cytotoxic cells, and altering the cellular membrane and vascular permeability of tumor cells.

Problems with Antibody Therapy

Significant problems that have impeded the progress of MoAbs use for the treatment of cancer include the following:

1. Antigenic specificity. No true tumor-specific antigens have been isolated; only tumor-associated antigens have been identified. Therefore it is critical that cross-reactivity with antigens on vital organs does not occur or at least that the antigen density is much lower on these organs than on tumors.
2. Antigenic modulation. The tumor cell surface antigen is shed or altered shortly after antibody administration. This effect may be overcome by the intermittent administration of the MoAb.
3. Antimouse antibodies. The human immune system recognizes mouse antibodies as foreign, triggers an immune response, and develops neutralizing antibodies to mouse immunoglobulin. Repeated treatments have confirmed that significant toxicity can result from the development of indigenous human antimouse antibodies.

Chimeric Antibodies

Murine MoAbs have dominated the field of antitumor antibodies since the inception of hybridoma technology. Recently, recombinant biologic techniques have been applied to develop a new type of antibody. The murine gene used to encode the portion of the antibody molecule that recognizes antigen is coupled with the human gene encoding the remainder of the immunoglobulin molecule. This antibody is then introduced into a system that is capable of producing the antibody in large amounts.

The chimeric antibody (a mixture of human and murine antibodies) is capable of mediating immunologic functions similar to the original murine antibody. Initial reports indicate that chimeric antibodies have a longer circulating half-life and are less immunogenic than murine MoAbs. In vivo testing has not yet occurred.

Clinical Toxicities

Although anaphylaxis occurs infrequently, the nurse must be prepared to deal immediately with this acute toxicity. Its onset is predicted by the presence of a generalized flush and/or urticaria followed by pallor and/or cyanosis. Patients may complain of a tickle in their throat or impending doom; complaints of bronchospasm also are common. If any of these symptoms are present, the MoAb infusion is stopped immediately, vital signs are assessed frequently, and the physician is alerted. Hypotension and unconsciousness may result.

Anaphylaxis is treated with 0.3 mL aqueous 1:1000 epinephrine injected subcutaneously if the patient is conscious and has a detectable blood pressure. Epinephrine 1:10,000 is given by intravenous push for patients who cannot be aroused. Additional therapeutic measures may include the use of oxygen; the administration of antihistamines, corticosteroids, and aminophylline; and possibly cardiopulmonary resuscitation.

Common toxicities seen with the administration of MoAbs include fever, chills, diaphoresis, rigors, malaise, pallor, weakness, generalized erythema, urticaria, pruritus, dyspnea, nausea, vomiting, diarrhea, and hypotension. Dillman[45] reports that the most common side effects of fever, rigors, chills, and diaphoresis occur within 2 to 8 hours after MoAb administration.

Serum sickness also may occur 2 to 4 weeks after MoAb therapy. The patient may have symptoms that include urticaria, pruritus, malaise, flulike symptoms, and generalized adenopathies and arthralgias. Pulmonary edema also may be present. Treatment depends on the symptoms experienced; it usually includes aspirin or acetominophen and in some cases corticosteroids. Obtaining information regarding onset and duration of symptoms is critical. Usually at this time a serum assay of immune complexes is obtained, as well as complement studies of heparinized blood. Once patients have serum sickness, further MoAb therapy is restricted.

CYTOKINES AND LYMPHOKINES

The most exciting BRMs in the treatment of cancer are the cytokines. Cytokines are substances that are released from activated immune system cells that affect the behavior of other cells. Lymphokines are cellular products released by antigen-activated T cells and originally thought to be produced only by lymphocytes. It is now clear, however, that lymphokines are not restricted to lymphoid cells as previously identified, and thus the general term *cytokines* is now used to refer to them.[46] These cellular products activate a variety of biologic activities that may alter the growth and metastasis of cancer cells, including their ability to augment the responsiveness of T cells to tumor-associated antigens, to enhance the effectiveness of B-cell activity, and to decrease suppressive functions of the immune system, thereby enhancing immune responsiveness. Lymphokines may be administered directly to patients for control of cancer, or they may be used to manipulate the immune response in vitro to generate products that are used to treat individuals with cancer. The most frequently studied agents are described in the next section.

Interferons

In the late 1940s virologists first noted that under certain conditions an infection of one virus protects for a time against infection by other viruses. In 1957, after much investigation, Isaacs and Lindemann[47] isolated a protein substance secreted by cells from a chicken embryo. Although this substance is not an antiviral agent itself, its presence appeared to interfere with virus activity in cells; it was called *interferon*. In the subsequent decade, researchers identified other properties of IFN, including its antiproliferative effects. Because isolation and preparation of interferon was difficult and costly, further information on its activity spectrum was limited until the 1980s when new genetic engineering processes made recombinant IFN available in sufficient quantities for large-scale clinical trials (Figure 14-2). Although hopes were high that IFN's antitumor activity would constitute a major breakthrough in cancer treatment, initial results were modest and disappointing.[48,49]

Types of interferons

The IFNs are a family of naturally occurring complex proteins that belong to the cytokine family. Three major types of human IFN have been isolated: α-IFN, β-IFN, and γ-IFN. Each type originates from a different cell and has distinct biologic and chemical properties.[50-53] Table 14-1 identifies the types of IFNs, the cells responsible for their natural production, and their major cellular effects. All three types are available in recombinant form.

Cellular effects

The activity of the IFNs has been documented in three areas: antiviral, immunomodulatory, and antiproliferative.[50-58] All three types of IFN exhibit these cellular effects in various degrees. Clearly, the antiviral activity is the best defined, having played a significant role in IFN's original

TABLE 14-1 Interferons

Type	Agents That Stimulate Production	Interferon-producing cells	Cellular effects
Alpha	B-cell mitogens, viruses, tumor cells	B cells, T cells, macrophages, and null cells	Antiviral,* antiproliferative,† immunomodulatory
Beta	Viruses	Fibroblasts	Antiviral, antiproliferative, immunomodulatory
Gamma	T-cell mitogens, specific antigens, interleukin-2	T lymphocytes	Immunomodulatory,* antiproliferative,† antiviral

*Strongest activity.
†Moderate activity.

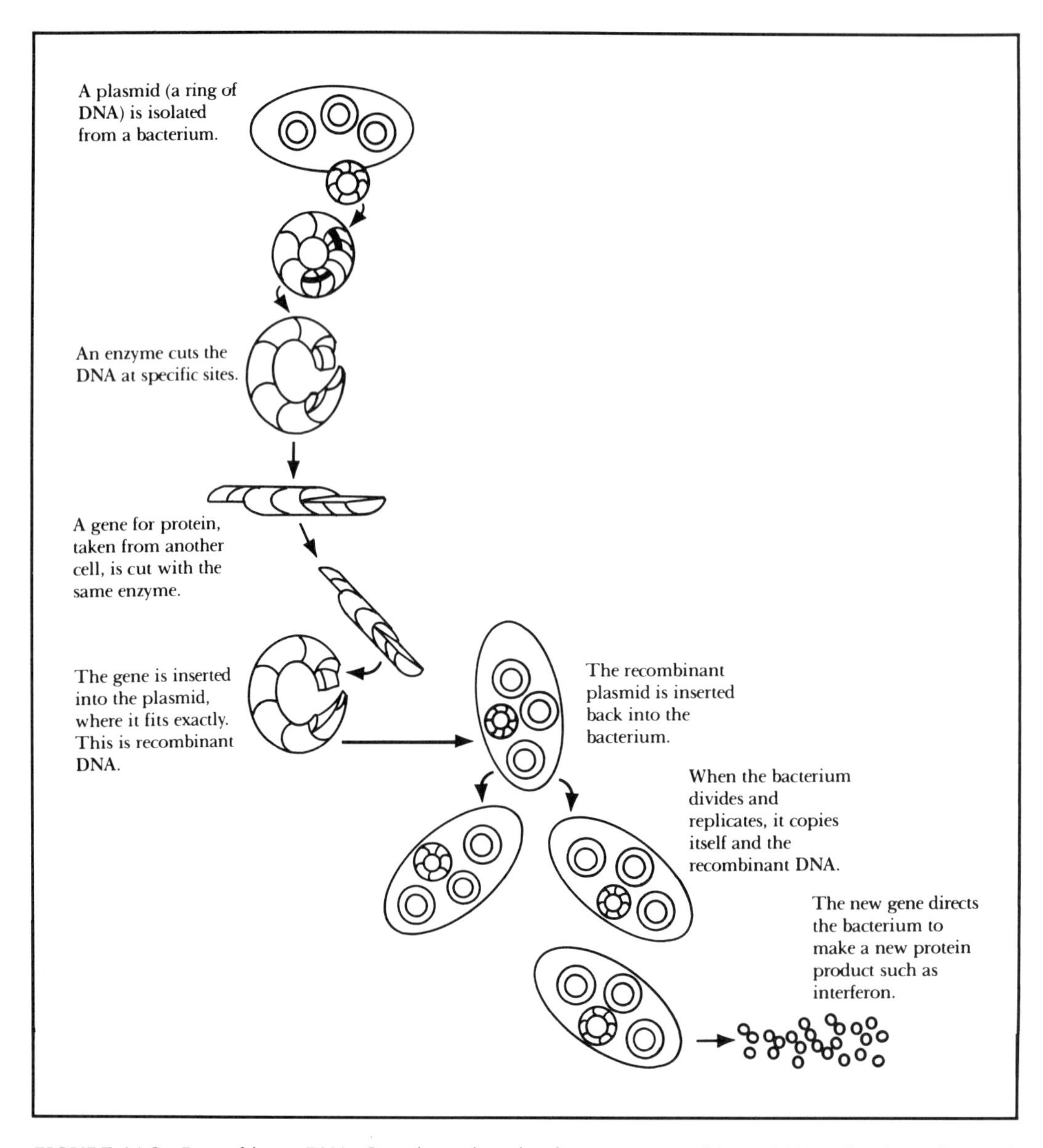

FIGURE 14-2 Recombinant DNA. Genetic engineering known as recombinant DNA technology allows scientists to pluck genes from one type of organism and combine them with genes of second organism, inducing cells to make large quantities of human proteins such as interferon or interleukins. Microorganisms also can be made to manufacture proteins from infectious agents such as the hepatitis virus or AIDS virus for use in vaccines. (Source: Schindler LW: Understanding the immune system. Bethesda, Md, US Department of Health and Human Services, NIH pub no. 88-529, July, 1988, p 27.)

identification. IFNs protect a virally infected cell from attack by another virus and, in addition, inhibit intracellular replication of viral DNA as part of a primary defense response. All nucleated cells of vertebrates produce IFN when exposed to a virus. IFN then binds to specific receptors on the infected cell's surface and induces enzyme production that damages the viral DNA strands.

IFNs exert profound effects on the immune system. Immunomodulatory effects result from direct interaction with T lymphocytes that stimulate the cellular immune response.[50,51,54,56,57] In vitro, the killing potential of natural killer (NK) cells is increased in the presence of IFN. The dose and route of IFN administration significantly affect NK cell activity.[54]

IFNs also exhibit an antiproliferative effect. Although the primary mechanism of the antiproliferative effect remains unclear, it is known that in tumor cells, IFN directly inhibits DNA and protein synthesis.[50,52,56,58] Furthermore, interferons increase tumor cell recognition by stimulating the expression of both human leukocyte antigens (HLA) and tumor-associated antigens on tumor cell surfaces. IFNs also act to increase all cell phases, prolonging the overall generation time and thus inhibiting the rate of cell growth. Potentially, this action is in itself antiproliferative.

Therapeutic uses/clinical trials

Most research to date has involved the use of recombinant α-IFN (r α-IFN), which received FDA approval in 1986 for use in hairy cell leukemia (HCL), and in 1989, its clinical indications were expanded to include AIDS-associated Kaposi's sarcoma. Two recombinant forms of α-IFN are available: Roferon-A (Roche Laboratories, Nutley, NJ) and Intron A (Schering Corp, Kenilworth, NJ). Clearly, hematologic diseases have responded best to IFN therapy, with measurable responses occurring in the lymphoproliferative malignancies, such as hairy cell leukemia, non-Hodgkin's lymphoma, and multiple myeloma and in chronic myelogenous leukemia and AIDS-associated Kaposi's sarcoma.[50,52,54,59-63]

Studies of solid tumors treated with IFN do not report as high objective response rates as those seen in the hematologic malignancies.[64] Tumors in which administration of systemic α-IFN has demonstrated good objective responses include renal cell carcinoma (15% to 20%),[65-67] malignant melanoma (10% to 15%),[68,69] and malignant carcinoid (47%).[70] A role for regional therapy with α-IFN exists such as intravesical use in low-grade carcinoma in situ bladder carcinoma (>50%),[71] intraperitoneal administration in minimal residual ovarian cancer (50%),[72] and intralesional therapy in cutaneous melanoma[73] and basal cell carcinoma.[74,75]

Clinical reports of the use of α-IFN in the treatment of viral hepatitis are beginning to appear in the literature.[75] Low-dose systemic α-IFN has demonstrated activity against the hepatitis B and non-A non-B virus by controling viral replication with patients demonstrating marked improvement in liver function tests.[76-78]

AIDS-associated Kaposi's sarcoma Kaposi's sarcoma (KS) is the most common malignancy in patients with acquired immunodeficiency syndrome (AIDS). Although non-AIDS-associated KS responds to standard chemotherapeutic agents, their use is prohibited in AIDS-associated KS because of the patient's compromised immune status. In the first clinical trial of α-IFN in AIDS-associated KS, Krown and colleagues reported that 5 of 12 patients demonstrated a partial or complete tumor response.[79] These data subsequently were confirmed in larger groups by other researchers who used various forms of r α-IFN.[80-83] Abrams and Volberding[84] reported a mean objective response rate approaching 30% with α-IFN doses of greater than 20 million U/m^2. Response rates appear to be highest when higher doses of α-IFN are administered.[81,83,85] To date, no substantial evidence exists that supports the use of chemotherapeutic agents with α-IFN to improve tumor response.[85]

In vitro, α-IFN has been shown to suppress human immunodeficiency virus (HIV) replication.[86] Interestingly, studies have described an increased tumor response to α-IFN in a subset of patients with AIDS-associated KS.[85] These patients with AIDS-associated KS have a helper T4 cell count of more than 200/cu mm^2, lack "B" symptoms (fever, weight loss, night sweats), and have no prior history of opportunistic infections. This suggests that in AIDS-associated KS α-IFN functions not only in an antiproliferative manner but also may be capable of modulating the patient's immune system. Thus it may be possible that interferon has a direct effect against HIV proliferation in individuals with AIDS.

On the basis of in vitro evidence of anti-HIV synergism, studies currently are under way that explore combinations of α-IFN with zidovudine (azidothymidine, AZT, Retrovir).[87] Preliminary data show that partial responses were observed; however, hematologic toxicity required dose reductions of α-IFN. Combined, these agents may be important in the treatment of AIDS and KS.

• • •

Phases I and II studies with the use of β- and γ-IFN are ongoing. Antitumor responses of γ-IFN have been reported for renal cell carcinoma, melanoma, non-Hodgkin's lymphoma, Hodgkin's disease, and leukemia; however, data are limited and the role of this agent in the therapy of any of these diseases has yet to be established.[88-91]

The search to find the optimal immunomodulating and/or antiproliferative IFN dose and route continues. Future studies will combine IFNs with chemotherapeutic agents and with other cytokines to obtain optimal tumor response.

Administration

With the exception of HCL and AIDS-associated KS, the best dose, route of administration, and frequency of IFN administration are yet to be determined. IFN cannot be given orally because it is a protein substance and digestive enzymes would destroy it. Therefore, viable administration routes include subcutaneous, intramuscular, intranasal, intravenous bolus, intravenous continuous infusion, intrathecal, intralesional, or intracavity. The route of administration of IFN has been shown to alter significantly the pharmacokinetics of this agent.[50,54] For example, the half-life of α-IFN administered intramuscularly or subcutaneously is approximately 2 to 4 hours, whereas the half-life of intravenous doses ranges from 6 to 8 hours.[55] Administration of IFN may cause local erythema and irritation at the injection site.

Alpha-IFN is supplied either as a sterile lyophilized powder that requires reconstitution with the accompanying diluent or sterile water, or as a prepared solution. All types of IFN require refrigeration storage at a temperature between 2°C to 8°C (36°F to 46°F). Data regarding shelf stability are still accumulating. Investigational IFN products (β and γ) do not contain preservatives, and therefore unused products should be disposed of within 3 to 8 hours after reconstitution or as designated per research protocol.

TABLE 14-2 Interferon Toxicities

Flulike syndrome	GI
Fevers*	Nausea
Chills,* severe rigors	Vomiting
Malaise*	Diarrhea
Fatigue	Anorexia*/weight loss
Myalgias	
CNS	**Hematologic**
Headache	Leukopenia
Lethargy	Thrombocytopenia
Somnolence	Anemia
Seizures	
Confusion	
Impaired concentration	
Renal/hepatic	**Cardiovascular**
Elevated transaminase	Hypotension
Proteinuria	Tachycardia
	Arrhythmias
	Myocardial ischemia
Reproductive	**Integumentary**
Impotence	Alopecia
Decreased libido	Irritation at injection site

*Most common toxicities experienced.
Source: Hahn MB, Jassak PF: Nursing management of patients receiving interferon. Semin Oncol Nurs 4:97, 1988.

Clinical toxicities

Multiple systemic toxicities occur with the administration of the various types of IFN.[92] It appears that most toxicities are dose-related; low doses of IFN are well-tolerated, with minimal measurable toxicity, whereas high doses often require cessation of therapy. A summary of potential toxicities is found in Table 14-2.

Flulike syndrome A common reaction to any type of IFN is the occurrence of fever, chills, fatigue, and malaise. These symptoms are grouped together and referred to as a flulike syndrome. When patients continue to receive doses of IFN, tachyphylaxis or tolerance develops. If, however, the dose or schedule is altered, symptoms may recur. Less notable tachyphylaxis has been reported with γ-IFN.[93] This syndrome can be acute, appearing within hours after IFN administration; it can be subacute, consistently present with mild severity; or it can become chronic. Fevers, which range from 38°C to 40°C, occur 2 to 4 hours after injection. Fatigue may become so severe that further therapy may be limited.

Musculoskeletal Patients commonly report the presence of myalgia, describing this as "aching" muscles. Low back pain also has been reported.

Gastrointestinal Nausea and vomiting occur less frequently and usually can be managed with conventional antiemetics. Weight loss associated with IFN therapy has been reported to be significant, frequently resulting in more than 5% loss of total body weight within a 4-week period.[94]

Cardiovascular Although rare, hypotension has been documented with α- and γ-IFN administration and may be dose-related.[53,95] Those at risk for cardiac toxicities, the elderly and patients with a history of cardiac disease, should be thoroughly evaluated and consistently monitored if IFN therapy is undertaken. Other cardiac toxicities reported include arrythmias, tachycardia, chest pain, and ischemia.

Renal/hepatic Increased hepatic enzymes, hyperbilirubinemia, proteinuria, and renal insufficiency have been documented. These toxicities appear to be dose-related and are monitored by laboratory studies.

Central nervous system (CNS) Symptoms that range from headache, mild confusion, somnolence, and seizure activity have been reported in patients receiving α-, β-, or γ-IFN. In most cases, patients return to baseline status within 96 hours after the IFN is discontinued. At doses above 15 million U/day, acute CNS toxicity occurs more frequently, and further IFN therapy may be withheld.

Hematologic Neutropenia and thrombocytopenia have been reported in the use of all types of IFN. These reactions are thought to be both dose-related and dose-limiting. Frequently, neutropenia requires a dose reduction, temporary cessation of therapy, or discontinuation of the IFN. Coagulopathies, although rare, have been reported with γ-IFN.[93]

Miscellaneous Other toxicities reported include dry mouth and inflammation at the subcutaneous injection site. In addition to toxicity, another limiting factor in IFN therapy may be the development of neutralizing antibodies.[96] Because IFN is a recombinant molecule, it is potentially antigenic and can induce antibody formation as part of the immune response. Steis and colleagues[97] indicate that many factors influence the antibody response, including the underlying disease state, treatment schedule, cumulative dose, treatment duration, route of administration, blood sampling time, source of protein, and assay method.[97] Renal cell carcinoma and KS have the highest incidence of antibody formation. What is not yet known is whether the presence of anti-IFN antibodies interferes with the biologic activity of IFN. Quesada et al[65] report that when neutralizing antibodies developed in patients with renal cell carcinoma, tumor responses ceased.[65] Figlin,[96] however, in summarizing the available data, cites variances in tumor response concomitant with antibody formation. Clearly, future studies must investigate this factor and determine its significance.

Interleukins

The ILs are among the most important regulatory substances produced by lymphocytes and monocytes. Seven types of ILs have been isolated and identified; however, other than IL-1, IL-2, and IL-3, little is known about their biologic effects. Presently only IL-2 and IL-3 are being studied actively in clinical trials.

Interleukin-1

IL-1, a lymphocyte-activating factor, is a glycoprotein produced by monocyte/macrophage fibroblasts and endothelial and smooth muscle cells. IL-1 serves an important immunoregulatory role through a variety of biologic activities, which include (1) activation of T cells to produce IL-2, (2) induction of fibroblast proliferation, (3) induction of fever, promotion of bone resorption, and initiation of acute phase protein synthesis, (4) enhancement of antibody responsiveness through stimulation of helper T cells and B cells, (5) enhancement of cytotoxicity of lymphocytes, (6) induction of tumor-cell markers, and (7) provision of radioprotective properties.[98,99] IL-1 is still in preclinical study. Potential clinical applications could involve use of this agent to promote wound healing (fibroblast growth) and to aid in protection against radiation-induced bone marrow failure. Both IL-1 and viable macrophages are necessary for the initial step in the activation of specific T cells.

Interleukin-2

IL-2, previously called T-cell growth factor, is a glycoprotein produced by helper T cells after stimulation by mitogens or specific antigens and IL-1. Researchers have learned much about this lymphokine since Morgan et al[100] first described it in 1976.

Cellular effects IL-2 binds to specific receptors on T lymphocytes and on certain malignant lymphocytes, which may account for the specificity of IL-2 action in the immune response.[101] IL-2, which is an essential factor in the growth of T cells, supports proliferation and augmentation of NK cells, is critical for the generation of LAK cells, and augments various other T-cell functions.[102-104] IL-2 also activates cytotoxic effector cells that produce a spectrum of secondary cytokines such as TNF and γ-IFN. It is hypothesized that these products play a significant role in the systemic toxicity of IL-2, although their antitumor effect is not yet known. Animal models have shown that administration of IL-2 can restore immunologic responsiveness in an immunodeficient host.

Pharmacokinetics The serum half-life of intravenous bolus IL-2 appears to be short, approximately 3 to 10 minutes.[105-108] However, when IL-2 is administered by means of intravenous infusions, the serum half-life significantly increases, ranging between 30 and 120 minutes.[106] This phenomenon of multicompartmental pharmacokinetics may be responsible for the differences in toxicities seen with different administration techniques.

Clinical trials IL-2 can be used as a single agent in a variety of doses and schedules, in conjunction with LAK cells or tumor-infiltrating lymphocytes (TILs), in combination with other cytokine agents, and in combination with chemotherapeutic agents. IL-2 therapy produces objective tumor responses in 20% to 50% of patients with renal cell carcinoma and malignant melanoma.

Initial studies in the use of naturally isolated IL-2 were reported in 1983 by Bindon et al.[109] At that time it took 150 L of source material to produce 0.1 mg of IL-2 from human peripheral blood lymphocytes and splenocytes, which was enough to study the half-life and toxicologic factors in only two patients. In 1984, 30 mg of IL-2 was derived from 10,000 L of material produced by stimulation of the Jurkat human T-cell tumor.[110] This was enough material to be used in a total of 16 patients with cancer or AIDS. In 1985 the emergence of recombinant technology made a significant impact on the ability to study the therapeutic uses of IL-2. IL-2 was successfully cloned in *Escherichia coli* with approximately 10 L of processed material generating 1 g of IL-2, which produced sufficient quantities for human investigation.[108]

IL-2 alone or combined with LAK cells At the same time phase I studies of IL-2 were ongoing with recombinant IL-2, Rosenberg and colleagues[111] at the National Cancer Institute (NCI) were investigating the use and therapeutic value of IL-2 and LAK cells. On the basis of the positive results obtained in murine models in which LAK cells were generated in the laboratory from lymphocytes plus IL-2 and then systemically administered, this regimen was administered to 25 patients with advanced metastatic cancer in whom standard therapy had failed. This treatment was termed *adoptive immunotherapy;* it required obtaining autologous lymphocytes by leukopheresis, incubating these cells with IL-2 to generate LAK cells, and then reinfusing the LAK cells in conjunction with additional doses of IL-2. Adoptive immunotherapy is an approach in which the tumor-bearing host passively receives cells that possess antitumor activity.

LAK cells are capable of selectively lysing tumor cells that are resistant to NK cells without affecting normal cells.[112] The adoptive transfer of these LAK cells plus recombinant IL-2 in individuals with advanced cancer resulted in regression of metastases from a wide variety of tumors, including melanoma, sarcoma, colon adenocarcinoma, and bladder cancer.[111] Objective responses, a reduction of more than 50% of disease volume, were seen in 11 of 25 patients. Complete tumor regression occurred in one individual with metastatic melanoma that was sustained for more than 10 months after therapy. Additional phase I and II studies of IL-2 substantiated the initially reported systemic toxicities and supported measurable clinical responses.[113-117]

The fact that this experimental therapy produced a high response rate in tumors previously unresponsive to standard therapy generated a tremendous amount of excitement and media attention in the scientific, consumer, and even business arenas. IL-2 was featured as a cover story in *Fortune* magazine, highlighting the "scientific breakthrough" and the potential business opportunities that this breakthrough would provide.[118] As a result of the exciting preliminary observations, NCI quickly established an IL-2/LAK extramural working group, which consisted of six centers across the country, to confirm or refute Rosenberg's initial findings. These phase II trials sought to further determine IL-2/LAK pharmacokinetics, toxicity, optimum dose schedule, and route of administration and to better define immunomodulatory effects and refine toxicity management.

The NCI extramural phase II study of renal cell carcinoma treated with the IL-2/LAK protocol confirmed the antitumor activity previously reported, with an overall objective response rate of 16%.[119] Two patients had complete responses and remained disease free at 9 and 12 months. Toxicity was severe but clinically manageable. A 19% overall objective response rate is reported for patients with metastatic malignant melanoma treated with the NCI extramural IL-2/LAK protocol.[120] Again, this phase II study confirms the activity of the IL-2/LAK regimen reported initially by Rosenberg and colleagues. It is clear that in both malignant melanoma and renal cell carcinoma the concept of adoptive immunotherapy is an important new treatment approach. Numerous reports of IL-2 clinical trials are now found in the literature.

Although far more knowledge of the therapeutic and immunologic activity spectrum of IL-2 must be obtained, a few key points can be summarized. Renal cell carcinoma and malignant melanoma are the solid tumors that have been studied extensively to date. Objective tumor responses have been reproduced, although many are partial responses and of short duration. It is important to note, however, that these tumors previously did not respond to standard therapy; thus these responses must be viewed as noteworthy. It remains unclear whether IL-2 should be administered by intravenous bolus or continuous infusion. Although higher doses of IL-2 can be administered through bolus intravenous infusion once or three times daily at equal daily doses, continuous infusions of IL-2 produce greater toxicity and exert greater immunobiologic effects.[121]

IL-2 and tumor-infiltrating lymphocytes A cell population obtained from tumor-bearing patients that appears to be more potent than LAK cells also was identified by Rosenberg and colleagues.[122,123] This subpopulation of lymphocytes, which are called tumor-infiltrating lymphocytes (TILs), infiltrate into tumors. Cultured with IL-2, TILs can be produced in large quantities and used to mediate the regression of metastatic tumors. TILs are functional without the administration of additional doses of IL-2, although low doses of IL-2 appear to enhance TIL's therapeutic efficacy.

Distinct from IL-2/LAK, therapeutic effectiveness of TILs depends on a state of immunosuppression in the host at the time of treatment, usually induced with either cyclophosphamide or total body irradiation. Initial reports of the clinical use of IL-2 with TILs document responses in patients with metastatic melanoma and renal cell carcinoma.[124,125] This promising technique may yield superior tumor control over IL-2/LAK therapy and provide critical information on the effect of IL-2/TILs therapy on the host/tumor relationship.

IL-2 in combination Numerous in vitro and preclinical animal studies have examined the use of various doses and schedules of IL-2 with other cytokines (including α-, β-, and γ-IFN, and TNF), MoAbs, and chemotherapeutic agents.[126-130] Many of these combinations have entered clinical trials. Rosenberg and colleagues[131] from the NCI surgical branch have the most extensive experience with IL-2. They present their experience in a summary analysis of the results of 652 patients treated with IL-2 alone or in combination with α-IFN, TNF, LAK cells, or TILs.

Clinical toxicities Administration of IL-2 results in multisystem toxicities that may be life-threatening. No organ system is spared. However, all side effects related to IL-2 administration are usually reversible; pretreatment laboratory values and physiologic states generally return within 24 to 96 hours after the cessation of therapy. These clinical toxicities are clearly related to dose and schedule. Although neither the mechanism for the induction of these toxicities nor their pathophysiology is well known, considerable evidence suggests the possibility that the IL-2–induced production of other cytokines, IFNs, and TNF either contributes to or is totally responsible for these toxicities.[101,108,132,133]

Central nervous system Confusion has been the major CNS toxicity observed. Patients are carefully monitored for any signs or symptoms of confusion or agitation and, if present, IL-2 doses are held or may be discontinued. Some patients may progress rapidly from confusion or agitation to somnolence, disorientation, or severe agitation, requiring the use of restraints. Although some studies have documented that neurotoxicity may progress even after therapy is stopped, generally these symptoms will resolve within 24 to 48 hours after the last dose of IL-2.[134]

Cardiovascular/pulmonary Marked cardiovascular and pulmonary toxicities occur when IL-2 is administered at a dose of 100,000 U/kg or greater.* At high doses, despite the expected occurrence of a capillary leak syndrome that causes marked extravascular fluid shifts, severe peripheral edema, ascites, or pleural effusions rarely occur. Respiratory dysfunction, however, is common. Patients may require oxygen therapy for dyspnea and, infrequently, temporary intubation. An average weight gain of between 5% and 10% of total body weight is observed, with 32% of patients experiencing weight gains of greater than or equal to 10% of their baseline weight. IL-2 causes peripheral vasodilation with a significant decrease in systemic vascular resistance and an increase in heart rate. Cardiac arrhythmias develop in approximately 10% of patients, mostly supraventricular in nature that respond to traditional medical management with digoxin or verapamil. Almost all patients experience hypotension, with a systolic blood pressure of less than 100 mm Hg, necessitating the use of albumin or vasopressors to facilitate continued administration of IL-2. Also a decrease of 5% or greater in the left ventricular ejection fraction has been documented, which suggests either a direct or indirect effect of IL-2 on the myocardium.[135] These changes appear to be limited and reversible. Transient cardiac ischemia also has been reported. Myocardial infarctions have occurred in four patients, one of which was fatal. Thus

*References 108,111,113,119,120,133-135.

patients with histories of cardiac or pulmonary dysfunction are not eligible for treatment with IL-2.

Renal Oliguria, anuria, azotemia, and elevations of serum creatinine and blood urea nitrogen levels have been documented with IL-2 therapy. In addition, Kozeny et al[136] noted a progressive respiratory alkalosis and the presence of hypophosphatemia, hypocalcemia, and hypomagnesemia. Azotemia and elevated creatinine levels have occurred in all patients. Episodes of anuria, defined as the presence of less than 10 mL of urine per hour, lasting longer than 8 hours, occur in 38% of patients. Normal renal function usually returns spontaneously after IL-2 therapy is stopped.

Gastrointestinal Nausea and vomiting can be controlled effectively with the administration of phenothiazines. Patients commonly experience diarrhea, which if severe may require administration of bicarbonate to correct deficiencies. Stomatitis frequently occurs but is not severe. Malaise and anorexia, although not treatment-limiting, are most likely caused by the presence of γ-IFN and TNF.[137]

Hepatic Increased levels of serum bilirubin and liver enzymes occur with IL-2 therapy, as does a progressive hypoalbuminemia. Mild to moderate hepatomegaly without tenderness in the right upper quandrant of the abdomen is also commonly reported.

Hematologic Anemia, severe enough to warrant the transfusion of packed red blood cells, occurs in 73% of patients who receive IL-2. Criteria for transfusions include not only the hemoglobin and hematocrit values but also consideration of the patient's cardiopulmonary status and the need for hemodynamic support not achieved with crystalloid or colloid solutions.[134] Thrombocytopenia (<50,000/mm^3) is common; however, platelet administration rarely is clinically indicated. No evidence of disseminated intravascular coagulation or other severe coagulopathies has been reported, although an increase in prothrombin time can be measured in most patients.

Integumentary A diffuse erythematous rash that is pruritic in nature and progresses to desquamation develops in all patients who receive IL-2. Skin desquamation can be severe, involving the soles of the feet, palms of the hands, and moist intertriginous areas.

Flulike syndrome Fever, chills, rigors, and malaise are universal symptoms in all patients who receive IL-2. These symptoms can be managed to a degree by prophylactic administration of acetaminophen, diphenhydramine, and indomethacin. When chills or rigors are present, meperidine, 25 to 50 mg intravenous push, is effective.

Endocrinologic Atkins et al[138] noted the development of hypothyroidism in 20% of patients who received high doses of IL-2/LAK. Other reported endocrine effects of IL-2 include increases in blood levels of adrenocorticotropic hormone, cortisol, prolactin, and growth hormone and the acute phase reactant C-reactive protein. This area of toxicity has not received much attention and only recently has been measured.

LAK cell reaction Mild to severe chills, followed by transient fever, have been reported within one half to 1 hour after the first administration of LAK cells.[134] These toxicities appear similar to those reported with granulocyte transfusions and therefore probably are directly related to LAK cell administration. Also noted is that patients generally report less severe reactions with subsequent LAK cell administration.

• • •

At this point, it is not known which of these toxicities are related to the immunomodulatory and antiproliferative effects of IL-2 and the subsequent production of other cytokines or purely toxic consequences of therapy that can and should be therapeutically altered.

Tumor Necrosis Factor

In 1975 Carswell et al[139] first identified TNF in the serum of mice injected with bacterial endotoxin (bacille Calmette-Guérin, or *C. parvum*) as the endogenous agent responsible for tumor necrosis. Further studies identified that TNF had cytotoxic or cytostatic in vitro effects on murine[139] and human[140,141] tumor cells with no effect on normal cells. TNF, a naturally occurring agent, is produced by activated macrophages.[142-144] The gene that encodes human TNF was identified, cloned, and expressed in *E. coli*.[145] This highly purified recombinant human TNF demonstrated the same biologic activity spectrum as the isolated natural agent and thus became available for human investigation.

Concomitantly, research was under way to understand the pathophysiology of cachexia, often seen in patients with chronic diseases. Beutler and colleagues[146] isolated a molecule they called *cachectin*, believed to be an etiologic agent of cachexia, and structurally similar to TNF. Subsequently, molecular cloning studies confirmed that cachectin and TNF are identical substances.

Cellular effects

TNF is produced by endotoxin activated macrophages; it travels through the blood stream and binds to designated receptors located on cell membranes. Once bound to cell membranes, TNF initiates its cellular action. Early laboratory research with the use of murine models identified that the immediate effect of TNF on tumor cells is cytostasis, producing cell arrest in the G2 phase of the cell cycle. Darzynkiewicz et al[147] found this effect to prevail during the first 4 hours after exposure to TNF, with extensive cell lysis measurable after 7 hours and nearly complete cell lysis occurring after 24 hours. Research has identified that approximately one third of human epithelial cancer cell culture lines are extremely sensitive to the cytolytic effects of TNF, whereas another one third demonstrate cytostasis without lysis and another third are basically resistant to TNF.[140,148] Normal cell activity is affected only by a 100- to 10,000-fold increase in TNF concentration. Thus TNF selectively attacks tumor cells while sparing normal cells.[139,148]

TNF possesses a broad range of biologic activity. In particular, TNF has been identified as a primary mediator of endotoxic shock.[149] Other biologic effects of TNF are

TABLE 14-3 Biologic Effects of Tumor Necrosis Factor

	Effect
Tumor cells	Produces cytostasis Induces cytolytic action
Normal cells	Promotes production and activation of hematopoietic cells Enhances function of effector cells Stimulates activation of vascular/coagulation system Induces secretion of other cytokines (GM-CSF, IL-1, IL-6) Induces synthesis of collagenase and prostaglandin E_2 Increased expression of several cell-surface antigens Induces secretion of small molecule mediators of inflammation

GM-CSF, Granulocyte-macrophage colony-stimulating factor.
IL, Interleukin.

summarized in Table 14-3.[150-158] The therapeutic significance of the biologic activity of TNF is under phase I and phase II clinical investigation.

Pharmacokinetics

Chapman et al[159] document that the serum half-life of intravenous bolus–administered recombinant TNF (rTNF) is approximately 20 minutes. Varying detectable serum TNF levels are reported for different routes of administration. With intravenous bolus TNF, serum levels were detectable at doses greater than 25 μg/m². Serum levels of rTNF were not detectable after subcutaneous administration except for one patient who received a dose of 250 μg/m². Jakubowski et al[160] could not detect serum TNF levels in patients treated with intramuscular doses of less than or equal to 100 μg/m². Much variability also exists in the time after injection that rTNF was detectable. This initial pharmacokinetic information suggests that the half-life of rTNF depends on the dose and route of administration.

Clinical trials

Since December 1985 more than 200 patients have participated in phase I studies of rTNF, receiving a fixed dose given repetitively by various routes and schedules.

Phase I studies of 30-minute intravenous infusions administered for 5 days every other week have established the maximum tolerated dose of rTNF to be 150 μg/m²/day. This is similar to the work of Jakubowski et al[160] in which rTNF was administered by intramuscular injection.

Phase II clinical trials are under way to determine further tumor response, immune system modulation, dosage, route of administration, and toxicities.

TABLE 14-4 Recombinant Tumor Necrosis Factor Systemic Toxicities

Flulike syndrome Fever, chills* Rigors* Headaches* Fatigue*	**Hematologic** Granulocytopenia Thrombocytopenia Increased circulating monocytes (monocytosis)
Pulmonary Dyspnea	**Hepatic** Increased bilirubin Increased ALT (SGOT) Increased alkaline phosphatase
Cardiovascular Hypotension Hypertension Supreventricular arrthymias	**Endocrine** Increased triglycerides Decreased cholesterol
CNS Seizures Confusion Aphasia	**Gastrointestinal** Anorexia Nausea Vomiting Diarrhea
	Integumentary Inflammation at injection site (intramuscular, subcutaneous)

*Most common.

Administration

In current clinical trials, rTNF is being administered by various routes, including intravenous bolus, continuous intravenous infusion, and subcutaneous and intramuscular injection. The optimal route and dosing schedule have yet to be established. Recombinant TNF is administered intravenously in a normal saline solution that contains human serum albumin at a concentration of 2 mg/mL. The intravenous tubing must be cleared with the admixture of normal saline and human serum albumin before the addition of rTNF so that rTNF is prevented from adhering to the tubing. Because rTNF is an investigational agent, administration must conform to each institution's standards and policies for the use of investigational drugs.

Clinical toxicities

Experience with rTNF indicates that most patients experience side effects similar to those observed with the interferons and IL-2. As with IFN, tachyphylaxis will develop, in which the flulike syndrome will decrease with subsequent doses of rTNF. Most toxicities appear to be dose-dependent and are reversible, resolving within 48 to 96 hours after the drug is discontinued.

Systemic toxicities of rTNF are summarized in Table 14-4. The most common toxicities are a flulike syndrome, which includes fever, chills, rigors, headaches, and fatigue, and a local reaction at the subcutaneous or intramuscular injection site.

Flulike syndrome Fever and chills generally occur within 1 to 6 hours after drug administration. Chapman et al[159] note that different patterns for the onset of fever, chills, or rigors depend on the route of administration. Rigors may occur within 10 minutes after intravenous bolus administration of rTNF, and temperature rises within 20 minutes, with peak spikes recorded 1 to 2 hours after injection. After subcutaneous administration, rigors were reported to be milder and fevers peaked at 4 to 8 hours. Increase in dose did not alter fever increases. Fever, chills, and rigors are treated with acetaminophen and meperidine. Mild to severe fatigue, which lasts up to 3 days after subcutaneous administration but fewer than 24 hours after intravenous administration, has been reported, necessitating changes in the patient's daily activities. Headaches, described as dull and aching, occur frequently and respond to acetaminophen or narcotic analgesics.

Gastrointestinal Gastrointestinal toxicities associated with rTNF administration have been reported but do not appear to be dose-dependent.[159,160] Anorexia, nausea, vomiting, and diarrhea may occur. Antiemetics, such as prochlorperazine, may be useful to control nausea. Significant weight loss has not been reported.

Cardiovascular Transient episodes of hypotension, in which the systolic blood pressure is 90 mm Hg or less, occur 1 to 11 hours after intravenous administration and 2 to 48 hours after subcutaneous administration at doses of 5 $\mu g/m^2$ or higher. This transient hypotension is treated effectively with intravenous saline infusions. Vasopressor agents have not been required. Hypertension also has been reported. It is believed that the hypertension episodes may be directly related to the presence of rigors that physiologically produce tachycardia and peripheral vasoconstriction. Supraventricular arrythmias, although rare, also have been reported.

Hematologic Hematologic toxicities of rTNF include granulocytopenia, thrombocytopenia, and increased circulating monocytes. These toxicities appear to be dose-related, with larger decreases from baseline values observed at doses greater than 100 $\mu g/m^2$/day. No consistent changes in coagulation factors have been identified. Thus no evidence currently exists that patients who receive rTNF are at risk for the development of disseminated intravascular coagulation. These hematologic toxicities occur independent of administration route. Patients' hematologic values return to baseline upon cessation of therapy.

Hepatic Moderate increases in liver enzymes and bilirubin have been reported.

Endocrine Increases in serum triglyceride levels were detectable at doses greater than 50 $\mu g/m^2$/day whereas cholesterol levels decreased during most treatment courses.

Central nervous system Although rare, transient focal neurologic toxicities such as seizures, confusion, and aphasia have been reported. Sherman and colleagues[161] describe aphasic episodes that subsequently resolved without adverse clinical effects. The cause is unknown.

Pulmonary Dyspnea has been reported in patients who receive rTNF. Morice et al[162] documented decreased gas exchange during treatment with rTNF, with return to near baseline values after therapy was discontinued. The cause of this toxicity is unknown but may be related to secondary alveolar endothelial damage.

Inflammation at injection site Subcutaneous and intramuscular injection of rTNF produces a local reaction at the injection site. Tenderness, erythema, induration, and vesiculation have been reported. This toxicity is dose-related, with increasing involvement and severity occurring at higher doses and increased symptoms with continued drug administration. Local treatment measures of dry heat, cold packs, or warm soaks have been used with variable therapeutic response. Infiltration or phlebitis have not been reported with intravenous injection sites.

Colony Stimulating Factors

Blood cell growth is regulated by a complex structure of hematopoietic growth factors that mediate the proliferation, maturation, regulation, and activation of granulocytes, monocytes, macrophages, lymphocytes, erythrocytes, and platelets.[163] These critical elements that regulate hematopoiesis are called CSFs. Haeuber and DiJulio[164] provide an excellent overview of the relationship of CSFs to normal hematopoiesis. CSFs acquired their name because in agar cultures, they stimulate the growth of colonies of maturing blood cells from their hematopoietic precursors. Modern techniques of molecular biology, biochemistry, and recombinant technology have been used to isolate these elements and produce sufficient quantities for clinical use.

CSFs are a group of naturally occurring glycoproteins (also classified as cytokines) that recently have received considerable clinical attention. In general, CSFs have been named for the major target cell lineage they affect. Thus granulocyte-macrophage CSF (GM-CSF) targets both the granulocyte and macrophage lineages; granulocyte CSF (G-CSF) targets only granulocytes; pleuripoietin IL-3 or multi-CSF targets the early cell lineage, and erythropoietin targets only the erythrocyte lineage. However, an overlap of the effects of one factor on other factors most probably occurs. CSFs hold great promise for the treatment of disease states in which myelosuppression, anemia, and thrombocytopenia prevail and limit therapeutic treatment options. CSFs may allow increased doses of chemotherapy to be given without the risk of long-term myelosuppression and may be used in other hematologic diseases in which abnormalities of blood cell components exist, such as congenital neutropenia and AIDS.

Therapeutic applications

Therapeutic applications of CSFs are currently under clinical investigation. Multiple clinical trials are investigating the growth factors involved in granulopoiesis, particularly GM-CSF and G-CSF, to determine therapeutic benefits in various myelosuppressive states that may be either disease-related (e,g, AIDS or leukemias) or treatment-induced by chemotherapeutic agents. Although both G-CSF and GM-CSF may prove to be of therapeutic value, each has distinct and different biologic characteristics.[165]

It appears that the regulatory function of G-CSF is lineage specific for the proliferation, maturation, and activation of neutrophil granulocytes. On the other hand, GM-CSF has a broader capability, which affects all levels of granulocytes and stimulates the production of monocytes and macrophages. It also functions to induce these cells to produce a number of cytokines. Gutterman[166] reports that GM-CSF also produces a multilineage effect in some patients, which decreases the requirement for platelet and red cell transfusions, in addition to its effects on granulocytes. Other factors such as thrombopoietin, although identified and isolated, have ill-defined functions and therefore have not been recombinantly produced.

Erythropoietin is the first CSF approved by the FDA in June 1989 and is available for clinical use. Erythropoietin has firmly established its role in the treatment of anemia caused by end-stage renal disease. When administered after dialysis treatments, erythropoietin is effective in stimulating erythropoiesis and either reducing or eliminating patient transfusion requirements.[167] Because patients with cancer generally have anemia related to chronic disease and/or blood loss, it seems highly unlikely that erythropoietin will play a major role in the supportive care of patients with cancer. Currently, patients with cancer with anemias that are treatment-induced are easily managed with minimal transfusions. However, clinical trials have been established to determine whether erythropoietin will provide an important function for patients with cancer.

The actual role CSFs play in the regulation of hematopoiesis is unknown. Research suggests that these factors may serve as emergency signals to accelerate the production of leukocytes in the presence of inflammation or infection.[168] Thus it is hypothesized that the physiologic role of the CSFs may be to augment production and function of mature granulocytes in pathologic disease states such as infection.

Clinical trials

Human trials with GM-CSF and G-CSF were initiated in the late 1980s. Either one or both of these factors demonstrated an increased production of leukocytes, with corresponding bone marrow changes in patients with AIDS, myelodysplastic syndromes, solid tumors, aplastic anemia, cyclic neutropenia, and congenital neutropenia (Kostmann's syndrome).[169-176] Studies also have shown that GM-CSF and/or G-CSF can significantly reduce or prevent myelosuppression caused by chemotherapy or bone marrow transplantation conditioning regimens.[166,169-171,176,177]

Multiple clinical trials have used various doses, schedules, and routes of administration of GM-CSF and G-CSF. Nonetheless, several specific treatment factors have emerged.[178] Therapeutically, the leukocyte response is dose-dependent, and the schedule and route of administration are important. Continuous intravenous infusion or subcutaneous administration appears preferable to intravenous bolus doses.[179] In patients with normal bone marrow function who receive high dose chemotherapy and either GM-CSF or G-CSF, the duration of severe neutropenia is reduced by 50% or more.

Neither GM-CSF or G-CSF affected the duration of thrombocytopenia. The CSF-induced leukocytosis appears to be reversible, with no evidence to date of subsequent marrow failure. Peters[173] reports a 17% decrease in the incidence of bacteremias with the use of GM-CSF or G-CSF in patients who receive autologous bone marrow transplants.[173] He believes that this is due to the early presence of increased numbers of circulating activated granulocyte neutrophils.

The effect of GM-CSF and/or G-CSF on leukemia remains unclear.[180] Laboratory research indicates that these CSFs are capable of inducing leukemic cell growth. It is possible that the use of CSFs in patients with acute leukemia accelerates cell entry into the synthesis (S) phase of cell division, making these cells more susceptible to treatment with S-phase chemotherapeutic agents such as cytosine arabinoside (ara-C).

Administration

Both G-CSF and GM-CSF have been administered by various routes, including intravenous push and subcutaneous injection, by either daily administration or continuous intravenous infusion. Groopman et al[169] reported that mild phlebitis occurred when GM-CSF was administered by continuous infusion through a peripheral vein. However, phlebitis did not occur when a central venous catheter was used. In one patient GM-CSF administered by subcutaneous injection produced a local skin reaction at the injection site.[177] This reaction consisted of an erythematous induration that persisted for 2 to 3 days after each injection. Maximum tolerated dosages for G-CSF have yet to be established. However, it appears that the maximum tolerated dosages for GM-CSF are in the range of 16 to 32 mg/kg/day.

Outpatients who require treatment with G-CSF or GM-CSF need instruction in administration techniques, drug stability, and storage and must be able to complete a daily symptom log to document toxicity trends.

Clinical toxicities

Minimal toxicity has been associated with G-CSF therapy. Studies cite occasional reports of transient bone pain.[171,181] Glaspy and Golde[182] propose that the cause of this bone pain may be the expansion of cells in the bone marrow. Negrin et al[183] report that some patients also experience a mild to moderate flulike syndrome and generalized rash.

GM-CSF therapy produces a wider array of systemic

toxicities than does G-CSF.[177,179] Herrmann et al[179] report facial flushing, mild myalgias, and bone pain with intravenous bolus administration. Commonly reported toxicities that appear to be route- and dose-related include low-grade fever with chills and/or rigors that occur 4 to 6 hours after administration. Patients experienced reversible dyspnea during the initial 2 to 6 hours of continuous intravenous infusion. The cause of this toxicity is believed to be the rapid sequestration of neutrophils within the lung.[179] Generalized rashes and fluid retention also were described.[181] These toxicities all have been reported to be reversible. Table 14-5 provides a summary of known toxicities for GM-CSF and G-CSF.

Clinical trials with CSFs have only begun to address the questions that will predict their future use. For example, does the increased number of granulocytes provide a clinical benefit; that is, are septic episodes decreased? Can doses of chemotherapeutic agents be increased to obtain a better tumor response rate that ultimately affects remission rates and overall survival? What long-term effect will CSFs have on the bone marrow? The initial trials are encouraging and lead to the conjecture that CSFs will have a significant impact on the patient with cancer or hematopoietic dysfunction.

TABLE 14-5 Colony-stimulating Factor (CSF) Toxicities

Granulocyte-macrophage CSF	Granulocyte CSF
Flulike syndrome Fever* Chills, rigors Myalgias* Headache Fatigue	**Flulike syndrome** Fever Myalgias* Headache
Integumentary Facial flushing Generalized rash Inflammation at injection site	**Integumentary** Generalized rash
Hematopoietic Leukocytosis Eosinophilia	**Miscellaneous** Bone pain*
Pulmonary Dyspnea	
Miscellaneous Bone pain* Fluid retention	

*Common toxicities reported.

NEW DEVELOPMENTS

Levamisole, a derivative of the synthetic drug tetramisole hydrochloride, which has been used as an anthelmintic in animals and humans, is a type of nonspecific immunomodulating agent. In the early 1970s it was noted that tetramisole increased the protective immunization effect of a *Brucella* vaccine in mice. This observation led to efforts to consider the effects of the drug on the immune system. Multiple physiologic effects have been described, but exact mechanisms are unknown. Data suggest an influence of levamisole on T lymphocytes and T-B lymphocytic interaction. Macrophage function also may be stimulated. One of the strongest impetuses for clinical trials with levamisole was the observation that levamisole augmented delayed hypersensitivity responses. This was shown by Tripodi and coworkers[184] in 1973 when patients with cancer whose test results were negative for dinitrochlorobenzene were challenged with orally administered levamisole for 3 consecutive days. Fourteen of the 20 individuals showed increased responsiveness to dinitrochlorobenzene (DNCB) or purified protein derivative (PPD); however, no one in a control group showed an augmented skin test response. Levamisole does not appear to overstimulate immunologic responses. It is active primarily in immunorestoration of deficient host mechanisms rather than immunostimulation of an already responsive host.[185]

Levamisole appears to have antiproliferative activity against metastatic foci rather than against primary tumors and demonstrates increased activity when a low tumor burden exists. Thus most clinical trials have evaluated the drug as an adjunct to chemotherapy, radiation, and/or surgery to increase survival. Extensive clinical studies in general have yielded marginal improvements in survival. Recent studies, however, have indicated moderate success for the use of levamisole in conjunction with fluorouracil as an adjunct to surgery in the treatment of patients with colon cancer whose regional lymph nodes show positive findings (modified Dukes' stage C disease). The drug is now available under Treatment Indications (INDs) from the National Cancer Institute for this specific use.[186] Side effects are relatively mild as compared with many BRMs. Nausea and vomiting sometimes occur. Diarrhea, malaise, headaches, and lightheadedness also have been reported. Levamisole causes reversible granulocytopenia.

Nonspecific active immunomodulatory agents that have undergone clinical trials include Picibanil (OK-432), Bestatin, Azimexon, muramyldipeptide (MDP), Tuftsin, Lentinan, Ned-137, immune RNA, cimetidine, Krestin, maleic anhydride-divinul ether (MVE-2), and prostaglandin inhibitors such as aspirin and indomethacin. Other new natural and synthetic agents are being evaluated continually in the laboratory and in animal models, and those that are active will move toward investigation in humans.[3]

NURSING MANAGEMENT

General Nursing Implications

Many biologic agents will be investigated in humans during the 1990s for their immunomodulatory and/or antiproliferative effects. The nurse has a professional obligation to obtain specific information about these agents.

Critical issues the nurse must address include the following:

1. What is the nature of this material? Does it contain tumor cells? Are they replicating? Does the material contain live organisms? Are they infectious? Does the material contain a foreign protein or other potentially allergenic substance?
2. Is this material standard or experimental? If experimental, is the material exactly equivalent to the preceding material? If not, how does it differ? Examples of differing materials might be interferons produced by different companies.
3. What equipment is needed, and what procedure should be followed to administer the agent? Does the agent require special admixture solutions? Does an antiseptic applied to the skin inactivate the bacteria in the vaccine? What handling and disposal precautions should be taken to protect the nurse and patient/family?
4. What is the nature of the expected response? Will there be an immediate hypersensitivity reaction? What type of toxicity or complications may be expected to occur?
5. What equipment and medication should be available to manage acute toxicities? What is an appropriate nurse-to-patient ratio to provide optimal observation and care?
6. Is an immune evaluation necessary?
7. How will this agent interact with other medication(s) the patient is receiving?
8. What additional information is needed by the nurse before information and guidance can be provided to the patient/family? Does this material cause potential danger to a family member who has intercurrent disease? An example of such danger is the administration of smallpox vaccine to the patient whose sibling has infantile eczema.

Nursing Interventions

Biotherapy is in the forefront of advancing medical science and merits personal study and consultation with medical investigators. The nurse has an obligation to obtain accurate knowledge concerning all phases of therapy so that appropriate patient and family planning and care through the nursing process may be achieved.

The physician obtains a detailed history from a patient before administration of any therapy. The patient and family are advised initially by the physician of the purpose of therapy, the course of treatment and necessary procedures, and the precautions to be taken to prevent adverse reactions. Because most BRM agents remain investigational, it is a medical responsibility to obtain a signed statement of informed consent from the patient for all research protocols. The nurse should be involved directly and integrally in these discussions with the patient and family so that their needs for care specifically in the areas of education and emotional support can be determined.[187]

Because of the investigational nature of BRMs, the patient must be encouraged to share information and observations concerning personal reactions to the treatment. The nurse as an astute listener may gain a wealth of information that is important to the ultimate evaluation of treatment efficacy and toxicities. This represents only one of many ways that nurses may play an indispensable role in the research process.

Although each BRM agent has distinct biologic and chemical properties, nursing interventions focus on common areas that most BRMs share. These include the nature of the biologic agent as a medication, the diversity of organ-system toxicities, and the presence of an acute or a chronic flulike syndrome.[188]

The toxicities of each BRM agent depend on the dose, route of administration, and schedule. Nurses must be familiar with the particular protocol in use, as well as the reported range of toxicities possible with each BMR agent in use. This knowledge allows the nurse to predict the severity of potential toxicities. Effective measures to manage or prevent these toxicities then can be readily available. This knowledge base also aids in patient and family education and reassurance.

Administration of BRMs results in diverse organ-system toxicities. In particular, certain biologic agents are associated with unique side effects. IL-2 produces a capillary leak syndrome that has not been observed with other cytokines.[189-191] The potential for anaphylactic or allergic reactions most commonly is associated with the administration of antibody therapy.[44,45,192] Administration of TNF causes a local irritation at the injection site.[193] Nursing assessment for organ toxicity involves establishing the patient's risk for development of such toxicity (in most cases, the eligibility criteria of research protocols will eliminate patients at increased risk for toxicities because of past or current medical history) and establishing baseline values for future comparison.

Interferon has been viewed as the prototypic BRM agent because of its constellation of toxicities, its biologic nature, and the presence of an acute and a chronic flulike syndrome.[189,194,195] An excellent review article of BRM-induced flulike syndrome is provided by Haeuber.[196] Management of this syndrome can be divided into three approaches: (1) treatment manipulation, ie, changing dose or schedule, (2) administration of effective medications to block or minimize the effect, eg, administration of meperidine at the onset of chills or rigors and premedication with acetaminophen and diphenhydramine, and (3) the practice of noninvasive nursing techniques such as imagery and/or relaxation therapy. These measures, undertaken either alone or in combination, provide patient comfort and decreased toxicity without adverse effects.

Finally, the patient will, without doubt, look to the nurse for psychosocial support during this new treatment endeavor. The nurse-patient relationship often is the critical factor in determining patient and family cooperation with the clinical trial. Continuous reassurance should be offered to patients being treated on an outpatient basis with no clinically obvious tumor. The element of patient responsibility and commitment to complete therapy, if at all feasible, should be emphasized. The oncology nurse frequently is a trend setter: the nurse's knowledge, capability, attitude, and expectations often are adopted by the patient undergoing BRM therapy. This awareness will guide the nurse to strive continually for excellence in planning and implementing each patient's care.

FUTURE PERSPECTIVES

The significant scientific and technologic breakthroughs represented by recombinant DNA and hybridoma techniques drastically have altered the nature of immunologic research. The ability to produce large quantities of purified biologic products and the ability to alter those products to generate more favorable cellular traits create unlimited therapeutic potential.

The ultimate success of biologic response modifiers as a fourth modality of cancer treatment lies in further understanding the unique complexities of the human immune system. Major research studies that involve BRM agents and components of the immune system are in progress; new paradigms are being proposed and constantly analyzed. These results stimulate hope that biotherapy will provide a means for the specific treatment of cancer without the problem of nonspecific toxicities. The future appears bright.

Oncology nurses with a major interest in biologic response modifiers share in the growing pains and opportunities of a new cancer modality. The clinical trials designed to define clearly more successful therapies for the treatment of patients with cancer will offer oncology nurses a multiplicity of new opportunities and challenges. In clinical practice the nurse will have the opportunity to make significant contributions. Sophisticated nursing care will be provided to individuals with complex organ toxicities.

Nurses will be active in developing and standardizing policies and procedures for monitoring patients receiving BRMs.[197] Suppers and McClamrock[198] point out that clinical trials of BRM agents demand different nursing approaches for nurses who are accustomed to clinical trials of cytotoxic drugs, inasmuch as an immunomodulatory and/or antiproliferative effect also will need to be measured.[198] In addition, toxicities of BRMs may be subjective or subtle, making them difficult to accurately observe, measure, and document. Acute observation skills will be needed by nurses to enable them to detect and analyze the individual's response to the agent being studied. The nurse's attention to detail, and observation of and communication with the patient, will be crucial factors to the success of BRM clinical trials.

The possibilities for nursing research in the field of biotherapy are limitless.[199] Oncology nurses have an obligation to investigate current methods of caring for individuals receiving BRM agents and to make recommendations for improving that care. As new agents become available, nursing research studies should be designed to explore their implications for nursing practice and patient care. Nurse investigators and experienced oncology nurses also must assume their professional responsibility to disseminate new concepts in cancer management to other nurses in order to improve patient care through research, presentations, and publications.

Nurses who care for persons with cancer need to understand this treatment modality and to participate actively in its further development. Progress will come. Oncology nurses must seek, earn, and nurture a role in the development of biotherapy.

REFERENCES

1. Oldham RK, Smalley RV: Immunotherapy: The old and the new. J Biol Res Mod 2:1-37, 1983.
2. Oldham RK: Biologicals and biological response modifiers: Fourth modality of cancer treatment. Cancer Treat Rep 68:221-232, 1984.
3. Mihich E: Future perspectives for biological response modifiers: A viewpoint. Semin Oncol 13:234-254, 1986.
4. Fauci AS, Rosenberg SA, Sherwin SA, et al: Immunomodulators in clinical medicine. Ann Intern Med 106:421-433, 1987.
5. Moertel CG: On lymphokines, cytokines, and breakthroughs, JAMA 256:3141-3142, 1986 (Editorial).
6. Durant JR: Immunotherapy of cancer: The end or the beginning? N Engl J Med 316:939-941, 1987 (Editorial).
7. Huffer TL, Kanapa DJ, Stevenson HC: Basic immunology for paramedical professionals. Bethesda, Md, Clinical Investigations Sections, Biological Response Modifiers Program, National Cancer Institute, National Institutes of Health, 1985.
8. Clark JW, Longo DL: Biological response modifiers. Mediguide Oncol 6:1-10, 1986.
9. Goodfield, J: Dr. Coley's toxins. Science 84:68-73, 1984.
10. Mathé G, Amiel JL, Schwarzenberg L, et al: Active immunotherapy for acute lymphoblastic leukemia. Lancet 1:697-699, 1969.
11. Terry WD, Rosenberg SA (eds). Immunotherapy of human cancer. New York, Excerpta Medica, 1982, pp 55-60.
12. Smalley RV et al: Biological response modifiers: Current status and prospects as anti-cancer agents, in Herberman RB (ed): Basic and Clinical Tumor Immunology. Boston, Martinus Nijhoff, 1986.
13. Kohler G, Milstein C: Continuous cultures of fused cells secreting antibody of predefined specificity. Nature 256:495-497, 1975.
14. Schindler LW: Understanding the immune system. Bethesda, Md: Office of Research Reporting and Public Response, National Institute of Allergy and Infectious Diseases and the National Cancer Institute, National Institutes of Health, 1988, pp 28, 29; NIH pub no. 88-529.
15. Kohler G: Derivation and diversification of monoclonal antibodies. Science 233:1281-1286, 1986.
16. Harris OT, Mastrangelo MJ: Serotherapy of cancer. Semin Oncol 16:180-198, 1989.
17. Ritz J, Pesando JM, Sallan SE, et al: Serotherapy of acute lymphoblastic leukemia with monoclonal antibody. Blood 58:141-152, 1981.
18. Dillman RO, Shawler DL, Dillman JB, et al: Therapy of CLL and cutaneous T-cell lymphoma with T101 monoclonal antibody. J Clin Oncol 2:881-891, 1984.
19. Dillman RO, Shawler DL, Sobol RE, et al: Murine mono-

clonal antibody therapy in two patients with chronic lymphocytic leukemia. Blood 59:1036-1045, 1982.
20. Foon KA, Schroff RW, Bunn PA, et al: Effects of monoclonal antibody therapy in patients with chronic lymphocytic leukemia. Blood 64:1085-1093, 1984.
21. Meeher TC, Lowder J, Maloney DG, et al: A clinical trial of anti-idiotype therapy for B cell malignancy. Blood 65:1349-1363, 1985.
22. Meeher TC, Lowder J, Cleary ML, et al: Emergence of idiotype variants during treatment of B-cell lymphoma with anti-idiotype antibodies. N Engl J Med 312:1658-1665, 1985.
23. Rankin EM, Hekman A, Somers R, et al: Treatment of two patients with B cell lymphoma with monoclonal anti-idiotype antibodies. Blood 65:1373-1381, 1985.
24. Miller RA, Maloney DG, McKillop J, et al: In vivo effects of murine hybridoma monoclonal antibody in a patient with T-cell leukemia. Blood 58:78-86, 1981.
25. Miller RA, Levy R: Response of cutaneous T cell lymphoma to therapy with hybridoma monoclonal antibody. Lancet 2:226-230, 1981.
26. Miller RA, Oseroff AR, Stratte PT, et al: Monoclonal antibody therapeutic trials in seven patients with T cell lymphoma. Blood 62:988-995, 1983.
27. Bertram JH, Gill PS, Levine AS: Monoclonal antibody T101 in T cell malignancies: A clinical, pharmakokinetic and immunologic correlation. Blood 68:752-761, 1986.
28. Sears HF, Atkinson B, Herlyn D, et al: The use of monoclonal antibody in a phase I clinical trial of human gastrointestinal tumor. Lancet 1:762-765, 1982.
29. Sobol RE, Dillman RO, Smith JD, et al: Phase I evaluation of murine monoclonal anti-melanoma antibody in man: Preliminary observations, in Mitchell MS, Ottgen HF (eds): Hybridomas in Cancer Diagnosis and Treatment. New York, Raven Press, 1982, pp 199-206.
30. Goodman GE, Beaumier P, Hellstrom I, et al: Pilot trial of murine monoclonal antibodies in patients with advanced melonoma. J Clin Oncol 3:340-352, 1985.
31. Oldham RK, Foon KA, Morgan AC, et al: Monoclonal antibody therapy of malignant melanoma: In vivo localization in cutaneous metastasis after intravenous administration. J Clin Oncol 2:1235-1244, 1984.
32. Vadhan-Raj S, Cordon-Cardo C, Carswell E, et al: Phase I trial of mouse monoclonal antibody against GD3 ganglioside in patients with melanoma: Induction of inflammatory responses at tumor sites. J Clin Oncol 6:1636-1648, 1988.
33. Dippold WG, Bernhard H, Dienes HP, et al: Treatment of patients with malignant melanoma by monoclonal ganglioside antibodies. Eur J Cancer Clin Oncol 24:S65-S67, 1988 (suppl 2).
34. Coit D, Houghton A, Cordon-Cardo C, et al: Isolation limb perfusion with monoclonal antibody R24 in patients with malignant melanoma. Proc Am Soc Clin Oncol 7:248, 1988.
35. Lichtin A, Iliopoulos D, Guerry D, et al: Therapy of melanoma with an anti-melanoma ganglioside monoclonal antibody: A possible mechanism of complete response. Proc Am Soc Clin Oncol 7:247, 1988.
36. Cheung N-KV, Lazarus H, Miraldi FD, et al: Ganglioside GD2 specific monoclonal antibody 3F8: A phase I study in patients with neuroblastoma and malignant melanoma. J Clin Oncol 5:1430-1440, 1987.
37. Vitetta ES, Uhr JW: Immunotoxin. Annu Rev Immunol 3:197-212, 1985.
38. Pastan I, Willingham MC, Fitzgerald DJP: Immunotoxins. Cell 47:641-648, 1986.
39. Spitler L, delRio M, Khentigan A, et al: Therapy of patients with malignant melanoma using a monoclonal antimelanoma antibody recin A chain immunotoxin. Cancer Res 47:1717-1723, 1987.
40. Halpern SE, Dillman RO: Problems associated with radioimmunodetection and possibilities for future solution. J Biol Response Mod 6:235-262, 1987,
41. Mach JA, Bucheggar F, Forni M, et al: Use of radiolabeled monoclonal anti-CEA antibodies for detection of human carcinomas by external photoscanning and tomoscintigraphy. Immunol Today 2:239-249, 1981.
42. Carrasquillo JA, Bunn PA Jr, Keenan AM, et al: Radioimmunodetection of cutaneous T-cell lymphoma with "Inlabeled T101" monoclonal antibody. N Engl J Med 315:673-680, 1985.
43. Order SE, Sleeper AM, Stillwagon GB, et al: Current status of radioimmunoglobulins in the treatment of human malignancy. Oncology 3:115-130, 1989.
44. Bucholtz JD: Radiolabeled antibody therapy. Semin Oncol Nurs 3:67-73, 1987.
45. Dillman JB: Toxicity of monoclonal antibodies in the treatment of cancer. Semin Oncol Nurs 4:107-111, 1988.
46. Dinarello CA, Mier JW: Current concepts, lymphokines. N Engl J Med 317:940-945, 1987.
47. Isaacs A, Lindemann JJ: Virus interference: The interferon. Proc R Soc Lond [Biol] 147:258-267, 1957.
48. Oldham RK, Smalley RV: The role of interferon in the treatment of cancer, in Zoon KC, Noguchi PD, Lui TY (eds): Interferon Research: Clinical Application and Regulatory Consideraton. New York, Elsevier-North Holland, 1984.
49. Toufexis A, Jecius A: The big IF in cancer. Time, March 31:60-66, 1980.
50. Oldham RK: Biologicals for cancer treatment: Interferons. Hosp Pract, Dec 15:71-91, 1985.
51. Borden EC: Interferons: Rationale for clinical trials in neoplastic disease. Ann Intern Med 91:472-479, 1979.
52. Kirkwood JM, Ernstoff MS: Interferons in the treatment of human cancer. J Clin Oncol 2:336-352, 1984.
53. Boonem EA, Oldham RK: Gamma-interferon: Physiology and speculation on its role in medicine. J Biol Response Mod 6:275-301, 1987.
54. Goldstein D, Laszlo J: Interferon therapy in cancer: From imaginon to interferon. Cancer Res 46:4315-4329, 1986.
55. Balmer CM: The new alpha interferons. Drug Intell Pharm 19:887-893, 1985.
56. Higgins PG: Interferons. J Clin Pathol 37:109-116, 1984.
57. Rinehart JJ, Young D, Laforge J, et al: Phase I/II trial of recombinant gamma-interferon in patients with renal cell carcinoma: Immunologic and biologic effects. J Biol Response Mod 6:302-312, 1987.
58. Harglum JE: Interferon: Mechanisms of action and clinical value. Clin Pharm 2:20-28, 1983.
59. Mitsuyasu RT: The role of alpha interferon in the biotherapy of hematologic malignancies and AIDS-related Kaposi's sarcoma. Oncol Nurs Forum 6:7-12, 1988 (suppl).
60. Spiegel RJ: Clinical overview of alpha interferon. Cancer 59:626-631, 1987.
61. Groopman JE: Therapeutic options in hairy-cell leukemia. Semin Oncol 12:30-34, 1985.
62. Roth MS, Foon KA: Alpha interferon in the treatment of hematologic malignancies. Am J Med 81:871-882, 1986.
63. Quesda JR, Gutterman JU, Hersh EV: Treatment of hairy-cell leukemia with alpha interferons. Cancer 57:1678-1680, 1986.
64. Figlin RA: Biotherapy with interferon in solid tumors. Oncol Nurs Forum 6:23-26, 1987 (suppl).
65. Quesada JR, Rios A, Swanson D, et al: Antitumor activity

of recombinant-derived interferon alpha in metastatic renal cell carcinoma. J Clin Oncol 3:1522-1528, 1985.

66. Umeda T, Niijima T: Phase II study of alpha interferon on renal cell carcinoma: Summary of three collaborative trials. Cancer 58:1231-1235,1986.
67. Buzaid AC, Robertone A, Kisala C, et al: Phase II study of interferon alfa-2a, recombinant (Roferon-A) in metastatic renal cell carcinoma. J Clin Oncol 5:1083-1089, 1987.
68. Legha SS, Papadopoulos NEJ, Plager C, et al: Clinical evaluation of recombinant interferon alpha-2A (Roferon-A) in metastatic melanoma using two different schedules. J Clin Oncol 5:1240-1246, 1987.
69. Creagan ET, Ahmann DL, Frytak S, et al: Recombinant leukocyte A interferon (rIFN-α-A) in the treatment of disseminated malignant melanoma: Analysis of complete and long-term responding patients. Cancer 58:2576-2578, 1986.
70. Oberg K, Norheim I, Lind E, et al: Treatment of malignant carcinoid tumors with human leukocyte interferon: Long-term results. Cancer Treat Rep 70:1297-1304, 1986.
71. Torti FM, Shortliffe LD, Williams RD, et al: Alpha-interferon in superficial bladder cancer. A northern California oncology group study. J Clin Oncol 6:476-483, 1988.
72. Berek JS, Hacher NJ, Lichtenstein A, et al: Intraperitoneal recombinant α-interferon for "salvage" immunotherapy in stage III epithelial ovarian cancer: A gynecologic oncology group study. Cancer Res 75:4447-4453, 1985.
73. Von Wussow P, Block B, Hartmann F, et al: Intralesional interferon-alpha therapy in advanced malignant melanoma. Cancer 61:1071-1074, 1988.
74. Greenway HT, Cornell RC, Tanner DJ, et al: Treatment of basal cell carcinoma with intralesional interferon. J Am Acad Dermatol 15:437-443, 1986.
75. Spiegel RJ: Additional indications for interferon therapy: Basal cell carcinoma, carcinoid, and chronic active hepatitis. Semin Oncol 15:41-45, 1988 (suppl 51).
76. Eddelston A: Interferons in the treatment of chronic hepatitis B virus infection. Med Clin North Am, May:25-30, 1986 (suppl).
77. LaBanda F, Moreno MR, Carreno V, et al: Recombinant α-interferon treatment in children with chronic hepatitis. Lancet 1:250, 1988.
78. Hoofnagle JH, Mullen KD, Jones B, et al: Treatment of chronic non-A, non-B hepatitis with recombinant human alpha interferon. N Engl J Med 315:1575-1578, 1986.
79. Krown SE, Real FX, Cunningham-Rundles S, et al: Preliminary observations on the effect of recombinant leukocyte A interferon in homosexual men with Kaposi's sarcoma. N Engl J Med 308:1071-1076, 1983.
80. Krown SE, Real FX, Krim M, et al: Recombinant leukocyte A interferon in Kaposi's sarcoma. Ann NY Acad Sci 437:431-438, 1984.
81. Real FX, Dettgen HF, Krown SE: Kaposi's sarcoma and the acquired immunodeficiency syndrome: Treatment with high and low doses of recombinant leukocyte A interferon. J Clin Oncol 4:544-551, 1986.
82. Groopman JE, Gottlieb MS, Goodman J, et al: Recombinant alpha-2 interferon therapy for Kaposi's sarcoma associated with the acquired immuno-deficiency syndrome. Ann Intern Med 100:671-676, 1984.
83. Rios A, Mansell PWA, Newell, GA, et al: Treatment of acquired immunodeficiency syndrome–related Kaposi's sarcoma with lymphoblastoid interferon. J Clin Oncol 3:506-512, 1985.
84. Abrams DI, Volberding PA: Alpha interferon therapy of AIDS-associated Kaposi's sarcoma. Semin Oncol 14:43-47, 1987 (suppl 2).
85. Krown SE: The role of interferon in the therapy of epidemic Kaposi's sarcoma. Semin Oncol 14:27-33, 1987 (suppl 3).
86. Ho DD, Rota TR, Kaplan JC, et al: Recombinant human interferon alpha-A, suppresses HTLV-III replication in vitro. Lancet 1:602-604, 1985.
87. Krown SE, Bundow D, Gansbacher B, et al: Interferon-alpha plus zidovirdine in AIDS-associated Kaposi's sarcoma: An ongoing phase I trial. Proc Am Soc Clin Oncol 7:1, 1988 (abstr 2).
88. Van der Berg M, Edelstein M, Gerlis L, et al: Recombinant interferon (Immuneron): Results of a phase I trial in patients with cancer. J Biol Response Mod 4:264-272, 1985.
89. Vadhan-Raj S, Al-Katib A, Bhalla R, et al: Phase I trial of recombinant interferon gamma in cancer patients. J Clin Oncol 4:137-146, 1986.
90. Thompson JA, Cos WW, Lindgren CG, et al: Subcutaneous recombinant gamma interferon in cancer patients: Toxicity, pharmacokinetics and immunomodulatory effects. Cancer Immunol Immunother 25:47-53, 1987.
91. Ernstoff MS, Trautman, T, Davis CA, et al: A randomized phase I/II study of continuous versus intermittent interferon gamma in patients with metastatic melanoma. J Clin Oncol 5:1804-1810, 1987.
92. Quesada JR, Talpaz M, Rios A, et al: Clinical toxicity of interferons in cancer patients: A review. J Clin Oncol 4:234-243, 1986.
93. Kirkwood JM, Ernstoff MS: A clinical update: The role of interferon in the biotherapy of solid tumors. Oncol Nurs Forum 6:3-6, 1988 (suppl).
94. Mayer D, Hetrick K. Riggs C, et al: Weight loss in patients receiving recombinant leukocyte A interferon (IFNrA): A brief report. Cancer Nurs 7:53-56, 1984.
95. Spiegel RJ: Intron A (interferon alpha-2b): Clinical overview and future directions. Semin Oncol 13:89-101, 1986 (suppl 2).
96. Figlin RA: Biotherapy with interferon—1988. Semin Oncol 15:3-9, 1988 (suppl 6).
97. Steis RG, Smith JW II, Urba WJ, et al: Resistance to recombinant interferon alpha-2a in hairy-cell leukemia associated with neutralizing anti-interferon antibodies. N Engl J Med 318:1409-1413, 1988.
98. Libby P, Ordovas JM, Birinyi LK, et al: Inducible interleukin-1 gene expression in human vascular smooth muscle cells. J Clin Invest 78:1432-1438, 1986.
99. Dinarello CA: Interleukin-1 and the pathogenesis of the acute-phase response. N Engl J Med 311:1413-1418, 1984.
100. Morgan DA, Ruscetti FW, Gallo R: Selective in vitro growth of T lymphocytes from normal human bone marrows. Science 193:1007-1008, 1976.
101. Ortaldo JR, Mason AT, Gerard JP, et al: Effects of natural and recombinant IL-2 on regulation of IFN production and natural killer activity: Lack of involvement of the TAC antigen for these immunoregulatory effects. J Immunol 133:779-783, 1984.
102. Ruscetti FW, Gallo RC: Human lymphocyte growth factor: Regulation of growth and function of T-lymphocytes. Blood 57:379-394, 1981.
103. Wanebo HS, Pace R, Hargett S, et al: Production of and response to interleukin-2 in peripheral blood lymphocytes of cancer patients. Cancer 57:656-662, 1986.
104. Ettinghausen SE, Lipford EH III, Mule JJ, et al: Systemic administration of recombinant interleukin-2 stimulates in vivo lymphoid cell proliferation in tissues. J Immunol 135:1488-1497, 1985.
105. Siegel JP, Lane HC, Stocks NI, et al: Pharmacokinetics of lymphocyte-derived and recombinant DNA-derived inter-

leukin-2 after intravenous administration to patients with the acquired immunodeficiency syndrome. J Biol Response Mod 4:596-601, 1985.
106. Donohue JH, Rosenberg SA: The fate of interleukin-2 after in vivo administration. J Immunol 130:2203-2208, 1983.
107. Chang AE, Hyatt CL, Rosenberg SA: Systemic administration of recombinant interleukin-2 in mice. J Biol Response Mod 3:561-572, 1984.
108. Lotze MT, Matory YL, Ettinghausen SE, et al: In vivo administration of purified human interleukin-2. II. Half-life, immunologic effects, and expansion of peripheral lymphoid cells in vivo with recombinant IL-2. J Immunol 135:2865-2875, 1985.
109. Bindon C, Czerniecki M, Ruell P, et al: Clearance rates and systemic effects of intravenously administered interleukin-2 (IL-2) containing preparations in human subjects. Br J Cancer 47:123-133, 1983.
110. Lotze MT, Frana LW, Sharrow SO, et al: In vivo administration of purified human interleukin-2. I. Half-life and immunologic effects of the Jurkat cell line–derived interleukin-2. J Immunol 134:157-166, 1985.
111. Rosenberg SA, Lotze MT, Mueel LM, et al: Observations on the systemic administration of autologous lymphokine-activated killer cells and recombinant interleukin-2 to patients with metastatic cancer. N Engl J Med 313:1485-1492, 1985.
112. Rosenberg SA: Immunotherapy of cancer by systemic administration of lymphoid cells plus interleukin-2. J Biol Response Mod 3:501-511, 1984.
113. Lotze MT, Matory YL, Rayner AA, et al: Clinical effects and toxicity of interleukin-2 in patients with cancer. Cancer 58:2764-2772, 1986.
114. Lotze MT, Chang AE, Seipp CA, et al: High-dose recombinant interleukin-2 in the treatment of patients with disseminated cancer. JAMA 256:3117-3124, 1986.
115. Atkins MB, Gould JA, Allegretta M, et al: Phase I evaluation of recombinant interleukin-2 in patients with advanced malignant disease. J Clin Oncol 4:1380-1391, 1986.
116. Rosenberg SA, Lotz MT, Mueel LM, et al: A progress report on the treatment of 157 patients with advanced cancer using lymphokine-activated killer cells and interleukin-2 or high dose interleukin-2 alone. N Engl J Med 316:889-897, 1987.
117. West WH, Tauer KW, Yannelli JR, et al: Constant-infusion recombinant interleukin-2 in adoptive immunotherapy of advanced cancer. N Engl J Med 316:898-905, 1987.
118. Bylinsky G: Science scores a cancer breakthrough. Fortune 112:16-21, 1985.
119. Fisher RI, Coltman CA, Doroshow JH, et al: Metastatic renal cancer treated with interleukin-2 and lymphokine-activated killer cells. Ann Intern Med 108:518-523, 1988.
120. Dutcher JP, Creekmore SP, Weiss GR, et al: A phase II study of interleukin-2 and lymphokine-activated killer cells in patients with metastatic malignant melanoma. J Clin Oncol 7:477-485, 1989.
121. Thompson MS, Kempf RA, Harel W, et al: Influence of dose and duration of infusion of interleukin-2 on toxicity and immunomodulation. J Clin Oncol 4:669-678, 1988.
122. Yron I, Wood TA Jr, Spiess P, et al: In vitro growth of murine T cells. The isolation and growth of lymphoid cells infiltrating syngeneic solid tumors. J Immunol 125:238-245, 1980.
123. Rosenberg SA, Spiess P, Lafreniere R: A new approach to the adoptive immunotherapy of cancer with tumor-infiltrating lymphocytes. Science 233:1318-1321, 1986.
124. Topalian SL, Solomon D, Avis FP, et al: Immunotherapy of patients with advanced cancer using tumor-infiltrating lymphocytes and recombinant interleukin-2. A pilot study. J Clin Oncol 16:839-853, 1988.
125. Rosenberg SA, Packard BS, Aebersold PM, et al: Use of tumor-infiltrating lymphocytes and interleukin-2 in the immunotherapy of patients with metasatic melanoma. N Engl J Med 319:1676-1680, 1988.
126. Winkelhake JL, Stampfl S, Zimmerman RJ: Synergistic effects of combination therapy with human recombinant interleukin-2 and tumor necrosis factor in murine tumor models. Cancer Res 47:3948-3953, 1987.
127. Papa MZ, Yang JC, Vetto JT, et al: Combined effects of chemotherapy and interleukin-2 in the therapy of mice with advanced pulmonary tumors. Cancer Res 48:122-129, 1988.
128. Munn DH, Cheun N-KV: Interleukin-2 enhancement of monoclonal antibody-mediated cellular cytotoxicity against human melanoma. Cancer Res 47:6600-6605, 1987.
129. Iigo M, Sakurai M, Tamura T, et al: In vivo activity of multiple injections of recombinant interleukin-2, alone and in combination with three different types of recombinant interferon, on various syngeneic murine tumors. Cancer Res 48:260-264, 1988.
130. Krigel RL, Padavic-Shaller KA, Rudolph AR, et al: A-phase I study of recombinant interleukin-2 plus recombinant β-interferon. Cancer Res 48:3875-3881, 1988.
131. Rosenberg SA, Lotze MT, Yand JC, et al: Experience with the use of high dose interleukin-2 in the treatment of 652 patients with cancer. Ann Surg (in press).
132. Herberman RB: Interleukin-2 therapy of human cancer: Potential benefits versus toxicity. J Clin Oncol 7:1-4, 1989 (Editorial).
133. Lee RE, Lotze MT, Skibber JM, et al: Cardiorespiratory effects of immunotherapy with interleukin-2. J Clin Oncol 7:7-20, 1989.
134. Margolin KA, Rayner AA, Hawkins MJ, et al: Interleukin-2 and lymphokine-activated killer cell therapy of solid tumors: Analysis of toxicity and management guidelines. J Clin Oncol 7:486-498, 1989.
135. Gaynor ER, Vitek L, Sticklin L, et al: The hemodynamic effects of treatment with interleukin-2 and lymphokine-activated killer cells. Ann Intern Med 109:953-958, 1988.
136. Kozeny GA, Nicolas JD, Creekmore S, et al: Effects of interleukin-2 immunotherapy on renal function. J Clin Oncol 6:1170-1176, 1988.
137. Parkinson DR: Interleukin-2 in cancer therapy. Semin Oncol 15:10-26, 1988.
138. Atkins MB, Mier JW, Parkinson DR, et al: Hypothyroidism after treatment with interleukin-2 and lymphokine-activated killer cells. N Engl J Med 318:1556-1563, 1988.
139. Carswell EA, Old LJ, Kassel RC, et al: An endotoxin induced serum factor that causes necrosis of tumors. Proc Natl Acad Sci USA 72:3666-3670, 1975.
140. Haranaka K, Satomi N: Cytotoxic activity of tumor necrosis factor (TNF) on the human cancer cells in vitro. Jpn J Exp Med 51:191-194, 1981.
141. Salmon SE, Young L, Scuderi P, et al: Antineoplastic effects on tumor necrosis factor alone and in combination with gamma-interferon on tumor biopsies in clonogenic assay. J Clin Oncol 5:1816-1821, 1987.
142. Old L: Tumor necrosis factor (rTNF). Science 230:630-632, 1985.
143. Currie GA, Basham C: Activated macrophages release a factor which lyses malignant cells but not normal cells. J Exp Med 142:1600-1605, 1975.
144. Mannel DN, Moore RN, Mergenhagen SE: Macrophages as a source of tumoricidal activity (tumor necrotizing factor). Infect Immun 30:523-530, 1980.

145. Aggarwal BB, Kohr WJ, Hass PE, et al: Human tumor necrosis factor: Production, purification, and characterization. J Biol Chem 260:2345-2354, 1985.
146. Beutler B, Milsark IW, Cerami A: Cachectin/tumor necrosis factor: Production, distribution, and metabolic fate in vivo. J Immunol 135:3972-3977, 1985.
147. Darzynkiewicz Z, Williamson B, Carswell EA, et al: Cell cycle–specific effects of tumor necrosis factor. Cancer Res 44:83-90, 1984.
148. Sugarman BJ, Aggarwal BB, Hass PE, et al: Recombinant tumor necrosis factor–alpha: Effects on proliferation of normal and transformed cells in vitro. Science 230:943-945, 1985.
149. Michie HR, Manogue KR, Spriggs DR, et al: Detection of circulating tumor necrosis factor after endotoxin administration. N Engl J Med 318:1481-1486, 1988.
150. Peetre C, Gullberg U, Nilsson E, et al: Effects of recombinant tumor necrosis factor on proliferation and differentiation of leukemic and normal hematopoietic cells in vitro. J Clin Invest 78:1694-1700, 1986.
151. Broxmayer HE, Williams DE, Lu L, et al: The suppressive influences of human tumor necrosis factors on bone marrow hematopoietic progenitor cells from normal donors and patients with leukemia: Synergism of TNF and gamma interferon. J Immunol 136:4487-4495, 1986.
152. Larrick JW, Graham D, Toy K, et al: Recombinant tumor necrosis factor causes activation of human granulocytes. Blood 69:640-644, 1987.
153. Nawroth PP, Stern DM: Modulation of endothelial cell hemostatic properties by tumor necrosis factor. J Exp Med 163:740-745, 1986.
154. Bevilacqua MP, Dober JS, Majeau GR, et al: Recombinant tumor necrosis factor induces procoagulant activity in cultured human vascular endothelium: Characterization and comparison with the actions of interleukin 1. Proc Natl Acad Sci USA 83:4533-4537, 1986.
155. Broudy VC, Kaushansky K, Segal GM, et al: Tumor necrosis factor type alpha stimulates endothelial cells to produce granulocyte/macrophage colony stimulating factor. Proc Natl Acad Sci USA 83:7467-7471, 1986.
156. Le J, Weinstein D, Gubler U, et al: Induction of membrane associated interleukin 1 by tumor necrosis factor in human fibroblasts. J Immunol 138:2137-2142, 1987.
157. Michie HR, Spriggs DR, Manogue KR, et al: Tumor necrosis factor and endotoxin induce similar metabolic responses in human beings. Surgery 104:280-286, 1988.
158. Bachwich PR, Chensue SW, Larrick JW, et al: Tumor necrosis factor stimulates interleukin 1 and prostaglandin E_2 production in resting macrophages. Biochem Biophys Res Commun 136:94-101, 1986.
159. Chapman PB, Lester TJ, Casper ES, et al: Clinical pharmacology of recombinant human tumor necrosis factor in patients with advanced cancer. J Clin Oncol 5:1942-1951, 1987.
160. Jakubowski AA, Casper ES, Gabrilove JL, et al: Phase I trial of intramuscularly administered tumor necrosis factor in patients with advanced cancer. J Clin Oncol 7:298-303, 1989.
161. Sherman ML, Spriggs DR, Arthur KA, et al: Recombinant human tumor necrosis factor administered as a five-day continuous infusion in cancer patients: Phase I toxicity and effects on lipid metabolism. J Clin Oncol 6:344-350, 1988.
162. Morice RC, Blick MB, Ali MK, et al: Pulmonary toxicity of recombinant tumor necrosis factor (rTNF). Proc Am Soc Clin Oncol 6:29, 1987.
163. Clark SC, Kamen R: The human hematopoietic colony-stimulating factors. Science 246:1229-1237, 1987.
164. Haeuber D, DiJulio JE: Hemopoietic colony stimulating factors: An overview. Oncol Nurs Forum 16:247-255, 1989.
165. Gabrilove JL: Introduction and overview of hematopoietic growth factors. Semin Hematol 26:1-4, 1989.
166. Gutterman J: Clinical studies of granulocyte-macrophage colony stimulating factor. Semin Oncol 15:52-53, 1988.
167. Eschbach J, Egrie J, Downing M, et al: Correction of the anemia of end-stage renal disease with recombinant human erythropoietin: Results of a combined phase I and II clinical trial. N Engl J Med 316:73-78, 1987.
168. Cannistra SA, Griffin JD: Regulation of the production and function of granulocytes and monocytes. Semin Hematol 25:173-188, 1988.
169. Groopman JE, Mitsuyasu RT, Deleo MJ, et al: Effects of recombinant human granulocyte-macrophage colony-stimulating factor on myelopoiesis in the acquired immunodeficiency syndrome. N Engl J Med 317:593-598, 1987.
170. Vadhan-Raj S, Keating J, LeMaistre A, et al: Effects of recombinant human granulocyte-macrophage colony-stimulating factor in patients with myelodysplastic syndromes. N Engl J Med 317:1547-1552, 1987.
171. Gabrilove JL, Jakubowski A, Scher H, et al: Effect of granulocyte colony-stimulating factor on neutropenia and associated morbidity due to chemotherapy for transitional-cell carcinoma of the urothelium. N Engl J Med 318:1414-1422, 1988.
172. Brandt BJ, Peters WP, Atwater SK, et al: Effect of recombinant human granulocyte-macrophage colony-stimulating factor on hematopoietic reconstruction after high-dose chemotherapy and autologous bone marrow transplantation. N Engl J Med 318:869-876, 1988.
173. Peters WP: The effect of recombinant human colony-stimulating factors on hematopoietic reconstitution following autologous bone marrow transplantation. Semin Hematol 26:18-23, 1989 (suppl 2).
174. Bronchud, MH, Scarffe JH, Thatcher N, et al: Phase I/II study of recombinant human granulocyte colony-stimulating factor in patients receiving intensive chemotherapy for small cell lung cancer. Br J Cancer 56:809-813, 1987.
175. Champlin RE, Nimer SD, Oette D, et al: Granulocyte-macrophage colony-stimulating factor (GM-CSF) treatment for aplastic anemia (AA) or agranulocytosis. Exp Hematol 6:238, 1988 (abstr).
176. Antman KS, Griffin JD, Elias A, et al: Effect of recombinant human granulocyte-macrophage colony-stimulating factor on chemotherapy-induced myelosuppression. N Engl J Med 319:593-598, 1988.
177. Thompson JA, Lee DJ, Kidd P, et al: Subcutaneous granulocyte-macrophage colony-stimulating factor in patients with myelodysplastic syndrome: Toxicity, pharmacokinetics, and hematological effects. J Clin Oncol 7:629-637, 1989.
178. Griffin JD, Hemopoietins in oncology: Factoring out myelosuppression. J Clin Oncol 7:151-155, 1989.
179. Herrmann F, Schulz G, Lindemann A, et al: Hematopoietic responses in patients with advanced malignancy treated with recombinant human granulocyte-macrophage colony-stimulating factor. J Clin Oncol 7:159-167, 1989.
180. Andreeff M, Welte K: Hematopoietic colony-stimulating factors. Semin Oncol 16, 211-229, 1989.
181. Morstyn G, Lieschke GJ, Sheridan W, et al: Clinical experience with recombinant human granulocyte colony-stimulating factor. Semin Hematol 26:9-13, 1989 (suppl 2).
182. Glaspy JA, Golde DW: Clinical applications of the myeloid growth factors. Semin Hematol 26:14-17, 1989 (suppl 2).

183. Negrin R, Haeuber D, Nagler A, et al: Treatment of myelodysplastic syndromes with recombinant human granulocyte colony-stimulating factor. Proceedings of the International Society of Experimental Hematology, August 1988 (abstr).
184. Tripodi D, Parks LC, Brugmans J: Drug induced restoration of cutaneous delayed hypersensitivity in anergic patients with cancer. N Engl J Med 289:354-357, 1973.
185. Oldham RK, Smalley RV: Biologicals and biological response modifiers, in Devita VT, Hellman S, Rosenberg SA (eds): Cancer: Principles and Practice of Oncology ed 2. Philadelphia, JB Lippincott, 1985.
186. Levamisole hydrochloride. AHFS Drug Information: suppl A, 26A-27A, 1989.
187. Lynch MT: The nurse's role in the biotherapy of cancer: Clinical trials and informed consent. Oncol Nurs Forum 15:23-27, 1988 (suppl).
188. Irwin MM: Patients receiving biological response modifiers: Overview of nursing care. Oncol Nurs Forum 14:32-37, 1987 (suppl).
189. Simpson C, Seipp CA, Rosenberg SA: The current status and future applications of interleukin-2 and adoptive immunotherapy in cancer treatment. Semin Oncol Nurs 4:132-141, 1988.
190. Padavic-Schaller K: IL-2: Nursing applications in a developing science. Semin Oncol Nurs 4:142-149, 1988.
191. Jassak PF, Sticklin LA: Interleukin-2: An overview. Oncol Nurs Forum 13:17-22, 1986.
192. Held J, McLaughlin P: Antiferritin immunoglobulin therapy for treatment of hepatoma. Oncol Nurs Forum 14:27-31, 1987.
193. Moldawer NP, Figlin RA: Tumor necrosis factor: Current clinical status and implications for nursing management. Semin Oncol Nurs 4:120-125, 1988.
194. Hahn MB, Jassak PF: Nursing management of patients receiving interferon. Semin Oncol Nurs 4:95-101, 1988.
195. Hood LE: Interferon. Am J Nurs 87:459-465, 1987.
196. Haeuber D: Recent advances in the management of biotherapy-related side effects: Flu-like syndrome. Oncol Nurs Forum 16:35-41, 1989 (suppl).
197. Carter P, Engelking C, Rumsey K, et al: Biological Response Modifier Guidelines. Recommendations for Nursing Education and Practice. Pittsburgh: Oncology Nursing Society, 1989.
198. Suppers VJ, McClamrock EA: Biologicals in cancer treatment: Future effects on nursing practice. Oncol Nurs Forum 12:27-32, 1985.
199. Strauman JJ: The nurse's role in the biotherapy of cancer: Nursing research of side effects. Oncol Nurs Forum 15:35-39, 1988 (suppl).

Chapter 15

Bone Marrow Transplantation

Patricia Corcoran Buchsel, RN, BSN

INTRODUCTION

Bone marrow transplantation (BMT) has evolved during the past 30 years from an experimental procedure to an established and effective treatment for selected patients. The number of recipients of marrow transplantation has increased over the last decade: more than 10,000 transplants have been performed worldwide in more than 200 marrow transplantation centers.[1] As BMT is used as a treatment for an expanding list of diseases, oncology nurses will care for larger numbers of marrow graft recipients and their donors and families. Clinical and technical nursing skills required to care for marrow recipients include proficiencies in oncology and hematology, pediatric nursing, ambulatory and home health nursing, critical care nursing, nursing research, and administration.[2]

HISTORY

The earliest description of marrow transplantation in humans was reported by Brown-Séquard in 1891 in the form of an extract of marrow given by mouth to patients with pernicious anemia and lymphadenoma.[3] In 1937 Schretzenmayr administered bone marrow intramuscularly. Although his studies were encouraging, they were not accepted by his peers.[4] These early attempts were soon followed, but without success, by the use of marrow given by the intramedullary and intravenous routes.[4]

After World War II, studies of radiation-induced bone marrow failure led to the treatment of patients with aplastic anemia and marrow failure after irradiation with infusions of bone marrow.[5] In 1949 and 1951, research in murine and canine models showed that animals given lethal doses of irradiation survived after parenteral infusion of bone marrow.[6] The first modern human marrow transplantations were conducted without success in patients with end-stage diseases. It was not until the mid-1960s that medical research focused on the importance of human tissue typing and applied these concepts to organ and marrow transplantation.[7] By the late 1960s, after the institution of histocompatible human leukocyte antigen (HLA) typing to identify suitable sibling donors, successful human allogeneic transplantations were carried out in increasing numbers. Simultaneously, the technology of platelet transfusions and methods of prophylaxis against infection were developed.[8,9] Today, intermediate post-transplantation care given in outpatient settings has been established as a safe and cost-effective method of caring for marrow recipients.[10] The number of long-term survivors of marrow transplantation (disease-free 1 year after BMT) has increased with advances in medical technology and the support of the immunosuppressed patient.

DISEASES TREATED WITH MARROW TRANSPLANTATION

Diseases treated with marrow transplantation fall into two categories: (1) malignant and (2) nonmalignant disease.[11] Table 15-1 summarizes results and long-term survival rates after allogeneic and autologous marrow transplantation.

Malignant Disease

Originally only patients with leukemia refractory to conventional therapy were considered for marrow transplantation. Successful marrow grafts now are performed in patients with a variety of hematologic and nonhematologic disorders. Hematologic malignancies are acute and chronic leukemias, myelosclerosis, and preleukemias. Nonhematologic diseases treated with BMT are lymphoma, multiple myeloma, hairy cell leukemia, neuroblastoma, and selected solid tumors.[9,12]

TABLE 15-1 Results of Marrow Transplantation

Disease	Disease State	Type of Transplant	Relapse Rate (%)	Long-Term Survival Rate (%)
Acute lymphocytic leukemia	Remission (second)	Allogeneic	30-50	25-50
	Relapse	Allogeneic	50-70	10-20
	Remission	Autologous	35	43
	Relapse	Autologous	>50	15
Acute nonlymphocytic leukemia	First remission	Allogeneic	10-40	40-70
	Second or more remission	Allogeneic	Unknown	20-50
	First relapse	Allogeneic	Unknown	20-34
	Second or more relapse	Allogeneic	50-70	25-30
	Remission	Autologous	32	40-48
	Relapse	Autologous	>50	30
Chronic myelogenous leukemia	Chronic phase	Allogeneic	12-25	45-60
	Accelerated phase	Allogeneic	40-60	15-29
	Blast crisis	Allogeneic	50-80	5-18
Preleukemic	N/A	Allogeneic	11-15	50-60
Metastatic neuroblastoma	N/A	Allogeneic	20	40
	N/A	Autologous	20	40
Aplastic anemia	Untransfused patient	Allogeneic	N/A	50-81
	Transfused patient	Allogeneic	N/A	40-75
Thalassemia	N/A	Allogeneic	N/A	75
Lymphoma (Hodgkin's or non-Hodgkin's)	Multiple relapses	Allogeneic	60	22
		Autologous	60	Not known
	First relapse or Second remission	Allogeneic	40	40
		Autologous	Not known	Not known
		Syngeneic	60	30

NA, Not applicable.

Nonmalignant Disease

Severe aplastic anemia, thalassemia major, and cyclic neutropenia are hematopoietic deficiencies that respond well to marrow transplantation therapy. Patients with severe aplastic anemia and thalassemia major have their immune systems ablated with immunosuppressive drugs to prevent marrow graft rejections.[6]

Immunologic deficiencies

Immunodeficiency diseases represent another category of life-threatening diseases that may be corrected by marrow transplantation. Cures have been reported in patients with severe combined immunodeficiency disease, Wiskott-Aldrich syndrome, and some rare inherited disorders.[11,12]

Inborn errors of metabolism

Diseases of inborn errors such as chronic granulomatous disease, osteoporosis, mucopolysaccharidosis, and lipidosis are treated with marrow transplantation.[5,7]

TYPES OF BONE MARROW TRANSPLANTATIONS

The type of bone marrow transplantation depends on the availability of a suitable donor, who is identified by histocompatibility typing, and on the disease being treated. There are three sources of donor marrow: autologous, syngeneic, and allogeneic.

Autologous

An autologous (self) marrow graft is a transplant in which a patient with a malignant disease receives his or her own marrow (collected and cryopreserved during remission) after preparation with high-dose preparative conditioning. Relapse of malignancy, which is a potential concern after autologous marrow transplantation, may be due to (1) failure of the pretransplantation conditioning therapy to successfully eradicate residual host tumor cells and (2) the presence of malignant cells that may contaminate the autologous marrow.

Syngeneic

A syngeneic marrow transplant is one in which the donor is an identical twin who by definition is a perfect HLA match. Conditioning regimens are determined by the disease being treated.[7] A higher incidence of leukemic relapse has been reported in syngeneic than in allogeneic marrow recipients because of the demonstrated antileukemic effect of graft-versus-host disease (GVHD).[7] This is known as graft-versus-leukemia effect and is discussed later in this chapter.

Allogeneic

Allogeneic marrow transplantation depends on the availability of an HLA-matched donor. GVHD, a complication unique to allogeneic marrow transplantation, is a major impediment to successful transplantation and is discussed later in this chapter. Intensive supportive care with protective environments, gut decontaminants, prophylactic and therapeutic antibiotics, and red cell, platelet, and granulocyte transfusions are required. Specialized nursing care is essential to manage the care of these patients.[13]

TISSUE TYPING

Human Leukocyte Antigen/Mixed Lymphocyte Culture

The basis for selection of the most appropriate donor begins with an understanding of the major histocompatibility complex in humans, which is composed of a series of closely linked genetic loci on chromosome 6. The antigens located at HLA-A and HLA-B loci are defined serologically, and those at the HLA-D locus are detected by the mixed leukocyte culture (MLC) test. A locus identical with or closely related to HLA-D, called HLA-DR, can be serologically typed by means of B lymphocytes. The chromosomal region is known as a haplotype. Every person inherits one haplotype from each parent, and within any given family there can be only four haplotypes. There is approximately a 25% chance for every patient to be HLA-matched with a sibling[14] (Figure 15-1). Until recent years most allogeneic transplantations were from HLA-identical siblings, but selected family members or unrelated phenotypically identical donors have been used successfully as marrow donors.[15]

ABO Typing

Major ABO-incompatible marrow grafting can be performed without significant hemolytic transfusion reaction.

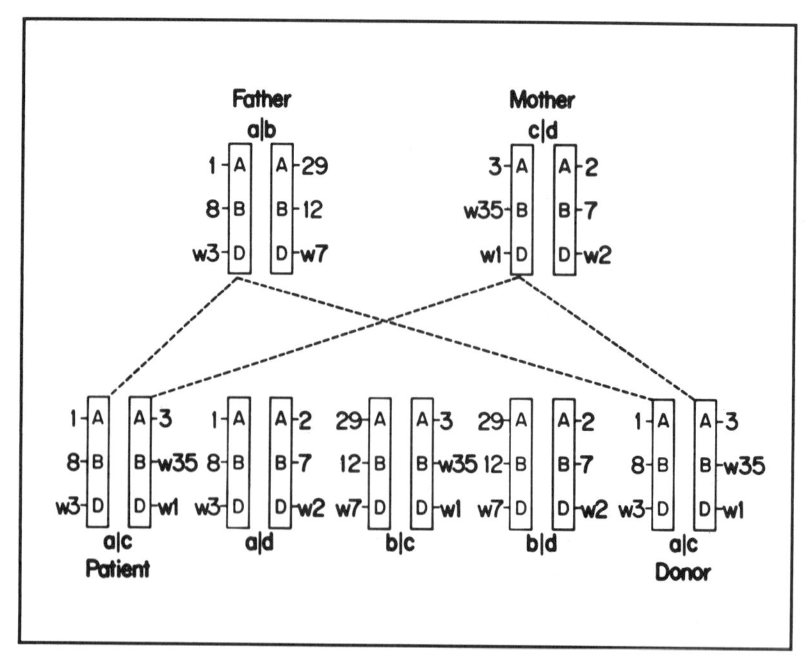

FIGURE 15-1 Diagram of the possible combinations of the human leukocyte antigen (HLA) region of chromosome 6 inherited from parents to siblings. The patient and donor have inherited the same haplotypes and are genotypically identical.

Effective techniques to remove red blood cells from donor marrow and plasma exchange of patient marrow have reduced the risk of acute hematologic transfusion reaction.[16] Blood group typing, however, must be done on patients and all potential donors.[17] If unmanipulated incompatible ABO marrow is transfused, it, like any incompatible blood product transfusion, will cause major hemolytic transfusion reaction, and these reactions can result in death. After transplantation the patient's ABO type will become the same as that of the marrow donor.

SELECTION OF THE MARROW DONOR

Donor selection is based on the availability of an appropriate donor who is suitably HLA- and MLC-matched.[18] Tissue typing is done on all family members. If there is not a match, or if the patient's disease is not treatable with an autologous graft, an unrelated donor search may be initiated.

National and international marrow registries involving more than 50 blood centers and more than 100,000 volunteer marrow donors hold promise for increasing the number of potential donors for transplantation. Research designed to further clarify tissue incompatibility will enlarge related and unrelated donor pools. Important ethical issues will emerge in terms of donor risks, protections, and reimbursements.[19,20]

Determination of serum cytomegalovirus (CMV) antibody status is performed for the patient and donor. For CMV-seronegative patients with seronegative marrow donors, CMV infection may be effectively prevented by exclusive use of CMV-seronegative blood products.[21]

A major impediment for wider application of allogeneic BMT is the limited number of HLA-identical siblings available to serve as donors. It has been possible to extend the donor pool by the use of selectively mismatched family member donors or matched unrelated donors.[19] Many of these recipients have achieved prolonged long-term survival.[22] As methods of GVHD prophylaxis improve and more volunteer donors are identified, the use of unrelated donors may increase.[18]

BONE MARROW TRANSPLANTATION PROCESS

Concepts of Bone Marrow Transplantation

The theory of replacing diseased marrow with healthy donor marrow is simple in concept but difficult to successfully implement because of the toxicities related to high-dose chemotherapy and irradiation in preparative regimens. Specialized medical and nursing care is required for supportive care. The concepts of the BMT process are as follows:

- The dose of most chemotherapeutic agents that may be administered to cure a patient's disease is limited as a result of marrow toxicity (conventional chemotherapy).
- The availability of donor marrow for marrow transplantation and subsequent engraftment makes it possible to administer chemoradiotherapy in supralethal doses in an effort to kill malignant cells (preparative regimens for BMT).
- The patient is then rescued with donor marrow to prevent iatrogenic death (bone marrow transplantation).
- The infused marrow will reconstitute the patient's (host's) hematopoietic and immunologic system, and the patient (host) will be rescued (engraftment).
- Complications that follow are the result of the high-dose chemotherapy and conditioning regimens that prepare the patient to receive the donor marrow (acute and chronic complications).

Table 15-2 provides the sequence and time of events in the process of allogeneic BMT.

Pretransplantation Evaluation and Preparation of the Patient

Marrow candidates require comprehensive evaluations to determine the patient's ability to sustain BMT. These evaluations, listed in Table 15-3, usually are done in the outpatient setting.

A family conference in the outpatient setting introduces the patient and family to the transplantation program. The purpose of the meeting is to explain the conditioning regimen and the risks of BMT and to discuss expected outcomes with the patient. Often the information given in this conference is new and may be inconsistent with the expectations of the patient; nurses must be prepared to support the family through this final decision-making process.[23]

Patient/family preparation for hospitalization can be conducted during the wait for hospital admission. Familiarizing the patient with the concepts of laminar air flow rooms, protective isolation, and various complex treatment and research protocols may decrease the patient's anxiety concerning the procedures.[23] All patients have double-lumen indwelling central catheters inserted before admission. Atrial catheters are essential to accommodate large volumes of parenteral fluids that will be required. Formal teaching programs with videotapes and booklets can be effective teaching measures.[24]

Gonadal failure is caused by high-dose chemotherapy and total body irradiation (TBI) used in preparative reg-

TABLE 15-2 Process of Allogeneic Bone Marrow Transplantation: Sequence and Time of Events

Event	Time
1. Diagnosis of patient with disease treatable with BMT	Days (AA) to years (CML, CP)
2. Identification of histocompatible donor	2 wk
3. Evaluation of patient and donor for BMT	2 wk
4. Placement of multiple-lumen Hickman line in patient	1 day
5. Admission to hospital for BMT	—
6. Initiation of pretransplantation conditioning regimen with high-dose chemoirradiation given either alone or in combination therapy	2-10 days
7. Admission of donor for marrow harvest	Day of BMT
8. Infusion of donor marrow into patient	Day of marrow harvest; several hour infusion
9. Engraftment	2-4 wk
Acute complications	Day 0 to 100 days after BMT
10. Discharge to outpatient setting	30-40 days after BMT
11. Outpatient care	30-100 days after BMT
12. Late acute and early chronic complications	30 days to 100 days after BMT
13. Return to referring health care team for continuing care	100 days after BMT
14. Chronic complications	100 days—4-5 yrs after BMT

AA, Aplastic anemia; *CML*, chronic myelogenous leukemia; *CP*, chronic phase.

TABLE 15-3 Pretransplantation Preparation and Evaluation of Candidate and Donor for BMT

Evaluation	Candidate	Donor
Clinical evaluation		
Histocompatible tissue typing (HLA, MLC, HLA-DR-RFLP)	X	X
ECG, possible cardiac ejection fraction	X	X
Complete history and physical examination	X	X
Immunization history	X	X
Diagnostic procedures (bone marrow aspiration, biopsies)	X	
Oral medicine examination	X	
Pulmonary function test, arterial blood gases	X	
Chest films	X	X
Informed consent	X	X
Nutritional evaluation	X	
Psychologic evaluation, if recommended	X	X
Appropriate consultations	X	X
Laboratory evaluation		
Complete blood count with differential and platelet count	X	X
Chemistry profile	X	X
Hepatitis screen	X	X
HIV antibody status	X	X
Serologic test for syphilis	X	X
ABO and RH groups	X	X
CMV antibody status	X	X
Preparation and intervention		
Placement of right atrial catheter	X	
Ferrous gluconate medication		X
Preoperative and postoperative teaching regarding marrow harvest	X (autologous)	X
Postoperative care and evaluation of marrow aspiration sites	X	X

RFLP, Restriction fragment length polymorphism.

imens for BMT; consequently, sperm banking should be considered before admission to the hospital in patients with adequate sperm counts.[23]

Preparation of the Donor

Although risks to marrow donors are minimal, donors are carefully evaluated for tolerance of general or spinal anesthesia for marrow harvest.[25] Donors also must be comprehensively evaluated before surgery (Table 15-3). To spare the donor the risks of blood transfusions, donors weighing more than 50 kg donate a unit of autologous whole blood to be reinfused intraoperatively at the time of marrow harvest.[23]

Several factors influence the amount of counseling and education a donor needs prior to marrow donation. These include not only the relationship the donor has with the patient and family but the donor's own life responsibilities as well.[26] Donors are required for platelet and granulocyte support for up to 3 months after marrow transfusion, and hardships can occur. Numerous studies have confirmed some long-term psychologic effects on marrow donors of patients who have died as a result of BMT.[27,28] Mood changes, lack of self-esteem, altered relationships, and guilt have been identified as long-term sequelae, which are based on the donor's perception of the success or failure of the BMT.[29] Donors and their families can be supported effectively through written and verbal educational programs directed toward providing sufficient information to minimize anxiety and to provide realistic expectations.[24]

Marrow donors are usually admitted to the hospital for marrow harvest the day of surgery and discharged 24 to 48 hours after surgery. Follow-up care for evaluation of donor aspiration sites for possible infection and other postoperative complications such as anemia, nausea, or pain is essential and provides psychologic support as well.[23]

Conditioning Regimens

Recipients of marrow transplantation usually are admitted to the hospital 1 day before the start of their conditioning regimen. The methods used to prepare patients for grafting differ according to the underlying disease. Patients receive high-dose chemotherapy alone or supralethal doses of chemoradiotherapy to eradicate malignant cells and to prevent graft rejection by the patient's own immune system.[30]

The most common chemotherapeutic agent used in the preparative regimen is cyclophosphamide because it provides tumor cell kill as well as immune ablation. Other drugs that may be used include daunomycin, busulfan, dimethyl busulfan, cytosine arabinoside, 6-thioguanine, and etoposide (VP-16).[31]

Total body irradiation (TBI) is delivered in varying doses from cobalt or linear accelerator units. TBI offers optimal tumor kill because of its ability to penetrate the central nervous system and other privileged sites.[32] Lung shielding sometimes is used in an effort to decrease the incidence of interstitial pneumonitis.

MARROW COLLECTION

Allogenic Transplantation

Donor marrow is harvested in the operating room under sterile conditions, with the donor anesthetized under general or spinal anesthesia. The marrow is obtained from the posterior iliac crests in 2 to 5 mL aspirates to a total of 10 to 15 mg/kg recipient body weight. If necessary, the anterior iliac crests and the sternum may be used. Although 150 to 200 aspirates are necessary to obtain sufficient marrow, only six to ten skin punctures are made because the aspiration needles are redirected to different sites under the skin.[9]

The heparinized marrow is screened through a series of progressively finer mesh screens to filter out bone particles and fat. Marrow then is placed in blood administration bags and infused into the patient within 2 to 4 hours.[5,9,13] The series of steps of marrow collection and harvest are outlined in Figure 15-2.

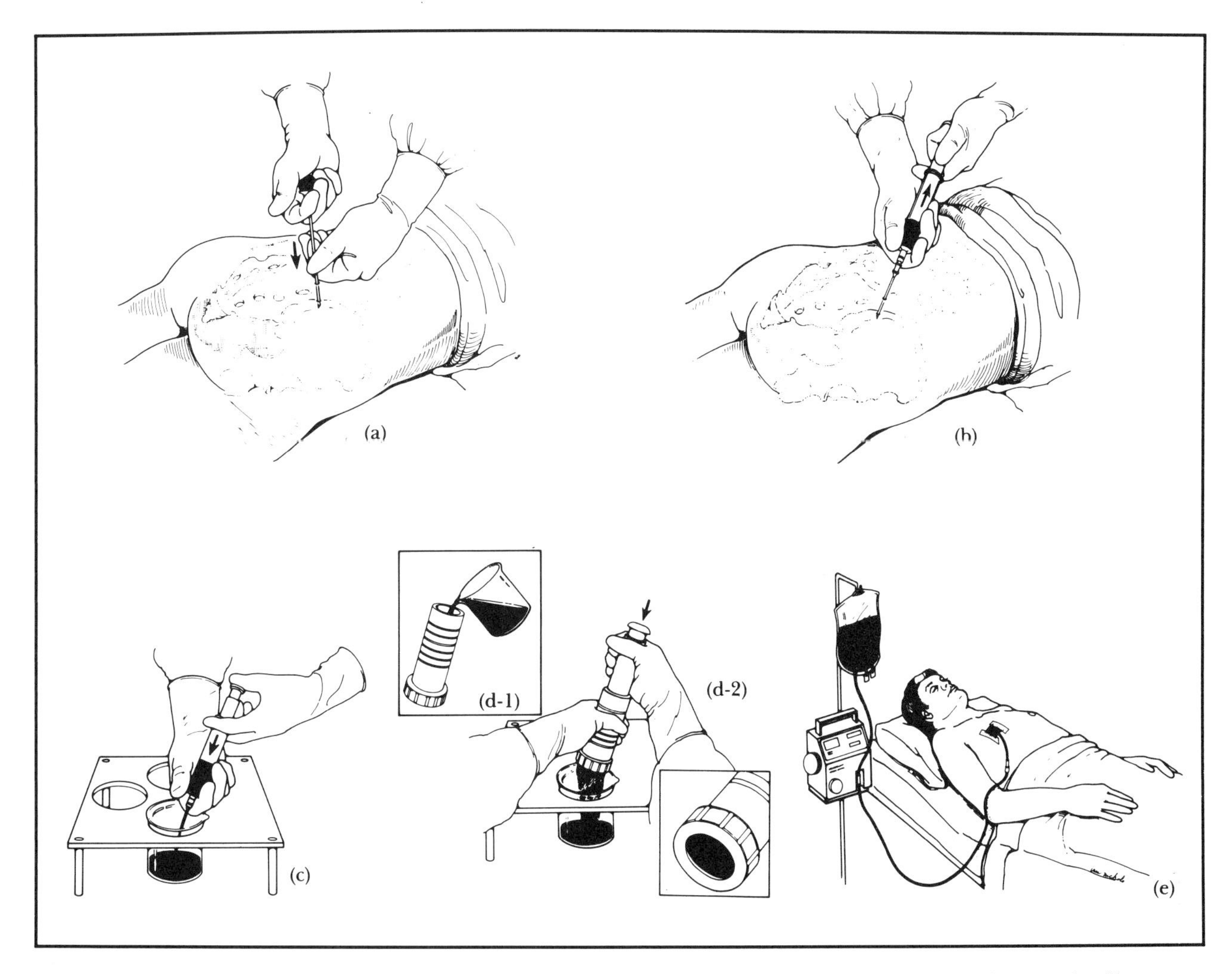

FIGURE 15-2 Series of steps in donor marrow aspiration and harvest. (a) Large bore needle placed in the posterior iliac crest. (b) Multiple aspirations. (c) Marrow drawn up in large syringe. (d-1) Marrow placed in collection beaker; (d-2) strained through metal grid. (e) Marrow placed in a blood administration bag and administered through multilumen catheter.

Autologous Transplantation

Aspirations for an autologous transplantation are obtained in a similar manner. This marrow may be incubated with chemotherapeutic drugs to purge tumor cells, cryopreserved for up to 3 years to use in the event that the patient relapses, or immediately infused after completion of the high-dose preparative regimen.[2,31,33]

There are three methods of purging marrow of the presence of malignant cells: (1) physical, (2) immunologic, and (3) pharmacologic. Physical purging requires separation of leukemic cells from marrow, whereas immunologic purging uses immunotoxins or monoclonal antibodies alone or in combination with magnetic immunobeads.[33] Pharmacologic purging uses potent agents of mercocyanine 540, mafosfamide (ASTA-2-7557), 4-hydroperoxycyclophosphamide, or alkyl-lysophospholipids.[33]

MARROW INFUSION

The day of marrow infusion is "day zero," with subsequent days numbered from this time. The actual marrow infusion is a procedure similar to a blood transfusion. The marrow is infused through a central line during the course of several hours. Marrow cells pass through the lung and home to the marrow cavity. Complications may include volume overload and pulmonary abnormalities as a result of fat emboli. Symptoms similar to blood transfusion reactions may occur, for example, chills, urticaria, and fever, and should be treated with antihistamines, antipyretics, or decreasing rate of infusion.[34]

Within 2 to 4 weeks the marrow graft becomes functional, and peripheral platelets, leukocytes, and red cells increase in number. Intensive nursing care is required to prevent complications until the recipient's marrow recovers.

COMPLICATIONS OF BONE MARROW TRANSPLANTATION

Although BMT holds potential cure for a number of diseases, acute and chronic toxicities may complicate the posttransplantation course. Complications are the result of (1) high-dose chemotherapy and irradiation for conditioning regimens, (2) GVHD (allogeneic), or (3) problems associated with the original disease.[23,35] The sequence of major complications following allogeneic BMT are identified in Figure 15-3. The major complications following autologous BMT are similar except for GVHD.

The interrelationships of BMT complications have been well defined as follows[13]:

- The chemoradiation therapy the patients receive would be fatal if the patients were not rescued with marrow infusion.
- The major complications in patients after transplantation usually are the result of the chemoradiation used to prepare for transplantation, or the marrow transplantation, not the original disease.
- The complications often occur simultaneously.
- Clinical manifestations of some complications, although often of sudden onset, may be subtle.
- The clinical manifestations of different complications can be the same; one complication can cause or exacerbate another.

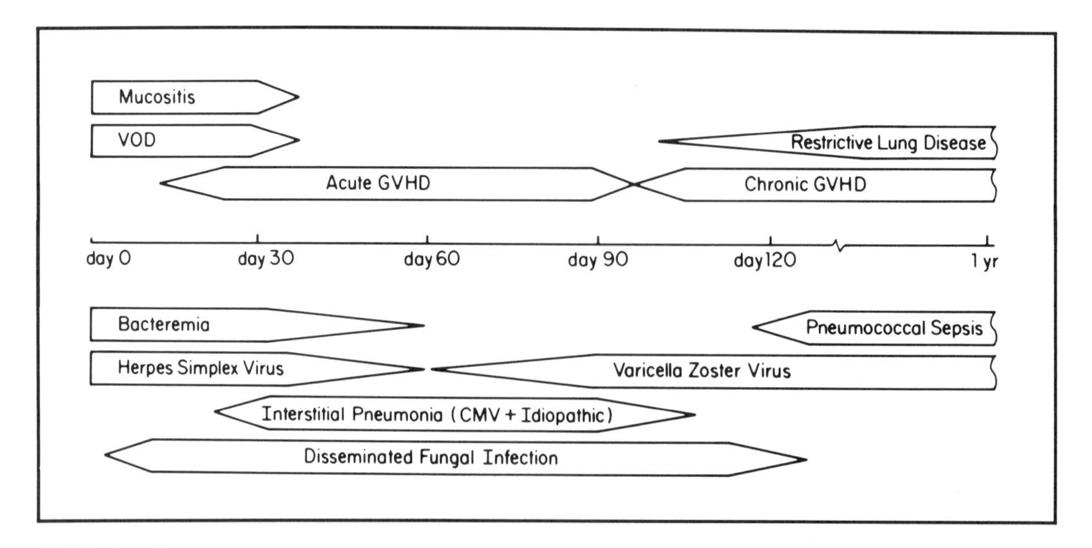

FIGURE 15-3 Temporal sequence of major complications after allogeneic bone marrow transplantation on day 0. (Source: Press OW, Schaller RT, Thomas ED: Complications of Organ Transplantation. New York, Marcel Dekker, 1987, Reprinted courtesy of Marcel Dekker, Inc.)

- The treatment of one complication can cause or exacerbate another.
- The prophylaxis or treatment for one complication may have to be modified or terminated because of the development of another complication.

Nursing care of marrow recipients requires an ability to organize procedures and therapies aimed at prevention and treatment of transplantation-related toxicities.[13] Patients and families experience anxiety because of the stress associated with this treatment, and nurses will require psychosocial nursing skills and the ability to interact with multidisciplinary teams.

Acute Complications

Acute complications are seen several days after BMT and affect multiple organ systems. Because pretransplantation chemoradiotherapy ablates all cell lines, complications will be most severe until early engraftment. See Table 15-4 for a detailed summary of the cause, incidence, onset, manifestations, and interventions associated with acute complications of BMT.

Gastrointestinal toxicity

Mucositis The gastrointestinal tract is affected by TBI and chemotherapy preparative conditioning. The major symptom is protracted pain, which usually is treated with intravenous morphine.[36] Mucositis is complicated by severe thrombocytopenia, and aspiration pneumonia can occur. Concomitant herpes simplex lesions can further damage the oral mucosa.[37] These problems resolve once engraftment occurs, and serious long-term problems are rare. Nursing care dictates maintenance of good oral hygiene with saline mouthwashes, and medical treatment consists of prompt institution of acyclovir and application of topical anesthetics.[13]

Nausea and vomiting Nausea and vomiting following chemotherapy and TBI present a consistent problem in patients who have BMT.[36] Protracted nausea and vomiting also may be caused by GVHD, CMV esophagitis, or gastrointestinal infections. Differential diagnosis must be made and may include endoscopy with duodenal biopsy.[36] Nursing care of the patient with nausea and vomiting includes administration of antiemetics, careful recording of intake and output of fluids, monitoring acid and electrolyte balances, and psychologic support.[13]

TABLE 15-4 Possible Acute Complications of Bone Marrow Transplantation

Complication	Cause	Incidence Rate (%)	Time of Onset after BMT (days)	Signs and Symptoms	Nursing Intervention	Medical Intervention
Gastrointestinal						
Oral mucositis	High-dose conditioning regimen of chemotherapy; TBI (immunosuppression) plus coexistent infection; HSV, methotrexate	100 Universal to chemotherapy and irradiation	0-28	Profuse, watery to thick ropy mucous, severe pain, bleeding ulceration, infection, potential airway obstruction, xerostomia	Assess nasal oral cavity for integrity of mucous membrane	Acyclovir for HSV infection; topical antibiotics: lidocaine, dyclonine
Esophageal mucositis	Same	100	Same	Esophageal dysphasia, bleeding, infection	Administer IV analgesic medication; provide frequent vigorous oral care	IV morphine sulfate; daily chest film and CBC; viral cultures; parenteral support
Gastric mucositis	Same	100	Same	Anorexia, nausea, vomiting, bleeding, infection	Monitor with care I & O, fluids, and management of pain	Parenteral nutrition, biopsy, appropriate antibiotic therapy
Intestinal mucositis	Same	100	Same	Watery diarrhea, cramping pain, ulcerations, infections	Monitor vital signs q4h; accurately measure I & O; manage pain	Surgical intervention; gut biopsy; antibiotic therapy

TABLE 15-4 Possible Acute Complications of Bone Marrow Transplantation (continued)

Complication	Cause	Incidence Rate (%)	Time of Onset after BMT (days)	Signs and Symptoms	Nursing Intervention	Medical Intervention
Gastrointestinal—cont'd						
Gastrointestinal lower bowel toxicity	High-dose TBIs and chemotherapy; GVHD	100	0-30	Nausea, vomiting, diarrhea	Monitor with care fluids and electrolytes, assessment of I & O; administer antiemetics, TPN	Antiemetics, fluid management, gut biopsy
Acute GVHD						
Skin	Reaction of immunocompetent donor T lymphocytes against immunoincompetent host	40-50	10-70; median onset day 25 after BMT	Maculopapular rash on trunk, palms, soles, ears; generalized erythoderma with desquamation	Assess integumentary system; understand side effects of drugs used in treatment; provide psychologic support of patient	Immunosuppressive therapy with methotrexate, cyclosporine; treated T-cell–depleted donor marrow before BMT; antithymocyte globulin; corticosteroids; skin biopsy
Liver	Same	40-50	Same	Elevated liver enzymes, alkaline phosphatase, right upper quadrant pain, heptatomegaly, jaundice	Monitor liver function tests	Liver biopsy
Gut	Same	40-50	10-70	Green watery diarrhea, abdominal cramping, anorexia, nausea, vomiting	Monitor guaiac stool test, weight, accurate I & O, central venous pressure, CBC, and electrolytes; administer antiemetics	Gut biopsy; differential diagnosis to rule out infection; VOD; gut rest, parenteral nutrition

TABLE 15-4 Possible Acute Complications of Bone Marrow Transplantation (continued)

Complication	Cause	Incidence Rate (%)	Time of Onset after BMT (days)	Signs and Symptoms	Nursing Intervention	Medical Intervention
Renal insufficiency	Nephrotoxins, amphotericin B, cyclosporine, methotrexate, aminoglycoside plus septic shock or cardiogenic shock or volume depletion because of diarrhea; hepatorenal syndrome of VOD	25	1-50	Decreased urine output, asymptomatic azolemia, proteinuria, hypertension, renal failure, thrombocytopenia purpura, thirst, dizziness; flat or distended neck veins, peripheral edema; doubling of baseline serum creatinine	Monitor vital signs, with postural BP; careful fluid management, accurate I & O; monitor serum creatinine, BUN, electrolyte levels; monitor urine electrolyte collections, specific gravity q4h; measure daily abdominal girth, weight; assess for peripheral edema; monitor patient during dialysis	Dialysis (5%-10% of BMT patients), removal or reduction of nephrotoxic drugs; correction of fluid electrolyte and acid base imbalance; treatment of infections
Veno-occlusive disease	High-dose conditioning regimens; patients with previous liver disease; patients >15 yr old	21 (6% mortality rate) aplastic anemia (rare)	6-15	Weight gain >12%, ascites, hepatic metabolism, bilirubin >20 mg/dL, SGOT >40 mU/mL; right upper quadrant pain; encephalopathy, hepatomegaly	Carefully and frequently assess fluid balance; monitor weight bid, vital signs with postural BP, accurate I & O; measure abdominal girth daily, restrict fluid, sodium; monitor narcotics and, if indicated, hemodynamics	No known treatment; maintain intravascular volume and renal profusion; restrict sodium; maintain hematocrit >35%; albumin; low-dose dopamine; supportive care

TABLE 15-4 Possible Acute Complications of Bone Marrow Transplantation (continued)

Complication	Cause	Incidence Rate (%)	Time of Onset after BMT (days)	Signs and Symptoms	Nursing Intervention	Medical Intervention
Infection		100	0-30	Neutropenia, oral fever >38° C, sepsis, cough, lethargy	Provide LAF rooms; prevent infection; use good handwashing techniques; wear mask in patient's room; provide surveillance, cultures, pan cultures; administer antibiotics; manage side effects of treatment drugs; regulate BP with pressor agents and hemodynamics monitoring; manage fluid and electrolyte acid-base balances; institute fever reduction measures	Prophylactic measures, protective isolation, LAF rooms, oral nonabsorbable antibiotics, low bacteria diet, TMP-SMX for pneumocystis, acyclovir prophylaxis for HSV, passive immunization with CMV-IG IGG, CMV blood product screening, surveillance chest films, total body skin cleaning, treatment with broad-spectrum prophylactic antibiotics; appropriate antibiotics for bacterial, viral, fungal, and protozoal infection
Bacterial		10				
Escherichia coli		5.5				
Staphylococcus epidermidis		35.9				
S. aureus		7.8				
Streptococcus sp.		6.3				
Viral						
Herpes simplex	Reactivation of latent virus	70-80	0-30	Pain, ulceration, bleeding, fever, infection	Provide vigorous mouth care; administer pain medication	Prophylaxis and treatment with IV acyclovir; analgesics
CMV pneumonia	Reactivation of latent virus	71	60-70	Dyspnea, infiltrates on chest film; abnormal ABGs, PFTs	Administer medication	Diagnostic bronchoscopy, DGHP, CMV-Ig

TABLE 15-4 Possible Acute Complications of Bone Marrow Transplantation (continued)

Complication	Cause	Incidence Rate (%)	Time of Onset after BMT (days)	Signs and Symptoms	Nursing Intervention	Medical Intervention
Infection—cont'd						
Fungal *Aspergillus (Candida)*	Immunosuppression caused by TBI and chemotherapy	10% unknown	0-30	Fever	Administer amphotericin B; monitor serum electrocytes, hydration status, side effects of amphotericin B; administer premedications to reduce drug reactions, for example, hydrocortisone, meperidine (Demerol), diphenhydramine (Benadryl)	Amphotericin B; endoscopic examination with biopsy
Alopecia	Highdose chemotherapy, TBI	100	7-10	Loss of body hair	Help patient cope with body image changes	Psychologic support

ABG, Arterial blood gas; *bid,* twice daily; *BP,* blood pressure; *BUN,* blood urea nitrogen; *CBC,* complete blood count; *CMV,* cytomegalovirus; *DHPG,* dihydroxyproproxymethylguanine; *HSV,* herpes simplex virus; *HZV,* herpes zoster varicella; *Ig,* immunoglobulin; *IgG,* immunoglobulin G; *I & O,* intake and output; *IV,* intravenous; *LAF,* laminar air flow; *PFT,* pulmonary function test; *SGOT,* serum glutamic oxaloacetic transaminase; *TBI,* total body irradiation; *TMP-SMX,* trimethorpim-sulfathoxazle (Bactrim); *TPN,* total parenteral nutrition.

Diarrhea In the first weeks after BMT, diarrhea occurs as a result of chemoradiotherapy but seldom persists beyond day 15. Oral magnesium and nonabsorbable antibiotics (vancomycin, tobramycin, and nystatin) can cause mild diarrhea. Diarrhea associated with acute GVHD and infections is seen as early as day 7 in mismatched BMT patients[36] and is discussed later in this chapter.

Hematologic complications

Recipients of grafts are at high risk for hemorrhage and must be supported with red blood cells and platelets until the donor marrow becomes fully engrafted and functional (Figure 15-4). Blood products must be irradiated to destroy T lymphocytes that can cause GVHD in the marrow recipient. Patients whose platelets become refractory to random platelet transfusions can receive HLA-matched platelets from family or community donors, and platelets that have undergone plasmapheresis from marrow donors yield optimal increments. Alloimmunization and platelet refractoriness contribute to a 1% case fatality rate from hemorrhagic complications.[36-38] Bleeding can occur from all body orifices and requires immediate intervention. Table 15-5 outlines clinical manifestations and interventions for management of hemorrhages.

Acute graft-versus-host disease

GVHD is an immunologic disease that is a direct consequence of allogeneic marrow transplantation and occurs in an acute and chronic form. Despite prophylaxis with postgrafting in vivo immunosuppression, this disease remains a major impediment to successful marrow grafting and occurs in 30% to 50% of HLA-identical recipients. GVHD is thought to be a graft-host response in which the grafted donor T lymphocytes recognize disparate non-HLA host cell antigens and initiate cytotoxic injury directed against host (patient) tissue.[38,39] Acute GVHD targets the skin, liver, and gut.[39] Symptoms, which range from mild to severe, are outlined in Table 15-6. GVHD-related

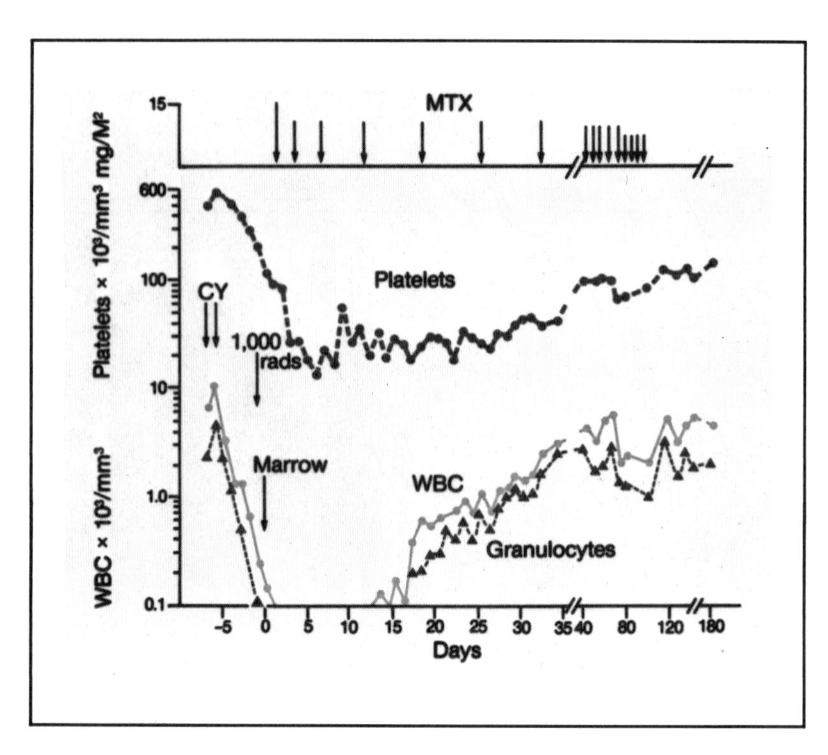

FIGURE 15-4 Return of a patient's platelet, white blood cell, and granulocyte counts from before transplantation to 180 days after BMT.

complications account for approximately 10% of all deaths from BMT.[40] Risk factors are highest for patients older than 30 years of age and for patients mismatched for two or more of the HLA loci on the unshared haplotype.[39]

Clinical manifestations Acute GVHD typically begins with a maculopapular erythema that may be pruritic and may cover 25% of the body. The disease can progress to a generalized erythroderma with frank desquamation and blistering similar to second-degree burns.[13,39]

Consistent with or subsequent to the onset of GVHD of the skin, GVHD may involve the liver. On abdominal examination patients may have pain in the right upper quadrant of the abdomen and hepatomegaly. In addition, increases in liver enzymes may be noted. Jaundice indicates progressive liver involvement.[13,36,39]

Gastrointestinal involvement of acute GVHD can result in nausea, vomiting, anorexia, abdominal cramping, and pain. A typical early symptom is green, watery diarrhea that may exceed 2 L/day.[13,36,39]

Diagnosis The diagnosis of GVHD may be difficult to distinguish from symptoms secondary to infection or the high-dose conditioning regimens. Differential diagnosis is imperative and usually is done by skin and liver biopsy and by clinical, laboratory, and x-ray data.[36]

Prophylaxis and treatment One of the most important concepts in transplantation medicine is the prevention of GVHD and its related symptoms. Prevention of infection by decontamination and laminar air flow room isolation can decrease the incidence, delay the onset of acute GVHD, and increase survival.[40] Immunosuppressive medications are aimed at removing or inactivating T lymphocytes that attack target organs.[6] Cyclosporine and methotrexate inhibit T lymphocytes that are believed to be responsible for acute GVHD. Used in combination, they are more effective than either agent used alone.[39] Newer prophylactic measures include T-cell depletion of donor marrow prior to transplantation with monoclonal antibodies, lectin agglutinin and sheep red cells, or T-cell immunotoxins.[31]

Nursing implications Nursing care of patients with acute GVHD requires skillful assessment and management of early complications of this problem.[41,42] Drugs given to treat or prevent GVHD may have adverse side effects.[13,42] Nursing care includes management of burnlike wounds, abdominal pain, and voluminous diarrhea.[42] Frequent clinical reassessment is required to monitor fluid replacement, hyperalimentation, transfusion, and antibiotic therapy.[43] Intensive nutritional assessment of the patient is mandatory because of the large volumes of diarrhea experienced by these patients[44] (Table 15-4).

Renal complications

Renal complications after BMT occur in more than 50% of marrow recipients and can be the result of one event or a combination of events.[7,45] Nephrotoxic drugs used for prevention and treatment of transplantation-related problems (eg, amphotericin B, cyclosporine, methotrexate, aminoglycosides) are implicated in renal toxicities. These toxicities superimposed on patients compromised with septic shock, volume depletion, or veno-occlusive disease (VOD) act in concert to further exacerbate renal hemodynamic complications.[36,45]

Clinical manifestations/monitoring Recipients of BMT in whom renal toxicities occur may initially have

TABLE 15-5 Prevention and Management of Hemorrhage in the Recipient of Bone Marrow Transplantation

Complication	Cause	Nursing Intervention	Medical Intervention
Nosebleed	High-dose chemotherapy and TBI (immunosuppression of megakaryocyte/erythrocyte lines)	Apply pressure and ice packs to nasal area; administer platelets; avoid invasive procedures	Daily CBC, blood product support, topical adrenalin and cocaine, ENT consult
Mouthbleed	Same as above	Assess airway for patency; provide vigorous mouth care, use toothettes, discourage toothbrushes; provide oral airway at bedside	Same; dental medicine consult
Cranial	Same as above	Frequent neurologic assessment for headache, seizure, confusion; lumbar puncture only with platelet count >50,000 U/L; avoid emesis and straining	Daily CBC; blood product support, neurologic consult; MRI, CT scans
Gastrointestinal	High-dose chemotherapy and TBI, mucosal irritation, infection, stress	Observe emesis and stools; avoid nasogastric tubes, enemas, rectal temperatures	Daily CBC; blood product support; endoscopy with platelets >50,000 U/L; coagulation studies
Invasive procedures	High-dose chemotherapy and TBI (immunosuppression of megakaryocyte/erythrocyte lines)	Place sandbags to surgical site after insertion of atrial catheters; avoid intramuscular injections	Platelet count >50,000 U/L; avoid cutdowns: use percutaneous procedures for Swan-Ganz catheters
Hemorrhagic cystitis	Same as above	Assess for blood in urine; irrigate bladder during administration of cyclophosphamide; use care in insertion of urinary catheters	Bladder irrigation; daily CBCs; IV hydration; blood product support
Menstrual bleeding	Same as above	Observe bleeding carefully (count number of sanitary pads); administer medroxyprogesterone acetate	Medroxyprogesterone acetate; daily CBCs; blood product support
Petachiae, bruising	Same as above	Turn patient frequently; avoid pressure sores; use eggshell mattress, sheepskin, alternating pressure mattress	

CBC, Complete blood count; *CT,* computerized tomography; *ENT,* ear, nose, and throat; *IV,* intravenous; *MRI,* magnetic resonance imaging; *TBI,* total body irradiation.

TABLE 15-6 Clinical Stages of Acute Graft-Versus-Host Disease

Stage	Skin	Liver	Gut
+ (mild)	Maculopapular rash <25% body surface	Bilirubin 2-3 mg/dL	Diarrhea 500-1000 mL/day
+ + (moderate)	Maculopapular rash 25%-50% body surface	Bilirubin 3-6 mg/dL	Diarrhea 1000-1500 mL/day
+ + + (severe)	Generalized erythroderma	Bilirubin 6-15 mg/dL	Diarrhea >1500 mL/day
+ + + + (life threatening)	Desquamation and bullae	Bilirubin >15 mg/dL	Pain or ileus

abrupt onset of anuria.[46] Acute tubular necrosis (ATN) or acute renal failure is heralded by anuria that may result from postrenal obstruction arising from cyclophosphamide-related hemorrhagic cystitis.[13] Renal failure that stems from tumor lysis as a result of high-dose chemotherapy may occur. Early symptoms are anuria with acid-base imbalances that result from the lack of elimination of nitrogenous wastes, water, electrolytes, and acids.[13,46,47]

Renal dysfunction in marrow recipients is usually mild, and care can be managed by medication dose adjustments and careful fluid regulation. After allogeneic transplantation, however, 5% to 10% of patients will require renal dialysis, and the mortality rate is 85% in this group.[38]

Nursing implications Nursing assessment for graft recipients at risk for acute tubular necrosis, which is aimed at recognition of the early symptoms of either prerenal or intrarenal failure, includes the monitoring of routine vital signs with postural blood pressures, determination of urine specific gravity, measurement of urine electrolytes, and determination of accurate intake and output of bodily fluids.[13,34] Complaints of thirst or dizziness, or indications of mental confusion, also are indicators of renal compromise. Observation of distended neck veins or peripheral edema must be noted. Correct determination of abdominal girth and daily weight is an important nursing assessment to distinguish between a prerenal and an intrarenal condition[13,48] (Table 15-4).

Pulmonary complications

Pulmonary complications are a major cause of morbidity and mortality, appearing as early and late sequelae of BMT, and they occur as a result of chemoradiotherapy toxicity or bacterial, viral, or fungal infection in severely immunosuppressed patients.[14,49,50] Early complications caused by severe mucositis can occur days after marrow transplantation, and aspiration of secretions and blood can lead to upper airway obstruction that requires intubation.[49] Pulmonary edema caused by sodium excess and cardiomyopathy, myocarditis, and volume overload from VOD can occur immediately after transplantation.[49] Interstitial pneumonia presents symptoms similar to those of adult respiratory distress syndrome and occurs early (before day 100) or late (after day 100) after transplantation.[49]

Clinical manifestations Manifestations of pneumonia may include nonproductive cough, dyspnea, hypoxemia, and fever. A chest radiograph may demonstrate evidence of interstitial infiltrates, and arterial blood gas levels may show hypoxia.[49,50] These symptoms have rapid onset in the compromised host, and the patient's condition deteriorates quickly.[13,38,49]

Differential diagnosis must be made rapidly to ensure appropriate treatment, but diagnosis often is hampered by unsatisfactory specimens or delays in results of sputum cultures and bronchoscopy washings. The most accurate diagnosis for isolating causative organisms is open lung biopsy.[50] Risks of performing invasive procedures in the compromised host, however, must be weighed against the benefits of an invasive surgical procedure.[13,38,49]

Interstitial pneumonia Interstitial pneumonia is a nonbacterial, nonfungal process that occurs in the interstitial spaces of the lungs. It occurs in approximately 35% of allogeneic marrow recipients and is the most frequent cause of death during the first 100 days after transplantation.[49] The overall mortality rate from interstitial pneumonia is approximately 20% in allogeneic recipients who have transplantation for advanced hematologic malignancy.[51]

Cytomegalovirus pneumonia CMV pneumonia is the leading cause of infectious pneumonia after BMT. It occurs in 20% of patients who receive allogeneic marrow transplantation and has a fatality rate up to 85%.[7,38,50]

The median time of onset for early CMV is greatest between 5 and 13 weeks after transplantation. High-risk factors include (1) patients older than 30 years of age, (2) severe GVHD, (3) TBI conditioning regimen, (4) CMV seropositivity in patients, and (5) advanced hematologic malignancies.[13,38,49]

The most effective prophylaxis against CMV pneumonia is avoidance of viral infection by infusing only CMV-negative blood products in cases in which both donor and patient demonstrated CMV seronegativity before BMT.[38,50] Patients who receive screened blood products must continue to do so through day 100 after BMT. Patients who are seropositive or whose donors are seropositive may benefit from the use of antiviral agents such as acyclovir or passive antibody prophylaxis with immunoglobulin.[50]

Historically, treatment of CMV pneumonia has been largely unsuccessful despite the use of various antiviral drugs and immunotherapeutic agents used alone or in combination therapy.[51] Treatment therapies, however, that use combination ganciclovir and intravenous cytomegalovirus immunoglobulin have demonstrated a 40% to 50% survival rate in marrow recipients whose diagnosis occurred during the initial episode of CMV pneumonia.[21,52]

Idiopathic pneumonia Idiopathic pneumonia accounts for 30% of all interstitial pneumonias in marrow recipients. It is believed to result from high-dose irradiation.[38,43] Idiopathic pneumonia is diagnosed when no specific organism is recovered in bronchial lavage washings or in lung biopsy tissue.[13,38,49]

Other pneumonias Other pneumonias may occur in patients who have BMT and may be caused by a virus (eg, adenovirus, herpes simplex, or varicella zoster), bacteria, or fungi.[50] These agents, which account for 15% of pneumonia in marrow recipients, may be treated successfully.[38,43] *Pneumocystis carinii* caused significant mortality in the early years of marrow transplantation but has been successfully prevented by the use of prophylactic trimethoprim-sulfamethoxazole (TMP-SMX) (Bactrim). Bacterial or fungal pneumonias are not a major cause of death in the marrow recipient.[49]

Nursing implications The median time of onset for interstitial pneumonias is 60 to 70 days after BMT, and typically patients have been discharged from the acute-care setting and are being followed up in a clinic or a physician's office.[50] Classic symptoms are related to the patient's inability to engage in daily activities and may manifest as fatigue, malaise, and/or dyspnea.[50] Patients must be routinely observed by chest films and thorough physical examination, including chest auscultation and determination of arterial blood gases in cases of suspected interstitial pneumonia. Readmission to the hospital is usually necessary, and patients may need respiratory support with mechanical ventilation.[50]

Neurologic complications

Leukoencephalopathy has been reported in the 7% of marrow recipients who have had prior cranial irradiation and intrathecal methotrexate.[53] Symptoms include lethargy, somnolence, dementia, coma, and personality changes. Patients who receive cyclosporine for posttransplantation immunosuppression have documented hypomagnesemia, which can result in neurologic sequelae such

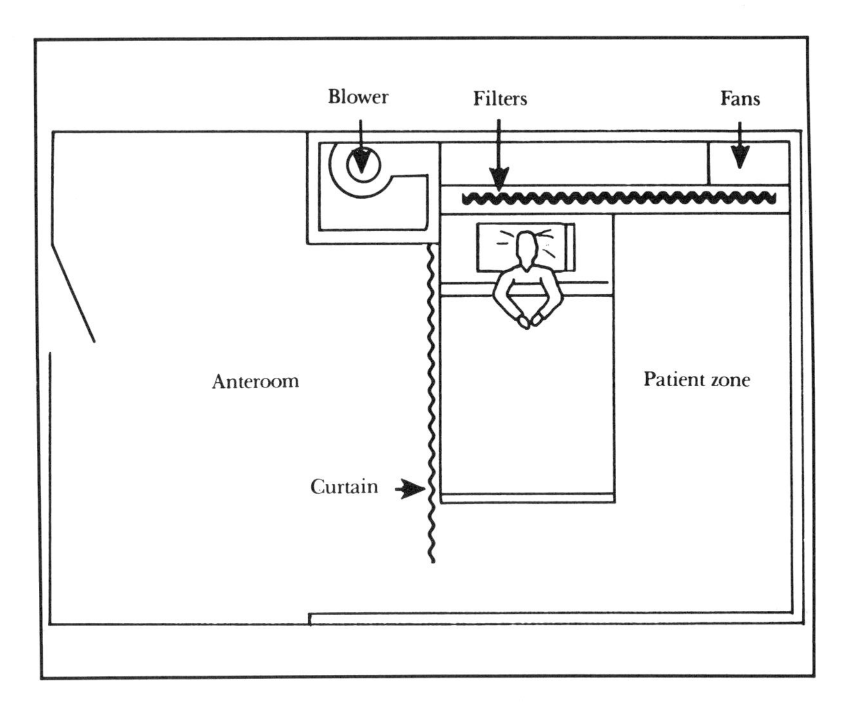

FIGURE 15-5 Diagram of a laminar air flow room. A plastic transparent curtain separates the sterile patient zone from the outer room. Patient decontamination occurs with drinking nonabsorbable antibiotics and application of antibiotic creams and powders to various body areas.

as seizure activity.[53] Neurologic nursing assessments must be incorporated into routine care of marrow recipients.[13]

Cardiac complications

Cardiac complications may develop within several days after administration of high-dose cyclophosphamide. Cardiomegaly, congestive heart failure, and fluid retention may develop, which can be managed with fluid balance to avoid iatrogenic pulmonary edema.[38] These symptoms usually resolve during the first 100 days after BMT and have a fatality rate of less than 1%.[38] Assessment of patients includes obtaining a history of previous therapy with cardiotoxic drugs (eg, doxorubicin) and monitoring cardiac function with routine electrocardiograms and cardiac ejection fractions during the first 100 days after BMT.[7]

Infection

Myeloablative therapy used in conditioning regimens, immunosuppressive prophylaxis, and GVHD renders marrow recipients profoundly susceptible to infection. Patients are at high risk for bacterial, viral, and fungal complications, which peak at predicted times after transplantation.[38,54]

The use of laminar air flow rooms, accompanied by gastrointestinal decontamination with oral nonabsorbable antibiotics, has been helpful in preventing infection in the granulocytopenic period[55] (Figure 15-5).

Clinical manifestations Fever is the cardinal symptom of infection.[46] The cytopenic condition of marrow recipients masks the classic infection-related symptoms of inflammation, pus formation, and elevated white blood cell counts. Consequently cultures of blood, throat, urine, stool, and sputum are necessary to identify and treat pathogenic organisms.[13,56] Risk factors associated with life-threatening infections, and measures to treat and prevent infections, are outlined in Table 15-7.

Treatment Prevention and treatment of infection in the marrow recipient are aimed at identifying the invasive organism and treating the accompanying infection with appropriate antibiotics. Antimicrobial therapy, including intravenous administration of acyclovir, has proven to be successful, whereas granulocyte transfusions seem to be less effective for treatment of infection.[50,55] The role of immunoglobulin therapy in marrow transplant recipients is being investigated and appears promising in preventing infection and correcting immunodeficiencies.[57] Routine surveillance criteria are useful adjuncts for identifying potential pathogens.

Nursing implications Astute nursing assessments are important in determining the onset and course of infectious problems. Fever may be associated with GVHD and administration of blood and drug products. Steroid administration in immunosuppressed patients masks fever, and nurses need to be alert to the subtle signs of infection[13] (Table 15-4).

Veno-occlusive disease of the liver

VOD is a serious problem that develops after BMT and is caused by the preparative chemoradiotherapy.[38,58] The incidence is 40% in adult patients, and 50% of persons with VOD have serious liver disease.[36,45,58] Approximately

TABLE 15-7 Infection in the Recipient of Bone Marrow Transplantation: Risks, Prophylaxis, and Treatment

Risk Factors
Older patients
Moderate or severe GVHD
CMV seropositivity before BMT
Antithymocyte therapy for GVHD
High-dose TBI
End-stage leukemia
Early neutropenia and colonization before or early in BMT
Extensive antibiotic use
Prophylactic Measures
Laminar air flow rooms
Protective isolation
Prophylactic systemic antibiotics
Trimethoprim-sulfamethoxazole
Acyclovir
Oral nonabsorbable antibiotics
Passive immunization with antibodies
CMV-negative blood products
Granulocyte transfusions
Leukocyte removal blood filters
Low bacterial/sterile diet
Routine hygiene: handwashing, mouth care, wearing a mask
Treatment Measures
Empiric broad spectrum antibiotics
Empiric amphotericin B
9-(1,3-dihydroxy-2-propoxymethyl) guanine (DHPG)
Hickman catheter removal
Acyclovir
Corticosteroids
Cyclosporine

30% of patients with VOD die of hepatic/renal complications. Patients at high risk for the development of VOD are those with hepatitis before transplantation, those who are older than 15 years of age, and those patients who receive grafts for hematologic malignancies.[36,38,58]

Clinical manifestations Liver damage caused by chemoradiotherapy involves two histopathologic processes: (1) venule occlusion and/or veno-occlusive process involving terminal hepatic venules and sublobular veins and (2) hepatocyte necrosis.[33] Clinical symptoms, which occur in the first weeks after transplantation, include fluid retention, sudden weight gain, pain in the right upper quadrant of the abdomen, jaundice, hepatomegaly, and encephalopathy. These symptoms are the result of sinusoidal obstruction and intrasinusoidal hypertension, and morbidity is 21%.[36,38,58]

Treatment Currently there is no prevention for VOD, but several promising studies are under way to test heparin prophylaxis in patients at risk for VOD. Treatment consists of fluid management with diuresis and restriction of sodium and water. Hematocrit levels should be kept above 35% to maintain intravascular volume and renal perfusion.[13,36] Of interest is the fact that most marrow recipients who require renal dialysis also have VOD because of liver-kidney hemodynamic interaction.[36]

Nursing implications Continuous and careful monitoring of the fluid status of the patient is a nursing responsibility and includes weighing the patient twice a day, taking daily abdominal girth measurements, and obtaining postural blood pressures.[13]

Discharge

Patients are discharged from the hospital when specific criteria are met,[23] including the following:

- Availability of 24-hour outpatient medical care provided by multidisciplinary BMT team
- Oral intake >50% of baseline nutrient requirements
- Requirement of no more than 2000 mL of parenteral fluid within 24 hours
- Nausea and vomiting controlled with oral medication
- Diarrhea controlled at <500 mL/day
- Afebrile and intravenous antibiotics discontinued for 48 hours
- Platelet count >15,000 mm^3 and supportable
- Granulocyte level >500 mm^3 for 48 hours
- Hematocrit level >30% for adults, 25% for children
- Toleration of oral medications for 48 hours, for example, narcotics, antihypertensives, cyclosporine, and prednisone
- Family support within the home

Ideally, patients and a strong support person need to reside near the transplantation center until 100 days after BMT when the immune system has recovered sufficiently. Comprehensive outpatient care of the transplant recipient consists of daily-to-weekly clinic visits to assess the patient's stability. Supportive care from a multidisciplinary team familiar with marrow transplantation is essential.[59] Blood products, parenteral nutrition, intravenous medications, research medications, and procedures can be delivered effectively in ambulatory care settings. The readmission rate is 50% for treatment of fever and neutropenia.[23] Clear, consistent patient/family teaching aimed at prevention and early recognition of transplantation-related problems must be emphasized. Patients and families are taught to prevent infections by avoiding crowds, school, and work for 1 year after BMT. Immunizations are recommended after 1 year in patients without chronic GVHD and only after testing of immune recovery in patients with chronic GVHD.[60]

Ambulatory/home health care

The role of ambulatory and home health care for the marrow recipient is gaining importance in the reduction of the high cost of marrow transplantation.[10,23] Medical technology allows for the safe delivery of many procedures in an ambulatory setting that traditionally have been given in inpatient settings. This care can be augmented by home health care. Research comparing the efficacy and cost for patients discharged early and supported with home health nursing studies with that for patients remaining in the hospital have been encouraging.[61,62] Similar studies are needed in BMT settings.

Late Complications

Late complications of BMT that are caused by conditioning regimens are defined as those developing 100 days or more after transplantation.[60,63] The incidence, time period, manifestations, and interventions of these late effects are outlined in Tables 15-8 and 15-9.

Late infectious complications

Infectious diseases may present major obstacles to the recovering bone marrow recipient. Varicella zoster virus (VZV) infections develop in 30% to 50% of long-term survivors within the first year of transplantation.[64] Patients with nonspecific suppressor cells and chronic GVHD may be at greater risk for VZV as a result of prolonged immunosuppression.[65] Intravenous acyclovir and analgesics are the treatment of choice and must be instituted immediately on diagnosis.[43,66]

Long-term survivors without chronic GVHD are remarkably free of infections after 1 year. In contrast, patients in whom chronic GVHD develops remain at high risk for bacterial pneumonia, septicemia, and sinusitis because their donor-derived immune systems have not matured and consequently cannot provide adequate protection against invasive organisms[65] (Figure 15-6).

Pulmonary complications

Restrictive pulmonary abnormalities rarely are observed in long-term survivors and are associated with chemoirradiation and recurrent pneumonias.[67] The incidence of restrictive disease peaks at 1 year. Obstructive pulmonary disease, which occurs in approximately 15% of long-term survivors in whom chronic GVHD develops, presents clinical and pathologic features of obliterative bronchiolitis. Late interstitial pneumonia occurs in 10% to 20% of

TABLE 15-8 Possible Late Effects of Bone Marrow Transplantation (BMT) Caused by High-Dose Chemotherapy and/or Irradiation in Conditioning Regimens

Late Effect	Incidence Rate	Time Post-BMT	Signs and Symptoms	Nursing Management	Diagnostic Tools	Medical Treatment
Late infectious complications						
Bacterial, viral, fungal infections with or without chronic graft-versus-host disease (GVHD)	>50%	100-365 days	Fever, wheezing, rales, postnasal drip, signs of infection	Preventive teaching Mask-wearing until 6 months post-BMT Good hand-washing techniques Avoid infectious persons (measles, chickenpox, mumps) Avoid school/work until 6 months post BMT Avoid hot tubs, public swimming pools until 6-9 months post BMT Limit number of sexual partners Avoid live virus vaccines	Positive blood culture for bacteria, fungus, virus Abnormal chest x-ray studies, pulmonary function tests (PFT) Pulmonary infiltrates Open lung biopsy Changes in CBC	Appropriate antibiotic support
Varicella zoster virus Without chronic GVHD With Chronic GVHD	 <50% >75%	100-365 days	Lesions, pain, malaise, tenderness, neurological manifestation	Relieve pruritus with calamine lotion Cool compresses Prevent secondary infection	Positive herpes zoster varicella (HZV) cultures	Strict isolation until lesions are crusting IV acyclovir, 10 mg/kg/dose, q8h × 7 days

TABLE 15-8 Possible Late Effects of Bone Marrow Transplantation (BMT) Caused by High-Dose Chemotherapy and/or Irradiation in Conditioning Regimens (continued)

Late Effect	Incidence Rate	Time Post-BMT	Signs and Symptoms	Nursing Management	Diagnostic Tools	Medical Treatment
Pulmonary complications						
Interstitial pneumonia Cytomegalovirus *Pneumocystis carinii*	70%	100-400 days	Fever, sepsis, hypotension, lethargy, cough	Anticipatory preventive teaching Routine vital signs Chest auscultation & percussion (A&P) Monitor PFT, arterial blood gases (ABG)	Chest x-ray studies, CBC, ABG, PFT Positive cultures for bacterial, fungal, and viral microorganisms Bronchoscopy IgA, IgG levels	Prophylactic trimethoprim-sulfamethoxazole Appropriate antibiotic therapy
Restrictive disease	5%		May be asymptomatic or Cough	Anticipatory teaching of pulmonary toilet Routine vital signs Chest A&P	Total lung capacity, diffusion capacity	Respiratory therapy Bronchodilation
Obstructive disease	11%		Decreased ability to perform daily living activities due to pulmonary insufficiency	Monitor PFT & ABG		
Cataracts						
Total body irradiation, fractionated	20%	1.5-5 years	Poor vision	Anticipatory teaching of BMT risk factors Ophthalmologist recommendation	Examination with slit lamp microscopy	Intraocular lens replacement
Total body irradiation, single dose	50%	1.5-5 years				
Neurologic complications						
Leukoencephalopathy	7%	1-5 months	Lethargy Somnolence Dementia Seizures Spastic quadriplegia Coma Personality changes	Early intervention Multidisciplinary approach with special education program Routine neurologic assessments	Periodic head computer assisted tomography (CAT) scans & psychometric evaluation	Symptomatic & supportive management
Psychologic complications	Unknown	Months to years	Depression, weight change Altered body image Survival syndrome Sibling rivalry	Allow patient/family to verbalize feelings Identify coping mechanisms, personal strengths Refer to mental health resources	Psychological testing	Mental health evaluation and treatment from appropriate source
Impaired growth in children						
Irradiation only	100%	Months to years	Subnormal growth and development	Anticipatory teaching to patients/parents Annual evaluation of growth pattern Serial height/weight	Adrenocortical function Growth hormone Thyroid hormone	Possible appropriate hormone replacement Long-term follow-up

Source: Corcoran-Buchsel P: Long-term complications of allogenic bone marrow transplantation: Nursing implications. Oncol Nurs Forum 13:61-70, 1986.

TABLE 15-9 Late Effects of Bone Marrow Transplantation: Chronic Graft-Versus-Host Disease (GVHD)

Late Effect	Incidence Rate	Time Post-BMT (Days)	Signs and Symptoms	Nursing Management	Diagnostic Tools	Medical Treatment
Skin	95%	100-400	Rough, scaly skin Malar erythema Generalized rash Hypo/hyperpigmentation Dyspigmentation Premature greying Alopecia Joint contractures Scleroderma Loss of sweating	Use of nonabrasive soaps, lotions, sunscreen Cosmetic support, makeup, wigs Range of motion activities Patient/family education Monitor compliance to treatment protocols	Skin biopsy positive for GVHD Karnofsky score	Lanolin-based creams Possible systemic immunosuppressive therapy with Cyclosporin A, prednisone, Imuran
Liver	30%	100-400	Jaundice	Infection precautions until differential diagnosis is made Monitor LFTS Low fat diet	Alkaline phosphatase SGOT Bilirubin	Possible systemic immunosuppressive therapy with Cyclosporin A, prednisone, Imuran
Oral	80%	100-400	Pain, burning, dryness, irritation, soreness, loss of taste Lichenoid changes, atrophy, erythema in oral cavity Candida infection Stomatitis Dental caries Xerostomia	Encourage soft, bland diet Dental hygiene education, soft toothbrush, flossing Saline rinses Dental medicine referral/recommendation Salivary gland stimulants, sugarless mints, artificial saliva	Labial mucosa biopsy positive for GVHD Secretory IgA levels Mouth culture positive for yeast organisms Mouth culture positive for bacterial and viral etiologies Radiographs	Possible systemic immunosuppressive therapy with Cyclosporin A, prednisone, Imuran Artificial saliva Clotrimazole touches or Nystatin Swish and Swallow Appropriate topical medication Topical flouride treatment Appropriate dental therapy
Ocular	80%	100-400	Grittiness, burning of eyes Dry eyes Sicca syndrome	Artificial tears Schirmer's tear test: if < 10 mm of wetting, refer to ophthalmologist	Keratoconjunctivitis Corneal ulceration Slit lamp microscopy	Lacriset plugs Soft contact lens Punctal ligation for obliteration of tear duct outflow Keratoplasty Tarsorrhaphies

TABLE 15-9 Late Effects of Bone Marrow Transplantation: Chronic Graft-Versus-Host Disease (GVHD) (continued)

Late Effect	Incidence Rate	Time Post-BMT (Days)	Signs and Symptoms	Nursing Management	Diagnostic Tools	Medical Treatment
GI tract, esophagus	36%	100-400	Anorexia Difficulty eating Painful swallowing Retrosternal pain Weight loss Vomiting	Serial weights High calorie food supplements Recommend nutritional counseling	Barium swallow of esophagus and small bowel follow-through	Esophageal dilatation Possible systemic immunosuppressive therapy with Cyclosporin A, prednisone, Imuran Parenteral nutrition
Vagina	20%	100-400	Inflammation Stricture formation causing obstruction of menstrual flow Adhesions Dry vagina Painful intercourse Marital problems	Water-soluble lubricants Recommend sexual counseling and therapy	Papanicolaou smear	Vaginal stints Estrogen cream Surgical intervention

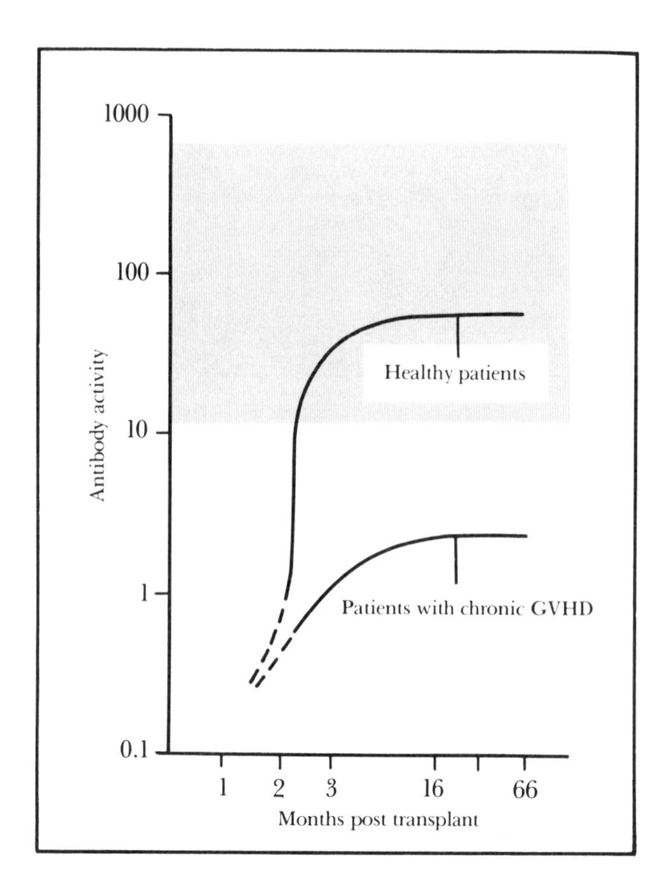

FIGURE 15-6 Effects of chronic graft-versus-host disease on the return of the immune system. (Source: Adapted from Witherspoon RP, Lum LG, Storb R: Semin Hematol 21:2-10, 1984.)

long-term survivors with chronic GVHD and carries a 50% mortality rate. Studies have identified specific pneumonias as idiopathic, CMV, varicella zoster, and *Pneumocystis* pneumonia.[39,50]

Complete nursing assessments of long-term survivors require careful histories and physical examinations. Determination of changes in activities of daily living must be made, chest auscultation and percussion performed, and pulmonary capacities and volumes monitored.[66]

Neurologic complications

Signs and symptoms of chronic leukoencephalopathy may not appear for months or years after transplantation. Learning disabilities in children have been reported, with abnormal motor, perceptual, behavioral, and language performance. Clinical signs and symptoms may be subtle and require careful observation of the behavior of the pediatric patient. Neurologic and developmental assessments are a vital part of follow-up care.[65]

Gonadal dysfunction and fertility

Most transplant recipients conditioned with TBI will demonstrate gonadal dysfunction.[68] Patients prepared with chemotherapy alone often demonstrate recovery of fertility and can successfully bear children.

The adverse effects of high-dose chemotherapy on gonadal function depends on the age of the patient at the time of BMT. Development is normal in girls and boys who are prepubertal at the time of BMT. Younger women (younger than 26 years of age) can expect return of menstrual periods, but only a few have borne children. Early menopause occurs in women older than the age of 26 years at BMT. Men, who usually have return of normal gonadotropin levels, have low-to-normal sperm counts and can father children.[68]

Studies have shown that primary ovarian failure and early menopause occur in female transplant recipients who received TBI, and primary gonadal failure with azoospermia develops in men who received TBI.[68,69] Most prepubertal girls who receive TBI have primary ovarian failure, do not achieve menarche, and do not develop secondary sexual characteristics. In a few prepubertal boys conditioned with TBI secondary sexual characteristics develop, but most have delayed onset of puberty. The most profoundly affected children are prepubertal boys who have received testicular irradiation before marrow conditioning. Testosterone therapy may be effective, but longer follow-up is needed.[68,69]

Sexual counseling before BMT is important for all candidates for marrow transplantation.[69] Women must be prepared for possible early menopause. Cyclic hormonal therapy has been successful for relief of menopausal symptoms.[68] In vitro fertilization and artificial insemination currently is not advised, and until further developments in this field it cannot routinely be recommended.[66] Sperm storage before BMT has been discussed.

Pediatric long-term survivors require special consideration in assessing possible gonadal dysfunction. Children who fail to reach puberty require neuroendocrine evaluation, and young adolescents who achieve puberty need information about possible sterility. Oncology nurses who work with these families may be important contributors to teaching and assessing needs of both parents and children.[66]

Growth in children

Children who undergo conditioning with high-dose cyclophosphamide alone have normal growth and development.[69] TBI used in conditioning regimens causes abnormalities of growth and development in children. All children have decreased growth rates after TBI, and those children who have chronic GVHD are the most significantly affected. Bone age does not seem to be as affected and often is consistent with chronologic age, but adrenocortical function, growth hormone levels, and thyroid function have been subnormal in some children, especially those given prior prophylaxis with cranial irradiation.[69]

Establishing parental awareness of the potential late effects of irradiation is a prime nursing function and should be addressed before and at regular intervals after transplantation. Growth patterns should be evaluated annually, and those who demonstrate a decreased growth rate should be referred to a pediatric endocrinologist. Careful long-term follow-up through puberty will be necessary.[69] Growth hormone replacement therapy may be indicated. Additionally, appropriate sex hormone therapy and thyroid hormone supplementation in selected children may be beneficial to growth and development.[69]

Cataract development

Cataract development is primarily related to TBI administration and/or long-term steroid therapy for GVHD. Recipients who undergo conditioning with single-dose TBI have a 80% probability of cataract development, as compared with a 20% probability among those who receive fractionated TBI.[70] Lens shielding is not employed during TBI because the eye is a potential site of leukemic relapse. Glucocorticoid therapy for treatment of GVHD increases the risk of cataract formation by 24% in patients who have had fractionated TBI or high-dose chemotherapy only.[70] Peak time for cataract formation is 3 to 6 years after transplantation. The treatment of cataracts with surgical extraction is highly successful. An important nursing function is to educate and prepare patients for the possibility of cataract development and its treatment and to encourage annual eye examinations[66] (Table 15-8).

Graft failure/rejection

Compared with unmodified HLA-identical marrow transplantation, graft failure is more frequent in patients who have had transplantation with HLA-nonidentical or T-cell-depleted marrow. Failure of sustained engraftment is seen in 5% of phenotypically HLA-identical mismatched pairs, 7% to 10% of one HLA-locus-mismatched pairs, and 15% to 25% of two- and three-HLA-locus-mismatched pairs.[6] Marrow recipients with graft failure are at substantial risk for fatal infection or hemorrhage.

Graft failure occurs in fewer than 1% of marrow recipients of unmodified HLA-identical marrow prepared with TBI. Marrow graft rejection is more frequent in patients with aplastic anemia not given TBI, primarily because of graft rejection that results from transfusion-induced sensitization.[71]

Current studies attempt to remove residual host T cells that mediate graft failure by increased intensity of chemoradiotherapy preparation and/or use of antithymocyte globulin or anti-T-cell antibodies given after grafting.[20,72] Administration of hematopoietic growth factors shows promise in speeding engraftment.[20,72]

Chronic graft-versus-host disease

Chronic GVHD is a major cause of morbidity after allogeneic BMT and occurs in 30% to 50% of long-term survivors.[63,73] Chronic GVHD is a multisystem disorder of the skin, liver, gut, esophagus, eyes, lungs, joints, vaginal mucosa, and serosal surfaces[73] (Figure 15-7). Clinical and pathologic findings resemble several naturally occurring autoimmune diseases such as scleroderma, lupus erythematosus, lichen planus, rheumatoid arthritis, or Sjögren's syndrome (sicca syndrome)[70,71] (Table 15-9).

Onset and classification Onset of chronic GVHD may be progressive, quiescent, or de novo. Progressive onset, which follows as a direct extension of acute GVHD, has the poorest prognosis. Quiescent onset develops in patients who have had a clinical resolution of acute GVHD,

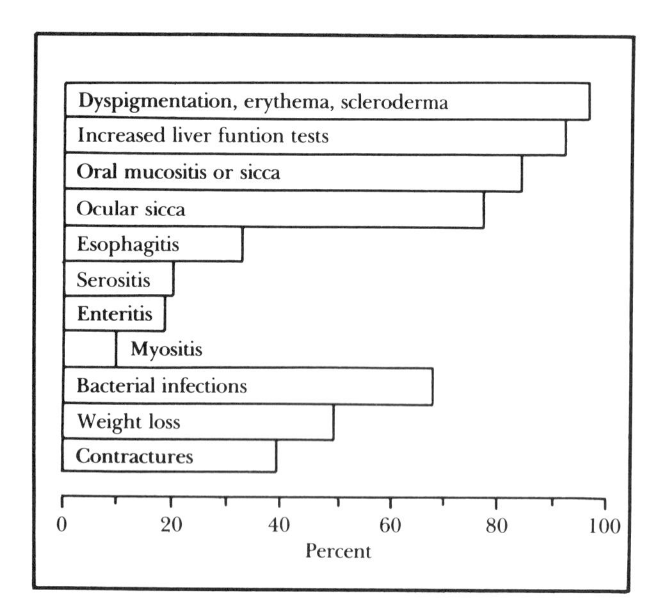

FIGURE 15-7 Frequency of clinical manifestations in patients with chronic GVHD. (Data from Sullivan KM, Parkman R: The pathophysiology and treatment of graft-versus-host disease. Clin Haematol 12:775-789, 1983.)

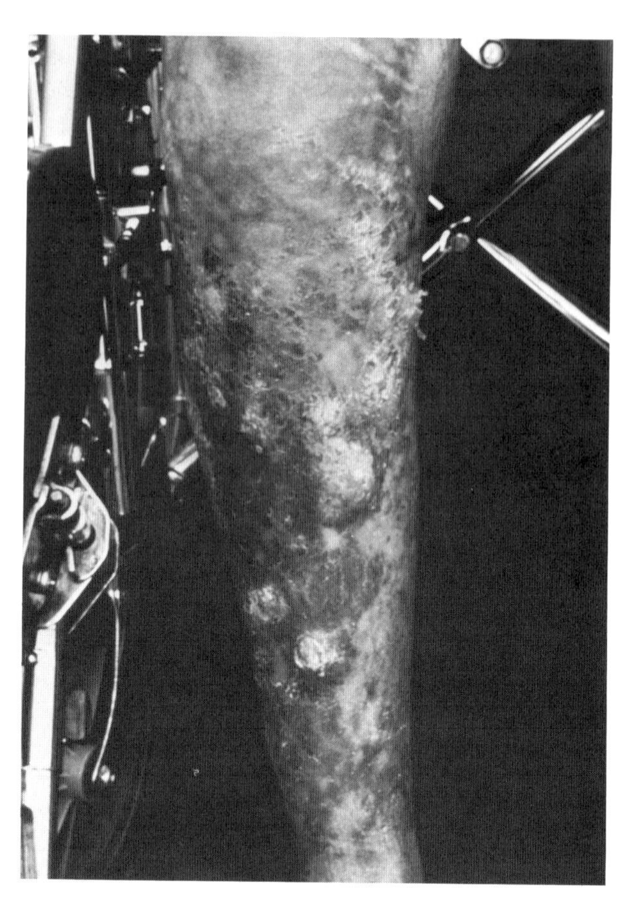

FIGURE 15-8 Chronic GVHD: patchy dyspigmentation, lichen planus–like papules, and papulosquamous plaques 210 days after transplantation.

and these patients have a fair prognosis. Patients with de novo onset have had no prior acute disease and have the best prognosis.[63,73] In addition, chronic GVHD may be limited or extensive. Limited disease targets only the skin and liver and has a favorable course even if untreated, whereas extensive disease affects numerous organ systems and can be fatal if not treated.[63,73] Risk factors associated with the development of chronic GVHD are an age greater than 18 years, a history of acute GVHD, and prior infusions of unirradiated donor buffy coat.[63,73]

Clinical manifestations of chronic GVHD The *skin* is affected in more than 95% of patients. Involvement may include the entire integument and produce alopecia and nail ridging (Figure 15-8). Initially patients will complain of itching and burning of the skin. Patchy hyperpigmentation, mottled-appearing skin, or dyspigmentation may occur. Some patients have a sudden onset of erythema that can be activated by exposure to the sun.[63,66,73]

Liver disorders are observed in about 90% of patients with chronic GVHD. Pathologic findings are characterized by damaged or absent small bile ducts with concomitant severe cholestasis that is similar to that seen in primary biliary cirrhosis.[36,63,74] Alkaline phosphatase, serum glutamic oxaloacetic transaminase (SGOT), and bilirubin levels are elevated. With treatment, bilirubin values return to normal within several weeks, but elevated alkaline phosphatase and SGOT may persist for months.[63,73,74] Nurses need to follow serial liver function laboratory values and be aware that jaundice in a patient 3 to 12 months after BMT may indicate liver involvement in chronic GVHD[66] (Table 15-9).

Oral mucosa involvement will develop in approximately 80% of patients with extensive GVHD (Figure 15-9). Xerostomia and stomatitis are common symptoms. Lichenoid lesions can be confused with candidiasis.[37,75] Labial mucosa biopsy is a major diagnostic tool to screen for the presence of chronic GVHD.[37,73] Salivary changes occur, and xerostomia may cause rampant tooth decay. Early subtle signs are patient complaints of changes in food tastes and burning after brushing teeth. The complete nursing assessment of the patient after transplantation must include examination of the oral cavity at each clinic visit[66] (Table 15-9).

Ocular involvement occurs in 80% of patients with extensive chronic GVHD.[76] Major symptoms include burning and itching of the eye and complaints of a "gritty" feeling in the eye. Unfortunately these symptoms usually appear after corneal stippling has occurred from lacrimal insufficiency. Schirmer's test may be employed to measure the tearing capacity of the eye. Supportive measures with artificial tear replacement will prevent keratitis sicca that can lead to corneal erosion, perforation, or scarring[66,73,74] (Table 15-9).

Esophageal abnormalities have been noted in 36% of patients whose diagnosis includes extensive chronic GVHD.[36,73,77] Symptoms include dysphagia, painful swallowing, and retrosternal pain caused by esophageal thinning. Patients may need to be readmitted to inpatient care for management of nutritional problems and pain.[36,66,74] Responsible nursing management requires early detection of nutritional deficiencies.[66]

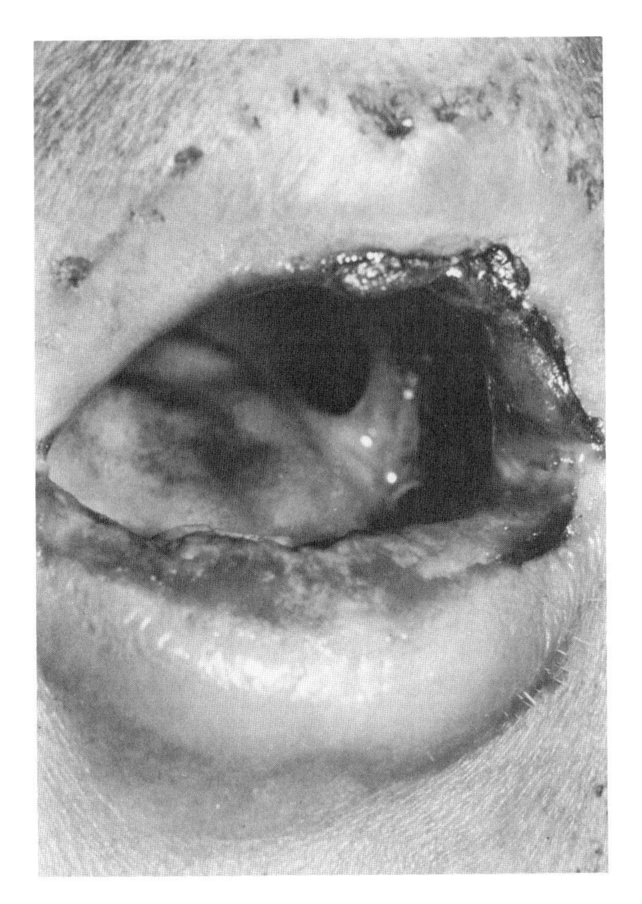

FIGURE 15-9 Significant cutaneous involvement (erythematous rash, hyperpigmentation, and leukoderma) in a patient with chronic GVHD 1 year after transplantation. (Source: Schubert MM, Sullivan KM, Truelove EL: Head and neck complications of bone marrow transplantation, in Peterson ED, Sonis ST, Elias EG (eds): Head and Neck Management of the Cancer Patient. Boston, Martinus Nijhoff, 1986, pp 399-424.)

Significant *vaginal* problems have been documented in women who have chronic GVHD. Vaginal inflammation, stricture formation, and adhesions are known complications that have occurred 1 to 3 years after transplantation.[78] Stricture formation can obstruct menstrual flow, causing abdominal distention and pain that require surgical intervention. Vaginal atrophy may cause painful intercourse leading to sexual dysfunction.[78] To identify real and potential problems a routine gynecologic examination should be incorporated into the care of female recipients of BMT.[66,78]

Problems in other organ systems will develop in 20% of patients with extensive chronic GVHD. The musculoskeletal system can be affected in a manner similar to the effects of rheumatoid arthritis and arthralgias, serosal effusions, joint contractures, and polymyositis.[79] Dyspnea may be a manifestation of bronchiolitis obliterans.[67]

Diagnosis and treatment of chronic GVHD Early detection and treatment of chronic GVHD are accomplished through screening studies performed at approximately day 100[23] (Table 15-10). Initial attempts at treating chronic GVHD were largely unsuccessful, and major studies are being directed toward identification of effective prophylaxis and treatment. Combination therapy of immunosuppressive, cytotoxic, and supportive antibiotics given over a period of 1 year to 18 months have improved morbidity and mortality rates.[80-82] The first encouraging studies demonstrated that combination immunosuppressive (prednisone) and cytotoxic (azathioprine) therapy held promising results and are precursors of current treatment measures.[81]

One study showed that, because of increased infections after combination treatment patients at normal risk who were treated with prednisone alone responded more favorably than those with combination immunosuppressive and cytotoxic therapy.[81] Cyclosporine, a nonmyelotoxic agent effective in treatment of acute GVHD, has been included in the pharmacopeia of immunosuppressive therapy for chronic GVHD, with minimal nephrotoxicity if managed efficiently.[82] Consequently, patients at normal risk can be treated with alternating-day tapering doses of immunosuppressive therapy (prednisone or cyclosporine) or tapering doses of either drug alone.[76] Supportive prophylactic TMP-SMX antibiotic treatment given alone or in combination with penicillin also is necessary to support the patient's recovering immune systems until treatment of chronic GVHD is resolved.[82] Patients in whom the initial treatment fails may be considered for further treatment with daily azathioprine and antibiotics.

High-risk patients (platelet counts <100,000 U/L) have been difficult to treat for reasons that are unclear.[82] There is increasing evidence that treatment with alternate-day dosing with cyclosporine and prednisone and twice-daily TMP-SMX appears to improve survival. Patients manifest few major medication toxicities.[82]

Patients who are on treatment therapy regimens must be monitored for possible toxicities associated with immunosuppressive agents. These complications may include nephrotoxicity, neurotoxicity, psychosis, hypertension, peptic ulcer disease, diabetes, osteoporosis, aseptic neurosis, and infection. Minor toxicities include tremors, mental depression, nausea, gingival hyperplasia, facial coarsening, cushingoid facies, and weight gain. Patient compliance may be a problem, and patients will need reassurance that these unpleasant side effects will disappear when treatment is complete.[66]

Clinical studies

Investigations are focused on identifying the ideal immunosuppressive therapy. Several research studies have used techniques to remove T cells, which are believed to be responsible for GVHD, from the donor marrow by means of monoclonal antibodies or immunotoxins. Although the incidence of GVHD was indeed lower, both graft rejection and leukemic relapse increased.[83,84] Current research is focused on the removal of T cells from the marrow inoculum by the use of lectin agglutination or monoclonal antibodies alone or bound to toxins.[72]

The combination of methotrexate and cyclosporine, given prophylactically to prevent GVHD, has led to 80% one-year survival rates in patients with early stage leukemia who were given HLA-identical marrow. It is considered the gold standard to which numerous research stud-

TABLE 15-10 Determination of Chronic Graft-Versus-Host Disease

Systems Affected	Clinical Evaluation	Signs and Symptoms
Skin	Physical examination and skin biopsy	Dry, flaky skin, scleroderma
Oral	Physical examination and lip biopsy	"White" patchy lichen planus lesions; taste changes
Eye	Schirmer's tear test OS/OD	Dry, scratchy eyes
Liver	Alkaline phosphatase/SGOT/total bilirubin	Laboratory values: alkaline phosphatase elevated, SGOT >41 mU/mL, bilirubin >1.2 mg/dL
Lungs	Pulmonary function tests	Obstructive/restrictive lung disease: abnormal PFTs
Immune system	ANA, AMA, ASMA, RA, GGT; IgA, IgM, IgE; C3, C4 (complement studies); immunoglobulin subclasses, immunoglobulin titers; direct Coombs' test	Serologic indicators of return of immune function
Vaginal	Gynecologic examination	Dry, constricted, striated vaginal tract; difficult intercourse

ANA, Antinuclear antibody; *AMA,* antimitochondrial antibody; *ASMA,* antismooth muscle antibody; *GGT,* gamma glutamyl transferase; *OD,* right eye; *OS,* left eye, *PFTs,* pulmonary function tests; *RA,* rheumatoid arthritis; *SGOT,* serum glutamic oxaloacetic transaminase.
Source: Corcoran-Buchsel P: Long-term complications of allogenic bone marrow transplantation: Nursing implications. Oncol Nurs Forum 13:61-70, 1986.

ies must be compared. Future treatments for GVHD under investigation include the use of methylprednisolone, antithymocyte globulin, monoclonal antibodies, and intravenous immunoglobulin and thalidomide.[20,85]

Graft-versus-leukemia effect

Recipients of allogeneic BMT in whom clinically significant GVHD develops have a lower relapse rate than those patients without GVHD.[7] Efforts at achieving the appropriate amount of GVHD by administering immunosuppressive agents that would control GVHD while permitting the graft-versus-leukemic effect are being studied.[83,84]

Secondary malignancy and relapse

Secondary malignancies have been observed in a small number of patients who receive BMT and are considered to be a late sequela of this treatment modality.[86] Long-term immunosuppressive therapy used in recipients of solid organ grafts also has given rise to secondary neoplasms and infectious agents such as Epstein-Barr virus infection that might predispose patients to secondary malignancies after transplantation.[65,71]

The success rate of BMT has increased during the past 10 years, but relapse remains a major problem. Most patients in whom relapse occurs have disease in host cells, which indicates that the conditioning regimen for transplantation was not sufficient to eradicate residual leukemic cells that found sanctuary in the marrow recipient. Late relapse in cells of donor origin has been detected by molecular analysis of donor and host DNA.[87] Patients in whom relapse occurs after BMT need intensive supportive care because families and patients feel that they have exhausted not only their medical options but also their psychologic and economic strengths. Options for these patients may include a second transplant; others may choose hospice care. Nurses who work with the families of patients who ultimately will die of their original disease or transplantation-related problems will be challenged to support patients and families in death and dying issues.[66]

Although marrow transplantation holds the promise of cure for many patients who would otherwise die of their disease, many problems exist and are the subject of ongoing research. Relapse of malignancy after marrow transplantation remains a significant impediment to successful transplantation. Conditioning protocols with new regimens of chemotherapeutic agents and hyperfractionated irradiation hold promise of obtaining optimal conditioning for BMT.[20]

Involved-field irradiation given in addition to TBI to patients with lymphoma may reduce both relapse rates and irradiation toxicity. This extra irradiation may be given before or after BMT and is being investigated in the hope of increasing tumor kill and lessening irradiation-related toxicities.[19] Monoclonal antibodies targeted to tumor or hematopoietic cells conjugated with radioisotopes or immunotoxins show encouraging early results.[19,28,88] Bone-seeking isotopes designed to ablate tumor cells in the marrow without creating additional toxicities to otherwise healthy organs may have application in BMT.[19,20]

Earlier transplantation for some patients also will reduce relapse rates.[19] Some patients who have refractory disease at diagnosis or have diseases in first remission (eg, acute lymphocytic leukemia and lymphoma) may not benefit from early transplantation because traditional treatment with chemoirradiation is curative in many patients.

SURVIVORSHIP

There has been little research on issues of survivorship in marrow recipients.[59] Marrow transplantation medicine has focused on treatment of long-term complications, which has been a major contribution in increasing the number of patients who are surviving disease-free.[60,66,89] Reports of guilt and discomfort about being a "survivor" and perceptions of altered body image have been described in long-term survivors of BMT.[90,91] Patients also report role changes, sibling rivalry, and marital and family problems.[91,92] Wolcott et al,[92] in a study of 26 young adult long-term survivors of BMT, indicated that 75% manifested normal psychosocial adaptation, and 15% to 20% reported low self-esteem and less than optimal life satisfaction. Anecdotal reports and observations of these patients and their families describe survival concerns that parallel long-term survivors of other diseases. Research aimed at identifying survivorship issues in bone marrow transplantation is being formulated to clarify specific stresses and recovery strategies.

PSYCHOSOCIAL ASPECTS OF BMT

Patient

Research on the psychosocial aspects of BMT as it relates exclusively to the patient is emerging.[93,94] Patients have consistently identified specific stresses associated with each phase of the BMT process (Table 15-11). Each phase is eclipsed by particular concerns and provides a framework for nurses who care for these patients to offer appropriate support through patient preparation and teaching.

TABLE 15-11 Patterns of Psychosocial Response During Bone Marrow Transplantation

Phase	Identified Stressful Events
1	Making the decision to undertake a BMT
2	Preadmission
3	The conditioning regimen
4	Immunosuppression and germ-free isolation
5	Transplantation and waiting for engraftment
6	Hospital discharge and outpatient treatment

Donor

Donors experience a variety of psychologic reactions before and after their marrow donation. Donor-related stresses are identified and reviewed earlier in this chapter.[26-29]

Family

Families may incur considerable psychologic, emotional, and social problems before and after marrow transplantation.[23] Transplantation centers often are located far from familiar support systems. Relocation of the family requires dramatic changes in every aspect of the family dynamics.[23] These changes include economic issues, as well as the stress involved in absorbing the enormity of medical consequences of marrow transplantation. Families need to confront the long-term issues of caring for a recovering family member until the physical sequelae of treatment have vanished.[60] The involvement of a strong social work team is beneficial in transplantation settings. Preparation of families for this experience and identification of ongoing community resources lessen the likelihood of anxiety-related dysfunctional family interactions.[23,27,28]

Staff

Provision of psychologic support for staff members who care for patients undergoing marrow transplantation is essential to the quality of nursing care provided to marrow recipients and their families. Inherent to BMT nursing is chronic stress related to caring for patients whose conditions may change rapidly. These nurses are challenged by family interactions as well as patient concerns, and they become part of a psychosocial team caring for acutely ill patients who may die. Excellence in patient care, staff retention, and emotionally healthy nurses can be the result of programs designed to support staff nurses. Implementation of successful programs has been described in the literature and requires a nursing administration committed to assist nurses in coping with the stresses of their environment.[27,95]

Ethical Issues

Marrow transplantation may involve complex moral and ethical considerations. Informed consent for experimental procedures is standard, but the effectiveness of these explanations is poorly understood. Moreover, concern about the rights of children continues to challenge medical and legal systems.[19,96] Broader societal issues such as allocation of resources need examination. Difficult questions of life support arise in light of irreversible organ failure.[27] These and other complex issues provide opportunities for multidisciplinary studies of some of the major biosocial issues of our time.

FUTURE APPLICATIONS

Stem Cell Technology

Research on techniques of separation of hematopoietic stem cells includes studies of sedimentation techniques, monoclonal antibodies, and immunoadsorption columns. Application of these processes might enable infusion of leukemia-free marrow in autologous transplantation.[19,20]

Two other sources of hematopoietic stem cells exist but have not had wide application in marrow transplantation.[19] These sources include peripheral blood and fetal liver cells. The use of peripheral blood imposes limitations because of the presence of a large number of T cells; fetal liver infusion, although rich in hematopoietic stem cells, currently has limitations. The use of peripheral blood treated in vitro with growth factors may one day allow marrow donors to contribute 5 to 10 mL of peripheral blood to be treated for marrow transplantation.[19]

Biologic Response Modifiers

Interferon may provide an antileukemic effect for some patients with chronic myelocytic leukemia and acute lymphocytic leukemia, and studies are showing some degree of efficacy.[97] Growth factors are emerging as a result of understanding and application of DNA recombinant technology.[19,20] The hematopoietic growth factors include erythropoietin, GM-CSF, G-CSF, and interleukins. These cytokines hold promise for stimulating marrow recovery and preventing graft failure. Growth factors may make it possible to grow stem cell in vitro. IL-2 may permit in vitro growth of donor T cells that may have an antiviral effect when given in conjunction with donor marrow.[19,20]

Gene Transfer

Gene transfer holds dramatic promise for future applications of BMT. Application of this technology may allow replacement of defective genomic material with healthy genes in patients who have genetic diseases and are candidates for marrow transplantation. Hematopoietic marrow stem cells would probably be used, and gene transfer techniques would use retroviral vectors.[98] The first diseases to be treated with gene transfer may be enzyme-linked immunodeficiency diseases such as adenosine deaminase deficiency.[98] Although this is a rare disorder, the first attempts will provide an arena of technologic challenges that, once hurdled, will provide wider application to other genetic diseases. Substantial preclinical improvements in transfer efficiency, however, are required before clinical studies are conducted.

CONCLUSION

The success of marrow transplantation is greatly influenced by the nursing care given to marrow recipients before and for months after marrow transplantation. Nurses are required to have in-depth knowledge of current practice in marrow transplantation and astute patient assessment and management skills.[2,13,66] Marrow transplantation nursing requires nurses who have strong clinical and technical skills, as well as psychosocial sensitivities to patients and family members. Methods of establishing unified goals between medical research and nursing care personnel will continue to challenge multidisciplinary teams. Nursing administrators are accountable for providing both staff education and an environment that will retain nurses in this arena.[99] As the number of patients undergoing marrow transplantation increases, the demand for nurses of highest professional caliber will increase.

• • •

Supported in part by grants No. CA18221 and No. CA15704 awarded by the National Cancer Institute, DHHS.

REFERENCES

1. Bortin MM, Rimm AA: Increasing utilization of bone marrow transplantation. Transplantation 42:229-234, 1986.
2. Corcoran-Buchsel P, Ford RC: Introduction. Semin Oncol Nurs 4:1-2, 1988.
3. Quine WE: The remedial application of bone marrow. JAMA 26:1012-1013, 1896.
4. Santos GW: History of bone marrow transplantation. Clin Haematol 12:611-639, 1983.
5. Thomas ED, Storb R, Clift RA, et al: Bone-marrow transplantation. N Engl J Med 292:832-843, 895-902, 1975.
6. Barnes DWH, Corp MJ, Loutit JL, et al: Treatment of murine leukaemia with x-rays and homologous bone marrow. Br Med J 2:96-99, 1956.
7. Weiden PL, Flournoy N, Thomas ED, et al: Antileukemic effect of graft-versus-host disease in human recipients of allogeneic-marrow grafts. N Engl J Med 300:1068-1073, 1979.
8. Doney KC, Buckner CD: Bone marrow transplantation: An overview. Plasma Ther Transfus Technol 6:149-161, 1985.
9. Thomas ED, Sargur M: Bone marrow transplantation, in Cerilli J (ed): Organ Transplantation and Replacement. Philadelphia, JB Lippincott, 1988, pp 608-616.
10. Stream P: Functions of the outpatient clinic. Nurs Clin North Am 18:603-610, 1983.
11. Storb R, Thomas ED: Allogeneic bone marrow transplantation. Immunol Rev 71:78-102, 1983.

12. Thomas ED, Buckner CD, Sanders JE: Marrow transplantation for thalassaemia. Lancet 2:227-229, 1982.
13. Ford R, Ballard B: Acute complications after bone marrow transplantation. Semin Oncol Nurs 4:15-24, 1988.
14. Hansen RA, Clift ED, Thomas CD, et al: Histocompatibility and marrow transplantation. Transplantation Proceedings 11:1924-1929, 1979.
15. Clift RA, Hansen JA, Thomas ED, et al: Marrow transplantation from donors other than HLA-identical siblings. Transplantation 28:235-242, 1979.
16. Buckner CD, Clift RA, Sanders JE, et al: ABO-incompatible marrow transplants. Transplantation 26:233-238, 1978.
17. Bensinger WI, Buckner CD, Thomas ED, et al: ABO-incompatible marrow transplants. Transplantation 33:427-429, 1982.
18. Beatty PG, Clift RA, Mickelson EM, et al: Marrow transplantation from related donors other than HLA-identical siblings. N Engl J Med 313:765-771, 1985.
19. Beatty PG, Anasetti C, Thomas ED, et al: Marrow transplantation from relatives other than HLA-identical siblings. UCLA Symposium Bone Marrow Transplantation—Current Controversy 1988, 1989, pp 619-624.
20. Thomas ED: The future of marrow transplantation. Semin Oncol Nurs 4:74-78, 1988.
21. Bowden RA, Sayers M, Flournoy N, et al: Cytomegalovirus immune globulin and seronegative blood products to prevent primary cytomegalovirus infection after marrow transplantation. N Engl J Med 314:1006-1010, 1986.
22. Appelbaum FR: Allogeneic marrow transplantation for malignancy: Current problems and prospects for improvement, in Magrath IT (ed): New Directions in Cancer Treatment. Heidelberg, Springer-Verlag, 1989, pp 143-165.
23. Corcoran-Buchsel P, Parchem C: Ambulatory care of the bone marrow transplant patient. Semin Oncol Nurs 4:41-46, 1988.
24. Holcombe A: Bone marrow harvest. Patient Education 14:63-65, 1987.
25. Buckner CD, Clift RA, Sanders JE, et al: Marrow harvesting from normal donors. Blood 64:630-634, 1984.
26. Dudjak LA: HLA typing: Implications for nurses. Oncol Nurs Forum 11:30-36, 1984.
27. Lesko LM, Hawkins DR: Psychological aspects of transplantation medicine, in Akhtar S (ed): New Psychiatric Syndromes: DSM-III and Beyond. New York, Aronson, 1983, pp 265-309.
28. Patenaude AF, Rappeport J: Psychological costs of bone marrow transplantation in children. Am J Orthopsychiat 49:409-422, 1979.
29. Ruggiero MR: The donor in bone marrow transplantation. Semin Oncol Nurs 4:9-14, 1988.
30. Thomas ED: Bone marrow transplantation: A lifesaving applied art. JAMA 249:2528-2536, 1983.
31. Freeman SE: An overview of bone marrow transplantation. Semin Oncol Nurs 4:3-8, 1988.
32. Thomas ED, Fefer A: Bone marrow transplantation, in DeVita VT, Hellman S, Rosenberg SA (eds): Cancer: Principles and Practice of Oncology (ed 2). Philadelphia, JB Lippincott, 1985, pp 2320-2325.
33. Schryber S, Lacasse CR, Barton-Burke M: Autologous bone marrow transplantation. Oncol Nurs Forum 14:74-80, 1987.
34. Phipps WJ, Long BC, Woods NF (eds): Medical-Surgical Nursing. St Louis, CV Mosby, 1979.
35. Sullivan KM, Storb R: Allogeneic marrow transplantation. Cancer Invest 2:27-38, 1984.
36. Wolford JL, McDonald GB: A problem-oriented approach to intestinal and liver disease after marrow transplantation. J Clin Gastroenterol 10:419-433, 1988.
37. Schubert MM, Sullivan KM, Truelove EL: Head and neck complications of bone marrow transplantation, in Peterson ED, Sonis ST, Elias EG (eds): Head and Neck Management of the Cancer Patient. Boston, Martinus Nijhoff, 1986, pp 401-427.
38. Press OW, Schaller RT, Thomas ED: Bone marrow transplant complications, in Toledo-Pereyra LH (ed): Complications of Organ Transplantation. New York, Marcel Dekker, 1986, pp 399-424.
39. Sullivan KM, Parkman R: The pathophysiology and treatment of graft-versus-host disease. Clin Haematol 12:775-789, 1983.
40. Meyers JD: Infection in bone marrow transplant recipients. Am J Med 81:27-38, 1986 (suppl 1A).
41. Nuscher R, Baltzer L, Repinec DA, et al: Bone marrow transplantation: A lifesaving option. Am J Nurs 764-772, 1984.
42. Parker N, Cohen T: Acute graft-versus-host disease in allogeneic marrow transplantation: A nursing perspective. Nurs Clin North Am 18:569-577, 1983.
43. Sullivan KM: Special care of the allogeneic marrow transplant patient, in Wiernik PH, Canellos G, Kyle RA, et al (eds): Neoplastic Diseases of the Blood. New York, Churchill Livingstone, 1985, pp 1117-1140.
44. Aker SN, Lenssen P, Darbinian J, et al: Nutritional assessment in the marrow transplant patient. Nutr Supp Serv 3:22-37, 1983.
45. McDonald GB, Sharma P, Matthews DE, et al: The clinical course of 53 patients with venoocclusive disease of the liver after marrow transplantation. Transplantation 39:603-608, 1985.
46. Anderson RJ, Schrier RW: Acute renal failure, in Braunwald E, Isselbacher KJ, Petersdorf RG, et al (eds): Harrison's Principles of Internal Medicine. New York, McGraw-Hill, 1987, pp 1149-1155.
47. Kennedy MS, Deeg HJ, Siegel M, et al: Acute renal toxicity with combined use of amphotericin B and cyclosporine after marrow transplantation. Transplantation 35:211-215, 1983.
48. Dixon BS, Anderson RJ: Nonoliguric acute renal failure. Am J Kidney Dis 6:71-80, 1985.
49. Buckner CD, Meyers JD, Springmeyer SC, et al: Pulmonary complications of marrow transplantation: Review of the Seattle experience. Exp Hematol 12:1-5, 1984 (suppl 15).
50. Sullivan KM, Meyers JD, Flournoy N, et al: Early and late interstitial pneumonia following human bone marrow transplantation. Int J Cell Cloning 4:107-121, 1986 (suppl 1).
51. Emanuel D, Cunningham I, Jules-Elysee K, et al: Cytomegalovirus pneumonia after bone marrow transplantation successfully treated with the combination of ganciclovir and high-dose intravenous immune globulin. Ann Intern Med 109:777-782, 1988.
52. Reed EC, Bowden RA, Dandliker PS, et al: Treatment of cytomegalovirus pneumonia with ganciclovir and intravenous cytomegalovirus immunoglobulin in patients with bone marrow transplants. Ann Intern Med 109:783-788, 1988.
53. Thompson CB, June CH, Sullivan KM, et al: Association between cyclosporine neurotoxicity and hypomagnesemia. Lancet 2:1116-1120, 1984.
54. Meyers JD, Thomas ED: Infection complicating bone marrow transplantation, in Rubin RH, Young LS (eds): Clinical Approach to Infection in the Immunocompromised Host. New York, Plenum, 1981, pp 507-551.
55. Lindgren PS: The laminar air flow room nursing: Practices and procedures. Nurs Clin North Am 18:553-561, 1983.
56. Buckner CD, Clift RA, Thomas ED, et al: Early infectious

complications in allogeneic marrow transplant recipients with acute leukemia: Effects of prophylactic measures. Infection 11:243-250, 1983.
57. Sullivan KM: Immunoglobulin therapy in bone marrow transplantation. Am J Med 83:34-45, 1987.
58. McDonald GB, Shulman HM, Sullivan KM, et al: Intestinal and hepatic complications of human bone marrow transplantation. Gastroenterology 90:460-477, 770-784, 1986.
59. Corcoran-Buchsel P: Ambulatory care of the bone marrow recipient: Pre and post transplant considerations. Puget Sound Quarterly 12(1): Winter, 1989.
60. Nims JW, Strom S: Late complications of bone marrow transplant recipients: Nursing care issues. Semin Oncol Nurs 4:47-54, 1988.
61. Brooten D, Kuman S, Brown LP, et al: A randomized clinical trial of early hospital discharge and home follow-up of very-low-birth-weight infants. N Engl J Med 315:934-939, 1986.
62. Donati MA, Guenette G, Auerbach H: Prospective controlled study of home and hospital therapy of cystic fibrosis pulmonary disease. J Ped 111:28-33, 1987.
63. Deeg HJ, Storb R, Thomas ED: Bone marrow transplantation: A review of delayed complications. Br J Haematol 57:185-208, 1984.
64. Atkinson K, Meyers JD, Storb R, et al: Varicella-zoster virus infection after marrow transplantation for aplastic anemia or leukemia. Transplantation 29:47-50, 1980.
65. Witherspoon RP, Storb R, Ochs HD, et al: Recovery of antibody production in human allogeneic marrow graft recipients: Influence of time posttransplantation, the presence or absence of chronic graft-versus-host disease, and antithymocyte globulin treatment. Blood 58:360-368, 1981.
66. Corcoran-Buchsel P: Long-term complications of allogeneic bone marrow transplantation: Nursing implications. Oncol Nurs Forum 13:61-70, 1986.
67. Clark JG, Schwartz DA, Flournoy N, et al: Risk factors for airflow obstruction in recipients of bone marrow transplants. Ann Intern Med 107:648-656, 1987.
68. Sanders JE, Pritchard S, Mahoney P, et al: Growth and development following marrow transplantation for leukemia. Blood 68:1129-1135, 1986.
69. Sanders JE, Buckner CD, Sullivan KM, et al: Growth and development in children after bone marrow transplantation. Hormone Research, 30:92-97, 1988.
70. Deeg HJ, Flournoy N, Sullivan KM, et al: Cataracts after total body irradiation and marrow transplantation: A sparing effect of dose fractionation. Int J Radiat Oncol Biol Phys 10:957-964, 1984.
71. Storb R, Prentice RL, Thomas ED, et al: Factors associated with graft rejection after HLA-identical marrow transplantation for aplastic anaemia. Br J Haematol 55:573-585, 1983.
72. Martin PJ, Hansen JA, Buckner CD, et al: Effects of in vitro depletion of T-cells in HLA-identical allogeneic marrow grafts. Blood 66:664-672, 1985.
73. Sullivan KM, Deeg HJ, Sanders JE, et al: Late complications after marrow transplantation. Semin Hematol 21:53-63, 1984.
74. Sullivan KM: Graft-versus-host disease, in Blume KG, Petz LD (eds): Clinical Bone Marrow Transplantation. New York, Churchill Livingstone, 1983, pp 91-129.
75. Schubert MM, Sullivan KM, Izutsu KT, et al: Oral complications of bone marrow transplantation, in Peterson DE, Sonis ST (eds): Oral Complications of Cancer Chemotherapy. Boston, Martinus Nijhoff, 1983, pp 93-112.
76. Jack MK, Jack GM, Sale GE, et al: Ocular manifestations of graft-vs-host disease. Arch Ophthalmol 101:1080-1084, 1983.
77. Shulman HM, Sullivan KM, Weiden PL, et al: Chronic graft-versus-host syndrome in man: A long-term clinicopathological study of 20 Seattle patients. Am J Med 69:204-217, 1980.
78. Corson SL, Sullivan K, Batzer F, et al: Gynecologic manifestations of chronic graft-versus-host disease. Obstet Gynecol 60:488-492, 1982.
79. Sullivan KM, Witherspoon RP, Storb R, et al: Chronic graft-versus-host disease: Recent advances in diagnosis and treatment, in Gale RP, Champlin R (eds): UCLA Symposia on Molecular and Cellular Biology (vol 91) (new series). New York, Alan R Liss, 1989, pp 511-522.
80. Loughran TP Jr, Sullivan KM: Early detection and monitoring of chronic graft-versus-host disease, in Burakoff SJ, Deeg HJ, Ferrara JLM, et al (eds): Graft-Versus-Host Disease. New York, Marcel Dekker (in press).
81. Sullivan KM, Witherspoon RP, Storb R, et al: Prednisone and azathioprine compared with prednisone and placebo for treatment of chronic graft-vs-host disease: Prognostic influence of prolonged thrombocytopenia after allogeneic marrow transplantation. Blood 72:546-554, 1988.
82. Sullivan KM, Witherspoon RP, Storb R, et al: Alternating-day cyclosporine and prednisone for treatment of high-risk chronic graft-v-host disease. Blood 72:555-561, 1988.
83. Sullivan KM, Weiden PL, Storb R, et al: Influence of acute and chronic graft-versus-host disease on relapse and survival after bone marrow transplantation from HLA-identical siblings as treatment of acute and chronic leukemia. Blood 73:1720-1728, 1989.
84. Sullivan KM, Storb R, Buckner CD, et al: Graft-versus-host disease as adoptive immunotherapy in patients with advanced hematologic neoplasms: A randomized study of short-course methotrexate vs. standard methotrexate vs. standard methotrexate plus donor buffy coat cells following allogeneic marrow transplantation. N Engl J Med 320:828-834, 1989.
85. Sullivan KM, Kopecky K, Jocom J, et al: Antimicrobial and immunomodulatory effects of intravenous immunoglobulin in bone marrow transplantation. Blood 72:410a, 1988 (suppl 1).
86. Deeg HJ, Sanders J, Martin P, et al: Secondary malignancies after marrow transplantation. Exp Hematol 12:660-666, 1984.
87. Witherspoon RP, Schubach W, Neiman P, et al: Donor cell leukemia developing six years after marrow grafting for acute leukemia. Blood 65:1172-1174, 1985.
88. Appelbaum FR, Badger C, Deeg HJ, et al: Use of Iodine-131-labeled anti-immune response-associated monoclonal antibody as a preparative regimen prior to bone marrow transplantation: Initial dosimetry. NCI Monogr 3:67-71, 1987.
89. Sullivan KM, Shulman HM, Storb R, et al: Chronic graft-versus-host disease in 52 patients: Adverse natural course and successful treatment with combination immunosuppression. Blood 57:267-276, 1981.
90. Patenaude AF, Rappeport JM: Surviving bone marrow transplantation: The patient in the other bed. Ann Intern Med 97:915-918, 1982.
91. Brown HN, Kelly MJ: Stages of bone marrow transplantation: A psychiatric perspective. Psychosom Med 38:439-446, 1976.
92. Wolcott DL, Wellisch DK, Fawzy FI, et al: Adaptation of adult bone marrow transplant recipient long-term survivors. Transplantation 41:478-488, 1986.
93. Haberman MR: Psychosocial aspects of bone marrow transplantation. Semin Oncol Nurs 4:55-59, 1988.

94. Mullan F: Seasons of survival: Reflections of a physician with cancer. N Engl J Med 313:270-273, 1985.
95. Sarantos S: Innovations in psychosocial staff support: A model program for the marrow transplant nurse. Semin Oncol Nurs 4:69-73, 1988.
96. Serota FT, O'Shea AT, Woodward WT Jr, et al: Role of a child advocate in the selection of donors for pediatric bone marrow transplantation. J Pediatr 98:847-850, 1981.
97. Myers JD, Flournoy N, Sanders JE, et al: Prophylactic use of human leukocyte interferon after allogeneic marrow transplantation. Ann Inter Med 107:809-816, 1987.
98. Cline MJ: Gene therapy: Current status. Am J Med 83:291-297, 1987.
99. Kelleher J, Jennings M: Nursing management of a marrow transplant unit: A framework for practice. Semin Oncol Nurs 4:60-68, 1988.

PART IV

PSYCHOSOCIAL DIMENSIONS OF CANCER

Chapter 16

Overview of Psychosocial Dimensions

Rose F. McGee, RN, PhD

INTRODUCTION

The focus of the psychosocial dimension of cancer care is the unique needs of the individual at risk for or with cancer and the social groups affected by that individual. Each individual brings to the cancer experience unique personality traits and a personal socialization pattern different from all others. Understanding the uniqueness of the individual is achieved only through study of the commonalities of the "personality and social psychological"[1] aspects of illness.

To separate the dimensions of health care into physical and psychosocial is artificial, yet it serves pragmatic purposes in narrowing the scope of the discussion. In fact, a whole body of literature exists on the study of psychosocial variables as a risk factor in carcinogenesis. Lickiss[2] noted that reviews of cancer research in the nineteenth century indicated that "while tissue and cellular changes were the characteristic phenomena of cancer, both inherent susceptibility and extrinsic influences played a part in the genesis of these phenomena—by mechanisms unknown" (p. 297). More recently, the study of psychosocial factors as independent variables has been focused on the study of the immune and endocrine systems as mechanisms of causation.[3] Thus the study of psychosocial variables as causative is an evolving area of study in oncology that may provide future clues to prevention.

In the meantime, professional commitment to quality of care and to holistic care has resulted in a focus on psychosocial aspects of illness as outcome variables of the cancer experience. Empirically, the prevalence of psychosocial distress in response to a diagnosis of cancer has been found to range from a rare occurrence to as high as 90% of all patients.[4] The burgeoning number of studies on variables that maximize self-actualization and minimize psychosocial distress offers new understanding about the meaning of the diagnosis of cancer and response patterns of individuals and groups to the actual or perceived threat.

The purpose of this chapter is to address the ubiquitous threat of cancer and to discuss the use of psychosocial resources to manage responses. To choose one theoretical orientation would be reductionistic, and to discuss the breadth of psychosocial theories is prohibitive; therefore, the chapter is of necessity an overview of selected concepts derived from the theoretical, empirical, and experiential body of knowledge of the psychosocial aspects of cancer and cancer care. A basic assumption of the following discussion is that psychosocial responses to the cancer experience are determined by the characteristics of cancer, the person with or at risk for cancer, and the social system of significance to the individual.

CANCER: THE UBIQUITOUS THREAT

The only certainty in oncology is that cancer is an actual or potential threat to all humans. Statistically, one in three persons and three of every four families will experience cancer. But statistics apply to groups and serve a minimal purpose in assessing individual risks. A small percentage of the population can personalize the risk further because of genetic predisposition to cancer, but for the majority, cancer risks are the product of unmeasurable, cumulative life-style and environmental exposure. Therefore to live in the current physical and psychosocial environment is to be at risk for cancer. The particular risk will vary with age, geographic location, and life-style choices, but no individual or social sector is exempt.

The threat or diagnosis of cancer can be characterized as follows:

1. The meaning to the individual is unique.
2. The disease and treatment are marked by uncertainty.
3. Cancer is a chronic illness.
4. Cancer results in a changed identity.
5. Cancer affects the entire social system of the person involved.

Cancer Is a Unique Experience

The stigma of cancer has been traced historically by Cassileth[5] from the naming of the disease by Hippocrates as *karkinos*, which means crab, to the seventeenth and eighteenth century notion that cancer was contagious, which led to the use of the word "tumor" or other euphemisms to minimize isolation of persons with the diagnosis. During the nineteenth century, "tumors" were classified as benign or malignant, and further pathologic delineation lead to the contemporary understanding of cancer as a composite of many diseases. Cassileth[5] described the last 50 years as an era in which cancer is no longer met with fearful retreat in Western cultures but is met with a more frontier-type spirit, as evidenced by the "war on cancer." Nevertheless, the stigma of cancer continues to exist with respect to social and individual perceptions. Insurance cancellations, job and military discrimination, and problems with reintegration into the school and workplace are manifestations of the persistent social stigma of cancer.

The prevailing Western view of cancer is that cancer is a treatable disease. The resulting societal expectation is that the individual will accept the diagnosis, seek care, and comply with a fighting spirit.[5] Nevertheless, to the individual, cancer has been described as the "ultimate existential crisis."[6] For most persons, cancer is among the most feared of all diseases.[7] Reasons listed for the fear of cancer include the occurrence without warning, uncontrollable spreading of the disease, incurability beyond a certain point, association with pain and discomfort, social and professional attitudes of hopelessness, difficulty of diagnosis, mutilative treatment, unknown causation, and the fact that cooperation with treatment does not necessarily lead to successful outcomes.[8]

In Western societies, health is a value and illness is experienced as a barrier to the achievement of valued goals; therefore the perceived threat of cancer includes a subjective evaluation of the threat to health in general and the threat of cancer in particular. Smith[9] provided a multidimensional and hierarchial description of health that is useful in studying the impact of cancer on health in general. According to Smith, perceptions of health range from the most primitive level of absence of pathology, to disruption of role functioning, to ability to adapt, to the highest level, which is self-actualization. Because of the problems of diagnosis and of determining spread or recurrence of disease, each dimension of health may be disrupted. A perceived absence of pathology with respect to cancer is never certain among both the general population and persons previously diagnosed with cancer; both ascribed and achieved roles are temporarily or permanently disrupted; the ability to adapt may be exceeded by the demands of the illness; and safety and survival needs may supercede self-actualization goals.

Cognitive appraisal[10] of the personal meaning of cancer and the impact on life goals determine the meaning of cancer to the individual. Knowledge of and past experiences with the disease are but two variables that influence psychosocial and behavioral responses. According to the health belief model,[11] necessary conditions for preventive or curative care include some knowledge of the disease, perceived vulnerability, motivation to seek help, and perceived benefits that exceed barriers to action.

In summary, the threat of cancer is a unique process determined by cognitive appraisal of the situation. Threat appraisal is subjective and includes evaluation of the adequacy of resources to deal with the perceived situation. Cohen and Lazarus[12] summarized patterns of cancer threat perceptions as follows:

1. Fear of dying
2. Changes in body integrity and comfort
3. Changes in self-concept and disruption of future plans
4. Inability to maintain emotional equilibrium
5. Lack of fulfillment of social roles and activities
6. Inability to adapt to new physical and social environments

Disease and Treatment Are Marked by Uncertainty

Experiential knowledge of delays in diagnosis, short illness trajectories, unpredictable prognoses, and early death in apparently healthy individuals compound the uncertainties associated with the cancer diagnosis and prognosis. Mishel[13] defined uncertainty as the "inability to determine the meaning of illness-related events" (p. 225). Uncertainty results from the inability to structure the meaning of illness-related stimuli to form a cognitive schema for the illness events perceived. Stimuli consist of symptom patterns, event familiarity, and event congruence between the expected and experienced patterns. The degree to which the specific malignancy fits the criteria for uncertainty outlined by Mishel is determined by the degree of:

1. Ambiguity concerning the state of the illness
2. The complexity of treatment and the system of care
3. Information held about the diagnosis and seriousness
4. Predictability of the course and prognosis.

Although these criteria are useful in determining the predicted degree of uncertainty of the specific cancer diagnosis, uncertainty is not inherent in the situation but is a perception of the individual. The cognitive capacity of the individual and perceived resources influence the outcomes of this appraisal process.[13] According to crisis theorists, the perception may be interpreted as a danger or as an opportunity for growth.

Cancer Is a Chronic Illness

Much has been written about the chronicity of cancer. Of significance with respect to management of psychosocial responses is the fact that simple crisis resolution models are not sufficient to address the scope of problems encountered with cancer. Mages and Mendelsohn[14] noted that people with cancer are confronted with a continuing series of stressors rather than with a single, time-limited crisis. The treatment is complex, often extended, and may cause irreparable damage to physical, mental, or social functioning. Patients identify the lifelong fear of recurrence as one of the most disruptive aspects of the illness.

Application of stress management theory to the cancer experience makes the health care professional attentive to the fact that the initial adaptive responses used by patients may be outmoded as the disease process and treatment change.[14] For example, denial may be adaptive in the early stages of the disease as a defense mechanism, allowing the individual to assimilate the impact of the illness in manageable increments of awareness. By the same token, persistent denial may block motivation of adaptive health behavior in later stages of the illness. Likewise, the preoccupation with self that is characteristic during diagnosis and recurrence may initiate problem-solving coping behaviors during these stressful events but may alienate the person's social and professional network if persistent.

A further implication of the usefulness of stress theory in understanding psychosocial responses is the consideration of the effect of cumulative stressors on the ability to adapt. Individuals come to the cancer experience with a history of stress responses. The individual who has been unsuccessful in resolving past stress situations, who is dealing with a number of stressors simultaneously, and who perceives minimal social support in the situation is at higher risk for psychosocial distress.

The Cancer Experience Results in a Changed Identity

The majority of individuals who encounter cancer report permanent changes in self-perception and future orientation. Weisman and Worden[15] used the Inventory of Current Concerns to accrue empirical data on changes in emotional responses and interpretation, in reactions to others and to one's immediate world, and in thoughts of life, death, and survival. The concept of "existential plight" was used to refer to this grouping of perceptions of self.

Some changes in identity are socially imposed, while others are internal in origin. Evans,[16] in describing a personal experience with cancer, related a vivid description of the interactional effects on identity:

> There I was. I had cancer—the big "C". . . . The initial period of discovering my cancer caused the most trauma with both family and friends. . . . I could not cope with that look in their eyes. I did not want their sympathetic glances, their hushed tones. I had not changed inside. I was still the same person. Yet suddenly I seemed to have become different; I had become a cancer victim, losing my personal identity at home and in the hospital. I tried to retain a normal life. . . . It was then that I decided a personal survival plan would help and support me. [The doctors] were great. They just listened. I just hoped that I had enough strength to fight long enough for my life. Then the waiting period. Another form of purgatory—to regain normality while waiting to see if the cure will be effective. I was fortunate to receive the constant support of my family, friends, doctors, and nurses. My role was to find the inner strength and determination to fight back. I hope if I was [sic] ever put to the test again I would be able to fight back—I know now I would try. Life is far more precious to me now (pp. 17-18).

Adaptive and defense mechanisms are means the individual uses to cope with the conflicts between the physiological, psychological and sociocultural demands of cancer. Repression, projection, reaction formation, situation avoidance, and transference have been observed in cancer patients coping with changes in identity inflicted by the diagnosis and treatment.[17]

The specific culture of the individual shapes the view of health in terms of the range of normal, cause and effect perceptions, and the language to describe deviations from normal. For example, in a culture in which life expectancy is short, cancer may be a less meaningful threat than in a culture in which the chronic diseases of aging are the leading causes of death.[18]

Finally, the culture, through socialization, shapes the more enduring aspects of the attitudes, beliefs, and values that constitute one's personality and that provide continuity in the reordering of the meaning of life and of one's relationship to a higher being. Cancer can challenge lifelong values and beliefs and may result in changed cognitive, affective, and behavioral responses.[18] Affective responses identified as occurring most frequently among cancer patients are anxiety and depression. No one response, per se, is either adaptive or maladaptive. The appropriateness of the response to the psychosocially constructed reality of the situation and adaptability of the social network in acquiring new patterns of response, as indicated, determine the adaptive potential of the specific response.

Cancer Affects the Social System of the Individual

Psychosocial responses may be categorized as a complex interaction of cognitive, affective, behavioral, and physical components. For example, a common cognitive response of patients and families is the "why me" phenomenon and a resultant search to make sense of a senseless situation. Causal attributions tend to cluster into the categories of self-blame and projection.[19] The cognitive search for causation may influence affective responses positively by dispelling some of the anxiety associated with the diagnosis or negatively by leading to self-doubt and hostility toward others. The behavioral response of continuously "telling one's story" may, in turn, lead to social rejection and further enhance physical feelings of distress.

Within the social milieu, the family may deal affectively with the problem of uncertain causation by blaming the patient and thus absolve personal guilt, while less intimate significant others or health care professionals may maintain cognitive beliefs in a "just world" by blaming the patient as well.[20] Thus a vicious cycle may emerge in which the person is held responsible for the illness by self or others, and the potential for psychosocial distress is heightened, especially if the disease is unrelenting or recurrent.

The level of perceived social support is a variable that is viewed as a buffer to the effects of stress on the health of the individual.[21] Postulated mechanisms of the buffering effect of perceived social support include diminishing the level of the perceived stress of the situation, facilitating coping effectiveness, and lessening the reactions of the individual to the stressors.[22]

THE SEARCH FOR PSYCHOSOCIAL RESOURCES

The search for psychosocial resources to deal with the actual or potential threat of cancer is generally initiated in terms of self-appraisal and can be conceptualized as expanding spheres to significant others and, finally, to members of the health care professions. Orem,[23] in emphasizing the self-care concept, heightened the awareness of the professional with respect to the fact that the initial help-seeking behaviors expand outward from the individual to the professional; likewise, the return to health should be manifest by the professional's returning the responsibility for health care to the family and ultimately to the patient. Fostering individual control, anticipatory socialization, and early discharge and rehabilitative planning are a few of the techniques that foster achievement of these goals.

In general, the primary objective of nursing intervention is to foster the coping responses of patients, significant others, and the health care team. According to stress theorists, coping may be emotion focused or problem-solving focused. Examples of emotion-focused interventions include fostering emotional expression through active listening; creating constructive release of affective responses through play therapy, music, or humor; fostering understanding of the impact of personal responses on others through role playing; and providing individual or group testing and counseling to facilitate insight into emotional needs and response patterns. Problem-solving interventions may include information giving on the subjective, environmental, and temporal features of diagnostic and treatment processes; anticipatory socialization to expected life stressors and processes, such as loss and grief; individual and group teaching based on assessment of learning needs; identification of resource information and personnel; and referral for more specialized or intensive therapy.

The taxonomy of nursing diagnoses developed in a series of National Conferences for Classification of Nursing Diagnosis (NANDA) reflects the commitment of the profession to addressing both patient and family responses to illness and treatment. Research findings that 65% to 75% of health care is provided by the patient or the family[24] and that the spouse is the primary mental health caregiver[25] attest to the appropriateness of nursing diagnoses specific to the individual and the family.

Finally, these diagnoses illustrate the fact that psychosocial responses include both the potential for distress and for growth. Nursing intervention to achieve the latter has been studied extensively, but methodologic problems and the complexity of human behavior hinder accumulation of definitive data on the relative effectiveness of each intervention. A recent review by Johnson and Lauver[26] of the theoretical and empirical relationships between preparatory information giving and coping with stressful treatment experiences is an example of the accrual of theoretical and empirical data that reflects both the progress and limitations in establishing the database needed to increase nursing effectiveness in dealing with the psychosocial aspects of cancer care.

CONCLUSION

The following two chapters provide models of more specific nursing approaches to the study of selected psychosocial responses to the actual or potential diagnosis of cancer. The focus of Chapter 17 is responses of the individual, and Chapter 18 addresses the interactional responses of the person and the social system. The final chapter in this section, Chapter 19, combines the responses of the person and the social network with respect to survivorship.

REFERENCES

1. Cooper C: The psychological precursors of cancer, in Cooper C (ed): Psychosocial Stress and Cancer. New York, John Wiley & Sons, 1984, pp 21-33.
2. Lickiss JN: The growing edge: Psychosocial aspects of cancer. Med J Aust 1:297-302, 1980.
3. Greer S: Psychological enquiry: A contribution to cancer research. J Psychol Med 9:81-89, 1979.
4. Farber JM, Weinerman BH, Kuypers JA: Psychosocial distress in oncology outpatients. J Psychosoc Oncol 2:109-118, 1984.
5. Cassileth BR: The evolution of oncology as a sociomedical phenomenon, in Cassileth BR (ed): The Cancer Patient: Social and Medical Aspects of Care. Philadelphia, Lea & Febiger, 1979, pp 3-16.
6. Brohn P: The Bristol Programme. London, Century Paperbacks, 1987.
7. Cox T: Stress: A psychophysiological approach to cancer, in Cooper CL (ed): Psychosocial Stress and Cancer. New York, John Wiley & Sons, 1984, pp 149-169.
8. Clark RL: Psychological reactions of patients and health professionals to cancer, in Cullen JW, Fox BH, Isom RN (eds): Cancer: The Behavioral Dimensions, New York, Raven Press, 1976, pp 1-10.
9. Smith JA: The idea of health: A philosophical inquiry. Adv Nurs Sci 3:43-50, 1981.
10. Folkman S, Schaefer C, Lazarus RS: Cognitive processes as mediators of stress and coping, in Hamilton V, Warburton DM (eds): Human Stress and Cognition. Chichester, England, John Wiley & Sons, 1979, pp 265-298.
11. Becker M, Haefner DP, Kasl SV, et al: Selected psychosocial models and correlates of individual health related behaviors. Med Care 15:27-46, 1977.
12. Cohen F, Lazarus RS: Coping with the stresses of illness, in Cohen F, Adler NE (eds): Health Psychology: A Handbook. San Francisco, Jossey-Bass, 1979, pp 217-254.
13. Mishel MH: Uncertainty in illness. Image: J Nurs Schol 20:225-232, 1988.
14. Mages NL, Mendelsohn GA: Effects of cancer on patient's lives: A psychological approach, in Cohen F, Adler NE (eds): Health Psychology: A Handbook. San Francisco, Jossey-Bass, 1979, pp 255-284.
15. Weisman AD, Worden JW: The existential plight in cancer: Significance of the first 100 days. Int J Psychiatr Med 7:1-5, 1976/1977.
16. Evans J: The cancer experience—a patient's view, in Pritchard AP (ed): Cancer Nursing: A Revolution in Care, Proceedings of the Fifth International Conference on Cancer Nursing. London, England, Macmillan Press, 1989, pp 17-18.
17. Westbrook MT, Viney LL: Psychological reactions to the onset of chronic illness. Soc Sci Med 16:899-905, 1982.
18. Haney CA: Psychosocial factors in the management of patients with cancer, in Cooper CL (ed): Psychosocial Stress and Cancer. New York, John Wiley & Sons, 1984, pp 201-227.
19. Bard MT: The price of survival for cancer victims, in Strauss AL (ed): Where Medicine Fails (ed 3). New Brunswick, NJ, Transaction Books, 1979, pp 225-236.
20. Lerner MJ: The desire for justice and reactions to victims, in Macaulay J, Berkowitz L (eds): Altruism and Helping Behavior. New York, Academic Press, 1970, pp 205-229.
21. Northouse LL: Social support in patients' and husbands' adjustment to breast cancer. Nurs Res 37:91-95, 1988.
22. House JS: Work, Stress and Social Support. Reading, Mass, Addison-Wesley, 1981.
23. Orem DE: Nursing: Concepts of Practice. New York, McGraw-Hill, 1985.
24. Levin L, Katz A, Hoist E: Self Care: Lay Initiatives in Health. New York, Prodist, 1976.
25. Oberst MT, James RH: Going home: Patient and spouse adjustment following cancer surgery. Topics Clin Nurs 7:46-57, 1985.
26. Johnson JE, Lauver DR: Alternative explanations in coping with stressful experiences associated with physical illness. Adv Nurs Sci 11:39-52, 1989.

Chapter 17

Psychosocial Dimensions: The Patient

Jane Clark, RN, MN, OCN

INTRODUCTION

Psychosocial responses to cancer are influenced by factors that create the perceived reality of cancer for the individual. The reality of the cancer experience is complex and uncertain and results in psychosocial responses that are dynamic, nonlinear, and nonhierarchial and that vary in severity. The complex intrapersonal and interpersonal reactions to the cancer experience mandate that health care professionals share a common concern and maintain a high index of suspicion for the occurrence of dysfunctional psychosocial responses. Focusing on systematic and continuous assessment for signs and symptoms of psychosocial responses, identification of dysfunctional responses, development of interdisciplinary interventions to facilitate adaptive psychosocial responses, and evaluation of the effectiveness and efficiency of selected interventions to meet identified needs can improve both the quantity and quality of survival for people with cancer.

What is the basis of psychosocial care in oncology? Historically, clinical case studies of individuals and groups experiencing cancer were used to identify the unique psychosocial responses to cancer, to describe the types of coping patterns among persons with cancer, and to guide health care professionals in assisting the person with cancer to adapt to the diagnosis, the demands of treatment, and the demands of living with a cancer diagnosis. Yet just as significant variability exists in physiologic responses to cancer of different sites as well as within the same site, the variability of psychosocial responses is multiplied by the fact that each individual brings his or her values, beliefs, attitudes, personality, resources, and coping patterns to the cancer experience.

Efforts of health care professionals to understand the unique psychosocial responses of persons with cancer have been enhanced through qualitative studies of the relationship of selected psychosocial variables to:

1. Physiologic factors, such as site of cancer, histology, grade, stage of disease, or treatment modality
2. Care settings, including primary, secondary, and tertiary care hospitals, outpatient clinics, and the home
3. Temporal elements of the disease trajectory, ranging from screening to diagnosis, primary treatment, recurrence or relapse, death, or long-term survival
4. Developmental stage of the individual, with emphasis on the responses of children and older adults

Yet the findings from qualitative studies often yielded conflicting results. Thus, health care professionals began to examine conceptual and theoretical inconsistencies of both clinical and empirical data. Recently researchers have focused on developing clarity and specificity in describing the psychosocial responses of persons with cancer. The development of instruments with acceptable reliability and validity estimates among persons with cancer, expansion of research methodologies to include qualitative methods, and development of advanced statistical modeling procedures to study the interaction of psychosocial responses both as dependent and independent variables have contributed to understanding complex psychosocial relationships.

The focus of this chapter is the psychosocial responses that are of high incidence among persons with cancer. Responses selected include anxiety, depression, hopelessness, and altered sexual health. An operational definition of each response has been developed. Selected research and clinical instruments to measure the response are described and a review of representative research articles addressing the incidence and relationship of the response to the cancer experience is presented. Finally, areas for future nursing research are suggested.

ANXIETY

Anxiety has been described, with depression, as the most common psychosocial reaction experienced by persons with cancer. However, limited data exist on the occurrence and patterns of anxiety in persons with cancer. Often associated with transitions in the course of the disease or treatment, anxiety is described as a recurring response, varying in levels of intensity throughout the cancer experience.

Operational Definition

Operationally, anxiety can be defined as follows:

- An individual exists with the ability to respond affectively to changes in the environment.
- The individual perceives certain beliefs, values, and conditions essential to a secure existence.
- The individual experiences a nonspecific internal or external stimulus that is perceived as a threat to the secure existence.
- *The individual responds to the perceived threat affectively with an increased level of arousal associated with vague, unpleasant, and uneasy feelings defined as anxiety.*

Measurement Instrument: State-Trait Anxiety Inventory

The instrument used most commonly to measure anxiety among persons with cancer is the State-Trait Anxiety Inventory (STAI).[1] The STAI consists of two scales, the A-trait and A-state. Subjects are asked to respond to 20 items (A-state) on a 4-point scale (not at all, somewhat, moderately so, and very much so). Responses are summed to measure how the subject feels at a particular moment. Scores indicate the level of transitory anxiety characterized by feelings of apprehension, tension, and autonomic nervous system–induced symptoms: nervousness, worry, and apprehension.

The trait inventory is designed to measure general level of arousal and predict anxiety proneness. Subjects are asked to respond to 20 items (A-trait) on a 4-point scale (almost never, sometimes, often, and almost always). Again, responses are summed to measure disposition to respond to a stressful situation with varying levels of A-state intensity and the degree to which presenting stimuli are perceived as dangerous or threatening. Scores range from 20 to 80 for each scale, with a higher score representing higher levels of anxiety.

Reliability estimates for the STAI have been reported in the alpha coefficient range of .83 to .92. Construct validity has been reported as point biserial ranges of .60 to .73 and alpha ranges of .83 to .94. Concurrent validity has been established with the Taylor Manifest Anxiety Scale (r = .79 to .83) and the Affect Adjective Checklist (r = .51 to .52). In addition, construct validity with the known groups technique has been established.[1]

Patterns of Occurrence

The occurrence of anxiety as a response to diagnosis and treatment of cancer was described in the literature by Lucente and Fleck,[2] who compared levels of anxiety between patients hospitalized with a diagnosis of cancer and with a nonmalignant condition. Findings indicated greater levels of anxiety in the group with a diagnosis of cancer. Similar findings have been reported by other researchers.[3,4]

Anxiety is increased at diagnosis and remains elevated in varying levels throughout the course of treatment regardless of treatment modality or setting. Surgery as a treatment modality in general elicits an anxiety response, yet when the surgery is for cancer, the response may be more severe. Morris and Royle[5] reported preoperative and postoperative levels of clinical anxiety among 20 patients with early breast cancer given a choice of surgery (simple mastectomy or wide excision and radiotherapy) and 10 patients not given a choice. Findings indicated that a significantly higher percentage of patients not offered a choice of surgery were clinically anxious preoperatively when compared with those patients given a choice ($p < .05$). For those patients offered a choice, no significant differences in clinical anxiety were found between those who had a simple mastectomy and those who had a wide excision and radiotherapy or between patients having surgery for benign breast disease (n = 31) and general surgical patients (n = 20).[5]

Oberst and Scott[6] reported no differences in anxiety scores among a group of patients with genitourinary cancer treated surgically with and without a resulting ostomy at five time periods from predischarge up to 180 days after discharge. Repeated measures ANOVA indicated that the pattern of anxiety scores were essentially linear with a significant time effect ($F(3,114) = 8.834$, $p < .0001$).[6]

To describe the emotional impact of surgical treatment for breast cancer within the first year after surgery, Gottschalk and Hoigaard-Martin[7] analyzed data collected from a collaborative study group supported by the National Cancer Institute. At 1 to 3 months after surgery, 118 women who had a unilateral mastectomy for stage I or II breast cancer had significantly higher mean death, mutilation, and total anxiety scores as measured by the Gottschalk-Gleser Content Analysis Scale than did 64 women who had a biopsy for benign breast disease, 69 women who had a cholecystectomy, and 78 women who had not had a major surgical intervention. However, significant reductions in mean mutilation, shame, and total anxiety scores ($p < .01$) were reported in the mastectomy group 10 to 12 months after surgery.[7]

Similar patterns of anxiety responses appear in the literature concerning radiation therapy as a treatment modality. In a study of 181 patients receiving external radiation therapy for cancer, Irwin et al[8] found that all patients, male and female, exhibited higher anxiety scores than nonpatient norms before treatment. Yet higher anxiety scores were reported among female versus male patients before initiation of treatment, 1 week after treatment was completed, and 2 months after completion of therapy. Patients in general reported significantly higher anxiety during rather than after treatment.[8]

In another study, anxiety was examined among patients (N = 45) receiving external radiation therapy for cancer.[9] A pattern of anxiety responses emerged. Patients with lower anxiety scores (STAI) before treatment exhibited significantly higher A-state scores after treatment; patients with moderate anxiety scores exhibited little change in A-state scores; and patients with high anxiety scores exhibited a significant decrease in A-state scores after treatment. No such patterns of change were found for A-trait scores among any group, supporting the hypothesis that changes in scores were related to situational factors rather than personality factors.[9]

Andersen et al[10] studied anxiety, as measured by the STAI, among 19 patients with gynecologic cancers receiving intracavitary radiation. A-state scores ranged in the 74th to 95th percentiles for all patients. As the time for treatment neared, anxiety increased for patients in both the low- and high-anxiety groups. When treatment was completed, high-anxiety patients had significantly lower A-state scores, while the low-anxiety patient group scores remained unchanged, indicating residual anxiety.

Anxiety related to chemotherapy and associated side effects has been implicated in the decision of patients either to reject treatment or to withdraw before completing the recommended therapy.[11] In a study of 78 stage II patients with breast cancer receiving adjuvant chemotherapy, anxiety was reported in 97% of the subjects, yet the levels of anxiety were represented by low scores, indicating mild distress.

Cassileth et al[12] administered the STAI to 378 patients with cancer and 379 matched relatives. Mean anxiety scores among the patient group (37.2) were similar to scores among other physically ill patient groups yet were lower than scores among patients who were being treated for depression. Of note was the trend for state and trait anxiety scores to increase among patients under follow-up care, active treatment, and palliative care, respectively.

In a sample of 60 men cured of Hodgkin's disease, Cella et al[13] studied the occurrence of persistent anticipatory nausea, vomiting, and anxiety after chemotherapy. Data generated from a semistructured interview revealed that 80% of the subjects who had completed chemotherapy at least 6 months before the study complained of anxiety when reminded of treatment.

In summary, increased levels of anxiety have been associated with a diagnosis of cancer. Patients treated with surgery, radiation therapy, and chemotherapy have also reported mild or moderate levels of anxiety. Yet anxiety at minimal or moderate levels may be motivating for the patient.

Impact of Anxiety on Patient Outcomes

Although increased levels of anxiety among persons with cancer have been documented, few researchers have studied the impact of increased anxiety on patient outcomes. Scott[4] studied the relationship of anxiety, critical thinking, and information processing during and after breast biopsy. Anxiety levels (STAI scores) among the 85 patients studied were extremely high and above group norms for acutely ill psychiatric patients. Women with high anxiety scores were found to have positively correlated critical thinking ability (Watson-Glaser Critical Thinking Appraisal) scores. In addition, critical thinking was substantially reduced at hospitalization when compared with 6 to 8 weeks after discharge.

Carey and Burish[14] studied the impact of anxiety as a predictor of behavioral therapy outcomes for 72 patients receiving chemotherapy. Findings indicated that pretreatment anxiety was associated with treatment outcome. Patients with low anxiety had significantly greater reduction in diastolic blood pressure, self-reported anxiety, and depression when compared with patients with moderate and high anxiety. However, pretreatment anxiety levels were not related to nausea levels.

Therefore, beginning empirical data indicate that anxiety is associated with selected patient outcomes. The strength and direction of the relationships between anxiety and selected psychosocial intervening and outcome variables remains to be defined.

Assessment Criteria

Anxiety has been recognized as an accepted nursing diagnosis category by the North American Nursing Diagnosis Association (NANDA).[15] As such, a preliminary definition, possible etiologies, and subjective and objective defining characteristics have been developed (Table 17-1).[15] Efforts have centered on developing specific criteria for deriving the diagnostic statement, yet the required clustering of signs and symptoms critical to the diagnosis are unclear. In addition, the criteria for fear and anxiety are remarkably similar except for the ability of the patient to identify the source of threat. Defining characteristics for anxiety include "fear"; defining characteristics of anticipatory anxiety include the designation of a "future/impending event perceived as a threat"; and contradiction exists over whether the consequences of the threat or the threat itself is the unspecified stimulus.

Consequently, the reliability and validity of the defining characteristics to predict the occurrence of anxiety are questioned. Thus, validation of the diagnosis with the perceptions of the patient is mandatory. Additional clinical research is needed to test the NANDA recommendations for definition and diagnostic criteria of anxiety. Critical characteristics to differentiate motivational versus dysfunctional anxiety also must be distinguished.

Nursing Interventions

Interventions are based on helping the patient to recognize the spectrum of manifestations of anxiety, to determine if the patient desires to do anything about the response, and to activate coping strategies to control anxiety levels.[16] Validation of observed manifestations of anxiety provides an opportunity for the patient to acknowledge or deny the presence of those manifestations and to prioritize the most disturbing responses. Although the manifestations may be classified by health care professionals as disturbing, the patient may perceive the level of anxiety experienced as positive and reject intervention.

However, if the patient expresses a desire to reduce the anxiety, the nurse has an opportunity to help the patient identify the threat, learn to modify responses to the stimuli, and channel the responses constructively. Based on the principles and assumptions of cognitive theory, the nurse may begin by exploring perceived patient concerns and helping the patient evaluate the concerns within the reality of the situation. Often the interventions of exploration and evaluation will result in the ability of the patient to focus on the threat or to appraise the stimuli in a different way, thus reducing anxiety.

Since the etiology of anxiety is defined as being nonspecific, interventions may focus on treating the symptoms by activating previously effective coping strategies or on teaching new strategies to control the anxiety. Each patient brings to the cancer experience a history of previous coping strategies that have been effective and ineffective in managing anxiety. The nurse has the opportunity to help the patient identify those strategies (Table 17-2)[17] used in the present milieu and evaluate the effectiveness of the strategies in reducing anxiety. For patients who desire to learn new strategies, the nurse may offer information through formal and informal education programs, assistance in problem solving through counseling, role modeling with anxiety-reducing techniques such as relaxation training or music therapy, or referral to support groups within the care institution and the community.

Few studies have been conducted among patients with cancer to determine the effectiveness of independent nursing interventions in reducing anxiety, yet available data indicate potential benefits for education programs,

TABLE 17-1 Nursing Diagnoses That Address Anxiety

Nursing Diagnosis	Definition	Defining Characteristics
Anxiety	Vague, uneasy feeling, the source of which is often nonspecific or unknown to the individual	Verbalizes apprehension, uncertainty, fear, distress, worry, verbalizes painful and persistent feelings of increased helplessness, inadequacy, regret, expresses concern (change in life events), fear of unspecified consequences, overexcited, rattled, jittery, scared, restlessness, focus on self, insomnia, increased perspiration, wariness, glancing about, poor eye contact, familial tension, voice quivering, increased tension, foot shuffling, hand and arm movements, trembling, hand tremor, shakiness
Mild Anxiety	Increased level of arousal associated with expectation of a threat (unfocused) to the self or significant relationships	Verbalizes feelings of increased arousal and concern, increased questioning, restlessness, increased awareness, attending, mild restlessness
Moderate Anxiety	Increased level of arousal associated with expectation of a threat (unfocused) to the self or significant relationships	Expressed feelings of unfocused apprehension, nervousness, or concern, verbalized expectation of danger, voice tremors, pitch changes, restlessness, increased rate of verbalization, pacing, hand tremor, increased muscle tension, narrowing focus of attention, diaphoresis, increased heart rate, respiratory rate, sleep or eating disturbances
Severe Anxiety (Panic)	Increased level of arousal associated with expectation of a threat to the self or significant relationships	Expressed feelings of unfocused, severe dread, apprehension, concern, or nervousness, inappropriate verbalization or absence of verbalizations, purposeless activity or immobilization, perceptual focus scattered, fixed, or inability to focus on reality, increased heart rate, hyperventilation, diaphoresis, increased muscle tension, dilated pupils, pallor
Anticipatory Anxiety	Increased level of arousal associated with a perceived future threat (unfocused) to the self or significant relationships	Indicators of anxiety (See Anxiety), future impending event perceived as a threat to physical or psychosocial self (unfocused)

Source: Gordon M: Manual of Nursing Diagnosis. New York, McGraw-Hill, 1987.

TABLE 17-2 Approach and Avoidance Coping Strategies

Approach Strategies	Avoidance Strategies
Information seeking	Denial of emotion
Participation in religious activities	Minimization of symptoms
Distraction	Social isolation
Expression of emotion and feeling	Passive acceptance
Positive thinking	Sleeping
Conservation of energy	Substance abuse
Maintenance of independence	Avoidance of decision making
Maintenance of control	Blame others
Goal setting	Excessive dependency

Source: Adapted from Miller JF: Coping with Chronic Illness: Overcoming Powerlessness. Philadelphia, FA Davis, 1983.

relaxation training, music therapy, and support groups. The following empirical studies are representative of the nursing literature with respect to the potential benefits of such interventions.

Johnson[18] reported on the effects of a patient education course on persons with a chronic illness. Fifty-two subjects were selected randomly from the patients with a first or recurrent diagnosis of cancer within a 12-month period. Preintervention measures of state anxiety (STAI), meaningfulness in life, and knowledge were obtained. Based on preintervention scores and demographic variables, subjects were paired. One subject from each pair was assigned randomly to the treatment group. Subjects in the treatment group attended eight educational sessions over a 4-week period. Content for the sessions included learning about the disease, managing daily health problems, communication, feeling good about oneself, living within physical limitations, and community resources. The experimental group had statistically significant lower anxiety scores than the control group.

Cotanch and Strum[19] reported on the effects of progressive muscle relaxation (PMR) on anxiety, nausea, and vomiting associated with cancer chemotherapy. Sixty patients were randomized into an experimental group (PMR), a placebo control group (relaxing music), and a true control group (no intervention). A statistically significant difference was found for trait anxiety scores across courses of chemotherapy within the different treatment groups; however, no statistical difference was found for state anxiety scores. This finding is perplexing in view of the theoretical constructs of state and trait anxiety and other research findings presented previously.

Frank[20] studied the effect of music therapy and guided visual imagery on anxiety associated with chemotherapy-induced nausea and vomiting. In a single group ($N = 15$), pretest- and posttest-designed study, musical tapes and visual imagery aided by a scenic poster were used beginning 15 minutes before chemotherapy and continuing through chemotherapy administration (2 hours). All subjects received antiemetic drugs before chemotherapy administration. State anxiety scores as measured by the STAI were reduced significantly ($p < .001$). In addition, a significant negative correlation was found between the length of time the subject listened to the music and the postchemotherapy state anxiety score ($r = -.4984$, $p < .05$).[19]

In summary, a variety of behavioral interventions have been used successfully to alleviate anxiety associated with a cancer diagnosis and treatment. Each intervention represents an independent nursing action to modify the anxiety response exhibited among persons with cancer.

Future Directions for Nursing Research

Anxiety has been reported to be present subjectively and objectively among patients diagnosed with cancer across the disease trajectory. The vague, uneasy feelings defined as anxiety may serve a protective or disabling function for the patient with cancer. However, assessment criteria used in collaboration with the perceptions of the patient to determine the individual level of anxiety at which interventions to reduce anxiety should be instituted lack reliability and validity.

Although beginning research efforts have focused on the effectiveness of a variety of independent nursing interventions in reducing anxiety among persons with cancer, studies have been limited by sample size and heterogeneity, cross-sectional designs, single measures of anxiety, use of anxiety as both an independent and a dependent variable, and lack of randomized control groups. Intervention studies for anxiety reduction among persons with cancer have concentrated on applying the intervention across cancer populations at a variety of points in the cancer trajectory, yet definition of criteria by which to select a specific intervention for a specific person may be impossible or, at best, subjective. Finally, the effect of anxiety reduction on patient outcomes such as information processing, physiologic responses to cancer and cancer therapy, psychosocial adaptation, and sense of control have not been corroborated.

DEPRESSION

Depression is a ubiquitous response to actual or potential loss. Since cancer represents a potential loss of not only life, but also body parts and functions, roles, and relationships, depression has been identified as one of the most common responses to cancer. Yet the differential diagnosis of depression among persons with cancer is complicated by the coexistence of signs and symptoms of disease and treatment that are similar to those of depression.[21] In addition, depression resulting from a predisposition within the personality must be differentiated from a depressed mood associated with an adjustment disorder as a result of changes caused by cancer.[22]

In either case, depression can influence the quality of life of persons with cancer and their significant others. However, empirical and clinical reports indicate that depression is an underdiagnosed response among persons with cancer and, probably more critical, undertreated.[23] In the following section, depression is defined, research on depression among persons with cancer is described, assessment criteria are discussed, and nursing interventions are outlined.

Operational Definition

The following operational definition of depression is presented:

- An individual exists with the ability to respond cognitively, behaviorally, and affectively to stimuli in the environment.
- The individual perceives certain goals for the future and attributes the possibilities for success to the self.
- The attempts of the individual to attain goals are blocked.
- The individual attributes the failure to attain goals to personal inadequacies.
- *The perceived loss of self-esteem results in a cluster of affective (worthlessness, hopelessness, guilt, sadness), behavioral (change in appetite, sleep disturbances, lack of energy, withdrawal, dependency), and cognitive (decreased ability to concentrate, indecisiveness, or suicidal ideation) responses defined as depression.*

Measurement Instruments

A variety of instruments is available to assess depression. The majority of these instruments were developed to assess depression in psychiatrically ill patients. Items cluster about the characteristics associated with major depression as described in the *Diagnostic and Statistical Manual of Mental Disorders-Revised* (DSM-III-R). Limited reliability and validity data with respect to use in oncology populations have been reported.

Hamilton Rating Scale for Depression

The Hamilton Rating Scale for Depression (HRS-D)[24] is a 17-item, self-report scale used to assess cognitive, behavioral, and physiologic signs and symptoms typical of depression. Each item is rated for severity from 0 to 2 or from 0 to 4. Scores on each item are summed to produce a total depression score. A total score of greater than 25 indicates severe depression; 18 to 24, moderate depression; 7 to 17, mild depression; and less than 6, no depression. Reliability and validity estimates for the instrument for nononcology populations include interrater reliability (r = .90); construct validity by factor analysis resulting in four factors (retarded depression, somatic symptoms, anxiety reaction, and insomnia).[24]

Beck Depression Inventory

The Beck Depression Inventory (BDI)[25] is a 21-item self-report scale used to assess symptoms of depression. Each item is composed of a set of statements, graduating in severity of symptoms, measured on a scale of 0 to 3, with a higher score representing a more severe symptom. The subject chooses the statement in the set that most closely describes his or her current feeling. Total scores for the BDI are based on the number and severity of symptoms experienced. Subjects scoring in the 0 to 4 range are classified as not or minimally depressed; in the 4 to 7 range, as mildly depressed; in the 8 to 15 range, as moderately depressed; and in the 16 to 42 range, as severely depressed. Reliability estimates among psychiatric populations include internal consistency (KR_{20} alpha coefficients ranging from .88 to .94).

Other instruments

In addition to the instruments presented, other personality and mood inventories with depression subscales have been used to quantify the level of depression. The Minnesota Multiphasic Personality Inventory (MMPI),[26] Psychosocial Adjustment to Illness Scale (PAIS),[27] and Profile of Mood States (POMS)[28] have been used most frequently in studies of depression among persons with cancer. Reliability and validity estimates for the total instrument as well as subscales are reported in administration and scoring manuals for each instrument.

Patterns of Occurrence

The occurrence of depression among persons with cancer has been described in the literature. Petty and Noyes[29] reported that moderate to severe depression was found in 17% to 25% of hospitalized cancer patients. At least 20% of adult cancer patients will have a clinically significant syndrome of depression during the course of the disease.[30-32]

Factors that affect the occurrence of depression among persons with cancer have been described. Andersen and Hacker[33] reported on the psychosexual adjustment of 15 patients treated surgically for vulvar cancer. Data were collected through a semistructured interview and battery of psychosocial questionnaires: Katz Social Adjustment Scale, Symptom Checklist-90, and Dyadic Adjustment Scale. A mean score of 12.3 on the BDI was obtained for the sample, indicating a mild to moderate level of depression among these patients. Activity scores were correlated significantly and negatively with the measures of psychologic distress.

Goldberg et al[34] reported on the relationship of the social environment and patient physical status to depression in 20 patients with lung cancer and their 18 spouses. Data were generated through a semistructured interview and a battery of psychological tests administered within 6 weeks of diagnosis and at 2-month intervals for 4 months. Physical status of the patient, as measured by the Karnofsky Scale, was related negatively to depressive symptoms as measured by POMS-D in patients.

The effects of age and marital status on emotional distress after mastectomy were studied by Metzger et al.[35] Data from interviews of 652 women who underwent a mastectomy 1 year before the study indicated that younger women were more likely to worry about disfigurement resulting from surgery but to have resources as buffers against depression. Married subjects were significantly less likely to worry about recurrence and experienced less depression.

Researchers have also attempted to differentiate depression associated with cancer from depression associated with a personality disorder. Robinson et al[36] conducted a study to determine if the degree of self-reported anxiety and depression that is attributed to having cancer differs from current or past history of anxiety and depression attributed to other life events in 57 patients presently being treated for cancer. Findings indicated that patients who reported a history of anxiety or depression for reasons other than cancer had significantly higher anxiety and depression scores than those who did not report preexisting anxiety or depression. Patients who reported a history of depression or anxiety due to the diagnosis of cancer had self-rating scores on anxiety and depression that did not differ significantly from those of patients who reported no problems or "normal" symptoms.

Evaluations for depression among 62 patients with a diagnosis of cancer were reported by Bukberg et al.[37] DSM-III-R criteria for major depressive episodes were used to evaluate the presence of depression.[38] Twenty-six patients (42%) met the criteria for major depression, 14% had depressive symptoms that did not meet the criteria for major depression, and 44% had no depressive affect. The factor most clearly associated with depression was physical performance as measured by the Karnofsky Scale. Qualitative differences between depression in psychiatric and cancer patients were found. No subjects were found to have psychotic depressive symptoms, melancholia, feelings of worthlessness, or suicidal ideation.

In addition to describing the occurrence of depression

among persons with cancer, researchers have studied the variations in occurrence and severity of depression across the disease trajectory. Layne et al[39] reported significant differences in levels of depression as measured by the MMPI-D among patients with a diagnosis of cancer in the terminal phase, patients with a diagnosis of cancer who had been told that they would survive for at least 5 years, family members of patients in the cancer groups, and a normal group. Depression scores for the terminal group were significantly greater than those of the family member and normal groups ($p < .05$). The nonterminal patient group also had depression scores greater than those of the family member and normal groups, although the differences were not statistically significant.

Depression also has been explored as a predictor of adjustment to a diagnosis of cancer. Morris et al[40] used standardized tests and structured interviews to identify factors that predicted psychological and social adjustment to mastectomy 2 years after surgery. High preoperative depression scores (HRS-D) were predictive of poor adjustment after mastectomy. Subjects who scored more than 10 on the HRS-D, with or without a history of depression, were significantly more likely to remain stressed by the mastectomy at 2 years ($p > .05$).

In summary, the focus of research related to depression among persons with cancer has been descriptive. The lack of assessment of preexisting depressive symptoms before the diagnosis of cancer, the presence of confounding physical and psychosocial responses related to the disease and treatment, and minimal reliability and validity estimates for instruments used among cancer populations result in significant limitations in previous research. Moreover, an emphasis on empirical studies that focus on independent nursing interventions to modify the depressive symptoms associated with the diagnosis of cancer is needed. With statistical modeling, knowledge of depressive responses within the context of other psychosocial variables inherent in the cancer experience may be enhanced.

Assessment Criteria

Reactive depression (situational) is defined as "an acute decrease in self-esteem or worth related to a threat to self competency" (p. 210).[15] Defining characteristics as established by NANDA are presented in Table 17-3.[15] Critical to establishing the diagnosis in physically ill persons is evaluation of selected defining characteristics commonly attributed to depression among the psychiatrically ill. Physiologic characteristics such as appetite disturbances, change in weight, sleep disturbance, and decreased energy are experienced frequently among persons with cancer as a result of disease or treatment. Furthermore, the psychosocial characteristics described for depression may occur in the person with cancer as a result of disease, treatment, or side effects (inability to concentrate, irritability, dependency, and anger). Therefore, the primary criteria for assessment of depression are that the characteristics are a change from previous functioning, are persistent, occur for most of the day, occur more days than not, and are present for at least 2 weeks (p. 219).[38]

TABLE 17-3 Defining Characteristics of Situational Depression

Expressions of hopelessness, despair
Inability to concentrate on reading, writing, conversation
Change in physical activities, eating, sleeping, sexual activity
Continual questioning of self-worth (self-esteem)
Feelings of failure (real or imagined)
Withdrawal from others to avoid possible rejection (real or imagined)
Threats or attempts to commit suicide
Suspicion and sensitivity to words and actions of others related to general lack of trust of others
Misdirected anger toward self
General irritability
Guilt feelings
Extreme dependency on others with related feelings of helplessness and anger

Source: Gordon M: Manual of Nursing Diagnosis. New York, McGraw-Hill, 1987.

Nursing Interventions

The selection of nursing interventions for the treatment of patients with depression is based on identification of stimuli that have resulted in a loss of self-esteem as well as the defining characteristics present for the particular patient. If the patient presents with a long-standing history of depression, referral to another member of the health care team may be appropriate. Otherwise, concentration on the psychological and behavioral responses associated with depression offer beginning cues for selection of nursing interventions.

The nurse may begin by helping the patient to acknowledge feelings of hopelessness, despair, failure, anger, or guilt and by giving permission to discuss those feelings. Because the expression of the feelings is associated with a degree of risk-taking for the patient, the nurse must be open and accepting of the feelings. Acceptance is demonstrated by attentive listening, acknowledgment of the feelings, and exploration of methods to deal positively with the feelings.

Sensitivity to potential increased vulnerability of the patient who shares feelings is a necessity. The nurse must assume the responsibility for emotional exposure of the patient and plan systematically for professional follow-up. Expression of depressive feelings may be both time-consuming and overwhelming for the patient and nurse; consultation with other health care personnel, namely, clinical nurse specialists in psychiatry, psychologists, and psychiatrists, may be indicated.

Besides giving permission for expression of feelings, the nurse has the opportunity to assist the patient to reappraise the situation cognitively with respect to aspects of the cancer experience and perceptions of self-esteem and self-competency. Accurate information about the plan of care and personal responses to treatment form the basis of cognitive reappraisal of the situation. Helping the patient focus on immediate goals of care often reduces the overwhelming feelings of powerlessness and helplessness associated with a chronic, life-threatening illness. Focusing on positive abilities of the patient, contracting short-term goals of care that the patient can achieve, and reinforcing patient attempts and successes to meet established goals provide the framework for effective nursing interventions in caring for the patient with depression.

In the milieu of the cancer experience, physical symptoms of the disease and treatment as well as lack of motivation accompanying depression may limit the ability of the patient to meet basic needs. Significant others as well as health care professionals may perceive the patient as generally helpless even in areas in which the patient is able to function independently. Enhancing self-competency and self-esteem may be accomplished by providing information about and role modeling self-care behaviors, negotiating goals for increasing independence in self-care as well as decision making, facilitating social interaction with others, and encouraging physical mobility.

Future Directions for Nursing Research

Although most persons with cancer are able to cope with the demands of illness and treatment with minimal psychosocial distress, criteria by which to predict those patients for whom the demands exceed interpersonal and intrapersonal resources are ambiguous. Furthermore, criteria to establish the diagnosis among medically versus psychiatrically ill patients are unclear.

Nursing interventions designed to effect positive outcomes for the patient diagnosed with depression are inherently time-consuming and may represent an unacceptable cost-benefit ratio in the acute care setting in light of the physical care demanded. However, if the goal of oncology care includes the quality as well as quantity of life, then intervention studies to compare both the effectiveness as well as costs of care in both inpatient and community settings for patients with depression are warranted.

HOPELESSNESS

Hopelessness is often described in the literature as a response of patients to the cancer experience; however, the response appears not to pervade the experience of the cancer patient but rather waxes and wanes with changes in perceived health, relationships, and spirituality. Described as both a unique response as well as one of a cluster of characteristics seen in other responses, hopelessness has been studied primarily within the framework of psychiatrically ill patients. Recently, however, health care professionals in general and nurses in particular have demonstrated increased interest in hopelessness and hope as both independent and dependent variables influencing the quantity and quality of the cancer experience.

Operational Definition

Operationally, hopelessness can be defined as follows:

- An individual exists within time and space.
- The individual has thoughts, feelings, and behaviors in response to stimuli in the environment.
- The responses an individual has to stimuli are based on the significance of the stimuli, potential responses identified, and calculated probabilities of success in creating a desired future.
- The individual, as an aspect of humanity, recognizes significant areas of life for which limited or no alternatives are identified or the probabilities of success in creating a desired future approach zero—the perceived reality for the individual.
- In an attempt to protect the individual against the despair generated by these areas of life, the individual seeks a personal or spiritual relationship, anticipating that interactions will lead to understandable, meaningful, or constructive outcomes in the future.
- *The interaction of thoughts, feelings, and behaviors resulting from the inability to mobilize internal and external resources sufficient to achieve a probability of success greater than zero or to create an understandable, meaningful, or constructive outcome in the future is defined as hopelessness.*

Measurement Instruments

Beck Hopelessness Scale

The Beck Hopelessness Scale (BHS)[41] is a 20-item, true-false scale designed to measure hopelessness in psychiatrically ill patients. Scores are calculated by summing the scores on each statement. Scores range from 0 to 20, with a higher score representing a higher level of hopelessness. Scores of 0 to 3 represent no or minimal hopelessness; 4 to 8, mild hopelessness; 9 to 14, moderate hopelessness; and 15 to 20, severe hopelessness. Reliability estimates for the instrument include internal consistency as measured by the KR_{20} reliability coefficient = .93 among a sample of suicide attempters; concurrent validity between clinical ratings of hopelessness and instrument ratings (r = .74, $p < .001$); face validity established by a panel of psychiatric experts; and construct validity through factor analysis resulting in three factors (feelings about the future, loss of motivation, and future expectations)[41] with Eigenvalues > 1.000.

Nowotny Hope Scale

Conceptualized as a polar opposite to hopelessness, hopefulness has been measured by a number of instruments developed by nurse researchers. The Nowotny Hope Scale (NHS)[42] is a 29-item scale designed to measure hope on six dimensions: confidence in outcomes, relates to others, possibility of a future, spiritual beliefs, active involvement, and comes from within.[42] For each of the positively and negatively worded statements, the subject is asked to respond on a 4-point, Likert-type scale (1 = strongly agree to 4 = strongly disagree). Reliability and validity estimates for the instrument include internal consistency as calculated by Cronbach's coefficient alpha = 0.90; item-total correlations ranging from 0.3 to 0.7; item to subscale correlations ranging from 0.4 to 0.8; concurrent validity with the BHS ($r = .47, p = .001$); and construct validity through factor analysis resulting in six factors with Eigenvalues ranging from 9.8 to 1.4.[42]

Herth Hope Scale

The Herth Hope Scale (HHS)[43] is a 32-item self-report scale to which subjects respond either "applies to me" or "does not apply to me" to each item. Responses on each item are summed to produce a total hope score ranging from 0 to 32, with a higher score representing higher levels of hope. Reliability and validity estimates among persons with cancer include internal consistency as determined by Cronbach's coefficient alpha = 0.89; and construct validity through factor analysis resulting in three factors—positive expectancies, sense of personal competency and mutuality, and temporality with future orientation.[43]

Patterns of Occurrence

In recent years, the interest of health care professionals in the relationship of hope and hopelessness to the cancer experience has resulted in numerous anecdotal articles, a few descriptive studies, and a limited number of intervention studies. As early as 1966, Schmale and Iker[44] conducted a study of 40 women with abnormal cervical cytology suspicious of cancer. To test the hypothesis that the experience of specific feelings may facilitate or permit the clinical appearance of disease,[44] the researchers conducted an interview and administered a battery of psychological tests the day after a cone biopsy was done under general anesthesia. Content analysis of interviews was compared with preestablished criteria for hopelessness potential. A determination of "cancer" or "no cancer" was made for each subject. Thirty-one subjects (77.5%) were assigned to the correct grouping (x_c^2, 7.343; df, 1; $p = .007$).

Subsequent studies of hope among persons with cancer were focused on concept clarification, describing levels of hope across the disease trajectory, or instrument development for measuring hope. Using a grounded theory methodology, Hinds[45] developed an empirically derived definition of hopefulness through interviews with healthy adolescents, inpatient adolescents on a substance abuse unit, and a diagnostically heterogeneous adolescent group with cancer.

TABLE 17-4 Induced Dimensions of Hopefulness Among Adolescents

Dimension	Definition
Forced effort	The degree to which an adolescent tries to take on artificially a more positive view
Personal possibilities	The extent to which an adolescent believes that second chances for the self may exist
Expectations of a better tomorrow	The degree to which an adolescent has a positive although nonspecific future orientation
Anticipation of a personal future	The extent to which an adolescent identifies specific and positive future possibilities for self

Source: Hinds PS: Adolescent hopefulness in illness and health. Adv Nurs Sci 10:79-88, 1988.

The induced definition of hopefulness had four dimensions that emerged from the data from the healthy and substance abuse adolescents (Table 17-4).[45] An additional attribute emerged from the adolescent cancer group, "the concern for and a focus on others in addition to self" (p. 85).[45] Thus, the resulting definition became "the degree to which an adolescent possesses a comforting or life-sustaining, reality-based belief that a positive future exists for self or others."[45] These data form the basis for additional study of the concept among adults.

In a similar study, the phenomena of hope and the hoping process were examined among 35 elderly patients with a diagnosis of cancer.[46] Hope was defined as a multidimensional dynamic life force characterized by confident yet uncertain anticipation of realistically possible and personally significant desirable future good having implications for action and for interpersonal relatedness (p. 380).[46] Two spheres of hope, generalized and particularized, were identified, and six dimensions of hope were described—affective, cognitive, behavioral, affiliative, temporal, and contextual.

In a report on the development of an instrument to measure hope after a stressful event, Nowotny[42] described levels of hope among a sample of 150 patients with cancer. Scores on the NHS for the cancer patient group were not significantly different from scores of a sample of 156 well adults. Data were not collected on type of diagnosis, length of time since diagnosis, or type of treatment for the cancer patient sample.

Zook and Yasko[47] found hope levels decreased as time since diagnosis increased among a group of 26 patients with cancer receiving chemotherapy. In contrast, Greene et al[48] reported no correlation between hope level and length of time since diagnosis.

The focus of more recent studies has been the description of the relationship of hope to other psychosocial variables in the cancer experience. Herth[43] reported a descriptive study to investigate the relationship between hope and coping in 120 adult patients with cancer undergoing chemotherapy in a variety of care settings. A significant relationship was found between level of hope and level of coping among subjects in hospital, outpatients, and home settings ($p < .05$). In addition, strength of religious convictions and performance of family role responsibilities, measured on one-item scales, were significantly related to the variables of hope and coping regardless of setting: subjects with a strong religious faith had significantly higher mean scores on the HHS than subjects with weak, unsure, or lost faith or who were without faith. Subjects who reported little or no interference in performing family role responsibilities had a significantly ($p < .05$) higher mean score on the HHS than did the group indicating severe interference.

Raleigh[49] studied 45 patients with cancer and 45 individuals with a nonthreatening chronic illness to describe the relationship between hope, locus of control, factors of illness, and personal factors. Raleigh reported no significant relationship between the level of hope and the identified personal and illness factors, yet these findings have been challenged.

To examine the relationship between hopelessness and locus of control, helpfulness of religious beliefs, and support from family and friends, Brandt[50] studied a sample of 31 women with breast cancer. Although all patients were receiving their first course of chemotherapy, variability existed in the time elapsed since initial diagnosis; that is, 42% of the sample had been diagnosed less than 6 months, while 26% of the sample had been diagnosed more than 24 months. Results indicate that the mean hopelessness score as measured by the BHS was 2.48, indicating minimal hopelessness. A statistically significant correlation ($r = .37$, $p < .05$) was found between hopelessness scores and locus of control scores (as measured by the Rotter I-E Locus of Control Scale). Patients who exhibited a more external locus of control expressed a greater level of hopelessness.[50] Perceived helpfulness of religious beliefs in coping with illness as measured by a one-item scale was found to be correlated significantly ($r = -.32$, $p < .05$) with lower levels of hopelessness. The author indicated minimal variability of scores on the religious beliefs question. Support from family and friends as measured by a one-item scale did not produce sufficient variability in scores to allow a Pearson correlation coefficient to be calculated.

Stoner[51] studied the relationship between personal and situational factors and hope in 58 white adults with cancer. Higher levels of hope ($p = .10$) were associated with being female, receipt of adequate information about disease and treatments, adherence by the subjects to their religious belief systems throughout illness, and lower socioeconomic status. Inability to carry out family role responsibilities, adverse effects of treatment, protracted illness, and greater severity of illness were not found to be associated with lower levels of hope.

In a subsequent study, Stoner and Keampfer[52] examined the effect of information with respect to life expectancy and phase of illness on levels of hope among a heterogeneous sample of 55 cancer patients. Although data indicated no significant differences in levels of hope between subjects according to the phase of illness (no evidence of disease, ongoing treatment, or terminal stage), a significant main effect for recalled life expectancy information on hope was shown ($F = 4.21$, $p < .05$). Subjects who did not remember receiving information about life expectancy had higher levels of hope than subjects who remembered receiving information.[52]

The relationship between hopefulness and participation styles with respect to treatment was studied among a sample of 256 patients with a diagnosis of cancer.[53] Selected findings of Stoner[52] were supported. The mean score on the BHS for the sample was 2.8, indicating minimal hopelessness. Levels of hope were found to correlate positively with medical status ($p < .05$); preference for active involvement in self-care ($p < .05$); and desire for as much information as possible ($p < .001$).

Hope as an intervening variable has been studied.[54] The relationship between locus of control, hope, and disease-free interval was examined among a convenience sample of 34 postmenopausal women with stage II breast cancer. Internal health locus of control was not found to be correlated significantly with disease-free interval; however, hope was found to be correlated positively and significantly ($p < .05$) with disease-free interval. Moreover, stressful life events were found to be intervening variables that had a significant negative correlation with disease-free interval.

Thus, hopefulness and hopelessness have been implicated in the development of cancer and in the quantity and quality of life after diagnosis of cancer. However, consistent conceptualization of hope and hopelessness remains elusive in the empirical studies reported. Ideally, future efforts in determining the relationship of hope and cancer will be targeted to demonstrate the biophysical-psychosocial connection between the variables.

Assessment Criteria

Hopelessness has been characterized by cognitive, affective, and behavioral responses (Table 17-5).[15] Few studies, however, have been conducted to establish the reliability and validity of the defining characteristics among clinical populations. Of even greater concern is the ability of the clinician to differentiate hopelessness from similar concepts such as depression and powerlessness using the accepted defining characteristics.

TABLE 17-5 Nursing Diagnosis: Hopelessness

Definition	A subjective state in which an individual sees limited or no alternative or personal choices available and is unable to mobilize energy on own behalf
Defining characteristics	Passivity Decreased verbalization Decreased affect Verbalization of despondent or hopeless content Lack of initiative Decreased response to stimuli Lack of involvement in care Turning away from speaker Closing eyes Shrugging in response to speaker Decreased appetite Increased sleep

Source: Gordon M: Manual of Nursing Diagnosis. New York, McGraw-Hill, 1987.

Nursing Interventions

Interventions for decreasing hopelessness and fostering hope among persons with cancer have been derived before development of conceptual and theoretical formulations. Based on conceptual models of the nature of hope and related variables, the following categories of interventions have been suggested: enhancing reality surveillance, fostering supportive relationships, enhancing personal power and abilities, and creating a future perspective.[55,56] Specific suggestions for implementation of each category are presented in Table 17-6.[55,56]

Future Directions for Nursing Research

Hope has been identified as a critical component of cancer care. As such, the necessity of conceptualizing hope and hopelessness within the context of the cancer experience, validating the defining characteristics of hope and hopelessness, describing the association of hope and hopelessness to other psychosocial variables, and evaluating the effectiveness of specific nursing interventions in fostering hope or protecting against hopelessness is apparent.

TABLE 17-6 Interventions to Foster Hopefulness

Category	Interventions
Assist with reality surveillance	Review changes in and current health status Seek perceptions of patient with respect to health Confirm accurate perception Correct misconceptions of reality Encourage discussion of reality with others in same situation
Reinforce personal power and ability	Review perceived strengths of patient and family Include patient in planning care, goals, schedules Encourage review of past successes in stressful times Reward approximations of goals Encourage value of use of needed external resources
Encourage supportive relationships	Review number, types, and availability of supportive relationships Assist in helping patient ask for support needed Encourage continued contacts with supportive persons Respect relationship of patient to higher being Encourage expression of faith, if applicable
Create a future perspective	Review past occasions for hope Discuss meaning of hope from patient perspective Establish short-term goals with patient and family Evaluate progress in achieving goals on routine basis Encourage expressions of hopes for future

Sources: Clark JC: Hope as a critical factor in the cancer experience, in Pritchard AP (ed): Cancer Nursing: A Revolution in Care, Proceeding of the Fifth International Conference on Cancer Nursing. London, Macmillan, 1989, pp 117-119. Dufault K, Martocchio BC; Hope: Its spheres and dimensions. Nurs Clin North Am 20:379-391, 1985.

ALTERED SEXUAL HEALTH

The diagnosis of cancer poses potential threats to sexuality, how one perceives the self, how one perceives how others see the self, and how one behaves as a sexual being. As the nature of cancer has changed from an acute to a chronic illness, concerns of health care providers have expanded beyond survival to include factors that affect the quality of survival. Sexual health is one such factor.

Operational Definition

Operationally, sexuality can be defined as follows:

- An individual exists who has the ability to express himself or herself physically, psychologically, and socially with other human beings.
- The ability of the individual to distinguish self from and express self with others based on anatomic, physiologic, developmental, and psychosocial factors is defined as sexuality.
- The satisfactory, consistent, and rewarding expression of and distinction by one's sexuality results in a state of sexual health for the individual.
- The individual perceives a stimulus that impairs distinction or expression of sexuality.
- *The inability to express one's sexuality consistent with personal needs and preferences is defined as altered sexual health.*

Measurement Instruments

Derogatis Sexual Functioning Inventory

The Derogatis Sexual Functioning Inventory (DSFI)[57] is a 245-item, self-report instrument designed to measure the multidimensional concept of sexuality. Reported reliability and validity estimates include test-retest reliabilities for 10 subscales ranging from 0.42 to 0.96; internal consistency coefficients ranging from 0.56 to 0.97; and construct validity through factor analysis that revealed seven factors (body image, psychologic distress, heterosexual drive, autoeroticism, gender role, sexual satisfaction, and sexual precociousness).[57]

Sexual Adjustment Questionnaire

The Sexual Adjustment Questionnaire (SAQ)[58] is a 108-item instrument designed to measure sexual adjustment over time among patients with head and neck cancers. The questionnaire is completed by the subject at three separate points in time: Section A (37 items), 4 to 6 weeks after treatment; Section B (30 items), retrospective assessment before the diagnosis of cancer; and Section C (39 items), 16 to 20 weeks after treatment. Items include some questions evaluated on a 5-point Likert scale, several open-ended questions, and questions that require an explanation from the subject. Each section is composed of 7 subsections: desire, relationship, activity arousal, orgasm, techniques, and satisfaction. Scores on each item are summed to produce a total score for the subsection. High scores indicate more positive feelings of functioning, greater variety of sexual methods and activities, or a long-term relationship with a single partner. Reliability and validity estimates for the instrument include: test-retest reliability (2 to 4 weeks and 10 to 12 weeks apart) with Pearson correlation coefficients for the subsections ranging from .5389 to .9374; content validity evaluation by a panel of experts; and construct validity established by known-group technique (healthy subjects would be expected to score higher than cancer patients).

Patterns of Occurrence

The sequelae associated with radical surgery, radiation, chemotherapy, and biotherapy may threaten the sexual health of persons with cancer. Early studies on the effects of cancer on sexual health focused on barriers to return to previous levels of sexual function or, more specifically, intercourse. Anecdotal reports and descriptive studies provided the basis for identifying the potential risks to sexual health for site-specific and treatment-specific patient populations. Recently, however, researchers have expanded the concept of sexual health and sexuality to include the issues of self-concept and perceptions and behaviors of significant others.

Sexual behaviors

Abitbol and Davenport[59] published data related to the impact of treatment for cervical cancer on sexual function. Subjects (28 treated with radiation therapy only, 32 treated with surgery, and 15 treated with a combination of surgery and radiation) were interviewed about their sexual life before disease, sexual life 1 year after treatment, and other changes in sexual functioning. Approximately 40% of patients ($N = 75$) reported a decrease or abstinence in sexual activity after treatment. The radiotherapy group had the highest percentage of subjects reporting a decrease in sexual activity (25%). Other changes in sexual functioning identified primarily by the radiotherapy group were lack of libido (43%), pain or discomfort with intercourse (39%), shortened or narrowed vagina (54%), and fear of recurrence (15%). The authors recommended that clinicians assume a proactive posture in addressing the sexual concerns of cancer patients treated with radiation therapy regardless of age.

Subsequently, Jenkins[60] discussed the self-reported sexual changes in 27 women treated for endometrial and cervical cancer with surgery and radiation therapy. A statistically significant ($p < .05$) negative change in the frequency of intercourse, frequency of desire, frequency of orgasm, and enjoyment of intercourse was reported after treatment. Additional significant findings of the study included that 59% of the sample had received no preparation or information about sexual functioning, the majority of sexual information given was verbal versus written, and nurses had not provided any of the information about sexual functioning.

These findings were supported in a study of 60 women newly diagnosed with gynecologic cancers.[61] Twenty-nine of the subjects were sexually active before diagnosis. However, none of these subjects continued to have sexual intercourse after diagnosis either on recommendation of the physician or fear that intercourse would increase the risk for vaginal bleeding or discharge.

Surgery also has been implicated in changes in sexual health among women with vulvar cancer. Andersen and Hacker[62] reported on the psychosexual adjustment of 15 patients treated surgically for vulvar cancer. Data were collected through a semistructured interview and battery of psychosocial questionnaires. Measures of sexual functioning indicated that the sample reported limited capacity for sexual arousal, considerable sexual anxiety, inadequate sexual relationships, a discrepancy between actual and ideal frequency of intercourse, and lower body image scores than reported for healthy women.

The sexual function and psychosocial reactions among 25 women who had undergone vulvectomy and 15 of their partners indicated that more than two thirds of the patients reported a decrease in frequency of intercourse from pretreatment levels.[63] Ten women ceased sexual intercourse completely. Half the women reported being dissatisfied with sexual relationships and the occurrence of low spirits, lack of respect for their body, and not feeling like a "proper woman." These data are consistent with the findings of Jenkins[60] in that between 25% and 33% of patients perceived the information given to them before treatment as inadequate.

However, findings from related studies among women with breast cancer have not been consistent with the changes reported among women with gynecologic cancers. Woods and Earp[64] reported on 49 patients cured of stage I and II breast cancer. Four years after therapy, 81% of the sample reported no differences in sexual frequency and 63% reported being satisfied with sexual relationships. These findings were supported by the work of Jamison et al[65] who interviewed 41 women with breast cancer. Seventy-six percent of the sample reported that the mastectomy had resulted in no difference or a positive effect on sexual satisfaction or orgasmic ability. Only 2.7% reported a decrease in sexual activity or interest.

In contrast, Taylor et al[66] reported changes in the levels of affectionate behavior in the marriage ($r = .51$, $p < .001$) and patient perception of frequency of intercourse ($r = .32$, $p < .03$) that were associated with poor psychosocial adjustment among 78 women diagnosed and treated for breast cancer. Patients treated with modified radical mastectomy had significantly higher concern about body disfigurement and were affected significantly more negatively with respect to marital affection and sexual intercourse levels than were patients treated with lumpectomy.

Thus, data indicate that women with gynecologic cancers in general and those treated with radiation therapy are at risk for changes in sexual activity. In contrast, the diagnosis of breast cancer and treatment with surgery do not appear to place the patient at increased risk for changes in the frequency of sexual intercourse but, rather, for changes in self-concept.

Although empirical data are available for evaluating the potential risks of cancer and treatment among females, such data for males are limited. Blackmore[67] reported on the impact of orchidectomy on the sexuality of men with testicular cancer. Self-report questionnaires were distributed to three groups of subjects: group I, 20 men with stage I germ cell testicular tumors treated with unilateral orchidectomy within 2 years before the study; group II, 10 men who had undergone unilateral orchidectomy within 2 years before the study for reasons other than cancer; and group III, 15 men who had no history of cancer or testicular problems. Five sections of the DSFI (sexual drive, symptoms, affect, body image, and sexual satisfaction) were used as the basis for data collection. No statistically significant differences were found on any outcome sexuality variables among the three groups. In contrast, Schover et al[68] found significant sexual morbidity among a sample of 84 men with a diagnosis of seminoma who were treated with radiation therapy. Problems reported included reduced semen volume (49%), reduced intensity of orgasm (33%), low rates of sexual activity (19%), low sexual desire (12%), erectile dysfunction (15%), difficulty reaching orgasm (10%), and premature ejaculation (14%).

Although treatment of prostatic cancer can affect sexual functioning (impotence and reduced frequency of intercourse and orgasm), limited empirical data are available to quantify the occurrence of sexual changes.[69] Banker[70] studied the preservation of potency among 100 men with prostate cancer treated with external radiation therapy. Subjects were interviewed before radiation therapy and again 1 year after treatment concerning frequency of intercourse, changes in sexual activity levels over the past 1 to 3 years, and ability to achieve and maintain a full erection. Forty-three percent of subjects ($n = 10$) who reported having intercourse with full erections less than three times per month before therapy maintained potency after treatment, compared with 73% of subjects ($n = 19$) who had intercourse with full erection more than three times per month.

In summary, researchers have identified the potential assaults to sexual health among males with genitourinary cancers, yet the data are limited with respect to threats to sexual health among persons with cancers of the head and neck, lung, and gastrointestinal tract. Also of interest is the lack of research related to the perceptions of significant others with respect to sexuality and perceptions of the patient with respect to self-concept.

Self-concept

Self-concept is defined as the total self-appraisal of appearance, background and origins, abilities, resources, attitudes, and feelings that culminate as a directing force in behavior.[71] Newman et al[72] reported on the effect of Hickman catheters on the self-esteem of patients with leukemia. Self-esteem was measured on admission, on day 5, and on day 30.[73] Consecutive patients admitted with acute nonlymphocytic leukemia (ANLL) were assigned to two groups based on adequacy of venous access. Thirty patients were assigned to each group. Patients who received a Hickman catheter had initial self-esteem scores similar to and even slightly higher than those who did not. Self-esteem in both groups remained similar over the 30-day study period. However, one may question the appropriateness of the use of the Purpose in Life test to measure the self-esteem concept.

In contrast to the minimal surgical incision involved with a Hickman catheter placement, Weddington et al[74] studied the psychological outcome of extremity sarcoma survivors undergoing amputation (n = 14) or limb salvage procedures (n = 19). No significant differences between group scores of cognitive capacity, symptoms, mood, body image changes, physical function, adjustment to illness and surgery, and lifetime prevalence of psychiatric disorders before or after surgery were noted.

Alopecia is one of the most common physiologic responses to chemotherapy. Baxley et al[75] studied the effect of alopecia on the body image of 40 patients with cancer receiving chemotherapy. Subjects were divided into two groups based on the presence of alopecia. Each subject completed the Body-Cathexis-Self-Cathexis (BC-SC) Scale.[76] Significant differences on body cathexis scores (t = 4.34, $p < .001$) and self-cathexis scores (t = 4.04, $p < .0001$) were found between patients with and without alopecia. In addition, comparisons of scores for female and male patients in the alopecia group indicated a significant difference (t = 2.91, $p < .0009$) in that men with alopecia scored higher, indicating that they had a lower self-image than women with alopecia.

Evaluation of the impact of radical versus conservative surgery on disease-related and adjustment-related outcomes has been studied. Kemeny et al[77] conducted a study of the differences in the psychosocial effects of mastectomy (n = 27) versus segmentectomy (n = 25) in women who were entered in a prospective randomized protocol for treatment of primary breast cancer. Questionnaires that were designed to evaluate psychosocial responses to treatment were sent to each subject who was at least 6 months past completion of treatment. Seven items were used to evaluate the emotional reaction to body image. Although responses to the items clustered around 3.0, "not sure," for the mastectomy patients, the segmentectomy patients had a significantly more positive assessment of themselves. Patients were asked to evaluate retrospectively changes in physical attractiveness before surgery, 6 months after surgery, and 6 months after completion of therapy. The mastectomy group rated themselves as significantly less physically attractive at 6 months after surgery ($p < .003$) and at the time of the questionnaire ($p < .04$). Mastectomy patients also had a significantly lower rating of femininity 6 months after surgery ($p < .01$) than patients in the segmentectomy group.[77]

In summary, the majority of empirical studies on the impact of cancer on sexual health have been descriptive in design and focused primarily on the effects of cancer and treatment on the frequency of sexual behaviors, particularly intercourse and orgasm, or on self-concept among females with gynecologic and breast cancer or on males with testicular and prostate cancer. However, the issues of perception of significant others' responses to the physical and psychological sequelae of cancer remain understudied. Additional empirical data are needed on the interaction of other variables, such as age, depression, and activity status, on the physical as well as psychosocial aspects of sexual health.

Assessment Criteria

Two nursing diagnoses related to sexual health have been approved by NANDA—sexual dysfunction and altered sexuality patterns.[15] Defining characteristics for each diagnosis are presented in Table 17-7.[15] Differential diagnosis of the two responses based on defining characteristics is conceptually ambiguous in that the defining characteristic for altered sexuality patterns (reported difficulties, limitations, or changes in sexual behaviors or activities) provides the broad categories of the defining characteristics for sexual dysfunction.

Although conceptualization of the diagnoses related to sexual health requires clarification, the defining characteristics do emphasize subjective as well as objective criteria for evaluation of sexual health. Like other responses described in this chapter, the subjective responses and per-

TABLE 17-7 Nursing Diagnoses: Altered Sexual Health

Nursing Diagnosis	Definition	Defining Characteristics
Altered sexual patterns	The state in which an individual expresses concern regarding sexuality	Reported difficulties, limitations, or changes in sexual behaviors or activities
Sexual dysfunction	Perceived problem in achieving desired satisfaction of sexuality	Verbalizations of problem in sexuality Alterations in achieving perceived sex role Actual or perceived limitation imposed by disease or therapy Conflicts involving values Alteration in achieving sexual satisfaction Inability to achieve desired sexual satisfaction Frequent seeking of confirmation of desirability Alteration in relationship with significant other Change of interest in self and others

Source: Gordon M: Manual of Nursing Diagnosis. New York, McGraw-Hill, 1987.

TABLE 17-8 Levels of Sexual Counseling: The PLISSIT Model

P (Permission)	LI (Limited Information)	SS (Specific Suggestions)	IT (Intensive Therapy)
Legitimize sexual concerns Express sexual concerns with partner and health care team	Anticipatory guidance with respect to sexual concerns Provide information needed for rehabilitation	Cognitive reappraisal Coping skills for changes experienced in communication, roles, relationships Modify behaviors to accommodate limitations imposed by cancer or treatment	Referral to professional therapist

Source: Adapted from Shipes E, Lehr S: Sexuality and the male cancer patient. Cancer Nurs 5:375-381, 1982.

ceptions of the individual and, in this case, significant others must be considered when identifying a problem and planning care.

Nursing Interventions

Interventions for alterations in sexual health are based on assessment of the subjective perceptions and objective responses of the patient and significant others and careful delineation of the etiology of the problem. From the review of the literature, one is able to identify the most common etiologies of alterations to sexual health related to a diagnosis of cancer and the primary categories of nursing interventions.[78-80] However, the specific approach, suggestions, and resources used to treat the problem must be guided by the etiology of the problem and the perceptions and motivations of the patient or significant other.

Annon[78] has described a simple hierarchy of interventions for sexual problems known as the PLISSIT model (Table 17-8).[80] The system implies that for many problems, the simple acknowledgement and discussion of the perception of change in sexual health may be sufficient to help the patient or significant other resolve the problem. For other problems, especially those that existed before the diagnosis of cancer, referral to a professional for intensive individual or couple therapy may be indicated. For a detailed discussion on this intervention, see Chapter 29, Altered Body Image and Sexuality.

Approaches to treatment of changes in sexual health identified in the literature include education and counseling, yet few empirical studies have addressed the effectiveness of such interventions in ameliorating the symptoms associated with altered sexual health. Capone et al[81] examined the effects of counseling on psychosocial rehabilitation in a study of 56 patients with gynecologic cancers and 41 patients who met the same criteria but served as controls. Forty-one (73%) of the experimental group and 25 (61%) of the control group were sexually active before initiation of treatment and not more than 6 weeks after diagnosis. Subjects in both groups were interviewed and completed a battery of psychological tests (Self-Rating Symptom Scale, Profile of Mood States, and Tennessee Self-Concept Scale). The experimental group received individual counseling based on crisis intervention principles. Counseling included helping the patient to shape reality-based expectations, facilitating adaptive changes in behaviors, enhancing reintegration of self, and teaching information-processing skills. Interviews and testing were repeated at 3, 6, and 12 months after treatment. Significant differences were found in comparative frequencies of intercourse between the counseling and control groups at 3 ($p < .04$), 6 ($p < .007$), and 12 ($p < .05$) months. Counseling was found to have a positive effect on the resumption of sexual intercourse during the first year after treatment.[81]

More recently, Cain et al[82] described the psychosocial benefits of a cancer support group for women with a diagnosis of gynecologic cancer. After a psychosocial assessment within 1 month of diagnosis, subjects were assigned to one of three counseling groups: standard mode ($n = 31$), thematic individual mode ($n = 21$), and thematic group ($n = 28$). Each intervention was conducted for 8 weeks. Postcounseling data at 2 weeks and 6 months were obtained. Before the intervention, many of the subjects had significant disruption in sexual relationships. Women in the thematic individual and group counseling categories described significantly better sexual relationships at 6 months compared with baseline data ($F = 4.10$, $p < .02$).[82]

The two studies described are examples of innovative approaches to modify the threat of cancer to sexual health. However, the outcomes by which the effectiveness of the interventions were measured focus primarily on resumption of sexual intercourse. One might question that if sexual health is determined by how individuals perceive themselves, how they perceive that others see them, and how they behave in relationships with others, why were significant others not included in the intervention?

A second concern with respect to the interventions described is the lack of screening of patients for participation. Resource consumption of personnel, time, physical facilities, and materials required by such programs must be weighed against the benefits of the program. Therefore, selection of high risk patients for sexual dysfunction to participate in the program may increase the likelihood that sexual morbidity would be reduced. Screening would increase the probability of identifying those patients and partners with preexisting problems that may require more intensive therapy. For more information on this subject, see Chapter 29.

Future Directions for Nursing Research

Although sexual health is important, health care professionals have assigned limited value to and assumed a limited perspective of sexual health in relation to cancer care. Increasingly complex, multimodal, and lengthy treatment for cancer increases the risks of changes in sexual health among people diagnosed with cancer and their significant others.

Development of clinical and research instruments that have established reliability and validity for assessment of sexual health dimensions among people with cancer are needed. In addition, multimethods of assessing sexual health not only in the patient but also from the perspective of significant others are required if the interrelationships of the complex factors that contribute to sexual health are to be understood.

Definition, labeling, and validation of changes in sexual health among persons with cancer that require professional intervention are mandated by the level of concept clarification that currently exists. In addition, the effectiveness of educational, counseling, and anticipatory guidance interventions for selected patient and significant other populations should be evaluated.

CONCLUSION

Cancer threatens both the quantity and quality of life for the person who is faced with complex treatment plans, the uncertainty of recurrence, and integration of changed concepts of self, roles, and relationships resulting from the disease and treatment. The responses discussed in this chapter represent high-incidence phenomena described in the literature. One can see how little professionals know and understand about the incidence, contributing factors, variations of response, and long-term consequences of responses for the individual experiencing cancer. Thus, interventions designed to minimize the dysfunctional effects of the experience of cancer are, by the nature of our understanding of the phenomena, limited to "shot-gun," trial-and-error efforts. The specificity of interventions to particular patients based on a systematic appraisal of intrapersonal, interpersonal, social, and economic resources awaits the future.

REFERENCES

1. Spielberger C, Gorsuch R, Lushene R: Manual for the state-trait anxiety inventory. Palo Alto, Calif, Consulting Psychologists Press, 1970.
2. Lucente FE, Fleck S: A study of hospitalization anxiety in 408 medical and surgical patients. Psychosom Med 34:304-312, 1972.
3. Gottesman D, Lewis MS: Differences in crisis reactions among cancer and surgery patients. J Consult Clin Psychol 50:381-388, 1982.
4. Scott DW: Anxiety, critical thinking, and information processing during and after breast biopsy. Nurs Res 32:24-28, 1983.
5. Morris J, Royle GT: Choice of surgery for early breast cancer: Pre- and postoperative levels of clinical anxiety and depression in patients and their husbands. Br J Surg 74:1017-1019, 1987.
6. Oberst MT, Scott DW: Post discharge distress in surgically treated cancer patients and their spouses. Res Nurs Health 11:223-233, 1988.
7. Gottschalk LA, Hoigaard-Martin J: The emotional impact of mastectomy. Psychiatr Res 17:153-167, 1986.
8. Irwin PH, Kramer S, Diamond NH, et al: Sex differences in psychological distress during definitive radiation therapy for cancer. J Psychosoc Oncol 4:63-75, 1986.
9. Andersen BL, Tewfik HH: Psychological reactions to radiation therapy: Reconsideration of the adaptive aspects of anxiety. J Personal Soc Psychol 48:1024-1032, 1985.
10. Andersen BL, Karlsson JA, Anderson B, et al: Anxiety and cancer treatment: Response to stressful radiotherapy. Health Psychol 3:535-551, 1984.
11. Redd WH, Andrykowski MA: Behavioral intervention in cancer treatment: Controlling aversion reactions to chemotherapy. J Consult Clin Psychol 50:1018-1029, 1982.
12. Cassileth BR, Lusk EJ, Walsh WP: Anxiety levels in patients with malignant disease. Hospice J 2:57-69, 1986.
13. Cella DF, Pratt A, Holland JC: Persistent anticipatory nausea, vomiting, and anxiety in cured Hodgkin's disease patients after completion of chemotherapy. Am J of Psychiatry 143:641-643, 1986.
14. Carey MP, Burish TG: Anxiety as a predictor of behavioral therapy outcome for cancer chemotherapy patients. J Consult Clin Psychol 53:860-865, 1985.
15. Gordon M: Manual of Nursing Diagnosis. New York, McGraw-Hill, 1987.
16. Scandrett S: Cognitive reappraisal, in Bulechek GM, McCloskey J (eds): Nursing Interventions: Treatments for Nursing Diagnosis. Philadelphia, WB Saunders, 1985, pp 49-57.
17. Miller JF: Coping with Chronic Illness: Overcoming Powerlessness. Philadelphia, FA Davis, 1983.
18. Johnson J: The effects of a patient education course on persons with a chronic illness. Cancer Nurs 5:117-123, 1982.
19. Cotanch PH, Strum S: Progressive muscle relaxation as antiemetic therapy for cancer patients. Oncol Nurs Forum 14:33-37, 1987.
20. Frank JM: The effects of music therapy and guided visual imagery on chemotherapy induced nausea and vomiting. Oncol Nurs Forum 12:47-52, 1985.
21. Davis T, Jensen L: Identifying depression in medical patients. Image: J Nurs Scholarship 20:191-95, 1988.
22. Robinson JK, Boshier ML, Dansak DA, et al: Depression and anxiety in cancer patients: Evidence for different causes. J Psychosom Res 29:133-138, 1985.

23. Neilson AC, Williams TA: Depression in ambulatory medical patients. Arch Gen Psychiatry 37:999-1004, 1980.
24. Hamilton M: A rating scale for depression. J Neurol Neurosurg Psychiatry 23:56-62, 1960.
25. Beck AT, Beamesderfer A: Assessment of depression: The depression inventory, in Pichot P, Olivier-Martin R (eds): Psychological Measurements in Psychopharmacology: Modern Problems in Pharmopsychiatry (Vol 7). Basel, Karger, 1974, pp 151-169.
26. Nelson LD: Measuring depression in a clinical population using the MMPI. J Consult Clin Psychol 55:788-790, 1987.
27. Derogatis LR, Melisaratos N: The DSFI: A multidimensional measure of sexual functioning. J Sex Marital Therapy 5:244-281, 1979.
28. McNair DM, Lorr M, Droppleman LF: Profile of mood states. San Diego, Calif, Educational and Industrial Testing Service, 1971.
29. Petty F, Noyes R: Depression secondary to cancer. Biol Psychiatry 16:1203-1220, 1981.
30. Derogatis LR, Morrow GR, Fetting J, et al: The prevalence of psychiatric disorders among cancer patients. JAMA 249:751-757, 1983.
31. Massie MJ, Holland JC: Diagnosis and treatment of depression in the cancer patient. J Clin Psychiatry 45:25-29, 1984.
32. Plumb M, Holland JC: Comparative studies of psychological function in patients with advanced cancer. II. Interviewer-rated current and past psychological symptoms. Psychosom Med 43:243-254, 1981.
33. Andersen BL, Hacker NF: Psychosexual adjustment after vulvar surgery. Obstet Gynecol 62:457-462, 1983.
34. Goldberg RJ, Wool MS, Glicksman A, et al: Relationship of the social environment and patients' physical status to depression in lung cancer patients and their spouses. J Psychosoc Oncol 2:73-80, 1984.
35. Metzger LF, Rogers TF, Bauman LJ: Effects of age and marital status on the emotional distress after a mastectomy. J Psychosoc Oncol 1:17-33, 1983.
36. Robinson JK, Boshier ML, Dansak DA, et al: Depression and anxiety in cancer patients: Evidence for different causes. J Psychosom Res 29:133-138, 1985.
37. Bukberg J, Penman D, Holland JC: Depression in hospitalized cancer patients. Psychosom Med 46:199-212, 1984.
38. Spitzer RL: Diagnostic and Statistical Manual of Mental Disorders-Revised (DSM-III-R). Washington, DC, American Psychiatric Association, 1987.
39. Layne C, Heitkemper T, Roehrig RA, Speer TK: Motivational deficit in depressed cancer patients. J Clin Psychol 41:139-144, 1985.
40. Morris T, Greer S, White P: Psychological and social adjustment to mastectomy: A two-year follow-up study. Cancer 40:2381-2387, 1977.
41. Beck AT, Lester D, Trexler L, et al: The measurement of pessimism: The hopelessness scale. J Consult Clin Psychol 42:861-865, 1974.
42. Nowotny ML: Assessment of hope in patients with cancer: Development of an instrument. Oncol Nurs Forum 16:57-61, 1989.
43. Herth KA: The relationship between level of hope and level of coping response and other variables in patients with cancer. Oncol Nurs Forum 16:67-72, 1989.
44. Schmale AH, Iker HP: The affect of hopelessness and the development of cancer. Psychosom Med 28:714-721, 1966.
45. Hinds PS: Adolescent hopefulness in illness and health. Adv Nurs Sci 10:79-88, 1988.
46. Dufault KJ: Hope of elderly persons with cancer (doctoral dissertation, Case Western Reserve University). Diss Abstr Intl 42:1820B, 1981.
47. Zook DJ, Yasko JM: Psychologic factors: Their effect on nausea and vomiting experiences by clients receiving chemotherapy. Oncol Nurs Forum 10:76-81, 1983.
48. Greene SM, O'Mahoney PD, Rungasamy P: Levels of measured hopelessness in physically-ill patients. J Psychosom Res 26:591-593, 1982.
49. Raleigh ED: An investigation of hope as manifested in the physically ill adult (doctoral dissertation, Wayne State University). Diss Abstr Intl 41:1313B, 1980.
50. Brandt B: The relationship between hopelessness and selected variables in women receiving chemotherapy for breast cancer. Oncol Nurs Forum 14:35-39, 1987.
51. Stoner M: Hope and cancer patients (doctoral dissertation, University of Colorado Health Sciences Center). Diss Abstr Intl 44:115-B, 1982.
52. Stoner M, Keampfer S: Recalled life expectancy information, phase of illness, and hope in cancer patients. Res Nurs Health 8:269-274, 1985.
53. Cassileth BR, Zupkis RV, Sutton-Smith K, et al: Information and participation preferences among cancer patients. Ann Intern Med 92:832-836, 1980.
54. Kerber A: Locus of control, hope, and disease-free interval (unpublished master's thesis), Emory University, Atlanta, Ga, 1985.
55. Clark JC: Hope as a critical factor in the cancer experience, in Pritchard AP (ed): Cancer Nursing: A Revolution in Care, Proceeding of the Fifth International Conference on Cancer Nursing. London, Macmillan, 1989, pp 117-119.
56. Dufault K, Martocchio BC: Hope: Its spheres and dimensions. Nurs Clin North Am 20:379-391, 1985.
57. Derogatis LR: Psychological assessment of psychosexual function. Psychiatr Clin North Am 3:113-131, 1980.
58. Waterhouse J, Metcalfe MC: Development of the sexual adjustment questionnaire. Oncol Nurs Forum 13:53-59, 1986.
59. Abitbol MM, Davenport JH: Sexual dysfunction after therapy for cervical carcinoma. Am J Obstet Gynecol 119:181-189, 1974.
60. Jenkins B: Patients' reports of sexual changes after treatment for gynecological cancer. Oncol Nurs Forum 15:349-354, 1988.
61. Cain EN, Kohorn EI, Quinlan DM, et al: Psychosocial reactions to the diagnosis of gynecologic cancer. Obstet Gynecol 62:635-641, 1983.
62. Andersen BL, Hacker NF: Psychosexual adjustment after vulvar surgery. Obstet Gynecol 62:457-462, 1983.
63. Andreasson B, Moth I, Jensen SB, et al: Sexual function and somatopsychic reactions in vulvectomy-operated women and their partners. Acta Obstet Gynecol Scand 65:7-10, 1986.
64. Woods NF, Earp JA: Women with cured breast cancer. Nurs Res 27:279-285, 1978.
65. Jamison KR, Wellisch DK, Pasnau RO: Psychosocial aspects of mastectomy. I. The woman's perspective. Am J Psychiatry 135:432-436, 1978.
66. Taylor SE, Lichtman RR, Wood JV, et al: Illness-related and treatment-related factors in psychological adjustment to breast cancer. Cancer 55:2506-2513, 1985.
67. Blackmore C: The impact of orchidectomy upon the sexuality of the man with testicular cancer. Cancer Nurs 11:33-40, 1988.
68. Schover LR, Gonzales M, von Eschenbach AC: Sexual and marital relationships after radiotherapy for seminoma. Urology 27:117-123, 1986.
69. Heinrich-Rynning T: Prostatic cancer treatments and their effects on sexual functioning. Oncol Nurs Forum 14:37-41, 1987.
70. Banker FL: The preservation of potency after external beam

irradiation for prostate cancer. Int J Radiat Oncol Biol Phys 15:219-220, 1988.
71. Labenne WD, Greene BI: Educational Implications of the Self-Concept Theory. Goodyear Publishing Company, 1969, p 10.
72. Newman KA, Schnaper N, Reed WP, et al: Effect of Hickman catheters on the self-esteem of patients with leukemia. South Med J 77:682-685, 1984.
73. Crumbaugh JC: Cross validation of purpose-in-life test based on Frankl's concepts. J Individual Psychol 24:74-81, 1968.
74. Weddington WW, Segraves KB, Simon MA: Psychological outcome of extremity sarcoma survivors undergoing amputation or limb salvage. J Clin Oncol 3:1393-1399, 1985.
75. Baxley KO, Erdman LK, Henry EB, et al: Alopecia: Effect on cancer patients' body image. Cancer Nurs 7:499-503, 1984.
76. Jourard S, Secord PF: Body cathexis and personality. Br J Psychol 46:130-138, 1955.
77. Kemeny MM, Wellisch DK, Schain WS: Psychosocial outcome in a randomized surgical trial for treatment of primary breast cancer. Cancer 62:1231-1237, 1988.
78. Annon JS: The Behavioral Treatment of Sexual Problems (vol 1). Honolulu, Mercentile Printing, 1974.
79. Lamb MA, Woods NF: Sexuality and the cancer patient. Cancer Nurs 4:137-144, 1981.
80. Shipes E, Lehr S: Sexuality and the male cancer patient. Cancer Nurs 5:375-381, 1982.
81. Capone MA, Good RS, Westie KS, et al: Psychosocial rehabilitation of gynecologic oncology patients. Arch Phys Med Rehabil 61:128-132, 1980.
82. Cain EN, Kohorn EI, Quinlan DM, et al: Psychosocial reactions to the diagnosis of gynecologic cancer. Obstet Gynecol 62:635-641, 1983.

Chapter 18

Psychosocial Dimensions: The Family

Jane Clark, RN, MN, OCN

INTRODUCTION

The diagnosis of cancer, although assigned to the individual, can precipitate significant changes in the lives of the individual, members of the family unit, and community. Although responses experienced vary among family members, across developmental stages of the family, with different illness demands, and with respect to economic and psychosocial resources, anecdotal data and clinical observations have substantiated the theoretical assumption that a change in one element of the social system, in this case the patient diagnosed with cancer, will result in a ripple effect throughout the system.

Predictability with respect to family routines, relationships, and communication patterns is threatened. Family members are challenged to learn new roles, self-care skills, and ways of relating and communicating to each other, friends, and members of the health care team as they cope with the chronic nature of the cancer experience. Life for families facing cancer becomes more complex. Although the demands of family members may be increased, few empirical studies have been conducted to describe the psychosocial responses of the family unit or individual members of the family unit to the cancer experience.[1]

Selected clinical and research instruments for evaluating the family will be described in this chapter. In addition, representative studies describing the responses of family members to the cancer experience, factors that place the family unit at risk for extreme responses, and effectiveness of selected interventions to modify responses of family members will be examined.

INSTRUMENTS TO EVALUATE THE FAMILY

The Family APGAR[2] is a screening questionnaire designed to assess family *A*daptability, *P*artnership, *G*rowth, *A*ffection, and *R*esolve from the perspective of the patient. The questionnaire consists of five questions to which the patient responds on a 3-point scale indicating the frequency of satisfaction on the dimensions measured (almost always = 2; some of the time = 1; or hardly ever = 0). Based on the definition of family as a "psychosocial group consisting of the patient and one or more persons, children or adults, in which there is a commitment for members to nurture each other" (p. 1232), the instrument does not assume the structural, institutional, or cultural boundaries of the traditional family. Reliability and validity data were not reported by the author.

The Family Functioning Index (FFI)[3] is a 15-item self-report instrument designed to assess the dynamics of family interaction. Questions assess areas of marital satisfaction, frequency of disagreement, communication, problem solving, and feelings of happiness and closeness.[4] Validity and reliability estimates for the instrument were determined by comparing scores on the FFI with clinical ratings by caseworkers and by resulting high positive correlations of husband and wife scores. Five-year test-retest reliability was reported as $r = .83$, $p<.001$.[4]

RESPONSES OF THE FAMILY TO PHASES OF THE CANCER EXPERIENCE

In the previous chapter, the individual responses of anxiety, depression, hopelessness, and altered sexual health were discussed with respect to the diagnosis of cancer. Surprisingly, the responses of family members have been shown to be similar to those of patients with cancer.

Responses of Family Members in General

Self-reported responses of family members to hospitalization of patients with cancer were described by Lovejoy.[5] Data were obtained from 105 subjects using a semistructured interview schedule. Content analyses of the interviews revealed five common responses to the hospitalization experience: shock, uncertainty, accommodation, immersion, and awareness. The responses were not unlike patient responses described by other researchers.

A comparison of psychological responses of patients with cancer and their next-of-kin ($N = 210$) was reported by Cassileth et al.[6] Patient and next-of-kin scores on three outcome measures—State-Trait Anxiety Inventory, Profile of Mood States, and Mental Health Index—were correlated significantly. Scores for both patients and next-of-kin indicated a decrease in psychological status related to the phase of the cancer experience; that is, the psychological status was better for patients and next-of-kin during follow-up care versus active treatment versus palliative care.

Responses of Spouses

Findings of Casselith et al[6] were supported by Oberst and James[7] in a study to determine the magnitude and pattern of crisis development among spouses of cancer patients ($N = 40$), to describe the effectiveness of crisis counseling, and to identify factors that predict crisis development (p. 48). Findings indicated that spouses experienced increased anxiety before the patient was discharged from the hospital, which was replaced by depression and anger at patients for egocentricity in the home care period. Depression and anger were succeeded eventually by guilt. Moreover, spouses reported distress, anger, and frustration about the lack of support from professionals and all sources (p. 56). Spouses also had a higher incidence of emotional problems than did the patients at 10, 30, 60, 90, and 180 days after discharge. In addition to the psychological responses to the demands of

TABLE 18-1 Perceived Spousal Caregiving Demands

Management of physical care
Management of household finances
Standing by
Alterations in caregiver's well-being and pattern of living
Unmet expectations from the health care system
Constant vigilance
Cancer
Anticipation of the future
Alterations in relationship with ill spouse

Source: Stetz KM: Caregiving demands during advanced cancer: The spouse's needs. Cancer Nurs 10(5):260-268, 1987.

TABLE 18-2 Psychosocial Problems Experienced by Family Members

Impaired relationships with the family or significant others
Impaired relationships with health care providers
Somatic side effects of disease and treatment
Difficulties in compliance with treatment
Mood disturbances
Difficulties in family roles
Difficulties in self-management
Financial difficulties
Transportation difficulties
Equipment difficulties
Significant concerns about body image
Denial
Cognitive impairment

Source: Wellisch DK, Fawzy FI, Landsverk J, et al: Evaluation of psychosocial problems of the home-bound cancer patient: The relationship of disease and the sociodemographic variables of patients to family problems. J Psychosoc Oncol 1:4-5, 1983.

the cancer experience, spouses reported disruption in many areas of lifestyle, including employment, home management, child care, social activities, and travel to and from hospital. Thus, the acute hospitalization period precipitates significant psychological responses among spouses of patients with cancer that continue through the postdischarge home care period and even into the terminal phase of illness.

The findings of Oberst and James[7] were extended to the terminal phase of illness in a study by Stetz[8] of 65 spouses of terminally ill adult cancer patients. Content analyses of semistructured interviews conducted in the home revealed nine categories of spouse caregiving demands (Table 18-1).[8] Gender differences were identified. Female caregivers had more difficulty with observing the physical deterioration of the spouse while male caregivers had more difficulty with home management.

The responses of spouses to home care demands were described by Wellisch et al.[9] Records of 447 homebound, married cancer patients were reviewed to determine the types of psychosocial problems experienced by family members (p. 1). A standardized instrument to abstract the frequencies of psychosocial problem areas (Table 18-2)[9] was used for review. Findings indicated that families of male patients were more likely to feel overwhelmed by the demands of home care (p = .0003) and were more likely to experience a severe mood disturbance (p = .0001) than were families of female patients.

Age had a significant impact on the family variables studied. Families of patients 70 years or older were more likely to be overwhelmed by home care demands (p = .0311). Role disturbances were more likely to occur in families of patients age 50 years or younger (p = .04), while mood disturbances were more likely to occur in families of patients 50 years or older (p = .02).

The findings of the study indicated that the type of cancer diagnosed, that is, lung, breast, or cervical cancer, had a specific impact on family outcome variables. The families of patients with lung cancer were more likely to exhibit significant mood disturbances (p = .001) and to be overwhelmed by the demands of home care (p = .003). In contrast, families of patients with cervical cancer were more likely to experience disturbances in family relationships (p = .01).

The findings of Goldberg et al[10] support the high incidence of depression amoung spouses (N = 18) of patients with lung cancer. Scores on the Profile of Mood States-Depression were measured within 6 weeks of diagnosis and at 2-month intervals for a total of 6 months. Spouses had elevated mean scores at diagnosis (Time 1 = 14.7), and the mean scores remained elevated throughout the data-collection period (Time 2 = 11.3, Time 3 = 10.6). In addition, scores of spouses on the Psychosocial Adjustment to Illness Scale (social environment subscale) were related significantly to the depression scores rather than to the physical status scores of the patient at all three time intervals.

Other psychosocial responses of spouses of patients with lung cancer were described by Cooper.[11] Fifteen patients with lung cancer and their spouses were interviewed to determine the effects of the diagnosis on the family. In content analyses of the interviews, the following effects were identified. Spouses experienced shock, fear, and depression at diagnosis. Spouses also reported more symptoms of stress (nervousness, sleeplessness, loss of appetite, inability to concentrate, and irritability) than did patients. Moreover, spouses reported feelings of aloneness and helplessness in response to the cancer experience.

Communication patterns between the patient-spouse dyads changed in that the spouses became protective of the patient with respect to discussing distressful information and reported not sharing their feelings with patients. Despite changed communication patterns, the majority of subjects reported increased closeness in patient-spouse and parent-child relationships.

Northouse and Northouse[12] reviewed 200 clinical papers and research studies printed over two decades to identify issues of communication among patients, health care professionals, and family members. The authors argue that although the number of articles on communication issues among family members of persons with cancer is limited, the potential impact of communication issues on the care of the patient and the well-being of family members is far-reaching.

Communication becomes a primary issue among family members as caregiving demands increase. Data indicate that although the responsibilities of care are being shifted to the family, family members express concern over the difficulty in obtaining necessary information.[13-15] Second, as the demands of care increase, mood disturbances among family members, particularly anxiety and depression,[7,16,17] become more prominent. However, professional concern for care of family members has been limited, and family members have not communicated their concerns and responses to health care professionals.

Responses of Adult and Adolescent Children

Just as data indicate that communication patterns can become strained between the patient and spouse facing cancer, indications are that communication patterns change between the parents and children within the family. Lichtman et al[18] interviewed 78 patients with a diagnosis of breast cancer to describe changes in the relationships between patients and their children and to examine the factors that influence these changes. In addition to structured interviews, the subjects completed the Profile of Mood States, Self-Esteem Scale,[19] Index of Well-Being,[20] and Marital Adjustment Scale.[21] Patients were also asked to provide the name of a significant other to be interviewed ($N = 63$).

Findings indicated 54% of patients ($N = 37$) reported changes in the relationships with children. The changes were characterized as improved (73%) and permanent (76%). Nineteen problem relationships were identified. Patients attributed the problems to changes in how the children were responding to the patient (28%) and how the patients were responding to the children (10%), changes in both response patterns (52%), and changes due to other reasons (10%). These findings were confirmed by interviews with identified significant others.

Deteriorated relationships were correlated significantly with a poor prognosis for the patient ($r = .32$, $p<.02$) as well as the severity of surgery ($r = .43$, $p<.001$). In addition, patient adjustment scores were predictive of perceived changes in relationships with children ($r = .20$, $p<.05$) in that patients with poor adjustment scores reported more changes and negative changes in relationships with children.

Changes in relationships with children differed significantly with respect to the gender of the child ($x^2(1) = 3.92$, $p<.05$). Although patients reported similar problems with fears related to prognosis, rejection, and refusal to discuss cancer in both mother-son and mother-daughter relationships, the frequency and magnitude of the problems were greater in the mother-daughter relationships.

The relationships with adult children can become more complex when the adult child is a health care professional. In a cross-sectional study by Baird[22] of 27 nurse/daughters, the subjects were interviewed and asked to compare their perceptions of family relationships before and after the diagnosis of cancer. Nurse/daughter perceptions of roles changed with the diagnosis of cancer in the following ways: roles expanded from that of information source to decision maker, intermediary, and caregiver. Even though the role changes were perceived as positive, nurse/daughters described role conflicts between daughter/nurse, sibling/nurse, and family member/nurse. However, positive changes in communication patterns were identified by 59% of the sample. Parents and family members were perceived to be more open, closer, and dependent after the diagnosis of cancer.

Loss of a parent during adolescence has been documented as a critical event in the life of a child. Berman et al[23] interviewed 10 adolescents and the surviving parent within 6 months to 2 years following the death of a parent of cancer to describe responses experienced. The adolescents described open information sharing among the family unit during the illness; however, after the death, communication patterns changed. The adolescent reportedly assumed the protector role in shielding the remaining parent from discussing distressful feelings. The adolescents, as did the spouses in the previous studies, indicated that the protector role was extremely stressful and that they lacked sufficient support during this period.

Discrepancies were reported between parents and adolescents in the changes in activities of daily living as well as in the sources of support for the adolescents. Adolescents perceived an increase in household responsibilities as well as more support from family and peers versus health care professionals and clergy.

EFFECT OF FAMILY RESPONSES ON PATTERNS AND OUTCOMES OF CARE

Whereas the majority of studies in the area of family responses to a diagnosis of cancer have been to describe the responses experienced in families of selected patient groups (site-specific or age-specific), limited data exist to quantify the impact of those responses on either outcomes or patterns of care. Hays[24] conducted a retrospective chart review of visits to 100 patients with cancer during the last 10 days of their lives to determine if the incidence of symptoms, family coping, and resources used were predictive of home and inpatient hospice use. The random sample of home care patients (group I, home care only; group II, home care/inpatient) were evaluated on physical symptoms of pain, nausea, vomiting, respiratory deficit, elimination, nutrition, and mental status; family coping patterns of anxiety and fatigue; and patterns of care including length and frequency of home visits, disciplines visited, telephone contacts, home care episodes, and place of death.

Patients who experienced more physical symptoms and more symptoms that were uncontrolled were more likely to require inpatient hospice services. Uncontrolled symptoms associated with increased anxiety and fatigue experienced by family members and demand for homecare services also increased the use of inpatient hospice services.

The relationships of family cohesion and adaptability (FACES II),[25] marital adjustment (Snyder Marital Disharmony and Disaffection Scales),[26] and psychosocial adjustment to illness (Psychosocial Adjustment to Illness Scale)[27] among 57 white women with breast cancer were explored by Friedman et al.[28] Based on the theoretical framework proposed by Olson et al,[29] the researchers examined if women who perceived that their families were balanced rather than extreme with respect to emotional connectedness and flexibility to change reported more positive levels of adjustment.

Findings supported the notion that family cohesion is a desirable quality among women faced with a diagnosis of breast cancer. In fact, 34% of the respondents expressed a desire for more cohesiveness within the family, while no respondent indicated that she desired less cohesiveness. Data analyses revealed that women who reported the highest levels of family cohesion also reported more positive adjustment to breast cancer. No significant relationship was found between reported family adaptability and adjustment to breast cancer. Although the findings are not consistent with the propositions of the model offered by Olsen et al,[29] the authors question if gender differences with respect to value of affection versus task orientation could have contributed to the differences seen in the study sample.

ASSESSMENT CRITERIA

The family is identified as a portion of four nursing diagnoses identified by the North American Nursing Diagnosis Association (NANDA): (1) Alteration in family processes, (2) Ineffective family coping: compromised, (3) Ineffective family coping: disabling, and (4) Family coping: potential for growth.[30] A comparison of each diagnosis is presented in Table 18-3.

The complexities of assessment measures of the family are detailed by Lewis.[1] Yet, the complexities of measures only reflect the complexities of the phenomena of study, in this case the family coping with the cancer experience. Thus the ideal assessment of families using multiple measures from multiple sources described by Lewis[1] offer the potential for collecting the most comprehensive and reliable data base on which to base family-level services.

However, the personnel and time demanded by such an extensive assessment precludes application to all families in the clinical setting. Yet, screening instruments described previously may serve to identify those families at high risk for dysfunctional responses to the cancer experience and to target families in need of a more comprehensive assessment.

FAMILY-LEVEL NURSING INTERVENTIONS

Selection of nursing interventions for families facing cancer is based on the needs of the individual family members as well as the needs expressed by the family unit. Family-level teaching with respect to the disease, treatment, rehabilitation, or prognosis; anticipatory guidance of family members throughout the cancer experience; single and multiple family group counseling; mobilization of health care or community resources; and referrals for intensive family therapy have been identified in the literature as strategies for family care.[31-35]

Although nursing interventions may be directed toward the individual members or the family unit, the majority of studies among families facing cancer have focused on the individual family members. Few empirical studies have been conducted to determine the effects of family-unit services. The effects of selected interventions on family outcomes will be discussed in the following section.

Spousal Support Groups

Sabo et al[36] studied the responses of husbands of 24 patients who had undergone a mastectomy ($N = 24$) and the effects of a 10-week support group intervention ($N = 6$) in modifying those responses. All subjects were interviewed and completed a 37-item self-report instrument to evaluate gender expectations, self-esteem, depression, sexual compatibility, frequency of verbal communication about the mastectomy, and supportive attitude toward the wife before the intervention. Six husbands elected to attend the support group.

Interview findings indicated that the husbands had strong reactions of disbelief, alarm, isolation, and anxiety related to the role of support-giver for the wife. After the surgery, the husbands described assuming the role of protector to shield the wife from both his and her emotional reactions to the cancer experience, which resulted in strained communication patterns, distrust, and resentment. Comparison of pre and post scores on the instrument revealed that husbands who had attended the support group communicated significantly more with their wives about mastectomy issues than did husbands who had not attended the group sessions.

TABLE 18-3 Comparison of Family-Related Nursing Diagnoses

Nursing Diagnosis	Definition	Defining Characteristics
Alteration in Family Processes	Inability of family system (household members) to meet needs of members, carry out family functions, or maintain communications for mutual growth and maturation	Inability of family members to relate to each other for mutual growth and maturation, failure to send and receive clear messages, poorly communicated family rules, rituals, symbols, unexplained myths, unhealthy family decision-making processes, inability of family members to express and accept wide range of feelings, inability to accept and receive help, does not demonstrate respect for individuality and autonomy of members, rigidity in functions and roles, fails to accomplish current or past family developmental tasks, inappropriate boundary maintenance, inability to adapt to change, inability to deal with traumatic or crisis experience constructively, parents do not demonstrate respect for each other's views on child-rearing practices, inappropriate level and direction of energy, inability to meet needs of members, family uninvolved in community activities
Ineffective Family Coping: Compromised	Usually supportive primary person providing insufficient, ineffective, or compromised support, comfort, assistance, or encouragement that may be needed by patient to manage or master adaptive tasks related to health challenge	Patient expresses concern or complaint about significant other's response to health problem, significant persons described preoccupation with personal reactions to patient's illness, disability, or other situational or developmental crisis, significant person describes or confirms inadequate understanding of knowledge base which interferes with effective assistive or supportive behaviors, significant person attempts assistive or supportive behaviors with less than satisfactory results, significant person withdraws or enters into a limited or temporary personal communication with client at time of need, significant person displays protective behavior disproportionate to patient's abilities or need for autonomy
Ineffective Family Coping: Disabled	Behavior of significant person disables own capabilities and patient's capacities to address effectively tasks essential to either person's adaptation to the health challenge	Neglectful care of patient in regard to basic human needs and/or illness treatment, distortion of reality regarding patient's health problem including extreme denial, intolerance, rejection, abandonment, desertion, carrying on usual routines disregarding patient needs, psychosomaticism, taking on illness signs of the patient, decisions or actions by family which are detrimental to economic or social well-being, agitation, depression, aggression, hostility, impaired restructuring of a meaningful life for self, impaired individuation, prolonged overconcern for patient, neglectful relationships with other family members, patient's development of helpless, inactive dependence
Family Coping: Potential for Growth	Family member has managed adaptive tasks involved with patient's health challenge effectively and is exhibiting desire and readiness for enhanced health and growth in regard to self and in relation to the patient	Family member attempts to describe growth impact of crisis on his/her own values, priorities, goals, or relationships, is moving in direction of health-promoting and enriching lifestyle which supports and monitors maturational processes, audits and negotiated treatment program and generally chooses experiences which optimize wellness, expresses interest in making contact on a one-to-one basis or on a mutual-aid group basis with another person who has experienced a similar situation

Source: Gordon M: Manual of Nursing Diagnosis 1986-1987. New York, McGraw-Hill, 1987.

Risk Counseling Interventions

To address the need of family members for information about the cancer of the patient as well as personal risks for cancer, Kelly[37] described a program of risk counseling designed specifically for relatives of persons with cancer. Based on the expressed concerns of the relative, elements of the program may include biologic and medical information about cancer risks or a review of individual personality, life-style, and environmental risks. In addition, relatives may be counseled on how to deal with tensions in the family, how to express concern for the family member with cancer, and how to deal with personal physical and psychosocial responses to the cancer experience. Data related to the outcomes of the program were not reported by the author.

FUTURE DIRECTIONS FOR NURSING RESEARCH

The issues of family responses to a diagnosis of cancer go far beyond those discussed in the previous chapter. Even though selected psychosocial responses have been identified for spouses, patient–significant other dyads, and children of adults with cancer, the effects of the interaction of those individual responses within the context of the family unit have not been studied systematically. The lack of data becomes even more critical when one considers the responses of nontraditional family units, multigenerational families, and culturally diverse families.

Obviously, family-level services are not needed nor available for every family faced with cancer. However, screening instruments with established reliability and validity among families facing cancer and delineation of critical defining characteristics that predispose the family to dysfunctional responses are areas requiring additional study.

Finally, given the identification of high-risk or dysfunctional families, individual and family-level services to address expressed dysfunctional responses among cancer families are minimal. Multiple services and programs designed to meet a spectrum of family needs are needed. In addition, the effectiveness of such services and programs in modifying the occurrence or resolution of dysfunctional responses in the family must be evaluated.

REFERENCES

1. Lewis FM: Family level services for the cancer patient: Critical distinctions, fallacies, and assessment. Cancer Nurs 6:193-200, 1983.
2. Smilkstein G: The family APGAR: A proposal for a family function test and its use by physicians. J Family Pract 6:1231-1239, 1978.
3. Pless IB, Satterwhite BB: A measure of family functioning and its application. Soc Sci Med 7:613-620, 1973.
4. Satterwhite BB, Zweig SR, Iker HP, et al: The family functioning index—five-year test-retest reliability and implications for use. J Comp Family Studies 7:111-116, 1976.
5. Lovejoy NC: Family responses to cancer hospitalization. Oncol Nurs Forum 13:33-37, 1986.
6. Cassileth BR, Lusk EJ, Strouse TB, et al: A psychological analysis of cancer patients and their next-of-kin. Cancer 55:72-76, 1985.
7. Oberst MT, James RH: Going home: Patient and spouse adjustment following cancer surgery. Topics Clin Nurs 7:46-57, 1985.
8. Stetz KM: Caregiving demands during advanced cancer: The spouse's needs. Cancer Nurs 10:260-268, 1987.
9. Wellisch DK, Fawzy FI, Landsverk J, et al: Evaluation of psychosocial problems of the home-bound cancer patient: The relationship of disease and the sociodemographic variables of patients to family problems. J Psychosoc Oncol 1:1-15, 1983.
10. Goldberg RJ, Wool MS, Glicksman A, et al: Relationship of the social environment and patients' physical status to depression in lung cancer patients and their spouses. J Psychosoc Oncol 2:73-80, 1984.
11. Cooper ET: A pilot study on the effects of the diagnosis of lung cancer on family relationships. Cancer Nurs 7:301-308, 1984.
12. Northouse PG, Northouse LL: Communication and cancer: Issues confronting patients, health professionals, and family members. J Psychosoc Oncol 5:17-46, 1987.
13. Krant MJ, Johnston L: Family members' perceptions of communication in late stage cancer. Int J Psychiatry Med 8:203-216, 1977-1978.
14. Morrow GR, Hoagland AC, Morse IP: Sources of support perceived by parents of children with cancer: Implications for counseling. Patient Counsel Health Ed 4:36-40, 1982.
15. Wright K, Dyck S: Expressed concerns of adult cancer patients' family members. Cancer Nurs 7:371-374, 1984.
16. Baider L, Kaplan De-Nour A, Atara K: Couples' reactions and adjustment to mastectomy: A preliminary report. Int J Psychiatry Med 14:265-276, 1984.
17. Northouse LL: The impact of cancer on the family: An overview. Int J Psychiatry Med 14:215-242, 1984.
18. Lichtman RR, Taylor SE, Wood JV, et al: Relations with children after breast cancer: The mother-daughter relationship at risk. J Psychosoc Oncol 2:1-19, 1984.
19. Rosenberg M: Society and the Adolescent Self-Image. Princeton, NJ, Princeton University Press, 1965.
20. Campbell A, Converse PE, Rodgers WL: The Quality of American Life: Perceptions, Evaluations, and Satisfactions. New York, Russell Sage Foundation, 1976.
21. Locke HF, Wallace KM: Short marital adjustment and prediction tests: Their reliability and validity. Marriage Family Living 21:251-255, 1959.
22. Baird SB: The effect of cancer in a parent on role relationships with the nurse/daughter. Cancer Nurs 11:9-17, 1988.
23. Berman H, Cragg CE, Kuenzig L: Having a parent die of cancer: Adolescents' reactions. Oncol Nurs Forum 15:159-162, 1988.
24. Hays JC: Patient symptoms and family coping: Predictors of hospice utilization patterns. Cancer Nurs 9:317-325, 1986.
25. Olson DH, Portner J, Bell R: Family Adaptability and Cohesion Evaluation Scales (FACES II). St. Paul, University of Minnesota, Family Social Science, 1982.
26. Snyder DK, Regts JM: Factor scales for assessing marital disharmony and disaffection. J Consult Clin Psychol 50:736-743, 1982.
27. Derogatis LR, Lopez MC: The Psychosocial Adjustment to Illness Scale (PAIS & PAIS-SR): Administration, Scoring, and

Procedures Manual-I. Baltimore, Md, Johns Hopkins University School of Medicine, 1983.
28. Friedman LC, Baer PE, Nelson DV, et al: Women with breast cancer: Perception of family functioning and adjustment to illness. Psychosom Med 50:529-540, 1988.
29. Olson DH, Sprenkle DH, Russell CS: Circumplex model of marital and family systems. I. Cohesion and adaptability dimensions, family types and clinical applications. Family Process 18:3-28, 1979.
30. Gordon M: Manual of Nursing Diagnosis 1986-1987. New York, McGraw-Hill, 1987.
31. Whitman HH, Gustafson JP: Group therapy for families facing a cancer crisis. Oncol Nurs Forum 16:539-543, 1989.
32. Giacquinta B: Helping families face the crisis of cancer. Am J Nurs 77:1585-1588, 1977.
33. Wellisch DK, Mosher MB, Van Scoy C: Management of family emotion stress: Family group therapy in a private oncology practice. Int J Group Psychother 28:225-231, 1978.
34. Edstrom S, Woehning Miller MW: Preparing the family to care for the cancer patient at home: A home care course. Cancer Nurs 4:49-52, 1981.
35. Heinricks RL, Coscarelli Schag C: Stress and activity management: Group treatment for cancer patients and spouses. J Consult Clin Psychol 53:439-446, 1985.
36. Sabo D, Brown J, Smith C: The male role and mastectomy: Support groups and men's adjustment. J Psychosoc Oncol 4:19-31, 1986.
37. Kelly PT: Risk counseling for relatives of cancer patients: New information, new approaches. J Psychosoc Oncol 5:65-79, 1987.

Chapter 19

Psychosocial Dimensions: Issues in Survivorship

Deborah Welch-McCaffrey, RN, MSN, OCN

Susan Leigh, RN, BSN

Lois J. Loescher, RN, MS

Barbara Hoffman, JD

INTRODUCTION

Early detection and effective multimodal therapies have increased significantly the numbers of cancer survivors to the extent that cancer is now considered a chronic, life-threatening illness rather than a terminal disease.[1] In 1989, over 5 million Americans had a history of cancer, with 3 million surviving 5 years or more.[2] Cancers with a high and continually increasing 5-year relative survival rate include testicular cancer (86%), endometrial cancer (85%), cutaneous melanoma (80%), breast cancer (74%), bladder cancer (73%), Hodgkin's disease (73%), prostate cancer (70%), and cervical cancer (67%).[2,3]

The health care community traditionally has been more concerned with the aggressive medical treatment of patients having cancers with a high survival rate than with the psychosocial aspects of long-term survivorship.[4] The burgeoning population of survivors, however, makes evident the need to address quality of survival and the psychosocial consequences of cancer and its therapies. Long-term survivors may experience problems ranging from minor short-term difficulties to major psychosocial crises.[5-7] Determining which individuals are at greatest risk for psychosocial morbidity is critical for clinicians.

DEFINITIONS OF SURVIVORSHIP

Survivorship as defined by *Webster's Ninth New Collegiate Dictionary* is summarized as the state of remaining alive or in existence (living on) and continuing to function or prosper despite life occurrences.[8] Medical definitions of long-term cancer survivorship are more limited in scope and are not yet fully agreed on by the health care community. Historically, cancer survivors have been defined as individuals "cured" of their disease, with the "cured" state commencing 5 years after diagnosis.[2] The term *cure* traditionally describes those individuals who have no evidence of disease with a minimal or nonexistent chance for recurrence.[9]

Controversial aspects of associating survivorship with cancer "cure" could be eliminated by basing the definition on the concept of control rather than "cure." Cancer itself constitutes many different diseases, each having distinct stages and behaviors and treated with a wide range of modalities. Some cancers, such as melanoma or early stages of breast cancer, are often "cured" once the cancer is physically removed. Other cancers, including stage I and stage II Hodgkin's disease, acute lymphocytic leukemias, and osteogenic sarcoma, may be considered cured following several courses of intensive multimodal therapy.[10] Individuals with these types of cancers may be, by definition, "cured" before the fifth year following diagnosis, but they are still not medically considered cured and, thus, a long-term survivor until the 5-year mark. Still other cancers such as multiple myeloma or chronic leukemia may not be "curable" but, with continued treatment, can be controlled, enabling patients to live for several years. Although these individuals are not "cured" in the medical sense, they are indeed survivors of a chronic disease. Finally, other cancers are initially labelled "incurable" or advanced at diagnosis, with expectations of inevitable death.[11] Exceptional patients who survive these cancers may be defined further as "miracle cures."

Vought et al[12] described a survival paradigm that allows health care providers to rank the importance of the issues a survivor might identify.[13] The six components of the paradigm are listed in descending order of importance but not in order of occurrence: (1) basic survival (food, shelter, medical care); (2) physiologic self-concept (attractiveness, fitness, physical function); (3) psychologic self-concept (self-respect, integrity, autonomy); (4) proximal affiliation (intimate relationships); (5) distal affiliation (social relationships); and (6) avocational component (recreation and play). Cancer-related barriers to the survival paradigm are listed in Table 19-1. Although physical self-concept has a higher importance rating, psychosocial components comprise the bulk of the model, indicating the overall importance of psychosocial issues.

SURVIVORSHIP AS A CONTINUUM

Using the control definition enables cancer survivorship to be viewed as a continual, ongoing process rather than as an explicit event occurring at a predetermined time period. Mullan[14] first proposed a continuum of survival stages or "seasons" in lieu of the word "cure." Seasons of survival apply to everyone diagnosed with cancer and consist of an acute, extended, and permanent survival stage. The acute survival stage begins at diagnosis, when patients must deal with immediate effects of therapy in addition to their mortality. Life modifications that will become part of their immediate and long-term future are begun. Social support of the patient is critical in this stage. Extended survival begins when the patient's disease has gone into remission or the patient has finished the primary treatment course and starts consolidation or adjuvant therapies. In this stage, patients begin to deal with issues such as altered body image or vocational changes. Psychosocial treatment is often lacking in the extended survival stage. Finally, Mullan[14] described the permanent survival stage that is most frequently associated with "cure" and evolves from the time when cancer activity or the chance of its return decreases and the disease can be arrested permanently. Economic problems often surface in this stage, along with concern for long-term and late effects of cancer treatment. This chapter will concentrate on psychosocial issues prevalent in the extended and permanent survival stages.

Agreement on a definition of survivorship will enable the adaptation or development of other survivorship models. Viewing cancer survivorship as an evolving process allows recognition of the fact that psychosocial issues of

TABLE 19-1 Components of a Cancer Survival Paradigm

Focus	Critical Elements	Cancer-Related Barrier
Basic survival	Concern about resources for food, shelter, medical care	Limited finances, loss of job benefits, lack of adequate follow-up medical care
Physical self-concept	Physical attractiveness, fitness, maintenance of body function	Any body image alteration, energy reserve impairment, residual physical disability
Psychological self-concept	Self-respect, integrity, autonomy	Use of self-blame, dependency, self-doubt, change in precancer life-style
Proximal affiliation	Relationships with family, lovers, and close friends	Fears about hereditary transmission, family stress related to illness, alterations in customary social support, sexual dysfunction, concern about disclosure
Distal affiliation	Relationships to coworkers and acquaintances	Shunning and isolationism, discriminatory practices, concern about disclosure
Avocational	Recreation, play, escape	Physical compromise, financial constraints, fear of distancing self from health care team

Source: Reprinted by permission of the publisher from Vought CA, Dintruff DL, Fotopoulos SS: Adaptations to the constraints of cancer: Motivational issues, in Ahmed P(ed): Living and Dying with Cancer. New York, Elsevier, 1981, pp 205-219. Copyright 1981 by Elsevier Science Publishing Co, Inc.

long-term survivorship can arise in any stage or phase of the survival continuum. Thus, in anticipation of long-term survivorship, psychosocial interventions should begin at diagnosis, rather than when the patient is considered medically "cured."

PSYCHOSOCIAL THEMES

Survivorship encompasses many aspects of psychobiologic functioning. Studies confirm, however, a relative lack of psychopathology in long-term survivors of cancer.[5,15-20] The major psychosocial themes that can be anticipated in significant cohorts of adults surviving cancer are (1) interrelationships between physiologic long-term effects and psychosocial outcomes, (2) fears of relapse and death, (3) dependence on health care providers, (4) survivor guilt, (5) uncertain sense of longevity, (6) social adaptation dilemmas, and (7) contagion effect—the family as survivor.

Interrelationships Between Physiologic Long-Term Effects and Psychosocial Outcomes

An individual's ability to cope within the trajectory of extended or permanent survival can be strongly influenced by physiologic compromise.[14,21] In a study of 49 women 4 years after mastectomy, Woods and Earp[22] noted that subjects with more symptom distress associated with their surgery had greater degrees of depressive symptoms. Rieker et al[23] studied 74 men 2 to 10 years after treatment for testicular cancer and found that those with resultant sexual impairment (ie, infertility, ejaculatory dysfunction) reported more psychologic symptomatology and strained intimate relationships than men without long-term sexual impairment. Fobair et al[6] noted the relationship of persistent energy loss and depression in 403 Hodgkin's disease survivors evaluated approximately 9 years after completion of therapy. Additional research that integrates the physical and psychosocial sequelae of surviving cancer will help identify those factors that enhance and detract from quality survival.

Fears of Relapse and Death

Probably the most common concern for all cancer survivors is the fear of cancer recurrence.[1,19,24-26] Not knowing when and if cancer will reappear often negatively affects the survivor's sense of control over his or her life.[27,28] Commonly referred to as the "Damocles syndrome," death anxiety often fluctuates in intensity as intermittent suspicious symptomatology is dealt with.[20] Fear of relapse may present in a variety of forms, ranging from general uneasiness about the etiology of mild to moderate somatic complaints to pronounced anxiety or panic attacks that interfere with daily life. Exaggerated worry over somatic distress is usually most intense within 2 years after completion of therapy.[4,24] As time passes, anxiety may lessen concerning relapse and recurrence. However, a heightened sense of vulnerability to illness is frequently a hallmark of the cancer survivor's long-term experience.[29]

Dependence on Health Care Providers

Both the survivor's need to determine the nature of suspicious symptomatology and the physician's need to evaluate the patient closely following cessation of therapy mandates an ongoing relationship between the patient and health care team. This reality often causes the patient to experience divergent reactions.

For many patients nearing the end of treatment, a significant ambivalence evolves. They are elated over the prospect of discontinuing therapy yet fear distancing themselves from the health care team who has helped them to get to this extended survival stage.[26,30] Mullan[25] also noted that the fear of recurrence along with the fear of the physician's finding disease can lead to behaviors such as hypochondriasis or avoidance of physicians. Routine checkups and yearly comprehensive examinations may engender pronounced anxiety.

Survivor Guilt

Waiting room scenarios may also poignantly depict the negative outcomes from cancer, closely followed by the introspection, "Will I end up that way, too?" The infrequently discussed phenomenon of survivor guilt may appear at this time as well.[31] As comparisons are made among patients, one may ponder, "Why am I doing well and they aren't?" Similar to questions arising around the time of initial diagnosis, attempts to justify "Why me?" or "Why not me?" may resurface. Hence, the survivor's ongoing involvement with follow-up care is characterized by mixed emotional reactions and multiple concerns.

Uncertain Sense of Longevity

Because of the prevailing perception that cancer results in a painful, lingering death, most patients' immediate reaction to the diagnosis is the expectation of a shortened lifespan. Once successful completion of therapy is achieved, hope for continued survival often supercedes thoughts of death. Many survivors, however, change their life-style as a reaction to the possibility of dying younger than expected.

A critical evaluation of life's meaning and priorities seems to take utmost importance. Survivors report greater appreciation of life and become more satisfied with life as a whole.[31] A significant value reassessment leads to heightened awareness of things taken for granted and lessened concern for the trivial. Mullan[14] characterized this phenomenon as "life re-kindled." This enhanced global acceptance of greater appreciation of life and improved quality of life for the present represent important secondary benefits of having survived cancer.

Social Adaptation Dilemmas

Attempts to minimize memories of the treatment experience and to "get on with life" are not often easy tasks for the survivor. The transition from a sick role to a healthy role can be compromised by persistent physical debility (despite cessation of therapy), negative expectations from within one's social support realm, personal concerns about one's ability to readjust, and social stigma. Shunning, a highly subjective phenomenon, may be a pervasive barrier to successful reorientation.[25]

Similar to the patient's ambivalent relationship with the health care team, confusing reactions to available social support may deter social adaptation. On the one hand, the survivor may not want to be treated like a patient, yet the survivor may also react negatively to withdrawal of the intense social support mobilized during the initial diagnosis phase.[26] Repeated explanations about one's health status to family, friends, acquaintances, employers, and insurors may drain the survivor's emotional responses. Constant scrutiny from these individuals can also be stressful. Dealing with relationships outside the immediate family unit becomes more difficult if internal family needs are not met successfully.

Contagion Effect—The Family as Survivor

A plethora of information exists about the plight of the family coping with the active phases of cancer. However, there is a paucity of information about families coping with extended or permanent survival.[32] Premorbid family style is an important assessment variable in determining postillness coping.[20] Even the most supportive family member is not immune to long-term psychologic stress throughout the extensive cancer continuum. The family's anxiety about the patient, that is, worry over potential relapse and unfavorable social situations, may be exhibited by overprotectiveness and pervasive anxiety. Marital discord and changes in sexual relationships can occur. Family members may not want to listen to or hear the survivor's concerns over potential relapse, since these can trigger their own sense of insecurity about continued long-term survival. Woods and Earp[22] identified the presence of "conversational isolationism" in families hesitant to discuss mutual concerns about the recurrence of cancer. As health care professionals acknowledge cancer as a family disease, they must be sensitive to the ramifications of survival for all members of the family unit.

EMPLOYMENT AND INSURANCE DISCRIMINATION

Many cancer survivors encounter ongoing socioeconomic impediments to full recovery. Concerns include regaining financial and work-related stability and maintaining medical insurance coverage. Access to insurance is usually through employment, but the issues of job discrimination and insurance-related problems are separate and complicated and therefore will be addressed individually.

Employment Discrimination

Survivors' employment problems can be attributed to three predominant myths about cancer: (1) cancer is a death sentence, (2) cancer is contagious, and (3) cancer survivors are an unproductive drain on the economy.[2,33-35] Meanwhile, current statistics indicate that more than half of all Americans diagnosed with cancer will survive their illness, that cancer is not contagious, and that cancer survivors have productivity rates similar to other workers.[2,36]

Categories of employment-related problems include (1) dismissal, demotion, and reduction or elimination of work-related benefits; (2) situations arising from coworkers' attitudes about cancer; and (3) problems related to survivors' attitudes about how they should be perceived by others in the workplace.[37] Discrimination can be as subtle as experiencing increased conflict with coworkers or as blatant as being terminated or rejected from a desired position.

Studies have confirmed that the work performance of cancer survivors differed little, if any, from the performance of others hired at the same age for similar assignments and that up to 80% of cancer patients returned to work after being diagnosed.[35,36,38,39] Yet an often troublesome effect of a cancer history continues to be "job-lock," where one fears leaving an undesirable position because of the potential loss of medical insurance and other benefits.[40]

Certain federal and state laws prohibit employment discrimination against qualified people with a history of cancer. Although the Federal Rehabilitation Act of 1973 is limited to those employers who receive federal funding, it can offer protection to those who qualify and feel discriminated against because of a real or perceived (by the employer) handicap.[41] Most states prohibit discrimination against the disabled in general, while a few states explicitly protect those with histories of cancer. There can be a problem, though, when the legal system attempts to label all cancer survivors as "handicapped or disabled" when there is often no visible evidence of their being either. This suggests the need for further clarification of terms through more explicit legislation.

Insurance Problems

With better access to treatment options, many cancer survivors are experiencing increased lifespans after receiving more sophisticated medical care. The availability of adequate health insurance is rarely guaranteed, and the problems created when attempting to secure or obtain these benefits can be financially and emotionally devastating. The numerous barriers to insurability include refusal of new applications, policy cancellations or reductions, higher premiums, waived or excluded preexisting conditions, and extended waiting periods.[42] These barriers may also affect the spouse or family member who carries the insurance policy. Studies suggest that 25% to 30% of cancer survivors experience some form of insurance discrimination.[42,43]

Because there is no state- or federally mandated "legal right" to health insurance, individuals should carefully examine the specific terms of their policies and the applicable state law to determine a legal violation. If an employer has more than 20 employees, it is required under COBRA, a federal law passed in 1986, to offer a continuance of group medical coverage to those whose circumstances warrant reducing or changing work hours or leaving the job.[44] The affected employee is eligible for extended coverage up to 18 months, while spouse and dependents receive these benefits for 36 months.

Other sources of assistance for insurance problems are state insurance commissions that regulate insurance rates, policy conditions, and all aspects of coverage and benefits. These state agencies are usually available to individuals with questions and complaints concerning existing policies and insurability. In addition, a number of states have introduced "high-risk pools" for those considered medically uninsurable.[45] By requiring the major insurance companies to share in the risks and expenses, more people with preexisting conditions have the opportunity to purchase comprehensive insurance plans, albeit at higher premiums. Nurses should be familiar with the available resources to assist the survivor who has employment or insurance problems. These resources are available on local, state, and national levels as described in Table 19-2.

TABLE 19-2 Local, State, and National Resources for Employment and Insurance Problems

Employment	Insurance
Local	
Disability and employment law attorneys	Insurance Department
Local survivor organizations	Social Security, local office
	Medicare
	Medicaid
	Group insurance plans
	Open enrollment periods
	Local survivor organizatons
State	
State Department of Labor, Civil Rights Division	State Insurance Commission
	"High-risk pools" (not applicable in all states)
National	
Rehabiiltation Act of 1973*	COBRA (Consolidated Omnibus Budget Reconciliation Act)†
ERISA (Employee Retirement and Income Security Act)†	National survivor organizations
National survivor organizations	

*Write to Department of Justice, Civil Rights Division, Coordination and Review Section, Washington, DC 20530.

†Write to Pension and Welfare Benefits Administration, U.S. Department of Labor, Room N-5658, 200 Constitution Avenue, NW, Washington, DC 20210.

TABLE 19-3 Foci and Objectives of a Comprehensive Assessment and Intervention Program for Adult Long-Term Cancer Survivors

Focus	Specific Considerations
Physical	Follow-up potential effects of cancer and multimodal therapies Recognize endurance, fatigue, energy reserve problems based on intensity of treatment Be aware of incidence of secondary malignancy from treatment along with second or third primary tumors
Emotional	Acknowledge potential chronic anxiety associated with fear of recurrence Be alert to reactions to social stigma, changes in interpersonal relationships Be sensitive to family's adaptation to the cancer experience Acknowledge the potential existence of survivor guilt
Sexual	Consider interplay of fertility issues with coping strategies Consider intimacy needs as a subset of sexual satisfaction Discuss disclosure options relative to potential partners Anticipate concern about health of offspring
Social	Discuss concerns about friends and acquaintances and reactions to cancer history Recognize that life goals may be reprioritized Relate social adaptation to health status Encourage integration of family, friends, hobbies, and vacation into long-range plans
Vocational	Acknowledge potential job-related stress and coworkers' responses to cancer history Educate about possible discrimination at work Assist with vocational rehabilitation if necessary
Economic	Consider possible long-term financial burden Provide resources for insurance problems Encourage a balance between long- and short-term goals

SUPPORTIVE CARE

Rehabilitation Framework

In considering the options for providing support for the long-term survivor of adult cancer, the concept of rehabilitation must be addressed. Veronesi and Martino[46] stated that rehabilitation is the bridge that leads the patient from the condition of diversity to a condition of normality. Mayer[47] noted that the concept of cancer rehabilitation encompasses the theme of quality survival—not how long a person lives, but how well he or she lives within the constraints of the disease. Watson[48] described rehabilitation as an appropriate umbrella concept applicable across the entire cancer continuum. The nurse's role in cancer rehabilitation is to help the patient reduce the extent to which the cancer-related disability becomes a handicap or interferes with the ability to function in everyday life, however long that life may be. Because there is a paucity of information available on the physiologic long-term effects of cancer therapy for adults, the residual end products of therapy are unclear.[31] However, as former patients cope with extended or permanent survival, many do not return to prior levels of functioning.[49] These survivors find that they must develop strategies to cope with new situations and alterations in health status and functional abilities.

Rehabilitation in cancer care is particularly relevant, since the number of cancer survivors is predicted to increase. The growing acknowledgement of the physical, emotional, sexual, social, vocational, and economic implications of surviving cancer suggests a more aggressive approach to both assessment and intervention planning for long-term survivorship (Table 19-3). To date, interest in this subset of people with a history of cancer has been negligible and certainly not comprehensive. The systematic follow-up of former active adult patients is virtually nonexistent in the United States. This nonpractice is incompatible with a model rehabilitative approach to cancer care that includes ongoing reassessment and redefinition of goals.[50] Groenwald and Thaney[51] described rehabilitation as a dynamic process, the antithesis of customary convalescence where a person is allowed passivity while nature takes its course. Preventive and restorative goal setting become critical parameters to the enhancement of a long-term survival trajectory that is characterized by minimal debilitation and a wellness orientation. Particular attention must also be paid to the ongoing and long-range implications of financial burden imposed by cancer.[52-54]

Significant policy statements have been made by key groups that encourage future investigation into the development of rehabilitation models of cancer care. Adult cancer survivors as a subset of people facing cancer would certainly benefit by policy implementation. In 1988, Deborah Mayer and the Oncology Nursing Society coordinated an invitational conference on "Addressing Barriers to Successful Cancer Rehabilitation."[55] Three of the fifteen proposed action items specifically addressed cancer survivors and included recommendations to (1) develop a system to identify cancer survivors, (2) develop a system for long-term follow-up and monitoring of cancer survivors, and (3) identify the needs of cancer survivors. Also in 1988, the Cancer Survivor's Bill of Rights was published by the American Cancer Society (ACS) (below). Finally, the Association of Community Cancer Centers stated that the provision of rehabilitation services to cancer patients and their families should be a basic standard of care in the community.[56] As increasing numbers of cancer patients survive, nurses can contribute to the quality and satisfaction of the survivors' lives by developing a philosophy that is both holistic and rehabilitative.[57]

American Cancer Society

THE CANCER SURVIVORS' BILL OF RIGHTS

A new population lives among us today—a new minority of 5 million people with a history of cancer. Three million of these Americans have lived with their diagnoses for five years or more.

You see these modern survivors in offices and in factories, on bicycles and cruise ships, on tennis courts, beaches and bowling alleys. You see them in all ages, shapes, sizes and colors. Usually they are unremarkable in appearance; sometimes they are remarkable for the way they have learned to live with disabilities resulting from cancer or its treatment.

Modern medical advances have returned about half of the nation's cancer patients of all ages (and 59 percent for those under the age of 55) to a normal lifespan. But the larger society has not always kept pace in helping make this lifespan truly "normal": at least, it has felt awkward in dealing with this fledgling group; at most, it has failed fully to accept survivors as functioning members.

The American Cancer Society presents this Survivors' Bill of Rights to call public attention to survivor needs, to enhance cancer care, and to bring greater satisfacton to cancer survivors, as well as to their physicians, employers, families and friends:

1. Survivors have the right to assurance of lifelong medical care, as needed. The physicians and other professionals involved in their care should continue their constant efforts to be:

- sensitive to the cancer survivors' lifestyle choices and their need for self-esteem and dignity;
- careful, no matter how long they have survived, to have symptoms taken seriously, and not have aches and pains dismissed, for fear of recurrence is a normal part of survivorship;
- informative and open, providing survivors with as much or as little candid medical information as they wish, and encouraging their informed participation in their own care;
- knowledgeable about counseling resources, and willing to refer survivors and their families as appropriate for emotional support and therapy which will improve the quality of individual lives.

2. In their personal lives, survivors, like other Americans, have the right of the pursuit of happiness. This means they have the right:

- to talk with their families and friends about their cancer experience if they wish, but to refuse to discuss it if that is their choice and not to be expected to be more upbeat or less blue than anyone else;
- to be free of the stigma of cancer as a "dread disease" in all social relations;
- to be free of blame for having gotten the disease and of guilt for having survived it;

3. In the workplace, survivors have the right to equal job opportunities. This means they have the right:

- to aspire to jobs worthy of their skills, and for which they are trained and experienced, and thus not to have to accept jobs they would not have considered before the cancer experience;
- to be hired, promoted and accepted on return to work, according to their individual abilities and qualifications, and not according to "cancer" or "disability" stereotypes;
- to privacy about their medical histories

4. Since health insurance coverage is an overriding survivorship concern, every effort should be made to assure all survivors adequate health insurance, whether public or private. This means:

- for employers, that survivors have the right to be included in group health coverage, which is usually less expensive, provides better benefits, and covers the employee regardless of health history;
- for physicians, counselors, and other professionals concerned, that they keep themselves and their survivor-clients informed and up-to-date on available group or individual health policy options, noting, for example, what major expenses like hospital costs and medical tests outside the hospital are covered and what amount must be paid before coverage (deductibles).

Resources and Interventions

Conflicting reactions to cancer survival can be a heavy burden for the strongest of individuals. Although grateful to be alive, these individuals may have difficulties adjusting to the tradeoffs of survival, that is, the possible long-term and potential unknown late effects of the disease and its treatment. As the health care profession's successes in controlling and eradicating disease increase, so too does its obligation to minimize the traumas of illness and medical interventions.

The availability of education, counseling, and supportive services becomes crucial in caring for those diagnosed with cancer. As more people live with cancer as a chronic illness, improvements in "quality of life" issues and survivor rights are a major concern. Even if support is available and adequate during the acute stage of care, an abrupt severance of this support can increase the trauma of readjusting to life as a nonhospitalized patient or cancer survivor. Although survival itself may be reward enough for some, others are seeking options to improve their current health status with hopes of preventing future problems.

From governmental agencies and medical institutions to grassroots organizations, the collective cancer survivor population is being heard as it organizes, networks, and advocates for the right to quality survival. Numerous model programs, encompassing both professional and peer support, are responding in a nationwide attempt to meet the changing needs of this growing group. However, before appropriate programs can be developed, in-depth interviews and studies must be undertaken to delineate the types of educational materials needed, the best methods for intervention, and the stages or timing to deliver information or interventions. Areas for consideration in planning interventions for long-term survivors of adult cancer include undertaking individualized needs assessments, addressing educational needs, engaging in research, and developing model programs.

Assessing individual needs

As in the acute phases of illness, it is imperative to continue assessing both the survivor's and the family's coping styles throughout the extended and permanent stages of survival. Included in this comprehensive and ongoing nursing assessment are strategies that help to resolve crisis intensity and enhance self-care. The survivor's age and developmental stage, socioeconomic background, type of cancer, prognosis, and treatment-related complications are important variables influencing his or her needs. Examples of nursing diagnoses related to an individual needs assessment include (1) ineffective patient or family coping related to ongoing surveillance for long-term effects from disease or treatment, (2) grieving related to loss of job after successful treatment for cancer, (3) alteration in sexuality related to difficulties in establishing intimate relationships, and (4) knowledge deficit related to the recognition of cancer recurrence symptomatology.

Addressing educational needs related to survivorship

During the development of educational resources for survivors, nurses must continue to acknowledge the different needs and information preferences of individuals and families. Researchers at Stanford University found that patients want to be well informed about potential or expected problems.[58] Individuals who seek much information may request specifics about cancer recurrence or anticipated problems relative to their diagnosis. Since fear of recurrence and worries about health are common among survivors, nurses can help reduce the stress associated with the unknown by anticipating crises points and sharing this information with survivors. Examples of time-related crises that may be experienced by survivors are anniversaries of diagnosis and treatment cessation, birthdays, holidays, yearly examinations, and waiting for the 5-year survival mark. Situation-specific crises include diagnosis disclosure to friends and coworkers, hearing stories about cancer, waiting for results of follow-up examinations, symptomatology assessment, revealing past medical history, and establishing intimate relationships. If a crisis becomes unmanageable or persistent, nursing referrals can be made for an appropriate intervention.

Survivors and their families may want to know about potential secondary benefits of the cancer experience.[46] These benefits, frequently emphasized by survivors themselves, may include a new-found zest for life, value reprioritization, and a greater sense of generalized well-being.

Promotion of a greater awareness of cancer survivorship issues should begin during basic nursing education. To sensitize student nurses to the continuing need for supportive care, interactions with long-term survivors are recommended.[47]

Engaging in research

Although the psychosocial ramifications were the first to be studied, relatively little systematic and longitudinal information on coping from diagnosis through "cure" has been obtained.[5] What is currently needed is a comprehensive assessment format to study the long-term needs of adult survivors, that is, a format similar to those available for studying children.[59] Areas for research include (1) the relationship of developmental stage to psychosocial sequelae, (2) description of survival trajectories, (3) family dilemmas during long-term survivorship, (4) the interrelationship of physical compromise and coping problems, (5) identification of the mediators of stress throughout survivorship, (6) association of the attitudes of the health care team with recurrence anxiety, and (7) how time influences fears of relapse.[29,31,57]

Developing model programs

Once survivor-specific assessments identify areas of individual need, a more general assessment of community resources already available for cancer survivors can then be performed. These two steps would logically precede the development of any formal survivor program. Including survivors themselves in dialogues concerning the planning and implementation of these programs will enhance program development and reliability. A variety of support options, whether individual or group related, allows one to better tailor interventions to the survivor's needs.

The success of any cancer survivor program will depend on (1) the commitment of the health care team to provide ongoing evaluation and planning for change as the subject lives with a history of cancer, (2) the identification of key individuals to coordinate activities within and among team members, (3) the involvement of the patient and family in the program from initial diagnosis, and (4) the effectiveness of communication among team members.[60] This approach encourages the early recognition of problems during therapy that is imperative for the possible prevention of long-term sequelae.[61]

The majority of long-term survivor programs are non–hospital-based programs and include national and local cancer hotlines, regional chapters of national organizations, and community networks that focus on peer support. The National Coalition for Cancer Survivorship (NCCS) (323 Eighth Street, SW, Albuquerque, NM 87102 [505]764-9956) serves as a resource to network individuals and groups concerned with cancer survivorship issues and has increased access to information, referrals, resources, educational opportunities, and professional and peer support. Refer to the Yellow Pages of this text for an extended list of resources.

Hospital- or community-based survivor programs can have multiple components. Comprehensive follow-up clinics provide surveillance for physical and psychological long-term effects. These clinics can be wellness-oriented, emphasizing the importance of proper nutrition, the need for individualized exercise programs, and disease-prevention behaviors. Another component can help to clarify misconceptions about cancer and address survivor limitations by providing information about cancer survival to coworkers and employers. This information should be provided by the treatment team before the survivor returns to the workplace. Some programs offer survivor reunions within hospitals or the community at large. Included in these reunions are those who continue to live with a history of cancer, their families and friends, and their health care providers.

All these options and approaches for long-term survivor program development become particularly important in light of the growing number of survivors. Programs must deal with all developmental stages, ranging from the elderly[32] to the growing number of younger adult survivors.

CONCLUSION

Long-term survivorship of adult cancers has many psychosocial ramifications. The definitions of survivorship, the concept of survivorship as a continuum, major psychosocial themes, employment and insurance discrimination, rehabilitation framework, and resources and interventions have been discussed.

Rosetta Poletti,[62] in her address to the Second European Conference on Clinical Oncology and Cancer Nursing, stated that "The goal of cancer nursing should be to assist the person to be a fully functioning person first and a cancer patient second." Within a framework of rehabilitation, support programs for cancer survivors can be developed in partnership with health care professionals and survivors and focus on delivering optimal care during all stages of survival. Nursing, with its dynamic, holistic focus, is in an ideal position to promote cancer survivor rehabilitation.

• • •

Funded in part by NIHCA 23074 and Arizona Disease Control Research Commission 33640000000-1-1-AP-6621.

REFERENCES

1. Cella DF, Lesko LM: Cancer survivors: Watch for signs of stress even years later. Oncology Rounds (Primary Care and Cancer), Burroughs-Welcome Co, 1988, pp 1-9.
2. American Cancer Society: Cancer Facts and Figures. Atlanta, Ga, The Society, 1988.
3. National Cancer Institute: Surveillance, Epidemiology, and End Results Program (SEER), Annual Cancer Statistics Review. Bethesda, Md, The Institute, November 1984.
4. Fobair P, Mages NL: Psychosocial morbidity among cancer patient survivors, in Ahmed P (ed): Coping With Cancer. New York, Elsevier, 1981, pp 285-308.
5. Cella DF: Cancer survival: Psychosocial and public issues. Cancer Invest 5:59-67, 1987.
6. Fobair P, Hoppe RT, Bloom J, et al: Psychosocial problems among survivors of Hodgkin's disease. J Clin Oncol 4:805-814, 1986.
7. Goldberg RJ, Tull RM: The Psychosocial Dimensions of Cancer. New York, The Free Press, 1983, pp 40-80.
8. Mish FC (ed): Webster's Ninth New Collegiate Dictionary. Springfield, Mass, Merriam-Webster, 1983.
9. Hammond GD: The cure of childhood cancers. Cancer 58:407-413, 1986.
10. Holland J: Psychological aspects of oncology. Med Clin North Am 61:737-748, 1977.
11. Roud PC: Psychosocial variables associated with the exceptional survival of patients with advanced malignant disease. J Natl Med Assoc 79:97-102, 1987.
12. Vought CA, Dintruff DL, Fotopoulos SS: Adaptations to the constraints of cancer: Motivational issues, in Ahmed P (ed): Living and Dying with Cancer. New York, Elsevier, 1981, pp 205-219.
13. Fobair P: A review of Smith K, Lesko L: Psychosocial problems in cancer survivors. Oncology 2:41-44, 1988.
14. Mullan F: Seasons of survival: Reflections of a physician with cancer. N Engl J Med 313:270-273, 1985.
15. Weddington WW, Segraves KB, Simon MA: Current and lifetime incidence of psychiatric disorders among a group of extremity sarcoma survivors. J Psychosom Res 30:121-125, 1986.

16. Shanfield SB: On surviving cancer: Psychological considerations. Comprehensive Psych 21:128-134, 1980.
17. Chang PN, Nesbit ME, Youngren N, et al: Personality characteristics and psychosocial adjustment of long-term survivors of childhood cancer. J Psychosoc Oncol 5:43-58, 1987.
18. Tebbi CK, Mallon JC: Long-term psychosocial outcome among cancer amputees in adolescence and early adulthood. J Psychosoc Oncol 5:69-82, 1987.
19. Schmale AH, Morrow GR, Schmitt MH, et al: Well-being of cancer survivors. Psychosom Med 45:163-169, 1983.
20. Smith K, Lesko LM: Psychosocial problems in cancer survivors. Oncology 2:33-44, 1988.
21. Gotay CC: Quality of life among survivors of childhood cancer: A critical review and implications for intervention. J Psychosoc Oncol 5:5-23, 1987.
22. Woods NF, Earp JL: Women with cured breast cancer: A study of mastectomy patients in North Carolina. Nurs Res 27:279-285, 1978.
23. Rieker PP, Edbril SD, Garnick MB: Curative testis cancer therapy: Psychosocial sequelae. J Clin Oncol 3:1117-1126, 1985.
24. Cella DF, Tross S: Psychological adjustment to survival from Hodgkin's disease. J Consult Clin Psychol 54:616-622, 1986.
25. Mullan F: Re-entry: the educational needs of the cancer survivor. Health Educ Q 10:88-94, 1984 (suppl).
26. Maher EL: Anomic aspects of recovery from cancer. Soc Sci Med 16:907-912, 1982.
27. Northouse LL: Mastectomy patients and the fear of cancer recurrence. Cancer Nurs 4:213-220, 1981.
28. Welch-McCaffrey D: Cancer anxiety and quality of life. Cancer Nurs 8:151-158, 1985.
29. Quigley KM: The adult cancer survivor: Psychosocial consequences of cure. Semin Oncol Nurs 5:63-69, 1989.
30. Gorsynski JG, Holland JC: Psychological aspects of testicular cancer. Semin Oncol 6:125-129, 1979.
31. Loescher LJ, Welch-McCaffrey D, Leigh SA, et al: Surviving Adult Cancers. I. Physiologic effects. Ann Intern Med 3:411-432, 1989; II. Psychosocial sequelae. Ann Intern Med 3:517-524, 1989.
32. Welch-McCaffrey D: Family issues in cancer care: Current dilemmas—future directions. J Psychosoc Oncol 6:199-211, 1988.
33. Hoffman B: Employment discrimination based on cancer history: The need for federal legislation. Temple Law Q 59:4-9, 1986.
34. Wasserman AL, Thompson ET, Wilmas A, et al: The psychosocial status of survivors of childhood/adolescent Hodgkin's disease. Am J Dis Child 141:626-631, 1987.
35. Crothers HM: Employment problems of cancer survivors: Local problems and local solutions, in Proceedings of the Workshop on Employment, Insurance and the Patient with Cancer. New Orleans, American Cancer Society, 1986, pp 51-57.
36. Wheatley GM, Cunnick WR, Wright BP, et al: Employment of persons with a history of treatment for cancer. Cancer 33:441-445, 1974.
37. Feldman F: Female cancer patients and caregivers: Experiences in the workplace, in Stellman S (ed): Women and Cancer. New York, Harrington Park Press, 1987, pp 137-153.
38. Stone RW: Employing the recovered cancer patient. Cancer 36:285-286, 1975.
39. Mellette SJ: The cancer patient at work. ACS Prof Ed Publ 35:6-8, 1985.
40. Greenleigh Associates: Report on the social, economic, and psychological needs of cancer patients in California, in proceedings of Western States Conference on Cancer Rehabilitation. Palo Alto, Calif, Bull Publishing Co, March 1982.
41. Rehabilitation Act of 1973. 29 U.S.C. (United States Code) 701 *et seq.*
42. Crothers H: Health insurance: Problems and solutions for people with cancer histories, in Proceedings of the 5th National Conference on Human Values and Cancer. San Francisco, American Cancer Society, 1987, pp 100-109.
43. Burton L, Zones J: The incidence of insurance barriers and employment discrimination among Californians with a cancer health history in 1983: A projection. Los Angeles, American Cancer Society (Calif division), 1982.
44. Consolidated Omnibus Budget Reconciliation Act (COBRA). 1986, 42 U.S.C. 300 bb *et seq.*
45. Trippler A: Comprehensive health insurance for high risk individuals: A state by state analysis. Fergus Falls, MN: Communicating for Agriculture, 1987.
46. Veronesi U, Martino G: Can life be the same after cancer treatment? Tumori 64:345-351, 1978.
47. Mayer NH: Concepts in cancer rehabilitation. Semin Oncol 2:393-398, 1975.
48. Watson PG: Rehabilitation philosophy: A means of fostering a positive attitude toward cancer. J Enterostom Ther 13:153-156, 1986.
49. Kudsk EG, Hoffman GS: Rehabilitation of the cancer patient. Primary Care 14:381-390, 1987.
50. Habeck RV, Romsaas EP, Olsen SJ: Cancer rehabilitation and continuing care: A case study. Cancer Nurs 7:315-320, 1984.
51. Groenwald SL, Thaney K: Rehabilitation, in Groenwald SL (ed): Cancer Nursing: Principles and Practice. Boston, Jones and Bartlett, 1987, pp 749-758.
52. Houts PS, Harvey HA, Simmonds MA, et al: Characteristics of patients at risk for financial burden because of cancer and its treatment. J Psychosoc Oncol 3:15-22, 1985.
53. McNaull FW: The costs of cancer: A challenge to health care providers. Cancer Nurs 4:207-212, 1981.
54. Baird SB: Economic realities in the treatment and care of the cancer patient. Topics Clin Nurs 2:67-80, 1981.
55. Mayer D: An invitational conference addressing barriers to successful cancer rehabilitation, in Proceedings of the 1988 Oncology Nursing Society President's Grant, Boston, August 1988.
56. Enck RE: ACCC standards: Past, present and future. J Cancer Progr Management 2:11-20, 1987.
57. Dudas S, Carlson CE: Cancer rehabilitation. Oncol Nurs Forum 15:183-188, 1988.
58. Fobair P, Hoppe R, Bloom J, et al: Psychosocial problems among survivors of Hodgkin's disease. J Clin Oncol 4:805-814, 1986.
59. Fergusson J, Ruccione K, Wasderwitz M, et al: Time required to assess children for the late effects of treatment. Cancer Nurs 10:300-310, 1987.
60. Broadwell DC: Rehabilitation needs of the patient with cancer. Cancer 60:563-568, 1987.
61. Andersen BL: Sexual functioning morbidity among cancer survivors. Cancer 55:1835-1842, 1985.
62. Poletti R: Living a full life with cancer, in Proceedings of the Second European Conference on Clinical Oncology and Cancer Nursing. Amsterdam, ECCO, November 1983.

PART V

MANIFESTATIONS OF CANCER AND CANCER TREATMENT

Chapter 20

Pain

Deborah B. McGuire, RN, PhD

Vivian R. Sheidler, RN, MS

INTRODUCTION AND BACKGROUND

Definitions of Pain

Over the years, pain has not been easy to define. During the seventeenth century, pain was viewed as a signal of bodily injury, with scant attention to its nonphysical aspects. This attitude persisted until the twentieth century, when researchers began to formulate concepts of pain that recognized and included not only the physical "alarm" aspect but other neurologic activities, cultural factors, and individual personality and experiential variables as well. Despite these broader concepts of pain, a precise definition eluded workers in the field for, as Livingston[1] wrote in 1943, "The chief difficulty encountered in a search for a satisfactory definition of pain is the fact that it can be considered from either a physiologic or psychologic approach. Any consideration of pain, by one approach alone, without due regard to the other, is incomplete."

Reconciliation of these two disparate approaches proved very difficult, since a single definition seemed unable to satisfy everyone. Melzack and Wall[2] highlighted this problem when they wrote in 1980: "Pain is such a common experience that we rarely pause to define it in ordinary conversation. Yet no one who has worked on the problem of pain has ever been able to give it a definition which is satisfactory to all of his colleagues." In their view, pain was a ". . . *category* of experiences, signifying a multitude of different, unique experiences having different causes, and characterized by different qualities varying along a number of sensory and affective dimensions."

The need for a standard definition of pain, however, prompted the International Association for the Study of Pain (IASP) to develop a definition acceptable to both clinicians and researchers. The major result, published in 1979, was the following: "Pain is an unpleasant sensory and emotional experience associated with actual or potential tissue damage, or described in terms of such damage."[3] This definition accounted for both sensory and emotional aspects of pain, as well as for pain of pathophysiologic and psychologic origin. It incorporated the essential elements of subjectivity and individual uniqueness in the pain experience.

In addition to the definition of pain, the IASP published a list of pain terms with their respective definitions (eg, *allodynia* and *causalgia*), which it viewed as a ". . . minimum standard vocabulary for members of different disciplines who work in the field of pain."[3] Bouckoms[4] wrote that the IASP definitions of pain and related terms provided a nontheoretic, relatively complete, valid taxonomy that was extremely useful to clinicians and researchers alike. It is probably safe to say that in the decade since the IASP definition of pain was published, it has become commonly accepted and used by most pain specialists.

Since 1979 the IASP has continued its work on a taxonomy, or classification system, for pain.[5] The intent of the IASP is, again, to foster acceptance and use of standard terminology and classification so that communication among members of the different disciplines who study and treat persons with pain can be enhanced.

Theories of Pain

Closely related to definitions of pain are theories of what pain is and how it occurs. Various theories have been proposed over the years and, as with definitions of pain, began with one or two simple anatomic or clinical aspects of pain and then expanded to include a multitude of anatomic, neural, physiologic, clinical, and psychologic variables. Until the mid–twentieth century, several traditional but opposing theories of pain were prominent. Price[6] reviewed these "classical" theories in a recent publication.

The *specificity theory* proposed that pain was a result of both a specific type of receptor and a specific central pathway. It considered pain as only one of four cutaneous stimuli—warmth, cold, touch, and pain—each of which had its own specific receptors and pathways leading to the perception of specific sensations. Although the theory was an oversimplification, two of its principles still hold true today: (1) that peripheral receptors are, in fact, specialized to respond to one or more types of stimuli and nociceptors are those that respond most optimally to noxious (painful) stimuli, and (2) that the eventual central nervous system destination of peripheral nerves and their ascending pathways is a key to distinguishing the type of peripheral stimulus that has occurred.

The *pattern theory* held that there were no specific nerve fibers or endings for pain. Instead, free nerve endings responded nonselectively to multiple different stimuli. Their responses, however, took the form of different patterns of impulses. The composition of these activated neurons would be different, depending on the different patterns (or energy). Increasing impulse frequencies were thought to be the critical factors in distinguishing painful from nonpainful sensory events. Little support has been found for any type of complex patterning of impulses from nociceptive afferent nerves, but the idea that impulse frequency is critical in pain perception has been retained in current theories of pain, since it is clearly involved in the overall input to ascending pain pathways.

Another classical theory proposed as an explanation for pain was the *summation theory* put forth by Livingston.[1] In addition to the ideas of specialized receptors, composition, and central destinations for afferent nerve pathways taken from previous theories, Livingston postulated that chronic pain could be triggered by brief painful episodes and could also become long standing because of reverberating circuits in the dorsal horn of the spinal cord. These circuits were viewed as closed loops of neurons that became activated following damage to peripheral nerves. Thus a central summative mechanism was the cause of such pain. Again, little support has been found for this theory exactly as it was proposed, but it is clear that there are mechanisms of slow temporal summation, spatial recruitment, and after-response.

Closely related to Livingston's theory is the *sensory interaction theory*, which proposed that there was a rapidly conducting system that could inhibit the transmission in a more slowly conducting nociceptive system. It was hypothesized that when pathologic pain developed, the fast conducting system lost its inhibitory control over the slow system, with the result, of course, being slow pain, burning pain, or hyperalgesia. Several researchers helped refine this theory by adding more specific types of interaction (for example, small afferent nerves carried impulse patterns for pain whereas large afferent nerves could inhibit these). The validity of these ideas has been confirmed over the last several decades. The most important contribution of this theory has been the knowledge that interactions between input from large myelinated nerve fibers and small unmyelinated nerve fibers determine both the presence and the severity of pain in persons with normal and pathologic pain states.

In addition to the classical theories that have been described, there are several current theories of pain.[6] Most notable of these is the *gate control theory of pain*, proposed by Melzack and Wall[7] in 1965 in an attempt to synthesize all the useful, documented tenets of the classical theories and to shed light on some as yet unexplained clinical pain phenomena.

There are five major tenets in the gate control theory, which can be summarized as follows. (1) Nerve impulses from afferent fibers to the transmission cells of the spinal cord are modulated in the dorsal horn of the cord by a gating mechanism. Input-output relationships between the impulses and the modulating mechanism are not one-to-one relays but, rather, involve central neural factors as well. (2) The gating mechanism in the dorsal horns is influenced by relative activity in the large- and small-diameter afferent nerve fibers. Activity in large fibers can "open" the gate, while activity in small fibers can "close" it. (3) Nerve impulses that descend from the central nervous system influence the gating mechanism in the dorsal horns. Many psychologic and related factors may be involved in this process. (4) A central control trigger system of large-diameter fibers conducts impulses rapidly and selectively activates certain cognitive processes that then have an influence, through descending fibers, on the gating mechanism's modulatory properties. (5) When the output of the transmission cells in the spinal cord exceeds a critical level, the action system is activated; it is composed of neural areas that are responsible for the complex, sequential patterns of experience and behavior that are the hallmark of pain itself.

Some of the theory's foundations were based on experimental neurophysiologic evidence that has never been confirmed.[8] Melzack and Wall,[2] however, have made attempts to incorporate new experimental and clinical research findings into their theory. In discussing these changes, they said: "Clearly, we do not imply that the gate theory is the final 'truth' about pain. However, a satisfactory alternative to the theory has not yet been proposed." Other pain specialists echo this sentiment,[6,9,10] and Price[6] in particular discussed the experimental evidence for and against support of the tenets. He concluded by saying: "The gate control theory and its accompanying schematic model thereby serves as an excellent first approximation of the neural interactions underlying the transmission of nociceptive information. . . . The tenets of the theory are not so much incorrect as they are too general."

Closely related to the gate control theory is the *parallel processing theory* of Melzack and Casey,[11] which evolved from the gate control theory. Those investigators proposed that the spinothalamic projection systems were divided functionally into two tracts. The neospinothalamic component was responsible for a sensory-discriminative dimension of pain, whereas the paleospinothalamic tract was responsible for the motivational drive and aversive reactions to pain. The affective-motivational sequelae of input into this system, then, were dependent on overall levels of neural activity; low levels caused approach responses, whereas higher levels provoked avoidance responses. The third part of this model consisted of higher central nervous system processes that were thought to have some evaluative reaction to the input that incorporated previous experience with pain and that could exert modulatory influences over the two processes mentioned above. All three processes interacted to produce the overall "experience" of pain. Although some of Melzack and Casey's proposals are supported in a general way by neuroanatomic and physiologic fact, a great deal of experimental evidence indicates that both pain sensations and cognitive processes serve together as causal links in affective reactions to pain and that the parallel processing suggested by Melzack and Casey does not occur.

In place of the parallel processing model, Price[6] proposed the *sequential processing theory*, which acknowledges that certain functions related to pain do occur in parallel, particularly sensory-discriminative responses, arousal, and some motor responses. The affective-motivational state, however, is dependent on sequential processes that involve cognitive processes. Neurophysiologic and psychologic observations support this thesis. The rationale for the theory is that ". . . an adequate psychological and neural model of pain is one that recognizes that a cognitive appraisal of the meaning of sensory-intensive and contextual factors have a direct causal role in pain-related affect."

Although the gate control theory is not perfect, it is the most comprehensive theory of pain yet proposed and serves an extremely useful purpose in explaining pain mechanisms for most health care givers. It is now abundantly clear that pain has a sensory component as well as a reactive (emotional) component. Much research is being conducted to elucidate the specific processes and phenomena that are responsible for producing the sensory and emotional puzzle called pain. While it is not possible to describe these efforts in any detail in this chapter, a brief overview of general mechanisms of pain is provided. The reader interested in more detail is referred to recent books by Price[6] and Fields.[10]

Mechanisms of Pain

Pain experienced by patients with cancer is, when considered strictly from the standpoint of the pathophysiologic and biochemical processes that cause it, no different from pain experienced by other persons. Etiologic, clinical, and psychosocial characteristics of both tumor- and treatment-related cancer pain, however, distinguish it from other types of pain. These differences will be elaborated in forthcoming sections; in this section the basic mechanisms of pain in general are considered.

The perception of and the response to pain are due to four distinct processes that operate simultaneously and are all required for pain to occur.[10] The first of these processes, *transduction,* begins when a noxious (painful or tissue-damaging) stimulus affects a peripheral sensory nerve ending, depolarizing it and setting off electrical activity that initiates the whole phenomenon of pain perception. *Transmission* is the next process; it consists of the series of subsequent neural events that carry the electrical impulses throughout the nervous system, from peripheral to central. *Modulation,* the third process, is a neural activity that controls pain-transmission neurons, either those originating in the periphery or those that originate in the central nervous system. The fourth process, *perception,* is less an actual physiologic/anatomic process than it is the vague subjective correlate (how the pain feels) of pain that encompasses complex behavioral, psychologic, and emotional factors that are little understood.

Transduction

Nerve endings that are specific to noxious stimuli are called nociceptors. Such nerve endings are located in skin, muscle, bone, visceral, and other tissues. It is in these afferent peripheral nociceptors that the process of transduction starts. Afferent nociceptors are defined and classified on the basis of their morphology, their conducting speed, and their responses to a variety of stimuli. There are three major afferent nerve fibers: large-diameter myelinated A alpha, small-diameter myelinated A delta, and even smaller unmyelinated C fibers. Most of the primary afferent nociceptors are A delta and C fibers, although each conducts impulses at different velocities and responds differentially to noxious stimuli. These two classes of nociceptors, however, are primarily responsible for perception of painful stimuli and, following transduction, for initiating the transmission process.

Two phenomena appear to be related to mechanisms of nociceptor depolarization following noxious stimulation.[10] First, the phenomenon of sensitization causes increased sensitivity in the nociceptors as the noxious stimulus is repeated. Second, hyperalgesia occurs as the effects of the noxious stimulus (that is, the painful sensation), spread past the initial site. Both of these phenomena are thought to be due in part to the presence of chemical substances located in the adjacent tissues. These substances, including prostaglandins, substance P, bradykinin, and histamine, are released and accumulate near nerve terminals following tissue damage. Most recently, Wall[12] provided evidence that when nerve injury occurs, new nerves or "sprouts" become active, responding to substance P and the activity of adjacent nerve fibers, and sending pain messages toward the spine, in a cascade effect. It appears that sensitization and hyperalgesia, although clearly related to transduction and thus to transmission, are still incompletely understood.

Transmission

After transduction, when the nerve fibers or afferent nociceptors begin to carry the pain impulses to the spinal cord, the process of transmission has begun. There are three components in this process. First, the peripheral sensory nerve fibers carry impulses to the spinal cord. Most of the afferent fibers enter the cord on the dorsal side, dividing by type (A delta and C) as they approach and then bunching together again as they enter. The spinal cord has six layers or laminae. Afferent nociceptors generally terminate in the first and second laminae. The second and third laminae are the substantia gelatinosa, hypothesized by the gate control theory of pain to be the site of the "gating" mechanisms that govern the transmission of pain impulses. In the fourth and fifth laminae are nerve fibers that project up to the first and second laminae. The incoming nociceptors synapse with these projecting apical dendrites, then decussate or cross over in the gray matter of the cord to the anterolateral side.

At this point, the second component of transmission begins; this consists of the network of relay neurons that go from the cord to the brain stem. Ascending nerve fibers travel upward through several tracts; the names vary, depending on the reference consulted,[6,10] but the generic term is *spinothalamic pathways.*[6] The neurons that originate in the spinal cord project to several different areas in the brain. One group of neurons can be divided into those that terminate in the medial thalamus and the ventroposterior lateral nucleus of the thalamus and those that terminate in both the medial and lateral areas of the thalamus. Another group of spinothalamic neurons have collateral axons to two areas of the midbrain—the central gray and the nuclei in the reticular formation. Since there are different patterns of ascending neuron projections, current thinking is that these ascending spinal nociceptive neurons participate in multiple functions related to the perception of, and response to, pain. In addition, the brain structures to which the spinal neurons project are also probably related to different aspects of the pain response.[6]

The third component of transmission has to do with the reciprocal connections between the thalamus and the cortex that are related to pain perception and response and the role of the cortex itself. Although little is known about this area, Price[6] summarized the evidence that different brain nociceptive neurons are related to pain, indicating that sensory-discriminative and affective-motivational-aversive reactions to pain are subserved by a variety of nociceptive neurons and their corresponding structures in the brain.

Modulation

The process of modulation is a central neural activity that controls the transmission of pain impulses and contributes to the variability seen in patients with pain. There are several mechanisms involved in modulation. First, the periacqueductal gray (PAG) in the midbrain has an important role in producing analgesia. Neurons originating in the PAG project downward to the rostral ventromedial medulla (RVM), which includes several areas involved in the transmission of pain impulses. Neurons from the RVM project to the dorsal horn of the cord, most commonly in the first and fifth laminae, which contain terminal afferent nociceptors. The neurotransmitters serotonin and substance P are released into these areas, thus contributing to the modulation of pain impulses.

Second, two classes of neurons that may have a modulatory function have been identified in experimental pain.[13] Cells of the first class—off-cells—are excited by the PAG and may inhibit nociceptive transmission in the cord; thus, when they are active, nociceptive impulses are blocked. Cells of the other class—on-cells—are also excited by stimulation of the PAG and appear to be active when off-cells are inactive. It is believed that on-cells facilitate transmission of nociceptive input, and it has been found that morphine inhibits on-cells. Although much more remains to be learned about off-cells and on-cells, their identification raises the possibility of both an endogenous analgesia system and a specific mechanism for enhancing the transmission of pain impulses.

The third modulatory mechanism involves three classes of opiate receptors (mu, delta, and kappa) that are located throughout the central nervous system. These receptors are molecule-recognition sites to which opiate and opiate-antagonistic analgesics bind. It is known that the majority of analgesic effects from opiate drugs are due to binding at the mu receptor sites in the PAG.

Finally, the fourth mechanism involved in modulation is the presence of the endogenous opioid peptides, which are pentapeptides that act at opiate receptors. Although there are three classes, only one (that which produces β-endorphin) produces opioid peptides that have potent analgesic effects in man. β-Endorphin is located chiefly in the central nervous system, but there is increasing evidence that it and other classes of endogenous opioids are located in the spinal cord and elsewhere. Exogenous opioid drugs mimic the action of the endogenous opioids through activation of the pain-modulation process in ways that are as yet unclear.

Perception

Perception is the fourth process necessary to the phenomenon of pain. The neural activities that occur in transmission and modulation culminate in a subjective correlate called "perception." This process is the least understood of all those related to pain. It is not known how it comes about or why seemingly objective noxious events produce such subjective responses.

Variability in responses to stimuli has been hypothesized to be due to several factors.[6] First, the pain-modulatory system may lower perceived intensity of pain through some of the mechanisms described above. Second, injury to the pain-transmission system, resulting in abnormal functioning, may contribute to lower pain intensity. Third, lesions of various areas in the central nervous system may actually cause an overreaction to incoming stimuli, thus raising perceived intensity. Finally, a tremendous variety of individual psychologic differences may result in unpredictable responses to a given stimulus.

Each of the sensory and affective aspects of pain that were mentioned earlier plays a role in the perception of pain. The sensory aspect of pain is uniform among patients with pain. The pain-detection threshold is a property of the sensory system that is related to a stimulus used to produce pain and, as defined by Fields,[10] ". . . is highly reproducible in different individuals and in the same individual at different times." The affective aspect of pain, on the other hand, is partially exemplified by the idea of pain tolerance, which is highly variable. Tolerance, according to Fields,[10] " . . . is a manifestation of a person's reaction to pain and it is highly dependent on psychological variables. Not only does it vary between different individuals in the same situation, but the same individual may react differently in different situations."

In summary, the four processes of transduction, transmission, modulation, and perception underlie the phenomenon we call pain. Figure 20-1 shows the pain pathway and demonstrates, in a schematic way, where transmission and modulation occur.

Cancer Pain as a Multidimensional Phenomenon

The notion of sensory and affective or physiologic and psychologic aspects of pain—developed through the gate control theory of pain—has been used to develop a conceptual framework for cancer pain. Ahles and colleagues[14] hypothesized five dimensions of the cancer pain experience: (1) *physiologic* (organic cause of pain); (2) *sensory* (intensity, location, quality); (3) *affective* (depression, anxiety); (4) *cognitive* (manner in which pain influences a person's thought processes, how he views himself, or the meaning of pain); and (5) *behavioral* (pain-related behaviors, such as medication intake or activity level). These investigators studied 40 cancer patients with tumor-related pain to assess each of the five dimensions. They used a variety of reliable and valid tools to assess the dimensions and found support for their conceptual model. When compared with

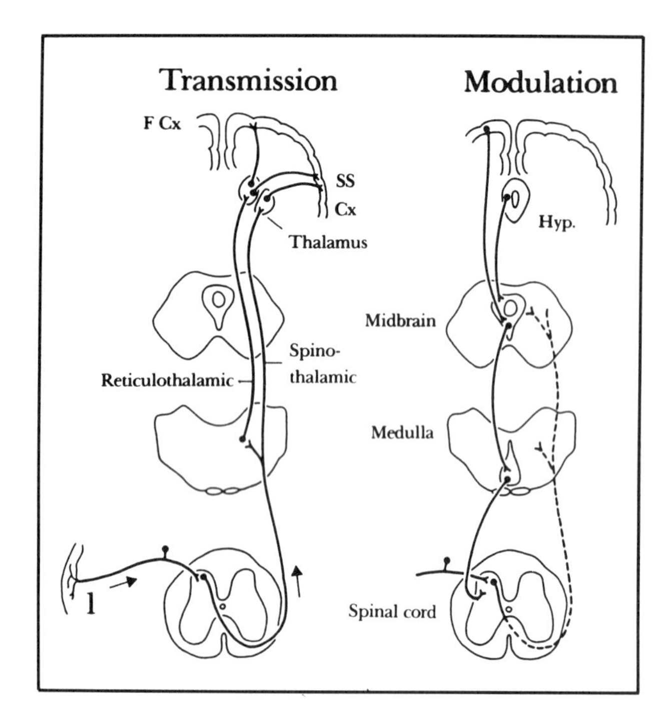

Left: Transmission system for nociceptive messages. Noxious stimuli activate the sensitive peripheral ending of the primary afferent nociceptor by the process of transduction (*1*). The message is then transmitted over the peripheral nerve to the spinal cord, where it synapses with cells of origin of the two major ascending pain pathways, the spinothalamic and spinoreticulothalamic. The message is relayed in the thalamus to both the frontal (*F Cx*) and the somatosensory cortex (*SS Cx*). **Right:** Pain modulation network. Inputs from frontal cortex and hypothalamus (*Hyp.*) activate cells in the midbrain, which control spinal pain transmission cells via cells in the medulla.

FIGURE 20-1 Pain transmission and modulation. (Source: Reprinted with permission from Fields HL: Pain. New York, McGraw-Hill, 1987.)

cancer patients who had no pain, the subjects in the study had more depression, were more irritable, engaged in less physical activity, and took more medications. Those who believed that pain indicated progression of cancer had higher depression and anxiety scores. As a result of their findings, Ahles and coworkers suggested that treatment for cancer pain should consist of specific therapeutic modalities targeted to each of the five dimensions.

McGuire[15] adapted Ahles' conceptual framework to conduct a descriptive study of 40 cancer patients with pain and 40 without pain. In general, support was found for the five dimensions of the model. Patients with pain had more depression, poorer physical function, and more psychosocial and other problems than the pain-free patients. Another finding was that individuals with cancer pain practiced a number of cognitive and behavioral coping strategies that they reported as moderately effective at reducing and controlling their pain.[16]

In addition to the five dimensions of the multidimensional model of cancer-related pain described, there is a sixth important area—the *sociocultural dimension,*[17] which involves various demographic, social, and cultural characteristics that are related to the experience of pain. The six dimensions contribute to the individual's perception of, and response to, pain. They are complex, interrelated, and as yet incompletely understood. Further discussion of each dimension follows.

Physiologic dimension

Ahles et al[14] originally described the physiologic dimension as consisting of the organic origin of pain, specifying such causes as a tumor that has metastasized to bone or infiltrated nerves or a hollow viscus. This definition was based on earlier work by researchers at the Memorial Sloan-Kettering Cancer Center in New York.

In 1979 Foley[18] described three types of pain in patients with cancer, each with a different cause: (1) pain associated with direct tumor involvement, (2) pain associated with cancer therapy, and (3) pain unrelated to either the tumor or its treatment. From this initial schema, a comprehensive listing of more specific causes of pain that fit within the first two categories was developed. Examples of pain due to direct tumor involvement are shown in Table 20-1.[19]

Additional work on the characterization of pain related to cancer therapy has been done.[20,21] The sources of pain associated with cancer treatment are many, ranging from initial diagnostic procedures that cause acute, short-term pain, to standard therapeutic modalities (surgery, radiotherapy, chemotherapy) that cause acute, short-term, and/or chronic long-term pain. Table 20-2 presents a comprehensive list of treatment-related pains.

The third type of pain described by Foley[18] was pain unrelated to either cancer or its treatment. She estimated that it accounted for 3% to 10% of the pain seen in cancer patients. Individuals with cancer pain are just as likely as the average individual to have pain from migraine headache, osteoarthritis, or degenerative disk disease. The presence of such pain, however, is important and should be carefully assessed to be sure that it is *not* related to cancer.

The work of Foley, Chapman, their colleagues, and others on the causes of cancer pain has led to a much greater understanding of the epidemiology and pathophysiology of cancer pain,[22-25] including three specific pain syndromes that occur in patients with cancer.[22,23] These syndromes of somatic, visceral, and deafferentation pain are characterized by pain of different qualities, located in different anatomic parts of the body, and caused by different mechanisms (Figure 20-2). All three syndromes are usually discussed in reference to tumor-related pain, but they apply equally well to treatment-related pain.[24] It is important to note that many cancer patients with pain will have one or more of these three syndromes simultaneously, and that each syndrome responds differently to different therapeutic modalities.

Related to the etiology of pain are two other characteristics. *Duration* of pain refers to whether pain is acute or chronic. Acute pain is generally due to tissue damage, is self-limited, and resolves when the tissue damage heals.

TABLE 20-1 Pain Associated with Direct Tumor Involvement

Direct Tumor Involvement	Signs and Symptoms
I. Tumor infiltration of bone	
a. Base of skull syndrome	Pain may precede neurologic signs and symptoms by weeks or months.
1. Jugular foramen metastases	Occipital pain, referred to vertex of head. Pain exacerbated by movement. Tenderness over the occipital condyle. Depending on nerves involved, may include hoarseness, dysarthria, dysphagia, neck and shoulder weakness, ptosis.
2. Clivus metastases	Vertex headache exacerbated by neck flexion. Lower cranial nerve dysfunction begins unilaterally, progresses to bilateral dysfunction.
3. Sphenoid sinus	Severe bifrontal headache (radiates to both temples). Intermittent retroorbital pain. Nasal stuffiness, fullness in head.
b. Vertebral body syndromes	Pain is an early symptom.
1. Odontoid process C1 involvement may result in pathologic fracture, subluxation, and spinal cord or brain stem compression.	Severe neck pain radiating over posterior aspect of the skull and vertex. Pain exacerbated by flexion. Progressive sensory and motor signs begin in upper extremities. Pain localized to adjacent paraspinal area.
2. C7-T1 Tumor spread may be hematogenous, or along nerves from tumor originating in brachial plexus or paravertebral space to contiguous vertebral body and epidural space.	Constant dull ache, radiating to both shoulders. Tenderness on percussion over spinous process at this level. Radicular pain, usually unilateral in posterior arm, elbow, and ulnar aspect of hand. Ptosis and miosis (Horner's syndrome).
3. L1	Dull, aching, mid-back pain. Exacerbated by lying or sitting, relieved by standing. Pain-radiating, girdle-like band anteriorly or to both paraspinal, lumbosacral area. May be referred to sacroiliac joint and/or superior iliac crest.
c. Sacral syndrome Most frequent in patients with gynecologic, genitourinary, or colon cancers.	Aching pain in low back or coccygeal area. Insidious onset. Exacerbated by lying/sitting, relieved by walking. Increasing pain with perianal sensory loss. Bowel, bladder dysfunction. Impotence.
II. Tumor infiltration of nerve	
a. Epidural spinal cord compression. Neurologic symptoms vary with site of disease. Considered a medical emergency.	Severe neck and back pain is initial symptom in 96% of patients. Motor weakness-paraplegia. Sensory loss with level. Loss of bowel/bladder function.
b. Peripheral nerve proximal infiltration occurs from paravertebral or retroperitoneal tumor.	Constant burning pain. Hypoesthesia and dysesthesia in area of sensory loss, early symptom.
c. Plexus 1. Brachial plexopathy Associated with lung (Pancoast), breast and lymphoma.	Pain radiating to ipsilateral shoulder and posterior aspect of arm and elbow (C8-T1 distribution). Pain and paresthesias in 4th and 5th fingers, may precede objective clinical signs by weeks or months. Paresthesias progress to numbness, weakness, C7-T1 distribution.
2. Lumbar plexopathy Result of extension of genitourinary, gynecologic and colon cancer.	Pain in L1-L3 distribution radiates to anterior portion of thigh or groin. Pain in L5-S1 distribution radiates down posterior aspect of leg to the heel. Paresthesias followed by numbness and dysesthesias. Progressive motor and sensory loss in plexus distribution.
3. Sacral plexopathy Occurs most frequently in patients with colon, genitourinary and gynecologic cancers.	Pain dull, aching, midline. Sensory loss beginning in perianal area. Sensory findings are at first unilateral. Progression to bilateral sacral sensory loss and autonomic dysfunction. Impotence, bowel and bladder dysfunction. Patient unable to lie or sit down.

TABLE 20-1 Pain Associated with Direct Tumor Involvement (continued)

Direct Tumor Involvement	Signs and Symptoms
II. Tumor infiltration of nerve—cont'd	
d. Root	
1. Leptomeningeal metastases Result of tumor infiltration of the leptomeninges with or without invasion of the parenchyma of the nervous system.	Pain occurs in 40% of patients. May be constant headache with or without stiff neck. May be localized low back and buttock pain.
III. Tumor infiltration of hollow viscus	
a. Infiltration of hollow viscus b. Compression of gastrointestinal tract or viscero-abdominal pain requires prompt diagnosis and treatment.	Pain may be local or referred, distortion, stretching, or inflammation of peritoneum may cause pain, obstruction to normal peristaltic flow results in hyperperistalsis and severe cramping colicky pain.

Source: Adapted with permission from Coyle N, Foley K: Prevalence and profile of pain syndromes in cancer patients, in McGuire DB, Yarbro CH (eds): Cancer Pain Management. Orlando, Fla, Grune & Stratton, 1987, pp 21-46.

There is a clear pattern of onset and resolution. When acute pain occurs, there may be hyperactivity of the autonomic nervous system, although this is not diagnostic of the presence of pain. Chronic pain also is usually, but not always, due to tissue damage. It may last 3 months or more,[5] and it is usually accompanied by adaptation, rather than hyperactivity, of the autonomic nervous system. There is not always a clear pattern of onset and resolution. Cancer pain, whether caused by tumor or by treatment, can be subdivided into acute and chronic types; sometimes both types occur simultaneously.

The second characteristic related to etiology of pain is the *pattern* that pain displays. Melzack[26] first described patterns of pain in a quantifiable way in his McGill Pain Questionnaire when he identified three separate patterns: (1) brief, momentary, or transient; (2) rhythmic, periodic, or intermittent; and (3) continuous, steady, or constant. The few researchers who have studied patterns of pain in cancer patients have found that about half of the patients experience pain that is constant, with just fewer than half experiencing intermittent pain and a very small number reporting brief or transient pain.[15,27,28,29] Most cancer patients experience two or more patterns simultaneously.

In summary, the physiologic dimension of cancer pain

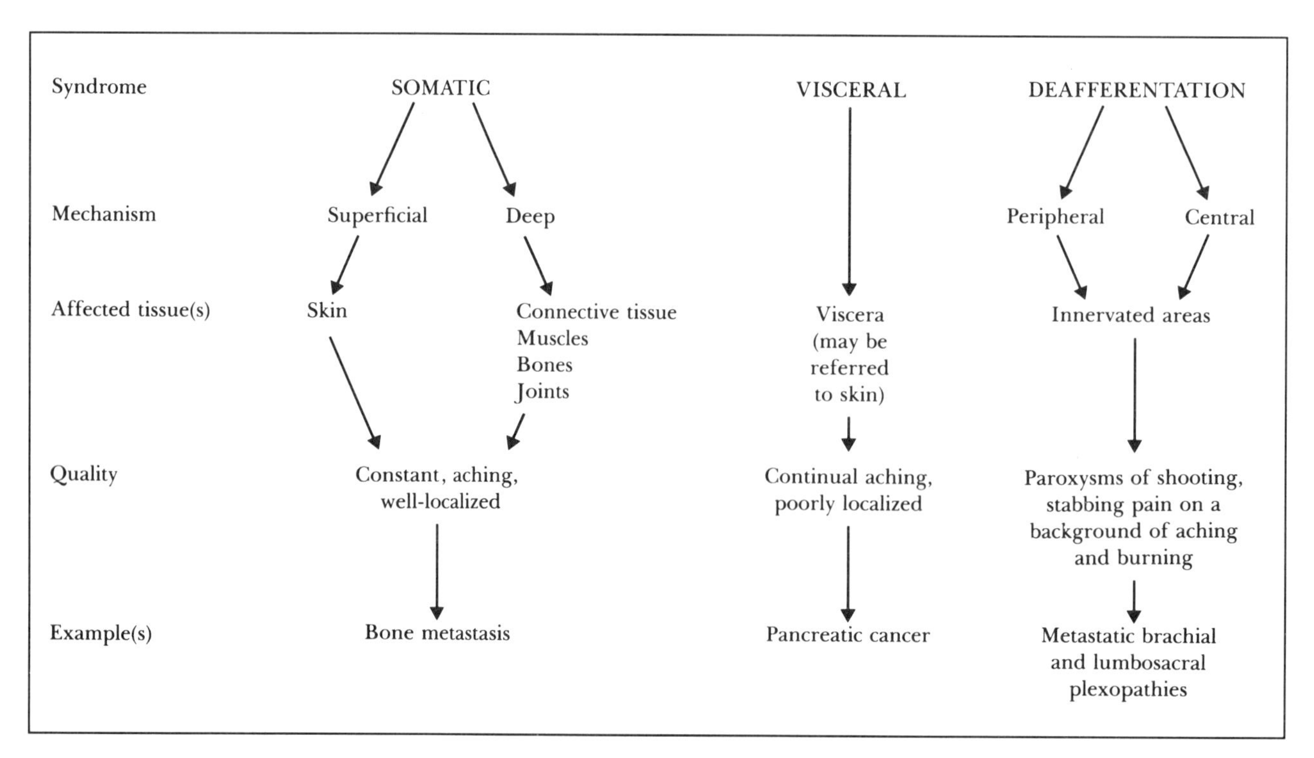

FIGURE 20-2 Pain syndromes in cancer.

TABLE 20-2 Sources of Pain Associated with Cancer Treatment

I. Diagnostic Procedures
  A. Lumbar punctures
  B. Blood samples
  C. Angiography
  D. Endoscopy
  E. Biopsies
II. Surgery
  A. Acute postoperative pain
  B. Chronic postoperative pain
    1. Mastectomy
    2. Radical neck resection
    3. Lymphedema
    4. Thoracotomy
    5. Phantom-limb
III. Chemotherapy
  A. Acute
    1. Gastrointestinal distress
    2. Mucositis
    3. Myalgia
    4. Joint pain
    5. Cardiomyopathy
    6. Pancreatitis
    7. Extravasation
  B. Chronic
    1. Peripheral neuropathy
    2. Steroid pseudorheumatism
    3. Aseptic osteonecrosis
IV. Radiation
  A. Acute
    1. Skin burn
    2. Gastrointestinal cramping
    3. Proctitis
    4. Mucositis
    5. Itching
  B. Chronic
    1. Osteonecrosis
    2. Fibrosis
    3. Keratitis
    4. Demyelination
    5. Pneumonitis
    6. Bowel ulceration or obstruction
    7. Myelopathy
V. Other Treatments and Treatment Complications

Source: Chapman CR, Kornell J, Syrjala K: Painful complications of cancer diagnosis and therapy, in McGuire DB, Yarbro CH (eds): Cancer Pain Management. Orlando, Fla, Grune & Stratton, 1987, pp 47-67.

includes organic etiology of the pain, which encompasses the specific anatomic sites affected. In addition, duration and pattern of pain are inherent in this dimension. Together, these factors constitute the physiologic portion of the multidimensional experience of cancer pain.

Sensory dimension

The sensory dimension of cancer-related pain is related to where the pain is located and what it feels like. Three specific components of this dimension are location, intensity, and quality.

First, location of pain is a critical component. Many cancer patients have been reported to have pain at two or more locations.[30,31] Given the patterns of metastasis or the sites of involvement of many solid tumors and some hematologic malignancies, this is not surprising. The number of separate locations of pain has clear implications for the sensory dimension as well as for the entire pain experience.

Intensity of pain, or how strong it feels, is the second important component of the sensory dimension. Intensity is a perceived and therefore subjective phenomenon, subject to individual pain threshold (the least stimulus intensity at which pain is perceived, according to Twycross and Lack[32]). Although intensity is primarily dependent on the cause of the pain, the individual threshold may be affected by a variety of factors, such as physical comfort, mood, medications, and social environment, that cause perceived intensity of pain to increase or decrease. Intensity is the most commonly assessed aspect of pain and is characterized by such words as *none, mild, moderate, severe, intolerable, excruciating, bad, intense,* and so on.

The third component of the sensory dimension is the quality of pain, which refers to how it actually feels. Melzack and Torgerson[33] were among the first to systematically study words that people used to describe pain. They composed a list of 102 words from the literature on pain and organized them into classes that described sensory, affective, and evaluative properties of pain. Words placed in the sensory category referred to temporal, spatial, pressure, thermal, and other aspects of pain. Examples of some of these words (sensations) are *pulsing, radiating, penetrating, burning,* and *aching,* respectively. This initial work provided the foundation for the McGill Pain Questionnaire,[26] the first multidimensional measure of pain.

A number of studies have revealed that patients with cancer pain use certain words more commonly than others to describe sensory aspects of their pain.[27-29,34-36] Words used by one third or more of patients in these studies include *sharp, tender, aching, throbbing, sore, stabbing, heavy, shooting,* and *gnawing*. Some authors distinguished between tumor- and treatment-related pain, but others did not; thus it is not entirely clear which words describe pain of which etiology. Nevertheless, the recurring word patterns found across time and in different groups of patients indicate that cancer pain is characterized by specific sensory qualities.

The sensory dimension of pain, as conceptualized by Ahles et al,[14] consists of location, intensity, and quality. The nature of and relationships among these three components are unique to each individual and undoubtedly have a strong impact on not only the entire experience of pain but the affective, cognitive, behavioral, and sociocultural dimensions as well.

Affective dimension

The affective dimension consists of depression, anxiety, or other psychologic factors or personality traits associated with pain.[14] Of the five dimensions proposed by Ahles, this one had the most support in the literature. In 1987 ten studies that examined relationships between pain in cancer patients and psychologic factors or personality traits were identified.[17]

Dalton and Feuerstein[37] reviewed the literature relating to biobehavioral factors in pain as well as affective, behavioral, and cognitive responses to pain. Although their review included both anecdotal and research reports relevant to the affective dimension of pain, it was clear that little research had been accomplished. Studies relevant to the affective dimension of pain are shown in Table 20-3.[14,38-58]

It is evident that parameters relevant to the affective dimension of pain range from specific personality traits (eg, neuroticism) to affective disorders (eg, depression) to vague general concepts, such as psychologic well-being. Taking into account the strong and weak points of each of the studies, it is possible to conclude the following: (1) specific personality traits are probably not related to the experience of cancer pain, (2) there is little evidence that affective disorders such as depression or anxiety are strongly related to pain, and (3) much more research on the relationships among these many psychologic parameters and the experience of cancer pain is needed.

Despite a limited body of research, it is quite clear from the clinical perspective that there is an affective component to the pain experience and that it influences the person's response to pain. The critical issue here is that psychologic variables important to a particular patient's pain experience must be identified and dealt with if pain is to be effectively managed.

Cognitive dimension

The cognitive dimension of cancer pain encompasses the manner in which the pain influences a person's thought processes or the manner in which he views himself. Ahles et al[14] found support for this dimension by assessing the meaning of each patient's pain. Almost two thirds believed their pain was an indicator of progressive disease, and these patients had significantly elevated anxiety and depression scores.

In patients with metastatic breast cancer, the belief that pain indicated worsening disease was significantly correlated with reports of more pain, more anxiety, and more depression.[38] Similarly, McGuire[15] found that 40% of patients considered pain an indicator of disease progression and that, although they were more depressed than those without this view, the difference was not statistically significant. In a different vein, Jacox and Stewart[50] found that cancer patients with pain had a decreased health self-concept. These studies were all related to the way an individual views himself or herself. Less clear is the area of how pain influences a person's thought processes; certainly, more research is needed.

Behavioral dimension

The behavioral dimension of pain includes a variety of observable behaviors related to pain. Until recently, there was little research supporting this dimension of the cancer pain experience. Ahles et al[14] focused on level of activity and intake of analgesics as manifestations of this dimension. They found that cancer patients with pain spent significantly less time walking or standing than those who did not have pain. Furthermore, 77% of the patients with pain reported that persons in their immediate environment could tell when they were in pain because of their facial expressions, changes in mood or activity, or verbal complaints.

Communication of pain to others was examined systematically by Bond and Pilowsky,[59] who studied the relationships among advanced cancer patients' subjective reports of pain, their communication of pain, and the reactions of nurses caring for them. About one quarter of their patients with pain did not communicate it to the nursing staff, and their pain scores were lower than those of patients who had pain and reported it or were offered analgesics by the nursing staff. There was a low correlation between pain intensity and amount of analgesic offered. In another study, these two researchers learned that patients who considered themselves "ill" reported considerable pain and tended to request analgesics frequently.[60]

Keefe and colleagues[61] conducted a study of the behavioral manifestations of pain in patients with head and neck cancer who were undergoing treatment of their disease. Guarded movements and grimacing were the major behavioral indicators of pain, with grimacing correlating significantly with patients' reports of pain intensity. Intake of analgesic medications increased significantly during therapy, as did use of nonpharmacologic pain-control methods. In addition, the amount of time patients spent walking or standing tended to decrease over the treatment period and time spent reclining increased. Finally, as treatment progressed, the number of simple daily activities that caused pain to occur increased significantly.

Another component of the behavioral dimension of pain consists of simple strategies or activities that patients engage in to control pain. Several studies have examined these activities. McGuire[27] noted that inpatients most frequently used analgesics, but one third also reported lying still, restricting movement, or positioning and moving affected body parts. In a survey of 351 hospitalized patients, some of whom had cancer, the most commonly cited (≥33%) pain-reduction methods involved medications, rest or lying down, heat, and distraction.[62] Several studies[57,63] found that cancer patients used an array of nonanalgesic, behaviorally oriented pain-control methods, including heat, distraction, position change, massage, nonnarcotic drugs, and exercise, to reduce pain. Wilkie and colleagues[64] attempted to correlate pain-control behaviors observed in cancer patients with pain intensity. The observed behaviors, many of which were validated by patients as pain-control methods, included positioning, distraction, pressure/manipulation, immobilization, guarding, and use of analgesics. McGuire[16] noted the use of a variety of behavioral and cognitive coping strategies by both inpatients and outpatients, who reported moderate effectiveness of these methods of relieving pain.

It is clear that the studies that have been described support the behavioral dimension of the cancer pain ex-

TABLE 20-3 Studies Relevant to the Affective Dimension of Cancer-Related Pain

Psychological Parameters	Author(s)	Relationship to Pain
Anxiety	Ahles et al[14]	None
	Spiegel and Bloom[38,39]	Positive correlation with increased pain
	Stam et al[40]	None
Depression	Ahles et al[14]	Elevated score
	Cleeland[41]	None
	Lansky et al[42]	Elevated score
	McGuire[43]	Elevated score
	Spiegel and Bloom[38,39]	Positive correlation with increased pain
	Stam et al[40]	None
	Woodforde and Fielding[44]	Elevated score
Ego strength	Fotopoulos et al[45]	Lower
Emotional distress	Cohen et al[46]	Lower than in patients with chronic benign pain
Extroversion	Bond[47]	Decreased correlation with greater use of analgesics
	Bond and Pearson[48]	Decreased correlation with greater use of analgesics
	Fotopoulos et al[45]	None
	Glynn[49]	Significantly related to diurnal variation
	Jacox and Stewart[50]	Negative correlation with pain intensity
Health locus of control (LOC)	Dalton[51]	Internal in patients taught self-control adjuvant analgesic techniques
	Fotopoulos et al[45]	Internal in males
	McKegney et al[52]	Higher LOC in patients closer to death
Health self-concept	Jacox and Stewart[50]	Decreased
Hostility	Ahles et al[14]	Elevated
Hypochondriasis	Bond[53]	Higher scores
Introversion	Glynn[49]	Significantly related to diurnal variation
	Jacox and Stewart[50]	Correlated with higher pain intensity
Mood disturbance	Cleeland[41]	Greater in depressed patients
	Cohen et al[54]	Decreased after treatment
	Shacham et al[55]	Positive correlation with severity of pain
	Spiegel and Bloom[38,39]	Positive correlation with increased pain
	Stam[40]	? unchanged when verbal report of pain changed
	Wallenstein[56]	Decreased after treatment
	Dorrepaal et al[57]	Associated with higher level of pain
Neuroticism	Bond[47]	Decreased after treatment
	Bond and Pearson[48]	Higher than in control patients
	Fotopoulos et al[45]	Lower than in tuberculosis patients
	Glynn[49]	Significantly related to diurnal variation
	Jacox and Stewart[50]	Increased compared to normal patients; negative correlation with pain intensity
Psychological well-being	Ferrell et al[58]	Significantly lower than in pain-free patients
Repression-sensitization	Fotopoulos et al[45]	None
Somatization	Ahles et al[14]	Elevated score

perience as conceptualized by Ahles et al.[14] The findings offer directions for therapeutic approaches as well, which will be examined in a subsequent section.

Sociocultural dimension

The sociocultural dimension of cancer pain consists of a variety of demographic, ethnic, cultural, spiritual, and related factors that influence a person's perception of and response to pain. There have been very few studies examining the relationships of any of these factors to cancer pain specifically, but the small body of research that has been conducted on sociocultural aspects of clinical pain is reviewed briefly here, since some of the findings may pertain to the individual with cancer pain.

A number of studies used experimentally induced laboratory pain to examine racial, age, religious, and ethnic differences in pain.[65] Although none of the studies reviewed in Wolf and Langley's paper[65] allowed definitive conclusions about differences in pain response due to the factors studied, a strong role of culturally determined attitudinal factors in pain perception and response was clearly supported. In an updated review, Wolff[66] lamented that little progress had been made in studying and understanding the important role that ethnocultural factors played in pain. He maintained, however, that cultural factors, such as majority/minority group status, seemed to be the most likely causes of differences in pain perception and response.

Lipton and Marbach[67] corroborated this idea in their study of interethnic differences and similarities in reported pain experiences of black, Irish, Italian, Jewish, and Puerto Rican patients with facial pain. All five groups were similar in their reported responses to pain, but the factors that *influenced* their responses were quite different. For example, Italians were most influenced by duration of pain, whereas Jews and Puerto Ricans were most influenced by level of psychologic distress. These researchers suggested that the relationship between ethnicity and pain experience should be viewed as a subtle continuum of behaviors, attitudes, and feelings.

A descriptive study of Arab-Americans' perceptions of and responses to pain emphasized that cultural characteristics heavily influenced individual behaviors.[68] For example, vehement, persistent, and perhaps exaggerated verbal messages were the norm for this group, and reporting of pain was included. Endurance of pain was not a priority since modern technology was available; endurance was easier if Arab-Americans understood that the consequences of pain would be more positive. Pain was generally perceived as unpleasant, to be avoided, and to be controlled by all means. Individuals with pain often displayed more behavioral manifestations of pain and were more vocal about it to family rather than to health care providers. Family members assumed a major role in trying to manage pain, primarily through usurping the decision-making related to care.

Age, sex, and race have been examined in relation to expression of pain. Females and older individuals were found to have increased verbal expressions of pain.[69,70] One study revealed that blacks used more moderate words than whites in describing pain,[69] but another study demonstrated no significant differences.[71]

Only a few studies have focused on cancer patients with pain, and the sociocultural variables studied have been mixed but have included sex, race, age, and cultural background. In a study of cancer inpatients, McGuire[27] noted that females and nonwhites had significantly lower scores on the McGill Pain Questionnaire than males and whites. In a subsequent study of inpatients and outpatients, she found that blacks and older patients had less pain (as measured by the McGill Pain Questionnaire) and depression.[15]

McMillan[72] found that cancer patients with pain who were older (over 55 years) reported less pain intensity than those who were younger. On the other hand, another study[73] found that the pain intensity of patients who were over 65 years of age was similar to that of those under 65.

Cleeland and associates,[74] using the Brief Pain Inventory (BPI), compared American and Vietnamese patients with cancer pain. Only items related to pain severity and interference of pain in several aspects of life (eg, activity, walking, sleep, work, relations with others, mood) were translated into Vietnamese. Their data suggested that these two groups of patients, from widely different cultural backgrounds, responded in a similar fashion to items related to pain and its interferences with daily living. The authors noted that Vietnamese patients, however, reported more severe pain despite fairly comparable cancers; it was hypothesized that this was due in part to the fact that 64% were receiving no analgesics at all whereas the remainder were taking nonnarcotic agents, specifically a benzodiazepine type of drug. Although the focus of this study was on instrument development, it was clear that the two areas of concern—pain severity and interference with daily life—were important cross-culturally.

The research literature supporting the sociocultural dimension of cancer is just beginning to emerge. Use of previous literature on noncancer populations, however, makes clear that ethnic and cultural factors are important in patients' perceptions of and responses to pain.

Implications of the multidimensional model

The multidimensional conceptualization of cancer pain, as initially defined by Ahles et al,[14] expanded by McGuire,[17] and supported by the research of many investigators, provides the organizing framework for this chapter. The six dimensions are highly appropriate for assessment and management of cancer pain; each contributes in its own way to various aspects of these two critical processes. In addition, the multidimensional framework allows the experience of cancer pain to be viewed as the complete, interrelated, interactive, and dynamic phenomenon that it is. The issue of "quality of life" is subsumed by the multidimensional model of pain, since the model incorporates the aspects of life that would be included in standard concepts of quality of life. Nursing assessment and management that are performed in a competent and multidisciplinary manner will ensure that individuals with cancer pain achieve optimal "quality of life" regardless of the status of their disease.

SCOPE OF THE CANCER PAIN PROBLEM

Organizations and agencies involved with the treatment of cancer are directing their efforts to improvement of overall pain management. The Oncology Nursing Society's (ONS) position paper on assessment and management of cancer pain[75] highlighted the fact that control of cancer pain is largely inadequate. Further, the ONS pointed out that individuals with cancer pain have the right to have pain recognized as a problem and dealt with expediently. Similarly, the World Health Organization has designated the relief of cancer pain as one of the goals of its Cancer Control Program. In addition, the National Institutes of Health consensus statement on an integrated approach to the management of pain[76] recommended the use of multiple treatment modalities to help control cancer pain. The positions and recommendations from these sponsoring groups have developed partly as a result of nearly two decades of documented evidence that unrelieved cancer pain is a significant clinical problem.

Prevalence

The American Cancer Society's 1989 statistics on cancer incidence[77] indicated that cancer will be diagnosed in more than 1 million persons in 1989 and that 500,000 will die of the disease. The prevalence of pain for all cancer diagnoses during all states of the disease, however, has been difficult to quantify.

Coyle and Foley[19] identified several problems affecting the accuracy of prevalence data: (1) lack of systematic data collection and pain-measurement techniques, (2) lack of documentation regarding the extent of patients' disease, (3) lack of identification of pain's cause, and (4) inclusion of multiple cancer diagnoses as a single group. In spite of these problems, however, researchers have examined the prevalence of cancer pain, with the majority of reports appearing during the last 15 years.

The prevalence of pain by clinical setting (Table 20-4), regardless of cancer diagnosis, indicates that patients in hospice and specialty units report a higher prevalence of pain than patients in other settings.[19,30,31,78-88] This observation can be understood when one recognizes that patients with advanced metastatic disease are often referred to these settings for terminal care. Patients with advanced disease report more severe pain than those who are in the early stages of their illness.[86-88] Foley[18] reported that 23 of 39 patients (60%) with terminal disease had significant pain. When McGuire[15] interviewed 40 patients with cancer pain, she found that 90% had metastatic disease and 10% had local or regional disease.

TABLE 20-4 Prevalence of Pain by Clinical Setting

Setting	Percentage	Reference
Hospice	58-84	Twycross[78] Wilkes[79] Baines[80]
Specialty unit	91	Twycross and Fairfield[31]
Inpatients	21-72	Foley[18] Donovan and Dillon[30] Dorrepaal et al[82] Gilbert and Grossman[85]
Outpatients	30-72	Trotter et al[81] Peteet et al[84] Ahles et al[87]
Inpatients/outpatients	56-65	Pannuti et al[83] Daut and Cleeland[86] Greenwald et al[88]

Even though types of assessment vary among studies, the severity of cancer pain, as opposed to merely having pain, has been used as a means of reporting prevalence data. In a study of 23 patients with metastatic prostate cancer, Pollen and Schmidt[89] found that 40% of the patients described their pain as mild to moderate and 60% described it as severe. Rankin[90] found that patients with advanced disease reported mild/moderate pain (10%) less often than they reported moderate/excruciating pain (88%). Conversely, Donovan and Dillon[30] reported that patients rated their pain mild to moderate more frequently (40%) than they did moderate to severe (11%).

In studying patients with pain in four different tumor types, Greenwald et al[88] reported moderate to very bad pain for all disease stages in from 38% to 60% of the patients. Daut and Cleeland[86] also studied patients with various tumor types, measuring pain on a scale of 0 (no pain) to 10 (extreme pain), but they found that for six cancers the percentage of patients who rated pain as more than 5 on the scale was only 0% to 34%. The 0% reflected the responses of a small number ($n = 6$) of patients with metastatic cervical cancer.

Examination of pain prevalence data by cancer diagnosis shows the likelihood of pain becoming a significant problem with the progression of disease. Table 20-5 shows prevalence data for cancers of the colon/rectum, pancreas, cervix, uterus, ovary, lymph system, bone, and prostate.[18,86-88]

Pain associated with several of the common solid tumor malignancies has been studied more extensively. Table 20-6 demonstrates five reports of pain in lung cancer.[18,87,88,91,92] Results from one study[88] indicated that the prevalence of pain in lung cancer increased with advancing disease, whereas those from another study[91] suggested

TABLE 20-5 Prevalence of Pain by Diagnosis and Stage

Site	Stage	Percentage	Reference
Colon/rectum	Metastatic	47	Daut and Cleeland[86]
	All stages	33	Ahles et al[87]
Pancreas	Local/regional	77	Greenwald et al[88]
	Distant	50	
Cervix	Local	35-41	Daut and Cleeland[86] Greenwald et al[88]
	Distant/metastatic	0-23	Daut and Cleeland[86] Greenwald et al[88]
Uterus	Nonmetastatic	14	Daut and Cleeland[86]
	Metastatic	40	
Ovary	Nonmetastatic	39	Daut and Cleeland[86]
	Metastatic	59	
Lymphoma	All stages	18-20	Foley[18] Ahles et al[87]
Primary bone	All stages	85	Foley[18]
Prostate	Local/nonmetastatic	30-35	Daut and Cleeland[86] Greenwald et al[88]
	Regional	26	Greenwald et al[88]
	Distant/metastatic	47-75	Daut and Cleeland[86] Greenwald et al[88]

TABLE 20-6 Prevalence of Pain in Lung Cancer

Stage	Percentage	Reference
Local (early)	40	Marino et al[92]
	53	Greenwald et al[88]
Regional	49	Greenwald et al[88]
Distant/metastatic	56	Greenwald et al[88]
All stages	33-51	Foley[18] Ahles et al[87] Greenwald et al[88]
At diagnosis	71	Turnbull[91]
During illness	18-65	Turnbull[91]

that a high percentage of patients reported pain at the time of diagnosis. In addition, a higher incidence of pain from lung cancer in patients 65 to 69 years of age has been noted.[92]

Patients with nonmetastatic breast cancer have pain-prevalence rates of 33% to 52%,[18,86,87] whereas in patients with metastatic breast cancer prevalence rates range from 56% to 68%.[38,86,93] An important finding was that even though patients had evidence of bone metastases, as documented by bone scan, nearly one third of them did not report pain.[93]

Taken together, the published studies of the prevalence of cancer pain indicate several important facts. First, our knowledge of cancer pain comes only from prevalence studies, as there are no published reports of the *incidence* of cancer pain. Second, pain is clearly more prevalent in those patients with advanced stages of disease and those being treated in hospice or specialty units. Third, certain common malignancies are more often associated with cancer pain, and it is these malignancies in which pain is better studied and understood.

Significance

Because of the complicated nature of cancer pain, with its different causes, varied presentations, multiple dimensions, and variety of treatments, and the previously mentioned problems with studying the incidence and prevalence of pain, one can speculate that the true prevalence is much greater than existing reports indicate. Although cancer pain is clearly a multidimensional phenomenon, the impact on patients who have it is as yet poorly understood.

The few published studies available indicate that behavioral manifestations are common[64] and that patients experience a wide variety of physical and psychosocial problems.[35,41,43,94,95] The effects of pain on a patient's friends and family are virtually unknown. Thus health professionals in general and nurses in particular are hampered by a lack of research-based knowledge about the real prevalence of pain and the impact it has on patients and others. In addition, there is a great deal of evidence to suggest that cancer pain is poorly managed worldwide by health professionals from a number of disciplines.

Professional Issues

If the preceding statements are true, it is logical to surmise that the published evidence supporting health care professionals' contributions to poor pain control does not represent the real magnitude of the problem. A number of issues that contribute to inadequate management of pain have been identified, but it is likely that they barely scratch the surface of the problem.

There are a number of obstacles to successful pain management (Table 20-7). Inaccurate knowledge of pharmacologic principles represents a major problem area, as documented by a number of studies. Questionnaires administered to nurses and physicians, as well as reviews of

TABLE 20-7 Obstacles to Successful Pain Management

Lack of understanding about pain
Expectation that pain should be present
Relief of pain not viewed as a goal of treatment
Inadequate or nonexistent assessment
Undertreatment with analgesics
Inadequate knowledge of analgesics and other drugs
Fears of addiction, sedation, and respiratory depression
Inadequate knowledge of other interventions for pain

patients' records, indicate that in the treatment of patients with cancer pain, there are problems such as prolonged dosing intervals (ie, not commensurate with the duration of action of the drug), lack of knowledge about equal analgesic doses, misconceptions about morphine's effectiveness as an oral analgesic, and use of doses that are too low to provide relief of pain.[96-101]

A related pharmacologic problem reflects nurses' decision making in administering narcotics. Cohen[102] found that patients received less narcotic than was ordered, as demonstrated by the fact that 75.2% reported moderate to marked distress from pain. Furthermore, nurses' decisions concerning amounts of narcotic administered appeared to be irrational. Sheidler and colleagues[97] found that when nurses were given hypothetical patient vignettes in which changes were made in drug, dose, route, or interval, very few were able to select the appropriate "new" order.

Issues surrounding addiction and potential toxicities of potent narcotics have also been cited as reasons for suboptimal pain control.[103-107] Although there is evidence that strongly suggests addiction is not a problem for persons who require narcotics,[108] nurses and physicians fear iatrogenically induced addiction and certainly overestimate its risk when narcotics are prescribed.

A more fundamental problem that nurses have exhibited is a deficiency in the assessment of pain. A lack of basic assessment skills, failure to acknowledge and document the existence of pain, and inaccurate documentation when the problem *is* known to exist prohibit patients from receiving the benefit of reasonable pain control.[30,98,109,110]

Several other problems have been identified as obstacles to successful management of pain. Perhaps most important are the perceptual differences between patients and professionals about the severity of existing pain.[60,107,111] Complete relief of pain has not been traditionally viewed as a treatment objective.[99,102,112] Little attention has been paid to beliefs, attitudes, and communication from patients and their friends and families with respect to pain.[32,113] Finally, the role of regulatory agencies in the prescribing of narcotics has created a whole set of additional problems.[114]

Inherent in all the problems identified with pain management is the fact that nurses' and physicians' attitudes and values with respect to pain and patients with pain affect their clinical judgments. When these judgments reflect a positive outcome for persons with cancer pain, then these individuals receive the quality of care they deserve. However, when clinical judgments reflect negative outcomes, then the professional behavior may be inexcusable and create needless suffering for patients.

Clinical experience may contribute to the development of negative attitudes toward specific types of patient.[115] Pilowsky and Bond[60] observed that potent narcotics were withheld from patients who complained about their pain and who regarded themselves as ill. Another example occurs when patients continue to report unrelieved pain, despite institution of pain-relief measures. Sometimes when the best efforts of health professionals are unsuccessful, placebos are ordered to help differentiate "real" pain from imaginary pain.[99,116] This unethical behavior arises from health professionals' frustration but may also reflect a not so subtle form of anger toward and punishment of the patient.

The value structure of health professionals is highlighted by how much pain they think patients should endure or be able to tolerate. In one study[99] nurses believed that patients should be encouraged to increase their tolerance of pain. In other words, the more pain a patient endured, the better a person he or she was. In a study of factors influencing physicians' behaviors toward patients with cancer pain, it was found that physicians with more "liberal" attitudes (favoring earlier interventions, more patient control over narcotics, and seeing lower levels of pain as acceptable relief) were younger and had more experience in specialized oncology settings.[117]

The behaviors displayed in the foregoing examples represent a complex process involving beliefs, values, and dispositions about pain. Altering this process to eradicate biases, ignorant attitudes, and misconceptions about pain is a major challenge. Educational programs *can* alter attitudes about pain. One study found that after a 3-hour educational program about cancer pain, nurses' knowledge and attitude scores were significantly higher on an attitude inventory and an analgesia knowledge test than those of a group of nurses who did not participate in the program.[106]

Sanford and Schlicher[118] developed a questionnaire to address biases about pain and related issues. Although it has not been proved a reliable and valid instrument, it could be used in educational programs to help nurses examine the effects of their attitudes and biases on their behavior and clinical judgments.

Nurses and physicians have acknowledged their educational deficiencies in the area of cancer pain and its management.[98,106,119] The need for structured educational content in basic educational programs of the health professions has been encouraged.[75,76,120] In nursing, Spross and colleagues[75] delineated positions involving not only basic and graduate nursing school education but continuing education as well. The intent behind the first two positions was that nursing education programs at both basic and graduate levels have a responsibility to provide their students with both theoretic and clinical content related to pain and its management and should specify some minimal behavioral outcomes related to this content. The intent behind the continuing education position was to support the idea that a professional nurse must continue to increase his or her knowledge base and change attitudes about pain if necessary to provide the best care possible for patients with cancer pain.

Formal educational programs may not be sufficient to change practice unless several other important factors are in place. First, there must be opportunities to apply newly acquired knowledge in the clinical environment. Weissman et al[121] described an educational format for the dissemination of pain information that involved a multidisciplinary team, patient consultations, and brief formal presentations about cancer pain. This approach allows nurses, house staff, attending physicians, and others to observe role models who place a high priority on cancer pain as an important clinical problem that requires resolution and to gain experience in applying what they have observed and learned.

A second major factor necessary for changing practice is the support of administration. The ONS addressed this problem in its position paper,[75] stating: "Effective management of cancer pain should be an organizational priority for nurse administrators including the establishment of lines of accountability and responsibility of nurses." Nursing and other administrators, by virtue of their control over budgets and allocation of resources, are in a position to make the assessment and management of cancer pain an important clinical priority of all staff members.

A third factor that is important in improving the management of patients with cancer pain consists of major multidisciplinary programmatic initiatives, such as the World Health Organization Cancer Control Program or the Wisconsin Cancer Pain Initiative, that are designed and implemented solely to improve pain control. To achieve this objective, legislative and health policy activities aimed at overcoming sociopolitical obstacles to adequate management of pain must be undertaken.[75] Further discussion of this area is beyond the scope of this chapter, but a recent volume edited by Hill and Fields[122] presented some excellent material on these issues.

PRINCIPLES OF ASSESSMENT AND MANAGEMENT

Effective clinical assessment and management of cancer pain rests on recognition and use of a number of critical principles. Foley[123] delineated several of these: (1) complete assessment of the history of the pain, (2) evaluation of the patient's psychosocial status, (3) careful medical and neurologic examinations, (4) use of appropriate diagnostic procedures to determine the nature of the pain, (5) early treatment with analgesics, (6) continual reassessment of the patient's response to prescribed therapy, (7) reassessment of the treatment approach or search for a new cause of the pain, and (8) continuity of care from diagnosis to treatment. While written primarily for physicians, many of these principles are applicable for nurses as well.

In addition, there are other principles of assessment and management and special considerations that are implicit in successful nursing management of cancer pain. These consist of the use of a multidisciplinary approach; a well-conceived scope-of-practice role for nurses; a thorough assessment and diagnosis; and consideration of patients' developmental, sociocultural, and terminal care needs. In the section that follows, each of these areas will be explored in turn, with emphasis on the specific roles and responsibilities of oncology nurses.

Multidisciplinary Approach

The multidimensional conceptualization of cancer pain clearly requires an approach to assessment and management that involves multiple health care disciplines. A casual perusal of some of the available texts on cancer pain[32,124-127] reveals quite clearly that treatment approaches include chemotherapy, radiotherapy, surgery, neurosurgery, neurologic techniques, anesthetic procedures, pharmacologic agents administered in a wide variety of ways, and cognitive/behavioral methods. Generally speaking, there is no one best way to treat cancer pain and no one best person to do it.

The many strategies available for managing pain can be easily conceptualized within the multidimensional framework. The *physiologic* dimension can be treated with surgical procedures, chemotherapy, or radiotherapy aimed at the organic cause of the pain. The *sensory* dimension can be modulated through the use of analgesics, neurostimulatory techniques, cognitive or behavioral interventions, or other modalities. The *affective* dimension can be managed by thorough assessment of its nature and scope and then by appropriate intervention, whether it be with antidepressive drugs, therapy sessions, or simply reducing the amount of pain. The *cognitive* dimension can be treated by giving the patient accurate and realistic information about pain and its meaning and by discussing possibilities for assessment and treatment. The *behavioral* dimension lends itself to well planning of activity, medication, and other behavioral strategies (eg, distraction, hypnosis) that will help reduce pain. Finally, the *sociocultural* dimension can be addressed by careful assessment of factors that influence the person's perception of and response to pain, including ethnic background, demographic variables, familial practices related to pain, and so on.

Whether these dimensions are treated singly or together, they all contribute to the overall pain experience, and all require input from different health care givers. Specific groups of health professionals that have a role in the assessment and management of cancer pain include nurses, pharmacists, social workers, occupational therapists, physical therapists, psychologists, and physicians from the specialties of anesthesiology, internal medicine, medical oncology/hematology, radiation oncology, general surgery and its subspecialties, neurosurgery, neurology, orthopedics, and psychiatry.

The concept of multidisciplinary pain-treatment programs is not a new one for specialists in the field of chronic, nonmalignant pain.[128] The entire concept of multidisciplinary approaches to help patients achieve relief from the pain of cancer has emanated from international and national programs.[129-131] Evaluation of these programs as well as of institution-specific multidisciplinary treatment programs has only recently begun.[54,121,132] Although the multidisciplinary approach to management of cancer patients' pain seems to be the most efficient, logical, and optimal route, its true efficacy still needs to be established through careful evaluation.[133]

Considerations for Nursing

Nurses are an integral and essential part of the multidisciplinary team approach to management of cancer pain. The Oncology Nursing Society position paper on cancer pain[75] delineated a number of positions related to the management of cancer pain and suggested strategies to accomplish the positions. Important components of the paper included the nurse's scope of practice relevant to pain and specific nursing responsibilities. Both of these key areas will be briefly summarized here; the interested reader is encouraged to read the original source.

Scope of practice

Oncology nurses, by virtue of their prolonged contact with cancer patients in a variety of settings and their relationships with these persons and their families, are best prepared to assume a leadership role in the assessment and management of cancer pain. Assumption of such a role is consistent with the ONS's mission of improving the care of persons with cancer. The 1986 National Institutes of Health consensus conference on the integrated management of people with pain[76] described and endorsed a pivotal role for professional nurses in the management of pain.

The ONS position paper[75] delineated a scope of practice for nurses with different levels of expertise (eg, nurse generalists, oncology nurse clinicians, and oncology clinical nurse specialists). These levels of expertise were made operational with the specific knowledge and skills associated with each level. For example, nurse generalists should be capable of basic assessment of pain, development of a care plan, evaluation of the plan, recognition of ineffective interventions, and reporting of problems to appropriate health care givers and/or supervisors. Clinical nurse specialists, on the other hand, should be able to perform sophisticated assessments, make appropriate nursing diagnoses, develop multidisciplinary treatment plans, coordinate contributions of the different disciplines, and evaluate and readjust the care plan as necessary.

Responsibilities

Two positions set forth in the ONS paper on cancer pain dealt with the ethical and practice responsibilities of nurses in managing pain. These positions, as well as all the others, were based on several assumptions: (1) patients have a right to relief of pain, (2) unrelieved pain causes significant and unnecessary suffering for patients, families, friends, and health professionals, (3) nurses and patients (ie, society) have a social contract in which alleviation of pain and suffering is a tenet, (4) nurses are often prevented from meeting this obligation because of inadequate education and a variety of sociocultural variables, (5) nurses have sustained contact with patients and their significant others over the course of a cancer illness that make them key providers of care, (6) cancer pain is an "orphan" problem with accountability for its relief unclear, and (7) cancer pain is a sociopolitical as well as a clinical problem.

It is clear that assumption of a leadership role in the effective management of cancer patients' pain is a nursing responsibility. The scope of nursing practice delineated in the ONS paper provided the foundation for positions relevant to nurses' ethical and practice responsibilities, defined below.

Ethics "Individuals with cancer pain have a right to optimal pain relief, and nurses caring for them have an ethical obligation to assure that everything possible to provide this relief is explored."[75] Included in this position are the beliefs that patients' pain must be recognized by nurses as a problem and its relief as a need, nurses must be knowledgeable about means to obtain relief, pain relief is a moral and ethical professional responsibility, nurses must help patients make their own decisions and determine their own actions regarding pain relief, and nurses must act with other health care providers to relieve patients' pain.

Practice "Nurses caring for individuals with cancer pain should exercise leadership in the identification and assessment of cancer pain while planning, implementing/coordinating, and evaluating the interdisciplinary management of cancer pain."[75] This position on nursing practice was based on the components of the nursing process and, in the ONS paper, was subdivided into five subpositions reflective of each of the components. Essentially, the subpositions stated that nurses were responsible for (at levels specified within their individual scope of practice) identifying pain as a problem in a given patient, assessing the pain, developing a plan of care that addressed nursing and collaborative responsibilities with other health care providers, implementing and coordinating the plan, and, finally, evaluating the plan and using the data to revise the plan as needed.

These subpositions describing the nursing role in relation to cancer pain serve as the framework for the remainder of this chapter, along with, of course, the view of cancer pain as a multidimensional experience. Assuming that a nurse has identified pain as a problem for a particular patient, careful assessment and diagnosis of the problem are the next steps.

Assessment and Diagnosis

The literature documenting nurses' problems with assessment of cancer pain has been discussed previously. In this section, the need and rationale for assessment, basic principles of assessment, and some examples of assessment tools are presented.

In the multidisciplinary section of this chapter, the physician's role in assessment and management of cancer pain was briefly described. The specific activities clearly imply that establishing and treating the cause of pain is the major goal, along with, of course, concomitant treatment of the pain itself.[57,123] The nursing role, however, is different in that, although nurses certainly contribute to the goals of the physician, the focus of their assessment and management activities is on the individual as a whole person and on the patient's response to the pain. In addition, nurses are interested in how pain affects an individual's significant others and support systems. The emphasis is on decreasing pain and increasing comfort rather than on the cancer itself.

Systematic nursing assessment of pain is important for several reasons.[134] First, it establishes a baseline from which to plan and begin interventions. Second, it assists in the selection of interventions. Third, it makes possible evaluation of the interventions. Assessment of pain is a critical process that aids in the clinical management of pain and, indeed, goes hand in hand with successful management. It is different from measurement of pain, which is generally carried out for research purposes.

The timing of assessments is critical as well. Any cancer patient with pain who enters any health care setting should have an initial or baseline assessment. After the initiation of interventions, continuous or ongoing assessment is necessary for evaluation and revision of treatment plans. This approach to the process of assessment is modeled on the nursing process. Collection of pain assessment data should be systematic and organized, just as the collection of general nursing data is.

Assessment

The need for a complete nursing assessment of pain and documentation of the assessment was highlighted in several studies.[109,110] In addition, there are some "pitfalls" in assessment of pain. They include (1) the belief that patients with pain will demonstrate changes in vital signs or display overt behavioral manifestations of pain; (2) the belief that all pain should have a documented organic cause; (3) the belief that pain in cancer patients may be of psychogenic origin ("all in the head"); (4) ascription of all pain in cancer patients to the tumor rather than to such "normal" problems as migraine headache or arthritis; and (5) feelings of being overwhelmed with clinical responsibilities and thus becoming insensitive to patients' pain and their related needs. Awareness and avoidance of these "pitfalls" should help nurses perform good pain assessments.

The range of assessment parameters is quite wide and represents each of the multiple dimensions of cancer pain. Parameters that require assessment in each dimension are described briefly below.

Physiologic parameters Physiologic parameters are assessed through the important act of obtaining a pain history. Relevant questions include the following: When did it start? What started it? How long has it been present? Is it acute or chronic? These questions provide information about the onset and duration of the pain and provide clues to its cause. While determining the specific cause of the pain is not the responsibility of the nurse, knowledge about it is helpful in the selection and planning of interventions. Likewise, knowledge of onset and duration assists in the same process.

Sensory parameters Location of pain is an essential part of the assessment, since it is well known that cancer pain can exist in more than one body area. The problem of referred pain is relevant to this assessment parameter as well. As discussed previously in the section on the physiologic dimension of pain, three cancer pain syndromes may occur simultaneously within the same person and are usually manifested in different anatomic locations. Interventions for the syndromes are different as well, and an accurate assessment of location helps determine the type(s) of pain present and the most appropriate interventions.

Intensity, or severity, of pain is perhaps the most important characteristic that requires assessment. The amount of pain a person is experiencing will usually be the predominant "pain complaint." Indeed, a study of 24 cancer patients documented that intensity was the most salient component of the pain experience.[135]

The quality of pain is a strong influencing factor in individuals' perception of and response to their pain. As mentioned previously, different cancer pain syndromes are characterized by different qualities, and cancer pain in general appears to be distinct from the pain associated with other disease processes. Thus specific qualities of pain, such as burning, stabbing, or throbbing, are important. Knowledge of these sensory properties of pain is used to establish a baseline against which interventions can be evaluated.

Pattern of pain is an essential component of the assessment, particularly when there are multiple sites of pain. Again, different patterns are characteristic of different cancer pain syndromes and require different approaches to management. For example, a patient with intermittent pain that occurs only with movement will need one set of interventions while someone with constant pain will require another.

Affective parameters As discussed with respect to the affective dimension, a striking number of psychologic factors are involved in the pain experience. Since clinical assessment is aimed at formulation and evaluation of interventions, the identification of specific problems, such as depression, anxiety, or mood disturbances, aids in the achievement of successful overall management.

Cognitive parameters Assessment of the meaning of pain for the patient will help in the approach to care. For example, if the patient has a great fear that cancer is recurring, such appropriate actions as explanation, reassurance, and emotional support can be offered.

Knowledge of the patient's previous coping strategies and their effectiveness are important in the formulation of a nursing care plan. Research has revealed that patients with cancer pain use a variety of coping mechanisms that are effective to some degree in relieving pain.[16,63] In addition, coping strategies that may not have been used previously but that may be beneficial can also be added to the care plan.

Similarly, knowledge of previous treatments individuals have experienced for their pain is an essential assessment parameter. The success or failure of previous interventions may influence individuals' beliefs and attitudes about certain interventions, as well as their willingness to try them again. For example, if a trial of a particular narcotic analgesic was inadequately carried out, and thus was unsuccessful in controlling pain, the effectiveness of that particular drug, or of narcotics in general, may be questioned by the individual. Such beliefs and attitudes may influence to some degree the success of a therapy. The challenge to the nurse is to determine any such potential problems through careful and systematic assessment and to devise strategies for overcoming them.

Behavioral parameters Cancer pain affects a number of aspects of patients' lives, and many of these aspects are behavioral areas that can be observed,[15,64] documented, and used in planning care. Effects of pain on activities of daily living range from interference with social interaction to interference with eating or mobility.[15] Also, persons with pain can cite many activities, behaviors, or other factors that increase or decrease the intensity of their pain[15,27,63] (eg, weather and humidity, food and drink, time of day, and amount of sleep).

Other specific parameters that require assessment are communication about pain, interaction with others (family, friends, health professionals), ambulation and physical activity, such pain behaviors as grimacing or nonverbal vocalizations, use of medications, and use of various self-intiated pain-control interventions. Again, this information is essential for an accurate, complete assessment of pain and for formulation of management strategies.

Sociocultural parameters Parameters that are important to assessment of the sociocultural dimension of pain actually encompass the entire psychosociocultural arena and include such areas as family and social life, work and home responsibilities, recreation and leisure activities, cultural background, and spiritual beliefs. Fong[136] presented a cultural assessment for nurses to use in identifying key aspects of an individual's cultural profile that may influence health practices. Areas she deemed important to assess included communication style, ethnic orientation, nutrition, family relationships, health beliefs, education, and religion.

The influence of family and friends on individuals' pain must be realized. For example, not only is an individual's style of expressing and coping with pain important,[137] but the family's views of pain expression and their influence on the patient are important as well. If verbal or nonverbal expressions of pain are deemed inappropriate (for whatever reason) by the family, a patient who complies with this wish presents a challenge for the nursing staff.

Similarly, the patient's own inherent willingness to report pain, take narcotic analgesics, and so on are important areas to assess. The existence and quality of patients' social support systems are additional examples of critical psychosociocultural information that the nurse needs. Since little research on the relationships among various psychosociocultural factors and cancer pain has been reported in the literature, it is difficult to recommend specific assessment parameters for all persons with pain. The guidelines suggested by Fong,[136] however, should prove helpful. Similar to the affective dimension is the idea that relevant psychosociocultural factors need to be assessed and then addressed in the care plan.

Nursing diagnoses

The outcome of a thorough baseline assessment of the cancer patient with pain should include a number of nursing diagnoses that serve to structure the design and implementation of the management plan. The North American Nursing Diagnosis Association (NANDA) has long included the diagnosis "Alteration in Comfort: Pain" in its taxonomy. In at least one clinical practice manual[138] this diagnosis has served as the conceptual framework for nursing management of patients with cancer pain. Recently Levin and colleagues[139] reported on a validation study of selected nursing diagnoses, including "Alteration in Comfort: Pain." Although this diagnosis was validated, nurse respondents indicated that critical defining characteristics included the patient's verbalization of pain and a facial mask of pain. The authors suggested that NANDA consider identifying these defining characteristics of pain as critical to the diagnosis.

Although the 1988 NANDA taxonomy of nursing diagnoses[140] included two diagnoses relevant to pain—"Pain" and "Chronic Pain"—McCaffery and Beebe[141] cited 18 other nursing diagnoses that the nurse should consider as part of the assessment process. These include anxiety, constipation, ineffective individual coping, diversional activity deficit, fatigue, fear, knowledge deficit (specify), impaired physical mobility, powerlessness, feeding self-care deficit, bathing/hygiene self-care deficit, dressing/grooming self-care deficit, toileting self-care deficit, sexual dysfunction, sleep pattern disturbance, social isolation, spiritual distress (distress of the human spirit), and altered thought processes. Certainly, the inclusion of *all* relevant nursing diagnoses can only serve to focus management efforts on the need for multiple disciplines to become involved in the treatment of a multidimensional phenomenon.

Assessment tools

There is an extensive literature on instruments to measure and/or assess clinical pain, including cancer pain.[142-145] A detailed discussion of these tools is beyond the scope of this chapter, but general information about types of tools and their appropriate uses should help the nurse select the best tool for a given situation.

Pain assessment tools can be classified by the number of dimensions they can be used to assess.[142] Unidimensional tools focus on one dimension of the pain experience, such as sensory, and within that dimension focus on a specific parameter, such as pain intensity. Ten-centimeter visual analog scales (VAS) (anchors of no pain and worst possible pain) or verbal descriptor scales (VDS) (none, mild, moderate, severe) are examples of unidimensional tools. Multidimensional tools focus on two or more dimensions of the pain experience. The McGill Pain Questionnaire[26] provides the major and best-known example.

The variety of unidimensional tools available for assessment of pain is limited. Most commonly used are the VAS and VRS scales to assess pain intensity. Although these scales have clearly documented reliability and validity in cancer-related pain,[142,145,146] they assess only one aspect of pain (even though it is a critical one). They can serve, however, as excellent ways to evaluate the success of specific interventions for pain, most notably analgesics[56] but also other interventions studied in randomized clinical trials.[147]

The variety of available multidimensional tools is far more extensive. The previously mentioned McGill Pain Questionnaire (MPQ), although originally developed to assess multidimensional aspects of pain in general, has been shown to be reliable and valid in a number of different cancer patient populations.[26-29,34,36,148] It measures sensory, affective, evaluative, and miscellaneous aspects of pain, pain intensity, pattern of pain, location of pain, and factors related to pain, such as sleep. The disadvantages of the MPQ include lengthy administration time and verbal descriptors of pain that are not understood by all patients. As a result, Melzack[149] developed the short-form version of the MPQ, which demonstrated beginning evidence of reliability and validity in his initial study. As of this writing, its use in patients with cancer pain has not been reported, but it appears to be a useful tool with applicability to the cancer pain patient population.

The Brief Pain Inventory (BPI) is another tool for assessment of multidimensional aspects of pain in general, but it has had fairly extensive use in cancer pain.[74,150,151] This tool includes location and intensity of pain as well as interference with mood, social relationships, walking ability, sleep, normal work, enjoyment of life, and other areas. The use of the BPI in the clinical setting of cancer pain by individuals who were not involved in its development has not been reported in the literature, so its reliability and validity are unclear. Nevertheless, it appears to be a tool that can be useful to nurses in the pain-assessment process, particularly because of its focus on areas that pain interferes with.

Recently devised multidimensional tools for the assessment of cancer pain provide a wider picture of an individual's pain than simply the intensity part of the sensory dimension; they are short, easy to administer, and thus more clinically useful. The Memorial Pain Assessment Card (MPAC) is one example.[152] It consists of three VASs designed to measure pain intensity, pain relief, and mood. In addition, it has a section of verbal descriptors of pain intensity (eg, just noticeable, mild, moderate, etc). The initial report suggested that the tool was reliable and valid for assessment of the pain of individual patients as well as for use as an outcome measure in clinical trials, but further work is clearly needed. Since it is short and easy to administer, it offers a clinically useful assessment method for monitoring responses to pain interventions; however, these characteristics make it less than ideal for baseline pain assessments.

McMillan et al[153] attempted to combine methods of baseline and ongoing assessment in an approach that included two tools for assessing and managing cancer pain. Their Pain Assessment Tool was designed to collect baseline subjectivity information from patients related to their pain history, intensity, location, quality, pattern, mitigating or exacerbating factors, and effects on other aspects of daily living, while their Pain Flow Sheet (PFS) was designed to collect continuous (ongoing) data on pain intensity, sedation level and other symptoms related to pain medications, use of alternative interventions for pain, and analgesic therapies. The PFS is based on the nursing process. Both tools show evidence of reliability and validity and appear to be clinically relevant for cancer patients. The authors have urged their use in clinical practice with adaptation to individual agencies as needed, according to a personal communication from S. McMillan (1989).

A similar approach was reported by Walker and colleagues,[154] who developed a chart for use in assessment and monitoring of chronic cancer pain. The chart provided for baseline information, including description of pain, pain intensity, mitigating and exacerbating factors, location of pain, and presence of pain during the night, at rest, or on movement. It also provided for ongoing assessment of pain intensity, location, analgesia, and patients' activities and comments. The authors recommended that the chart be considered for use primarily in patients with straightforward pain problems rather than those with unresolved or intractable pain, since they believed its use in the latter instance served "only as a reminder of the problem to both patient and staff." Although this is certainly open to debate, the usefulness of the chart, especially when used by *all* health professionals involved in pain management, was indisputable.

Children with cancer pain represent a unique challenge. Because of children's developmental characteristics, many of the assessment parameters discussed above are inappropriate. For example, infants and very young children lack verbal skills and therefore cannot tell others what their pain feels like, where it is located, and what makes it better or worse. According to Beyer and Levin,[155] the "most pressing problem impacting on pain control to date has been the lack of valid and reliable methods to measure or assess pain intensity in children."

Several instruments designed to measure pain in children 3 years of age and older have shown evidence of reliability and validity.[155] These tools included the Oucher Scale[155] and the Children's Hospital of Eastern Ontario Pain Scale (CHEOPS), which is a behavioral scale for rating postoperative pain.[156] Additional tools recommended for assessment of pain intensity include numerical scales (for ages 10 and older), the Wong/Baker Faces Rating Scale, the Eland Color Scale, and the Hester Poker Chip Scale.[141] A discussion of each of these tools is beyond the scope of this chapter, but the reader who needs more information is referred to the sources cited.

Because of children's varying developmental levels, cognitive skills, and behavioral manifestations of pain, nurses are urged to use a multidimensional approach to assessment of pain.[141] This approach includes conducting discussions about pain with child and family, obtaining a self-report from the child if possible, identifying the presence of pathologic conditions that could cause pain, observing behavioral manifestations of pain such as vocalizations or facial expressions, and considering a trial of analgesics with careful attention to the child's responses.

The choice of which tool or tools to use for assessment of pain in both adults and children depends on several factors, including purpose (baseline or ongoing evaluation); the information that is required (unidimensional or multidimensional); patient characteristics, such as age, cognitive abilities, type of pain, level of acuity, and physical function; environmental variables, such as type of clinical setting (inpatient, outpatient, home, hospice); and, finally, available time and/or skills of the nursing staff. Less important than the actual tool used for assessment is the performance of a thorough baseline assessment followed by regular, systematic ongoing assessments. Also of importance is the need for nurses to document their assessments in a manner appropriate for their clinical settings. These processes of assessment and documentation are critical to successful management of pain in cancer patients, regardless of their clinical setting or demographic and clinical characteristics.

Developmental Issues

Since cancer is a group of diseases that affects individuals across the lifespan, the pain associated with it likewise occurs in different age groups. Two populations—children and the elderly—require special consideration in the areas of pain assessment and management. This need was highlighted by a statement issued by the presidents of the International Pain Foundation and the International Association for the Study of Pain, which stated, in part: "We are appalled, too, by the fact that pain is most poorly managed in those most defenseless against it—the young and the elderly."[157] There are specific considerations relevant to the assessment and management of pain in these two groups that, in general, have been neglected in the nursing literature on cancer pain.

Children

While the incidence of cancer per se in children is not exceedingly high as compared to that in adults, cancer is the second leading killer of children 1 to 14 years of age.[77] The incidence and prevalence of cancer-related pain (due to tumor or treatment) in children of all ages are generally unknown. One study, conducted in a tertiary referral, clinical research setting found that 48% of inpatients and 27% of outpatients were experiencing pain.[158] When only patients with pain were examined, relapse of cancer was found to be related to the pain in 46% of the inpatients and 26% of the outpatients. Interestingly, the majority of patients with pain had treatment-related pain, most commonly due to mucositis, surgery, or neuropathic causes.

Pain has also been studied as a presenting symptom in children and young adults with newly diagnosed cancers.[159] Of 92 patients with leukemia, lymphoma, or sarcomas of soft tissue or bone, 72 (78%) were observed to have pain at initial presentation. For 31 of them, pain was the only symptom of their cancer at the time of diagnosis. Similarly, a survey in an Italian pediatric cancer population indicated that a majority of children with cancer experienced pain at some point during their illness.[160]

Assessment and management of pain in children with cancer have received little attention in the research arena.[161] The reasons for the paucity of published research are not entirely clear, but Stevens et al[162] proposed that they included theories of pain that were inadequate to explain children's pain, methodologic and measurement difficulties, and clinical dilemmas brought about by differences in interpretation of children's behaviors coupled with nurses' and children's personal beliefs, values, fears, and pain experiences.

The majority of existing research deals with the pain and distress of treatment-related procedures, such as bone marrow aspirations.[155,163] In fact, Eland[164] commented that nurses really knew very little about the experience of pain itself in children. It certainly is not at all clear whether the multidimensional nature of cancer pain described here applies to children's cancer pain.

What is known, however, is that the developmental level of children is directly related to how they perceive, interpret, and respond to pain, regardless of its cause.[165] Children's developmental stages have a number of implications for the assessment and management of their pain and, in fact, can be used to help clarify a number of misconceptions that are held by health professionals and others about children with pain.

Generally speaking, the facts about children's pain can be represented by the following statements[141]: There is significant evidence to indicate that neonates, including premature ones, do feel pain. Children who are verbally fluent may deny they have pain when, in fact, they *do* have it; this occurs when they have certain fears about pain, or when they have adapted to it and do not realize it is worsening. Children's lack of willingness or ability to express pain or request treatment for it does *not* mean they do not have it. The child who sleeps, plays, or is otherwise distracted may still have a good deal of pain; such distractions are a common coping method used by children with pain. Children do *not* tolerate pain better than adults do. Narcotics may be used safely in children, provided there is an understanding of the pharmacokinetics and the children are properly observed; their use in all age groups, including teenagers, is generally safe. Pain is *not* a harmless entity in children, without side effects or life-threatening potential; it has been documented that the presence of pain in neonates may be harmful because of stressful reactions, which can include prolonged crying leading to hypoxemia and increased heart rate and blood pressure.[166] There is also a possibility of long-term effects of having pain.[155]

The realities of children's highly variable responses to pain contribute to the challenge of assessing the phenomenon. These responses call for a multidimensional, multimethod approach to assessment. It is extremely important that parents be involved in the process and that the methods used be tailored to the child's age and developmental status.

The issue of undertreatment of children with pain is an important one. Although the evidence is not as massive as that documenting undertreatment of adults, there is clearly a problem in the pediatric arena. It was demonstrated that children who were hospitalized for surgery received very little of the analgesic medication ordered for them and that they received 26 times *less* than adults who had the same diagnoses.[167] Similarly, Schechter et al[168] demonstrated that hospitalized children and adults with the same diagnoses were treated differently with respect to administration of narcotics. Children were likely to have less narcotic than adults. One of the reasons suggested for the findings included the possibility that beliefs and attitudes of nursing and medical staff affected administration of drugs.

In a follow-up study of the attitudes of physicians toward pain in children, Schechter and Allen[169] found that although 75% of the sample believed that children experienced adultlike pain by the age of 2, 35% were somewhat or significantly concerned about the risks of addiction when narcotics were used. Pediatricians were significantly more likely than other specialists to view children as having adultlike pain and to prescribe narcotics to younger children. While this study provided some explanation for differences in how adult versus pediatric patients with pain are treated, there are probably other as yet unelucidated reasons.

Interventions for pain in children with cancer should be tailored to the type of pain they are experiencing.[161] Pain that is acute in nature and related to operative procedures may be treated in the same manner as adult postoperative pain (ie, with narcotics, including patient-controlled analgesia if the patient is old enough). It is important to note that children metabolize narcotics more quickly than adults do, so their doses may need to be scheduled more frequently.[161] Since needles and shots are uniformly hated by children, the intravenous route in the immediate postoperative period followed by the oral route when possible is the preferred strategy. Management of other types of treatment-related pain, such as that caused by esophagitis or oral mucositis, can be successfully implemented through the use of continuous intravenous and subcutaneous infusions of morphine.[170]

The treatment of acute, procedure-related pain is different. This type of pain is usually transient but is accompanied by a great deal of anxiety and fear. Interventions range from pharmacologic approaches (eg, sedatives) to cognitive and behavioral techniques (eg, relaxation or hypnosis). Sedatives, particularly the combination of meperidine, promethazine, and chlorpromazine (DPT) should be used with caution, since they do not decrease pain and anxiety[161] and they may cause respiratory depression.[171] Patterson and Klopovich[161] recommended the use of premedications for such procedures as bone marrow aspiration combined with cognitive/behavioral techniques as the procedure progressed. The efficacy of several techniques has been documented.[172,173]

Finally, the management of the pain associated with terminal cancer is a challenging area, since the goal is pain relief without undue sedation. Oral analgesics, administered around the clock, are often very helpful. Since children metabolize narcotics more quickly than adults, drugs with a longer duration of action, such as methadone, are advisable and have been shown to provide adequate pain relief.[174,175] When pain remains intractable, however, the parenteral route should be considered. A series of studies clearly demonstrated that continuous intravenous or subcutaneous infusions of morphine are safe and effective ways of relieving the pain of terminal cancer in children.[176,177]

In summary, the prevalence of cancer pain in children is inadequately documented but is clearly a significant clinical problem. Dispelling the misconceptions and misinformation that surround the assessment and management of pain in children is essential to the achievement of success. Although the research base of knowledge in this area is still limited, good assessment tools are continually being developed, and adequate interventions exist. The nurse caring for the pediatric cancer patient with pain plays a key role in managing this challenging problem.

The elderly

The elderly population in the United States (persons 65 years of age and older) more than doubled between 1950 and 1980 (from 12.3 million to 25.5 million), and one projection for the year 2030 is that the elderly population will increase to 64.3 million.[178] As this population increases in number, one would expect to see a corresponding increase in the incidence of cancer and cancer-related deaths. Current statistics indicate that 53% of all cancer deaths are in individuals between the ages of 55 and 74 and 34% are in individuals 75 years of age or older.[77]

The problem of cancer pain in elderly patients has been grossly neglected,[179,180] and prevalence surveys of pain are nonexistent. Ferrell[181] recently reviewed 11 textbooks on geriatric medicine and found that only two had chapters on pain in the elderly, with negligible content about cancer-related pain. Research in this area has been limited, and much of what is known about pain in the elderly is based on empirical observations and anecdotal reports.

A misconception that lay persons have about pain and the elderly is that pain is a normal sequela of aging.[141] As a result of this belief, elderly patients may not report pain as a problem since it is considered "normal." In one study of "younger" elderly versus "older" elderly, there was a trend for the older elderly to report pain less often.[182] Similarly, if health care professionals are told about pain by elderly patients, they may dismiss the complaint as insignificant since pain becomes a manifestation of the aging process. Although it may be true that people develop more chronic diseases as they age,[183] the experience of pain does not have to be an expectation.

The normal process of aging creates unique problems in the management of cancer pain, especially as related to assessment. With the prevalence of more chronic diseases, there will potentially exist multiple causes of the same complaint. The elderly experience greater alterations in the musculoskeletal system and are more vulnerable to acute and soft tissue pain.[184] Chronic problems, such as arthritis, degenerative disk disease, osteoporosis, and peripheral neuropathy, may confuse the pain problem for individuals who also have cancer-related pain.

Another unique problem is that the elderly may experience significant sensory and cognitive impairment.[141,180,184,185] The symptoms associated with these potential impairments alert the health care professional to be especially astute in obtaining a careful, detailed pain history.[141,178,180,184] The risk of inadequate histories due to underreporting of symptoms, memory deficits, and concomitant depression-related symptoms may lead to an inaccurate pain diagnosis and inappropriate treatment. A very important piece of assessment data to obtain in a history of the elderly patient is any change from baseline behaviors, usual routines, and social interactions. A gradual loss of physical health, changes in family structure, limited economic resources, and a loss of social status can greatly influence the pain problem.[141,178,186] Newton[184] stated: ". . . elderly patients have a considerable morbidity due to inadequately treated pain which includes confusion, withdrawal, agitation, anorexia, immobility, depression, and (perhaps) a predisposition to develop chronic pain."

A third major unique problem is the issue of the sensitivity of elderly patients to both perception of pain and sensitivity to pharmacologic interventions. The literature about perceptual sensitivity reveals contradictions. Bayer et al[187] reviewed symptoms of acute myocardial infarction in elderly patients and found that chest pain was reported less frequently than other symptoms, especially by patients more than 85 years of age. They proposed several explanations to account for this finding: higher pain threshold, autonomic dysfunction, or cortical failure from neurologic disease. McMillan[72] found that younger cancer patients (less than 55 years of age) reported significantly more intense pain than older patients (over 55 years). Conversely, another study found no statistically significant differences in pain intensity in cancer outpatients less than 60 years of age.[35]

TABLE 20-8 Age-Related Changes and Drug Pharmacologic Properties

Absorption	↑ Gastric pH, ↓ absorptive surface and ↓ splanchnic blood flow Change in GI motility
Distribution	↑ Fat, ↓ lean body mass, total body water, and serum albumin
Metabolism	↓ Liver mass, liver blood flow, enzyme activity, and inducibility
Excretion	↓ Renal blood flow, glomerular filtration rate, tubular secretory function
Receptor sensitivity	Altered receptor number and affinity, second messenger function, and cellular responses

Source: Reproduced with permission from Ouslander JG: Drug therapy in the elderly. Ann Intern Med 95:711-722, 1981.

Issues related to sensitivity and response to pharmacologic interventions have been examined by several investigators. Physiologic responses to medication in light of changes in absorption, distribution, metabolism, and excretion of drugs are a major concern in the elderly population.[141,178,185,188-190] Table 20-8 depicts age-related changes in these four pharmacologic properties of drugs. The changes reflect the contribution of the gastrointestinal system, nutritional composites, and hepatic and renal function and relate to studies demonstrating that, with increasing age, the elderly reported an increase in pain relief when given the same narcotic (at the same dose) as younger patients.[191,192] If increasing age is associated with a decrease in morphine clearance,[191] then the toxic effects of narcotics and other drugs are potentially much greater.

An issue related to toxicity is whether the elderly are at greater risk of adverse drug reactions. Problems with study design and definitions of adverse reaction have contributed to the conflicting evidence in this area.[193] Since the elderly have more chronic diseases and take more medications for these illnesses, the risk of adverse drug reactions may be higher solely because of increased drug intake. The interactions of multiple drug therapies are also an important issue related to toxicities.

A fourth and final issue relevant to pain in the elderly follows naturally from the issues already discussed. If assessment of cancer pain in the elderly is complicated by the possibility of multiple causative factors, sensory and cognitive impairment, differences in sensitivity, and pain relief because of normal physiologic aging, does this population of patients receive adequate analgesic management? Several reports indicate that the elderly are prescribed fewer narcotic analgesics than younger patients.[180,194,195] Portenoy[179] raised a very important issue. If the elderly perceive pain less often, indicating a lower prevalence of pain, then less frequent prescribing of analgesics is appropriate. If, however, the elderly experience pain similar to that of the younger population of patients and choose not to report it, or if they respond more slowly to painful stimuli, indicating a higher prevalence of pain, then underprescribing creates needless suffering. As in other areas related to cancer pain, more well-controlled, epidemiologic studies of the prevalence of pain in the elderly are needed to help answer this question about appropriate analgesic management.

In summary, the problem of cancer pain in the elderly population is very important. As individuals enter the later stages of life the risk of cancer increases, and thus cancer pain increases. Specific attention to the unique physiologic, pharmacologic, psychologic, and sociologic issues for these individuals is crucial for appropriate, successful management of cancer pain. Listed below are general recomendations for management of medications in the elderly[189]:

1. Evaluate carefully for treatable, underlying conditions.
2. Avoid interactions between drugs.
3. Begin with smallest dose of specific drug.
4. Adjust dosage to accommodate for hepatic and renal abnormalities.
5. Individualize and simplify regimens.
6. Consider visual, auditory abilities/disabilities when giving instructions and labeling medications.
7. Address compliance issue by assuring patients can afford the medications, can obtain the medication from a pharmacy, and can open the containers.
8. Monitor for toxicity, efficacy, and compliance.
9. Use caution in drugs with long half-life.
10. Be aware of added toxicity from adjuvant analgesics.

Sociocultural Issues

Sociocultural factors that affect nurses' assessment and management of the individual with cancer pain can include a wide range of variables. For the purpose of the following discussion, attention is focused on two specific areas—(1) sociocultural variables that influence the nurse's own perception of and response to the individual with pain and (2) approaches for dealing with individuals whose ethnocultural backgrounds are different from that of the nurse.

Nurses' responses to individuals with pain

Reactions of nurses to the pain and suffering of patients may influence subsequent interactions and interventions. Davitz and Davitz [196,197] reported on a series of studies over a 12-year period to examine factors related to nurses' inferences of physical pain and psychologic distress, collectively termed *suffering*. Nurses of different cultural backgrounds inferred different degrees of suffering and in general believed that psychologic distress caused more suffering than physical distress.[198,199] Cross-culturally, nurses tended to infer less psychologic distress in children than in adults and more pain in females than in males.[199] In a study of the influence of cultural background on nurses' attitudes and care of the oncology patient,[200] data on questions related to pain revealed that African Zulu nurses perceived males as experiencing more pain whereas South African English and American nurses perceived the opposite. Other data indicated, however, that the type and severity of the illness and the patient's age and sex differentially influenced the nurse's inferences of suffering.[201]

The influence of nursing specialty area and length of nursing experiences on inferences of suffering has been studied, but results are conflicting.[196,198,201-203] Age, educational preparation, shift assignment, and relative job satisfaction of nurses do not appear to be related to inferences of suffering.[196,201,203] In one study, black nurses inferred higher degrees of psychologic distress than white nurses, and nurses who had experienced physical pain themselves inferred higher degrees of physical pain.[196] A recent study[204] found that the intensity of a nurse's personal pain experience significantly influenced assessment of the patient's pain, in that nurses who had experienced pain themselves were more sensitive to pain in their patients.

Various patient characteristics have also been studied in relation to nurses' inferences of suffering. Type, severity, and stage of disease affect nurses' inferences, with worse illnesses (eg, cancer, trauma) receiving higher scores.[196,198,201,202] One study[205] revealed that the presence of physical disease positively affected the nurses' assessments of patients' pain while duration of pain had a negative effect. In addition, nurses' judgments of pain based on the presence or absence of nonverbal indicators of pain (eg, groaning, thrashing) may not correspond with patients' self-reports of pain.[206] Patients' behavioral manifestations of pain have been interpreted differently by nurses of different cultural backgrounds as well. Martin and Belcher[200] found that a disproportionately high number of American nurses thought that screaming indicated the most severe pain, while South African English nurses thought that quietness indicated the most pain. Relationships between patients' age, sex, socioeconomic status, ethnic background, and nurses' inferences of pain remain unclear, since the literature provides conflicting findings, indicating a clear need for researchers to continue to pursue these lines of investigation.[196,198,201,203,207]

The above information should be useful to the nurse because it makes clear the many possible factors that may influence how the nurse responds to the patient with cancer pain.

Approaches to sociocultural differences

"The American health care system, its philosophies, and its practices have their roots in white, middle-class values and beliefs."[208] This quotation makes the point that in the American system of health care, provision is frequently not made for even acknowledging the person's ethnocultural perspective, let alone understanding or using it in the planning of health care interventions. There is a tendency on the part of nurses and other health care providers to take an ethnocentric approach (ie, to believe that their own health practices are superior to those of others).[136] Since nurses espouse the notion of care tailored to individuals' unique and specific needs, the idea of not only accepting cultural diversity but incorporating it into plans for care is essential to actually achieving care.

With respect to pain in particular, it is important to realize that different ethnic groups express pain and suffering differently, as was noted earlier in this chapter. The nurse's interpretation of individuals' behaviors and verbalizations with respect to pain should be based on knowledge of how the patient's culture views responses to pain.[136] Respect for cultures other than one's own, and for the fact that people have specific beliefs and behaviors that emanate from their cultural background, is known as cultural sensitivity. Although providing nursing care for people of other cultures can be extremely challenging, the nurse's commitment to care and to supporting a patient's integrity and dignity can be exemplified by attempts to learn as much as possible about the individual's ethnocultural background and its influences on beliefs and behaviors with respect to health and illness.[209]

Several authors have made recommendations that should be useful to nurses caring for individuals of different backgrounds. Fong[136] discussed the importance of developing rapport as the foundation of successful nursing interventions. She urged the use of good manners, a broad and open attitude, and maintenance of flexibility. Kagawa-Singer[209] highlighted the importance of developing good communication with patients and their families, followed by facilitation of their integrating the disease process and its treatment into their lives. A key principle is the use of negotiation to achieve feasible treatment plans and to enlist the patient's and family's participation in reaching treatment goals. Similarly, Louie[210] made a number of recommendations to help avoid culture-related conflicts in the care of Chinese patients. These recommendations, however, should be generically quite useful and included identification and achievement of mutual goals, compromise and integration of different health care practices into the care plan, identification and discussion of nursing interventions with patient and family, stressing the importance of health education, use of vital teaching materials if language is a problem, and seeking of additional information and assistance from cultural organizations and resources when necessary.

Although very little has been written specifically on dealing with cancer pain, or even with pain in general, in individuals of different cultural backgrounds, there is some literature on ethnocultural nursing practice that should prove helpful in dealing with specific cultural groups who have cancer pain. Fong's general discussion of ethnicity and nursing practice is extremely good, particularly with respect to cultural assessment.[136] Kagawa-Singer[209] provided an excellent discussion of oncology nursing in people of Hispanic and Japanese-American backgrounds. Reizian and Meleis,[68] as mentioned earlier, described the responses of Arab-Americans to pain and gave recommendations for nursing care, particularly in the critical care setting. Further information about persons with Middle Eastern backgrounds is given in another paper.[211] Louie[210] gave an excellent presentation of nursing care of the patient of Chinese background and, finally, Capers[212] wrote about Afro-Americans and implications for the care of these individuals.

Related to the area of sociocultural differences is the national problem of drug abuse, which creates unique and different management challenges for health care professionals when a recovered substance abuser or an active abuser has cancer pain. For the recovered substance abuser, opioid analgesics may contribute to a reversion to previous addictive behavior; thus the patient should be asked whether the use of narcotics will be detrimental to his or her recovery. Similarly, the patient should be asked whether he or she has any concerns about using narcotics for pain relief. The use of aggressive nonnarcotic approaches should be maximized in this population.[141]

The active substance abuser may be more of a concern to physicians and nurses. Twycross and Lack[32] discussed errors that may occur with this population: (1) Pain may be discounted so that, no matter what the patient says, it is unlikely that adequate medication will be provided, or (2) the patient may be treated as a nonaddict, receiving higher doses than actually needed.

With this group of patients, it is important that an adversarial relationship does not begin or escalate between the patient and the staff. As with any other patient, the substance abuser's report of pain should not be questioned or doubted.[141] Withholding of appropriate medications should not be used as a form of punishment.[141] Communication between all members of the health team, including the patient, about how pain will be managed should be instituted early in the course of contact with the patient. The assistance of a professional person experienced in dealing with substance abuse may be helpful.[213]

Twycross and Lack[32] recommend changing from parenteral administration of analgesics to use of oral or rectal routes so that the association between street drugs and pain relief is not present. Regardless of a patient's history of substance abuse, he or she is entitled to receive reasonable, adequate care for a concomitant cancer pain problem. Obstacles to the achievement of this goal need to be discussed, examined, and resolved to assure pain relief.

One final important area for nurses to include in their care of the sociocultural dimension of individuals' pain is that of spirituality. Little has been written about spirituality in the nursing literature, but the subject is beginning to receive more attention, particularly as it relates to sociocultural differences, the nursing process, chronic illness, and dying.[214] Of special importance for oncology nursing is Jacik's excellent chapter on the spiritual care of the dying adult,[215] in which (among many other important things) she emphasizes the need for measures to keep the individual free of pain as death approaches.

Terminal Care

Twycross[216] wrote: "The aim of terminal care is to help the patient, despite the cancer and increasing physical limitations, to go on having a good quality of life until he dies." In essence, this aim underlies all approaches to terminal care, regardless of setting. It is the responsibility of the health care professional to create an environment for the dying patient that allows a peaceful death.[217]

Philosophical, organizational, and practical aspects of caring for terminally ill individuals with cancer pain have been described for inpatient and home hospice settings,[215,218-220] the home care setting,[32,81] extended care facilities,[221] and the special situation of children and adolescents.[222] There are several key aspects of caring for these individuals, and these need to be considered by nurses.

The focus of terminal care is on relief of pain and other symptoms, as well as psychologic support of both the patient and the family.[216] Teamwork is a requisite to the success of these efforts.[216,218] Death is often accompanied by great fear, a normal human response that is part of the survival instinct.[216] In the care of terminal illness, not only are the dying afraid of death, but the living are as well. Withdrawal from those who are dying is a common reaction; yet remaining with the individual is one of the most important aspects of terminal care. Jacik[215] wrote: "Human presence is a priceless source of comfort to dying persons." For those dying with pain, the knowledge that health care providers and others are not only present but continually focusing on relieving the pain gives great comfort.

Related to continual efforts at relieving pain are the issues of assessment and treatment, particularly when pain worsens or new pain appears. The goal of minimizing pain and increasing comfort in the terminally ill patient must not obstruct the normal response to complaints of pain or restrict the range of interventions that might be considered or attempted. There is no reason why terminally ill persons with worsening or new symptoms of pain should be evaluated, diagnosed, and treated any differently than nonterminally ill persons with cancer pain. For example, the development of new and painful metastatic lesions of the bone in a home hospice patient should not preclude use of radiotherapy if appropriate, even if it means that the patient must be moved. The goal is increased comfort, and all possible means to achieve it should be considered.

A flexible and adjustable care plan to meet the patient's changing needs as the disease progresses is essential.[217] Such tailoring involves the use of multiple interventions, including pharmacologic therapy, and the expertise to use these interventions properly. Often there is inadequate knowledge of pharmacokinetics, neurology, and medical oncology.[223] Similarly, underutilization of narcotics can erode the patients' confidence in the medical system and bring their dying into sharper focus.[218] Indeed, adjuvant drugs have not been used as often as they could be in the terminal care setting.[224] Although nonpharmacologic, noninvasive interventions for pain are appropriate in the terminal cancer patient, their use and evaluation have not been addressed in the literature. Since these interventions often are instituted by nurses, carefully planned studies of their effectiveness seem indicated.

In some clinical settings, such as hospice or home care, adjustments or modifications of interventions need to be made to accommodate the setting[32,218] (eg, the formulation of rectal diazepam or the provision of such systems as reminder cards and special containers for home administration of narcotics). Considerable creativity may go into devising methods for patients and their families to manage interventions on their own. These activities, as well as the ongoing need for assessment of pain and coordination of pain management, are well within the scope of practice for oncology nurses who care for the terminally ill.

In summary, a number of basic principles and special considerations need to be employed by nurses who care for all cancer patients with pain—the multidisciplinary approach, understanding the scope of nursing practice, accurate assessment and diagnosis, developmental issues, sociocultural issues, and terminal care issues. Awareness and use of the information presented above will help the nurse identify and assess cancer pain and plan, implement, coordinate and evaluate its interdisciplinary management.[75] Specific approaches to the management of cancer pain follow.

INTERVENTIONS

Methods of managing cancer pain can be categorized into three major approaches (Figure 20-3). In the first, treatment is aimed at the underlying pathologic condition or the organic cause of the pain. In most cases, this approach consists of attempts to reduce or eradicate the tumor. The second approach is used to change the individual's perception or sensation of pain. A wide variety of techniques are available to help achieve this goal. Finally, the third approach consists of a number of interventions that are aimed at diminishing the suffering component of pain. It is important to realize that interventions from each of these three approaches may be, and usually are, used simultaneously in the treatment of a given individual.

It is also important to realize that a multidisciplinary treatment strategy is clearly the optimal approach to effective management of pain. In the sections that follow, specific interventions and the role of the nurse within each of the three major treatment approaches are discussed.

Treatment of Underlying Pathology

Chemotherapy, radiotherapy, and surgery are the major modalities used to treat cancer when cure is the intent, but they can also be useful when palliation is the goal. Hormonal therapy is a fourth treatment modality used for palliative treatment of certain tumors and will be discussed along with chemotherapy.

Chemotherapy and hormonal therapy

In 1979 Bonadonna and Molinari[225] wrote: "The specific impact of medical treatment on pain produced by

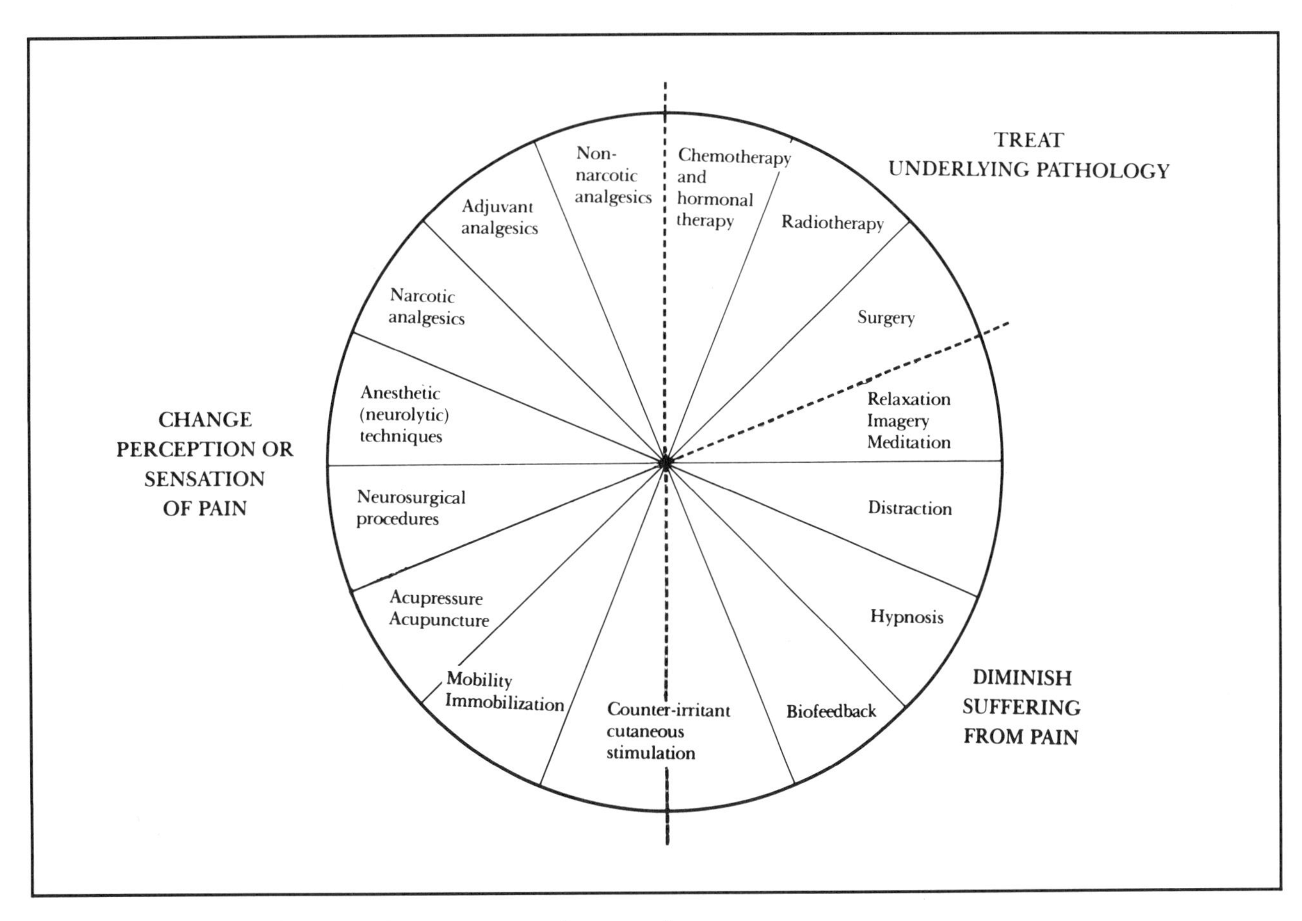

FIGURE 20-3 Three major approaches to treatment of cancer pain.

advanced cancer has not yet been the subject of a detailed report." They proposed that the main reason was that responses to antineoplastic drugs were generally considered significant only if tumor regression was documented objectively. Improvement of subjective clinical phenomena such as pain was not regarded as meaningful. In 1983 Russell[226] commented that "few reports on the results of chemotherapy give details of how pain relief is measured. . . ." In 1989 MacDonald[227] reported that in a review of 24 phase II-III studies in patients with esophagus, stomach, pancreas, and non–small-cell lung cancer published in the *Journal of Clinical Oncology* in 1986-1987, he found that not one of them measured the impact of the chemotherapy on patients' pain. In only one study was pain even mentioned, and in that one it was viewed as a factor that could influence patients' responses to chemotherapy!

An argument was made for the importance of measuring pain relief as an outcome in cancer clinical trials, particularly those in individuals with poor-prognosis tumors such as those of the lung, pancreas, stomach, and esophagus.[227] Others[225] held the same view and stressed the importance of measuring pain relief when effective first-line chemotherapeutic regimens were used. The challenges of standardizing and measuring pain in such endeavors may be partly addressed through the use of a clinical staging system for cancer pain, developed to include all the known prognostic factors for response to treatment.[228]

In the years since 1979, however, some evidence has accumulated to suggest that various chemotherapeutic drugs have some beneficial effects on cancer pain. Anecdotal data indicate that patients with breast and prostate cancer and some with leukemia and lymphoma experienced very good to complete relief of pain from their chemotherapy.[225] In a very small sample of persons with colorectal cancer, Estes et al[229] reported that intra-arterial 5-fluorouracil, with or without whole-body hyperthermia, was beneficial in helping to control pelvic pain. In a review of seven studies of single drugs, it was found that one study reported pain relief in women with breast cancer after treatment with doxorubicin.[226] In 11 studies in which combination chemotherapy was used for bone metastases from breast cancer, pain relief ranging from 40% to 94% was reported as an outcome in all of them.[226]

Thus it appears that some chemotherapeutic agents may provide some relief of pain in some types of tumors. It has been suggested that, for gastrointestinal cancers, lung cancer, esophageal and prostate cancers, sarcomas, and melanoma, where chemotherapy was unlikely to significantly increase survival time, it might palliate symptoms. Further research is needed, however, to document the efficacy of chemotherapeutic regimens in relieving cancer pain.

Hormonal therapy has been used for many years to treat breast and prostate cancer; it provides palliation with fewer side effects and may afford significant relief of pain, sometimes even for prolonged periods of time.[230] Investigators have reported good responses in patients with painful bone metastases from breast and prostate cancers to a variety of therapeutic agents, including estrogen, androgen, progestin, aminoglutethimide, and corticosteroids.[83,231]

Radiotherapy

Radiation has long been used to treat painful bone metastases, most often in cancers of the breast, lung, and prostate.[225,230,232] In addition, it may be helpful in relieving pain due to epidural cord or nerve root compression, brain metastases or primary brain tumors, hepatic metastases, and advanced gynecologic, gastrointestinal, or upper aerodigestive cancers.[230] There appears to be no standard prescribed doses of radiation for specific tumor problems, and there appears to be little correlation between dose of radiation and extent of relief or between dose required for relief and the histologic tumor type. Relief of pain can begin to occur within 24 to 48 hours after initiation of radiotherapy.[230]

The evidence of the efficacy of radiotherapy in relieving cancer pain caused by bone metastases is quite convincing. Ford and Yarnold[232] reviewed 11 studies and found that in 10 of them patients reported pain relief. Abrams and Hansen[230] cited several studies in which patients with cancer of the prostate, lung, and breast experienced significant relief of their pain following radiotherapy. A study by the Radiation Therapy Oncology Group (RTOG) indicated that 90% of individuals with bone metastases experienced some relief of their pain; 54% had complete relief, although initial pain intensity and site of the primary lesion affected responses to some degree.[233] A second RTOG study revealed that 73% of the patients who had multiple symptomatic bone lesions experienced some relief of pain and 20% had complete relief when treated with half-body radiation.[234] The advantages of this method of delivery included faster pain relief and less evidence of recurrence of pain in the treated area than with conventional delivery methods.

Surgery

Surgery as a modality for treating cancer pain can take many forms, but the primary goal is palliation. Direct palliative surgery either helps resolve oncologic emergencies or other serious clinical situations, such as epidural spinal cord compression or bowel obstruction,[235] or it helps improve the therapeutic effects of the previous two modalities by reducing tumor burden. Indirect palliative surgery involves ablation of endocrine glands in endocrine-related tumors (eg, ovariectomy for advanced breast cancer). Two other forms of palliative surgery for individuals with pain consist of procedures to provide direct access to areas of tumor (eg, implants of infusion pumps or radiation seeds) and procedures performed on various areas of the CNS to interrupt the pain pathway (see below).

Although very little data are available to indicate the success of these various surgical approaches in relieving pain, in many clinical situations there is anecdotal relief of pain. Chalmers,[236] for example, described a number of orthopedic procedures useful in dealing with skeletal metastases. Table 20-9 shows clinical conditions and tumors that may benefit from various types of palliative surgery; relief of pain from these conditions is obviously an outcome of the surgical procedures.

The treatment modalities described offer one approach to the relieving of cancer pain—treatment of the underlying pathology. Nursing responsibilities in relation to these methods are fairly standard and quite similar to those associated with use of the same methods in first-line, curative therapy. In the second major approach to treatment of cancer pain, the role and responsibilities of the nurse assume greater proportions.

Change in Perception and Sensation of Pain

As can be seen in Figure 20-3, the number of interventions in this approach is quite extensive. The most effective and commonly used techniques are included here in some detail. Techniques used less frequently, and with a lesser nursing role, are discussed briefly. Pharmacologic therapy—consisting of nonnarcotics, adjuvant drugs, and narcotics—is a major responsibility of nurses and, as discussed previously, is an area about which much more knowledge and skill are needed.

Pharmacologic therapy

The pharmacologic management of cancer pain accounts for the major source of pain treatment. Yet the problem of inadequate and undertreatment of cancer pain is a major issue related to pharmacologic management. Regardless of *when* a patient has a pain problem as a result of cancer or its treatment, the use of various pharmacologic strategies should be incorporated into the plan of care.

During the past 11 years there have been a number of publications addressing the overall issue of pharmacologic management of cancer pain,[32,123,141,237-248] This noninclusive, selected list of resources gives health care professionals ample opportunity to have access to information about pharmacologic management of cancer-related pain. The sections that follow include the main pharmacologic therapies used in drug treatment approaches to cancer pain.

Nonnarcotics The World Health Organization (WHO) recently developed and has been promoting a "ladder" for cancer pain management that includes nonopioids in all three of its steps.[249] In the first step, these drugs are used as the primary therapy. In the second step they are used in conjunction with a weak opioid, and in the last step they are suggested only as an option.

TABLE 20-9 Major Clinical Conditions Requiring Palliative Surgery for Pain

Clinical Condition	Tumor	Type of Palliative Surgery
Breast tumor	Ulcerating Fungating	Simple mastectomy
Abdominal cancer		
Intestinal occlusion	Colorectal carcinoma ovarian, peritoneal carcinomatosis	Colostomy GI bypass
Intractable pelvic pain	Colorectal carcinomas	Intra-arterial infusion (5FU, Nitrogen mustard)
Serious ascites	Breast, ovarian cancer	Peritoneovenous shunt
Acute urinary tract occlusion	Upper tract: flank and retroperitoneal tumor Pelvic tract: cancer of cervix, prostate, rectum	Nephrostomy Cutaneous ureterostomy Cystostomy
Rectovesical fistula		Colostomy
Rectovaginal fistula		Colostomy
Tumors of the extremities		
Large lesions	Sarcomas, epithelial tumors, metastatic visceral tumors	Reductive surgery (amputation) Disarticulation
Pathological fracture	Metastases from lung, breast, prostatic, renal, thyroid carcinomas Primary advanced bone and soft tissue tumors	Amputation Prostheses Pins
Axial nervous system involvement		
Spinal cord compression	Metastases from lung, breast, prostatic, renal, thyroid carcinomas Lymphomas, sarcomas	Decompressive laminectomy

Source: Azzarelli A, Crispino S: Palliative surgery in cancer pain treatment, in Swerdlow M, Ventafridda V (eds): Cancer Pain. Lancaster, England, MTP Press, 1987, pp 97-103.

Although nonnarcotic drugs are different in their chemical structure and have many different classifications, they are often presented in two distinct categories: (1) nonsteroidal anti-inflammatory drugs (NSAIDS), which include aspirin, and (2) acetaminophen. The similarities between categories is that both have antipyretic and analgesic properties. Their site of action is the peripheral nervous system, and even though there have been reports of central nervous system (CNS) toxicities,[250] they generally do not affect the CNS.[251] In addition, the nonnarcotic agents do not produce physical dependence, tolerance, or addiction, and they have a maximum ceiling effect for analgesic potential. Except for acetaminophen, nearly all the NSAIDs have antiplatelet properties as well. This potential hematologic problem is caused by irreversible acetylation of platelet cyclooxygenase, which inhibits platelet aggregation.[10]

The mechanism of action for these drugs has been well described. The NSAIDs inhibit cyclooxygenase in peripheral tissues, which prevents arachidonic acid from converting to prostaglandin.[10,251] This action alters transduction in primary afferent nociceptors. Prostaglandins are associated with pain, which results from injury or inflammation, and they can sensitize pain receptors to mechanical and chemical stimulation.

The indication for using nonnarcotic drugs in patients with cancer is pain that is mild to moderate in its intensity. Non-cancer-related pain, such as that caused by arthritis, primary dysmenorrhea, muscle sprains, orthopedic injuries, and toothache are commonly treated with nonnarcotic drugs. In cancer-related pain, NSAIDs are useful for (1) metastatic bone pain, (2) pain from mechanical compression of tendons, muscles, pleura, and peritoneum, and (3) nonobstructive visceral pain.[252]

Studies of NSAIDs in persons with cancer pain indicate that the drugs are efficacious in providing pain relief. Moertel et al[253] found aspirin (ASA), 650 mg, to be superior to three other nonnarcotic agents (acetaminophen, phenacetin, mefenamic acid), three weak narcotics (pentazocine, codeine, propoxyphene), and one phenothiazine (promazine). ASA and naproxen provided equal pain relief, with statistically significant improvement from baseline pain for both drugs.[254] In a study that examined two different dosing schedules of naproxen, Levich et al[255] reported that both schedules provided pain relief in approximately 80% of the patients after the same initial dose, but that the higher-dose group had greater pain relief without a significant increase in adverse side effects. A drug recently approved by the Food and Drug Administration, diclofenac, was compared to ASA/codeine combinations and nefopam (not available in the United States). Although patients in all three groups had improved pain relief, side effects were less frequent with diclofenac than with the other two analgesics.[256]

The combination of nonnarcotics and narcotics administered simultaneously is designed to enhance analgesia and decrease toxicity.[257] One of the earliest studies with cancer patients demonstrated the beneficial effect of aspirin and morphine over morphine alone.[258] Another nonnarcotic agent, ibuprofen, was the drug of choice in two studies, the first involving two different doses of methadone[259] and the second involving a variety of scheduled narcotics.[260] Both studies showed increased analgesic efficacy with the ibuprofen/narcotic combination compared with the narcotic alone.

The major toxic effect of NSAIDs involves potential gastrointestinal disorders (nausea, vomiting, epigastric pain, ulcers, bleeding, diarrhea, constipation).[251] The loss of the cytoprotective effect of prostaglandin on the gastrointestinal epithelium contributes to these problems.[261] Other potential toxicities include renal dysfunction, sodium and water retention, skin rashes, and headaches.[251,256,261,262]

The selection of a nonnarcotic drug for a patient is often based on trial and error. As Table 20-10 indicates, the variety of drugs to choose from creates a problem for the practitioner. Aspirin is considered by some to be a first-line nonnarcotic because it is relatively inexpensive and very efficacious.[32,249] Mannix and Rawlins[261] developed an algorithm for using NSAIDs in patients with pain from bone metastasis (Figure 20-4.). They selected naproxen as their initial drug of choice because it is reasonably effective, moderately toxic, comes in three forms (tablet, suspension, and suppository), and can be given on a twice-a-day schedule to simplify drug administration.

Table 20-11 lists problems related to nonnarcotic administration, as well as possible choices of drug. The usual recommended doses are reasonable starting points; increases should be based on efficacy and the presence or absence of toxicity. Portenoy[263] recommended a maximum ceiling of one and one-half to two times the recommended starting dose and continuation of the drug for 2 to 3 weeks.

It is important to realize that the benefits of nonnarcotic agents in patients who have pain of severe intensity and require high doses of opioid narcotics have not been established. When analgesic regimens are designed for these individuals, however, nonnarcotics should be considered, either alone or as part of an opioid combination.

Adjuvant analgesics Adjuvant analgesics are defined as those medications that enhance the action of pain-modulating systems.[10] In general, adjuvant analgesics are indicated primarily for uses other than pain management. The following categories of drugs are considered to be adjuvant analgesics: antidepressants, anticonvulsants, psychostimulants, corticosteroids, phenothiazines, and antihistamines. Each category is discussed briefly.

Antidepressants The use of antidepressant medications for individuals with endogenous depression is considered standard treatment. These drugs act by inhibiting the uptake of neurotransmitters into nerve terminals.[264] They have been used in the treatment of many types of chronic nonmalignant pain, such as postherpetic neuralgia, diabetic neuropathy, and migraine headaches.[265] In cases of cancer pain, where their mechanism of action is not clear, their use has been for neuropathic pain, which is often due to tumor infiltration of nerves.[266] This type of pain can be described as having a continuous, dysesthetic, burning quality.

Walsh[267] reviewed nine studies involving antidepres-

TABLE 20-10 Nonnarcotics Used in Cancer Pain

Salicylate
Acetylsalicylate (aspirin)
Salicylsalicylate acid (salsalate)
Choline salicylate
Choline magnesium trisalicylate
Diflunisal
Acetic acids
Phenylacetic acid
Diclofenac
Indoles
Indomethacin
Sulindac
Pyroles
Tolmetin
Fenamic acids
Mefanemic acid
Meclofenamate
Propionic acids
Ibuprofen
Naproxen
Fenopren
Oxicams
Piroxicam
Pyrazolon derivatives
Phenylbutazone
Oxyphenbutazone
Para-aminophenol derivatives
Acetaminophen

Source: Data from Twycross and Lack,[32] Flower et al,[251] Kantor,[262] and Portenoy.[266]

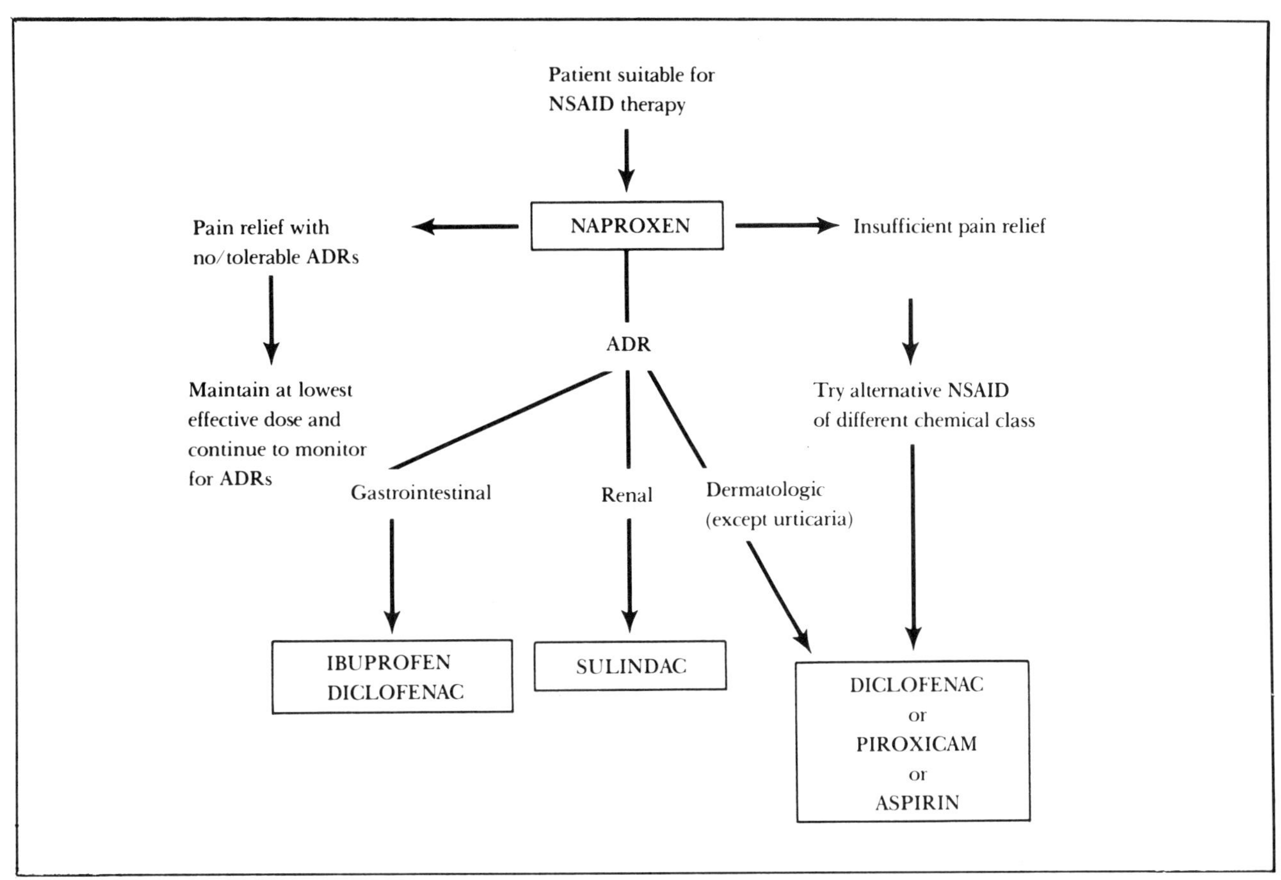

FIGURE 20-4 Algorithm for the use of NSAIDs in osseous metastases. *ADR*, Adverse drug reaction. (Source: From Mannix KA, Rawlins MD: The management of bone metastases: Nonsteroidal anti-inflammatory drugs. Palliat Med 1:128-131, 1987.)

TABLE 20-11 Considerations in the Use of Nonnarcotic Analgesics

Problem	Suggested Nonnarcotic
Need for strong anti-inflammatory activity	All drugs except acetaminophen
Risk of thrombocytopenia or other hematologic disorder	Acetaminophen, choline magnesium trisalicylate
Impaired renal function	Acetaminophen, diflunisal, sulindac
Altered gastrointestinal function	Acetaminophen, choline magnesium trisalicylate, salsalate
Compliance	Diflunisal, naproxen, piroxicam (longer half-lives)
Risk of significant adverse side effects	Avoid indomethacin, phenylbutazone, oxyphenbutazone
Need for chronic drug	Avoid mefenamic acid, meclofenamate
Cost	Aspirin, acetaminophen

sants and cancer pain. He found that these drugs were often used in an attempt to decrease opiate use. Although these studies were beset with significant design and methodologic problems, he concluded that the drugs were useful in an opiate-potentiating role in cancer pain.

Two more recent studies using antidepressants in combination with other analgesics showed that patients' pain intensity decreased and analgesia improved, but the contribution of the antidepressants to improved pain was unclear.[268,269] Amitriptyline (25 to 75 mg), methadone, and a nonnarcotic agent (aspirin, acetaminophen, or ibuprofen) were used in 14 patients for a duration of 14 days, and patients reported a 74% decrease in pain intensity.[268] Doxepin, in a starting dose of 25 mg (titrated upward to a maximum of 225 mg), and piroxicam, a nonsteroidal anti-inflammatory drug, were used concomitantly. In this study patients reported analgesia within 48 to 72 hours.

In a randomized double-blind trial, Ventafridda et al[269] compared trazadone and amitriptyline for patients with deafferentation pain. The analgesic efficacy of the drugs was similar. A partial list of antidepressants with starting and usual doses for cancer-related pain is presented in Table 20-12. Dose changes, in increments of 25 mg, at 1- to 2-day intervals are recommended for these drugs.[270] The pain-relieving doses for antidepressants are often lower than the amount needed for treatment of depression. If patients do not experience a therapeutic benefit

TABLE 20-12 Antidepressants for Cancer-Related Pain

Tricyclics	Usual Starting Dose (mg)	Usual Daily Dose (mg)
Amitriptyline	10-25	75-150
Nortriptyline	25-50	75-100
Imipramine	10-25	50-200
Desipramine	10-25	75-200
Doxepin	25-50	75-150
Second generation		
Trazadone	50 t.i.d.	150-250
Maprotiline	25	75-100

Source: Data from Baldessarini,[264] and Massie and Holland.[270]

within a few weeks, then another drug should be considered.

The major side effects from antidepressants are anticholinergic. Sedation, dry mouth, constipation, postural hypotension, and urinary retention can be troublesome, especially if a patient is already receiving opioid analgesics and is experiencing similar problems.

Anticonvulsants The site and mechanism of the effectiveness of anticonvulsants for cancer-related pain are not well understood. They are primary treatment agents for the pain caused by trigeminal neuralgia and have also been used for diabetic neuropathy and postherpetic neuralgia. Their effectiveness in chronic malignant pain has been supported by clinical observations and anecdotal experiences.

For patients who have neurogenic or neuropathic pain that is described as lancinating or stabbing, anticonvulsants may be beneficial.[271] Swerdlow and Cundill[272] studied 170 patients who had pain of the lancinating type from a variety of causes. Each patient received four anticonvulsants (carbamazepine, clonazepam, phenytoin, valproate), proceeding from one to another after toxicity or lack of efficacy was demonstrated. On the basis of this study, the authors suggested that clinicians use carbamazepine or clonazepam as their first choices in the treatment of the lancinating type of pain.

Carbamazepine was used for 6 weeks in 13 patients with neurogenic pain caused by brachial plexus injury, peripheral nerve injury, and postherpetic neuralgia.[273] Toxicities from ataxia and rash caused six patients to withdraw from the study early, but five of seven patients reported pain relief at a maximum dose of 1200 mg/day. The patients in this study had pain for a duration of 6 months to 8 years.

A recent case report of a patient who had neurogenic pain from a Pancoast tumor of the lung demonstrated the benefit of oral carbamazepine and hydromorphone.[274] The patient eventually received epidural hydromorphone but continued to receive oral carbamazepine as part of the analgesic regimen. Table 20-13 lists common doses and toxicities of four anticonvulsants.[10,275-277] The use of one over another is based primarily on clinical judgment.

Psychostimulants Psychostimulants are useful in counteracting the sedation that accompanies opioid analgesics. If the sedation is present without any other CNS problems, such as delirium and confusion, and if pain occurs when the narcotic dose is lowered, then psychostimulants may be indicated.

The two psychostimulants that are used for opioid-related sedation are amphetamines and methylphenidate. Amphetamines are a more powerful CNS stimulant than methylphenidate. They both decrease the central depression caused by other drugs. Their effects may be from cortical stimulation and/or reticular activating system stimulation.[278]

The more desirable side effects are increased alertness, increased ability to concentrate, mood elevation, euphoria, and an increase in motor and speech activity. The unpleasant side effects include confusion, agitation, dysphoria, apprehension, and fatigue.[278]

In a double-blind, single-dose study involving morphine (3, 6, and 12 mg) and dextroamphetamine (0, 5, and 10 mg) postoperative patients reported increased pain relief with dextroamphetamine.[279] It has been only in the past few years that the use of methylphenidate has been studied in cancer patients. In a controlled trial Bruera et al[280] demonstrated an increased analgesic effect and decreased sedation when methylphenidate (15 mg/day) was compared with a placebo. In a subsequent study, Bruera and colleagues[281] found that 91% of their patients reported improvement in somnolence 48 hours after treatment. They also found that patients became tolerant of the methylphenidate with an initial dose of 15 mg/day and a mean maximal daily dose of 42 ± 6 mg after 39 ± 20 days.

The limited trials with psychostimulants in patients with opioid-induced sedation indicate that the sedation becomes less of a problem when psychostimulants are used. As in other areas of pharmacologic management, more research is needed to clearly outline the benefits of these agents.

Phenothiazines/antihistamines According to Dundee and Moore,[282] the origin of the myth of the potentiation of analgesics with promethazine came from "... observations after its [promethazine's] use with large doses of pethidine [meperidine] or other analgesics, and erroneously attributing reductions in barbiturate dosage and side effects during anaesthesia to the promethazine." Even though promethazine was reported to be antianalgesic to meperidine almost 30 years ago[282] the potentiation myth is still a widely held belief today. Similarly, Keats et al[283] found that promethazine did not increase analgesic efficacy, meperidine-induced respiratory depression, or prevent meperidine-induced nausea and vomiting but that it *did* increase the sedative effects of meperidine. There is, however, one phenothiazine (methotrimeprazine) that has demonstrated analgesic properties,[284, 285] but its use is not

TABLE 20-13 Anticonvulsants for Pain Management

Drug	Dose	Therapeutic Level	Toxicities
Phenytoin	150-200 mg b.i.d.	15-25 μg/mL	Drowsiness, dizziness, diplopia, ataxia
Carbamazepine	100-200 mg b.i.d. increase q.o.d. until pain free or side effects, total daily dose 600-1200 mg/day	5-10 μg/mL	Drowsiness, dizziness, unsteadiness, gastric distress, anorexia, nausea
Clonazepam	0.5-1.5 mg/day, maximum 3-4 mg/day	20-80 ng/mL	Sedation, ataxia, behavioral disturbances
Valproic acid	15 mg/kg, maximum 3000 mg/day	50-100 μg/mL	Nausea, vomiting, indigestion, sedation

Source: Data from Fields,[10] Fromm,[275] McEvoy,[276] and Rall and Schleifer.[277]

recommended because of toxicity and because it is not available as an oral agent.

Hanks et al[286] dispelled the myth about haloperidol potentiation with a retrospective review of 424 patients who received different doses of haloperidol and experienced no opiate-sparing effect.

Perhaps one of the best examples of erroneous application of research to clinical practice involves hydroxyzine. Beaver and Feise[287] compared the effects of 100 mg intramuscular (IM) hydroxyzine alone, 8 mg IM morphine alone, a combination of both drugs, and placebo in postoperative patients. In this *single-dose* study, the combination of morphine and hydroxyzine was superior to the other three groups. Hydroxyzine by itself was superior to placebo but less efficacious than morphine alone. Hydroxyzine seems to have analgesic properties, but it is not a potentiator of opioids; nor has it been shown to be less efficacious at a lower dose or as an oral substitute (ie, 25 mg orally twice a day).

Steroids Steroids are essential for managing the pain caused by epidural cord compressions, but their use as adjuvant analgesics is based on a very limited amount of information. Bruera et al[288] compared methylprednisolone, 32 mg/day, with placebo in a 14-day randomized double-blind study to evaluate relief of pain and other associated symptoms. Pain was reduced significantly more with the methylprednisolone than with the placebo. They found an improvement in appetite (77%) and daily activity (68%), a decrease in depression (71%), and a decrease in analgesic consumption (57%).

The known toxicities from steroids, particularly an increase in appetite and elevation of mood, may be desirable in some patients, but the use of these agents as adjuvant analgesics early in the course of a patient's pain problem is not recommended.

Narcotics To understand pharmacologic management with narcotics, one must be familiar with the terminology used in describing analgesics (Table 20-14).[289] These terms are especially important for an understanding of the actions of opioid drugs.

Opioid analgesics, which interfere with the perception of pain in the CNS, are classified into three groups:

TABLE 20-14 Terminology in Analgesics

Term	Definition
Efficacy	Degree of analgesia provided by a given dose of an analgesic administered under a particular set of conditions
Dose response	Increases in doses accompanied by increases in effectiveness
Relative analgesic potency	Ratio of doses of two drugs
Relative analgesic potential	The relationship between efficacy and adverse effects
Half-life	The time it takes a drug to fall to half of its concentration in the blood
Opiate receptors	Specific recognition sites on which opioids produce their actions

Source: Data from McCaffery and Beebe,[141] Catalano,[245] and Pasternak.[289]

(1) Morphine-like opioid agonists bind with mu and kappa receptors (mu receptors affect supraspinal analgesia, respiratory depression, euphoria, and physical dependence; kappa receptors affect spinal analgesia, miosis, and sedation); this group includes such drugs as codeine, hydromorphone, meperidine, morphine, and methadone. (2) Opioid antagonists have no agonist receptor activity; naloxone is a pure opioid antagonist. (3) The last group includes opioid agonists-antagonists and partial agonists; the former, which includes such drugs as pentazocine, butorphanol, and nalbuphine, acts competitively at different receptor sites, and the latter, which includes buprenorphine, acts at only one receptor site (mu).[290] It is generally accepted by cancer pain experts that opioid agonist-antagonist drugs have very limited usefulness in the man-

TABLE 20-15 Relative Potencies of Commonly Used Analgesics

	Mild to Moderate Pain			Oral Dose (mg)*
	Codeine			30
	Meperidine			50
	Propoxyphene			65
	Acetaminophen			650
	Sodium salicylate			1000
Severe Pain	**IM (mg)†**	**PO (mg)†**	**Plasma Half-life (hr)**	**Average Duration of Action (hr)**
Codeine	130	200	2.5-3	3-5
Meperidine	75	300	3-5	2-4
Oxycodone	15	30	2-3	3-5
Hydromorphone	1.5	7.5	2-3	3-6
Morphine	10	60*	2-3.5	4-5
Levorphanol	2	4	11-16	4-5
Methadone	10	20	15-30	4-6
Oxymorphone	1	–	2-3	4-5

*Approximately equal to aspirin 650 mg.
†Approximately equivalent to morphine 10 mg IM.
These values were determined from and based on clinical experience and single-dose studies of patients in acute pain.
For chronic dosing, some pain experts[32,123,309] believe that the oral morphine dose is approximately 20 to 30 mg, but this has not been demonstrated in any controlled trial.
Source: Data from Foley,[123] Inturrisi,[248] Jaffe and Martin,[290] Houde,[293] Walsh,[311] and Houde.[313]

agement of cancer pain because of their propensity to induce narcotic withdrawal. Consequently, these drugs will not be discussed in this chapter.

There is certain information that physicians and nurses must have before they prescribe and administer opioids. The specifics include the mechanism of action, purpose and category, common starting doses and equivalences of other analgesics when needed, duration of effect, half-life, available routes, and unique side effects.[123,245,266] Table 20-15 contains information about the relative potencies of analgesics commonly used for mild to moderate pain and for severe pain.

All opioid analgesics share common effects as a result of their action. Central nervous system, respiratory, cardiovascular, gastrointestinal, genitourinary, and dermatologic effects of these drugs are included in Table 20-16. The four most common side effects, however, are sedation, respiratory depression, nausea and vomiting, and constipation. The problem of sedation has been addressed in the discussion about psychostimulants.

If respiratory depression occurs, it can be easily and successfully treated with naloxone. The amount of naloxone a patient receives should be titrated to changes in respiratory rate. Rapid bolus injections of naloxone should be avoided in opioid-tolerant patients, so as not to precipitate an abstinence syndrome (nausea, vomiting, agitation, diaphoresis, intense pain). Respiratory depression is a matter of concern when patients who have been maintained on opioid agonist drugs undergo an anesthetic procedure that may totally eliminate their pain. The stimulus of pain on respiratory function is eliminated, which places the patient at risk of respiratory depression.

The chemoreceptor trigger zone (CTZ) in the brain is sensitive to chemical stimuli, such as opiates. Similar to the effect of chemotherapy-related nausea and vomiting, the CTZ and the vomiting center are stimulated to produce eventual nausea and vomiting.

If a patient experiences opiate-related nausea and vomiting, there are many options that can be used. Phenothiazines such as prochlorperazine and thiethylperazine, given on a scheduled basis, may help alleviate symptoms. Other antiemetics that may be useful include haloperidol and metoclopramide. After a reasonable trial of antiemetic agents, if a patient continues to experience nausea and vomiting, a different analgesic should be given.

Constipation can become a significant clinical problem for patients who are taking opioid analgesics if preventive measures are not instituted. Detailed guidelines for man-

TABLE 20-16 Common Side Effects of Opioid Analgesics

System	Side Effect
Central nervous	Sedation, drowsiness, mental clouding, euphoria, analgesia, nausea, vomiting, ↓ physical activity, lethargy, mood changes
Respiratory	↓ Respiratory rate, ↓ ventilatory minute volume, ↓ tidal exchange, ↓ P_{O_2}, ↑ P_{CO_2}
Cardiovascular	Hypotension from peripheral vasodilation or histamine release
Gastrointestinal	Stomach: ↓ motility; small intestine: ↓ propulsive contractions, delayed digestion from ↓ biliary and pancreatic secretions; large intestine: ↓ or absent propulsive peristaltic waves causing delay in passage of contents; biliary tract: ↑ pressure from morphine-like drugs, causing epigastric distress to biliary colic
Genitourinary	↑ Tone and amplitude of ureter contractions, ↑ tone of bladder muscles→urgency, ↑ tone of vesical sphincter
Dermatologic	Vasodilation of cutaneous blood vessels→ ↑ warmth and flushing of skin on face, neck, and upper thorax, sweating, pruritus

Source: Data from Jaffe JH, Martin WR: Opioid analgesics and antagonists, in Goodman AG, Goodman LS, Rall TW, et al (eds): Goodman and Gilman's The Pharmacological Bases of Therapeutics (ed 7). New York, Macmillan, 1985, pp 491-531.

agement of constipation are available.[32,141,291] At the very least, patients should be encouraged to increase their intake of fluids and dietary fiber. The use of stool softeners and bulk laxatives is an initial step in a bowel regimen. The addition of stronger contact cathartics or osmotic cathartics needs to be incorporated as indicated.

There are inherent properties in opioids that can create potential problems for patients if health care professionals do not understand the distinctions among them. The definitions of tolerance, physical dependence, and addiction are as follows[290]:

1. *Tolerance*—A pharmacologic phenomenon that develops when a given dose of a drug produces a decreased effect or when larger doses must be given to obtain the effects observed from the original dose.
2. *Physical dependence*—An altered physiologic state produced by the repeated administration of a drug, which necessitates the continued administration of the drug to prevent the appearance of withdrawal.
3. *Addiction*—A behavioral pattern of drug use, characterized by overwhelming involvement with the use.

Tolerance requires that doses of specific analgesics need to be adjusted to accommodate the pharmacologic phenomenon. Physical dependence is an issue when patients no longer require opioids for pain control and must be tapered slowly off the opioids. It is also an issue if a patient inadvertently receives an opioid agonist-antagonist drug that causes acute withdrawal or if he or she requires naloxone to slowly reverse opioid-induced respiratory depression. The problem of addiction has been addressed elsewhere in this chapter. To reiterate, addiction is not a problem for patients who require opioids for justifiable medical indications.

Specific drug selection A wide variety of narcotics and combination narcotics are available (Table 20-17). Various factors contribute to a specific opioid selection for an individual patient. One very important factor is the knowledge that has been gained through research on analgesia. For example, meperidine is a drug that can produce significant CNS toxicities (agitation, tremors, myoclonus, seizures) as a result of normeperidine accumulation in plasma.[292] In addition, meperidine has poor oral efficacy[293] and should not be used for long-term analgesic management. Another example of an opioid that has limited usefulness is heroin. Supporters of the Compassionate Pain Relief Act (HR 5290) believe that heroin should be legalized for management of cancer pain, as it is in England. The emotionalism associated with this issue supersedes the data that show heroin is no better than morphine in providing pain control.[294,295] Although heroin may be twice as potent as morphine and have a faster onset of analgesic effect, morphine in equal analgesic doses exhibits similar effects.[296] Equally important is the fact that morphine is a product of heroin metabolism,[297] indicating again that heroin probably offers no advantage over morphine.

In the sections that follow, selected drugs are discussed because they require special considerations when used to manage cancer pain.

Morphine Morphine is probably the most frequently used opioid analgesic for moderate to severe pain. It is recommended as the drug of choice according to the World Health Organization ladder.[249] It is available in a variety of preparations, as can be seen in Table 20-17. One of the more recent contributions in the field of analgesics is the use of long-acting morphine, which provides patients with every-12- or every-8-hour doses, as opposed to 4-hour dosing. Numerous studies, both controlled and uncontrolled, have demonstrated the efficacy and safety of the long-acting preparations.[298-304] Portenoy et al[305] reported that with a 100 mg tablet, which is not yet available in the United States, pain relief, side effects, and use of extra doses were similar to those associated with three 30 mg tablets. These studies were similar in design. Patients were switched from their prestudy analgesic to short-acting morphine, the dose was titrated to achieve adequate pain relief for 24 to 48 hours, and then the short-acting morphine was replaced with long-acting morphine.

Even though morphine is considered an effective oral analgesic,[32,306-308] its oral absorption rate is variable. Sawe et al[309] demonstrated that oral morphine's bioavailability is 15% to 64%. A related issue is the oral/parenteral ratio

TABLE 20-17 Commonly Used Opioid Agonist Drugs and Commercially Available Dose Forms

Drug	Dose Form	Availability (mg)
Codeine	I	15, 30, 60 mg/mL
	T	15, 30, 60
	SO	3 mg/mL
Codeine combinations		
with acetaminophen 300 mg	T	7.5, 15, 30, 60
with acetaminophen 325 mg	C	15, 30, 60
with acetaminophen 325 mg, butalbital 50 mg	C	30
with acetaminophen 325 mg, butalbital 50 mg, caffeine 40 mg	C	30
with acetaminophen 500 mg	C	15, 30
with acetaminophen 500 mg	T	15, 30
with acetaminophen 500 mg, caffeine 30 mg	T	8, 15, 30
with acetaminophen 500 mg, butalbital 50 mg	C	15
with acetaminophen 650 mg	T	30
with acetaminophen 120 mg/5mL	SUS, E	12 mg/5 mL
with aspirin 325 mg, butalbital 50 mg, caffeine 40 mg	C	30
with aspirin 325 mg	T	15, 30 60
with aspirin 325 mg, butalbital 50 mg, caffeine 40 mg	T	30
with aspirin 325 mg, carisoprodol 200 mg	T	16
with aspirin 250 mg, acetaminophen 400 mg	T	30
Hydrocodone combinations		
with acetaminophen 500 mg	C	5
with acetaminophen 500 mg	T	2.5, 5, 7.5
with acetaminophen 650 mg	T	7.5
with aspirin 224 mg, caffeine 32 mg	T	5
with aspirin 500 mg	T	5
with aspirin 120 mg/5 mL	SO	2.5 mg/5 mL
Hydromorphone	I	1, 2, 3, 4, 10 mg/mL
	T	1, 2, 3, 4
	SO (cough syrup)	1 mg/5 mL
	SUP	3
	P	as desired
Levorphanol	I	2 mg/mL
	T	2
Meperidine	I	25, 50, 75, 100 mg/mL
	SO	10 mg/mL
	T	50, 100
Meperidine combinations		
with promethazine 25 mg	I	25 mg/mL
with atropine 0.4 mg/mL	I	50, 75 mg/mL
with acetaminophen 300 mg	T	50
with promethazine 25 mg	C	50
Methadone	I	10 mg/mL
	T	5, 10
	TD	40
	SO	1, 2, 10 mg/mL
Morphine sulfate	I	1, 2, 4, 5, 8, 10, 15 mg/mL
	T	15, 30
	TS	10, 15, 30
	TSR	30, 60
	SO	2, 4, 20 mg/mL
	SUP	5, 10, 20, 30
	IN	0.5, 1 mg/mL
Oxycodone	T	5
	SO	1 mg/mL
Oxycodone combinations		
with acetaminophen 325 mg	T	5
with acetaminophen 500 mg	C	5
with acetaminophen 325 mg/5 ml	SO	1 mg/mL
with aspirin 325 mg	T	2.25, 4.5
Oxymorphone	I	1, 1.5 mg/mL
	SUP	5
Propoxyphene hydrochloride	C	32, 65
Propoxyphene hydrochloride combinations		
with aspirin 325 mg	C	32
with aspirin 389 mg, caffeine 32.4 mg	C	32, 65
with acetaminophen 650 mg	C	65
Propoxyphene napsylate	T	100
	SUS	10 mg/mL
Propoxyphene napsylate combinations		
with acetaminophen 325 mg	T	50
with acetaminophen 650 mg	T	100
with aspirin 325	T	100

Code: *C*, Capsule; *E*, elixir; *I*, injection; *IN*, intraspinal; *P*, powder; *SO*, solution; *SUP*, suppository; *SUS*, suspension; *SYR*, syrup; *T*, tablet; *TD*, tablet, disket; *TS*, tablet, soluble; *TSR*, tablet, slow-release.

Source: Data from McEvoy GK (ed): American Hospital Formulary Service, Bethesda, Md, American Society of Hospital Pharmacists, Inc., 1989.

of morphine. The oral/parenteral ratio of 6:1 (60 mg orally = 10 mg intramuscularly) was determined from a single-dose, postoperative study.[310] This number has been challenged by clinicians[32,123,244,311] who believe that, on the basis of clinical experience only, the ratio is 2:1 to 3:1 (20 to 30 mg orally = 10 mg intramuscularly) in long-term dosing. One possible explanation for this analgesic effect of oral morphine in long-term dosing relates to a product of morphine metabolism, morphine-6-glucuronide. This by-product may be a potent analgesic.[246] The issue will be best resolved by a well-controlled clinical trial.[312]

Methadone and levorphanol Both methadone and levorphanol have prolonged plasma half-lives (see Table 20-15), which do not correspond with the average duration of action. When patients are initially placed on fixed schedules of these opioid analgesic drugs, they are at risk of significant sedation and respiratory depression as the level in their plasma rises.[313,314] Houde[313] has continued to recommend that patients initially receive methadone on an as-needed basis to determine the optimal dose and schedule. Clinicians must be aware of the potential toxicities associated with analgesics that have long plasma half-lives.

Routes of opiate administration Just as there is no one best opioid agonist for all patients, there is no one best route for all patients. Six different routes of administration with important advantages and disadvantages are listed in Table 20-18[315] and each is discussed briefly below.

Oral The oral route should be used before any parenteral or intraspinal route. In addition to the reasons listed in Table 20-18, oral analgesics are less expensive than the other routes, provide patients with a less complicated regimen, and allow more control over care. With the exception of oxymorphone, all of the opioid agonist drugs are available as oral preparations (see Table 20-17).

The scheduling of oral medications should be on a fixed-interval basis[32,249] except in a few circumstances, including (1) initial dose titration for methadone and levorphanol,[313] (2) concomitant treatment such as radiation and chemotherapy, which may reduce the need for opioid analgesics, and (3) simultaneous scheduling with round-the-clock administration to provide for incident or breakthrough pain (this also applies to continuous infusions). Even though one study with a small sample and methodologic problems showed no difference in pain relief in fixed-interval scheduling versus as-needed scheduling of oral analgesics,[316] and there is a lack of studies supporting round-the-clock scheduling, it is considered standard practice to deliver medications in this manner.

Patients with acute pain, such as postoperative pain, usually receive intermittent intramuscular or subcutaneous injections. For cancer-related pain, if a patient requires immediate relief, does not have a peripheral intravenous line in place, and does not have a central venous access device, then an occasional intramuscular or subcutaneous injection would be indicated. For prolonged administration of analgesics, these two routes should be replaced by other routes that do not involve pain when drugs are administered.

TABLE 20-18 Advantages and Disadvantages of Routes of Opiate Administration for Patients With Cancer Pain

Route	Advantages	Disadvantages
Oral	Convenient Practical Safe Self-administered	Slow onset Unpredictable absorption
Intermittent intramuscular-subcutaneous	Requires no venous access Safe Faster onset than oral	Unpredictable absorption Trauma to tissue Abscess formation Increased risk of bleeding Lack of suitable injection sites in cachectic patient Peak and trough effect "Clock watching" when dependent on others to administer narcotic on time
Intravenous bolus	Rapid onset	Requires venous access Shorter duration Peak and trough effect Presence of "clock watching"
Continuous intravenous infusions	Provides steady blood level of narcotic Improved control Eliminates "clock watching" Avoids need for repeated injection	Requires maintenance of IV line Potential for infection, sepsis Requires special infusion pump Need for greater patient monitoring

TABLE 20-18 Advantages and Disadvantages of Routes of Opiate Administration for Patients With Cancer Pain—(continued)

Route	Advantages	Disadvantages
Continuous subcutaneous infusions	Provides steady blood level of narcotic Improved control Less potential for complications than continuous intravenous route Eliminates "clock watching" Venous access not required Avoids need for repeated injections Safety of use in home setting with portable pump established	Requires infusion device Local irritation Limited use in patients requiring large volumes of drug
Intrathecal/epidural administration	Lower doses of narcotic required via intrathecal route Longer duration of analgesia Selective analgesia with intrathecal route Fewer side effects than with systemic opiates	Risk of respiratory depression Rostral redistribution of drug limiting selective analgesia Rapid development of tolerance Presence of cross tolerance; patients tolerant to systemic opiates do not benefit greatly Invasive procedure; requires skilled professional Requires special subcutaneous implantable reservoir or rebolus device

Source: Reprinted by permission of Elsevier Science Publishing Co., Inc. from Advances in cancer pain management: A review of patient-controlled analgesia by G. Barkas and M.E. Duafala. Journal of Pain and Symptom Managment, vol. no. 3, pp 150-160. Copyright 1987 by the U.S. Cancer Pain Relief Committee.

Intravenous Intravenous bolus is a reasonable alternative to intramuscular or subcutaneous injections. If scheduled bolus doses of intravenous opioids produce significant peak and trough effects, or if doses need to be given every 2 hours or less, then continuous parenteral infusion may be considered. Additional indications for infusional therapy are gastrointestinal problems, such as uncontrollable vomiting or obstruction; inability to take the quantity of oral analgesic liquids or pills needed for pain relief; inadequate pain relief or unacceptable toxicities from intermittent bolus injections; and impracticality of frequent repeated injections.

The safety and efficacy of continuous intravenous infusions have been demonstrated with only a limited number of reports and studies. In addition to the findings presented in Table 20-19,[170,213,317-324] Stuart et al[325] reported in a retrospective review of 79 patients that all patients achieved baseline control of their pain but 54% needed additional analgesics. The median duration of the infusion was 7 days (range, 24 to 162 days), and the morphine dose range was 0.5 to 300 mg per hour. Fourteen patients experienced toxic effects, which included hallucinations, sedation, respiratory depression, and diaphoresis.

In a review of the literature on continuous intravenous infusions, Portenoy[326] provided guidelines for initiating and managing opioid analgesics delivered by this method. Although the guidelines are not based on controlled studies, they provide much needed assistance for clinicians who already use this route to manage pain. The guidelines are detailed in Table 20-20.

Continuous subcutaneous Continuous subcutaneous infusions are alternatives to intermittent intramuscular or subcutaneous injections and to continuous or bolus intravenous infusions if venous access is a problem. With the availability of new infusion devices, continuous subcutaneous infusions have become a common means of analgesic delivery. Since 1981 there have been at least 14 reports of studies concerning subcutaneous infusions in cancer patients with pain.[327-340]

For patients who are unable to use the oral route because of nausea or obstruction and lack of control with the oral route, and those in whom there is no venous access, this delivery system offers a reasonable alternative. The system is efficacious and safe. Toxic effects have included local skin irritation, leakage, swelling, and discomfort at the needle site. Bruera et al[340] reported that patients preferred the system for analgesic administration because they achieved better pain control, had increased mobility, and found it easy to administer.

In addition to the technical aspects outlined in Table 20-21, other factors that one needs to be concerned with are the drug concentration and the volume infused per 24 hours. Morphine and hydromorphone can be reconstituted to make concentrations as high as 60 mg/mL and 100 mg/mL, respectively.[341,342] The volume per 24 hours without the addition of such substances as hyaluronidase

TABLE 20-19 Studies of Continuous Intravenous Infusion of Narcotics

Report	Age	Dose Range/ Hour	Duration of Infusion	Side Effects	Comments	Drug Preparation
Boyer[321]	NR	1-20 mg/hr	NR	Less lethargic, more coherent less short of breath, less anxious. Also noted decreased respiratory rate and slightly increased P_{CO_2}	One case was fully described; this patient was pain-free, mentally alert with a normal respiratory rate; this patient's pain, probably due to a pulmonary embolus, eventually resolved and she was discharged on oral analgesia	50 mg morphine added to 500 mL D5W via rate-controlled infusion pump
DeChristoforo et al[322]	19 yr	Increased to maximum dose of 275 mg/hr	52 d; highest dose given for 4 d	Somnolence	Patient received IV push morphine, methadone, radiotherapy, diazepam, diphenhydramine, and other therapies to help control her symptoms; the effect of the preservative used in the preparation of morphine was explored and considered as a possible etiology for the patient's somnolence	Continuous infusion of morphine diluted in 150 mL D5W
Citron et al[323]	32-60 yr	20-359 mg/hr	1-80 d	Somnolence reduced respiratory rate	A majority of the 13 patients studied experienced significant pain relief; patients were generally able to walk, eat, and talk without difficulty; in some trials, adequate analgesia was not achieved for over 7 days	Morphine infusion via IVAC pump
Portenoy et al[324]	1.5 yr to 67 yr	4-480 mg (mean maximum dose) Various narcotics used (see text)	1-45 d	Sedation and confusion, nausea/vomiting, constipation, myoclonus, dizziness; respiratory depression in one patient	Side effects were difficult to assess because the patients in this survey were experiencing advanced cancer and concomitant medical problems; sedation occurred with greatest frequency; respiratory depression occurred in 1 patient also receiving intrathecal morphine	NR
Holmes[317]	NR	40-95 mg/hr	30-70 d	NR	Reasonably alert and coherent, good pain control	500 mg morphine sulfate in sterile water added through 0.22 micron filter of 500 mL D5W resulting in 1 mg/mL; an infusion pump employed

TABLE 20-19 Studies of Continuous Intravenous Infusion of Narcotics (continued)

Report	Age	Dose Range/ Hour	Duration of Infusion	Side Effects	Comments	Drug Preparation
Entsworth[318]	NR	5-144 mg/ hr	1 pt, 6d; 1 pt, at least 5 d	Local phlebitis Agitation Restlessness Nightmares, tremors and diaphoresis in one patient	Both patients were alert; one patient free of pain	Initial drug preparation: 240 mg morphine sulfate and 50 mg chlorpromazine added to 482 mL of D5W, resulting in a concentration of 0.48 mg/mL; an infusion pump was not used; 100 mL of solution was administered by volutrol using a microdrip
Kowolenko[319]	NR	NR	NR	NR	Patients described as more coherent and less lethargic	Infusion pump essential; caution about use of narcotic antagonists; suggests respiratory depression should be treated by mechanical means
Miser et al[176]	3-16 yr	0.8 to 80 mg/hr	1-16 d	Constipation, mild drowsiness, decrease in respiratory rate to 10 breaths per minute	Satisfactory pain relief; the physician, nurse, patient and parent(s) determined the rate of infusion based on achievement of maximal pain relief with minimal drowsiness. Side effects easily controlled	Continuous infusion in a dextrose-saline vehicle via an infusion pump
O'Donnell and Papciak[320]	Adults (aged 41, 74)	0.4-3.2 mg/ hr	1-2 d	Sedated, respiratory rate of 6-10; one patient described as restless	One patient was experiencing liver failure and small bowel obstruction prior to initiation of IV morphine infusion; the second patient did not receive an adequate trial because of an administrative decision	100 mg morphine in 250 mg D5W via an infusion pump

Source: Howard-Ruben J: Issues in cancer pain management, in McGuire DB, Yarbro CH (eds): Cancer Pain Management. Orlando, Fla, Grune & Stratton, 1987, pp 69-104.

has been reported as high as 48 ml/day.[340] Bruera et al[336] recently reported on the successful use of hyaluronidase with a dextrose/saline solution to deliver subcutaneous hydration and opioid analgesics. The rate of infusion was 20 to 100 mL/hour.

Intraspinal The identification of opiate receptors in the brain and spinal cord[343] and the results of early animal experiments with spinal opiates[344] provided the basis for the use of intraspinal opioid administration for control of cancer pain. One of the earliest studies demonstrated complete pain relief for a mean of 15 hours after a single 0.5 mg injection of morphine,[345] indicating that epidural opiates could provide analgesia without sensory, motor, or sympathetic involvement. Subsequent studies revealed similar findings for low-dose administration and prolonged pain relief. Many later studies have demonstrated that patients require higher doses of opioid to achieve pain relief[346-348] and that not all patients respond to intraspinal administration.[348-350] Patients reported initial pain relief, but after 6 months there was a trend toward increased dosages and a need for systemic narcotics and neurodestructive procedures.[347]

Max et al[350] gave possible explanations for their patients' receiving pain relief of brief duration: (1) the patients had been on high doses of systemic analgesics prior to intraspinal administration and (2) the patients also had

TABLE 20-20 Guidelines for the Management of Continuous Intravenous Infusion (CII) of Opioid Drugs

1. CII should be indicated (bolus effect, nursing considerations, or rapid titration of dose).
2. Select an appropriate drug (consider the efficacy of current analgesic, prior opioid exposure, and pharmacokinetic factors such as half-life).
3. Choose the infusion device (flow-calibrated infusion pump should be used).
4. Convert the current total daily opioid consumption to intramuscular equivalent mg.
5. If the current drug is used, infuse this quantity over the next 24 hours.
6. For CII with a drug different from the current one, convert the daily quantity of opioid into intramuscular equivalent mg of the new drug and infuse one-half this amount over the next 24 hours.
7. Administer a loading bolus at the start and with each increase in infusion rate (10-15 morphine equivalent mg of a short half-life drug if the maintenance rate is 15 morphine equivalent mg per hour or less; an amount equalling that infused over one hour if the maintenance rate is between 15-30 morphine equivalent mg per hour; and 30 morphine equivalent mg if the maintenance rate is greater than 30 morphine equivalent mg per hour).
8. Increase infusion rate until analgesia or intolerable side effects (if close monitoring is available, repeat the bolus injection and increase the infusion rate by 10-20 per cent every few hours; if close monitoring is not available, offer a "rescue dose," that is, a dose of a short half-life drug equivalent to the loading dose administered every two hours as needed, and increase the infusion rate after 12-24 hours by either 10-20 per cent or an amount equivalent to the total of the "rescue doses" during the preceding period).
9. Take vital signs every 30 minutes for four hours after a loading dose accompanied by an increase in the infusion rate and every 30 minutes for two hours after a "rescue dose."
10. If possible, control side effects with adjuvant drugs; if not, an alternative method of analgesia, such as CII with a different drug, should be considered.

Source: Portenoy RK: Continuous intravenous infusion of opioid drugs, Med Clin North Am 71:237, 1987.

TABLE 20-21 Continuous Subcutaneous Infusions: Technical Summary

Device	Syringe driver, disposable ambulatory infusor, computerized ambulatory pump
Drugs	Morphine, hydromorphone, diamorphine, levorphanol, methadone
Needle	21-, 23-, 25-, 27-gauge
Location	Deltoid, anterior chest, abdomen

deafferentation pain problems, which historically do not respond well to opioids.

Arner and Arner[348] presented a hierarchy of responses to intraspinal analgesia from different pain problems. From best response to least response, these are (1) somatic continuous pain, (2) visceral continuous pain, (3) somatic intermittent pain, (4) visceral intermittent pain, (5) neurogenic pain, either intermittent or continuous, and (6) cutaneous pain.

Many clinicians will place temporary catheters prior to permanent placement of catheters and always before placement of implantable pumps to determine the likelihood of a response.[351-353] Penn et al[352,353] evaluated response to temporary catheter placement by assessing (1) decrease in systemic narcotics, (2) degree of pain relief, and (3) improvement in activity level. Responses are categorized as excellent, good, poor, or failure.

Intraspinal opioids can be administered by an externally placed catheter, a subcutaneous catheter with a reservoir, or a port for injection (either a bolus injection or continuous infusion), and a totally implantable pump for continuous infusion. Combined toxicities from these different techniques may include equipment-related problems, such as dislodgement, obstruction/occlusion, breakage, or leakage from the catheter, or leakage of cerebrospinal fluid, or they may include such drug-related problems as urinary retention, pruritus, nausea, vomiting, and respiratory depression.

Usually patients who receive intraspinal opioids have been given various systemic opiates initially and have experienced poor relief or unacceptable side effects. In these cases, one would expect the tolerant patient to exhibit less toxicity than the opioid-naive patient. Pfeifer et al[354] demonstrated significant differences in ventilatory minute volume, P_{CO_2}, and pH in patients with and without morphine exposure before epidural analgesics. There were no differences in heart rate, blood pressure, P_{O_2}, and pain scores. It is important to note that even the tolerant patients experienced hypoventilation and concomitant respiratory acidosis.

Baggerly[355] identified the goal of temporary catheter placement as achievement of pain control and the goals

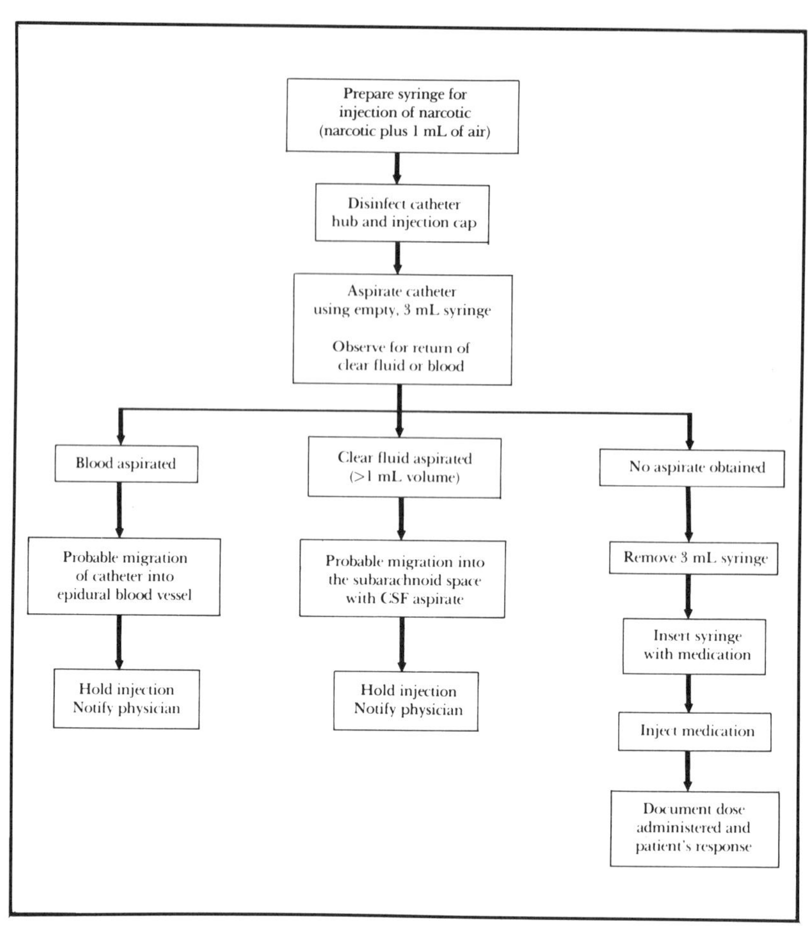

FIGURE 20-5 Schematic for epidural narcotic injection technique. (Source: From Olsson GL, Leddo CG, Wild L: Nursing management of patients receiving epidural narcotics. Heart Lung 18:130-138, 1989.)

of permanent placement as maintenance of pain relief, maintenance of asepsis, and helping the patient become independent in home care on hospital discharge. In a discussion of nursing management of patients with epidural narcotics, Olsson et al[356] developed a care plan that included nursing diagnoses, patient outcomes, and nursing interventions. The nursing diagnoses were (1) potential alteration in respiratory function; (2) potential alteration in comfort related to pruritus, nausea, vomiting, pain on injection, and inadequate pain relief; (3) potential alteration in elimination (urine); (4) knowledge deficit regarding epidural analgesia; and (5) potential infection at catheter site. Figure 20-5 is a schematic portrayal of a technique of epidural narcotic injection.

Intraventricular In addition to epidural and intrathecal opioid administration, the intraventricular route has also been used. A catheter is placed in the frontal horn of the lateral ventricle, and an Ommaya reservoir is used for the injection site. Patients obtain effective pain relief without significant respiratory depression.[357-360] Pain relief usually occurs in between 5 and 60 minutes. Initial daily doses have been 0.1 to 0.3 mg, with final doses as high as 8 mg/24 hours.[358] Toxicities have included somnolence, disorientation, hallucinations, pruritus, nausea, vomiting, and dizziness.

Patient-controlled analgesia Patient-controlled analgesia (PCA) has been used in postoperative patients since 1968,[361] but its use in cancer patients has been limited primarily to the last several years. PCA is designed to allow the patient to self-administer analgesics within preset guidelines from special infusion pumps. Originally developed as a response to inadequate analgesic management in postoperative patients, PCA gives patients some independence in their health care, allows individual response to analgesics to determine the amount of drug a patient will receive, and eliminates the usual lag time inherent in nurse-administered analgesics.

PCA is designed to avoid the peaks and troughs of conventional prn parenteral administration. Figure 20-6 shows a schematic diagram of conventional and patient-controlled analgesia.[362] PCA can be used in two ways: (1) bolus dosing only and (2) bolus dosing and continuous infusion. Some pumps can provide continuous infusion only as an option, which would be similar to standard infusion pumps.

The routes for PCA can be intravenous, subcutaneous, and intraspinal. Citron et al[363] used intravenous PCA and subcutaneous PCA in 12 patients and found it to be safe and effective for both inpatients and outpatients. Bauman et al[364] used PCA requirements to switch three of eight

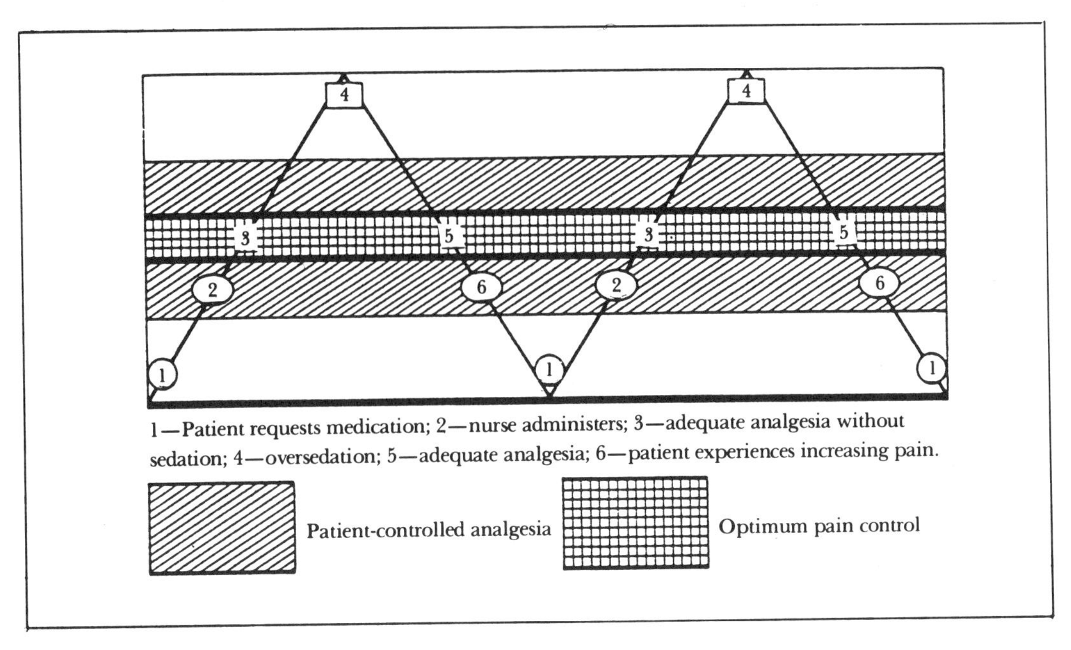

FIGURE 20-6 Schematic of conventional and patient-controlled analgesia. (Source: From Sheidler VR: Patient-controlled analgesia. Curr Concepts Nurs 1:13-16, 1987.)

patients to oral analgesic regimens. They also found PCA to be a safe and efficacious system. Even though patients used PCA more in the first 4 hours of administration than at any other time period, Citron et al[363] reported no significant respiratory depression and sedation during the initial 4 hours. PCA has also been used to treat severe mucositis pain resulting from bone marrow transplantation, and it is considered a safe alternative to continuous intravenous infusion.[365] Bruera et al[366] reported similar efficacy and toxicity in 22 patients when they compared subcutaneous PCA with subcutaneous continuous infusions. Each PCA bolus dose was equivalent to 4 hours of the infusion. The total dose for the PCA group was 168 ± 197 mg and 181 ± 234 mg, which was not significant. Kerr et al[367] reported that patients had greater pain control when PCA was used with subcutaneous and intravenous narcotic infusions. Maximum hourly doses for the narcotics in the study were hydromorphone 60 mg, morphine 80 mg, and meperidine 50 mg. Another study[368] used PCA to examine an unrelated research question concerning the duration of analgesia between intravenous methadone and morphine. The time between a patient's request and administration of the analgesic by a nurse needed to be eliminated as a variable in the study.

The pumps for PCA are designed for both inpatient and outpatient use. The technology has undergone rapid changes since the pumps were first introduced into the market. There is even one disposable PCA pump on the market, along with pumps that have sophisticated computer technology. All the devices have a lock-out period during which a patient may not receive a dose of drug. Lock-out intervals can be set as low as 3 minutes and as long as 199 minutes, depending on the device used.

Although the use of PCA in the cancer pain population has increased within the last few years, specific research issues have not been addressed. Does PCA provide better pain control than other forms of parenteral analgesic administration? Is there an optimal bolus dose in light of a concomitant continuous infusion? Are there specific patient characteristics that make some individuals better candidates for PCA than others?

Other routes Other routes of opioid administration that are available include rectal, sublingual/buccal, and transdermal. Table 20-17 indicates that morphine, hydromorphone, and oxymorphone are available in suppository form. Very little research has been performed on the use of this route. The benefit of sublingual opioid administration is that the first-pass effect from the portal circulation is avoided.[369] Even though there is a limited absorption area on which the drug can be placed, the mouth has a rich vascular and lymphatic supply. Buprenorphine, morphine, methadone, and heroin have been studied as sublingual preparations. None of these opioids are approved for sublingual use in the United States. Unpleasant taste and local irritation have been reported as side effects of sublingual preparations.

One of the newest opioid delivery systems is transdermal administration. Miser et al[370] reported on five cancer patients treated with fentanyl, which is 75 times more potent than morphine. Patients initially received an intravenous fentanyl infusion and then transdermal patches were placed on the chest, back, or upper arm. The patches were changed every 24 hours. Even though the patch system provided adequate pain relief, there were two problems: (1) delay in obtaining steady-state levels, and, therefore, pain relief, and (2) a prolonged effect after the patch was removed because of the prolonged terminal half-life of fentanyl. Toxicities included somnolence, respiratory depression, and vomiting (which was a prestudy symptom). Certainly, this delivery system offers exciting pos-

TABLE 20-22 Nurse's Power and Responsibility in Relation to Medication for Pain Relief

Nurse is Expected to:	Comments
1. Determine whether the analgesic is to be given and, if so, when.	1. Many analgesics are on PRN basis (PRN means use clinical judgment). Assess and apply knowledge. Based on this assessment, a PRN analgesic order may be given around the clock (ATC), on a regular basis, for example, q3h.
2. Choose the appropriate analgesic(s) when more than one is ordered.	2. More than one analgesic is often available. Which one does the nurse give? Two at the same time? Avoid one? This decision is based on pharmacological knowledge along with skills in assessment and evaluation.
3. Be alert to the possibility of certain side effects as a result of the analgesic.	3. Nurse plays a key role in identifying life-threatening side effects, for example, respiratory depression. Identifies constipation, which can seriously influence patient's comfort as much as pain itself.
4. Evaluate effectiveness of analgesic at regular frequent intervals following each administration, but especially the initial dose.	4. This is a vital step in ensuring effective pain control. Assessment and evaluation are continuous processes. A flow sheet is recommended.
5. Report promptly and accurately to the physician when a change is needed.	5. Every new prescription of analgesic for the individual patient is merely a guess that must be evaluated. Too small a dosage should be changed as quickly as too large a dosage.
6. Make suggestions for specific changes, for example, drug, route, dosage, and interval.	6. The nurse has unique blend of knowledge: pharmacological information and direct observation of patient. The result is that nurse is in ideal position to make an educated guess about what may work better for the individual patient.
7. Advise the patient about the use of analgesics, both prescription and nonprescription.	7. Nurse has a key educational role about dosage, side effects, addressing misconceptions, preventive schedule, and how to talk with physician or nurse about questions or problems with drug.

Source: Adapted by permission from McCaffery M, Beebe A: Pain: Clinical Manual for Nursing Practice. St. Louis, 1989, The C.V. Mosby Co.

sibilities, but more research is needed on the administration of opioids by means of transdermal patches.

Regardless of the medication a patient receives or the route of administration, nurses have a pivotal role in assuring adequate management. Table 20-22 delineates nurses' power and responsibility in relation to medication for pain relief. It assumes that nurses have a solid background in pharmacology, including analgesic selection, dosing schedules, and identification of side effects. It also assumes that nurses have effective communication skills in conveying appropriate information to physicians, other nurses, patients, and other health care providers. The ONS position paper on cancer pain assessment and management[75] makes similar recommendations about the nurse's role in analgesic administration. The need for the nurse to have a thorough understanding of the pharmacology of the medications and then to apply this knowledge in clinical practice cannot be overemphasized. Phrases such as "it's not time yet" would become obsolete if knowledge about pain and pharmacology were being properly applied.

Anesthetic and neurosurgical treatment

Anesthetic or nerve-block procedures for cancer-related pain help modulate a patient's neural responses to noxious stimuli.[371] According to Swerdlow,[372] proper use of analgesic drugs should necessitate the use of nerve blocks in 20% of patients with cancer pain. Local anesthetic agents prevent generation and conduction of nerve impulses. The use of these agents, in addition to agents used for neurolytic blocks, comprises the major focus of anesthetic interventions.

Nondestructive nerve blocks serve two functions: (1) They are used for treatment of intractable pain, such as neuropathic pain caused by invasion or compression of intraspinal nerve roots, and (2) they are used for prognostic/diagnostic purposes in which they help differentiate between visceral and somatic pain, demonstrate neural pathways for individual problems, and help predict the efficacy of more permanent neuroablative procedures.[371]

Neurolytic (destructive) nerve blocks can lead to more prolonged pain relief than nondestructive nerve blocks. They are used in conjunction with other forms of therapy, since they often do not provide complete pain relief.[372]

Three categorical criteria can be used for determining the appropriateness of a neurolytic block for a patient: (1) *Physiologic*—evaluate the extent of disease, know the pathophysiology of the pain syndrome; (2) *cognitive*—explain risks and benefits to both the patient and the family; and (3) *functional*—know the benefit of loss of function as a result of the procedure.[373] The choices of neuroablative procedures based on anatomy and type of pain (nociceptive versus deafferentation) are listed in Table 20-23.

Destructive neurosurgical procedures are most often used when standard pharmacologic and nonpharmacologic strategies are no longer effective. Patients are carefully selected for these procedures because of the potential motor and sensory losses associated with them. Common neurosurgical procedures are as follows[374]:

TABLE 20-23 Choice of Neuroablative Procedures for Cancer Pain

	Nociceptive Pain	Deafferentation Pain
Face and oral cavity	Block of trigeminal ganglion and its branches	Upper and middle cervical ganglion block
Neck	Cervical plexus block $C_{2\text{-}3\text{-}4}$ somatic nerve block	Upper and middle cervical ganglion block
Shoulder and upper extremities	Cervical epidural or intrathecal block C_2-T_1	Stellate ganglion block
Chest wall	Intercostal nerve block or thoracic epidural T_1-T_8	Thoracic epidural T_2-T_8
Abdominal wall	Intercostal nerve block T_8-T_{12}	Thoracic epidural T_8-T_{12}
Abdominal viscera	Celiac plexus block	Celiac plexus block
Pelvic/perineum		
Absent bladder/bowel function	Intrathecal phenol	Intrathecal phenol
Intact bladder/bowel function	Epidural morphine	Epidural morphine
Lower extremities	Intrathecal phenol (L_1-L_5) or percutaneous chordotomy	Lumbar sympathetic block

Source: Ferrer-Brechner T: Neurolytic blocks for cancer pain, in Abram SE (ed): Cancer Pain. Boston, Kluwer, 1988, pp 111-124.

1. *Peripheral neurotomy*—destroys sensory modalities from particular nerve, not recommended for pain in extremities.
2. *Rhizotomy*—eliminates all sensation entering dorsal spinal cord; preserves motor function; percutaneous procedure an option for debilitated patients.
3. *Cordotomy*—involves interruption of ascending pain and temperature fibers in anterolateral spinal cord; preserves major sensory function; good for unilateral pain.
4. *Myelotomy*—interrupts pain and temperature fibers as they cross before reaching opposite spinothalamic tract; used for bilateral pain.

The first segment of Figure 20-7 shows the anatomic locations in relation to these procedures.[374]

The nurse's responsibilities for patients undergoing anesthetic and neurodestructive procedures include knowledge of (1) the purpose of the procedure and how

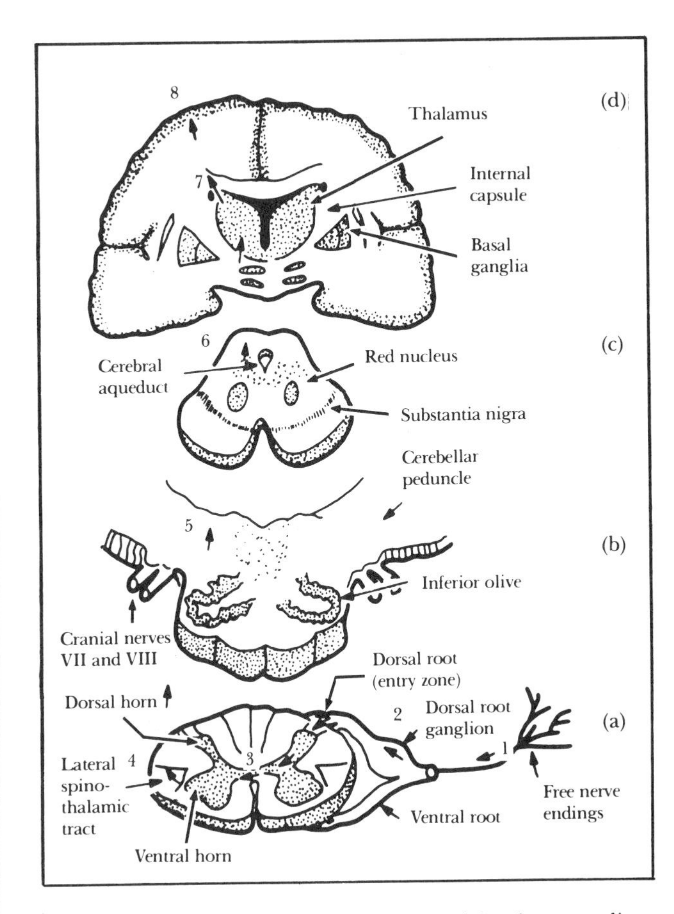

(a) Afferent pain pathway from the level of peripheral nerve endings to the contralateral lateral spinothalamic tract, and (b) continuing in the lower brainstem, (c) in the upper brainstem, and (d) at and above the diencephalic level. In all four segments the short noncaptioned arrows represent the afferent pain flow. The numbers indicate portions of the pain pathway amenable to surgical intervention for pain relief as follows: *1*, peripheral neurotomy; *2*, rhizotomy; *3*, myelotomy; *4*, cordotomy; *5*, medullary tractotomy; *6*, mesencephalic tractotomy and deep brain stimulation; *7*, thalamotomy; *8*, gyrectomy.

FIGURE 20-7 Anatomic locations for neurodestructive procedures. (Source: From Carson B: Neurologic and neurosurgical approaches to cancer pain, in McGuire DB, Yarbro CH (eds): Cancer Pain Management. Orlando, Fla, Grune & Stratton, 1987, pp 223-244.)

it is performed; (2) potential complications based on type of block, agent, and location; and (3) potential benefit of the procedure. An efficient way of obtaining some of this information is to participate in the explanation of the procedure to the patient and talk with the anesthesiologist or the neurosurgeon. Since this requisite information is based on the patient's individual pain problem, standard reference materials may provide incomplete information.

Diminishing the Suffering Component of Pain

Interventions included in this approach to management of cancer pain are those that do not affect the underlying pathology or alter the perception or sensation of pain but, rather, help in a variety of ways to decrease the suffering caused by pain. Thus they are strategies that help patients cope with their pain in a positive and proactive way. Several issues surround the use of these techniques in the health care environment.

It has long been known that both physicians and nurses have little information about such interventions; in fact, a recent survey[84] revealed that individuals with cancer had a greater awareness of them than did their health care providers. The same survey also indicated that respondents found the techniques helpful in reducing pain.

Aside from being little understood or used, the efficacy of these interventions has rarely been studied in a controlled way in the clinical environment.[375] Most evidence of their usefulness in treatment of cancer pain comes from anecdotal reports. Although there are a number of methodologic and logistic difficulties inherent in conducting psychologic/behavioral intervention studies with cancer patients,[376] there is still a need to describe and evaluate (in a systematic way) their usefulness in management of cancer pain. In particular, information is lacking about how they are best used in conjunction with pharmacologic approaches to therapy.

The role of these techniques is clearly that of an adjuvant to standard pharmacologic therapy.[377] Drugs are used to treat the somatic (physiologic and sensory) effects of pain, while these methods are aimed at treating the affective, cognitive, behavioral, and sociocultural effects of pain. The benefits of many of the techniques are that they may increase the sense of personal control, reduce feelings of helplessness, provide opportunities to become actively involved in care, reduce stress and anxiety, elevate mood, raise the pain threshold, and thereby reduce pain.

Mayer[378] reviewed a number of nonpharmacologic interventions, stressing that many of them were ideal components of nursing practice because they were within the scope of the average nurse's qualifications, did not require special equipment, were not subject to a physician's prescription or approval, did not interfere with standard medical therapy, and did not require informed consent. Indeed, these types of intervention are the major foci of clinical nursing texts that deal with pain management.[141,379,380]

Treatment strategies aimed at diminishing the suffering component of pain can best be classified as cognitive, behavioral, and cognitive/behavioral techniques. Cognitive methods are those that attempt directly to modify thought processes in order to attenuate or relieve pain; they can be applied to thoughts, images, and attitudes. Examples include information, distraction, imagery, calming self-statements, and identification of detrimental responses to pain. Behavioral methods are those that modify physiologic reactions to pain or behavioral manifestations of pain. Examples include relaxation, meditation, music therapy, biofeedback, hypnosis, and various desensitization strategies. Sometimes cognitive and behavioral techniques are used simultaneously. Relaxation with guided imagery is one example.

Another group of interventions includes those that provide counterirritant cutaneous stimulation. Examples include menthol ointments, heat, cold, and massage. Although these methods technically fall into the major treatment approach of changing perception/sensation of pain, they are placed in this section because they can also be considered behavioral interventions and are clearly actions that nurses should consider using or teaching to patients. A fourth category of interventions, also considered behavioral, uses mobility and/or immobilization as the basis of nursing actions. Following are brief discussions of selected techniques from these four categories and the research evidence supporting their efficacy in cancer patients with pain.

Counterirritant cutaneous stimulation

Counterirritant cutaneous stimulation is thought to help relieve pain by somehow physiologically altering the transmission of nociceptive stimuli; these methods are based on the gate control theory of pain. Mentholated ointments are rubbed onto the skin in a painful area; heat is applied with hot packs, a heating pad, a hot water bottle, or a shower or bath; cold is applied with cold packs, cold cloths, ice, gel packs, or cold water; massage is applied with fingers, hands, or various devices; transcutaneous electrical nerve stimulation (TENS) is administered by placement of electrodes on selected areas of the body, depending on location of pain. Some of these methods are "home remedies" that are used frequently by many people with pain, and combinations are common (eg, massage with mentholated ointment). The relief that is achieved may outlast the actual application of the counterirritant.

Immobilization/mobility

Even when good pharmacologic therapy has been instituted, some patients may still experience pain on movement. Such methods as complete or partial immobilization of the body or parts of the body and positioning of specific body parts may be quite helpful. In other circumstances, mild exercise such as joint range of motion and stretching may help decrease pain. Finally, rest or lying down may help in some instances, perhaps partly because of the relaxation that occurs.

Distraction

Distraction is ". . . directing one's attention away from the sensations or emotional reactions produced by a noxious stimulus; block awareness of the pain stimulus or its effects."[381] Distraction can be significantly helpful in reducing pain. A classic example are the focusing exercises (accompanied by relaxation techniques) taught in childbirth education classes. There are many individual distraction techniques and strategies; examples include conversation, verbalization to self or others, deep thinking, visualization and imagery, mind-body separation, routines/rituals, breathing exercises, counting, reading, and watching television.

A trap that nurses and others may fall into is that individuals using some of these strategies do not appear to be in pain. The fact is that the strategy being used may be effectively diverting the patient from his or her pain, causing the appearance of a pain-free state. Nurses and others do not always realize the broad scope and variety of distractive strategies; some may work for one person and not for another.

The research that examines the methods just described falls into two categories—studies that asked patients to report what they used to help control cancer pain and studies that used structured scales or questionnaires. In the first group, several studies[15,30,62-64,84] of both inpatients and outpatients with cancer pain revealed that such means as heat, cold, distraction (including reading and television), relaxation, position change, exercise, inactivity, and massage helped to reduce pain to some degree. In one study that used a structured questionnaire to ascertain coping strategies,[16] patients with cancer pain used a variety of cognitive and behavioral coping techniques (ignoring pain, reinterpreting the sensation, increasing physical activity, etc.) and rated them as moderately effective at reducing pain.

The use of TENS in management of cancer pain has been studied infrequently; only two studies were found. In one study[382] beneficial effects were noted in two thirds of the patients initially, but over time efficacy diminished. In the other study[383] 37 patients were studied for a maximum of 30 days. There was a 96% marked reduction in pain intensity intially, but after 30 days there was only an 11% reduction. They reported that TENS was more effective in patients with head and neck pain and phantom limb pain.

Relaxation and guided imagery

Relaxation training helps produce physiologic and mental relaxation. The two most common methods are progressive muscle relaxation, which is the systematic tensing/relaxing of 16 muscle groups, and autogenic relaxation, which is the passive, quiet, and still use of autogenic phrases such as "my arms are warm and heavy." Training usually occurs in six to ten sessions with a therapist. Audiotapes can be used at home afterward, and individuals are encouraged to practice and use their new skills. Guided imagery, in which an individual visualizes pleasant places or things, is frequently used in conjunction with relaxation.

The literature on the use of these techniques in the cancer patient population is scanty. Bayuk[384] provided anecdotal evidence of the helpfulness of relaxation in a group of bone marrow transplant patients. In addition, she emphasized the importance of establishing rapport before using the technique, educating patients, involving friends and family, and giving advice in the practice and use of skills. One study of relaxation as an intervention[94] found that patients who use relaxation or relaxation in combination with distraction reported mild to quite good or complete relief of pain. Another study[385] found that taped transcripts that used guided imagery or progressive muscle relaxation were equally effective in reducing pain and distress. These two studies involved small samples and had methodologic problems, so there is still a need to investigate the efficacy of these methods for reducing cancer pain, particularly when used with narcotic analgesics.

Biofeedback

Biofeedback is "... a process in which a person learns to reliably influence physiological responses of two kinds: either responses that are not ordinarily under voluntary control or responses that ordinarily are easy to regulate but regulation has broken down because of trauma or disease."[386] There are several biofeedback techniques, of which electromyography is the most common. It is taught in six to ten sessions and is often combined with relaxation. The purpose of the technique is to decrease muscle tension and/or sympathetically mediated responses, such as vasoconstriction, which may produce or worsen pain. A decrease in variables that amplify pain (eg, anxiety) may occur as well. Only a few studies have systematically examined the effects of biofeedback; one of them dealt with relaxation as well.[45,387,388] Although biofeedback appeared helpful in the hospital setting, patients found it difficult to use at home, and the merits of its use are still unclear.

Hypnosis

Hypnosis is "... a state of aroused, attentive focal concentration with a relative suspension of peripheral awareness."[389] It is a technique that has been used for many years to relieve pain, relax muscles, and facilitate healing. When it is used as a psychotherapeutic tool it can help alleviate symptoms, uncover forgotten memories, and facilitate behavioral changes. While an individual is hypnotized, there are perceptual, motor, and cognitive alterations. With the help of a therapist or on one's own, several hypnotic strategies can be used for management of cancer pain: block the pain from awareness, substitute another sensation, move pain to a smaller or less important area, change the meaning of pain, increase pain tolerance, or dissociate part of the body from awareness.[390]

Although hypnosis has been in use for many years, the studies supporting its efficacy are fairly old, hindered by small sample sizes and nonexperimental designs. In a review of these studies, Twycross and Lack[32] concluded that most patients showed reduced pain when hypnosis was used. The only prospective, controlled study to date[39] was conducted in women with pain caused by metastatic breast cancer. When self-hypnosis training was used in conjunction with a psychologic support group, pain decreased and mood improved. This study was fraught with attrition problems and variable pain experiences (eg, 41% of the patients had no pain at the start of the study but developed it later), but it did provide beginning evidence of the helpfulness of hypnosis. More research is clearly needed.

TABLE 20-24 Use of Common Nursing Interventions for Pain

Intervention	Advantages/Disadvantages	Techniques
Cutaneous stimulation	*Adv:* Many methods available; eliminates or decreases pain sometimes after stimulation has stopped; produces relaxation and distraction *Disadv:* May be viewed as curative; effects underestimated; tissue damage could occur; mild stimulation yields only mild pain relief	Superficial massage Pressure massage Vibration Superficial heat and cold Ice application and massage Menthol application to skin Transcutaneous electrical nerve stimulation (TENS)
Distraction	*Adv:* Increases pain tolerance; makes quality of pain more acceptable; improves mood and allows focusing on other things; gives sense of control *Disadv:* Effective use can cause others to doubt presence of pain; pain may recur or increase when distraction ceases, along with more fatigue and irritability; patient needs pain relief measure that allows rest (eg, analgesic) and staff may be reluctant to give	Reading, watching TV, talking, singing/humming, rhyming, counting, word games, tactile/touch, rhythm, music, coping self-statements, try for auditory, visual, tactile, kinesthetic methods to stimulate all sensory modalities
Relaxation	*Adv:* Decreases oxygen consumption, respiratory rate, heart rate, and muscle tension, helps maintain normal blood pressure, increases alpha waves, aids sleep, helps decrease stress, improves problem-solving, increases confidence and self-control, decreases fatigue, distracts from pain, increases effects of other pain treatments, elevated mood, decreases distress *Disadv:* People think they are relaxed when they are not, some have trouble accepting it or connect it with "psychologic" pain; it is *not* a substitute for drugs; it may not help with very severe pain; must be highly individualized for patient; and sometimes will not work at all	Deep breathe/tense, exhale relax; yawn; humor for relaxation; heartbeat breathing; jaw relaxation; slow rhythmic breathing; peaceful past experiences; meditative relaxation script; progressive relaxation script; simple touch, massage or warmth
Imagery	*Adv:* Forms and strengthens nurse-patient relationship, assists expressions about pain, exploration/understanding of pain and illness beliefs; increases confidence in ability to control pain; increases effects of other measures; decreases intensity or pain or changes sensation to more acceptable one *Disadv:* May connect it with "psychologic" pain; not a substitute for standard measures; not well accepted by all health care givers; unwanted side effects can occur; trial and error; does not work for all; time-consuming; emotionally exhausting	Subtle conversation; simple, brief symptom substitution; standardized imagery techniques; systematically individualized imagery techniques

Source: Adapted by permission from McCaffery M, Beebe A: Pain: Clinical Manual for Nursing Practice. St. Louis, 1989, The C.V. Mosby Co.

Comprehensive cognitive/behavioral methods

Several individuals have proposed comprehensive cognitive and behavioral "treatment" packages for cancer pain. These proposals are based on cognitive and social learning models in which pain can be described in terms of objective qualities (eg, location and intensity) and psychologic significance. In Turk and Rennert's cognitive-social learning approach,[391] the goal is to help individuals modify thoughts, beliefs, or actions or behaviors that may exacerbate pain, depression, and anxiety and to provide them with specific skills for coping with pain. Unfortunately, there are no data as yet on the efficacy of this treatment approach. In Fishman and Loscalzo's cognitive-behavior "specialized psychological approach,"[392] therapists provide short-term therapeutic interventions that are adaptable to the individual patient, with goals similar to those of Turk and Rennert.[391] Fishman and Loscalzo stated that their approach "can be very useful for both short-term and prolonged supportive care of cancer patients with pain" but provided only one case study as evidence.

Summary and nursing implications

In summary, the available evidence indicates that the techniques described here may be useful in the management of cancer pain, although the number of studies is small and more work is needed. The majority of the techniques may be easily used by nurses who practice in a variety of settings. Some of the methods, such as the counterirritant cutaneous stimulation techniques or actions to immobilize or mobilize, are second nature to nurses. Other methods, such as music therapy, are relatively new to those who deal with cancer pain and require more evaluation.[393-395] Still other techniques are somewhat familiar but must be learned and practiced before they can be effectively used with patients.[14] A number of resources are available to help nurses learn and understand these methods, which include heat, cold, and other cutaneous measures,[141,396,397] relaxation and imagery,[141,398-401] and distraction.[141] Finally, such interventions as hypnosis, biofeedback, and comprehensive cognitive social-learning approaches require specialized training and/or specific equipment and are best left to individuals who have or can obtain such training and equipment. Table 20-24 demonstrates the most commonly used nursing interventions for decreasing the suffering component of pain, along with their advantages and disadvantages and information on specific techniques. For more detail and clinical examples, the reader is referred to McCaffery and Beebe's excellent clinical manual on pain[141] (see especially Chapters 5 to 8).

CONCLUSION

In this chapter the multidimensional phenomenon of cancer pain has been presented, with special reference to the physiologic, sensory, affective, cognitive, behavioral, and sociocultural aspects of the experience. The importance of a multidisciplinary approach to management has been emphasized, with particular attention to the pivotal role of the nurse in this process. Various strategies for managing cancer pain have been presented, some of which call for more nursing involvement than others. Clearly, a great deal of information is readily available for nurses and other health professionals to use in achieving the best possible care for individuals with cancer pain. The challenge for the future is to use this knowledge to its fullest, to continue experimenting with new ways to treat pain, and to share the information gained with colleagues.

REFERENCES

1. Livingston WK: Pain Mechanisms: A Physiologic Interpretation of Causalgia and Its Related States. New York, Macmillan, 1943, p 62.
2. Melzack R, Wall PD: The Challenge of Pain. New York, Basic Books, 1982, pp 9, 71, 235.
3. International Association for the Study of Pain Subcommittee on Taxonomy: Pain terms: A list with definitions and usage. Pain 6:249-252, 1979.
4. Bouckoms AJ: Recent developments in the classification of pain. Psychosomatics 26:637-642, 645, 1985.
5. International Association for the Study of Pain: Pain terms: A current list with definitions and notes on usage. Pain 3:S216-221, 1986.
6. Price DD: Psychological and Neural Mechanisms of Pain. New York, Raven, 1988, p 221, 228.
7. Melzack R, Wall PD: Pain mechanisms: A new theory. Science 150:971-979, 1965.
8. Nathan PW: The gate-control theory of pain: A critical review. Brain 99:123-158, 1976.
9. Weisenberg M: Pain and pain control. Psychol Bull 84:1008-1044, 1977.
10. Fields HL: Pain. New York, McGraw-Hill, 1987.
11. Melzack R, Casey KL: Sensory, motivational, and central control determinants of pain: A new conceptual model, in Kenshalo D (ed): The Skin Senses. Springfield, Ill, Thomas, 1968, pp 423-443.
12. Wall PD: Physiology of pain, in Pain: An Educational Update on Assessment and Management for Nurses. Sponsored by the International Pain Foundation, Toronto, Canada, Nov 10, 1988.
13. Fields HL: Sources of variability in the sensation of pain. Pain 33:195-200, 1988.
14. Ahles TA, Blanchard EB, Ruckdeschel JC: The multidimensional nature of cancer-related pain. Pain 17:277-288, 1983.
15. McGuire DB: Cancer-related pain: A multidimensional approach. Unpublished doctoral dissertation, University of Illinois at Chicago, Health Sciences Center, 1987.
16. McGuire DB: Coping strategies used by cancer patients with pain. Oncol Nurs Forum 14:123, 1987 (suppl).
17. McGuire DB: The multidimensional phenomenon of cancer pain, in McGuire DB, Yarbro CH (eds): Cancer Pain Management. Orlando, Fla, Grune & Stratton, 1987, pp 1-20.
18. Foley KN: Pain syndromes in patients with cancer, in Bonica JJ, Ventafridda V (eds): Advances in Pain Research and Therapy, vol 2. New York, Raven, 1979, pp 59-75.
19. Coyle N, Foley K: Prevalence and profile of pain syndromes in cancer patients, in McGuire DB, Yarbro CH (eds): Cancer Pain Management. Orlando, Fla, Grune & Stratton, 1987, pp 21-46.
20. Chapman CR, Kornell J, Syrjala K: Painful complications of cancer diagnosis and therapy, in McGuire DB, Yarbro CH (eds): Cancer Pain Management. Orlando, Fla, Grune & Stratton, 1987, pp 47-67.
21. Schreml W: Pain in the cancer patient as a consequence of therapy (surgery, radiotherapy, chemotherapy). Recent Results Cancer Res 89:85-99, 1984.
22. Payne R: Anatomy, physiology, and neuropharmacology of cancer pain. Med Clin North Am 71:153-167, 1987.
23. Portenoy RK: Cancer pain: Epidemiology and syndromes. Cancer 63:2298-2307, 1989.
24. Payne R: Cancer pain: Anatomy, physiology, and pharmacology. Cancer 63:2266-2274, 1989.
25. Wall PD: Neurological mechanisms in cancer pain. Cancer Surv 7:127-140, 1988.
26. Melzack R: The McGill Pain Questionnaire: Major properties and scoring methods. Pain 1:277-299, 1975.
27. McGuire DB: Assessment of pain in cancer inpatients using the McGill Pain Questionnaire. Oncol Nurs Forum 11(6):32-37, 1984.
28. Nicholson B, McGuire DB, Maurer VE: Assessment of pain in head and neck cancer patients using the McGill Pain Questionnaire. The Journal (official journal of the Society of Otorhinolaryngology and Head-neck Nurses) 6(3):8-12, 1988.
29. Graham C, Bond SS, Gerkovich MM, et al: Use of the McGill Pain Questionnaire in the assessment of cancer pain: Replicability and consistency. Pain 8:377-387, 1980.
30. Donovan MI, Dillon P: Incidence and characteristics of pain in a sample of hospitalized cancer patients. Cancer Nurs 10:85-92, 1987.
31. Twycross RG, Fairfield S: Pain in far-advanced cancer. Pain 14:303-310, 1982.

32. Twycross RG, Lack SA: Symptom Control in Far Advanced Cancer: Pain Relief. London, Pitman, 1983.
33. Melzack R, Torgerson WS: On the language of pain. Anesthesiology 34:50-59, 1971.
34. Dubuisson D, Melzack R: Classification of clinical pain descriptions by multiple group discriminant analysis. Exp Neurol 51:480-487, 1976.
35. Bressler LR, Hange PA, McGuire DB: Characterization of the pain experience in a sample of cancer outpatients. Oncol Nurs Forum 13(6):51-55, 1986.
36. Zimmerman L, Duncan K, Pozehl B, et al: Pain descriptors used by patients with cancer. Oncol Nurs Forum 14(4):67-71, 1987.
37. Dalton JA, Feuerstein M: Biobehavioral factors in cancer pain. Pain 33:137-147, 1988.
38. Spiegel D, Bloom J: Pain in metastatic breast cancer. Cancer 52:341-345, 1983.
39. Spiegel D, Bloom J: Group therapy and hypnosis reduce metastatic breast carcinoma pain. Psychosom Med 45:333-339, 1983.
40. Stam H, Goss C, Rosenal L, et al: Aspects of psychological distress and pain in cancer patients undergoing radiation therapy, in Fields HL (ed): Advances in Pain Research and Therapy, vol 9. New York, Raven, 1985, pp 569-573.
41. Cleeland CS: The impact of pain on the patient with cancer. Cancer 54:2635-2641, 1984.
42. Lansky SB, List MA, Hermann CA, et al: Absence of major depressive disorder in female cancer patients. J Clin Oncol 3:1553-1560, 1985.
43. McGuire DB: A multidimensional approach to cancer-related pain. Abstract session, Key Aspects of Comfort: Management of Pain, Fatigue, and Nausea. Chapel Hill, NC, 1988.
44. Woodforde JM, Fielding JR: Pain and cancer. J Psychosom Res 14:365-370, 1970.
45. Fotopoulos SS, Graham C, Cook MR: Psychophysiologic control of cancer pain, in Bonica JJ, Ventafridda V (eds): Advances in Pain Research and Therapy, vol 2. New York, Raven, 1979, pp 231-243.
46. Cohen RS, Brechner TF, Pavlov A, et al: Comparison of cancer pain and chronic benign pain patients on dimensions of pain intensity, affect, and approach to treatment. Clin J Pain 1:205-209, 1986.
47. Bond MR: Personality studies in patients with pain secondary to organic disease. J Psychosom Res 17:257-263, 1973.
48. Bond MR, Pearson IB: Psychological aspects of pain in women with advanced cancer of the cervix. J Psychosom Res 13:13-19, 1969.
49. Glynn CJ: Factors that influence the perception of intractable pain. Med Times, March:11s-26s, 1980.
50. Jacox A, Stewart M: Psychosocial Contingencies of the Pain Experience. Iowa City, University of Iowa, 1973 (monograph).
51. Dalton JA: Pain relief for cancer patients. Cancer Nurs 11:322-328, 1988.
52. McKegney FP, Bailey LF, Yates JW: Prediction and management of pain in patients with advanced cancer. Gen Hosp Psychiatry 3:95-101, 1981.
53. Bond MR: The relation of pain to the Eysenck Personality Inventory, Cornell Medical Index, and Whiteley Index of Hypochondriasis. Br J Psychiatr 119:671-678, 1971.
54. Cohen RS, Ferrer-Brechner R, Pavlov A: Prospective evaluation of treatment outcomes in patients referred to a cancer pain center, in Fields HL (ed): Advance in Pain Research and Therapy, vol 9. New York, Raven, 1985, pp 655-662.
55. Shacham S, Reinhardt LC, Raubertas RF, et al: Emotional states and pain: Intraindividual and interindividual measures of association. J Behav Med 6:405-414, 1983.
56. Wallenstein SL: Measurement of pain and analgesia in cancer patients. Cancer 53:2260-2266, 1984 (suppl).
57. Dorrepaal KL, Aaronsen NK, van Dam FSAM: Pain experience and pain management among hospitalized cancer patients: A clinical study. Cancer 63:593-598, 1989.
58. Ferrell BR, Wisdom C, Wenzl C: Quality of life as an outcome variable in the management of cancer pain. Cancer 63:2321-2327, 1989.
59. Bond MR, Pilowsky I: Subjective assessment of pain and its relationship to the administration of analgesics in patients with advanced cancer. J Psychosom Res 10:203-208, 1966.
60. Pilowsky I, Bond MR: Pain and its management in malignant disease: Elucidation of staff-patient transactions. Psychosom Med 31:400-404, 1969.
61. Keefe FJ, Brantley A, Manuel G, et al: Behavioral assessment of head and neck cancer pain. Pain 23:327-336, 1985.
62. Donovan MI: Nursing assessment of cancer pain. Semin Oncol Nurs 1:109-115, 1985.
63. Barbour LA, McGuire DB, Kirchhoff KT: Non-analgesic methods of pain control used by cancer outpatients. Oncol Nurs Forum 13(6):56-60, 1986.
64. Wilkie D, Lovejoy N, Dodd M, et al: Cancer pain control behaviors: Description and correlation with pain intensity. Oncol Nurs Forum 15:723-731, 1988.
65. Wolff BB, Langley L: Cultural factors and the response to pain: A review, in Weisenberg E (ed): Pain: Clinical and Experimental Perspectives. St. Louis, CV Mosby, 1975, pp 144-151.
66. Wolff BB: Ethnocultural factors influencing pain and illness behavior. Clin J Pain 1:23-30, 1985.
67. Lipton JA, Marbach JJ: Ethnicity and the pain experience. Soc Sci Med 19:1279-1298, 1984.
68. Reizien A, Meleis AI: Arab-Americans' perceptions of and responses to pain. Crit Care Nurs 6:30-37, 1986.
69. Miller JF, Shuter R: Age, sex, race affect pain expression. Am J Nurs 84:981, 1984.
70. Swanson DW, Maruta T: Patients complaining of extreme pain. Mayo Clin Proc 55:563-566, 1980.
71. Flannery RB, Sos J, McGovern P: Ethnicity as a factor in the expression of pain. Psychosomatics 22:39-40, 1981.
72. McMillan S: The relationship between age and intensity of cancer-related symptoms. Oncol Nurs Forum 16:237-241, 1989.
73. Ferrell BA, Ferrell BR: The experience of pain and quality of life in elderly patients. Gerontologist 28:76A, 1988 (suppl).
74. Cleeland CS, Ladinsky JL, Serlin RC, et al: Multidimensional measurement of cancer pain: Comparisons of US and Vietnamese patients. J Pain Sympt Manag 3:23-27, 1988.
75. Spross JA, McGuire DB, Schmitt R: Oncology Nursing Society position paper on cancer pain assessment and management (in preparation).
76. National Institutes of Health Consensus Statement. The integrated approach to the management of pain. Bethesda, Md, National Institutes of Health, vol 6, no 3, 1986.
77. Silverberg E: Cancer statistics, 1989. CA 39:3-20, 1989.
78. Twycross RG: Clinical experience with diamorphine in advanced malignant disease. Int J Clin Pharmacol Ther Toxicol 9:184-198, 1974.
79. Wilkes E: Some problems in cancer management. Proc Roy Soc Med 67:23-27, 1974.
80. Baines MJ: Cancer pain. Postgrad Med J 60:852-857, 1984.
81. Trotter JM, Scott R, MacBeth FR, et al: Problems of the oncology outpatient: Role of the liaison health visitor. Br Med J 282:122-124, 1981.

82. Dorrepaal KL, Schimmel HB, van Dam FSAM: Pain experience and pain management: A descriptive study among cancer patients. Proceedings of the American Pain Society. Washington, DC, The Society, 1986.
83. Pannuti F, Martoni A, Rossi AP, et al: The role of endocrine therapy for relief of pain for advanced cancer, in Bonica JJ, Ventafridda V (eds): Adv Pain Res Therapy 2:145-165, 1979.
84. Peteet J, Tay V, Cohen G, et al: Pain characteristics and treatment in an outpatient cancer population. Cancer 57:1259-1265, 1986.
85. Gilbert MR, Grossman SA: Incidence and nature of neurologic problems in patients with solid tumors. Am J Med 81:951-954, 1986.
86. Daut RL, Cleeland CS: The prevalence and severity of pain in cancer. Cancer 50:1913-1918, 1982.
87. Ahles TA, Ruckdeschel JC, Blanchard EB: Cancer-related pain. I. Prevalence in an outpatient setting as a function of stage of disease and type of cancer. J Psychosom Res 28:115-119, 1984.
88. Greenwald HP, Bonica JJ, Bergner M: The prevalence of pain in four cancers. Cancer 60:2563-2569, 1987.
89. Pollen JJ, Schmidt JD: Bone pain in metastatic cancer of prostate. Urology 13:129-134, 1979.
90. Rankin MA: Use of drugs for pain with cancer patients. Cancer Nurs 5:181-190, 1982.
91. Turnbull F: The nature of pain that may accompany cancer of the lung. Pain 7:371-375, 1979.
92. Marino C, Zoppi M, Morelli F, et al: Pain in early cancer of the lungs. Pain 27:57-62, 1986.
93. Front D, Schneck SO, Frankel A, et al: Bone metastasis and bone pain in breast cancer: Are they closely related? JAMA 242:1747-1748, 1979.
94. Norvell K, Zimmerman L: Psychological variables and cancer pain. Oncol Nurs Forum 16:160, 1989 (suppl).
95. Ferrell BR, Schneider C: Experience and management of cancer pain at home. Cancer Nurs 11:84-90, 1988.
96. Grossman SA, Sheidler VR: Skills of medical students and house officers in prescribing narcotic medications. J Med Educ 60:552-557, 1985.
97. Sheidler VR, McGuire DB, Gilbert MR, et al: Nurses' (RNs) inabilities to recognize safe narcotic orders. Oncol Nurs Forum 16(2):195, 1989 (suppl) (abstr).
98. Fox LS: Pain management in the terminally ill cancer patient: An investigation of nurses' attitudes, knowledge, and clinical practice. Milit Med 147:455-460, 1982.
99. Watt-Watson JH: Nurses' knowledge of pain issues: A survey. J Pain Sympt Manag 2:207-211, 1987.
100. Charap AD: The knowledge, attitudes, and experience of medical personnel treating pain in the terminally ill. Mt Sinai J Med 45:561-580, 1978.
101. Schauer PK, Wetterman TL, Schauer AR: Physicians' attitudes and knowledge about the management of cancer-related pain. Conn Med 52:705-707, 1988.
102. Cohen FL: Postsurgical pain relief: Patients' status and nurses' medication choices. Pain 9:265-274, 1980.
103. Morgan JP: American opiophobia: Customary underutilization of opioid analgesics, in Hill CS, Fields WS (eds): Advances in Pain Research and Therapy, vol 11. New York, Raven, 1989, pp 181-195.
104. Marks R, Sachar E: Undertreatment of medical inpatients with narcotic analgesics. Ann Intern Med 78:173-181, 1973.
105. Hauck SL: Pain: Problem for the person with cancer. Cancer Nurs 9:66-76, 1986.
106. Myers JS: Cancer pain: Assessment of nurses' knowledge and attitudes. Oncol Nurs Forum 12(4):62-66, 1985.
107. Weis OF, Sriwatanakul K, Alloza JL, et al: Attitudes of patients, housestaff, and nurses toward post-operative analgesic care. Anesth Analg 62:70-74, 1983.
108. Porter J, Jick H: Addiction rare in patients treated with narcotics. N Engl J Med 302:123, 1980.
109. Camp LD: Comparison of medical, surgical and oncology patients' descriptions of pain and nurses' documentation of pain assessments. J Adv Nurs 12:593-598, 1987.
110. Dalton JA: Nurses' perceptions of their pain assessment skills, pain management practices, and attitudes toward pain. Oncol Nurs Forum 16:225-231, 1989.
111. Grossman SA, Sheidler VR, Swedeen K, et al: Perceptual differences between health care providers and patients about pain intensity. Manuscript submitted, 1989.
112. Rankin MA, Snider B: Nurses' perceptions of cancer patients' pain. Cancer Nurs 7:149-155, 1984.
113. Cleeland CS: Barriers to the management of cancer pain: The role of patient and family. Wis Med J 87(11):13-15, 1988.
114. Hill CS: Pain management in a drug oriented society. Cancer 63:2382-2386, 1989.
115. Lisson EL: Ethical issues in pain management. Semin Oncol Nurs 5:114-119, 1989.
116. Goodwin JS, Goodwin JM, Vogel AA: Knowledge and use of placebos by house officers and nurses. Ann Intern Med 91:106-110, 1979.
117. Cleeland CS, Cleeland LM, Dar R, et al: Factors influencing physician management of cancer pain. Cancer 58:796-800, 1986.
118. Sanford KD, Schlicher CM: Pain management: Are your biases showing? Nurs Life 6(5):47-51, 1986.
119. Pritchard AP: Management of pain and nursing attitudes. Cancer Nurs 11:203-209, 1988.
120. Pilowsky I: An outline curriculum on pain for medical school. Pain 33:1-2, 1988.
121. Weissman DE, Abram SE, Haddox AD, et al: Educational role of cancer pain rounds. J Cancer Educ 4:113-116, 1989.
122. Hill CS, Fields WS (eds): Advances in Pain Research and Therapy, vol 11. New York, Raven, 1989.
123. Foley KM: The treatment of cancer pain. N Engl J Med 313:84-95, 1985.
124. McGuire DB, Yarbro CH (eds): Cancer Pain Management. Orlando, Fla, Grune & Stratton, 1987.
125. Abram SE (ed): Cancer Pain. Boston, Kluwer, 1989.
126. Kanner R: Diagnosis and Management of Pain in Patients With Cancer. Basel, Karger, 1988.
127. Swerdlow M, Ventafridda V (eds): Cancer Pain. Lancaster, England, MTP Press, 1987.
128. Crue BL: Multidisciplinary pain treatment programs: Current status. Clin J Pain 1:31-38, 1985.
129. Stjernsward J: WHO cancer pain relief programme. Cancer Surv 7:195-208, 1988.
130. MacDonald N: Canada and the WHO cancer pain relief program. J Palliat Care 1(2):31, 1986.
131. Joranson DE, Dahl JL, Engber D: Wisconsin initiative for improving cancer pain management: Progress report. J Pain Sympt Manag 2:111, 1987.
132. Ventafridda V, Tamburini M, Caraceni A, et al: A validation study of the WHO method for cancer pain relief. Cancer 59:850-856, 1987.
133. Mohide EA, Royle JA, Montemuro M, et al: Assessing the quality of cancer pain management. J Palliat Care 4:9-15, 1988.
134. Donovan MI: Clinical assessment of cancer pain, in McGuire DB, Yarbro CH (eds): Cancer Pain Management. Orlando, Fla, Grune & Stratton, 1987, pp 105-131.

135. Clark WC, Ferrer-Brechner T, Janal MN, et al: The dimensions of pain: A multidimensional scaling comparison of cancer patients and healthy volunteers. Pain 37:23-32, 1989.
136. Fong CM: Ethnicity and nursing practice. Top Clin Nurs 7(3):1-10, 1985.
137. Copp LA: Pain coping model and typology. Image: J Nurs Schol 17:69-71, 1985.
138. McNally MC, Stair JC, Somerville ET (eds): Guidelines for Cancer Nursing Practice. Orlando, Fla, Grune & Stratton, 1985, pp 78-84.
139. Levin RF, Krainovitch BC, Bahrenburg E, et al: Diagnostic content validity of nursing diagnoses. Image: J Nurs Schol 21:40-44, 1989.
140. North American Nursing Diagnosis Association: Proceedings of the Eighth National Conference NANDA, St. Louis, 1988.
141. McCaffery M, Beebe A: Pain: Clinical Manual for Nursing Practice. St. Louis, CV Mosby, 1989.
142. McGuire DB: Measuring pain, in Frank-Stromborg M (ed): Instruments for Clinical Nursing Research. Norwalk, Appleton & Lange, 1988, pp 333-356.
143. Ross DM, Ross SA: Assessment of pediatric pain: An overview. Iss Compr Ped Nurs 11:73-91, 1988.
144. Syrjala KL: The measurement of pain, in McGuire DB, Yarbro CH (eds): Cancer Pain Management. Orlando, Fla, Grune & Stratton, 1987, pp 133-150.
145. Deschamps M, Band PR, Coldman AJ: Assessment of adult cancer pain: Shortcomings of current methods. Pain 32:133-139, 1988.
146. Ahles TA, Ruckdeschel JC, Blanchard EB: Cancer-related pain. II. Assessment with visual analogue scales. J Psychosom Med 28:121-124, 1984.
147. Machin D, Lewith GT, Wylson S: Pain measurement in randomized clinical trials. Clin J Pain 4:161-168, 1988.
148. Kremer EF, Atkinson JH, Ignelzi RJ: Pain measurement: The affective dimensional measure of the McGill Pain Questionnaire with a cancer pain population. Pain 12:153-163, 1982.
149. Melzack R: The short-form McGill Pain Questionnaire. Pain 30:191-197, 1987.
150. Daut RL, Cleeland CS, Flanery RC: Development of the Wisconsin brief pain questionnaire to assess pain in cancer and other diseases. Pain 17:197-210, 1983.
151. Cleeland CS: Measurement and prevalence of pain in cancer. Semin Oncol Nurs 1:87-92, 1985.
152. Fishman B, Pasternak S, Wallenstein SL, et al: The Memorial Pain Assessment Card: A valid instrument for the evaluation of cancer pain. Cancer 60:1151-1158, 1987.
153. McMillan SC, Williams FA, Chatfield R, et al: A validity and reliability study of two tools for assessing and managing cancer pain. Oncol Nurs Forum 15:735-741, 1988.
154. Walker, VA, Dicks B, Webb P: Pain assessment charts in the management of chronic cancer pain. Palliat Med 1:111-116, 1987.
155. Beyer JE, Levin CR: Issues and advances in pain control in children. Nurs Clin North Am 22:661-676, 1987.
156. McGrath PJ, Johnson G, Goodman J, et al: The Children's Hospital of Eastern Ontario Pain Scale (CHEOPS): A behavioral scale for rating postoperative pain in children, in Fields HL, Dubner R, Cervero F (eds): Advances in Pain Research and Therapy, vol 9. New York, Raven, 1985, pp 395-402.
157. Liebeskind JC, Melzack R: The International Pain Foundation: Meeting a need for education in pain management. Pain 30:1-2, 1987.
158. Miser AW, Dothage JA, Wesley RA, et al: The prevalence of pain in a pediatric and young adult cancer population. Pain 29:73-83, 1987.
159. Miser AW, McCalla J, Dothage JA, et al: Pain as a presenting symptom in children and young adults with newly diagnosed malignancy. Pain 29:85-90, 1987.
160. Cornaglia C, Massimo L, Haupt R, et al: Incidence of pain in children with neoplastic diseases. Pain 2:S28, 1984.
161. Patterson KL, Klopovich PM: Pain in the pediatric oncology patient, in McGuire DB, Yarbro CH (eds): Cancer Pain Management. Orlando, Fla, Grune & Stratton, 1987, pp 259-272.
162. Stevens B, Hunsberger M, Browne G: Pain in children: Theoretical, research, and practice dilemmas. J Pediatr Nurs 2:154-166, 1987.
163. Broome ME, Lillis PP: A descriptive analysis of the pediatric pain management research. Appl Nurs Res 2:744-781, 1989.
164. Eland JM: The role of the nurse in children's pain, in Copp L (ed): Recent Advances in Nursing: Perspectives on Pain. London, Churchill Livingston, 1985, pp 29-45.
165. Katz ER, Kellerman J, Siegel SE: Behavioral distress in children with cancer undergoing medical procedures: Developmental considerations. J Consult Clin Psychol 48:356-365, 1980.
166. Beaver PK: Premature infants' response to touch and pain: Can nurses make a difference? Neonatal Network 6(Dec):13-17, 1987.
167. Eland JM, Anderson JE: The experience of pain in children, in Jacox AK (ed): Pain: A Sourcebook for Nurses and Other Health Professionals. Boston, Little, Brown, 1977, pp 453-476.
168. Schechter NL, Allen DA, Hanson K: Status of pediatric pain control: A comparison of hospital analgesic usage in children and adults. Pediatrics 77:11-15, 1986.
169. Schechter NL, Allen D: Physicians' attitudes toward pain in children. J Dev Behav Pediatr 7:350-354, 1986.
170. Miser AW, Moore L, Greene R, et al: Prospective study of continuous intravenous and subcutaneous morphine infusions for therapy-related or cancer-related pain in children and young adults with cancer. Clin J Pain 2:101-106, 1986.
171. Nahata MC, Clotz MA, Krogg EA: Adverse effects of meperidine, promethazine, and chlorpromazine for sedation in pediatric patients. Clin Pediatr 24:558-560, 1985.
172. Kuttner L: Favorite stories: A hypnotic pain-reduction technique for children in acute pain. Am J Clin Hypn 30:289-295, 1988.
173. Kuttner L, Bowman M, Teasdale M: Psychological treatment of distress, pain, and anxiety for young children with cancer. J Dev Behav Pediatr 9:374-381, 1988.
174. Martinson IM, Nixon S, Geis D, et al: Nursing care in childhood cancer: Methadone. Am J Nurs 82:432-435, 1982.
175. Miser AW, Miser JS: The use of oral methadone to control moderate and severe pain in children and young adults with malignancy. Clin J Pain 1:243-248, 1986.
176. Miser AW, Miser JS, Clark BS: Continuous intravenous infusion of morphine sulfate for control of severe pain in children with terminal malignancy. J Pediatr 96:930-932, 1980.
177. Dothage JA, Arndt C, Miser AW: Use of a continuous intravenous morphine infusion for pain control in an infant with terminal malignancy. J Assoc Pediatr Oncol Nurs 3(4):22-24, 1986.
178. Gilford DM (ed): The Aging Population in the Twenty-first Century: Statistics for Health Policy. Washington, DC, National Academy Press, 1988.

179. Portenoy RK: Optimal pain control in elderly cancer patients. Geriatrics 42:33-44, 1987.
180. Ferrell BA, Ferrell BR: Assessment of chronic pain in the elderly. Geriatr Med Today 8(5):134, 1989.
181. Ferrell BA: Pain in the elderly, in Focus on Geriatric Care and Rehabilitation. Frederick, Md, Aspen, 1990.
182. Thomas MR, Roy R: Age and pain: A comparative study of the "younger and older" elderly. Pain Management 1:174-179, 1988.
183. Office of Technology Assessment: Technology and Aging in America. Washington DC, Publication, OTA-BA-264, 1985.
184. Newton PA: Chronic pain, in Cassel KY, Walsh JR (eds): Geriatric Medicine, vol II, Fundamentals of Geriatric Care. New York, Springer-Verlag, 1984, pp 236-274.
185. Lamy PP: Pain management, drugs, and the elderly. J Am Health Care Assoc 10:32-36, 1984.
186. Harkins SW, Kwentus J, Price DD: Pain in the elderly, in Bendetti C, Chapman CR, Morrica G (eds): Advances in Pain Research and Therapy, vol 7. New York, Raven, 1984, pp 103-121.
187. Bayer AJ, Chadha JS, Farag RR, et al: Changing presentations of myocardial infarction with increasing old age. J Am Geriatr Soc 34:263-266, 1986.
188. Schmucker DL: Drug disposition in the elderly: A review of the critical factors. J Am Geriatr Soc 32:144-149, 1984.
189. Ouslander JG: Drug therapy in the elderly. Ann Intern Med 95:711-722, 1981.
190. Amadio P, Cummings DM, Amadio PB: Pain in the elderly: Management techniques. Pain Management 1:33-41, 1987.
191. Kaiko RF, Wallenstein SL, Rogers AG, et al: Narcotics in the elderly. Med Clin North Am 66:1079-1089, 1982.
192. Bellville JW, Forrest WH, Miller E, et al: Influence of age on pain relief from analgesics: A study of postoperative patients. JAMA 217:1835-1841, 1971.
193. Nolan L, O'Malley K: Prescribing for the elderly. Part I. Sensitivity of the elderly to adverse drug reactions. J Am Geriatr Soc 36:142-149, 1988.
194. Faherty BS, Grier MR: Analgesic medication for elderly people post-surgery. Nurs Res 33:369-372, 1984.
195. Portenoy RK, Kanner RM: Patterns of analgesic prescription and consumption in a university-affiliated community hospital. Arch Intern Med 145:439-441, 1985.
196. Davitz JR, Davitz LL: Inferences of Patients' Pain and Psychological Distress: Studies of Nursing Behaviors. New York, Springer, 1981.
197. Davitz LL, Davitz JR: Nurses' Responses to Patients' Suffering. New York, Springer, 1980.
198. Davitz LJ, Pendleton SH: Nurses' inferences of suffering. Nurs Res 18:100-107, 1969.
199. Davitz LJ, Sameshima Y, Davitz J: Suffering as viewed in six different cultures. Am J Nurs 76:1296-1297, 1976.
200. Martin BA, Belcher JV: Influence of cultural background on nurses' attitudes and care of the oncology patient. Cancer Nurs 9:230-237, 1986.
201. Dudley SR, Holm K: Assessment of the pain experience in relation to selected nurse characteristics. Pain 18:179-186, 1984.
202. Lenburg CB, Burnside H, Davitz LJ: Inferences of physical pain and psychological distress. III. In relation to length of time in the nursing education program. Nurs Res 19:399-401, 1970.
203. Mason DJ: An investigation of the influences of selected factors on nurses' inferences of patients' suffering. Int J Nurs Stud 18:251-259, 1981.
204. Holm K, Cohen F, Dudas S, et al: Effect of personal pain experience on pain assessment. Image: J Nurs Schol 21:72-75, 1989.
205. Taylor AG, Skelton JA, Butcher J: Duration of pain condition and physical pathology as determinants of nurses' assessments of patients in pain. Nurs Res 33:4-8, 1984.
206. Teske K, Daut RL, Cleeland CS: Relationships between nurses' observations and patients' self-reports of pain. Pain 16:289-296, 1983.
207. Davitz LJ, Davitz JR: How do nurses feel when patients suffer? Am J Nurs 75:1505-1510, 1975.
208. Donnelly GF, Sutterley DC: From the editors (editorial). Top Clin Nurs 7(3):v, 1985 (entire issue on cultural diversity and nursing practice).
209. Kagawa-Singer M: Ethnic perspectives of cancer nursing: Hispanics and Japanese-Americans. Oncol Nurs Forum 14(3):59-65, 1987.
210. Louie KB: Providing health care to Chinese clients. Top Clin Nurs 7(3):18-25, 1985.
211. Lipson JG, Meleis AI: Culturally appropriate care: The case of immigrants. Top Clin Nurs 7(3):48-56, 1985.
212. Capers CF: Nursing and the Afro-American client. Top Clin Nurs 7(3):11-17, 1985.
213. Howard-Ruben J: Issues in cancer pain management, in McGuire DB, Yarbro CH (eds): Cancer Pain Management. Orlando, Fla, Grune & Stratton, 1987, pp 69-104.
214. Carson VB: Spiritual Dimensions of Nursing Practice. Philadelphia, WB Saunders, 1989.
215. Jacik M: Spiritual care of the dying adult, in Carson VB (ed): Spiritual Dimensions of Nursing Practice. Philadelphia, WB Saunders, 1989, pp 254-288.
216. Twycross RG: Terminal care: Organization and technical aspects, in Swerdlow M, Ventafridda V (eds): Cancer Pain. Lancaster, England, MTP Press, 1987, pp 173-184.
217. Wanzer SH, Federman DD, Adelstein SJ, et al: The physician's responsibility toward hopelessly ill patients. N Engl J Med 320:844-849, 1989.
218. Burchman SL: Hospice care of the cancer pain patient, in Abram SE (ed): Cancer Pain. Boston, Kluwer, 1989, pp 153-169.
219. Kane RL, Bernstein L, Wales J, et al: Hospice effectiveness in controlling pain. JAMA 253:2683-2686, 1985.
220. Austin C, Cody CP, Eyres PJ, et al: Hospice home care pain management: Four critical variables. Cancer Nurs 9:58-65, 1986.
221. Degner LF, Fujii SH, Levitt M: Implementing a program to control chronic pain of malignant disease for patients in an extended care facility. Cancer Nurs 5:263-268, 1982.
222. Milch RA, Freeman A, Clark E: Palliative Pain and Symptom Management for Children and Adolescents. Alexandria, Children's Hospice International, 1985.
223. Mount B: Challenges in palliative care (keynote address). Am J Hosp Care 2:22-29, 1985.
224. Steitz AM: Analgesic utilization patterns in a hospice. Oncology April: 33-36, 1987, (suppl).
225. Bonadonna F, Molinari R: Role and limits of anticancer drugs in the treatment of advanced cancer pain, in Bonica JJ, Ventafridda V (eds): Advances in Pain Research and Therapy, vol 2. New York, Raven, 1979, pp 131-138.
226. Russell JA: Cytotoxic therapy—Pain relief and recalcification, in Stoll BA, Parbhoo S: Bone Metastasis: Monitoring and Treatment. New York, Raven, 1983, pp 354-368.
227. MacDonald N: The role of medical oncology in cancer pain control, in Hill CS, Fields WS (eds): Advances in Pain Research and Therapy, vol 11. New York, Raven, 1989, pp 123-130.
228. Bruera E, MacMillan K, Hanson J, et al: The Edmonton

staging system for cancer pain: Preliminary report. Pain 37:203-209, 1989.
229. Estes NC, Morphis JG, Hornback NB, et al: Intraarterial chemotherapy and hyperthermia for pain control in patients with recurrent rectal cancer. Am J Surg 152:597-601, 1986.
230. Abrams RA, Hansen RM: Radiotherapy, chemotherapy and hormonal therapy in the management of cancer pain: Putting patient, prognosis, and oncologic options in perspective, in Abram SE (ed): Cancer Pain. Boston, Kluwer, 1989, pp 49-66.
231. Stoll BA: Hormonal therapy—Pain relief and recalcification, in Stoll BA, Parbhoo S (eds): Bone Metastasis: Monitoring and Treatment. New York, Raven, 1983, pp 321-342.
232. Ford HT, Yarnold JR: Radiation therapy—Pain relief and recalcification, in Stoll BA, Parbhoo S (eds): Bone Metastasis: Monitoring and Treatment. New York, Raven, 1983, pp 343-354.
233. Tong D, Gillick L, Hendrickson FR: The palliation of symptomatic osseous metastases: Final results of the study by the Radiation Therapy Oncology Group. Cancer 50:893-899, 1982.
234. Salazar OM, Ruben P, Hendrickson FR, et al: Single-dose half-body irradiation for palliation of multiple bone metastases from solid tumors: Final Radiation Therapy Oncology Group report. Cancer 58:29-36, 1986.
235. Azzarelli A, Crispino S: Palliative surgery in cancer pain treatment, in Swerdlow M, Ventafridda V (eds): Cancer Pain. Lancaster, England, MTP Press, 1987, pp 97-103.
236. Chalmers J: The management of bone metastases: Orthopaedic procedures. Palliat Med 1:121-127, 1987.
237. Houde RW: Systemic analgesics and related drugs: Narcotic analgesics, in Bonica JJ, Ventafridda V (eds): Advances in Pain Research and Therapy, vol 2. New York, Raven, 1979, pp 263-272.
238. Shimm DS, Logue GL, Moltbie AA, et al: Medical management of chronic cancer pain. JAMA 241:2408-2412, 1979.
239. Lipman AG: Drug therapy in cancer pain. Cancer Nurs 3:40-46, 1980.
240. Beaver WT: Management of cancer pain with parenteral medication. JAMA 244:2653-2657, 1980.
241. Moertel CG: Treatment of cancer pain with orally administered medications. JAMA 244:2448-2450, 1980.
242. Foley KM: The practical use of narcotic analgesics. Med Clin North Am 66:1091-1104, 1982.
243. McGivney WT, Crooks GM: The care of patients with severe chronic pain in terminal illness. JAMA 251:1181-1188, 1984.
244. Levy MH: Integration of pain management into comprehensive cancer care. Cancer 63:2328-2335, 1989.
245. Catalano RB: Pharmacologic management in the treatment of cancer pain, in McGuire DB, Yarbro CH (eds): Cancer Pain Management. Orlando, Fla, Grune & Stratton, 1987, pp 151-201.
246. Hanks GW: Opioid analgesics in the management of pain in patients with cancer: A review. Palliat Med 1:1-25, 1987.
247. Twycross RG: Opioid analgesics in cancer pain: Current practice and controversies. Cancer Surv 7(1):29-53, 1988.
248. Inturrisi CE: Management of cancer pain: Pharmacology and principles of management. Cancer 63:2308-2320, 1989.
249. World Health Organization. Cancer Pain Relief. Geneva, WHO, 1986.
250. Goodwin JS, Regan M: Cognitive dysfunction associated with naprosyn and ibuprofen in the elderly. Arthritis Rheum 25:1013-1015, 1982.
251. Flower RJ, Moncada S, Vane JR: Analgesic—anti-pyretics and anti-inflammatory agents: Drugs employed in the treatment of gout, in Gilman AG, Goodman LS, Rall TW, et al (eds): Goodman and Gilman's The Pharmacological Basis of Therapeutics (ed 7). New York, Macmillan, 1985, pp 674-715.
252. Ventafridda V, Fochi V, DeConno D, et al: Use of non-steroidal anti-inflammatory drugs in the treatment of pain in cancer. Br J Clin Pharmacol 10:3435-3465, 1980.
253. Moertel CG: Treatment of cancer pain with orally administered medications. JAMA 244:2448-2450, 1980.
254. Turnbull R, Hills LJ: Naproxen versus aspirin as analgesics in advanced malignant disease. J Palliat Care 1(2):25-28, 1986.
255. Levich S, Jacobs C, Loukas DF: Naproxen sodium in treatment of bone pain due to metastatic cancer. Pain 35:253-258, 1988.
256. Minotti V, Patoria L, Roila F, et al: Double-blind evaluation of analgesic efficacy of orally administered diclofenac, nefopam, and acetylsalicylic acid (ASA) plus codeine in chronic cancer pain. Pain 36:177-183, 1989.
257. Beaver WT: Aspirin and acetaminophen as constituents of analgesic combinations. Arch Intern Med 141:292-300, 1981.
258. Houde RW, Wallenstein SL, Rogers A: Clinical pharmacology of analgesics: A method of assaying analgesic effect. Clin Pharmacol Ther 1:163-174, 1960.
259. Ferrer-Brechner T, Ganz P: Combination therapy with ibuprofen and methadone for chronic cancer pain. Am J Med 77:78-83, 1984.
260. Weingart WA, Sorkness CA, Earhart RH: Analgesia with oral narcotics and added ibuprofen in cancer patients. Clin Pharm 4:53-58, 1985.
261. Mannix KA, Rawlins MD: The management of bone metastases: Nonsteroidal anti-inflammatory drugs. Palliat Med 1:128-131, 1987.
262. Kantor TG: Control of pain by nonsteroidal anti-inflammatory drugs. Med Clin North Am 66:1053-1059, 1982.
263. Portenoy RK: Drug treatment of pain syndromes. Semin Neurol 7:139-149, 1987.
264. Baldessarini RJ: Drugs and the treatment of psychiatric disorders, in Gilman AG, Goodman LS, Rall TW, et al (eds): Goodman and Gilman's The Pharmacological Basis of Therapeutics (ed 7). New York, Macmillan, 1985, pp 387-445.
265. Hollister LE: Tricyclic anti-depressants. N Engl J Med 16:1106-1109, 1978.
266. Portenoy RK: Practical aspects of pain control in the patient with cancer. CA 38:327-352, 1988.
267. Walsh TD: Antidepressants for chronic pain. Clin Neuropharmacol 6:271-295, 1983.
268. Richlin DM, Jamron LM, Novich NC: Cancer pain control with a combination of methadone amitriptyline and non-narcotic analgesic therapy: A case series analysis. J Pain Sympt Manag 2:89-94, 1987.
269. Ventafridda V, Caraceni A, Saita L, et al: Trazadone for deafferentation pain: Comparison with amitriptyline. Psychopharmacology 95:544-549, 1988.
270. Massie MJ, Holland J: The cancer patient with pain: Psychiatric complications and their management. Med Clin North Am 71:243-258, 1987.
271. McQuay HJ: Pharmacologic treatment of neuralgia and neuropathic pain. Cancer Surv 7:141-159, 1988.
272, Swerdlow M, Cundill JG: Anti-convulsant drugs used in the treatment of lancinating pain: A comparison. Anaesthesiology 36:1129-1132, 1981.
273. Rapoport WG, Rogers KM, McCubbin TD, et al: Treatment of intractable neurogenic pain with carbamazepine. Scottish Med J 29:162-165, 1984.
274. Tanelian DL, Cousins MJ: Combined neurogenic and no-

ciceptive pain in a patient with Pancoast tumor managed by epidural hydromorphone and oral carbamazepine. Pain 36:85-88, 1989.
275. Fromm GF: Trigeminal neuralgia and related disorders, in Portenoy RK (ed): Pain: Mechanisms and Syndromes. Neurol Clin 7:305-320, 1989.
276. McEvoy G (ed): Amer Hosp Formulary Service. Bethesda, Md, American Society of Hospital Pharmacy, Inc, 1989.
277. Rall TW, Schleifer LS: Drugs effective in the therapies of epilepsies, in Gilman AG, Goodman LS, Rall TW, et al (eds): Goodman and Gilman's The Pharmacologic Basis of Therapeutics (ed 7). New York, Macmillan, 1985, pp 446-472.
278. Weiner N: Norepinephrine, epinephrine and sympathomimetic amines, in Gilman AG, Goodman LS, Rall TW, et al (eds): Goodman and Gilmans' The Pharmacological Basis of Therapeutics (ed 7). New York, Macmillan, 1985, pp 145-180.
279. Forrest WH, Brown BW, Brown CR, et al: Dextroamphetamine with morphine for treatment of post-operative pain. N Engl J Med 296:712-715, 1977.
280. Bruera E, Chadwick S, Brenneis C, et al: Methylphenidate associated with narcotics for the treatment of cancer pain. Cancer Treat Rep 71:67-70, 1987.
281. Bruera E, Brenneis C, Patterson AH, et al: Use of methylphenidate as an adjuvant to narcotic analgesics in patients with advanced cancer. J Pain Sympt Manag 4:3-6, 1989.
282. Dundee JW, Moore J: The myth of phenothiazine potentiation. Anaesthesia 16:95-96, 1961.
283. Keats AS, Telford J, Kurosu Y: "Potentiation" of meperidine by promethazine. Anesthesiology 22:34-41, 1961.
284. Beaver WT, Wallenstein SL, Houde RW, et al: A comparison of the analgesic effect of methotrimeprazine and morphine in patients with cancer. Clin Pharm 7:436-446, 1966.
285. Bloomfield S, Simard-Savoie S, Bernier J, et al: Comparative analgesic activity of levomepromazine and morphine in patients with chronic pain. Can Med Assoc J 90:1156-1159, 1964.
286. Hanks GW, Thomas PJ, Trueman T, et al: The myth of haloperidol potentiation. Lancet 2:523-524, 1983.
287. Beaver WT, Feise G: Combination of analgesic effects of morphine sulfate, hydroxyzine and their combinations in patients with postoperative pain, in Bonica JJ, Albe-Fessard D (eds): Advances in Pain Research and Therapy, vol 1. New York, Raven, 1976, pp 553-557.
288. Bruera E, Roca E, Cedaro L, et al: Action of oral methylprednisolone in terminal cancer patients: A prospective randomized double blind study. Cancer Treat Rep 69:751-754, 1985.
289. Pasternak GW: Biochemistry and pharmacology of multiple mu opioid receptors, in Foley KM, Inturrisi CE (eds): Advances in Pain Research and Therapy, vol 8. New York, Raven, 1986, pp 337-344.
290. Jaffe JH, Martin WR: Opioid analgesics and antagonists, in Goodman AG, Goodman LS, Rall TW, et al (eds): Goodman and Gilman's The Pharmacological Basis of Therapeutics (ed 7). New York, Macmillan, 1985, pp 491-531.
291. Portenoy RK: Constipation in the cancer patient: Causes and management. Med Clin North Am 71:303-311, 1987.
292. Kaiko RF, Foley KM, Grabinski PY, et al: Central nervous system excitatory effects of meperidine in cancer patients. Ann Neurol 13:180-185, 1983.
293. Houde RW: Systemic analgesics and related drugs: Narcotic analgesics, in Bonica JJ, Ventafridda V (eds): Advances in Pain Research and Therapy, vol 2. New York, Raven, 1979, 263-272.
294. Kaiko, RF, Wallenstein SL, Rogers AG, et al: Analgesic and mood effects of heroin and morphine in cancer patients with postoperative pain. N Engl J Med 304:1501-1505, 1981.
295. Twycross RG: Choice of strong analgesic in terminal cancer: Diamorphine or morphine? Pain 3:93-104, 1977.
296. Kaiko RF, Wallenstein SL, Rogers A, et al: Clinical analgesic studies of intramuscular heroin and morphine in postoperative and chronic pain, in Foley KM, Inturrisi CE (eds): Advances in Pain Research and Therapy, vol 8. New York, Raven, 1986, pp 107-116.
297. Inturrisi CE, Max MB, Foley KM: The pharmacokinetics of heroin in patients with chronic pain. N Engl J Med 310:1213-1217, 1984.
298. Homesley HD, Welander CE, Muss HB, et al: Dosage range study of morphine sulfate controlled release. Am J Clin Oncol 9:449-453, 1986.
299. Meed SD, Kleinman PM, Kantor TG, et al: Management of cancer pain with oral controlled-release morphine sulfate. J Clin Pharmacol 27:155-161, 1987.
300. Savarese JJ, Shepherd L, Krant MJ: Long-acting oral morphine in cancer pain analgesia. Clin J Pain 3:177-181, 1987.
301. Brescia FJ, Walsh M, Savarese JJ, et al: A study of controlled-release oral morphine (MS Contin) in an advanced cancer hospital. J Pain Sympt Manag 2:193-198, 1987.
302. Khojasteh A, Evans W. Reynolds RD, et al: Controlled release oral morphine sulfate in the treatment of cancer pain with pharmacokinetic correlation. J Clin Oncol 5:956-961, 1987.
303. Thirwell MP, Sloan PA, Maroun JA, et al: Pharmacokinetics and clinical efficacy of oral morphine solution and controlled-release morphine tablets in cancer patients. Cancer 63:2275-2283, 1989.
304. Goughnour BR, Arkinstall WW, Stewart JH: Analgesic response to single and multiple doses of controlled-release morphine tablets and morphine oral solution in cancer patients. Cancer 63:2294-2297, 1989.
305. Portenoy RK, Maldonado M, Fitzmartin R, et al: Oral controlled-release morphine sulfate: Analgesic efficacy and side effects of a 100 mg tablet in cancer pain patients. Cancer 63:2284-2288, 1989.
306. Walsh TD, Kadam BV: Morphine steady-state levels during repeated oral administration. Br J Clin Pharmacol 17:232, 1984.
307. Walsh TD, Grabinski PY, Kaiko RF: Clinical implications of morphine plasma levels in advanced cancer, in Foley KM, Inturrisi CE (eds): Advances in Pain Research and Therapy, vol 8. New York, Raven, 1986, pp 31-35.
308. Ventafridda V, Oliveri E, Caraceni A, et al: A retrospective study on the use of oral morphine in cancer pain. J Pain Sympt Manag 2:77-81, 1987.
309. Sawe J, Dahlstrom B, Rase A: Morphine kinetics in cancer patients. Clin Pharmocol Ther 30:629-635, 1981.
310. Houde RW, Wallenstein SL, Beaver WT: Clinical measurement of pain, in de Stevens G (ed): Analgetics. New York, Academic Press, 1965, pp 75-122.
311. Walsh TD: Oral morphine in chronic cancer pain. Pain 18:1-11, 1984.
312. Kaiko R: Controversy in the management of chronic cancer pain: Therapeutic equivalents of im and po morphine. J Pain Sympt Manag 1:42-45, 1986.
313. Houde RW: Misinformation: Side effects and drug interactions, in Hill CS, Fields WS (eds): Advances in Pain Research and Therapy, vol 11. New York, Raven, 1989, pp 145-161.
314. Ettinger DS, Vitale PJ, Trump DC: Important clinical considerations in the use of methadone in cancer patients. Cancer Treat Rep 63:457-459, 1979.
315. Barkas G, Duafala ME: Advances in cancer pain manage-

ment: A review of patient-controlled analgesia. J Pain Sympt Manag 3:150-160, 1988.
316. McGuire DB, Barbour L, Boxler J, et al: Fixed-interval v as-needed analgesics in cancer outpatients. J Pain Sympt Manag 2:199-205, 1987.
317. Holmes AH: Morphine intravenous infusion for chronic pain (letter). Drug Intell Clin Pharm 12:556-557, 1978.
318. Entsworth S: Morphine IV infusion for chronic pain (letter). Drug Intell Clin Pharm 13:297, 1979.
319. Kowolenko M: An additional comment on IV morphine infusion (letters). Drug Intell Clin Pharm 14:296-297, 1980.
320. O'Donnell L, Papciak B: Continuous morphine infusion for control of intractable pain. Nursing 81 11:69-72, 1981.
321. Boyer M: Continuous drip morphine. Am J Nurs 82:502-504, 1982.
322. DeChristoforo R, Corden BJ, Hood JC, et al: High-dose morphine infusion complicated by chlorobutanol-induced somnolence. Ann Intern Med 98:335-336, 1983.
323. Citron M, Johnston-Early A, Fossieck B, et al: Safety and efficacy of continuous intravenous morphine for severe cancer pain. Am J Med 77:199-204, 1984.
324. Portenoy RK, Moulin DE, Rogers A, et al: IV infusions of opioids for cancer pain: Clinical review and guidelines for use. Cancer Treat Rep 70:575-582, 1986.
325. Stuart GJ, Davey EB, Wight SE: Continuous intravenous morphine infusions for terminal pain control: A retrospective review. Drug Intell Clin Pharm 20:968-972, 1986.
326. Portenoy RK: Continuous intravenous infusion of opioid drugs. Med Clin North Am 71:233-241, 1987.
327. Campbell CF, Mason JB, Weiler JM: Continuous subcutaneous infusion of morphine for the pain of terminal malignancy. Ann Intern Med 98:51-52, 1983.
328. Coyle N, Mauskop A, Maggard J, et al: Continuous infusions of opiates in cancer patients with pain. Oncol Nurs Forum 13:53-57, 1986.
329. Dickson RJ, Howard B, Campbell J: The relief of pain by subcutaneous infusion of morphine, in Wilkes E (ed): Advances in Morphine Therapy, The 1983 International Symposium on Pain Control, Royal Society of Medicine International Congress and Symposium Series 64. London, Royal Society of Medicine, 1983 pp 107-110.
330. Dickson RJ, Russell PSB: Continuous subcutaneous analgesics for terminal care at home (letter). Lancet 1(8264):165, 1982.
331. Hutchinson HT, Leedham GD, Knight AM: Continuous subcutaneous analgesics and antiemetics in domiciliary terminal care (letter). Lancet 1(8258):1279, 1981.
332. MacDonald N, Bruera E, Chadwick S, et al: Treatment of cancer pain with a portable disposal device. Proc Am Soc Clin Oncol 5:252, 1986 (abstr).
333. Miser AW, David DM, Hughes CS, et al: Continuous subcutaneous infusions of morphine in children with cancer. Am J Dis Child 137:383-385, 1983.
334. Moss H: Subcutaneous continuous infusion narcotics at home. Oncol Nurs Forum Suppl 12:128, 1986 (abstr).
335. Smith JM, Bulich R: Continuous subcutaneous infusion morphine sulfate: A report of 40 patients. Oncol Nurs Forum Suppl 13:87, 1986 (abstr).
336. Bruera E, Legris MA, Kuehn N, et al: Hypodermoclysis for the administration of fluids and narcotic analgesics in patients with advanced cancer. J Natl Cancer Inst 81:1108-1109, 1989.
337. Drexel H, Dzien A, Spiegel RW: Treatment of severe cancer pain by low dose continuous subcutaneous morphine. Pain 36:169-176, 1989.
338. Bruera E, Michaud M, Brenneis C, et al: A radomized cross-over trial of patient controlled subcutaneous analgesia (PCSA) versus continuous subcutaneous infusion (CSCI) in patients with cancer pain. Proc Am Soc. Clin Oncol 7:285, 1988 (abstr).
339. Brenneis C, Michaud M, Bruera E, et al: Local toxicity during subcutaneous infusion of narcotics: A prospective study. Cancer Nurs 10:172-176, 1987.
340. Bruera E, Brenneis C, Michaud M, et al: Continuous sc infusion of narcotics using a portable disposable device in patients with advanced cancer. Cancer Treat Rep 71:635-637, 1987.
341. The Merck Index (ed 9). Rahway, NJ, Merck, 1976.
342. The United States Pharmacopeia, 21st rev. Rockville, Md, The United States Pharmacopeial Convention, 1984.
343. Pert CB, Snyder SH: Opiate receptor demonstration in nervous tissue. Science 179:1011, 1973.
344. Yaksh TL, Rudy TA: Analgesia mediated by a direct spinal action of narcotics. Science 192:1357-1358, 1976.
345. Wang JK, Nauss CA, Thomas JE: Pain relief by intrathecally applied morphine in man. Anesthesiology 50:149-151, 1979.
346. Zenz M, Schappler-Scheele B, Neuhaus R, et al: Long term peridural morphine analgesia in cancer pain. Lancet 1:91, 1981.
347. Coombs DW, Maurer LH, Saunders RL, et al: Outcomes and complications for continuous intraspinal narcotic analgesia for cancer pain control. J Clin Oncol 2:1414-1420, 1984.
348. Arner S, Arner B: Differential effects of epidural morphine in the treatment of cancer-related pain. Acta Anaesthesiol Scand 29:32-36, 1985.
349. Wang JK, Intrathecal morphine for intractable pain secondary to cancer of pelvic organs. Pain 21:99-102, 1985.
350. Max MB, Inturrisi CE, Kaiko RF, et al: Epidural and intrathecal opiates: Cerebrospinal fluid and plasma profiles in patients with chronic cancer pain. Clin Pharmacol Ther 38:631-641, 1985.
351. Krames ES, Gershow J, Glassberg A, et al: Continuous infusion of spinally administered narcotic for the relief of pain due to malignant disease. Cancer 56:696-702, 1985.
352. Penn RD, Paice JA, Gottschalk W, et al: Cancer pain relief using chronic morphine infusion: Early experience with a programmable implanted drug pump. J Neurosurg 61:302-306, 1984.
353. Penn RD, Paice JA: Chronic intrathecal morphine for intractable pain. J Neurosurg 67:182-186, 1987.
354. Pfeifer BL, Seinaker HC, Ter Horst UM: Pain scores and ventilatory and circulatory sequelae of epidural morphine in cancer patients with and without prior narcotic therapy. Anesth Analg 67:838-842, 1988.
355. Baggerly J: Epidural catheters for pain management: The nurse's role. J Neurosci Nurs 18:290-295, 1986.
356. Olsson GL, Leddo CC, Wild L: Nursing management of patients receiving epidural narcotics. Heart Lung 18:130-138, 1989.
357. Leavens ME, Hill CS, Cech DA, et al: Intrathecal and intraventricular morphine for pain in cancer patients: Initial study. J Neurosurg 56:241-245, 1982.
358. Lobato RD, Madrid JL, Fatela LV, et al: Intraventricular morphine for control of pain in terminal cancer patients. J Neurosurg 59:627-633, 1983.
359. Su CF, Liu MY, Lin MT: Intraventricular morphine produces pain relief, hypothermia, hyperglycaemia and increased prolactin and growth hormone levels in patients with cancer pain. J Neurol 235:105-108, 1987.
360. Lazorthes Y, Verdi JC, Caute B, et al: Intracerebroventri-

cular morphinotherapy for control of chronic cancer pain. Prog Brain Res 77:395-405, 1988.
361. Sechzer PH: Objective measurement of pain. Anesthesiology 29:209-210, 1968.
362. Sheidler VR: Patient-controlled analgesia. Curr Concepts Nurs 1:13-16, 1987.
363. Citron ML, Johnston-Early A, Boyer M, et al: Patient-controlled analgesia for severe cancer pain. Arch Intern Med 146:734-736, 1986.
364. Bauman TJ, Batenhorst RL, Graves DA, et al: Patient-controlled analgesia in the terminally ill cancer patient. Drug Intell Clin Pharm 20:297-301, 1986.
365. Hill HF, Saeger LC, Chapman CR: Patient-controlled analgesia after bone marrow transplantation for cancer. A special report. Postgrad Med 28:33-40, 1986.
366. Bruera E, Brenneis C, Michaud M, et al: Patient-controlled subcutaneous hydromorphone versus continuous subcutaneous infusion for the treatment of cancer pain. J Natl Cancer Inst 80:1152-1154, 1988.
367. Kerr IG, Sone M, DeAngelis C, et al: Continous narcotic infusion with patient controlled analgesia for chronic cancer pain in outpatients. Ann Intern Med 108:554-557, 1988.
368. Grochow LB, Sheidler VR, Green L, et al: Duration of analgesia between methadone and morphine. Pain 38:151-157, 1989.
369. Payne R: Novel routes of opioid administration, in Hill CS, Fields WS (eds): Advances in Pain Research and Therapy, vol 11. New York, Raven, 1989, pp 319-338.
370. Miser AW, Narang PK, Dothage JA, et al: Transdermal fentanyl for pain control in patients with cancer. Pain 37:15-21, 1989.
371. Abram SE: The role of non-neurolytic blocks in the management of cancer pain, in Abram SE (ed): Cancer Pain. Boston, Kluwer, 1989, pp 67-76.
372. Swerdlow M: Role of chemical neurolysis and local anesthetic infiltration, in Swerdlow M, Ventafridda V (eds): Cancer Pain. Lancaster, England, MTP Press, 1987, pp 105-128.
373. Ferrer-Brechner T: Neurolytic blocks for cancer pain, in Abram SE (ed): Cancer Pain. Boston, Kluwer, 1988, pp 111-124.
374. Carson B: Neurologic and neurosurgical approaches to cancer pain, in McGuire DB, Yarbro CH (eds): Cancer Pain Management. New York, Grune & Stratton, 1987, pp 223-244.
375. Ahles TA: Psychological techniques for the management of cancer-related pain, in McGuire DB, Yarbro CH (eds): Cancer Pain Management. Orlando, Fla, Grune & Stratton, 1987, pp 245-258.
376. Ahles TA, Cohen RE, Blanchard ED: Difficulties inherent in conducting behavioral research with cancer patients. Behav Ther 7:69-70, 1984.
377. Breitbart W: Psychiatric management of cancer pain. Cancer 63:2336-2342, 1989.
378. Mayer DK: Non-pharmacologic management of pain in the person with cancer. J Adv Nurs 10:325-330, 1985.
379. McCaffery M: Nursing Management of the Patient With Pain (ed 2). Philadelphia, JB Lippincott, 1979.
380. Yasko J: Guidelines for Cancer Care: Symptom Management. Reston, Va, Reston Publishing, 1983.
381. McCaul KD, Malott JM: Distraction and coping with pain. Psychol Bull 95:516-533, 1984.
382. Avellanosa AM, West CR: Experience with transcutaneous electrical nerve stimulation for relief of intractable pain in cancer patients. J Med 13:203-213, 1982.
383. Ventafridda V, Sganzerla EP, Fochi C, et al: Transcutaneous nerve stimulation in cancer pain, in Bonica JJ, Ventafridda V (eds): Advances in Pain Research and Therapy, vol 2. New York, Raven, 1979, pp 509-515.
384. Bayuk L: Relaxation techniques: An adjunct therapy for cancer patients. Semin Oncol Nurs 1:147-150, 1985.
385. Graffam S, Johnson A: A comparison of two relaxation strategies for the relief of pain and its distress. J Pain Sympt Manag 2:229-231, 1987.
386. Blanchard EB, Epstein LH: A Biofeedback Primer. Reading, Pa, Addison-Wesley, 1978.
387. Fleming U: Relaxation therapy for far-advanced cancer. Practitioner 229:471-475, 1985.
388. Fotopoulos SS, Cook MR, Graham C, et al: Cancer pain: Evaluation of electromyographic and electrodermal feedback. Prog Clin Biol Res 132D:33-53, 1983.
389. Spiegel D: The use of hypnosis in controlling cancer pain. CA 35:4-14, 1985.
390. Barber J, Gitelson J: Cancer pain: Psychological management using hypnosis. CA 30:130-136, 1980.
391. Turk DC, Rennert K: Pain and the terminally ill cancer patient: A cognitive-social learning perspective, in Sobel HJ (ed): Behavior Therapy in Terminal Care: A Humanistic Approach. Cambridge, Ballinger, 1981, pp 95-123.
392. Fishman B, Loscalzo M: Cognitive behavioral interventions in management of cancer pain: Principles and applications. Med Clin North Am 71:271-287, 1987.
393. Munro S, Mount B: Music therapy in palliative care. Can Med Assoc J 4:1029-1034, 1978.
394. Spross JA: Behavioral intervention, in Baird SB (ed): Decision Making in Oncology Nursing. Toronto, Decker, 1988, p 72.
395. Beck SL: The therapeutic use of music for cancer pain. Oncol Nurs Forum 16(2):169, 1989 (suppl).
396. McAlary P: Relieving pain with heat or cold. Nursing 88 17:64K-64N, 1988.
397. Spross JA: Cutaneous measures for pain, in Baird SB (ed): Decision Making in Oncology Nursing. Toronto, Decker, 1988, p 74.
398. Mast D, Meyers J, Urbanski A: Relaxation techniques: A self-learning module for nurses: Unit I. Cancer Nurs 10:141-147, 1987.
399. Mast D, Meyers J, Urbanski A: Relaxation techniques: A self-learning module for nurses: Unit II. Cancer Nurs 10:217-225, 1987.
400. Cobb SC: Teaching relaxation techniques to cancer patients. Cancer Nurs 7:157-161, 1984.
401. Donovan MI: Relaxation with guided imagery: A useful technique. Cancer Nurs 3:27-32, 1980.

Chapter 21

Infection

Paula R. Klemm, RN, MS, DNSc Candidate

Susan Molloy Hubbard, RN, BA

INTRODUCTION

Infection is the major cause of death in individuals diagnosed with cancer. This may be due to the underlying disease, intensive treatment modalities, or prolonged hospitalization. To understand why individuals with cancer are so susceptible to infection, it is necessary to understand how the cancer and its treatment impair normal host defense systems. Specific concepts, principles of cancer treatment, and the known interrelationships among disease treatment, underlying immune defects, and epidemiologic factors are addressed in this chapter.

NORMAL HOST DEFENSES

Integumentary, Mucosal, and Chemical Barriers

Intact skin constitutes the most important physical barrier against invasion by both exogenous and endogenous organisms. The cornified layers of epithelial cells that cover the body protect tissues against dehydration and invasion by harmful bacteria. However, environmental microbes and those that normally inhabit hair follicles and sebaceous glands may enter the body and cause infection when a break in the skin occurs.

A second major defense against infection is the mucociliary activity found in the mucous membranes. The cilia of the epithelial cells that line the respiratory tract beat rhythmically to propel mucus and its entrapped foreign particles toward the nose and throat. In the gastrointestinal tract the cilia propel bacteria and foreign particles to be removed in the feces. Microorganisms constitute up to 60% of the weight of the stool; therefore an intact mucous membrane is essential to the prevention of infection.

The acid pH of the skin discourages the growth of harmful bacteria, whereas the acid pH of the stomach kills most bacteria it contacts. The low pH of urine renders it essentially sterile. Prostatic fluid contains bactericidal elements, whereas the low pH of the vagina acts to decrease the growth of pathogenic organisms.

Leukocytes

Important lines of defense against infection and/or trauma are the cells produced by the bone marrow. In relation to infection the most important of these is the leukocyte series. Suppression of leukocyte production and/or abnormalities in leukocyte function compromises the host's ability to prevent and/or combat infection. Table 21-1 classifies white blood cells by subtype and provides the range of normal values for each. The normal values for erythrocytes (red blood cells) and platelets also are provided. *Leukopenia*, a reduction in the total number of white blood cells, and *granulocytopenia*, the reduction in the number of granulocytes, are common consequences of myelotoxic cancer therapy, which predisposes the person with cancer to infectious complications.

Macrophages

Macrophages are cells of the reticuloendothelial network that engulf and destroy foreign material or debris within

TABLE 21-1 Normal Blood Values

Hematocrit (Hct)		
Men	45% (38–54%)	
Women	40% (36–47%)	
Hemoglobin (Hgb)		
Men	14–18 g/dL	
Women	12–16 g/dL	
Children	12–14 g/dL	
Blood Counts	**Per Cubic Millimeter**	**Percentage**
Erythocytes (RBC)		
Men	5 (4.5–6) × 10	100%
Women	4.5 (4.3–5.5) × 10	100%
Reticulocytes		0–1%
Total leukocytes (WBC)	5000–10,000	100%
Polymorphonuclear leukocytes*	2500–6000	40–60%
Bands	0–500	0–5%
Lymphocytes	1000–4000	20–40%
Eosinophils	50–300	1–3%
Basophils	0–100	0–1%
Monocytes	200–800	4–8%
Platelets	200,000–500,000	100%

* Granulocytes, segmented neutrophils, polymorphonuclear cells

the body. Macrophages are found in the loose connective tissues and various other tissues of the body (Table 21-2). Through the process of phagocytosis, macrophages capture, process, and present antigen to lymphocytes, which triggers the lymphocytes to initiate a full immunologic response. Antigen that is not processed by macrophages in this way may only stimulate a weak immune response or no response. Activated macrophages are capable of inhibiting or killing intracellular pathogens nonspecifically; therefore the presence of activated macrophages appears to be an important factor in host resistance to infection.[1] The mature macrophage is more resistant to cytotoxic chemotherapy than is the mature polymorphonuclear granulocyte and appears to provide an important phagocytic capability even during periods of severe granulocytopenia. The activated macrophage is an important defense against *Mycobacterium*, *Listeria*, and *Brucella* organisms, several of the fungi, the protozoans, and the viruses.[1,2]

Interferons

Interferons are species-specific proteins that are produced by most cells of the body, especially lymphocytes and macrophages in response to viral infection. Interferons protect virally infected cells from infection by other viruses and produce general antiviral, antiproliferative, and immu-

TABLE 21-2 Macrophages

Type	Tissue
Alveolar macrophage or dust cell	Lung
Kupffer's cell	Liver
Histiocyte	Loose connective tissue
Microglia	Spinal cord and brain
Monocyte	Peripheral blood
Macrophage	Peritoneal cavity, pleural cavity, bone
Splenocyte	Spleen

nomodulatory activity. Although interferons may play an important role in the body's defense against viruses, they are not specific agents but act against a variety of different viruses. Interferons can act directly on T lymphocytes to stimulate cellular immune responses. Finally, interferons have an antiproliferative effect on tumor cells by interfering with protein synthesis and replication of DNA.[1,3,4]

IMPAIRMENT OF HOST DEFENSES IN CANCER

Granulocytopenia

There is a quantitative relationship between the level of circulating polymorphonuclear leukocytes and infection. Individuals whose granulocyte count is less than 1000/mm^3 are considered to have granulocytopenia. Incidence of infection begins to rise when the absolute granulocyte count falls to 500/mm^3 or less (Figure 21-1). When the granulocyte count is less than 100/mm^3, bacteremia predominates the clinical picture. As the length of therapy and duration of granulocytopenia increase, so does the incidence of superinfection.[5,6]

Because of the short life span of circulating granulocytes, their number must be determined on a daily basis, especially in individuals with severe granulocytopenia. The absolute number of granulocytes is determined by obtaining a total white blood cell count and a differential count, which specifies the relative number of normal white blood cells by type (segmented granulocytes, bands, lymphocytes, monocytes, eosinophils, and basophils), as well as any abnormal or premature forms that are observed microscopically. By multiplying the fraction (percentage) of granulocytes times the total number of white blood cells (WBC), the absolute number of granulocytes can be determined. The absolute number of granulocytes (poly-

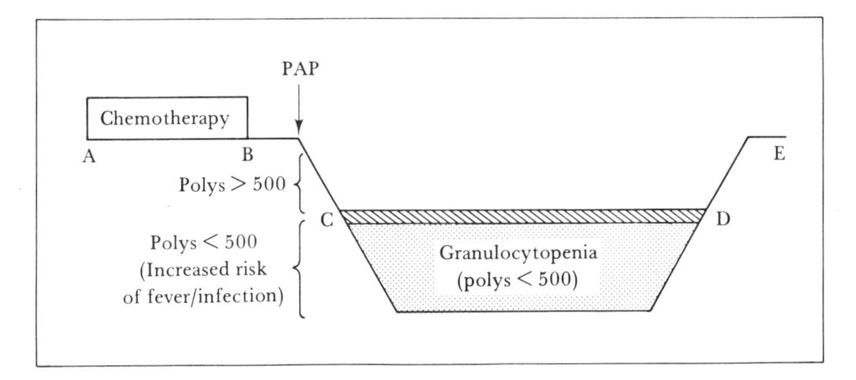

FIGURE 21-1 Chemotherapy cycle. Days of risk vary from drug to drug and person to person. The period of administration of myelotoxic chemotherapy is indicated by points *A* to *B*. The period between the end of therapy (*B*) and the onset of granulocytopenia (*C*) is illustrated as a sloping line that falls from point *B* to point *C*. This downward slope indicates the fall in the granulocyte count, which may begin a few days after therapy or may be delayed for 1 to 2 weeks. The duration of the granulocytopenia, depicted as the line extending from point *C* to point *D*, may last a few days, a week, or longer. If an oral prophylactic antibiotic program (*PAP*) is to serve as an effective "bridge" against infection during this period of risk (*C-D*), the antibiotic program must be established before the onset of severe granulocytopenia and should continue until the granulocyte count rises above 500/mm^3. The increase in the granulocyte count illustrated by the line that rises from point *D* to point *E* (>500 polys/mm^3) is associated with a decreased risk of infection and signals that the prophylactic antibiotic treatment may safely be discontinued.

morphonuclear leukocytes [polys]) is calculated by the use of the following formula when the results of the blood count are known:

Total WBC × percentage of granulocytes (polys/bands)
= Absolute number of granulocytes for that day
For example: Total WBC = 2500 cells/mm^3

The differential is as follows:

38% polys } = 50% granulocytes
12% bands }
45% lymphocytes
1% eosinophils
1% basophils
3% monocytes

Polys and bands are categories of granulocytes; therefore 50% of the WBCs are granulocytes. To obtain the absolute number, multiply 50% or 0.50 times the total WBC of 2500:

2500 × 0.50 = 1250 = The absolute number of granulocytes for that day

The WBC count and percentage of granulocytes change every day. The total WBC count may be the same (eg, 2500 cells/mm^3), but the percentage of granulocytes may vary tremendously over several days. Therefore the WBC count alone will not always provide enough information to determine whether the person has granulocytopenia. A person with fewer than 500 granulocytes/mm^3 has severe granulocytopenia and an increased risk of infection.

Fever

Febrile episodes occur frequently in individuals diagnosed with cancer. Although fever may be caused by the underlying cancer, the majority of fevers result from infection, especially when patients have granulocytopenia. Lymphomas, hypernephromas, and tumors of gastrointestinal origin that have metastasized to the liver may cause fever unrelated to infection. In addition, tumor masses that cause local obstruction or compromise the blood supply to normal tissue can predispose tissue to necrosis, local infection, and fever. Fever caused by an underlying cancer cannot be distinguished from fever caused by infection on the basis of duration or the degree of temperature elevation.[6,7] Excluding febrile episodes related to the administration of blood products and chemotherapeutic agents, which will resolve spontaneously, there remain a large number of febrile episodes of unknown cause that occur in individuals with cancer in whom infection must be ruled out. Nursing assessment of the febrile patient includes careful physical examination to identify a potential source of infection and an evaluation of disease and treatment-induced compromise of host defenses.

Causes of Immunosuppression

Infection

Infection can occur as a result of depression of the cell-mediated immune system. Depression of lymphocyte function in vitro has been associated with certain infections, including (1) viral infections such as influenza and infectious mononucleosis, (2) live vaccine, for example, measles, mumps, and rubella, (3) bacterial infections such as tuberculosis, leprosy, syphilis, and bacterial pneumonia, and (4) fungal infection such as candidiasis and coccidioidomycosis. It appears that both lymphocyte and monocyte functions may be abnormally depressed during and after acute infections, thereby extending susceptibility beyond the acute episode.

Acquired immunodeficiency syndrome

Acquired immunodeficiency syndrome (AIDS) is caused by a human retrovirus and is characterized by loss of T4 cells, which leads to progressive loss of immune system competency with development of opportunistic infections, impairment of the central nervous system, chronic wasting, and often malignancy. The virus that causes AIDS has been called by a variety of names since its discovery: human T-lymphotrophic virus type III (HTLV-III), lymphadenopathy-associated virus (LAV), and human immunodeficiency virus (HIV); it is referred to here as HIV. HIV has been isolated in blood, saliva, tears, urine, cerebrospinal fluid, semen, vaginal secretions, and breast milk. However, only blood, semen, and intrauterine exposure (possible vaginal secretions and breast milk) are known vectors.[8-11]

Infection with HIV is not synonymous with AIDS. AIDS is part of a continuum of illnesses that is related to the HIV virus. Persons infected with HIV may have no symptoms, they may display some symptoms of immune deficiencies, or they may have physical manifestations of AIDS. Many persons with primary HIV infection are asymptomatic even though they show seropositivity for antibodies to HIV. Others may have symptoms that include fever, rigors, arthralgias, rash, abdominal cramping, and diarrhea 2 to 6 weeks after infection. These symptoms may be accompanied by mild immunologic deficiencies, including leukopenia, thrombocytopenia, and lymphopenia.[12]

Lymphadenopathy syndrome or persistent generalized lymphadenopathy, terms used to describe an immunologic deficiency, refer specifically to chronic, nonmalignant diffuse enlargement of lymph nodes in at least two extrainguinal sites. Nodes must be at least 1 cm in diameter and remain swollen for at least 3 months. Other symptoms, in addition to swollen lymph nodes, include pain and fever, night sweats, weight loss, and splenomegaly.

Aids-related complex (ARC) is a term for an HIV infection in a person who displays two symptoms of immunodeficiency and at least two laboratory-verified abnormalities. ARC may remain in a mild form or progress to AIDS. Immune thrombocytopenic purpura (ITP) is a second AIDS-related diagnosis related to HIV infection. Symptoms include easy bruising, petechiae, mucosal bleeding, and varying degrees of lymphadenopathy. Both ARC and ITP lie midway along the continuum of HIV infection.[12,13]

AIDS is characterized by underlying cellular immunodeficiency and absence of other disease known to cause immunodeficiency. Common opportunistic infections associated with AIDS include cytomegalovirus (CMV), herpes simplex, herpes zoster, *Candida albicans*, *Cryptococcus* organisms, *Pneumocystis carinii*, *Toxoplasma gondii*, *Cryptosporidium* organisms, *Mycobacterium avium-intracellulare*, and tuberculosis.[8-13]

Infections related to tumor-associated abnormalities

The types of infections that occur in persons diagnosed with cancer are somewhat predictable. The abnormal cell-mediated immunity in Hodgkin's disease is associated with an increased incidence of intracellular pathogens, including herpes zoster virus, *Cryptococcus neoformans*, *Brucella* species, *Mycobacterium tuberculosis*, *Listeria monocytogenes*, *Salmonella* species, and *Toxoplasma gondii*.[14,15]

Other malignancies are associated with a decreased sensitivity and decreased ability to respond to the challenging antigen, for example, advanced lung cancers, intracranial tumors, and other specific solid tumors. It is interesting to note that individuals with malignancies other than those of the reticuloendothelial system who have not been immunosuppressed appear to have normal cell-mediated immunity.[14-16]

Individuals who are asplenic as a result of trauma, staging laparotomy for malignant lymphoma, hypersplenism, or sickle cell disease have impaired opsonization that can increase susceptibility to infection.[17] The risk of overwhelming sepsis and death in those with asplenia, especially persons with Hodgkin's disease, is at least 50 times greater than in the normal population. Baccarani et al,[18] however, have noted that patients with Hodgkin's disease in complete remission have a 2.30% cumulative risk of the development of an overwhelming postsplenectomy infection, whereas the percentage increased to 15.25% for those patients in whom relapse had occurred.

Nutrition

Cancer can affect an individual's nutritional status in several ways. The tumor can interfere with the functional capacity of gastrointestinal structures or organs and may cause inlet or outlet obstruction. Chronic obstruction can compromise the blood supply to surrounding tissue, especially if vascular impairment is severe or prolonged. The resulting necrosis and ulceration will predispose the affected areas to hemorrhage and infection.

Cachexia, a state of malnutrition and wasting, is often a debilitating manifestation of cancer (see Chapter 24). The exact mechanisms responsible for cachexia are not well understood. The rate of wasting does not appear to be related to the histologic findings of the tumor, the stage of the disease, or the specific sites of involvement. The severity of the syndrome may be unrelated to the quantity or quality of calories consumed, inasmuch as cachexia often develops without evidence of malabsorption.[19] Bengoa[20] noted that the host's normal cells seem to atrophy while cancer cells grow, possibly indicating a growth advantage in cancer cells.

There appears to be an interaction between malnutrition and infection; even subclinical malnutrition seems to lower a person's resistance to infection. Infection compromises nutritional status by decreasing appetite, increasing the metabolic rate as a result of fever, and decreasing gastrointestinal absorption. Protein-calorie malnutrition decreases the host's resistance to infection by interfering with both cellular and humoral immunity.

Immune defects related to nutritional deficiencies appear to be corrected by nutritional support, and cell-mediated immunity may return to normal when malnourished persons receive either oral or intravenous hyperalimentation.[20]

Cancer therapy

Surgery Surgery is commonly employed in the diagnosis, staging, and treatment of patients diagnosed with cancer. Various factors can increase the incidence of infectious complications in the individual undergoing surgery, including the length of preoperative hospitalization; the extent of the surgery; the length of the procedure; the degree of hemorrhage and decreased tissue perfusion; the age, sex, and nutritional status of the patient; prior cytotoxic chemotherapy or corticosteroid administration; and, most important, the presence of infection or wound contamination during surgery. Patients who undergo surgical intervention for treatment of cancer often receive preoperative prophylactic antibiotics in dosages to provide adequate serum levels of antibiotic during the operative risk period. The choice of antibiotic is based on the site of operation, potential pathogens, presence of a prior infection, or heavy colonization with particular microorganisms.[21] Teaching patients respiratory hygiene techniques before surgery and ensuring that they comply with this practice after surgery can significantly reduce the incidence of postoperative pneumonia.

The surgical wound is the most common site of infection during the postoperative period. Wound infections range in severity from minor inflammatory responses to deep infections that may be life threatening. Distinctive patterns of microorganisms usually are seen in different hospital environments, and each hospital's microbial surveillance team will monitor infection patterns, trends, and incidence of specific microorganisms that cause infections. Special concern must be directed toward the detection of resistant microorganisms, which may develop with astonishing rapidity and cause severe morbidity in the hospital environment.

Certain types of surgery are more likely to precipitate sepsis. Surgical instrumentation of the genitourinary and gastrointestinal tracts carries considerable risk of morbidity and mortality for the general patient population and a formidable risk for individuals with compromised host defense mechanisms. Any incision, intubation, injection, or infusion increases the risk of infection, and any hospitalization increases the opportunities for nosocomial transmission of pathogenic organisms. Prevention of infection through strict aseptic techniques is one of the most important nursing responsibilities.

Radiotherapy and chemotherapy Infection is the leading cause of death in cancer patients who receive myelotoxic therapy. Radiotherapy and chemotherapy can interfere with the essential metabolic functions of the cell and may cause inflammation and ulceration of normal tissues, thus predisposing individuals to infection. The doses of chemotherapy and/or radiotherapy that can be safely administered are determined and limited by the toxicities to normal tissue. Fractionation of radiation doses and administration of chemotherapy in intermittent cycles have been effective in enhancing therapeutic benefits while limiting toxicity.[22] The major risks associated with therapeutic radiation and cytotoxic chemotherapy relate to the induction of granulocytopenia and immunosuppression. For example, Figure 21-1 illustrates the sequence of events that can follow the administration of a myelotoxic form of chemotherapy given to a person with an adequate granulocyte and platelet count. Those on a prophylactic antibiotic program who take all their prescribed medications without missing any doses have fewer fevers, infections, and hospitalizations than those who miss one or more doses of prophylactic antibiotics.

Chemotherapy may induce immunologic defects that lead to bacterial, fungal, parasitic, and viral infection (Table 21-3). Not all chemotherapeutic agents, however, produce immunologic compromise. The potential effects and side effects of each agent should be reviewed and incorporated into the patient's plan of care and assessment (see Chapter 13 for specific information concerning chemotherapy).

Hematologic competency can be adversely affected by radiation therapy. Leukocytes will be decreased first, followed by thrombocytes and then hemoglobin. Blood counts should be monitored during radiation, especially if a large area is treated or if significant areas of the bone marrow are included in the radiation field.

Depending on the total dose and type of radiation, the skin and mucous membranes may be affected.[22,23] Radiation reactions may include epilation, erythema, dry desquamation, and moist desquamation. Some common oral complications associated with radiation to the head and neck region include xerostomia, dental caries, oral mucositis, taste loss, osteoradionecrosis, oral infection trismus, and nutritional stomatitis. Because an intact integumentary system is a major defense against infection, aggressive therapeutic measures should be taken to maintain the skin and mucous membranes in maximal condition. The skin and oral mucosa should be inspected and assessed daily for signs of inflammation, ulceration, infection, and moisture.[22-25] Management of the person receiving radiation is discussed in Chapter 12.

TABLE 21-3 Immune Defects and Infectious Organisms in the Patient with Cancer Who Is Immunocompromised

Defect	Cause	Bacteria	Fungi	Parasites	Viruses
Granulocytopenia	Chemotherapy used to treat acute leukemia Chronic myelocytic leukemia in blast crisis Chemotherapy used to treat lymphoma Chemotherapy used to treat solid tumors (eg, lung, testicular, ovarian)	*Pseudomonas* *Escherichia coli* *Klebsiella* *Staphylococcus aureus* *Staphylococcus epidermidis*	*Candida* *Aspergillus*		
Cell-mediated immune system suppression	Lymphoma Chemotherapy used to treat Hodgkin's disease, acute lymphocytic leukemia	*Mycobacterium* *Norcardia asteroides* *Legionella* *Salmonella*	*Cryptococcus* *Histoplasma* *Coccidioides* *Candida* *Aspergillus* *Mucor*	*Listeria* *Pneumocystis carinii* *Toxoplasma gondii*	Varicella zoster Cytomegalovirus
Humoral defect	Multiple myeloma Chronic lymphocytic leukemia Splenectomy	*Streptococcus pneumoniae* *Haemophilus influenzae* *Neisseria meningitidis* *Klebsiella pneumoniae* *Staphylococcus aureus*	*Rickettsia* *Toxoplasma gondii* *Pneumocystis carinii*	Herpes zoster	

Nosocomial Infections

Unperturbed, the endogenous microbial flora exist as a carefully balanced synergistic microenvironment within the host. Although the majority of the infections that occur in persons with cancer arise from endogenous microbial flora, nearly 50% of the infectious organisms are nosocomial.[6] The classic highly virulent bacteria, as well as organisms considered "normal flora," are capable of causing sepsis and other serious infections.[21,26] The most frequent bacterial isolates that cause nosocomial infections are gram-positive *Staphylococcus aureus* and gram-negative *Escherichia coli* and *Klebsiella pneumoniae.* Although gram-negative isolates still predominate as the source of infection at most cancer centers, gram-positive bacteria, especially *Staphylococcus epidermidis,* have increased in recent years, whereas infections caused by *Pseudomonas aeruginosa* have decreased.[5] Nosocomial infections are caused by common endogenous organisms that become pathogenic when disease impairs host defenses, when antibiotics create an imbalance in the microenvironment of the host, or when invasive procedures allow a portal of entry. Many sources in an individual's external environment may contribute to the acquisition of potentially harmful microorganisms, but the significant sources appear to be staff-patient and patient-patient transmission.[26]

The concept of infection control was first introduced by Semmelweis in the mid-1800s to the physicians and students of his day. He stressed the importance of the simple act of handwashing between patient contacts.[27,28] Surprisingly, although handwashing generally is considered to be the single most important procedure in the prevention of nosocomial infections, motivating hospital personnel to wash their hands consistently before and after every patient contact remains difficult.

When an infection occurs, hospitalization may be necessary or extended and the costs of health care increase. Up to $10 billion in annual hospital costs can be attributed to nosocomial infections.[26,29] It is estimated that 6% of patients (2 to 4 million persons) acquire infections while in the hospital and that the majority of these infections are in the urinary tract or in surgical wounds.[26,29]

Urinary tract infections associated with catheterization

Of the infections that occur in hospitalized persons 30% to 40% are urinary tract infections associated with the use of urinary catheters.[2,28] In fact, the most frequent cause of gram-negative sepsis is the urinary catheter. Adherence to the basic principles of catheter management will dramatically reduce catheter-related infections. These include (1) restriction of urinary catheterization to conditions of clinical necessity, not convenience, (2) use of sterile, closed drainage systems, especially in prolonged catheterization or in individuals susceptible to infection, (3) insertion of urinary catheters by means of careful aseptic technique, and (4) removal of catheters as soon as they are no longer required.

Infections associated with vascular access

Intravenous catheters Although risk associated with contaminated needles and syringes has been reduced by the use of individually packaged disposable units, hazards associated with intravenous therapy continue to represent a major threat to individuals with pancytopenia and immunosuppression. Contamination of intravenous fluids can occur as a result of improper technique during the addition of fluid supplements, during "breaks" in aseptic technique, during assembly of the infusion, during blood sample withdrawals through three-way stopcocks, during flushing, and during the prolonged use of single intravenous cannula.

It is generally recommended that intravenous needles be changed every 48 hours.[30] Because patients with cancer often have fragile superficial veins, careful assessment of their condition may indicate less frequent changing of the intravenous needle unless there are signs of infection or infiltration. With frequent and careful assessment of the puncture site, vein, and surrounding area for phlebitis, infiltration, or other signs of potential infection, the needle may be left in place for longer periods. If early signs of an infectious complication are detected, the intravenous infusion should be discontinued, the needle or catheter should be withdrawn and cultured, and blood should be drawn for culture to identify the causative organism.

Venous access catheters and devices Indwelling right atrial catheters and vascular access devices have revolutionized the administration of chemotherapy and supportive care of the person with cancer by providing long-term venous access. However, the immunosuppressive effect of the therapy administered to these individuals increases the risk of infection and sepsis associated with indwelling catheters and devices. When a fever of unknown origin occurs in a patient with an indwelling catheter or port, this device must be considered a potential source of infection.

Even though the incidence of catheter-associated sepsis is somewhat higher with indwelling catheters, most infections can be treated successfully with antibiotics without catheter removal.[19] For the patient who needs frequent venipuncture or has limited vascular accessibility, the advantages of an indwelling catheter or vascular access device appear to outweigh the risk of infection.

Other nosocomial infections

Although the overall incidence of gram-negative infection has decreased over the years, pneumonia caused by these organisms is still a serious problem in individuals with cancer. Gram-negative bacteria, both exogenous water-borne species and hospital-acquired oropharyngeal flora, readily bypass bacterial clearance mechanisms when introduced into the lower respiratory tract by contaminated equipment used for respiratory support or aerosol administration.[2,21] Contaminated respiratory equipment, including nebulizers, ventilators, tracheal catheters, and suction equipment, have been implicated as a source of infections in hospitalized persons.

Other causes of infection are contaminated intravascular instruments, including cardiac catheters and adapters, oxygenator or heart-lung machines, plastic parts of the hemodialyzer, and various liquids, including hand and skin lotions, saline eye irrigation solutions, and pooled water in flower vases. The reduction of nosocomial infections depends heavily on improved and careful methods for the control and elimination of external sources of infection, as well as on the thoughtful protection and handling of infected individuals so that infections are not carried from patient to patient by hospital personnel.[2,31]

TYPES OF INFECTIONS

Any microorganism can cause disease in a compromised host. The porta of entry determines the type of infection and some of its characteristics. Microorganisms may be inhaled, ingested, inoculated through the skin, or introduced through invasive procedures. Organisms may cause local infections or may be transported to distant sites. Several major groups of microorganisms are responsible for infection and disease in individuals with cancer: bacteria, fungi, viruses, and protozoa.

Bacteria

Bacteria are single-cell organisms with well-defined cell walls. All bacteria are capable of independent growth on artificial media and do not require assistance from other living cells. Bacteria are classified as aerobic or anaerobic and gram-positive or gram-negative (Table 21-4). Bacteria that cause disease in humans include spherical forms (cocci) and rod-shaped forms (bacillae). Streptococci are a primary cause of pharyngitis, wound infection, localized skin infection, sepsis, and scarlet fever. Other cocci include meningococci, which cause the epidemic form of bacterial meningitis; pneumococci, which cause pneumococcal pneumonia; and staphylococci, which cause skin infection, sepsis, and nosocomial infections. The rod-shaped bacteria or bacilli, shigellae and salmonellae, are the causative agents of bacillary dysentery and the enteric fevers, including typhoid fever. The coliform bacilli are normal endogenous organisms that are found in the gastrointestinal tract. Coliform bacilli usually function in harmony with the host by providing necessary vitamins and certain factors that contribute to infection resistance and by help-

TABLE 21-4 Bacteria That Cause Disease in Humans

	Gram-Positive		Gram-Negative		
Bacteria	**Cocci**	**Bacillae**	**Cocci**	**Bacillae**	**Anaerobic/Aerobic**
Actinomyces spp		Yes			Anaerobic
Bordetella pertussis				Yes	Aerobic
Brucella spp				Yes	Aerobic
Campylobacter jejuni				Yes	Aerobic
Clostridium tetani		Yes			Anaerobic
Corynebacterium diphtheriae		Yes			Aerobic
Enterobacter spp				Yes	Aerobic
Escherichia coli				Yes	Anaerobic
Klebsiella spp		Yes			Aerobic
Legionella pneumophilia				Yes	Aerobic
Listeria		Yes			Aerobic
Salmonella spp				Yes	Anaerobic
Mycobacterium tuberculosis		Yes			Aerobic
Mycoplasma pneumoniae		Yes			Anaerobic
Neisseria meningitidis			Yes		Aerobic
Pneumococci	Yes				Aerobic
Proteus				Yes	Anaerobic
Salmonella typhi		Yes			Anaerobic
Shigella spp				Yes	Anaerobic
Staphylococcus aureus	Yes				Aerobic
Streptococcus pneumoniae	Yes				Aerobic
Streptococcus pyogenes	Yes				Aerobic
Streptococcus viridans	Yes				Aerobic

ing to maintain the host's normal intestinal flora; however, these gram-negative enteric bacteria can become serious pathogens in the person who is immunosuppressed, who has granulocytopenia, or is recovering from gastrointestinal surgery.

Mycoplasmas

Mycoplasmas resemble bacteria in that they are capable of life on an artificial medium, but they lack the rigid cell wall of bacteria and are more selective in their growth requirements. *Mycoplasma pneumoniae* is a serious respiratory infection that may be difficult to diagnose in the person with cancer.

Rickettsiae

Rickettsiae are smaller than true bacteria, are located within the cells of the host, and require living cells for growth and multiplication. Although their cell walls resemble gram-negative bacteria, they really are intracellular parasites.[2] Rickettsiae are responsible for typhus, Rocky Mountain spotted fever, and rickettsialpox.

Legionella pneumophilia

Legionella pneumophilia may be responsible for a significant but unrecognized number of fatal pneumonias in persons with cancer who are immunosuppressed. The bacterium has a predilection for immunocompromised hosts and appears to multiply intracellularly in human monocytes, rendering them incapable of their normal protective function.[32] Monocytes represent a major line of defense against infection in individuals with leukopenia; therefore, exposure to *L. pneumophilia* in those with cancer who are receiving cytotoxic therapy can be expected to produce a high risk of life-threatening infection.

Of the eight species of *Legionella* organisms that have been identified, *L. micdadei* shows the strongest tendency to appear in immunosuppressed hosts. A prodromal syndrome that consists of malaise, myalgias, and headache may be seen. These symptoms may be accompanied by watery diarrhea, nausea, vomiting, and confusion. Most patients begin with a dry, nonproductive cough coupled with bloody sputum production, and 25% complain of pleuritic chest pain. Almost all patients have a high unremitting fever, often accompanied by recurrent rigors. Sputum cultures and Gram's stains are not specific for differential diagnosis. Blood cultures are normal. Proteinuria, hematuria, hepatic enzyme abnormalities, and leukocytosis are common. Radiologic findings show the pneumonia to be bilateral and multilobular, although the chest radiogram may appear to be clear at the onset of dyspnea, which often is the only initial symptom. Cavitation can occur but has been seen only in immunocompromised persons. Pleural effusions are present in 40% of cases. The most common cause of death is respiratory failure and shock. Specific diagnosis of legionellosis can be made after seroconversion, which takes at least 2 weeks. Most physicians use open lung biopsy for definitive diagnosis of *Legionella* pneumonia, because diagnosis by tracheal aspiration, bronchoscopy, or percutaneous needle biopsy yields results less than 50% of the time.[32]

L. pneumophilia has been isolated from water and from various heat exchange and air conditioning units, as well as from streams, lakes, showers, tap water, and cooling towers. Nosocomial infection has been documented.[28,33] Although the infection is usually multisystemic in nature, the lung seems to be the primary target organ in most cases. Successful treatment depends on early diagnosis and administration of erythromycin, 2 to 4 g/day for at least 3 weeks, to completely eliminate the offending organism. Doxycycline is the drug of choice when erythromycin cannot be given. Even with prompt treatment the mortality rate may reach almost 25%.[34]

Nursing measures include close assessment of the patient for signs of respiratory compromise, including monitoring vital signs, arterial blood gases, level of consciousness, signs of cyanosis in the buccal membranes, and signs and symptoms of shock. Supportive treatment may include fluid and electrolyte replacement, treatment with antipyretics, oxygen, and circulatory support with pressor drugs.

Viruses

Viruses are the smallest known infectious microorganisms and are visible only with the aid of a microscope. Viruses are replicated by host cell mechanisms after invasion of the cell by a single virus particle. The primary virus invades the cell and initiates the formation of similar particles by the host cell itself. The organisms have no intrinsic energy systems; they consist only of a deoxyribonucleic acid (DNA) or a ribonucleic acid (RNA) nucleus surrounded by a protein coat. Common viruses cause measles, mumps, rubella, respiratory infections, colds, and bronchitis.

Varicella

Infection with the varicella virus (chickenpox) can cause a serious vesicular eruption in individuals with cancer, especially children, and results in a mortality rate of about 7%. The major complication is visceral dissemination, which occurs in about 30% of cases, with a resulting mortality rate near 20%.[35] Pneumonia occurs in almost 80% of persons with visceral varicella, generally presenting as "fluffy," nodular-appearing infiltrates on a chest radiograph.[33] Other target organs that become involved when varicella infection disseminates include the lungs, liver, spleen, central nervous system, gastrointestinal tract, bone marrow, and lymph nodes. Varicella dissemination frequently is complicated by secondary bacterial infections. The risk of varicella visceral dissemination is increased in persons who are receiving chemotherapy at the time of infection, especially if lymphopenia occurs (<500 lymphocytes/mm^3).

Reye's syndrome also has been associated with varicella, inasmuch as varicella has been noted to precede up to 30% of all cases of this syndrome.[35] In both these infections severe brain swelling is noted, making it difficult to distinguish between varicella and Reye's syndrome.

Because of the severity of varicella infection in individuals with cancer, infected patients have been treated with varicella-zoster immune globulin (VZIG). When administered within 72 hours of exposure to varicella virus, VZIG generally modifies the infection to a subclinical or mild form. Management of persons with cancer who are seronegative and who have been exposed to varicella includes the interruption of all chemotherapy and the administration of VZIG. Whenever possible, chemotherapy should not be reinstituted until the end of the incubation period, which is approximately 21 days. When clinical evidence of varicella infection occurs in persons with cancer, they should not receive immunosuppressive agents until all skin lesions have dried and scabbed.

Radiotherapy can increase a person's risk of the development of varicella zoster, especially those with advanced Hodgkin's disease who are anergic. The dermatomes that become involved with varicella zoster lesions usually have been encompassed in the radiation field before the infection.

Varicella is highly contagious and the risk of spread to other seronegative, immunosuppressed persons is substantial, especially in adults with Hodgkin's disease and children with leukemia. Seronegative persons should be warned to avoid exposure to those with known cases of

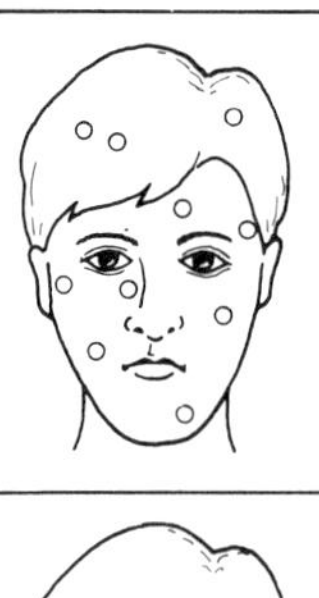

1. **Person with chickenpox (varicella)**
   Other individuals may "catch" chickenpox from this person if they have not had the infection before. The person is infectious for about 7 days. (Two days before the pox are noticeable and about 5 days after the first pox appears.)

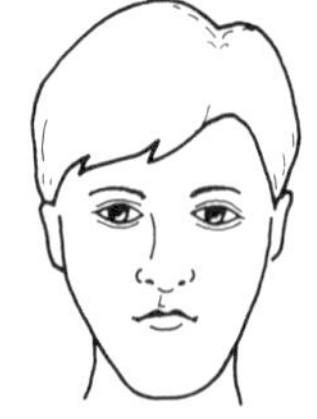

2. **Person after recovery from chickenpox (varicella)**
   The varicella virus remains inactive in the previously infected individual. The person is no longer infectious and is "immune" to chickenpox. The person can develop varicella zoster from varicella virus remaining in the body. This is an "endogenous" infection, "from within," and may occur in individuals receiving chemotherapy.

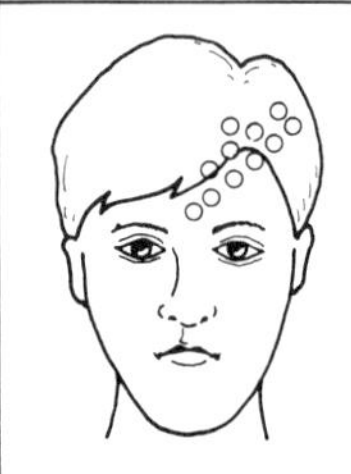

3. **Person with varicella zoster**
   The person has a history of a prior chickenpox infection. The pox are distributed in a limited pattern along nerve endings on the individual's body. Viral cultures are positive. Varicella zoster patients of any age are infectious. Individuals who have not had chickenpox can "catch" it from patients with varicella zoster (shingles).

FIGURE 21-2 Varicella-zoster infection.

varicella infection or those who have been exposed (most exposures occur inadvertently in the infectious period 2 days before the appearance of skin eruptions) (Figure 21-2). To reduce the possibility of contracting the disease and transmitting it to others, staff members who have not previously had chickenpox should avoid caring for infected individuals. Although varicella is not common in adults, its highly contagious nature and the serious infection it can cause necessitate isolation of hospitalized persons with varicella. Staff members should wear gowns and gloves while in the patient's room. Nasal and oral discharges are carefully discarded into plastic bags to minimize contamination of bed linens and other objects in the room. Disinfection of the hospital or clinic room is advisable before reuse.

Reactivation of varicella zoster virus (shingles) can occur in seropositive individuals because varicella virus from a primary varicella infection remains dormant in the spinal ganglia. Varicella zoster is an endogenous infection; however, varicella zoster in an affected person can cause chickenpox (primary varicella) in others who have not previously had the infection.

The diagnosis of zoster is based on a history of chickenpox, the characteristic distribution of vesicular lesions with a dermatomal distribution, and positive culture results of the lesions. Skin lesions (vesicles) may become confluent, and meticulous local skin care is needed to avoid the development of secondary bacterial infections. Supportive treatment is based on symptoms. Skin care and pain control measures can provide some relief during the acute phase of the infection.

Dissemination of zoster outside the original dermatome, as well as visceral involvement of the lungs, gastrointestinal tract, and central nervous system, may occur. Treatment of zoster with VZIG in immunodeficient children who are at high risk has been useful. Acyclovir has been effective in bringing about negative culture results, in decreasing the appearance of new lesions, and in promoting the crusting of lesions already present on the skin. Acyclovir has shown to be effective in reducing pain and facilitating the healing of lesions.[35] In addition, some success has been reported with the use of human leukocyte interferon to treat varicella in children with malignancies.[33]

Herpes simplex virus

Herpes simplex viruses cause serious infections in persons with cancer. Severe infections can occur with primary exposure to the virus or when the latent virus is activated. Major sites of infection are the oral mucosa, esophagus, eyes, skin, and urogenital tract. When the virus disseminates, which is relatively rare, pulmonary, central nervous system, and hepatic involvement may be seen. Oral lesions may be painful for the patient with herpes simplex. Comfort measures include relief of pain with analgesics, cool liquids, ice pops, and a soft, nonirritating diet. Antipyretics are administered as necessary. Gloves are worn to avoid contact with lesions.

Vidarabine has been shown to reduce mortality and morbidity in herpes simplex encephalitis.[36] Gastrointestinal and neurologic side effects, however, have been noted with the use of vidarabine. Tremors, paresthesias, ataxia, and seizures may appear several days after initiation of therapy and require astute and ongoing neurologic assessment. Gastrointestinal effects most often include anorexia and nausea.[36]

Acyclovir has been useful in the management of mucosal and cutaneous herpes simplex infections in immunocompromised adults and children. Parenteral acyclovir therapy decreases the duration of pain and itching, the duration of positive cultures and viral shedding, and the time required for crusting and healing of lesions.[36]

Cytomegalovirus

CMV is a ubiquitous virus that is a member of the herpes virus family. Infection is generally a consequence of viral reactivation, and immunosuppressive chemotherapy appears to be a factor in this reactivation. Dissemination to visceral organs can occur but usually is seen only in the terminal phase of disease. CMV appears to predispose individuals to superinfections with other pathogens. Cytomegalopneumonia, frequently observed in persons who have undergone bone marrow transplantation, characteristically occurs within 3 months of transplantation and often is fatal.[37] 9-(1,3-dihydroxy-2-propoxymethyl) guanine (DHPG) has been useful in the treatment of CMV in immunosuppressed patients who have had bone marrow transplantation and in persons with AIDS. This drug, however, has significant toxicities associated with its use. Because CMV is present in bodily secretions, the health care provider should wear gloves when handling urine, saliva, or other body secretions.[38]

Hepatitis virus

Hepatitis in individuals with cancer can occur as a primary infection with one of the hepatitis viruses (A, B, or non-A, non-B) or from visceral dissemination of other viral organisms. Hepatitis B virus (HBV) and the non-A, non-B virus are the major causative organisms in transfusion-related hepatitis. Specific viral antigens generally can be detected in the sera of infected individuals.

Viral hepatitis can occur as an acute or a chronic infection. Asymptomatic carriers may have nondetectable hepatic dysfunction. Although transfusions of blood products constitute the major route of hepatitis transmission, nonparenteral transmission occurs through contaminated saliva, urine, and feces and also may occur through sexual relations. Venipunctures, culture specimens, and stool and urine from infected persons must be handled according to the universal precautions outlined by the Centers for Disease Control (CDC)[38] (Figure 21-3). Under this system of control every patient is approached as if he was infected with hepatitis.

The risk of infection to the hospital staff is high when a patient has hepatitis. Because the presence of hepatitis is not always known during early patient contact, the nursing staff should adhere strictly to universal precaution guidelines. Adhering to the principles of proper hand washing and handling of dressings, linen, discharges, and culture specimens as outlined by the CDC will effectively protect the hospital staff, patients, and laboratory personnel from preventable infections.

1. Never recap, bend, break, or clip needles.
2. Place needles and sharps promptly in an approved puncture-resistant container designated for needle disposal.
3. Use approved disposal containers in all areas.
4. Do not overfill containers.
5. Close container securely when three quarters full.
6. Bag closed containers in red bags.
7. Protect open wounds from coming in contact with potentially infected materials.
8. Be sure to cover properly any broken skin surfaces.
9. Gloves are necessary when:
   a. drawing blood
   b. handling specimens that have obvious blood in them
   c. starting intravenous infusions (IVs)
   d. cleaning blood spills
   e. during cardiopulmonary resuscitation (CPR)
   f. suctioning (especially a new tracheostomy)
   g. changing dressings
10. Wear mask, gloves, and protective eyewear when:
   a. blood splattering may occur
   b. inserting or maintaining arterial lines
   c. doing oral care
   d. doing emergency procedures
   e. doing invasive procedures
   f. doing hemodialysis or hemapheresis
   g. doing peritoneal dialysis
11. Change gloves between patients.
12. Wash hands thoroughly before leaving the patient's room.

FIGURE 21-3 Universal Precautions for Prevention of Transmission of Human Immunodeficiency Virus, Hepatitis B Virus, and Other Blood-Borne Pathogens (Source: Center for Disease Control: Universal precautions for prevention of transmission of human immunodeficiency virus, hepatitis B virus, and other blood-borne pathogens. MMWR 37 (June 24): 377-387, 1988.)

Treatment

Vidarabine is a purine nucleoside that interferes with viral DNA synthesis, especially in varicella zoster and herpes simplex infections. It is administered over 5 to 10 days as a 12- to 24-hour infusion at doses ranging from 10 to 15 mg/kg. Therapy is most effective when initiated early in the infection. Patients with disseminated disease generally do not benefit from vidarabine therapy. In cases where the disease is disseminated, treatment with acyclovir acts to halt further progression of the infection. Because it penetrates into the cerebrospinal fluid, vidarabine is useful in the treatment of herpes simplex encephalitis. Vidarabine toxicity includes bone marrow depression, hepatic dysfunction, and neurologic disturbances such as tremor, confusion, and ataxia.

The solubility of vidarabine in intravenous infusion fluids is limited. A maximum of 450 mg of the drug can be dissolved in 1 L of intravenous infusion fluid. It is absolutely essential that only completely clear solutions be administered. The presence of particulate matter in the fluid indicates incomplete solubilization and necessitates that the solution be discarded. Persons who receive vidarabine should be assessed for nausea, vomiting, diarrhea, anorexia, and weight loss, which are the most frequent side effects of the drug. These reactions are usually mild and subside in 1 to 4 days without discontinuing or decreasing the dose. Increased asparate aminotransferase (AST, formerly transaminase serum glutamic-oxaloacetic transaminase, or SGOT) is a common side effect; however, it is transient.

The development of acyclovir, a synthetic purine nucleoside, is a major breakthrough in the management of mucocutaneous herpes simplex infections. Acyclovir is preferentially taken up and selectively converted by the virus to its active antiviral form in herpes-infected cells. This conversion, which does not occur to any significant degree in normal cells, accounts for acyclovir's relative lack of toxicity to normal cells. Once activated in the herpes-infected cells, acyclovir interferes with the synthesis of viral DNA, which is essential for the assembly of new virus particles. Acyclovir has been shown to provide significant prophylaxis against recurrent herpes infection in immunocompromised individuals, especially those who have had allogeneic bone marrow transplantation, and it is a safe and effective treatment for those in whom mucocutaneous herpes infections develop.[36] Treatment with acyclovir is associated with decreased viral shedding from infected cells, accelerated healing of lesions, and decreased pain.

Intravenous acyclovir is usually given at a dosage of 7 mg/kg or less every 8 hours, which is infused over a period of at least 60 minutes. Because acyclovir is water soluble, it can be given in smaller volumes of fluid than vidarabine. Acyclovir ointment 5% is used for the management of mucocutaneous herpes symptoms in immunocompromised persons. Acyclovir also has been noted to have a beneficial effect in immunocompromised children who have chickenpox if treatment is initiated early in the disease.

In general, adverse reactions to acyclovir are minimal. Persons who receive this drug, however, should be assessed for local reactions at the injection site (eg, pain, inflammation, or phlebitis). Transient increases in blood urea nitrogen or serum creatinine may occur, especially with rapid intravenous injection or infusion that runs less than 10 minutes. Other side effects that have been noted are headache, nausea, vomiting, and diarrhea.

Alpha-interferon has been used in the management of herpes simplex and herpes zoster with some success. Side effects of interferon most often include a flulike syndrome (fever, chills, malaise, and myalgias), which affects up to 90% of patients and lasts 5 to 9 days. The onset of chills usually occurs 3 to 6 hours after administration of the drug and may be accompanied by fever and elevated blood pressure. Severe rigors are treated with morphine to decrease muscle contractions. Fever usually peaks about 30 minutes to 1 hour after the onset of chills and may reach 38.2° to 40° C (102° to 104°F). Fever can be controlled effectively by the administration of acetominophen before and after the administration of interferon. Tachyphylaxis usually develops after several injections of interferon. If the dose is increased or the administration schedule is changed, side effects may recur. Patients and families should be prepared for the rapid onset of side effects and be reassured that these are expected and temporary in nature.[39-41]

Fungi

In humans fungi can exist in harmony with other endogenous flora in a carefully balanced synergistic microenvironment. However, alterations in this environment as a result of the disruption of integumentary and mucosal barriers, disease, treatment-induced granulocytopenia, and immunosuppression, as well as alterations in the microbial flora because of the administration of antibiotics, can lead to invasive fungal infections. Fungal infections have become an increasingly important cause of morbidity and mortality in persons with cancer, especially those with hematologic and lymphoreticular neoplasms. In the 1950s fungal infections accounted for only 5% of infections in patients diagnosed with leukemia. Now, fully 37% of fatal infections are fungal in nature. This tremendous increase is due to the development and use of better antibiotics that have resulted in decreased mortality rates from bacterial infection. These advances are coupled with an intensification of leukemia therapy, which has led to prolonged myelosuppression and higher incidence of fungal infection.[42]

The six most common sources of fungal infections in cancer patients are *Candida, Aspergillus, Cryptococcus, Histoplasma,* Phycomycetes, and *Coccidioides* organisms. Two major problems in the treatment of fungal infection are (1) the difficulty associated with culturing organisms from infected tissues and (2) the limited number of effective agents available to manage severe fungal infections.

Candida

Candida organisms are the most common cause of invasive fungal infection. The presence of *Candida* in sputum, the mouth, or throat cannot be definitively correlated with infection because *Candida* can reside harmlessly in the healthy host. The immunosuppressed person, however, is at the greatest risk for candidiasis because normal granulocytes and cell-mediated immunity form the major line of defense against a severe *Candida* infection. Broad-spectrum antibiotics limit normal bacterial growth; thus individuals treated with these antibiotics may be at greater risk for the development of a fungal infection.

Skin infections caused by *Candida* occur most frequently in the groin and perianal area. Oral candidiasis (thrush) is a common yeast infection that can disseminate throughout the gastrointestinal tract. If candidal esophagitis, documented by barium swallow or esophagogram, develops in the person with granulcytopenia, treatment with intravenous amphotericin B is warranted. Although antemortem confirmation of candidal infection is difficult, disseminated candidiasis often involves the lungs, kidneys, bones, joints, and central nervous system. Immunosuppressed persons in whom new or progressive pulmonary infiltrates develop while they receive broad-spectrum antibiotics present major problems for differential diagnosis and a fungal infection of *Candida* must be considered.[16,17,21]

Aspergillus

Aspergillus is another common fungal organism that causes serious infections in individuals with cancer.[16] Among opportunistic fungi, aspergilli are the most common cause of pneumonia.[43] Granulocytopenia and the administration of immunosuppressive drugs, especially corticosteroids, are associated with *Aspergillus* infection. Aspergilli enter the host through the upper airway and frequently cause a pulmonary or sinus infection. Nosocomial transmission of aspergilli has occurred in hospitals in which aspergilli spores contained in construction materials were disseminated through the ventilation system.

Aspergillosis is characterized by blood vessel invasion, which can lead to thrombosis and infarction of pulmonary arteries and veins. Blood cultures are rarely positive, even in disseminated aspergillosis. The infection is difficult to diagnose, often necessitating aggressive treatment with amphotericin before documentation of the infection. Without prompt and aggressive treatment with amphotericin, *Aspergillus* pneumonia is almost always fatal in persons with granulocytopenia.[16,21,44]

Cryptococcus

Cryptococcus neoformans is a yeast that is found in soil and pigeon excreta and generally is acquired by inhalation. The infection appears most frequently in individuals with advanced Hodgkin's disease and other lymphomas. It occurs most commonly as an insidious meningoencephalitis. Headache, vomiting, and diplopia without fever are the most common symptoms. Cerebrospinal fluid examination reveals mononuclear pleocytosis and a low glucose level. Intrathecal administration of antifungal agents may be required in individuals whose cerebrospinal fluid does not clear with intravenous therapy. As with other fungi, cryptococcosis also can occur in the lungs and disseminate to visceral organs.[16,21]

Histoplasma

Histoplasmosis generally occurs as a pulmonary infection, usually in individuals with lymphoreticular neoplasms. The infection frequently is disseminated, causing adenopathy and hepatosplenomegaly, which may be confused with the underlying neoplasm.[2] Dissemination of histoplasmosis can occur in persons whose cancer is in remission, as well as in those with active disease; therefore histologic examination of biopsy material for *Histoplasma* is necessary when this organism is suspected as a cause of infection. Amphotericin B is the treatment of choice for histoplasmosis.

Phycomycetes

The Phycomycetes (*Mucor, Rhizopus,* and *Absidia*) are opportunistic fungi that are widespread in dust and air. The lungs, nasal sinuses, and gastrointestinal tract are the three major sites of infection. After the fungi are inhaled into the lungs, the disease may disseminate to other sites in the body. Person-to-person infection is rare. Amphotericin B is the treatment of choice.

Coccidioides

Coccidioides organisms are found in the soil of the southwestern United States and enter the host by inhalation. The organism is rapidly phagocytosed in persons who have a competent immune system and may cause no symptoms. Immunocompromised persons, however, are susceptible to the development of serious pulmonary infections.[16,21,45]

Treatment

Amphotericin B is an effective antibiotic in the treatment of systemic fungal infections such as histoplasmosis, coccidioidomycosis, cryptococcosis, aspergillosis, phycomycosis, blastomycosis, and disseminated moniliasis. Its administration, however, is associated with a significant degree of toxicity. Side effects include fever, chills, rigors, nausea, vomiting, hypotension, bronchospasm, and, occasionally, seizures. The premedication of persons with acetaminophen and the addition of hydrocortisone sodium succinate to the intravenous solution generally reduces the reactions associated with the drug. Intravenous meperidine (1 mg/kg) can be used to ameliorate the fever and chills that frequently accompany the initial administration of amphotericin.[46] The fever and chills tend to diminish with continued daily therapy. Patients who receive amphotericin should be kept warm and quiet and be reassured that the side effects will be managed with effective measures and will abate with continued medication.

The major limiting toxicity of amphotericin is nephrotoxicity, and with continued administration, elevated levels of creatinine and azotemia, in addition to mild renal tubular acidosis, may become evident. Electrolyte imbalances invariably occur. Hypokalemia can be managed effectively by potassium replacement therapy and careful monitoring of serum electrolytes and intravenous fluids. Individuals with meningeal candidiasis may in rare cases require intrathecal administration of amphotericin B, and those with bladder candidiasis may be treated with bladder instillations of amphotericin. Because amphotericin B is a colloid, it should be mixed with dextrose and water and protected from light.

5-Fluorocytosine is another major antifungal agent commonly used in the treatment of fungal infections such as those caused by *Cryptococcus* and *Candida* organisms. The drug has little or no activity against *Coccidioides* or *Histoplasma* organisms. The major limitation to its use is the rapid onset of drug resistance. The drug is well absorbed orally, and its side effects include nausea, vomiting, myelosuppression, and hepatotoxicity. 5-Fluorocytosine and amphotericin B appear to be synergistic in cryptococcal meningitis and may be recommended as combination therapy in severe disseminated infections. Because both these drugs may have adverse effects on renal function, patients should be closely monitored for signs of renal compromise.

Ketoconazole is a synthetic, imidazole-derived, and orally administered antifungal drug. Cerebrospinal fluid concentration is unpredictable after oral administration; thus ketoconazole is given in conjunction with other antifungal agents in the treatment of fungal meningitis. Ketoconazole has been used to treat fungal infections caused by disseminated coccidiodomycosis, candidiasis, histoplasmosis, and pulmonary or disseminated paracoccidioidomycosis. The most frequent side effects of ketoconazole are nausea and vomiting. Transient elevations of serum AST and ALT have been reported, in addition to rare instances of hepatotoxicity.

Miconazole is a synthetic antifungal that exerts its activity by altering cellular membranes and interfering with intracellular enzymes. It is effective against most fungi and some gram-positive bacteria. Although the drug can be administered orally or intramuscularly, it usually is administered by slow intravenous infusion when systemic infection is suspected. In the treatment of meningitis, miconazole may be given intrathecally. With bladder infections the drug can be either instilled or used as an irrigation. Adverse effects of miconazole are mild in comparison to amphotericin B, with oral doses being well tolerated. The most common adverse reactions to intravenous administration are phlebitis and pruritus.

Flucytosine, given orally, is used to treat severe fungal infections caused by *Candida* and *Cryptococcus* organisms. The most common side effects are nausea, vomiting, and diarrhea.[15-17,21]

Protozoa

Protozoa include organisms responsible for amebiasis and malaria. Although malaria is rare, it can be transmitted by contaminated blood transfusions. *Giardia lamblia* causes giardiasis, which is characterized by severe abdominal cramps, fever, and diarrhea. Giardiasis is especially common in malnourished children and persons with cancer who are immunosuppressed.

Pneumocystis carinii

Pneumocystis carinii is a protozoa that causes an infection that develops in malnourished infants, in children with primary immunodeficiency disorders, in individuals with AIDS, and in those with cancer who are undergoing chemotherapy, especially patients receiving corticosteroids. *Pneumocystis* is a ubiquitous organism that often is detected in symptom-free persons. *Pneumocystis* pneumonia commonly develops in those whose disease is in complete remission and who do not have granulocytopenia. The clinical manifestations of the infection include fever, nonproductive cough, tachypnea with intercostal retractions, and respiratory compromise, which may be life threatening. Rales are absent. Chest radiographs show hazy, bilateral alveolar infiltrates, and open-lung biopsy may be necessary to confirm the diagnosis. Untreated *Pneumocystis* pneumonia is fatal in individuals with cancer. Those with respiratory insufficiency should receive aggressive respiratory support until the infection is under control.[47]

Even with therapy the mortality is high in patients with infections caused by *Pneumocystis carinii.* Treatment of choice is trimethoprim-sulfamethoxazole. The side effects associated with trimethoprim-sulfamethoxazole include rash, nausea, vomiting, hepatotoxicity, and myelosuppression. Renal function is monitored in persons with preexisting renal function abnormalities while they are receiving this antibiotic. A history of sulfonamide sensitivity contraindicates the use of trimethoprim-sulfamethoxazole.[21]

Pentamidine isethionate has been found effective in treating *P. carinii* in some patients whose infection has not responded to trimethoprim-sulfamethoxazole. This drug, however, may cause troublesome side effects, including azotemia, hypocalcemia, and hepatotoxicity. When given intramuscularly, pentamidine isethionate can cause local pain and sterile abscess formation. Intramuscular administration in persons with thrombocytopenia is contraindicated; it can necessitate intravenous administration, which may cause flushing, tachycardia, syncope, vomiting, and respiratory depression.

Toxoplasma gondii

Toxoplasma gondii is an obligate intracellular parasite that is found in soil and cat excreta or is ingested in improperly cooked meat products. It can remain encapsulated in host tissues, and reactivation of latent organisms often causes infection. Central nervous system involvement occurs in 90% of infected individuals but the infection rarely is restricted to the central nervous system.[17,47] Cysts may be found in symptom-free persons. The diagnosis is made by histologic examination of biopsy material, by culture results, or by serologic findings. Treatment with pyrimethamine in combination with sulfadiazine has been effective in immunocompromised patients.[48]

ASSESSMENT OF THE PATIENT AT RISK OF DEVELOPING INFECTION

The early detection of infection in the person with cancer who is immunosuppressed depends on a high index of professional sensitivity and frequent patient assessment for subtle evidence of infection. The classic signs and symptoms of infection are often not evident because of the absence or decreased number of granulocytes.

Physical Examination

Assessment of the person with cancer who is at risk of the development of infection is not a one-time activity but an ongoing nursing responsibility. Initial assessment provides a baseline from which to make future decisions.

A general review of body systems is conducted to detect any important symptoms that have not yet been identified. In assessing the patient for the presence or absence of infection, special attention is given to the results of physical and laboratory data.

Skin

Skin is examined for evidence of rashes or eruptions that may signify infection and any disruptions in the skin's surface that would predispose the patient to infection. The presence of petechiae and/or bruising should raise concern about myelosuppression, leading the nurse to consider infection even in afebrile individuals. Skin temperature and turgor are evaluated. Any deficiencies in personal hygiene should receive high priority. If the appearance of skin lesions changes or new lesions appear, the primary physician is notified and lesion specimens are cultured for bacterial, fungal, or viral pathogens.

Eyes, ears, and nose

Eyes, ears, and nose assessment includes examination of the sclera for icterus, which may indicate the presence of hepatitis, and the conjunctiva and eyelids for evidence of inflammatory changes as a result of infection. The external ears are included in the physical examination. Symptoms of sinusitis or ear pain may indicate a bacterial or fungal infection.

Oral cavity

The oral cavity sometimes sustains tissue injury from certain chemotherapeutic agents, especially the antimetabolites and antitumor antibiotics. Local infections can occur when inflamed or injured mucosal surfaces become colonized with bacteria, and these local infections may lead to systemic infections. Teeth in poor repair can be a source of sepsis during periods of granulocytopenia. By the time individuals experience oral discomfort, stomatitis may be so severe that the potential for serious systemic infection has increased. Because severe stomatitis can necessitate the interruption of chemotherapy, compromise nutritional status and fluid intake, and lead to serious systemic infection, consistent and routine examination of the oral cavity is essential in the nursing management of patients receiving any therapeutic regimens that have the potential to cause mucositis.

Gastrointestinal tract

When a patient with granulocytopenia who is receiving broad-spectrum antibiotics for a fever of unknown origin or a documented infection complains of dysphagia and/or retrosternal burning pain, candidal infection or herpes simplex esophagitis must be considered. Abdominal pain, distention, and diarrhea can be symptoms of an intraabdominal infection caused by gram-negative bacilli or other opportunistic organisms that reside in the bowel. Any gastrointestinal infection in these patients is likely to represent a serious medical and nursing problem.

Perirectal region

Perirectal and other soft tissues can be sites of serious infection in the person with cancer. Small ulcerations or fissures in the rectal mucosa represent a porta of entry for gram-negative bacteria. The perirectal area is examined frequently, particularly in those with granulocytopenia, with symptoms of perineal itching, tenderness, constipation, or with pain during defecation that may indicate the beginning stages of perirectal cellulitis. Enemas, rectal temperatures, rectal suppositories, and rectal examinations are contraindicated when granulocytopenia is present. A suspected infection is treated with broad-spectrum antibiotics after specimens from the area have been cultured for routine and fungal examination. Nursing care of the person with perirectal infection includes meticulous skin and perineal care, warm sitz baths, and soothing compresses. Stool softeners, low-residue diets, antidiarrheal agents, and pain medications help alleviate the problems associated with the immediate infection and may prevent the development of secondary problems. Treatment of other soft tissue infections may include incision, drainage, and continued antibiotic therapy until the period of risk has abated and the infection has cleared.

Lung

The lung is the most frequent site of serious infectious complications. Individuals with granulocytopenia may have little radiographic evidence of pneumonia, and purulent sputum may not be produced despite the presence of pulmonary infection. If the patient has fever and granulocytopenia and the physical findings suggest the possibility of a pulmonary infection, broad-spectrum antibiotics often are instituted empirically after routine cultures are performed. When an interstitial pneumonia develops in a person free of granulocytopenia who exhibits the symptoms of fever, tachypnea, cough, cyanosis, alkalosis, or severe hypoxemia, the differential diagnosis must include *Pneumocystis* pneumonia.[17] The patient may require an open-lung biopsy to identify the causative agent; therefore oncology nurses will be caring for patients after thoracic surgery and must be skilled in respiratory care. The need for open-lung biopsy has been reduced by the successful use of trimethoprim-sulfamethoxazole in the treatment of patients suspected of having *Pneumocystis* pneumonia. Radiographic evidence of improvement is required before open-lung biopsy is ruled out.

If a tracheostomy is performed, nursing care is focused on pulmonary hygiene, suctioning procedures, and care of the stoma. Sterile technique is mandatory in all contact with the person's stoma and suctioning equipment.

Nursing care of the debilitated patient concentrates on

pulmonary care, especially the need for frequent deep breathing. Visitors and staff members with respiratory infections should be kept away from patients with granulocytopenia, and patients should be warned to avoid people with these infections when they are released from the hospital.

Urinary tract

Urinary tract infections are common in hospitalized persons, especially those with cancer who have fever and granulocytopenia. Clean-catch urine specimens are obtained routinely during febrile episodes. The risk and incidence of bladder infections are increased during catheterization; therefore this procedure should be avoided whenever possible. If catheterization is required, strict aseptic technique is used throughout the procedure. In the event that a prolonged catheterization is necessary, closed sterile drainage systems rather than open drainage systems reduce the incidence of catheter-related infections.

Muscles and joints

Muscle or joint pain may indicate infection in the person with cancer or may represent a new site of tumor involvement. Any erythema or tenderness should be evaluated to determine the significance and possible treatment.

Central nervous system

Central nervous system infections have been documented in persons whose spleens have been removed and in those with leukemia or lymphoma. Subtle changes in neurologic functioning may signify the onset of an infection or progression of the malignancy. Whenever a lumbar puncture is performed on a patient with cancer, the cerebrospinal fluid is examined visually and microscopically and cultured for bacteria and fungi. Any abnormality in neurologic functioning demands immediate attention.

The assessment of individuals diagnosed with cancer is most effective when the approach is consistent and routine. Because of the potential for serious infectious complications in immunosuppressed patients, the nurse assesses minor complaints and physical findings and acts without delay on the patient's behalf. Prevention of serious infection is possible. Nurses do not need to perform a full physical examination to recognize important and reportable signs and symptoms in their patients. They need only to pay attention to the most likely sites for infections that have been briefly reviewed to make major contributions in the prevention and early detection of infection.

Laboratory Studies

The hematologic status of the person with cancer is an important component of daily patient assessment. Nongranulocytopenic individuals with infections often demonstrate leukocytosis and an increased percentage of bands and nonsegmented forms in the differential blood count because large numbers of immature neutrophils are stimulated and released from the bone marrow. By contrast, with granulocytopenia, the WBC count may remain low during periods of fever and infection because marrow production of neutrophils often is impaired and the available granulocytes will be defending the host against the infection in tissue. Bone marrow recovery and successful eradication of an infection often occur simultaneously in persons with granulocytopenia.

PREVENTION OF INFECTION

In the acute care setting, it is essential that all health care personnel understand the principles of medical asepsis and consistently employ aseptic techniques, especially when caring for patients with cancer who are at risk of serious infection. The key to sound aseptic technique is simplicity and consistency. Policies and procedures for all patient care areas and personnel should be standardized, reviewed frequently, and reinforced through in-service programs.[49]

Specimens for blood cultures are collected in duplicate, one anaerobic and aerobic culture in each set, to increase the likelihood of recovering and identifying the infecting microorganism. Laboratory personnel must be protected from contaminated cultures and specimen containers by strict adherence to universal precautions.

There is no single way to control nosocomial infections. Each infection is associated with different predisposing factors and requires different preventive measures. A carefully planned patient assessment and treatment care plan for the prevention and management of infection is the most effective nursing measure. Many infection control programs have concentrated on staff education in preventing nosocomial transmission of infection by conducting frequent seminars on all shifts for personnel who are in contact with patients so that information is consistent and reaches everyone involved in patient care.

Nurses who specialize in infection control will monitor and investigate infection espisodes within a given agency. These nurses are instrumental in providing staff members with patient management information and in preventing further infection by ensuring that procedures and techniques are being performed safely and effectively. Nurses perform an important service when they teach and reinforce the basic principles of infection prevention to patients, families, and medical personnel. In general, noncompliance with accepted practices by the professional staff is related to a poor understanding of how staff members personally contribute to nosocomial transmission by contaminating themselves, others, and communal objects in the hospital environment.

When patients with cancer are admitted to isolation rooms to prevent them from transmitting infection to others or to reverse isolation rooms to protect them from infections, patients and their families are thoroughly informed about the isolation procedures. Additional support measures and assessment of the patient's coping mechanisms and family dynamics are often needed when serious infections develop. By taking the time to explain, support, and reassure patients and their families, nurses can help them to actively participate in their medical care.

In the ambulatory or home setting, special precautions can be taken by the patient and family to reduce the potential risk of infection. The critical component of infection control is good hand washing by patient, family members, and health care providers. Additional simple and practical measures to minimize risk include the avoidance of unnecessary exposure to large crowds and infected people, adequate circulating room air, and good nutritional and fluid intake. When persons with cancer are receiving chemotherapy, they probably will be more susceptible to infection during the nadir period of the drug cycle. This is the period when hematologic and immune compromise may be greatest. Caution should be exercised to avoid exposure to sources of infection.

Early detection of an impending infection can lead to easier control of the infection and less trauma to the patient. Persons at risk for infection should check and record their temperature on a daily basis at a standard time. Temperatures of 38.3°C (101°F) or greater or temperature elevations that last more than 12 hours should be reported immediately. The person with cancer should be suspicious for signs of infection: inflammation of the skin or mucous membranes, pulmonary congestion, or pain on urination.

TREATMENT OF INFECTION

Antibiotics: Mechanisms of Action

The penicillins, cephalosporins, and vancomycin act by interfering with cell wall synthesis. When *Staphylococcus* organisms are exposed to a cephalosporin, the first change noted is the extrusion of globular material believed to be particles of the cell wall and membrane of the bacteria. Defects then occur on the cell surface, giving the bacterial cells a raspberry appearance. When multiple defects occur, the cell wall is no longer able to maintain cell size and shape, and the cell enlarges until it bursts. Penicillin affects *Streptococcus* organisms by causing an enlargement and defect at midcell, giving the microorganism an apple core–like appearance. When *Escherichia coli* is exposed to certain penicillins, the first change is elongation of the bacteria as a result of interference with cell division, but cell growth is not affected. As the cell wall defects occur, the weakening at midcell causes a bulge, which enlarges until the rod-shaped bacteria have been converted into spherical ones (spheroblasts), which finally collapse, causing cell death. These morphologic alterations do not occur in all microorganisms to the same extent because any cell population is composed of varying numbers of bacterial cells with varying antibiotic sensitivities. Some cells are exquisitely sensitive to the antimicrobial agents and will lyse immediately, whereas others are highly resistant and may show no effect at all.

Polymyxin, nystatin, and amphotericin B act by interfering with cell membrane function and appear to alter permeability of cell membranes. These changes in cell membrane permeability allow leakage of potassium ions and other cellular components and can cause electrolyte abnormalities. Theoretically, by affecting cellular permeability, amphotericin B may potentiate the effects of other drugs when given in combination. Data suggest that amphotericin B may be able to reverse resistance to chemotherapy. Although the exact mechanism of action remains unknown, increased transmembrane transport could account for the increased therapeutic effect.[2]

The aminoglycosides (gentamicin, amikacin, and tobramycin), the tetracyclines, and chloramphenicol interfere with intracellular protein synthesis at different levels. Cell surface morphologic alterations induced by these agents are identical to those induced by agents that interfere with cell wall synthesis. It has been shown that interference with intracellular protein synthesis is manifested through changes at the cell surface. The sulfonamides and certain other drugs (eg, isoniazid) interfere with specific reactions of intermediate metabolism and folic acid production. They are structural analogues of para-aminobenzoic acid (PABA), a component of folic acid used in purine synthesis. The sulfonamides are competitive antagonists of PABA and form "false" folic acid. Antibiotic agents that interfere with intermediary metabolism also produce alterations in the cell surface morphology that are almost identical to the changes brought about by agents that interfere with cell synthesis[21] (Table 21-5).

Aminoglycosides have the narrowest therapeutic-to-toxic ratio among the commonly used antimicrobials; therefore aminoglycoside levels are assayed at the initiation of antibiotic therapy and at least once a week thereafter. When assay results indicate that the levels are low, dosage increases are necessary. Conversely, when the assay results indicate that the levels are too high, dosage decreases are necessary to optimize the therapeutic value and minimize the risk of nephrotoxicity. When dosage adjustments are made, the levels should again be assayed until the results indicate a safe and therapeutic dose of the antibiotic. Therapeutic ranges in the antibiotic assays vary from institution to institution and should be determined by the laboratory responsible for performing the assay, the pharmacists, and the physicians. A consistent, coordinated procedure for drawing blood samples before and after the antibiotic infusion will ensure that each assay level is being compared with an accurate standard. If blood samples are being drawn at arbitrary times, the assay results will be meaningless for interpretation and dosage regulation.

Approach to the Patient Without Granulocytopenia

Individuals with cancer who are not immunosuppressed or granulocytopenic can be treated with appropriate antibiotic therapy when a specific infectious etiologic agent is identified. The drug of choice is based on in vitro sensitivity testing. Treatment with a broad-spectrum antibiotic

TABLE 21-5 Antibiotics Used in the Treatment of Bacterial Infections

Drug	Side Effects	Nursing Considerations
Penicillins		
Methicillin	Eosinophilia, vein irritation, thrombophlebitis	Use cautiously in patients with other drug allergies, especially cephalosporins; mixing penicillins with aminoglycosides in solution can result in considerable inactivation of the aminoglycoside.
Nafcillin	Nausea, vomiting, diarrhea, vein irritation, thrombophlebitis, hypersensitivity	See Methicillin
Oxacillin	Granulocytopenia	See Methicillin
Ampicillin	Nausea, vomiting, diarrhea, hypersensitivity	See Methicillin
Carbenicillin	Bleeding with high doses, thrombocytopenia, convulsions, hypokalemia, hypersensitivity	See Methicillin
Ticarcillin	Hypokalemia, hypersensitivity	
Cephalosporins		
Cephalothin	Headache, nausea, vomiting, diarrhea, nephrotoxicity	Pain at injection site, hypersensitivity; watch for penicillin-cephalosporin cross-sensitivity.
Cefazolin	Headache, nausea, vomiting, diarrhea, rash	See Cefazolin
Cefatoxime	Headache, nausea, vomiting, diarrhea, nephrotoxicity, rash, urticaria	See Cefazolin
Moxalactam	Headache, nausea, vomiting, diarrhea, rash, urticaria	See Cefazolin
Aminoglycosides		
Gentamicin	Nausea, vomiting, ototoxicity, nephrotoxicity, rash, urticaria	Monitor serum levels of drug.
Tobramycin	See Gentamycin	See Gentamycin
Amikacin	See Gentamycin	See Gentamycin
Miscellaneous		
Chloramphenicol	Aplastic anemia, headache, nausea, vomiting	Penicillins antagonize antibacterial effect; give 1 hr apart. Acetaminophen elevates chloramphenicol level. Use with caution in persons with impaired renal or hepatic function.
Erythromycin	Decreased hearing with high doses, abdominal pain, cramping, nausea, vomiting, diarrhea, vein irritation, thrombophlebitis with intravenous administration, anaphylaxis	Contraindicated in persons with hepatic disease.
Clindamycin	Nausea, vomiting, diarrhea, bloody or tarry stools, rash, pain at injection site, anaphylaxis	Antagonism between erythromycin and clindamycin; monitor hepatic, renal, hematopoietic functions.
Vancomycin	Tinnitus, ototoxicity, nausea, nephrotoxicity, pain at injection site, anaphylaxis	Contraindicated when patient is receiving other ototoxic or nephrotoxic agents.
Trimethoprim-sulfamethoxazole	Hypersensitivity, nausea, vomiting, rash, pruritis, exfoliative dermatitis	Use cautiously in persons with hepatic or renal impairment.

may be initiated, however, when rapidly developing serious infections occur. In these situations the physician must choose an antibiotic known to be effective even if the causative organism is unknown. If possible, cultures are performed before initiation of therapy and the antibiotics appropriately changed when the results of sensitivity testing are known.

Approach to the Patient with Fever and Granulocytopenia

Persons with cancer who have fever during periods of granulocytopenia will have a careful physical examination, chest radiograph, and complete microbiologic body cultures and be started on empirical broad-spectrum antibiotic therapy, even when the origin of fever has not been determined (Figure 21-4). Antibiotic combinations to treat gram-negative infections have been used extensively in patients with granulocytopenia. Combination therapy provides a synergistic effect that one drug cannot accomplish. Fungal infections may require the administration of amphotericin B, miconozole, ketoconazole, or nystatin, depending on the site and extent of infection. Therapy for disseminated viral infections includes treatment with acyclovir, adenine arabinoside (vidarabine), DHPG, or interferon.

Persons with granulocytopenia may not manifest any clinical evidence of infection because the granulocytopenia prevents the mounting of an inflammatory response. The result is high risk of morbidity and mortality from an untreated infection inasmuch as infection may not be apparent until evidence of septic shock appears. Therefore patients with granulocytopenia must be evaluated at frequent intervals for subtle signs and symptoms of infection.

The morbidity and mortality rates of infection are clearly reduced when empiric broad-spectrum antibiotic therapy is initiated immediately after the diagnostic evaluation of the person with fever and granulocytopenia, regardless of whether a bacterial infection can be documented. The mortality associated with an untreated infection in the person with severe granulocytopenia makes early diagnosis and empiric antibiotic treatment critical. Because the median survival time with inappropriate therapy is less than 3 days, broad-spectrum combination antibiotics must be started at once. In addition, intravenous antibiotic therapy should be given in full dosage and maintained until the period of risk, that is, fever and granulocytopenia, has abated.[6] Most combination antibiotic therapy includes the use of an aminoglycoside because of the bactericidal activity against most gram-negative rods and some gram-positive cocci like *S. aureus*.

Microbial cultures

Microbial cultures are performed routinely before the administration of antibiotics in the patient with fever and granulocytopenia. Specimens for blood cultures are obtained in duplicate (separate venipunctures, if possible) and placed in appropriate media, including media that will sustain anaerobes. Culture specimens of skin lesions, sputum, throat, urine, and stool also are obtained before the initiation of antibiotics.

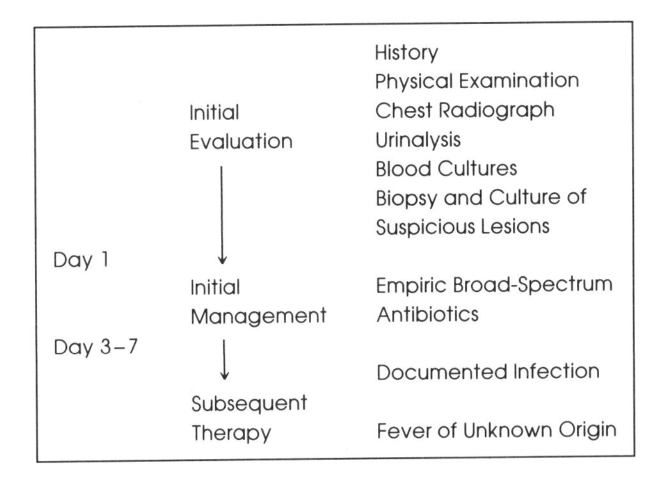

FIGURE 21-4 Approach to the patient with fever and granulocytopenia.

Empiric antibiotics

Empiric antibiotic therapy in the patient with fever and granulocytopenia reduces the number of infections that become severe enough to be demonstrated by microbiologic culture or clinical documentation. The decreasing incidence of septic shock in this high-risk patient population suggests that prompt aggressive antibiotic therapy is effective in reducing the serious morbidity associated with gram-positive sepsis.[5] The particular antibiotic regimen selected for the empiric therapy of the patient with fever and granulocytopenia should satisfy the following criteria: the drug combination should provide broad-spectrum coverage for the major pathogenic microorganisms; the combination should be synergistic and contain one bactericidal agent; and the agents should have the least organ toxicity, be well absorbed by the route given, be metabolized effectively, be distributed to infected tissue consistently, and be appropriately excreted.[5,16] Drug levels should be monitored on a regular basis while the patient is receiving the antibiotic, and dosage adjustments should be made when indicated to maintain safe, therapeutic levels throughout the period of treatment.

Treatment with a two- or three-drug combination that consists of an aminoglycoside plus a semisynthetic penicillin generally is used to provide synergistic activity against susceptible organisms. Other options include the use of trimethoprim-sulfamethoxazole in combination with an aminoglycoside or an antipseudomonal penicillin. Newer semisynthetic penicillins such as azlocillin and pipercillin have a broader spectrum of antibacterial activity than some of the older penicillins. These newer drugs also can be combined with an aminoglycoside to provide even greater coverage against infection. The disadvantage of this last approach is that hypokalemia may develop from the penicillins and ototoxicity and nephrotoxicity from the aminoglycoside. Patients are continuously assessed for these adverse effects throughout their antibiotic treatment.

Protection of highly compromised individuals from infection

Persons with cancer who are receiving intensive therapeutic regimens with total body irradiation, steroids, and chemotherapy are significantly more susceptible to infection than those receiving less intensive therapy. These severely immunocompromised patients often are placed on "protective" regimens intended to reduce the risk of infection. One such regimen, routine protective isolation, does not appear to reduce the risk of infection any more than does consistent and frequent hand washing during patient care. Routine protective isolation may fail to reduce the risk of infection in severely immunocompromised patients because of infection by endogenous microorganisms or by colonization and infection by microorganisms transmitted by the contaminated hands of medical personnel.[26]

Efforts to exclude all microorganisms by the use of patient isolator units (usually laminar air flow rooms), nonabsorbable prophylactic antibiotics to eradicate endogenous gastrointestinal flora, and sterilization of the person's food and water may prevent or delay the onset of some infections. Therefore these procedures have been recommended by some investigators for immunocompromised persons who have a predictable period of high risk.[50] These precautions do not appear warranted for routine patient care.

Personnel who care for immunocompromised individuals perform thorough hand washing before and after contact with each patient if they wish to minimize infectious complications. Hand washing is the single best method of decreasing the incidence of nosocomial infections. Another precaution that appears to prevent nosocomial infections is the protection of immunocompromised persons from those who are infected. Private rooms are preferred for immunocompromised patients.[6]

Laminar air flow rooms

Protected environment systems were developed to protect the compromised host from exogenous and endogenous sources of infection. In this sophisticated isolation system, air is circulated through high-efficiency particulate air filters that are capable of removing particles from the air larger than 0.3 μm with a greater than 99.7% efficiency. The unidirectional (laminar) air flow significantly reduces air turbulence, which decreases the potential of microbial contamination in the consistently clean, protected environment. Semiportable units with horizontal air flow can be installed in regular hospital rooms.

To create an environment that is as free of microorganisms as possible, patients undergo cutaneous and gastrointestinal decontamination with oral nonabsorbable antibiotics before entry into the room; all objects that enter the room are sterilized by steam or gas, and food is semisterile. Anyone who enters the room wears gloves, mask, cap, and gown if the patient is to be touched. The drawbacks of laminar air flow rooms are that the protected environment is elaborate, cumbersome, and expensive. In addition, the patient may experience psychotic episodes because of sensory deprivation. Although laminar air flow rooms reduce incidence of infection and improve short-term survival, long-term survival has not been affected.

Approach to the Patient with Gram-Negative Sepsis

Shock develops in approximately 25% of patients with gram-negative bacteremia.[51] Septic shock causes inadequate blood perfusion and circulatory collapse. The mortality rate in septic shock approaches 80% unless vigorous treatment is begun at once. This clinical syndrome is a result of a number of interrelated factors that include direct effect of bacterial endotoxin on the cardiovascular system, activation of the protein cascade systems, hydration status of the patient, and the nature of the underlying disease. Signs and symptoms depend on the stage of shock, the causative organism, and the age of the patient. The first sign of impending septic shock in a person with cancer who is immunosuppressed may be limited to a shaking chill and/or hypotension (Table 21-6). Early recognition of sepsis and aggressive medical and nursing management are essential if irreversible damage to vital organs and subsequent death are to be averted (Figure 21-5).

TABLE 21-6 Early Warning Signs of Septic Shock

Clinical Features	Laboratory Findings	Hemodynamic Features
Fever ± chills	Respiratory alkalosis	High cardiac index/output
Warm, dry skin	Lactic acidosis	Relative hypotension
Confusion	Low serum potassium	High central venous pressure
Rapid breathing	Elevated white blood count	Low peripheral resistance
Rapid pulse	Urine output decreased Urine concentration increased	Narrowing arteriovenous oxygen difference

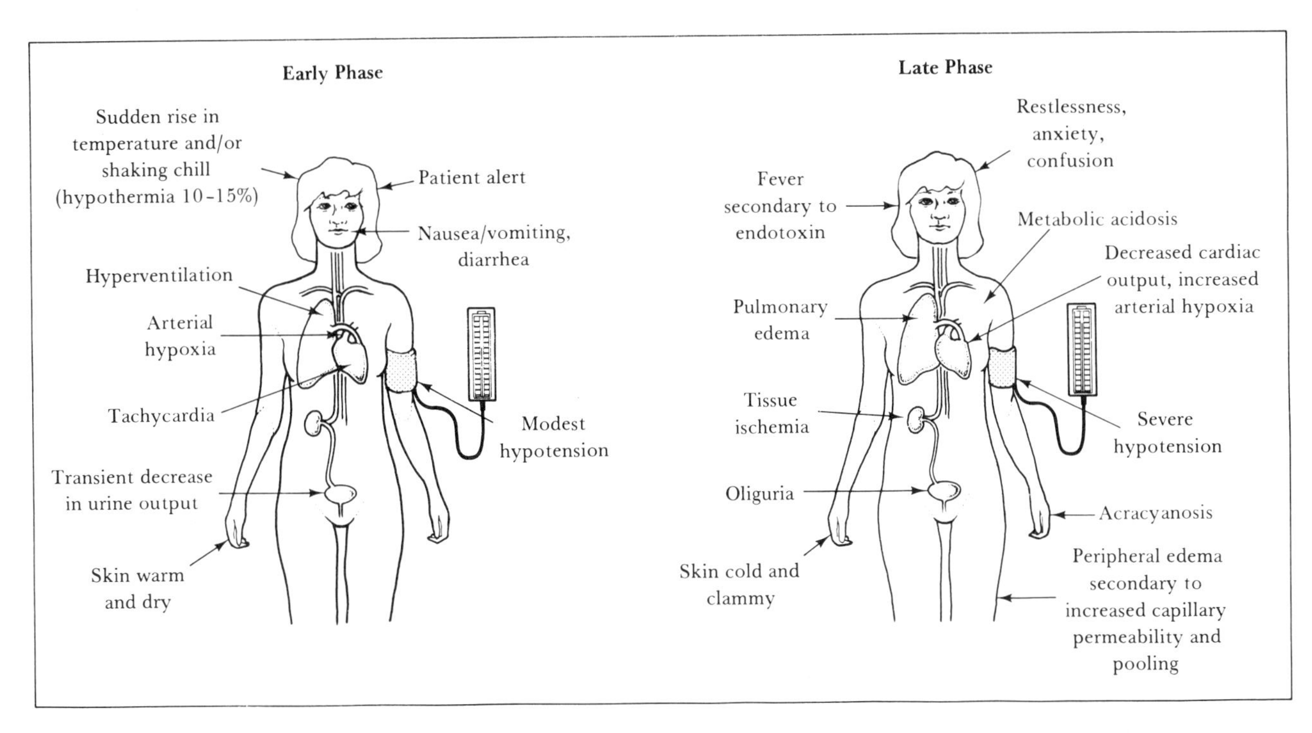

FIGURE 21-5 Sepsis and septic shock.

Early (warm) septic shock

Septic shock evolves through two distinct phases that are characterized by different hemodynamic patterns: an early and a late phase.[51] The early phase consists of vasodilation, decreased peripheral vascular resistance, normal to increased cardiac output, and mild hypotension. The signs of overt shock are not present in this phase. The patient may appear flushed, with warm extremities and adequate urinary output. The central venous pressures are generally low, as is left ventricular and diastolic pressures, and respiratory alkalosis is present. This is the phase of peripheral vasodilation and loss of fluid to the interstitial spaces. If myocardial function and fluid replacement are adequate, the syndrome may not progress, provided immediate and appropriate antibiotic therapy is instituted. The duration of this early phase may vary from 30 minutes to 16 hours; however, if myocardial function is poor and volume replacement is inadequate or if there is delay in initiating appropriate antibiotic therapy, severe (late phase) shock may develop. Immediate treatment may be lifesaving.

Late (cold) septic shock

The late phase of septic shock is characterized by a profound reduction in cardiac output, increased peripheral vascular resistance, oliguria, and metabolic acidosis. These factors create a cycle of vasoconstriction, ischemia, and vasodilation, which can cause irreversible damage to the heart, vascular system, kidney, liver, and vasomotor center of the brain.

Treatment of septic shock

The management of septic shock begins with recognition of the process, a thorough patient evaluation, routine cultures, the immediate institution of broad-spectrum antibiotics, volume replacement with electrolyte (crystalloid) solutions, and vasoactive agents if hypotension persists despite fluid replacement. Dopamine is the vasoactive agent of choice. It increases arterial blood pressure without causing significant vasoconstriction and selectively increases renal, coronary, cerebral, and mesenteric blood flow.[52,53]

The treatment of septic shock is based on two objectives: to reverse the shock and to treat the underlying sepsis. Treatment first must support the patient's defense against shock and immediately thereafter control the underlying infectious process. Individuals in shock must have an adequate airway and supplemental oxygen, effective blood circulation and tissue perfusion, intravenous nutrition restoration, and immediate, appropriate broad-spectrum antibiotic support.

Monitoring devices, including central venous pressure lines, Swan-Ganz catheters, arterial lines, and urinary catheters, increase the risk of further infection, but this risk is to be balanced against the acute situation at hand. Prevention of septic shock is a challenge to the medical and nursing staff and is far more effective than the treatment of shock in either the early or the late phase. The recognition of the high-risk patient and the procedures and clinical conditions that may increase the potential for shock, as well as continued measures to prevent shock, are important responsibilities for health professionals. Pa-

TABLE 21-7 Complications of Septic Shock

Complication	Manifestation
Disseminated intravascular coagulation	Abnormal bleeding
Renal failure	Oliguria, increased specific gravity
Heart failure	Dyspnea, edema, tachycardia, distended neck veins
Gastrointestinal ulcers	Hematemesis, melena
Hepatic abnormality	Jaundice, hypoprothrombinemia, hypoalbuminemia

tients with serious infection and a potential for shock and those already in shock need immediate, vigorous medical intervention until the situation is under control and the person is out of danger.

Nurses should be familiar with the signs of impending septic shock and should not rely on technical aids to assess the patient's status. Any change in blood pressure, mental status, or urinary output in high-risk patients alert the nurse to the probability of early septic shock. Once treatment has been initiated, nurses closely monitor serum levels of aminoglycosides such as gentamicin. In addition, patients are assessed for complications of septic shock: disseminated intravascular coagulation, renal failure, heart failure, gastrointestinal ulcers, and hepatic abnormalities (Table 21-7).

Finally, care is taken to meet the psychosocial needs of patients with septic shock and their families. The critical nature of septic shock coupled with the intensive treatment regimen can be overwhelming. Patients may face not only a fear of death but loss of control and feelings of dependence. The role of the oncology nurse in this situation is to provide honest information, education, assurance, and explanations to both patients and families.

Granulocyte transfusions

Patients with gram-negative sepsis and persistent granulocytopenia often will respond to antibiotic therapy alone provided the initial choice of antibiotics is appropriate and instituted promptly. The choice of initial antibiotics can determine the ultimate recovery status, and it is the prompt institution of those antibiotics that can prevent septic shock and its complications. Granulocyte transfusions are unnecessary for the majority of patients although they may be beneficial to those with prolonged aplasia, gram-negative sepsis, and an inadequate clinical response to antibiotics.[17,30]

Gram-negative sepsis is a serious infection associated with a poor prognosis in the presence of granulocytopenia. The controversy that surrounds granulocyte transfusions focuses on data that suggest that the administration of granulocyte transfusions does not influence survival. Some physicians believe that individuals with cancer, granulocytopenia, and documented gram-negative sepsis should be treated with the combination of broad-spectrum antibiotics and granulocyte transfusions from compatible donors until a controlled, randomized study can be conducted that compares the efficacy of antibiotics alone versus a combination of granulocyte transfusions and the same antibiotics.

Severe pulmonary reactions have occurred in persons with cancer who are receiving combination treatment with amphotericin B and granulocyte transfusions. These reactions are characterized by sudden dyspnea, hypoxia, and diffuse interstitial infiltrates appearing on chest radiographs.[54] It is hypothesized that the granulocyte transfusions cause changes in the lungs that result in severe pulmonary distress when amphotericin B is added to the regimen.[54] Caution and close monitoring are indicated when these treatments are used in combination.

Approach to the Patient with HIV Infection: Opportunistic Infections

The nursing management of persons who are positive for HIV presents a unique challenge. These individuals are threatened with an increased risk of opportunistic infections not only because of the HIV but also the chemotherapeutic agents used to treat the concomitant malignancies of HIV and AIDS.

Nurses need to exercise extra care when they conduct a baseline assessment of persons with HIV. The assessment will be the basis for subsequent evaluation and follow-up for these high-risk individuals. Patients are taught the signs and symptoms of infection. In addition, thorough hand washing and personal hygiene are stressed to help decrease the chances of infection from both exogenous and endogenous organisms. Good nutrition and proper preparation of food to aid in prevention of food-borne infections are a part of the care plan.

Persons with active HIV infection and AIDS present a special challenge to nurses who care for them. Although their nursing and medical care is comparable to that for others with opportunistic infections acquired as a result of cancer, a diagnosis of AIDS frequently carries with it a heavy burden. The progression of AIDS leads to severe dementia, malnutrition, pain, anorexia, cachexia, nausea, and vomiting. Infection in a patient with HIV and advanced AIDS is a life-threatening complication because of severe defects in both humoral and cell-mediated immunity.[55] The challenges are great for both the patient and the health professionals. Knowledge, communication, and caring are required. Because HIV and AIDS are escalating health problems, research results are of major importance to guide health professionals who care for persons with one of these diagnoses.

CONCLUSION

Persons with cancer are especially prone to the development of infections that result from impairment of host defense mechanisms. Immunosuppression in this patient population may be due to infection, tumor-associated abnormality, nutrition, or the cancer treatment itself. As a result, these persons are particularly vulnerable to bacterial, fungal, viral, and protozoal infections that may be difficult to treat. Nurses have a primary role in the prevention, detection, and treatment of infection. Until there are significant improvements in the field of oncology, the prevention and management of infections and their complications will continue to be among the most serious and complex problems.

REFERENCES

1. Abernathy E: How the immune system works. Am J Nurs 87:456-458, 1987.
2. Larson E: Clinical Microbiology and Infection Control. Boston, Blackwell Scientific Publications, 1984.
3. Budesheim Neuberger G, Reckling JB: Immunologic problems, in Cahill, M (ed): Nurse Review. Springhouse, Pa, Springhouse Corp, 1989, pp 1-160.
4. Goldstein D, Laszlo J: The role of interferon in cancer therapy: A current perspective. CA 38:258-277, 1988.
5. Klastersky J: Concept of empiric therapy with antibiotic combinations. Am J Med 80:2-12, 1986 (suppl).
6. Schimpff SC: Empiric antibiotic therapy for granulocytopenic cancer patients. Am J Med 80:13-20, 1986.
7. Rosenberg SA: Hodgkin's disease, in Calabresi P, Schein PS, Rosenberg SA (eds): Medical Oncology: Basic Principles and Clinical Management of Cancer. New York, Macmillan, 1985, pp 457-475.
8. Gallo RC: Retroviruses that cause human disease, in Wyngaarden JB, Smith LH (eds): Textbook of Medicine (ed 18). Philadelphia, WB Saunders, 1988, pp 1794-1798.
9. Groopman JE: The acquired immunodeficiency syndrome, in Wyngaarden JB, Smith LH (eds): Textbook of Medicine (ed 18). Philadelphia, WB Saunders, 1988, pp 1799-1808.
10. Lovejoy NC: The pathophysiology of AIDS. Oncol Nurs Forum 15:563-571, 1988.
11. Waldman TA: Immunodeficiency diseases: Primary and acquired, in Samter M (ed): Immunological Diseases (ed 4). Boston, Little, Brown and Co, 1988, pp 411-466.
12. Flaskerud JH: AIDS/HIV Infection: A reference guide for nursing professionals. Philadelphia, WB Saunders, 1989.
13. Levy JA: AIDS: Pathogenesis and Treatment. New York, Marcel Dekker, 1989.
14. Hellman S, Jaffe ES, DeVita VT: Hodgkin's Disease, in DeVita VT, Hellman S, Rosenberg SA (eds): Cancer: Principles and Practice (ed 3). New York, JB Lippincott, 1989, pp 1696-1740.
15. Gurevich I, Tafuro P: The compromised host: Deficit-specific infection and the spectrum of prevention. Cancer Nurs 9:263-275, 1986.
16. Schimpff SC: Infections in patients with cancer, in Moossa AR, Robson MC, Schimpff SC (eds): Comprehensive Textbook of Oncology. Baltimore, Williams & Wilkins, 1986, pp 367-377.
17. Armstrong D: Infection in the patient with neoplastic disease, in Wittes RE (ed): Manual of Oncologic Therapeutics. Philadelphia, JB Lippincott, 1989/90, pp 517-534.
18. Baccarani M, Fiacchini M, Galiene P: Meningitis and septicaemia in adults splenectomized for Hodgkin's disease. Scand J Haematol 36:492-498, 1986.
19. Thom AK, Daly JM: Nutritional support of the cancer patient, in Wittes RE (ed): Manual of Oncologic Therapeutics, Philadelphia, JB Lippincott, 1989/90, pp 517-534.
20. Bengoa JE: Malnutrition in the cancer patient, in Moossa AR, Robson MC, Schimpff SC (eds): Comprehensive Textbook of Oncology. Baltimore, Williams & Wilkins, 1986, pp 379-385.
21. Cohn I, Bornside GH: Infections, in Schwartz SI, Shires GT, Spencer FG (eds): Principles of Surgery. New York, McGraw-Hill, 1989, pp 181-213.
22. Lewis F, Levita M: Understanding radiotherapy. Cancer Nurs 11:174-185, 1988.
23. Shank B: Radiotherapy: Implications for general patient care, in Wittes RE (ed): Manual of Oncologic Therapeutics. Philadelphia, JB Lippincott, 1989/90, pp 82-93.
24. Parker RG, Rice DH, Casciato DA: Head and neck cancers, in Casciato DA, Lowitz BB (eds): Manual of Clinical Oncology (ed 2). Boston, Little, Brown and Co, 1988, pp 93-114.
25. Hilderley LJ: Nursing considerations in cancer, in Calabresi P, Schein PS, Rosenberg SA (eds): Medical Oncology: Basic Principles and Clinical Management. New York, Macmillan, 1985, pp 1446-1461.
26. Lynch P, Jackson MM, Cummings JM, et al: Rethinking the role of isolation practices in the prevention of nosocomial infections. Ann Intern Med 107:243-245, 1987.
27. Larson E: Skin cleansing, in Wenzel, RP (ed): Prevention and Control of Nosocomial Infections. Baltimore, Williams & Wilkins, 1987, pp 250-256.
28. Wenzel RP: Prevention and treatment of hospital-acquired infections, in Wyngaarden JB, Smith LH (eds): Textbook of Medicine (ed 18). Philadelphia, WB Saunders, 1988, pp 1541-1549.
29. Mann JJ: Fevers of obscure origin, in Harvey AM, Johns RS, McKusick VA (eds): The Principles and Practice of Medicine (ed 22). Norwalk, Conn, Appleton & Lange, 1988, pp 566-575.
30. Zinner SH, Klastersky J: Infectious considerations in cancer, in Calabresi P, Schein PS, Rosenberg SA (eds): Medical Oncology: Basic Principles and Clinical Management of Cancer. New York, MacMillan, 1985, pp 1327-1354.
31. Browne MJ, Dinndorf PA, Perek D, et al: Infectious complications of intraventricular reservoirs in cancer patients. Pediatr Infect Dis J 6:182-189, 1987.
32. Murphy PA: Pneumonia, in Harvey AM, Johns RS, McKusick VA (eds): The Principles and Practice of Medicine (ed 22). Norwalk, Conn, Appleton & Lange, 1988, pp 599-613.
33. Pizzo PA, Meyers J: Infections in the cancer patient, in DeVita VT, Hellman S, Rosenberg SA (eds): Cancer: Principles and Practice of Oncology (ed 3). New York, JB Lippincott, 1989, pp 2088-2133.
34. Fraser DW: Legionellosis, in Wyngaarden JB, Smith LH (eds): Textbook of Medicine (ed 18). Philadelphia, WB Saunders, 1988, pp 1570-1572.
35. Brunell PA, Varicella-zoster virus, in Mandell ML, Douglass

RG, Bennett J (eds): Principles and Practice of Infectious Diseases (ed 2). New York, Wiley, 1985, pp 952-960.
36. Hirsch MS: Herpes simplex virus, in Mandell ML, Douglass RG, Bennett JE (eds): Principles and Practice of Infectious Diseases (ed 2). New York, Wiley, 1985, pp 945-950.
37. Lang DJ: Cytomegalovirus infection, in Wyngaarden JB, Smith LH (eds): Textbook of Medicine (ed 18). Philadelphia, WB Saunders, 1988, pp 1784-1786.
38. Centers for Disease Control: Universal precautions for prevention of transmission of human immunodeficiency virus, hepatitis B virus and other blood-borne pathogens. MMWR 37 (June 24):377-387, 1988.
39. Edwards Hood L: Interferon: getting in the way of viruses and tumors. Am J Nurs 87:459-464, 1987.
40. Foon KA: Advances in immunotherapy of cancer: Monoclonal antibodies and interferon. Semin Oncol Nurs 4:112-119, 1988.
41. Hahn MB, Jassak PF: Nursing management of patients receiving interferon. Semin Oncol Nurs 4:95-101, 1988.
42. Anaissie E, Kantarjian H, Ro J, et al: The emerging role of *Fusarium* infections in patients with cancer. Medicine 67:77-83, 1988.
43. Nishiura T, Miyazaki Y, Oritani K, et al: *Aspergillus* vegetative endocarditis complicated with schizocytic hemolytic anemia in a patient with acute lymphocytic leukemia. Acta Haematol (Basel) 76:60-62, 1986.
44. Karp JE, Burch PA, Merz WG: An approach to intensive antileukemia therapy in patients with previous invasive aspergillosis. Am J Med 85:203-206, 1988.
45. Robbins SL, Cortran RS, Kumar V: Pathogenic Basis of Disease (ed 3). Philadelphia, WB Saunders, 1988.
46. Galpin JE: Infectious diseases in cancer patients, in Casciato DA, Lowitz BB (eds): Manual of Clinical Oncology (ed 2). Boston, Little, Brown & Co, 1988, pp 507-526.
47. DeJongh CA, Schimpff SC: Infection in the compromised host, in Samter M (ed): Immunological Diseases (ed 4). Boston, Little, Brown & Co, 1988, pp 963-977.
48. Masur H: Toxoplasmosis, in Wyngaarden JB, Smith LH (eds): Textbook of Medicine (ed 18). Philadelphia, WB Saunders, 1988, pp 1875-1884.
49. Kozier B, Erb G: Fundamentals of Nursing (ed 2). Menlo Park, Calif, Addison-Wesley, 1983.
50. Wade JC, Schimpff SC: Epidemiology and prevention of infection in the compromised host, in Rubin RH, Young LS (eds): Clinical Approach to Infection in the Compromised Host (ed 2). New York, Plenum Medical Book Co, 1988, pp 5-40.
51. Barry SA: Septic shock: Special needs of patients with cancer, Oncol Nurs Forum 16:31-35, 1989.
52. Sheagren JN: Shock syndromes related to sepsis, in Wyngaarden JB, Smith LH (eds): Textbook of Medicine (ed 18). Philadelphia, WB Saunders, 1988, pp 1538-1541.
53. Sande M, Root RR: Septic Shock: Newer Concepts in Pathophysiology and Treatment. New York, Churchill Livingstone, 1985.
54. Conte JE, Barriere SL: Manual of Antibiotics and Infectious Diseases (ed 6). Philadelphia, Lea & Febiger, 1988.
55. Kovacs JA: Diagnosis, treatment, and prevention of pneumocystis carinii pneumonia in HIV-infected patients. AIDS Updates (vol 2, no. 2). Philadelphia, JB Lippincott, 1989.

Chapter 22

Bleeding

Barbara Holmes Gobel, RN, MS

INTRODUCTION

Bleeding represents one of the most complex clinical challenges in the supportive care of the person with cancer. The numerous and unique complications of each neoplasm, combined with the often toxic effects of various cancer treatments, create a difficult problem in the diagnosis and management of a bleeding disorder. Appropriate supportive measures are a vital aspect of the total care of the patient with a bleeding disorder. Supportive care actually may represent the difference between survival and death.

Multiple hemostatic abnormalities may be involved in bleeding associated with cancer. Considerable differences exist in the presentation, proper management, and implications of these clinical problems. Minor bleeding may be the initial symptom that leads to the diagnosis of cancer. Severe bleeding may indicate the onset of a progressive or terminal disease. Because the morbidity and mortality connected with many bleeding problems are significant, prevention of the problem is clearly the best management plan. Rapid recognition, assessment, and knowledgeable treatment of the hemorrhagic complications of cancer will improve significantly the quality of life and the possibility of survival for the person with cancer.

This chapter includes a review of both normal platelet physiology and hemostasis, a discussion of the etiologic factors of bleeding associated with cancer, and patient assessment. Care of the individual with cancer who is experiencing bleeding, including both nursing and medical support, is addressed. Finally, future perspectives on the issue of bleeding associated with cancer are discussed.

PLATELET PHYSIOLOGY

Platelets, also known as thrombocytes, are anucleated, disk-shaped fragments of large marrow cells or megakaryocytes. The megakaryocyte, precursor of the platelet, matures in the bone marrow and is derived from the bone marrow pleuripotent stem cell. In a mature megakarocyte the cytoplasm fragments to form platelets. These cytoplasmic fragments are released in the marrow and then into the blood stream. The nuclei of the platelets are removed by the reticuloendothelial system. This maturing and budding process takes approximately 10 days.

This process of platelet formation is controlled by a regulatory hormone called *thrombopoietin*. Under normal circumstances any reduction in the platelet count causes an increased production of megakaryocytes and platelets in the bone marrow.

Platelets remain in the vascular system and are not found in extravascular fluid. Normally about two thirds of the total platelet mass circulates in the blood stream, and the rest are concentrated in the spleen. Platelets move freely between these two pools. In a patient who has had a splenectomy, the platelet count will rise sharply but transiently. In a patient with an enlarged spleen, however, the platelet count is reduced greatly as the platelets become trapped in the spleen. Platelets survive on the average for about 10 days and then die.

Circulating platelets perform several functions. First and most important is hemostasis, or the formation of a mechanical hemostatic plug. A second function is that platelets furnish a phospholipid surface necessary for a component of hemostasis, that is, interaction of the clotting factors of the intrinsic system. Finally, platelets are responsible for fibrinolysis, or lysis of the fibrin clot and vessel repair.

HEMOSTASIS

Hemostasis is the process by which the fluid nature of blood becomes altered so that a solid clot develops. This process is initiated by vascular or tissue injury and culminates in the formation of a firm mechanical barrier, a platelet plug, which prevents free escape of blood from the damaged vessels. Hemostasis is the end result of two dynamic processes. The first is the vascular-platelet phase. In this phase vessel wall damage causes accumulation of platelets and plug formation at the site of the injury. In the second phase, or biochemical phase, a more stable fibrin clot is formed. This clot seals the vessel, and repair of the vessel is facilitated. Both processes are required to arrest bleeding, regardless of the cause.

Vascular-Platelet Phase

When blood vessel injury occurs, vasoconstriction initially provides a minimal degree of bleeding control. Within seconds the primary hemostatic mechanism is called into play. Platelets are attracted to and adhere to collagen fibers of the exposed subendothelial tissue. This adherence is restricted to one layer of platelets. Platelets then release a number of components, including calcium, serotonin, proteolytic enzymes, cationic proteins, and nucleotide adenosine diphosphate (ADP). ADP causes platelets to swell and platelet membranes to become "sticky." This stickiness causes increased adherence of platelets to one another. Increasing levels of ADP lead to clot contraction, degranulation, and ultimate fusion of the platelets. The end result of ADP-mediated platelet accumulation is the formation of large platelet aggregates, or a hemostatic plug. This initial phase of hemostasis depends on platelet number and function and the ability of the blood vessels to constrict. The primary hemostatic mechanism can produce only temporary cessation of bleeding.

The consolidation and degranulation of platelets are believed to initiate chemical activation of the biochemical phase of coagulation. A complex of lipoproteins, identified as platelet factor 3, is released from the granules on platelet membranes. This factor in turn contributes to the interaction of the plasma coagulation proteins (Table 22-1). It also contributes to the formation of intrinsic prothrombin activation, which is a vital link in ultimate thrombin production.[1]

Biochemical Phase

The biochemical phase, or the phase of coagulation, consists of a biochemical cascade of enzyme activation that ultimately activates fibrin. This fibrin clot is the final product of hemostasis. Activation of this coagulation mechanism may be initiated through one of two independent sequences, the intrinsic (blood) pathway or the extrinsic (tissue) pathway. Each system is equally potent in its activity.

The intrinsic pathway (Figure 22-1) is initiated by contact activation after endothelial injury (thus "intrinsic" to the blood vessel itself). Factor XII activates the processes of the intrinsic system inasmuch as contact occurs between the damaged vessel wall and the plasma protein. The specific factor or substance that stimulates the activation of coagulation factor XII, as well as its function, is uncertain.[2] Factors VIII, IX, and XI all function as part of the intrinsic system until it converges with the common pathway.

TABLE 22-1 Blood Coagulation Factors

Factor	Synonym
I	Fibrinogen
II	Prothrombin
III	Tissue factor, tissue thromboplastin (extrinsic prothrombin activator)
IV	Calcium
V	Proaccelerin, accelerator globulin
VI	Not assigned
VII	Proconvertin, serum prothrombin conversion accelerator (SPCA)
VIII	Antihemophilic globulin (AHG), antihemophilic factor (AHF)
IX	Plasma thromboplastin component (PTC), Christmas factor
X	Stuart-Prower factor
XI	Plasma thromboplastin antecedent (PTA)
XII	Hageman factor
XIII	Fibrin stabilizing factor (FSF)

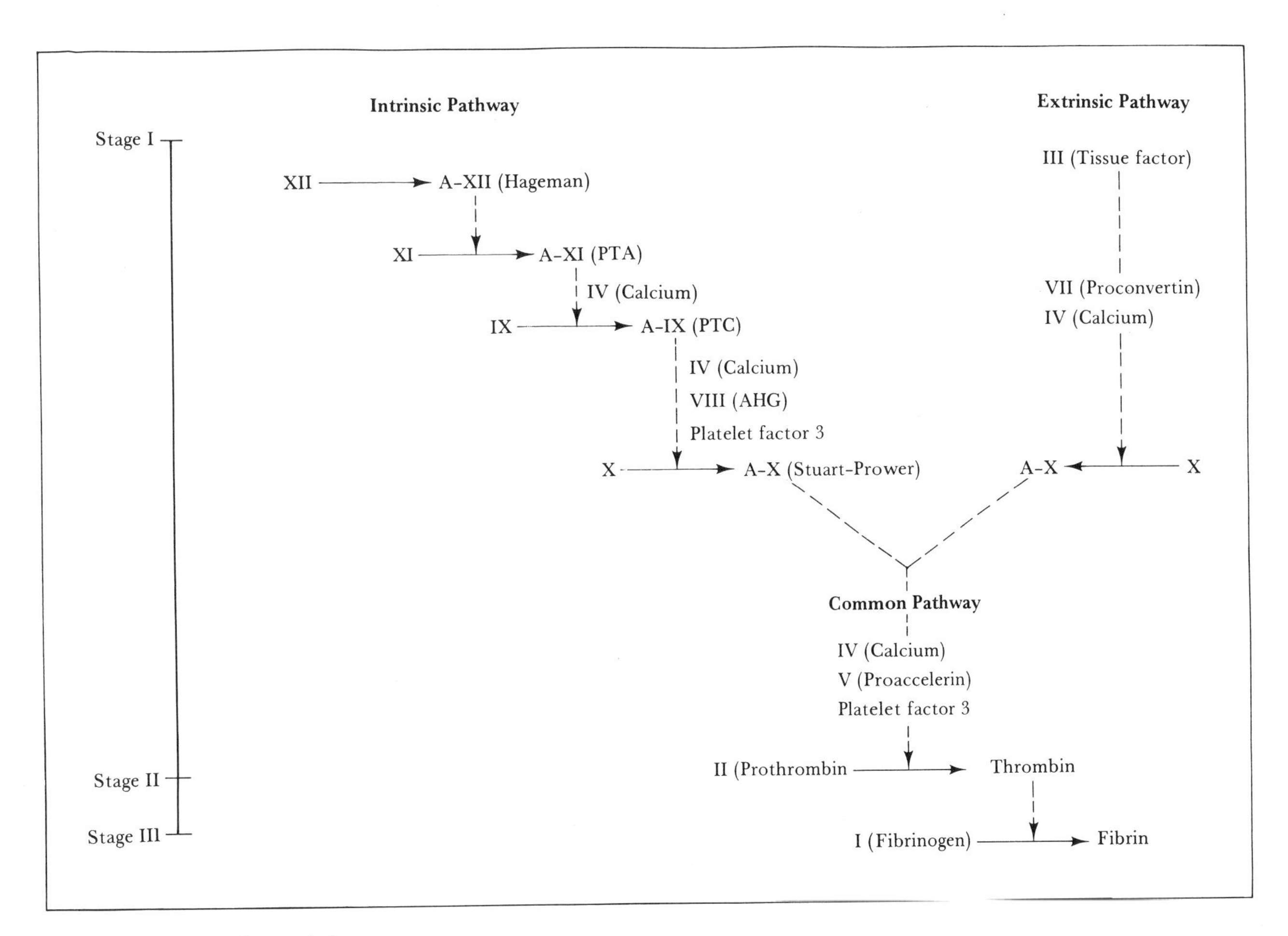

FIGURE 22-1 Blood coagulation.

The extrinsic pathway is initiated by lipoprotein or tissue thromboplastins (tissue factor III). Tissue factor III reacts with factor VII and calcium, resulting in marked coagulant activity.[2] These factors are released from damaged vessel walls during periods of significant tissue injury (thus "extrinsic" to vessel walls). Factors III, VII, and IV function as part of the extrinsic system, then converge with the common pathway.

Once activated, each system leads to the development of thromboplastic activity, an essential factor for prothrombin-thrombin conversion. The interaction of these factors involved in the intrinsic pathway and/or the extrinsic pathway leads to the stimulation of factor X. At this point, thromboplastin formation is complete. This represents the first stage of biochemical coagulation. The second stage occurs when the intrinsic and extrinsic pathways merge into the common pathway. In this stage prothrombin is converted to thrombin by thromboplastin. Thrombin is the most powerful of the coagulation enzymes. Finally thrombin acts on fibrinogen to form fibrin. This fibrin network is an essential portion of a clot. The clot is soluble until it becomes polymerized by factor XII (fibrin stablizing factor), which converts it into a stable (insoluble) fibrin clot. Hemostasis is complete when the fibrin network alone is able to resist the hydrostatic pressure in the vessel.[3]

Fibrin formation is an essential component of hemostasis, inflammation, and tissue repair. It is, however, a temporary reaction to an inciting stimulus. The fibrin clot must be remodeled and removed to restore normal tissue structure and function, as well as to restore normal blood flow. This is done by the fibrinolytic system that controls the enzymatic degradation of fibrin.

Fibrinolysis

Fibrinolysis, or clot dissolution, is initiated by enzymes that are present in most body fluids and tissues. These enzymes are known as plasminogen activators. They activate plasminogen, which converts to plasmin in the presence of thrombin. It is plasmin that is responsible for the lysis of fibrin clots. The breakdown of fibrinogen and fibrin results in polypeptides known as X, Y, D, and E fragments. These fragments are called collectively *fibrin degradation products* (FDPs). FDPs are powerful anticoagulant substances that have the ability to neutralize thrombin, inhibit fibrin polymerization, and interfere with normal platelet production.[4] This process is summarized in Figure 22-2.

Under usual conditions of homeostasis the processes of coagulation and fibrinolysis are localized strictly at the sites of injury. The fragmentation and dilutional effect of continuous blood flow on the activated coagulation factors, combined with the inhibitory effect of certain biochemical control mechanisms and the rapid removal of coagulation components from the body by means of the liver, prevent a generalized hemostatic response. A delicate balance between the processes of fibrin clot formation (coagulation) and clot dissolution (fibrinolysis) is necessary for effective hemostasis.

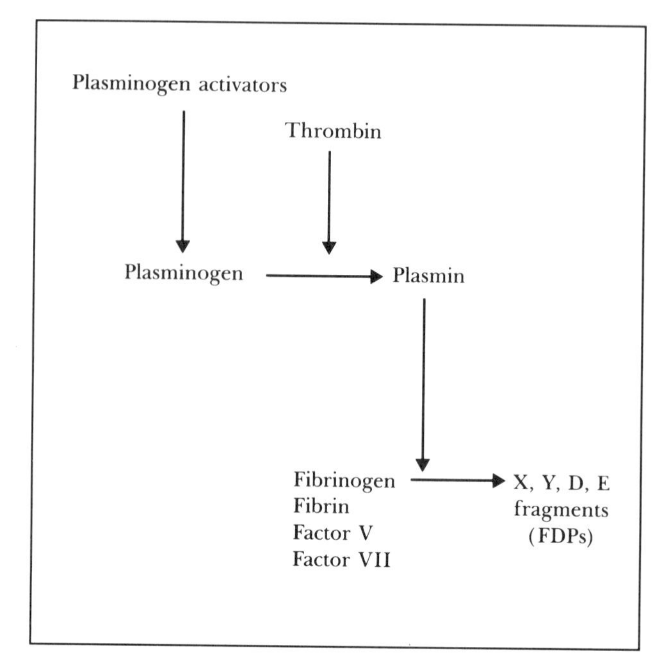

FIGURE 22-2 Fibrinolysis.

CAUSES OF BLEEDING IN CANCER

Structural Abnormalities

Etiology and pathogenesis

Most organs affected by tumors are susceptible to bleeding. Bleeding may be one of the presenting symptoms of the diseases of cancer, or it may be evidence of tumor extension. Bleeding as a symptom of cancer generally is due to the mechanical pressure of tumors on organs and interference with vasculature. Bleeding has been found to be one of the common presenting symptoms of cancer. For example, painless hematuria is the first symptom in 75% of patients with bladder carcinoma.[5] The initial symptom of renal cell carcinoma in 40% of patients is gross hematuria, with another 35% displaying this symptom at some time during the course of the disease.[6] Acute gastrointestinal bleeding may be the presenting symptom of prostate cancer, although it is not a common manifestation.[7] Bleeding may occur as excessive pinkish, viscid sputum, typical of bronchoalveolar cell carcinoma, or as frank blood in the stool with cancer of the left-side of the colon.

The most obvious and frequently the most dramatic cause of bleeding in the person with cancer is the inability to maintain the integrity of the vital circulatory system structures. This loss of integrity most commonly is due to the erosion and rupture of vessels precipitated by tumor invasion or tumor pressure, with resultant tissue ischemia. Any tumor involvement of vascular tissue or any tumor lying in close proximity to major vessels is seen as a threat of bleeding. For example, cancers of the large bronchi or lung may erode into the bronchial artery or branches of the pulmonary artery. Hemoptysis from tumor erosion into the pulmonary blood vessels may appear as streaks or dots to gross blood loss. Head and neck tumors are another cause of serious hemorrhage. Large ulcerative tumors of the larynx and hypopharynx may cause blood-streaked sputum to gross hemoptysis. Other invasive neoplasms, particularly at the base of the tongue, can erode branches of the external carotid artery. Massive vaginal bleeding in women with pelvic tumor masses that invade major pelvic vessels is commonly seen in cervical carcinoma. Vaginal bleeding also may be seen occasionally with endometrial or ovarian carcinoma.

Structural causes of bleeding other than from direct tumor involvement that frequently occur in the individual with cancer include cavitational and ulcerative effects of local infections at sites of vessels, destructive effect of radiotherapy on normal structures in the radiation field, and denuded remains of vessels at the site of radical cancer surgery. One example of a surgical cause of bleeding is the potential of a carotid artery rupture after a radical neck dissection. Ischemic necrosis of the neck skin flap also may occur, further exposing the blood vessel.[8] This may occur particularly when the patient has received preoperative radiotherapy.

Minor incidents of vascular bleeding that eventually are expressed as chronic occult blood loss occur in individuals whose neoplasms produce abnormal proteins of very high viscosity. These paraproteins are common in individuals with myeloma and Waldenström's macroglobulinemia. This macroglobulinemia creates a circulating backflow in small vessels, thereby causing vascular rupture with resultant microscopic hemorrhage. A similar phenomenon is seen in individuals with acute leukemia who have high white blood cell counts. Leukostasis, a potential complication of leukocytosis, results in aggregation and clotting of white blood cells in the microvasculature. This condition may mechanically stimulate obstruction, degeneration, and eventual disruption of small vessels, which results in bleeding.

TABLE 22-2 Tumor Involvement Causing Bleeding in Cancer

Site	Common Manifestations
Head and neck	Hemoptysis: mild to gross blood loss; carotid artery rupture
Thyroid	Hemoptysis
Lung	Hemoptysis: mild to massive
Breast	Bloody nipple discharge (occasionally a result of intraductal papillary carcinoma)
Liver	Hematemesis: mild to severe blood loss
Esophagus	Hematemesis: mild to severe
Stomach	Symptomatic anemia from occult blood loss; hematemesis; melena
Large bowel	Melena: occult or frank
Rectum	Rectal bleeding; melena; blood on surface of stool
Anus	Surface bleeding; melena
Kidney	Hematuria, frequently gross
Renal pelvis and ureters	Hematuria
Bladder	Painless hematuria
Ovary	Vaginal bleeding
Fallopian tube	Abnormal vaginal bleeding
Endometrial	Abnormal vaginal bleeding; watery blood streaked to frank blood (uncommon in women after menopause)
Cervix	Abnormal vaginal bleeding, usually from contact irritation
Vagina	Abnormal vaginal bleeding or staining
Penis	Penile discharge

Manifestations

Bleeding in cancer may appear as symptoms that range from minor incidents of vaginal bleeding to gross blood loss (Table 22-2). Direct injury to vital vascular structures may well lead to acute bleeding and a true oncologic emergency. Specific symptoms depend on the site and extent of damage. Internal bleeding may occur as massive hemoptysis, severe hematemesis, vaginal hemorrhage, loss of consciousness, or hypovolemic shock.

More gradual bleeding that involves smaller circulatory structures is usually less obvious and therefore more difficult to diagnose. Melena caused by colorectal carcinoma or the microscopic bleeding of macroglobulinemia may persist undetected until manifested by iron-deficiency anemia. A continual loss of 6 to 8 mL of blood per day eventually will precipitate classic iron deficiency because the compensatory need for cell production exceeds the iron-producing capacity of the normal adult diet. A definitive diagnosis depends on demonstration of absent stainable iron stores in the patient's marrow. Other methods used to aid in the diagnosis of iron deficiency anemia include the determination of the plasma iron levels, the unsaturated iron-binding capacity (UIBC), and the analysis of the serum ferritin level. The clinical picture of iron deficiency anemia reflects a decreased plasma iron level, an increased UIBC, and a low serum ferritin level.[9] The homeostatic mechanisms in the body provide such remarkable compensatory adaptation that iron deficiency anemia may be serious before significant symptoms develop. It is important to remember therefore that the onset of symptoms may better reflect the rate of progression of the anemia rather than the severity. Fatigue, weakness, irritability, dyspnea, and tachycardia are typical clinical symptoms of anemia.

Management

Acute bleeding caused by the interruption of vascular structures by tumor infiltration is best managed by prevention. Tumors lying near or on major vasculature generally are treated aggressively to avoid complications. Surgery, radiotherapy, and chemotherapy are treatment methods used to shrink or completely remove the neoplasm, if possible. If the wound breakdown is in the neck area and carotid exposure occurs, generally wound debridement followed by a skin or skin-muscle flap carrying its own blood supply is done.[10] Prophylactic arterial ligation may be performed to minimize the risk of carotid hemorrhage. The patient who undergoes a bilateral ligation of the external carotid arteries runs the risk of a stroke. Small transient bleeding usually occurs before vessel rupture. Therefore careful observation may assist the caregiver in predicting and controlling such a complication (see Chapter 41, Head and Neck Cancer).

If vascular integrity is threatened by infection, antibiotic therapy generally is initiated. Preventing and treating infection are crucial in minimizing the potential for bleeding in the patient with cancer.

If acute bleeding does occur, direct methods to halt the hemorrhage are instituted immediately. Direct and steady pressure at the site of bleeding is applied. Mechanical pressure may be used if the site of bleeding is not directly exposed. Examples of mechanical pressure include insertion of an occlusion balloon catheter into the bronchus or the use of nasal packing during epistaxis. Iced saline gastric lavages or enemas may help to control gastrointestinal bleeding. Hypovolemic shock must be avoided in situations of acute hemorrhage. Whole blood is the blood component of choice to restore or maintain blood volume in acute hemorrhage.[11] Whole blood restores circulatory volume and oxygen-carrying capacity simultaneously.

Minor vascular bleeding as a result of capillary destruction is best controlled by treating the underlying malignancy. If iron deficiency has occurred, oral or parenteral iron supplements are indicated. Because iron stores are replenished slowly, iron therapy should be continued for a prolonged period of time even after the malignancy has been treated.[9] If the hemoglobin level drops below 8 to 10 g/dL, blood replacement may be considered. Generally, blood replacement therapy is based on concurrent cardiac, pulmonary, or other conditions that may impair a person's tolerance to anemia. At times, the decision is based on the intention of improving the patient's clinical condition by increasing the blood's oxygen-carrying capacity. Packed cells usually are the therapy of choice. The advantage of packed red blood cells is that they provide more than 70% of the hematocrit of whole blood with only one third of the plasma. This prevents unnecessary volume, electrolyte load, and anticoagulants that may otherwise be transfused.

Platelet Abnormalities

Abnormalities of platelet production, function, survival, and metabolism frequently occur in persons with cancer. These abnormalities may be due to a variety of causes. Generally, they result from mechanical or humoral effects of the tumor itself or from tumor-induced abnormalities in the host.

Quantitative abnormalities

Thrombocytosis Thrombocytosis is a disorder in which there is an increased number of circulating platelets. This disorder commonly is associated with all types of neoplasms. It is particularly common in the myeloproliferative disorders such as chronic granulocytic leukemia. It also is seen frequently in lung, ovarian, pancreatic, breast, kidney and gastrointestinal carcinomas, in Hodgkin's disease, and in persons who have had splenectomies. Thrombocytosis often is associated with widespread cancer.

Generally, the platelet count is only mildly elevated in thrombocytosis caused by cancer (400,000 to 600,000 cells/mm^3) but may on occasion be markedly elevated (800,000 cells/mm^3).[12] The mechanism by which this disorder occurs is unknown. Individuals with thrombocytosis usually have no symptoms and do not require treatment, but thrombosis occurs in a small proportion of cases. Even though no data link the likelihood of complications to the platelet count in thrombocytosis, levels greater than 1 million cells/mm^3 are considered dangerous because of the threat of catastrophic bleeding and thrombosis.[13]

Symptomatic thrombocytosis may be treated by thrombocytopheresis, which rapidly removes large numbers of circulating platelets. A platelet count can be reduced by 50% or more within a few hours. Concurrent with apheresis, the patient is begun on marrow-suppressive therapy. Alkylating agents and ionizing radiation frequently are used to suppress the hyperproliferative marrow. These agents have a high leukemogenic potential.[14] Hydroxyurea also may be given to lower platelet counts, particularly to younger patients without symptoms. This agent too may have leukemogenic potential.[15,16] A new drug for treating thrombocytosis in myeloproliferative diseases currently is being studied. Anagrelide is an agent with a powerful antiaggregating effect on platelets. This drug has been found to lower the platelet count without altering the leukocyte count or the hemoglobin level. It is nonmutagenic and is not known to be leukemogenic.[17]

Thrombocytopenia Thrombocytopenia is the most frequent platelet abnormality associated with cancer and can lead to life-threatening bleeding. The platelet count is considered to be the single most significant factor for predicting bleeding in the individual with cancer. The risk of life-threatening hemorrhage is inversely proportional to the quantity of circulating platelets in patients with acute leukemia. Patients with platelet counts below 20,000 cells/mm^3 have a greater than 50% chance of bleeding.[18] It generally is accepted that if the platelet count in an individual with cancer drops below 20,000 cells/mm^3 or the patient is bleeding, platelet support is given. Other factors such as concomitant infections or the rapidity with which the platelet count is falling are important influences on the risk of bleeding in individuals with cancer who have thrombocytopenia.

Platelet production The most common cause of thromocytopenia in patients with cancer is a decreased production of platelets in the bone marrow. This decrease in platelet production generally is due either to tumor involvement or to the consequences of cancer therapy on the marrow. The low platelet count is directly proportional to the degree of bone marrow infiltration by tumor cells. The decreased production of platelets is believed to be a response to the physical "crowding out" of normal marrow elements by the neoplastic process, the competitive use of nutrient substrate by invading cells, or the production by the invading cells of metabolic end products that are toxic to the normal marrow elements. Marrow infiltration may represent metastatic disease or an intrinsic neoplastic proliferation of marrow elements as occurs in leukemia.

Bone marrow suppression is a common side effect and is the major dose-limiting toxicity associated with chemotherapy.[19,20] It is especially prominent with the alkylating agents. The platelets and the leukocytes are the marrow cells most often affected by the cytotoxic effects of chemotherapy. The megakaryocytes generally are affected 1 to 2 weeks after exposure, but a decrease in the platelet count may be seen even earlier. Early-onset thrombocytopenia has been identified in patients treated with vinblastine for testicular cancer. The platelet count decreases significantly from the start of vinblastine administration.[21] Radiation therapy, particularly if given in combination with chemotherapy, also will produce some degree of bone marrow suppression because the stem cells in the marrow are highly radiosensitive. All cell lines are affected, the megakaryocytes being affected 1 to 2 weeks after exposure. Of the cell lines, platelets take the longest to recover, generally within 2 to 6 weeks. If tumor infiltration or bone marrow suppression is the basis for the thrombocytopenia, megakaryocytes will be decreased or absent in the marrow.

Platelet sequestration Thrombocytopenia caused by an abnormal distribution of platelets that results in increased platelet sequestration may occur in patients with splenomegaly as part of the neoplastic disease process. An enlarged spleen may sequester up to 90% of the platelet population. Tumor metastasis to the spleen, particularly that caused by cancers of the lung, breast, prostate, colon, and stomach and lymphomas, are known to cause platelet sequestration. Splenic enlargement as a result of tumor involvement in the liver, which causes portal hypertension and congestive splenomegaly, may precipitate secondary platelet sequestration.

Sequestration of platelets with resultant bleeding may occur within the vascular channels of some tumors, such as giant hemangiomas. Surgical removal of the tumor or shrinkage of the tumor by low-dose radiation therapy is necessary for recovery of the platelet count.[22] Denuded areas because of surgery, mucositis that results from chemotherapy and/or microbial toxins, and necrotic tumor may cause platelet aggregation and a decrease in circulating platelets.

If the primary cause of thrombocytopenia is platelet sequestration, the bone marrow will contain normal to increased numbers of megakaryocytes. This is due to the attempt of the bone marrow to compensate for the decreased number of circulating platelets. When splenomegaly is accompanied by marrow infiltration by the tumor, the degree of thrombocytopenia is compounded inasmuch as the compensatory production of platelets will be inadequate.

Platelet destruction Thrombocytopenia also may be due to rapid platelet destruction characterized by a dramatically shortened platelet life span and an abundance of megakaryocytes in the bone marrow. Although the platelet normally survives 8 to 10 days, it may live as little as a few hours. This type of thrombocytopenia is seen in two situations.

The first situation in which rapid platelet destruction occurs is in immune thrombocytopenia, or idiopathic thrombocytopenic purpura. This disorder occurs most frequently in individuals with lymphoproliferative diseases such as chronic lymphocytic leukemia and lymphoma. Idiopathic thrombocytopenia also has been found in association with extragonadal germ cell cancer, although it is seen rarely in disseminated cancers.[23] The use of alpha-interferon therapy for patients with cancer also has been identified with the development of immune thrombocytopenia.[24] The rapid destruction of platelets is due to an autoimmune process in which antibodies are formed against the person's own platelets.

The second type of rapid platelet destruction is seen in conditions of increased platelet consumption. This may be observed in various clinical syndromes with intravascular coagulation. Disseminated intravascular coagulation is discussed in depth in this chapter (see the section on coagulation abnormalities). In any condition that involves increased platelet destruction, increased numbers of megakaryocytes will be present in the marrow as the body attempts to compensate for this abnormal state.

Platelet dilution Dilution is another factor that leads to thrombocytopenia. It is believed that rapid reconstitution of the intravascular volume by the use of stored platelet-poor blood dilutes thrombocytes already present. Whole blood can be stored up to 21 days with a minimal decrease of erythrocyte survival. The platelets in the whole blood, however, lose considerable effectiveness after 24 hours at usual storage temperatures of 4°C. This dilutional effect of platelets occurs in direct proportion to the amount of blood transfused.

Multiple-donor transfusions, possibly with incompatible platelet antigens, may stimulate an isoantibody response in the recipient. Studies of persons with posttransfusion purpura have demonstrated the presence of platelet antibodies in the plasma, as well as the occurrence of microaggregation and lysis of platelets.[25]

Management Although thrombocytopenia may be the immediate cause of bleeding in individuals with platelet disorders, the target of therapy is the underlying cause of the decreased platelet level. When the decreased platelet production is due to marrow infiltration with tumor, the best therapy is treatment of the tumor itself. The hematologic complications will remain or worsen as long as the marrow involvement persists. Platelet transfusions often are given to maintain a safe level of circulating thrombocytes until tumor regression occurs and marrow function returns. If platelet production has been depressed by chemotherapy or radiotherapy, the dosage or administration schedule may be altered.

Platelet sequestration within a spleen that is enlarged because of malignancy is treated most effectively by aggressive tumor therapy. Chemotherapy and radiotherapy usually are most effective. Sequestration of platelets is at times reversible by the administration of epinephrine. Epinephrine causes a release of trapped platelets from an enlarged spleen.[12] Transient control of sequestration also has been achieved with corticosteroid therapy. Steroids have a capillary-stabilizing effect that is important in minimizing the bleeding potential of thrombocytopenia.[26]

High-dose intravenous immunoglobulin therapy has been advocated as a treatment choice for patients who have active bleeding and in whom alloimmunization to human leukocyte antigen (HLA)–matched platelets has occurred.[27] Immunoglobulins provide a quick rise in the platelet count with a radical decrease in bleeding. In the absence of active bleeding the use of high-dose intravenous methylprednisone has been found as effective as high-dose intravenous immunoglobulins for the treatment of autoimmune thrombocytopenia.[28] Splenectomy may be considered if other methods fail to control the sequestration of platelets.

Platelet destruction by an autoimmune reaction rarely is treated by platelet transfusions. This therapy generally is ineffective and has the risk of a serious transfusion reaction. Should patients require red cell therapy, it is recommended that they receive extensively washed red cells or frozen deglycerolized red cells. These preparations may provide less antigenic material.[29]

Qualitative abnormalities

Patients with cancer may at times have bleeding despite normal platelet counts and coagulation factors. Alterations in platelet function may cause the bleeding. The major abnormality noted is a decrease in the procoagulant activity of platelets, which is a measure of platelet factor 3. This deficiency has been demonstrated in patients with chronic lymphocytic leukemia, acute leukemia, multiple myeloma, and macroglobulinemia.[12] Decreased platelet adhesiveness and decreased aggregation in response to ADP have been reported, especially in persons with leukemia.[3] Abnormal platelet function also has been described in patients with thrombocytosis associated with the myeloproliferative disorders. This may help to explain the increased incidence of hemorrhage in patients with an increased platelet concentration.

These abnormalities may be due to the malignancy itself or to a partial release of the platelet contents after contact with malignant tissue.[12] Another pathogenic factor may be the increased activation of coagulation factors in individuals with cancer. Intravascular coagulation followed by fibrin breakdown results in significant increases in circulating fibrin degradation products. These substances coat the surfaces of platelets and interfere with their functioning. In the malignant paraprotein disorders (eg, macroglobulinemia), the interaction of the platelet membrane with the abnormal proteins prevents the release of platelet factor 3.[12]

TABLE 22-3 Drugs That Affect Platelet Function

Drug	Reference No.
Nonsteroidal antiinflammatories: aspirin, indomethicin, phenylbutazone, meclofenamic acid	31
Plasma expanders (dose related): dextran, hydroxyethal starch	31
Antidepressants: chlorpromazine, promethazine, reserpine, imipramine, amitryptyline	3
Miscellaneous: ethanol, local and general anesthetics, phenothiazine, antihistamines, dipyridamole, clofibrate, vitamine E, ticlopidine, furosemide, vasodilators (hydralazine and nitroprusside)	31
Semisynthetic penicillins (dose related): pencillin, ticarcillin, carbenicillin, ampicillin	32

Drug-induced platelet dysfunction probably is underestimated in individuals with cancer. Numerous pharmacologic agents are known to be associated with impaired hemostasis. Probably the best known drug that affects platelet function (decreases platelet adhesiveness) is acetylsalicylic acid (aspirin). Platelet function is impaired by other nonsteroidal anti-inflammatory agents as well, including indomethicin, phenylbutazone, and meclofenamic acid.[31]. (Table 22-3 lists several other drugs that affect platelet function[3,31,32]). Qualitative platelet changes frequently stimulate an increased production of megakaryocytes in an attempt to compensate for their poor functioning.

Management of hemorrhagic disorders caused by platelet malfunction is aimed at the underlying cause. The effects of malignancy are counteracted by aggressive antineoplastic therapy. The development of fibrin degradation products are minimized by correction of the specific hypercoagulation disorder that stimulated their formation. Anticoagulation therapy usually is instituted. Drug-induced platelet abnormalities are managed best by avoidance of the aggravating agent. Platelet transfusions often are given during periods of thrombocytopenia to avoid hemorrhage.

Coagulation Abnormalities

Hypocoagulation

Etiology and pathogenesis Malignancy or the metabolic alterations that frequently accompany malignancy may precipitate an imbalance in the coagulation factors, leading to decreased hemostasis. In 1974 Slichter and Harker[33] showed that these imbalances were related directly to tumor burden. Successful tumor therapy brought about a normalization of coagulation values. The most significant factor that leads to a state of hypocoagulability is liver disease. Liver disease may be due to tumor invasion, chemotherapy, infection, or surgical resection. Liver disease interferes with the synthesis of plasma coagulation factors I, II, V, VII, IX, and X. In addition to decreasing the production of these factors, liver disease also may interfere with their functioning. For example, failure of the liver to neutralize inhibitors of specific coagulation factors will create a constant state of decreased hemostasis. Diminished liver clearance of fibrin degradation products and activated clotting factors further inhibits the coagulation mechanism.

A deficiency of vitamin K also may cause a hypocoagulation syndrome that may be seen in patients with neoplastic disease in which there is a dietary lack of vitamin K, biliary obstruction, malabsorptive states, or intestinal sterilization as a result of antibiotic administration. A deficiency of vitamin K results in a greatly reduced chemical activation of vitamin K–dependent proteins, factors II, VII, IX, and X.

Laboratory studies of patients who receive large amounts of frozen plasma during massive transfusions demonstrate a prolonged prothrombin time and prolonged partial thromboplastin time, which may occur when patients undergo extensive surgical procedures[4]. Frozen plasma has deficient levels of factors V and VIII.

A nonspecific plasma antagonist of several coagulation proteins has been described in various disease states, including neoplastic disease. These anticoagulants have been identified in acute leukemias, lymphocytic lymphomas, and other disease states in which white cell turnover is rapid. These inhibitors have been found to be highest at the onset of chemotherapy when there is lysis of white cells and in disease relapse when there is a large tumor burden.[4]

Isolated factor deficiencies also are reported in neoplastic disease. Acquired von Willebrand's syndrome (deficiency of factor VII) has been identified in a number of neoplastic diseases including solid tumors, hematologic malignancies, macroglobulinemia, and lymphoproliferative disorders.[34] Factor VIII deficiency generally is due to acquired inhibitors of coagulation proteins.[35] These inhibitors have also been demonstrated in monoclonal IgG gammopathies, lymphosarcoma, and macroglobulinemia.[4] The exact relationship between the specific inhibitors and the underlying neoplastic disease is unclear. Factor XIII deficiency is another factor commonly affected by malignancy and liver disease.

Manifestations Conditions of decreased coagulability are less common than other types of hemostatic alterations discussed in this chapter. Although any type of coagulation abnormality can lead to bleeding, decreased coagulability less frequently causes serious bleeding when it occurs. Hemorrhages tend to develop in the deeper areas of the body such as the subcutaneous or intramuscular tissue. Bleeding into the joints, especially of the distal extremities, also is seen in the hypocoagulability states.[36] Acquired von Willebrand's syndrome is characterized by clinical and laboratory features similar to those of congenital von Willebrand's disease. These patients are characterized clinically by mucosal bleeding. The laboratory data demonstrates a prolonged bleeding time and diminished or absent factor VIII procoagulant activity (factor VIII:C), von Willebrand factor antigen (vWF:Ag), and ristocetin cofactor activity.[34] A deficiency of any factor leads to abnormal fibrin formation, which provides an ineffective matrix for normal fibroblastic proliferation and wound healing.

Management Successful tumor therapy combined with infection control generally is the best means of controlling hypocoagulability abnormalities. Production of coagulation factors by the liver can be augmented by fresh-frozen plasma or prothrombin complex concentrates. Prothrombin complex (containing prothrombin and factors VII, IX, and X) is often given to shorten a prolonged prothrombin time, particularly before a needle biopsy of the liver.[37] Specific replacement of diminished factors is difficult because of the complex nature of these abnormalities. Generally, the treatment of specific inhibitors of coagulation factors depends on the severity of the abnormality. Patients in whom factor VIII is deficient are infused with factor VIII concentrates that contain von Willebrand's protein. These concentrates may include fresh-frozen plasma and cryoprecipitate, along with packed red cell and platelet concentrate to control the bleeding.[34,38] When factors V and VIII are deficient because of infusion of large amounts of frozen plasma, the infusion of several units of fresh plasma may correct the disorder.[4] Factor VIII deficiency (fibrin stabilizing factor deficiency) is readily treated by replacement therapy with plasma or cryoprecipitate.

Administration of parenteral phytonadione (Aquamephyton) is used to correct the protein defects when vitamin K is deficient. If absorption of vitamin K is not a problem, the patient is instructed regarding the dietary sources of vitamin K. The ingestion of green leafy vegetables such as spinach, kale, and cabbage is encouraged.

Hypercoagulability

Disseminated intravascular coagulation (DIC) is the most common serious hypercoagulable state that occurs in persons with cancer. It represents an inappropriate and exaggerated overstimulation of normal coagulation in which thrombosis and hemorrhage may occur simultaneously. This seemingly paradoxical situation results in hypercoagulation, in which multiple small clots are formed in the microcirculation of many organs, and in fibrinolysis, in which there is consumption of clots and clotting factors. Ultimately the body becomes unable to respond to vascular or tissue injury through stable clot formation, and hemorrhage ensues. DIC always is secondary to an underlying disease process such as malignancy, septicemia, obstetric accidents, or similar systemic stressors.

Although DIC is considered to be a common problem associated with malignancy, the incidence rate is difficult

TABLE 22-4 Common Causes of Disseminated Intravascular Coagulation in Cancer

Neoplasms
Acute leukemia (promyelocytic, monocytic, myelocytic)
Solid tumors (lung, prostate, colon, stomach, breast, gallbladder, ovary, melanoma)
Chemotherapy administration
Infections
Gram-negative sepsis (endotoxin)
Gram-positive sepsis
Viremias (varicella)
Hepatic failure
Intravascular hemorrhage
Multiple transfusions of whole blood
Hemolytic transfusion reaction

to estimate. The syndrome often remains undetected until severe hemorrhage occurs, and frequently it is discovered only at the time of autopsy. Rickles and Edwards[39] reported that of the routine blood coagulation tests up to 92% of patients with cancer show abnormal results that are compatible with DIC. DIC contributes strongly to morbidity and mortality in patients with cancer, particularly in those with thrombosis or bleeding in the lung, central nervous system, or the gastrointestinal tract.[40] The mortality rate of DIC is in the range of 54% to 68%, increasing with age, number of clinical manifestations, and severity of laboratory abnormalities.[41]

Etiology The most common cause of DIC is infection. It is believed that bacterial endotoxins, released in gram-negative bacteremia, activate the Hageman factor (XII). This factor initiates coagulation by means of the intrinsic pathway of hemostasis and stimulates fibrinolysis.[41] DIC also is seen in the presence of gram-positive bacteremia and in viremias (Table 22-4 lists common causes of DIC in cancer).

Tumors themselves have been identified as stimulators of intravascular coagulation. The most commonly associated cancers include acute promyelocytic leukemia and the adenocarcinomas. Acute promyelocytic leukemia has a very high correlation with DIC. A procoagulant substance has been identified on the promyelocytic blast cells that is similar to thromboplastin and is believed to initiate the clotting response.[42] The solid tumors most often associated with DIC are the adenocarcinomas. It is suggested that the mucin formed by adenocarcinoma may stimulate both intrinsic and extrinsic pathways of coagulation by means of factor X activation.[43] Tumors also may cause intravascular coagulation through their erosive properties that lead to exposure of vascular subendothelium and resultant hemostatic stimulation. In addition, DIC is associated with the administration of cytotoxic agents used to treat this malignancy. The cytotoxic drugs cause destruction of the blast cells, which then release the procoagulant substance.

Pathogenesis DIC always results from an underlying disease process. The pathophysiology of DIC involves an extensive triggering of the coagulation system by the underlying disease, which results in abnormal activation of thrombin formation. This triggering mechanism may be direct, as with tissue thromboplastin associated with acute promyelocytic leukemia, or indirect because of endotoxins from gram-negative sepsis. Excess circulating thrombin may abnormally activate both coagulation and fibrinolysis, which upsets the balance of hemostasis.

Thrombin cleaves fibrinogen that easily combines with circulating fibrin degradation products to form a soluble form of fibrin. At times this combination forms insoluble clots that deposit in the microvasculature of various organs. These fibrin thrombi are considered to be the hallmark of DIC. The lodged clots further trap circulating platelets, which results in the thrombocytopenia associated with DIC.[44] This entrapment of platelets impedes blood flow, which leads to tissue ischemia, hypoxia, and necrosis of multiple organs, along with consumption of clots and clotting factors.

The abnormal activation of thrombin results in increased fibrinolysis. Thrombin acts not only to convert fibrinogen to fibrin but also to assist in the conversion of plasminogen to plasmin. Plasmin is responsible for the breakdown of fibrinogen and fibrin. This breakdown of fibrinogen and fibrin causes increased circulating fibrin degadation products (FDPs) that have strong anticoagulant properties. The FDPs interfere with fibrin clot formation and aid in the consumption of clotting factors and platelets. The bleeding manifestations of DIC are caused by the combination of the consumption of platelets and certain clotting factors, plasmin's fibrinolytic properties, and the anticoagulant properties of the FDPs.

Manifestations DIC can occur as a chronic coagulation disorder or an acute hemorrhagic diathesis, or it can be detected through various laboratory studies. Clinical symptoms may be similar to those of other thrombocytopenic conditions.

In chronic DIC the patient is not critically ill. It may produce minimal or no clinical manifestations. Easy and spontaneous bruising may be present. Mild petechiae, ecchymosis, gingival bleeding, and minor gastrointestinal bleeding may be noted. Laboratory tests may vary but generally show minor coagulation abnormalities. Neurologic dysfunction may occur occasionally in chronic DIC as a result of small episodic cerebral bleeding. It is often mistaken, however, for metabolic encephalopathy or metastasis.

Acute DIC occurs rapidly over hours to days and always results from the disease process. Widespread purpura and significant gastrointestinal and genitourinary hemorrhage may occur. Overt hemorrhage that involves multiple unrelated sites is not uncommon. The patient

TABLE 22-5 Clotting Studies of Disseminated Intravascular Coagulation

Test	Abnormality	Cause
Prothrombin time*	Prolonged	Elevated fibrin split products; decreased plasma clotting factor levels
Partial thromboplastin time	Prolonged	Elevated fibrin split products; decreased plasma clotting factor levels
Platelet count*	Decreased	Platelet consumption
Plasma fibrinogen*	Low	Consumption of fibrinogen by the clotting cascade and by fibrinolysis
FDP assays	Increased	Fibrinogen destruction by plasmin
Factor assays	Decreased	Consumption of clotting factors
Antithrombin III assay	Decreased	Consumption of clotting factors
Protamine paracoagulant	Negative	Severe hypofibrinogenemia

*Classic triad of tests.
FDP, Fibrin degradation product.

may display signs of shock and associated organ hypoxia. Hemoptysis, intraperitoneal hemorrhage, and intracranial bleeding may be life threatening to the patient with DIC.

There is no specific laboratory finding that is absolutely diagnostic of DIC. A battery of laboratory tests in conjunction with clinical evidence must be used to confirm the diagnosis and to monitor response to treatment. A number of clinical conditions affect these tests, which makes their interpretation even more difficult. Multiple blood product transfusions dilute clotting factors or platelets; liver disease with portal hypertension may lead to thrombocytopenia and the activation of the fibrinolytic system.

A classic triad of tests generally are done to help support the diagnosis of DIC (Table 22-5). These tests include determination of prothrombin time (PT), the platelet count, and the plasma fibrinogen level. In DIC the PT usually is less than 15 seconds, which reflects decreased levels of clotting factors II and V and of fibrinogen. The platelet count drops below 150,000 cells/mm^3. A low platelet count is considered to be a cardinal diagnostic finding in DIC. The count is below 50,000 cells/mm^3 in about one half of all cases of DIC.[45] A low plasma fibrinogen level (<150 mg/dL) results from the consumption of fibrinogen because of thrombin-induced clotting and from fibrinolysis in DIC. Other laboratory tests that are used frequently to detect DIC include FDP assays (increased in DIC), factor assays (decreased), partial thromboplastin time (PTT) (prolonged), antithrombin III assay (decreased), and protamine paracoagulant determination (which shows negative results in DIC with severe hypofibrinogenemia).

Management Treatment of the underlying malignancy is vital in treating the patient with a hypercoagulability abnormality, inasmuch as the tumor is the ultimate stimulus. All other therapy, although effective on a short-term basis, provides only an interval of symptomatic relief.

Early detection of the signs and symptoms of DIC may allow for prompt diagnosis and treatment. Bleeding with resultant hemorrhage is the most common complication of DIC. It may be the first sign of underlying pathologic disease. Measures to detect bleeding and further prevent blood loss are covered in the section on physical examination and general nursing considerations in this chapter.

Thrombus formation often occurs simultaneously with bleeding in DIC. Thrombi generally form in the superficial and smaller veins and may be clinically undetectable. Subtle signs and symptoms of thrombi include red, indurated, tender areas in multiple organ sites. When thrombosis occurs, the signs and symptoms include focal ischemia, acral cyanosis, superficial gangrene, altered sensorium, ulceration of the gastrointestinal tract, and dyspnea that may lead to acute respiratory distress syndrome. Continuous assessment is done to determine progression or regression of signs and symptoms.

Heparin therapy often is the primary treatment for DIC in malignancy, yet its use remains controversial.[37] The controversy stems from the lack of randomized trials of heparin therapy use in patients with DIC as a result of malignancy. There also is a controversy as to whether high-risk patients (eg, a patient with promyelocytic leukemia who is undergoing chemotherapy) should be treated prophylactically with heparin therapy. The problem lies in the potential for unnecessarily exposing the patient to a risk of bleeding.

Heparin inhibits the formation of new clots and may decrease the consumption of clotting factors. Heparin therapy for DIC generally is maintained until symptoms disappear and laboratory values return to normal. Large doses of heparin often are required to overcome intravascular clotting. A bolus of 10,000 U or more may be given, followed by intermittent intravenous injections or continuous intravenous infusion.[45]

Another drug that may be used with DIC is epsilon-amino caproic acid (EACA; Amicar). This drug may be used when the fibrinolysis of DIC has been resolved but uncontrolled bleeding persists. Epsilon-amino caproic acid prevents the binding of plasminogen or plasmin to fibrin or fibrinogen.[46] The drug may be given intravenously or orally, and the maintenance dose is 0.5 to 1.0 g/hour.[47]

Blood component therapy often is necessary in DIC. Platelets may be given if the platelet count drops below 30,000 cells/mm^3. Packed red cells may be given if hemorrhaging occurs. Fresh frozen plasma contains all the clotting factors, including antithrombin III, and also is given for volume expansion. Antithrombin III is a coagulation factor that also may be given; it neutralizes thrombin, plasmin, and activated forms of factors XII, XI, X, and VII.[41] Cryoprecipitate may be given for severe hypofibrinogenemia, which often occurs in DIC. It is a concentrated source of fibrinogen and factor VIII.

Prevention of further complications is another important goal in managing DIC. Any tight or restrictive clothing is removed if thrombophlebitis is suspected or apparent. Edema, if present, is measured daily. Elastic support stockings may help to minimize stasis and promote venous return. Other measures to decrease stasis and promote venous return include assisting the patient with leg lifts and/or elevating the legs 15 to 20 degrees at intervals and teaching the patient to wiggle the toes and perform ankle circles frequently while in bed. Compression to the knee vessels is minimized by having the patient avoid placing anything under the knees while in bed (eg, pillows and knee gatches), crossing the knees or legs, and dangling the legs over the side of the bed.

Patient education is a necessary component of care for the patient at risk for DIC. Patients and families are taught to report any bleeding or unusual and abnormal symptoms. They are taught to save all excreta for the nurse to examine for blood. Finally, the patient and family need excellent psychosocial support should the paradoxical hemorrhage and thrombus formation of DIC develop.

ASSESSMENT

Patient assessment begins with a thorough history and physical examination. Either component of the assessment may be comprehensive, for example, during the interview of a patient suspected of having a malignancy, or cursory, for example, during the care of a person with acute blood loss because of the malignancy. The information gathered in the assessment is instrumental in planning an appropriate plan of care for the patient.

Patient and Family History

The patient and family history is a vital component of the complete assessment. Because bleeding is a common problem in many malignancies, one must remain alert to findings that suggest hemostatic disorders. Patients may respond more openly and with greater ease if questions are focused on activities of daily living, for example, excessive bleeding while the person shaves or prolonged bleeding after minor cuts and scrapes while the person cooks or cleans. Key aspects of a comprehensive history for patients at risk for bleeding include the following:

1. Bleeding tendencies, such as easy bruising, excessive nosebleeds, gingival bleeding, presence of petechiae, change in color of stools or urine, stomach discomfort, vision problems, or painful joints
2. Family history of any bleeding abnormalities
3. Drugs and chemicals taken that may interfere with the coagulation mechanism or that may uncover an important symptom for which the person is taking medication
4. General performance status that helps to identify the effects of the disease or the presence of complications
5. Current blood component therapy, including reason for and response to therapy
6. Nutritional status to identify vitamin K or C deficiency or generalized malnutrition that will affect the person's hematologic system
7. Presence of any signs or symptoms of anemia that may signify undetected long-term bleeding

Physical Examination

Observation is the most important measure in early detection of bleeding. Diagnostic signals may be subtle, including skin petechiae that may be noticed while bathing the person, traces of blood during tooth brushing, oozing from venipuncture sites or sites of injections, and traces of blood on the rectal thermometer. These are examples of the types of information that can lead to early diagnosis of hemostatic problems and that may prevent an incident of spontaneous hemorrhage.

The major problem associated with active bleeding is hemorrhage. Although bleeding can occur from any part of the body, common sites of hemorrhage include the gums, nose, bladder, gastrointestinal tract, and brain. A systematic examination is done on a routine basis for any patient known to have a bleeding disorder.

Integumentary system

A thorough skin assessment, including intertrigonous areas, is undertaken routinely. Bruising, petechiae, purpura, and any areas of ecchymosis are noted carefully and documented: the location, size, and pattern of distribution for all skin changes. Acrocyanosis that appears as irregularly shaped cyanotic patches on the periphery of arms and legs may be detected in hemorrhage because of DIC. (It results from fibrin deposition in the microcirculation and may lead to gangrene). The clinician inspects for any oozing from venipuncture sites or injections, catheters, or nasogastric tubes.

Eyes

The eyes are checked for any visual disturbances, increased injection on the sclera, periorbital edema, or subconjunctival hemorrhage (homogeneous red color that is sharply outlined on the sclera). Bleeding in the optic fundus can lead to permanent vision impairment.

Nose

The patient is observed for petechiae on the nasal mucosa, signs of excessive nosebleeds, or bloody discharge from the nose.

Mouth and throat

The mucous membranes of the mouth and throat are checked for petechiae or oozing of blood, and the gums are checked for tenderness or bleeding.

Lungs and thorax

The patient is assessed for crackles, wheezes, stridor, dyspnea, tachypnea, cyanosis, and hemoptysis. All may be signs of bleeding in the lungs.

Cardiovascular system

The patient is assessed frequently for changes in vital signs and peripheral perfusion. The color and temperature of all extremities is checked and the peripheral pulses monitored.

Gastrointestinal system

The patient is assessed for abdominal discomfort, blood around the rectum, tarry stools, and frank or occult blood in the stools. All body excretions are checked for occult blood in the patient who is at risk for bleeding.

Renal system

Fluid intake and output is routinely monitored. If the urine output drops below 30 mL/hr it may be due to acute tubular necrosis as a result of thrombi, hemorrhage, or hypovolemia.[45] Occult blood in the urine is monitored routinely.

Musculoskeletal system

The patient should be assessed for painful joints during the performance of active or passive range of motion, which may indicate bleeding into the joints.

Central nervous system

Intracranial hemorrhage or impaired tissue perfusion may be detected by mental status changes, including restlessness, confusion, lethargy, obtundation, seizures, or coma.

Screening Tests

Several screening tests provide information regarding hemostatic function. These groups of tests give information about both phases of hemostasis and fibrinolysis. The hematologic alterations leading to bleeding are complex, and test results will vary depending on the degree of original coagulation dysfunction and the cascading effect of related hemostatic mechanisms.

A brief discussion regarding some of the most common screening tests of hemostatic function follows, as well as a more comprehensive list in Table 22-6.

TABLE 22-6 Tests of Hemostasis

Test	Measures	Normal Value
	PLATELET FUNCTION	
Bleeding time	Platelet plug formation; response of small vessels to injury	1-9 minutes
Platelet count	Number of circulating platelets	150,000-400,000/mm^3
Clot retraction	Ability of platelets to support retraction of a clot	50% retraction within 1 hour; compare with normal value
Platelet aggregation	Ability of platelets to aggregate	Compare with normal control
Platelet phospholipid (factor 3) availability	Availability of platelet factor 3 for coagulation	Compare with normal control
	COAGULATION	
Partial thromboplastin time (PTT)	Intrinsic and common pathways	Varies; compare with normal control (usually 30-40 seconds)
Prothrombin time (PT)	Extrinsic and common pathways	Varies; compare with normal value
Thrombin time	Fibrinogen concentration; structure of fibrinogen; presence of inhibitors	Varies; compare with normal value
Specific factor assays	Concentration of functional factor in plasma	50%-150% activity in pooled normal plasma
	FIBRINOLYSIS	
Assay of fibrinogen or fibrin degradation products (FDP)	Presence of FDP in serum	1:8, 10 mg/mL; 1:4, 0-8 mg/mL (10 mg/mL)

Bleeding time

Bleeding time measures the time that it takes for a small skin incision to stop bleeding. The results of the test depend on the platelet number and function and the ability of the capillary wall to constrict. The time varies between 1 to 9 minutes. The bleeding time is prolonged when there is a lack of platelets or in diseases that affect the blood vessel walls. Examples of disease states in which a prolonged bleeding time may be found include thrombocytopenia, von Willebrand's disease, infiltration of the marrow by tumor, and consumption of platelets in DIC, and in the use of drugs that affect platelet function, such as acetylsalicylic acid.

Platelet count

Platelet count measures the actual number of circulating platelets per cubic millimeter of blood. Normal counts are considered to be 150,000 to 400,000 cells/mm^3. Counts below 100,000 cells/mm^3 are considered to be a sign of thrombocytopenia. Spontaneous hemorrhage generally is not a concern until the platelet count drops below 15,000 cells/mm^3. Thrombocytosis occurs when the count rises above 400,000 cells/mm^3.

Whole blood clot retraction test

Whole blood clot retraction test measures the speed and extent of blood clot retraction in a test tube. The test is done to determine the degree of platelet adequacy. A normal clot shrinks to one half its normal size in 1 to 2 hours and completely retracts in 24 hours. Clot retraction is slower and will stay soft and watery with thrombocytopenia or with abnormally functioning platelets.

Prothrombin time

The PT is determined by adding tissue thromboplastin and ionized calcium to citrated plasma and recording the time required for clotting. The test is measured against the time needed for a normal sample of blood to clot. The PT is a measure of the factors involved in the extrinsic and common pathways in the clotting mechanism. Test results usually are given as the actual time in seconds and also compared with a normal or control value. When the clotting factors exist in diminished quality, the PT is prolonged. Prolonged PT values also are seen in liver disease (eg, hepatitis and tumor involvement), obstructive biliary disease (eg, bile duct obstruction as a result of tumor), and coumarin ingestion.[48]

Partial thromboplastin time (activated)

The activated PTT is determined by adding phospholipid reagents to plasma in the presence of calcium chloride. The test is a sensitive measure of the intrinsic and common pathways of the clotting mechanism. The normal activated PTT is 30 to 40 seconds. A prolonged activated PTT is evidenced when any of the factors exist in inadequate quantities, as with consumptive coagulopathy, liver disease, biliary obstruction, and circulating anticoagulants such as heparin.[49]

The PT and PTT taken together can give a fair indication of the nature of the clotting defect. If both the PT and PTT are normal, the vessels or platelets are probably defected. The defect is likely to be in the clotting mechanism if either the PT or PTT is prolonged. If both are prolonged, the defect is most likely in the common pathway.

Fibrin degradation product test

The FDP test is determined by adding peripheral venous blood to serum that contains antifibrinogen degradation fragments. The measurement of FDPs provides an indication of the activity of the fibrinolytic system. Agglutination is demonstrated if the patient's blood contains the degradation fragments. FDP levels greater than 10 mg/mL indicate increased fibrinolysis such as that seen in DIC and primary fibrinolytic disorders. No agglutination occurs if degradation products are absent in the patient's blood.

GENERAL NURSING CONSIDERATIONS

The physical safety of the patient is always ensured to prevent trauma in those with diminished thrombocytic activity. Potential threats of injury in the environment are identified and then reduced or eliminated. Bumps or falls may be dangerous or even fatal in the person with a low platelet count. Shoes or slippers with good soles are worn to help avoid breaks in the skin and to aid in ambulation. Patients may require assistance with ambulation, particularly if they are known to have an unsteady gait. Disoriented or confused patients may require some type of restraint while in bed. Side rails of the bed and any sharp protruberances are padded should the platelet count drop below 10,000 cells/mm^3. The cooperation of the patient and family, who are educated regarding all safety measures, is vital in ensuring the patient's physical safety.

Diligent measures to maintain skin integrity are instituted. Electric razors are used to prevent cuts during shaving. The mouth and gums, which are easily damaged when the platelet count drops, become a significant potential source of infection. Soft-bristled toothbrushes help to avoid trauma to sensitive gums. When the platelet count drops below 20,000 to 30,000 cells/mm^3, bristled toothbrushes are avoided and mouth swabs or toothettes are used. A nonirritating (alcohol-free) mouthwash is recommended. When the mouth and gums are irritated, dentures should not be replaced, particularly if they are ill-fitting. Patients who require oxygen therapy by means of a nasal cannula or an endotracheal tube are assessed for irritation to the mucosa.

All unnecessary procedures are avoided, including intramuscular or subcutaneous injections, rectal temperatures or suppositories, and indwelling catheters. If the patient requires parenteral administration of medication, the intravenous route is used whenever possible. Intramuscular and subcutaneous injections place the patient at risk for the development of hematomas. Hematomas may become sites of infection when granulocytopenia is present. Injections, if unavoidable, are administered with a needle of the smallest possible gauge. Pressure to the injection site is applied for several minutes, followed by the application of a pressure bandage to avoid hematomas. Similar care is taken at venipuncture sites.

Severe uterine hemorrhage may be a complication in women menstruating with thrombocytopenia. Menses can be suppressed by pharmacologic agents, generally progestational medications. In women whose menses are not suppressed, careful napkin counts are done during menstrual bleeding to help determine the volume of blood loss.

Forceful coughing, sneezing, or nose blowing may lead to bleeding. Epistaxis may be life threatening in a person with thrombocytopenia. The patient with epistaxis is placed in high Fowler's position. Ice packs, nasal packing, or topical epinephrine (adrenaline) to decrease bleeding caused by small vessel rupture within the nasal mucosa also may be used. Bowel strain caused by constipation can initiate rectal bleeding; stool softeners may be prescribed. Instruction regarding proper diet and exercise to avoid constipation also are appropriate.

Hygiene is clearly a problem in the patient who has active bleeding. The patient may require frequent baths and linen changes to feel and smell better. A room deodorizer may be needed because blood exposed to air is malodorous.

Physical and emotional rest is essential to the patient when active bleeding occurs. Rest helps to decrease pulse rate and blood pressure, allowing for clot formation to occur. A state of active bleeding is frightening and anxiety-producing for the patient and family. A calm approach and reassurance are in order in the management of active bleeding. Sedation also may be used to allow for a decreased level of anxiety and a decreased metabolic rate.

PLATELET THERAPY

The use of platelet transfusions has proved to have tremendous therapeutic value in controlling and preventing hemorrhage in individuals with cancer. The incidence of fatal hemorrhage fell from 70% to less than 25% when platelet support was used in individuals with leukemia associated with severe thrombocytopenia.[50] Generally, the patient is transfused when there is actual bleeding associated with thrombocytopenia, when the platelet count is greater than 20,000 cells/mm^3 yet bleeding is present, and when patients with abnormally functioning platelets have bleeding. Prophylactic platelet transfusions may be given in the absence of clinical hemorrhage to maintain a platelet count greater than 20,000 cells/mm^3 or during periods of intense chemotherapy to prevent spontaneous hemorrhage into the brain. Other factors that determine appropriateness of transfusion therapy are determined on an individual basis. The presence of infection or a rapid decrease in circulating platelets make the patient far more susceptible to thrombocytopenia.

Preservation Techniques

Platelets can be given in fresh whole blood, platelet-rich plasma, or platelet concentrates. The concentrated method is the most widely used today. The use of fresh whole blood generally is used only in emergency situations in which there is severe and rapid hemorrhage. Platelet concentrates can be obtained from one donor and suspended in minimal plasma by plateletpheresis techniques of closed-bag collection systems or by a blood cell separator. One unit of platelets is routinely obtained from 500 mL of fresh whole blood. Theoretically, one unit of platelets should increase the recipient's peripheral blood platelet level by 10,000 to 12,000 cells/mm^3. An attempt usually is made to maintain the patient's platelet count greater than 20,000 cells/mm^3. This necessitates frequent transfusions in the patient with leukemia, in whom the platelet life span is greatly shortened because of conditions such as fever, infection, and incidents of vascular bleeding.

Random donor platelet concentrate

Platelet concentrate from random donors is harvested from fresh whole blood. A random concentrate consists of four bags or units of platelets, each from different donors. When random donor platelets are used, the patient-recipient is exposed to multiple tissue antigens. Over time these tissue antigens initiate an antigen-antibody formation that leads to platelet refractoriness. This is the time that the transfusion of a unit of platelets fails to achieve an effective or expected increase in the platelet count. Patients who require platelet transfusions over an extended period of time often are switched to single donor or HLA-matched platelets because of this refractoriness. The patient also is at an increased risk of transmission of hepatitis when pooled products are used. Random donor platelets can be used fresh, frozen, or after cryopreservation. Frozen or cryopreserved platelets have limited application because their recovery is less than half that of fresh platelets. They generally are used in an emergency when fresh platelets are unavailable.[51]

Single donor platelet concentrate

Single donor platelet concentrate is taken from one donor. One unit of platelets has a volume of 35 to 50 mL. Single donor platelets are generally more effective than random donor platelets when refractoriness to random donor platelets occurs. Because only one donor is used, patients are not exposed to multiple antigens. Patients who are severely immunosuppressed, such as those who have undergone bone marrow transplantation, may receive only single donor platelets or HLA-matched platelets during their treatment period, which minimizes their exposure to multiple antigens as they require long-term platelet support. Platelets are most effective if used fresh, with maximal effectiveness 6 hours after donation. A pheresis can be done frequently (up to every other day) if it is found that the donor's platelets provide the patient with good platelet count increases.

Human leukocyte antigen–matched platelet concentrate

HLA-matched platelets are used in the event of refractoriness to random donor or single donor platelets. They are obtained from a single donor who has been determined by a blood test to be compatible at the HLA complex. This complex is found on all blood cells and acts as a "genetic monogram." HLA-matched platelets minimize the exposure of the recipient to foreign antigens. These platelets generally provide much more effective increments than random donor or single donor platelets.

Platelet Survival

Several factors have been identified as important in determining posttransfusion platelet survival in a patient. Failure to achieve adequate increments in the circulating platelet count often are due to infection, fever, DIC, and splenomegaly. Infection may enhance the consumption of platelets and increase the occurrence of hemorrhage. Patients with hemorrhage may require more frequent transfusions at shorter intervals.[51] If platelets are being transfused while the person has active bleeding, increased increments will not be detected by laboratory data. Their effectiveness, however, may be measured by clinical improvement and control of bleeding.

In an attempt to minimize platelet destruction, patients with fever caused by infection may receive premedication with antipyretics before platelet transfusion. When a fever is caused by the platelet transfusion, that is, febrile reaction to the transfusion, premedication may consist of antipyretics, corticosteroids, and/or antihistamines. Certain antimicrobial drugs also have been found to cause occasional platelet refractoriness as a result of drug-induced antibodies. Drug-induced antibodies have been demonstrated against trimethoprim-sulfathoxazole, amphotericin B, and certain semisynthetic penicillins.[51]

Platelet survival is decreased greatly when refractoriness to the platelet transfusion develops. Because of repeated exposure of patient/recipient platelets to the HLA antigens on the donor's platelets, patients eventually may become refractory to random donor platelets.

Platelet increments may be affected negatively by leukoagglutinin reactions directed at non-HLA leukocyte antigens. In this situation donor platelets are contaminated with granulocytes.[27] After transfusion there is subsequent antibody formation that causes allergic symptoms, including hives, skin flush, fever, and chills. These reactions can be avoided by leukocyte depletion from the platelet concentrate during preparation. The leukocyte-depletion process requires fresh platelets.[41] Patients also may receive premedication with antipyretics, corticosteroids, and antihistamines to minimize this reaction.

The preparation and storage of platelets are important factors in determining the quality of the platelet transfusion. Platelets must be fresh and metabolically active to be most effective. Maximum effectiveness remains up to 6 hours after being obtained. Storage longer than 24 hours at 22° C causes significant loss of platelet function because of release of ADP and alterations of platelet membrane permeability.[52]

Transfusion Complications

Complications of platelet transfusions are similar to those of any blood product. These reactions may be immediate in onset, occurring within a few minutes or hours after the start of the transfusion, or delayed by days or weeks after the transfusion. Immediate transfusion reactions include hemolytic transfusion reactions, febrile and allergic reactions, shock or sepsis caused by bacterial contamination, and circulatory overload. Delayed reactions include infections (eg, viral hepatitis), graft-versus-host disease, and delayed hemolysis.

Platelets generally can be transfused across incompatibilities of the major red blood cell antigen (ABO) unless there is gross red blood cell contamination into the transfusion pack. If significant spillage has occurred, the donor and recipient are matched by A, B, and O antigens. If matching is not done when spillage occurs, hemolytic reactions are likely.[27]

Bacterial contamination of platelets, although rare, can lead to infection in the host. The storage of platelets at 22° C, although important for cell survival, increases the possibility of microbial survival and growth.

Another serious transfusion complication in patients with significant immunosuppression is the risk of the development of graft-versus-host disease after the transfusion of blood products that contain viable lymphocytes. The donor-competent T lymphocyte immunologically attacks the immunocompromised host tissue after transfusion. This disease generally is manifested in the skin, liver, and gastrointestinal tract and can be fatal.[53] It generally is recommended that all blood products given to the severely immunocompromised host be exposed to irradiation before transfusion.[54] Irradiation of platelets is done to inhibit proliferation of lymphocytes without impairment of platelets, red cells, or granulocytes.[55]

CONCLUSION

Bleeding in the individual with cancer is the result of multiple factors. Bleeding can occur as a result of the neoplastic disease itself or the therapies used in treating the malignancy. Bleeding can be occult, causing no immediate danger to the patient, or it can be acute and life threatening as in the hemorrhage and clotting of DIC. Each hematologic entity must be therapeutically approached according to its cause, the person's condition, and the health goals that have been set for each patient.

The increasing survival rates in individuals with cancer is due in large part to multiagent treatment protocols currently being used. The success of many of these treatment protocols has been possible through the great achievements that have been reached in intensive care support. Yet it must be emphasized that early detection of the signs and symptoms of various complications during treatment such as bleeding may allow for prompt diagnosis and treatment of the disorder. As survival rates and cure rates increase, patients and families continue to need support. This support includes physical, emotional, and spiritual help. The identification of the most appropriate methods of providing patient care to the person with cancer who is at risk for bleeding is an area of potential research.

• • •

The material in this chapter is adapted in part from the original work by Susan Gross Fisher.

REFERENCES

1. Eastham RD: Bleeding, clotting, and transfusion, in Eastham RD (ed): Clinical Hematology. Bristol, England John Wright and Sons, 1984, pp 239-399.
2. Williams WJ: Sequence of coagulation reactions, in Williams WJ, Beutler E, Erslev AJ, et al (eds): Hematology (ed 3). New York, McGraw-Hill, 1983, pp 1238-1247.
3. Wintrobe MM: Clinical Hematology (ed 8). Philadelphia, Lea & Febiger, 1981.
4. Rosenberg RD, Green DM: The hemostatic process in neoplastic disease, in Holland JF, Frei E III (eds): Cancer Medicine. Philadelphia, Lea & Febiger, 1982, pp 1326-1338.
5. Prout GR, Garnick MB, Canellos GP: The bladder, in Holland JF, Frei E III (eds): Cancer Medicine. Philadelphia, Lea & Febiger, 1982, pp 1896-1912.
6. Prout GR, Garnick MB: The kidney and ureter, in Holland JF, Frei E III (eds): Cancer Medicine. Philadelphia, Lea & Febiger, 1982, pp 1880-1896.
7. Doll DC, Kerr DM, Greenberg BR: Acute gastrointestinal bleeding as the presenting manifestation of prostate cancer. Cancer 58:1374-1377, 1986.
8. Shedd DP: Cancer of the head and neck, in Holland JF, Frei E III (eds): Cancer Medicine. Philadelphia, Lea & Febiger, 1982, pp 1671-1685.
9. Beutler D: The common anemias. JAMA 259:2433-2437, 1988.
10. Riley WB, Larson DL: Reconstruction in head and neck oncology, in Copeland EM (ed): Surgical Oncology. New York, John Wiley & Sons, 1983, pp 189-206.
11. Masouredis SP: Preservation and clinical use of erythrocytes and whole blood, in Williams WJ, Beutler E, Ersler AJ, et al (eds): Hematology. New York, McGraw-Hill, 1983, pp 1529-1549.
12. Lazlo J: Hematologic effects of cancer, in Holland JF, Frei E III (eds): Cancer Medicine. Philadelphia, Lea & Febiger, 1982, pp 1275-1288.
13. Silverstein MN: Diagnosis and treatment of polycythemia vera, agnogenic myeloid metaplasia, and primary thrombocytopenia, in Wiernik PH, Canellos GP, Kyle RA, et al (eds): Neoplastic Diseases of the Blood. New York, Churchill-Livingston, 1984, p 135.
14. Adamsom JW: Wither the platelet. N Engl J Med 318:1331-1332, 1988 (editorial).
15. Donovan PB, Kaplan ME, Goldberg JD, et al: Treatment of polycythemia vera with hydroxyurea. Am J Hematol 17:329-334, 1984.
16. Schimke RT, Sherwood SW, Hill AB, et al: Overreplication and recombination of DNA in higher eukaryocytes: Potential consequences and biological implications. Proc Natl Acad Sci USA 83:2157-2161, 1986.
17. Silverstein MN, Petitt RM, Solberg LA, et al: Anagrelide: A new drug for treating thrombocytosis. N Engl J Med 318:1292-1294, 1988.
18. Gaydos LA, Freirich EJ, Mantel N: The quantitative relation between platelet count and hemorrhage in patients with acute leukemia. N Engl J Med 266:905-909, 1962.
19. Haskell CM: Principles of cancer chemotherapy, in Haskell CM (ed): Cancer Treatment (ed 2). Philadelphia, WB Saunders, 1985, pp 21-43.
20. VanZandwijk N, ten Bokkel-Huinink WW, Wanders J, et al: Dose finding studies with carboplatin (JM8), ifosphamide (IFO), etoposide (VP16) and mesna in non small cell lung cancer (NSCLC), Proceedings of the Annual Meeting of the American Society of Clinical Oncology, vol. 7. Chicago, WB Saunders, 1988, p A757.
21. Steurer G, Kuzmits R, Pavelka M, et al: Early onset thrombocytopenia during combination chemotherapy in testicular cancer is induced by vinblastine. Cancer 63:51-58, 1989.
22. Dachman AH, Ros PR, Shekitka KM, et al: Colorectal hemangioma: Radiologic findings. Radiology 167:31-34, 1988.
23. Garnick MB, Griffin JD: Idiopathic thrombocytopenia in association with extragonadal germ cell cancer. Ann Intern Med 98:926-927, 1983.
24. McLaughlin P, Talpaz M, Quesada JR, et al: Immune thrombocytopenia following alpha-interferon therapy in patients with cancer. JAMA 254:1353-1354, 1985.
25. Kickler TS, Herman JS, Furihata TJ, et al: Identification of Bak^b, a new platelet-specific antigen associated with post-transfusion purpura. Blood 71:894-898, 1988.
26. Aster RH: Thrombocytopenia due to enhanced platelet destruction, in Williams WJ, Beutler E, Erslev AJ, Lichtman MA (eds): Hematology. New York, McGraw-Hill, 1983, p 1323.
27. Deisseroth A, Wallerstein R: Use of blood and blood products, in DeVita VT, Hellman S, Rosenberg SA (eds): Cancer Principles and Practice of Oncology. Philadelphia, Lippincott, 1989, pp 2045-2059.
28. von dem Borne: High dose IV methylprednisolone or high dose IV gammaglobulin for autoimmune thrombocytopenia. Br Med J 296:249-250, 1988.
29. Vogelsang N, Kickler TS, Bell WR: Post-transfusion purpura: A report of five patients and a review of the pathogenesis and management. Am J Hematol 21:259-267, 1986.
30. Cowan DH, Haut MJ: Platelet function in acute leukemia. J Lab Clin Med 79:893-905, 1972.
31. Weiss HJ: Acquired qualitative platelet disorders, in Williams WJ, Beutler E, Erslev AJ, et al (eds): Hematology. New York, McGraw-Hill, 1983, pp 1355-1363.
32. Brown CH III, Bradshaw MW, Natelson EA, et al: Defective

platelet function following the administration of penicillin compounds. Blood 47:949-956, 1976.
33. Slichter SS, Harker LA: Hemostasis in malignancy. Ann NY Acad Sci 230:252-261, 1974.
34. Rao KPP, Kizer J, Jones TL, et al: Acquired von Willebrand's syndrome associated with an extranodal pulmonary lymphoma. Arch Pathol Lab Med 112:47-50, 1988.
35. Shapiro SS, Hultin M: Acquired inhibitors to the blood coagulation factors. Semin Thromb Hemost 1:366, 1975.
36. Williams WJ: Congenital deficiency of factor XIII (fibrin-stabilizing factor), in Williams WJ, Beutler E, Ersler AJ, et al (eds): Hematology. New York, McGraw-Hill, 1983, pp 1410-1412.
37. Johnson AJ, Aronson DL, Williams WJ: Preparation and clinical use of plasma and plasma fractions, in Williams WJ, Beutler E, Ersler AJ, et al (eds): Hematology. New York, McGraw-Hill, 1983, pp 1410-1412.
38. Roussi JH, Houbouyan LL, Alterescu R, et al: Acquired von Willebrand's syndrome associated with hairy cell leukemia. Br J Haematol 46:503-506, 1980.
39. Rickles FR, Edwards RL: Activation of blood coagulation in cancer: Trousseau's syndrome revisited. Blood 62:14-31, 1983.
40. Bunn PA, Ridgway EG: Paraneoplastic syndromes, in DeVita VT, Hellman S, Rosenberg SA (eds): Cancer Principles and Practice of Oncology. Philadelphia, JB Lippincott, 1989, pp 1916-1923.
41. Siegrist CW, Jones JA: Disseminated intravascular coagulopathy and nursing implications. Semin Oncol Nurs 1:237-243, 1985.
42. Sakuragawa N, Takahashi K, Hoshiyma M, et al: Pathologic cells as procoagulant substance of DIC syndrome in acute promyelocytic leukemia. Thromb Res 8:263-273, 1976.
43. Caprini J, Selner S: Altered coagulability in cancer patients. Cancer 32:162-172, 1982.
44. Rooney A, Haviley C: Nursine management of disseminated intravascular coagulation. Oncol Nurs Forum 12:15-22, 1985.
45. Griffin JP: Be prepared for the bleeding patient. Nurs 86 16(6):34-40, 1986.
46. Marder VJ, Butler FO, Barlow GH: Antifibrinolytic therapy, in Coleman RW, Hirsh J, Marder VJ, et al (eds): Hemostasis and Thrombosis: Basic Principles and Clinical Practice. Philadelphia, JB Lippincott, 1982, p 640.
47. Marder VJ, Francis CW: Clinical aspects of fibrinolysis, in Williams WJ, Beutler E, Ersler AJ, et al (eds): Hematology. McGraw-Hill, 1983, pp 1462-1473.
48. Pagana KD, Pagana TJ: Diagnostic Testing and Nursing Implications (ed 2). St Louis, CV Mosby, 1986.
49. Beare PG, Rahr VA, Ronshausen CA: Nursing Implications of Diagnostic Tests (ed 2). Philadelphia, JB Lippincott, 1985.
50. Hersh EM, Bodey GP, Nies BA, et al: Causes of death in acute leukemia. JAMA 193: 99-103, 1965.
51. Brand A, Claas FHJ, Falkenburg JHF, et al: Blood component therapy in bone marrow transplantation. Semin Hematol 21:141-153, 1984.
52. Yankee RA, Sherwood GK: Platelet transfusions, in Holland JF, Frei E III (eds): Cancer Medicine. Philadelphia, Lea & Febiger, 1982, pp 1319-1325.
53. Parker N, Cohen T: Acute graft-versus-host disease in allogeneic marrow transplantation. Nurs Clin North Am 18:569-577, 1983.
54. Cohen D, Weinstein H, Mihm M: Nonfatal graft-versus-host disease occurring after transfusion with leukocytes and platelets obtained from normal donors. Blood 53:1053-1057, 1979.
55. Weiden PL, Zuckerman N, Hansen JA, et al: Fatal graft-versus-host disease in a patient with lymphoblastic leukemia following normal granulocyte transfusions. Blood 57:328-332, 1981.

Chapter 23

Fatigue

Lillian M. Nail, RN, PhD

INTRODUCTION

At one time or another, everyone has experienced fatigue. One popular view of the function of fatigue is that it serves to protect individuals from harm by keeping them from engaging in excessive amounts of physical or mental activity. Feelings of fatigue usually are attributed to physical exertion, psychological stress, and inadequate sleep and rest. People complain that fatigue changes their appearance, interferes with concentration, impairs physical performance, and makes them tense and irritable. Fatigue can interfere with all aspects of day-to-day life.

Acute fatigue is a relatively temporary state that is relieved by rest, although one night of undisturbed sleep may not provide complete relief. When fatigue persists over time, it is known as chronic fatigue or chronic fatigue syndrome.[1] Individuals with cancer may experience both acute and chronic fatigue as a result of the disease, as a side effect of treatment, and as a result of the psychological distress produced by the diagnosis of a potentially life-threatening condition.[2-6] The incidence of fatigue reported by cancer patients treated with surgery, radiation therapy, chemotherapy, or biologic response modifiers reached 90%.[7-13] Despite the prevalence of fatigue in cancer patients and the extent to which it can interfere with daily activities, there is limited research describing the time of onset, duration, pattern, and severity of fatigue, identifying factors that contribute to fatigue, or testing interventions designed to prevent or ameliorate fatigue.

DEFINITION OF FATIGUE

Fatigue is a complex concept that has been associated with many other terms such as tiredness, exhaustion, weariness, drowsiness, malaise, weakness, asthenia, somnolence, lack of energy, and feeling "bushed" or "beat." Fatigue has been defined in terms of both objective performance and subjective experience. Early fatigue research focused on individuals' jobs or athletic performances. The aim of this research was to identify the causes of fatigue and find ways to improve performance. In this approach to understanding fatigue, an objective indicator of the point at which performance declines, such as exercise endurance or accuracy of completion of a mental task, is used to define fatigue.[14] Weakness is related to the objective view of fatigue, since it also represents a muscular performance deficit demonstrated on objective testing.

In the subjective experience approach, fatigue is conceptualized as involving both a feeling state and the impact of that state on the individual's perception of his or her ability to engage in usual activities.[4,6] In contrast to weakness, defined as the *inability* either to initiate or to maintain specific muscular activities, subjectively defined fatigue has a voluntary component, since individuals may push themselves to engage in a highly valued activity.

The subjective view of fatigue is most relevant to the concerns of nurses caring for individuals with cancer. The actions individuals take in response to fatigue will be based on their perceptions rather than on the results of a performance test or an evaluation of the individual's level of fatigue made by another person. Some individuals will define their fatigue in terms of sensations, while others will define it in terms of their perception of their ability to engage in usual activities. Nursing care focuses on helping those who are at risk for fatigue or experiencing fatigue to plan for and deal with the experience.[1-4,6]

PATHOPHYSIOLOGY OF FATIGUE

Theories of Causation

Although causes of fatigue have been explored in numerous studies, no clear support for any of the major hypotheses has emerged. The majority of the research was conducted before 1970 using normal human subjects in performance test situations. Specific hypotheses about fatigue in cancer patients remain untested. The extent to which findings from research on fatigue in healthy normal subjects or trained athletes apply to individuals with cancer is not known.

Accumulation hypothesis

Early research on fatigue led to the accumulation hypothesis, which proposed that a buildup of waste products in the body produces fatigue. This hypothesis was supported when rapid accumulation of lactic acid, pyruvic acid, and other metabolic products was found during strenuous exercise, although subsequent research failed to relate the accumulation of waste products to the occurrence of fatigue.[15] Although it is common for fatigue in cancer patients receiving radiation treatment or chemotherapy to be attributed to the presence of by-products of cell death, to date no research has been conducted to test this hypothesis.

Depletion hypothesis

The depletion hypothesis was based on the idea that muscular activity is impaired when certain substances, such as carbohydrates, fats, proteins, adenosine triphosphate (ATP), and adrenal hormones are not readily available.[15] The relationship between nutrition and muscular activity is complex, involving both the supply and use of nutrients. When carbohydrates or fats are available for conversion into glycogen, protein is spared. With sustained muscle activity, glycogen is depleted, leading to fatigue.

The nutritional problems many cancer patients experience may lead to inadequate intake of nutrients; the way the body uses nutrients may change in the presence of cancer; and the tumor may successfully compete with normal tissues for available nutrients.[16] Therefore, indicators of changes in nutritional status, such as weight loss or changes in the nutrients available at the cellular level, should be associated with fatigue if the depletion hypothesis explains fatigue. However, the limited research in this area does not provide adequate support for this line of reasoning. For example, although weight loss was positively correlated with subjective postoperative fatigue in a group of general surgery patients, including some cancer patients, there was no association between fatigue and changes in specific muscle or plasma amino acids.[17]

The fatigue produced by anemia can also be thought of as an example of the depletion mechanism. Anemia decreases the blood's oxygen-carrying capacity, inhibiting the delivery of essential nutrients to the cells and decreasing the energy available to the organism. When anemic individuals who have experienced fatigue are treated with transfusions and subsequently demonstrate improvement in their hematocrit or hemoglobin values, they generally report a concurrent decrease in the severity of fatigue. However, not all individuals with cancer who have anemia experience fatigue.[18]

Biochemical and physiochemical phenomena

Changes in the production, distribution, use, balance, and movement of substances such as muscle proteins, glucose, electrolytes, and hormones may be important factors influencing the experience of fatigue.[15,19] Changes in the production and balance of hormones are central components of the Selyé syndrome of stress response and may contribute to the fatigue experienced by individuals with cancer during physical or psychological stress.[20] Many of the drugs used to treat cancer or to manage side effects of treatment also can produce biochemical and physiochemical changes related to those believed to produce fatigue.[5]

Central nervous system control

In a 1970 review of the research on fatigue in animals and healthy human subjects, Grandjean concluded that central control of fatigue is vested in the reticular formation.[21] In Grandjean's neurophysiologic model of fatigue, the level of fatigue is determined by the balance between two opposing systems: the activating system and the inhibiting system. The reticular activating system, located in the reticular formation, controls alertness or wakefulness by stimulating the cerebral cortex and responding to both sensory stimulation and feedback from the cerebral cortex. The inhibitory system, believed to involve the cerebral cortex and the brain stem, depresses the activity of the reticular activating system. In Grandjean's model, both internal stimuli, such as thoughts and perceptions, as well as external stimuli (eg, noise and light) stimulate the reticular activating system and promote wakefulness or alertness. The sustained arousal or wakefulness that occurs after environmental stimulation may be produced by release of adrenergic substances from the adrenal glands. Feelings of sleepiness or tiredness occur when the level of cortical stimulation of the reticular activating system is low, when there is little or no sensory input, or when the level of activity of the inhibitory system is high.

The neurophysiologic model of fatigue may explain the occurrence of fatigue in conditions of low stimulation, such as immobility produced by bed rest, even when there is little expenditure of energy. It also accounts for rapid decreases in feelings of fatigue when danger or excitement is perceived or a sudden increase in intensity or change in the nature of environmental stimuli occurs.

Adaptation and energy reserves

Selyé's approach to fatigue is that every individual has a certain amount of superficial energy available for adaptation and that fatigue occurs when that energy supply is depleted. Rest allows time for energy to be replenished from the individual's deep reserves so that adaptation can continue.[20] As the reserves of adaptation energy are consumed, fatigue eventually leads to exhaustion and then to death. Selyé's ideas incorporate accumulation, depletion, biochemical-physiochemical changes, and central nervous system (CNS) control, since all these may be involved in the individual's response to stressors.

Summary

Acute fatigue is an expected outcome of strenuous physical and mental activity and is believed to serve the same sort of protective effect as acute pain. However, fatigue in individuals with cancer is more likely to resemble chronic fatigue than acute fatigue in that it may not respond to rest, persists over time, and often interferes with performance of usual daily activities.[22] Although there are many different hypotheses about the causal mechanisms of fatigue, none has been adequately tested in a population of cancer patients. However, all are potentially relevant to explaining at least some aspects of the fatigue experienced by individuals with cancer. Presently, the most reasonable approach to exploring the etiology of fatigue in individuals with cancer is to consider multiple factors, as illustrated in Figure 23-1.

Individuals with cancer experience biologic factors such as tumor burden, the physical stress of treatment, environmental changes during hospitalization, psychological factors such as fear of death, changes in social relationships and roles, nutritional changes, and side effects of treatment or symptoms of the disease. In addition to the energy expenditure required to deal with symptoms or side effects, individuals with cancer may also experience disruption in their usual restorative activities when nausea, pain, or urinary frequency interferes with sleep and rest.

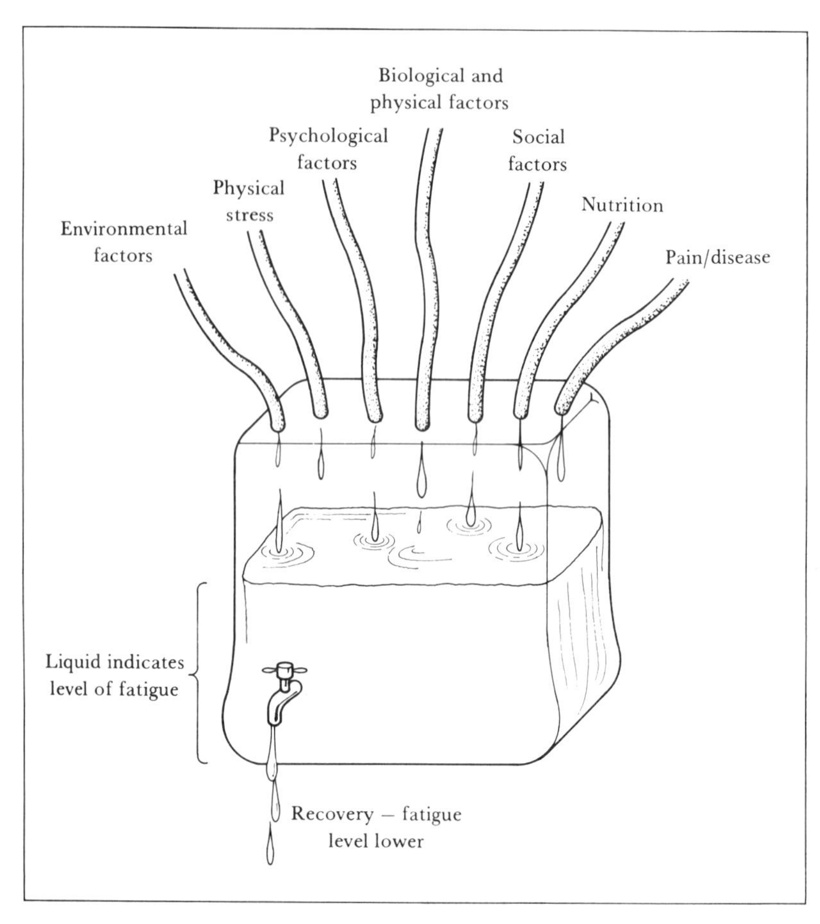

FIGURE 23-1 Fatigue in cancer pictured as the level of liquid in a container. Effects of various sources pour in; recovery is the outflow. (Source: Adapted from Grandjean EP: Fatigue: Its physiological and psychological significance. Ergonomics 11:427-436, 1968.)

CANCER AND FATIGUE: PATHOPHYSIOLOGY AND PATHOPSYCHOLOGY

Treatment Effects

Surgery

Patients undergoing surgery experience direct tissue damage as well as the effects of anesthesia and analgesics. Fatigue is a consistent finding in patients who are recovering from surgery and is generally assumed to have multiple causes.[7,17,23,24] Fatigue may persist up to 6 months following surgery.[24] Since it is not unusual for patients to undergo several surgical procedures for diagnosis and initial treatment of cancer, the possible cumulative effects of multiple surgical procedures on fatigue are of concern to those who care for oncology patients. The effects of multiple surgical procedures on the severity and duration of postoperative fatigue have not been examined.

Radiation treatment

The majority of the side effects of radiation treatment are local and predictable based on the site of the treatment field. For example, individuals receiving radiation treatment to a pelvic field experience diarrhea, while those receiving treatment to the neck experience a sore throat. Fatigue is one of the only systemic side effects of local radiation treatment and has been reported to be the most severe side effect of radiation during the last week of treatment.[11,12,25,26] In a sample of 30 patients who received radiation therapy and completed the Pearson Byars Fatigue Feeling Checklist daily throughout the course of their treatment, the mean level of fatigue increased over the course of treatment, with decreases in level of fatigue over the weekends (when patients were not treated).[11] A subgroup of the sample, consisting of patients with lung cancer, entered treatment with higher levels of fatigue than the other subjects and reported declines in fatigue before the end of treatment.

Weekly interviews of 96 patients undergoing radiation

treatment revealed that fatigue was reported by 93% of the patients receiving treatment for lung cancer, 68% of the patients treated for head and neck cancer, 65% of the men treated for genitourinary cancer, and 72% of the women treated for gynecologic cancer. Among the patients with lung cancer, 60% reported fatigue at the first week of treatment compared with 5% to 35% of the patients in the other three groups. In all four groups, fatigue declined gradually over the 3 months following treatment. Subjects reported that the fatigue was intermittent early in treatment but that it became continuous by the end of treatment, was worse in the afternoon or evening, and that resting or sleeping in the afternoon was helpful.

The difference between the pattern of fatigue before and during radiation treatment reported by patients with lung cancer when compared with patients with other cancer diagnoses may be related to the characteristics of the disease. The high incidence of fatigue at the beginning of radiation treatment in patients with lung cancer may be explained by the increased energy expenditure required for breathing through partially obstructed airways. In research with healthy volunteers, decreases in airway diameter were associated with increased work of breathing.[27] If radiation treatment is successful in decreasing tumor size, individuals who enter treatment with some degree of airway obstruction are likely to experience some relief of fatigue as a result of the treatment.

The research on cancer patients' perceptions of fatigue as a side effect of radiation treatment is limited to patients receiving local radiation treatment. The experience of patients who receive total body irradiation in preparation for bone marrow transplantation has not been examined. Since patients who receive total body irradiation also receive a variety of drugs and undergo multiple medical procedures, their fatigue cannot be attributed to a single treatment modality and may be much different from that experienced by patients receiving local radiation treatment.

Chemotherapy

In general, the nature and severity of the side effects of cancer chemotherapy vary according to the type of drug(s) prescribed and the dose of the drug(s) (see Chapter 13, Chemotherapy). Despite the variation among treatment regimens, fatigue is one of the most frequently reported side effects of chemotherapy.[8-10,28-37] In a prospective study of 66 patients with advanced colon or rectal cancer receiving either intravenous or intraperitoneal 5-fluorouracil (5-FU), 90% of the patients receiving intravenous 5-FU and 85% of the patients receiving intraperitoneal 5-FU reported fatigue on a questionnaire completed at home following each cycle of chemotherapy.[8] In patients with lung cancer receiving combination treatment with radiation plus either of two drug regimens, fatigue increased compared with pretreatment levels in 68% of the patients in one group and 76% in the other at the completion of treatment.[31] Seventy-five percent of 61 patients with malignant lymphoma, 90% of whom were receiving treatment at the time of interview, reported fatigue as a side effect of chemotherapy.[10] In addition, fatigue was related positively to emotional distress.

Women receiving adjuvant chemotherapy for breast cancer have provided a great deal of information about side effects of treatment and quality of life during cancer chemotherapy. Forty-eight (96%) of 50 women receiving adjuvant chemotherapy for stage II breast cancer reported fatigue as a side effect of treatment, and many reported fluctuations in the level of fatigue depending on the phase of the treatment cycle.[35] Anecdotal data from these subjects characterize the fatigue as a lack of ambition, a feeling of slowness, and continuous feelings of tiredness.[34,35] Among 50 women receiving adjuvant chemotherapy for breast cancer and 28 women who had completed this treatment, fatigue received the highest physical distress rating among women currently receiving treatment and the second highest rating among those who had completed treatment.[9] Although fatigue produced the most distress of any of the physical symptoms reported by the women under treatment, the mean level of distress fell between 2 and 3 on a scale of 1 (no distress) to 5 (great distress). The finding of a low level of physical distress among women with breast cancer was replicated in a sample of 107 subjects who completed a self-administered questionnaire, with the mean level of distress from fatigue, insomnia, nausea, and pain falling between 2 and 3 on the same 5-point scale described above.[36]

Among 128 women beginning a course of daily aminoglutethimide and medroxyprogesterone acetate for advanced metastatic breast cancer, fatigue appeared in 50% of the subjects and gradually disappeared during the first 6 weeks of treatment.[36] In a group of 56 patients with a variety of types of cancer beginning their first cycle of chemotherapy, 46 (82%) of the patients reported experiencing fatigue by the completion of the second treatment cycle.[32] Fatigue was the second most distressing symptom, after pain, reported by 26 patients with a variety of solid tumors who participated in a phase I clinical trial, with the level of distress produced by fatigue similar to that reported by patients receiving adjuvant chemotherapy for breast cancer.[30]

These studies indicate that fatigue is the most prevalent side effect experienced by patients receiving chemotherapy for cancer. Fatigue is an important problem regardless of cancer diagnosis and type of drug treatment, although the time of onset, duration, pattern, and severity of the fatigue associated with chemotherapy and differences in the pattern of fatigue specific to individual drug regimens are not well documented.

Biologic response modifiers

Fatigue is described as the most important dose-limiting side effect of interferons.[38,39] In a small sample of patients with leukemia (n = 11) given two different types of interferon, 50% of the patients who received beta interferon and 60% of the patients who received gamma interferon experienced fatigue.[40] Findings of a phase I study of beta interferon demonstrated a positive relationship between dose and fatigue, with the incidence of fatigue reaching 100% at the highest dosage level administered in the protocol.[41] Findings of this study also suggest that patients may develop tolerance to some of the side effects of beta interferon, including fatigue. Interleukin-2 produces multiple systemic toxicities such as fatigue, chills, fever, and headaches that resemble those produced by the interferons.[42]

Based on the limited information available on the incidence and characteristics of fatigue associated with the use of biologic response modifiers, it appears that this cancer treatment modality is likely to produce fatigue that is more severe than that associated with surgery, radiation treatment, and the most commonly used chemotherapy regimens. The severity of the fatigue may exceed the individual's level of tolerance, either in terms of the sensation of fatigue or the impact of the fatigue on day-to-day activities, causing the person to terminate treatment. Since fatigue is a dose-limiting side effect of biologic response modifiers, a high priority for nursing care of individuals receiving this form of treatment is preventing and ameliorating fatigue.

Combined modality treatment

The majority of cancer patients who present for adjuvant chemotherapy or radiation treatment already have undergone a surgical procedure. Some patients receive concurrent radiation treatment and chemotherapy, while others receive radiation and biologic response modifiers. Research to determine whether the fatigue produced by sequential or combined modality treatment exceeds that produced by the most toxic treatment alone is needed to predict the responses of patients who receive multiple forms of cancer treatment.

Other Etiologic Factors

In addition to the direct effects of treatment, cancer patients experience a variety of problems that may produce fatigue.[2,4,6,43-45]

Physical factors

Physical problems such as pain, pruritus, urinary frequency, diarrhea, nausea, and vomiting may interfere with patients' ability to rest or sleep. Nutritional deficits, changes in nutrient metabolism, and alteration in fluid and electrolyte balance are produced by anorexia, taste changes, nausea, vomiting, stomatitis, esophagitis, mucositis, xerostomia, diarrhea, use of a restricted diet as part of an unproven method of cancer treatment, inappropriate use of a weight-reduction diet, hepatic and renal damage, side effects of medications, changes in absorption due to surgery, or diabetes. Bone marrow depression can produce anemia, bleeding, and increased susceptibility to infection, all of which are believed to produce fatigue. Some physical conditions increase energy expenditure, such as amputation of a limb or a neurologic deficit requiring the use of assistive devices for ambulation, weakness due to prolonged bed rest, a sensory deficit producing a need for increased vigilance, dyspnea, and decreased cardiac reserve. Alcohol and the use of prescription or nonprescription drugs also can contribute to feelings of fatigue, especially when the individual is using narcotics, sedatives, hypnotics, or antihistamines.

Psychosocial factors

Fatigue is often viewed as a symptom of anxiety and depression. Anxiety is associated with feelings of panic or tension and can produce agitated behavior, while depression is a state of low energy and low levels of activity.[46] Receiving a diagnosis of cancer is certainly a frightening and stressful experience, and confronting a life-threatening disease can lead to depression. Conversely, feelings of anxiety and depression can result from the disruption in life-style produced by fatigue. When severe fatigue experienced as a side effect of cancer treatment forces the individual to decrease participation in social activities, transfer family responsibilities to others, and limit work activities, the person's response may include anxiety or depression as a result of the loss of usual social roles or inability to reach desired goals. The impact of the severity of fatigue and associated changes in activity depends on the individual's perception of what limitations are acceptable to the self and the family as well as these limitations' expected duration. These value judgments will differ substantially from person to person, with some individuals finding a week of fatigue following chemotherapy to be unacceptable and others regarding it as a perfectly acceptable experience.

For those who strive to maintain all their usual activities in addition to dealing with the demands of cancer treatment, fatigue may be the result of expending too much energy. For example, a person who maintains a full-time work commitment while commuting 1 or 2 hours a day for radiation treatment may experience fatigue as the daily commute is added to an already full schedule. Individuals who deny the effects of their illness and its treatment may find it difficult to set priorities for their activities and consequently may experience more fatigue than those who curtail some activities. The relationship between level of daily activities and fatigue in individuals undergoing cancer treatment has not been systematically examined.

NURSING CARE OF THE CANCER PATIENT WITH FATIGUE

The goal of nursing care for the patient with cancer who is experiencing fatigue is to assist the patient to maintain the highest quality of life. To reach this goal, the nurse must understand the possible causes of the person's fatigue and his or her values, coping resources, usual activities, and perception of fatigue.

Assessment

Level of fatigue

Since the patient's perception of fatigue will influence decisions about activities, participation in treatment, and overall quality of life, so-called objective ratings of fatigue made by health care professionals are less relevant to the patient's situation than assessments made by the patient. Fernsler found that when the problems reported by cancer patients receiving chemotherapy were compared with their nurses' reports of the problems they perceived the patients to be experiencing, patients reported three times the incidence of problems related to activity and rest than did their nurses.[47] In research on side effects of cancer treatment, various self-report measures have been used to obtain patients' ratings of the severity of fatigue or the distress produced by fatigue.[9,11,12,23,28] The measurement approaches used in these studies range from a single simple yes-no question to multiple adjective checklists. Although the multiple-item instruments are more likely than the single-item measures to be subjected to psychometric testing to assess their reliability and validity, the longer instruments are not readily incorporated in clinical interviews.[48,49] Clinicians often find it useful to ask if the person has experienced fatigue and then ask those responding affirmatively to rate the severity of their fatigue on a 5-point scale ranging from not at all to extremely severe.

The measures of fatigue based on health care providers' judgments or observations depend on observations of the individual's appearance, level of consciousness, activity level while in the hospital or during an outpatient visit, or patient reports of activity level. Using any measure of activity level as an indicator of fatigue is problematic in that it may represent a response to a variety of problems, such as nausea and pain, rather than a report of the sensation of fatigue. Measures of level of consciousness and appearance also are likely to represent multiple causes other than fatigue. In addition, this type of measure may not be very sensitive, since it is unlikely that the majority of patients experiencing fatigue will demonstrate marked changes in level of consciousness. The use of motor or mental task performance tests such as those used in research with healthy individuals has limited relevance to the clinical assessment of individuals with cancer.

Level of fatigue should be assessed at multiple points in time. Individuals who do not have fatigue when they begin treatment are likely to experience it at some point during treatment, and those whose fatigue does not gradually decrease once treatment is completed may require evaluation to determine if their fatigue is something other than an expected side effect of treatment. To assist patients in planning ways to deal with fatigue, the nurse must obtain information about both the daily pattern of fatigue and variations in fatigue in relation to the treatment cycle.

1. Are you fatigued? (If yes, ask questions 1a through 1c.)
   - 1a. How severe is the feeling of fatigue (on a scale of 1 = not at all severe to 5 = extremely severe)?
   - 1b. What time of day is the feeling of fatigue the lowest? What time of day is the feeling of fatigue most severe? How does the feeling of fatigue relate to your treatment? (How many days after chemotherapy, how many hours after radiation, etc?)
   - 1c. What things have you tried to relieve the fatigue, and how well did each action work?
2. Please describe a typical day for you over the past week, beginning when you get up in the morning.
3. How does the day you just described differ from your usual day *before this illness or before this treatment*? (Probe: What additional things are you doing now that you did not do before? What things have you stopped doing or do less?)
   - 3a. If activities have decreased, ask: Which of the changes you mentioned were made because of the fatigue?
4. For the things you are doing now, which ones are the most important for you to continue because they must be done? Which of these could be done by someone else?
5. What activities that you are now doing or stopped doing are things you really like to do?

FIGURE 23-2 Questions used to assess the cancer patient's level of fatigue and pattern of usual activities.

Usual activities

Information about the type and intensity of the individual's usual activities can be obtained by asking the patient to describe a typical day. The description should include the time the patient arises and retires, the number of times the patient awakens during the night, physical and mental activities performed during the day, the extent to which naps or rests are taken during the day, and a comparison of the current level of activity to the individual's level of activity before this episode of illness or the beginning of the present course of treatment. Individuals who report fatigue should be asked to describe what they do about it and to indicate the extent to which their self-care activities are effective in relieving their fatigue.

To assist the person to plan ways of modifying daily activities, the nurse determines who might be available to assume some of the individual's usual responsibilities and gains understanding of the meaning and value of each of the individual's activities. For example, a person who highly values maintaining his or her usual work role and places a lower value on recreation and entertainment will probably find it acceptable to suspend participation in sports and social events temporarily rather than take a leave of absence from work when experiencing fatigue as a side effect of cancer treatment. Figure 23-2 contains a list of questions that can be incorporated in an interview to obtain information about fatigue and daily activities.

Additional assessment data

The assessment includes information about potential causes of fatigue. Chronic diseases such as diabetes, congestive heart failure, chronic obstructive pulmonary disease, Addison's disease, hyperthyroidism, hypopituitarism, renal or liver failure, anemia, and a variety of neurologic disorders as well as infection, pain, acute CNS changes, sleep disruption, overexertion, dehydration, electrolyte imbalances, malnutrition, anxiety, and depression may contribute to fatigue.[50-52] A careful review of the patient's medical and social history, including previous and current cancer treatment, laboratory data, and a thorough physical assessment, are essential in obtaining information about potential causes of fatigue.

Interventions

Despite the prevalence of fatigue as a side effect of cancer treatment, little attention has been given to determining the efficacy of the self-care activities patients use to deal with fatigue or to developing and testing new approaches to the problem. The types of interventions that are suggested for dealing with fatigue include providing preparatory information, decreasing activities, increasing sleep or rest, adjusting schedules to allow rest periods between activities, planning activities to coincide with the time the individual feels the most energetic, and encouraging exercise.[3,4,37,53]

Preparatory information

Preparatory information is used to structure the person's expectations about receiving chemotherapy or radiation therapy. In one type of preparatory information, individuals are told about the pattern of fatigue expected as a side effect of treatment based on data collected from patients who have had the same treatment. Preparatory information, combined with suggestions about planning for rest periods, has had positive effects on patients' maintenance of usual activities when combined with similar information about various aspects of the experience of receiving radiation treatment for prostate cancer.[54] Although there are many other reports of research on the effects of providing other types of preparatory informational interventions in samples of patients receiving cancer treatment, none of them includes dependent variables relevant to level of performance of usual activities.

Rest and sleep

Rest is the most frequently recommended intervention for cancer patients who experience fatigue. Rest may take the form of a nap, a period of inactivity, a lower level of activity than usual, or a momentary respite from contact with others. Increasing the length of nighttime sleep may be considered a form of rest. However, increased sleep or rest may not improve fatigue for all individuals. Some have reported that sleep helps with fatigue only because they do not notice the fatigue while they are asleep, while others find sleep and rest to be extremely effective in relieving fatigue. Symptoms or treatment side effects that interfere with sleep and rest should be controlled to the extent possible. For example, when pain is not adequately controlled, the nurse can advocate for adequate pain control. Establishing a schedule for medication administration that does not interfere with the individual's desired rest time may also be helpful. The use of medication to induce sleep or relieve anxiety that interferes with sleep or rest may be appropriate for some individuals.

Rearranging activities

Rearranging activities to allow for rest periods or to shorten the time that high-energy output is required is another approach to dealing with limitations imposed by fatigue. Individuals may rearrange their weekly errands so they are spread throughout the week or schedule strenuous or high-priority activities at the time of day or week when they have the most energy. Some activities will be abandoned, performed in a different way, or shifted to another person. Rhodes et al[37] have provided a rich description of these changes in patients' lives as part of their research on self-care for the side effects of chemotherapy. Tiredness and weakness was the side effect that most interfered with self-care. The subjects limited energy expenditure through careful planning and scheduling, decreasing activities, and depending on others to complete some activities.

Exercise

Although some individuals have reported that exercise relieves fatigue, the effects of exercise on perceptions of fatigue have not been tested in cancer patients. However, aerobic exercise decreased reports of nausea and improved functional status in women receiving adjuvant chemotherapy for breast cancer.[55,56] Further research is needed to determine the effects of exercise on perceived fatigue in cancer patients. Individuals for whom exercise is not contraindicated can be encouraged to try short walks or their usual exercise to see if it relieves their fatigue.

Manipulating the environment

Manipulating the environment to allow undisturbed time for sleep and rest as well as providing adequate stimulation to prevent boredom-related fatigue are nursing interventions used both in the hospital and the home. For the severely fatigued individual, it may be preferable for the nurse or a family member to perform activities of daily living for the person, even when the person can do them, so that he or she can conserve energy for other activities. The provision of care and opportunities for socialization should be scheduled individually to allow appropriate periods of rest and organized to take advantage of times of high energy for the activities the individual desires the most.

Posttreatment fatigue

When fatigue is experienced as a side effect of treatment, it does not disappear immediately once treatment ends. Individuals who have experienced fatigue during cancer treatment should be warned to expect a gradual lessening of fatigue over the months following treatment. The interventions that helped with fatigue during treatment may need to be continued, and activities should be resumed gradually. Individuals with advanced cancer may complete treatment and subsequently experience worsening of their fatigue. For these individuals, the side effects of pain medications and immobility may contribute to the fatigue. The use of assistive devices such as wheelchairs and grab rails, systematic planning of activities to include those most valued by the individual, and careful conservation of energy to ensure that adequate energy is available for highly valued activities are important in enabling the individual to maintain the best possible quality of life.[52]

Summary

Further research is needed to identify and test interventions designed to prevent or ameliorate fatigue. Eliminating problems or situations that produce fatigue or interfere with sleep and rest, rearranging or omitting some usual activities, providing information about fatigue so individuals view it as an expected side effect of treatment, increasing sleep and rest, and encouraging exercise are all possible interventions for cancer patients experiencing fatigue. Finding ways to deal with fatigue has the potential to improve the quality of life of cancer patients.

CONCLUSION

Fatigue is an important problem in the care of cancer patients. Although a number of hypotheses have been proposed to explain the causes of fatigue experienced as a symptom of cancer or a side effect of cancer treatment, none has been adequately tested. Among the many side effects of cancer treatment, fatigue is the most prevalent but may be the most poorly understood.

The existing research on fatigue documents the incidence of fatigue among individuals receiving varying forms of cancer treatment. However, the measures of fatigue used in these studies represent a mix of patients' perceptions and those of physicians and nurses. Since the subjective view of fatigue is most relevant to patient care, both clinical assessment and further research should focus on obtaining the patient's assessment of the experience. To plan nursing care for the patient who is experiencing fatigue, the patient's pattern of usual activities and the relative importance or value of each activity must also be understood. In addition, data also should be obtained on a variety of physical and psychosocial factors that are expected to produce fatigue.

The interventions routinely suggested to patients to lessen fatigue focus on increasing rest and decreasing the expenditure of energy. The specific activities suggested include naps, lengthening periods of sleep, rearranging schedules to spread strenuous activities over longer periods, and eliminating those activities that are unnecessary or are judged to be too taxing. Although some patients report using exercise to relieve fatigue, this intervention is not usually included in the clinical literature. Providing individuals with cancer with information about expected side effects of treatment, including fatigue, and assisting those who experience fatigue to plan alterations in their daily activities are important in helping individuals with cancer deal with their experience.

• • •

The preparation of this chapter was partially supported by grants from the National Cancer Institute, NIH, Nos. SP30-11198 and R01-CA48333, and the American Cancer Society, No. PBR-20.

REFERENCES

1. Potempa K, Lopez M, Reid C, et al: Chronic fatigue. Image 18:165-169, 1986.
2. Alistars J: Fatigue in the cancer patient: A conceptual approach to a clinical problem. Oncol Nurs Forum 14:25-30, 1987.
3. Britton D: Fatigue, in Yasko JM (ed): Guidelines for Cancer Care: Symptom Management. Reston, VA, Reston, 1983, pp 33-37.
4. Nail LM, King KB: Fatigue. Semin Oncol Nurs 3:257-262, 1987.
5. Piper BF: Fatigue, in Carrieri VK, Lindsey AM, West CM (eds): Pathophysiological Phenomena in Nursing: Human Responses to Illness. Philadelphia, WB Saunders, 1986, pp 219-234.
6. Piper BF, Lindsey AM, Dodd MJ: Fatigue mechanisms in cancer patients: Developing nursing theory. Oncol Nurs Forum 14:17-23, 1987.
7. Christensen T, Hjortso NC, Mortensen E, et al: Fatigue and anxiety in surgical patients. Acta Psychiatr Scand 73:76-79, 1986.
8. Gianola FJ, Sugarbaker PH, Barofsky I, et al: Toxicity studies of adjuvant versus intraperitoneal 5-FU in patients with advanced primary colon or rectal cancer. Am J Clin Oncol 9:403-410, 1986.
9. Knopf MT: Physical and psychologic distress associated with adjuvant chemotherapy in women with breast cancer. J Clin Oncol 4:678-684, 1986.
10. Nerenz DR, Leventhal H, Love RR: Factors contributing to emotional distress during cancer chemotherapy. Cancer 50:1020-1027, 1982.
11. Haylock PJ, Hart LK: Fatigue in patients receiving localized radiation. Cancer Nurs 2:461-467, 1979.
12. King KB, Nail LM, Kreamer K, et al: Patients' descriptions of the experience of receiving radiation therapy. Oncol Nurs Forum 12:55-61, 1985.
13. Recombinant Human Interferon Gamma (S-6810) Research Group on Renal Cell Carcinoma: Phase II study of recombinant human interferon gamma (S-6810) on renal cell carcinoma: Summary of two collaborative studies. Cancer 60:929-933, 1987.
14. Grandjean EP: Fatigue: Its physiological and psychological significance. Ergonomics 11:427-436, 1968.
15. Simonson E: Physiology of Work Capacity and Fatigue. Springfield, Ill, Charles C Thomas, 1971.
16. Lindsey AM: Cancer cachexia, in Carrieri VK, Lindsey AM, West CM (eds): Pathophysiological Phenomena in Nursing: Human Responses to Illness. Philadelphia, WB Saunders, 1986, pp 122-136.

17. Christensen T, Kehlet H, Vesterberg V, et al: Fatigue and muscle amino acids during surgical convalescence. Acta Chir Scand 153:567-570, 1987.
18. Maxwell MB: When the cancer patient becomes anemic. Cancer Nurs 7:321-326, 1984.
19. Taylor LA, Rachman SJ: The effects of blood sugar level changes on cognitive function, affective state, and somatic symptoms. J Behav Med 11:279-291, 1988.
20. Selye H: Stress without Distress. Philadelphia:JB Lippincott, 1974.
21. Grandjean EP: Fatigue. Am Ind Hyg Assoc J 31:401-411, 1970.
22. Holmes GP, Kaplan JE, Gantz NM, et al: Chronic fatigue syndrome: A working case definition. Ann Intern Med 108:387-389, 1988.
23. Rhoten D: Fatigue and the postsurgical patient, in Norris CM (ed): Concept Clarification in Nursing. Rockville, Md, Aspen, 1982, pp 277-300.
24. Rose EA, King TC: Understanding postoperative fatigue. Surg Gynecol Obstet 147:97-102, 1978.
25. Peck A, Boland J: Emotional reactions to radiation treatment. Cancer 40:180-184, 1977.
26. Andersen BL, Tewfik HH: Psychological reactions to radiation therapy: Reconsideration of the adaptive aspects of anxiety. J Pers Soc Psychol 48:1024-1032, 1985.
27. Shapiro M, Wilson K, Casar G, et al: Work of breathing through different sized endotracheal tubes. Crit Care Med 14:1028-1031, 1986.
28. McCorkle R, Young K: Development of a symptom distress scale. Cancer Nurs 1:373-378, 1978.
29. Meyerowitz BE, Watkins IK, Sparks FC: Psychosocial implications of adjuvant chemotherapy. Cancer 52:1541-1545, 1983.
30. Strauman JJ: Symptom distress in patients receiving phase I chemotherapy with Taxol. Oncol Nurs Forum 13(5):40-43, 1986.
31. Silberfarb PM, Holland JCB, Anbar D, et al: Psychological response of patients receiving two drug regimens for lung carcinoma. Am J Psychiatry 140:110-111, 1983.
32. Cassileth BR, Farber JM, Lusk EJ, et al: Chemotherapeutic toxicity—the relationship between patients' pretreatment expectations and post-treatment results. Am J Clin Oncol 8:419-425, 1985.
33. Wander HE, Nagel GA, Blossey HC, et al: Aminoglutethimide and medroxyprogesterone acetate in the treatment of patients with advanced breast cancer. Cancer 58:1985-1989, 1986.
34. Meyerowitz BE, Watkins IK, Sparks FC: Quality of life for breast cancer patients receiving adjuvant chemotherapy. Am J Nurs 83:232-235, 1983.
35. Meyerowitz BE, Sparks FC, Spears IK: Adjuvant chemotherapy for breast carcinoma: Psychosocial implications. Cancer 43:1613-1618, 1979.
36. Ehlke G: Symptom distress in breast cancer patients receiving chemotherapy in the outpatient setting. Oncol Nurs Forum 15:343-346, 1988.
37. Rhodes VA, Watson PM, Hanson BM: Patients' descriptions of the influence of tiredness and weakness on self-care activities. Cancer Nurs 11:186-194, 1988.
38. Quesada JR, Talpaz M, Rios A, et al: Clinical toxicity of interferons in cancer patients: A review. J Clin Oncol 4:234-243, 1986.
39. Krown SE: Interferons and interferon inducers in cancer treatment. Semin Oncol 13:207-217, 1986.
40. Tamura K, Makino S, Araki Y, et al: Recombinant interferon beta and gamma in the treatment of adult T-cell leukemia. Cancer 59:1059-1062, 1987.
41. Grunberg SM, Kempf RA, Venturi CL, et al: Phase I study of recombinant beta interferon given by four-hour infusion. Cancer Res 47:1174-1178, 1987.
42. Jassak PF, Sticklin LA: Interleukin-2: An overview. Oncol Nurs Forum 13:17-22, 1986.
43. Chen MK: The epidemiology of self-perceived fatigue among adults. Prev Med 15:74-81, 1986.
44. Minden SL, Reich P: Nervousness and fatigue, in Blacklow RS (ed): MacBryde's Signs and Symptoms (ed 6). Philadelphia, JB Lippincott, 1983, pp 591-621.
45. Silberfarb PM, Hauri PJ, Oxman TE, et al: Insomnia in cancer patients. Soc Sci Med 20:849-850, 1985.
46. Garber J, Miller SM, Abramson LY: On the distinction between anxiety and depression: Perceived control, certainty, and probability of goal attainment, in Garber J, Seligman MEP (eds): Human Helplessness. Orlando, Fla, Academic Press, 1980, pp 131-169.
47. Fernsler J: A comparison of patient and nurse perceptions of patients' self-care deficits associated with cancer chemotherapy. Cancer Nurs 9:50-57, 1986.
48. McNair DM, Lorr M, Droppleman LF: Profile of Mood States Manual. San Diego, EdITS, 1971.
49. Lorr M, McNair D: Profile of Mood States: Bi-Polar Form. San Diego, EdITS, 1982.
50. Minden SL, Reich P: Nervousness and fatigue, in Blacklow RS (ed): MacBryde's Signs and Symptoms: Applied Pathologic Physiology and Clinical Interpretation (ed 6). Philadelphia, Lippincott, 1983, pp 591-621.
51. Bruera E, MacDonald RN: Overwhelming fatigue in advanced cancer. Am J Nurs 88:99-100, 1988.
52. Billings JA: Weakness and fatigue, in Billings JA (ed): Outpatient Management of Advanced Cancer. Philadelphia, Lippincott, 1985, pp 125-130.
53. Spross JA: Fatigue, in Baird SB (ed): Decision Making in Oncology Nursing. Philadelphia, Decker, 1988, pp 76-77.
54. Johnson JE, Nail LM, Lauver D, et al: Reducing the negative impact of radiation therapy on functional status. Cancer 61:46-51, 1988.
55. MacVicar M, Winningham M: Effect of aerobic training on functional status of women with breast cancer. Oncol Nurs Forum 11:62, 1984 (abstr).
56. Winningham ML, MacVicar MG: The effect of aerobic exercise on patient reports of nausea. Oncol Nurs Forum 15:447-450, 1988.

Chapter 24

Nutritional Disturbances

Debra J. Szeluga, RD, PhD

Susan L. Groenwald, MS, RN

Debra K. Sullivan, RD, MS

INTRODUCTION

Nutritional complications are a common consequence of cancer or its treatment. Malnourished individuals are more susceptible to infection and are less likely to tolerate or derive optimal benefits from therapy. In some studies malnutrition has been shown to be an important prognosticator of morbidity and survival.[1-4] Malnutrition also is an important issue in the quality of life of individuals with cancer.

In recognition of the serious consequences of malnutrition in cancer patients, scientists have examined a variety of problems related to nutrition to gain information for use in improving patient care. Among the most popular areas of inquiry are the role of nutrition in carcinogenesis; the effect of cancer on host metabolism; the use of parenteral infusates to improve the nutritional status of individuals with cancer; the identification of taste changes that alter eating habits; causes of anorexia in cancer; nutritional consequences of cancer therapy; and the impact of culture, values, and other societal factors on the eating patterns of individuals. Much has been learned, but even more remains to be learned to establish nutritional therapy as a means of improving survival and the quality of life for individuals with cancer.

PATHOPHYSIOLOGY OF MALNUTRITION IN CANCER

Protein-calorie malnutrition occurs when the protein-calorie composition of the diet does not meet the individual's physiologic requirements. When dietary calories and protein are insufficient, adipose reserves and muscle are catabolized for energy. Thus the first sign of malnutrition may be a reduction in fat stores and loss of muscle mass.

In cancer local and systemic tumor effects result in a tremendous demand for nutrients. Dietary intake of protein and calories, regardless of quantity, may be insufficient to meet the demands of the tumor. Body stores of fat and protein are used. This parasitic process leads to loss of muscle protein, which results in weakness and debilitation; loss of subcutaneous fat, predisposing the individual to skin breakdown; impaired cellular and humoral immunity, increasing the individual's risk of infection; poor wound healing; apathy; and depression.

A variety of factors affect the development and severity of malnutrition related to cancer.[5]

Metabolic Effects of the Tumor

The most severe syndrome of malnutrition in cancer is cancer *cachexia*, which is characterized by profound and progressive loss of body weight, fat, and muscle. One half to two thirds of all individuals with cancer experience cachexia.[6] Progressive cachexia is one of the major causes of mortality in individuals with advanced cancer. Donaldson[7] reports that in a series of autopsies of 500 individuals with cancer, cachexia was the only identifiable cause of death in 22% of cases. Most frustrating about this devastating syndrome is the fact that little correlation has been made between cachexia and tumor extent, type, or location.

Research data suggest that cancer cachexia may be partially a result of paraneoplastic syndromes arising from the abnormal production of peptides by cancer cells.[8-10] In paraneoplastic syndromes, cells that do not normally produce certain peptides or hormones are altered by the cancer process. Genes responsible for hormone production that are usually repressed during the process of cell differentiation are depressed in cancer cells. Peptides or hormones comparable in their biologic activity to endorphins, such as enkephalins, somatostatin, neurotensin, and cholecystokinin, are released by some tumors, causing a number of metabolic alterations that result in profound nutritional consequences to the host.[11]

Altered carbohydrate metabolism

Carbohydrate metabolism in individuals with cancer is characterized by a number of aberrations.

Anaerobic glycolysis Normally, glucose is metabolized through the Embden-Meyerhof pathway to yield pyruvate; it proceeds either to glycolysis, of which lactic acid is the end product, or respiration, where the pyruvate is oxidized to carbon dioxide and water. Anaerobic glycolysis produces two adenosine triphosphate (ATP) molecules from each glucose molecule, whereas complete oxidation of glucose to carbon dioxide and water yields 36 ATP molecules. Thus, anaerobic glycolysis is far less efficient in energy production than oxidative respiration.

Tumors predominantly use anaerobic glycolysis in glucose metabolism. The tumor uses glucose for its own growth, demanding increasing amounts as it enlarges.[12]

Increased rate of gluconeogenesis The lactic acid produced by anaerobic glycolysis is recruited back into glucose production (gluconeogenesis). This cycle of glucose to lactic acid and back to glucose is called the *Cori cycle* and is an energy-consuming process that occurs at an increased rate in individuals with cancer.[13] The energy required for gluconeogenesis cannot be supplied by lactic acid alone, so host reserves of amino acids and other sources make up the energy deficit. Young [14] estimates that the Cori cycle may account for a 10% increase in energy expenditure for an individual with cancer. As the tumor enlarges, a tremendous drain on body reserves to meet the excessive nutritive needs of the growing tumor results in vast depletion of body tissues.

Glucose intolerance A third aberration of carbohydrate metabolism present in individuals with cancer is glucose intolerance, which is evidenced by delayed clearing of intravenously or orally administered glucose. Glucose intolerance may be due to a defect of insulin response to hyperglycemia or a lack of tissue responsiveness to insulin.[15] However, because a number of clinical conditions are associated with glucose intolerance, such as bed rest, sepsis, and starvation, it is not possible to establish the tumor as the specific cause of the intolerance.[16]

Altered protein metabolism

Abnormalities of protein metabolism are common in individuals with cancer, especially those with cachexia. In the healthy adult, approximately 50 g of nitrogen is synthesized and broken down every day; only 10 g of nitrogen is excreted per day.[17] Most of the amino acids that result from the breakdown of protein are reincorporated into protein synthesis.

Although an individual can lose 30% of body fat without serious consequences, loss of 30% of protein content will cause death.[18] This is why cancer cachexia and the resulting loss of lean muscle mass present a serious hazard to the person with cancer. Protein depletion is a common occurrence in individuals with cancer. Protein depletion is a common occurrence in individuals with cancer. One of the most common nonspecific abnormalities that occurs in individuals diagnosed with cancer is hypoalbuminemia. In a study of serum albumin levels of 222 individuals with cancer at various stages of disease, the mean concentration of serum albumin was 2.9 g/dL, compared with 4.0 g/dL in healthy adults.[19] A number of factors may be responsible for the protein depletion seen in individuals with cancer.

Increased uptake of amino acids by the tumor The apparent capacity of tumors to gain weight while the rest of the body wastes led some researchers to call the tumor a "nitrogen trap."[20] In its need for increasing amounts of glucose, the tumor draws on the host's protein reserves for gluconeogenesis.[21] The result is progressive muscle wasting. The amino acids taken up by the tumor are converted to lactic acid through the Cori cycle and are returned to glucose through gluconeogenesis.

Decreased protein synthesis Protein synthesis is decreased in individuals with cancer.[22] Although the decreased protein synthesis may be explained partially by poor intake and malnutrition, tumor factors also may play a role because protein synthesis is decreased even in individuals with normal food intake, possibly due to a decreased rate of synthesis of serum albumin.

Increased protein degradation Goodlad et al[23] have demonstrated that muscle protein breakdown is accelerated in the tumor-bearing animal. Other researchers have demonstrated increased muscle protein degradation in humans with cancer.[24] Skeletal muscle is preferentially affected as opposed to cardiac muscle.

Protein loss Loss of protein through abnormal excretion or leakage can contribute significantly to depletion of protein stores and decreased muscle mass. In protein-losing enteropathies associated with some types of cancers such as gastric, colon, and esophageal carcinomas or carcinoid syndrome, release of an ectopic hormone causes ulceration of the mucosa of the gastrointestinal tract and loss of protein-rich exudate.[25] Fistulas, decubitus ulcers, or other exudative lesions also may be sources of protein loss.

Use of protein for energy needs In starvation in the healthy adult, adaptive processes cause the body to conserve protein and use body fat for energy needs. All stored energy in humans is in the form of adipose tissue. During fasting or starvation, fat depots are the first to be used to meet energy needs. In the case of cancer cachexia, however, such adaptation does not occur. Protein use by the tumor continues independent of the host's nutritional intake.

Altered lipid metabolism

There are conflicting laboratory observations regarding the degree to which lipid metabolism is altered in individuals with cancer. Theologides[6] hypothesizes that cancer cells synthesize and secrete a lipid-mobilizing factor that increases plasma fatty acids to meet the tumor's increased caloric requirements. Goodlad and Clark[26] provided evidence that mobilization of lipids from host tissues (hyperlipemia) occurs as a result of the tumor's excessive energy needs. The tumor exhausts its glucose supply and is forced to use fatty acids as an additional energy source.

Axelrod and Costa,[27] however, observed decreased mobilization of fat in individuals with cancer. They attribute the decreased fat mobilization to a normal homeostatic response to reduced caloric intake whereby the body conserves energy by decreasing its metabolism of fat. Waterhouse[28] corroborates Axelrod and Costa's observations through studies that demonstrated that normal control mechanisms for inhibiting free fatty acid mobilization following ingestion of carbohydrates are intact in individuals with cancer.

Fluid and electrolyte disturbances

Tumors can affect renal function directly or indirectly through fluid and electrolyte abnormalities resulting from the action of ectopic hormones. The following are a few of the more common tumor-related fluid and electrolyte abnormalities that occur in individuals with cancer.

Hypercalcemia In some tumors, such as parathyroid, lung, kidney, ovary, or colon tumors, an ectopic parathyroidlike hormone causes deposition of calcium in renal tubules or other genitourinary structures and may result in a gradual or sudden onset of renal failure. Hypercalcemia also may cause a concentrating defect that leads to polyuria and water depletion (see Chapter 25).

Hyperuricemia In some leukemias and lymphomas, a rapid neoplastic cell growth phase is accompanied by increased catabolism of cellular nucleic acids. Hyperuricemia, hyperphosphatemia, and hyperkalemia occur as a result of the release of electrolytes from the resultant cellular breakdown. This situation also occurs in tumor lysis syndrome in which cells are rapidly destroyed as a result of chemotherapy for lymphoproliferative diseases such as leukemia.

Hyperuricemia involves a sudden increase of uric acid in the plasma. Urate crystals may be deposited in the kidney, causing renal damage. The combined electrolyte disturbances may result in renal failure and cardiac arrest.

Hyponatremia A common presentation of some occult tumors, especially bronchogenic and oat cell carcinomas, is the syndrome of inappropriate antidiuretic hormone secretion (SIADH). SIADH secretion of ectopic antidiuretic hormone (ADH) by tumor cells is characterized by persistent urinary loss of sodium and excessive retention of water by the renal tubules. This produces a water excess characterized by reduced levels of serum sodium and serum osmolality but no edema.

Hypokalemia Renin-secreting tumors such as hypernephromas and renal juxtaglomerular cell tumors cause increased secretion of aldosterone, resulting in hypokalemic alkalosis. Aldosterone causes sodium and water retention in exchange for potassium and hydrogen ion excretion in the renal tubules. Prolonged hypokalemia damages the renal tubules, causing inability to concentrate urine. Polyuria and nocturia are clinical signs of hypokalemia.

Increased energy expenditure

Because of the excessive energy requirements of tumors, individuals with cancer cachexia have a greater energy expenditure then their normal counterparts.[15] Protein turnover and gluconeogenesis are energy-requiring metabolic processes that are increased in individuals with cancer, causing a tremendous drain on energy reserves.

Warnold et al[30] assessed heart rate (as a function of oxygen consumption) to measure energy expenditure of individuals with cancer cachexia. They found that both the resting metabolic expenditure and daily energy expenditure were significantly greater in individuals with cancer cachexia than in individuals who had similar degrees of cachexia due to other disease processes.

In starvation in otherwise healthy adults, the body adapts by lowering its basal metabolic rate to conserve energy. In cancer, however, increased basal metabolic rate may be a frequent feature of advanced disease, even when food intake is significantly decreased.[31,32]

Altered taste

Taste changes occur frequently in individuals with cancer. In a study of 35 individuals with cancer, 25 complained of a general reduction in taste perception, or *hypogeusesthesia.*[33] Twenty-two (88%) of the 25 respondents complained of aversion to meat. This perverted sense of taste, called *dysgeusia,* caused the individuals to refuse meat, fish, poultry, eggs, foods fried in oil or fat, and tomatoes. DeWys and Walters[34] reported that individuals with cancer have a decreased threshold for bitter, making bitter foods such as those high in protein less palatable, and an increased threshold for sweet, making sweet foods more difficult to taste.

Although the exact mechanisms responsible for taste changes in individuals with cancer remain unknown, nutritional deficiencies may play a role. Deficiencies of zinc, copper, nickel, niacin, and vitamin A have been implicated in decreased or altered taste sensations.

Recent research has focused on learned aversions as a major factor in the taste changes that occur in cancer. Learned food aversions develop when a food is associated with unpleasant symptoms such as nausea and vomiting, pain, and so forth.[35] Aversions seem to develop most rapidly to new and novel foods, but even the most familiar and favored foods may become aversive over time. Smith and Blumsack[36] report that "more than 50 different substances have been proven to be effective in producing these profound aversions, including amphetamine, apomorphine, cyclophosphamide, ethanol, lithium and pentobarbital."

In children receiving chemotherapy, Broberg and Bernstein[37] have shown that the use of a scapegoat food item (eg, a coconut or rootbeer Lifesaver) effectively reduced the impact of chemotherapy on the preference for normal menu items. Mattes et al[38] have also demonstrated that the development of aversions to usual foods was reduced when adults consumed scapegoat foods just before their first course of therapy. Additional clinical research and application theories related to learned food aversions may produce other intervention possibilities.

Anorexia

It is well recognized that individuals with cancer experience metabolic abnormalities that induce or aggravate loss of appetite, or *anorexia*, which compounds the cachexia and weight loss associated with cancer. Anorexia is an initial symptom of cancer and is sometimes the first evidence of recurrence or progression. It is a nonspecific symptom of cancer that plagues almost all individuals with cancer at some point during their illness. Various factors contribute to loss of appetite and reduced food intake in individuals with cancer.

Central mechanisms The previously described metabolic alterations evoked by the tumor may cause appetite suppression by creating a false interpretation of satiety by the hypothalamus as a result of increased circulating lipids and peptides.[39] For example, the lactic acid produced by tumor metabolism or ketones resulting from lipolysis may be anorexigenic.

Neurotransmitters In recent years a variety of neurotransmitters have been investigated for their role in anorexia in cancer. Krause et al[40] (1981) found that tumor-bearing animals have increased brain levels of the amino acid tryptophan and serotonin metabolites. Because decreased brain levels of tryptophan and serotonin seem to be associated with increased food intake in animals, these researchers hypothesized that the increased tryptophan levels and serotonin metabolism found in the brains of tumor-bearing animals may be responsible for the decreased food intake. Similar studies have been conducted on endorphins.[41] Although studies of the role of tryptophan and endorphins in cancer anorexia and cachexia offer exciting possibilities for clinical intervention through dietary and metabolite manipulation, definitive research is yet to be conducted.

Taste changes Taste changes lead to altered dietary habits and disinterest in food. Recent research has indicated that learned aversions to food may play a major role in the decreased food intake of individuals with cancer.[42] A positive taste experience is important in stimulating a variety of physiologic factors that contribute to the ingestion and digestion of food.[33] The volume and character of saliva and gastric secretions partially depend on the individual's taste experience. When food aversions or unpleasant taste changes occur, the taste stimulus may be insufficient to stimulate the physiologic responses necessary for effective ingestion and digestion of food, contributing to anorexia.

Physical discomfort Physical discomfort of any type may depress appetite and lead to reduced food intake. In addition, because eating is a motor activity that requires the expenditure of energy, a person who is immobile or fatigued may have loss of appetite or be unable to perform the motor functions necessary for eating.

Immunosuppression

The progressive growth of most neoplasms is accompanied by profound immunologic disturbances. Early in the disease process, the immune system is reasonably intact. As the disease advances and disseminates, alterations in humoral and cellular immunity occur.

Malnutrition has a number of deleterious effects on the immune system.

Decrease in lymphoid tissues Lymphatic structures of the immune system, such as the spleen, lymph nodes, thymus, tonsils, and adenoids, are decreased in size, weight, and structure in malnourished individuals.[43] Because lymphatic structures participate directly in the immune response and also contribute to the number and function of immune cells, decrease in their size contributes to immunosuppression.

Decreased phagocytic activity Phagocytic activity and function are decreased in malnutrition. This decreased phagocytic activity apparently is due to deficiency of the protein necessary for synthesis of the neutrophils responsible for phagocytosis. The result is ineffective killing of bacteria.

Decreased T-lymphocyte function Malnutrition results in a decreased number of T lymphocytes in the peripheral circulation. T lymphocytes are responsible for the delayed hypersensitivity response to antigens, a response that is depressed in malnutrition. The greater the degree of malnutrition, the greater the deficiency of T lymphocytes and the lack of delayed hypersensitivity response. A total absence of delayed hypersensitivity response is called *anergy*.

Decreased B-lymphocyte function The percentage of B lymphocytes and the levels of immunoglobulins in the peripheral blood of malnourished individuals are frequently normal or elevated. Normal or elevated levels of B lymphocytes and immunoglobulins may be the result of repeated infections that occur as a result of the immune deficiency associated with malnutrition. As malnutrition progresses to severe, the percentage of B lymphocytes may decrease.

The complement system that participates with immunoglobulins in the destruction of bacteria is compromised in malnutrition, apparently as a result of a deficiency of protein necessary to synthesize the complement factors. Suppression of the complement system increases the individual's susceptibility to bacterial infection.

The degree of immunologic impairment is affected by

the type of tumor, its extent, and the methods that are used to treat it. Cancer prognosis seems to be closely related to the degree of immunosuppression, and the degree of immunosuppression is related to the degree of malnutrition. The immune system works in concert with cancer treatment methods to destroy and eliminate tumor cells. Therefore, preservation of both nutritional status and immune system function are important considerations in cancer therapy. Dudrick et al[44] demonstrated improved therapeutic response in individuals whose immune status improved because of nutritional support.

Mechanical Effects of the Tumor

The nutritional consequences of tumor destruction of local tissue depend on tumor location, type, and extent. A particularly invasive type of tumor may be more damaging to local tissue than an encapsulated tumor. However, if the encapsulated tumor is located within a constricted area, the pressure caused by tumor expansion will have more severe consequences. Table 24-1 shows some of the nutritional consequences of expanding tumors.

Nutritional Consequences of Cancer Treatment

Maintenance of adequate nutrition may become a problem if the person's ability to eat or absorb food is compromised by physiologic reactions to the treatment regimen. The following are the most common nutritional problems that result from cancer treatment.

Anorexia

All the treatments for cancer may cause anorexia. The classic nausea and vomiting associated with many chemotherapeutic agents eliminates any interest in food for fear of the consequences. Constipation, immobility, dysphagia, odynophagia, fatigue, infection, and stomatitis—all consequences of cancer treatments—contribute to decreased interest in and sometimes aversion to food. Decreased food intake contributes to general weakness and weight loss.

Constipation

Constipation and adynamic ileus are major complications of the drug vincristine. Surgical procedures involving the alimentary tract may produce a transient constipation until bowel function is restored. Immobility and/or the administration of narcotics for pain contribute to constipation. Whatever the cause, constipation creates a full abdominal feeling and discomfort and contributes to anorexia.

Diarrhea

Diarrhea is most commonly the result of chemotherapy or abdominal radiation. The diarrhea associated with chemotherapy is part of general mucosal toxicity. The rapidly proliferating cells of the intestinal mucosa are highly susceptible to the effects of chemotherapy. Diarrhea is particularly severe after the administration of actinomycin D and 5-fluorouracil (5-FU) but also frequently occurs after the administration of thioguanine, methotrexate, floxuridine, hydroxyurea, the nitrosoureas, and 5-azacytidine. In severe cases the diarrhea may be accompanied by proctitis, ulceration, fistulas, and bleeding, which lead to dehydration, electrolyte imbalances, and malnutrition. In rare cases diarrhea may be so severe as to cause perforation of the bowel.

Abdominal irradiation also causes diarrhea as a result of mucosal toxicity. Altered function of the bowel and malabsorption occur during therapy but usually disappear when radiotherapy is stopped. In some cases symptoms of late radiation changes may occur within 1 year and up to 10 or more years following abdominal irradiation and include diarrhea, ulceration, fibrosis, fistula formation, and obstruction. Bowel resection may be required in severe cases.

Fistulas

In many cases surgery precedes the development of a fistula. The fistula may develop as a result of technical defects such as inadequate closure, unrecognized damage to internal structures, lack of blood supply to an anastomosis, or tension on an anastomosis. In cancer, fistulas may develop as a result of tissue necrosis adjacent to an expanding tumor or tissue destruction caused by chemotherapy or radiotherapy.

The complications of fistulas include loss of fluids and electrolytes, infection, and malnutrition due to loss of nutrients. The higher in the gastrointestinal tract the fistula is located, the more serious the complications and the higher the mortality rate.

Fluid and electrolyte imbalances

Fluid and electrolyte disturbances occur frequently as a result of cancer therapy. Vomiting, diarrhea, and fistulas may induce profound fluid and electrolyte imbalances through losses in excreta. Fluid volume is depleted, and sodium, chloride, and potassium are lost. Metabolic alkalosis may occur.

Surgical procedures may evoke fluid and electrolyte disturbances as a result of body fluid losses. In addition, surgical procedures may alter hormone secretion, indirectly affecting fluid and electrolyte homeostasis. For example, surgical manipulation of the hypothalamus may cause a lack of vasopressin, or ADH, and result in the excretion of dilute urine.

Treatment measures may indirectly alter fluid and electrolyte homeostasis as a result of kidney damage. In hyperuricemia resulting from a sudden increase in the release of uric acid after cytotoxic chemotherapy of lymphoproliferative diseases, urate crystals may be deposited in the kidney, resulting in renal shutdown and subsequent fluid and electrolyte disturbances.

TABLE 24-1 Nutritional Consequences of the Mechanical Effects of an Expanding Tumor

System	Local Tumor Effect	Nutritional Consequences	
Integument	Ulceration Decubiti Fistulas	Loss of fluid and electrolytes Loss of cellular components and nutrients Pain Infection—increased energy requirements Odor	Fluid, electrolyte, and protein disturbances; loss of appetite; loss of weight
Hematologic/immunologic	Inflammation; infection	Increased basal metabolic rate and energy requirements lead to weight loss	
	Bone marrow invasion	Infection increases energy requirements; anemia leads to fatigue and loss of appetite	
Cardiovascular	Hemorrhage	Loss of blood components and fluids; anemia causes fatigue and loss of appetite	
	Vascular obstruction	Ischemia; necrosis; inflammation; infection; edema; increased blood pressure; increased heart rate	
	Lymphatic obstruction	Edema; loss of protein; infection	
	Congestive heart failure	Edema; fatigue; shortness of breath	
Respiratory	Obstruction	Congestive heart failure; shortness of breath; edema; fatigue; effusions	
	Effusion	Shortness of breath; fatigue; loss of fluid and cellular components	
	Decreased lung capacity	Shortness of breath; increased energy requirements; loss of appetite; infection	
Genitourinary	Obstruction	Increased blood urea nitrogen; uremia; fluid and electrolyte disturbances	
	Ascites	Early satiety; hypoalbuminemia; fluid and electrolyte disturbances	
	Renal injury	Renal failure; fluid, electrolyte, and protein disturbances	
Gastrointestinal	Vomiting	Fluid and electrolyte disturbances	
	Mucositis	Pain; inability to swallow and eat	
	Obstruction	Impaired ingestion, digestion, and absorption; nausea, vomiting, and pain; nutritional deficiencies; jaundice	
	Constipation	Loss of appetite; nausea, vomiting, and pain	
	Diarrhea	Fluid and electrolyte disturbances	
	Fistulas	Loss of fluid and electrolytes; malabsorption	
	Liver dysfunction	Hypoalbuminemia; loss of fluid and electrolytes; malabsorption, ascites, and jaundice	
	Decreased digestive enzymes	Malabsorption; impaired digestion	
Central nervous	Pain	Loss of appetite	
	Confusion, somnolence	Missed meals	
	Increased intracranial pressure	Nausea and vomiting lead to fluid and electrolyte disturbances	
	Hypothalamic destruction	Hypernatremia; diabetes insipidus	
Endocrine			
Hypothalamus	Lack of vasopressin	Diabetes insipidus leads to polyuria and dehydration	
	Somnolence	Missed meals	
	Increased body temperature	Increased basal metabolic rate; increased energy requirements	
Pituitary	Lack of ADH	Diabetes insipidus leads to polyuria and dehydration	
	Increased ACTH secretion	Cushing's syndrome—hyperglycemia, osteoporosis, hypertension, weight gain	
	Decreased ACTH secretion	Addison's disease—loss of appetite, decreased blood pressure, weight loss, hypoglycemia, hyperkalemia	
Adrenal	Adrenal hypersecretion	Cushing's syndrome	
	Adrenal insufficiency	Addison's disease	
Thyroid	Deficiency	Decreased metabolic rate; anemia	
	Hypersecretion	Increased basal metabolic rate; weakness	
Parathyroid	Deficiency	Hypocalcemia	
	Hypersecretion	Hypercalcemia	
Pancreas	Deficiency	Lack of pancreatic enzymes; malabsorption; hyperglycemia	
	Hypersecretion	Hypoglycemia	
Ovarian	Ascites	Hypoalbuminemia; early satiety; fluid and electrolyte disturbances	
Musculoskeletal	Pain, immobility, weakness, bone destruction	Loss of appetite; hypercalcemia; osteoporosis	

Infection

All techniques used in cancer treatment predispose individuals to infection by suppressing the immune system. Chemotherapy and radiotherapy to sites of hematopoiesis damage hematopoietic tissue, impose neutropenia, and place the individual at risk for infection. Infection increases the metabolic demands on the host and may facilitate malnutrition.

Malabsorption

Intestinal malabsorption may occur as a result of several factors:

1. Interruption of the structure of the bowel. Surgical procedures such as intestinal resection reduce the absorptive surface of the gastrointestinal tract.

2. Damage to the absorptive surface of the bowel. Cytotoxic drugs and radiotherapy injure the epithelial cells that line the intestine. Damage to these epithelial cells flattens the intestinal villi and reduces the absorptive surface of the bowel, resulting in malabsorption of fat, protein, carbohydrate, vitamins, and minerals as well as loss of fluid.

3. Lack of the substance necessary for the absorption of nutrients. In liver dysfunction arising from surgical procedures, chemotherapy, or immunotherapy, lack of bile impairs the absorption of fats from the duodenum. Pancreatectomy eliminates the digestive enzymes that are important for the absorption of nutrients. Gastrectomy reduces or eliminates the gastric secretions that aid in the breakdown of foods to prepare for digestion and absorption. Bilateral vagotomy required in conjunction with esophagectomy induces significant malabsorption of fat and the clinical manifestation of steatorrhea.

Mucositis

The rapid turnover of epithelial cells of the mucous membranes makes them vulnerable to the toxicities of chemotherapy and radiotherapy. Because chemotherapy is a systemic treatment, all mucous membranes are at risk; however, the most common sites of mucositis are the oral cavity and the esophagus. Drugs that contribute to nutritional deterioration by rendering the person unable to eat because of painful oral mucosal toxicities include bleomycin, mitomycin, actinomycin D, methotrexate, mercaptopurine, thioguanine, vinblastine sulfate, daunorubicin, doxorubicin, and 5-FU.

Radiotherapy that includes mucosal tissue in the radiation field will lead to mucositis of the irradiated tissue. The development and severity of mucositis following radiation therapy depend on the dose of radiation and the method of administration. Mucositis usually disappears when therapy is discontinued; however, fibrosis with esophageal stricture may occur as a delayed effect of radiotherapy.

Nausea and Vomiting

Nausea and vomiting are most commonly associated with the administration of antineoplastic drugs. The nausea and vomiting following chemotherapy are mediated by the chemoreceptor trigger zone located in the area postrema of the brain's fourth ventricle. Nausea and vomiting occur with many anticancer drugs and may be anticipatory.

As a result of the administration of some drugs, vomiting may be so severe as to require the dosage of the drug to be reduced or the chemotherapy to be interrupted. Drugs that may cause severe and prolonged nausea and vomiting include dacarbazine, daunorubicin, streptozotocin, actinomycin-D, cisplatin, doxorubicin, and mechlorethamine. The nutritional consequences of prolonged vomiting are profound. Present antiemetic therapy is not wholly effective in preventing or treating the nausea and vomiting associated with chemotherapy. (Detailed discussion of the nausea and vomiting of chemotherapy and its treatment may be found in Chapter 13.)

Taste changes

Individuals receiving some antineoplastic drugs complain of experiencing a metallic taste during the intravenous administration of these agents. Drugs implicated include nitrogen mustard, cisplatin, and cyclophosphamide. Some individuals become so sensitized by this taste that they begin vomiting at the mere thought of the drug administration, even as they enter the waiting room of the outpatient clinic. Other taste changes have been documented in relation to the administration of specific drugs. 5-FU has been documented to cause decreased sensitivity to salty and sweet tastes.[45]

Radiotherapy to the head and neck region destroys taste buds and cells responsible for the secretion of saliva, resulting in a condition called *xerostomia*. The volume of saliva is decreased, and the saliva that is produced is viscid, acidic, and high in organic content. Individuals complain that food tastes like cardboard or cotton. Decreased taste perception and difficult mastication are the consequences, compounding the preexisting functional problems that result from extensive surgical procedures in the head and neck region.

Additionally, dental caries commonly result from the xerostomia and alteration in bacterial flora in the mouth.

Psychosocial Effects of Cancer on Nutritional Status

Several phases during a person's experience with cancer have been identified as stressful periods during which anorexia may be secondary to psychologic distress: initial diagnosis, diagnosis of recurrent disease, and during periods of pain and discouragement. In addition, aversions may develop to foods consumed during a period of discomfort or immediately preceding it because of behavioral conditioning.[42]

Moreover, individuals with cancer, especially those receiving cancer treatment, may feel they have lost control over their life. Refusing or limiting food intake often gives these individuals some feeling of control.

A host of psychologic factors determine an individual's ability or willingness to eat. These factors must be included in the evaluation of the causes of malnutrition in the person with cancer.

NUTRITIONAL ASSESSMENT

Nutritional assessment is the critical first step in developing a plan to improve or maintain the nutritional status of the individual with cancer. The nutritional assessment should identify individuals at risk of becoming malnourished, provide baseline data for the clinician to develop a nutritional therapy plan for the malnourished person, and provide ongoing data with which the clinician can evaluate therapy. Nutritional assessment is important for both hospitalized individuals and those receiving ambulatory care.

Physical Signs

The physical signs and symptoms of malnutrition do not become evident until malnutrition is advanced. The clinical manifestation and physical effects of cancer may make it difficult for the clinician to distinguish the signs of nutritional deficiencies.

Nevertheless, the nurse conducting a general physical examination of the person with cancer should pay particular attention to the condition of the mucous membranes, skin, eyes, lips, oral cavity, nails, subcutaneous tissues, and muscles as indexes of nutritional status. Common manifestations of malnutrition include sparse, thin hair; pallor; dry, flaky skin; dull, sunken eyes; apathy; mouth lesions; muscle and tissue wasting; and edema. Also important to evaluate is the individual's mental status and performance level. Can the patient feed himself or herself, prepare meals, or follow the directions of a nutrition care plan?

Dietary History

During the nutritional assessment, it is important to elicit information about the person's usual dietary habits. The nurse should explore with the person the type and quantity of food consumed, likes and dislikes, location of meals, times of meals, family living situation, difficulty with chewing or swallowing, nausea, vomiting, or diarrhea, and changes in diet as a result of illness or treatment.

The two most common methods of assessing a person's nutritional intake are dietary recall and weighing and recording the food eaten.

Dietary recall

During a dietary recall, the person is asked to recall specific types and quantities of food eaten over a particular span of time, usually 24 hours. The interviewer may use a checklist of common foods to stimulate the person's memory. The person reports all foods, snacks, dressings, and condiments; the quantities in which they are used; and the time of day they are consumed.

The advantage of the dietary recall is that it is easy to use. However, the accuracy depends on the individual's memory, communication skills, and degree of motivation. The recall reported may not be representative of the individual's usual dietary patterns, however. In addition, the quantities of food reported by the person are only estimates of the actual quantities consumed.

Weighed inventory

If a more accurate dietary history is required the individual may be requested to weigh and measure food. If the person is hospitalized, the nurse or dietician may do the recording. The person who is at home may use standard household measures to record intake.

Weighing and recording of food is far more accurate than the dietary recall. However, this method requires a high degree of motivation on the person's part. It can be tedious, and the individual may alter intake to avoid having to weigh and record the food.

• • •

With both the dietary recall and weighed inventory methods of obtaining a dietary history, standard food tables are used to analyze the person's nutrient intake. Deficits are recognized, and areas for potential nutritional intervention identified. Dietary history also helps the clinician to tailor a nutritional plan to the person's preferences and habits.

Anthropometric Measurements

Anthropometric measurements are physical measurements of the human body that provide important information about an individual's nutritional status. Standard anthropometric measurements for adults include height, weight, midarm circumference, and skinfold thickness.

Height and weight

Height should be measured whenever possible but may be obtained from the personal interview or patient chart.

Body weight is one of the most important measures of the nutritional assessment. Several investigators have demonstrated that increased morbidity and mortality are associated with significant weight loss. Johnston et al[46] found that dysgeusia, xerostomia, dysphagia, and mouth pain associated with head and neck radiation were greater and lasted longer in individuals with weight losss. DeWys[47] demonstrated that the median survival of individuals with cancer who experienced weight loss before receiving chemotherapy was half that of individuals who had not lost weight. Hickman et al[48] found that individuals who weighed 20% less than their ideal weight had a complication rate of over 70% and a mortality rate of 42% after surgery for colorectal cancer. DeWys et al[1] demonstrated that weight loss alone was a powerful independent prognosticator of survival of women with breast cancer. Thus, weight is an important factor in assessing nutritional status and possibly in predicting the outcome of therapy.

The person should be weighed without shoes, using a lever balance or beam scale. Weight should be recorded to the nearest 0.5 kg. The person's current weight is then evaluated against ideal weight and usual preillness weight.

Ideal body weight corresponding to the person's height and sex is derived from standard weight tables. The percentage of ideal body weight is calculated as follows:

$$\text{Percentage of ideal body weight} = \frac{\text{Actual weight}}{\text{Ideal weight}} \times 100$$

Although the percentage of ideal body weight may be an indicator of weight loss, there are several limitations to using it as a standard. The index may not be an accurate measure of nutritional status. For example, the actual weight of a formerly obese individual may be close to the ideal weight; however, the person's present weight is significantly lower than the preillness weight. The person may be malnourished, even though he or she is at ideal weight.

Gray and Gray[49] have criticized the standards for weight because the commonly used table was derived from a population studied from 1935 to 1954. The data are probably no longer relevant because the average size of individuals has increased since that time. In addition, the Metropolitan Life Insurance Table was developed using a select group of individuals who applied for insurance from 1935 to 1954 and does not represent a random sampling of the American population. The table is also limited because it does not allow for differences in body frame or for stature changes that occur as a result of the aging process.

A more sensitive index of nutritional status is percent weight change, which is calculated as follows:

$$\text{Percent weight change} = \frac{\text{Actual weight} - \text{usual weight}}{\text{Usual weight}} \times 100$$

The percent weight change indicates the extent of tissue loss as a result of inadequate nutrition. Questions that can be asked of an individual to accurately assess preillness weight include: "How much did you weigh when you got married? How much did you weigh 10 years ago? 5 years ago? 1 year ago?" The questions asked should provide a frame of reference and reveal whether weight loss occurred gradually over a long period or rapidly over a short period. Table 24-2 provides a means of evaluating weight loss on percent weight change.

TABLE 24-2 Evaluation of Weight Change*

Time	Significant Weight Loss	Severe Weight Loss
1 week	1–2%	>2%
1 month	5%	>5%
3 months	7.5%	>7.5%
6 months	10%	>10%

* Values charted are for percent weight change.
Percent weight change =

$$\frac{\text{Usual weight} - \text{actual weight}}{\text{Usual weight}} \times 100.$$

Source: Blackburn GL, Bistrian, BR, Maini, BS, et al: Nutritional and metabolic assessment of the hospitalized patient. J Parent Ent Nutr 1:17, 1977.

The factors that should be considered in weights recorded for an individual on a serial basis are:

1. Calibration and accuracy of the scale. It is best to use the same scale for each weighing. The zero point should be checked daily or more often if the scale is moved, and the scale should be calibrated regularly (every few months) against the reference weight to maintain accuracy.

2. Presence and degree of edema or dehydration. Fluid composition of the body can have a profound effect on weight fluctuations from day to day.

Skinfold measurement

The skinfold thickness measurement is the best single determinant of the degree of subcutaneous fat in body tissues. Although the distribution of subcutaneous fat varies substantially from individual to individual, variations within an individual as a result of dietary alterations appear to occur proportionately throughout the body.[50] Therefore, a measurement of subcutaneous fat will reflect changes in total body fat.

The skinfold thickness measurement is relatively reproducible provided that it is conducted by a trained individual who does all the measurements on the same individual.

The procedure requires a great deal of practice to obtain a reproducible measure. Therefore, many clinicians feel that it is not a reliable measure of nutritional status.

Skinfold thickness measurements can be taken from the subscapular or pectoral areas, abdomen, triceps, or biceps. The actual measurement obtained is the double thickness of the pinched skin plus the subcutaneous adipose tissue. The measuring instrument is a caliper, commonly the Lange (Cambridge Scientific Industries, Cambridge, MD) or Harpenden (British Indicators, St. Albans, Herfordshire, England) model.

Midarm muscle circumference

Arm muscle circumference has been shown to be a sensitive index of protein status that correlates significantly with serum albumin levels.[51] Once again, it is important that the same person who has been trained in the technique perform all measurements for one person to avoid errors in measurement. It has been estimated that measurements of midarm circumference of the same person by different persons can vary as much as 5%. The methodology has been described elsewhere.[52] From measured arm circumference and triceps skinfold thickness, arm muscle circumference (in centimeters) can be calculated.

$$\text{Arm muscle circumference (cm)} = \text{Arm circumference (cm)} - [0.314 \times \text{triceps skinfold (mm)}]$$

These anthropometric measurements are taken when an individual with cancer is initially examined and serially to evaluate nutritional therapy or to diagnose nutritional problems resulting from cancer or its treatment.

Biochemical Measurements

Biochemical data provide important information about the actual deficiencies of specific substances in the body. Biochemical data are the most specific of the assessment parameters, detecting covert nutritional deficiencies and thus allowing early intervention.

The major biochemical parameters for assessing nutritional status can be divided into those that measure the visceral protein compartment and those that measure lean body mass.

Visceral protein compartment

Standard measurements of the visceral protein compartment include the serum albumin, serum transferrin, and prealbumin. Albumin has a half-life of 20 days, transferrin has a half-life of 8 days, and prealbumin has a half-life of 2 days. Therefore, serum albumin, transferrin, and prealbumin measurements assess the individual's visceral protein status on a long-term, intermediate, and short-term basis, respectively.

Several investigators have found decreased plasma albumin levels to be associated with increased complication rates after cancer treatment.[53,54] Mullen et al[55] observed that when the level of serum albumin was less than 3.0 g/dL, individuals had a postoperative complication rate that was 2.5 times greater than that of individuals with a higher serum albumin concentration. Thus, serum protein measurements can be used to identify an individual's risk of developing complications before therapy so that nutritional therapy can be instituted to prevent those complications.

The plasma concentration of proteins measures the net result of protein synthesis versus protein degradation. However, plasma protein concentration is also affected by changes in the amount and distribution of body fluids, changes in capillary permeability, external losses, and ineffective lymphatic return. Therefore, hypoalbuminemia may be the result of a number of physiologic processes, including malnutrition.

Lean body mass

Forbes and Bruining[56] demonstrated that urinary creatinine is an excellent index of lean body mass. All muscle produces creatinine; therefore the proportion of creatinine produced is directly proportional to the amount of muscle in the body. Creatinine excretion is fairly constant in an individual with normal renal function. In the individual with cancer or other malnourished individuals, creatinine excretion is decreased as muscle protein is degraded and used to meet energy requirements.

Twenty-four-hour urine collections are used to measure urinary creatinine for nutritional assessment. For reliable results, three collections are needed. Creatinine excretion is compared with ideal creatinine excretion for height to determine the *creatinine height index,* as follows:

$$\text{Creatinine height index} = \frac{\text{Actual urinary creatinine excretion}}{\text{Ideal urinary creatinine excretion}} \times 100$$

Ideal creatinine excretion is determined as 23 mg/kg of ideal body weight for males and 18 mg/kg of ideal body weight for females.[62]

Immunologic Measurements

Immune function is a critical measure of nutritional status. Cell-mediated immunity orchestrated by T lymphocytes is especially vulnerable to the effects of malnutrition. The degree of T-lymphocyte depresson correlates in an almost linear fashion with the degree of protein-calorie malnutrition.[57] Protein-calorie malnutrition places the individual at greater risk of infection and results in a poorer response to cancer therapy. Daly et al[58] showed that individuals without an immune response averaged over 20 kg greater weight loss than individuals whose immune systems were functioning.

Two measurements are commonly used to evaluate immune function in relation to nutritional status: total lymphocyte count and skin sensitivity tests to recall antigens. The total lymphocyte count is derived from a complete blood count and calculated as follows:

$$\text{Total lymphocyte count} = \frac{\text{Percent lymphocytes}}{100} \times \text{WBC}$$

The total lymphocyte count is decreased in individuals with protein-calorie malnutrition.

The second major test of immune response is the skin sensitivity test. When cell-mediated immunity is impaired, there is a diminished or lack of response to antigens to which the individual was previously exposed. This lack of response is called *anergy*.

An individual may be tested with a variety of antigens. The most common antigens are streptokinase-streptodornase (SK-SD), dinitrochlorobenzene (DNCB), mumps, and *Candida*. The antigen is injected just under the skin. The induration is measured in millimeters at 24 hours and 48 hours.

Dionigi and colleagues[59] demonstrated that the skin test was an important prognosticator of postoperative complications in individuals with cancer undergoing surgery. Septic complications occurred in 37% of normoergic, 46% of hypoergic, and 83% of anergic individuals.

Several factors may limit the usefulness of the skin test in assessing nutritional status. Technical difficulties such as improper method of administration, reader variability, lack of previous exposure to the antigen, and so on may alter the individual's response to the antigen and provide false information. Concomitant diseases or therapies may be immunosuppressive and cause a lack of response. For example, because of general anesthesia, cell-mediated immunity can be depressed for as long as 2 to 3 weeks after surgery. In addition, immune components have high metabolic priority and thus are reduced only in severe malnutrition. Because of these limitations, several investigators do not recommend skin testing to measure immune status in a nutritional assessment.[60,61]

Summary

Table 24-3 summarizes the components of the nutritional assessment and provides a guide for collecting and evaluating both subjective and objective data. Once malnutrition is diagnosed, a therapeutic plan is established and implemented on the basis of the data obtained from the nutritional assessment. After the therapeutic plan is implemented, periodic reassessment should be done to evaluate the effects of therapy. Blackburn et al[62] recommend the following protocol for evaluating the efficacy of nutritional therapy:

1. Daily—body weight
2. Twice weekly—nitrogen balance (urinary creatinine, creatinine height index, serum albumin)
3. Weekly—total lymphocyte count
4. Every 3 weeks—anthropometrics, serum transferrin, skin tests

NUTRITIONAL MANAGEMENT

Malnutrition was once considered to be an inevitable consequence of advanced cancer. With the advent of relatively safe methods of delivering aggressive nutritional support and an increasing body of research demonstrating the positive effects of nutritional support on the quality and quantity of life for the person with cancer, clinicians now consider malnutrition an unnecessary and often preventable consequence of cancer. Aggressive nutritional therapy for individuals with cancer has been shown to decrease the morbidity and mortality of cancer and its therapy by preventing weight loss, maintaining or improving nutritional status, increasing responsiveness to therapy, minimizing side effects of therapy, improving the individual's sense of well-being, and improving the quality of life. The discussion of nutritional management in this section is concerned with the treatment of existing nutritional deficiencies as well as the prevention of deficiencies in the high-risk individual.

Controversies in Nutritional Support for Individuals with Cancer

Despite advances in the effectiveness of nutritional support therapies, controversy exists over whether nutritional therapy is contraindicated in some individuals with cancer because it permits or even encourages tumor growth by improving the supply of nutrients. As discussed earlier in this chapter, the energy requirements of a rapidly growing tumor take precedence over the individual's nutritional needs. Some researchers report that although the person benefits temporarily from long-term total parenteral nutrition, it does not sustain positive nitrogen balance[63] or increase the lean muscle mass of individuals with cancer.[64] Nixon et al[64] studied individuals with lung cancer, a population of people who have been shown to lose weight regardless of nutritional intake, apparently because of the paraneoplastic effects of lung tumors.[10] These data indicate that nutritional therapy is not a panacea in cancer care. Brennan[65] stated, "The best nutritional support is a full, complete response to cancer therapy such that normal substrate intake and body composition restoration can take place."

Although tumor growth is stimulated in rats as a result of exogenously administered nutrients,[66] it is unclear whether the same phenomenon occurs in humans. Research demonstrates that even if tumor stimulation does occur, the benefits to the individual in terms of outcome and well-being warrant the benefits to the tumor. For example, Copeland et al[67] demonstrated that intravenous hyperalimentation improved immune hypersensitivity response in individuals with cancer, resulting in fewer complications of surgery, radiation, and chemotherapy. Other similar studies have shown that individuals with cancer who receive nutritional support have less chemotherapeutic toxicities, are able to tolerate larger doses of drugs, achieve positive nitrogen balance and weight gain, and live longer (for those who respond to treatment).[68,69] In addition, improvement of the tumor's nutritional supply may stimulate the proliferation of malignant cells, inducing a more favorable response to chemotherapy or radiotherapy.[66]

Torosian et al[70] have demonstrated in an animal model that parenteral protein (with or without hypertonic dextrose) potentiates the tumor response to methotrexate without increasing host toxicity. One possible explanation for the enhanced tumor response to cycle-specific che-

TABLE 24-3 Components of the Nutritional Assessment

Medical History	Physical Examination
Duration and type of malignancy Frequency, type, and severity of complications (infections, draining lesions, etc.) Type and duration of therapy Specific chemotherapeutic agents used Radiation sites Antibiotics used Other drugs used Surgical procedures performed (site, type, date) Side effects of therapy (diarrhea, anorexia, nausea and vomiting) Concomitant medical conditions (diabetes, heart disease, liver failure, kidney failure, infection)	General appearance Condition of hair Condition of skin Condition of teeth Condition of mouth, gums, and throat Edema Performance status Identification of nutritionally related problems (fistula, pain, stomatitis, xerostomia, infection, constipation, diarrhea, nausea and vomiting, obstruction)
Dietary History	**Socioeconomic History**
24-hour recall of foods eaten, including snacks Composition of food taken in 24 hours (calories and protein, caffeine, liquor) Time of day meals and snacks eaten Past or current diet modifications Self-feeding ability Special cancer diet Vitamins, minerals, or other supplements Modifications of diet or eating habits as a result of treatment or illness Foods withheld or given on the basis of personal or religious grounds (kosher, vegetarian, etc.) Food preferences Food allergies or intolerances	Number of persons living in the home (ages and relationships) Kitchen facilities Income Food purchased by Food prepared by Amount spent on food per month Outside provision of meals
Anthropometric Data	**Biochemical Data**
Height Weight Actual weight as percentage of ideal Weight change as percentage of usual Triceps skinfold measurement Actual triceps skinfold as percentage of standard Midarm circumference Midarm muscle circumference Actual midarm muscle circumference as percentage of standard	Hematocrit Hemoglobin Serum albumin Serum transferrin Creatinine Creatinine height index Total lymphocyte count Delayed hypersensitivity response—skin testing Nitrogen balance Blood urea nitrogen Sodium, potassium, carbon dioxide, chloride Glucose

motherapy is increased induction of tumor cells into S-phase (synthesis), where the drug acts.[71]

Thus, nutritional support, when used in conjunction with curative or palliative cancer therapies, may have a significant impact on survival and the quality of life.

Establishing the Nutritional Therapy Plan

Identifying the goal of nutritional therapy

The first factor to be considered in selecting a nutritional therapy plan is the goal of the therapy. Is the goal of nutritional therapy weight gain? Weight maintenance? Restoration of immune function? Improvement of the person's sense of well-being? Prolongation of life? The therapeutic goal will determine the most effective method. The individual and family must participate in establishing the therapeutic goal.

Establishing the individual's caloric requirements

The average resting adult requires approximately 1200 to 1800 kcal/day (18 to 22 kcal/kg body weight) to maintain the basal metabolic rate (BMR). Any condition that increases energy expenditure, such as advanced cancer, sepsis, a healing wound, a draining fistula, or even simple exercise, increases the individual's caloric needs. Weight loss occurs when the energy expended is in excess of the calories consumed. The caloric intake necessary to maintain an individual's weight or cause the individual to gain weight must be determined on the basis of the nutritional assessment, and the results of nutritional therapy must be evaluated regularly so that any adjustments needed to achieve the desired goals can be made.

BMR is a measure of the amount of energy required to sustain life in a fasting, resting individual. BMR is determined primarily by an individual's body size; however, age, sex, and the stress of illness are also factors. Investigators found that energy requirements vary in individuals with cancer.[72,73] Not every individual is hypermetabolic. In fact, 25% to 35% of patients are hypometabolic, 40% to 50% are normometabolic, and only 25% are hypermetabolic. Therefore, because energy expenditure cannot be predicted accurately in cancer patients, measurement of energy expenditure by indirect calorimetry ("metabolic cart"), when available, may be valuable for individualizing the caloric prescription.

When indirect calorimetry is not possible, Bell et al[74] recommend the following forumula based on the BMR calculated from the Harris-Benedict equations (1919):

$$\text{Calories} = 1.2 - 1.3 \times \text{BMR where}$$
$$\text{BMR (men)} = 66 + 13.8(\text{weight, kg}) + 5.0(\text{height, cm}) - 6.8(\text{age, yr})$$
$$\text{BMR (women)} = 655 + 9.6(\text{weight, kg}) + 1.9(\text{height, cm}) - 4.7(\text{age, yr})$$

These formulas do not apply to obese individuals because BMR is correlated with lean body mass. For obese individuals, ideal body weight is substituted for actual body weight in the formulas for BMR.

Activity level is the major variable in the energy requirements of individuals. A more active individual will require more calories per day to maintain or gain weight. Long et al[75] estimated that the average hospitalized individual requires an addition of 20% to the BMR to adjust for minimal activities such as short walks, turning in bed, and walking from bed to chair. For the outpatient, caloric intake must be adjusted according to activity levels.

Once caloric needs have been established, the composition of the diet and method of feeding may be determined.

Composition of the diet

Carefully planned dietary intake is important in providing the individual's energy requirements and the nutrients necessary to maintain important physiologic processes. Energy requirements are supplied primarily from carbohydrates and fat; lean tissue anabolism is supported by proteins, minerals, and vitamins. Energy requirements, present nutritional deficits, allergies, individual preferences, and conditions that affect digestion or absorption all must be considered.

Because there is no body protein reserve for energy as there is for fat in adipose tissue and carbohydrate in liver glycogen, the main aim of nutritional therapy is to protect or restore body protein. Nitrogen balance is an index of protein balance in the body. A positive nitrogen balance implies that body protein is intact; a negative nitrogen balance implies that body protein is being depleted.

An individual must take in both calories and protein to maintain a positive nitrogen balance. In the normal individual, at least 7% to 8% of the total calories taken in must be provided by protein to maintain a positive nitrogen balance.[76] For the hypermetabolic individual, protein requirements will double and should be 15% to 20% of the total calories or 1.5 to 2.0 g protein/kg body weight. In patients with liver and/or renal dysfunction, protein may need to be limited.

Selecting the method of feeding

Several factors must be considered when selecting the method of feeding an individual:

1. The person's ability to chew and swallow
2. Function of the gastrointestinal tract
3. Severity of the nutritional problem
4. Potential complications
5. Cost
6. Duration of the therapy
7. Acceptability to the individual
8. Expertise available

Enteral Nutrition

It has been demonstrated that the nutritional benefits to individuals of enteral and parenteral hyperalimentation are comparable; the major factor in choosing one over the other is bowel function.[77,78] Therefore, if the gastrointestinal tract is normal and patent, enteral alimentation is the treatment of choice.

It has been estimated that of all individuals requiring active nutritional care, two thirds can be supported by enteral feeding and one third by parenteral feeding.[79] Enteral alimentation encompasses both oral and tube feeding.

Oral feeding

If the individual is able to consume an adequate quantity of foods orally, a regular diet composed of the appropriate amount of protein and calories is preferred. The dietary plan is determined primarily by the individual's needs and preferences. In addition to protein and calories supplied by the diet, vitamin and mineral suppplements may be necessary. If the person is unable to eat an adequate amount of regular food, the diet may be supplemented or replaced with liquid nutritional formulas. The monotony of liquid formulas generally prohibits their use as the sole source of oral intake. Liquid formulas allow flexibility in use for oral intake or tube feedings.

Composition of the diet may need to be altered based

on the symptoms the individual experiences as a result of the tumor or cancer treatments. Individuals who have stomatitis or difficulty chewing or swallowing may require a mechanically soft diet. It may be necessary to provide foods more frequently than the standard three times per day due to limited appetite or early satiety. Individuals with stomatitis may require a bland diet to prevent discomfort. Individuals undergoing abdominal or pelvic irradiation frequently are unable to tolerate milk because of a lack of the enzyme lactase necessary for digestion of lactose. It has been demonstrated that use of gluten-free, lactose-free, low-residue diet in children receiving radiation resulted in complete prevention of acute and chronic radiation enteritis.[80]

It is generally the nurse's responsibility to observe and record the person's tolerance of his or her diet and the quantities of food consumed. The nurse, in conjunction with other members of the nutritional support team, will monitor and assess whether the person is maintaining adequate nutritional status with the foods ingested. If the therapeutic goals are not being met, alternative forms of feeding will be considered.

It is often necessary for the nurse to use creative and persuasive talents in encouraging individuals with cancer to eat. These individuals often are unwilling rather than unable to eat because of discomfort, anorexia, and so on. Figure 24-1 provides a number of suggestions for encouraging oral feeding. Some individuals may choose starvation and refuse to eat. In such cases the nutritional support team faces ethical and moral dilemmas as they make decisions about the person's therapy.[81]

Dysphagia

- Eat soft or liquid foods
- Blenderize recipes
- Eat lubricating foods such as creams, oils, gravies
- If dysphagia is associated with pain, eat bland foods that are smooth and tepid

Nausea/Vomiting

- Avoid acid foods such as citrus juice and tomatoes
- Eat salty foods
- Avoid overly sweet, greasy, or high-fat foods
- Drink clear, cool beverages
- Drink carbonated beverages
- Eat dry foods such as toast or crackers, especially after getting up in the morning
- Eat slowly and chew food thoroughly
- Eat small, frequent meals
- Popsicles or gelatin increase fluid intake and are satisfying
- Rest with the head elevated after eating
- Avoid sweet, rich foods
- Wear loose clothing
- Avoid favorite foods during chemotherapy to avoid developing an aversion to them
- Use antiemetics—anticholinergics, antihistamines such as diphenhydramine (Benadryl), promethazine (Phenergan), and trimethobenzamide (Tigan) as needed
- Use tranquilizers—chlorpromazine (Thorazine), haloperidol (Haldol), prochlorperazine (Compazine), and thiethylperazine (Torecan) as needed

Early Satiety

- Eat five or six small meals per day
- Keep nutritious snacks available for eating throughout the day
- Eat foods high in calories, low in fats
- Avoid greasy foods such as butter and rich sauces
- Chew foods slowly
- Avoid liquids with meals. Take ½ hour before meals
- Be sure any liquids taken are nutritious such as juices, milk shakes, or milk

Pancreatic Insufficiency

- Take digestive enzyme supplements
- Follow diet high in calories and protein, low in fat
- Take commercial products for protein and carbohydrate supplementation

Anorexia

- Eat small frequent meals
- Make changes in diet or surroundings. Try new recipes or foods, eat with friends, go to a favorite restaurant
- Stimulate appetite with light exercise
- Coincide meals with "best time" during the day
- Eat snacks high in protein (cheese, milk) often during the day. Avoid "empty calories" such as cakes, coffee
- Use high-calorie foods with which to take medications such as a cold chocolate protein drink
- Use grains or nuts in desserts and add 4–6 tbsp of powdered milk to cookie and cake recipes to increase protein content
- Drink wine or a small glass of fruit juice before meals to stimulate appetite
- Avoid fatty foods
- Try fresh, cold fruits
- If hospitalized, have the family bring favorite foods from home

Dumping Syndrome

- Eat foods low in carbohydrate, high in protein, and moderate in fat
- Eat six small, dry meals per day
- Eliminate fluids during meals. Take fluids 30–45 minutes prior to or after meals
- Avoid concentrated sweets, including sugar
- Limit milk to a maximum of 4 oz/day
- If tube feeding, dilute one-quarter to one-half strength initially, gradually increase to patient tolerance

FIGURE 24-1 Suggested approaches to problems that interfere with normal nutrition.

Continued.

Constipation

- Increase fluids to 2 L/day
  Set aside 2 L at beginning of day. Drink 8 oz glass every waking hour
- Eat foods high in fiber such as fruits, vegetables, whole grain breads and cereals, bran, dried fruits, and nuts
- Engage in light, regular exercise
- Utilize previously successful bowel stimulants

Diarrhea

- Drink plenty of fluids to avoid dehydration
- Decrease solid foods
- Eliminate milk products
- Drink Gatorade to provide electrolytes
- Follow low-fiber, high-protein diet
- Avoid high-fat, spicy, and gas-forming foods
- Eat foods rich in potassium
- Eat foods at room temperature

Dyspepsia

- Avoid spicy foods
- Avoid fatty foods
- Elevate the upper trunk following meals
- Use antacids

Stomatitis

- Softer consistency of food—avoid rough and irritating foods such as citrus fruit or acid foods
- Use warm saline irrigations to cleanse
- Popsicles taste good and numb pain
- Drink tepid tea
- Person may only be able to tolerate liquids

Taste Changes

- Marinate red meat with sweet marinades or soy sauce
- Substitute poultry, fish, eggs, and cheese for red meats
- Serve meats chilled rather than hot—chicken salad or cold roast beef sandwich
- If person is averse to all meats and protein foods no matter how prepared, substitute sweet, high-protein, high-calorie foods such as milk shakes, puddings, and ice cream with various flavorings
- Acid foods (if tolerated) stimulate the taste buds
- Use extra seasoning, spices, onions, garlic
- Rinse mouth with carbonated water before meals to clear the taste buds
- Try sucking on a lemon wedge before eating
- Lemonade, tea with lemon, citrus fruits and drinks, and pickled foods all stimulate taste buds
- Foods that were previously not liked may now be acceptable because taste is altered. Keep experimenting.

Xerostomia

- Eat moistened foods—use gravies and sauces
- Use artificial saliva preparations for comfort and to facilitate swallowing
- Use blender or food processor to make foods easier to eat
- Soak foods in coffee, tea, milk, cocoa, or warm beverages
- Avoid dry foods
- Take a swallow of liquid with each bite
- Use a humidifier or steam kettle in the room

General

- Drink lots of fluids
- Pleasant surroundings—out of bed, nice restaurant, company of people the person likes to be with
- Serve food attractively—use garnishes
- Experiment with recipes, flavorings, spices, types and consistencies of food. Likes may change from day to day.
- Do not take in empty calories—eat high-protein foods such as dry skim milk powder, eggs, cheese, evaporated milk, peanut butter, nuts, etc.
- Take advantage of the best time during day for eating; especially early in the day when not fatigued
- Keep nutritious snacks handy to make it easy
- Eat nutritious foods whenever hungry
- Make use of time savers such as meals in a dish or frozen foods

FIGURE 24-1, cont'd.

The nurse should also be aware that individuals with cancer may be following unconventional diets purported as "cures" by the media. Among the dietary therapies commonly tried are the macrobiotic diet (primarily grains and miso, a soybean product), laetrile, and megadoses of vitamins. None of these diets has been proven to cure cancer. Additionally, these diets are often expensive, unpalatable, and deficient in many essential nutrients and calories, predisposing the individual to malnutrition. For more information, see Chapter 56, Unproven Methods of Treatment.

Tube feeding

If oral intake cannot prevent weight loss, or if the person's physical condition prevents oral intake for prolonged periods, tube feeding may be required. Gastrointestinal function must be intact for tube feeding. The advent of Silastic and polyethylene tubes has made tube feedings more tolerable to people than they were when only rubber tubes were available. The newer tubes are lighter, have a finer bore, and are more flexible, making them more suitable for nasogastric placement. Larger polyethylene or rubber tubes often are used for gastrostomies or jejunostomies. Tube feedings may be administered by nasogastric intubation, esophagostomy, gastrostomy, or jejunostomy. See Rombean and Caldwell[82] for procedures for administering tube feedings.

Diarrhea is the most common side effect of tube feedings. Diarrhea can be caused by bacterial contamination of the formula, high osmolarity of the fluid, lactose intolerance, rapid administration, or broad-spectrum antibiotic therapy. The most common factor contributing to diarrhea is the rate of delivery because even hyperosmolar feedings introduced slowly are quickly diluted in the large volume of intestinal fluid. Diarrhea is treated by decreasing the volume or rate of delivery. If decreasing the rate does not help diminish the diarrhea, the concentration of the liquid is adjusted to decrease osmolarity. If the person continues to experience diarrhea and is not positive for *Clostridium difficile* toxin, antidiarrheal medications may be prescribed. Alternatively, a formula containing nondigestible fiber can be used.

Fluid and electrolyte disturbances such as hypernatremia, hyperchloremia, azotemia, and dehydration may occur as a result of excessively high concentrations of electrolytes and protein in the formula, inadequate fluid intake, or renal insufficiency. The person should be weighed daily and observed and monitored for fluid and electrolyte status.

Blood and urine glucose levels are monitored regularly for glucose intolerance. Urine is tested by the nurse daily; hyperglycemia is treated with sliding scale insulin regimens. Diabetic individuals may have increased insulin requirements.

Liquid formulas for enteral nutrition

Many individuals with cancer at some time require supplementation or replacement of solid foods with nourishing liquids either by mouth or by tube. The advantage of liquid feedings is that they can be ingested and digested more easily than solid foods. The major disadvantages to liquid diets are their monotony and the lack of satisfaction associated with chewing foods of various textures.[83]

Liquid foods may be prepared from regular food sources or commercially prepared. Commercially prepared formulas are more convenient and ensure consistent nutritional composition and microbiologic safety. However, psychologic acceptance may be better if the individual and family are able to control what foods go into the preparation. Knowledge that the feeding is composed of regular food may be important for the person's satisfaction.

Commercially prepared liquid formulas provide approximately 1 to 2 kcal/mL. The dozens of formulas available differ significantly in their composition and nutrient sources and especially in their osmolarity. Specific individual needs should be considered in selecting the appropriate formula. For example, if the person has lactose intolerance, the formula should be low in lactose. If the person has impaired fat digestion, a formula containing easily absorbed medium-chain triglycerides (MCT) may be indicated. Because the quality and effectiveness of commercial preparations improve regularly, it is advisable for the nurse to keep a product information file and update it frequently for clinical reference.

Evaluation

The efficacy of an enteral feeding is evaluated primarily by the individual's ability to gain or maintain weight and an improvement in the individual's nitrogen balance as measured by urinary urea nitrogen or creatinine tests. In addition to the objective measures of response to enteral nutritional therapy, many individuals have subjective responses such as improved mood, return of appetite, and improved sense of well-being.

Parenteral Nutrition

Before the 1970s, parenteral administration of nutrients was limited to peripheral administration of 5% to 10% dextrose solutions (usually providing less than 1000 kcal/day). Attempts to increase the concentration of the solutions resulted in thrombophlebitis of the peripheral vein. The average adult requires 1200 to 1800 calories/day to maintain the basal metabolic rate. Standard intravenous therapy is clearly ineffective in providing the dietary constituents necessary to maintain adequate nutrition.

Total parenteral nutrition (TPN) is the intravenous infusion of a concentrated mixture of proteins, glucose, fluid, vitamins, minerals, electrolytes, and trace elements (iodine, copper, fluoride, zinc, manganese, and chromium) into a central vein, usually the superior vena cava. The large diameter of the superior vena cava and its great blood flow allows concentrated solutions to be infused relatively safely without causing thrombophlebitis.

The TPN solution provides nitrogen in the form of essential and nonessential amino acids. Nonprotein caloric requirements are supplied by dextrose. Essential fatty acids, which are important in many metabolic processes, are often infused with the TPN solution in a 10% or 20% soybean or safflower oil emulsion.

In 1981, an estimated 150,000 to 200,000 individuals in the United States received TPN: one third of these individuals had cancer.[84] The initial success of TPN in producing dramatic results in malnourished individuals stimulated its wide, untested use. However, clinicians are now taking a more moderate approach to the use of TPN. It is felt that TPN probably has been misused and overused. Researchers are now carefully studying the benefits, costs, and complications of TPN.[85] When used for an appropriate group of individuals, TPN improves response to primary cancer therapy and improves the quality of life by restoring or maintaining nutritional status.[70,86]

Indications of total parenteral nutrition for the individual with cancer

Total parenteral nutrition is indicated when it becomes impractical or impossible to administer food through the gastrointestinal tract or when other feeding methods fail to provide the individual with sufficient calories and nutrients to meet metabolic needs. For example, for individuals with cancer of the head and neck region, caloric intake is frequently limited for prolonged periods because of mechanical interference by the tumor, major ablative or reconstructive surgical procedures, edema and ulceration due to irradiation of the head and neck region, nausea, vomiting, or anorexia. TPN may provide the individual with adequate nutrition to allow for healing of surgically disrupted tissue or to enable the individual to complete a prescribed course of radiotherapy.

Individuals with cancer of the gastrointestinal tract often face partial or total obstruction of the gastrointestinal tract as a result of expanding tumor, altered bowel function resulting from surgical manipulation, malabsorption syndromes because of irradiation to the bowel, dehydration, or cachexia as a result of fluid and electrolyte loss from fistulas. In the past, fistulas were a major cause of mortality for persons with gastrointestinal cancers. In addition, many persons were unable to complete a full course of cancer therapy because of malnutrition. The advent of TPN has vastly improved the outcome for individuals with gastrointestinal cancers. TPN allows the bowel to rest, promoting healing of surgically disrupted tissue or allowing fistulas to close spontaneously, and provides rapid total nutrient buildup to enable the individual to receive aggressive therapy more safely. TPN also helps prevent secondary complications of cancer therapy such as infection and anemia.

Benefits of total parenteral nutrition to the individual with cancer

Deitel at al[68] demonstrated that TPN is worthwhile for individuals with cancer, achieving significant palliation and improvement in the quality of life. These researchers were able to prevent postoperative complications in a group of individuals who would otherwise be prone to significant morbidity and decrease postoperative mortality in another group of individuals who had already developed significant complications. Other researchers have shown that instituting TPN during preoperative and postoperative periods for individuals undergoing surgery for cancer reduces septic complications.[87,88] However, using meta-analysis, Klein et al[85] demonstrated that there is a statistically significant increase in the infection rate in patients who are receiving both chemotherapy and TPN.

Copeland et al[89] demonstrated that anorexia, nausea, and vomiting disappeared in individuals experiencing enteritis during radiation who were treated with TPN for an average of 34 days. When those same individuals tried to eat, their symptoms recurred. All individuals were able to complete the planned course of therapy because of TPN and the bowel rest it affords. Decreased morbidity from radiation as a result of TPN has also been demonstrated.[90]

Several researchers have demonstrated improved response or decreased morbidity when TPN was included with chemotherapy in the management of individuals with cancer.[70,91] TPN improves the nutritionally depleted state of these individuals and allows more extensive chemotherapy. Lean body weight increases, and tolerance for chemotherapy is enhanced.

Because of data such as these, nutritional experts believe that TPN is a valuable supportive therapy that is to be used when enteral nutrition fails and nutritional rehabilitation is essential for the effective delivery of antineoplastic treatment or to recover from the malnutrition imposed by cancer and cancer therapy.[86,91]

TPN has been shown to have little or no benefit for well-nourished individuals because the weight gain experienced is due to fat and water as opposed to lean muscle tissue. In addition, TPN is not indicated for the person whose life would be prolonged needlessly by its use. In fact, ethical decisions regarding the initiation or withdrawal of nutritional support in terminally ill cancer patients have challenged the medical community. Ethical decisions are reached by carefully considering factors including physiologic benefits and risks, patient preference, quality of life, cost, family concerns, and previous legal decisions.[92]

Criteria for selecting individuals to receive total parenteral nutritional therapy

TPN therapy is not without risks. Individuals are carefully selected on the basis of well-defined criteria. Generally, a person is considered eligible for TPN therapy if enteral therapy has failed or is inappropriate and if any two or all of the following criteria have been met[65]:

- Weight loss of 10% or more from the usual
- A serum albumin level below 3.5 g/dL
- Immunoincompetence to a battery of recall skin test antigens

Establishing a goal for use of total parenteral nutrition therapy

Before TPN therapy is instituted, it is important for the nutritional support team to establish a measurable goal for the outcome of therapy. Examples of goals include continuation of TPN until the person gains a certain amount of weight, completes a regimen of chemotherapy or radiotherapy, or until a fistula heals. Establishment of a goal will enable the team to evaluate the effects of nutritional therapy and will allow the individual receiving TPN to participate in attaining the goal or assessing the progress made toward it.

The plan for TPN therapy should be discussed thoroughly with the individual and family. The goals of therapy should be discussed with the individual, as well as what to expect regarding catheter insertion, monitoring studies and their purposes, dressing changes, care of the infusion equipment, possible complications, and the expected duration of therapy.

Complications of total parenteral nutrition

Mullen[84] states, "Most TPN-related complications are iatrogenic, avoidable, and, in reality, an indictment of the quality of care rather than the technique itself." Mullen suggests that the risks associated with TPN and their frequency, severity, and outcome depend on the following:

1. Patient population—nutritional status, histologic type of tumor, stage of disease, rate of progression, and concomitant therapy
2. Competence of the nutritional support team
3. Competence of the institutional core staff—physicians, nurses, pharmacists, and house staff
4. Rapidity with which innovations are used
5. Organizational management of the nutritional support team

Three categories of complications are associated with TPN therapy: infectious, mechanical, and metabolic.

Infectious complications The incidence of infectious complications associated with TPN therapy has decreased substantially in the last decade as a result of attention to the importance of a regular program of catheter care involving strict aseptic technique. The incidence of infection decreases when there is an organized approach to TPN care such as through the services of a TPN team. Ryan et al[93] studied 200 patients who had 355 catheters in 4492 hospital days. The sepsis rate of these individuals was only 3% when strict aseptic technique was maintained. When catheter care protocols were violated, the sepsis rate rose to 20%.

Individuals with cancer are frequently immunosuppressed as a result of malignancy. The added insult of immunosuppressive therapy such as chemotherapy or radiotherapy makes the individual vulnerable to overwhelming infection. The introduction of TPN through a central or peripheral line creates a real risk of infection. In addition, glucose and protein-rich TPN solutions provide an excellent medium for bacterial and fungal growth.

Infection results from contamination of the TPN solution, insertion site, or the equipment used or, more rarely, from seeding of the catheter tip by blood borne infection. Skin microorganisms are the most frequent cause of sepsis. Offending organisms are either bacterial or fungal. Bacterial organisms include *Staphylcoccus aureus, Staphylococcus epidermidis,* and gram-negative bacteria such as *Klebsiella. Corynebacterium* has been recognized as an organism causing infection in individuals receiving TPN. Its incidence is increasing, expecially in severely immunosuppressed individuals, such as those who have undergone bone marrow transplantation.

Also commonly implicated in TPN-related sepsis are the fungi *Candida albicans* and *Candida parapsilosis.*

Early detection of sepsis is an important nursing responsibility. The first sign of sepsis may be sudden glycosuria (or hyperglycemia) in the previously stable individual, which may precede any other clinical signs by as much as 24 hours.

Glycosuria is easily detected by the nurse who is conducting urine tests every 6 hours. Clinical signs of sepsis include fever, hypotension, tachycardia, and tachypnea.

In the presence of a temperature spike, peripheral blood and blood drawn from the catheter are cultured for bacteria and fungi. If both are positive, the catheter is the presumed source of the infection and should be removed.

If the individual's condition deteriorates or the fever persists, the catheter cannula is most likely the source of infection and must be removed. The distal portion of the catheter is cultured for bacteria and fungi. If the catheter is found to be the source of the infection, symptoms of infection usually subside within 12 to 24 hours of catheter removal. If symptoms persist, other sources of infection are investigated. A new catheter cannot be inserted until all blood cultures are negative unless the lack of nutrients is deemed life threatening[95] or intravenous access is essential but peripheral access is unavailable. If blood cultures and the catheter tip culture are negative and no other source of infection is identified, yet the patient becomes afebrile without antibiotics, the catheter is the presumed site of infection. Sepsis resulting from bacterial infection is treated with antibiotics; fungal infections are treated with a fungicidal agent such as amphotericin B.

Mechanical complications Mechanical problems can result from improper functioning of the central line due to blockage of the line from catheter crimping or thrombosis, malfunction of the infusion pump, or failure of the infusion set. Such mechanical problems can be minimized if the personnel caring for and using the equipment are knowledgeable and skilled and if there is a standardized protocol for care of the TPN equipment.

Thromboses are the most common mechanical problems associated with TPN therapy. Thrombosis of the catheter lumen is common, especially in individuals receiving intermittent feedings or when continuous infusions are interrupted. The incidence of thrombosis is reduced by the use of a heparin lock when the catheter is not in use.

If the lumen of the catheter becomes obliterated with a clot, patency may be restored by applying gentle negative pressure to the barrel of a sterile syringe that is fitted snugly into the catheter hub. If the clot is not dislodged by this method, the physician may choose either to irrigate the catheter gently or to instill streptokinase for clot lysis.

Thrombosis of the central vein is a rare but serious complication, requiring prompt removal of the catheter and administration of sodium heparin. Signs and symptoms of central vein thrombosis or thrombophlebitis include erythema, edema of the catheter insertion site, pain along the course of the vein, ipsilateral swelling of the arm, neck, or face, fever, tachycardia, tachypnea, and malaise.

Air embolism is a rare but potentially fatal complication of TPN therapy. A fatal bolus of air is 15 mL/kg of body weight although lesser amounts can occlude smaller vessels.[97]

Air embolism can be prevented by assisting the individual to maintain a supine or Trendelenburg position and hold his or her breath or perform the Valsalva maneuver whenever the catheter cannula is exposed to the atmosphere. In addition, all intravenous tubing junctions should be taped securely to prevent air from entering the system. The infusion system should be inspected regularly for leaks or cracks as part of the standard TPN protocol.

If the individual develops a significant air embolus, signs of sudden vascular collapse will be manifested by chest pain, apprehension, tachycardia, hypotension, and cyanosis progressing to seizures, loss of consiousness, and

TABLE 24-4 Metabolic Complications of Total Parenteral Nutrition

Complications	Possible Causes
Glucose metabolism	
Hyperglycemia, glycosuria, osmotic diuresis, hyperosmolar, nonketotic dehydration and coma	Excessive total dose or rate of infusion of glucose; inadequate endogenous insulin; glucocorticoids; sepsis
Postinfusion (rebound) hypoglycemia	Persistence of endogenous insulin production secondary to prolonged stimulation of islet cells by high carbohydrate infusion
Amino acid metabolism	
Hyperchloremic metabolic acidosis	Excessive chloride content of crystalline amino acid solutions
Prerenal azotemia	Excessive amino acid infusion
Calcium and phosphorus metabolism	
Hypophosphatemia	Inadequate phosphorus administration; redistribution of serum phosphorus into cells and/or bone
Hypocalcemia	Inadequate calcium administration; hypoalbuminemia
Hypercalcemia	Excessive calcium administration; excessive vitamin D administration
Essential fatty acid metabolism	
Serum deficiencies of phospholipid linoleic and/or arachidonic acids	Inadequate essential fatty acid administration; inadequate vitamin E administration
Miscellaneous	
Hypokalemia	Inadequate potassium intake relative to increased requirements for protein anabolism; diuresis
Hyperkalemia	Excessive potassium administration; renal decompensation
Hypomagnesemia	Inadequate magnesium administration relative to increased requirements for protein anabolism and glucose metabolism
Hypermagnesemia	Excessive magnesium administration; renal decompensation
Anemia	Iron deficiency; folic acid deficiency; vitamin B_{12} deficiency; copper deficiency
Bleeding	Vitamin K deficiency
Elevations of SGOT, SGPT, and serum alkaline phosphatase	Enzyme induction secondary to accelerated glucose metabolism; possible hepatotoxicity secondary to amino acid imbalance; excessive glycogen and/or fat deposition
Zinc, copper, or chromium deficiency	Inadequate trace metal administration

Source: Adapted from Cupit GC: Total parenteral nutrition of the cancer patient. Cancer Nurs 2:66, 1979.

cardiac arrest. Englert[95] recommends that even if the person must be resuscitated, the immediate emergency nursing action should be to position the person on the left side with the head down to allow the air to dissipate gradually through the pulmonary artery. This action may take several minutes, but it eliminates the vascular obstruction.

Precipitation of minerals, most commonly calcium phosphate, can occlude catheters when the concentration infused exceeds its solubility limit. Thus, the nurse should not coinfuse calcium and phosphate riders; riders should be hung consecutively, after flushing, and preferably into separate ports of the catheter.

Metabolic complications A variety of metabolic complications have been associated with TPN administration. Some of the most common complications are listed in Table 24-4. Most metabolic requirements are satisfied by the volume and content of the TPN solution. However, metabolic complications do occur. Weinsier et al[96] reported that 67% of their 220 patients experienced at least one metabolic complication during TPN therapy.

The most common metabolic complication of TPN therapy is hyperglycemia which occurs in approximately 15% of all individuals receiving TPN therapy.[84] Hyperglycemia results when the TPN infusion is too rapid, if insulin response is inadequate, or when there are increased insulin demands on the individual, such as occurs in sepsis.

Hyperglycemia is easily monitored by the nurse with the use of fractional urine tests or finger sticks for blood glucose every 6 hours. Clinical symptoms of hyperglycemia include dry mouth, flushed skin, thirst, malaise, polyuria, nausea, or vomiting. If untreated the hyperglycemia increases serum osmolality, causing fluid to shift from the intracellular to extracellular space. Osmotic diuresis occurs, with urine output as much as 800 to 900 mL in 1 to 2 hours, and results in dehydration. Hyperosmolar, hyperglycemic dehydration, if untreated, leads to convulsions, coma, and death.

Hyperglycemia is best treated by the addition of crystalline insulin to each TPN solution. Initial doses are 10 U/L, with gradual increases until the desired blood glucose level is achieved.

Occasionally, when hyperglycemia is significant (blood glucose 300 to 400 mg/dL) and not well controlled with sliding scale insulin, an insulin drip may be necessary to achieve "normoglycemia" (blood glucose 100 to 200 mg/dL). To prevent life-threatening hypoglycemia, the insulin drip must be held when the TPN solution is not being infused.

Hypoglycemia occurs when too much insulin is administered or when the TPN infusion is interrrupted or discontinued shortly after sliding scale insulin is given. In the patient on a stable TPN regimen (even those with insulin as a component of the TPN mixture), the infusion usually can be stopped abruptly without significant hypoglycemia; however, the infusion should be tapered for an hour or two before discontinuation, if time permits. This is possible for patients receiving insulin as a component of the TPN mixture because intravenously administered insulin is only effective for a few minutes.

Symptoms of hypoglycemia include headache, drowsiness, dizziness, tachycardia, and tremor. Hypoglycemia is corrected when the TPN infusion is balanced against insulin administration.

Essential fatty acid deficiency occurs as a result of a prolonged reduction of fat intake. The symptoms of essential fatty acid deficiency include scaling of the skin over the lower calf and dorsum of the foot, alopecia, delayed wound healing, increased capillary fragility, and thrombocytopenia. Lipid emulsion should be administered regularly to individuals who receive TPN for longer than 14 days without dietary fat intake. DeWys and Kubota[97] recommend that a minimum of two to three bottles (250 or 500 mL per bottle) per week should be infused. Lipid emulsions prevent essential fatty acid deficiency, provide a concentrated energy source, are isotonic and therefore do not damage venous endothelium, and do not require insulin to promote nitrogen. Finally, provision of 25% to 35% of the individual's calorie requirements as lipid may help reduce carbon dioxide production, which may be clinically significant in individuals with chronic obstructive pulmonary disease or those ventilator-dependent patients who retain carbon dioxide.[98]

Animal studies suggest that regimens with a high level of fat may have some metabolic advantages for cancer-bearing hosts.[99] Most clinicians continue to recommend that lipids should not exceed 60% to 80% of the total daily caloric intake (Intralipid product circular, Cutter Laboratories[97]).

The following is a list of guidelines for lipid emulsion infusion:

- Do not use the emulsion if the color or texture is inconsistent.
- Do not shake the container excessively.
- *Nothing* should be added to the lipid infusion—additives crack the emulsion.
- Infuse in the same line as the TPN solution using a Y-connector located near the infusion site.
- The lipid infusion should be hung higher than TPN or it will run up the TPN line.
- Do not use a filter.
- The initial maximum rate of infusion is 1 mL/min for the first 30 minutes. If no untoward reactions occur, increase the infusion rate to 500 mL over 4 to 12 hr.
- Observe the individual for untoward effects such as allergic reactions, dyspnea, cyanosis, nausea, vomiting, headache, flushing, fever, chills, pain in the chest or back, irritation at the infusion site, and diaphoresis.
- Discard any solution remaining in the container. Do not store it for later use.

If the individual experiences any of the untoward effects just mentioned, the lipid infusion should be discontinued. If the symptoms are a result of fat overload, the individual may receive sodium heparin intravenously to clear plasma lipids. Overall tolerance to the lipid infusion is monitored with routine serum triglyceride and cholesterol measurements.

Most of the other metabolic complications are deficiency states that can be avoided by appropriate replacement in the TPN solution. Trace metals have emerged as important factors in deficiency states resulting from long-term TPN therapy. However, most standard TPN solutions contain trace metals and vitamins.

Pharmacologic Treatment of Cachexia

Hormonal treatment of malignancy has recently received attention because of the potential for therapeutic efficacy with relatively little toxicity. Megestrol acetate is a synthetic derivative of progesterone that is used often in the hormonal treatment of patients with advanced breast cancer and prostrate cancer. Weight gain (10 or 20 pounds or more) and increased appetite are common side effects, even when the drug is administered at conventional doses (120 to 160 mg/day).[100-105] Regardless of the patient's pretreatment weight, type of cancer, extent of disease or response to therapy, weight gain is observed and is not due to edema. Although megestrol acetate is a potent inducer of lipocyte differentiation,[106] the mechanism by which megestrol acetate exerts its effects on appetite and anabolism has not been determined and is under investigation.

The use of megestrol acetate as a possible treatment for cachexia due to cancer or human immunodeficiency virus (HIV) has been proposed[107-110] because of the initial anecdotal observations. The therapeutic efficacy and most effective dose of megestrol acetate are under investigation in several clinical trials of patients with cachexia due to cancer or HIV.

Nutritional Therapy at Home

Many individuals are now able to carry out their own nutritional program at home. Home nutritional support is indicated especially for individuals who would otherwise not need to be hospitalized.

Tube feedings generally can be accomplished at home with little difficulty if the individual and family receive sufficient instruction. It is important that the regimen be as simple as possible. It should be written out for the individual and family, including goals for caloric intake and the desired weight gain. Instruction should include insertion of the tube (if applicable), preparation of the feeding, administration of the feeding, care and use of the equipment, documentation of intake, potential complications or side effects, and management of complications and equipment problems.

The individual and family have the opportunity to decide whether they would like to use blenderized home dietary formulas or commercially prepared formulas. The former are less expensive and give the individual and family more control in the food the individual receives and therefore more satisfaction. However, it is more difficult to ensure a nutritionally complete diet when a home formula is used. In addition, the risk of bacterial contamination is increased. Nonetheless, the individual's and family's ability to participate in decisions made about dietary intake plays an important role in their acceptance of the dietary regimen.

If the individual and family are intimidated by an electronic infusion pump, they should be encouraged to use continuous drip by gravity for the feedings. Feedings should be administered during family mealtimes to encourage the socialization that is associated closely with eating. If appropriate, feedings can be infused over night, allowing the individual freedom from the pump during the day. In addition, during the hiatus, the individual may develop an appetite and be able to enjoy small meals with the family.

Follow-up by a visiting nurse and regular visits to the outpatient department will reassure the individual and family that the therapy is being conducted properly. In addition, it allows the physician or nurse to evaluate the therapy and make necessary modifications.

Parenteral nutrition in the home is much more complicated and requires that the individual and family be capable of learning the technique, possess a high degree of motivation, and have adequate family support. Home TPN is indicated for individuals with fistulas, short bowel syndrome, severe radiation enteritis, or obstruction.

The individual who will be receiving long-term TPN at home will have a Broviac or Hickman type of catheter. The person must be instructed about catheter care and the infusion procedure in its entirety. If individuals are properly instructed and catheter care is meticulous, catheters may last up to 1 year or longer. The most frequent complication of home TPN is sepsis, requiring removal of the catheter.

For the person at home, the TPN fluid volume is 1000 to 2500 mL/24hr. The total volume of TPN fluid often is administered overnight while the person is asleep to allow for mobility during waking hours. The solution is tapered during the last 2 hours of administration to prevent hypoglycemia on discontinuation.

The cost of home TPN is high but significantly lower than comparable therapy received in a hospital. A 1982 report showed that monthly expenses for individuals receiving TPN in the hospital averaged approximately $12,400 as compared with $3300 for individuals receiving TPN at home.[100] The major component of this difference was the cost of the hospital room. Most major insurance companies and state medical aid programs reimburse individuals for home TPN.

Close follow-up and evaluation by the TPN support team or visiting nurse are critical to the success of a home TPN program. Further information on home TPN is provided in Chapter 51.

FUTURE TRENDS

Significant advances have been made in the last few decades regarding our knowledge about nutrition and cancer. Nutritional intervention has achieved the status of an important adjunct to cancer therapy through the premise that nutritional intervention supports and sustains the individual while the cancer therapy is destroying the tumor. Despite the tremendous gains in knowledge, however, much more remains to be learned.

The future of knowledge to be gained through nutritional research is promising. Health care professionals can look forward to the identification of factors that cause altered nutrition in individiuals with cancer and new ways of applying this knowledge toward improving the quality of life for persons whose normal eating patterns are altered by cancer. For example, the brain peptides that are thought to cause anorexia in individuals with cancer are shown to play a role in cancer cachexia; antagonists to these peptides administered therapeutically may prevent the anorexia of cancer.

Mullen[84] states that the major question yet to be answered in research about cancer and malnutrition is whether nutritional depletion on the individual with cancer is purely a manifestation of cancer that will resolve spontaneously after succesful cancer therapy or whether nutritional intervention will actually improve treatment success. The challenge is for research to define areas where nutritional support will result in a measurable improved response to cancer therapy. More careful documentation of nutritional deficits at the beginning of nutritional and cancer therapy is needed so that changes can be measured. A concomitant need is for the identification of assessment parameters that can measure response to nutritional therapy. The goal is for nutritional assessment to be a prognosticator of outcome of cancer. Nurses must take a leadership role on behalf of individuals with cancer in this most important quest for improved patient care.

REFERENCES

1. DeWys WD, Begge C, Band P, et al: The impact of malnutrition on treatment results in breast cancer. Cancer Treat Rep 65:87-91, 1981 (suppl 5).
2. Freeman M, Frankenman C, Beck J: Prognostic nutrition factors in lung cancer patients. J Parent Ent Nutr 6:122-127, 1982.
3. Rickard KA, Detamore CM, Coates TD, et al: Effect of nutrition staging on treatment delays and outcome in stage IV neuroblastoma. Cancer 52:587-598, 1983.
4. Meguid MM, Meguid V: Preoperative identification of the surgical cancer patient in need of postoperative supportive total parenteral nutrition. Cancer 55:258-262, 1985.
5. Heber D, Byerley LO, Chi J, et al: Pathophysiology of malnutrition in the adult cancer patient. Cancer 58:1867-1873, 1986.
6. Theologides A: Cancer cachexia. Curr Con Nutr 6:75-94, 1977.
7. Donaldson SS: Nutritional consequences of radiotherapy. Cancer Res 37:2407-2413, 1977.
8. Costa G: Cachexia, the metabolic component of neoplastic disease. Cancer Res 37:2327-2335, 1977.
9. Theologides A: Cancer cachexia, Cancer 43:2004-2012, 1979.
10. Costa G, Donaldson S: The nutritional effects of cancer and its therapy. Nutr Cancer 2:22-29, 1980.
11. Theologides A: Anorexia in cancer: Another speculation on its pathogenesis. Nutr Cancer 2:133-135, 1981.
12. Gold J: Cancer cachexia and gluconeogenesis. Ann NY Acad Sci 230:103-110, 1974.
13. Waterhouse C: How tumors effect host metabolism. Ann NY Acad Sci 230:86-93, 1974.
14. Young VR: Energy metabolism and requirements in the cancer patient. Cancer Res 37:2336-2347, 1977.
15. DeWys WD: Pathophysiology of cancer cachexia: Current understanding and areas for future research. Cancer Res 42:721s-726s, 1982 (suppl).
16. Holroyde CP, Reichard GA: Carbohydrate metabolism in cancer cachexia. Cancer Treat Rep 65:55-59, 1981, (suppl 5).
17. Waterlow JC, Jackson AA: Nutrition and protein turnover in man. Brit Med Bull PS37PS:5-10, 1981.
18. Stein TP: Nutrition and protein turnover: A review. J Parent Ent Nutr 6:444-454, 1982.
19. Mider GB, Alling EL, Morton JJ: The effect of neoplastic and allied diseases on concentrations of the plasma proteins. Cancer 3:56-65, 1950.
20. Fenninger LD, Mider GB: Energy and nitrogen metabolism in cancer. Adv Cancer Res 2:229-253, 1954.
21. Munro HN: Metabolic integration of organs in health and disease. J Parent Ent Nutr 6:271-279, 1982.
22. Lundholm K, Edstrom S, Ekman L, et al: Metabolism in peripheral tissues in cancer patients. Cancer Treat Rep 65:79-83, 1981 (suppl 5).
23. Goodlad GAJ, Tee MK, Clark CM: Leucine oxidation and protein degradation in the extensor digitorum longus and soleus of the tumor-bearing host. Biochem Med 26:143-174, 1981.
24. Jeevanandam M, Tracey KJ, Schiller WR, et al: Effect of total parenteral nutrition on whole body protein kinetics in cachetic patients with benign or malignant disease. J Parent Ent Nutr 12:229-236, 1988.
25. Waldmann TA, Broder S, Strober W: Protein-losing enteropathies in malignancy. Ann NY Acad Sci 230:306-317, 1974.
26. Goodlad GAJ, Clark CM: Protein metabolism in the tumor-bearing host. Acta Chir Scand 498:137-140, 1980 (suppl).
27. Axelrod L, Costa G: The contribution of fat loss to weight loss in cancer. Nutr Cancer 2:81-83, 1980.
28. Waterhouse C: Oxidation and metabolic interconversion in malignant cachexia. Cancer Treat Rep 65:61-66, 1981 (suppl).
29. Knox LS, Crosby LO, Feurer ID, et al: Energy expenditure in malnourished cancer patients. Ann Surg 197:152-162, 1983.
30. Warnold I, Lundholm K, Shersten T: Energy balance and body composition in cancer patients. Cancer Res 38:1801-1807, 1978.
31. Arbeit JM, Lees DE, Corsey R, et al: Resting energy expenditure in controls and cancer patients with localized and diffuse disease. Ann Surg 199:292-298, 1984.
32. Lindmark L, Beenegård K, Edén E, et al: Resting energy expenditure in malnourished patients with and without cancer. Gastroenterology 87:402-408, 1984.
33. DeWys WD: Abnormalities of taste as a remote effect of neoplasm. Ann NY Acad Sci 230:427-434, 1974.
34. DeWys WD, Walters K: Abnormalities of taste sensation in cancer patients. Cancer 36:1888-1896, 1975.
35. Bernstein IL: Etiology of anorexia in cancer. Cancer 58:1881-1886, 1986.
36. Smith JC, Blumsack JT: Learned taste aversion as a factor in cancer therapy. Cancer Treat Rep 65:37-42, 1981 (suppl 5).
37. Broberg DJ, Bernstein L: Candy as a scapegoat in the prevention of food aversions in children receiving chemotherapy. Cancer 60:2344-2347, 1987.
38. Mattes RD, Arnold C, Boraas M: Management of learned food aversions in cancer patients receiving chemotherapy. Cancer Treat Rep 71:1071-1078, 1987.
39. Theologides A: Pathogenesis of cachexia in cancer. Cancer 29:484-488, 1972.
40. Krause R, Humphrey C, Von Meyenfeldt M, et al: A central mechanism for anorexia in cancer: A hypothesis. Cancer Treat Rep 65:15-21, 1981 (suppl).
41. Lowy MT, Yim GKW: Similar feeding profiles in tumor-bearing and dexamethasone-treated rats suggest endorphin depletion in cancer cachexia. Neurosci Abst 6:518, 1980.
42. Bernstein IL: Physiological and psychological mechanisms of cancer anorexia. Cancer Res 42:715s-720s, 1982 (suppl).
43. Dionigi R, Campani M: Nutritional and immunological abnormalities in malignant disease. Acta Chir Scand 507:435-474, 1981 (suppl).
44. Dudrick SJ, Copeland EM III, Daly JM: Cancer and immunocompetence. Acta Chir Scand 498:146-150, 1980 (suppl).
45. Carson JS, Gormican A: Taste acuity and food attitudes of selected patients with cancer. J Am Diet Assoc 70:361-364, 1977.
46. Johnston CA, Keane TJ, Prudo SM: Weight loss in patients receiving radical radiation therapy for head and neck cancer: A prospective study. J Parent Ent Nutr 6:399-402, 1982.
47. DeWys WD: Nutritional care of the cancer patient. J Am Med Assoc 224:374-376, 1980.
48. Hickman DM, Miller RA, Rombeau JL, et al: Serum albumin and body weight as predictors of postoperative course in colorectal cancer. J Parent Ent Nutr 4:314-316, 1980.
49. Gray GE, Gray LK: Validity of anthropometric norms used

in the assessment of hospital patients. J Parent Ent Nutr 3:366-368, 1979.
50. Bastow MD: Anthropometrics revisited. Proc Nutr Soc 41:381-387, 1982.
51. Bistrian BR: Nutritional assessment and therapy of protein-calorie malnutrition in the hospital. J Am Diet Assoc 71:393-397, 1977.
52. National Center for Health Statistics: Anthropometric and Clinical Findings. Rockville, Md, DHEW pub no. (HRA) 75-1229, 1975.
53. Hickman DM, Miller RA, Rombeau JL, et al: Serum albumin and body weight as predictors of postoperative course in colorectal cancer. J Parent Ent Nutr 4:314-316, 1980.
54. Kokal WA: The impact of antitumor therapy on nutrition. Cancer 55:273-278, 1985.
55. Mullen JL, Gertner MH, Buzley GP, et al: Implications of malnutrition in the surgical patient. Arch Surg 114:121-125, 1979.
56. Forbes GB, Bruining GJ: Urinary creatinine excretion and lean body mass. Am J Clin Nutr 29:1359-1366, 1976.
57. Neuman CG, Jelliffe DB, Zerfas A, et al: Nutritional assessment of the child with cancer. Cancer Res 42:6995-7125, 1982 (suppl).
58. Daly JM, Dudrick, SJ, Copeland EM, III. Evaluation of nutritional indices as prognostic indicators in the cancer patient. Cancer 43:925-931, 1979.
59. Dionigi R, Gnes F, Bonera A, et al: Delayed hypersensitivity response (DHR) and infections in surgical cancer patients. Brit J Surg 66:900, 1979.
60. Miller CL: Immunological assays as measurements of nutritional status: A review. J Parent Ent Nutr 2:554-566, 1978.
61. Twomey P, Ziegler D, Rombeau J: Utility of skin testing in nutritional assessment: A critical review. J Parent Ent Nutr 6:50-58, 1982.
62. Blackburn GL, Bistrian BR, Moini BS, et al: Nutritional and metabolic assessment of the hospitalized patient. J Parent Ent Nutr 1:11-22, 1977.
63. Dudrick SJ, Wilmore DW, Vars HM, et al: Long-term total parenteral nutrition with growth, development and positive nitrogen balance. Surgery 65:134-142, 1968.
64. Nixon D, Rudman D, Heymsfield S, et al: Abnormal hyperalimentation response in cachectic cancer patients. Proc Am Assoc Cancer Res Am Soc Clinic Oncol 20:173, 1979 (abstr).
65. Brennan MF: Nutritional support, in Devita VT, Hellman S, Rosenberg SA, eds. Cancer principles and practice of oncology. Philadelphia, Lippincott, 1985.
66. Steiger E, Oram-Smith J, Miller E, et al: Effects of nutrition on tumor growth and tolerance to chemotherapy. J Surg Res 18:455-461, 1975.
67. Copeland EM III, MacFadyen BV Jr, Dudrick SJ: Effect of intravenous hyperalimentation on established delayed hypersensitivity in the cancer patient. Ann Sur 184:60-64, 1976.
68. Deitel M, Vasic V, Alexander M: Specialized nutritional support and cancer. J Parent Ent Nutr 2:671-675, 1978.
69. Kishi T, Iwasawa Y, Itoh H, et al: Nutritional responses of tumor-bearing rats to oral or intravenous feeding. J Parent Ent Nutr 6:295-300, 1982.
70. Torosian MH, Mullen JL, Miller EE, et al: Enhanced tumor response to cycle specific chemotherapy by parenteral amino acid administration. J Parent Ent Nutr 7:337-345, 1983.
71. Torosian MH, Tsou KC, Daly JM, et al: Alteration of tumor cell kinetics by pulse total parenteral nutrition. Cancer 53:1409-1415, 1984.
72. Dempsey DW, Mullen JL: Macronutrient requirements in the malnourished cancer patient. Cancer 55:290-294, 1985.
73. Merrick HW, Long CL, Grecor GP, et al: Energy requirements for cancer patients and the effect of total parenteral nutrition. J Parent Ent Nutr 12:8-14, 1988.
74. Bell SJ, Coffey LM, Blackburn GL: Use of total parenteral nutrition in cancer patients. Top Clin Nutr 1:37-49, 1986.
75. Long CL, Schaffel N, Geiger JW, et al: Metabolic response to injury and illness: Estimation of energy and protein needs from indirect calorimetry and nitrogen balance. J Parent Ent Nutr 3:452-456, 1979.
76. MacBurney MM: Determination of energy and protein needs in the hospitalized patient. Am J Int Ther Clin Nutr (February)10:18-27, 1983.
77. McArdle AH, Palmason C, Morency I, et al: A rationale for enteral feeding as the preferable route for hyperalimentation. Surgery 90:616-623, 1981.
78. Burt ME, Gorschboth CM, Brennan MF: A controlled, prospective randomizing trial evaluating the metabolic effects of enteral and parenteral nutrition in the cancer patient. Cancer 49:1092-1105, 1982.
79. Jones BJ, Payne S, Silk DB: Indications for pump-assisted enteral feeding. Lancet 1:1057-1058, 1980.
80. Donaldson SS, Lenon RA: Alterations of nutritional status: Impact of chemotherapy and radiation therapy. Cancer 43:2036-2052, 1979.
81. Fry ST: Ethical aspects of decision-making in the feeding of cancer patients. Semin Oncol Nurs 2:59-62, 1986.
82. Rombeau JL, Caldwell MD: Enteral and Tube Feeding. Philadelphia, WB Saunders, 1984.
83. Padilla GV, Grant MM: Psychosocial aspects of artificial feeding. Cancer 55:301-304, 1985.
84. Mullen JL: Complications of total parenteral nutrition in the cancer patient. Cancer Treat Rep 65:107-113, 1981 (suppl 5).
85. Klein S, Simes J, Blackburn GL: Total parenteral nutrition and cancer clinical trials. Cancer 58:1378-1386, 1986.
86. Nixon DW: The value of parenteral nutrition support. Cancer 58:1902-1903, 1986.
87. Williams RHP, Heatley RV, Lewis MH, et al: A randomized controlled trial of preoperative intravenous nutrition in patients with stomach cancer. Brit Surg 63:667, 1976.
88. Chwals WJ, Blackburn GL: Perioperative nutritional support in the cancer patient. Surg Clin North Am 66:1137-1165, 1986.
89. Copeland EM III, Dudrick SJ: The importance of parenteral nutrition as an adjunct to cancer treatment, in Johnston IDA (ed): Advances in parenteral nutrition, Lancaster, England, MTP Press, 1978, pp 473-496.
90. Pezner R, Archambeau JO: Critical evaluation of the role of nutritional support for radiation therapy patients. Cancer 55:263-267, 1985.
91. Copeland EM III: Intravenous hyperalimentation and chemotherapy: An update. J Parent Ent Nutr 6:236-239, 1982.
92. Repka FR: Ethical considerations in nutritional support of cancer patients. Top Clin Nutr 1:50-55, 1986.
93. Ryan JA Jr, Abel RM, Abbott WM, et al: Catheter complications in total parenteral nutrition: A prospective study of 200 consecutive patients. N Eng J Med 290:757-761, 1974.
94. Allen JR: Prevention of infection in patients receiving total parenteral nutrition. Acta Chir Scand 507:405-418, 1981 (suppl).
95. Englert D: The role of the nurse in intravenous hyperalimentation in the United States. Acta Chir Scand 507:298-313, 1981 (suppl).
96. Weinsier RL, Bacon J, Butterworth CE, Jr: Central venous

alimentation: A prospective study of the frequency of metabolic abnormalities among medical and surgical patients. J Parent Ent Nutr 6:421-425, 1982.
97. DeWys WD, Kubota TT: Enteral and parenteral nutrition in the care of the cancer patient. J Med Assoc 246:1725-1727, 1981.
98. MacFie J: Metabolic properties of intravenous rat emulsions during total parenteral nutrition (TPN). Nutrition 3:27-28, 1987 (suppl).
99. Buzby GP, Mullen JL, Stein TP, et al: Host tumor interaction and nutrient supply. Cancer 45:2940-2948, 1980.
100. Bonomi P, Pessis D, Bunting N, et al: Megestrol acetate used as primary hormonal therapy in stage D prostate cancer. Semin Oncol 12:36-39, 1985 (suppl).
101. Morgan LR: Megestrol acetate v. tamoxifen in advanced breast cancer in postmenopausal patients. Semin Oncol 12:43-47, 1986 (suppl).
102. Aisner J, Tchekmedyian NS, Moody M, et al: High-dose megestrol acetate for the treatment of advanced breast cancer: dose and toxicities. Semin Oncol 14:48-55, 1987 (suppl).
103. Tchekmedyian NS, Tait N, Abrams J, et al: High-dose megestrol acetate in the treatment of advanced breast cancer. Semin Oncol 15:44-49, 1988 (suppl).
104. Sikic BI, Scudder SA, Ballon SC, et al: High-dose megestrol acetate therapy of ovarian carcinoma: A phase II study by the Northern California Oncology Group. Semin Oncol 13:26-32, 1986 (suppl).
105. Creagan EG, Ingle JN, Schutt AJ, et al: A prospective, randomized controlled trial of megestrol acetate among high-risk patients with resected malignant melanoma. Semin Oncol 12:152-155, 1989 (suppl).
106. Hamburger AW, Parnes H, Gordon GB: Megestrol acetate induced differentiation of 3T3-L adipocytes in vitro. Semin Oncol 15:76-78, 1988 (suppl).
107. Tchekmedyian NS, Tait N, Moody M, et al: Appetite stimulation with megestrol acetate in cachectic cancer patients. Semin Oncol 13:37-44, 1986 (suppl).
108. Tchekmedyian NS, Tair N, Moody M, et al: High-dose megestrol acetate: A possible treatment for cachexia. J Am Med Assoc 257:1195-1198 1987.
109. von Roenn JH, Murphy RL, Weber KM, et al: Megestrol acetate for treatment of cachexia associated with human immunity virus (HIV) infection. Ann Intern Med 109:840-841, 1988.
110. Aisner J, Tchekmedyian NS, Tait N, et al: Studies of high-dose megestrol acetate: Potential applications in cachexia. Semin Oncol 15:68-75, 1988 (suppl).
111. Weiss SM, Worthington PH, Prioleau M, et al: Home total parenteral nutrition in cancer patients. Cancer 50:1210-1213, 1980.

Chapter 25

Hypercalcemia

Jennifer M. Lang-Kummer, RN, MN

INTRODUCTION

Incidence

Primary hyperparathyroidism and malignancy are responsible for 90% of all cases of hypercalcemia (Table 25-1).[1] Overall, the incidence of primary hyperparathyroidism is twice that of malignancy-associated hypercalcemia and is most commonly described as a stable, asymptomatic disorder in an outpatient population of mostly elderly women.[2,3] In hospitalized populations, hypercalcemia due to malignancy is much more common because of more severe symptomatology and the progressive nature of the syndrome when associated with cancer.[4] Since the hypercalcemia of malignancy frequently is associated with a high tumor burden and end-stage disease, hospitalizations for malignancy-associated hypercalcemia tend to be recurrent.

Hypercalcemia is a frequent complication of malignancy. About 10% to 20% of cancer patients will develop hypercalcemia at some point during the course of their disease,[5] but not all cancer patients are at the same risk of developing hypercalcemia. Patients with lung cancer account for 25% to 35% of reported cases, while 20% to 40% of cases occur in patients with breast cancer. Cancers of the stomach, duodenum, colon, rectum, biliary tract, and prostate are rare causes of hypercalcemia.[1,3,4,6,7] The reported frequencies of malignancy-associated hypercalcemia by tumor type are summarized in Table 25-2.

Tumor histology is also a factor in the development of hypercalcemia in cancer patients. Although rare in patients with small cell lung cancer, 23% of patients with squamous epidermoid carcinoma of the lung and 13% of

TABLE 25-1 Causes of Hypercalcemia

Hyperparathyroidism

Malignancy
- Humoral hypercalcemia of malignancy
- Local osteolysis (cell-mediated)
- Mixed humoral and local factors

Granulomatous disorders
- Sarcoidosis
- Tuberculosis
- Other granulomatous diseases

Immobilization
- Spinal cord injury
- Paget's disease
- Fractures

Endocrine
- Hyperthyroidism
- Adrenal insufficiency
- Pheochromocytoma

Drug induced
- Thiazides
- Vitamin D intoxication
- Vitamin A
- Total parenteral nutrition
- Lithium

Renal dialysis and transplantation

TABLE 25-2 Frequency of Malignancy-Associated Hypercalcemia*

Tumor Type	Fisken et al[4] (1980)	Fisken et al[1] (1981)	Mundy and Martin[3] (1982)	Blomqvist[6] (1986)	Combined Data	
					No.	%
Lung	54	24	25	24	127	27.3
Breast	44	20	18	33	115	25.7
Multiple myeloma	14	7	5	8	34	7.3
Lymphoma/leukemia	9	3	5	3	20	4.3
Head and neck	15	7	4	6	32	6.9
Renal	7	6	2	5	20	4.3
Prostate	3	1	2		6	1.3
Gastrointestinal	9	4	4	2	19	4.1
Esophagus	13	4		2	19	4.1
Ureters, bladder, urethra	15				15	3.2
Female genital	14	2			16	3.4
Others	12	4	2	2	20	4.3
Unknown primary	10	7	5		22	4.7
Total patients	219	89	72	85	465	

*Data have been combined from references 1, 3, 4, and 6 as follows: a 1-year prospective general hospital review,[1] a prospective general hospital review,[3] a 32-month retrospective general hospital review,[4] and a 1-year prospective oncology hospital review.[6]

those with large-cell anaplastic carcinoma of the lung will develop hypercalcemia.[8] Squamous histology also is the predominant feature for esophageal, head and neck, and many female reproductive system tumors, together making up 20% of cases.[9,10]

The high frequency of breast and lung cancer diagnoses among patients with hypercalcemia is related to the high overall incidence of these two types of cancers. Multiple myeloma, a relatively rare cancer, is the underlying cause in 10% of malignancy-associated hypercalcemia cases. However, one third of patients with multiple myeloma develop hypercalcemia, a high frequency rate for a disease with low prevalence.[10]

Hypercalcemia of malignancy is usually progressive, causes unpleasant symptoms, can cause the patient to deteriorate rapidly, and may be the cause of death in patients refractory to treatment. In the early stages, symptoms may be vague and nonspecific and can be confused with symptoms resulting from treatments such as radiation therapy, chemotherapy or biologic response modifiers, brain metastases, or progressive disease. The pathophysiology of hypercalcemia is complex and heterogeneous and usually involves a combination of both bone resorption and decreased renal calcium clearance. Treatment approaches are numerous and vary with the degree of hypercalcemia and associated symptomatology, the underlying malignancy, and the patient's overall physical status and prognosis. Nurses play an important role in recognition of patients at risk, patient and family teaching, early recognition and monitoring of symptoms and response to treatment, and, when all else fails, assisting the patient and family in the terminal phases of illness.

Definition

The normal range of serum calcium in adults is 8.5 to 10.5 mg/dL (2.13 to 2.63 mmol/L). Hypercalcemia is considered to exist when the serum calcium level exceeds 11.0 mg/dL (2.75 mmol/L).

Physiology of Calcium Metabolism

Calcium is essential for the maintenance of bones, teeth, clotting mechanisms, and intracellular metabolism. Extracellular calcium plays an important role in influencing cell membrane permeability. As a result, alterations in extracellular calcium levels will affect nerve excitability and muscle contractility. The majority of calcium (99%) is found in bone combined with phosphate. The remaining 1% is divided evenly in the plasma between protein-bound (primarily albumin) and freely ionized forms. It is the freely ionized form that is biologically active, that is, available to influence such physiologic functions as clotting or cell membrane permeability.

Extracellular calcium levels are controlled tightly within a narrow range, primarily through the effects of three systemic hormones: parathyroid hormone (PTH), 1,25-dihydroxyvitamin D, and calcitonin. The secretion of each of these hormones is influenced by circulating levels of ionized calcium through three negative-feedback loops.[11] Calcitonin, secreted by thyroid parafollicular cells, appears to play a minor role in calcium homeostasis, since abnormalities in calcium levels do not occur in the absence of the thyroid gland.[11] PTH and 1,25-dihydroxyvitamin D exert their effects on extracellular calcium levels by controlling movement of calcium across three organs: bone, kidney, and small intestine.

Although 99% of the body's calcium is stored in the skeleton, bone makes little contribution to calcium homeostasis in the healthy adult. The ability to control extracellular calcium levels is influenced primarily by the rate of calcium absorption from the intestine and the kidney's threshold for calcium.[3] Renal regulation of calcium is controlled by PTH and intestinal calcium absorption by 1,25-dihydroxyvitamin D. Only when pathologic states involving increased bone resorption (eg, some malignancies, Paget's disease) occur do other homeostatic mechanisms come into play.

Parathyroid hormone and vitamin D

Secreted by the parathyroid glands, PTH is responsible for minute-to-minute maintenance of calcium homeostasis through direct action on the kidney and indirect action on the intestine. Like other polypeptide hormones, PTH actions are due to binding with hormone-specific receptors on target tissue cell membranes. This interaction generates the production of adenosine 3′:5′-cyclic monophosphate (cAMP), the intracellular mediator for hormonal action.[12] This fact will later be important to the understanding of malignancy-associated hypercalcemia.

The direct effect of PTH on the kidney is used to rapidly regulate and fine tune calcium balance.[3] Normally, the kidneys filter approximately 10 g of calcium each day, 98% of which is reabsorbed by the tubules, resulting in a net excretion of approximately 150 to 200 mg/day.

PTH produces different actions at different sites along the nephron. In the proximal tubule, PTH has at least three activities important in calcium homeostasis: production of nephrogenous cAMP, stimulation of 1-alpha-hydroxylase activity, and inhibition of phosphate resorption. PTH activates PTH-sensitive adenylate cyclase in renal plasma membranes to produce nephrogenous cAMP (NcAMP), which serves as a second messenger influencing calcium transport. PTH's actions on the kidney occur through the formulation and action of NcAMP.[12] PTH-stimulated 1-alpha-hydroxylase activity converts 25-hydroxyvitamin D (the primary form of circulating Vitamin D) to 1,25-dihydroxycholecalciferol (1,25-dihydroxyvitamin D), which influences intestinal calcium absorption, resorption of calcium in the distal tubule, and bone calcium mobilization. In the proximal tubule, calcium is resorbed in parallel with sodium and water rather than under the influence of PTH. Since phosphate resorption is inversely related to calcium resorption, PTH's actions in the proximal tubule are directed at inhibition of water, sodium, calcium, bicarbonate, and phosphate resorption.[12]

PTH-mediated resorption of calcium occurs in the ascending limb of the loop of Henle and in the distal tubule. PTH's effect on fine regulation of calcium resorption, which takes place in the distal tubule, is enhanced by 1,25-dihydroxyvitamin D.[11,12]

In the skeleton, PTH plays a mediating role in bone resorption by stimulating the number and activity of bone osteoclasts, leading to release of calcium and phosphate into the circulation.[12]

A drop in extracellular calcium stimulates release of PTH from the parathyroid glands; this in turn stimulates renal hydroxylation of the precursor 25-hydroxyvitamin D to form 1,25-dihydroxyvitamin D. The actions of 1,25-dihydroxyvitamin D tend to produce an intestinal calcium-binding protein, absorb intestinal calcium and thus elevate serum calcium levels. On a daily basis, the net intestinal absorption of calcium is roughly equivalent to the amount excreted by the kidneys (150 to 250 mg).

Homeostatic responses to increased calcium loads

With an increased calcium load, the secretion of PTH is suppressed; this decreases physiologic calcium release from bone and inhibits intestinal calcium absorption. This inhibitory effect occurs as a result of decreased renal synthesis of 1,25-dihydroxyvitamin D. In addition, decreased PTH results in increased urinary calcium excretion. The kidney is the principal route by which a calcium load can be cleared.[10] To protect against an increased extracellular fluid calcium level of hypercalcemic proportions, the kidney can increase calcium excretion approximately fivefold. Renal adaptation to an excess calcium load is limited to an excretion rate of approximately 600 mg/day.[11] Mild hypercalcemia impairs glomerular filtration and urinary concentrating ability, creating a polyuric state. This predisposes a patient to dehydration and prerenal azotemia. Once the renal compensatory mechanisms are exceeded, further renal insufficiency enhances calcium resorption and phosphate wasting in the proximal tubule, further exacerbating the development of hypercalcemia and renal failure.[10]

Bone remodeling

Skeletal bone serves as the body's calcium reservoir. In the healthy adult before middle life, bone resorption and formation are in balance and occur as a renewal process in response to the need for repair and to local mechanical factors such as weight bearing and fluid pressure.[11,13] The bone cells primarily concerned with the process of bone formation and resorption, known as bone remodeling, are the osteoclasts, osteocytes, and osteoblasts (Table 25-3). Incitement of bone remodeling is thought to be directed at the osteocyte, which prepares the bone surface for osteoclastic activity and liberates chemical messengers that not only attract osteoclasts but also initiate osteoblast precursor proliferation.[13] Thus, normal bone remodeling activity can be said to be "coupled"; bone resorption is coupled with bone formation. "Uncoupling" refers to the failure of bone formation to follow the resorption process.[14]

TABLE 25-3 Cells Responsible for Bone Remodeling*

Cell	Origin	Function
Osteoblasts	Undifferentiated mesenchymatous cells	Bone forming cells that secrete collagen; differentiation is promoted by PTH
Osteocytes	Osteoblasts buried within osteocytic lacunae in bone matrix	Responsive to PTH; liberates collagenase, which prepares bone surface for osteoclast resorption; communicates with osteoclasts through liberation of prostaglandin E
Osteoclasts	Mononuclear* bone marrow cells	Multinuclear bone cells that erode and resorb previously formed bone; chemotactic factors attract to osteocyte prepared bone; differentiation and fusion promoted by IL-1, 1,25-dihydroxyvitamin D; function inhibited by calcitonin

*Osteoclast precursors are mononuclear cells that fuse to form large multinuclear units.

PTH, parathyroid hormone.

Source: Adapted from Taylor BM, Weller LA: Hypercalcemia, in Groenwald SL (ed): Cancer Nursing: Principles and Practice (ed 1), 1987, p 292.

The location and frequency of bone remodeling activity is influenced by mechanical factors such as weight bearing, by the activity of the osteotropic hormones PTH, 1,25-dihydroxyvitamin D, and calcitonin, and by the presence of local factors such as prostaglandins, regulatory proteins, and constituents of the organic matrix (Table 25-4).[13] The action of PTH, mediated by intracellular cAMP, promotes the cellular differentiation of osteocytes, osteoblasts, and their precursors, while 1,25-dihydroxyvitamin D promotes the differentiation and fusion of osteoclasts. At physiologic levels of these hormones, bone remodeling takes place in an orderly and coupled manner (Figure 25-1). High levels of PTH and 1,25-dihydroxyvitamin D, on the other hand, stimulate large volumes of osteocytic and osteoclastic bone breakdown and resorption of calcified matrix.[12] The presence of an elevated serum acid phosphatase can indicate the presence of osteoclastic bone catabolism, as seen in metastatic skeletal involvement as well as other disease states. An elevated serum alkaline phosphatase indicates osteoblastic activity, which can be seen in states of high bone turnover: Paget's disease, prostate cancer with blastic skeletal involvement, or healing of a bone fracture.

Since normal bone remodeling is a "coupled" process,

TABLE 25-4 Local Factors Influencing Bone Remodeling*

Factor[a]	Source	Action
IL-1	Monocyte/ macrophages	Stimulates production and fusion of osteoclast precursors (action inhibited by calcitonin but not PGE)
PGE	Tumor cells Monocytes Osteocytes	Stimulate osteoclast bone resorption, shape change, collagenase release Mediate release of PDGF, EGF, stimulate lymphokine OAF
TNF-alpha (cachectin)	Monocytes	Stimulate osteoclast activity through an intermediate cell (?)
TNF-beta (lymphotoxin)	Lymphocytes	Stimulate osteoclast activity
IFN-γ	Lymphocytes	Inhibit cytokine-mediated bone resorption
CSF-GM	Lymphocytes	Simulate monocyte-macrophage precursors; increase proliferation of osteoclast precursors
CSF-1, CSF-M	Monocytes	Stimulate monocyte-macrophage precursors; increase proliferation of osteoclast precursors

*Although all the local factors described have been shown to mediate bone remodeling, the precise role each factor plays in the hypercalcemia of malignancy is uncertain.

CSF-1, CSF-M, colony-stimulating factor-1; *CSF-GM,* Granulocyte-macrophage colony-stimulating factor; *EGF,* epidermal growth factor; *IFN-γ,* interferon gamma; *IL-1,* Interleukin-1; *OAF,* osteoclast-activating factor; *PDGF,* platelet derived growth factor; *PGE,* prostaglandin E; *TNF,* tumor necrosis factor.

Source: Data derived from Mundy,[11] Broadus et al,[16] Mundy et al,[17] and Gowen et al.[18]

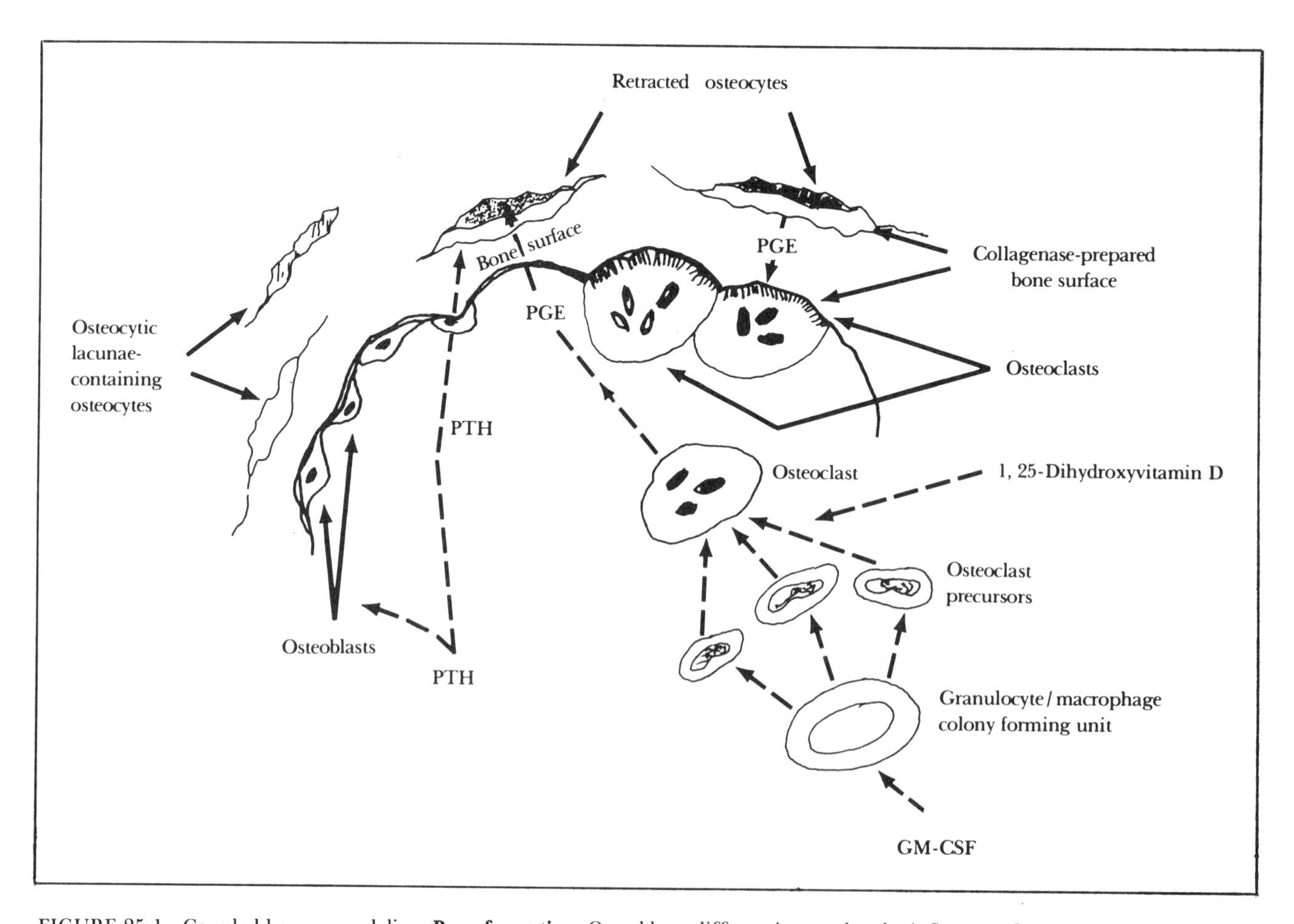

FIGURE 25-1 Coupled bone remodeling. **Bone formation:** Osteoblasts differentiate under the influence of PTH, secreting collagen and mineralizing bone. Some osteoblasts become buried within osteocytic lacunae during bone-forming process to become osteocytes. Osteoblasts recycle C^{2+} liberated during bone resorption process to mineralize new bone. **Bone resorption:** Osteocytes retract within lacunae under influence of PTH-liberating collagenase and messengers such as PGE. Collagenase prepares bone surface for osteoclast resorption. PGE attracts osteoclasts to bone surface. Osteoclast precursors, derived from granulocyte/macrophage colony forming units under influence of GM-CSF, differentiate and fuse to form multinuclear osteoclasts under influence of 1,25-dihydroxyvitamin D. (*GM-CSF,* Granulocyte/macrophage colony stimulating factor; *PGE,* prostaglandin E; *PTH,* parathyroid hormone.)

TABLE 25-5 Humoral Factors Influencing Bone Remodeling

Factor	Source	Action
PTH	Parathyroid glands	Stimulates cellular differentiation of osteoblasts, osteocytes; promotes coupled remodeling; affects lymphocyte proliferation and lymphokine production; stimulates renal-1-alpha-hydroxylase activity*; physiologic NcAMP excretion
Parathyroid-like hormone	Tumor cells, usually squamous histology	↑ Osteocyte and osteoclast activity; ↓ osteoblast activity (uncoupled); no stimulation of renal-1-alpha-hydroxylase activity; ↑ renal tubular calcium reabsorption; ↑ NcAMP excretion and renal phosphate wasting
1,25-dihydroxyvitamin D	Renal hydroxylation of 25-hydroxyvitamin D; Some lymphoma cells produce 1-alpha-hydroxylase; also produced by macrophages	Enhances intestinal Ca^{2+} transport; promotes differentiation and fusion of osteoclast precursors and macrophages; inhibits lymphocyte mitogenesis and IL-2 production; ? stimulation of IL-1
Calcitonin	Thyroid parafollicular cells	Inhibits osteoclasts ? by inhibiting IL-1; affects lymphocyte proliferation and lymphokine production
Transforming growth factor-alpha† TGF-alpha	Most solid tumors	Binds to EGF; stimulates production of osteoclast progenitors; ? produces PGE

*1-alpha-hydroxylase is released from renal plasma membrane in response to PTH and acts on the circulating form of Vitamin D (25-hydroxyvitamin D) to form 1,25-dihydroxyvitamin D, the mediator of intestinal calcium transport.

†There is circumstantial, but not confirmatory, evidence that TGF plays a role in human humoral hypercalcemia of malignancy.[11]

EGF, Epidermal growth factor; *IL-1,* interleukin-1; *PGE,* Prostaglandin E; *PTH,* parathyroid hormone; *TGF,* transforming growth factor.

skeletal calcium generally plays an insignificant role in calcium homeostasis. Although not important to the understanding of calcium homeostasis in the healthy adult, local and humoral factors that influence the liberation of calcium from bone in pathologic states assume more significance.

PATHOPHYSIOLOGY

In the 1960s, malignancy-associated hypercalcemia was thought to be a simple paraneoplastic syndrome caused either by an excess of circulating PTH or by bone resorption mediated by primary or metastatic tumor cells in direct contact with bone.[2,11,16] We now know that malignancy-associated hypercalcemia is not related to either of the two mechanisms above but is a complex metabolic complication in which bone resorption exceeds both bone formation and the kidney's ability to excrete extracellular calcium.[11] Several mechanisms are involved that implicate abnormalities in calcium transport in bone, kidney, and intestine at both the humoral and local level.[11]

Humoral, or tumor-produced, circulating factors that have been implicated in the pathophysiology of malignancy-associated hypercalcemia include a parathyroid hormone–like factor, transforming growth factors, and 1,25-dihydroxyvitamin D. Local factors implicated include a family of cytokine *osteoclast-activating factors.*

Humoral Hypercalcemia of Malignancy

Parathyroid hormone–like factors

Hypercalcemia that develops in patients with solid tumors without bone metastases is thought to be due to a circulating tumor–produced parathyroid hormone–like factor (Table 25-5). Patients with humorally mediated hypercalcemia (formerly known as pseudohyperparathyroidism) do not manifest the same biochemical profile and bone remodeling abnormalities as patients with primary hyperparathyroidism. In primary hyperparathyroidism, a parathyroid gland adenoma secretes excessive PTH, which stimulates intestinal and renal calcium absorption and renal phosphate wasting. Bone remodeling activity is accelerated, with a "coupled" increase in both osteoclastic and osteoblastic activity.[19] Hypercalcemia occurs due to the combined action of PTH and 1,25-dihydroxyvitamin D on bone and kidney; 1,25-dihydroxyvitamin D acts on the gut.

The two primary biochemical markers associated with hyperparathyroidism are increased secretion of NcAMP and elevated levels of 1,25-dihydroxyvitamin D, reflecting the action of parathyroid hormone on renal PTH receptors. Patients with humoral hypercalcemia of malignancy (HHM) are similar to patients with primary hyperparathyroidism in that they do secrete high levels of NcAMP, but, conversely, they do not have elevated levels of 1,25-dihydroxyvitamin D and do not have increased intestinal calcium absorption rates. Additionally, HHM is accompanied by an "uncoupling" of osteoblastic and osteoclastic activities such that bone resorption exceeds bone formation, and hypercalcemia and hypercalciuria occur to a greater degree than in primary hyperparathyroidism.[20]

The peptide responsible for humoral hypercalcemia of malignancy, identified in 1987, is highly homologous to but not exactly like PTH and therefore could bind to some but not all PTH receptors.[21-23] This could explain the differences between the intestinal calcium transport mechanisms in patients with HHM and patients with hyperparathyroidism. In addition, the PTH-like factor appears to be more effective in stimulating bone osteoclastic activity than is PTH.[21,22] Whether this PTH-like factor is singularly responsible for HHM has not been established.[25] Other factors have been implicated in HHM (Table 25-6).

Transforming growth factors

Several authors have postulated that perhaps the PTH-like factor is responsible for the renal effects of HHM, while another agent such as transforming growth factor alpha (TGF-alpha) may be responsible for bone-resorbing activity.[10,11,23,26] In vitro evidence indicates that TGF-alpha plays an important role in increased bone resorption in some solid tumors.[11]

1,25-dihydroxyvitamin D

Hypercalcemia in patients with Hodgkin's and non-Hodgkin's lymphomas historically has been attributed either to the direct action of skeletal metastases on bone cells or to the production of an osteoclast-activating factor.[2] However, several investigators have reported the presence of elevated levels of circulating 1,25-dihydroxyvitamin D in hypercalcemic patients with Hodgkin's disease and non-Hodgkin's lymphoma without bony metastases that resolved with effective treatment of the primary disease.[27-30] A proposed mechanism of action is tumor production of 1-alpha-hydroxylase, which acts on the circulating substrate 25-hydroxyvitamin D to produce, independent of parathyroid hormone, high circulating levels of 1,25-dihydroxyvitamin D that enhance bone resorption and increased intestinal calcium transport.[30,31]

Concomitant hyperparathyroidism

Although hypercalcemia is associated with malignancy in most cancer patients, primary hyperparathyroidism has been reported to occur rarely in patients with cancer.[32] On the other hand, humoral hypercalcemia of malignancy is rarely a presenting finding in patients with occult carcinomas. Hypercalcemia of malignancy generally is associated with large tumor masses and is easily diagnosed.[33]

TABLE 25-6 Humoral Hypercalcemia of Malignancy

Tumor Type	Implicated Factor	Features
Squamous cell carcinoma Lung Head and neck Bladder Ovary Renal Prostate Pancreas Some breast T-cell leukemia due to HTLV-1 Pheochromocytoma	PTH-like factor ?± TGF-alpha	Uncoupled bone resorption ↑ Excretion of NcAMP ↑ Renal Ca^{2+} absorption ↑ Renal phosphate wasting; low serum levels of 1,25-dihydroxyvitamin D
Some Hodgkin's and non-Hodgkin's lymphomas	Tumor production of 1,25-dihydroxyvitamin D	↑ Bone resorption and ↑ intestinal Ca^{2+} transport due to ↑ levels of 1,25-dihydroxyvitamin D

HTLV-1, Human T-cell leukemia/lymphoma virus 1; *NcAMP,* nephrogenous cyclic AMP; *PTH,* parathyroid hormone; *TGF,* transforming growth factor.

Local Osteolytic Hypercalcemia

The original theory that hypercalcemia in cancer patients with skeletal involvement such as breast cancer, lymphoma, and multiple myeloma occurred due to the direct osteolytic effect of tumor cells on bone matrix has been replaced. The current consensus is that the causes of hypercalcemia in patients having cancers with skeletal metastases are more heterogeneous, particularly in breast cancer.[34,35] Many cancers invoke their hypercalcemic effect through a combination of humoral and local cell-mediated mechanisms (Table 25-7). Among the implicated factors are prostaglandins of the E series (PGE), TGF-alpha, and the cytokines known as osteoclast-activating factor.[10,11,16]

Prostaglandins

PGE_2 is a potent osteoclast stimulator and has been demonstrated to mediate hypercalcemia by stimulating bone resorption in several animal models.[11] A prostaglandin synthesis inhibitor, indomethacin, was shown to alleviate hypercalcemia in animals, but similar results have not been found in humans. Fewer than 10% of patients with hypercalcemia have been found to be responsive to optimal doses of indomethacin.[10,11,25]

Breast cancer

Hypercalcemia occurs in up to 40% of women with breast cancer.[35] Although the majority of patients with hypercalcemia have widespread skeletal metastases, not all patients with metastases develop hypercalcemia.[34,35] Cultured breast cancer cells were once thought to be capable of direct bone resorption without participation of osteoclasts, but new evidence indicates that osteoclasts do par-

TABLE 25-7 Local Osteolytic Hypercalcemia

Tumor Type	Implicated Factor	Features
Most breast carcinomas with skeletal involvement	? Production of PGE_2	↑ Osteoclastic bone resorption with ↓ excretion of NcAMP; ↓ 1,25-dihydroxyvitamin D production
Some estrogen-receptor-positive breast cancer with skeletal involvement	PGE release mediated by tamoxifen, androgens, or estrogens	Self-limiting hypercalcemia within 1 month of starting therapy—"tumor flare"
Multiple myeloma	OAFS: IL-1, TNF-alpha, TNF-beta, CSF-GM, CSF-1, ? mediated by PGEs	↑ Osteoclastic bone resorption without bone formation; ↓ GFR; ↓ intestinal Ca^{2+} absorption; Normal renal Ca^{2+} resorption except as influenced by ↓ GFR
T-cell leukemias and lymphomas with skeletal involvement; Hodgkin's disease	? Combination of OAF and 1,25-dihydroxyvitamin D; other lymphokines	↑ osteoclastic bone resorption; ± synthesis of 1,25-dihydroxyvitamin D

CSF-GM, Granulocyte/macrophage colony-stimulating factor; *GFR,* glomerular filtration rate; *HTLV-1,* human T-cell leukemia/lymphoma virus 1; *IL-1,* interleukin-1; *NcAMP,* nephrogenous cyclic adenosine monophosphate; *OAF,* osteoclast activating factor; *PGE_2,* prostaglandin E_2.

ticipate in vitro and in vivo.[17] Therefore, bone resorption due to PGE-mediated osteolysis is thought to be a more likely cause than direct bone resorption. Unfortunately, hypercalcemia in breast cancer patients is generally unresponsive to prostaglandin inhibitors, making understanding of the precise role of PGE in the pathogenesis of hypercalcemia difficult.

Some patients with estrogen-receptor-positive breast cancers suddenly develop hypercalcemia that may be associated with bone pain within 1 month of starting estrogens, androgens, or tamoxifen. Known as tumor-flare, it is associated with a temporary period of accelerated tumor growth shortly after beginning additive hormonal therapy. Tamoxifen-induced hypercalcemia occurs 4 to 10 days after the initiation of hormonal therapy and has a rapid onset.[36] Tumor flare is generally self-limiting and is thought to indicate a hormonally responsive tumor. The hypercalcemia is probably due to tumor release of PGE, which accelerates bone resorption. A decision to withdraw the hormone temporarily or to treat the patient with indomethacin or glucocorticoids (one of the few situations in which indomethacin may be effective) without terminating the hormonal agent is usually influenced by the degree of hypercalcemia and its responsiveness to therapy.[9,11,36]

PTH-like hormone factors appear to play a greater role in the pathogenesis of hypercalcemia in breast cancer patients with and without skeletal metastases than was previously appreciated. Isales et al[35] reported that four of 17 patients followed prospectively developed hypercalcemia in the absence of skeletal metastases and six of 17 hypercalcemic breast cancer patients had elevations of NcAMP. Using current criteria (elevated NcAMP excretion), 35% of the patients in this study developed humoral hypercalcemia of malignancy.

Hematologic malignancies

Multiple myeloma accounts for 10% of all hypercalcemia in malignancy, while the lymphomas account for 3%.[10] HTLV-I- and HTLV-II-associated T-cell lymphoma/leukemias are very commonly associated with hypercalcemia.[37] In lymphomas, hypercalcemia usually is seen in patients with bone involvement.[10]

Again, the possible causative factors are diverse. Osteoclast-activating factors IL-1 and tumor necrosis factors alpha and beta have been implicated as causes of hypercalcemia in patients with multiple myeloma as well as those with some lymphomas. Other candidates are bone-resorbing substances such as CSF-GM and CSF-1 (CSF-M).

Humoral factors also play a part in multiple myeloma and lymphoma. As previously discussed, elevated 1,25-dihydroxyvitamin D levels have been found in lymphoma patients without bone metastases. Secretion of NcAMP also has been demonstrated in half of patients with myeloma and in some patients with leukemia.[20] Hypercalcemia in patients with myeloma is almost always accompanied by renal insufficiency due to impaired glomerular filtration caused by Bence Jones protein, uric acid nephropathy, pyelonephritis, or occasionally amyloidosis, which results in an inability to clear ultrafilterable calcium through the glomerulus.[11,36]

Other factors

Immobilization, dehydration, poor nutrition, inappropriate use of diuretics, and generalized wasting all play an important role in the pathogenesis of malignancy-associated hypercalcemia.

Local mechanical forces such as weight bearing are important to stimulate bone formation. Individuals with a preexisting state of high bone turnover are more likely to experience increased hypercalciuria and bone resorption when immobilized.[10] Passive range-of-motion exercises may be useful in maintaining muscle and joint mobility but are not helpful in preventing hypercalcemia due to immobilization. Weight bearing is more important.

Dehydration occurs as a result of diminished fluid intake (due to nausea, vomiting, and anorexia) as well as polyuria and inability to concentrate urine due to hypercalcemic interference with the effects of antidiuretic hormone (ADH) on the renal tubules.

Thiazide and potassium-sparing diuretics act on the

TABLE 25-8 Symptoms of Hypercalcemia

System	Mechanism	Signs and Symptoms
Gastrointestinal	Depressed smooth muscle contractility causes delayed gastric emptying and decreased intestinal motility	Early: Nausea, vomiting, anorexia, constipation Late: Obstipation and ileus; weight loss
Neuromuscular	Depressed excitability of neurons	Early: lethargy, drowsiness; restlessness, mood changes Mid: mental status changes, poor calculation, decreased attention span, somnolence Late: psychotic behavior, marked confusion, slurred speech, stupor, coma
	Impaired electrical conduction and cell membrane permeability in skeletal muscles	Early: muscle weakness, fatigue Late: profound muscle weakness, hypotonia
	? PGE-mediated bone resorption	Bone pain
Renal	Interference with action of ADH on renal collecting tubules → inability to concentrate urine and then volume contraction followed by ↓ GFR	Early: polyuria Mid: polydipsia Late: prerenal azotemia
Cardiovascular	Impaired electrical conduction and cell membrane permeability; altered intracellular metabolism; arterial vasoconstriction	Early: hypertension Mid: sinus bradycardia, prolonged PR interval, shortened QT interval, dysrhythmias especially in digitalized patients Late: Prolonged QT interval due to widened T wave, coving of ST segment, AV block, asystole

ADH, Antidiuretic hormone; *Early,* mild hypercalcemia (<12 mg/dL); *GFR,* glomerular filtration rate; *Late,* severe hypercalcemia (>15 mg/dL); *Mid,* moderate hypercalcemia (12 to 15 mg/dL); *PGE,* prostaglandin E.

distal tubule to enhance calcium but not sodium reabsorption. Thus administration of such diuretics not only produces volume depletion but a hypercalcemic effect.

CLINICAL MANIFESTATIONS

The clinical presentation of hypercalcemia is variable, influenced not only by the degree of hypercalcemia, the rapidity of onset, and the patient's general physical and mental condition, but also by the kidney's ability to maintain calcium homeostasis. Hypercalcemia that develops slowly and gradually is associated with few if any symptoms. Conversely, a rapidly expanding tumor burden associated with a progressively increasing rate of bone resorption may suddenly overwhelm renal compensatory mechanisms, producing a rapid and symptomatic rise in serum calcium levels. This is particularly true in HHM.

Signs and Symptoms

Because of calcium's role in maintaining cell membrane permeability, hypercalcemia produces symptoms in almost all organ systems. Symptoms are numerous, vague, and nonspecific. Since many cancer patients with hypercalcemia have large tumor burdens and will die in 3 to 6 months (particularly those with HHM), symptoms of hypercalcemia may be confused with those of end-stage disease.[3] Recognition of symptoms is important for early identification and treatment of the syndrome to reduce the risk of coma, irreversible renal failure, or a terminal cardiac event. Common symptoms of hypercalcemia are nausea, vomiting, polyuria, polydipsia, anorexia, weakness, fatigue, and confusion (Table 25-8).

Gastrointestinal

Elevated extracellular calcium levels depress smooth muscle contractility, leading to delayed gastric emptying and decreased gastrointestinal motility. Anorexia, nausea, and vomiting are early and common symptoms in hypercalcemic patients.[39] Constipation may also occur. These symptoms may be exacerbated by the disease itself or by cytotoxic therapy.[3] The development of obstipation and ileus are late findings associated with high serum calcium levels and are probably exacerbated by dehydration.

Neuromuscular

Elevated extracellular calcium levels depress the excitability of central nervous system (CNS) neurons, leading primarily to alterations in mental status.[39] Some of the neuromuscular symptoms of hypercalcemia are weakness, confusion, lethargy, drowsiness, and personality change. Patients with rapidly advancing hypercalcemia may lapse into a stupor or coma, usually at serum calcium levels greater than 15 mg/dL. Neuromuscular manifestations usually are much more prominent in the elderly and may persist for several days after normalization of serum calcium levels.

Personality changes at first occur subtly and are often unnoticed by the individual or family. Extreme restlessness, irritability, overt confusion, and progressive deterioration in cognitive function may develop. In a study of hospitalized patients with hypercalcemia, Mahon[39] reported increasing problems with memory span, ability to calculate, attention span, inappropriate conversation, slow mentation, and inappropriate behavior in patients with corrected serum calcium levels greater than 12.1 mg/dL.

Impairment of skeletal muscle electrical conduction and cell membrane permeability leads to profound muscle weakness and hypotonia, usually with severe hypercalcemia.[40]

Renal

Hypercalcemia interferes with the action of ADH on the kidney's collecting tubules, causing an inability to concentrate urine and polyuria (a syndrome similar to nephrogenic diabetes insipidus). Subsequent volume contraction, which is exacerbated by nausea and vomiting, decreases the glomerular filtration rate (GFR). Decreased GFR stimulates sodium and water resorption in the proximal tubule. Since sodium and calcium are absorbed in parallel, hypercalcemia is exacerbated. In addition, evidence indicates that TGF-alpha also acts on the kidney's proximal tubule to enhance the resorption of calcium, while distal tubular calcium resorption is influenced by PTH-like factors.[11] The downward spiral continues with the development of nitrogen retention, acidosis, and eventual renal failure. Renal failure is most common in patients with multiple myeloma.[11]

Cardiovascular

Calcium ions affect not only smooth, skeletal, and cardiac muscle contractility and cell membrane permeability but also influence conduction of electrical impulses within the heart. Hypertension may occur due to the direct effect of hypercalcemia on arterial smooth muscle.[40] Hypercalcemia results in bradycardia, shortened QT intervals in moderate hypercalcemia, and prolonged QT intervals with calcium levels above 16 mg/dL. Prolonged QT intervals are actually due to widening of the T wave, with coving of the ST segment.[40,42] Prolonged PR intervals and significant dysrhythmias may also occur, particularly in patients taking digitalis.[41] Since the effects of digitalis are mediated partly by membrane-bound calcium, digitalis toxicity may be potentiated.[40] Atrioventricular block and asystole may occur when the serum calcium level reaches 18.0 mg/dL.[39]

Laboratory Assessment

An elevated serum calcium (corrected for abnormal protein values) is diagnostic. Calcium is found in the serum in three forms: 45% protein bound (primarily to albumin), 45% freely ionized, and 10% complexed to anions such as sulfate, phosphate, or citrate. It is the freely ionized form that is biologically active. Normally, freely ionized calcium is in equilibrium with protein-bound calcium. When there is an abnormality in serum protein levels, serum calcium determinations may not represent true ionized calcium levels. Rarely, in multiple myeloma, a monoclonal protein may have an affinity for calcium and be associated with elevated protein-bound but normal ionized calcium levels, thus creating an illusion of an elevated serum calcium level.[3]

The more common finding in cancer patients is hypoalbuminemia, in which more calcium may be ionized due to low levels of serum albumin available for binding. Ionized serum calcium levels provide a more accurate means of measuring calcium when serum proteins are abnormal. A normal serum calcium is 8.5 to 10.5 mg/dL (2.13 to 2.63 mmol/L), while a normal serum ionized calcium level is 4.2 to 5.2 mg/dL (1.05 to 1.3 mmol/L). When ionized calcium levels are not available, total serum calcium levels can be corrected to reflect more accurately ionized serum calcium. A frequently used formula is:

$$\text{Corrected calcium (mg/dL)} = \text{Measured calcium} + [4 - \text{albumin (g/dL)}] \times 0.8$$

or

$$\text{Corrected calcium (mmol/L)} = \text{Measured calcium} + [40 - \text{albumin (g/dL)}] \times 0.02$$

Where, in the first example, 0.8 mg/dL of calcium is added (to the laboratory determination of serum calcium) for every 1 g/dL the reported serum albumin is less than 4.0. Four is used as the mid-range normal value for serum albumin.[40]

TREATMENT

Hypercalcemia results from a combination of excessive bone resorption and impaired renal calcium excretion. Treatment therefore must be directed at both causes. Most important initially is improving renal calcium excretion by correcting those factors impairing renal function, usually dehydration and diminished GFR. Second, bone resorption must be inhibited either by eliminating the underlying cause (treating the primary tumor) or by inhibiting osteoclast function to prevent recurrence of hypercalcemia. Unless the primary tumor or skeletal metastases can be controlled, all other interventions tend to be palliative. Although there currently are several pharmacologic approaches to treatment of patients with hypercalcemia, there is little scientific evidence to support the efficacy of one intervention program over another, nor are there any

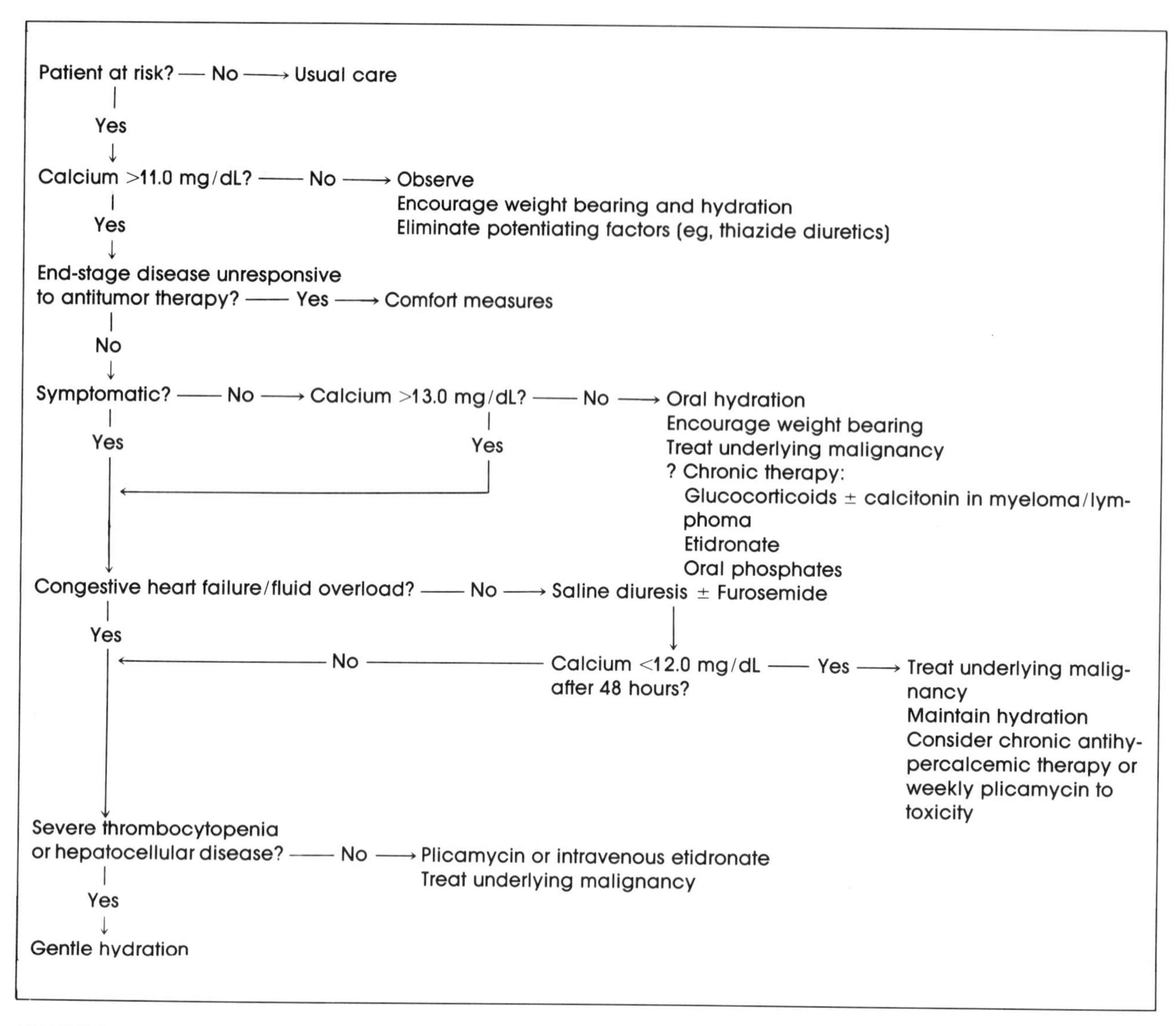

FIGURE 25-2 A medical approach to the management of hypercalcemia. This algorithm is intended to demonstrate a rational approach to hypercalcemia for the benefit of planning nursing interventions. It should not be considered a guideline for medical practice.

clear guidelines that indicate whether certain patients require more specific therapy.[3,43] A general approach to management of hypercalcemia is summarized in Figure 25-2.

The degree of urgency with which the hypercalcemia is treated depends on the serum calcium level and the patient's symptomatology. Patients with corrected serum calcium levels above 13.0 mg/dl or symptomatic patients with a calcium level less than 13.0 mg/dl should be treated aggressively, whereas asymptomatic patients with lower calcium levels require specific but less urgent treatment.[3,11]

In patients with recurrent humoral hypercalcemia and end-stage disease where all cancer treatment options have been exhausted, physicians may, after discussion with the patient and family, elect not to treat further episodes of hypercalcemia, allowing the patient to lapse into a coma and, shortly thereafter, die.

General Measures

Initial measures should include correcting volume contraction and removing factors that may exacerbate hypercalcemia such as thiazide diuretics, vitamins A and D, and, in some breast cancer patients, hormonal agents. Discontinuation of tamoxifen is not always indicated. Medications whose actions are potentiated by hypercalcemia, such as digoxin, should be adjusted.

Mobilization in an effort to promote weight bearing should be encouraged whenever possible. Except in some patients with lymphoma in whom elevated levels of 1,25-dihydroxyvitamin D enhance intestinal calcium absorption, restriction of dietary calcium is without scientific basis. However, calcium supplementation in intravenous hyperalimentation formulas should be discontinued because of the intravenous route of administration.

Hydration and Saline Diuresis

The cornerstone of all hypercalcemic therapy is to expand volume, correct dehydration and renal insufficiency, and promote calciuresis. In patients with mild hypercalcemia and normal renal function, oral hydration may be all that is required.[44] In symptomatic patients, intravenous hydration is indicated. Since sodium and calcium are excreted in parallel, calciuresis can be promoted by administering high volumes of normal saline, usually at 250 to 300 mL/hr, until corrected serum calcium levels are less than 12 mg/dL. Measurement of fluid intake and output, body weight, and frequent assessment for signs of fluid overload are important. Patients with compromised cardiovascular function or renal failure may need central venous pressure and cardiac monitoring during therapy. Hypokalemia, hypomagnesia, and hypophosphatemia may occur.[3] Hyperosmolar states due to some patients' inability to excrete high sodium loads have been observed.[3]

Loop Diuretics

Once rehydration has been established, loop diuretics such as furosemide may be used to enhance calcium excretion. Use of such diuretics, which block calcium and sodium reabsorption across the ascending limb of Henle's loop, is controversial. Mild to moderate hypercalcemia can usually be managed by saline diuresis alone, and the benefit of adding furosemide to saline diuresis has not been documented.[3,11] There is a difference between the diuretic and the calciuretic doses of furosemide.[3] Doses of 20 mg every 4 to 6 hr are usually sufficient to manage overhydration in patients with compromised cardiovascular or renal function.[44]

To achieve a calciuretic effect, the recommended dose of furosemide is 80 to 100 mg every 1 to 2 hr.[40] Patients treated with high doses of furosemide must be monitored in an intensive care setting to ensure that fluid and electrolyte losses are carefully replaced and that extracellular fluid volume is not depleted. Depletion of extracellular fluid volume in the hypercalcemic patient ensures reabsorption of calcium from the proximal tubule and further exacerbation of hypercalcemia. Side effects of high-dose furosemide are severe potassium and magnesium loss, but calcium levels can be decreased 2 to 4 mg/dL in 24 to 48 hours with this approach.[40]

Calcitonin

Calcitonin, a 32 amino acid polypeptide normally produced by the parafollicular cells of the thyroid gland, produces transient (24 to 72 hours) inhibition of bone resorption. Onset of action is rapid, with declines in serum calcium within 4 to 6 hours of the first dose. It is the preferred treatment when saline diuresis or plicamycin (Mithracin) therapy is contraindicated (eg, thrombocytopenia, renal or cardiac failure). Best responses are seen in patients with multiple myeloma and other hematologic neoplasms.[3] Unfortunately, inhibition of bone resorption is short and "escape" from the therapeutic effect limits its usefulness, but use of calcitonin can buy time while antineoplastic therapy is started. Administration in combination with glucocorticoids appears to be more effective.[44] Other disadvantages include the expense of the preparation (approximately $100/day) and the need for parenteral injections. Synthetic calcitonin is administered subcutaneously at a starting dose of 4 to 12 units/kg body weight every 8 to 12 hours.

Glucocorticoids

Glucocorticoids (prednisone and hydrocortisone) are most effective in hypercalcemia associated with multiple myeloma, other hematologic diseases, and sometimes breast carcinoma. Hypercalcemia associated with other solid tumors is responsive only 30% of the time.[44] Glucocorticoids may be effective in hypercalcemia due to myeloma because they inhibit bone resorption mediated by osteoclast-activating factors or because they cause a decrease in calcium either by a direct tumor cytolytic effect or by inhibiting tumor production of prostaglandin.[40] Glucocorticoids also increase urinary calcium excretion and decrease intestinal calcium absorption. This latter effect may be important in those lymphomas that can hydroxylate 25-hydroxyvitamin D to produce high circulating 1,25-dihydroxyvitamin D levels, which stimulate intestinal calcium absorption. The benefits of long-term use of glucocorticoids outweigh potential side effects, including Cushing's syndrome and osteomalacia.

Glucocorticoids used alone are not as effective as when used with calcitonin.[44] Both can be used in patients with renal or cardiac failure who are dehydrated, and they therefore are useful for treatment of hypercalcemia when saline diuresis is contraindicated. The advantages to combined use are a more rapid response and prevention of the "escape" phenomenon encountered with use of calcitonin alone.[3,40] Calcitonin-glucocorticoid combinations have been recommended as first-line therapy for hypercalcemia but have the disadvantages discussed earlier.[40]

Plicamycin

Although plicamycin is an effective antihypercalcemic agent that probably acts through osteoclast inhibition, it has a slow onset of action (24 to 30 hours) and therefore is not indicated for emergency treatment of hypercalcemia.[3] Plicamycin has been associated with thrombocytopenia and with renal and hepatic toxicity. Nausea, vomiting, and toxic effects are related to cumulative dosage and rarely occur with the first or second dose. Since the drug is excreted through the kidneys, toxicity is more likely in patients with impaired renal function. Hypocalcemia and tetany also have been reported. Although some authors recommend use of this agent only when other less toxic regimens have failed,[11,40,44] its ease of administration in the ambulatory setting as well as cost constraints encourage its use as a first-line approach to moderate hypercalcemia.

Plicamycin is administered intravenously at a dose of 25 μg/kg (maximum dose 1500 mg) either as a slow bolus injection or as a 4-hour infusion. Bolus injections are associated with a higher incidence of nausea and vomiting. The dose may be repeated if no detectable lowering of serum calcium is seen within 48 hours. Once the serum calcium is lowered, the duration of action is variable and may last from 3 days to 1 week or more. Treatment is not repeated until hypercalcemia returns.[40,44] Extravasation is associated with local irritation and cellulitis at the injection site. A change in the injection site and application of warm compresses are recommended by the manufacturer should extravasation occur (Miles Laboratories package insert).

Phosphates

Intravenous administration of inorganic phosphates rapidly decreases extracellular fluid calcium concentration by promoting skeletal calcification. Unfortunately, extraskeletal calcification also occurs and is associated with, among other things, impairment of renal function due to nephrocalcinosis. Intravenous phosphates should not be employed except as a last resort.[44]

Oral phosphates are less toxic in patients with normal renal function and serum phosphorus levels less than 4.0 mg/dL and are useful for chronic treatment of hypercalcemia. Phosphates prevent intestinal calcium absorption by forming poorly soluble $Ca\text{-}PO_4$ salts in the intestinal lumen, which make less calcium available for absorption, and also by impairing the conversion of 25-hydroxyvitamin D to 1,25-dihydroxyvitamin D (a major stimulator of intestinal calcium transport). In addition, phosphates inhibit mineral and bone matrix resorption. Soft tissue and skeletal calcification also occurs to a lesser extent than with intravenous phosphates, but lung and renal calcification has been documented with chronic administration.[3] The most common and also the most limiting side effect is diarrhea, since phosphates are administered in the form of either sodium or potassium salts, Fleet Phospho Soda being one of the preparations most commonly prescribed. Despite an initial response, chronic administration is often accompanied by a loss of effectiveness.[3] No randomized prospective studies have evaluated the efficacy of oral phosphates. Phosphates are contraindicated in patients with renal failure or serum phosphorus levels greater than 3.8 mg/dL.

Prostaglandin Inhibitors

Aspirin, indomethacin, and nonsteroidal anti-inflammatory drugs have been tried, but only on occasion is there an antihypercalcemic response.

Bisphosphonates

Bisphosphonates inhibit the action of osteoclasts on bone. Sodium etidronate (EHDP) currently is available for treatment of patients with Paget's disease. Two other bisphosphonates are still undergoing clinical trials in the United States but are available in Europe: aminohydroxypropane bisphosphonate (AHPrBP), and clodronate (Cl_2MDP). All three agents are known to be potent osteoclastic inhibitors. EHDP has also been found to inhibit or retard bone mineralization causing osteomalacia. This effect limits chronic oral use to 3 months or less.[45]

Intravenous EHDP is given in 500 mL of normal saline over 3 hours at a dose of 7.5 mg/kg daily for 5 days. Three liters of saline are also administered daily. Serum calcium levels are usually significantly reduced by the third day of therapy. EHDP is then continued orally at a dose of 10 mg/kg/day. Other than inhibition of bone mineralization, few side effects have been reported.[46] EHDP is contraindicated in patients with renal failure.

AHPrBP shows more promise as being a safe and effective therapy with few side effects and without inhibition of osteoid mineralization. In two recent studies, AHPrBP demonstrated a rapid onset of action with normalization of serum calcium levels within 4 to 6 days and a duration of action longer than that seen with currently available therapies.[47,48]

Cl_2MDP may not be introduced into the United States, since acute leukemia has been documented in several patients treated with this agent.

Gallium Nitrate

Another osteoclastic inhibitor, gallium nitrate, recently was compared with calcitonin. In a randomized double-blind trial 50 patients received either a 5-day infusion of gallium nitrate or intramuscular injections of salmon calcitonin every 6 hours for 5 days. Eighteen of the 24 patients receiving gallium nitrate achieved normocalcemia, compared with 8 of the 26 patients receiving calcitonin. Median duration of normocalcemia before other cytotoxic or hypocalcemic therapy was 6 days with gallium nitrate and 1 day with calcitonin.[49]

CONCLUSION

Hypercalcemia is a common metabolic complication of malignancy with vague symptoms that often can be confused with those of other paraneoplastic syndromes as well as those of end-stage disease. Nurses caring for cancer patients must be cognizant both of patients at risk and of their associated risk factors. In an exploratory study of hospitalized and ambulatory hypercalcemic patients, 88% of the patients were not aware that hypercalcemia might occur, and 80% to 95% were not aware of the various symptoms of hypercalcemia.[50] Counseling of patients and families regarding prevention and recognition of early symptoms enables therapy to commence before extreme debilitation develops. Patient and family education regarding the purposes and goals of therapy promotes coping with yet another complication of cancer. Meticulous monitoring of fluid and electrolyte balance is essential for effective medical treatment. If hypercalcemia becomes refractory to treatment, nursing measures that facilitate coping with issues related to death and dying are essential.

Although theoretical knowledge regarding humoral and local factors associated with hypercalcemia is advancing, current therapies are nonspecific, aimed at osteoclast inhibition rather than at the mediating bone-resorbing factor itself. The development of a parathormone antagonist to prevent humoral hypercalcemia would help treatment of hypercalcemia immensely.

REFERENCES

1. Fisken RA, Heath DA, Sommers S, et al: Hypercalcaemia in hospital patients: clinical and diagnostic aspects. Lancet 1:202-207, 1981.
2. Mundy GR, Ibbotson KJ, D'Souza SM, et al: The hypercalcemia of cancer: Clinical implications and pathogenic mechanisms. N Engl J Med 310:1718-1727, 1984.
3. Mundy GR, Martin TJ: The hypercalcemia of malignancy: Pathogenesis and management. Metabolism 31:1247-1277, 1982.
4. Fisken RA, Heath DA, Bold AM: Hypercalcaemia—a hospital survey. Q J Med 49:405-418, 1980.
5. Blomqvist CP: Malignant hypercalcemia—a hospital survey. Acta Med Scand 220:455-463, 1986.
6. Myers WP: Hypercalcemia associated with malignant disease, in Endocrine and nonendocrine producing tumors. Sixteenth Annual Clinical Conference on Cancer, M.D. Anderson Hospital and Tumor Institute. Chicago, Year Book Medical Publishers, 1973, pp 147-171.
7. Monno S, Nagata A, Furuta S: Hypercalcemia of cancer in the digestive tract. J Clin Gastroenterol 9:78-82, 1987.
8. Bender RA, Hansen H: Hypercalcemia in bronchogenic carcinoma: A prospective study of 200 patients. Ann Intern Med 80:205-208, 1974.
9. Stewart AF, Romero R, Schwart PE, et al: Hypercalcemia associated with gynecologic malignancies: Biochemical characterization. Cancer 49:2389-2394, 1982.
10. Strewler GJ, Nissenson RA: Nonparathyroid hypercalcemia. Adv Intern Med 32:235-258, 1987.
11. Mundy GR: The hypercalcemia of malignancy. Kidney Int 31:142-155, 1987.
12. Habener JF, Rosenblatt M, Potts JT: Parathyroid hormone: Biochemical aspects of biosynthesis, secretion, action and metabolism. Physiol Rev 64:985-1040, 1984.
13. Peck WA, Rifas L, Cheng SL, et al: The local regulation of bone remodeling. Adv Exp Med Biol 208:255-259, 1986.
14. Taylor BM, Weller LA: Hypercalcemia, in Groenwald SL (ed): Cancer Nursing: Principles and Practice (ed 1). Boston, Jones & Bartlett, 1987.
15. Meunier PJ: Cellular mechanisms of bone remodeling evaluated at the intermediary level of organization of bone. Adv Exp Med Biol 208:247-254, 1986.
16. Broadus AE, Mangin M, Ikeda K, et al: Humoral hypercalcemia of cancer: Identification of a novel parathyroid hormone-like peptide. N Engl J Med 319:556-563, 1988.
17. Mundy GR, Ibbotson KJ, D'Souza SM: Tumor products and the hypercalcemia of malignancy. J Clin Invest 76:391-394, 1985.
18. Gowen M, MacDonald BR, Hughes DE, et al: Immune cells and bone resorption. Adv Exp Med Biol 208:261-273, 1986.
19. Burtis WJ, Wu TL, Insogna KL, et al: Humoral hypercalcemia of malignancy. Ann Intern Med 108:454-457, 1988.
20. Stewart AF, Horst R, Deftos LJ, et al: Biochemical evaluation of patients with cancer-associated hypercalcemia: Evidence for humoral and nonhumoral groups. N Engl J Med 303:1377-1383, 1980.
21. Burtis WJ, Wu T, Bunch C, et al: Identification of a novel 17,000-dalton parathyroid hormone-like adenylate cyclase–stimulating protein from a tumor associated with humoral hypercalcemia of malignancy. J Biol Chem 262:7151-7156, 1987.
22. Mangin M, Webb AC, Dreyer BE, et al: Identification of a cDNA encoding a parathyroid hormone-like peptide from a human tumor associated with humoral hypercalcemia of malignancy. Proc Natl Acad Sci 85:597-601, 1988.
23. Ikeda K, Mangin M, Dreyer BE, et al: Identification of transcripts encoding a parathyroid hormone-like peptide in messenger RNAs from a variety of human and animal tumors associated with humoral hypercalcemia of malignancy. J Clin Invest 81:2010-2014, 1988.
24. Moseley JM, Kubota M, Diefenbach-Jagger H, et al: Parathyroid hormone-related protein purified from a human lung cancer line. Proc Natl Acad Sci USA 84:5048-5052, 1987.
25. Ralston SH: The pathogenesis of humoral hypercalcaemia of malignancy. Lancet 2:1443-1446, 1987.
26. Jacobs JW, Simpson E: Hypercalcemia of malignancy. Adv Exp Med Biol 208:357-366, 1986.
27. Mercier RJ, Thompson JM, Harman GS, et al: Recurrent hypercalcemia and elevated 1,25-dihydroxyvitamin D levels in Hodgkin's disease. Am J Med 84:165-168, 1988.
28. Breslau NA, McGuire JL, Zerwekh JE, et al: Hypercalcemia associated with increased serum calcitriol levels in three patients with lymphoma. Ann Intern Med 100:1-7, 1984.
29. Rosenthal N, Insogna KL, Godsall JW, et al: Elevations in circulating 1,25-dihydroxyvitamin D in three patients with lymphoma associated hypercalcemia. J Clin Endocrinol Metab 60:29-33, 1985.
30. Mudde AH, van den Berg H, Boshuis PG, et al: Ectopic production of 1,25-dihydroxyvitamin D by B-cell lymphoma as a cause of hypercalcemia. Cancer 59:1543-1546, 1987.
31. Fetchik DA, Bertolini DR, Sarin PS, et al: Production of 1, 25-dihydroxyvitamin D_3 by human T-cell lymphotrophic virus-1-transformed lymphocytes. J Clin Invest 78:592-596, 1986.
32. Strodel WE, Thompson NW, Eckhauser FE, et al: Malignancy and concomitant hyperparathyroidism. J Surg Oncol 37:10-12, 1988.
33. Coggeshall J, Merrill W, Hande K, et al: Implications of hypercalcemia with respect to diagnosis and treatment of lung cancer. Am J Med 80:325-328, 1986.
34. Percival RC, Yates AJ, Gray RE, et al: Mechanism of malignant hypercalcemia in carcinoma of the breast. Br Med J (Clin Res) 291:776-779, 1985.
35. Isales C, Carcangiu ML, Stewart AF: Hypercalcemia in breast cancer: Reassessment of the mechanism. Am J Med 82:1143-1147, 1987.

36. Legha S, Powell K, Budzan A, et al: Tamoxifen-induced hypercalcemia in breast cancer. Cancer 47:2803-2806, 1986.
37. Kiyokawa T, Yamaguchi K, Takeya M, et al: Hypercalcemia and osteoclast proliferation in adult T-cell leukemia. Cancer 59:1187-1191, 1987.
38. Mundy GR: Pathogenesis of hypercalcaemia of malignancy. Clin Endocrinol 23:705-714, 1985.
39. Mahon SM: Signs and symptoms associated with malignancy induced hypercalcemia. Cancer Nurs 12:153-160, 1989.
40. Fields ALA, Josse RG, Bergsagel DE: Metabolic emergencies: Hypercalcemia, in DeVita VT, Hellman S, Rosenberg SA (eds): Cancer Principles and Practice of Oncology, Philadelphia, Lippincott, 1985, pp 1866-1872.
41. Coward DD: Cancer-induced hypercalcemia. Cancer Nurs 9:125-132, 1986.
42. Poe CM, Radford AI: The challenge of hypercalcemia in cancer. Oncol Nurs Forum 12:29-34, 1985.
43. Warrell RP: Questions about clinical trials in hypercalcemia. J Clin Oncol 6:759-761, 1988 (editorial).
44. Fetchick DA, Mundy GR: Hypercalcemia of malignancy: Diagnosis and therapy. Comprehen Ther 12:27-32, 1986.
45. Schiller JH, Rasmussen P, Benson AB 3d, et al: Maintenance etidronate in the prevention of malignancy associated hypercalcemia. Arch Intern Med 147:963-966, 1987.
46. Carlson HE, Casciato DA, Lowitz BB: Metabolic and electrolyte complications, in Casciato DA, Lowitz BA (eds): Manual of Clinical Oncology. Boston, Little, Brown, 1988, pp 411-415.
47. Coleman RE, Rubens RD: 3(Amino-1,1-hydroxypropylidene) bisphosphonate (APD) for hypercalcemia of breast cancer. Br J Cancer 56:465-469, 1987.
48. Thiebaud D, Jaeger AF, Jacquet AF, et al: Dose-response in the treatment of hypercalcemia of malignancy by a single infusion of the bisphosphonate AHPrBP. J Clin Oncol 6:762-768, 1988.
49. Warrell RP Jr, Israel R, Frisone M, et al: Gallium nitrate for acute treatment of cancer-related hypercalcemia: A randomized, double-blind comparison to calcitonin. Ann Intern Med 108:669-674, 1988.
50. Coward D: Hypercalcemia knowledge assessment in patients at risk of developing cancer induced hypercalcemia. Oncol Nurs Forum 15:471-476, 1988.

Chapter 26

Hormonal Disturbances

Ada M. Lindsey, RN, PhD

INTRODUCTION

Abnormal hormone secretion can occur as a consequence of malignant neoplastic growth.[1-8] For example, ectopic secretion of adrenocorticotropic hormone (ACTH) from lung tumors is one of the more commonly observed hormonal abnormalities. In normal circumstances ACTH is secreted from the anterior pituitary gland in response to stimulation from corticotropin-releasing hormone released from the hypothalamus and in response to circulating levels of glucocorticoids (eg, cortisol) released from the adrenal cortex. However, in some cases of lung cancer, as well as in other cancers, with the alterations that occur with malignant cell growth these nonendocrine cells synthesize and secrete specific hormones. What is unusual is that normally these cells are from organs and tissues, such as lung tissue, that are not endocrine glands, but when they become transformed, some will synthesize hormone(s) or other peptides. The release of hormone from nonendocrine tissue is termed *ectopic hormone secretion.* In some cases the hormone molecules that are produced by the malignant nonendocrine cells are exactly like the biologically active hormone that normally is produced by the respective endocrine gland. In some cases only fragments of a hormone or the precursor may be produced. In that circumstance, if the fragments or precursor is not capable of producing a biologic response in the target organs, there would be no clinical evidence of this ectopic hormone secretion. If, however, the hormone produced by the malignant cells is biologically active, the target organ for the specific hormone will respond. If the hormone is produced in sufficient quantity, this abnormal secretion will become clinically evident as an endocrine syndrome. For example, there have been cases of lung cancer in which the initial or presenting symptoms reflected a Cushing's syndrome that resulted from excess glucocorticoid production by the adrenal glands in response to the ectopic production of ACTH from the lung tumor. These syndromes also may occur some time after the cancer has been diagnosed.

In normal circumstances, hormone secretion is very finely controlled and regulated; however, what is unusual in the ectopic secretion of hormones is that the malignant nonendocrine cells that produce these hormones are not sensitive to the control or regulatory feedback systems that exist for the endocrine glands. Thus the ectopic production of the hormone goes unchallenged by the usual regulatory mechanisms, resulting in excess secretion of the hormone. Depending on the hormone produced, some of the resulting endocrine abnormalities may be more immediately life threatening than the cancer itself. It is imperative to recognize the variety and the significance of hormonal disturbances that may result from the ectopic production of hormones by malignant tumors of nonendocrine origin.

It has been recognized that most tumors synthesize protein or polypeptide molecules. Some of these are hormones or hormone fragments, others have become known as tumor markers such as alpha-fetoprotein and carcinoembryonic antigen (CEA), and investigations on others are still in progress. The systemic effects of these tumor products are referred to as *paraneoplastic phenomena.* For example, cancer cachexia is believed to be a paraneoplastic syndrome. As tumor products are identified and assays are developed or improved—that is, have increased sensitivity and specificity—measurement of these tumor products can be used for cancer detection, diagnosis of disease recurrence, and assessment of tumor response to treatment.

Tumors also can arise in endocrine glands and may result in hormonal abnormalities. In contrast to ectopic secretion the release of hormone from endocrine cells is termed *entopic.* The hormonal disturbances that occur with endocrine gland malignancies are presented in Chapter 37.

ANATOMY, PHYSIOLOGY, AND SCIENTIFIC PRINCIPLES

Understanding the normal anatomic structures and physiologic regulation and functions of the neuroendocrine system provides the basis for elucidating and interpreting the hormonal alterations that can occur with ectopic secretion from nonendocrine malignant tissue. Significant scientific advances in delineating the mechanisms of action and regulation, as well as in the measurement of hormones, have been made. These advances, in addition to those made in the field of genetics, have contributed to the development of knowledge about the endocrine syndromes observed in association with cancer.

Neuroendocrine Structures

The major central neuroendocrine structures include the hypothalamus, the pituitary, and the connecting hypothalamic-pituitary stalk. The hypothalamus and the pituitary are in close proximity; the vascular connections, that is, the hypophysial-portal system between the two structures, are located in the stalk. The hormones released via these structures directly enter the blood stream and circulate to the peripherally located target endocrine glands. The hormones from the hypothalamus are produced and released via neurons whereas those from the pituitary are produced and released by endocrine cells. The majority of the hypothalamic hormones have a stimulatory or an inhibitory action on the anterior pituitary gland cells. Two hypothalamic hormones, antidiuretic hormone (ADH) and oxytocin, are released via hypothalamic neurons in the posterior pituitary where they enter the circulatory system. The secretion rates of hormones are not constant. The hypothalamus is influenced by circadian rhythms, and as a result some of the hormones have a characteristic diurnal secretory pattern. Some hormones are secreted in a pulsatile rhythm, and others such as those involved in ovulation and menstruation have a complicated secretory pattern. All the hypothalamic and pituitary hormones are derived from amino acids and thus are classified as polypeptide or protein hormones.

The target organs, the peripherally located endocrine glands, respond to the centrally released hormones by producing and releasing another hormone or by exhibiting some other biologic response. The release of glucocorticoids, for example, cortisol, by the adrenal cortex in response to the pituitary release of ACTH is one example, whereas the conservation of water by the renal tubules illustrates the example of a biologic response, in this case to the release of the hypothalamic ADH, or vasopressin.

Most peripheral endocrine glands are regulated primarily through the hypothalamic pituitary neuroendocrine axis. Some peripheral endocrine glands, however, have other regulatory mechanisms; these include the parathyroid glands, the insulin-producing islets of the pancreas, the thymus gland, and the gastrointestinal endocrine cells. For example, the circulating levels of calcium influence the secretion of parathormone whereas the circulatory levels of glucose influence the secretion of insulin.

Some of the hormones produced by these target organs are polypeptides, for example, insulin; some such as cortisol, estrogen, testosterone, and aldosterone are steroids; the thyroid hormones are classified as iodothyronines, and epinephrine and norepinephrine are catecholamines.

The neuroendocrine structures of major importance include the hypothalamus, the connecting hypophysial-portal system, the pituitary gland, and the target endocrine glands and tissues. The hormones produced by the endocrine cells and some hypothalamic neurons are the chemical signals that are transported by the circulatory system to their specific sites of action.

Neuroendocrine Regulation and Function

The regulation of neuroendocrine function is based on a responsive feedback system that involves stimulation and inhibition. The hormones secreted from the hypothalamus will be used as a beginning point. Some of these, such as thyrotropin-releasing hormone (TRH), stimulate production of anterior pituitary hormones; others such as somatostatin are inhibitory. If the hormones are stimulatory in nature, the specific anterior pituitary hormone will be released, and it in turn will stimulate the release of hormone from its peripherally located target endocrine gland. Thus TRH stimulates thyroid-stimulating hormone (TSH) from the anterior pituitary gland, which in turn stimulates release of thyroxine and triiodothyronine from the thyroid gland. In many cases the end product, such as cortisol (resulting from corticotropin-releasing factor [CRF] stimulation of ACTH and subsequent production of cortisol from the adrenal cortex), acts in an inhibitory way on the hypothalamus and on the anterior pituitary, which results in decreased release of CRF. Figure 26-1 shows a diagrammatic representation of this feedback system of regulation.

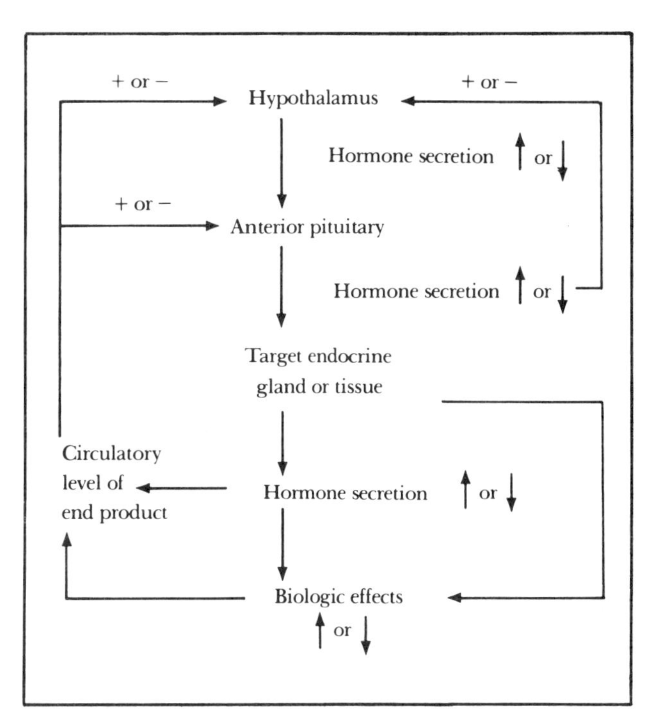

FIGURE 26-1 Diagrammatic representation of neuroendocrine feedback regulation mechanisms. (+ Stimulatory; − inhibitory; ↑ increase; ↓ decrease.)

There are other models of regulation. For example, ADH secretion by the hypothalamic neurons is sensitive to osmotic pressure, blood volume, and blood pressure. Pain, stress, and emotional states also influence ADH secretion. ADH plays a role in the conservation of water and in the maintenance of plasma osmolality, blood pressure, and volume. The renin-angiotensin-aldosterone system also is involved in the control of the internal fluid and electrolyte environment. Although the model for regulation of this system is different from that shown in Figure 26-1, in each case feedback mechanisms are involved in regulation. The biologic effects that result from the initial hormone stimulation serve as the inhibitory mechanisms, resulting in a decrease in hormone release. For example, when sufficient quantities of water have been conserved by the renal tubule cells in response to ADH, the change in osmotic pressure, blood volume, and/or blood pressure acts to result in a decrease in the release of ADH from the hypothalamic neurons that end on blood vessels in the posterior pituitary.

The regulation of the gonadotropin-releasing hormone (GnRH) or luteinizing hormone-releasing hormone (LHRH), follicle-stimulating hormone (FSH), luteinizing hormone (LH), estrogen, and progesterone system is even more complex than other endocrine regulatory systems and is not completely elucidated. Secretions occur in cyclic patterns and change over the life span.

Trophic hormones have several general functions. Many stimulate the synthesis of their specific cell receptors, some induce differentiation of cells, some stimulate cell mitosis, and some stimulate other cell functions. Thus the stimulation of target tissue may result in an increase of cells' sensitivity to the hormone, an increase in the number of functional cells, and an increase in other specific cell activities.

From this very brief overview, it is apparent that many factors are involved in the normal regulation of neuroendocrine function. The factors vary, depending on the system. The regulation, however, includes the capacity to sense minute environmental changes in the internal milieu and in some cases in the external world. The regulation includes the ability of the system, in response to changes, to increase or decrease synthesis and release hormones or other biologic effects. The regulatory systems involve a chain of events that result in modulation of the system.

In the case of ectopic hormone production by malignant cells, the regulatory system is not effective. The ectopic production of the hormone is not a result of trophic hormone stimulation but occurs as the result of gene expression in the undifferentiated, transformed malignant cells, and these cells are not responsive to a decrease in the trophic (stimulating) hormone. They produce the hormone autonomously without regard to the normal regulatory feedback mechanisms to which normal endocrine cells respond. Thus ectopic hormones are produced in excess and are not subject to usual control mechanisms. There have been some cases reported in which there is evidence that the releasing hormone and the stimulatory or trophic hormone both have been synthesized by the same malignant tumors.[9,10]

Glands

The hypothalamus, although not considered a gland, synthesizes and secretes hormones that stimulate the synthesis and secretion of the pituitary gland trophic hormones. The target glands for these trophic hormones include the pineal gland, the thyroid gland, the adrenal gland, the ovary, and the testis. Other hormone-secreting tissues include the pancreatic A and B cells, the parathyroid, the adrenal medulla, the C cells of the thyroid, the gastrointestinal hormone-secreting cells, and the placenta. In addition to the endocrine cells in these glands or tissues, each is comprised of other structural and functional components. One common feature is that the hormones are released directly into the circulatory system.

Hormones

Hormones known to be produced by neurons that originate in the hypothalamus include TRH, GnRH or LHRH, somatostatin (somatotropin-release inhibiting factor [SRIF]), ADH, and oxytocin. These last two are released directly into the circulation at the posterior pituitary and the preceding hormones are released into the hypophysial-portal system that goes to the anterior pituitary. There is evidence of the release of other hormones from the hypothalamus such as CRF; however, because additional research is needed, these substances are called factors rather than hormones.

Hormones produced by the pituitary include growth hormone ([GH] or somatotropin), ACTH, TSH, luteinizing hormone (LH in females and interstitial cell-stimulating hormone [ICSH] in males), prolactin (PRL), and melanocyte-stimulating hormone (MSH). ACTH is synthesized in the form of a large precursor molecule, which contains MSH, B-lipotropin, β-endorphin, and met-enkephalin; these latter two peptides have morphinelike properties.[1]

Some of the peptide hormones generally characterized as originating from gastrointestinal-secretory cells have been found to occur in extrahypothalamic areas of the brain. These hormones include gastrin, substance P, and cholecystokinin (CCK). Some of the hypothalamic and pituitary hormones also have been found in other discrete locations within the central nervous system. These include TRH, SRIF, ACTH, and GnRH.

Other hormones are released from the peripheral target glands and tissues, for example, epinephrine from the adrenal medulla, aldosterone and glucocorticoids from the adrenal cortex, thyroxine from the thyroid, calcitonin from the C cells of the thyroid, insulin from the pancreatic B cells, glucagon from pancreatic A cells, estrogens from the ovary, and testosterone from the testis. Hormones are released from the placenta and also from the gastrointestinal tract secretory cells; the liver and kidney are the major source for the cholecalciferol metabolites (vitamin D).

Hormones are classified by their primary chemical composition. The four major classifications are (1) the amine group, which includes the catecholamines, norepinephrine and epinephrine, (2) the iodothyronines, that is, thyronine and triiodothyronine, (3) the peptide, protein, and glycoprotein group that includes a large number of hormones, and (4) the steroids. Examples of the peptide hormones are ADH or vasopressin, oxytocin, TRH, GnRH, SRIF, and the angiotensins. Insulin, glucagon, prolactin, calcitonin, and ACTH are protein hormones; examples of glycoprotein hormones are follicle-stimulating hormone, luteinizing hormone, and thyroid-stimulating hormone. Peptides are small chains of amino acids whereas proteins are larger chains of amino acids; that is, polypeptide chains are linked to create larger structures. Glycoproteins are created intracellularly by the addition of sugars to various specific locations on the protein structure. The peptide/protein class of hormones is synthesized by intracellular DNA-RNA actions. The synthesis of the steroid class of hormones such as estrogens, progesterone, testosterone, glucocorticoids (eg, cortisol), and aldosterone also occurs intracellularly but through a complicated orderly sequence of enzymatic steps. Iodothyronines also are synthesized through a series of enzymatic steps.

What is of significance and interest is that of the ectopic production of hormones observed to occur with malignant tumors, all the hormones have been of the peptide/protein class in which the synthesis occurs via DNA-RNA direction.

Because a number of specific enzymatic steps are involved sequentially in the synthesis of other classes of hormones, this synthetic process is much more difficult and thus unlikely to occur as a paraneoplastic phenomenon. The end result in some circumstances of ectopic hormone production, however, is the excess secretion of some nonprotein hormones such as cortisol. For example, Cushing's syndrome that occurs with the excess unregulated cortisol secretion is the result of the ectopic production of the protein hormone, ACTH, by nonendocrine malignant cells. The excess ACTH stimulates the cortisol production by the adrenal cortex.

Normally, hormone production and release are highly regulated. Some hormones are produced as larger molecules and are called *precursor* molecules, or *prohormones*. These larger molecules must be cleaved or separated to yield the biologically active hormone. Such is the case for ACTH, which is part of the larger proopiomelanocortin molecule, and for insulin, which also is initially part of a larger molecule. This separation is required for biologic activation. In the case of glycoprotein hormones, sugars are added to their protein structure to confer their biologic activity.

Most hormones are transported in the circulatory system attached to carrier proteins specific for the hormone such as the sex hormone–binding globulin that carries estrogen and testosterone. Many hormones also are carried by binding to albumin. It is only the free, or unbound, hormone, however, that is available as the biologically active molecule and that is free to interact with its cell-specific receptors. Thus many factors influence the biologic activity of hormones. Hormones are effective in low concentrations; they have a physiologic range of 10^{-7} to 10^{-12} mol/L. The time frame of action of hormones is generally comparable to their chemical classification. The amines, epinephrine and norepinephrine, are effective in milliseconds; peptides such as angiotensin and ADH within minutes; proteins and glycoproteins such as insulin, calcitonin, and thyroid-stimulating hormone within minutes to hours; steroids such as estrogen, cortisol, and aldosterone within hours; and iodothyronines such as thyroxine are effective over days. The hormones are the chemical signals. These chemical substances, which are carried in the bloodstream, serve as the highly specialized messengers for their respective target tissue sites.

Target Tissues and Receptors

Because hormones circulate in the bloodstream, they are virtually accessible to all tissues. What conveys the specificity of hormone "recognition" is the presence of receptors in the target tissues. These receptors recognize the hormone specific for the particular target tissue. Some hormones have receptors in many types of tissues whereas some have specific receptors in only one or a few types of tissue. For example, receptors specific for growth hormone are found in almost all cells whereas receptors for antidiuretic hormone are localized in renal tubule cells. Some hormone-specific receptors are located on the cell surface, and others are located intracellularly. In the case of the peptide/protein hormones, the hormone-specific receptors are located on the cell surface. When the hormone is bound to the receptor, a series of actions evolve; depending on the target organ, the result could be the synthesis and release of a hormone, as is true for ACTH action on the adrenal cortex, which stimulates release of the glucocorticoids. Alternately, some protein hormones, when they bind with their specific target cell receptors, result in other types of biologic activity such as occurs with insulin that interacts with peripheral tissues, effecting entry of glucose and decrease of lipolysis. In the case of the steroid hormones the specific receptors are located intracellularly. The lipid hormones cross cell membranes and interact with a cytosol receptor; this hormone-receptor complex moves into the cell nucleus where the cascade of hormone action begins.

The receptors for all hormones, whether they are on the cell surface or intracellular, are protein structures; these receptors are specific for their respective hormone. The number of receptors and the amount of hormone binding to the receptors influence the magnitude of the hormone response. There is evidence that the number and the binding capacity of receptors is regulated. Thus, in addition to the amount of circulating biologically active free hormone, the receptors have a major role in specific hormone action.

Definitions

Entopic refers to the production of hormones by endocrine cells. *Ectopic* hormone production occurs in malignant cells that are of nonendocrine origin. *Paraneoplastic syndromes* is the term used when the tumor produces biologically active substances, and these tumor by-products enter the circulation and cause remote effects. They result in some physiologic alteration. The remainder of this chapter is focused primarily on examples of ectopic hormone production observed in association with cancer.

PATHOPHYSIOLOGY

All cells in an individual have the same genetic material, the entire genome. Through the processes of cellular differentiation and specialization depending on the tissue, specific genes will be expressed whereas others are not expressed. These processes are what convey the differences in cells. It is believed that in the malignant transformation of cells, some of the genes that are not ordinarily expressed in the normal differentiated cell are, in fact, expressed or become activated in the malignant cells.[2,3,4,8] This can account for the expression of genes that code for the synthesis of the peptide/protein hormones in the nonendocrine malignant cells. The only hormones produced ectopically are the peptide class. No steroid hormones nor catecholamines have been found in ectopic production.[2] All the polypeptide hormones, however, have occurred in ectopic production from tumors of nonendocrine origin. Some of the peptides synthesized by the malignant cells are exactly like the normally secreted hormone from endocrine cells, and some are only fragments or deviate in other ways. It is only in those cases in which the tumor product has sufficient biologic activity that a clinical syndrome will become evident.

In addition to hormones, tumors are known to elaborate other biologically active substances that enter the circulation and result in remote or systemic effects. In cases in which these effects result in some recognized physiologic alteration, they are known as paraneoplastic syndromes. In some cases, on the basis of associated clinical evidence, the biologically active substance is presumed to exist, but specific substances have not been identified for all paraneoplastic syndromes such as cancer cachexia, anorexia, and hypertrophic pulmonary osteoarthropathy. It is estimated that at some time during the course of cancer at least half the individuals will be affected by some paraneoplastic phenomenon.[2] The systemic effects may be a greater problem than that resulting from the local tumor growth. As is true of ectopic hormone secretion, some paraneoplastic syndromes may precede the diagnosis of the malignancy or may occur at any time after the diagnosis. In both situations the syndromes will be reversed only when the tumor treatment is effective. Symptom management may be possible for some of these syndromes when treatment of the malignancy fails.

The expression of the oncofetal proteins, CEA and alpha-fetoprotein, has occurred with several different malignancies. Although these abnormally produced proteins do not result in a syndrome, measurement of the tumor proteins has been used to monitor response to anticancer therapies.

Originally it was believed that the malignant cells that produced ectopic hormones had a common embryonic origin. Cells that originate from the neural crest are characterized by their capacity for *a*mine *p*recursor *u*ptake and *d*ecarboxylation and thus have been referred to as *APUD cells*.[11] These cells, which are widely distributed, were believed to result in the ectopic hormone production. This concept, however, no longer explains all the ectopic hormone production that has been observed to occur in many other morphologic cell types.[2,4,8,12,13] Also, there is evidence to suggest that all the neuroendocrine cells may not have a common embryologic origin. Thus the concept of activation of some genetic expression in malignant cells, ordinarily not expressed in normally differentiated cells, as already described, is the more widely accepted explanation for the occurrence of paraneoplastic syndromes, including ectopic hormone production. There is evidence now, however, that suggests that some hormones are produced in small quantities by nonendocrine cells.[6] On the basis of these new findings, other explanations for the production of hormones by nonendocrine malignant cells may be forthcoming.

MANIFESTATIONS

The clinical manifestations of the paraneoplastic syndromes vary, depending on the type of ectopic product(s) produced by the malignant tumor. More than one hormone or product may be produced by a tumor. It is known that many peptides are produced by malignant cells. In many cases, no clinical syndrome will occur because the tumor product is not biologically active; these may be hormone fragments or prohormones (larger precursor molecules) in which cleavage of the larger molecule did not occur, or the hormone structure may be altered. Only those products that are biologically active and that are secreted in sufficient excess result in a clinical syndrome. Paraneoplastic syndromes have been reviewed in detail.[1-8] The syndromes that result from the more commonly occurring ectopically produced hormones are described in the following section.

Glands

Malignancies arising in endocrine glands may or may not result in hormonal disturbances. If a malignancy occurs, the hormonal secretions may be increased or decreased; however, the secretion is entopic. The affected gland may remain responsive to the regulatory feedback mechanisms, or this control may be compromised. When the malignancy arises in an endocrine gland, the hormonal changes observed may be variable from patient to patient. Multiple endocrine neoplasias (MEN) have been reported.[8] Several endocrine glands are involved, and the result is alteration in secretion of hormones from the multiple affected glands. The more common malignancies arising in endocrine glands are described in Chapter 37.

Endocrine glands also are affected when the malignancy arises in nonendocrine tissue and the malignant cells produce hormones ectopically. The ectopic hormone, if biologically active, will affect its specific target tissue. Some tumors secrete more than one hormone ectopically; thus, in those cases, more than one endocrine gland or endocrine responsive tissue will be affected.

Hormones, Target Tissues, and General Manifestations

The hormones that are produced ectopically by malignant tumors are in the peptide/protein class. These hormones, however, may be trophic to an endocrine gland that secretes a steroid hormone, and thus the clinical syndrome results from increased ectopic steroid hormone production from the endocrine gland that was stimulated by the ectopically produced peptide hormone. An example is Cushing's syndrome in which the entopic production of cortisol results from stimulation of the adrenal cortex by the ectopically produced peptide hormone, ACTH.

The list of hormones and hormone precursors that have been observed to be secreted in association with tumors is long.[1,2] These include ACTH, CRF, ADH, growth hormone-releasing hormone, prolactin, chorionic gonadotropin, calcitonin, glucagon, somatostatin, and many others.[1,2,6] The hormone disturbances from the ectopic production and the resulting clinical syndromes observed more commonly in association with malignant tumors are described next.

Ectopic adrenocorticotropic hormone production

Ectopic production of ACTH occurs most often in association with small cell lung cancer and in carcinomas of the pancreas or thymus.[1,6] It also has been observed in other lung cancer types and in a variety of other tumors such as medullary carcinoma of the thyroid, carcinoma of the breast, ovary, testis, stomach, colon, prostate, and other sites, especially those neoplasms originating from neural crest tissue such as pheochromocytoma and neuroblastoma.

The ACTH molecule is part of a larger structure, proopiomelanocortin, which also contains the melanocyte-stimulating hormone and endorphin.[6] Thus clinical evidence of ectopic secretion may include increased pigmentation. Clinical evidence of ectopic ACTH that is biologically active results from the ACTH stimulatory effect on the adrenal cortex and the subsequent increased glucocorticoid production. Symptoms include muscle weakness and atrophy, edema, hypertension, and psychosis. High serum ACTH (§150 pg/mL) and plasma cortisol (§35 mg/dL) levels, hyperglycemia, abnormal glucose tolerance, elevated urinary cortisol and urinary 17-hydroxycorticoid levels, and hypokalemia are diagnostic of ectopic ACTH production.[1,3] Other classic features of Cushing's disease such as centripetal obesity, moon facies, buffalo hump, and cutaneous striae are seen infrequently in those with ectopic secretion except when the tumor grows slowly.[2,8] If the tumor is growing rapidly, the characteristics of Cushing's syndrome may not appear, but in cases in which the tumor growth is less rapid, the symptoms that appear may range from a few abnormalities to the entire group of classic features of the syndrome.

In ectopic ACTH production, use of dexamethasone (8 mg/day) most often will not result in suppression of ACTH nor of plasma cortisol.[2,8,10] This dexamethasone suppression test is used to distinguish between an endocrine pathology in which suppression of secretion occurs and ectopic production in which suppression usually does not occur.[6,14] Cases have been reported in which suppression has occurred in those with ectopic production; in some there is evidence that the tumor is producing the CRF.[4,9,10,15] Responses to the administration of metyrapone and ovine CRF also are used in making the differential diagnosis of ectopic ACTH production.[14-17] Measurement of ACTH levels in specimens aspirated from intrathoracic tumors has been used to identify the ectopic production of ACTH.[18] If tumor therapy is not effective, levels of cortisol can be decreased with the administration of agents that inhibit cortisol production such as aminoglutethimide, metyrapone, and ketoconazole.[1,2,8,19]

Ectopic antidiuretic hormone production

Vasopressin (ADH) is produced ectopically most often in carcinomas of the lung (small cell) and colon.[1,2,6,8,20] It also has occurred with other lung cancer types, in carcinoma of the adrenal cortex, pancreas, colon, prostate, and other tissues, and in Hodgkin's disease. Clinically these patients may have hyponatremia (sodium < 130 mEq/L) and inappropriate high urine osmolality (≥500 mOsm/kg) resulting from renal sodium loss (>20 mEq/L) and water retention. There may be no symptoms if the individual does not take in excess fluids. However, if there is an excessive fluid intake, with water intoxication, symptoms of the syndrome of inappropriate antidiuretic hormone (SIADH) will occur. Neurologic and behavioral symptoms include lethargy, agitation, altered mental status, including confusion and psychotic behavior. Seizures and coma also may occur; in some cases death may result.[1,20,21] The treatment is directed at the tumor. Fluid restriction to 500 mL/day or less may be necessary to control hyponatremia. If chemotherapy requires hydration, it may need to be postponed for several days to allow plasma osmolality to increase by means of fluid restriction; this will occur over a week or more.[1]

Infusion of 3% hypertonic saline and furosemide (1 mg/kg) may be used if the patient has severe symptoms or is comatose as a result of SIADH.[2,20] The goal is to increase serum sodium and to decrease retention of water to raise plasma osmolality to 270 mOsm/kg. If cancer treatment fails and there is recurrence of SIADH, demeclocycline can be used to block the action of ADH on the renal tubule cells. Orally administered urea also has been used to create obligatory diuresis.[1]

Vasopressin normally is secreted from the hypothalamic neurons with a carrier protein, neurophysin. Neurophysin also has been found in ectopic secretion.[1,6] Researchers have used the measurement of neurophysin to determine tumor response to therapy and suggest that it may be an effective tumor marker particularly in patients with small cell lung cancer.

Ectopic gonadotropin production

The three hormones classified as gonadotropins are FSH, LH, and human chorionic gonadotropin (HCG). FSH, LH, and HCG all have common alpha subunits but distinct beta subunits, and in each case, biologic activity requires the presence of combined alpha and beta subunits.[6,8] FSH and LH levels vary normally over time and age, and ectopic production has not been well documented yet. HCG normally is produced by the placenta; thus in cases in which an ectopic gonadotropin hormone production is suspected, the measurement of HCG is the more commonly used approach. It also has been used to monitor therapy. Although HCG normally is produced by the placenta by means of radioimmunoassays (RIA) and radioreceptor assays, an HCG-like material has been found in extracts from all tissues.[1,6,8] The HCG-like material differs from that produced by the placenta and by tumors in that it has no or few carbohydrates attached to the protein structure whereas the placental HCG is a glycoprotein. The HCG that does not have the sugars attached is much less biologically active and is rapidly cleared from the blood stream. The biologically active HCG that has been produced ectopically by tumors has resulted in gynecomastia in men, oligomenorrhea in premenopausal women, and precocious puberty in children.[1,8,22] Tumors in addition to those in the pituitary gland found to secrete HCG include germ cell tumors of the ovary and testis, those arising from extragonadal sites, and gestational trophoblastic tumors such as hydatidiform mole and choriocarcinoma. HCG secretion also has been reported for other tumors such as cancer of the lung, breast, pancreas, gastrointestinal tract, and prostate. The types of cancer in which ectopic HCG occurs are relatively uncommon, and thus the expression of the clinical syndromes resulting from HCG production also is less common. Treatment is directed at the tumor.

Ectopic calcitonin production

Increased calcitonin levels have occurred in patients with lung (especially small cell) cancer, with breast, gastric, and colon cancer, and with carcinoid tumors. Normally it is produced by the C cells of the thyroid and frequently is increased in individuals with medullary carcinoma of the thyroid. Calcitonin action results in the release of calcium from the bone and an increase in the urinary excretion of calcium and phosphate. Although calcitonin participates in the regulation of serum calcium, there is to date no recognized clinical syndrome that results from the ectopic production.[1,6]

Ectopic parathyroid hormone production and hypercalcemia

Hypercalcemia (serum calcium§11 mg/dL) that occurs with malignancy results from several mechanisms. In addition to bone metastases, one of the earlier mechanisms proposed is the ectopic production of parathyroid hormone (PTH) by malignant tumors.[8] Ectopic production of growth hormone or vitamin D also could influence serum calcium levels because absorption of calcium from renal tubules and the gastrointestinal tract is stimulated by growth hormone, vitamin D, and PTH. There is controversy about whether PTH production results in hypercalcemia.[1,6,23] Current evidence suggests that hypercalcemia is rarely the result of ectopic PTH; however, other tumor-produced factors that have parathyroid-like hormone activity have been reported.[1,6,23,24] A parathyroid hormone–like substance, an osteoclast activating factor (OAF), and prostaglandins (PGE) 1 and 2 have been produced by tumors and can result in hypercalcemia.[1,24] The resulting effect is stimulation of osteoclastic bone resorption, and for some of the factors inhibition of renal excretion of calcium also occurs. Hypercalcemia that is not a result of metastasis to bony structures is associated more frequently with carcinoma of the lung, head, and neck, ovary, and kidney. It also occurs with lymphomas and leukemias that have been shown to produce osteoclast-activating factors.[2,23] Symptoms associated with hypercalcemia include anorexia, nausea, vomiting, lethargy, weakness, and mental confusion.[24] Treatment to decrease these symptoms is directed at decreasing serum calcium levels; the initial approach is the administration of 2 to 3 L saline per day and furosemide. Drugs that block or inhibit bone resorption may be used; these include calcitonin, mithramycin, and etidronate.[23,25] Hypercalcemia is discussed in detail in Chapter 25.

Ectopic growth hormone-releasing hormone production

A number of tumors have produced growth hormone-releasing hormone (GHRH). These include carcinoid tumors, pancreatic islet cells, small cell lung cancer, thyroid medullary carcinoma, and endometrial cancer.[6,8] In some cases there is no evidence of clinical abnormality, but there are cases in which GHRH has stimulated the secretion of growth hormone and the classic features of acromegaly have resulted.[4,26-30] This is particularly true for slow-growing bronchial carcinoid tumors. Acromegaly induced by ectopic GHRH production is rare, but it does occur. The treatment is directed at the tumor, and signs of acromegaly will regress with tumor regression. If the cancer treatment fails, an analog of somatostatin can be used to control acromegaly. It decreases circulating levels of growth hormone and somatomedin C.

Other paraneoplastic syndromes

Syndromes other than those resulting from ectopic hormone production have been associated with a variety of malignancies, for example, cachexia, fever, and neurologic and dermatologic syndromes.[2] These paraneoplastic syndromes are believed to result from tumor-produced factors that have not yet been identified or specified. Examples of neurologic syndromes include subacute cerebellar degeneration and subacute motor neuropathy. These and other less frequently occurring paraneoplastic phenomena such as dermatomyositis and paraneoplastic skin lesions are reviewed elsewhere in more detail.[1,2,6]

Ectopic production

There is evidence that some polypeptide hormones are found normally in small amounts in nonendocrine tissue; this new information somewhat changes the meaning of ectopic production.[1,4,6] Hormones that presumably are synthesized in normal nonendocrine tissue include chorionic gonadotropin, growth hormone, and insulin.[6] Thus the question is whether the hormones produced by nonendocrine tumors really are ectopic. One general characteristic, however, is that the ectopic hormone production appears to be autonomous. The hormone synthesis by malignant nonendocrine tissue does not respond to the regulatory feedback mechanisms such as occurs for hormones produced entopically.

ASSESSMENT

In some cases the paraneoplastic syndrome may be the presenting symptoms for which the individual seeks medical attention.[3,17] The syndromes can occur at any time during the course of the cancer illness. Thus the nurse needs to be alert to signs and symptoms that are associated with the specific ectopic hormone production.[3,31] It is also important to be knowledgeable about the tumors that are more frequently associated with ectopic hormone production and the more commonly observed syndromes. For example, many paraneoplastic syndromes have occurred in association with small cell lung cancer. When the cancer is treated effectively, the syndrome also will diminish.

History

If the paraneoplastic syndrome occurs after the cancer is diagnosed, usually the history will have been recorded previously. If the diagnosis of cancer has not been made, a careful history is taken. In taking the individual's history, the usual procedure is followed. Questions about the specific symptoms focus on onset, duration, and severity, for example, when the symptoms were first apparent, under what circumstances they occur, and whether there have been changes in severity. It also is important to identify any other known diseases. If the individual has symptoms characteristic of an endocrine syndrome and also has symptoms frequently associated with cancer, the history is focused on questions that may help to identify or rule out a possible malignancy. The history elicits any evidence of weight loss, changes in diet, fatigue, weakness, and other changes in usual patterns. For the person with a known malignancy, the history includes information about the type, stage, treatment used, and evidence of any paraneoplastic syndromes. The history provides information that can guide the physical examination and the diagnostic studies.

Physical Examination

The primary focus of the physical examination is derived from the history and presenting symptoms. Hypertrophy or other structural changes in the endocrine gland, such as a nodule, may be found during the physical examination. Hyperplasia or hypertrophy may result from excess trophic hormone stimulation of the endocrine gland. Tumor growth within the gland can change the structure. Recognition of these changes during the examination depends on the location of the affected tissue. For example, testicular and thyroid gland changes are more easily determined because of their accessibility for palpation. The location of the gland also influences whether the individual will notice sensations associated with glandular hypertrophy. In cases of thyroid enlargement the individual may feel a tightness in the neck or a pressure sensation on the trachea. If the pituitary gland is enlarged, the symptoms may include a bilateral loss of the temporal visual field and headache. Because the pituitary is almost surrounded by bone and dura, enlargement causes pressure on the optic nerve chiasm, which results in the visual loss.

The physical examination also identifies changes that may be associated with ectopic hormone syndromes such as hyperpigmentation or gynecomastia. Results of the examination provide direction for selecting appropriate diagnostic tests.

Diagnostic Studies

First it is determined if there are alterations in secretion of the suspected hormone(s). Radioimmunoassay techniques have been developed to measure hormone precursor molecules, hormone fragments, and subunits, as well as the biologically active hormone. Because hormones circulate in very low concentrations, the assays need to be sensitive to very minute amounts of specific hormone. A number of hormones or their metabolites are excreted in the urine. Thus in addition to determination of blood levels of specific hormones, urine may be collected for measurement of selected hormones or their metabolic products.

When excess hormone production is identified, it is important to determine if the alteration is a paraneoplastic syndrome, if it is due to a malignancy of an endocrine gland, or if it is the result of a benign change in endocrine tissue.[4,7,32] Serial monitoring of hormone levels over time may be included in the diagnostic evaluation inasmuch as the typical secretory pattern for specific hormones may not be apparent with ectopic production.

Determination of an abnormally high level of the suspected hormone by radioimmunoassay is necessary for the diagnosis of ectopic production. Measurement of the hormones involved in the feedback control mechanisms of the specific hormone in question also is necessary. Responses to the administration of stimulatory and/or inhibitory hormones are useful in determining if the hormone production is ectopic.[14,15] Because ectopic hormones are produced autonomously, it is unusual for changes in hormone level to occur in response to stimulation or inhibition of the hormones involved in the feedback regulatory system. Other evidence that the secretion is ectopically produced is that the hormone level decreases with tumor removal or other successful tumor therapy. High concentrations of the hormone in the tumor or a difference in hormone concentration across the arteriovenous gradient of the tumor tissue are evidence of hormone production by the tumor.[1,4,17,18]

In all cases, diagnostic procedures are used that allow differentiation between an ectopic paraneoplastic syndrome and some other plausible diagnosis. For example, diuretics and some chemotherapeutic agents such as cyclophosamide and vincristine can result in hyponatremia; thus it is important to determine whether the hyponatremia is associated with these agents or reflects SIADH.[1,20,21] When patients with small cell lung cancer are treated with high doses of cyclophosamide and are hydrated, SIADH, if present, may be exaggerated.

Monitoring levels of the specifically identified hormone(s), as well as other tumor products such as CEA, is useful in determining tumor response to therapy. The presence of a known tumor marker suggests malignancy.

When the excess hormone secretion is believed to be paraneoplastic and the cancer has not been diagnosed, other procedures are used. For example, radiographic and imaging techniques can be used for determining tumor site and extent. Computed tomography (CT) scans and magnetic resonance imaging techniques have been useful in diagnosing cancer (see Chapter 9 for information pertinent to cancer diagnosis).

The nurse's role includes explaining the specific diagnostic procedures to the patient and family, ensuring accurate collection of specimens such as urine, and assisting the patient and family to cope with all the attendant circumstances associated with the diagnostic procedures.[3,31] The nurse may be involved in the administration of the stimulatory or suppressive test agents. Recording the specific times of administration is imperative for correct interpretation.

TREATMENT

If the paraneoplastic syndrome is life threatening, treatment must be directed at correcting or altering the hormonal disturbance. The most effective therapy for paraneoplastic syndromes, however, is the ablation of the tumor and metastases. When tumor therapy is effective, the excess ectopic hormone secretion is alleviated and most usually there is regression of the syndrome. The various treatment strategies for managing malignancies are described in Part III.

If tumor therapy is not effective, other symptom-reducing strategies may be used. For example, fluid restriction may be necessary for ameliorating symptoms associated with SIADH. (Other therapies for SIADH have already been described.) Use of drugs that block hormone receptors or that block hormone synthesis may be necessary. The aims of therapy are to prevent the synthesis of excess hormone or to prevent hormone-receptor interaction. The best resolution of paraneoplastic syndromes occurs with tumor regression.

FUTURE TRENDS

There is need for more specific and sensitive assays for known hormones and tumor markers. There is need for increased understanding of malignant cell aberrations that result in the abnormal (or normally repressed) synthesis of peptides. There is need to develop techniques to identify other factors that are believed to occur as a result of synthesis by tumor cells. There is need to develop agents that are selectively effective in blocking the actions of these factors or in preventing their synthesis. The greatest need is for effective anticancer therapies.

All of these areas require laboratory research and clinical trials. Nurses will continue to increase their participation in these efforts. One current challenge for nurses is to continue to test effectiveness of various nursing therapies in assisting the patient and family to alleviate or diminish the distressing consequences of these syndromes and of the cancer experience.

REFERENCES

1. Bunn PA Jr, Minna JD: Paraneoplastic syndromes, in DeVita V, Hellman S, Rosenberg SA (eds): Cancer Principles and Practice of Oncology. Philadelphia, JB Lippincott, 1985, pp 1797-1842.
2. Griffin TW, Rosenthal PE, Costanza ME: Paraneoplastic and endocrine syndromes, in Cody B (ed): Cancer Manual. Boston, American Cancer Society Massachusetts Division, 1986, pp 373-390.
3. Lindsey AM, Piper BF, Carrieri V: Malignant cells and ectopic hormone production. Oncol Nurs Forum 8:13-15, 1981.
4. Melmed S, Rushakoff RJ: Ectopic pituitary and hypothalamic hormone syndromes. Endocrinol Metab Clin 16:805-821, 1987.
5. Mundy GR: Ectopic hormonal syndromes in neoplastic disease. Hosp Pract April 15:179-194, 1987.
6. Odell WD: Humoral manifestations of cancer, in Wilson JD, Foster DW (eds): Williams Textbook of Endocrinology. Philadelphia, WB Saunders, 1985, pp 1327-1344.
7. Root AW, Diamond FB, Duncan JA: Ectopic and entopic peptide hormone secreting neoplasms of childhood. Adv Pediatr 32:369-415, 1985.
8. Stolinsky DC: Paraneoplastic syndromes. West J Med 132: 189-208, 1980.
9. Suda T, Kondo M, Totani R, et al: Ectopic adrenocorticotropin syndrome caused by lung cancer that responded to corticotropin-releasing hormone. J Clin Endocrinol Metab 63:1047-1051, 1986.
10. Schteingart DE, Lloyd RV, Akil H, et al: Cushing's syndrome secondary to ectopic corticotropin-releasing hormone-adrenocorticotropin secretion. J Clin Endocrinol Metab 63:770-775, 1986.

11. Pearse AGE: Endocrine tumors of neural crest origin: Neurolophomas, apudomas and the APUD concept. Med Biol 52:3, 1974.
12. Odell WD, Wolfsen AR: Hormones from tumors: Are they ubiquitous? Am J Med 68:317-318, 1980.
13. Stevens R, Moore G: Inadequacy of APUD concept in explaining production of peptide hormones by tumors. Lancet 1:118-119, 1983.
14. Nieman LK, Chrousos GP, Oldfield EH, et al: The ovine corticotropin-releasing hormone stimulation test and the dexamethasone suppression test in the differential diagnosis of Cushing's syndrome. Ann Intern Med 105:862-867, 1986.
15. Malchoff CD, Orth DN, Abboud C, et al: Ectopic ACTH syndrome caused by a bronchial carcinoid tumor responsive to dexamethasone, metyrapone and corticotropin-releasing factor. Am J Med 84:760-764, 1988.
16. Cagliero E, Lorenzi M: The corticotropin-releasing factor test in the diagnosis of ectopic ACTH secretion. West J Med 146:614-615, 1987.
17. Findling JW, Tyrrell JB: Occult ectopic secretion of corticotropin. Arch Intern Med 146:929-933, 1986.
18. Doppman JL, Loughlin T, Miller DL, et al: Identification of ACTH-producing intrathoracic tumors by measuring ACTH levels in aspirated specimens. Radiology 163:501-503, 1987.
19. Farwell AP, Devlin JT, Stewart JA: Total suppression of cortisol excretion by ketoconazole in the therapy of the ectopic adrenocorticotropic hormone syndrome. Am J Med 84:1063-1066, 1988.
20. List AF, Hainsworth JD, Davis BW, et al: The syndrome of inappropriate secretion of antidiuretic hormone (SIADH) in small-cell lung cancer. J Clin Oncol 4:1191-1198, 1986.
21. Poe CM, Taylor LM: Syndrome of inappropriate antidiuretic hormone: Assessment and nursing implications. Oncol Nurs Forum 16:373-381, 1989.
22. Wurzel RS, Yamase HT, Nieh PT: Ectopic production of human chorionic gonadotropin by poorly differentiated transitional cell tumors of the urinary tract. J Urol 137:502-504, 1987.
23. Canfield RE: Rationale for diphosphonate therapy in hypercalcemia of malignancy. Am J Med 82:1-5, 1987 (suppl 2A).
24. Chevinsky AH, Berelowitz M, Hoover HC: Adenosquamous carcinoma of the colon presenting with hypercalcemia. Cancer 60:1111-1116, 1987.
25. Singer FR, Fernandez M: Therapy of hypercalcemia of malignancy. Am J Med 82:34-41, 1987 (suppl 2A).
26. Barkan AL, Shenker Y, Grekin RJ, et al: Acromegaly due to ectopic growth hormone (GH)–releasing hormone (GHRH) production: Dynamic studies of GH and ectopic GHRH secretion. J Clin Endocrinol Metab 63:1057-1064, 1986.
27. Roth KA, Wilson DM, Eberwine J, et al: Acromegaly and pheochromocytoma: A multiple endocrine syndrome caused by a plurihormonal adrenal medullary tumor. J Clin Endocrinol Metab 63:1421-1426, 1986.
28. Sano T, Saito H, Yamasaki R, et al: Production and secretion of immunoreactive growth hormone-releasing factor by pheochromocytomas. Cancer 57:1788-1793, 1986.
29. Boizel R, Halimi S, Labat F, et al: Acromegaly due to a growth hormone–releasing hormone-secreting bronchial carcinoid tumor: Further information on the abnormal responsiveness of the somatotroph cells and their recovery after successful treatment. J Clin Endocrinol Metab 64:304-308, 1987.
30. Garcia-Luna PP, Leal-Cerro A, Montero C, et al: A rare cause of acromegaly: Ectopic production of growth hormone-releasing factor by a bronchial carcinoid tumor. Surg Neurol 27:563-568, 1987.
31. Lind JM: Ectopic hormonal production: Nursing implications. Semin Oncol Nurs 1:251-258, 1985.
32. Freeman DA: Steroid hormone-producing tumors in man. Endocr Rev 7:204-220, 1986.

Chapter 27

Edema and Effusions

Claudette G. Varricchio, RN, DSN, OCN

Nancy Miller, RN, MS

Mary Pazdur, RN, MS

INTRODUCTION

Although edema, fluid accumulation, or a serous effusion may be the first sign of malignant disease, its presence indicates the need for intervention to remove the fluid and control the underlying disease. Edema and lymphedema are not life threatening. Effusions often signify advanced disease or metastases. The prognosis for an individual with a malignant effusion depends on several factors: type of cancer and responsiveness to systemic therapy, mechanisms of fluid production, and efficacy of local therapy used to treat the effusion.

The presence of an effusion in a person with neoplastic disease is not always due to the underlying malignancy. Nonmalignant causes include infection, cirrhosis, tuberculosis, congestive heart failure, peritonitis, nephrosis, pancreatitis, pneumonia, atelectasis, pulmonary embolus, trauma, connective tissue disease, Meigs' syndrome, pericarditis, uremia, myxedema, drug effects, anemia, previous irradiation, and rheumatic fever.[1] Therefore an accurate diagnostic assessment is essential.

This chapter addresses the physiology of fluid accumulation and the specific situations that are common in malignant processes. The causes, clinical manifestations, assessment, treatment, and nursing interventions are presented for each type of effusion.

PHYSIOLOGY OF FLUID EQUILIBRIUM

The hydrodynamic balance between plasma and interstitial fluid is complex and involves a variety of factors. The capillary membrane's permeability to various substances and its relative impermeability to plasma proteins is the basis of a fundamental homeostatic mechanism that governs the distribution and exchange of fluid between plasma and interstitial fluid.[2]

Four forces regulate fluid equilibrium in normal states: (1) colloid osmotic pressure of plasma, (2) colloid osmotic pressure of interstitial fluid, (3) capillary hydrostatic pressure, and (4) interstitial fluid hydrostatic pressure. These forces effect the transfer of fluid volume from plasma to interstitial fluid. This filtration effect is counterbalanced by lymphatic drainage.[2]

Increased capillary membrane permeability may result from damage to the capillary endothelium, for example, burns, allergic reaction, or toxins. Increased capillary permeability causes a fluid shift from the intravascular to the interstitial compartment. This shift also may be the result of a change in plasma protein concentration from conditions such as plasmapheresis, malnutrition, liver disease, burns, and nephrosis.[2] Venous obstruction is a cause of increased capillary hydrostatic pressure.

Normal Fluid Equilibrium

Two different pressure gradients determine fluid flow across the capillary membrane. The first is the gradient of hydrostatic pressure (pressure of fluids) between the intravascular and interstitial spaces. The second gradient is that which results from the difference in protein concentration between the plasma and the interstitial fluids (osmotic or oncotic pressure). Hydrostatic pressure in the capillary is greater than hydrostatic pressure in the interstitial spaces, forcing fluid out of the capillaries into tissues. Osmotic pressure (also greater within capillaries) serves to absorb fluid. Fluid equilibrium is achieved by the balance of these opposing gradient forces and is described in the Starling equation as follows[3]:

$$F = k([P_{cap} - P_{if}] - [O_{cap} - O_{if}])$$

where
F = Fluid movement
k = Permeability constant in mL/sec/cm^2 of water
P_{cap} = Capillary hydrostatic pressure
P_{if} = Pericapillary interstitial fluid hydrostatic pressure (or effusion hydrostatic pressure)
O_{cap} = Plasma osmotic pressure
O_{if} = Interstitial fluid osmotic pressure (or effusion osmotic pressure)

In addition, lymphatic drainage aids in the removal of proteins that leak into the interstitial spaces, thereby keeping the interstitial osmotic pressure low. The continual movement of the heart and the lungs augments fluid return to the lymphatic system and prevents accumulation.

Alterations in pressures or lymphatic drainage can result in "edema" of potential spaces in exactly the same manner as edema develops in tissue spaces. Edema of a potential space is called an *effusion.*

PATHOPHYSIOLOGY OF ABNORMAL FLUID ACCUMULATION

An effusion may be defined as an excessive accumulation of fluid within a body space such as the pleural space, peritoneal cavity, or pericardial space. These spaces normally contain a small amount of fluid. Pathophysiologic processes can change the volume and characteristic composition of fluids within the body's spaces, resulting in interference with function.

Effusions are a common complication for the individual with cancer. Effusions compromise bodily functions, resulting in pain and discomfort, and add to the physical and emotional stresses facing the individual with cancer. Treatment for effusions is palliative and includes surgery, chemotherapy, and radiotherapy. The nurse assumes an active role in caring for the person with a malignant effusion through accurate assessment, assistance in therapeutic interventions, performing physical comfort measures, and helping the person to cope. Three serous cavities are commonly subject to the development of effusions: the pleural space, the peritoneal cavity, and the pericardial space.

Edema is an excess of body water with an increase in sodium, which leads to retention of excess fluid in the extracellular compartments. This state may be caused by increased capillary fluid pressure, decreased capillary oncotic pressure, increased interstitial oncotic pressure, or increased aldosterone in the circulating blood.[4]

Movement of fluid into a body space other than the intracellular or extracellular compartments is referred to as fluid in a *third space*. This may refer to fluid accumulations in the bowel as a result of obstruction or to fluid collected in the peritoneal cavity.

Causes of Fluid Shifts

An increase in capillary fluid pressure can result from overloading of the vascular compartment. This causes fluid to be shifted to the surrounding interstitial spaces. Overloading may be caused by administering too much fluid within a short period of time to a person who cannot process the excess volume. Retention of sodium or water also is a common cause of volume overload. Volume overloading is a risk when plasma, plasma expanders, albumin, or blood are given in therapeutic regimens. This same mechanism can cause fluid to collect in spaces between two membranes that normally contain only traces of fluid.[4] Any deviation from normal fluid control mechanisms may be responsible for the production of fluid in the two major types of effusions. The identification of the source of pathogenesis is critical to the selection of treatment to be used to resolve the effusion.

There are two categories of effusions: transudates and exudates. A transudate is a fluid that has passed through a membrane for reasons other than a change in vascular permeability. An exudate is material such as cells or cellular debris that has escaped from blood vessels and has been deposited in tissues or on tissue surfaces. Exudative effusions originate from serous membrane linings.

Transudate Effusions

Malignant transudate effusions result from venous or lymphatic obstruction. This type of effusion usually is associated with large tumors such as lymphomas. Transudate effusions have a protein level of less than 3 g/dL, specific gravity less than 1.016, and few tumor cells.[5]

The obstruction or obliteration of lymph channels or restriction of venous flow causes congestion in the circulation of fluids, which leads to fluid buildup in the tissues and protein leakage from the capillaries. This will result in localized edema from transudates.

Exudate Effusions

Malignant effusions caused by irritation of the serous membrane by sloughed cancer cells or from solid tumor implants are known as exudates. Exudates are the most common type of malignant effusions. Characteristics of exudates include protein levels greater than 3 g/dL, specific gravity greater than 1.016, and a tumor cell count of 50 to 1000 cells/mm^3.[5]

Exudates and transudates also may be differentiated on the basis of simultaneous measurement of lactic dehydrogenase (LDH) and protein in serum and effusion.[5] An exudate is defined by one or more of the following criteria: a fluid protein to serum protein ratio greater than 0.5; a fluid LDH to serum LDH ratio greater than 0.6; and a fluid LDH greater than 200 IU. Using these criteria Light and colleagues[3] were able to correctly classify 148 of 150 pleural effusions as exudates or transudates.

ASCITES

Etiology

Ascites, broadly defined, is the abnormal accumulation of fluid in the abdominal cavity that is not reabsorbed into the systemic circulation. This accumulation also may be referred to as *peritoneal effusion*. Ascites usually is the result of a transudative process. A change in the vascular permeability to large molecules accounts for the elevated protein levels associated with malignant ascites. Portal system obstruction as a result of intra-abdominal carcinomas and obstruction of diaphragmatic lymphatics often are cited as the primary etiologic process in the formation of malignant ascites.[6]

Ascites is associated with a number of different tumors. The following comprise more than 80% of tumors associated with ascites: ovarian, endometrial, breast, colon, gastric, and pancreatic. Rarer tumors associated with ascites include primary mesothelioma, testicular and lung cancers, lymphoma, sarcoma, multiple myeloma, and melanoma.[7]

Ascites may occur in ovarian carcinoma as an exudate. It is caused by seeding of the tumor along the peritoneal surfaces. The ascites of ovarian carcinoma may be further increased if the tumor obstructs the abdominal lymphatic vessels.

Clinical Manifestations

The formation of malignant ascites has been recognized as an adverse prognostic sign. Despite the limited survival of many of these patients, discomfort and overall well-being are sufficient reasons to justify palliative therapy.[6]

Abdominal distention, weight gain, and general discomfort are presenting signs of ascites. Increased intra-abdominal pressure may result in early satiety, indigestion, and reduced bladder capacity. Decreased bowel mobility from ascites and carcinomatosis may lead to bowel obstruction. Dyspnea, orthopnea, or tachypnea may result from the fluid accumulation, causing an elevated diaphragm, or from an associated pleural effusion.

Clinical Assessment

The physical signs of ascites are a tender, distended abdomen with tightly stretched skin, everted umbilicus, and bulging flanks. Fluid wave and flank dullness that shift with changes in the person's position also can be observed.

Diagnostic tests include an abdominal radiograph, which will show fluid between bowel loops, potential areas of small bowel obstruction, and decreased psoas and kidney shadow. A computed tomography (CT) scan is useful in evaluating the liver, spleen, and retroperitoneum for the presence of a tumor.[8]

A diagnostic paracentesis is essential to establish the presence of malignant cells in the ascitic fluid. Benign causes of ascites must be ruled out even in individuals with a history of cancer. The ascitic fluid is cultured to rule out infection. The fluid is examined for protein because 75% of individuals with cancer have ascitic fluid with protein values greater than 2.5 g/dL. Cirrhosis and nephrosis rarely cause increased protein. Cytology and cell block examinations are performed routinely.[7] Lowenstein and colleagues[9] indicate that carcinoembryonic antigen (CEA) evaluations help distinguish malignant from nonmalignant ascites. In their studies 50% of individuals with malignant disease had CEA levels above 12 ng/mL, and no individuals with nonmalignant ascites had CEA levels greater than 12 ng/mL.

Treatment

Several methods are used to treat malignant ascites: systemic chemotherapy, intraperitoneal radioisotopes, intraperitoneal and intra-abdominal chemotherapy, and surgery.

Systemic chemotherapy is indicated if the underlying disease is responsive to the drugs. Breast and ovarian tumors and lymphoma are most likely to respond to chemotherapy.

Intraperitoneal administration of radioactive gold (^{198}Au) and colloidal chromic phosphate (^{32}P) produce a response rate of 47% and 31%, respectively.[10,11] These therapies are well tolerated with only mild anemia and leukopenia as late effects,[10,11] but they are difficult to use because of the required radiation safety precautions.

Intraperitoneal chemotherapy is being studied extensively. The rationale for this therapy is based on the premise that a high concentration of drug can be delivered directly to the tumor site without exposing the rest of the tissues to the same concentration of drug and toxicities experienced with systemic chemotherapy.

Intra-abdominal chemotherapy has been used in the treatment of malignant ascites. Reduction or complete cessation of the accumulation of peritoneal fluid has been reported in 35% of individuals treated with 5-fluorouracil, 36% of those treated with bleomycin, 32% of those treated with thiotepa, and 53% of those treated with nitrogen mustard. The major side effects are mild leukopenia and fever.[7]

For intraperitoneal chemotherapy a Tenckhoff catheter or comparable type of catheter is inserted using local anesthesia. The actual procedure is performed in a manner similar to that used for peritoneal dialysis, except that chemotherapeutic agents are in the infusion. Chemotherapeutic agents under study include methotrexate, 5-fluorouracil, doxorubicin, and cisplatin with systemic thiosulfate protection.

The most commonly used method for relieving ascites is a peritoneovenous shunt (LeVeen and Denver). The shunt is surgically placed using local anesthesia. The LeVeen shunt extends from the abdominal cavity through the peritoneum under subcutaneous tissue into the superior vena cava (Figure 27-1). The shunt drains the ascites directly into the circulatory system. The LeVeen shunt contains a pressure-sensitive one-way valve that permits flow when intraperitoneal pressure exceeds the central venous pressure by 3 to 5 cm of water pressure. This one-way system prevents the backflow of blood from the venous system into the peritoneum. Complications of the therapy include shunt clotting, pulmonary edema, fever, infection, disseminated intravascular coagulation, ascitic fluid leak, emboli, and pulmonary dissemination of the tumor. The LeVeen shunt originally was designed for nonmalignant ascites but currently is being used for malignant ascites. Most patients achieve palliation of ascites for longer than 3 months or until death.[12]

The Denver shunt is somewhat like the LeVeen shunt. It has a valve mechanism placed inside a compressible chamber, which is placed in the subcutaneous tissue over the ribs. The system can be flushed manually by compressing the chamber to clear debris or clots. The complications are similar to those of the LeVeen shunt, but the Denver Shunt seems to have a lower mechanical failure rate in malignant ascites therapy.[13]

Figure 27-2 summarizes the treatment of malignant ascites.[7] The use of diuretics and paracentesis is often ineffective. Peritoneovenous shunts, intraperitoneal radioisotopes, and chemotherapy are all useful. The choice of treatment depends on the experience of the physician and the institution's ability to administer the selected therapy.

Nursing Care

The nursing care of an individual with malignant ascites focuses on maintenance of fluid and electrolyte balance, nutrition, skin care, comfort measures, and assessment of bowel obstruction. To evaluate the rate of ascites accumulation, daily weight and daily abdominal girth measurements are obtained. To control the formation of ascites the patient may be placed on a sodium-restricted diet and given diuretics. Strict monitoring of fluid intake and output is essential, as is observation for symptoms of hypokalemia, hyponatremia, and hypoproteinemia.

Hypoalbuminemia caused by malignant tumors, liver disease, or other conditions may result in generalized edema. In addition to the ascites, the edema can become so severe that the patient is unable to walk or sit up. Nursing interventions for an immobilized individual include prevention of skin breakdown, contractures, and muscle deterioration. Positioning and passive exercises can be helpful.

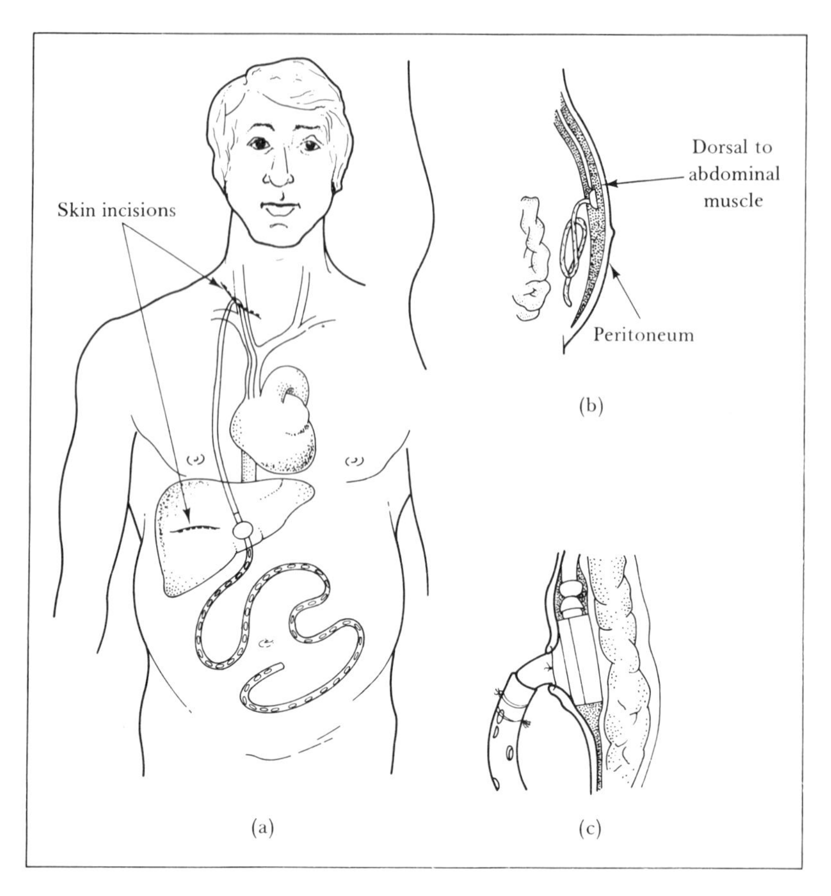

FIGURE 27-1 LeVeen shunt.

Respiratory assessment is essential because pleural effusion often is associated with ascites formation. The signs of effusion are dullness to percussion, diminished breath sounds, and egophony.

Another factor that contributes to hypoalbuminemia is malnutrition. The patient should have a high-protein, high-caloric diet with or without sodium restriction. The patient usually will have anorexia, early satiety, and constipation, which can influence intake. Consultation with a nutritionist or nutritional support team may be indicated to determine the best schedule, type of foods, and supplements to offer the patient. Enteral tube feedings may be instituted if the oral route is unsuccessful. Stool softeners, laxatives, and enemas are used to relieve constipation. The nurse assesses bowel sounds and monitors regularity of bowel function.

A paracentesis always is performed in the diagnostic phase. Complete removal of the fluid may be done. The patient should void before the procedure to prevent potential bladder puncture. The patient is placed in Fowler's position with back, arms, and feet supported. The nurse explains that the procedure is uncomfortable but not painful. The rate of fluid removal is not a significant factor. Carey and colleagues[14] rapidly removed large amounts of ascitic fluid from 27 subjects with cirrhosis without hemodynamic, renal, or electrolyte abnormalities. After the procedure, a sterile dressing is applied, vital signs are monitored, and the dressing is observed for potential ascitic fluid leakage. The patient is encouraged to drink fluids to counterbalance orthostatic changes and to ambulate carefully to avoid dizziness or falls.

Intraperitoneal chemotherapy is administered in a manner similar to peritoneal dialysis. The solution is delivered into the abdominal cavity through a Tenckhoff catheter (similar to a Broviac catheter) or a Port-A-Cath. These devices are placed in the abdominal cavity using local anesthesia.

After surgical insertion of the catheter, several exchanges are performed by means of heparinized dialysate without chemotherapy to prevent the formation of fibrin clots and to assess the patient's tolerance of dialysis. When the fluid is clear (it will be bloody at first), the Tenckhoff catheter is flushed with heparinized dialysate, capped, and the site dressed by means of aseptic technique. The Port-A-Cath is flushed with saline, and no dressing is required.

The daily exchanges of heparinized dialysate continue for 7 to 10 days after catheter placement. When the surgical incision has healed, chemotherapy can begin. The chemotherapeutic agent is placed in the dialysis solution and infused into the abdomen. The number of exchanges,

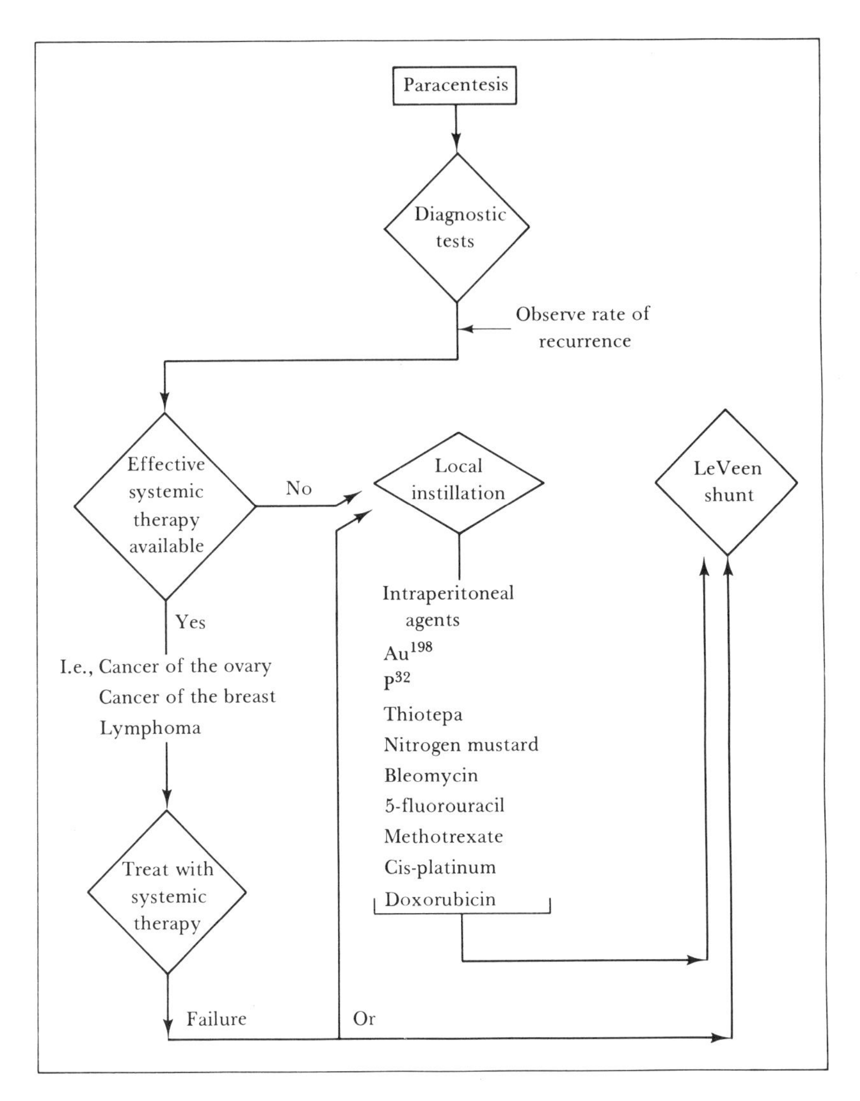

FIGURE 27-2 Management of malignant ascites. (Source: Mauch PM: Treatment of malignant pleural effusions, in DeVita VT, Hellman S, Rosenberg SA (eds): Cancer: Principles and Practice of Oncology. Philadelphia, JB Lippincott, 1982, p 1575.)

fluid dwelling time, and treatment schedules vary according to institution or protocol.

Nursing care is comparable to that of a person receiving peritoneal dialysis, including careful monitoring of the exact amount of fluid instilled, the times of each exchange, the exact amount drained, and the patient's tolerance of the entire procedure. If the patient has a Tenckhoff catheter, the site is examined daily when the sterile dressing change is performed. The patient is taught how to change the dressing before discharge.

The most common complication of intracavity dialysis is abdominal pain or discomfort. This can be caused by peritoneal irritation, incomplete drainage of dialysate, failure to warm the dialysate to body temperature, chemical peritonitis, or bacterial peritonitis.[15]

The nurse's role is critical in managing the dialysis treatment, maintaining the catheter, and teaching the patient how to care for the catheter. The patient will need emotional support to cope with the frequent hospitalizations and the discomfort experienced during the treatments.

The nursing care of patients with LeVeen shunts incorporates that of caring for persons with ascites plus some special considerations. Before surgery the patient is instructed about the importance of wearing an abdominal binder when the shunt is inserted. The special breathing exercises that will activate the shunt are demonstrated. The patient takes deep breaths against resistance for 15 minutes four times a day. This can be done by breathing in through a tube inserted into a bottle filled with 5 to 8 mL of water or by using an incentive spirometry apparatus. Inspiration increases intraperitoneal pressure, which causes the one-way valve to open.

After surgery, daily measurements of weight and abdominal girth are essential. Within 24 hours of shunt placement, the patient should have a tight abdominal binder in place and be assisted in the special breathing exercises that stimulate the valve function of the shunt.

For self-care teaching, the nurse emphasizes the importance of wearing the abdominal binder, continuing the breathing exercises, keeping a chart of daily weight and abdominal girth, and adhering to the prescribed diet. In addition, the nurse will reinforce teaching to recognize the signs of potential complications, such as abdominal pain, fever, sudden weight gain, increased abdominal girth, bleeding, or infection.

PULMONARY EDEMA

Etiology

Risk factors for the development of pulmonary edema in association with cancer include chemotherapy-induced cardiomyopathy, rapid administration of blood and blood products in the presence of low serum albumin, and administration of high osmolarity solutions in the presence of low serum albumin.[16] Kuhn et al[17] reported pulmonary edema related to a venous air embolism after the removal of a subclavian catheter.

Pulmonary edema can be caused by capillary hypertension or altered barrier permeability. Capillary hypertension most often is related to congestive heart failure. Permeability-related pulmonary edema may be secondary to an acute rise in microvasculature pressure. More commonly, permeability-related pulmonary edema is the result of chemical mediators released after local or systemic insults. This usually is described as adult respiratory distress syndrome. In this condition there is extravasation of protein.[18]

Clinical Manifestations

The primary clinical signs of pulmonary edema are tachypnea, increased respiratory effort, and dyspnea. Interstitial lung tissue changes may be seen on chest radiographs. With interstitial edema there usually are not overt signs of compromised pulmonary function as reflected by arterial blood gases (ABG) and pulmonary functions tests.[18] In the early stages there is dry cough that progresses to the production of large quantities of sputum. With progressive interstitial pulmonary edema there is airway obstruction and alveolar flooding and collapse. Arterial carbon dioxide pressure ($PaCO_2$) rises, and respiratory acidosis ensues.

Clinical Assessment

Chest radiographs and assessment of effective gas exchange are the principal means of diagnosis. Arterial blood gas determination is the standard method of monitoring alterations in pulmonary status. Regular assessment of respiratory rate and depth, lung sounds, use of accessory muscles, skin color, and behavior provide additional data.[18]

Treatment and Nursing Care

Medical and nursing interventions are aimed at eradicating the underlying neoplasm. Depending on the tumor, aggressive radiation, chemotherapy, or surgery may be indicated to resolve the underlying cause. The immediate goals of therapy for pulmonary edema are to maintain adequate lung function and oxygenation and to reverse the process of edema formation. Oxygen administration can improve hypoxemia; however, oxygen does not change the restrictive effects of pulmonary edema on the lungs nor ease the work of breathing. Position change may relieve the respiratory distress caused by accumulation of the extravasated fluid. No pharmaceutical agents have been clearly shown to restore pulmonary barrier permeability to normal. The use of high-dose corticosteroids remains controversial.[18] Positive end-expiratory pressure (PEEP) has been used to prevent and reverse atelectasis. There is little evidence that PEEP forces fluid from the alveoli to the interstitium. Therapy typically includes proper positioning in semi-Fowler's position; sedation to alleviate anxiety, promote sleep, decrease pulmonary reflexes, and reduce venous return; oxygen therapy; digitalization if there is an underlying cardiac problem; diuresis; relief of bronchospasm; reduction of blood volume; and management of hydration status.[16]

The psychologic status of the patient requires continuous attention, and every effort should be made to reduce anxiety. Acute pulmonary edema is a medical emergency. Treatment may be palliative or more rigorous depending on the overall prognosis and the treatment plan for the cancer.

PLEURAL EFFUSION

Etiology

Malignancy is the major cause of pleural effusion. It is one of the most common symptomatic complications of cancer, occurring in up to 50% of all individuals with cancer. Malignant pleural effusions most commonly result from primary tumors of the lung, breast, and hematopoietic system. A pleural effusion will develop at some time during the course of the disease in as many as one half of individuals with breast or lung cancer.[19] Metastases from genitourinary and gastrointestinal malignancies can cause pleural effusion, as well as less common malignancies such as mesotheliomas, sarcomas, and melanomas.

The presence of abnormal amounts of fluid in the pleural space may be caused by increased hydrostatic pressure in the microvascular circulation, decrease in oncotic pressure in the microvascular circulation, decreased pressure in the pleural space, increased permeability of the microvascular circulation, impaired lymphatic drainage from the pleural space, and movement of fluid from the peritoneal space.[20,21]

Malignant pleural effusion, the presence of malignant cells in the pleural space, may occur from direct extension of a primary lung tumor to the pleura, involvement of the pleural surfaces by primary mesothelioma, or by a variety of metastatic diseases. Malignant involvement of the pleural surface can shed cells into the pleural space, which can then seed unaffected visceral or parietal pleura. Irritation of these surfaces results in an inflammatory response and increased capillary permeability. Obstruction of lung or pleural lymphatic vessels by lymphoma or breast cancer impairs reabsorption of fluid and protein. Obstruction of the pulmonary vein by the tumor increases the capillary hydrostatic pressure, thus reducing the gradient between the visceral and parietal pleura.[20-23]

Pleural effusions may be caused by the effects of radiation therapy on mucosal surfaces of the thoracic cavity: radiation pleuritis and systemic venous hypertension or lymphatic obstruction from mediastinal fibrosis. Pleural effusions also may be a late effect of mediastinal radiation and may occur 1 to 2 years after therapy.[20]

Clinical Manifestations

The onset of a pleural effusion may be sudden or evolve over time. As many as 25% of individuals may be asymptomatic upon presentation with a pleural effusion.[23,24] Dyspnea is the most common symptom of a pleural effusion. Dyspnea is caused by the compression of a significant amount of underlying lung parenchyma. Cough is the second most common symptom, but the exact pathogenesis is not clear. Pathogenesis may be related to compression of bronchial walls by fluid, thus stimulating the cough reflex. Chest pain with a pleural effusion is usually caused by increased intrapleural or intraparenchymal pressure stimulating the sympathetic nervous system. Fever also may be present. Other symptoms are likely related to the underlying cancer rather than to the effusion.[22,23]

No symptoms distinguish a malignant pleural effusion from a benign disorder. Malignant pleural effusions often have an insidious onset, with relatively minor symptoms gradually increasing over a period of months. Pleural effusions from nonmalignant causes usually have an abrupt onset of symptoms.[1]

Clinical Assessment

Physical examination of the chest may reveal dullness to percussion, diminished or absent breath sounds, and egophony on the affected side. A pleural friction rub occasionally is heard. Before abnormal physical findings can be detected, 300 to 500 mL of fluid must have accumulated.[25]

A thoracentesis and withdrawal of a minimum of 25 to 30 mL of fluid is needed for an accurate cytologic diagnosis.[21,23] Pleural fluid can be a transudate effusion when it is the result of the alteration of mechanical factors that influence fluid movement. An exudate results from the inflammation of the pleural surface or from seeding of tumor.[23] Most malignant pleural effusions are exudates. Ruckdeschel[22] reported that increased levels of protein or lactic dehydrogenase (LDH), elevated fluid to serum ratio of the same markers, and combinations of the two are all that are required for near-certain distinction of an exudate from a transudate.[20,21]

Radiologic examination yields further evidence of pleural fluid accumulation. On chest radiograph, blunting of the costophrenic angle and fluid density along the lateral chest wall may be observed. Lateral decubitus radiographs, taken with the patient lying on the side, demonstrate free-flowing fluid versus loculated (pocket) effusion. This view can detect as little as 100 mL of pleural fluid.[20,26]

Other diagnostic tests include pleural fluid aspiration for cytologic examination and pleural biopsy. Salyer and associates[27] found that cytologic examination confirms the diagnosis in 50% of individuals. If the examinations are repeated two, three, or four times, the yield increases to 64%, 69%, and 73%, respectively. Pleural biopsies alone produce positive results 50% to 60% of the time. The combination of cytologic examination and pleural biopsy, however, establishes the diagnosis in 90% of patients. It is important to remember that an absence of malignant cells does not rule out a neoplastic process.[20,21]

Specimens of the pleural fluid also should be cultured to rule out tuberculosis or other infection. Several chemical tests may be performed: LDH level, the ratio of pleural fluid LDH to serum LDH, and the ratio of pleural fluid protein to serum protein.[3,21] These tests help to determine if the fluid is an exudate, the most common classification of malignant pleural effusion.

Further confirmation of malignancy can be obtained through pleural fluid CEA levels. Elevated CEA levels rarely are associated with benign effusions. A comparison is made between the CEA level of the pleural fluid and the CEA level of the serum. Thus, elevated levels are pathognomonic for malignancy, but normal levels do not rule out malignancy.[20,21,25]

The presence of malignant pleural fluid does not necessarily mean the person has entered the terminal phase of illness. Mauch and Ultmann[28] cited two studies that show that median survival times after diagnosis of malignant pleural effusions have varied from 3 months to more than 19 months. Aggressive control of the accumulation of pleural fluid can alleviate symptoms, lengthen survival time, and improve the quality of life for the person with cancer.

Treatment

The optimal treatment of a pleural effusion not only removes pleural fluid but prevents its reaccumulation. A variety of systemic therapies are given concomitantly with local treatments to control the malignant effusion. If the underlying tumor is responsive to chemotherapy, effective systemic therapy improves response to local therapy for malignant effusions. In a responsive tumor, systemic therapy alone may be effective in eliminating a small effusion.

Thoracentesis is performed to remove fluid from the intrapleural space and relieve immediate symptoms of dyspnea. Reaccumulation of the fluid is common, even within days. Repeat thoracentesis may cause anxiety and pain for the patient. Hypoproteinemia, pneumothorax, empyema, and fluid loculation are potential untoward effects of thoracentesis.[26,29] For these reasons thoracentesis is of limited value in the treatment of recurrent malignant effusions. However, for diagnosis, palliation for an individual in the terminal stages of cancer, or relief of acute respiratory distress, thoracentesis is an effective procedure.[21-23]

Alternative treatments to thoracentesis are the insertion of chest tubes for drainage or the combination of chest tube drainage followed by the instillation of a sclerosing agent. Chest tubes attached to continuous suction ensure complete evacuation of fluid to promote adherence of the pleural surfaces. Theoretically, the negative intrathoracic pressure created by suction causes an obliterative pleuritis; thus fluid should not recur. Pleural drainage alone is only minimally effective for long-term control of malignant pleural effusions.[30,31] The addition of various intrapleural sclerosing agents appears to improve the likelihood of an effective response.

Sclerosing agents are instilled into the pleural space after thoracostomy drainage. Chemotherapeutic agents such as nitrogen mustard, bleomycin, thiotepa, and 5-fluorouracil have been used. Beneficial results vary from 25% to 100%.[28] Tetracycline, talc, nitrogen mustard, and various biological agents are known to cause a dense fibrosis. The effects of bleomycin and 5-fluorouracil are less clear. Many other agents previously used as sclerosing agents have been abandoned.[22,29,32] Biologic agents are being studied for the treatment of pleural effusion. Promising results have been obtained in current trials.

Sherman et al[33] reported that, among the numerous agents advocated to achieve pleurodesis, tetracycline is the agent of choice. Memon and Zawadski[25] indicated that the best approach appears to be intrapleural tetracycline, which irritates the pleura because of its low pH in solution, in conjunction with thoracostomy drainage. It is effective (83% to 100%), has low morbidity, and is well tolerated by the individual. Tetracycline is inexpensive, readily available, does not interfere with concurrent chemotherapy, and has minimal systemic side effects.[33]

Intracavitary chemotherapy is given in doses similar to those for systemic administration: nitrogen mustard, 10 to 40 mg; thiotepa, 30 to 45 mg; 5-fluorouracil, 2 to 3 mg; and bleomycin, 15 to 240 mg.[28] Effects on the effusion are related more to the creation of a pleurodesis, preventing effusion reaccumulation, than to any antineoplastic effect.[34]

Talc poudrage is a silicate that is closely related to asbestos and causes an intense pleuritis and obliteration of the pleural space. Of those individuals treated with talc 90% require no additional therapy.[28] Treatment with intrapleural talc causes severe local pain. Special techniques are required for application. The procedure often is done with the use of general anesthesia, which increases mortality and morbidity. Talc is recommended in patients with recurrent malignant pleural effusion after two or more sclerosing attempts with other agents.[21]

Factors that contribute to the successful use of sclerosing agents for intracavitary instillation are complete drainage of pleural effusion before instillation (residual fluid dilutes the agent instilled and limits the inflammatory reaction), sufficient volume of the sclerosing agent (approximately 30 to 40 mL), proper positioning of the patient to promote adequate distribution, and complete reexpansion of the lung before the chest tube is removed.

The sclerosing agent is instilled into the pleural space through a chest tube, which then is clamped. The patient's position is changed approximately every 30 minutes during a period of 2 to 6 hours to ensure contact of the sclerosing agent with the entire pleural surface. These positions include prone, left side, supine, right side, and knee-chest. At the end of the specified period of clamping, the chest tube is reconnected to a closed water-seal drainage system to completely evacuate the pleural space and promote reexpansion of the lung. Chest radiographs are taken to verify complete reexpansion; then the chest tube is removed.[29]

External beam radiotherapy is recommended for the treatment of mediastinal tumors (lymphoma and lung). Neither mediastinal nor pleural irradiation are recommended as first-line management of pleural effusions.[21,34]

Radioactive colloidal gold or colloidal chromic phosphate have been instilled through a thoracostomy tube into the pleural cavity for the treatment of malignant effusions. Response rates of 50% to 60% with minimal toxic side effects have been achieved. The disadvantages, however, are cost and inconvenience. These radioactive substances are not readily available, have short half-lives that make storage difficult, and require special precautions in preparation and use to prevent radiation contamination.[28] Because equally effective treatment alternatives are available, intrapleural radiotherapy is infrequently used.

Pleurectomy, or mechanical pleurodesis, has been shown to be highly effective (about 99%) for individuals with malignant effusions. Pleurectomy is used infrequently because of the success of sclerotherapy. Pleurectomy usually is considered only for individuals who have not responded to intrapleural agents and who are good surgical candidates. Mortality from pleurectomy is about 10%, and morbidity is about 20% (from persistent pneumonia, empyema, and bronchopleural fistula).[21,28,29,34]

Pleuroperitoneal shunting has been described in isolated reports and is used when sclerotherapy has failed. It can be effective in selected patients if palliation is the goal of treatment. This treatment has a potential risk of pneumothorax and air emboli.[29,35,36]

The ideal treatment for a recurrent malignant pleural effusion should be effective, safe, and convenient. Thoracostomy drainage is used to ensure that the pleural space is fully evacuated before instillation of a sclerosing agent. On the basis of effectiveness and decreased risk of morbidity, the agent of choice is tetracycline. Pleurectomy is effective but is associated with an unacceptably high morbidity and mortality rate. A sample treatment schema is outlined in Figure 27-3.

Nursing Care

Several nursing considerations are needed for accurate assessment and intervention. Dyspnea motivates the patient to seek medical attention. The presence of a pleural effusion may lead to an initial diagnosis of primary malignancy or a recurrence.

A thoracentesis usually will be performed in the diagnostic phase. Before the procedure the nurse explains the process to the patient and family, assembles the equipment, and positions the person properly. Patient education includes an explanation of the procedure and the rationale, emphasizing the importance of not moving or coughing during the procedure and reassuring the patient that the discomfort is minimal. The nurse explains that if pain is felt, the patient should mention it so that more local anesthetic can be given. Premedication usually is not indicated unless the patient is very anxious. Positioning is crucial. Thoracentesis is best performed with the person sitting upright (so that the pleural fluid will accumulate at the base of the chest), with the neck and dorsal spine flexed and arms and shoulders raised (which elevates and separates the ribs, making needle insertion easier).

The nurse remains at the patient's side during the procedure to assess and to reassure the person. The patient's pulse and respirations are monitored several times during the procedure. The patient is observed for chills, pain, nausea, coughing, pallor, dyspnea, weakness, increased respiratory rate, and diaphoresis. The physician is advised if these symptoms develop.

After thoracentesis, manual pressure is applied to the site, a sterile dressing is applied, and the patient is positioned on the unaffected side. This position minimizes fluid seepage into the pleural space and allows the pleural puncture site to seal. The nurse observes the patient for signs of complications or fluid reaccumulation. Shock is rare but can occur as a result of fluid shifting into the pleural space from the vascular space. The dressing is checked for leakage. The person is observed for signs of pneumothorax, mediastinal shift, or tension pneumothorax.

Treatment of pleural effusion usually consists of an indwelling thoracostomy tube and chemical sclerosing. Nursing care of individuals with chest tubes requires knowledge of the mechanics of breathing, the chest tube systems available, and the ability to assess and remedy any malfunctions in the system.[37,38]

Patient care during preparation and insertion of a chest tube is similar to that for individuals who require thoracentesis. Before insertion of a chest tube, however, the patient usually receives premedication with a narcotic analgesic plus a tranquilizer. Despite local anesthesia, chest tube insertion can be a lengthy, painful procedure. After the tube is inserted and connected to water-seal drainage, the patient takes deep breaths and exhales completely. This helps to reexpand the lung and drain the pleural space.

Before insertion of the sclerosing agent, the patient receives premedication with a narcotic analgesic. The sclerosing agent is injected into the pleural space only after the space has been completely drained (ie, chest tube output <150 mL/day). After injection, the chest tube is clamped with two clamps (each clamped in an opposite direction to ensure total occlusion). The patient must change position every 30 minutes. Rotation to prone, left, supine, right, and knee-chest positions is essential to distribute the sclerosing agent over the entire pleural surface. Otherwise, loculated areas of effusion can form. After 2 to 6 hours, the clamps are removed and a closed water-seal drainage system is applied to the chest tube for several days until there is no more drainage. Patient care after removal of the chest tube is similar to patient care after thoracentesis.

Patients undergoing pleurectomy require the same preoperative and postoperative care as a patient undergoing thoracotomy. This includes care of chest tubes and knowledge of complications (mediastinal shift, bleeding, cardiac dysrhythmias, and respiratory complications).

Nursing care of patients with malignant pleural effusions is challenging. Some oncology nurses may have limited experience with chest tubes. Management of malignant pleural effusions provides an opportunity for medical and surgical nurses to consult each other. Individuals with pleural effusion also need psychosocial support to deal with the initial diagnosis or recurrence of cancer signaled by the pleural effusion.

CEREBRAL EDEMA

Etiology

Cerebral edema often is a complication of late-stage intracranial neoplasms or metastases. Metastatic brain tumors, malignant astrocytoma, and meningioma are asso-

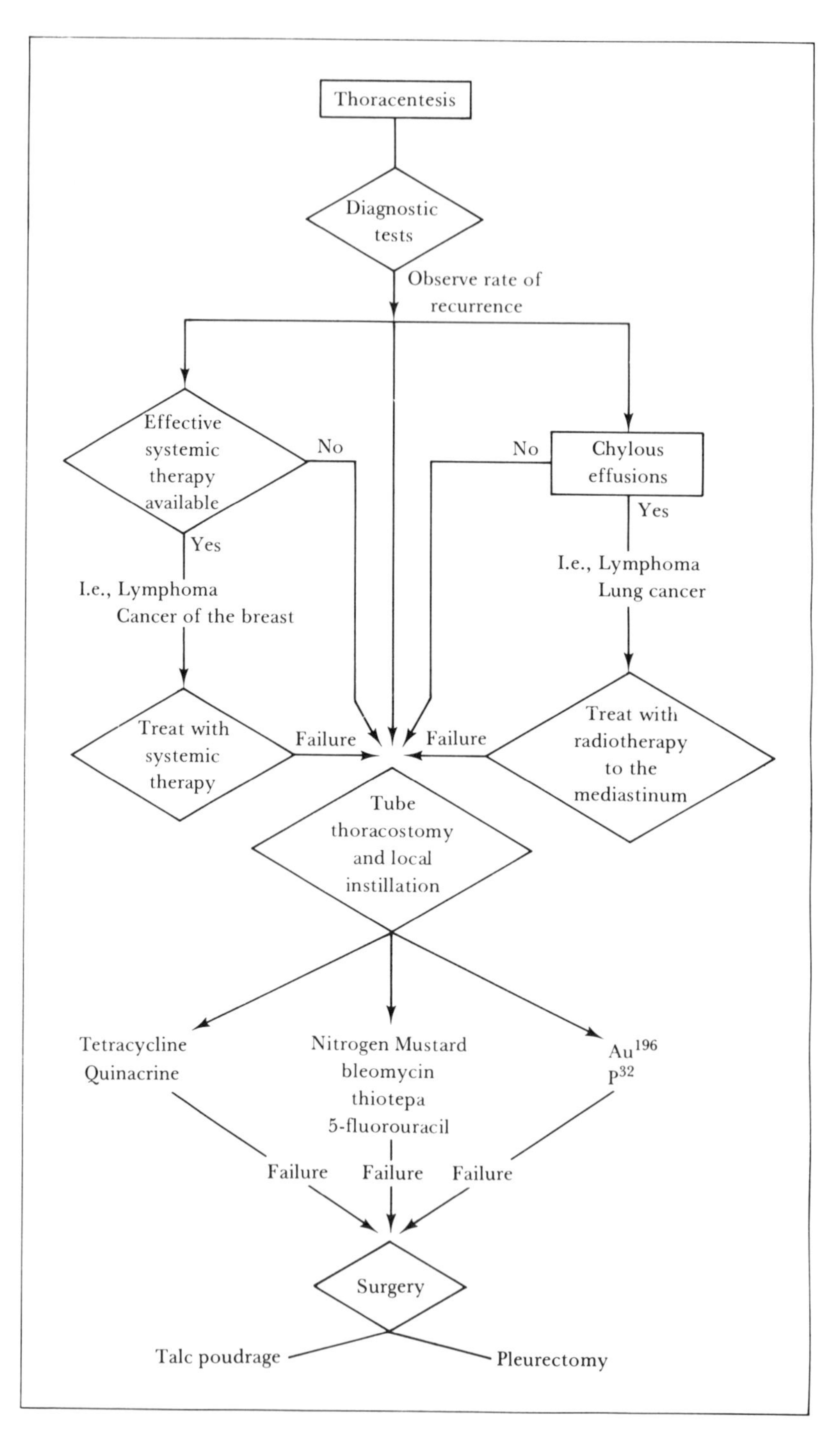

FIGURE 27-3 Treatment of malignant pleural effusions. (Source: Mauch PM: Treatment of malignant pleural effusions, in DeVita VT, Hellman S, Rosenberg SA (eds): Cancer: Principles and Practice of Oncology. Philadelphia, JB Lippincott, 1982, p 1570.)

ciated with cerebral edema.[39,40] Cerebral peritumoral edema is one of the most serious complications of intracranial tumors.

Vasogenic edema, the most common type of cerebral edema, occurs in association with localized brain tumors. Vasogenic edema is believed to involve a defect in the junctions of the capillary endothelial cells and the normal barrier functions of these cells. As a result, proteins, sodium, and other large molecular solutes are allowed to enter the brain as transudates.[18]

The exact pathogenesis of cerebral peritumoral edema is not known although it usually is of the vasogenic type.[40,41] It is generally accepted that edema secondary to brain tumors is the result of extravasates from leaky vessels within the tumor into the extracellular space of the surrounding white matter, with the transcapillary hydrostatic pressure as the driving force. The ultimate event is believed to be the breakdown of the blood-brain barrier with leakage of plasma.[41,42] Challa[41] suggested that possible causal factors for cerebral edema associated with intracranial tumors may be multifactorial: the size of the tumor in relationship to the rate of edema formation, tumors that secrete edemogenic substances, tumor metabolites, and compression of superficial veins and venous sinuses. Cerebral edema also may be a complication of external beam radiation therapy for brain metastases from a variety of tumors.[43] It is suggested by Jagadha and Deck[39] that edema in the brain may contribute more to patient morbidity than the effects of direct compression by the tumor itself.

Clinical Manifestations

Cerebral edema generally adds to the increasing intracranial pressure produced by the tumor mass. As the edema increases, the blood supply to the brain is compromised and carbon dioxide is retained. Blood vessels will then dilate in an effort to increase the oxygen supply, which subsequently causes increased pressure and can lead to rapid deterioration.[2] Signs related to cerebral edema are general impairment of cerebral function, changes in level of consciousness, seizure, and changes in parasympathetic regulation. Papilledema is a relatively late sign of increased intracranial pressure. When the edema exceeds the compensatory mechanisms, the irreversible outcome is cerebral herniation.

Clinical Assessment

Assessment is focused both on the effects of an intracranial neoplasm and on the changes in intracranial pressure. The signs and symptoms of cerebral edema may resemble and coexist with those of the brain tumor. Headache may be related to increased intracranial pressure. Signs of increased intracranial pressure are changes in level of consciousness, pupillary response, blood pressure, pulse, respiration, and visual acuity. Other signs related to the specific neoplasm or the specific area of the brain affected may be observed. Assessments of localized neurologic effects are reviewed in Chapter 36.

CT scan and radionuclide scans of the brain are used to localize the tumor and monitor the rate of tumor growth and changes associated with cerebral edema. Lumbar puncture is avoided if cerebral edema is suspected because of the risk of brainstem herniation.[2] With vasogenic edema, there is a characteristic increase in cerebrospinal fluid protein, which is normal in cytotoxic edema.[18]

Treatment

Treatment focuses on reducing the cerebral edema and eradicating underlying neoplasm. A combination of treatment approaches, including drugs, surgery, and radiation, often is used. Reducing the pressure on the brain tissue may be accomplished by surgical removal of the tumor, creation of a shunt to drain excess fluid, and radiation or chemotherapy, or both, to reduce tumor mass. The aggressiveness of the therapy correlates with the severity of the underlying malignant disease.

External beam radiation commonly is used in the treatment of primary and metastatic brain tumors. Cerebral edema is a side effect of radiation to the brain. Corticosteroids, begun 48 to 72 hours before radiation, are widely used to reduce the incidence of radiation-induced cerebral edema.[43] Dexamethasone has been the drug of choice. Other drugs used to relieve the symptoms of cerebral edema are hyperosmotic agents such as mannitol, urea, furosemide, and barbiturates.[44] Hormones are given if there is reduced production because of tumor location or involvement.[44]

Nursing Care

Nursing care centers on observing and monitoring neurologic status. Determining changes in the neurologic status is essential to the course of therapeutic interventions. Specific nursing care measures are indicated by the underlying cause of the cerebral edema and the medical or surgical interventions. Teaching patient and family to recognize and promptly report changes is essential.

PERICARDIAL EFFUSION

Etiology

The incidence of malignant pericardial effusion usually is underestimated. An autopsy series indicated that up to 21% of individuals with cancer have a varying degree of pericardial effusion.[45] A variety of tumors have been reported to metastasize to the pericardium. The tumors most commonly reported include lung, breast, leukemia, lymphoma, melanoma, gastrointestinal, and sarcoma. Certain primary tumors of the heart may cause pericardial effusions, including sarcoma and mesothelioma. Metastatic involvement of the pericardium may occur from direct invasion by an adjacent primary tumor or by lymphatic or hematogenous spread.[46] Cancer has been documented to be the single most common cause of pericardial effusion leading to cardiac tamponade.[47]

Pericardial effusion in patients with diagnosed malignancies is not always caused by the primary tumor. The effusion may be drug induced or associated with other nonmalignant pathologic conditions such as tuberculosis, rheumatic fever, trauma, uremia, collagen vascular diseases, myxedema, or previous irradiation.[29,46]

Obstruction of venous and lymphatic drainage of the heart disrupts the equilibrium that exists among capillary filtration and hydraulic and osmotic forces. This results in excessive accumulation of pericardial fluid. Metastatic implants on the pericardial serosal surface cause fluid exudation.[47] The effects of pericardial fluid accumulation are largely dependent on the rate of exudation and the physical compliance capacity of the pericardial cavity. It is not the absolute quantity of pericardial fluid but the rapidity with which the effusion accumulates and the pericardial compliance that determines progression to cardiac tamponade.[48] If the fluid accumulation is gradual, the pericardium can stretch to accommodate as much as 4 L of fluid, despite the fact that the normal amount of pericardial fluid is 50 mL. Rapid accumulation of 150 to 200 mL may trigger an oncologic emergency.[29]

Pericardial effusion interferes with cardiac function because the fluid accumulates and occupies space, thereby reducing the volume of the heart in diastole. Systemic circulatory effects are a decrease in cardiac output and impaired venous return, which results in congestion.

Clinical Manifestations

Small pericardial effusions cause no specific symptoms and often are detected only at autopsy.[48] The most frequently occuring symptoms, dyspnea, cough, and chest pain, are nonspecific (Table 27-1).[49] There is not one clinical manifestation that alone would indicate the presence of a pericardial effusion. Symptoms depend on the rate of fluid accumulation.

Effusive, constrictive pericarditis is characterized by a thickened pericardium and a pericardial effusion that develops under pressure. Constrictive pericarditis occurs when a dense, thickened, somewhat fibrotic pericardium encases the heart, causing restriction of filling of all four chambers. It more commonly occurs with lung and breast cancers and can appear months or years after thoracic radiotherapy.[48,50]

TABLE 27-1 Clinical Manifestations of Pericardial Effusion

Decreased cardiac output
Tachycardia
Tachypnea
Vasoconstriction
Low systolic blood pressure
Diminished pulse pressure
Dyspnea
Impaired consciousness
Shock
Distended pericardial sac
Precordial dullness to percussion
Distant weak heart sounds
Chest discomfort
Venous congestion
Jugular vein distention
Ascites
Hepatomegaly
Peripheral edema

Source: Adapted from Miller SE, Campbell JB: Malignant pericardial effusions, in Polomano RC, Miller SE (eds): Understanding and Managing Oncologic Emergencies. Columbus, Ohio, Adria Laboratories, 1987, pp 19-26.

Clinical Assessment

The simplest, safest, and most reliable diagnostic study for the assessment of a pericardial effusion is the echocardiogram. If the patient is hospitalized, this test can be done at the patient's bedside and can be used to follow the progress of the effusion. Echocardiogram also can be used as an adjunct to pericardiocentesis.

Chest radiographs may show an increased heart size or a change in the contour of the heart shadow. A normal radiograph does not exclude the possibility of effusion. Electrocardiogram changes often are minimal but may show voltage decreases, sinus tachycardia, diffuse ST and T wave abnormalities. Large effusions or tamponade may produce electrical alternans (variation in size of the QRS complex).[29]

CT scans have become an important tool in diagnosing pericardial effusions. Whether or not the patient has symptoms, the volume of fluid can be estimated rapidly so that appropriate therapy can be initiated.[51]

Pericardiocentesis must be performed to determine if the effusion is malignant. With the use of the echocardiogram as a guide, the needle can be placed more accurately and without serious complications.[52] Pericardial fluid should be examined for infectious causes, particularly in immunocompromised patients. Pericardial fluid may be serous, serosanguinous, or hemorrhagic. There is a high percentage of false-negative cytologic results. Negative results do not rule out malignancy as the source of the effusion. In general, levels of LDH and protein and cell count are not particularly important in distinguishing malignant effusion from other causes.[48] Often symptoms and clinical manifestations are the definitive factors that lead to aggressive therapy.

Treatment

Management of malignant pericardial effusions depends on the biologic behavior of the underlying cancer and the clinical presentation of the effusion. The treatment plan often includes local control measures and more systemic management of the underlying disease.[29] Pericardial effusions can progress to pericardial tamponade, which is life threatening and must be treated immediately.

If the patient has symptoms, supportive therapy may be needed first, which includes the administration of saline and colloids, oxygen, and drugs to increase cardiac output and blood pressure. Emergency pericardiocentesis then can be performed. If no further therapy is undertaken, rapid fluid reaccumulation may occur. Various therapeutic approaches include surgery, local instillation of chemotherapeutic agents or radioisotopes, and external radiotherapy.

The most effective immediate intervention is the prompt withdrawal of fluid, which can be accomplished by pericardiocentesis or creation of a pericardial window. Dramatic improvement in clinical status can occur with the removal of 50 to 100 mL of fluid.[29,47]

Surgical treatment includes pericardial window or pericardiectomy. A pericardial window can be performed using local anesthesia through a subxiphoid incision. Drainage tubes are placed in the pericardium and attached to water-seal drainage. The tubes are removed when the drainage is less than 50 mL/day. There are few complications, and the procedure provides effective local control by the formation of adhesions, which prevent fluid accumulation. Pericardiectomy is effective but requires a thoracotomy, has a higher morbidity rate, and therefore may not be justified.[53,54]

Various agents have been instilled into the pericardial cavity as sclerosing agents. These include tetracycline, bleomycin, thiotepa, nitrogen mustard, cisplatin, vinblastine, and 5-fluorouracil. Sclerosis is approximately 50% effective in decreasing fluid formation. Side effects include nausea, chest pain, and transient fever.[46] Intrapericardial instillation of tetracycline seems to be the treatment of choice. It is most effective and has the fewest side effects.[54,55] ^{198}Au and ^{32}P have been used with good results, but problems in handling make them difficult to use.[46] Most clinicians have abandoned radioisotopes for use in managing pericardial effusions.

Before sclerosing agents are instilled, a large catheter is placed in the pericardium and attached to a closed water-sealed drainage system. The sclerosing agent is injected through the catheter in a manner similar to that used in treating malignant pleural effusions.[56] The agent must be instilled slowly while the patient's cardiac status is carefully monitored.

External radiation can be used in the long-term management of pericardial effusions in selected tumors that are radiosensitive (leukemia, lymphoma, and oat cell carcinomas). Fifty percent of cases will respond to doses in the range of 2500 to 3000 cGy.[47]

Depending on the type of tumor, systemic therapy is initiated in addition to local approaches to control the effusion. In responsive tumors such as lymphoma and breast cancer, results may be satisfactory.

Nursing Care

A pericardial effusion that progresses to tamponade is a life-threatening emergency. Nursing care involves monitoring the cardiovascular system, restoring optimal cardiac function, and providing patient reassurance. Reassurance and emotional support are essential because compromised cardiac function and metastatic disease are extremely stressful to the individual and family.

When a pericardiocentesis is planned, the patient will receive premedication with a narcotic analgesic and a tranquilizer. The head of the bed is raised 60 degrees and electrocardiographic leads applied. If a pericardial catheter is left in place for continuous drainage, strict asepsis is required during the changing of the dressing or the flushing of the catheter. The nurse monitors the pericardiocentesis site for signs of bleeding and auscultates the heart to detect muffling sounds that indicate fluid accumulation. Assessment of respiratory status is important to detect pneumothorax if the pleural cavity was penetrated.

During insertion, injection, or removal of the catheter the patient must be monitored for cardiac dysrhythmia. Emergency equipment must be available in case cardiac arrest occurs.

LYMPHEDEMA

Etiology

The lymphatic system is a network of vessels that serve to return lymph and proteins from the tissue spaces to the circulatory system. The rate of lymph flow is determined by three factors: the continual rhythmic contraction of each vessel, the motion of the tissues, and the pressure of the interstitial fluid. Interstitial fluid protein is one of the major factors in controlling the equilibrium of capillary exchange. When the protein concentration decreases, lymph flow is slowed and fluid enters the interstitial spaces as a transudate and is reabsorbed.[57]

Lymphedema of the extremities may be divided into two types: primary and secondary. Primary lymphedema has an insidious onset, and its cause is obscure. Secondary lymphedema may result from surgery, irradiation, infection, or neoplastic replacement.[58] In secondary lymphedema, the lymphatic channels are blocked, absent, or not patent. Fluid transport is insufficient and swelling results. Radical mastectomy is considered the major cause of secondary lymphedema, with incidence rates reported as high as 50%. Modified radical mastectomy has an incidence of lymphedema reported at 5% to 10%.[57] Therapeutic groin dissection of the lymph nodes also may lead to lymphedema.[59]

Clinical Manifestations

Accumulation of lymph in the extremities results in physical discomfort and cosmetic disfigurement. It may lead to cellulitis or lymphangitis. Lymphedema characteristically is firm, rubbery, and nonpitting. The edema may be somewhat soft and become fibroblastic as the interstitial fluid protein concentration rises. The weight of the extremity contributes to limitations in function. This in turn causes contraction of the unused muscle, which results in pain.[57] Karakousis et al[59] reported that important factors related to the appearance of lymphedema were the location of the primary tumor and compliance with the prophylactic program to avoid lymphedema. They reported that lymphedema associated with groin dissection increased gradually with time and reached over 80% after the fifth postoperative year.[59]

Clinical Assessment

Assessments for edema include measurement of the circumference of the limb, condition of the skin, and mobility of the extremity, signs of infection, nutritional status, impairment of circulation, and constriction caused by clothing or other objects. These assessments should be made before surgery, before discharge, and at each follow-up visit.[57,60] Acute lymphedema occurs within 6 weeks of surgery and usually resolves with full function of the extremity. Chronic edema is a persistent swelling that may occur weeks or years after surgery.[57]

Treatment and Nursing Care

The initial interventions for lymphedema are aimed at prevention. These measures include elevation of the limb for the first 24 to 48 hours after surgery and prevention of trauma and infection by avoiding venipuncture, administration of medication by the intravenous route, and measurement of blood pressure on the affected side. Appropriate exercises to prompt the pumping action of the muscles and reduce the potential of lymph stagnation are recommended.[57,60]

Secondary interventions for the symptoms of lymphedema include patient education for the monitoring and reporting of signs and symptoms of lymphedema, position of the limb to promote effective drainage, massage by manual or mechanical means, application of elastic (antiembolism) stocking or sleeves, progressive exercise of the limb, and management of pain.[57,58,60,61] Care is taken to prevent skin breakdown as a sequela of infection, irritation, burns, or other threats to skin integrity.

General precautions for the person who is vulnerable to lymphedema include the avoidance of cuts, scratches, pinpricks, insect bites, and burns; the avoidance of injections or blood drawing on the affected arm; and the avoidance of tight straps, garters, and carrying heavy objects on the affected side.

CONCLUSION

Abnormal fluid accumulation may develop in any person with a malignancy. Goals of treatment are removal of fluid, palliation of symptoms, and prevention of reaccumulation of the transudate or exudate. Effusion usually is a manifestation of advanced disease. Edema may be a transient manifestation that has no influence on the overall prognosis of the person. Lymphedema, a related phenomena, is not life threatening but may cause severe reduction in the quality of life. Control of the abnormal fluid accumulation may afford the person several months of palliation and an improved quality of life.

REFERENCES

1. Lowell J: Pleural effusions: A comprehensive review. Baltimore, University Park Press, 1977.
2. Fundamentals of Fluid and Electrolyte Imbalances. Deerfield, IL, Travenol Laboratories, 1981, pp 85-96.
3. Hausheer F, Yarbro JW: Malignant effusions as oncologic emergencies. Prog Clin Biol Res 132D:347-360, 1983.
4. Soltis B, Cassmeyer VI: Fluid and electrolyte imbalance, in Phipps WJ, Long BC, Woods NF (eds): Medical Surgical Nursing. St Louis, CV Mosby, 1987, pp 215-228, 867.
5. Light RW, MacGregor MI, Luchsinger PC, et al: Pleural effusions: The diagnostic transudates and exudates. Ann Intern Med 77:507-513, 1972.
6. Garrison RN, Kaelin LD, Heuser LS, et al: Malignant ascites. Ann Surg 203:644-651, 1986.
7. Mauch PM, Ultmann JE: Treatment of malignant ascites, in DeVita VT, Hellman S, Rosenberg SA (eds): Cancer: Principles and Practice of Oncology. Philadelphia, JB Lippincott, 1985.
8. Callen PW, Marks WM, Filly RA: Computed tomography and ultrasonography in the evaluation of the retroperitoneum in patients with malignant ascites. J Comput Assist Tomogr 3:581-584, 1979.
9. Lowenstein MS, Rittgers RA, Feinerman AE, et al: Carcinoembryonic antigen assay of ascites and detection of malignancy. Ann Intern Med 88:635-641, 1978.

10. Jacobs ML: Radioactive colloidal chromic phosphate to control pleural effusion and ascites. JAMA 166:597-599, 1958.
11. Dybecki J, Balchum, OJ, Meneely GR: Treatment of pleural and peritoneal effusion with intracavitary colloidal radiogold (198Au). Arch Intern Med 104:802-815, 1959.
12. Straus AK, Roseman DL, Shapiro TM: Peritoneovenous shunting in the management of malignant ascites. Arch Surg 114:489-491, 1979.
13. Reinhold RB, Lokich JJ, Tomashefski J, et al: Management of malignant ascites with peritoneovenous shunting. Am J Surg 145:455-457, 1983.
14. Carey WD, Kohne JC, Leatherman J, et al: Ascitic fluid removal: Does it cause renal or hemodynamic decompensation? Cleve Clin Q 50:397-400, 1983.
15. Jenkins JF, Hubbard SM, Howser DM: Managing intraperitoneal chemotherapy: A new assault on ovarian cancer. Nursing 12:76-83, 1982.
16. Varricchio C, Jassak P: Acute pulmonary disorders associated with cancer. Semin Oncol Nurs 1:269-277, 1985.
17. Kuhn M, Fitting JW, Leuenberger P: Acute pulmonary edema caused by venous air embolism after removal of a subclavian catheter. Chest 92:364-365, 1987.
18. Skov P, Muwaswes M: Edema, in Carrieri VK, Lindsey AM, West CM (eds): Pathophysiological Phenomena in Nursing: Human Responses to Nursing. Philadelphia, WB Saunders, 1986, pp 68-98.
19. Leff A, Hopewell PC, Costello J: Pleural effusion from malignancy. Ann Intern Med 88:532-537, 1978.
20. Sahn SA: State of the art. The pleura. Am Rev Respir Dis 138:184-234, 1988.
21. Hausheer FH, Yarbro JW: Diagnosis and treatment of malignant pleural effusion. Cancer Metastasis Rev 6:23-40, 1987.
22. Ruckdeschel JC: Management of malignant pleural effusion: An overview. Semin Oncol 15:24-28, 1988 (suppl 3).
23. Gobel BH, Lawler PE: Malignant pleural effusions. Oncol Nurs Forum 12(4):49-54, 1985.
24. Chernow B, Sahn S: Carcinomatous involvement of the pleura. Am J Med 63:695-702, 1977.
25. Memon A, Zawadski ZA: Malignant effusions: Diagnostic evaluation and therapeutic strategy. Curr Probl Cancer 5:3-30, 1981.
26. Austin EH, Flye MW: The treatment of recurrent malignant pleural effusion. Ann Thorac Surg 28:190-203, 1978.
27. Salyer WR, Eggleston JC, Erozan YS: Efficacy of pleural needle biopsy and pleural fluid cytopathology in the diagnosis of malignant neoplasm involving the pleura. Chest 67:536-539, 1975.
28. Mauch PM, Ultmann JE: Treatment of malignant pleural effusions, in DeVita VT, Hellman S, Rosenberg SA (eds): Cancer: Principles and Practice of Oncology. Philadelphia, JB Lippincott, 1985.
29. Miller SE, Campbell DB: Pleural effusions in malignant disease, in Polomano RC, Miller SE (eds): Understanding and Managing Oncologic Emergencies. Columbus, Ohio, Adria Laboratories, 1987, pp 11-18.
30. Hewitt JB, Janssen WR: A management strategy for malignancy-induced pleural effusion: Long-term thoracostomy drainage. Oncol Nurs Forum 14(5):17-22, 1987.
31. Greenwald DW, Phillips C, Bennett JM: Management of malignant pleural effusion. J Surg Oncol 10:361-368, 1978.
32. Ostrowski MJ: An assessment of the long-term results of controlling the reaccumulation of malignant effusions using intracavity bleomycin. Cancer 57:721-727, 1986.
33. Sherman S, Grady KJ, Seidman JC: Clinical experience with tetracycline pleurodesis of malignant pleural effusions. South Med J 80:716-719, 1987.
34. Malden LT, Tattersall MHN: Malignant effusions. Q J Med (NS) 58(227):221-239, 1986.
35. Little AG, Ferguson MK, Golomb HM, et al: Pleuroperitoneal shunting for malignant pleural effusions. Cancer 58:2740-2743, 1986.
36. Cimochowski GE, Joyner LR, Fardin R, et al: Pleuroperitoneal shunting for recalcitrant pleural effusions. J Thorac Cardiovasc Surg 92:866-870, 1986.
37. Saum M: Taking the mystery out of chest tubes. J AORN 32:86-100, 1980.
38. Erikson R: Chest tubes: They're really not that complicated. Nursing 11:34-43, 1981.
39. Jagadha V, Deck JHN: Massive cerebral edema associated with meningioma. J Can Sci Neurol 14:55-58, 1987.
40. Shinonaga M, Chang CC, Suzuki N, et al: Immunohistological evaluation of macrophage infiltrates in brain tumors. J Neurosurg 68:259-265, 1988.
41. Challa VR: Cerebral edema associated with intracranial tumors. Surg Neurol 27:68, 1987.
42. Ito HJ, Tomita H, Ikeda J, et al: Formation and propagation of brain oedema fluid around human brain metastases. A CT study. Acta Neurochir (Wien) 90:35-41, 1988.
43. Datz FL: Cerebral edema following iodine-131 therapy for thyroid carcinoma metastatic to the brain. J Nucl Med 27:637-640, 1986.
44. Abels L, Belcher A, Russo BL: The nervous system, in Abels L (ed): Critical Care Nursing, A Physiologic Approach. St Louis, CV Mosby, 1986, pp 328-329.
45. Theologides A: Neoplastic cardiac tamponade. Semin Oncol 5:181-192, 1978.
46. Mauch PM, Ultmann JE: Treatment of malignant pericardial effusions, in DeVita VT, Hellman S, Rosenberg SA (eds): Cancer: Principles and Practice of Oncology. Philadelphia, JB Lippincott, 1985.
47. Press OW, Livingston R: Management of malignant pericardial effusion and tamponade. JAMA 257:1088-1092, 1987.
48. Kralstein J, Frishman WH: Malignant pericardial diseases: Diagnosis and treatment. Cardiol Clin 5:583-589, 1987.
49. Miller SE, Campbell DB: Malignant pericardial effusions, in Polomano RC, Miller SE (eds): Understanding and Managing Oncologic Emergencies. Columbus, Ohio, Adria Laboratories, 1987, pp 19-26.
50. Missri J, Schechter D: When pericardial effusion complicates cancer. Hosp Pract April 15:277-281, 1988.
51. Tomada H, Mitsumoto H, Furuya H, et al: Evaluation of pericardial effusion with computed tomography. Am Heart J 99:701-708, 1980.
52. Callahan JA, Seward JB, Tajek AJ, et al: Pericardiocentesis assisted by two-dimensional echocardiography. J Thorac Cardiovasc Surg 85:877-879, 1983.
53. Hankins JR, Satterfield JR, Aisner J, et al: Pericardial window for malignant pericardial effusions. Ann Thorac Surg 30:463-469, 1980.
54. Shepherd FA, Morgan C, Evans WK, et al: Medical management of malignant pericardial effusion by tetracycline sclerosis. Am J Cardiol 60:1161-1166, 1987.
55. Davis S, Rambotti P, Grignani F: Intrapericardial tetracycline sclerosis in the treatment of malignant pericardial effusion: An analysis of twenty-three cases. J Clin Oncol 2:631-636, 1984.
56. Wei JY, Taylor GJ, Achuff SC: Recurrent cardiac tamponade and large pericardial effusion: Management with an indwelling pericardial catheter. Am J Cardiol 42:281-282, 1978.

57. Getz DH: The primary, secondary, and tertiary nursing interventions of lymphedema. Cancer Nurs 8:177-184, 1985.
58. Lerner R, Requena R: Upper extremity lymphedema secondary to mammary cancer treatment. Am J Clin Oncol 9:481-487, 1986.
59. Karakousis CP, Heiser MA, Moore RH: Lymphedema after groin dissection. Am J Surg 145:205-208, 1983.
60. North Central New Jersey Chapter of Oncology Nursing Society: Mobility, impaired physical, related to lymphedema, in McNally JC, Stair JC, Somerville ET (eds): Guidelines for Cancer Nursing Practice. Orlando, Fla, Grune & Stratton, 1985, pp 195-199.
61. Gray B: Management of lymphedema in advanced cancer. Nurs Times 83:(49): 39-41, 1987.

Chapter 28

Sexual and Reproductive Dysfunction

Linda U. Krebs, RN, MS, OCN

INTRODUCTION

Sexual and reproductive dysfunctions often have been dismissed as normal side effects of cancer and cancer therapy about which the caregiver can do little or nothing. More often, however, the dysfunctions have gone undiagnosed or underrated, or both, because of lack of concern, information, or knowledge on the part of the caregiver and fear or discomfort on the part of the patient or family. Unfortunately, of all the complications associated with cancer, difficulties in the ability to be sexually intimate or to bear children have remained major problems that affect all aspects of the patient's and family's lives, sometimes influencing choices for therapy.[1,2] For some patients, sexual or reproductive dysfunctions may be temporary, with full recovery expected when therapy is completed. For many others, however, alterations in sexual or reproductive function is permanent, requiring adaptations in the management of intimate relationships and life-long plans to bear and raise children. Even short-term, temporary alterations can have long-term effects on the patient and family, affecting life-styles and life choices.

Various factors may affect the cancer patient's sexuality, including the biologic process of cancer, the effects of treatment, the alterations caused by cancer and treatment, and the psychologic issues surrounding the patient and family.[3] Physiologic problems of infertility and sterility, changes in body appearance, and the inability to have intercourse are enhanced by the psychologic and psychosexual issues of alteration in body image, fears of abandonment, loss of self-esteem, alterations in sexual identity, and concerns about self. Without appropriate education, counseling, and support, it may be difficult for the patient and family to adapt to the alterations that cancer may produce.

PHYSIOLOGY OF GONADAL FUNCTION

Gonadal function is regulated by the pituitary and the hypothalamus. The pituitary is divided into two distinct parts, the anterior and posterior portions. The pituitary is attached to the hypothalamus by the pituitary or hypophysial stalk through which runs a minute blood vessel system, the hypothalamic-hypophysial portal vessels.[4,5]

The secretion of hormones by the anterior pituitary is controlled by hormones called *hypothalamic-releasing or -inhibiting hormones*. These are secreted within the hypothalamus and then spread via the portal vessel system to the anterior pituitary where they act to influence glandular secretion. These hormones, when produced in appropriate amounts, institute a feedback mechanism that shuts off hormonal secretion at the hypothalamus and/or pituitary level.[1,4-6]

In gonadal function, luteinizing hormone-releasing hormone (LHRH), or gonadotropin-releasing hormone (GnRH), is secreted by the hypothalamus and stimulates the anterior pituitary to produce luteinizing hormone (LH) and follicle-stimulating hormone (FSH). These stimulate the testis or ovary to produce the appropriate hormones. When blood levels of these hormones are adequate, the hormones exert a negative feedback on the pituitary, thus decreasing secretion.[1,4-6]

FSH and LH play major roles in the control of male sexual function. LH acts on the interstitial Leydig cells to produce testosterone, whereas FSH, in conjunction with testosterone, is responsible for the conversion of spermatogonia into spermatocytes. To keep the level of hormones stable, there is a reciprocal inhibition of hypothalamic/anterior pituitary secretion of gonadotrophic hormones by testicular hormones. In this system the hypothalamus secretes GnRH, which causes the anterior pituitary to secrete LH. LH stimulates the Leydig cells to produce testosterone. The testosterone then negatively feeds back to the hypothalamus, inhibiting production of

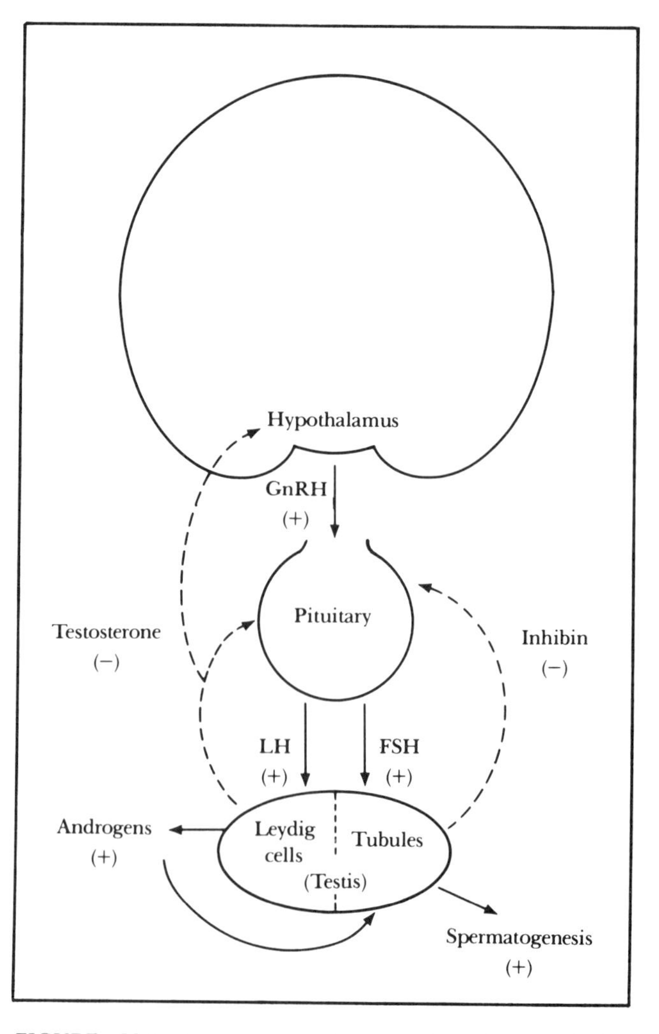

FIGURE 28-1 Normal testicular function. *FSH*, Follicle-stimulating hormone; *GnRH*, gonadotropin-releasing hormone; *LH*, luteinizing hormone. (Source: Adapted from Yarbro and Perry,[1] Guyton,[4] and Gill.[5])

GnRH. Spermatogenesis is controlled in much the same manner, with FSH stimulating the Sertoli cells to convert spermatides into sperm. The Sertoli cells then secrete a hormone called *inhibin* that, through negative feedback, causes a decrease in FSH production, thus keeping spermatogenesis at a constant rate[1,4-6] (Figure 28-1).

The female hormonal system, like the male, consists of three levels of hormones: GnRH from the hypothalamus, LH and FSH from the anterior pituitary, and estrogen and progesterone from the ovary. In the nonpregnant woman, monthly rhythmic changes in the rates of secretion of female hormones and responding change in the sexual organs result in the female sexual (menstrual) cycle. As a result a single mature ovum is released from an ovary and the endometrium of the uterus is prepared for implantation. FSH is responsible for growth of the ovarian follicle that eventually will become the mature ovum. At the beginning of menstruation, FSH and LH increase, causing rapid cellular growth in about 20 follicles. Eventually one follicle begins to outgrow the others, causing atresia of the remaining follicles. During follicle growth, estrogen is secreted, probably causing a positive feedback that results in a surge of LH. This surge of LH, which occurs 2 days before ovulation, is necessary for follicular growth and ovulation. Around the time of ovulation, the ruptured follicle, under the stimulation of LH, becomes the corpus luteum that secretes both estrogen and progesterone. After several days the estrogen and progesterone create a negative feedback to decrease secretion of FSH and LH. The corpus luteum, which also secretes inhibin, slowly degenerates, creating a loss of the feedback mechanism and an associated rise in secretion of FSH and LH, beginning a new ovarian cycle and leading to menstruation[1,4-6] (Figure 28-2).

Ovarian failure and germinal aplasia may occur as a result of disease, therapy, psychologic factors, or any combination of these. Ovarian failure also is related to age; as women near menopause ovarian failure is more likely. In failure, damage to ovarian follicles causes decreased levels of estrogens and progesterones. This results in increased levels of LH and FSH with no compensating feedback mechanism. In addition, inhibin may be produced and react further to alter FSH production. Ovulation ceases, menstruation becomes erratic or ceases, and early menopause often results[1,4-7] (Figure 28-3). In the male, damage to the Leydig cells results in decreased testosterone pro-

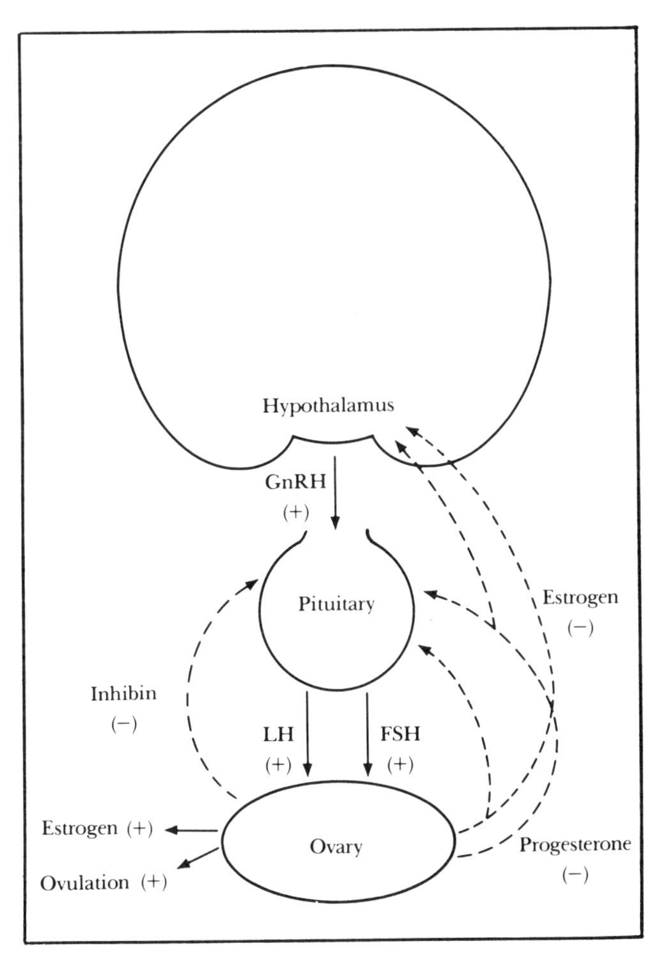

FIGURE 28-2 Normal ovarian function. *FSH*, Follicle-stimulating hormone; *GnRH*, gonadotropin-releasing hormone; *LH*, luteinizing hormone. (Source: Adapted from Yarbro and Perry,[1] Guyton,[4] and Gill.[5])

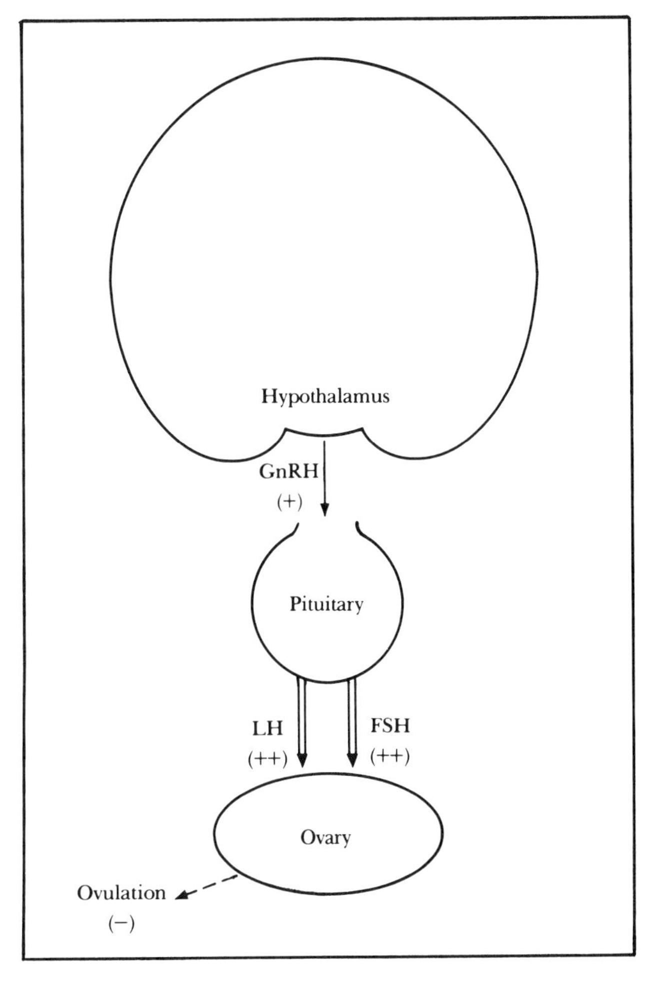

FIGURE 28-3 Ovarian failure. *FSH*, Follicle-stimulating hormone; *GnRH*, gonadotropin-releasing hormone; *LH*, luteinizing hormone. (Source: Adapted from Yarbro and Perry,[1] Guyton,[4] and Gill.[5])

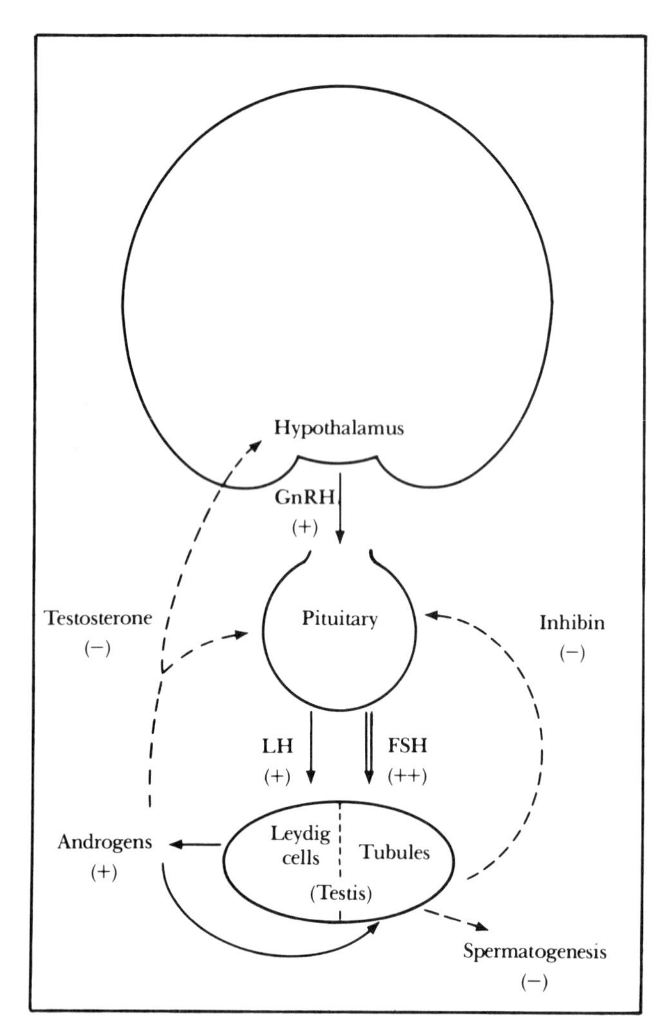

FIGURE 28-4 Germinal aplasia. *FSH*, Follicle-stimulating hormone; *GnRH*, gonadotropin-releasing hormone; *LH*, luteinizing hormone. (Source: Adapted from Yarbro and Perry,[1] Guyton,[4] and Gill.[5])

duction. Initially, Leydig cell activity may be compensated enough to produce adequate amounts of testosterone, but continued damage results in temporary, but more often permanent, sterility[1,4-7] (Figure 28-4).

EFFECT OF CANCER THERAPY ON GONADAL FUNCTION

Surgery

Some surgical procedures for cancer of the gastrointestinal and genitourinary tracts cause sexual dysfunction through the removal of sexual organs, through damage to nerves that enervate sexual organs, or through alteration in normal function. In addition, surgery on head and neck areas and on the breast or amputations may alter body image and affect sexual identity. Organ dysfunction, either through loss or alteration in normal function, is most common in cancers of the colon, rectum, bladder and associated urinary structures, and male and female genital tracts. Even when organs are not removed, normal function may be disrupted through the removal of tumorous tissue surrounding an organ, through lymph node dissection, or through associated physiologic and psychologic abnormalities related to the type of surgery.

Cancer of the colon and rectum

Surgery for cancer of the colon or rectum may cause sexual dysfunction in both men and women. In general, sexual dysfunctions in women are more commonly related to psychosocial issues, whereas in men dysfunctions may be both organically and psychosocially caused. The most common surgery for colon cancer is some degree of colectomy with or without a colostomy. Whenever possible, primary anastomosis is performed. Cancer of the rectum, however, may require anterior or abdominoperineal resection (APR). If possible, sphincter-preserving surgery without need for an ostomy may be done but only for midrectal or high rectal lesions. In general, the type of surgery depends on tumor location.[8]

For the patient who requires an APR, sexual dysfunction may be related to the placement of a colostomy, to dysfunctions related to removal of or interference with sexual organ function, or some combination of the two. A colostomy has been associated with sexual dysfunction because of the patient's negative changes in body image and self-esteem, as well as the responses by family and friends. In a study by MacDonald and Anderson[9] of 420 patients with rectal cancer, 265 had a permanent colostomy. Of these individuals 16% felt severely stigmatized because of the colostomy. Of those who were married or widowed since surgery, 48% of men and 27% of women younger than 65 years old ($n = 116$) felt that their married life had suffered as a result of the colostomy.

For the woman with an APR (in addition to colostomy) the ovaries or uterus also may be removed at the time of surgery, thus causing dysfunction from primary inability to bear children or from alterations in normal hormonal patterns. In addition, women may have part of the vagina removed, or healing of the perineal wound may result in vaginal scarring that causes painful or incomplete vaginal intercourse. A decreased incidence of orgasm, a decrease in vaginal lubrication, and decreased libido have been noted.[8,10-12]

For the man who has an APR, sexual dysfunction is more severe, with a suggestion that permanent sexual dysfunction may be as high as 80%.[13] Although men may lose the ability to obtain or maintain an erection, 30% to 50% maintain the ability to have an orgasm and 25% to 50% maintain the ability to ejaculate.[14,15] Age appears to be a factor, with the older patient more likely to suffer complete or incomplete erectile impotence.[16] This most likely is due to damage to parasympathetic and sympathetic nerves that control both erection and ejaculation. In addition to erectile dysfunction, decreased amount and/or force of ejaculation or retrograde ejaculation may occur. This occurrence may be temporary or permanent and adds to the trauma of this surgery because of its unpredictable outcome. For all patients the removal of rectal tissue appears to be the most common denominator to organic sexual dysfunction. If the rectum remains intact, there rarely is an associated sexual dysfunction without direct tumor invasion.[17-19]

Cancers of the genitourinary tract

Bladder cancer The treatment of bladder cancer may alter sexual function in men and women but only if the cancer is advanced or radical treatment is required. Transurethral resection or partial cystectomy may result in mild pain or dyspareunia; however, normal sexual function should not be altered.[20] Radical cystectomy results in sexual dysfunction for both men and women because of organ removal and/or enervation. In men, radical cystectomy consists of removal of the bladder, prostate, seminal vesicles, pelvic lymph nodes, and occasionally the urethra.[20] It has been noted that about 15% of men who undergo radical cystectomy will recover full erection potential and that men older than 60 years of age are more likely to be negatively affected. Retrograde or no ejaculation may result.[15] For these men the increasing availability and use of penile prostheses and the ability to perform revascularization of the penis have made erectile dysfunction a more manageable problem.[11,21] For the woman who has radical cystectomy, the surgery usually includes removal of the bladder and urethra, the uterus, ovaries, fallopian tubes, and the anterior portion of the vagina. Although vaginal reconstruction usually is performed, the resulting vaginal canal may be narrow and shallow and provide less lubrication than before surgery. In addition, the removal of the ovaries with associated estrogen loss leads to dryness, inelasticity of the vagina, dyspareunia, and menopausal symptoms. Vaginal dilation and the liberal use of lubrication may provide relief.[21-23] For both sexes, urinary diversion is a necessity with radical cystectomy. In the past the ileal conduit, which necessitated the continuous use of an ostomy appliance, was the most common method for urinary diversion. Today the surgical development of a Kock pouch, or continent reservoir, has become more widely employed, decreasing some assault to body image.[20]

Penile cancer/cancer of the male urethra Cancer of the penis is rare, with fewer than 500 cases in the United States in 1989.[24] Treatment includes total or partial penectomy, radiation therapy, or topical chemotherapy, with radiation therapy or chemotherapy used for small, early lesions. Partial penectomy does not result in loss of erectile, ejaculative, or orgasmic abilities whereas erectile ability obviously is absent with total penectomy. Orgasmic ability and ejaculation (through perineal urethrostomy) should continue. New techniques to create a penis have been used after total penectomy. A semirigid or inflatable prosthesis restores the ability to have intercourse.[20,21,25] A Mayo Clinic study reported a successful placement rate of 90% to 95% and an 8% mechanical failure rate in the 3-year study period of patients with penile implants. Eighty-nine percent of subjects and mates felt satisfied with function and appearance.[26]

Testicular cancer Testicular cancer, which represents about 1% of all cancers in men, is the leading cause of cancer in young men.[24] The treatment of testicular cancer includes an orchiectomy and possibly retroperitoneal lymph node dissection and/or removal of a pelvic mass. Unilateral orchiectomy will not result in infertility or sexual dysfunction providing that the contralateral testis is normal and the individual is fertile at diagnosis. Infertility before any definitive therapy is well documented and may be related to hormonal imbalance or the result of subacute chronic illness.[27-29] If bilateral orchiectomy is performed, sterility and decreased libido, related to loss of testosterone, will result. Retroperitoneal lymph node dissection, done for staging or as treatment for stage II disease, may result in temporary or permanent loss of ejaculation, whereas potency and the ability to have an orgasm remain.[20,21,27,29] Narayan et al[29] reported that 100% of 55 patients who underwent peritoneal lymphadenectomy reported loss of ejaculation, with 45% regaining function within 3 years after surgery. Nerve-sparing procedures with careful adherence to surgical boundaries and identification of sympathetic fibers has resulted in an almost 80% preservation or return of ejaculation after lymphadenectomy.[27] Retrograde ejaculation has been noted in 25% of patients, whereas decreased libido, decreased pleasure at orgasm, and erectile dysfunction have occurred in 10% to 38% of these men.[11,20,21,25,30] For those individuals who desire to maintain fertility, sperm banking should be arranged before therapy.

Prostate cancer Prostate cancer, because it generally occurs in men older than 50 years of age, often is not considered in terms of its potential to cause sexual dysfunctions. However, because sexual concerns are not necessarily related to age and therapy for prostate cancer frequently causes sexual dysfunction, counseling and management of potential problems need to be addressed. Therapy for prostate cancer consists of various combinations of surgery, chemotherapy, radiation therapy, and hormonal manipulation, all of which have a potential to alter sexual function. Surgical treatment of prostate cancer includes prostatectomy accomplished through transurethral, perineal, or transabdominal approaches or bilateral orchiectomy. Transurethral resection of the prostate generally does not cause impotence or erectile dysfunction; however, retrograde ejaculation occurs in approximately 90% of all patients. Transabdominal resection of the prostate results in retrograde ejaculation in 75% to 80% of patients and may cause erectile dsysfunction. The perineal approach, or radical prostatectomy, includes removal of the prostate, seminal vesicles, and vas deferens and may result in permanent damage to erectile function with concomitant loss of emission and ejaculation.[17,20,31] Eggleston and Walsh[32] evaluated 100 patients who had had radical prostatectomies that incorporated surgical techniques and reported that potency was maintained in approximately 86% of patients. Bilateral orchiectomy causes sexual dysfunction through gradual diminution of libido, impotence, gynecomastia, and penile atrophy.[11,20] Penile prostheses may restore erectile potential; however, it is suggested that the patient wait at least 6 months after surgery to see if function will be restored.[20,21] With new techniques, sterility previously found in individuals with retrograde ejaculation is not as frequent. Because of the ability to separate sperm from urine, artificial insemination of the mate may be possible.[33]

Gynecologic malignancies

Surgical management of gynecologic malignancy includes surgery of the vulva, vagina, uterus and uterine cervix, ovary and fallopian tube, or pelvic exenteration. Although the majority of gynecologic surgeries most commonly are invisible assaults to femininity, sexual identity, as well as sexual functioning, often are affected permanently. It is imperative that sexual and reproductive counseling be provided to the patient and family before surgical intervention because most surgeries permanently alter fertility and may alter sexuality.

Vulvar cancer Vulvar cancer represents 1% of all cancers found in women, with approximately 85% occurring in postmenopausal women.[34] Treatment for carcinoma in situ or preinvasive disease may include simple vulvectomy, wide local excision, skinning vulvectomy, topical 5-fluorouracil cream, or laser therapy. In general, good cosmetic results occur for all but the simple vulvectomy, which removes the labia and subcutaneous tissue, with retention of the clitoris. Introital stenosis may result but should be easily managed. Radical vulvectomy, which removes the labia minora and majora and the clitoris, and usually includes a groin node dissection, frequently results in altered body image, abnormalities in sensory perception of the genital area, leg edema, and decreased range of motion in lower extremities, altered orgasmic potential, and introital stenosis.[11,34,35]

Vaginal cancer Vaginal cancer is less common. Surgery for the majority of gynecologic cancers results in some abnormality and/or need for reconstruction of the vagina. A shortened vagina can cause considerable sexual dysfunction because of vaginal length and width, lack of lubrication, or pain on intercourse. Total vaginectomy without reconstruction precludes vaginal intercourse; however, there are multiple techniques for vaginal reconstruction. It has been noted that in 30% to 70% of patients who have reconstruction there is a return of orgasmic sensations if they existed before surgery.[36]

Cervical cancer and endometrial cancer Invasive cancer of the uterine corpus and cervix are the first and second most common gynecologic malignancies, representing 10% of all cancers in women.[24] Treatment for cervical intraepithelial neoplasia and carcinoma in situ includes conization, laser therapy, cryosurgery, or simple hysterectomy. All but the last usually do not affect fertility (conization may result in cervical stenosis or incompetence), nor should they cause any physiologic sexual dysfunction. Simple hysterectomy precludes further childbearing but should not affect sexual functioning, although numerous authors have noted that altered sexual identity and/or body image may result in sexual dysfunction.[17,37-39] Treatment for invasive disease usually is radical hysterectomy, consisting of removal of the uterus and cervix, supporting structures, and upper third of the vagina and pelvic lymph nodes. For cancer of the endometrium, the ovaries and fallopian tubes also may be removed. If oophorectomy is included, menopausal symptoms with hot flashes and decrease in vaginal lubrication and elasticity may severely alter sexual functioning.[17] Zussman et al[39] noted that 33% to 46% of women who had a radical hysterectomy, including oophorectomy, reported decreased sexual desire, whereas Jenkins[40] noted alterations in frequency of desire, orgasm, and frequency and enjoyment of intercourse in women who had had abdominal hysterectomy and bilateral salpingo-oophorectomy and had received pelvic radiation for cervical or endometrial cancer. Although sexual feeling should not be altered after a radical hysterectomy, it should be remembered that many women measure femininity by the ability to bear children. If this ability is removed, sexual dysfunction may occur.[17]

Ovarian cancer Ovarian cancer represents approximately 25% of gynecologic cancers and frequently is seen in the premenopausal female. Initial treatment is surgery, usually consisting of a radical hysterectomy with bilateral salpingo-oophorectomy and omentectomy. Fertility is lost and the associated menopausal symptoms occur. In the young woman with ovarian teratoma, it is possible to maintain fertility if disease is confined to one ovary and is of low grade; however, it is most common for radical surgery to be performed.[41,42] Treatment usually continues with combination chemotherapy, thus further compounding sexual and reproductive dysfunctions.

Pelvic exenteration

Although pelvic exenteration may be performed in the man or woman with advanced colorectal or bladder cancer, the most common indication for this procedure is a locally advanced gynecologic malignancy. A pelvic exenteration that is anterior preserves the rectum, whereas a posterior exenteration preserves the bladder. A total pelvic exenteration involves removing the vagina, uterus, ovaries, fallopian tubes, bladder, and rectum (in the man, the prostate, seminal vesicles, and vas deferens are removed).[23,37,43,44] In patients with total pelvic exenteration a urinary conduit and colostomy also are created; a neovagina may be constructed.[23,43] In the woman reproductive and sexual dysfunction is profound. Dysfunction related to removal of all pelvic organs with resulting ostomies is obvious. In addition, body image, sexual identity, and self-esteem are disturbed, and appropriate interventions and education need to be provided. In the woman with vaginal reconstruction intercourse will be possible; however, the physiologic and psychologic ramifications of this surgery may result in inability and/or lack of desire to participate in sexual activities.[45]

Breast cancer

Although some surgeries may not be strictly related to sexual functioning, they may cause dysfunction as a result of the psychologic issues related to the particular body part. Probably the most likely assault to body image and sexual identity with resultant sexual dysfunction is surgical removal of all or part of the breast. Although fertility is not altered by mastectomy or lumpectomy, the inability or difficulty in breast-feeding should pregnancy be accomplished may be a major assault to the woman's femininity. In addition, the removal or partial removal of a breast may result in sexual dysfunction because of fear of rejection, physical discomfort, anxiety about initiating sexual activities, feelings of being defective or different, or any combination of these factors.[46,47]

The use of breast-preserving surgery (lumpectomy) has been shown to cause significantly less alteration in body image, sexual desire, and frequency of intercourse.[46,47] It should be considered when possible. If breast-preserving surgery is not an option, breast reconstruction can be considered. The ability to have breast reconstruction has been shown to bolster sexual self-esteem and decrease negative reactions to body image alterations.[48] If such options are limited, sexual dysfunction that should be temporary may become permanent.

Radiation Therapy

Radiation therapy can cause sexual and reproductive dysfunction through primary organ failure (eg, ovarian failure and testicular aplasia), through alterations in organ function (eg, decreased lubrication and impotence), and through the temporary or permanent effects of therapy unassociated with reproduction (eg, diarrhea and fatigue). Permanent effects most commonly are related to total dose, location, and prior fertility status.[33,49] In the woman, fertility depends on follicular maturation and ovum release. Radiation therapy to the ovaries has its most direct effect on the intermediate follicle. If these follicles are damaged by radiation and insufficient small follicles remain, permanent sterility results.[50] In the man, although the Leydig cell and mature sperm are relatively radioresistant, immature sperm and spermatogonia are extremely radiosensitive. Small doses of radiation will begin the process of infertility, which, depending on total dose, may be permanent.[5]

In women, temporary or permanent sterility is related to the dose of radiation, the volume of tissues radiated, the time period the ovaries are exposed to radiation, and the woman's age.[51,52] Because a woman has fewer oocytes as she nears menopause, radiation injury is more likely to be permanent. Balducci et al[33] and Hilderley[50] noted that a radiation dose of 600 to 1200 cGy is capable of inducing menopause; however, younger women appear to be more resistant to this effect. In addition, although age is an important factor, doses <400 cGy may result in temporary sterility whereas doses >400 cGy often result in permanent sterility. The number of oocytes is one of the most important factors in permanent sterility, with 95% of young women becoming sterile with a radiation dose >2000 cGy. In women older than 40 years of age, 600 cGy often is associated with subsequent menopause.[53]

For women, movement of the ovaries out of the radiation field (oophoropexy) either to the iliac crests or behind the uterus, with appropriate shielding, has helped maintain fertility even when relatively high doses of radiation have been given. In a study by Horning et al[54] 8 of 19 patients treated with total lymphoid irradiation for Hodgkin's disease had reversible amenorrhea and 7 eventually became pregnant. Even with oophoropexy and appropriate shielding, 30% to 50% of all patients who receive more than 600 to 1000 cGy will have permanent menstrual cessation.[55,56]

In men, temporary or permanent azoospermia also is a function of age, dose, tissue volume, and exposure time. When the testis is exposed to radiation, a reduction in sperm count begins within 6 to 8 weeks and continues for up to 1 year after completion of therapy. Doses of <500 cGy usually are associated with temporary sterility whereas doses >500 cGy usually result in permanent sterility.[50] The return of normal spermatogenesis is related to total testicular dose, with a dose of <100 cGy taking 9 to 12 months for recovery, whereas 200 to 300 cGy may take 2 to 3 years and 400 to 600 cGy more than 5 years to infinity.[57] Kinsella et al[58] reported on 27 male adults with soft tissue sarcoma who were treated with high-dose radiation therapy. The testes were not in the primary field and were shielded; however, significant scatter radiation still was received. In 11 of 27 patients who received <50 cGy, no abnormalities resulted, whereas in 6 patients with exposures of 50 to 150 cGy, FSH was elevated 200% and testosterone was decreased. In the 10 patients who received >150 cGy, FSH was increased whereas LH and testosterone were decreased; thus testicular function was inadequate to support spermatogenesis.

In addition to sterility or transient infertility, radiation therapy can produce other sexual dysfunctions that may be temporary or permanent. Decreases in sexual enjoyment, ability to attain orgasm, libido, and frequency of intercourse and sexual dreams, as well as vaginal stenosis or shortening and decreased lubrication and sensation, have been reported in women treated with radiation therapy. Painful intercourse and menstrual changes also have been reported.[35,52,59-63]

The majority of men treated by external beam for prostate cancer have temporary or permanent impotence. Impotence is believed to be caused by fibrosis of pelvic vasculature or radiation damage of pelvic nerves. Herr[64] reported that 40 of 41 patients treated by lymphadenectomy remained potent if interstitial therapy was used, whereas Carlton et al[65] noted that only 25% of patients treated with internal and external therapy plus lymphadenectomy became impotent, which suggests that interstitial therapy may be less likely to cause impotence. In patients treated for testicular cancer, Schover and von Eschenbach[66] noted that 10% of 121 patients reported erectile dysfunction whereas 38% experienced a decrease in pleasure of orgasm. The inability to gain and maintain an erection may begin as early as 2 weeks into treatment and may last several weeks after treatment.[63] Occasionally impotence does not occur until after radiation therapy is completed, and in these patients the effects usually are not reversible.[67] In addition to difficulty in gaining or maintaining erection, a decreased libido, inability to ejaculate, inability to lubricate, inability to achieve orgasm, and decreased sexual pleasure are common findings in men who receive radiation to the pelvis.

Along with direct assaults to sexual and reproductive function by radiation therapy, the general side effects and the accompanying psychologic effects frequently can alter sexual function. Severe fatigue can limit all activity. Nausea, vomiting, and diarrhea can decrease energy, sexual desire, and feelings of desirability and can interfere with a sense of general well-being. Inflammation, pain, and limited range of motion may make sexual activities difficult or impossible. In addition to physical limitations, fear, depression, anxiety, stress, body image alterations, and lowered self-esteem may be additional burdens.[51,68-72] The appropriate use of energy-conserving strategies, medications, lubricants, prostheses, time, and counseling may alleviate side effects, promote a sense of well-being, and improve sexual function.

Chemotherapy

Chemotherapy-induced reproductive and sexual dysfunction is related to the type of drug, dose, length of treatment, age, and sex of the individual receiving treatment and the length of time after therapy. In addition, single versus multiple agents and drugs given to combat side effects of chemotherapy also play a role in infertility or sexual dysfunction.

Infertility and sterility after chemotherapy have been noted since the early 1970s, with reports of amenorrhea and azoospermia after single-agent or combination therapy.[73] Adult men are more likely to experience long-term side effects regardless of age, whereas women are more apt to have permanent cessation of menses as they near the age of 40 years.[74,75] The primary agents that induce infertility are the alkylating agents, but other drugs have been implicated, in particular cytosine arabinoside, 5-fluorouracil, vinblastine, vincristine, and procarbazine. Combinations of these drugs appear to prolong infertility[74,76-78] (Table 28-1).

TABLE 28-1 Chemotherapeutic Agents That Affect Sexual or Reproductive Function

Agent	Complication
Alkylating	
Busulfan Chlorambucil Cyclophosphamide Melphalan Nitrogen mustard	Amenorrhea, oligospermia, azoospermia, decreased libido, ovarian dysfunction, erectile dysfunction
Antimetabolites	
Cytosine arabinoside 5-Fluorouracil Methotrexate	As for alkylating agents
Antitumor antibiotics	
Doxorubicin Plicamycin	As for alkylating agents
Plant products	
Vincristine	Retrograde ejaculation, erectile dysfunction
Vinblastine	Decreased libido, ovarian dysfunction, erectile dysfunction
Miscellaneous	
Procarbazine	As for alkylating agents
Androgens	Masculinization (women)
Estrogens	Gynecomastia, acne
Progestins	Menstrual abnormalities, change in libido
Corticosteroids	Irregular menses, acne

Source: Data from Yasko,[52] Dodd,[63] Schilsky and Erlichman,[74] Tenenbaum,[76] Skeel,[77] and Carter et al.[78]

Men

Infertility occurs in men primarily through depletion of the germinal epithelium that lines the seminiferous tubules. On testicular biopsy the interstitial Leydig cells appear normal, whereas the tubules are abnormal, contain Sertoli's cells, and have depleted or absent germinal epithelium. Clinically, testicular volume decreases, oligospermia or azoospermia occurs, and infertility results.[79]

Single-agent and combination chemotherapy have been reported to cause germinal aplasia, with alkylating agents the most extensively studied. Richter et al[80] reported that doses of chlorambucil <400 mg cause progressive oligospermia whereas doses >400 mg have caused azoospermia and permanent germinal aplasia. They also studied cyclophosphamide and noted that dosages as low as 50 to 100 mg/day for 2 months resulted in azoospermia. Recovery time related to total dose and length of time since the completion of treatment. Nijman et al[30] studied the gonadal function of 54 patients with testicular cancer who received chemotherapy with cisplatin, vinblastine, and bleomycin (PVB) after surgery. They noted, as have others,[27-29] that 72% of these men were infertile before treatment. Two years following therapy 48% remained infertile, with increased levels of LH and FSH. Drasga et al[81] reviewed 69 patients with disseminated testicular cancer treated with PVB ± doxorubicin; 41 patients were part of a prospective study and 28 were part of a retrospective study. In the prospective group only 6.6% of patients were able to meet sperm banking requirements; the others had severe oligospermia or azoospermia. With a median of 17 months' follow-up, 100% of these men continue to be infertile. In the retrospective group 46% had a normal sperm count at the time of evaluation. Thirty-two percent (8 of 25) have successfully impregnated their wives. Fertility may improve with time.

The most widely studied combination chemotherapy has been mechlorethamine, vincristine, procarbazine, and prednisone (MOPP) used in the treatment of Hodgkin's disease. Chapman[75] reported frequent sexual dysfunction and decreased fertility in men treated with MOPP. This is corroborated by Cunningham et al[82] who noted that only 1 in 10 men receiving MOPP and 1 in 13 men receiving MOPP plus pelvic radiation were able to impregnate. Viviani et al[83] reported that azoospermia developed in only 54% of patients treated with doxorubicin, bleomycin, vinblastine, and dacarbazine (ABVD) whereas azoospermia occurred in 97% of patients treated with MOPP. In addition, 100% of those treated with ABVD had complete restoration of spermatogenesis whereas only 14% of those treated with MOPP had return of spermatogenesis. Although ABVD is less toxic to the germinal epithelium, the long-term effects on cardiac function of doxorubicin also must be considered.

Hormonal manipulation and treatment with estrogens are well known as causes of sexual dysfunction. The majority of patients who receive antiandrogen therapy experience a major reduction in interest in sexual intercourse and are unable to attain or maintain an erection.[84] Decreases in libido, sexual excitement, and ability to achieve sexual fulfillment and the development of gynecomastia are significant problems.[52,76,85]

Women

Women experience sexual and reproductive dysfunction from chemotherapy as a result of hormonal alterations or direct effects that cause ovarian fibrosis and follicle destruction. FSH and LH levels are elevated and estradiol is decreased, leading to amenorrhea, menopausal symptoms, dyspareunia, and vaginal atrophy and dryness.[1,79]

As in men, women experience reproductive dysfunction from both single-agent and combination chemotherapy; however, age appears to play a more significant role in infertility in women than in men, with women younger than 35 years old able to tolerate much higher doses of chemotherapy without resultant infertility. Amenorrhea has been noted in women with breast cancer who receive 40 to 120 mg/day of cyclophosphamide.[86] Busulfan, which may be used to treat chronic myelogenous leukemia also induces amenorrhea.[87] Chapman et al[88] reported that amenorrhea developed in 49% of patients treated with MOPP, 34% experienced irregular menses, and 17% maintained normal menses. Of those with irregular or normal menses, 30% later had irreversible amenorrhea. Other investigators[82,89] have also reported that permanent amenorrhea occurred in 26% to 50% of women treated with MOPP combination chemotherapy and that permanent amenorrhea and early menopause were more common with advancing age. It was noted in a study of ABVD plus radiation therapy versus MOPP plus radiation therapy that 50% of women older than 30 years of age treated with MOPP plus radiation therapy had prolonged amenorrhea.[90] In contrast, none of the women younger than 30 years and none of the women receiving ABVD plus radiation therapy noted this side effect. Other combination therapy also has been reviewed with similar results.[91]

It appears that any combination of drugs that contain an alkylating agent is apt to cause infertility, and as women near menopause, permanent cessation of menses is more likely. When hormonal manipulation includes androgens, not only are sexual and reproductive functions affected but also body image and feelings of sexual identity. Appropriate support should be provided.

Children

Chemotherapy and gonadal dysfunction have been studied in children. Effects of chemotherapy appear to be age related. Prepubescent boys seem to be minimally affected by chemotherapy and progress into and through puberty without major difficulty. Young men treated during puberty, however, appear to be more likely to have gonadal dysfunction with profound effects on both germ cell production and Leydig cell function, with a resultant increase in FSH and LH and a decrease in testosterone levels.[92,93] Little information is available about prepubertal or pubertal girls; however, the majority of girls treated with combination therapy have normal ovarian function.[1,94]

Other issues

No discussion of gonadal dysfunction from chemotherapy is complete without acknowledgment that drugs used to manage chemotherapy side effects can alter sexual function. Impotence, decreased sexual desire, decreased sense of sexual fulfillment, and decreased ability to achieve orgasm all have been associated with these agents[52,74,76,85,95,96] (Table 28-2).

Biological Response Modifiers

Little information presently is available on the sexual and reproductive dysfunctions associated with the biologic response modifiers. In part, this lack of information is due to the experimental nature of the agents and their use primarily in advanced cancer patients. As use of these agents becomes more frequent in individuals who are less ill, the effects on gonadal function will become more apparent.

Some information is available with the use of the interferons, in particular alpha-interferon, alone or in combination with other agents. A decrease in libido has been reported with alpha-interferon, and animals exposed to interferon have demonstrated an increased rate of spontaneous abortion.[97] In patients with chronic myelogenous leukemia and melanoma treated with alpha-, gamma-, or alpha plus gamma–interferon, Mangold and Robinson (personal communication, 1988) stated that patients have reported decreased sexual desire and pleasure and difficulty in attaining and maintaining an erection. In addition to drug-induced dysfunction, the usual side effects of fatigue and flulike symptoms affect interest in and comfort with sexual activities.

TABLE 28-2 Cancer-Associated Drugs That Affect Sexual and Reproductive Function

Agent	Complication
Antiemetics/sedatives/tranquilizers	
Prochlorperazine Chlorpromazine Diazepam Lorazepam Metoclopramide	Sedation, orgasm without ejaculation, impotence, decreased sexual interest, decreased intensity of orgasm
Antihistamines	
Diphenhydramine	Sedation, decreased sexual interest
Antidepressants	
Amitriptyline Imipramine	Impotence, altered libido
Narcotics	
Morphine Hydromorphone Codeine	Decreased libido, sedation, impaired potency
Steroids (see Table 28-1)	

Source: Data from Yasko,[52] Schilsky and Erlichman,[74] Tenenbaum,[76] Kaempfer,[85,95] and Brager and Yasko.[96]

FERTILITY CONSIDERATIONS AND PROCREATIVE ALTERNATIVES

Mutagenicity

Mutagenicity is the ability to cause an abnormality in the genetic content of cells, resulting in cell death, alteration(s) in growth and replication, or no noticeable alteration in cell function. Mutagenicity following radiation therapy in mice has been documented; however, the mutagenic effects after radiation therapy or chemotherapy in humans are less clear.[98] Possible germ cell mutations may not be evident for generations of offspring.[99,100]

Numerous researchers have investigated pregnancy outcomes of children and adolescents exposed to chemotherapy or radiation therapy as a method to adequately assess mutagenicity following therapy.[101-105] Mulvihill et al[102] reviewed 12 retrospective case series of pregnancies in survivors of cancer. There were 1573 pregnancies and 1240 live-born infants with 46 (4%) birth defects (which is comparable to the rate among the general population). The researchers noted only two instances of possible mutants. In all studies it has been difficult to specifically implicate germ cell mutations as the cause of adverse outcomes to pregnancies. Follow-up over several generations of patients and their offspring willl be needed before definitive answers are obtained.

Teratogenicity

Teratogenicity is the ability of a toxic compound to produce alterations in the fetus following its exposure to that compound. Both chemotherapy and radiation therapy are known to have teratogenetic effects on the fetus, causing spontaneous abortion, fetal malformation, or fetal death. Low-dose radiation has also been implicated in fetal malignancy.[99,100,106,107] Mulvihill et al,[102] in their study of fetal exposure to radiation therapy or chemotherapy during gestation, noted a 28% abnormal outcome (spontaneous abortion or birth defects) of five conceptuses exposed only to radiation therapy. Two were electively aborted, one was stillborn, and two were carried to term. All had some form of congenital malformation.

Fetal damage probably does not occur at doses <10 cGy and is only rarely reported at doses <50 cGy.[33] Radiation exposure during the first trimester represents the greatest risk to the fetus with exposure ≥ 100 cGy resulting in fetal death, microcephaly, eye anomalies, and intrauterine growth retardation. In the second or third trimester fetal death is unlikely, but growth retardation, sterility, and cataracts are common findings.[106]

Chemotherapy, particularly during the first trimester, has been related to congenital abnormalities, with approximately 10% of fetuses experiencing some type of anomaly. In general, the alkylating agents and antimetabolites most often have been associated with fetal malformations. Chemotherapy during the second or third trimesters may cause premature birth or low birth weight infants, but congenital abnormalities are not increased over the normal pregnancy incidence[107,108] (Table 28-3).

TABLE 28-3 Teratogenetic Effects of Chemotherapy

Agent	Complication
Alkylating	
Busulfan Chlorambucil Cyclophosphamide Nitrogen mustard	Spontaneous abortions, skeletal malformations
Antimetabolites	
Cytosine arabinoside 6-Mercaptopurine 5-Fluorouracil Methotrexate	Spontaneous abortions, skeletal malformations
Miscellaneous	
Procarbazine	Atrial/septal defects
Glucocorticoids	Spontaneous abortions
Daunorubicin	Spontaneous abortions
Vinblastine	Spontaneous abortions

Source: Data from Balducci et al,[33] Tenenbaum,[76] Kaempfer,[99] Robinson and Krebs,[107] and Accola and Sommerfield.[108]

Reproductive Counseling

Discussions concerning fertility and reproduction issues need to be held before the onset of therapy and should continue well into the posttreatment and follow-up stages. Kaempfer[109] suggests that current fertility status, desire for future childbearing, and contraception practices should be investigated during initial assessment. Potential alterations should be openly discussed and referrals made as appropriate. Birth control methods need to be implemented to minimize the possibility of an unplanned pregnancy during therapy. In addition, methods to maintain fertility during therapy should be investigated.

For those who receive radiation therapy, appropriate shielding of the testes or ovaries or oophoropexy to position the ovaries outside the radiation field may be of benefit. For those who receive chemotherapy it has been suggested that birth control pills in women and gonadotropin-releasing hormone analogues in men may protect the germ cells from damage by chemotherapeutic agents.[110,111]

Because it is often difficult to predict when an individual who is receiving chemotherapy is infertile, it is extremely important that methods to prevent pregnancy are discussed and appropriate drugs or devices provided. It also has been suggested that after cancer therapy an individual should wait a minimum of 2 years before attempting conception. This suggestion is made both to prevent pregnancy during the time recurrence is most likely and to allow for the recovery of spermatogenesis or ovarian function if it has been temporarily altered by therapy.[107,109,112]

Sperm Banking

Semen storage for use in artificial insemination has been available for many years. Although initially used to establish pregnancy in infertile couples, sperm banking also has been used more recently to preserve procreation abilities in men undergoing cancer therapy. The option to bank sperm unfortunately will not be available to every man undergoing cancer therapy. As has been previously noted, many men will be subfertile or infertile at the time of diagnosis. In addition, because sperm banking needs to be completed before initiation of therapy, anyone with rapidly progressing disease frequently cannot delay the start of therapy to complete the cryopreservation process. Redman et al[113] investigated 79 men treated for Hodgkin's disease who had pretreatment semen analysis. Of these individuals 28% were considered to be infertile at diagnosis. Of these men 44 were followed post therapy, and only 20% had normal sperm counts at a median of 27 months' follow-up. Eleven couples attempted pregnancy, using the cryopreserved semen; thus far only three inseminations have been successful.

Kaempfer et al[114] noted that even if artificial insemination is never completed, the knowledge that semen has been banked and is available when needed can provide a significant psychologic boost for the male undergoing cancer therapy. They also stated that all aspects of the sperm banking process, from initial visit through the completion of the insemination, be fully discussed so that informed decisions can be made.

In Vitro Fertilization and Embryo Transfer

In vitro fertilization, used for male infertility because of low sperm counts or for female infertility as a result of severe endometriosis, immunologic infertility, or absent or damaged fallopian tubes, has undergone remarkable technologic advances with more than 30,000 fertilization cycles undertaken each year.[115] In vitro fertilization requires ovarian stimulation followed by ova retrieval via ultrasound-guided needle aspiration of the preovulatory follicles. Laparoscopy also may be used. The retrieved oocytes then are incubated with sperm for 5 to 26 hours. Following incubation these embryos then are transferred to the uterus and released. The woman remains hospitalized on a bed-rest regimen for about 6 hours. After discharge, she is encouraged to rest for 48 to 72 additional hours. Initial results of a single oocyte-retrieval procedure have resulted in a pregnancy rate of 10% to 16%. It has been shown, however, that after four to six attempts, the rate of successful pregnancies may approximate 50% to 60%.[115,116]

PREGNANCY AND CANCER

Although pregnancy complicated by a diagnosis of cancer is a rare event, it creates multiple problems for all concerned. Uncertainty about the prognosis of mother and fetus, the rigors of treatment, and the long-term sequelae of cancer for patient, infant, and family compound events that normally are surrounded by myriad conflicting emotions. Only with comprehensive care by many health care and ancillary individuals can a positive outcome for mother, fetus, and family be anticipated.

Cancer is the second leading cause of death in the reproductive years. It is estimated that cancer complicates about 1 in 1000 pregnancies, and approximately 1 in 118 women with cancer also have a concomitant pregnancy. The most commonly associated cancers are those of the breast, cervix, ovary, and colorectum and lymphoma, leukemia, and malignant melanoma, which reflect those cancers most commonly seen during the reproductive years.[42]

In general, most cancers do not adversely affect a pregnancy nor does the pregnancy adversely affect the cancer outcome, although it is possible that the treatment necessary to manage the cancer may have an adverse affect on the pregnancy. Therapeutic abortion has not been shown to be of benefit in altering disease progression and should not be considered unless continued pregnancy will compromise treatment and thus prognosis. The wishes of the patient and family must be considered, with therapeutic options, including prognosis for mother and fetus, fully explained.[42,107]

It was previously believed that cancer associated with pregnancy was more aggressive and the outcome for all patients poor. It now is recognized that delay in diagnosis may be a more likely cause of advanced disease at the time of diagnosis. Because diagnosing cancer during a pregnancy is difficult, signs and symptoms of the disease may be misconstrued or underestimated. Treatment options should be evaluated as though the patient were not pregnant and therapy should be instituted when appropriate.[42,107,112]

Medical Management of Commonly Associated Cancers

Breast cancer

Breast cancer is the cancer most commonly associated with pregnancy, representing one cancer for every 3000 pregnancies.[42,107,112] Parente et al[117] noted that collected series show a range from one to seven breast cancers per 10,000 pregnancies. In terms of all women with breast cancer, 1 in 35 will be pregnant at the time of diagnosis[42,108,112]

Breast examination should be part of the initial prenatal visit. Although breast enlargement during pregnancy makes examination difficult, it is essential that all women have a thorough examination. If the woman does not practice breast self-examination (BSE), BSE education should be included. If a mass is felt, prompt evaluation is necessary. Although a mammogram is difficult to interpret because of breast density, it may safely be undertaken if appropriate fetal shielding is used. Even if the mammogram shows negative results, a breast mass must be investigated until a definitive diagnosis is made.[42,107]

Treatment of breast cancer should proceed as in the nonpregnant patient. Biopsy with the patient under local anesthesia has not been shown to cause fetal harm and should be performed without delay.[118] Once a definitive diagnosis is made, further therapy can be tailored to time of gestation, physician recommendations, and patient wishes. In general, modified mastectomy with lymph node sampling is the standard treatment for early disease. Depending on gestational age, adjuvant chemotherapy often can be delayed until after delivery. For the woman who desires breast-conserving surgery, lumpectomy with lymph node sampling may be done if she is close to term. Radiation therapy and chemotherapy will be delayed until delivery. For advanced disease, surgery and chemotherapy should be undertaken without delay. Therapeutic abortion may be suggested during the first trimester to prevent chemotherapy exposure to the fetus.[42,108,118-120]

The chance for survival has been considered poor, with Peters[121] reporting a 30% overall survival rate and Nujent and O'Connell[122] reporting a survival rate of 57%. Most authors note that when patients are matched stage for stage with nonpregnant control subjects, there appears to be no differences in survival rates.[42,108,118-122]

Further pregnancies after a diagnosis of breast cancer have been considered controversial. Some authors[112,117] suggest that all women refrain from any pregnancies, whereas others[121,123] suggest that a further pregnancy may actually protect against recurrence. Those who do not believe that another pregnancy is contraindicated suggest a waiting period of 2 to 5 years after completion of all therapy inasmuch as recurrence is most likely during this time period.[42,108,118,119,124]

Breast-feeding after breast cancer diagnosis also has been highly debated. On the basis of breast cancer in mice, some authors[120,125] believe that breast-feeding is contradicted; however, no information on human beings is available. Hassey[126] stated that breast-feeding should no longer be discouraged and, in fact, should be recommended if the woman desires. For the woman who has received primary breast radiation, it has been suggested that breast-feeding occur only on the nonirradiated side, primarily because of the possible increase in mastitis associated with breast-feeding in the irradiated breast.

Cancer of the cervix

The second cancer most commonly associated with pregnancy is cancer of the cervix, which occurs in 1 in 400 pregnancies. Approximately 1 in every 100 women diagnosed with cervical cancer will be pregnant at the time of diagnosis. Carcinoma in situ is most commonly found, with invasive disease seen in only 2% to 5% of all cases. Signs and symptoms are similar to those found in the nonpregnant patient, with the majority of pregnant patients experiencing vaginal bleeding or discharge.[127] Diagnosis is most commonly made by Papanicolaou smear. If the smear is abnormal, colposcopy with appropriate biopsies should be undertaken. Cone biopsy should be avoided because it is associated with a 30% complication rate, including hemmorhage, premature delivery, and infection.[42,107,118,119,123]

For carcinoma in situ the pregnancy may be allowed to continue. Biopsy should be repeated every 6 to 8 weeks and, unless there is progression, definitive therapy delayed until after delivery. If frank invasion is found, treatment, consistent with standard practice for the nonpregnant women, should not be delayed. During the first two trimesters, surgery or radiation therapy, without therapeutic abortion, usually is undertaken. Early-stage disease (IA and IB) may be treated with radical hysterectomy and pelvic lymph node dissection, whereas in advanced disease radiation therapy is the most common treatment. During the third trimester, fetal viability usually can be awaited and the baby delivered by cesarean section, after which the appropriate cancer therapy can be given.[42,107,123,125,127,128]

Controversy exists over the safety of vaginal delivery. Some researchers[123,125] suggest that vaginal delivery may disseminate the cancer or cause hemmorhage or infection. Thus cesarean section is recommended. Others have suggested that vaginal delivery actually may be associated with an improved overall survival and should be allowed if possible. To date, no definitive answer is available.[123,125,129]

Ovarian cancer

Ovarian masses are common during pregnancy, occurring once in every 81 pregnancies. In general only 2% to 5% of these are malignant, for an estimated 1 in 9000 to 1 in 25,000 case ratio. Most patients are asymptomatic, with an adnexal mass noted at the first prenatal visit.[107,116,118] There are a variety of ways to approach a pelvic mass during pregnancy. Orr and Shingleton[120] suggest that a mass >5 cm that lasts into the second trimester should be explored. Roberts[127] suggests that any mass >6 cm or symptomatic be immediately evaluated, whereas Barber[123] states that a unilateral, encapsulated, movable mass <10 cm can wait until the second trimester for evaluation.

If malignancy is diagnosed, treatment should proceed as in the nonpregnant patient. Early disease (stage IA) of low-grade histologic findings can be managed by unilateral oophorectomy and biopsy of the other ovary. The pregnancy may be allowed to continue. For all other stages, standard therapy of radical hysterectomy, omentectomy, node biopsy, and peritoneal washings should be carried out. If the patient is near term, a cesarean section, followed by the appropriate therapy, may be performed. Unfortunately, 30% to 50% of all patients will be diagnosed with stage III or IV disease. Although recent management of stage III disease has resulted in improved survival, in general, a prognosis of long-term survival is poor.[118,120,123,125,127] As in the treatment of all cancers, the wishes of the patient must be considered. It is not uncommon for a pregnant woman with advanced disease to delay treatment until the fetus is viable. Palliative treatment should be instituted at the earliest possible time.

Malignant melanoma

Malignant melanoma is one of the most rapidly increasing cancers, with a predicted incidence of 1 in 100 Caucasians by the year 2000. It occurs most often in a preexisting mole in fair-haired individuals with blue or green eyes and an inability to tan when exposed to the sun, and the peak incidence is during the third and fourth decades.[120,130]

It has been suggested[131] that melanoma arising during pregnancy is associated with a poor prognosis because it is hormonally influenced and thus exacerbated by pregnancy. At present this has yet to be definitively proven. What is known is that melanoma that occurs during pregnancy more often is found on the trunk, a melanoma site associated with a poor prognosis. In addition, all pigmented areas darken during pregnancy, thus making diagnosis of early changes more difficult. Biopsy and removal of questionable lesions are indicated. There appears to be no difference in the survival rate between the pregnant and nonpregnant woman with melanoma.[131-133]

Treatment consists of wide excision with skin graft if necessary. Lymph node dissection remains controversial. Adjuvant therapy is being investigated; however, no definite answers are available, although chemotherapy does not appear to be of benefit (WA Robinson, personal communication, 1988). It is unknown if biologic response modifiers will prove beneficial. For patients with advanced disease, therapeutic abortion followed by palliative chemotherapy is advised. For the patient with brain metastasis, surgery or radiation therapy with appropriate fetal shielding may be undertaken.[118,120,133]

Malignant melanoma is known to metastasize to the placenta and fetus. The placenta should be carefully evaluated at delivery and the baby monitored for development of melanoma. Because of the controversy surrounding hormonal influence, further pregnancies should be discouraged and birth control pills avoided.[42,107,118,133-135]

Lymphomas

Both non-Hodgkin's lymphoma (NHL) and Hodgkin's disease occur with pregnancy, although the incidence is rare, with Hodgkin's disease occurring in 1 in 6000 pregnancies and NHL rarely associated.[125] Hodgkin's disease usually occurs as asymptomatic lymphadenopathy of the cervical, supraclavicular, or mediastinal regions. Disease confined to the neck or axilla usually can be treated with radiation therapy used with fetal shielding. Because more extensive disease requires combination chemotherapy, a therapeutic abortion is suggested during the first half of pregnancy. During the last half of pregnancy therapy will be defined by the stage of the pregnancy. If viability is imminent, therapy may be delayed or single-drug treatment instituted and delivery awaited. For rapidly progressing disease, combination chemotherapy should be instituted immediately.[42,107,125]

Fewer than 50 cases of NHL and pregnancy have been reported in the literature. Steiner-Salz et al[136] reported on six cases of NHL that complicated pregnancy, and they reviewed an additional 22 cases. Therapy consisted of chemotherapy or radiation therapy, or both. Seventeen patients died within 9 months of delivery, six infants died shortly after birth, and the remaining patients and offspring are believed to be alive and well. Although NHL is known to metastasize to the placenta and fetus and thus requires careful observations at delivery, NHL has not developed in these infants.[134,135]

Leukemia

Leukemia occurs in 1 in 75,000 pregnancies. Diagnosis often is made on routine complete blood cell count. Treatment should be instituted immediately unless the fetus is viable or near viability. If the fetus is viable, delivery should not be delayed. If the fetus is near viability, leukapheresis may be utilized until delivery is possible. Therapeutic abortion is suggested in the first trimester to avoid fetal exposure to chemotherapy.[137] Aviles and Niz[138] reported on 20 children born of 18 women with acute leukemia. One infant was stillborn, and two others died within 90 days of birth. Five of the 18 women remain alive; the other 13 died of recurrent leukemias. The 17 remaining children developed normally without apparent psychologic or physiologic abnormalities. In another report[139] perinatal mortality was as high as 50%, with 75% of mothers dying within 7 months of delivery. Leukemia also may spread to the placenta and fetus; thus placental and fetal monitoring are important aspects of delivery and postpartum care.[134,135]

Effects of Treatment and Malignancy on the Fetus

Surgery

Maternal surgery can be safely accomplished with minimal risk to the fetus.[118,120,125] Pelvic surgery is more easily accomplished during the second trimester. There is little risk to the fetus from short exposure to anesthetic agents after the first trimester. Adequate ventilation and prevention of hypotension are of prime importance.[120] As long as competent surgeons and anesthesiologists with appropriate fetal monitoring equipment are available, no harm to the fetus should occur.[112]

Radiation

Radiation doses >250 cGy during pregnancy have been associated with fetal damage, for example, mental retardation, skin changes, and spontaneous abortions (depending on stage of gestation). Low doses of radiation associated with diagnostic x-ray studies (<0.5 cGy) probably are not harmful if adequate fetal shielding is provided. Radiation to the pelvis should be avoided.[140,141] Long-term effects of low-dose radiation remain unknown, but the concerns of chromosomal aberrations and an increase in childhood cancer in children exposed in utero remain. Follow-up over many generations may be necessary to determine the exact effects.[125,141]

Chemotherapy

Chemotherapy has been administered prior to and concurrent with pregnancy.[142] As previously noted, chemotherapy during the first trimester has been associated with fetal wastage, malformations, and low birth weight. Many studies indicate that the incidence of fetal malformations is low (<10%) and may be minimized or avoided with careful selection of agents. Latent effects are still unknown and offspring need continuous evaluation.

Maternal-fetal spread

Only a few cancers spread from the mother to the fetus, with melanoma, NHL, and leukemia the most common. Because few series have been compiled, the exact incidence is unknown. Rothman et al[134] reviewed 11 cases and Potter and Schoeneman[135] reported 24 cases of maternal cancer that metastasized to the infant. Seventeen of the 35 women had metastatic melanoma. Fifteen infants died of cancer, and an additional six died of events unrelated to cancer. Because of the rare incidence of metastatic involvement to the infant, evaluation of the placenta and fetus is essential in women with disseminated cancers.

Nursing Management of the Pregnant Patient

Nursing management of the pregnant patient with a concomitant diagnosis of cancer can be extremely complicated. Interventions to include psychosocial, educational, and ethical considerations must be developed and implemented. It has been suggested that pregnancy and cancer be treated as a high-risk event with all the associated needs.[42] Careful explanations of all aspects of care, with special emphasis on support of the patient and her family, need to be included. Normal activities of pregnancy may be delayed or prevented by disease or treatment, and fears of fetal demise, cancer therapy, and death may prevent resolution of ambivalence toward pregnancy and establishment of emotional affiliation to the growing child. Ethical considerations become apparent as plans for pregnancy are contrasted with needs for therapy. In some instances therapeutic abortion may be necessary for optimal treatment; in other instances therapy delays may be requested to provide for the safety of the fetus. Nonjudgmental care by health care personnel is essential during these difficult times.

Although extremely complex, nursing care of the woman with cancer and her baby is of utmost importance. With a focus on educational interventions, psychologic support, and coordination of care, the nurse has an important role in the final outcome. Treatment plans, coordination of follow-up, education about cancer, pregnancy, and treatment, and emotional support of the patient and significant others are integral components of the comprehensive care needed by the pregnant woman with cancer. Without these essential elements, it may not be possible to provide the necessary care for a positive or improved maternal and fetal outcome.

CONCLUSION

Sexual and reproductive dysfunction in cancer patients occurs much more frequently than previously recognized. Almost every patient exposed to cancer or cancer treatment has the possibility of experiencing some form of sexual dysfunction at some point during the illness. With cancer survival rates improving and with the understanding that sexual and reproductive function are important to all individuals, it is essential that sexuality and sexual function be assessed and evaluated prior to therapy and that appropriate interventions are implemented throughout treatment and the follow-up period.

REFERENCES

1. Yarbro CH, Perry MC: The effect of cancer therapy on gonadal function. Semin Oncol Nurs 1:3-8, 1985.
2. Yasko JM, Green P: Coping with problems related to cancer and treatment. CA 37:107-125, 1987.
3. Fisher SG: The psychosexual effects of cancer and cancer treatment. Oncol Nurs Forum 10(2):63-68, 1983.
4. Guyton AC: Endocrinology and reproduction, in Human Physiology and Mechanism of Disease (ed 4). Philadelphia, WB Saunders, 1987, pp 563-654.
5. Gill GN: Endocrine, in West JB (ed): Best and Taylor's Physiological Basis of Medical Practice (ed 11). Baltimore, Williams & Wilkins, 1985, pp 844-933.
6. Emslie-Smith D, Paterson CR, Schratcherd T, et al (eds): Reproduction, in Textbook of Physiology. Edinburgh, Churchill Livingstone, 1988, pp 323-335.
7. Marieb EN: Reproductive system, in Essentials of Human Anatomy and Physiology. Menlo Park, Calif, Addison-Wesley, 1987, pp 311-333.
8. Wicks LJ: Treatment modalities for colorectal cancer. Semin Oncol Nurs 2:242-248, 1986.
9. MacDonald LD, Anderson HR: Stigma in patients with rectal cancer: A community study. J Epidemiol Community Health 38:284-290, 1984.
10. Dobkin KA, Broadwell DC: Nursing considerations for the patient undergoing colostomy surgery. Semin Oncol Nurs 2:249-255, 1986.
11. Lamb MA, Woods NF: Sexuality and the cancer patient. Cancer Nurs 4:137-144, 1981.
12. Donovan MI (ed): Teaching the patient about sexuality, in Cancer Care: A Guide for Patient Education. New York, Appleton-Century-Crofts, 1981, pp 257-289.
13. de Bernardinis G, Tuscano D, Negro P, et al: Sexual dysfunction in males following extensive colorectal surgery. Int Surg 66:133-135, 1981.
14. Hurney C, Holland J: Psychosocial sequelae of ostomies in cancer patients. Cancer 35:170-183, 1985.
15. Shipes E, Lehr S: Sexuality and the male cancer patient. Cancer Nurs 5:375 381, 1982.
16. Danzi M, Ferulano GP, Abate S, et al: Male sexual function after abdominoperineal resection for rectal cancer. Dis Colon Rectum 26:665-668, 1983.
17. Glasgow M, Halfin V, Althausen AF: Sexual response and cancer. CA 37:322-333, 1987.
18. Williams JJ, Slack WW: A prospective study of sexual function after major colorectal surgery. Br J Surg 67:772-774, 1980.
19. Burnham WR, Leonard-Jones JE, Brook BN: Sexual problems among married ileostomists. Gut 18:673-677, 1977.
20. Bachers ES: Sexual dysfunction after treatment for genitourinary cancer. Semin Oncol Nurs 1:18-24, 1985.
21. Schover LR, vonEschenbach AC, Smith DB, et al: Sexual rehabilitation of urologic cancer patients: A practical approach. CA 34:66-74, 1984.
22. Watt RC: Nursing management of a patient with a urinary diversion. Semin Oncol Nurs 2:265-269, 1986.
23. Schover LR, Fife M: Sexual counseling of patients undergoing radical surgery for pelvic or genital cancer. J Psychol Oncol 3(3):21-41, 1986.
24. Cancer Facts and Figures—1989. New York, American Cancer Society, 1989.
25. Donovan MI, Girton SE: Self concept, in Cancer Care Nursing (ed 2). Norwalk, Conn, Appleton-Century-Crofts, 1984, pp 506-556.
26. Furlow WL: Sexual consequences of male genitourinary cancer: The role of sex prosthetics, in Vaeth J N, (ed): Frontiers of Radiation Therapy and Oncology. Basel, Karger, 1980, pp 104-107.
27. Lange PH, Chang WY, Fraley EE: Fertility issues in the therapy of nonseminomatous testicular tumors. Urol Clin North Am 14:731-747, 1987.
28. Blackmore C: The impact of orchiectomy upon the sexuality of the man with testicular cancer. Cancer Nurs 11:33-40, 1988.
29. Narayan P, Lange PH, Fraley EE: Ejaculation and fertility after extended retroperitoneal lymph node dissection for testicular cancer. J Urol 127:685-688, 1982.
30. Nijman JM, Koops HS, Kremer J, et al: Gonadal function after surgery and chemotherapy in men with stage II and III nonseminomatous testicular tumors. J Clin Oncol 5:651-656, 1987.
31. Heinrich-Rynning T: Prostatic cancer treatments and their effects on sexual functioning. Oncol Nurs Forum 14:37-41, 1987.
32. Eggleston JC, Walsh PC: Radical prostatectomy with preservation of sexual function: Pathological findings in the first 100 cases. J Urol 134:1146-1148, 1985.
33. Balducci L, Phillips DM, Gearhart JG, et al: Sexual complications of cancer treatment. Am Fam Physician 37(3):159-172, 1988.
34. Lamb M: Vulvar cancer. Patient information booklet. Oncol Nurs Forum 13(6):79-82, 1986.
35. Lamb M: Sexual dysfunction in the gynecologic oncology patient. Semin Oncol Nurs 1:9-17, 1985.
36. Hubbard JL, Shingleton HM: Sexual function of patients after cancer of the cervix treatment. Clin Obstet Gynecol 12:247-264, 1985.
37. Morgan S: Sexuality after hysterectomy and castration. Women Health 3:5-10, 1978.
38. Masters WF, Johnson VE (eds): Human Sexual Response. Boston, Little, Brown & Co, 1966.
39. Zussman L, Zussman S, Sunley R, et al: Sexual response after hysterectomy-oophorectomy: Recent studies and reconsideration of psychogenesis. Am J Obstet Gynecol 140:725-729, 1981.
40. Jenkins B: Patients' reports of sexual changes after treatment for gynecologic cancer. Oncol Nurs Forum 15:349-354, 1988.
41. Lamb MA, Bargman C, Brozovich K: Ovarian cancer. Patient information booklet. Oncol Nurs Forum 12:83-88, 1985.
42. Krebs LU: Pregnancy and cancer. Semin Oncol Nurs 1:35-41, 1985.
43. Hampton BG: Nursing management of a patient following pelvic exenteration. Semin Oncol Nurs 2:281-286, 1986.
44. Hubbard SM, Jenkins J: An overview of current concepts in the management of patients with testicular tumors of germ cell origin. II. Treatment and strategies by histology and stage. Cancer Nurs 6:125-139, 1983.
45. McKenzie F: Sexuality after total pelvic exenteration. Nurs Times 84:27-29, 1988.
46. Schain WS: The sexual and intimate consequences of breast cancer treatment. CA 38:154-161, 1988.
47. Schain WS: Breast cancer surgeries and psychosexual sequelae: Implications for remediation. Semin Oncol Nurs 1:200-205, 1985.

48. Andersen BL: Sexual functioning morbidity among cancer survivors: Current status and future research directions. Cancer 55:1835-1842, 1985.
49. Witt ME, McDonald-Lynch A, Grimmer D: Adjuvant radiotherapy to the colorectum: Nursing implications. Oncol Nurs Forum 14(3):17-21, 1987.
50. Hilderley LJ: Radiotherapy, in Groenwald S (ed): Cancer Nursing Principles and Practice. Boston, Jones & Bartlett, 1987, pp. 320-347.
51. Yasko JM: Sexual dysfunction, in Care of the Client Receiving External Radiation Therapy. Reston, Va, Reston Publishing Co, 1982, pp 192-231.
52. Yasko JM: Sexual and reproductive dysfunction, in Guidelines for Cancer Care: Symptom Management. Reston, Va, Reston Publishing Co, 1983, pp 269-287.
53. Johnston CH, Stair JC: Sexual dysfunction: Infertility, in McNally JC, Stair JC, Sommerville ET (eds): Guidelines for Cancer Nursing Practice. Orlando, Fla, Grune & Stratton, 1987, pp 273-277.
54. Horning SJ, Hoppe RT, Kaplan HS, et al: Female reproductive potential after treatment for Hodgkin's disease. N Engl J Med 304:1377-1382, 1981.
55. Ray GR, Trueblood HW, Enright L, et al: Oophoropexy: A means of preserving ovarian function following pelvic megavoltage radiotherapy for Hodgkin's disease. Radiology 96:175-180, 1970.
56. Baker JW, Peckham MJ, Morgan RL, et al: Preservation of ovarian function in patients requiring radiotherapy for paraaortic and pelvic Hodgkin's disease. Lancet 1:1307-1308, 1972.
57. Rowley MJ, Leach DR, Warner GA, et al: Effects of graded doses of ionizing radiation on human testes. Radiat Res 59:665-678, 1974.
58. Kinsella TJ, Shapiro E, Fraass BA, et al: Testicular injury following high dose conventionally fractionated irradiation. Int J Radiat Oncol Biol Phys 9:136-137, 1983 (suppl).
59. Seibel MM, Freeman MG, Graves WL: Carcinoma of the cervix and sexual function. Obstet Gynecol 55:484-487, 1980.
60. Fisher SG: Sexuality, in Johnson BL, Gross J (eds): Handbook of Oncology Nursing. New York, John Wiley & Sons, 1985, pp 363-379.
61. Jenkins B: Sexual healing after pelvic irradiation. Am J Nurs 86:920-922, 1986.
62. Shell JA, Carter J: The gynecological implant patient. Semin Oncol Nurs 3:54-66, 1987.
63. Dodd MJ: Managing side effects of chemotherapy and radiation therapy: A guide for nurses and patients. Norwalk, Conn, Appleton and Lange, 1987.
64. Herr HW: Preservation of sexual potency in prostatic cancer patients after iodine implantation. J Am Geriatr Soc 27:17-19, 1979.
65. Carlton CE, Hudgins PT, Guerriero WG, et al: Radiotherapy in the management of stage C carcinoma of the prostate. J Urol 116:206-210, 1976.
66. Schover LR, von Eschenbach AC: Sexual and marital counseling with men treated for testicular cancer. J Sex Marital Ther 10:29-40, 1984.
67. Goldstein I, Feldman M, Deckers P, et al: Radiation-associated impotence. JAMA 251:903-910, 1984.
68. Nevidjon B: Sexuality, in McIntire SN, Cioppa AL (eds): Cancer Nursing: A Developmental Approach. New York, John Wiley & Sons, 1984, pp 257-276.
69. Brown MH, Kiss ME, Outlaw EM, et al: Standards of Oncology Nursing Practice. New York, John Wiley & Sons, 1986.
70. Howard-Ruben, J: Sexual dysfunction related to disease process and treatment, in McNally JC, Stair JC, Sommerville ET (eds): Guidelines for Cancer Nursing Practice. Orlando, Fla, Grune & Stratton, 1987, pp 268-273.
71. Hassey KM: Radiation therapy for rectal cancer and the implications for nursing. Cancer Nurs 10:311-318, 1987.
72. Aistars J: Fatigue in the cancer patient: A conceptual approach to a clinical problem. Oncol Nurs Forum 14(6):25-30, 1987.
73. Longo DL, Fisher RI: Medical problems in long-term survivors of Hodgkin's disease. Internal Med Spec 4(1):165-171, 1983.
74. Schilsky RL, Erlichman C: Late complications of chemotherapy: Infertility and carcinogenesis, in Chabner B (ed): Pharmacologic Principles of Cancer Treatment. Philadelphia, WB Saunders, 1982, pp 109-128.
75. Chapman RM: Effect of cytotoxic therapy on sexuality and gonodal function. Semin Oncol 9:84-94, 1982.
76. Tenenbaum L: Effects on sexuality, in Tenenbaum L (ed): Cancer Chemotherapy—A Reference Guide. Philadelphia, WB Saunders, 1989, pp 195-204.
77. Skeel RT (ed): Handbook of Cancer Chemotherapy (ed 2). Boston, Little, Brown, 1987.
78. Carter SK, Bakowski MT, Hellman K: Chemotherapy of Cancer (ed 3). New York, John Wiley & Sons, 1987.
79. Schilsky RL, Lewis BJ, Sherins RJ, et al: Gonadal dysfunction in patients receiving chemotherapy for cancer. Ann Intern Med 93:109-114, 1980.
80. Richter P, Calamera JC, Morgenfeld MC, et al: Effect of chlorambucil on spermatogenesis in the human with malignant lymphoma. Cancer 25:1026-1030, 1970.
81. Drasga RE, Einhorn CH, Williams SD, et al: Fertility after chemotherapy for testicular cancer. J Clin Oncol 1:179-183, 1983.
82. Cunningham J, Mauch P, Rosenthal DS, et al: Long-term complications of MOPP chemotherapy in patients with Hodgkin's disease. Cancer Treat Rep 66:1015-1022, 1982.
83. Viviani S, Santoro A, Bon Pante V, et al: Gonadal toxicity after combination chemotherapy for Hodgkin's disease: Comparative results of MOPP vs ABVD. Eur J Cancer Clin Oncol 21:601-605, 1985.
84. Rousseau L, Dupont A, Labrie F, et al: Sexuality changes in prostate cancer patients receiving antihormonal therapy combining the antiandrogen flutamide with medical (LHRH agonist) or surgical castration. Arch Sex Behav 17:87-98, 1988.
85. Kaempfer SH: Male sexual dysfunction, in Baird SB (ed): Decision Making in Oncology Nursing. Toronto, BC Decker, 1988, pp 164-165.
86. Warne GL, Fairley KF, Hobbs JB, et al: Cyclophosphamide-induced ovarian failure. N Engl J Med 289:1159-1162, 1973.
87. Belohorsky B, Siracky YJ, Sandor L, et al: Comments on the development of amenorrhea caused by Myleran in cases of chronic myelosis. Neoplasma 4:397-402, 1960.
88. Chapman RM, Sutcliffe SB, Malpas JS: Cytotoxic-induced ovarian failure in women with Hodgkin's disease. II. Effects on sexual function. JAMA 242:1171-1181, 1979.
89. Andrieu JM, Ochoa-Molina ME: Menstrual cycle, pregnancies and offspring before and after MOPP therapy for Hodgkin's disease. Cancer 52:435-438, 1983.
90. Santoro A, Bonadonna G, Valagussa P, et al: Long-term results of combined chemotherapy-radiotherapy approach in Hodgkin's disease: Superiority of ABVD plus radiotherapy versus MOPP plus radiotherapy. J Clin Oncol 5:27-37, 1987.

91. Gershenson DM: Menstrual and reproductive function after treatment with combination chemotherapy for malignant ovarian germ cell tumors. J Clin Oncol 6:270-275, 1988.
92. Rivkees SA, Crawford JD: The relationship of gonadal activity and chemotherapy-induced gonadal damage. JAMA 259:2123-2125, 1988.
93. Blatt J, Poplack DG, Sherins RJ: Testicular function in boys after chemotherapy for acute lymphoblastic leukemia. JAMA 304:1121-1124, 1981.
94. Byrne J, Mulvihill JJ, Myers MH, et al: Effects of treatment on fertility in long-term survivors of childhood or adolescent cancer. N Engl J Med 317:1315-1321, 1987.
95. Kaempfer SH: Female sexual dysfunction, in Baird SB (ed): Decision Making in Oncology Nursing. Toronto, BC Decker, 1988, pp 162-163.
96. Brager BL, Yasko J: Sexual and reproductive dysfunction, in Care of the Client Receiving Chemotherapy. Reston, Va, Reston Publishing, 1984, pp 287-297.
97. Roferon A (package insert). Nutley, NJ, Roche Laboratories, 1987.
98. Mulvihill JJ, Byrne J: Genetic counseling of the cancer survivor. Semin Oncol Nurs 5:29-35, 1989.
99. Kaempfer SH: The effects of cancer chemotherapy on reproduction: A review of the literature. Oncol Nurs Forum 8(1):11-18, 1981.
100. Kaempfer SH, Wiley FM, Hoffman DJ, et al: Fertility considerations and procreative alternatives in cancer care. Semin Oncol Nurs 1:25-34, 1985.
101. Li FP, Gimbere K, Gelber RD, et al: Outcome of pregnancy in survivors of Wilms' tumor. JAMA 257:216-219, 1987.
102. Mulvihill JJ, McKeen EA, Rosner F, et al: Pregnancy outcome in cancer patients—experience in a large cooperative group. Cancer 60:1143-1150, 1987.
103. Holmes GE, Holmes FF: Pregnancy outcome of patients treated for Hodgkin's disease—a controlled study. Cancer 41:1317-1322, 1978.
104. Mulvihill JJ, Myers MH, Connelly RR, et al: Cancer in offspring of long-time survivors of childhood and adolescent cancer. Lancet 2:813-817, 1987.
105. Leonard MA, Waskerwitz MJ: Late effects in adolescent survivors of childhood cancer. Semin Oncol Nurs 2:126-132, 1986.
106. Earley WC: Risks of radiation exposure, in Abrams R, Wexler P (eds): Medical Care of the Pregnant Patient: Concepts and Management. Boston, Little, Brown, 1983, pp 89-98.
107. Robinson WA, Krebs LU: Oncologic disease, in Abrams R, Wexler P (eds): Medical Care of the Pregnant Patient: Concepts and Management. Boston, Little, Brown, 1983, pp 307-319.
108. Accola KM, Sommerfeld DP: Helping people with cancer consider parenthood. Am J Nurs 79:1580-1583, 1979.
109. Kaempfer SH: Reproductive planning, in Baird SB (ed): Decision Making in Oncology Nursing. Toronto, BC Becker, 1988, pp 166-167.
110. Chapman RM, Sutcliffe SB: Protection of ovarian function by oral contraceptives in women receiving chemotherapy for Hodgkin's disease. Blood 58:849-851, 1981.
111. Glode LM, Robinson W, Gould SF: Protection from cyclophosphamide-induced testicular damage with an analog of gonadotropin releasing hormone. Lancet 1:1132-1134, 1981.
112. Lowitz BB: Pregnancy and sexual function, in Casciato DA, Lowitz BB (eds): Manual of Clinical Oncology (ed 2). Boston, Little, Brown, 1988, pp 403-410.
113. Redman JR, Bajoruna DR, Goldstein MC, et al: Semen cryopreservation and artificial insemination for Hodgkin's disease. J Clin Oncol 5:233-238, 1987.
114. Kaempfer SH, Hoffman DJ, Wiley FM: Sperm banking: A reproductive option in cancer therapy. Cancer Nurs 6:31-38, 1983.
115. Speirs AL: The changing face of infertility. Am J Obstet Gynecol 158:1390-1394, 1988.
116. Seibel MM: A new era in reproductive technology: In vitro fertilization, gamete intrafallopian transfer, and donated gametes and embryos. N Engl J Med 318:828-834, 1988.
117. Parente JT, Amsel M, Lerner R, et al: Breast cancer associated with pregnancy. Obstet Gynecol 71:861-864, 1988.
118. Donegan WL: Cancer and pregnancy. CA 33:194-214, 1983.
119. Mitchell MS, Capizzi RL: Neoplastic disease, in Burrow GN (ed): Medical Complications during Pregnancy (ed 3). Philadelphia, WB Saunders, 1988, pp 540-569.
120. Orr JW, Shingleton HM: Cancer in pregnancy. Curr Probl Cancer 8:1-50, 1983.
121. Peters MV: The effect of pregnancy in breast cancer, in Forrest APM, Kunkler PB (eds): Prognostic Factors in Breast Cancer, Edinburgh, Livingston, 1968, pp 65-89.
122. Nugent P, O'Connell TX: Breast cancer and pregnancy. Arch Surg 120:1221-1224, 1985.
123. Barber HRK: Manual of Gynecologic Oncology. Philadelphia, JB Lippincott, 1980, pp 51-63.
124. Cooper DR, Butterfield J: Pregnancy subsequent to mastectomy for cancer of the breast. Ann Surg 171:429-443, 1970.
125. DiSaia PJ, Creasman WT: Clinical Gynecologic Oncology. St Louis, CV Mosby, 1981, pp 376-400.
126. Hassey KM: Pregnancy and parenthood after treatment for breast cancer. Oncol Nurs Forum 15:439-444, 1988.
127. Roberts JA: Management of gynecologic tumors during pregnancy. Clin Perinatol 10:369-382, 1983.
128. McGee JE: Management of cervical dysplasia in pregnancy. Nurs Pract 12(3):36-42, 1987.
129. Lee RB, Neglia W, Park RC: Cervical carcinoma in pregnancy. Obstet Gynecol 58:584-589, 1981.
130. Rifkin RN, Thomas MR, Mughal TI, et al: Malignant melanoma—profile of an epidemic. Western J Med 149:43-46, 1988.
131. Riberti C, Marola G, Bertani A: Malignant melanoma: The adverse effect of pregnancy. Br J Plast Surg 34:338-339, 1981.
132. Shiu MH, Schohenfeld D, Maclean B, et al: Adverse effect of pregnancy on melanoma: A reappraisal. Cancer 37:181-187, 1976.
133. Houghton AN, Flannery J, Viola MV: Malignant melanoma of the skin occurring during pregnancy. Cancer 48:407-410, 1981.
134. Rothman LA, Cohen CJ, Astarloa J: Placental and fetal involvement by maternal malignancy: A report of rectal carcinoma and a review of the literature. Am J Obstet Gynecol 116:1023-1024, 1973.
135. Potter JF, Schoeneman M: Metastasis of maternal cancer to the placenta and fetus. Cancer 25:380-388, 1970.
136. Steiner-Salz D, Yahalom J, Samuelov A, et al: Non-Hodgkin's lymphoma associated with pregnancy: A report of six cases, with a review of the literature. Cancer 56:2087-2091, 1985.
137. Henderson ES: A selected overview, in Gunz FW, Henderson ES (eds): Leukemia (ed 4). Orlando, Fla, Grune & Stratton, 1983, pp 785-798.
138. Aviles A, Niz J: Long-term follow-up of children born to mothers with acute leukemia during pregnancy. Med Pediatr Oncol 16:3-6, 1988.

139. Lilleyman JS, Hill AS, Anderkon KJ: Consequences of acute myelogenous leukemia in early pregnancy. Cancer 40:1300-1303, 1977.
140. Dekaban AS: Abnormalities in children exposed to x-radiation during various stages of gestation: Tentative timetable of radiation injury to the human fetus. Part I. J Nucl Med 9:471-477, 1968.
141. Jankowski CB: Radiation and pregnancy: Putting the risks in proportion. Am J Nurs 86:260-265, 1986.
142. Schapira DV, Chudley AE: Successful pregnancy following continuous treatment with combination chemotherapy before conception and throughout pregnancy. Cancer 54:800-803, 1984.

Chapter 29

Altered Body Image and Sexuality

Susan Dudas, RN, MSN

INTRODUCTION

Self-image is a significant factor in the recovery and rehabilitation of the person with cancer. Body image and sexuality are integral parts of a person and must be given as much attention in a nursing care plan as other physical, emotional, and spiritual needs. How changes in body image should be managed depends primarily on the patient's perception of these changes and the reactions of those persons who are important to the patient. The nurse needs to accurately assess the impact of an altered body image and the significance of sexuality to ensure that the patient is given the information and attention necessary to cope with these concerns.

This chapter is concerned with the assessment of changes in body image and sexuality in the person with cancer. Interventions to help the patient cope with body image changes and sexuality issues will also be discussed.

CONCEPT OF BODY IMAGE

Carlson[1] has defined self-concept as "all unconscious and conscious perceptions, cognitions, information, feelings, goals, and evaluation that refer to the self." Self-esteem includes all evaluative aspects of the self-concept: perceptions of self, self-acceptance, self-approval, and self-expectations. Basic to self-esteem and self-concept is the concept of body image; body image includes those elements that refer to the physical self. Concepts of body image and self-concept are, according to Klopp,[2] "dynamic constructs which are developed and changed both by private perceptions and social feedback." The attitudes and beliefs that a person has about self are influenced by significant others and significant events in one's life. Norris[3] cites body image as the intrapersonal experience of feelings and attitudes toward one's body but also acknowledges body image as a "social creation." This view is reflected in the way cultural and societal attitudes, as well as those of significant others, influence body image. Schilder[4] also extended the body image concept to include a sociologic meaning for both the individual and society as well as the individual's personal or psychologic investment in his or her body and body parts.

Early concern with body image phenomena occurred in psychiatry and neurologic practice. Kolb[5] reported that body-image phenomena (in general clinics) were viewed as either "a healthy psychophysiological reaction or psychological and emotional maladaption." The concept of body image disturbance developed in the sixteenth century with recognition by the French surgeon Paré of the phantom limb phenomenon after amputation.[5] The concept of "disturbances in body image" was derived from observation of individuals who failed to perceive changes in their bodies and their body parts and failed to adapt to them as they actually existed (ie, when the basic body image persisted despite the visible loss of a body part). In addition to acute disturbances in body image occurring as a result of traumatic or surgical dismemberment, similar disturbances were noted with radical excision of the face, head and neck, thoracoplasty, polio, sudden paraplegia and hemiplegia, and body distortions associated with endocrine dysfunction.[5]

The most commonly used definition of body image is that of Schilder,[4] who refers to body image as the "picture of our body, formed in the mind's eye." This picture involves interpersonal, environmental, and temporal factors and includes how our bodies look and how they function.[6] Schilder also recognized body image as a part of normal psychology and noted the impact of sensory input on body image. Feelings about intelligence, mobility, and physical capacity to endure pain and stress are also part of body image.[7] Thus body image is affected by physical factors and sensations as well as emotional and social reactions; body image relates to one's actual appearance and body function as well as to how one perceives the self and what one perceives as an "ideal" body or image. In current American society, an "ideal" body, for example, often emphasizes youth, beauty, and slimness.

Secord and Jourard[8] described *body cathexis* as the degree of satisfaction or dissatisfaction with the various parts or processes of the body. They developed a scale, Body Cathexis—Self Concept (BC-SC), to appraise body cathexis and found a strong relationship between body cathexis with various parts or processes of the body and one's self-concept. Body image is a multidimensional construct that requires multimethods approach for study.[7]

Kolb[5] has described five broad classifications of human states that significantly threaten one's body image and may lead to body image disturbance. These include (1) neurologic disorders that affect any part of the sensory or motor system connected with movement and posture; (2) acquired or induced toxic or metabolic disorders that result in changes in body structure; (3) somatic disorders that lead to progressive deformity either early or late in life; (4) acute dismemberment resulting from trauma or surgical procedures as either a planned or an emergency event; and (5) disorders of personality development, such as psychoses and psychoneuroses. Cancer, its treatment, and its progression can actually be used very readily to illustrate the first four items in this classification.

CANCER AND BODY IMAGE

Cancer, its treatment, and resulting changes in appearance, disabilities, and loss of function often cause a change in body image and can negatively affect a person's self-esteem. Emphasis on physical attractiveness places an additional burden on individuals who must sustain disfigurement or dysfunction from illness such as cancer. Changes in body image that are not realistically integrated into the patient's self-concept hinder adaptation and adjustment. Such body image changes are viewed as threats or major losses. Any alteration to the body is a threat to the body image as perceived by the individual patient and can result in the patient's feeling worthless as a person, physically unattractive or even repulsive, and unable to be valued or loved.[9] As patients go through a process of mourning these losses, they may express their feelings as anger, depression, pessimism, or withdrawal.[9]

Problems in coping with changes in body image caused by cancer affect the patient's ability to learn, to be motivated for self-care, and to resume the role in the family that he or she held before the cancer diagnosis. Nurses should be concerned with body image factors in order to help cancer patients be comfortable and realistic about their physical selves. They cannot make assumptions about a patient's reactions to cancer and its sequelae without verifying these perceptions with the patient.[10] Nursing assessment of the state of the patient's self-esteem and perspective of his or her body image is important; awareness of these aspects is necessary to foster the cancer patient's potential for rehabilitation and improved quality of life. Frank-Stromborg and Wright[11] found that more than half of the 323 ambulatory cancer patients in their study perceived the diagnosis and treatment of cancer as changing their physical appearance and that these changes made them feel worse; in addition, the majority felt moderately or strongly negative about these changes. These patients primarily referred to changes in their body image or changes in their emotional outlook as factors affecting their changed feelings about themselves.

Damage or alteration to the body usually causes conflict between the image that has been established over time and current reality.[12] If the patient does not change the image of his or her physical self, self-esteem may decrease because the patient may still have some expectations that can no longer be met. Changing of self-assessments in ways that are congruent with reality is a necessary part of the adjustment process.[1] Norris[3] has identified factors that contribute to the ability of persons to adapt to changes in the appearance, structure, or function of the body: (1) the nature of the threat, (2) the meaning that the change has for the person, (3) the person's own coping ability, (4) the responses from significant others, and (5) the help available to the patient and his or her family. Additional factors are the time available to prepare for and absorb the meaning of the change and to experience and accept the changes in the body.

Certain types of cancer are more likely to affect body image. For example, breast cancer that results in a mastectomy or changes related to radiation therapy, head and neck cancer that results in residual defects, colorectal or bladder cancer that requires an ostomy, gynecologic cancer that affects the woman's genitalia or organs that are involved in reproductive function, and prostate or testicular cancers are the major cancers associated with altered body appearances and functions that may result in body image disturbances. Changes in reproductive functioning, such as fertility problems associated with cancer chemotherapy or radiation therapy, effects of chemotherapeutic agents on gonadal function and pregnancy, parenting issues, and alternative options, such as sperm banking, are discussed elsewhere in this book and will not be covered in this chapter.

Breast Cancer

In today's society, the breast is valued in terms of fertility and femininity and is symbolic of sexuality. Women who undergo mastectomy for the treatment of breast cancer may suffer manifestations of psychologic maladjustment that cause them to feel rejected, sexually mutilated, and depressed.[13] These feelings may contribute to a poor self-image, a sense of worthlessness, difficulties in interpersonal relationships, a decline in sexual activity, and, in some cases, deterioration of marriage.[13] Many patients with breast cancer become socially isolated and withdraw from social contacts.[14] One cannot assume that age is a factor, making the younger woman more vulnerable to body image disturbances than the older woman. Factors other than chronologic age are more likely to be the issue. For example, mastectomy for a woman who has a strong marital relationship that has lasted over many years is not as likely to be as threatening as for a young divorcee who depends on her physical appearance to initiate new relationships with men.[15]

Changes in treatment methods for breast cancer, such as the use of lumpectomy in lieu of modified mastectomy in selected patients and the use of radiation therapy, have been oriented to improving the cosmetic outcome of therapy. However, nurses should not assume that body image changes are not as significant with these techniques as with mastectomy. Although women undergoing radiation therapy generally have fewer negative feelings regarding body image changes,[16,17] it is necessary to consider their perspective of the situation. Although the breast is retained in these techniques, radiation therapy, for example, can cause changes in the texture of the breast tissue and the contour of the breast, thickening of the skin, discoloration of the skin, and, in the case of simultaneous chemotherapy, it may cause severe skin reactions, which can have an impact on the patient's perception of body image.[16,17] Side effects, such as alopecia, weight gain, and early menopause, are commonly encountered in women with breast cancer who are receiving adjuvant chemotherapy, and these side effects often result in a lowered body image.[13] Even though the nurse may view a lumpectomy and axillary resection as less traumatic for the woman with breast cancer, it is important to remember that "any visual or perceived change in the breast affects the woman's perception of her 'self' as well as her physical being."[16] Foltz[18] has concluded from her review of studies related to body image and cancer that, although generally lesser surgery or immediate cosmesis does reduce distress related to altered body image in the immediate posttreatment period, the concerns and distress of all patients are similar at 1 year, regardless of the extent of surgical intervention.

Confrontation with an altered body image occurs at different times with different people and also may occur unexpectedly, even when someone perceives that he or she has handled a situation well. A female patient, for example, on being informed that she had breast cancer decided definitively that a modified mastectomy was appropriate for her. She was very confident before and after the operation and verbalized her reasons for this decision, handling the loss of her breast in a matter-of-fact manner. However, when she went to purchase a breast prosthesis, she faced herself in a full-length mirror and felt particularly vulnerable. She expressed how surprised she felt by her sad and anxious feelings on being measured for the prosthesis and viewing herself in the mirror; she had thought that she had accepted her mastectomy in a very realistic and positive way with no display of regret or sadness prior to this time.

Because of advances in plastic and reconstructive surgery, breast reconstruction is an option for women with mastectomy. The goal is to provide symmetry and preserve body image.[16] This procedure can be done at the time of the mastectomy or later. Winder and Winder[19] have concluded from a review of multiple studies that women seek breast reconstruction to increase their self-esteem, to improve their appearance, to eliminate their need for a prosthesis, and to permit them to wear more attractive clothing. They also found that some of the barriers to women's considering reconstruction as an option included the cost of the procedure, the fear of another surgical experience (if not done at time of the mastectomy), and the concern about others' reactions to their having the cosmetic procedure. In her review of studies on self-concept, Foltz[18] noted that reconstruction may not always, for example, be seen by marital partners as a positive action. Nurses also need to be sure that their own views about breast reconstruction do not bias them in working with patients with mastectomy. For example, if they do not provide information about breast reconstruction because they do not believe it is important or necessary, the patient is denied knowledge on which to base a decision. The choice for or against reconstruction, however, cannot be made until the patient both cognitively and emotionally recognizes that the breast is gone.[19] The time required for this acknowledgment to occur varies considerably among individual patients.

Head and Neck Cancer

Facial appearance is an important component of body image. Aversion to visible deformities, especially in the face, is well documented.[20] Aggressive treatment of head and neck cancer, because of removal of large portions of bony and soft tissue from the head and neck, results in extensive defects, often causing professionals as well as the patient to wonder if the result is worth it. These visible defects, which affect both appearance and functions (ie, speech, eating, swallowing, salivary control, and chewing), result in alterations in body image that require sensitive nursing care to assure patients that they need not expect rejection, loss of sexual appeal, or even repulsion as a result of the defects.[21] Unless patients adjust to an altered body image, they will not be successfully rehabilitated in spite of the restoration of cosmetic appearance and function.

Dropkin and colleagues[20] have developed a Disfigurement/Dysfunction Scale to quantitatively measure the perception of visible disfigurement and dysfunction after head and neck surgery for treatment of cancer. The scaling technique measured others' perceptions of the relative severity of 11 common disfigurements and 8 commonly associated dysfunctions. Their study documented that procedures viewed as "most severe were associated with major structural alteration in the center of the face or that region that provides the greatest audiovisual stimuli in interaction with others" (ie, orbital exenteration and radical maxillectomy). The scale was used as a way to determine patients' ability to cope with disfigurement and dysfunction by measuring the impact of specific alterations in body image through observation of self-care and "social affiliation behaviors."[22]

Cancers Resulting in Ostomies

Frequently cited as patients with disturbances of body image are those with surgically constructed stomas, either colostomies or urostomies, for the treatment of cancer. Klopp[2] examined the relationship between body image and self-concept at varying lengths of time after ostomy surgery and reported that, because control of elimination is learned as a private, controlled function, the necessity of an ostomy and the loss of sphincter control result in a changed body image. She further explains that if the body image is unacceptable to the individual, an alteration in how that individual views and values self may also occur; conversely, how the individual views self overall may affect body image. Klopp[2] has stated that "the person with a stoma is faced with psychosocial adjustment to the stoma, and to the new or accentuated sensory phenomena (ie, involuntary noise of passage of flatus in absence of sphincter and odor) created by it, into his or her body image and self-concept."

Other authors[10,23-25] have also noted that persons with stomas often have poor psychosocial outcomes, which range from failure to return to occupations, withdrawal from social and intimate contacts, depression, and anxiety. These patients are concerned with the visibility of urine or stool on their bodies and on the potential visibility (or detectability) to others' during social or intimate contact. Behaviors that are often associated with the construction of a stoma, which is seen as an undesirable change in body structure and function, include social isolation, sexual dysfunction, anxiety, and dependency.[2,10,23-25]

Oberst and Scott,[26] in their study of surgically treated cancer patients, found that patients with ostomies were slower to return to preillness functional levels and had greater psychologic distress than nonostomy patients.

Side Effects of Chemotherapy

Even if no anatomic alterations occur, body image disturbances may be encountered as a result of side effects of cancer treatments. These side effects may also result in distressing symptoms that interfere with the patient's body image. These symptoms include alopecia, pain, nausea, vomiting, diarrhea, weakness, fatigue, muscle atrophy, and neurologic changes. Women may feel unattractive when loss of hair from the head, axilla, and pubic area results from therapy. One study[27] of 44 cancer patients found that, regardless of sex, alopecia negatively affected a person's body image. Appropriate wigs in styles worn perviously, hats, turbans, or attractive scarves can be used effectively, but with some patients this intervention may not be adequate and the patients withdraw from social interactions.

It is important for the nurse working with cancer patients to realize that the impact of changes in body image may fluctuate during the cancer experience. Priorities are variable at different times for different individuals. Nurses cannot assume that body image changes mean the same to each person.

A female patient who had ovarian cancer and was to receive chemotherapy that would result in alopecia sobbed uncontrollably when she was informed that she would lose her stunning black hair. For someone who valued her beautiful hair to the degree she did, this was viewed as a cruel and unjust experience. She, who had been stoic and courageous in having four major surgical procedures in the treatment of her cancer, was devastated by the potential experience of alopecia. However, after several months when her cancer progressed in spite of chemotherapy, she inadvertently went out to her garden without her wig, talking with her neighbors without realizing that she did not have her wig on. When she came into the house and looked in the mirror and saw her bald head, she simply laughed. Her priority at this time was to have a day without pain; somehow her views about her alopecia had decreased in importance. This is also an illustration of the time factor that Norris[3] has identified as being important in the experiencing and acceptance of changes in the body.

The self-esteem of some patients is dependent on physical strength, endurance, and productivity, and these patients may have increased difficulty when side effects of fatigue and weakness occur. Because productivity is so important to them, they may exceed their capacity for work and become ill from exhaustion. Sometimes nurses may actually foster this by their emphasis on all the patients are able to do in spite of therapy, putting even higher expectations on the patients. Nurses may believe that the patient has no problem in this area, because he or she is able to keep up with considerable activity; from the patient's perspective, however, productivity and activities may have changed so drastically from the premorbid style that the patient actually feels like a worthless failure. The nurse does not have a complete picture of the person's premorbid life-style, but the patient compares the current situation with the preillness pattern of activity and productivity. If the patient's pattern of activity and his or her attitude about the changes that are occurring as a result of the cancer are not determined, opportunities for identifying body image disturbances may be missed. Emphasizing the individual patient's remaining abilities rather than the disabilities is an important focus of the nurse in promoting acceptance of an altered body image.

PROMOTING THE ADJUSTMENT TO AN ALTERED BODY IMAGE

The goal of promoting a healthy and realistic attitude requires support for the patient who has to accept a new or changed body image. To reach this goal, the nurse helps prevent disturbances in body image by providing emotional support as patients grieve the loss of a body part or a body function. Patients need assurance that such grieving is appropriate and normal. Attentive listening is a major intervention in this process. Touching, spending calm and unrushed time with patients, and conveying sincere interest are ways to convey acceptance and caring. Providing information and teaching them to appropriately manage procedures involved with body changes will help patients gain control; this also will enhance body image and self-concept. Enabling patients to manage necessary procedures or care in an efficient way may also be helpful in ensuring that the body change does not become the focus of their lives. This principle is a major aspect of rehabilitation protocols after head and neck surgery. Dropkin et al[20] emphasize that the patient's taking over irrigation and self-care techniques after head and neck surgery helps improve body image perceptions. Support for their self-esteem may help the patients accept and adapt to changes. It is important for nurses to avoid pushing or forcing patients to accept change. Readiness is an important factor to assess. Acceptance of change takes time; just as adjusting to grief and loss varies widely in terms of time and manner, so does adjustment to changes in body image vary.

Alteration in body image may be associated with loss; thus a process of mourning and grief occurs. The nurse can play an influential role in helping patients express anger and grief and cope with these feelings. Assisting patients to deal with the change and not make it the focus of their lives reinforces their self-esteem. Patients need to understand the full situation to avoid placing undue restrictions on themselves because of cancer or its treatment. Some may also need help to not use cancer as an excuse for unsuccessful relationships but, instead, to resume social relationships satisfactorily.[10]

Watson[28,29] studied the effects of short-term counseling on ostomy patients' self-concept. Participants cited the following feelings about their experiences: (1) anger at having the ostomy and the change in physical condition; (2) grief and revulsion at losing bowel or bladder control; (3) fears regarding their sexuality; (4) feelings of ugliness because of the presence of the ostomy; and (5) feelings of worthlessness caused by the need for the ostomy. She demonstrated that patients who were counseled with empathetic understanding, positive regard, genuineness, and concreteness (based on the Carkhuff Helping Model) achieved independence and competence in ostomy care, an improved self-concept, and social involvement outside the home more readily than did a control group. In addition, problem-solving skills were developed to facilitate a positive adaptive response. Thus attention paid to self-concept (and potential or actual body image disturbances) with provision of counseling and teaching was beneficial for these patients.

The role of the family cannot be overemphasized in terms of sustaining the person with cancer, but this support can be more freely given and be more realistic if the spouse, partner, or significant others are prepared for the patient's changes. It is important to remember that there has to be an ongoing assessment of the family's response to the patient's illness, treatment, and changes. Northouse,[30] for example, has documented the need for an ongoing assessment of patients with breast cancer and of their husbands. She found that difficulties in psychosocial adjustment are not confined to the early phase of illness but persist over time for both patients and husbands. Spouses need to be involved and informed about ways to support cancer patients' self-esteem. The family must be prepared for any physical changes resulting from cancer or its treatment; it is necessary to help the family avoid displaying fear or revulsion to physical changes that may have occurred. Children can be particularly helpful in this situation if they have a secure and special relationship with the patient. This author has seen grandchildren unconcerned with their grandfather's facial disfigurement after head and neck surgery, because they responded to the grandparent as the same person they had always known. These positive reactions helped the grandfather adjust more readily to body image changes. Admittedly, some children may be fearful of these changes and avoid the person; such children need guidance and reassurance from the person who has had the radical surgery and body changes.

Orienting patients and their families to mutual self-help groups, such as the United Ostomy Association, Reach to Recovery, CanSurMount, and I Can Cope, can be very helpful to patients who are adjusting to changes in body image. Sharing concerns with others who have had similar experiences and have resolved some of their negative reactions to body changes may help patients make their own adjustments. Nurses need to be cautious, however, that they do not force patients to participate in these groups. Not everyone benefits from such activities. Some patients have adequate opportunities to express their concerns with family members and significant friends and do not desire to make their altered body and cancer the focus of their lives by socializing only with others who have had similar illnesses.

One of the areas in which psychologic factors, such as body image changes and altered self-concept, can adversely affect relationships in the family and with significant others is in the area of sexual relationships. A person's perception of his or her body image affects self-esteem and is closely linked to sexuality. Body image changes, therefore, may contribute to feelings of sexual inadequacy.[31]

ALTERATION IN SEXUAL FUNCTIONING

Closely tied to the concepts of self-esteem, self-concept, and body image is the aspect of sexuality. Sexuality, or sexual health, is defined by the World Health Organization[32] as the integration of somatic, emotional, intellectual, and social aspects of sexual being in ways that are positively enriching and that enhance personality, communication, and love. Sexuality is concerned with the biologic, psychologic, sociologic, spiritual, and cultural aspects of life.[33] Since sexuality is an integral part of living and an essential part of a person's personality and behavior, it should be a significant part of any nursing care plan.[10,34]

Because of the nature of cancer, which may threaten the biopsychosocial status of a person, oncology nurses often work with patients who have concerns about their sexuality. Cancer and cancer therapy may temporarily or permanently affect behavior used to express sexual identity. Cancer of the bladder, prostate, testes, and penis, for example, may affect libido, erection, orgasm, and ejaculation in the male patient.[24] Sexuality, however, involves more than the single act of intercourse.[34] Changes in appearance and physiologic changes that affect function may cause patients to doubt their masculinity or femininity.[31] Side effects of treatments for cancer may result in anxiety, depression, dependency, and anger, which may interfere with sexual desire and the maintenance of satisfactory relationships. Thus adverse effects on sexual functioning may occur as a result of the stress associated with the cancer experience itself. Foltz,[18] in her review of studies related to effects of cancer and cancer treatment on sexual aspects of self-concept, has concluded that the incidence, magnitude, and duration of sexual dysfunction are mediated by the site of disease, treatment-associated injury determined by disease site, treatment modality, marital status, and age. She further suggests that sexual disability may be determined less by body-image alteration (defined as perceived sexual attractiveness) than by other psychosexual and treatment-related physiologic changes.

Sexuality has been recognized as a significant part of nursing care of patients with cancer as documented by the fact that sexuality is the ninth standard developed by the Oncology Nursing Society.[35] It identifies the importance of maintaining sexual identity because of the threat of cancer to sexuality.

BARRIERS TO INTERVENTIONS FOR SEXUALITY

There are varieties of sexual expression, as well as sexual preferences, and patients must receive the right kind of information for their situation. Feelings about body acceptability, sexual ability, libido, partners' enjoyment, and rejections are not unusual, especially in new relationships. However, persons experiencing cancer and body changes that threaten their sexuality are even more vulnerable to these fears and stresses related to sexual functioning.

Nurses may be reluctant to discuss sexuality with their patients or even to include sexuality as part of an assessment. They often do not see sex as a priority topic for discussion with cancer patients compared with information on treatments or medications. They often think patients are too concerned with other health problems to be concerned with sexual issues. Nurses may be uncomfortable discussing sexual matters because they feel inadequately informed or because their beliefs regarding sex may be rigid and they do not think such a discussion is appropriate. They may feel that other health professionals can handle this aspect. It may be difficult for nurses to not base their actions on their own values regarding sexuality. They may feel that they do not wish to invade the patient's privacy, since sexuality is very personal and the patient may be offended. Yet, these same nurses may not hesitate to ask patients about other personal factors, such as bowel and bladder function or hygiene values and beliefs. Avoiding inquiries into sexuality may convey to patients the impression that sex is no longer appropriate for them. Nurses need to listen carefully to what their patients say, because there may be subtle cues that patients desire to discuss these sexual concerns.

Williams and coworkers[36] studied nurses' attitudes toward sexuality in cancer patients. They found, in their sample of 211 registered nurses at a continuing education program in nursing, that only 3% responded "always" and 27% responded "never" to a question concerning how often they had offered to discuss sexual concerns with patients in the past month. Thirty-three percent responded "seldom" or "sometimes" to this question, while 19% responded "frequently" or "very frequently." The majority of the nurses in this study did not feel sexual counseling was part of their role or that addressing the sexual needs of cancer patients was a major component of nursing care. There was no investigation into the reasons for these attitudes, but the findings are significant in drawing attention to the need for greater emphasis on sexual aspects in the assessment and care of cancer patients and to the need for educating nurses about sexual issues in the provision of nursing care.

Fisher and Levin[37] also investigated the sexual knowledge and attitudes of 120 professional nurses specifically caring for oncology patients. They found that the nurses had significantly lower knowledge scores and more conservative attitudinal scores related to heterosexual relations, masturbation, and abortion than medical students and graduate nurses who had been tested a decade before. They suggested "that the nurses sampled recently are less knowledgable regarding human sexuality and more conservative in their attitudes toward sexuality" than those tested previously, which was a surprising finding in an era of increased sexual education and publicity.

NURSING CARE ISSUES REGARDING SEXUALITY

Nurses need to be aware of and comfortable with their own sexuality, and they need to examine their own values regarding sex and sexuality in order to provide assistance to the patient who is experiencing problems in this area. Nurses should recognize their own biases regarding sexuality to be assured that they are not forcing their own attitudes and biases on the patient or that they are not informing the patient of other options because the options do not fit into the realm of their own value systems. Determining whether their values are in conflict with the values of their patients is a necessary process for nurses. If there is a conflict of values, they need to refer these patients to other persons who may be more helpful, rather than omit opportunities for assistance. They cannot deny patients the information they need to function in satisfying sexual relationships. They also need to consider the sociocultural factors on which the person's sexual value system is based.[38] Age, religious and ethnic background, education, and specific illness ramifications are other factors that should be taken into consideration to determine their impact on the patient's sexuality. Issues on sexual morality are taught differently among different religions; yet members of a specific religious denomination may also have different beliefs and practices.[38] Therefore when they identify the religion of their patients nurses cannot assume that these patients abide by traditional teachings. Again, it is important to obtain the patient's specific views on these matters and to not act on assumptions.

One of the first ways a nurse can affirm the view that the patient is still a sexual being is to discuss sexual issues with that patient, who may be reluctant to bring the topic up for discussion. Bringing up the topic in a matter-of-fact manner is an interaction that acknowledges the patient as a sexual person. The nurse's behavior should communicate to patients that their sexual concerns are respected and justified; nurses must reflect open-mindedness and tolerance, regardless of their personal sexual beliefs and practices. Nurses cannot assume that patients no longer are interested in sex because they are older. Nor can they assume that all persons are interested in sex; for example, some persons may not have valued sex previously and may use cancer as an excuse for reducing sexual activity in their relations with their partners.

It is important for nurses to recognize their own preconceived notions about age, gender, and expectations about sexual behavior. Nurses cannot assume that all patients follow their sexual behavior or practices. Interviews can be conducted to discover the patient's feelings about sexual aspects of life after experiencing cancer, its treatment, and its effect on themselves and their families.

It is also important not to make assumptions about sexual preference or behavior and not to press for information if it is not readily given. Stevens and Hall[39] reviewed studies on the interactions of lesbians with health care providers, citing that lesbians found them to be judgmental, nonsupportive, and negatively responsive when their identity as lesbians became known. In fact, these persons often did not identify themselves as lesbians because they feared it would hinder the quality of their health care. They described being responded to with ostracism, invasive personal questioning, shock, embarrassment, and fear, and they also believed that their partners had been mistreated and their confidentiality breached. The respondents also noted that questions asked by health care providers assumed that their female clients were heterosexual, that their partners were male, and that their sexual activity involved intercourse. They often felt "forced to make an announcement" of their lesbian identity. These researchers concluded that lesbians often do not feel comfortable about seeking health care because of experiences with nonempathetic responses when they did and that they even feel at risk of harm in some health care situations.

Sexual concerns are probably most often discussed after ostomy surgery, because there is evidence that sexual problems frequently occur after this type of surgery. Impotence, for example, has been reported as occurring in 33% to 100% of patients after abdominoperineal resection for rectal cancer and in 85% of patients after radical cystectomy.[40] Erectile impotence, the persistent inability to achieve or maintain a penile erection to permit coitus, is of deep concern to male patients after these surgical procedures.[40] Impairment of sexual function also may occur after orchidectomy for treatment of testicular cancer and can have profound effects on self-image, masculinity, and sexual identity.[41] This is particularly significant since cancer of the testicle is the most common malignancy in men between 25 and 34 years of age.[15] Fear of venereal spread of cancer or cancer as a punishment for past sexual conduct and concern about future sexual dysfunction may come to the forefront when patients are allowed to explore sexual concern.[15,42]

Gloeckner[43] studied the impact of sexuality and body image disturbances on patients with ostomies and found that 60% of the participants reported that they felt a decrease in sexual attractiveness. It is difficult to separate sexuality from feelings of attractiveness and desirability. The loss of body functions is a source of anxiety about sexual functioning as well as about interpersonal relationships. Fear of sexual or social rejection may be a factor that leads some cancer patients to isolate themselves and avoid taking the risks necessary to develop intimate relationships.[6] It should be obvious that to ignore discussions of sexuality with patients who have ostomies is to omit a significant aspect of the nursing care plan.

Less often is concern for sexuality issues displayed in more subtle situations. For example, peripheral neuropathy can result from the use of antineoplastic agents, such as vincristine or cisplatin. The effects of these drugs can affect sexual functioning because sensations of touch, loss of muscle control and proprioception, and discomfort, as well as loss of strength and endurance, can interfere with sexual activity.[44] For these patients, there is a need to identify appropriate alternative means of expressing sexuality and receiving sexual pleasure.

Patients who have undergone radical surgery may feel threatened in their self-worth if they sense that care givers are withdrawing or are uncomfortable about coping with their changes. Patients who have undergone head and neck surgery have described the negative impact of facial appearances on their sexual relationships, citing deficits caused by tongue changes, misshapen mouths, interference by nasogastric tubes, and facial disfigurement.[21] Sexual counseling should focus on helping patients understand their own abilities and disabilities so they can make knowledgeable choices and decisions regarding sexual aspects of their illness. It is important to not allow patients to place undue restrictions on themselves because of having cancer or to use cancer as an excuse for insecure relationships.[45]

INTERVENTIONS TO ENHANCE SEXUAL FUNCTIONING

Nurses can increase their knowledge by reviewing films, attending sexuality conferences and workshops, and reading books and such journals as *Medical Aspects of Human Sexuality* to broaden their knowledge base and views on sexuality. They also need to review or obtain a sound knowledge base in anatomy and physiology of normal sexual responses to be able to understand alterations resulting from cancer and its treatment. Oncology units may help their nursing staffs by obtaining the services of a qualified consultant to help nurses cope with the sexual needs of their patients and also to discuss specific issues involving selected patients.

As stated previously, assessment is the first step in determining the need for interventions related to sexuality. This requires interviewing the patient regarding sexual issues. Open-ended and direct questions may be used, along with active listening, reflection techniques, and avoidance of judgmental comments that can close the discussion quickly. Table 29-1 provides examples of questions that can be integrated into an overall nursing assessment interview to obtain information on sexuality and sexual concerns of the patient.[46-51] These interviews should begin with the least sensitive sexual matters, usually starting with general questions.[42] Questions and approach should be based on the patient's specific diagnosis and treatment issues, on the type of relationship the nurse has with the patient, and on how comfortable the nurse is in seeking information on sexuality. For example, when an atmosphere of trust and comfort has been created, discussion of the more intimate aspects of sexuality can begin.[15] Determining the patient's views on sexuality can help clear the air for further discussions or for referral to other persons who may be able to handle the specific problem or issue more effectively. Assessment also includes an awareness of when the time is appropriate for counseling; planning by the nurse may include a time 2 days later, but a sexual issue may come earlier than planned. During assessment of knowledge and attitudes, teaching strategies can be used to clarify information, impart facts, and dispel

TABLE 29-1 Nursing Assessment of Sexuality Issues in the Cancer Patient: Options for Questions*

Goals	Options for Questions
To determine the patient's self-concept and feelings of body image and To determine the extent of stress imposed by symptoms (eg, alopecia, fatigue, etc)	What currently makes you feel good about yourself?[51] How do you see yourself since your surgery or treatment?[31,51] How do you think others see you?[51] Has there been any change in the way you feel about your personal appearance?[49] Do you think there has been any change in you personally since you had your surgery (or were diagnosed with cancer)?[49] Do you see yourself differently as a result of your surgery or cancer treatment?
To provide opportunity for initial discussion regarding effect of cancer on sexuality and To facilitate exploration of sexual concerns	Please describe changes you have made in your life as a result of your cancer. What changes do you anticipate making as a result of having cancer (or cancer surgery)?[49,50] Has treatment affected the way you feel about yourself as a woman (man)?[46] Has the cancer (or treatment) interfered with you being a mother, father, or spouse?[33] How has the diagnosis of cancer altered how you feel about being a young man or a young woman?[47] Some other single women who have had a mastectomy (or other surgery) often have concerns about how they will handle telling significant men in their lives about the mastectomy (or other surgery). They have been reluctant to start new relationships. How do you think you would handle this if it should happen to you? Has treatment affected your roles as a wife, mother or worker (husband, father, worker)?[46] How has your cancer, surgery, treatment, affected your relationships (ie, with spouse, significant other, family, children)?
To obtain specific information on patient's sexual interest, practices, and concerns	Have you had any difficulties in sexual relationships prior to getting this diagnosis? Has this changed any since your diagnosis/treatment? Other patients often wonder if there will be changes in their sexual relationships with their spouse after this type of surgery/treatment. Tell me a little about the place that sexuality has in your relationship with your spouse or significant other.[42] Some couples have intercourse every day, some a couple of times a week, and still others not at all. About how often do you have intercourse?[48] Frequently, men are concerned about sexual activity after a prostatectomy (or other surgery). How has the cancer diagnosis affected your sex life so far?[42] Are you currently active with a partner? How often do the two of you have some sexual activity together?[42] Have you had changes in your breast tissue or breast sensation since radiation therapy that may have had an effect on satisfaction with foreplay or intercourse?[50] Has your sexual activity changed during treatment?[46] Have you experienced a change in sexual desire, excitement, or orgasm?[46] Do you have difficulty obtaining or maintaining an erection?

*These are options for questions or comments to facilitate discussion with the patient. The nurse varies the order or choice of question, depending on the comfort level of the nurse and the patient with each other as well as with the type of question. The nurse needs to observe the patient's appearance, body language (including posture and tone of voice), and any change in affect such as withdrawal, crying, or inappropriate responses or unwillingness to discuss questions. The nurse should note the language the patient uses in sexual discussion. If a specific problem is identified, then questions explore the onset, history of the problem, and perceptions about the cause and treatment events.

myths. These misconceptions may include, for example, the belief that cancer is transmitted sexually or that sex caused the cancer.[46]

A sexual-adjustment questionnaire (SAQ), originally designed for use with head and neck patients, has been modified for use with other postsurgical patients. The authors[52] believe the information gained from use of the SAQ could help clarify the kinds and frequency of sexual problems experienced by cancer patients and identify patients at higher risk of postoperative sexual problems.

When it is expected that the cancer and its treatment are likely to affect sexual functioning, a thorough assessment requires that the nurse determine the patient's level of understanding about sexual functions in general and learn how important sexual functioning is in the person's life. The nurse should take into consideration the patient's previous level of sexual activity and ascertain previous methods of sexual expression.[45] Nurses can erroneously assume that sexuality is not an important element, for example, when they are working with older patients and later learn that, in reality, sexuality was a major concern and required attention that was not given. It is important to listen to the patient's real concerns.[45] Just as it is inappropriate to avoid sexual discussions, it is also inappropriate to make assumptions about the person's sexual status and to emphasize sexual activities to a patient who has placed minimal significance on sexual activity in the past.[10] Some patients may not wish to discuss their sexual views or behavior, and they should not be forced to do so.

Mobility limitations, positioning, changes in body image, and increased dependence on others for hygiene and personal care are all factors that affect the patient's confidence in sexual relationships.[45] Patients who are receiving chemotherapy may not have the energy necessary to engage in even limited sexual activities. Fatigue and other symptoms may interfere with sexual relationships when, for example, the patient is too fatigued and weak and unable to be a partner in the sexual act. Couples can be advised that intimacy can be expressed by close body contact, lying together, showing a caring approach, and touching; the actual exertion of sexual intercourse is not the only expression of sexual experience. Leiber and coworkers[53] studied 38 patients receiving chemotherapy for advanced cancer and found that patients and spouses of both sexes experienced simultaneously an increase in desire for physical closeness (ie, simple proximity, holding hands, embracing, and kissing) and a decrease in the desire for sexual intercourse.

Alterations in sexual patterns can result from the cancer or its symptoms or from its treatment (eg, chemotherapy or radiation), or they may occur when there is a change in appearance after radical surgery that affects the person's self-concept. Feminization resulting from hormonal therapy, for example, may have a negative effect on body image of the male patient and result in a decreased desire for sexual activities.

Further assessment requires investigation into a patient's perspectives on how illness will affect or has affected sexuality and how the patient and significant others have responded to these changes. To determine any other possible causes of alterations in sexual functioning, questions should be raised regarding any medications that the patient is taking. For example, large amounts or chronic use of cocaine, narcotics, or marijuana inhibit sexual performance, and alcohol in large amounts inhibits performance and desire. In addition, antihypertensives, tranquilizers, sedatives, antidepressants, some antihistamines, and some antispasmotics are known to affect sexuality.[33] Awareness of the effects of drugs and specific illnesses on sexuality is essential if the nurse is to ask appropriate questions in any sexual assessment.

Timing of counseling on sexuality varies; for some persons, it may be an immediate concern, while for others the diagnosis, the prognosis, and the surgery itself have to be assimilated before the person is ready to discuss sexual concerns.[54] This author recalls a female patient whose first question of the nurse after an emergency transverse colostomy was, "Will this affect my having sex?" The depth of discussions should be guided by the patient's needs at the specific time.

Another patient with familial polyposis refused to have surgery in spite of the fact that his father had died of colon cancer and he was informed of the definite likelihood of his having cancer if surgery and an ileostomy were not performed. This patient walked out of the hospital rather than have surgery, when he learned that his sexual functioning would be altered by the procedure.

SEXUAL COUNSELING AS AN INTERVENTION FOR NURSES

The PLISSIT model, a commonly used counseling model for sexuality, consists of four stages of interventions used in sexual counseling. Permission, limited information, specific suggestions, and intensive therapy are the stages that form the acronym, P-LI-SS-IT.[55] As implicated in their names, the first three tend to require brief therapy whereas the last requires longer and more intensive therapy. Nurses usually may assist patients with the first three levels of interventions, but the last stage requires more expertise unless they have had additional education and experience.[54] Zalar[56] believes that the graduate professional nurse should be able to competently assist patients with needs involving "permission" and "limited information" because they are viewed as preventive interventions. The nurse may be better able than other health professionals to establish the trusting relationships necessary to do brief sexual counseling because of their frequent and lengthy contacts with patients and their families in hospitals and in communities.[55] It is appropriate to refer patients to other nurses or other personnel at any of the levels if the nurse is not comfortable with dealing with the needs of patients or believes that someone else may be able to respond to the patient more effectively. Nurses need to recognize their abilities, limitations, biases, and knowledge bases in working with patients and to determine which level of sexual counseling is needed for specific patients.

Permission

At the first level of counseling, the discussion of sexual concerns is promoted by creation of a permissive atmosphere or introduction of the topic in such a way as to suggest that it is one that can be discussed. Permission is first promoted when the nurse asks patients about their sexual concerns or suggests that it is an appropriate topic for discussion. This level indicates to the patient that sexual concerns are normal and expected. Providing time to discuss sexual concerns is an appropriate activity at this level. In the case of the cancer patient, it is characterized by discussion of the impact of cancer and its treatment on sexuality. An attitude is conveyed that sexual concerns, needs, and feelings related to sexual function are appropriate for discussion and that the nurse is willing to discuss these aspects with the patient, spouse, or significant others. Active listening on the part of the nurse helps the patient explore the problem.

Limited Information

The second level of counseling continues to convey the willingness to discuss sexuality, but, in addition, the nurse provides specific factual information to help clarify concerns the patient may have as well as to eliminate myths and clarify misconceptions. Anticipated changes related to the surgery or other treatments are aspects to be discussed, with provision of specific suggestions for actions. For example, fear of hurting the patient or making the cancer worse (especially when the genitalia are involved in the cancer) are often areas of concern that need clarification. Information about results of the surgery (for example, the loss of vaginal lubrication resulting from oophorectomy) is warranted at this point. If surgery or other therapy causes loss of sensation in essential areas, the couple may require more information on how to continue to enjoy physical intimacy. In cases in which sexual intercourse is no longer possible, patients and partners can be helped to recognize the importance and effectiveness of touching. It is important to encourage open communication and honest sharing of feelings and concerns between partners so that patients can let partners know their desires and fears and to allow enough time for both partners to become accustomed to the loss of a body part or change in appearance.[10,50]

Specific Suggestions

The third level of sexual counseling is appropriate when support and limited information are not adequate for the particular patient. Specific suggestions are given and follow-up is assured in order to monitor the effectiveness of the suggestions. For example, a patient who has had neurologic changes from a spinal tumor, resulting in paraplegia, needs specific information about management of the urinary catheter and preparation for sexual intercourse, depending on the level of injury and whether the patient is a female or a male. The use of sexual foreplay, erotic literature, alternatives to vaginal intercourse, the use of masturbation, and the finding of other effective erogenous zones on the body may be advised as a means for a couple to achieve sexual gratification. Any interventions that are recommended, however, should be within the framework of the patient's religious and spiritual beliefs and practices to avoid inciting distrust and distress in the patient and partner.[38] This requires nurses to intervene with sensitivity, compassion, and respect for beliefs and values that may be different from their own.[38]

Changes of position to increase comfort or decrease fatigue is another aspect to discuss. It is important to be sensitive in discussing alternate methods because some couples will not wish to have this information and may think it is inappropriate for them.

There are several strategies for enhancing sexual expression after the patient and partner express their goals for sexual activity. For some, increasing their willingness to communicate their feelings about sexual activity with the partner may be sufficient to help the couple work together to resolve the issues. Other partners may need encouragement to experiment with various methods, such as fantasy, activation of erogenous zones, changing positions, and finding alternative methods to achieve sexual satisfaction. For some patients, teaching ways to stimulate and maintain erections or referral for penile implants may be the appropriate intervention. Others may benefit from planned schedules to capitalize on times of peak energy for sexual pleasure. Patients can be advised to alternate positions so that they can choose the position that requires the least expenditure of energy. Advising the use of water-based lubrication for the woman who has had surgery, chemotherapy, or radiation therapy that interferes with vaginal lubrication may be helpful. For the patient with an ostomy, guidance on managing ostomy appliances to prevent leakage during sexual activity and ways to avoid odor and noise from the ostomy may be the appropriate intervention.

Possible solutions are considered and should take into consideration the patient's and the partner's values and attitudes toward sexual relationships. For example, consideration must be given to a homosexual patient's lifestyle in the proposal of resolutions or suggestions regarding appropriate activities based on the patient's physical status. If sexual concerns remain unresolved, intensive therapy and referral to an expert are the most appropriate form of intervention. It is important to recognize, however, that a trusting relationship that supports the patient's gender identity and promotes a positive body image is the essential factor necessary for effective discussions on sexual concerns.

Intensive Therapy

The fourth level requires referral when adequate progress is not being made at the other levels and when more depth in counseling is needed for complex needs. Nurses should recognize when there is a need for more competent and expert sexual therapists to obtain adequate and appropriate support for the patient and partner. Referral to a qualified therapist can be one of the nurse's most important functions.[54] Intensive therapy, for example, may be necessary to deal with sexual problems that existed prior to the cancer experience. Extensive psychologic counseling may be necessary, for example, when reconstructive surgery of genitalia is needed or when the use of prosthetic devices, such as penile implants, may be necessary.

The level of the nurse's participation in the PLISSIT model is based on the nurse's knowledge, experience, and own comfort level with sexual discussions. Shipes and Lehr[24] propose that approximately 70% of all sexual concerns can be dealt with in all types of settings by nurses using the first three levels (PLISS) of the model and that the remaining 30% require referral to a qualified therapist for intensive therapy (IT). However, the nurse should be careful not to delve into alternate methods of sexual experiences without gaining permission from the patient. A full assessment of the couple's attitudes is necessary to determine their values and comfort level. Some expectations regarding alternate methods may be very threatening to some couples; in some cases, the discussion is inappropriate and can actually increase the sexual concerns of the couple. Keen sensitivity to the needs of individual patients is extremely important. A knowledgeable, nonjudgmental nurse with good communication skills can play an important role, through effective sexual counseling, in enhancing a patient's quality of life.[50,51]

Shipes[54] has identified several factors necessary for effective counseling about sexuality. Although developed for working with ostomy patients, these factors are applicable to other cancer patients as well. Factors that require attention during counseling include the following:

1. Use of patient's language, speaking in terms that are clearly understood
2. The need to remember that age, physical and emotional health, previous sexual activity, and enjoyment of sex affect rehabilitative outcomes
3. Awareness that many conditions affect sexual function
4. Awareness that many medicines decrease sexual responsiveness
5. Focusing on the positive aspects

CONCLUSION

In this time of shorter hospital stays, increased demand on nurses, increased acuity of hospitalized patients, and the intensity of the clinical setting, there needs to be an increased awareness of psychosocial needs of patients in the area of body image and sexuality if quality care is to be achieved. For continuity of care, nurses must relay sources of concern to those providing follow-up care. If these issues are not adequately addressed in the hospital situation, they should at least not be lost to future health care givers. Since cancer patients are surviving for longer periods, it is important for nurses to include more interventions regarding the aspects of adjustment to body image and altered sexual functioning related to cancer in order to help improve the quality of their lives.

Research is needed to determine the relationship between cancer and its treatment and the impact on body image and sexuality. Research is also needed to develop effective techniques for assessing those persons at high risk of body image disturbances and sexual difficulties. These techniques will be helpful in identifying those persons who are most vulnerable and in need of specific interventions. Research into the most helpful approaches and interventions for working with patients with body image disturbances and sexual dysfunction will be valuable in improving the quality of life of our patients with cancer.

REFERENCES

1. Carlson CE: Psychosocial aspects of neurological disability. Nurs Clin North Am 15:309-320, 1980.
2. Klopp AR: Body Image and Self-Concept in Persons with Stomas. Unpublished doctoral dissertation, University of Illinois at Chicago, December 1989. (Available on microfilm through Dissertation Abstracts International.)
3. Norris CM. Body image: Its relevance to professional nursing, in Carlson CE, Blackwell B (eds): Behavioral Concepts and Nursing Interventions (ed 2). Philadelphia, JB Lippincott, 1978, pp 5-36.
4. Schilder P: The Image and Appearance of the Human Body. London, Kagan, Paul, Trench, Trubner, 1935.
5. Kolb LC: Disturbances of the body image, in Arieti S (ed) American Handbook of Psychiatry (ed 2). Vol IV. Organic Disorders and Psychosomatic Medicine. New York, Basic Books, 1975, pp 810-837.
6. Bogle JE, Shaul SL: Body image and the woman with a disability, in Bullard DG, Knight SE (eds): Sexuality and Physical Disability: Personal Perspectives. St. Louis, CV Mosby, 1981, pp 91-96.
7. Fawcett J, Frye S: An exploratory study of body image dimensionality. Nurs Res 29:324-327, 1980.
8. Secord PF, Jourard SM: The appraisal of body cathexis: Body cathexis and the self. J Consult Psychol 17:343-347, 1953.
9. Shipes E: Psychosocial issues: The person with an ostomy. Nurs Clin North Am 22:291-302, 1987.
10. Dudas S: Psychosocial aspects of patient care, in Smith D, Johnson DE (eds): Ostomy Care and the Cancer Patient. Orlando, Fla, Grune & Stratton, 1986, pp 93-102.
11. Frank-Stromborg M, Wright P: Ambulatory cancer patients' perception of the physical and psychosocial changes in their lives since the diagnosis of cancer. Cancer Nurs 7:117-130, 1984.
12. Dudas S, Carlson CE: Cancer rehabilitation: Implications for nursing. Oncol Nurs Forum 15:183-188, 1988.
13. Kriss R: Self image and sexuality after mastectomy, in Bullard DG, Knight SE: Sexuality and Physical Disability: Personal Perspectives. St Louis, CV Mosby, 1981, pp 185-192.
14. Wellisch DK: The psychologic impact of breast cancer on relationships. Semin Oncol Nurs 1:196-199, 1985.
15. von Eschenbach AC, Schover LR: Sexual rehabilitation of cancer patients, in Gunn AE (ed): Cancer Rehabilitation. New York, Raven Press, 1984, pp 155-173.

16. Knobf MKT: Primary breast cancer: Physical consequences and rehabilitation. Semin Oncol Nurs 1:214-224, 1985,
17. Rutherford DE: Assessing psychosexual needs of women experiencing lumpectomy: A challenge for research. Cancer Nurs 11:244-249, 1988.
18. Foltz AT: The influence of cancer on self-concept and life quality. Semin Oncol Nurs 3:303-312, 1987.
19. Winder AE, Winder BD: Patient counseling: Clarifying a woman's choice for breast reconstruction. Patient Educ Counsel 7:65-75, 1985.
20. Dropkin MJ, Malgady RG, Scott DW, et al: Scaling of disfigurement and dysfunction in postoperative head and neck patients. Head Neck Surg 6:559-570, 1983.
21. Metcalfe MC, Fischman SH: Factors affecting the sexuality of patients with head and neck cancer. Oncol Nurs Forum 12(2):21-25, 1985.
22. Dropkin MJ: Rehabilitation after disfigurative facial surgery. Plast Surg Nurs Winter:130-134, 1985.
23. Dyk RB, Sutherland AM: Adaptation of the spouse and other family members to the colostomy patient. Cancer 9:123-138, 1956.
24. Shipes E, Lehr S: Sexuality and the male cancer patient. Cancer Nurs 5:375-381, 1982.
25. Sutherland AM, Orbach CE, Dyk RB, et al: The psychological impact of cancer and cancer surgery. Part I. Adaptation to the dry colostomy: Preliminary report and summary of findings. Cancer 5:857-872, 1952.
26. Oberst MT, Scott DW: Postdischarge distress in surgically treated cancer patients and their spouses. Res Nurs Health 11:223-233, 1988.
27. Baxley KO, Erdman LK, Henry EB, et al: Alopecia: Effect on cancer patients' body image. Cancer Nurs 7:499-503, 1984.
28. Watson PG: The effects of short-term post-operative counseling on cancer/ostomy patients. Cancer Nurs 6:21-29, 1983.
29. Watson PG: Postoperative counseling for cancer ostomy patients. J Enterost Ther 10 (3):84-91, 1983.
30. Northouse L: A longitudinal study of the adjustment of patients and husbands to breast cancer. Oncol Nurs Forum 16:511-515, 1989.
31. Cooley ME, Cobb SC: Sexual and reproductive issues: Hodgkin's disease. Part I. Cancer Nurs 9:189-193, 1986.
32. World Health Organization Technical Report Series (No. 572): Education and Treatment in Human Sexuality: The Training of Health Professionals. Geneva, World Health Organization, 1975.
33. Woods NF: Human Sexuality in Health and Illness (ed 3). St. Louis, CV Mosby, 1984.
34. Smith DB: Sexual rehabilitation of the cancer patient. Cancer Nurs 12:10-15, 1989.
35. Oncology Nursing Society and American Nurses' Association, Division on Medical-Surgical Nursing Practice: Outcome Standards for Cancer Nursing Practice. Kansas City, Mo, American Nurses' Association, 1979.
36. Williams HA, Wilson ME, Hongladarom G, et al: Nurses' attitudes toward sexuality in cancer patients. Oncol Nurs Forum 13(2):39-43, 1986.
37. Fisher SG, Levin DL: The sexual knowledge and attitudes of professional nurses caring for oncology patients. Cancer Nurs 6:55-58, 1983.
38. Hogan RM: Influences of culture on sexuality. Nurs Clin North Am 17:365-375.
39. Stevens PE, Hall JM: Stigma, health beliefs, and experiences with health care in lesbian women. IMAGE 20(2):69-73, 1988.
40. van Driel MF, de Vries AT, Mensink HJA: Intracavernous self-injection of papaverine in the treatment of erectile impotence after major pelvic surgery. J Enterost Ther 14:101-104, 1987.
41. Blakemore C: The impact of orchiectomy upon the sexuality of the man with testicular cancer. Cancer Nurs 11:33-40, 1988.
42. Schover LR: Sexual rehabilitation of the ostomy patient, in Smith D, Johnson DE (ed): Ostomy Care and the Cancer Patient. Orlando, Fla, Grune & Stratton, 1986, pp 103-119.
43. Gloeckner MR: Perceptions of sexual attractiveness following ostomy surgery. Res Nurs Health 7(2):87-92, 1984.
44. Holden S, Felde G: Nursing care of patients experiencing cisplatin-related peripheral neuropathy. Oncol Nurs Forum 14(1):13-19, 1987.
45. Dudas S: Rehabilitation concepts of nursing. J Enterost Ther 11:6-15, 1984.
46. Cooley ME, Yeomans AC, Cobb SC: Sexual and reproductive issues for women with Hodgkin's disease. II. Application of PLISSIT model. Cancer Nurs 9:248-255, 1986.
47. Klopovich PM, Clancy BJ: Sexuality and the adolescent with cancer. Semin Oncol Nurs 1:42-48, 1985.
48. MacElveen-Hoehn P: Sexual assessment and counseling. Semin Oncol Nurs 1:69-75, 1985.
49. Morris CA: Self-concept as altered by the diagnosis of cancer. Nurs Clin North Am 20:611-630, 1985.
50. Schwarz-Appelbaum SJ, Dedrick J, Jusenius K, et al: Nursing care plans: Sexuality and treatment of breast cancer. Oncol Nurs Forum 11(6):16-24, 1984.
51. Swanson B, Cronin-Stubbs D, Sheldon JA: The impact of psychosocial factors on adapting to physical disability: A review of the research literature. Rehabil Nurs 14:64-68, 1989.
52. Waterhouse J, Metcalfe MC: Development of the sexual adjustment questionnaire. Oncol Nurs Forum 13(3):53-59, 1986.
53. Leiber L, Plumb MM, Gerstenzang ML, et al: The communication of affection between cancer patients and their spouses. Psychosom Med 38:379-388, 1976.
54. Shipes E: Sexual function following ostomy surgery. Nurs Clin North Am 22:303-310, 1987.
55. Annon JS: The Behavioral Treatment of Sexual Problems. Honolulu, Mercantile Printing, 1974.
56. Zalar MK: Role preparation for nurses in human sexual functioning. Nurs Clin North Am 17:351-363, 1982.

Chapter 30

Integumentary and Mucous Membrane Alterations

Jean Lydon, RN, MS

Sandra Purl, RN, MS

Michelle Goodman, RN, MS

INTRODUCTION

Regardless of the setting, the oncology nurse commonly is faced with the challenge of how to care for the patient with skin and mucous membrane complications, especially those caused by cancer treatment. This chapter discusses how these complications come about and how to manage them. The problem of extravasation of vesicant chemotherapeutic agents is discussed in Chapter 13 (Chemotherapy) and will not be addressed here. On the other hand, malignant tumor wounds, although not necessarily treatment related, are discussed later in this chapter.

ANATOMY AND PHYSIOLOGY

Integument

Skin

The skin forms a protective, pliable covering over the entire surface of the body. It is the largest organ of the body, receiving approximately one third of the heart's oxygenated blood. The skin of an adult has a surface area of approximately 1.8 m^2 (3000 sq in) and makes up about 15% of total body weight.[1,2] The skin is composed of three layers: epidermis (outer layer), dermis, and subcutaneous tissue (deepest layer) (Figure 30-1). The epidermis is the thin outer covering of the skin that renews itself continually through cell division in its deepest layer (the basal layer) and undergoes keratinization to produce scales that are shed from the outer layer (stratum corneum). It is avascular, receiving its nutrient support from the underlying dermis. The epidermis is a stratified (multiple layer) squamous epithelium that arises from the outer germ layer, the ectoderm. The thickness of the epidermis varies in different parts of the body. For example, the epidermis on the palms of the hands and the soles of the feet is usually thicker than the epidermis in other areas of the body.

The functions of the skin are many and include protection, regulation of body temperature, sensory perception, vitamin D production, and expression.

The skin provides protection against ever-changing and often adverse environmental conditions. Intact skin is the first line of defense against bacteria and foreign substances, physical trauma, heat, or rays. If this barrier is weakened for any reason, permeability to bacteria, drugs, rays, and so on is increased. Protection against the environment is accomplished by (1) eccrine gland sweating, (2) insulation by the skin and the subcutaneous tissue, (3) regulation of cutaneous blood flow (vasoconstriction and vasodilation), and (4) muscle activity (eg, shivering). Receptors for heat, cold, pain, and touch are present in the skin, making it possible for the skin to receive sensory stimuli. Another function of the skin is excretion. For example, loss of water and salt through excessive sweating

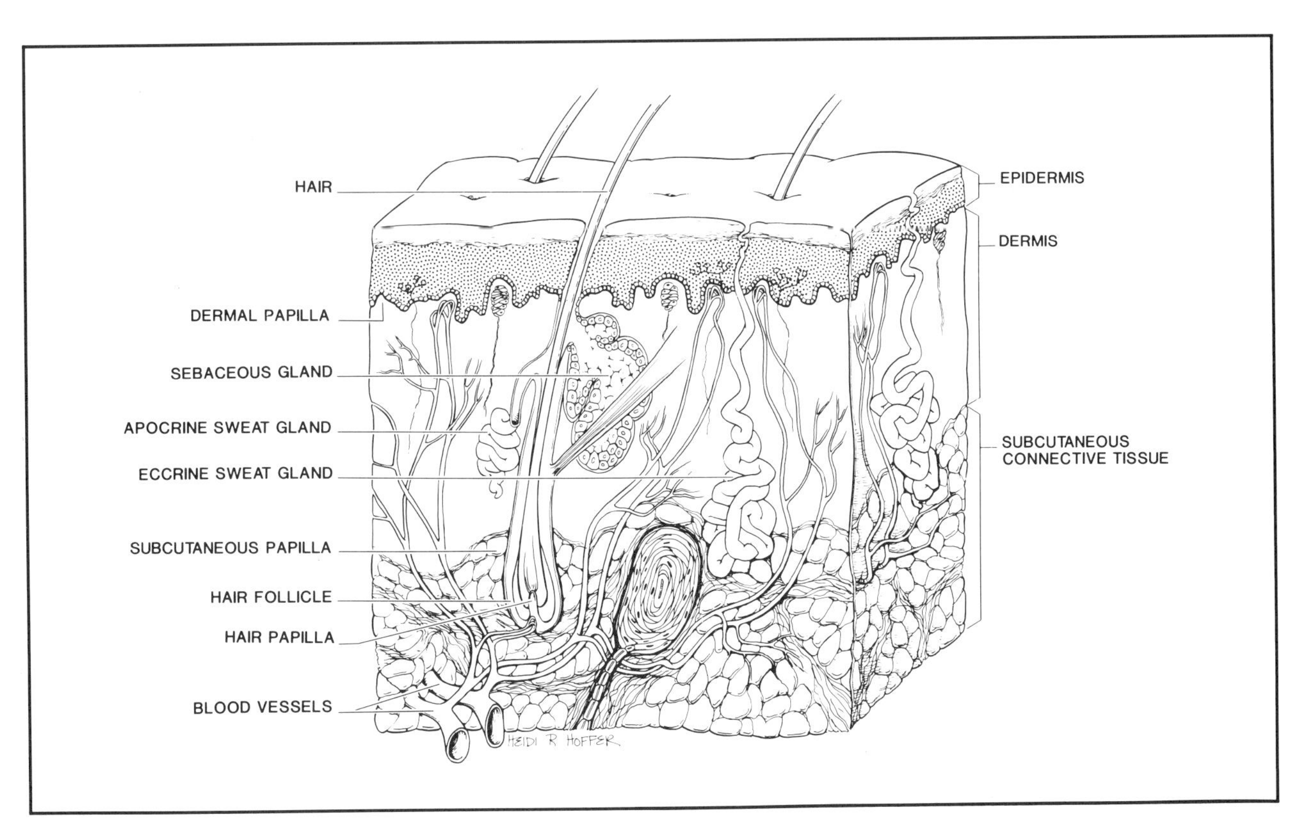

FIGURE 30-1 The structures of the skin.

is important in maintaining water balance in the body. Vitamin D necessary for bone and tooth formation is made in the skin by the effect of sunlight (ultraviolet [UV] rays). Finally, because the skin is the part of the body visible to others, it is a way of communicating feelings and is largely involved in an individual's body image.

The appendages of the skin are the hair, nails, apocrine and eccrine sweat glands, and sebaceous glands. The anatomy and physiology of each appendage will be discussed briefly.

Hair

Hair, a product of the epidermis, is composed of tightly fused keratinized cells. Hairs are distributed widely over all body surfaces, being absent only on the lips, palms of the hands, soles of the feet, and nipples of the breast. Hair varies in thickness, length, and color in different parts of the body and among different people.

Each body hair develops from a hair follicle (a follicular involution of the epidermis) (see Figure 30-1). The full portion of the hair projecting from the surface of the skin is the hair shaft; the portion under the skin is the hair root. At the base of the root is the hair bulb, which is lodged in the hair follicle. At the hair bulb, the dermis pushes up to form the dermal papilla, through which the blood and nerve supply reach the hair. Over the surfaces of the dermal papilla lie the rapidly dividing stem cells (regeneration time of 24 hours) that give rise to the hair.

Hair growth and loss in humans occur randomly so that hair loss is continuous, unlike in other mammals in which hair growth and loss are seasonal. There are three phases in the hair growth cycle: anagen, catagen, and telogen. Duration of each phase varies depending on body location of hair.

The anagen phase is the metabolically active period involving the growth of a hair from a follicle. The average hair root produces 0.35 mm of hair shaft daily or 1 cm in 28 days. An average of 85% to 90% of scalp hairs are in this anagen growth phase at any one time, but this may vary from 35% to 100%. Scalp hair remains in anagen for 2 to 6 years or an average of 3 years.[3] Approximately 3% of scalp hairs enter the catagen or transitional phase at any one time. Hair growth is slow or intermittent during this 2- to 3- week period in which involution of the hair root occurs. During the telogen or resting phase all activity ceases. About 12% of scalp hairs are in this phase, which lasts approximately 3 months. It is normal to lose 25 to 100 telogen hairs each day and even more when the hair is washed.[3]

In contrast to scalp hair, hairs located elsewhere on the body (legs, eyelashes, pubic area) have a shorter anagen phase and longer catagen and telogen phases, which explains why these hairs remain short. For example, the eyebrows actively grow for up to 30 to 60 days and then rest for approximately 105 days.[4]

The function of hair is both physical and psychosocial in humans. Physically, hair plays a less important role in humans than in most mammals by protecting the surface of the skin and offering temperature regulation by conserving body heat. Specifically, scalp hair decreases exposure of the scalp to UV rays and minimizes loss of body heat from the head. Eyelashes and hairs lining the nose and ears help to filter out insects, dusts, and other airborne contaminants.

Psychosocially, hair contributes greatly to body image and is closely associated with secondary sexual characteristics. It is a major component of an individual's physical appearance and is often taken for granted. Throughout the ages, hair has meant strength, power, wealth, and beauty. Its very color and style defines each person's identity and feelings and shapes self-image.[5]

Nails

The nail is a specialized epidermal structure made of keratinized cells cemented together. Specifically, nails are modifications of the stratum corneum and lucidum of the epidermis. Nails are found on the dorsal surfaces of the terminal phalanges of the fingers and toes. They rest on the nail bed, composed of the germinal layer of the epidermis and the underlying dermis. The visible part of the nail, called the body, is highly vascular, resulting in the pink color seen through the semitransparent structure. The nail shapes the fingers and greatly enhances the coordinated fine motion of the fingers.

Glands

In humans there are two types of sweat glands: apocrine and eccrine. Apocrine glands have a duct that opens into a hair follicle, whereas eccrine glands have a duct that opens onto the skin surface independent of a hair follicle. Most of the apocrine sweat glands regress during embryonal life and are found only in limited areas in adults: axillae, nipples, periumbilical region, perineum, and genitalia. These glands do not become functional until just before puberty. Apocrine sweat glands are odiferous and increase evaporative heat loss.[6]

Some 1.6 to 4 million eccrine sweat glands are present over the entire body. These glands are especially plentiful in the palms, soles, and axillae and least abundant on the back. Eccrine sweat glands are simple coiled tubules that extend down into the reticular layer of the dermis and occasionally into the subcutaneous tissue. The main function of these glands is to cool the body through secretion of water and its evaporation. Eccrine sweat glands secrete a thin watery solution, primarily composed of sodium chloride and some sulfates, phosphates, and urea, known as perspiration or sweat.[7]

The sebaceous glands are small, sacculated granular organs located in the dermis. Although not grossly visible, sebaceous glands are found in most parts of the skin, particularly on the face, scalp, upper chest, and back. They are not found on the palms or soles. The size and number of sebaceous glands vary from area to area. Each gland opens directly into a hair follicle and is lined by a cuboidal epithelium. Sebaceous glands continually secrete a mixture of fat, fatty acids, and cell remnants called sebum. Sebum keeps the skin and hair lubricated, pliable, and waterproof.[8]

Mucous Membranes

Epithelial membranes are formed in the body by epithelia combined with connective tissue. The major epithelial membranes are the serous membranes, mucous membranes, and the cutaneous membrane or skin. Serous membranes line the body cavities that *do not* open to the exterior, such as the peritoneum; whereas mucous membranes line the body cavities and hollow organs that open to the exterior, such as organs of the respiratory, digestive, excretory, and reproductive tracts. The skin is continuous with the mucous membranes. The function of the mucous membranes depends on their location in the body but may include absorption, transport, or secretion of mucus for lubrication of tissue surfaces. The rapidly proliferating cells of the epithelial layer of the mucous membranes make these membranes sensitive to the effects of both radiation and chemotherapy.

The *oral mucosa* is the body organ that forms a continuous lining of the oral cavity from the mucocutaneous junction of the lips to the oropharynx. The oral mucosa separates the interior of the oral cavity from the complex underlying organs. Because the oral mucosa is exposed to an aggressive environment in which injury and cell death are an everyday occurrence, the epithelial lining of the mucosa constantly renews itself, with cell production meeting cell replacement needs.[1,2] Maintenance of the integrity of the oral mucosa depends on continuous stem cell replication at the basement membrane. Epithelial cells produced at the basement membrane migrate upward to the mucosal surfaces to replace cells lost as a result of normal sloughing. It has been estimated that the average time of the sequential phases of skin cell mitosis of the oral mucosa is as follows: M (mitotic division), 8 hours; G_1 (mitotic resting phase), 14 hours; S (DNA synthesis phase), 10 to 11 hours; and G_2 (mitotic resting phase), 10 to 19 minutes, for a total of approximately 32 hours.[1] Complete replacement of the epithelial layer occurs approximately every 7 days.[9]

The mucous membranes of the oral mucosa play a vital role in maintaining homeostasis. The primary function of the oral mucosa is to provide a first line of defense against infection. This is accomplished primarily by the epithelial lining of the mucosa. If, however, the integrity of the mucosa is altered and does not succeed in barring unwanted substances, the lamina propria of the connective tissue will provide a second line of defense. Similar to the skin, the oral mucosa can both receive and transmit stimuli from the environment (eg, heat, cold, pain, touch, and pressure). Sensory innervation of the oral mucosa is provided largely by the connective tissue component.

ALTERATIONS TO THE INTEGUMENT

Skin

Radiation effects

The sensitivity of a cell or tissue to radiation and the rate at which radiation injury is manifested are, at least in part, directly linked to the rate of turnover of target cells and their progeny. Radiation-induced death of a cell is a result of damage to the cell's reproductive integrity and is expressed only if the cell attempts division. The rapidly proliferating cells and tissues (eg, hematopoietic stem cells, basal skin cells) are more sensitive to radiation than mature tissues with slow or nondividing cells (eg, muscle and nerve cells). In radiosensitive tissues where cells divide regularly, radiation damage is exhibited early, within weeks to a few months after irradiation, whereas in radioresistant tissues where cells never or infrequently divide, expression of radiation damage requires longer periods (months to years after irradiation).[10,11]

The response of normal tissue to radiation has been classified in a variety of ways.[12,13] For the purposes of this chapter, radiation effects will be classified as either acute or chronic. Acute effects may occur during treatment or several weeks after completion of treatment. Chronic effects may occur several months or years later.[11] The severity of acute and chronic changes depends on dose-time-volume factors; that is, the greater the dose, the shorter the time, and the larger the volume of treatment, the more severe the reaction.[14]

Acute reactions depend more on dose-time factors (total number of cGy in a total number of days) than total dose delivered.[15] The pathogenesis of acute reactions results from depletion of the parenchymal or stromal cells.[11] Depletion of actively proliferating cells in a renewing cell population stimulates noncycling cells to proliferate and greatly reduces their cell cycle time.

Every acute radiation reaction is followed by some degree of permanent or late change. The severity of chronic effects, however, cannot be assessed adequately from acute reactions, since late complications such as tissue necrosis or dense fibrosis can occur despite the lack of acute reaction.[10] Chronic radiation reactions depend on dose-fractions and total dose.

Acute reactions With few exceptions, radiation therapy techniques by necessity include normal skin and vascular connective tissue within the treatment field. With technologic advances and the widespread use of megavoltage equipment, it is rare to see the serious and severe skin reactions of the past. Despite the skin-sparing effect of megavoltage equipment, certain skin reactions from radiation are normal and expected. The degree of skin reaction from radiation depends on several factors[14-17]:

1. The dose, number of fractions, and time in which given
2. The energy or particular beam-quality machine used, which influences the surface or skin dose
3. Anatomic location of the irradiated area (eg, intertriginous skin folds may increase reaction)
4. Use of bolus material
5. Tangential fields
6. Concomitant chemotherapy
7. Radiosensitivity of various structures of the skin

The major acute skin reactions associated with radiation include erythema, changes in pigmentation (eg, perifollicular pigmentation, hyperpigmentation), dry desquamation, and moist desquamation.

Erythema Erythema that occurs during radiation is the result of vascular changes. The erythema generally appears in two phases. An acute, faint erythema, often unrecognized, may appear within hours or days after the start of treatment. This phase of erythema is short lived, fading within a few days, but reoccurs if radiation treatment continues. Although the cause of this erythema is unknown, it is probably a vascular response to extracapillary cell injury.[14] The second phase of erythema, erythema proper, is seen during the third or fourth week of standard fractionated radiation treatment and may last 20 to 30 days. This is the more typical erythema associated with radiation that clearly outlines the treatment field. A rise in skin temperature and edema of the affected area usually accompany erythema proper. The rise in skin temperature in the irradiated field results from an increase in blood flow through the dermis. This capillary vasodilitation is accompanied by endothelial swelling and increased capillary permeability, resulting in tissue edema. From the third or fourth week of treatment to one or two weeks following completion of treatment, the skin is red, warm, edematous, and tender to the touch. The peak intensity of erythema results from capillary damage and congestion and occurs during the desquamative phase of the reaction.[14,18]

Hyperpigmentation Hyperpigmentation results from stimulation of the melanocytes (cells that produce melanin pigment) located at the junction of the epidermis and dermis. The melanocyte passes the melanin to the basal layer of the epidermis where it can be incorporated into new cells. During radiation, these basal cells become cornified, carrying the melanin into the more superficial layers of the epidermis and resulting in the characteristic "tanned" appearance. There is an increased number of melanocytes present initially in the skin of black people; therefore hyperpigmentation of skin will be greater in blacks than in whites. Following radiation, some degree of hyperpigmentation may be permanent.

During the second or third week of standardized radiation therapy, perifollicular pigmentation frequently occurs and is characterized by brown spots of several millimeters within the irradiated area. Perifollicular pigmentation is due to pigmentation of the epithelial cells surrounding the hair follicles.

Dry desquamation A dry flaking or peeling of the skin, known as dry desquamation, usually occurs at the start of the fourth or fifth week of treatment and continues for one or two weeks following treatment. Dry desquamation is characterized by scaling, dryness, and pruritis of the skin. This skin reaction occurs because the basal cells of the epidermis are quite sensitive to radiation. Each dose of radiation destroys a fixed percentage of basal cells. Intermediate doses of radiation will kill many but not all basal cells. In less than 3 to 4 weeks, dry desquamation results, whereby the dermis is not exposed.[14,18]

Moist desquamation With skin doses of 4000 rad (cGy) or more, basal cell division is stopped and the superficial epidermal cells are not replaced as they shed. This leads to a skin reaction called moist desquamation in which the dermis is exposed and a serous exudate oozes from the surface. It is characterized by a brilliant erythema and often significant pain from exposed nerve endings. Moist desquamation is comparable to a second-degree burn in histology, appearance, and sensation. When moist desquamation occurs, radiation treatment is discontinued temporarily until reepithelialization of the denuded skin is evident. This usually occurs within 10 days as epithelial cells around the hair follicle proliferate to cover the denuded area. By 3 months, the skin may have a normal appearance aside from a change in pigmentation.

Chronic reactions The pathogenesis of chronic effects has not been clearly established. Many believe chronic radiation reactions result from vascular or connective tissue damage.[11] However, others propose that the pathogenesis of both acute and chronic changes is related to the depletion of parenchymal or stromal cells and that they differ only in the rate of turnover of their respective target cells.[10] Whereas acute reactions may require time off from radiation, the possibility of chronic reactions limits the total dose that can be delivered to a tumor, which in turn may affect cure.

Factors that may affect the development of chronic radiation reactions include the physical properties of radiation (eg, skin dose delivered), radiobiologic factors (eg, size of dose per fraction, volume treated), and the anatomic and physiologic integrity of the tissue.[19] In some cases, disturbance of tissue integrity by surgery before radiation results in increased chronic complications.[20]

Chronic radiation reactions of the skin include atrophy, changes in pigmentation, fibrosis, telangiectasia, and rarely ulceration and necrosis.

Atrophy Following radiation, the new epidermis is very thin, fragile, and pink; although it thickens over time, it never attains its normal thickness. This results in atrophy of the skin.

Pigmentation changes Hypopigmentation is a chronic effect of radiation, whereas hyperpigmentation can be either acute or chronic. Hypopigmentation or depigmentation results from destruction of melanocytes from exposure to radiation. Radiation doses necessary to eradicate a cancer frequently destroy the melanocytes so that irradiated skin is unable to form pigment. The term *radiation-induced achromia* is used to describe this condition. Hyperpigmentation was discussed previously in the section on acute radiation reactions.

Fibrosis The development of fibrosis is due to chronic changes in connective tissue. The papillary dermis, reticular dermis, and subcutaneous tissues become replaced by a very dense, irregular, fibrotic tissue. The resultant fibrosis gives the skin a hard and uneven texture. If extensive, fibrosis can cause considerable induration. Certain anatomic areas such as the lower abdominal wall and the upper cervical and paramandibular areas are particularly susceptible to fibrosis.

Telangiectasia The development of telangiectasia is a result of chronic changes in the vascular supply. Chronic vascular changes follow an orderly sequence: (1) increased permeability of material through capillary walls and edema and dilatation of blood vessels with hyperemia, (2) occlusion of capillaries, (3) reduction in the number of functioning small vessels, (4) increased pressure of blood flow through remaining underground superficial blood vessels, and (5) telangiectasia. Telangiectasia, which is simply a dilatation of existing capillaries, causes the skin to have a spidery appearance. Telangiectasia will progress for up to 8 years after radiation therapy. The progression rate is clearly dose and fraction size dependent.

Ulceration Ulceration with subsequent necrosis may occur approximately 2 weeks after the first or only exposure to radiation, or be delayed up to 10 to 20 years after radiotherapy. Early ulcers usually heal but may recur. In contrast, delayed ulcers rarely heal, generally worsen over time, and may persist for years.

Radiation ulceration or radionecrosis is an infrequent, chronic complication of radiation. In the past, radiation ulcers occurred because of poor radiotherapy techniques as well as the use of orthovoltage machines that delivered high doses of radiation to the skin.

Although radiation techniques have improved and the supervoltage machines in use have skin-sparing effects, chronic ulcerations of the skin continue to develop. These ulcerations may develop secondary to trauma but often occur spontaneously. Characteristically, radiation ulcers are exceptionally painful with red raised edges and a shaggy necrotic base, and they show little or no tendency to contract or epithelialize. With time, these ulcers tend to get deeper and more painful, frequently enlarging despite local treatment.[21-23] Because of these characteristics, radiation ulcers produce significant morbidity to the patient and are difficult to manage.

Traditionally, chronic radiation skin damage and ulceration have been attributed to tissue ischema caused by obliterative endarteritis of the microvasculature. However, recent electron microscopic studies demonstrate that microsvascular occlusion occurs only occasionally in radiation-damaged tissue.[22-25] Furthermore, these studies suggest that ulceration may be due to direct cellular injury, particularly damage to fibroblasts, rather than being secondary to vascular compromise caused by blood vessel occlusion. Atypical fibroblasts now known as "radiation fibroblasts" have long been a recognized feature of chronic radiation wounds. The nuclei of these radiation fibroblasts typically are large, irregular, hyperchromic, and rarely in mitosis. Although atypical fibroblasts are not a new finding, their role in the pathogenesis of late radiation injury has only recently been appreciated. Permanent damage to fibroblasts and their stem cells may prevent these cells from providing new blood vessels and contractile fibroblasts necessary for wound contraction and healing.[22]

Treatment of radiation ulcers continues to be challenging. As with any other chronic problem wound, consideration is given to the benefit versus cost ratio of the treatment. The initial step is conservative treatment to correct systemic factors, remove necrotic tissue, reduce bacteria, and drain any areas of abscess. Dietary intake and nutritional status of these patients are often poor as a result of the relentless pain associated with a radiation ulcer. If the ulcer is in the head and neck area, loss of taste, xerostomia, or trismus may further complicate nutritional status. Successful wound healing depends in part on the presence of adequate stores of protein, carbohydrates, fat, vitamins, and minerals. Analgesics to control the pain, nutritional counseling, and possibly hyperalimentation are ways to improve a patient's nutritional status. As nutritional deficiencies are being corrected, local wound treatment is initiated, usually consisting of judicious debridement of obvious necrotic tissue and topical antibiotic therapy to control the infection. Total debridement of necrotic tissue is deferred until the surgeon can accomplish simultaneous wound closure.[21-24]

The use of debriding agents such as half-strength Dakin's solution applied as a wet-wet dressing may be useful for debriding shallow ulcers. However, it will not penetrate deeply into necrotic tissue.[21] Chronic radiation ulcers are heavily colonized with bacteria; therefore obtaining qualitative or quantitative bacteriologic studies of these wounds is not useful. The infection is responsible for the bad odor associated with radiation ulcers. Once the infection is under control, the odor of these wounds greatly improves. Systemic antibiotics generally are not helpful because they fail to reach the ulcer area in sufficient concentrations to control the infection.[24] Therefore, topical antibacterial agents including sulfadiazine (Silvadene), mafenide (Sulfamylon),[21,23,24] and more recently metronidazole (Flagyl)[26] have been used to treat the infection. Hyperbaric oxygen may contribute to more rapid wound healing in ischemic tissues; however, clinical experience with this modality in the treatment of radiation ulcers is limited.[27]

Definitive debridement of the ulcer and the underlying contaminated fibrotic bed and closure of the would are done following conservative treatment. Usual methods of would closure are often unsuccessful for the following reasons: (1) radiation tissue is fibrotic and unyielding, making it prone to dehiscence, (2) healthy tissue often cannot be reached because the ulcers are so deep, and (3) radiation injury extends beyond the ulcer to surrounding areas.[21-24]

When radiotherapy was given by orthovoltage machines, ulcers were more superficial and closure could be achieved successfully by split-thickness skin grafts. Modern radiotherapy using higher voltage machines causes deeper tissue injury that requires alternate closure techniques. Myocutaneous flaps are the preferred method for closure of radiation ulcers because they provide a rich vascular supply to ischemic tissue and have greater resistance to infection than other flaps in contaminated wounds.[21-24] Once the wound is closed, the patient has dramatic relief of pain.

Care of irradiated skin

Assessment The oncology nurse has a critical role in assessing skin integrity, educating the patient and family on skin care to be followed during and after radiation, and managing alterations in skin integrity secondary to radiation. This requires knowedge of the normal anatomy and physiology of the skin, the acute and chronic effects of radiation on the skin, and factors that can affect the degree of skin reaction.

Initially, a comprehensive skin assessment is done to

TABLE 30-1 Systems of Categorizing Impaired Skin Integrity

	I	II	III	IV	V
McNally	Potential	Dry or moist desquamation	Severe—large, open, draining, purulent skin lesions	—	—
Yasko	Erythema Slight edema Inflammation	Inflammation and dry desquamation Itching and slight burning sensation	Edema Moist desquamation Inflammation	Depilation of hair, suppression of sebaceous and sweat gland function Atrophy Telangiectasis Lymphedema	—
RTOG	No change	Follicular Dull redness Epilation Dry desquamation	Moderate edema Moist Bright erythema	Moist pitting edema	Necrotic ulceration hemorrhage

Source: McNally,[28] Yasko,[29] and Radiation Therapy Oncology Group.[30]

determine baseline status of the skin before radiation. Age-related skin changes, nutritional status, history of chronic sun exposure, medical conditions, and medications (especially chemotherapy) that can affect the skin and treatment-related factors are documented. A careful physical examination, particularly of the treatment area including the exit site, is done to evaluate the current condition of the skin. To assess skin changes associated with radiation, a scale or system of categorizing impaired skin integrity is used. Table 30-1 shows three such scales or systems of categorizing impaired skin.[28-30] Oncology nurses should use one of these scales on a consistent basis. Skin assessment is done at least weekly during radiation, 1 to 2 weeks following completion of treatment, and every few months thereafter.

Management Before initiation of external radiation therapy, the nurse discusses with the patient and family the anticipated skin reactions, a probable time frame for each reaction, and skin care guidelines to be followed during and after treatment. Because the patient is usually anxious and fearful before starting treatment, written information regarding skin reactions and skin care is provided. The patient is informed that he or she will usually not experience any discomfort during the first 2 weeks of standard fractionated radiotherapy. However, as treatment continues, the anticipated skin reactions of itching, dryness, erythema, hyperpigmentation, or dry desquamation will probably occur.

Dryness and itching of the skin occurs due to impaired function of sweat and sebaceous glands. During radiation treatments, cornstarch is recommended for relief of itchiness. It should be used for dry desquamative reactions, since cornstarch on moist areas promotes fungal growth and increases the risk of a secondary infection. The use of a mild lubricant such as Natural Care Gel (Catalina Co.) or Carrington Wound Gel (Carrington Laboratories, Inc.) can be helpful in decreasing pruritus, increasing comfort, and preventing cracking and fissure formation from dry skin. The use of topical steroids, which also can increase comfort and reduce itching, generally is avoided, since they can cause diffuse thinning of the epidermis, thereby making the skin more susceptible to injury.[31] Following completion of radiation, a hydrophilic lotion or cream such as Eucerin, Lubriderm, or Aquaphor is recommended for dryness and itching and to lubricate the skin.

Although basic skin care instructions during radiation therapy are more or less standard, ways of managing an acute skin reaction such as moist desquamation vary.[28-30] Moist desquamation is characterized by a brilliant erythema, pain or burning sensation from exposed nerve endings, and a serous exudate that oozes from the dermal surface. Intertriginous skin folds such as the axilla, inframammary fold, perineum, groin, abdomen, and perirectal area are particularly at risk for this reaction due to frequent friction, high moisture content, and less air circulation. If moist desquamation occurs, radiation treatments usually are suspended until there is evidence of reepithelialization in the denuded areas.

The goals of nursing care are to prevent fluid loss and infection and increase comfort. Using a weak astringent soak such as the Domeboro solution (Miles Laboratory) is useful to prevent or minimize fluid loss and infection as well as to promote comfort. To make a weak solution, one Domeboro tablet or packet is mixed with one quart of water rather than a pint as suggested on the package. The patient is instructed to dip gauze into the solution, lightly wring out, and apply to area of moist desquamation for 15 to 20 minutes three or four times a day. Application of moist astringent soaks decreases oozing and aids in reducing inflammation by forming a protective film over the denuded area. An alternative to Domeboro solution is irrigating or soaking with a solution of one third hydrogen peroxide and two thirds normal saline.

A hydrogel primary wound dressing such as Vigilon (Bard Pharmaceuticals) or Geliperm (Fougera) may be used to protect the denuded area, maintain a moist environment, and increase comfort level. These dressings are semitransparent, nonadhesive, absorbent, moisture vapor permeable, and comfortable. They are composed of 98% water and 2% cellulose fiber. These dressings can promote healing and decrease the patient's complaints of pain or burning. Disadvantages of these dressings include high cost and potential for bacterial proliferation, leakage, and maceration of the skin. Other moisture vapor-permeable dressings such as Tegaderm or Opsite have been used in managing moist desquamation with increased healing and relief of discomfort. Unfortunately, few of these methods have emerged from scientific study, highlighting the need for further nursing research. Table 30-2 shows guidelines for skin care before, during, and after radiation and the rationale for these instructions.[32]

Nursing care also is directed toward educating the patient and family on the chronic effects of radiation on the skin and its appendages. Although chronic effects of radiation are discussed before initiating treatment, this information usually is not remembered after completion of treatment. Therefore, the nurse discusses these chronic effects after finishing treatment and monitors these effects with each follow-up visit. The nurse also educates the patient regarding the vulnerability of irradiated tissue and the need to protect this area from injury and infection.

The patient should understand that the radiation treatment is an important aspect of the medical history and should be shared with other physicians, particularly surgeons. To assist the patient in this endeavor, it is often helpful for the nurse to provide the patient with pertinent written information regarding treatment.

Unfortunately, the incidence and management of chronic radiation reactions are not always clearly documented in the literature. Oncology nurses can participate in research studies designed to evaluate chronic effects of radiation. Development of a close, trusting relationship with the patient and communication and collaboration with other health care professionals caring for the patient will assist the nurse in maintaining close follow-up of the patient to assess and document these chronic changes.

TABLE 30-2 Guidelines for Skin Care Before, During, and After Radiotherapy

Guidelines	Rationale
BEFORE THERAPY	
Discuss with patient and family anticipated skin reactions: Itching Dryness Increased pigmentation Erythema Dry desquamation The possibility that moist desquamation may occur	Anticipatory guidance is an important measure in allaying patient's fears. Occurrence of the reactions without prior discussion may cause the patient to believe that treatment is not being administered properly. Skin care is focused on maintaining skin integrity and decreasing the incidence of trauma and irritation.
Instruct patient to avoid heating pads, hot water bottles, heat lamps, sun lamps, and ice bags on the treated area of skin.	These methods may further compromise vascular reactions in capillaries in the treatment area. There is potential injury to the irradiated skin due to decreased temperature sensitivity in the irradiated area.
Instruct patient to avoid exposing the irradiated skin to the sun. Application of sunscreen should precede any anticipated sun exposure.	The body's ability to protect the skin from sunburn is decreased secondary to destruction of melanocytes in the irradiated epidermis and the slower rate of melanin production in new epidermal cells.
Instruct patient to wear cotton undergarments as much as possible (if the treatment area includes the perineal or axillary area).	Cotton undergarments allow for air exchange and decrease moisture buildup.
Instruct patient to avoid wearing tight-fitting clothing that constricts skin in the treatment area. The use of tape in the treatment area should also be avoided.	Mechanical irritation of the treatment area should be reduced or avoided to decrease further trauma to the sensitive irradiated skin.
Instruct patient not to shave the skin in the treatment field during treatment and for at least 2 weeks after treatment.	Shaving increases loss of superficial cells, potentially resulting in desquamation earlier. Shaving may also result in small lacerations, providing an avenue for infection.
Instruct patient to increase daily fluid intake to 3000 mL unless contraindicated.	Radiation to the skin, sweat, and sebaceous glands causes dryness and itchiness of the skin. This is characterized by dehydration of the stratum corneum, the water-retaining layer of the skin. Increased fluid intake replaces water lost from radiation therapy.

TABLE 30-2 Guidelines for Skin Care Before, During, and After Radiotherapy (continued)

Guidelines	Rationale
DURING THERAPY	
Dry desquamation	
Cornstarch may be applied to the skin in the treatment area to decrease itching.	Cornstarch relieves itchiness and reduces moisture buildup, especially in areas of skin folds. It should be used only on areas of *dry* desquamation. Use of cornstarch on moist areas promotes fungal growth (through formation of a glucose-rich environment), thereby increasing risk of infection.
During radiation therapy treatments, mild skin lubricants such as Natural Care Gel or Carrington Wound Care Gel may be applied to prevent cracking and fissure formation. These products are hydrophobic and contain no heavy metal ions. Deodorant, cosmetics, cologne, creams, and lotions should not be applied to irradiated skin.	Substances that contain heavy metal ions enhance skin reactions that occur during external beam radiation therapy. Hydrophobic preparations are not well absorbed, are insoluble in water, and are difficult to remove. Perfumes, cosmetics, creams, and lotions contain chemicals that irritate the sensitive irradiated skin.
The treated area may be cleansed gently with tepid water and patted dry. A mild soap that does not contain perfume (such as Basis) may be used on the area if desired. Vigorous rubbing of the treated skin should be avoided.	Soap helps to decrease the incidence of folliculitis and local skin infections. Perfumed soaps contain chemicals and heavy metal ions that enhance skin reactions due to external beam radiation therapy.
Moist desquamation	
Apply moist astringent soaks or irrigate the affected area with an astringent solution (Domeboro's solution) for 15 to 20 minutes three to four times a day.	Astringents aid in decreasing oozing from denuded areas. They also result in the formation of a protective film over the denuded area due to a slight protein-coagulation effect. This aids in reducing inflammation.
Keep the area covered with a hydrogel dressing (Vigilon).	Hydrogel dressings prevent tissue loss through dehydration and scab formation; they also decrease pain in the area by providing a cushion for exposed nerve endings. A moist tissue environment enhances the migration of leukocytes and epithelial cells to denuded areas, thus promoting healing.
Discuss use of oral pain medications as needed with the physician and patient.	Pain occurs in the denuded areas as a result of exposed nerve endings.
AFTER THERAPY	
Apply hydrophilic substances that do not contain any perfumes, such as Eucerin cream or lotion, Aquaphor, or Lubriderm lotion two or three times a day on the irradiated area.	The skin may become dry and itchy due to impaired function of sebaceous and sweat glands. Hydrophilic lubricants will put back moisture into the skin and prevent cracking and fissure formation.
Instruct the patient not to shave or use deodorants, cosmetics, or cologne in the irradiated area for several weeks following treatment.	Irradiated skin is highly susceptible to injury. Shaving can result in small lacerations, thereby increasing risk of infection. Deodorants, cosmetics, cologne, and so on can be irritating to the sensitive irradiated skin.
Instruct the patient to avoid exposing the irradiated skin to the sun. If avoiding the sun is not possible, sunscreen with an SPF of 15 or greater should be applied to the irradiated skin. These recommendations should be followed for life.	The body's ability to protect the skin from sunburn is decreased secondary to destruction of melanocytes in the irradiated epidermis and the slower rate of melanin production in new epidermal cells. The irradiated skin remains vulnerable to injury and infection for many years after completion of therapy.

Source: Adapted with permission from Coleman J: Unpublished manuscript, 1988.

Chemotherapy effects

Hyperpigmentation Numerous chemotherapeutic agents can cause hyperpigmentation or hypopigmentation of the skin and mucous membranes with varying patterns and presentations. Patients receiving busulfan often experience a generalized darkening of the skin that usually subsides following completion of treatment. Hyperpigmentation also has been noted following chronic 5-fluorouracil (5-FU) therapy, especially in those patients who receive high-dose weekly infusions for colon carcinoma. Areas of the skin exposed to sunlight will appear more tan in these patients. Bleomycin and 5-FU also will cause a change in pigmentation over the veins into which the drug is given. A painful exfoliation of the tissues over the veins has been observed with 5-FU infusion therapy. A similar reaction has not been seen when 5-FU is given as a low-dose injection.[33] Hyperpigmentation with 5-FU is further enhanced by radiation exposure. Hyperpigmentation is most prominent in olive-complexioned individuals and blacks. Widespread cutaneous hyperpigmentation also has been reported in patients receiving cyclophosphamide, hydroxyurea, and methotrexate.[34]

More localized cutaneous hyperpigmentation has been seen in patients receiving doxorubicin, busulfan, cyclophosphamide, 5-FU, and thiotepa. Hyperpigmentation over pressure points (elbows) can occur with bleomycin. Linear streaks of hyperpigmentation on the skin has been reported with bleomycin administration. Rubbing the patient's skin during bleomycin infusion or scratching the skin can produce hyperpigmented lesions, which fade with time. It is thought that local trauma, pressure, or heat can cause vasodilation, which causes an increased concentration of bleomycin in the skin resulting in hyperpigmentation. It does not appear to be inflammatory and cannot be reproduced by scratching.[35] Doxorubicin, busulfan, cyclophosphamide, and 5-FU have been associated with hyperpigmentation of the oral mucosa and tongue, especially in blacks (Color plate 1). Doxorubicin and 5-FU may also cause skin darkening over the interphalangeal and metacarpophalangeal joints (Color plate 2). The mechanism of this effect is not known, but the darkening decreases once therapy is terminated.[33]

Hypersensitivity Hypersensitivity reactions to chemotherapy occur infrequently but have been reported with L-asparaginase and cisplatin. Other drugs producing uticaria and angioedema include chlorambucil, daunorubicin, melphalan, methotrexate, and thiotepa. Erythema multiforme has been reported in patients receiving hydroxyurea and mechlorethamine.[34] An allergic vasculitis associated with fever and flulike syndrome has been reported with hydroxyurea.[36]

Dactinomycin folliculitis presents as diffuse erythematous papules over the face and trunk resembling acne, appearing approximately 5 days after therapy. The rash usually resolves in 3 to 5 days. Folliculitis also has been reported following administration of high-dose methotrexate.[37]

Patients receiving chemotherapy commonly report dry skin and scaling, most likely due to the drugs' effect on sebaceous and sweat glands.[33]

Hand-foot syndrome Erythema, scaling, and epidermal sloughing from the palms of the hands and soles of the feet followed by desquamation and reepithelialization of the skin has been reported with continuous infusion of 5-FU, doxorubicin, and high-dose cytarabine.[38] This condition, called the hand-foot syndrome or acral erythema[35] (palmar-plantar erythrodysesthesia syndrome), is characterized by painful intense erythema of the palms and soles, particularly the distal phalanges (Color plate 3).Therapy is usually suspended until the symptoms subside. Chemotherapy generally is resumed at a lower dose. However, the symptoms usually reappear, necessitating cessation of therapy.

Pruritus

Etiology Pruritus can be defined as a sensation that leads to a desire to scratch. Many medical conditions, both benign and malignant, may be associated with pruritus. Infrequently, pruritus can occur in association with the following malignancies: lymphoma (particularly Hodgkin's disease), leukemia, sarcoma, and carcinoma. The carcinomas most likely to be associated with pruritus include squamous cell carcinoma of the vulva, carcinoid tumors, lung carcinoma, primary or metastatic malignant obstructive biliary disease, and intracranial neoplasms. Additionally, patients with cancer can experience pruritus as a symptom of infection, a side effect of radiation therapy, a reaction to antibiotics, analgesics, or chemotherapy.[39] Pruritus associated with radiation therapy is due primarily to dry desquamation of the skin. Dryness or pruritus may occur at an accumulated dose of approximately 2000 to 2800 cGy. This skin reaction is due to obliteration of the sebaceous glands in the treatment field.[40] Pruritus associated with chemotherapy generally is due either to a hypersensitivity reaction to the drug or to dry skin and scaling caused by the drug's effect on sebaceous and sweat glands.

Assessment Assessment requires an accurate and thorough history and physical examination. The oncology nurse ascertains the following information: (1) localization, onset, duration, and intensity of itching; (2) prior history of pruritus; (3) past or present cancer, cancer treatment, noncancer systemic diseases, or use of analgesics or antibiotics; and (4) presence of infection. The oncology nurse carefully examines all areas of the skin for any obvious sign of infection or drug reaction as well as for anything in the environment (eg, tight clothes, hot and humid conditions) that may contribute to pruritus. Any areas of redness or dryness or signs of injury secondary to scratching are recorded. Additionally, the nurse checks the patient's skin turgor and hydration status.

Management Nursing care focuses on three areas: skin care, environmental control, and administration of therapeutics.[39] Knowledge of factors that alleviate or aggravate pruritus in these three areas will help the nurse in addressing this distressing symptom[39-41] (Table 30-3). Although pruritus is not a life-threatening symptom, it causes the patient great distress, discomfort, and anxiety. Nurses who have knowledge of pruritus and its relationship to cancer and cancer treatment, and are willing to take time to try different approaches to relieve pruritis, will greatly increase patient comfort and prevent alteration in the skin's protective mechanism.

Photosensitivity

There are three main types of ultraviolet radiation: ultraviolet A (UVA), ultraviolet B (UVB), and ultraviolet C (UVC). Most of the sun's effect on the skin is caused by

TABLE 30-3 Factors that Alleviate and Aggravate Pruritus

Alleviating Factors	Aggravating Factors
Basic skin care measures	
Daily fluid intake of 3000 mL	Increased fluid loss secondary to fever, diarrhea, nausea and vomiting, decreased fluid intake
Application of emollient creams (eg, Eucerin, Nivea) or lotions (eg, Lubriderm, Alpha Keri, Nivea)	Ointments (eg, petroleum, mineral oil)
Bathe with tepid water	Bathe with hot water
Use mild soaps or soaps made for sensitive skin (eg, Neutrogena, Basis, Dove)	Use of soaps that contain detergents
Limit bathing to ½ hour every day or every other day	Frequent baths (eg, twice a day), increase duration of bath to greater than ½ hour
Oil added toward the end of the bath or Aveeno (a colloidal oatmeal treatment) added early to the bath	Oil added early to the bath
Cornstarch to areas of irradiated skin after the bath	Genital deodorants or bubble baths
Environmental control	
Humid environment (eg, humidifier)	Dry environment
Cotton flannel blankets if needed	
Sheets, clothing, undergarments washed in mild soaps for infant clothing (eg, Dreft)	Sheets and clothing laundered with detergents
Loose-fitting clothing; clothing made of cotton or other soft fabrics	Restrictive tight clothing; clothes made of wool or other harsh fabrics
Use of distraction, relaxation, positive imagery, cutaneous stimulation	Emotional stress
Medications	
Antibiotics if pruritus secondary to infection	Opium alkaloids, morphine, and antibiotics may cause pruritus
Oral antihistamines (with increased dose at bedtime)	
Topical mild corticosteroids except for pruritus secondary to radiation therapy	

Source: Dangel,[39] Hassey and Rose,[40] and Campbell.[41]

UVB. UVB penetrates only as far as the epidermis, and therefore a sunburn that primarily affects the epidermis is the manifestation of overexposure to UVB. UVA, now used in tanning salons, is able to penetrate deeper into the dermis than UVB and may be just as (if not more) damaging to the skin as UVB. UVC usually does not affect the skin because it is absorbed in the upper atmosphere and does not reach the earth.[42]

Photosensitivity, the enhanced skin response to UV light, is caused by a variety of topical or oral medications such as analgesics, antidepressants, antimicrobials, diuretics, antihistamines, nonsteroidal anti-inflammatory agents, and cytotoxic drugs as well as certain sunscreens.[43] Table 30-4 lists some agents that may cause photosensitivity reactions.[44] Patients with cancer often are taking several different prescription and nonprescription medications, many of which can cause photosensitivity reactions. This fact highlights the importance of oncology nurses' obtaining a complete list of all medications that the patient has taken or is taking.

Melanin protects the skin in two ways: it absorbs UVB and acts as a sponge that mops up free radicals.[42] Following radiation therapy, the skin's ability to protect itself from UV rays from the sun is decreased as a result of destruction of melanocytes in the irradiated epidermis and the slower rate of melanin production in new epidermal cells. The new and thinner epidermis after radiation is more easily damaged and is susceptible to all types of injuries: infectious, chemical, or physical.[14]

Photosensitivity reactions caused by radiation therapy

TABLE 30-4 Some Agents that may Cause Photosensitivity Reactions

Anticancer drugs

*Dacarbazine (DTIC–Dome)
Fluorouracil (Fluoroplex and others)
Methotrexate (Mexate and others)
Procarbazine (Matulane)
Vinblastine (Velban)

Antidepressants

Amitriptyline (Elavil and others)
Amoxapine (Asendin)
Desipramine (Norpramin, Pertofrane)
Doxepin (Adapin, Sinequan)
Imipramine (Trofranil and others)
Isocarboxazid (Marplan)
Maprotiline (Ludiomil)
Nortriptyline (Aventyl, Pamelor)
Protriptyline (Vivactil)
Trimipramine (Surmontil)

Antihistamines

Cyproheptadine (Periactin)
Diphenhydramine (Benadryl and others)

Antimicrobials

*Demeclocycline (Declomycin and others)
Doxycycline (Vibramycin and others)
Griseofulvin (Fulvicin-U/F and others)
Methacycline (Rondomycin)

Diuretics

Acetazolamide (Diamox)
Amiloride (Midamor)
Bendroflumethiazide (Naturetin and others)
Benzthiazide (Exna and others)
Chlorothiazide (Diuril and others)
Cyclothiazide (Anhydron)
Furosemide (Lasix)
Hydrochlorothiazide (HydroDIURIL and others)
Hydroflumethiazide (Diucardin and others)
Methyclothiazide (Aquatensen, Enduron)
Metolazone (Diulo, Zaroxolyn)
Polythiazide (Renese)
Quinethazone (Hydromox)
Trichlormethiazide (Metahydrin and others)

Hypoglycemics

Acetohexamide (Dymelor)
Chlorpropamide (Diabinese, Insulase)
Glipizide (Glucotrol)
Glyburide (DiaBeta, Micronase)
Tolazamide (Tolinase)
Tolbutamide (Orinase and others)

Nonsteroidal anti-inflammatory drugs

Ketoprofen (Orudis)
Naproxen (Naprosyn)
Minocycline (Minocin)
*Nalidixic acid (NegGram)
Oxytetracycline (Terramycin and others)
Phenylbutazone (Butazolidin and others)
Piroxicam (Feldene)
Sulfacytine (Renoquid)
Sulfadoxine-pyrimethamine (Fansidar)
Sulfamethazine (Neotrizine and others)
Sulfamethizole (Thiosulfil and others)
Sulfamethoxazole (Gantanol and others)
Sulfamethoxazole-trimethoprim (Bactrim and others)
Sulfasalazine (Azulfidine and others)
Sulfathiazole
Sulfisoxazole (Gantrisin and others)
Sulindac (Clinoril)
Tetracycline (Achromycin and others)

Antiparasitic drugs

*Bithionol (Bitin)
Pyrvinium pamoate (Povan)
Quinine (many manufacturers)

Antipsychotic drugs

Chlorpromazine (Thorazine and others)
Chlorprothixine (Taractan)
Fluphenazine (Permitil, Prolixin)
Haloperidol (Haldol)
Perphenazine (Trilafon)
Piperacetazine (Quide)
Prochlorperazine (Compazine and others)
Promethazine (Phenergan and others)
Thioridazine (Mellaril)
Thiothixene (Navane)
Trifluoperazine (Stelazine and others)
Triflupromazine (Vesprin)
Trimeprazine (Temaril)

Sunscreens

6-acetoxy-2, 4,–dimethyl-m-dioxane (preservative in sunscreens)
Benzophenones (Aramis, Clinique, and others)
Cinnamates (Aramis, Estee Lauder, and others)
Oxybenzone (Eclipse, PreSun, and others)
PABA esters (Eclipse, Block Out, Sea & Ski, and others)
Para-aminobenzoic acid (PABA–Pabagel, Pabanol, PreSun, and others)

Others

*Amiodarone (Cordarone)
*Bergamot oil, oils of citron, lavender, lime, sandalwood, cedar (used in many perfumes and cosmetics; also topical exposure to citrus rind oils)
Benzocaine
Captopril (Capoten)
Carbamazepine (Tegretol)
Contraceptives, oral
Disopyramide (Norpace)
Gold salts (Myochrysine, Solganol)
Hexachlorophene (pHisoHex, and others)
Isotretinoin (Accutane)
6-methylcoumarin (used in perfumes, shaving lotions, and sunscreens)
Musk ambrette (used in perfumes)
Quinidine sulfate and gluconate

*Reactions occur frequently.
Source: Drugs that can cause photosensitivity. Med Letter Drugs Therapeutics 28:51-52, 1986.

occur in the area treated with radiation following unprotected sun exposure. Photosensitivity also has been reported following chemotherapy administration. An enhanced erythema over the skin exposed to UV light has been seen after administration of 5-FU, dacarbazine, vinblastine, and high-dose methotrexate.

Nurses are responsible for educating patients on the dangers of exposure to UV radiation following treatment with radiation or certain chemotherapeutic agents. Clearly, the most effective way to reduce the risk of enhanced skin reactions to ultraviolet light is to avoid exposure to all sources of UV radiation. For most people, particularly those who enjoy the sun and outdoor recreational activities, avoiding sun exposure is a difficult task. Verbal and written information on the consequences of sun exposure and ways to reduce the risk of developing a photosensitivity reaction are given to the patient. Oncology nurses instruct patients to avoid tanning booths and to limit their exposure to direct sunlight, particularly between 10 AM and 3 PM, when the sun's rays are the most intense. Because clouds allow nearly 80% of the sun's UV light to reach the earth's surface, patients are reminded that they are still vulnerable to UV light on cloudy days. Tightly woven protective clothing or a hat may be worn to protect areas of irradiated skin.

Most important, nurses provide instructions regarding the proper use of a sunscreen. To determine which sunscreen is best for a specific individual, consideration is given to the person's skin type and to the sun protection factor (SPF) and composition of the product.[45] An individual's skin type is based on skin color and the acute and chronic responses to UV radiation. There are six basic types of skin: type I, very fair skin that always burns easily and never tans, through type VI, brown-black skin that never burns or is deeply pigmented (eg, blacks).[42,46]

SPF, a rating assigned to sunscreens, defines the ratio of the time it takes to develop erythema with the sunscreen applied compared with the time it takes to develop erythema without the sunscreen.[47] For example, an individual who can only be in the sunlight for 30 minutes without erythema may, by applying a sunscreen with an SPF of 8, remain outside for 240 minutes (30 × 8) without burning. The higher the SPF number, the more complete the sun protection. Initially, 15 was the highest SPF available; however, now many products have SPFs into the high 30s. For most situations in the continental United States, a sunscreen product with an SPF of 15 provides complete protection. Products with an SPF higher than 15 are generally recommended for use in a tropical climate or for protecting skin following chemotherapy or radiotherapy.[48]

Nurses also encourage patients to examine the composition of a sunscreen product, since it contains potent chemicals, many of which can irritate the skin. One of the original sunscreen chemicals was PABA (para-aminobenzoic acid). PABA is rarely used today because it caused skin reactions and tended to wash off and stain clothing. Today, most sunscreen products contain PABA derivatives such as octyl dimethyl PABA or cinnamates, benzophenones, or salicylate. Patients are told to stop using a particular sunscreen if their skin becomes red or itchy, and to switch to another sunscreen that contains different active ingredients.

Two additional but equally important factors for the oncology nurse to discuss with the cancer patient at risk for developing photosensitivity are the amount and the frequency of sunscreen applications. Recent studies indicate that most people use approximately half as much sunscreen as necessary for complete protection.[48] In general, adults will get the labeled SPF protection by using about 5 1/2 teaspoons of sunscreen product. Sunscreen should be applied at least 15 to 30 minutes before sun exposure to maximize its effectiveness.[49] Sunscreen also must be applied frequently because it can be removed by water and perspiration. Most products are labeled water-resistant or waterproof. Water-resistant products will provide protection for up to 40 minutes of continuous water exposure, while waterproof products will protect for up to 80 minutes of continuous water exposure. Either type of product, however, will wipe off with a towel; therefore, to be effective, sunscreens must be reapplied as often as indicated by activities in which the individual is engaged.

In summary, patients at high risk for development of photosensitivity reactions, especially those patients treated with radiation therapy or certain chemotherapeutic agents, need information about the dangers of exposure to UV radiation and specific ways to prevent such a reaction. It is not enough for the nurse to tell a patient "protect yourself from the sun." Rather, it is important to inform and counsel patients on the recommended sun precautions and the appropriate use of a sunscreen, ideally for life.

Hair

Radiation effects

Hair follicles are radiosensitive and therefore are susceptible to radiation damage. The radiosensitivity of the hair follicle is due to the high growth rate or mitotic activity of the epithelial cells in the root of the hair. Radiation affects hair growth in two distinct ways: (1) change in the normal hair cycle and (2) disruption of the mitotic cycle.[50] In the normal adult scalp, approximately 90% of hairs are in an actively growing phase (anagen) and 10% are in a resting phase (telogen). Under these conditions, no obvious changes in the amount of scalp hair can be seen. However, radiation to the scalp causes the hair shafts in anagen to be converted prematurely to telogen, with subsequent loss of these hairs. Radiation also affects hair growth by disrupting the mitotic cycle. Unlike chemotherapy, which primarily inhibits a specific phase of the cell cycles, radiation inhibits all phases of the cell cycle. This inhibits growth of new hairs and increases the hair shaft's susceptibility to breakage.[50]

Factors that affect radiation-induced alopecia include an individual's growth rate of hair, area or volume treated, dose per fraction, and total dose. The more rapidly an individual's hair growth, the more radiosensitive the hair follicle. Lacassagne and Gricouroff[51] ranked the radiosensitivity of hair in decreasing order as scalp hair, male beard, eyebrows, axilla, pubis, and fine hair of the body.

The degree and duration of hair loss depend on the area being treated, the dose per fraction, and the total dose. Hair loss can be either complete or partial. Whole brain irradiation, used to treat primary or metastatic disease of the brain, results in complete hair loss. Partial hair loss occurs when a region of the scalp rather than the entire scalp is irradiated. For example, patients with a pituitary tumor, a lymphoma or carcinoma of the head or neck, or Hodgkin's disease receiving mantle irradiation may experience partial or regional alopecia.

Radiation-induced alopecia follows a typical pattern. At approximately 2500 to 3000 cGy fractionated over 2 to 3 weeks, the patient will notice excessive amounts of hair in the brush or comb. This gradual thinning of hair continues for 2 to 3 weeks, and then quite suddenly the remaining hair comes out, with the patient finding the remainder of the hair on the pillow. The duration of hair loss can be either temporary or permanent. A low dose of radiation (3000 cGy) will produce temporary hair loss, whereas a high dose (4500 to 5500 cGy) will produce permanent hair loss. Following low-dose radiation, hair may grow again, but not with its former growth rate or density. The new hair may have a different color or texture and is usually finer than the previous hair. Regrowth of hair begins approximately 8 to 9 weeks after completion of treatment. Chances for hair regrowth diminish with age and higher doses of radiation.[52] If alopecia persists for 6 months or longer, regrowth is extremely unlikely.

Unfortunately, hair loss is an unavoidable sequela of irradiation to the scalp. Unlike chemotherapy, there is no way to prevent hair loss secondary to radiation therapy. The only treatment for permanent radiation alopecia is hair transplantation by a flap or punch graft technique. The use of hair transplantation for radiation-induced alopecia is controversial. It is reported that although the grafts take, the number of hairs per graft is poor, presumably due to the compromised or poor vascularity of irradiated skin.[53] Thus, some clinicians feel that the benefit of the treatment does not outweigh the cost or time of the transplantation sessions. However, successful case reports of treating radiation-induced alopecia by the punch graft technique have been reported.[54-55] In these case reports, good technical and cosmetic results were achieved, improving the quality of life for these patients.

Chemotherapy effects

Alopecia Alopecia is the most common cutaneous side effect of chemotherapy and often one of the most distressing.[5,33,56] Extent of hair loss may range from thinning of the scalp to total body hair loss. Although certainly not a life-threatening event, loss of hair has a profound psychological impact on the patient and the patient's acceptance of treatment. Some patients may even refuse potentially curative therapy for fear of this side effect.[57]

Hair follicles are susceptible to the effects of chemotherapy because of their high metabolic and mitotic activity. These drugs produce an anagen alopecia by interfering with hair growth at the proliferative (anagen) phase. At any given time, 85% of scalp hair follicles are in the anagen phase of cell growth, while the majority of other body hair follicles (eyebrows, pubic, axilla) are in the resting (telogen) phase.[58] This explains why scalp hair loss is a more common and severe occurrence than the loss of other body hair.

Chemotherapy-induced alopecia occurs by two different mechanisms, either affecting the hair root or the hair shaft. Higher doses of chemotherapy or more potent epilators destroy enough cells to cause complete atrophy of the root and loss of the hair root bulb. Hair falls out spontaneously or is lost easily when combed or washed. Drugs of less intensity slow the cellular mitotic rate, causing partial atrophy of the bulb and narrowing of the hair shaft. Narrow, weakened hair shafts break off easily at the point of constriction. However, the root remains intact in the scalp and active, leaving a thinning pattern of hair.[58] Unlike natural hair loss, chemotherapy-induced alopecia occurs rapidly and becomes apparent over a 2- to 3-week period following a dose of chemotherapy. Assuming the human scalp is composed of an average of 100,000 hairs, alopecia is clinically evident when 25% of hair is lost.[59] Chemotherapy-induced hair loss is essentially reversible and temporary. After discontinuation of the epilating drugs, regrowth generally begins in 1 to 2 months. Regrowth may even start during active treatment, but this is most often not appreciable because of chemotherapy's continuing insult to hairs recruited into anagen. Hair that grows back is often a different texture, color, and thickness and is often curlier; these changes are temporary, since hair usually will return to normal once therapy ends.[60]

Several drug and patient-related factors affect the degree of chemotherapy-induced alopecia. Contrary to patient perceptions, the majority of antineoplastic drugs do not cause hair loss. Rather, hair loss is a common side effect of several drugs that are used frequently in cancer treatment. The degree and duration of hair loss depend on the drug or combination of drugs, pharmacokinetics, dose of the drug, and method of administration. For example, doxorubicin (doses greater than 50 mg/m^2) and cyclophosphamide (doses greater than 500 mg/m^2) particularly are known to induce epilation after two cycles.[61] Combination therapy with both drugs almost always produces severe alopecia.[62] Other agents with the potential to cause alopecia when given alone or in combination with other drugs include bleomycin, dactinomycin, daunorubicin, etoposide, 5-FU, hydroxyurea, ifosphamide, methotrexate, mitomycin, mitoxantrone, melphalan, and vincristine.[33,63] It has been noted that methotrexate does not cause alopecia when leucovorin rescue is instituted.[33]

Bolus intravenous administration of chemotherapy results in immediate peak serum levels with subsequent exposure and damage of sensitive growing hairs. Infusions over several hours or longer are associated with a greater likelihood of alopecia. Some authors suggest, however, that the risk of alopecia is decreased with low-dose continuous infusion.[63] This may be related to the fact that high peak serum levels are necessary to cause hair loss.

Since the liver is the organ of metabolism for most drugs, hepatic dysfunction can result in prolonged serum levels of drug. Abnormal hepatic function has been associated with severe hair loss in patients treated with doxorubicin even when preventive measures were used.[64-66]

Patient-related factors that may result in differences in the degree of hair loss include variability of scalp hair growth. Scalp hairs in anagen at any one time may vary from 35% to 100%.[58] Therefore, individuals who have relatively few hairs growing will be less sensitive to the epilatory effects of chemotherapy. Additionally, the condition of a patient's hair before treatment is another factor that must be considered; damaged hair may potentiate alopecia.

It is important to remember that other noncytotoxic drugs (ie, heparin, propranolol, ibuprofen) and medical conditions (ie, malnutrition, chronic stress, hypothyroidism) may be factors that contribute to or cause alopecia in the cancer patient.[63]

Efforts to decrease or prevent chemotherapy-induced alopecia have included the use of two methods: scalp tourniquet and scalp hypothermia. Since the 1960s, varying creative approaches with these methods have been employed, ranging from rubber bands to inflatable cuffs around the head to thermocirculator units.

Scalp tourniquet Success in the use of scalp tourniquets was reported first in 1966 by Hennessey,[67] who reported a significant decrease in alopecia in patients with breast cancer receiving intravenous cyclophosphamide after using an inflatable scalp tourniquet. However, the claims were not validated in subsequent attempts, and this method was discontinued in the early 1970s.[68] In theory, rationale for use of the scalp tourniquet is that pressure from the tourniquet causes a temporary constriction of the superficial veins of the scalp. The result is a decrease in the amount of drug uptake by hair follicles, thereby minimizing the loss of scalp hair.[57,68]

Two types of scalp tourniquets have been described in the literature: one using a tube tourniquet (Penrose drain) and the other using an inflatable cuff. Refer to guidelines by Brager and Yasko[69] for correct application of these tourniquets. The pneumatic cuff appears to be more advantageous because the amount of pressure over the underlying tissue can be controlled and more evenly distributed compared with the tube tourniquet.[70] Although early successes with the use of scalp tourniquets were encouraging,[67,71,72] other researchers found the method ineffective.[70,73] It is difficult to compare findings as a whole or draw conclusions from these studies because of variability in study designs. Inconsistencies are noted in the wide range of reported tourniquet pressures and variance in tourniquet timing schedules. Other limitations include small sample size and, in most cases, nonrandomized samples, variance in chemotherapy drugs and doses, and lack of consistent assessment and measurement parameters for alopecia.

Scalp hypothermia Scalp hypothermia may be more advantageous than scalp tourniquet in hair preservation because it not only causes scalp vasoconstriction, but it also reduces cellular uptake of drug by hair follicles that are temperature dependent.[62] Additionally, scalp hypothermia may lower the metabolic rate of cells, making hair follicles less susceptible to the epilatory effects of chemotherapy.[74]

Doxorubicin-induced alopecia has been the focus of research on scalp hypothermia because of the high incidence of reported hair loss with its widespread and routine clinical use in a number of cancers. Further, doxorubicin has a short initial distribution phase with a rapid fall in plasma concentration during the first 15 to 30 minutes following injection[75]; therefore it is possible to minimize the amount of hair loss with this drug.

The earliest study on scalp hypothermia was reported by Luce et al.[76] A plastic helmet was attached to a room air conditioner to cool patients' scalps to 18° to 28°C 5 minutes before, during, and 10 to 20 minutes after doxorubicin administration. The control group lost 80% of hair compared to 30% hair loss in the experimental group. Subsequent studies using an ice cap method of cooling the scalp[62,77,78] demonstrated that cooling the scalp to 25°C or less can reduce and sometimes prevent alopecia. Some researchers have practiced wetting the hair before applying cooling in an effort to minimize trapped air and thereby improve the efficacy of the cooling device.[78,79] Reports indicate that scalp hypothermia is less effective with high doses of doxorubicin[79] and when used in combination with cyclophosphamide.[80,81]

More recently, research has addressed the effectiveness of scalp cooling in patients receiving high-dose cyclophosphamide, a practice not considered viable in the past. Cyclophosphamide is activated when metabolized by the liver and has a plasma half-life of 4 to 6.5 hours. Parker[82] used a commercially available cooling cap on patients with breast cancer receiving combination cyclophosphamide (600 mg/m^2) 10 minutes before, during, and 60 minutes after intravenous administration. Patients in the control group had significantly greater hair loss than those in the experimental group.

Two studies combined the use of scalp tourniquet and scalp hypothermia. Kennedy et al[74] reported no significant difference in hair loss between control and experimental groups. However, Satterwhite and Zimm[83] reported that the combination appears to be more effective. Acceptable hair loss (not requiring a wig or hat) was seen in 75% of the experimental group compared with 80% in the control group.

The use of hair preservation techniques is not indicated for all patients. Such techniques currently are not recommended for use in patients with hematologic malignancies[84] or in those with solid tumors that have a high incidence of scalp metastases.[85,86] Opponents caution that methods used to decrease blood flow to the scalp during chemotherapy administration could create a drug sanctuary, thereby minimizing exposure of tumor cells to cytotoxic therapy. Others report that the risk of cutaneous metastases as first site of recurrence is minimal (ie, 0.025% with breast cancer). They routinely recommend scalp hypothermia for a number of solid tumors including breast, ovarian, and osteosarcoma.[84] The benefits versus the risks of scalp micrometastases and possibility of developing scalp metastases at a later date should be discussed with the patient when considering hair preserving techniques during treatment.

High-dose tocopherol In addition to the application of a scalp tourniquet and scalp cooling, ingestion of high-dose tocopherol (vitamin E) has been suggested to prevent doxorubicin-induced alopecia. Wood[87] claimed that 1600 IU of tocopherol given daily during treatment with doxorubicin was effective in preventing alopecia in 11 out of 16 evaluable patients (69%). Of the five patients who developed alopecia, three had taken the tocopherol less than 72 hours before starting doxorubicin, suggesting longer than 72 hours was needed. Attempts to duplicate these results were unsuccessful,[88] and researchers therefore concluded that high-dose vitamin E has no protective activity in doxorubicin-induced alopecia.

Nursing care Hair contributes greatly to body image and is associated closely with one's sexuality. How hair looks plays an important role in shaping self-image and sexual identity and is often taken for granted. Consequently, the sudden loss of one's hair can have a devastating emotional impact on a patient. Both women and men suffer from loss of hair and find their self-image shattered by the physical changes.[5]

The nurse has a vital role in assisting the patient to adapt to alopecia. Adequate preparation can minimize the negative effects of hair loss. The nurse addresses with the patient the possibility of alopecia, when it will occur, its relationship to self-concept and body image, and measures to minimize the loss and other potential problems secondary to alopecia[89](Table 30-5).

Some clinicians advise patients to cut their hair short in anticipation of hair loss to decrease the weight of the hair and to prevent tangling of exfoliated hairs with those still attached to the scalp. This is controversial, as is the use or nonuse of hair care practices such as blow drying, teasing, perming, or coloring. Some claim these practices make the hair brittle and cause it to fall out faster during chemotherapy, while others have not found these practices to be related to postchemotherapy hair loss.[82] Further nursing research is needed in this area. Every effort must be made by the health care team to give accurate information and correct misconceptions.

Hirsutism Androgens are efficacious in the treatment of patients with breast cancer.[90] Hirsutism (an increase in body hair) is a troublesome side effect for women being treated with androgen hormonal therapy. An increase in body and facial hair occurs, accompanied by loss of hair in the frontotemporal portion of the scalp. The intensity of this side effect depends on the amount of drug used, with distribution of hair returning to normal after the drug is discontinued.

Nursing intervention is aimed at providing emotional support for altered body changes. Excess hair can be removed by tweezing or shaving; however, electrolysis is not recommended because of the increased possibility of skin irritation and infection. If the hair is fine, bleaching may mask the condition.

Nails

The radiosensitivity of a nail is similar to that of a hair follicle. With low doses of radiation (1200 to 1500 cGy), as seen with total body irradiation, the patient does not lose the nail(s). However, with higher doses of radiation (3000 cGy), as seen with treatment of mycosis fungoides, the patient can lose the nails(s). Radiation to the nail causes decreased production or growth rate, and ridges develop as the nail attempts to grow out.

Changes in the fingernails and toenails are commonly seen during chemotherapy. Pigmentation is seen most commonly and occurs with more regularity and intensity in black patients than in whites. The pigment generally is deposited at the base of the nail, causing transverse dark bands that correlate with the times the drug was administered (Color plate 4). This reaction occurs most commonly with doxorubicin and cyclophosphamide but has been reported with melphalan, 5-FU, daunomycin, and bleomycin. If continuous infusion therapy of these drugs is given, the nails darken evenly.

Beau's lines (a transverse white line or depression of the nail) (Figure 30-2) indicate a reduction or cessation of mitotic activity in the nail that can be expected with cytotoxic therapy. A partial separation of the nail plate (onycholysis) can be seen with 5-FU and bleomycin therapy.

Glands

The apocrine and eccrine sweat glands are only moderately sensitive to radiation. This is because the cells lining the glands and ducts do not divide rapidly, undergoing mitosis only occasionally. Complete and permanent destruction of sweat glands requires doses greater than 3000 cGy in 3 weeks. Irradiated skin receiving such a dose does not perspire and becomes noticeably dry. Doses less than 3000 cGy result in incomplete destruction, with recovery of sweat gland function in months.[14]

Sebaceous glands are more sensitive to radiation than are sweat glands. Absence of sebaceous glands contributes to the changed texture of irradiated skin. Loss of oil from the skin leaves it dry and susceptible to fissuring and may thereby increase the risk of infection.[14]

No drugs are known to specifically affect glands. However, some drugs may cause damage to glandular cells, manifested by dry itchy skin not associated with hypersensitivity.

ALTERATIONS OF THE MUCOUS MEMBRANES

Mucositis is a general term used to describe inflammation of the mucous membranes. Mucositis may affect any mu-

TABLE 30-5 Nursing Diagnoses Related to Alopecia

Diagnosis	Expected Outcome	Nursing Interventions
Knowledge deficit regarding alopecia related to inexperience with chemotherapy and/or radiation therapy	Patient and significant others will verbalize understanding of hair loss and its temporary nature	Instruct patient and significant others regarding alopecia: Why hair falls out and stops growing Onset may be gradual or sudden Variable extent or hair loss: scalp, eyebrows, eyelashes, pubic hair, general body hair Duration and temporary nature of hair loss related to chemotherapy cycles and radiation therapy Color and texture of hair may change as regrowth occurs Financial aid may be available through various forms of reimbursement such as a cancer society
Potential disturbance in self-concept related to alopecia as evidenced by: Verbalization of feeling vulnerable, rejected, or "different" Withdrawn, nonsocial behavior	Patient will: Verbalize feelings regarding hair loss and anticipated method of coping before hair loss Identify negative and positive feelings before hair loss Demonstrate interest in self by: Wearing own clothes Looking in mirror Verbalizing positive feelings Maintaining social contacts	Assess degree of importance of hair to patient and significant others. Encourage patient to describe feelings regarding: General appearance "Best" feature Role of hair in appearance on scale of 1 to 10 (1 being of no importance and 10 being of major importance); focus on psychosocial aspects accordingly Perception of significant others' reaction to hair loss Encourage patient to describe himself or herself without hair before hair loss, ie, tie tight scarf around head and look in mirror Encourage patient to cut long hair before scalp hair loss (inform patient about availability of hairdresser) Have patient identify possible measures to take during hair loss: Use of wig, scarf, hat, or turban Use of cosmetics to highlight other features Use of baseball cap or cowboy hat for males Encourage verbalization of feelings about alopecia: Have patient discuss feelings Identify patient's negative references to appearance Clarify negative references, ie, "I'm not sure what you feel is 'bad' about yourself" Identify patient's tendency to generalize negative feelings about alopecia to entire body image Review patient's positive perceptions of self: What is your best quality? What do you like about yourself? What do others like about you? Encourage patient to speak with other patients who have adjusted to alopecia Keep pillow and bed clothes free from hair Encourage patient to maintain personal identity by: Wearing own clothes Placing items of interest and meaning in environment, eg, posters Retaining social contacts
Potential alteration in skin integrity related to total loss of hair	Patient will verbalize knowledge of scalp care when hair loss is evident	Instruct patient to: Use baby shampoo or wash scalp with mild soap Use a soft-bristle hair brush to minimize pulling on hair Use mineral oil or vitamin A&D ointment to lubricate scalp and reduce itching Use a sunscreen with a sun protection factor of 15 or more and wear a hat when exposed to the sun
Potential for eye injury related to eyelash and eyebrow loss	Patient will identify measures for eye protection	Inform patient of the protective mechanisms of eyelashes Instruct patient regarding methods of protecting eyes, that is, use of eyeglasses, hat with a wide brim

Source: Adapted from Didonato K: Standards of clinical practice: Alopecia. Cancer Nurs 8:76-77, 1985.

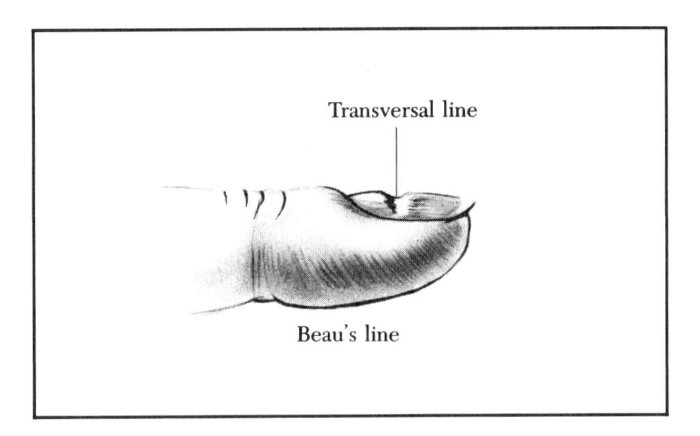

FIGURE 30-2 Beau's line.

cous membrane in the gastrointestinal (GI) tract from mouth to anus or the vagina, progressing to painful ulceration, hemorrhage, and secondary infection.

Gastrointestinal Mucositis

Epithelial cells of the mucosa renew frequently (every 12 to 24 hours), enabling them to replace cells lost from general wear and tear that occurs when food is eaten, digested, and eliminated from the body. Toxicity results when cells damaged by the cytotoxic effects of cancer treatment are not able to replace this normal cell loss. Manifestations of GI toxicity include oral mucositis (stomatitis), esophagitis, and enteritis.

Stomatitis

The oral cavity is a frequent site for development of complications resulting from cancer treatment. As many as 40% of patients being treated with chemotherapy and radiation therapy develop some degree of oral epithelial denuding (stomatitis) during treatment.[91] This excludes those patients with cancer of the head and neck region, in whom the frequency of stomatitis is greater.

As treatment becomes more complex and intense (ie, bone marrow transplantation, concomitant chemotherapy and radiation therapy), these complications increase. In patients undergoing allogeneic bone marrow transplantation, severe oral complications have been reported in up to 70% of patients; however, they are decreased and of shorter duration with syngeneic and autologous transplantations.[92]

The oral mucosa is composed of stratified, squamous, nonkeratinizing epithelium forming a continuous lining of the oral cavity from the mucocutaneous junction of the lips to the oropharynx. It provides a first line of defense against infection. Since turnover rate of the oral epithelium is one of the most rapid in the body, it is particularly vulnerable to the toxic effects of radiotherapy and chemotherapeutic agents.

Radiation-induced stomatitis The stratified squamous epithelial lining of the oral cavity is moderately sensitive to the effects of radiation. The radiosensitivity of the epithelial lining is not the same throughout the oral cavity. Desquamation of the soft palate usually occurs first, followed in order by desquamation of the hypopharynx vallecula, floor of mouth, cheeks, medial aspect of the mandible, laryngeal surface of the epiglottis, interarytenoid area, base of tongue, vocal cords, and last the dorsum of the tongue. Tissue reactions of the oral mucosa secondary to radiation therapy depend on several factors: type of radiation, fraction per dose, total dose, time between fractions, type of tissues irradiated, field size or volume, overall treatment time, introduction of rest periods during treatment, anatomic structures exposed, and the individual's physiologic and psychological status.[93,94]

Patients with acquired immune deficiency syndrome (AIDS) are at increased risk for substantial toxicity when radiotherapy is delivered to the oral cavity. Possible explanations for this enhanced toxicity include the presence of subclinical candidiasis, tumor involvement, immunologic deficits, or an intrinsic property of the tissue.[95] When external radiation is given to a large tissue volume, most or all of the anatomic structures of the oral cavity are at risk for tissue damage. However, if interstitial brachytherapy is used, only the immediately exposed structures are at risk for radiation damage.[94]

Several different reactions of the oral mucosa become apparent during radiation therapy. Early in the course of treatment, after approximately 1000 cGy or more is delivered, the oral mucosa will appear white. This results from a decrease in mitotic activity and retention of the superficial cells, allowing these cells to continue to a higher degree of keratinization. As these superficial cells are lost, the epithelial stem cells are unable to replace them adequately, resulting in thinning of the mucosa. Increasing erythema also is present due to inflammatory changes in the submucosa. With standard fractionated therapy (200 cGy/day), radiation mucositis occurs after 2000 to 2500 cGy have been delivered to the oral cavity.[96] However, mucositis can be seen earlier if the area being treated is near a tooth filling or if the patient continues to use alcohol or tobacco during treatment. As radiation treatment continues, mucositis progressively worsens, with a marked increase in swelling of the mucosa from hyperemia and edema. Additionally, a fibrinous exudate composed of serum and dead cells may cover some of the irritated areas, creating the appearance of a tan or white glistening membrane. This membrane can be removed easily; once it is removed, ulceration develops.[93]

Initially, patients with oral mucositis from radiotherapy complain of tenderness, swelling, and discomfort of the oral cavity and increased sensitivity to certain liquids (eg, acidic juices) and foods (eg, spicy or rough-textured foods). As radiation therapy continues, patients experience pain and burning in the mouth associated only with eating at first; this later becomes a continuous sensation. Oncology nurses are actively involved in managing problems resulting from radiation-induced mucositis including pain, anorexia, weight loss, dehydration, and infection. If mucositis and the accompanying problems become too severe, additional radiation treatments may be suspended temporarily. Radiation mucositis usually resolves 2 to 3 weeks after completion of treatment; however, continued use of alcohol or tobacco greatly aggravates the mucosa, delaying resolution of the mucositis.

Following radiation to the oral cavity, a thin and fragile epithelium forms that is more susceptible than normal to chemical and mechanical injury. The mucosa may eventually appear pale and telangiectatic. Several months after completion of radiotherapy, progressive fibrosis is seen in all subepithelial tissues; thus there is perivascular and periglandular fibrosis. The degree of fibrosis can vary from a small induration to a hard stony fibrosis depending on the dose and method of administration of radiation. Over time, these fibrotic tissues contract and shrink the irradiated tissue.

An infrequent late side effect of irradiation to the oral cavity is soft tissue necrosis. Progressive fibrosis and a diminished blood supply of the irradiated tissue decrease its ability to heal and ward off infection, thus resulting in necrosis. The incidence of necrosis increases with higher doses and larger treatment volumes. Additionally, the potential to develop necrosis appears to vary depending on the anatomic site. For example, late necrosis develops in the floor of the mouth more often than in the buccal mucosa or the tongue. Resolution of soft tissue necrosis can vary from months to years. The diagnosis of soft tissue necrosis should be made early and conservative treatment started promptly. First, any local irritant such as ill-fitting dentures must be removed. Appropriate antibiotics and, if necessary, analgesics should be prescribed. Education of patients regarding proper oral hygiene techniques is important if self-inflicted trauma to the oral mucosa by hard or improper brushing is to be avoided and frequent oral hygiene measures performed. Oncology nurses must provide nutritional counseling for these patients, emphasizing high-calorie, high-protein soft foods and the avoidance of tobacco, alcohol, and rough or spicy foods. Finally, these patients need close and frequent evaluation to ensure healing and to rule out the presence of active tumor.[97]

Chemotherapy-induced stomatitis Chemotherapy affects the oral mucosa either directly at the cellular level where the drugs are destroying actively proliferating cells (direct stomatotoxicity) or indirectly as a result of reduced myeloproliferation (indirect stomatotoxicity).[98,99] (Figure 30-3).

Direct stomatotoxicity Direct stomatotoxicity results from the cytotoxic action of drugs on the oral epithelium, causing a decrease in the rate of cell renewal. The sequelae are a thinned atrophic mucosa and initiation of an inflammatory response (stomatitis). Most common areas of occurrence include the buccal and labial mucosa, tongue, soft palate, and floor of the mouth. Rarely is the gingiva or hard palate involved.[99]

Histologic changes including dry mucosa, tongue, or lips; burning sensation in the oral cavity; and increased salivation can occur within 5 to 7 days of drug exposure.

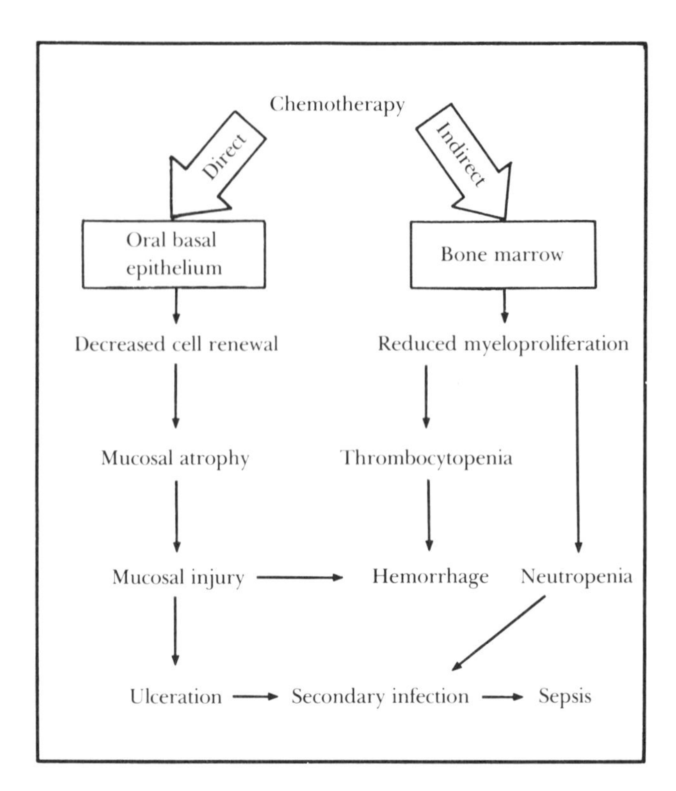

FIGURE 30-3 Stomatotoxic effects of chemotherapy. (Source: Adapted with permission from Lockhart PB, Sonis ST: Relationship of oral complications to peripheral blood leukocyte and platelet counts in patients receiving cancer chemotherapy. Oral Surg 48:26, 1979.)

Visible signs of inflammation and oral ulceration can be seen 7 to 14 days following therapy. Observable mucosal changes noted on days 7 to 10 include a reddened mucosa, decreased salivation, swollen tongue with protective white coating, and isolated ulcerations. Taste perceptions may be diminished. Severe stomatitis results when the body's adaptive resources are exhausted (days 10 to 14) and is characterized by an intense inflammation of the oral mucosa and tongue, painful confluent ulcerations, and taste alterations. Without complications and further insult from repeated drug administration, stomatitis is self-limiting and gradually reverses itself within 2 to 3 weeks. However, if a break in mucosal integrity occurs, secondary infection leading to sepsis can readily occur.[100,101]

The risk of developing chemotherapy-induced stomatitis is not the same for all cancer patients, nor is it equal in similar drug regimens. Table 30-6 lists factors contributing to stomatitis in patients with cancer.[100,102] Patient- and drug-related variables are by far the most important in determining the incidence and severity of stomatitis.

Patient-related factors include:

- Type of disease
- Age of patient
- Condition of oral cavity before therapy
- Level of care given during treatment

TABLE 30-6 Factors Contributing to Stomatitis in the Cancer Patient

Poor oral hygiene	Dehydration
Dental caries	
Ill-fitting dental prostheses	
Peridontal disease	Malnutrition
Exposure to irritants	Radiation therapy
Chemical (tobacco, alcohol)	Head and neck area
Physical (coarse foods)	
Thermal (extremes of food temperature)	Surgical manipulation
Drug therapy	Immunosuppression and myelosuppression
Antibiotics	
Chemotherapy	Cancer
Steroids	Cancer therapy

Source: Beck SL and Yasko JM: Guidelines for Oral Care. Cary, Ill, Illinois Sage Products Inc., 1984. Daeffler RJ: Mucous membranes, in Johnson BL and Gross J (eds): Handbook of Oncology Nursing. Bethany, Conn, Fleschner Publishing, 1985, pp 253-274.

The frequency of oral problems is two to three times higher in patients with hematologic malignancies (eg, leukemias—69%) than it is for solid tumors (eg, GI tumors—20%). Further, poor oral hygiene (eg, dental caries, tobacco and alcohol use) and periodontal disease predispose patients to an increased risk of oral ulcerations. Local irritants such as jagged teeth and ill-fitting dental prostheses may aggravate mucositis.[103,104] Oral complications can be reduced or eliminated by meticulous oral assessment and interventions before, during, and between courses of chemotherapy.[104,105]

Drug-related factors influencing stomatitis include:

- The drug
- Dose of drug
- Scheduling of administration
- Concomitant therapy

Most important is the choice of cytotoxic agent. Numerous chemotherapy drugs can produce direct stomatotoxicity and are listed in Table 30-7.[33,106] The antimetabolites and antitumor antibiotics are most commonly associated with stomatitis. Although stomatotoxicity generally is dose related and is more common with higher doses, patients differ in their ability to tolerate a given dose of a specific drug or combination. Those who develop stomatitis with their initial cycle of therapy will almost assuredly develop similar side effects in subsequent courses unless the drugs or doses are changed.

The administration schedule also can influence the toxicity pattern of the drug. For example, when the antimetabolite 5-FU is given by continuous infusion, stomatotoxicity becomes the dose-limiting toxicity, whereas a daily bolus administration schedule causes dose-limiting bone marrow toxicity.[107] Drugs used in combination or combined with radiation also can increase the risk.

In addition, prolonged stomatitis may occur as a complication of the body's inability to adequately eliminate a stomatotoxic drug. For example, the body's ability to excrete methotrexate is compromised by renal dysfunction, and doxorubicin excretion is compromised by liver dysfunction.[102]

Oral pain is the major clinical problem associated with direct stomatotoxicity. Pain results from inflammation of the oral mucosa and ulceration. Treatment is palliative, and a variety of products are available. When pain is not controlled, systemic pain medication may be necessary.

Indirect stomatotoxicity Chemotherapeutic drugs can affect not only the cells of the oral mucosa but also other cell pools, especially those in the bone marrow, causing indirect stomatotoxicity. Myelosuppression is manifested by neutropenia and thrombocytopenia; infection and hemorrhage secondary to myelosuppression can then occur.[98,99]

Since leukocytes and oral mucosal cells have similar cell renewal rates, it is not surprising that stomatitis is most frequently observed near the nadir of leukocytes. However, resolution of the oral mucositis often precedes bone marrow recovery by 2 to 3 days.[98] Consequently, improvement in the status of the oral mucosa is predictive of recovery of the white blood cell count.

The oral cavity is susceptible indirectly to infection because of neutropenia resulting from chemotherapy-in-

TABLE 30-7 Chemotherapeutic Drugs with Potential to Cause Stomatotoxicity

Antimetabolites	Alkylating Agents
Cytosine arabinoside	Cyclophosphamide
Floxuridine	Nitrogen mustard
*5-Fluorouracil	
6-Mercaptopurine	**Plant Alkaloids**
*Methotrexate	Vinblastine
6-Thioguanine	Vincristine
Antibiotics	**Miscellaneous**
*Bleomycin	Hydroxyurea
*Dactinomycin	Procarbazine
Daunomycin	
*Doxorubicin	
Mitomycin	

*Frequently associated.

Source: Dunagin WG: Clinical toxicity of chemotherapeutic agents: Dermatology toxicity. Semin Oncol 9:14-22, 1982. Levine N, Greenwald ES: Mucocutaneous side effects of cancer chemotherapy. Cancer Treat Rev 5:67-84, 1978.

duced myelosuppression. The most frequent sites of occurrence are the areas of the marginal, papillary, and attached gingivae. Spread to other areas of the mucosa can occur once this initial breakdown of the gingivae takes place. Secondary infection and bleeding are common. Indirect stomatotoxicity can result from any drug with toxic effects on the marrow.[98,99]

Patients with a leukocyte count less than 1000/mm^3 have a greater than 50% chance of developing an opportunistic infection—bacterial, viral, or fungal.[108] It is important to remember that when a patient's granulocyte count is significantly reduced, classic signs of inflammation may be absent.

Oral bleeding and hemorrhage are indirect stomatotoxic sequelae resulting from chemotherapy-induced thrombocytopenia. Bleeding results when the oral mucosa is traumatized or because of underlying periodontal disease and may occur anywhere in the mouth. Bleeding from the gingivae is the most common source for oral hemorrhage. The lower the platelet count, the greater the possibility of bleeding. Spontaneous gingival bleeding may occur whenever the platelet count is less than 15,000 to 20,000/mm^3 and generally is more severe in patients with preexisting periodontal disease or poor oral hygiene. Bleeding precautions should be exercised with oral hygiene measures for these patients. Management with topical thrombin-soaked gauzes held under pressure is often helpful if gingival bleeding occurs. When local measures fail, platelet transfusions may be necessary.[99,109]

Nursing Care

Assessment Identification and treatment of oral mucositis secondary to chemotherapy or radiation therapy must be based on a comprehensive assessment of the physical condition of the oral mucosa and the patient's perception of any changes in oral sensations. Assessment of the oral cavity requires adequate knowledge of the anatomy and physiology and the effects of radiation and chemotherapy on the structure and function of the oral mucosa. Nurses must know which chemotherapeutic agents commonly cause mucositis and the dose, route of administration, and schedule of these agents, since these factors influence the incidence and severity of stomatitis. Nurses caring for patients receiving radiation to the head and neck must be knowledgeable about the clinical manifestations and time of occurrence of the acute and chronic effects of radiation.

Pretreatment assessment of the oral cavity to determine the patient's oral and dental status and the presence of preexisting infection or tissue breakdown is necessary for baseline measurement. Assessing the status of the oral mucosa requires adequate lighting, removal of dentures or appliances, and inspection and palpation of the oral cavity.

An in-depth patient interview should be conducted to ascertain information regarding the patient's (1) oral hygiene practice, (2) risk factors, (3) life-style patterns (eg, tobacco, alcohol use, occupation, culture), (4) nutritional status and regular diet, (5) previous and concurrent cancer therapies, (6) knowledge of cancer, cancer treatment, and its potential side effects, and (7) self-care abilities.

Oral cavity changes secondary to radiotherapy or chemotherapy must be quantified through the use of a clear, concise, reliable, valid, and clinically useful tool. Adequate clinical assessment tools to assess the status of the oral cavity will allow oncologists and nurses to evaluate the effectiveness of different oral care regimens and interventions as well as identify stomatotoxic treatment protocols. Additionally, an assessment tool that narratively describes mucosal changes and grades the severity of stomatitis will ensure that all caregivers are "speaking the same language," thereby facilitating initial and ongoing assessment.

A number of clinical tools for oral assessment and grading scales for stomatitis have been developed. Unfortunately, many problems have been associated with these tools, including (1) lack of reliability and validity data, (2) lack of terminology necessary for accurate description of the mucosal changes, (3) complexity and time required to use tool, thereby decreasing its clinical usefulness, and (4) lack of patient's perception of mucosal changes.

Management Early research documented the value of general oral care intervention in patients with stomatitis of noncancer etiology. Ginsberg[110] observed that the frequency and regularity of nursing care were the most important variables in preventing stomatitis in a study population of patients with acute renal failure. Furthermore, nursing omission of oral hygiene care for 2 to 6 hours negated past benefits. Van Drimmelen and Rollins[111] researched the effects of two different oral hygiene agents on oral tissue of 136 nursing home patients. They validated previous findings that attention to oral care of the patient, rather than the specific agents used most, influences the general condition of the patient's oral mucosa.

Few studies exist on oral care measures with cancer patients receiving chemotherapy. Lindquist et al[112] studied 20 patients with breast cancer receiving FAC (5-FU, adriamycin, cyclophosphamide) to determine if a relationship exists between dental plaque and the development of stomatitis. They concluded that there was significantly less stomatitis and for a shorter time when dental plaque was absent during chemotherapy administration. Initiation of dental scaling and prophylactic cleaning before chemotherapy was then recommended as a measure to minimize stomatitis.

Beck[105] was the first to publish research on nursing interventions for stomatitis after chemotherapy. A systematic protocol for oral care was developed and shown to improve significantly the oral status of patients when used, even though patients' perceptions did not change significantly. Stomatitis is a significant complication of chemotherapy and radiation therapy. More studies addressing this problem and validating interventions that may influence the treatment of stomatitis resulting from cancer therapy are needed. Oral care is initiated with the goals of decreasing morbidity, maintaining good oral hygiene, minimizing infection, and managing pain. A comprehensive team approach, including dental services, is involved in this care.

The method of mouth care is individualized according to the degree of stomatitis and the patient's overall physical condition. Although stomatitis is often described as mild, moderate, or severe, a grading scale is more specific in monitoring the toxicity and response to treatment. A grading scale for stomatitis developed by Capizzi et al[113] is as follows:

Grade 1	Erythema of oral mucosa
Grade 2	Isolated small ulcerations (white patches)
Grade 3	Confluent ulcerations (white patches) covering more than 25% of oral mucosa
Grade 4	Hematologic ulceration

The value of oral hygiene in reducing oral mucositis has been substantiated in the literature.[100,112,114] A systematic protocol for oral care is used. The type of oral hygiene is determined by the condition of the patient's mouth. Table 30-8 identifies oral hygiene measures for varying degrees of stomatitis.[115]

The treatment of stomatitis remains palliative and symptom oriented. However, there is some research evaluating oral hypothermia techniques as preventive measures. Preliminary results of a study by Gainey and Dose[116] suggest that the use of ice chips to cool the buccal mucosa before, during, and after 5-FU administration may minimize the known toxicity of stomatitis.

Most pretreatment as well as oral hygiene protocols aimed at preventing or minimizing the oral complications of therapy require diligent patient adherence to prescribed oral hygiene procedures. Patient and family education is essential for the success of these strategies. Patient teaching includes the rationale for the regimen, proper oral hygiene, signs and symptoms to report, and measures to control pain and ensure adequate food and fluid intake.

In addition to oral hygiene, various topical formulations have been administered to relieve the pain and inflammation of stomatitis. Few studies have been reported comparing the effectiveness of various oral care agents. As stated earlier, it appears that the process of giving care is more important than the specific agent. There is no evidence that commonly used symptomatic treatments are effective, but many have been reported to provide subjective relief. A review of oral care agents in use and their applicability in stomatitis management is discussed in detail elsewhere.[103,114,117]

Maintenance of nutrition during this period is also essential. A diet high in calories and protein is needed to promote healing. Nutritional supplements may be indicated. Irritating food should be avoided. Bland foods and warm, rather than hot, foods are recommended. Cold, soft foods such as yogurt or ice cream are soothing and well tolerated. Dehydration can occur when severe stomatitis develops, and total enteral or parenteral nutritional support may be necessary until stomatitis resolves.

Stomatitis can have a great impact on a patient's quality of life and compliance with therapy. A standard of nursing care to assess, plan, intervene, and evaluate is necessary to prevent or minimize this distressing side effect, to decrease the incidence of infection, and to prevent nutritional deficits.

Infection of the oral cavity Infection is one of the most common complications of mucositis secondary to chemotherapy or radiation therapy. It occurs primarily because of damage to the mucosal barrier, poor oral hygiene, poor nutritional state, or depression of the immune system. Certain chemotherapeutic agents and radiation to the head and neck are directly toxic to the oral mucosa causing numerous changes that lead to a breakdown of the integrity of the epithelial barrier, resulting in an overgrowth of the normal oral microorganisms and the invasion of pathogenic organisms. The discomfort and pain associated with mucositis from either treatment modality often result in compromised oral hygiene practices and decreased intake of food and fluids. It has been shown that as oral hygiene measures are decreased, the presence of microbial populations increases. Depletion of protein stores and malnutrition increase the risk of infection by altering the integrity of the mucosal barrier and depressing the immune system. Data from Dudjak's study[93] suggest that adequate nutritional status as evidenced by normal serum albumin levels and optimal pretherapy weight may decrease the rate of oral infection. Immunosuppression due to treatment of cancer or the cancer itself further increases a patient's susceptibility to oral infection. Specifically, immunosuppression depresses phagocytic activity, interferes with the inflammatory responses, abolishes antibody production, and inhibits the development of delayed hypersensitivity.

Infections of the oral cavity are most frequently caused by candidiasis, herpes simplex, or gram-negative bacteria.[118] Each infection has certain clinical features, such as the white or "cottage cheese" appearance of *Candida albicans* or the painful vesicular lesions of herpes simplex, that assists in identification of the pathogen. However, this task is difficult at times, particularly when one is trying to differentiate between therapy-induced lesions and those caused by pathogenic organisms. Ultimately, proper identification of the responsible pathogen requires culture.

Patients at high risk for development of an infection often are treated prophylactically. Treatment varies depending on the pathogenic organism. Fungal infections often are treated with topical antifungal agents such as Nystatin or Clotrimazole troches. The Nystatin liquid is swished in the mouth for 1 minute and then swallowed, or mixed with flavored syrup and frozen in ice cups and taken four times a day. The Clotrimazole troche is sucked until it dissolves. It will take a longer time to dissolve the troche (eg, 20 to 30 minutes) if xerostomia secondary to radiation is present. Two factors must be kept in mind when using these topical agents. First, because they work

TABLE 30-8 Stomatitis: Oral Hygiene Measures

I. Potential stomatitis
  1. Prophylactic oral care regimen after meals and at bedtime
     a. Floss every 24 hours with unwaxed dental floss
     b. Brush with soft toothbrush and nonabrasive toothpaste after meals and at bedtime
     c. Avoid mouthwashes with high alcohol content
     d. Remove dentures or bridge; cleanse and replace after oral care
     e. Provide fluoride treatment for patients with xerostomia and those receiving concurrent radiation and chemotherapy
  2. Use oxidizing agent for thick, tenacious mucus
     a. H_2O_2 ¼ strength—swish, gargle and expectorate
        or
     b. Sodium bicarbonate solution (eg, 1 tsp in 8 oz water)—swish, gargle, and expectorate
     c. Rinse with warm water or saline
     d. Remove mucus with a swab as needed
  3. Apply lip lubricant (eg, Blistex, lanolin)
  4. Evaluate need for dental consult
  5. Use prophylactic chlorhexidine swish, gargle and expectorate every 8 hours for high risk populations

II. Mild or moderate stomatitis (Grade 1 or Grade 2)
  1. Follow oral care regimen (see section I, above) every 2 hours while awake and every 6 hours during the night
     a. Normal saline mouthwash if no crusts are present
     b. Oxidizing agent every 4 hours if crusts are present
     c. Alternate oxidizing agent rinse with warm saline mouthwash every 2 hours
     d. Brush with soft toothbrush and nonabrasive toothpaste
     e. Floss if bleeding does not occur
     f. Rinse with saline
     g. Remove dentures or bridge; do not replace except for meals
  2. Apply lip lubricant (eg, Blistex, lanolin)
  3. Culture oral cavity—prophylactic use of oral antifungal, antibacterial, or antiviral per physician's order if needed
  4. Local pain control
     a. Lidocaine HCl viscous 2% or 5% oral swish every 2 hours before meals; swallow if throat is sore (Note: May cause decreased or absent gag reflex)
     b. Apply Orabase emollient (Davies, Rose-Hoyt) for local pain control
     c. Cetacaine spray and dyclonine (0.5% or 1%) every 2 hours as needed
     d. "stomatitis cocktail"—mixture equal parts lidocaine viscous, diphenhydramine HCl elixir (12.5 mg/mL), and Maalox; swish and spit 30 mL every 4 hours as needed; may swallow if throat is sore (Note: may cause decreased or absent gag reflex)
     e. If xerostomia is not present: 50% Kaopectate and diphenhydramine HCl elixir equal parts, 15 to 30 mL oral swish every 4 hours as needed
     f. Zilactin-hydroxypropyl cellulose topical application
  5. Mild analgesic every 3 hours as needed
  6. Avoid irritants
     a. Chemical (citrus fruits, spicy foods)
     b. Thermal (extremes in food temperature)
     c. Physical (coarse foods)
     d. Tobacco and alcohol
  7. Provide appropriate nutritional intake
     a. Bland foods
     b. Foods high in protein
     c. Consult dietician
  8. Oral lubricants or "artificial salivas" (Xero-Lube, OraLube, Salivart, and Moi-Ster) may be helpful for patients with xerostomia

III. Severe stomatitis (Grade 3 or 4)
  1. Assess patient for infection and culture suspicious ulcerations
  2. Institute aggressive and timely systemic antimicrobial therapy as ordered
  3. Alternate warm saline mouthwash with antifungal or antibacterial oral suspension every 2 hours while awake and every 4 hours at night
  4. Use oxidizing agent for thick mucus every 4 hours followed by saline rinse
  5. Gently brush teeth every 4 hours—avoid trauma to gums; use soft foam toothettes for cleaning if bleeding occurs or brushing is too painful
  6. Apply lip lubricant every 2 hours
  7. Apply warm saline soaks to bleeding or ulcerated lips every 4 hours for 20 minutes
  8. Remove dentures or bridge—do not replace
  9. Local pain control measures as in section II, above
  10. Systemic analgesia as needed, especially before meals
  11. Provide appropriate nutritional and fluid intake
     a. Liquid or pureed diet
     b. Prevent dehydration with intravenous fluids or enteral feedings

Source: Adapted from Goodman M, Stoner C: Mucous membrane integrity impairment of: Stomatitis, in McNally J (ed): Guidelines for Cancer Nursing Practice (ed 2). Orlando, Fla, Grune & Stratton, 1990 (in press).

on contact, cleansing of the mucosa should be done before administering the agent to permit drug contact with the mucosal surfaces. Second, for the agent to be effective, it must remain in place for a certain period. Therefore, patients are instructed not to rinse or drink for at least 15 minutes after application. For disseminated or resistant fungal infections, systemic agents such as ketaconazole or amphotericin are given. A disadvantage of these agents is the potential toxicity to both kidneys and liver.

Herpes simplex is the most common viral infection in the oral cavity. For patients with limited tissue involvement, acyclovir ointment can be applied topically every 3 to 6 hours while awake. Oncology nurses should instruct patients to use gloves or cotton swabs when applying ointment, since autoinoculation with the virus can occur. Patients with extensive tissue involvement require systemic acyclovir therapy either by mouth or intravenous infusion.

The vast majority of bacterial infections are due to

TABLE 30-9 Stomatitis: Sites of Oral Infections

Site	Clinical Presentation	Treatment	Comment
Gingivae	Necrosis of papillary gingivae around teeth Pain Fever Lymphadenopathy	Parenteral antibiotics Aggressive oral hygiene	Risk is increased in patients with preexisting periodontal disease and in presence of thrombocytopenia (<20,000/mm^3)
Mucosal Bacterial 35% (Gram$^-$ 25%) (Gram$^+$ 10%)	Ulceration with deep yellow core Fever Pseudomonas lesions are necrotizing and enclosed by a reddened halo	Aggressive oral hygiene Broad-spectrum antibiotics may be necessary	Ulceration is an ideal nidus for infection
Fungal 50%	*Candida albicans* presents as raised pearly white spots over oral epithelium; if scraped off, underlying mucosa often bleeds	Prophylactic antifungal agents are used when aggressive antineoplastic therapy is begun For mild candidal infection, treat with topical Nystatin, clotrimazole or ketoconazole More extensive candidal infections require amphotericin B therapy	Oral *Candida* can spread to esophagus and lung
Viral 15% Herpes simplex varicella zoster	Herpes simplex gingivitis and mucosal vesicles begin as painful itching areas around the lips and circumoral region Fever, anorexia, and malaise may be present Varicella presents as unilateral vesicular lesion along trigeminal nerve	Acyclovir (Zovirax ointment) Keep extra-oral lesions moist with saline soaks	Acyclovir helps to prevent secondary bacterial infection Crust formation disrupts healing A moist dressing promotes healing
Odontogenic	Tooth pain May present as fever of unknown origin	Extraction of affected tooth Fluoride treatment Parenteral broad-spectrum antibiotics to cover opportunistic and normal flora	Dental examination and extraction of affected teeth are appropriate before therapy

Source: Goodman M: Side-effects of chemotherapy. Semin Oncol Nurs 5:29-52, 1989 (suppl 1).

gram-negative bacteria. Commonly isolated organisms include *Pseudomonas, Klebsiella, Enterobacter, Serratia,* and *Proteus* species and *Escherichia coli.* Systemic antibiotic therapy is the treatment for gram-negative bacterial infections. Table 30-9 outlines the sites, clinical presentations, and treatment of oral infections.[119]

Esophagitis

The mucosal lining of the esophagus histologically is the same as the oral cavity and is lined with stratified squamous epithelial cells. Destruction and inadequate replacement of these epithelial cells by radiotherapy or chemotherapeutic agents results in an inflammatory response called *esophagitis.* Similarly to stomatitis, esophagitis can progress to include ulceration, hemorrhage, and secondary infection and can cause sufficient pain to make eating very difficult. Treatment may be discontinued temporarily to allow recovery of these cells, which parallels recovery of the white blood cell count.

Most common early symptoms of esophagitis include dysphagia (difficulty in swallowing), odynophagia (painful swallowing), and epigastric pain. Esophageal pain that worsens and becomes continuous and substernal indicates progressing esophagitis.[120,121]

Radiation-induced esophagitis Similar to the oral mucosa, the esophagus is lined with stratified squamous epithelium and is moderately radiosensitive. This epithelium, along with the thin submucosa and muscularis mucosa, forms the longitudinal folds of the esophagus. When radiation is given to the esophagus for treatment of esophageal cancer, to the mediastinum for treatment of lung or breast cancer, or for Hodgkin's disease, the esophagus receives a sufficient dose of radiation to produce esophagitis. Esophagitis is the acute but transient effect of radiation to the esophagus and is due to epithelial loss of the esophageal mucous membrane.

It is characterized by edema, inflammation, and mucositis of the esophagus and moderate to severe dysphagia. The clinical spectrum may range from a mild substernal burning to severe dysphagia and an anginalike chest pain usually triggered by swallowing.[122] Initially, the patient will experience difficulty in swallowing solids, often described as "a lump in the throat." In the second or third week of treatment, after receiving approximately 2000 to 3000 cGy, the patient will begin to experience some mild to moderate dysphagia and substernal burning.[123] As treatment continues, the esophagitis can be so severe as to require a prolonged rest period from radiation. Infrequently, hospitalization is necessary to correct dehydration and electrolyte imbalances and to improve nutritional status.

The acute reaction of esophagitis usually will subside 2 to 3 weeks after completion of irradiation.[123] Because of the rapid cell renewal properties, reepithelialization of the mucosa occurs within weeks after radiation therapy and is usually complete 3 months to 2 years after irradiation.[124]

Chronic effects of irradiation to the esophagus often include thicker than normal epithelium, small-vessel telangiectasia, and moderate to severe fibrosis of the muscle layer and connective tissues. Ulceration, fistula formation, and stenosis also are chronic effects of esophageal irradiation but occur less frequently.

Factors that influence the frequency and severity of esophageal complications secondary to radiation include cancer of the esophagus, total dose, and concurrent chemotherapy.[123,125,126] If radiation is being used to treat carcinoma of the esophagus, ulceration, perforation, and a fistula may occur during treatment. To anticipate this complication, an esophagram may be done before initiating radiation.

The incidence and degree of severity of esophagitis increase with increasing doses of radiation. The esophagus generally can withstand doses up to 6000 to 6500 cGy in 6 to 7 weeks.[123] However, if doses reach a level of 7500 cGy, there is a 50% chance of ulceration or stricture in 5 years.[126] Late stenosis or narrowing of the esophageal lumen results from submucosal fibrosis and generally occurs 1 to 5 years after treatment. This complication often requires repeated dilation of the esophagus and occasionally gastrostomy.

Chemotherapy-induced esophagitis Mucositis has been observed as a treatment-related side effect of many chemotherapy drugs, particularly the antimetabolites and antitumor antibiotics (see Table 30-7). Therefore, any patient who develops stomatitis while taking these drugs is at risk for progression of the mucositis to the esophageal mucosa. Patients frequently complain of epigastric pain and heartburn, which can be managed with antacid therapy. It is not uncommon for the stomatotoxic agent (eg, methotrexate) to be discontinued for the duration of radiation therapy to the chest region and begun again once radiation is complete. Local analgesic therapy may be helpful if esophagitis should occur.

Other causes Both infectious and noninfectious causes may result in clinically significant esophagitis. In immunocompromised patients who have been granulocytopenic and receiving antibiotics, an infectious esophagitis is most common. Fungal, viral, and bacterial organisms can all be responsible. *C albicans* is the most likely cause and can be fatal if disseminated systemically. Herpes simplex should be considered in the differential diagnosis. Patients who have received extensive chest wall or mediastinal radiation treatments can present with symptoms clinically identical to an infectious esophagitis.[127]

Multimodal therapy Of greatest concern is the increased incidence and severity of esophageal complications from combined chemoradiotherapy. Initial concern was caused by the study of Brereton et al[128] in which intensive chemotherapy was used concomitantly with high doses of radiation therapy for treatment of small-cell carcinoma of the lung. Results of this study revealed that more than 50% of the patients developed moderate to severe esophagitis and 56% developed esophageal strictures. Further studies have substantiated the high incidence of severe esophagitis and esophageal stricture in patients who received either simultaneous chemoradiotherapy or chemotherapy within 1 week after completion of irradiation.[129,130] Doxorubicin, known to enhance radiation effect on the esophagus, was felt to be the cause for the increased esophageal toxicity. When concomitant doxorubicin-containing regimens were used, severe esophagitis developed with even low doses of radiation.[125] In addition, the "recall phenomenon" may occur in patients receiving a doxorubicin-containing chemotherapy regimen and thoracic radiation therapy.[129,131] The recall phenomenon occurs when subsequent courses of chemotherapy are given, and in the majority of patients the esophagitis is more severe than that experienced during combined modality treatment.[125]

These findings led to the recommendation that doxorubicin-containing regimens and thoracic radiation therapy should not be given together so that serious and potentially fatal esophageal toxicity can be prevented.[132] However, subsequent studies have reported the concomitant use of doxorubicin-containing chemotherapy regimens and thoracic radiotherapy without a high incidence of esophageal complications.[133,134] Variables such as volume of the area treated, dose rate of both types of cytotoxic therapy, type of chemotherapy, and sequence of treatment may account for these findings.[125,135] Regardless, this problem requires further investigation. Communication between oncology nurses in the radiation and medical oncology departments is necessary to anticipate and manage the enhanced esophageal reaction secondary to combined modality therapy.

Nursing care The nurse plays an important role in preparing the patient for the possibility of the development of esophagitis by discussing its nature, time of occurrence, and management. It is essential to determine the cause of esophagitis so that appropriate therapy may be given. Reports indicate that endoscopy is more accurate than radiographic examination of the esophagus in identifying the correct cause in immunocompromised patients.[120,136] Culture and biopsy and histologic examination is necessary for definitive diagnosis. Documentation of the incidence and severity of esophagitis must be done weekly. In one study, the degree of esophagitis was quantified as follows:[125]

None	No symptoms and no difficulty swallowing
Mild	Mild symptoms of difficulty or painful swallowing, but not enough to limit the intake of solid foods
Moderate	Marked difficulty swallowing, leading to inability to ingest solid food, able to drink liquids
Severe	Marked difficulty swallowing, preventing the ingestion of solids and liquids

With a grading scale such as this, the nurse not only defines a particular patient's esophageal toxicity but also assists researchers in discovering the true incidence of esophageal complications secondary to a particular treatment.

Treatment is mainly symptomatic and supportive. Therapy may be suspended. Nursing interventions are aimed at minimizing trauma to the mucosal membrane and promoting comfort and healing. Nutritional management often is required with diet manipulation. Bland, soft, cool (room temperature) foods and liquids are recommended. Irritating foods (eg, thermally [too hot], chemically [too acidic or spicy], or physically [too hard or rough]) are avoided. Tobacco and smoking also can irritate the mucosa and therefore are avoided. Depending on the extent of esophagitis, food should be soft, cooked well, and high in calories and protein such as milk shakes, puddings, and ice cream. Sauces and gravies added to food help to moisten and provide comfort and ease in swallowing. Pureed foods or liquid supplements high in calories may be necessary if severe esophagitis occurs.

Pain associated with esophagitis can be managed locally with topical anesthetics such as xylocaine viscous 2% (Lidocaine), 15 mL swallowed 3 to 4 hours as needed or 15 minutes before meals. Caution should be taken when swallowing because the gag reflex may be decreased. Over-the-counter preparations, including Aspergum (Plough, Inc, Memphis, TN) and Maximum Strength Sucrets with dyclonine (Beecham Products, Pittsburgh, PA) may offer temporary relief. If pain becomes moderate to severe, systemic analgesics are provided every 3 or 4 hours or as needed.

Because mild to moderate esophagitis commonly occurs in patients receiving mediastinal irradiation, a considerable number of studies to evaluate both local and systemic agents have been conducted. Nifedipine, an antispasmodic, was reported to be effective in relieving esophagitis associated with chemotherapy and radiation therapy. This agent was chosen on the basis that esophageal spasm may contribute to the pain of radiation esophagitis. Because nifedipine can cause hypotension, blood pressure is carefully monitored.[122] Nicolopoulos and associates[137] investigated the prophylactic use of indomethacin for irradiation esophagitis. Results of the data revealed a statistical difference in the endoscopic findings, favoring the group that received indomethacin. In addition, and perhaps most important, symptomatology based on a 4-point grading scale was milder in the patients receiving indomethacin.

Encouraging data emerged when sucralfate suspension (carafate) was used to treat chemotherapy or radiation-induced stomatitis and radiation-induced esophagitis. Sucralfate, an aluminum salt of a sulfated disaccharide, traditionally has been used to treat patients with duodenal and gastric ulcers. Based on its mechanism of action, it was postulated that sucralfate also may bind to oral and esophageal ulcers, thereby protecting the oral cavity and esophagus from ulcer formation and possibly promoting healing of these areas. The ingredients of this sucralfate suspension are as follows: sucralfate, 12 g dissolved in 60 mL water; Benylin syrup, 60 mL; and Maalox suspension, to a total of 180 mL. Patients are instructed to swish for approximately 2 minutes and then swallow 15 mL of the sucralfate suspension four times a day—after meals and at bedtime.[138-140] Although nifedipine, indomethacin, and sucralfate suspension have been reported to be helpful in alleviating esophagitis, further research is needed to establish their efficacy in the treatment of patients with radiation-induced esophagitis.

Finally, narcotic elixirs such as Tylenol no. 3 or 4 or morphine may be given to patients with moderate to severe dysphagia. The alcohol content of various narcotic elixirs and other medications the patient may be taking should be assessed, since a high alcohol content will further irritate the esophageal mucosa. A primary nursing responsibility is to assess and document the effectiveness of interventions to relieve esophagitis. In addition, nurses can take a more active role in conducting research studies to evaluate measures to alleviate esophagitis.

The patient with esophagitis must modify the diet, substituting high-calorie, high-carbohydrate, and protein liquids and soft bland foods for regular meals. Blenderized foods from the patient's regular diet also may be tried. Quite often, patients will need commercially prepared nutritional supplements and instant liquid meals (eg, Carnation Instant Breakfast) or homemade eggnogs and milk shakes in between meals or every few hours when solids or soft meals cannot be taken. Nurses or a nutritionist may provide nutritional counseling for these patients. Verbal and written information clearly outlining dietary modifications and an assortment of nutritional supplements are given to the patient. Nurses often obtain daily calorie counts and review this information with the patient, making any necessary dietary changes. Weight loss, hematologic and biochemical parameters, and skin turgor are monitored closely to prevent significant dehydration and electrolyte imbalances.

Finally, nurses assess for *Candida* infection of the esophagus, since it has become increasingly prevalent in patients with cancer. Patients with a predisposition to *Can-*

dida esophagitis include those with a lymphoreticular or hematologic malignancy or disseminated carcinoma, those receiving corticosteroids or radiation therapy, or those having chronic mucocutaneous candidiasis, diabetes mellitus, polyendocrine deficiency syndromes, and other immunodeficiences (eg, AIDS).[141] Patients with *Candida* esophagitis may be symptomatic or asymptomatic. Symptoms such as dysphagia, odynophagia, awareness of the passage of food, and retrosternal pain occur in approximately 50% of patients, particularly those with advanced involvement.[142]

Esophageal candidiasis may be managed with antifungal agents. Nystatin oral suspension, 4 to 6 mL (100,000 U/mL) "swish and swallow" 4 times daily is the classic treatment; however, the taste is not always well tolerated by patients. The addition of dyclone, 5 mL, to the Nystatin helps minimize the sting. Clotrimazole troche, 10 mg dissolvable in the mouth, is an alternative and is taken 3 times a day for prevention and 5 times a day for treatment. Ketaconazole, 200 to 400 mg/day, another alternative, must be taken on a full stomach and is indicated in disseminated candidiasis.

Most important, the oncology nurse emphasizes the temporary nature of the esophagitis and provides continual encouragement and emotional support to the patient and family.

TABLE 30-10 Radiation Tissue Tolerance for Various Anatomic Sites of the Gastrointestinal Tract

Patients at Risk: Cancer Site	Radiation Dosages Required for Development of Enteritis
Cervix	4000 rad + radium implant
Uterus	4000-5000 rad + radium implant
Ovary	3000-4000 rad
Testes	2400-4000 rad
Hodgkin's disease	4000-5000 rad
Prostate	5000-6500 rad
Rectum and sigmoid	3000-5000 rad
Bladder	4000-5000 rad
Renal	4000-5000 rad
Abdominal lymph nodes	3000-5000 rad

Source: O'Brien PH, Jenrette JM, Garvin AJ: Radiation enteritis. Am Surg 53:501-504, 1987.

Enteritis

The epithelial cells lining the intestinal mucosa are continually renewing to balance cells lost from normal wear and tear occuring during the passage of stool through the colon. These cells have a short life span and need a rapid mitotic rate (generation time 24 hours) to replace the cells that are destroyed. In the intestinal tract renewal rate is shortest in the small intestine (2 days) and longest in the distal portion of the large intestine (2 to 6 days).

Radiation-induced enteritis Radiation-induced enteritis is a disorder of intestinal function resulting from radiation therapy to the abdomen or pelvis. During treatment to patients with malignancies of the abdomen or pelvis, radiation enteritis occurs easily because of the narrow therapeutic ratio. With higher doses of radiation (4500 to 6000 cGy), the probability of tumor control is increased; however, the risk of injury to critical normal tissue is also increased.[143] Patients at risk and the dosages required for development of radiation-induced enteritis are reviewed in Table 30-10.[144] In a study by O'Brien et al,[144] patients at greatest risk for developing severe radiation enteritis were those receiving high-dose irradiation for cervical cancer.

Radiation-induced enteritis can be classified as acute or chronic. Acute radiation enteritis occurs during the course of radiation therapy and usually improves within 6 weeks after completion of treatment.[145] Chronic radiation-induced enteritis is defined as the persistence of significant GI symptoms for 3 months or more.[143]

Factors known to influence the severity of GI injury include the total dose, duration of radiation, volume of area treated, daily incremental amount, technique employed, and sensitivity of the tissue irradiated.[143,146] The risk of developing significant chronic radiation-induced enteritis correlates with the severity of the acute syndrome. However, the absence of severe acute syndrome does not preclude the development of chronic radiation-induced enteropathy.[147,148] Factors that predispose to radiation enteritis include abdominal surgery or peritonitis before radiation, pelvic inflammatory disease (PID), diabetes, atherosclerosis, hypertension, inadequate nutrition, and concomitant radiation and chemotherapy.[149]

Previous abdominal surgery or PID can cause adhesion formation, resulting in fixation of loops of bowel within the radiation field. The presence of small-vessel disease due to diabetes or atherosclerosis will exacerbate radiation damage and is thought to be the reason for the long latency period between radiation and the onset of symptoms. There are conflicting reports on whether chemotherapy given with radiation therapy increases the incidence of radiation enteritis. Stein[150] suggests an increased incidence of radiation injury to the bowel with the use of dactinomycin and doxorubicin, whereas the Gastrointestinal Tumor Study[151] group did not report an increased incidence with 5-FU and methyl CCNU (semustine).

The diagnosis of acute radiation-induced enteritis is essentially clinical and straightforward. The diagnosis of chronic radiation-induced enteritis is more difficult because it can occur years after radiation and because the clinical features can be attributed to recurrent malignant disease.[143] However, the diagnosis of chronic radiation-induced enteritis is suspected in any patient who has received previous radiation to the abdomen or pelvis.[152] Unfortunately, there are no sensitive and specific noninvasive screening tests currently available for accurately diagnosing chronic radiation enteritis; therefore the diagnosis often is delayed. The initial diagnostic test is a contrast roentgenographic study (small bowel follow-through). The radiologic changes of radiation-induced enteritis in the small intestine have been described as subtle, even in the presence of severe clinical symptoms.[153,154] Additionally, results of these studies frequently are normal.[155]

The single-contrast barium infusion technique has been shown to be superior to the conventional follow-through examination in diagnosing chronic radiation enteritis. The advantage of this technique is its ability to distend the small intestine maximally, providing a closer examination of mucosal patterns. Using this technique, the most frequent radiologic change was submucosal thickening of the valvulae conniventes or mural thickening. Despite its sensitivity, this technique is not specific for diagnosing radiation-induced enteritis because these changes can be seen in patients with Crohn's disease, carcinoid tumors, lymphoma, ischemia, neoplastic infiltration, and intramural hemorrhage. Therefore, correlation of radiologic findings with the clinical history and presentation is necessary for a correct diagnosis.[156]

Biochemical and hematologic testing such as plasma calcium, vitamin B_{12}, and folate can be performed but are also nonspecific for the diagnosis of chronic radiation-induced enteritis. Disturbances of intestinal functioning such as lactose intolerance and malabsorption of bile acid and vitamin B_{12} secondary to radiation-induced enteritis can be determined by specific tests. The diagnostic tests and management of these problems are presented in Table 30-11.[155-158]

The pathogenesis, histology, symptomatology, and treatment of acute and chronic radiation-induced enteritis is different; therefore each will be discussed separately.

Acute radiation-induced enteritis The acute effects of radiation in the small intestine are due to the rapidly proliferating cells of the intestinal mucosa. The proliferative area of mucosal epithelium is in the crypts of Lieberkühn. Acute radiation-induced enteritis is due to depletion of these cells along the crypts of Lieberkühn, decreased mitosis of the cells of the bowel, and loss of villi in the small gut. Destruction of the mucosal epithelium is reversible.[159]

Histologic features associated with acute radiation-induced enteritis include transient mucosal atrophy and dense infiltration of the lamina propria with polymorphonuclear leukocytes and plasma cells. Histologic changes of acute radiation-induced enteritis do not always correlate with a patient's symptomatology. For example, extensive histologic changes seen on a biopsy specimen may be associated with few or no symptoms.[159]

In acute radiation-induced enteritis, diarrhea with or without colicky abdominal pain or cramps occurs during or soon after pelvic or abdominal radiation. Nausea and vomiting are also common symptoms, particularly if the whole abdomen is being treated. Frequent sequelae of diarrhea and nausea and vomiting are anorexia and weight loss. Malabsorption of lactose, fat, bile acids, and vitamin B_{12} can occur, presumably due to mucosal damage.[149,159]

The onset of these symptoms occurs earlier in the treatment when the volume of the intestine in the radiation field is increased or the daily incremental dose is increased. Symptoms of acute radiation-induced enteritis are usually greatly improved within 6 weeks of finishing radiation. However, these symptoms can be severe enough to interrupt treatment in up to 20% of patients.[160]

Treatment of acute radiation enteritis is medical management with antidiarrheal drugs, anticholinergics, antispasmodic agents, antiemetics, opiate drugs, or a bile salt sequestrating agent such as cholestryamine.[151,161] Occasionally a decrease in the daily fraction or a break from radiation treatment is necessary. Dietary changes, specifically a low-fat, lactose-free, or low-fiber diet, are often very helpful.[143] The use of an elemental diet during radiation therapy has been found by some to decrease the prevalence and severity of radiation-induced diarrhea.[162] However, others have found no significant benefit in increasing tolerance to radiation with an elemental diet.[163] The value of an elemental diet during radiation remains controversial and is an area in which further research is needed.

Chronic radiation-induced enteritis Although acute radiation-induced enteritis is almost inevitable from irradiation of the pelvis or abdomen, the incidence of chronic radiation-induced enteritis is uncertain. Incidence rates for chronic radiation enteritis range from 0.5% to 36%, with the majority reporting a 5% to 15% incidence rate.[164-166] The magnitude of the problem of chronic radiation-induced enteritis, both in terms of morbidity and mortality, reportedly is underestimated for the following reasons[143]:

1. The majority of studies are retroactive
2. Data often do not reflect those who died or were lost to follow-up
3. The majority of patients do not seek medical help until a severe complication (eg, perforation, stricture, chronic blood loss) occurs secondary to radiation enteritis.

Chronic radiation-induced enteritis usually occurs 6 months to 5 years after completion of radiation. However, it has occurred as early as 6 weeks and as late as 29 years.[149] Unlike acute radiation-induced enteritis, chronic radiation-induced enteritis is a progressive, disabling disease of long duration causing both morbidity and mortality. The most common sites affected by chronic radiation-induced enteritis are the sigmoid colon and rectum, whereas the terminal part of the ileum and small intestine are less frequently involved. Although the small bowel is the most sensitive viscera to radiation, the effect of radiation is decreased by the mobility of the small bowel within the peritoneal cavity.

Chronic radiation-induced enteritis is thought to be due to progressive irreversible ischemia, resulting in diffuse collagen deposition, atrophy of the mucosa, and fibrosis in the submucosa and subserosa of the muscle coat.[144] Histologic features of chronic radiation-induced enteritis include submucosal fibrosis, lymphatic dilatation,

TABLE 30-11 Diagnostic Tests and Management of Radiation-Induced Enteritis

Problem	Test/Diagnosis	Management	Comments
Increased small bowel transit time	Hydrogen (solid meal) breath test: patient eats a meal containing unabsorbable carbohydrate (eg, baked beans) and breathes into a machine at 10-minute intervals First sustained rise over baseline indicates abnormality	Exclusion of single (monosaccharides and disaccharides) carbohydrate from diet (in the absence of fistula or short bowel) Medications (eg, loperamide or codeine phosphate)	Test helps to distinguish small bowel diarrhea from colonic diarrhea; used to assess "gut hurry" or short bowel syndrome May be misleading in presence of bacterial overgrowth in small bowel
Lactose intolerance	Hydrogen breath test using a 50-g lactose meal Sustained rise over baseline levels with symptoms indicate lactose intolerance Alternate tests include a blood glucose measurement every 15 minutes after lactose meal	Lactose-free diet	Diet may need to be followed temporarily (as with acute radiation-induced enteritis or possibly permanently in chronic radiation-induced enteritis)
Bile acid malabsorption	SeHCAT test uses a synthetic gamma-labelled bile acid and measures its absorption by a variety of counting techniques	Medication (cholestyramine) (8 to 24 g daily) (bile acid sequestrating agent)	Sensitive and specific test of terminal ileal function Unaffected by small bowel bacteria overgrowth (unlike bile acid breath test) Cholestyramine tastes unpleasant and requires careful titration of dosage
Bile acid deconjugation	Bile acid breath test (c-glycocholate given orally); expired carbon dioxide measured hourly A rise in 8-hour profile indicates abnormality	Broad-spectrum antibiotics (eg, tetracycline, ampicillin, or co-trimoxazole)	Bile acid breath test not specific unless small bowel radiography or SeHCAT test is given with it
Steatorrhea	Bile acid breath test Ideally diagnosis is made by aspiration of postprandial jejunal contents and measurements of pH and bile acid concentration	Low fat diet Histamine H_2 receptor antagonist before meals	
Malabsorption of vitamin B_{12}	Schilling test	Supplements of fat soluble vitamin B_{12}	Vitamin B_{12} malabsorption is common but seldom manifest May be due to either bacterial overgrowth or terminal ileal mucosal damage

Source: Ludgate and Merrick,[155] Mendelson and Nolan,[156] Zentler-Munro and Bessel,[157] and Beer et al.[158]

and obliterative endoarteritis of the small vessels in the intestinal wall.[167] Additionally, mucosal ulceration or necrosis of the intestinal wall may be seen.

The signs and symptoms of chronic radiation-induced enteritis include diarrhea, steatorrhea, abdominal cramping, nausea and vomiting, abdominal pain or discomfort, malabsorption of fat, lactose, bile salts, and vitamin B_{12}, and obstruction. Mucosal ulceration and necrosis can result in luminal narrowing, perforation, fistula formation, and chronic blood loss. Injury to the intestinal wall with edema, loss of collagen, and obliterative vascular injury results in progressive fibrosis, shortening, constriction, and stenosis of the irradiated portion of the bowel. Adhesions occur between the loops of bowel, causing further functional and obstructive symptoms. Partial or complete obstruction of the small intestine is the most frequent serious manifestation of chronic radiation-induced enteritis. These complications can lead to severe disturbances of intestinal function including steatorrhea, lactose deficiency, and intestinal failure requiring nutritional support.

Treatment of chronic radiation-induced enteritis often involves both medical and surgical intervention. Unless a patient presents with an acute surgical problem (eg, perforation) that requires emergency surgery, conservative medical management is the initial treatment.[164] Antidiarrheal medications (eg, loperamide [Imodium], and diphenoxylate [Lomotil], antispasmodics (eg, belladonna, phenobarbital), a bile-sequestrating agent (cholestyramine), broad-spectrum antibiotics, and salicylazosulfapyridine have been used with some success to relieve the obstructive and malabsorptive symptoms.[149] Specialized diets such as low-fat, low-residue, gluten-free, lactose-free, and elemental diets have been reported to be beneficial.[157,158,161] Partial bowel obstruction occurs frequently in chronic radiation-induced enteritis. Conservative management of this complication involves hospitalization, decompression with a nasogastric tube, and support with parenteral fluids. Following this initial treatment, the patient often is discharged on a liquid-soft diet. Although conservative nonsurgical treatment frequently can control enteritis symptoms for a short time, it does nothing for the underlying pathologic condition. Therefore, a majority of these patients return to their physician with recurrent symptoms, anytime from 1 to 18 months after initial treatment. Repeated episodes of partial small bowel obstruction secondary to radiation-induced enteritis cause further nutritional deprivation and deterioration of the patient's status. Some clinicians now believe that these patients with chronic intermittent bowel obstruction are treated conservatively far too long before definitive surgical intervention is initiated.

It has been estimated that 10% to 20% of patients with disabling symptoms from chronic radiation-induced enteritis will require surgery. The most frequent indication for surgery is small bowel obstruction and intractable diarrhea, with abdominal pain as the second most common indicator.[152] Surgical management of chronic radiation-induced enteritis is extremely difficult because the irradiated intestine is susceptible to complications from inadvertent injury; wound healing after the operation is often delayed, requiring prolonged parenteral feeding. If possible before surgery, sepsis should be controlled, metabolic abnormalities and acid-base imbalances corrected, and nutritional support given by administration of hyperalimentation. In a study by Haddad et al,[152] total parenteral nutrition before surgery greatly reduced morbidity and mortality in patients with prolonged periods of incomplete bowel obstruction, malabsorption, multiple surgical procedures, and peritonitis.

The choice of surgical procedure remains controversial. Some favor resection of the radiation-injured section of bowel,[168,169] whereas others[164,170] recommend leaving the injured section of bowel in place and bypassing it because of the lower surgical mortality (10%) compared with resection and primary anastomosis (21%) and a lower incidence of anastomotic dehiscence (36% vs. 6%). The high morbidity and mortality associated with resection was found to be due to the use of irradiated bowel for the anastomosis. This caused a high incidence of anastomotic breakdown or leakage. The current surgical resection technique requires that at least one end (ideally both ends) of bowel anastomosed is free of disease, outside the radiation field, and has an adequate blood supply. Using this surgical technique, Galland and Spencer[145] reportedly achieved a low anastomotic leakage rate with no operative deaths. In part, the choice of surgical procedure depends on the presenting problem as well as the findings at surgery. For example, if a patient presents with intestinal perforation and peritonitis, the preferred surgical management is removal of the perforated segment and drainage.[149] If extensive disease is found at surgery, a bypass procedure is recommended; whereas if there is only a single discrete area of radiation-induced enteritis, resection and primary anastomosis is the preferred treatment.[171]

Prevention of chronic radiation-induced enteritis The frequent use of pelvic or abdominal irradiation for the treatment of certain malignancies and the high morbidity and mortality associated with chronic radiation-induced enteritis require that every attempt is made to reduce the prevalence of this serious complication. Careful patient selection for radiation treatment is the first step toward decreasing the incidence of chronic radiation-induced enteritis. The benefit of radiation treatment must be balanced carefully against the risk of a serious complication such as radiation-induced enteritis.

Significant damage to the small intestine can be minimized by treating a volume of 14 × 14 cm with a dose of less than 4000 cGy delivered over 4 to 5 weeks.[144] However, this is not always feasible if the goal of treatment is to eradicate the tumor totally. Other techniques have been proposed to minimize the amount of small intestine within the radiation area. These techniques include reconstruction of the pelvic floor by an omental sling or by side-side reapproximation of the peritoneum and the use of prone treatment position and bladder distention during radiation treatment.[172] A technique using a polyglycolic acid mesh sling sewn above the pelvic inlet has been reported to be successful in preventing the small bowel from descending into the true pelvis. In addition, various chemical treatments and special diets (eg, elemental diet) have been tried with varying degrees of success.[172,173]

Optimally, the use of pretreatment contrast studies of the small intestine and computer-assisted planning to provide more individualized dosimetry, will decrease the prevalence of chronic radiation-induced enteritis. Further research of the pathogenesis, diagnosis, and treatment of chronic radiation-induced enteritis is necessary if significant advances are to be made in the management and prevention of radiation-induced enteropathy.

Chemotherapy-induced enteritis Since it is known that chemotherapeutic drugs affect rapidly proliferating cells, cells in the small intestine (villi and microvilli) are more vulnerable to destruction than are cells in the sigmoid colon, which have a longer cell cycle time. Slavin et al[174] observed that epithelial damage histologically occurs in 3 stages:

- Initial injury (cellular atypia and maturation arrest)
- Progressive injury (cellular necrosis and epithelial denuding)
- Regeneration (resumption of mitotic activity and mucosal repair)

These alterations due to chemotherapy cause inadequate digestion and absorption of nutrients and result in rapid passing of intestinal contents—diarrhea.

Diarrhea and cramping most often result from the cytotoxic effects of the antimetabolites (cytosine arabinoside, methotrexate, and 5-FU) as well as hydroxyurea, actinomycin D, and doxorubicin.[175,176] The degree and duration of diarrhea depend on the drug, dose, scheduling, and duration of therapy. For example, weekly administration of 5-FU causes less toxicity than if the drug is given over 5 consecutive days.[177] Bloody diarrhea may occur with mucositis when high-dose 5-FU is given, and is considered a grave complication of chemotherapy.[175]

Other contributing factors for diarrhea in the patient receiving chemotherapy include radiation therapy to the abdominal-pelvic region, antibiotic therapy, GI tumors, fecal impaction, anxiety or increased stress, diet, and bowel infection. Once the etiology is known, intervention can be planned to manage the problem and prevent complications, including fluid and electrolyte imbalances.

GI candidiasis is another problem reported following chemotherapy administration. It is most prevalent in individuals with lymphoma and leukemia and is unusual in patients with solid tumors. The role of chemotherapy in the development of candidiasis is not proven because many other variables such as concomitant antibiotic therapy and steroids may be present. GI candidiasis should be suspected in any patient receiving any combination of chemotherapy, radiation therapy, corticosteroids, and antibiotics. A negative fungal culture of the oropharynx should not rule out involvement distally in the GI tract.

The incidence of GI bleeding secondary to chemotherapy-induced enteritis is rare.[175] Exposure to gastric irritants such as aspirin or steroids may cause hemorrhagic gastritis. The bleeding usually stops when the irritant is discontinued.

Pseudomembranous colitis, most often associated with *Clostridium difficile* and the use of certain antibiotics, has been reported in patients receiving chemotherapy who have had no antibiotic exposure. Neutropenia may be responsible for the increased incidence of *C difficile* in individuals with leukemia. Neutropenic enterocolitis is a rare condition that can occur with treatment of hematologic malignancies, mainly lymphomas and leukemias; however, it may occur in any patient who is neutropenic and receiving chemotherapy. Clinical symptoms are nonspecific and include fever, abdominal pain located in the right lower quadrant, diarrhea, and bloody stools.[178]

Nursing care The role of the nurse includes assessment, symptom management, and nutritional counseling. Assessment includes a history of the normal pattern of elimination and changes in this pattern, identification of contributing factors, and description of associated pain, appearance, consistency and frequency of stool in relation to treatments. Determination of personality, level of stress, and nutritional status may facilitate the diagnosis. An abdominal examination as well as assessment of skin in the rectal area are done.

The nurse discusses with the patient and family the potential side effects of treatment (eg, diarrhea, nausea and vomiting) and the time in which these side effects usually occur. For example, nausea or vomiting can occur after only one radiation treatment, but diarrhea usually begins after 2 or 3 weeks of treatment. In acute radiation-induced enteritis, diarrhea with or without abdominal cramping is the predominant symptom.

Diarrhea, by definition, is the passage of loose, fluid stools more frequently than the individual's usual pattern of bowel elimination. If the nurse is to report that a patient is experiencing diarrhea, he or she must first establish the patient's usual bowel habits. Before initiating treatment, the nurse obtains information on the patient's usual bowel patterns, noting the frequency and character of stool (color, amount, odor, consistency) and the frequency and type of laxatives used. Recent changes in factors that contribute to adequate bowel elimination such as fluid intake, activity level, stress, and changes in diet are also noted. Additionally, the nurse assesses for factors known to influence the severity of GI injury and those that predispose the patient to enteritis.

Physical assessment parameters to be monitored include abdominal tenderness, bowel sounds, skin turgor, and weight. A physical examination is done before initiating treatment to determine baseline status and is then continued weekly or more frequently if symptoms warrant during treatment. Additionally, laboratory parameters such as complete blood count, platelet count, and electrolytes are checked before and during treatment.

If diarrhea is treatment related, therapy may need to be temporarily stopped until the condition improves. Management is aimed at preventing fluid and electrolyte imbalances and promoting comfort. Diet is adjusted to minimize overstimulation of the GI tract. Dietary alterations include having the patient:

- Eat a low-residue diet high in calories and protein (ie, bananas, rice, applesauce)
- Avoid foods that irritate or stimulate the GI tract (ie, popcorn, raw vegetables, fresh and dried fruit, cold liquids)

- Avoid tobacco and alcohol
- Avoid milk and milk products to prevent lactose-intolerance symptoms
- Drink 8 to 10 glasses of liquid daily (Gatorade, meat broth or bouillon, weak tea)

Antidiarrheal medications are given to reduce urgency, frequency, and volume of stool and include:

- Non-prescription agents containing kaolin, pectin, or bismuth (ie, Kaopectate, Pepto-Bismol, Donnagel) per instructions on bottle
- Diphenoxylate (Lomotil), 2.5 mg orally, 1 to 2 tablets every 4 hours, up to 20 mg daily
- Loperamide (Imodium) 2 mg orally, 1 to 2 tablets every 4 hours, up to 16 mg daily

For severe diarrhea, opiates can be used to decrease peristalsis and include:

- Opium tincture, 0.5 to 1.0 mL orally every 4 hours
- Paregoric elixir, 4 mL orally every 4 hours
- Codeine, 15 to 30 mg orally every 4 hours

Temporary bed rest is suggested for a patient with acute or severe diarrhea because decreased physical activity will decrease peristalsis, thereby preventing diarrhea. The impact of diarrhea on the patient's life-style must not be forgotten, and emotional support must be given continually until this side effect resolves.

Nursing care also focuses on skin care in the perianal area to prevent skin breakdown and increase patient comfort. As soon as diarrhea develops, the patient is instructed to take sitz baths three times a day. If desquamation should occur in the perianal area, the addition of aluminum subacetate (Domeboro) (one package to 1 quart of water) to the sitz bath is recommended. For irritation or discomfort outside the rectum, a topical anesthetic such as Hurricaine (Beutlich, Inc., Niles, IL) may be helpful. If hemorrhoids are a problem or if a patient is experiencing discomfort or irritation inside the rectum, Preparation H (hydrocortisone acetate 1% and pramoxine hydrochloride 1% topical aerosol) or Proctofoam (Reed and Carnrick, Piscataway, NJ) can be used, with some relief usually noted. If these measures are ineffective, a low-dose steroid may be prescribed.

Complications of diarrhea such as dehydration, anorexia, weight loss, and electrolyte imbalance require active replacement of fluids and electrolytes, further dietary instructions, and a suspension of treatment.

The patient with chronic enteritis and the family need continual encouragement and support. The nurse can provide the necessary teaching regarding symptom management and diet and the emotional support during this difficult time. Patients who are cured of their cancer yet have a chronic side effect of the treatment such as enteritis, often experience a wide variety of emotions such as fear, anxiety, anger, and grief. The nurse can help the patient and family deal with these emotions by listening, correcting any misconceptions, emphasizing the necessity of cancer treatment, and providing new or alternate coping strategies. If necessary, the nurse can encourage the patient to consult a psychologist or psychiatrist.

Vaginal Mucositis

The vagina consists of three principal layers: an outer fibrous layer, a middle muscular layer, and an inner mucosal layer. Similar to the oral mucosa, the mucosa of the vagina undergoes rapid cellular division and is thus sensitive to the effects of radiation and chemotherapy.

Radiation-induced vaginitis

High-dose pelvic irradiation for gynecologic or colorectal malignancies frequently results in erythema, inflammation, mucosal atrophy, inelasticity, and ulceration of the vaginal tissues. This can progress to adhesion formation and stenosis, resulting in partial or complete vaginal agglutination (occlusion) and occasionally tissue necrosis of the vagina. This sequence is sometimes referred to as postirradiation vaginitis. Patients receiving radiation therapy for carcinoma of the cervix are particularly at risk for this complication, since high doses of ionizing radiation (10,000 cGy or greater) are given to the cervix and upper vagina in an effort to eradicate the tumor. Despite greater skills and improved equipment of modern radiotherapy, the incidence of postradiation changes in the upper vagina and cervix has reportedly not diminished.[179]

Vaginal effects of radiotherapy for carcinoma of the cervix result from a combination of three factors: physical trauma to the vaginal mucosa produced by radium applicators and packs, direct effects of radiation on the vaginal mucosa, and estrogen deprivation from radiation castration. The most serious changes are attributed to the direct effects of irradiation on the vagina. A cytologic and histologic study by Pitkin and Bradbury[180] described the sequential changes in the vagina as a direct and immediate response to radiation. Initially, there was loss of virtually all epithelium in areas receiving maximal surface radiation (eg, vaginal fornices and ectocervix), and this persisted for 3 to 6 months after radiation. Following this period, there was gradual epithelialization that became progressively more complete during the second year after radiation. Two years following radiation, the epithelium was nearly normal, although a fully developed stratified squamous epithelium was not observed. Knowledge of the vaginal effects of radiotherapy will in part explain the predominant clinical features of postirradiation.

Clinical symptoms of postirradiation vaginitis include vaginal discharge, spontaneous and contact bleeding, dyspareunia, pruritis, dysuria, or pain. Objective signs of vaginitis secondary to radiation include erythema, inflammation, a white radiation membrane, ulceration, adhesions, atrophy, stenosis, or necrosis. The erythema of the vaginal mucosa remains for weeks or months following radiation. Over several months, the vaginal mucosa assumes a pale appearance and telangiectasia develops. Ulceration can lead to formation of adhesions. Adhesions tend to develop at the sites of maximum irradiation (eg, between the ectocervix and mucosa of the vaginal vault, anterior and posterior surfaces of the upper third of the vagina). Adhesions, if not broken up soon after their formation, often result in permanent closure or stenosis. Stenosis can cause partial or total agglutination (stenosis is generally limited to the upper third of the vagina). Following pelvic irradiation, it has been estimated that more than 80% of women have at least partial vaginal stenosis and occlusion.[181] This, in turn, causes constriction of the submucosal tissues and pronounced vaginal shortening.

Vaginal vault necrosis, resulting from severe vascular compromise, is the most serious complication following high-dose pelvic irradiation. Vault necrosis may respond to local measures such as estrogen cream and antiseptic douches, or it may progress relentlessly, resulting in anorexia, weight loss, malaise, and severe pain that is unresponsive to narcotics. Life-threatening hemorrhage or bowel or urinary tract fistulas may occur. Treatment options for vaginal vault necrosis include conservative management with hyperalimentation, antibiotics, debridement, and douching or surgical management with a diverting procedure and, rarely, a total pelvic exenteration.

Treatment for postirradiation vaginitis includes early vaginal dilatation, either by frequent sexual intercourse or the use of a dilator, and estrogen cream. Early vaginal dilatation prevents fibrous tissue or adhesions from narrowing the capacity of the vagina, maintaining patency for sexual intercourse and pelvic examinations. Studies examining the value of estrogen cream in the treatment of postirradiation vaginitis have documented promotion of epithelial regeneration, leading to improved gross and histologic appearance of the vagina.[182,183] These changes are evident particularly in those patients in whom 3 or more months have elapsed since radiation. In addition, patients treated with estrogen cream prophylactically on completion of radiation had significantly less bleeding, dyspareunia, and narrowing of vaginal caliber.[184] Discontinuation of estrogen cream reverses the appearance of the vagina microscopically to pretreatment patterns in approximately 6 months. The use of estrogen cream in the treatment of postirradiation vaginitis appears to be safe and relatively easy for the patient to administer. There has been only one case report of gynecomastia from exposure to vaginal estrogen cream.[184]

Vaginal estrogen cream preparations (eg, Premarin, Estrace) are absorbed systemically and result in sustained high estrogen levels in the systemic circulation. Therefore, if systemic estrogen is contraindicated for either oncologic (eg, estrogen-dependent tumors, endometrial cancer) or general medical reasons, the use of vaginal estrogen cream preparations should be avoided.[185]

Vaginitis and infection Vaginitis is an inflammation of the vulvar and vaginal tissues. It generally is associated with changes in the usual distribution of microbes, changes in the vaginal environment, or the presence of abnormal pathogenic organisms. The normal, noninfected vagina is maintained by four factors[186]:

1. Secretion of normal estrogen levels necessary to maintain the epithelial lining
2. Availability of glycogen in vaginal tissue
3. Presence of adequate numbers of lactobacilli to produce lactic acid
4. Adequate lactic acid to maintain acidity of vagina (pH 4 to 4.5)

A change in one or more of these factors can lead to vaginitis. High-dose pelvic irradiation results in estrogen deprivation, which in turn causes mucosal atrophy and loss of the epithelial lining of the vagina. Atrophic conditions of the vagina in which the epithelium is compromised lead to changes in the distribution of normal flora. These changes in the normal flora allow an overgrowth of pathogenic bacteria. Organisms most commonly associated with vaginitis are *C albicans, Trichomonas vaginalis,* and *Gardnerella vaginalis.* Less frequently, vaginitis is associated with the herpes virus or other sexually transmitted diseases such as Chlamydia or gonorrhea.

Subjective symptoms of vaginitis generally include pruritis, odor, discharge, dyspareunia, dysuria, or burning. Vaginitis symptoms may be continuous or intermittent and vary depending on the specific vaginal infection. Table 30-12 identifies symptom patterns in specific vulvovaginal infections.[187] Treatment of vaginitis requires proper identification of the organism, since the treatment will differ according to the type of infection present (Table 30-13).[188]

Nursing care Nursing care focuses on the prevention or management of postirradiation vaginitis. Vaginal dilatation, either by frequent sexual intercouse or vaginal dilators, and the administration of estrogen are recommended. The nurse must be comfortable with his or her own sexuality and develop a trusting and caring relationship with the patient and significant other if these preventative measures are to be followed. Good rapport between the patient and nurse will allow the nurse to discuss openly the patient's sexual practices and how radiation to the pelvic region can affect sexual function. Unfortunately, compliance with these measures is often poor. Reasons cited for this poor compliance include the fear of spouse's contracting malignancy from the patient, fear of aggravating the disease, dyspareunia or bleeding, and connotation of masturbation associated with the use of a mechanical dilator.[189] The nurse can also correct misconceptions that may contribute to poor compliance with the recommended regimen. Patients must understand that vaginal dilators and the use of estrogen can alleviate symptoms, decrease the incidence and severity of postirradiation vaginitis, and preserve sexual function. Additionally, the nurse emphasizes the importance of maintaining a patent vagina for pelvic examinations, smears, and, if necessary, biopsy. Although this last reason is a practical one,

TABLE 30-12 Symptom Patterns in Specific Vulvovaginal Infections

Symptom	*Candida*	*Trichomonas*	*Gardnerella*	Herpes	Gonococcus	*Chlamydia*
Pruritis	Intense Painful	Sometimes	Seldom	Sometimes		
Lesions				Vesicles	Abscess of Bartholin's glands	
Pain				Tender groin nodes	Right upper quadrant pain	
Discharge	White, curdlike	Yellowish green	Grayish yellow		Mucopurulent from cervix	Mucopurulent from cervix
Odor		Foul	Fishlike			
Dyspareunia	Present					
Dysuria	Present			Present	Present	Present
Fever				Moderate		
Asymptomatic		25%	50%		70%-80%	50%

Source: Grant MM, Davidson SB: Assessment of vaginitis, in Stromberg MF (ed): Instruments for Assessing Clinical Problems. East Norwalk, Conn, Appleton & Lange, 1988, pp 401-414.

TABLE 30-13 Treatment of Vaginitis

Infection	Organism	Treatment
Candidiasis	*Candida albicans* (a fungus)	Improvement in general health (if patient is debilitated) Control of predisposing factors (eg, weight loss if patient is obese, stabilization of diabetes, avoidance of excessive moisture) Topical applications of antifungal agents (eg, miconazole nitrate cream or Nystatin)
Trichomoniasis	*Trichomonas vaginalis* (a flagellated protozoa)	Topical treatments unsuccessful Administration of a systemic antiprotozoan agent (eg, metronidazole [Flagyl])
Gardnerella	*Gardnerella vaginalis* (a gram-negative bacillus)	Topical agents (eg, oxytetracycline [Terramycin]) vaginal tablets, often used concurrently with a topical antifungal agent (eg, mycostatin), since Terramycin predisposes to fungal infections Administration of a systemic antibiotic (eg, ampicillin, cephalexin [Keflex] or cephradine [Anspor]); oral tetracyclines are partially effective If trichomoniasis is present too, administration of metronidazole (Flagyl) for both infections
Herpes genitalis	Herpes virus	Oral acyclovir is effective for first episode cases but does not seem to prevent virus latency or recurrent disease
Chlamydia	*Chlamydia trachomatis*	Administration of a broad-spectrum antibiotic; Tetracycline is presently the treatment of choice
Gonorrhea	*Neisseria gonorrhoeae*	Administration of penicillin or ampicillin; some strains are resistant to these medications

Source: Kaufman RH: Anatomy of the vulva and vagina, in Gardner HL, Kaufman RH (eds): Benign Diseases of the Vulva and Vagina (ed 2). Boston, GK Hall, 1981.

it is also crucial for careful follow-up of the patient and one with which the patient and family is concerned and readily understands. Discussion of these measures begins before completion of treatment and continues with each follow-up visit indefinitely.

If vaginal dilatation is to be achieved by use of a dilator, both verbal and written information on how to use the dilator should be provided. "Vaginal Dilatation Post-Pelvic Irradiation: A Patient Education Tool" by Richards and Hiratzka is very helpful.[190] If possible, vaginal dilators are given to the patient by the radiation oncology department to minimize the embarrassment for many women buying one. Patients are shown how to lubricate the vaginal dilator with a water-soluble lubricant such as K-Y jelly and how to insert the dilator. Vaginal dilatation is recommended on a regular basis. Although the schedule varies somewhat 15 minutes three times a week for the first year is fairly standard.

Finally, nurses must be aware that patients who receive radiation to the pelvic area are more susceptible to developing infections of the vagina. Knowledge of the factors associated with maintenance of the noninfected vagina and how radiation changes one or more of these factors will assist the nurse to identify patients at risk for infection. Parameters used to assess infections of the vagina include identification of pathogenic organisms, complaints of subjective symptoms, and observation of objective signs. A careful and thorough assessment of these parameters by the nurse may lead to earlier recognition and referral to a physician for treatment, thereby alleviating patient discomfort and promoting healing.

Chemotherapy-induced vaginitis

Potentially any drug known to cause oral mucositis may also be associated with painful irritation and inflammation of the vagina (eg, the antimetabolites 5-FU and methotrexate). As with stomatitis, symptoms may occur 3 to 5 days after chemotherapy and resolve 7 to 10 days later. The nurse should inquire as to whether the patient is experiencing any discomfort because she might not volunteer such information.

Because the vagina is near the vulva, women may experience both vulvar and vaginal irritation (vulvovaginitis). They may report symptoms of vaginal discharge, itching, odor, pain, or bleeding. Other factors contributing to vaginitis besides cytotoxic therapy include radiation therapy exposure, antibiotics, and change in pH of the vagina. The importance of recognizing specific treatable causes such as monilial vaginitis must be emphasized.

Prevention includes instructing the patient on good hygiene measures. The perineum should be cleansed with a mild soap after each bowel movement. The patient is also instructed to use a water-based lubricant during vaginal intercourse to avoid mucosal irritation. Management includes providing comfort measures such as cold compresses or cool sitz baths for relief of pruritis and warm compresses for severe inflammation. Patients are instructed to wear cotton underpants and to avoid tight-fitting clothing and panty hose. Topical medications are applied based on cause (eg, miconazole nitrate [Nystatin] cream and suppositories for monilial vaginitis). Vaginal intercourse is avoided in the presence of vaginitis.

EFFECTS OF COMBINED MODALITY TREATMENT ON SKIN AND MUCOUS MEMBRANES

Combined modality therapy using radiation and chemotherapy is increasingly being used to manage a number of types of malignancies. The goals of combined modality therapy are to (1) improve local tumor control or prevent or reduce the risk of development of metastatic disease and (2) improve the cure rate while minimizing treatment-related complications (eg, improve the therapeutic ratio).[191]

The combined use of radiation therapy and chemotherapy has led to more severe skin reactions and mucositis. This enhanced response is due in part to the fact that both radiation and chemotherapeutic agents produce death and depletion of stem cells in rapidly proliferating tissues (eg, skin and mucous membranes). One of the first documented enhanced skin reactions due to combined modality therapy is the "recall skin reaction" observed in children treated for Wilms' tumor.[192] The recall skin reaction occurred in patients who had prior radiotherapy and who subsequently were given courses of actinomycin D. The recall phenomenon only occurred in the radiation portal and was usually more severe than the skin reaction seen during the original treatment. Phillips[192] proposes that this skin reaction is not an actual recall of the damage but rather the addition of chemotherapeutic cell kill to that already caused by radiation in the stem cell population in the basal layer. It appears that the number of stem cells remain depleted long after radiation. Therefore, if a certain chemotherapeutic agent such as actinomycin D, doxorubicin, or dacarbazine is given before this depletion is restored, the result is erythema or desquamation of the skin in the irradiated portals.

Chemotherapy and radiation can be administered sequentially or concomitantly, with the order of administration varying by protocol and type of malignancy. Chemotherapy agents associated with enhanced skin effects in combination therapy, according to the time of administration, are found in Table 30-14.[193] Except for the recall phenomenon, the majority of enhanced skin reactions occur when chemotherapy and radiation are administered concurrently. This enhanced effect is best illustrated in patients with breast cancer who received concurrent post-operative radiation and adjuvant chemotherapy. In a study by Hahn et al,[194] 26 patients with stage I or II breast cancer who received cyclophosphamide, methotrexate, and 5-FU with radiation had an 81% incidence of acute skin reactions, compared with 33% among 43 patients in a control group who received only radiation. In another study, severe skin reactions and unexpected skin necrosis were observed in patients with breast cancer who received

TABLE 30-14 Chemotherapeutic Agents Associated with Enhanced Skin Effects in Combination Therapy

Time of Drug Administration	Chemotherapeutic Agent
Concurrent with radiation	Actinomycin D Doxorubicin Bleomycin 5-Fluorouracil Hydroxyurea Methotrexate Doxorubicin-cyclophosphamide combination
Seven days or more after radiation	Actinomycin D Doxorubicin 5-Fluorouracil Methotrexate Doxorubicin-cyclophosphamide combination
Seven days or more before radiation	Methotrexate Doxorubicin-cyclophosphamide combination

Source: O'Rourke ME: Enhanced cutaneous effects in combined modality therapy. Oncol Nurs Forum 14:31-35, 1987.

postoperative doxorubicin and cyclophosphamide with radiation.[195] Specifically, these patients experienced moist desquamation in 50% to 80% of the treated areas and an increase in chronic radiation effects including fibrosis, skin atrophy, and telangiectasia. From this study and others, it became apparent that skin reactions could be either enhanced or reduced depending on the time interval between radiation and chemotherapy. For example, the risk of skin reaction was minimized when the time interval between administration of doxorubin and radiation was increased to 7 or more days.

In addition to enhanced skin reaction, the frequency and severity of mucositis is greater in patients receiving both chemotherapy and radiation than in those receiving either modality alone. This reaction has been demonstrated in patients receiving combined modality therapy for head and neck cancers.[118,196] The specific agents associated with enhanced responses, the degree of enhancement, and the time of maximum drug and radiation reaction for skin and mucous membrane are found in Table 30-15.[192]

Certain drugs, such as bleomycin, 5-FU, hydroxyurea, methotrexate, and doxorubicin, are known radiation-sensitizers and are associated with undesirable reactions in the skin, esophagus, GI tract, and lung. When patients receive radiation, these drugs generally are held until radiation is completed unless the drugs (5-FU or doxorubicin) are specifically used to enhance the effect of the radiation.

Dactinomycin, doxorubicin, and high-dose methotrexate can severely damage tissues that have received radiation exposure. This "radiation recall" can occur months after completion of radiation therapy but generally occurs within 7 days of radiation.[197]

The nursing care of patients receiving combined modality therapy is directed toward anticipating the potential for enhanced reactions and educating the patient and family regarding early recognition of treatment-related side effects and self care interventions. This can only be accomplished through frequent and open communication and collaboration between nurses in radiation therapy and

TABLE 30-15 Combined Modality: Enhanced Response on Skin and Mucous Membranes

Drug or Combination	Degree of Modification	Timing
Skin		
Actinomycin D	+ +	C, A
Adriamycin	+ +	C, A
Bleomycin	+	C
5-Fluorouracil	+	C, A
Hydroxyurea	+	C
Methotrexate	+ +	B, A
Adriamycin and cyclophosphamide	+ +	C
Adriamycin and cyclophosphamide	0	B, A >7 days
Mucosa (acute mucositis)		
Bleomycin	+ +	C
5-Fluorouracil	+, + +	C
Hydroxyurea	+	C
Methotrexate	+, + +	B, C
6-Mercaptopurine	+	C
Vincristine, actinomycin D, and cyclophosphamide	+, + +	C, A
Vincristine, bleomycin, cyclophosphamide (methotrexate)	+ +	B, C
Bleomycin, and cisplatin	+	B

+, definitely enhanced; + +, markedly enhanced; + + +, fatal.

C, concurrent; *B*, before radiation, usually weeks or months; *A*, after radiation, usually more than 7 days, weeks, or months.

Source: Philips TL: Tissue toxicity of radiation—drug interactions, in Sokol GH, Maickel RP (eds): Radiation Drug Interactions in the Treatment of Cancer. New York, Wiley, 1980, pp 175-200.

hematology-oncology departments. Before initiation of therapy, the nurse systematically assesses the patient's integumentary system, noting the color, texture, moisture, and temperature of skin and mucous membranes. In addition to a comprehensive physical assessment, the nurse must be aware of the patient's total treatment protocol and assess for other factors that may place the patient at greater risk for severe reaction (eg, elderly or poorly nourished patients, large surface volume that includes intertriginous skin folds).

Before discussing the possible treatment-related side effects with the patient and family, the nurse must assess the patient's understanding of the diagnosis and treatment plan as well as ability to read and comprehend the teaching material. Once this is accomplished, the nurse can begin to teach the patient and family about possible side effects, when these reactions can occur, and ways to manage the skin reaction. The use of printed materials or handwritten notes along with weekly conversations with the patient is helpful to reinforce initial teaching. Patients who receive combined modality therapy must understand that they have a greater risk of developing a severe skin reaction or mucositis and that occasionally this requires a temporary cessation of treatment. Because enhanced reactions can occur after the administration of radiation or chemotherapy or both, patients must understand what symptoms must be reported to the health care team and the importance of close follow-up with their physician and nurses in the radiation and hematology-oncology departments. Nurses are also responsible for managing these enhanced reactions, the goals of which are to alleviate discomfort, minimize further trauma and irritation, prevent infection, and promote healing. General skin and mouth care, management of severe skin reactions, and mucositis have been discussed previously.

In summary, the use of combined modality therapy involving radiation and chemotherapy offers a specific therapeutic advantage by providing enhanced tumor destruction. However, the synergism of these modalities may also enhance normal tissue toxicity. Regardless of the timing of combined modality therapy, it is clear that enhanced skin reactions may occur and that severity of these reactions will occur at a lower accumulated radiation dose with greater frequency.

MALIGNANT TUMOR WOUNDS

Ulcerating skin lesions can occur secondary to cancerous infiltration of the epithelium (Color plate 5) or by metastasis to the skin (Color plates 6 and 7). Metastatic skin lesions most commonly are associated with breast cancer but also can occur in cancers of the head and neck, lung, stomach, kidney, uterus, ovary, colon, and bladder as well as in lymphoma and melanoma. Metastatic skin lesions develop from local extension or tumor embolization into the epithelium and its lymph and blood vessels. As the cancer grows locally into the skin and its supporting structures, the tumor mass increases and loses its vascularity. Subsequently, capillary rupture, necrosis, and infection occur, resulting in wounds that are purulent, friable, malodorous, and sometimes itchy and painful.[198] These ulcerating skin lesions are a source of acute and chronic blood loss, protein and electrolyte loss, and a portal for life-threatening systemic infections. The development of severe skin involvement secondary to cancer causes significant morbidity to the patient so affected. In addition to the physical factors, these chronic wounds have a profound psychological impact on the patient and family, often causing embarrassment, fear, self-repugnance, withdrawal, depression, hopelessness, and fear that the condition will not be controllable.

Definitive cancer treatment, either local or systemic, is necessary to manage the problem. Local measures include radiotherapeutic sterilization and surgical excision of the ulcerated area. In breast cancer, radiation therapy or surgery has been used to treat such major problems as obstruction of regional vessels, invasion of the brachial plexus, and bleeding, necrotic, ulcerated areas of the chest wall. Because skin lesions indicate metastatic disease, systemic treatment (chemotherapy) is usually given concurrent with radiation. The success rate of radiation depends highly on the dose (higher doses yield better tumor control), the size of the field, and the number and size of the tumor recurrences treated.[199,200] Radiation can be particularly beneficial in eliminating the bleeding of tumor wounds. Doses of 200 to 400 cGy are given on a daily basis until bleeding is stopped.[201]

Surgical resection can offer good palliation for patients who present with ulcerated breast cancer as well as those with locally recurrent breast cancer or osteoradionecrosis. McKenna et al[202] define indications and contraindications for chest wall resection in patients with breast cancer. Indications include local symptoms such as pain, infection and ulceration, tumor recurrence despite radiotherapy, and infection that precludes chemotherapy. Relative contraindications are liver, lung, and bone metastasis and malignant pleural effusions. Absolute contraindications are brain metastasis, bone marrow involvement, bulky disease in two or more organs, and lack of response to several different chemotherapy regimens. One further absolute contraindication may be evidence of pericardial metastasis, since these patients rarely survive more than 3 months. In one series of 43 patients,[202] chest wall resection significantly reduced morbidity and improved quality of life by relieving pain, controlling infection, removing drainage and odor, and allowing chemotherapy for metastatic disease. However, survival benefit from chest wall resection in patients with locally recurrent breast cancer has not been established.

Systemic therapy involves initiating or changing drug or hormonal therapy. This occurs after the treatment of choice for widely disseminated local breast cancer or distant metastasis. Most commonly the patient will receive chemotherapy either during or following local treatment (radiation). In patients with breast cancer, continuous infusion of 5-FU or doxorubicin will act not only to treat presumed or proved distant disease but potentiate the cytotoxic effects of radiation by sensitizing the tumor cells in the radiation portal.

More recently, the carbon dioxide laser and hyperthermia have been used to manage ulcerating skin lesions. The carbon dioxide laser has been reported to excise contaminated and purulent wounds (benign and malignant), allowing safe wound closure in even the most highly contaminated situations.[203]

Hyperthermia combined with either chemotherapy or radiation has been helpful in decreasing the pain, bleeding, and drainage associated with these lesions as well as decreasing the size of tumor lesions. Significant differences in tumor regression were found in patients with 1-to 3-cm tumors of the chest wall who received greater than 3000 to 4000 cGy. There was no difference in tumor regression for radiation alone or with hyperthermia in lesions greater than 3 cm. There may be a definite role for hyperthermia in the management of these lesions; however, current technical difficulties and patient tolerance limit its usefulness at present.[201]

When definitive cancer treatment is not successful or appropriate, management of these ulcerating skin lesions becomes a nursing responsibility. In this situation, the goal of nursing care is not to heal the lesions but rather to improve a patient's quality of life by minimizing infection, odor, drainage, bleeding, and pain. Six nursing activities have been identified when caring for a patient with ulcerating metastatic lesions: (1) cleansing, (2) debridement, (3) reduction of superficial bacterial flora, (4) control of bleeding, (5) reduction of odor, and (6) teaching patients to manage the wound and dressing changes. In most situations the patient can be taught to cleanse the area using a mild soap (Basis) and rinsing in the shower or using a handheld irrigation device. If crusting is present over the wound, a dilute solution of hydrogen peroxide (1%) can be used to irrigate the wound, followed by a water or saline rinse. The goal is not debridement but rather cleansing. Mechanical debridement with wet-to-dry saline dressings or Betadine dressings is counterproductive. Such measures cause bleeding, which indicates disruption of whatever reepithelialization has occurred. For these wounds to heal there must first be adequate tumor control. A tumor does not "heal." Debridement of a tumor wound only leads to bleeding. The best that can be accomplished is healing of tissues around the tumor and maintenance of skin integrity. The goal is to maintain a clean, moist environment to promote wound healing. Granulating cells create a basement membrane for reepithelialization of tumor tissue. A dry wound that is mechanically debrided is continuously disrupted in its healing effort. However, if the wound has areas where necrotic tissue through dermis exists, then no amount of cleansing will promote healing. Provided that tumor therapy is at least controlling disease, then surgical debridement is indicated. Once the necrotic eschar is removed, the healing surface is kept clean and moist to promote granulation.

To maintain a moist (not wet) wound, the patient can be taught to apply moist saline dressings following the cleansing procedure and cover with a dry dressing. Water dressings such as Vigilon (see Color plate 7) will also keep the wound moist and clean and minimize odor. However, these dressings, because they absorb wound exudate, must be changed frequently and are very expensive. For patients who complain of itching over the lesion and neighboring skin, placing the Vigilon in the refrigerator before application eases the itching and is quite soothing. A number of dressings, gels, and ointments have proved useful in the management of ulcerating tumor wounds. See the appendix to this chapter.

REFERENCES

1. The integument (skin), in Crouch JE (ed): Functional Human Anatomy (ed 4). Philadelphia, Lea & Febiger, 1985, pp 74-84.
2. Cutaneous anatomy and physiology, in Rosen T, Lanning MB, Hill MJ (eds): The Nurse's Atlas of Dermatology. Boston, Little, Brown, 1983, pp 1-7.
3. Hair disease, in Habif TP (ed): Clinical Dermatology: A Color Guide to Diagnosis and Therapy. St Louis, CV Mosby, 1985, pp 493-504.
4. Johnson E: Cycles and patterns of hair growth, in Jarrett E (ed): The Hair Follicle. London, Academic Press, 1977, pp 1237-1249.
5. Baxley KO, Erdman LK, Henry EB, et al: Alopecia: Effect on cancer patients' body image. Cancer Nurs 7:499-503, 1984.
6. Robertshaw D: Biology of apocrine sweat glands, in Fitzpatrick TB, Eisen AZ, Wolff K, et al (eds): Dermatology in General Medicine (ed 3). New York, McGraw-Hill, 1987, pp 209-212.
7. Sato K: Biology of eccrine sweat glands, in Fitzpatrick TB, Eisen AZ, Wolff K, et al (eds): Dermatology in General Medicine (ed 3). New York, McGraw-Hill, 1987, pp 195-208.
8. Downing DT, Stewart ME, Strauss JS: Biology of sebaceous glands, in Fitzpatrick TB, Eisen AZ, Wolff K, et al (eds): Dermatology in General Medicine (ed 3). New York, McGraw-Hill, 1987, pp 185-190.
9. The skin, in Nasemann T, Sauerbrey W, Burgdorf WHC (eds): Fundamentals of Dermatology. New York, Springer-Verlag, 1983, pp 1-14.
10. Thames HD, Withers HR, Peters LJ, et al: Changes in early and late radiation responses with altered dose fractionation: Implications for dose-survival relationships. Int J Radiat Oncol Biol Phys 8:219-226, 1982.
11. Withers HR, Peters LJ, Thames HD, et al: Responses of normal tissues to dose fractionation. Cancer Bull 34:182-185, 1982.
12. Lever WF, Schaumburg-Lever G (eds): Histopathology of the Skin, Philadelphia, JB Lippincott, 1975.
13. Tessmer CF: Radiation effects in skin, in Berdjis CC (ed): Pathology of Irradiation. Baltimore, Williams & Wilkins, 1971, pp 146-170.
14. Chahbazian CM: The skin, in Moss WT, Co JD (eds): Radiation Oncology, Rationale, Techniques, Results (ed 6). St Louis, CV Mosby, 1989, pp 83-111.
15. Bloomer W, Hellman S: Normal tissue responses to radiation therapy. N Engl J Med 293:8-83, 1975.
16. Hilderley LJ: Radiotherapy, in Groenwald SL (ed): Cancer Nursing: Principles and Practice. Boston, Jones & Bartlett, 1987, pp 320-347.

17. Walker VA: Skin care during radiotherapy. Nurs Times 12:2068-2070, 1982.
18. Fajardo L-G LF: Skin, in Pathology of Radiation Injury. New York, Masson Inc., 1982, pp 186-200.
19. Stone HB, Milas L: Enhancement of radiation-induced normal tissue damage by a fibrosarcoma. Int J Radiat Oncol Biol Phys 13:1721-1724, 1987.
20. Fletcher GH: Textbook of Radiotherapy. Philadelphia, Lea & Febiger, 1980.
21. Rudolph R: Radiation ulcers, in Rudolph R, Noe JM (eds): Chronic Problem Wounds. Boston, Little, Brown, 1983, pp 87-94.
22. Reinisch JF, Puckett CL: Management of radiation wounds. Surg Clin North Am 64:795-802, 1984.
23. Luce EA: The irradiated wound. Surg Clin North Am 64:821-829, 1984.
24. Shack RB: Management of radiation ulcers. South Med J 75:1462-1466, 1982.
25. Rudolph R, Arganese T, Woodward M: The ultrastructure and etiology of chronic radiotherapy damage in human skin. Ann Plast Surg 9:282-292, 1982.
26. Khanna AK, Khanna A, Asthana AK: Post irradiation ulcer and topical metronidazole. Cancer Invest 6:123-124, 1988.
27. Kivisaari J, Mirrikaski J: Effects of hyperbaric oxygenation in prolonged hypoxia on the healing of open wounds. Acta Chir Scand 141:14-19, 1975.
28. McNally JC: Skin integrity, impairment related to radiation therapy, in McNally JC, Stair JC, Somerville ET (eds): Guidelines for Cancer Nursing Practice. Orlando, Fla, Grune & Stratton, 1985, pp 174-177.
29. Yasko JM: Skin reaction, in Yasko JM (ed): Care of the Client Receiving External Radiation Therapy (ed 2): Reston Va, Reston, 1982, pp 114-117.
30. Radiation Therapy Oncology Group.
31. Harvey SC, Withrow CD: Hormones, in Gennaro AR (ed): Remington's Pharmaceutical Sciences (ed 17): Pennsylvania, Mack, 1985, pp 951-1001.
32. Coleman J: Unpublished manuscript, 1988.
33. Dunagin WG: Clinical toxicity of chemotherapeutic agents: Dermatologic toxicity. Semin Oncol 9:14-22, 1982.
34. Hood AF: Cutaneous side-effects of cancer chemotherapy. Med Clin North Am 70:187-209, 1986.
35. Kerker BJ, Hood AF: Chemotherapy-induced cutaneous reactions. Semin Dermatol 8:173-181, 1989.
36. Moschella SL, Greenwald MA: Psoriasis with hydroxyurea: An 18 month study of 60 patients. Arch Dermatol 107:363-368, 1973.
37. Jaffe N, Paed D, Farber S, et al: Favorable response of metastatic osteogenic sarcoma to pulse high dose methotrexate with citrovorum rescue and radiation therapy. Cancer 31:1367-1373, 1973.
38. Lokich JJ, Moore C: Chemotherapy associated palmar-plantar erythrodysesthesia syndrome. Ann Int Med 101:798-800, 1984.
39. Dangel RB: Pruritis and cancer. Oncol Nurs Forum 13:17-21, 1986.
40. Hassey KM, Rose CM: Altered skin integrity in patients receiving radiation therapy. Oncol Nurs Forum 9:44-50, 1982.
41. Campbell J: Management of pruritis in the cancer patient. Oncol Nurs Forum 8:40-41, 1981.
42. Mallory SB, Watts JC: Sunburn, sun reactions, and sun protection. Pediatr Annu 16:77-84, 1987.
43. Hawk J: Sunlight and the skin. Occup Health 38:60-62, 1986.
44. Drugs that can cause photosensitivity. Med Lett Drugs Therapeutics 28:51-52, 1986.
45. Stewart DS: Indoor tanning: The nurse's role in preventing skin damage. Cancer Nurs 10:93-99, 1987.
46. Schreiber MM: Exposure to sunlight: Effects on the skin. Compr Ther 12:38-42, 1986.
47. Pathak MA: Sunscreens. Dermatol Clin 4:321-334, 1986.
48. Sunscreens. Consumer Reports 54:370-374, 1988.
49. DeSimone EM: Sunscreen and suntan products, in Handbook of Nonprescription Drugs (ed 7). Washington, DC, American Pharmaceutical Association, 1982, pp 499-511.
50. VanScott EJ: Drug induced alopecia, in Orfanos CE, Montagna W, Stuttgen G (eds): Hair Research Status and Future Aspects. Heidelberg-Berlin, Springer-Verlag, 1981, pp 469-474.
51. Lacassagne A, Gricouroff G: Action des radiations ionisanks sur l'organisme. Paris, Masson, 1956.
52. Cancer, cancer therapy, and hair. Lancet (Nov 19):1177-1178, 1983 (editorial).
53. Ayres S: Hair transplantation, in Epstein ED (ed): Skin Surgery (ed 6). Philadelphia, WB Saunders, 1987, pp 198-279.
54. Jacobs JB, Monell C: Treatment of radiation induced alopecia. Head Neck Surg 2:154-159, 1979.
55. Nordstrom REA, Holsti LR: Hair transplantation in alopecia due to radiation. Plast Reconstruct Surg 72:454-458, 1983.
56. Coates A, Abraham S, Kaye SB, et al: On the receiving end—patient perception of the side effects of cancer chemotherapy. Eur J Clin Oncol 19:203-208, 1983.
57. Cline BW: Prevention of chemotherapy-induced alopecia: A review of the literature. Cancer Nurs 7:221-228, 1984.
58. Crounse RG, VanScott EJ: Changes in scalp hair roots as a measure of toxicity from cancer chemotherapeutic drugs. J Invest Dermatol 35:83-90, 1960.
59. Kligman AM: Pathologic dynamics of human hair loss. Arch Dermatol 83:175-198, 1961.
60. Dorr RT, Fritz WL: Cancer Chemotherapy Handbook. New York, Elsevier, 1980.
61. Seipp CA: Adverse effects of treatment: Hair loss, in DeVita VT Jr, Hellman S, Rosenberg SA (eds): Cancer Principles and Practice of Oncology (vol 3). Philadelphia, JB Lippincott, 1989, pp 2135-2136.
62. Dean JC, Solomon SE, Griffith KS: Prevention of doxorubicin-induced hair loss with scalp hypothermia. N Engl J Med 301:1427-1429, 1979.
63. Keller JR, Blausey LA: Nursing issues and management in chemotherapy-induced alopecia. Oncol Nurs Forum 15:603-607, 1988.
64. Symonds RP, McCormick CV, Maxled KJ: Adriamycin alopecia prevented by cold air scalp cooling. Am J Clin Oncol 9:454-457, 1986.
65. David J, Speechley V: Scalp cooling to prevent alopecia. Nurs Times 83:36-37, 1987.
66. Johansen LV: Scalp hypothermia in the prevention of chemotherapy-induced alopecia. Acta Radiol (Oncol) 24:113-116, 1985.
67. Hennessey JD: Alopecia and cytotoxic drugs. Br Med J 2:1138, 1966 (letter).
68. Tierney AJ: Preventing chemotherapy-induced alopecia in cancer patients: Is scalp cooling worthwhile? J Adv Nurs 12:303-310, 1987.
69. Brager BL, Yasko J: Alopecia in Care of the Client Receiving Chemotherapy. Reston, Va, Reston, 1984, pp 211-221.
70. Lovejoy NC: Preventing hair loss during adriamycin therapy. Cancer Nurs 2:117-121, 1979.

71. Lyons A: Prevention of hair loss by headband during cytotoxic therapy. Lancet 1:354, 1974.
72. Pesce A, Cassuto JP, Joyner MV, et al: Scalp tourniquet in the prevention of chemotherapy-induced alopecia. N Engl J Med 298:1204-1205, 1978.
73. Maxwell M: Scalp tourniquets for chemotherapy-induced alopecia. Am J Nurs 80:900-903, 1980.
74. Kennedy M, Packard R, Grant M, et al: The effects of using Chemocap on occurrence of chemotherapy-induced alopecia. Oncol Nurs Forum 10:19-24, 1982.
75. Hunt JM, Anderson JE, Smith IE: Scalp hypothermia to prevent adriamycin-induced hair loss. Cancer Nurs 5:25-31, 1982.
76. Luce JK, Raffetto TJ, Crisp IM, et al: Prevention of alopecia by scalp cooling of patients receiving adriamycin. Cancer Chemo Rep 57:108-109, 1973 (abstr).
77. Guy R, Parker H, Shah S, et al: Scalp cooling by thermocirculator. Lancet 1:937-938, 1982.
78. Anderson JE, Hunt JM, Smith IE: Prevention of doxorubicin-induced alopecia by scalp cooling in patients with advanced breast cancer. Br Med J 282:423-424, 1981.
79. Wheelock JB, Myers MB, Krebs HB, et al: Ineffectiveness of scalp hypothermia in the prevention of alopecia in patients treated with doxorubicin and cisplatin combinations. Cancer Treat Rep 68:1387-1388, 1984.
80. Middleton J, Franks D, Buchanan RB, et al: Failure of scalp hypothermia to prevent hair loss when cyclophosphamide is added to doxorubicin and vincristine. Cancer Treat Rep 69:373-375, 1985.
81. Knobf T, Kalm D, Mealia M: Clinical observations of scalp cooling in patients receiving multidrug chemotherapy. Oncol Nurs Forum 16:abstr 288, 1989 (suppl).
82. Parker R: The effectiveness of scalp hypothermia in preventing cyclophosphamide-induced alopecia. Oncol Nurs Forum 14:49-53, 1987.
83. Satterwhite B, Zimm S: The use of scalp hypothermia in the prevention of doxorubicin-induced hair loss. Cancer 54:34-37, 1984.
84. Dean JC, Griffith KS, Cetas TC, et al: Scalp hypothermia: A comparison of ice packs and the Kold Kap in the prevention of doxorubicin-induced alopecia. J Clin Oncol 1:33-37, 1983.
85. Wittman G, Cadman E, Chen M: Misuse of scalp hypothermia. Cancer Treat Rep 65:507-508, 1981.
86. Seipp CA: Scalp hypothermia: Indications for precautions. Oncol Nurs Forum 10:12, 1983 (letter).
87. Wood LA: Possible prevention of adriamycin-induced alopecia by tocopherol. N Engl J Med 312:1060, 1985.
88. Perez JE, Macchiavelli M, Leone BA, et al: High-dose alphatocopherol as a preventive of doxorubicin-induced alopecia. Cancer Treat Rep 70:1213-1214, 1986.
89. Didonato K: Standards of clinical nursing practice: Alopecia. Cancer Nurs 8:76-77, 1985.
90. Allegra JC, Hamm JT: Hormonal therapy for cancer, in Wittes RE (ed): Manual of Oncologic Therapeutics. Philadelphia, JB Lippincott, 1989, pp 170-176.
91. Sonis ST, Sonis AL, Lieberman A: Oral complications in patients receiving treatment for malignancies other than the head and neck. J Am Dent Assoc 97:468-472, 1978.
92. Carl W. Higby DJ: Oral manifestations of bone marrow transplantation. Am J Clin Oncol 8:81-87, 1985.
93. Dudjak LA: Mouth care for mucositis due to radiation therapy. Cancer Nurs 10:131-140, 1987.
94. Marcial VA: The oral cavity and oropharynx, in Moss WT, Cox JD (eds): Radiation Oncology, Techniques, Results (ed 6). St Louis, CV Mosby, 1989, pp 112-163.
95. Cooper JS, Fried PR: Toxicity of oral radiotherapy in patients with acquired immunodeficiency syndrome. Arch Otolaryngol Head Neck Surg 113:327-328, 1987.
96. Blozis C. Robinson JE: Oral tissue changes caused by radiation therapy and their management. Dent Clin North Am 12:643-656, 1968.
97. Engelmeier RL, King GE: Complications of head and neck radiation therapy and their management. J Prosthet Dent 49:514-522, 1983.
98. Lockhart PB, Sonis ST: Relationship of oral complications to peripheral blood leukocyte and platelet counts in patients receiving cancer chemotherapy. Oral Surg 48:21-28, 1979.
99. Sonis ST: Epidemiology, frequency, distribution, mechanisms and histopathology, in Peterson DE, Sonis ST (eds): Oral Complications of Cancer Chemotherapy. The Hague, The Netherlands, Martinus Nijhoff, 1983, pp 1-12.
100. Beck S, Yasko JM: Guidelines for Oral Care. Cary, IL, Sage Products, 1984.
101. Engelking C: Managing stomatitis: A nursing process approach, in Supportive Care for the Patient with Cancer. New York, Medical Marketing Interaction, 1988, pp 20-28.
102. Daeffler RJ: Mucous membranes, in Johnson BL, Gross J (eds): Handbook of Oncology Nursing. Bethany, Conn, Fleschner, 1985, pp 253-274.
103. Daeffler R: Oral hygiene measures for patients with cancer. I. Cancer Nurs 3:347-356, 1980.
104. Hickey AJ, Toth BB, Lindquist JB: Effect of intravenous hyperalimentation and oral care on the development of oral stomatitis during cancer chemotherapy. J Prosthet Dent 47:188-193, 1982.
105. Beck S: Impact of a systematic oral care protocol on stomatitis after chemotherapy. Cancer Nurs 2:185-189, 1979.
106. Levine N, Greenwald ES: Mucocutaneous side effects of cancer chemotherapy. Cancer Treat Rev 5:67-84, 1978.
107. Seifert P, Baker LH, Reed ML, et al: Comparison of continuously infused 5-fluorouracil with bolus injection in treatment of patients with colorectal adenocarcinoma. Cancer 36:123-128, 1975.
108. Carl W: Oral manifestations of systemic chemotherapy and their management. Sem Surg Oncol 2:187-199, 1986.
109. Lockhart PB: Dental management of patients receiving chemotherapy, in Peterson DE, Sonis ST (eds): Oral Complications of Cancer Chemotherapy, The Hague, The Netherlands, Martinus Nijhoff, 1983, pp 113-149.
110. Ginsberg MK: A study of oral hygiene nursing care. Am J Nurs 61:67-69, 1961.
111. Van Drimmelen J, Rollins HF: Evaluation of a commonly used oral hygiene agent. Nurs Res 18:327-332, 1969.
112. Lindquist SF, Hickey AJ, Drane JB: Effect of oral hygiene on stomatitis in patients receiving cancer chemotherapy. J Prosthet Dent 40:312-314, 1978.
113. Capizzi RL, DeConti RC, Marsh JC, et al: Methotrexate therapy of head and neck cancer: Improvement in therapeutic index by the use of leucovorin "rescue." Cancer Res 30:1782-1788, 1970.
114. Daeffler R: Oral hygiene measures for patients with cancer. III. Cancer Nurs 4:29-35, 1981.
115. Goodman M, Stoner C: Mucous membrane integrity impairment of Stomatitis, in McNally J (ed): Guidelines for Cancer Nursing Practice (ed 2) Orlando, Fla, Grune & Stratton, 1990 (in press).
116. Gainey D, Dose AM: The use of ice chips to minimize stomatitis in patients receiving 5-fluorouracil plus leucovorin. Oncol Nurs Forum 16:173, 1989 (abstr).
117. Daeffler R: Oral hygiene measure for patients with cancer. II. Cancer Nurs 3:427-432, 1980.

118. Lustig RA, Demari P, Kramer S: Adjuvant methotrexate in radiotherapeutic management of advanced tumors of the head and neck. Cancer 37:2703-2708, 1976.
119. Goodman M: Side-effects of chemotherapy. Semin Oncol Nurs 5:29-52, 1989 (suppl 1).
120. Auguste LJ, Nava H: Postchemotherapy esophagitis: The endoscopic diagnosis and its impact on survival. J Surg Oncol 33:254-258, 1986.
121. Nunnally C, Donoghue M: Esophagitis, in Yasko JM (ed): Nursing Management of Symptoms Associated with Chemotherapy. Adria Laboratories, 1986, pp 53-55.
122. Finkelstein E: Nifedipine for radiation and oesophagitis. Lancet 1:1205-1206, 1986 (letter).
123. Stevens KR: The esophagus, in Moss WT, Cox JD (eds): Radiation Oncology, Rationale, Techniques, Results (ed 6). St Louis, CV Mosby, 1989, pp 351-361.
124. Berthrong M, Fajaroo LF: Radiation injury in surgical pathology. II. Alimentary tract. Am J Surg Pathol 5:153-178, 1981.
125. Umsawasdi T, Valdivieso M, Barkley HT, et al: Esophageal complications from combined chemoradiotherapy (cyclophosphamide + adriamycin + cisplatin + XRT) in the treatment of non–small cell lung cancer. Int J Radiat Oncol Biol Phys 11:511-519, 1985.
126. Rubin P, Casarett GW: Clinical Radiation Pathology (vols 1 and 2). Philadelphia, WB Saunders, 1968.
127. Pizzo PA, Meyers J: Infections in the cancer patient, in DeVita VT Jr, Hellman S, Rosenberg SA (eds): Cancer Principles and Practice of Oncology, Philadelphia, JB Lippincott, 1989, pp 2088-2133.
128. Brereton HD, Kent CH, Johnson RE: Chemotherapy and radiation therapy for small cell carcinoma of the lung. A remedy for past therapeutic failure, in Progress in Cancer Research and Therapy (vol 2). New York, Raven Press, 1979, pp 575-586.
129. Chabora BM, Hopfan S, Wittes R: Esophageal complications in the treatment of oat cell carcinoma with combined irradiation and chemotherapy. Radiology 123:185-187, 1977.
130. Kent CH, Brereton HD, Johnson RE: "Total" therapy for oat cell carcinoma of the lung. Int J Radiat Oncol Biol Phys 2:427-432, 1977.
131. Greco FA, Brereton HD, Kent H, et al: Adriamycin and enhanced radiation reaction in normal esophagus and skin. Ann Intern Med 85:294-298, 1978.
132. Feld R: Complications in the treatment of small cell carcinoma of the lung. Cancer Treat Rev 8:5-25, 1981.
133. Greco FA, Richardson RL, Schulman SF, et al: Treatment of oat cell carcinoma of the lung: Complete remissions, acceptable complications, and improved survival. Br Med J 2:10-11, 1978.
134. Eagan RT, Lee RE, Carr DT: Adriamycin and radiation reaction. Ann Intern Med 85:243, 1971.
135. Abeloff MD, Klaskersky J, Drings PD, et al: Complications of treatment of small cell carcinoma of the lung. Cancer Treat Rep 67:21-26, 1983.
136. Slee GR, Wagner SM, McCullough FS: Odynophagia in patients with malignant disorders. Cancer 55:2877-2879, 1985.
137. Nicolopoulos W, Mantidis A, Stathopoulos E, et al: Prophylactic administration of indomethacin for irradiation esophagitis. Radiother Oncol 3:23-25, 1985.
138. McGraw BF, Caldwell GE: Investigational drug information: Sucralfate. Drug Intell Clin Pharmacol 15:578-580,1981.
139. Ferraro JM, Mattern JQA: Sucralfate suspension for stomatitis. Drug Intell Clin Pharmacol 18:153, 1984 (letter).
140. Parashos PJ, Bell PL, Poland JM, et al: Comment: Revised treatment of ulcerative stomatitis. Drug Intell Clin Pharmacol 19:139, 1985 (letter).
141. Eras P, Goldstein MJ, Sherlock P: *Candida* infections of the gastrointestinal tract. Medicine 51:367-375, 1972.
142. Koose BE, Wickremesingle PC, Kozinn PJ, et al: *Candida* esophagitis—a prospective study of 27 cases. Gastroenterology 71:715-719, 1976.
143. Yeoh EK, Horowitz M: Radiation enteritis. Surg Gynecol Obstet 165:373-379, 1987.
144. O'Brien PH, Jenrette JM, Garvin AJ: Radiation enteritis. Am Surg 53:501-504, 1987.
145. Galland RB, Spencer J: Surgical management of radiation enteritis. Surgery 99:133-138, 1986.
146. Mulholland MW, Levitt SH, Song CW, et al: The role of luminal contents in radiation enteritis. Cancer 54:2396-2402, 1984.
147. Kline JC, Buchler DA, Boone ML, et al: The relationship between reactions to complications in the radiation therapy of cancer of the cervix. Radiology 105:413-416, 1972.
148. Bourne RG, Kearsley JH, Grove WD, et al: The relationship between early and late gastrointestinal complications of radiation therapy for carcinoma of the cervix. Int J Radiat Oncol Biol Phys 9:1445-1450, 1983.
149. Steven KR: The stomach and intestine, in Moss WT, Cox JD (eds): Radiation Oncology, Rationale, Techniques, Results (ed 6). St Louis, CV Mosby, 1989, pp 362-380.
150. Stein RS: Radiation-recall enteritis after actinomycin-D and adriamycin therapy. South Med J 72:960-961, 1978.
151. Thomas PRM, Lindblad AS, Stablein DM, et al: Toxicity associated with adjuvant postoperative therapy for adenocarcinoma of the rectum. Cancer 57:1130-1134, 1986.
152. Haddad GK, Grodinsky C, Allen H: The spectrum of radiation enteritis: Surgical considerations. Dis Colon Rectum 26:590-594, 1983.
153. Mason GR, Dietrich P, Friedland GW, et al: The radiological findings in radiation induced enteritis and colitis: A review of 30 cases. Clin Radiol 21:232-247, 1970.
154. Rogers F, Goldstein HM: Roentgen manifestations of radiation to the gastrointestinal tract. Gastrointest Radiol 2:281-291, 1977.
155. Ludgate SM, Merrick MV: The pathogenesis of post irradiation chronic diarrhea: Measurement of SeHCAT and B12 absorption for differential diagnosis determines treatment. Clin Radiol 36:275-278, 1985.
156. Mendelson RM, Nolan DJ: The radiological features of chronic radiation enteritis. Clin Radiol 36:141-148, 1985.
157. Zentler-Munro PL, Bessell EM: Medical management of radiation enteritis—an algorithmic guide. Clin Radiol 38:291-294, 1987.
158. Beer WH, Fan A, Halsted CH: Clinical and nutritional implications of radiation enteritis. Am J Clin Nutr 41:85-91, 1985.
159. Trier JS, Browning TH: Morphologic response of the mucosa of human small intestine to x-ray exposure. J Clin Invest 45:194-204, 1966.
160. Joslin CAF, Smith CW, Malik A: The treatment of cervix cancer using high activity Co-60 sources. Br J Radiol 45:257-270, 1972.
161. Arlow FL, Dekovich AA, Priest RJ, et al: Bile acids in radiation-induced diarrhea. South Med J 80:1259-1261, 1987.
162. McArdle AH, Reid EC, Laplante MP, et al: Prophylaxis against radiation injury. Arch Surg 121:879-885, 1986.
163. Brown MS, Buchanan RB, Karren SJ: Clinical observations on the effects of elemental diet supplementation during irradiation. Clin Radiol 31:19-20, 1980.

164. Wobbes T, Verschueren RCJ, Lubbers EJC: Surgical aspects of radiation enteritis of the small bowel. Dis Colon Rect 27:89-92, 1984.
165. Kwitko AO, Pieterse AS, Hecker R, et al: Chronic radiation injury to the intestine: A clinico-pathological study. Aust NZ J Med 12:272-277, 1982.
166. Schofield FF, Holden D, Carr HD: Bowel disease after radiotherapy. JR Soc Med 76:463-466, 1983.
167. Wellwood JM, Jackson BT: The intestinal complications of radiotherapy. Br J Surg 60:814-818, 1973.
168. DeCosse JJ, Rhodes RS, Wentz WB, et al: The natural history and management of radiation induced injury of the gastrointestinal tract. Ann Surg 170:369-384, 1969.
169. Smith ST, Seski JC, Copeland LJ, et al: Surgical management of irradiation-induced small bowel damage. Obstet Gynecol 65:563, 1985.
170. Lillemore KD, Brigham RA, Harmon JW, et al: Surgical management of small-bowel radiation enteritis. Arch Surg 118:905-907, 1983.
171. Smith DH, Decosse JJ: Radiation damage to the small intestine. World J Surg 10:189-194, 1986.
172. Green N, Iba G, Smith W: Measures to minimize small intestine injury in the irradiated pelvis. Cancer 35:1633-1640, 1975.
173. Devereux DF, Kavanah MT, Feldman MI, et al: Small bowel exclusion from the pelvis by polyglycolic acid mesh sling. J Surg Oncol 26:107-112, 1984.
174. Slavin RE, Dias MA, Saral R: Cytosine arabinoside induced gastrointestinal toxic alterations in sequential chemotherapeutic protocols. Cancer 42:1747-1759, 1978.
175. Mitchell EP, Schein PS: Gastrointestinal toxicity of chemotherapeutic agents. Semin Oncol 9:52-57, 1982.
176. Basch A: Changes in elimination. Sem Oncol Nurs 3:287-292, 1987.
177. Horton J, Olson KB, Sullivan J, et al: 5-Fluorouracil in cancer: An improved regimen. Ann Intern Med 73:896-900, 1970.
178. Fainstein V, Bodey GP, Fekety R: Relapsing PMC associated with cancer chemotherapy. J Infect Dis 143:865, 1981.
179. Byfield JE, Lacey C: Principles of radiation therapy, in Morrow CP, Townsend DE (eds): Synopsis of Gynecologic Oncology (ed 3). New York, Wiley, 1987, pp 459-520.
180. Pitkin RM, Bradbury JT: The effect of topical estrogen on irradiated vaginal epithelium. Am J Obstet Gynecol 92:175-182, 1965.
181. Poma PA: Post-irradiation vaginal occlusion: Non-operative management. Int J Obstet Gynecol 18:90, 1980.
182. Pitkin RM, VanVoorhis LW: Post-irradiation vaginitis: An evaluation of prophylaxis and topical estrogen. Radiology 99:417-421, 1971.
183. Goldstein F, Khomy J, Thorton JJ: Treatment of chronic radiation enteritis and colitis with salicylazofulfapyridine and systemic corticosteroids. Am J Gastroenterol 65:201-208, 1979.
184. DiRaimondo CV, Roach AC, Meador CK: Gynecomastia from exposure to vaginal estrogen cream. N Engl J Med 302:1089-1090, 1980 (letter).
185. Martin PL, Yen SSC, Burnier AM, et al: Systemic absorption and sustained effects of vaginal estrogen creams. JAMA 242:2699-2700, 1979.
186. King J: Vaginitis. J Obstet Gynecol Nurs 13:413, 1984 (suppl).
187. Grant MM, Davidson SB: Assessment of vaginitis in Stromberg MF (ed): Instruments for Assessing Clinical Problems. East Norwalk, Conn, Appleton-Lange, 1988, pp 401-414.
188. Kaufman RH: Anatomy of the vulva and vagina, in Gardner HL, Kaufman RH (eds): Benign Diseases of the Vulva and Vagina (ed 2). Boston, GK Hall, 1981.
189. Hartman P, Diddle AW: Vaginal stenosis following irradiation therapy for carcinoma of the cervic uteri. Cancer 30:426-429, 1970.
190. Richards S, Hiratzka S: Vaginal dilatation post-pelvic irradiation: A patient education tool. Oncol Nurs Forum 12:89-91, 1986.
191. Howes AE, Coleman CN, Phillips TL, et al: Combined modality therapy using cytotoxic agents and radiation therapy. Am J Clin Oncol 11:304-312, 1988.
192. Phillips TL: Tissue toxicity of radiation-drug interactions, in Sokol GH, Maickel RP (eds): Radiation Drug Interactions in the Treatment of Cancer. New York, Wiley, 1980, pp 175-200.
193. O'Rourke ME: Enhanced cutaneous effects in combined modality therapy. Oncol Nurs Forum 14:31-35, 1987.
194. Hahn P, Hallberg O, Virkerlof KJ: Acute skin reactions in postoperative breast cancer patients receiving radiotherapy plus chemotherapy. Am J Radiol 130:137-139, 1978.
195. Aristizabel SA, Manning MR, Miller RC, et al: Combined effects of chemotherapy and radiotherapy on normal tissue tolerance, in Frontiers of Radiation Therapy and Oncology (vol 13), New York, Basel Karger, 1979, pp 103-112.
196. Peterson DE, Sonis ST (eds): Oral Complications of Cancer Chemotherapy. Boston, Martinus Nijhoff, 1983.
197. Aristizabal SA: Complications from combination chemotherapy and irradiation in oat cell lung cancer. JAMA 237:1824, 1977.
198. Foltz A: Nursing care of ulcerating metastatic lesions. Oncol Nurs Forum 7:8-13, 1980.
199. Levitt SH, Perez CA: Breast cancer, in Perez CA, Brady LW (eds): Principles and Practice of Radiation Oncology. Philadelphia, JB Lippincott, 1987, pp 730-792.
200. Wilson JF: The breast, in Moss WT, Cox JD (eds): Radiation Oncology Rationale, Technique, Results (ed 6). St Louis, CV Mosby, 1989, pp 312-350.
201. Perez CA, Emami BN, Kuske RR, et al: Irradiation and hyperthermia in the treatment of recurrent carcinoma of the breast in the chest wall: MIR and RTOG Experience 1987-1988. Radiation Oncology Scientific Report. St Louis, Mo, pp 278-287.
202. McKenna RJ, McMurtrey MJ, Larson DL, et al: A perspective on chest wall resection in patients with breast cancer. Ann Thoracic Surg 38:482-487, 1984.
203. Hinshaw JR, Kerrera HR, Lanzafame RJ, et al: The use of carbon dioxide laser permits primary closure of contaminates and purulent lesions and wounds. Lasers Surg Med 6:581-583, 1987.

APPENDIX Survey of Commercial Products for Wound Care

Wound Cleansing/ Irrigating Solutions	Advantages	Disadvantages	Comments	Indications for Use	Method of Application
Hydrogen peroxide commercial strength—3%	Inexpensive, readily available	Unstable; poor penetrability; interferes with granulation if used full strength; May damage normal tissue; Toxic in vitro to human fibroblasts at concentrations greater than 0.03%	Never to be used full strength; decomposes rapidly in the presence of slight traces of impurities and on exposure to bright light	Oxidizing agent that mechanically loosens tissue, has brief germicidal activity at full strength	Irrigate wound with large-tip (60 mL) syringe or soak gauze with solution and apply to skin; protect normal skin with petroleum or zinc-based ointment; if soak is allowed to dry, it will adhere to wound bed
Betadine (povidone iodine; Purdue-Frederick, Norwalk, CT) commercial strength—1%	Effective against broad spectrum; long-lasting action	May damage fibroblasts; stains skin an intense yellowish brown color; painful on open wounds; solution may not be stable	Hypersensitivity can occur in patients with iodine allergy; may cause contact dermatitis; incidence of allergic reactions is 12% to 20% and may occur in the absence of sensitivity to iodine solutions; available in a variety of formulas (spray, foam, vaginal gel); germicidal action	Disinfectant useful in disinfecting intact skin; avoid detergent formula (Scrub); nonfibroblast toxic and bactericidal 0.001 concentrate	Irrigate wound with large-tipped (60 mL) syringe or soak gauze with solution and apply to skin; protect normal skin with petroleum or zinc-based ointment; if soak is allowed to dry, it will adhere to wound bed
Dakin's solution (sodium hypochlorite) standard strength—0.5%	Loosens, dissolves, and deodorizes necrotic tissue; has bactericidal, sporicidal, fungicidal, and protozoacidal effects	Dissolves clots and delays clotting; hypochlorite is inactivated by organic matter; may cause burning	Irritating to healthy skin and must be rinsed promptly; protect solution from light; solutions are relatively unstable and must be prepared daily	Debride and dissolve necrotic tissue; reduce odor	Recommend diluting solution to 0.005% strength for wound irrigation or soak gauze and apply to skin; protect normal skin with petroleum or zinc-based ointment; do not allow soak to become dry, since it will adhere to wound bed
(Chlorhexidine) Hibiclens (Stuart Pharmaceuticals, Wilmington, DE)	Potent antiseptic activity; rapidly bactericidal to gram-positive and some gram-negative bacilli	Inactive against bacterial spores at room temperature; prolonged repetitive use may cause contact dermatitis	pH dependent (5.5 to 7.0 optimum range); pH for optimal wound healing is 4.5 to 5.5; active residue (26%) remains on skin after 29 hours; available in liquid and detergent formulas	Avoid or use with extreme caution; retards epithelialization; Avoid detergent formula (Scrub)	

Biolex wound cleanser (Catalina Biomedical, Duarte, CA)	Nontoxic; nonharmful to proliferating fibroblasts; does not contain sodium lauryl, sulfate, or harsh antiseptics		Spray nozzle has various settings (stream to gentle moisturizing spray); does not need to be rinsed from wound bed.	Aids in the removal of wound debris and slough; helps facilitate softening and removal of eschar	Spray entire wound bed and ½ in (1 cm) margin of good tissue; or soak gauze pad to wound bed and spray until completely saturated
Cara-Klenz (Carrington Laboratories, Dallas, TX)	Contains a blend of moisturizers and wetting agents; nonirritating to tissues; will not harm fibroblast cells		Spray nozzle adjusts from fine mist to powerful jet spray; does not need to be rinsed from wound bed	Assists in debridement and removal of particulate matter; assists in softening of eschar	Spray entire wound bed and ½ in (1 cm) margin of good tissue; or soak gauze pad to wound bed and spray until completely saturated

Tissue Necrosis/ Debriding Agents	Advantages	Disadvantages	Comments	Indications for Use	Method of Application
Granulex (Trypsin, 1.0 mg, balsam of peru, 72.5 mg, and castor oil, 650 mg) (Hickam, Sugarland, TX)	Easy to apply; reduces odor; reduces premature epithelial cell damage by providing a protective covering	Causes occasional burning; wound must be cleansed before application	Balsam of Peru is an effective capillary stimulant used to increase circulation within the wound bed and has a mild bacteriostatic action; can dissolve clots	Topical debridement of small amounts of eschar and necrotic tissue	Aerosal spray; should be applied at least twice daily
Elase (fibrinolysin and deoxyribonuclease) (Parke-Davis, Morris Plains, NJ)	Can be used as a debriding agent in a variety of inflammatory and infected lesions	Localized redness; inactivated by plasma, serum, urea, and heat	Hypersensitivity can occur in patients with bovine and mercury allergy; fibrinolysin acts primarily on fibrin in blood clots and exudates; deoxyribonucleasae attacks DNA in devitalized tissue and disintegrates cells; enzymatic debridement is directed primarily against denatured protein and dead tissue, leaving normal tissue relatively unaffected; solutions must be prepared daily	Topical debridement of eschar and necrotic tissue	Solution must be prepared fresh daily; loss of potency is delayed somewhat by refrigeration; wound must be cleansed before application; dense eschars should be removed surgically before therapy is initiated; dressings should be changed at least once a day, preferably two or three times daily; solution: mix vial of powder with 10 mL saline; saturate gauze with solution and pack in wound; allow gauze to dry 6 to 8 hours; wound is mechanically debrided when dried gauze is removed; repeat three to four times daily Ointment: Cleanse wound and gently pat dry with gauze; apply a thin layer of ointment and cover with nonocclusive dressing

APPENDIX Survey of Commercial Products for Wound Care (continued)

Tissue Necrosis/ Debriding Agents	Advantages	Disadvantages	Comments	Indications for Use	Method of Application
Travase (Sutilains) (Flint, Deerfield, IL)	Enzymatic activity of sutilains selectively digests necrotic soft tissue, hemoglobin and purulent exudate	Mild transient burning, paresthesia, bleeding, and dermatitis	Optimal activity at pH range 6.0 to 6.8 in a moist wound; if bleeding or dermatitis occurs, therapy should be discontinued; store in refrigerator at 2° to 8°C (35° to 40°F); action is adversely affected by detergents and metallic ion compounds (silver mercury); if hydrogen peroxide is used to cleanse the wound, it should be used before application of sutilains	Topical debridement of eschar and necrotic tissue; action is unaffected by presences in wound of topical bacitracin, gentimycin, neomycin, penicillin, sulfadiazine, streptomycin, or systemic anti-infectives; allergic reactions to sutilains have not been reported; such symptoms should suggest reaction to another agent being used concomitantly	Apply ointment 3 or 4 times daily; onset of action occurs after 1 hour, and optimal effects occur during the first 6 hours; thoroughly cleanse and moisten wound area and apply a very thin layer (a small dab will cover an area as large as the back of the hand); cover wound and extend ointment ¼ to ½ in beyond areas being debrided; cover with loose nonadherent dressing; maximum effect in wound ulcers is usually achieved in 8 to 12 days
Santyl (collagenase) (Kaall, Whippany, NJ)	Enzymatic activity derived from fermentation of clostridium histolyticum. Able to liquify necrotic tissue without affecting collagen in newly formed granulation	Lacks direct anti-infective properties; may cause local pain, burning, redness, and irritation	Optimal activity at pH range 6.0 to 8.0; action is adversely affected by detergents, hexachlorophene, and metallic ion compounds (silver, mercury). Normal saline, hydrogen peroxide, modified Dakin's solution, neomycin, bacitracin, polymyxine, and streptomycin do not interfere with collagenase activity	Topical debridement of eschar and necrotic tissue	Apply to wound every other day or more frequently if the dressing becomes soiled; collagenase should be discontinued when necrotic tissue has been debrided and healthy granulation tissue is present, generally in 7 to 14 days
Silvadene (silver sulfadiazine) (Marion, Kansas City, MO)	Broad microbial activity including many gram-negative and gram-positive bacteria and yeast; does not alter pH or electrolyte balance	Topically applied proteolytic enzymes may be inactivated by the silver in the silver sulfadiazine; silver sulfadiazine reacts with most heavy metals, with possible release of silver and darkening cream	Hypersensitivity can occur in patients with sulfa or silver allergy; pain, burning, itching, rash, and reversible leukopenia are possible side effects	Short-term treatment of wound infection	Apply once or twice daily to a thickness of approximately 1⁄16 in (0.16 cm)

Bacitracin ointment (polymyxin B-bacitracin ointment) (Quad, Indianapolis, IN)	Broad microbial activity against many gram-positive organisms	Ineffective against most gram-negative organisms; prolonged use may result in overgrowth of nonsusceptible organisms, especially *Candida albicans*	Hypersensitivity can occur to any ingredient in the formulation	Short-term treatment of wound infection	Wound must be cleansed before application; apply thin layer of ointment and cover with a nonadherent dressing
Neosporin Ointment (neomycin-polymyxin B sulfate-bacitracin-zinc) (Burroughs-Wellcome, Research Triangle Park, NC)	Aminoglycoside antibiotic with broad-spectrum antibacterial activity against gram-negative and some gram-positive organisms	May be absorbed systemically; prolonged use may result in overgrowth of nonsusceptible organisms, especially *Candida albicans*	A high incidence of allergic dermatitis is associated with topical neomycin; hypersensitivity may occur to neomycin or any ingredient in the formulation	Short-term treatment of wound skin infection	Wound must be cleansed before application. Apply thin layer of ointment 1 to 3 times a day; duration of treatment should be limited to 7 to 10 days

Local Bleeding/ Hemostatic Agents	Advantages	Disadvantages	Comments	Indications for Use	Method of Application
Silver nitrate pencils (silver nitrate, toughened)	Cauterizes small bleeding vessels within the wound bed and friable surface tumors	Cannot control extensive bleeding	If healthy skin is accidentally touched, wash area with normal saline; skin stains usually persist indefinitely or disappear very slowly	Effective in controlling oozing of blood from capillaries and small vessels within the wound bed	Before applying, cleanse area to be treated; dip pencil in water and apply to the area until bleeding stops; the treated area will appear grayish black (silver stain)
Gelfoam (absorbable gelatin) (Upjohn, Kalamazoo, MI)	Can absorb and hold within its mesh many times its weight of whole blood	Use of Gelfoam is not recommended in the presence of infection	When applied to bleeding areas in wound, liquifies within 2 to 5 days; by absorbing fluid, Gelfoam may expand and impinge on neighboring structures; avoid overpacking in cavities or closed tissue spaces; since gelatin sponge is completely absorbed, removal is unnecessary	Effective in controlling frank bleeding from blood vessels within the wound bed	Cut to desired size (minimal amount is applied to cover area); apply to bleeding area with moderate pressure for 10 to 15 seconds; may be moistened with sterile isotonic saline or thrombin solution. Squeeze to remove air bubbles and reimmerse in solution—sponge should swell to original size and shape; if not, knead vigorously until all air is removed and reimmerse in solution; wet piece may be blotted with gauze before application to bleeding area; apply moderate pressure for 10 to 15 seconds

APPENDIX Survey of Commercial Products for Wound Care (continued)

Local Bleeding/ Hemostatic Agents	Advantages	Disadvantages	Comments	Indications for Use	Method of Application
Thrombostat (Thrombin) (Parke-Davis, Morris Plains, NJ)	Can be used as a solution, in dry form, or by mixing thrombin with blood plasma to form fibrin "glue"; may be used in conjunction with absorbable gelatin sponge	Intravascular clotting and death if thrombin is allowed to enter large vessels	Hypersensitivity can occur in patients with bovine allergy; thrombin activity affected by dilute acids, alkali, heat, and salts of heavy metals	Effective in controlling oozing of blood from capillaries and small vessels within the wound bed	Sponge area free of blood before applying thrombin powder; a spray may be used on the surface of the wound; may be flooded using a sterile syringe and small gauge needle; the most effective hemostasis results when thrombin mixes freely with the blood as soon as it reaches the surface

Dressings/Occlusive Hydrocolloid	Advantages	Disadvantages	Comments	Indications for Use	Method of Application
DuoDerm (Squibb, Convatec, Princeton, NJ) (Made of gelatin, pectin and carboxymethyl-cellulose; sodium incorporated in polysobutylene) Comfeel Ulcer Care Dressing (Kendall, Mansfield MA) (made of carboxymethylcellulose particles embedded in an elastic mesh) Restore (Hollister, Libertyville, IL) (Made of cross-linked synthetic elastaniers and hydrocolloids with flexible foam–impermeable outer layer)	Promotes rapid epithelialization; stimulates debridement and healing of chronic ulcers; adheres securely to dry or moist skin; reduces or eliminates wound pain and absorbs fairly large volumes of wound fluid; dressings can remain in place for up to 7 days, thereby reducing frequency of dressing changes, making it less expensive and easy to apply and remove; not penetrated by bacteria, which isolates the wound against further bacterial contamination	Produces a yellow-brown colorless fluid that usually becomes malodorous and contains many bacteria and may be mistaken as an infection; opaque	If leakage or infection is present, change dressing immediately to nonocclusive absorbent dressing, which is available in several sizes—4 × 4, 6 × 8, 8 × 8, 8 × 12. When dressing, press down on skin and carefully lift all edges of the dressing and lift carefully from wound, if wound is nondraining, small amounts of sterile saline during removal of dressing may be helpful; dressing should extend 1 ¼ in (2.5 cm) beyond the wound margin so it can be attached to healthy skin	Useful in the management of acute and chronic wounds; useful for chronic wounds that are malodorous and have moderate amounts of exudate	Remove silicone-release paper from dressing, gently but firmly apply in a rolling motion, not stretching unnecessarily; may need to press down to conform to a body part or "dart" to a skin fold; tape edges using 1-in (½-cm) hypoallergenic tape

Occlusive/ Transparent Films	Advantages	Disadvantages	Comments	Indications for Use	Method of Application
Op-Site (Acme United, Bridgeport, CT) Tegaderm (3M, Eagon, MN) Bioclusive (Johnson & Johnson, New Brunswick, NJ) (Made of a thin, transparent, and adherent polyurethane)	Water-repellent so can be worn in shower or bath; bacteria cannot penetrate the polyurethane; highly elastic and conforms to body contours; comfortable	Will not stick to wet surfaces, new epithelium is sometimes stripped away when film is removed; bacteria can enter the wound through channels that frequently develop at the edges of the dressings; nonabsorbent	Some practice is required to apply these films skillfully, particularly Op-Site, with safe technique; fluids can be aspirated with a small (20-gauge) needle and film will reseal, or else hole may be patched with additional dressing material	Acute or chronic wounds with little drainage or wound fluid; superficial wounds, intravenous sites	Each film has a distinctive system of application: all should be applied unstretched to wound and extended to cover ½ in (1 cm) margin of normal skin; Op-Site: Hold green nonadherent edges while pulling away its slightly rigid, facing paper; gently press edge around wound; green portion of film can be carefully cut off after dressing is in place; Tegaderm; peel off separate full facing paper of the film; then peel off the paper liner exposing the adhesive surface and apply dressing; then pull remaining facing paper away from the edges

Occlusive/Hydrogels	Advantages	Disadvantages	Comments	Indications for Use	Method of Application
Vigilon (Bard Home Health, Berkley Heights, NJ) (Made up of hydrogel between two polyethylene films; the middle portion is a thick gelatinous polyethylene oxide and >95% water gel)	Semitransparent, relieves wound pain; absorbs up to twice its weight in fluid epithelialization; easy to apply and remove; provides moist wound healing environment; very comfortable to patients with skin irritations	Does not exclude bacteria; nonadherent and must be taped in place; difficult to keep on wound in certain body parts (groin, axilla); expensive and difficult to obtain in some areas	Available in sterile and nonsterile form: hyperemic wounds will cause dressings to "dry up" because dressings will evaporate more quickly; removing both polyethylene films will increase the rate of water vapor transmission; dressings can be removed and reapplied for routine wound cleansing; change dressings before they "dry up" and stick to skin	Useful for chronic wounds with little or no odor	Remove the film from one side of the dressing and place the hydrogel portion on the wound or skin; place nonadherent dressing (Telfa, Kendall Company; Mansfield, MA) or gauze over the outer film and use hypoallergenic tape to secure in place

APPENDIX Survey of Commercial Products for Wound Care (continued)

Occlusive/Absorptive	Advantages	Disadvantages	Comments	Indications for Use	Method of Application
Bard Absorptive Dressing (Bard, Berkley, NJ) (Made of dry polysaccharide derivative made by graft copolymerization of carboxyl and carboxanide groups into cornstarch; particle size may range from 0.2 to 4 mm; when partially hydrogenated, it forms a moldable hydrogel)	Hydrophilic properties can absorb bacteria and bacteria toxins from wound surface; absorbs large quantities of wound exudate (up to 30 times its dry weight); provides moist environment for wound healing; large absorption capacity results in continuous cleansing of wound surface	Not a debriding agent; difficult to mix in the package, pain of short duration reported with changing Bard Absorptive Dressing	Frequency of dressing change will depend on the amount of wound drainage; do not tightly pack wound bed	Cleanses, deodorizes, and protects secreting tissues; used for chronic wounds with large quantities of wound fluid	Peel open the outer package and remove inner dressing package; squeeze water chamber until seal is broken and water empties into the powder chamber, continue to squeeze until seal of dispensing chamber is broken, and knead dressing until all powder is absorbed by the water; tear notch at bottom of dispensing chamber and dispense dressing directly into wound; fill wound to a depth approximately ½ in (1 cm) or a level no higher than the surrounding skin; apply nonadherent dressing over the Bard Absorptive Dressing
Debrisan (Dextranomer) (Johnson & Johnson, New Brunswick, NJ)	Absorbs tissue exudate in draining wounds. Effective in removing bacteria and protein. Shortens healing time by retarding eschar formation (scab) and by reducing inflammation and edema		Do not use occlusive dressings because maceration of tissue surrounding wound may result; dextranomer has no debriding action; not effective for cleaning nondraining wounds	Effective for cleaning and draining wounds	Apply to clean, moist wound; pour dextranomer into a wound to at least 6 mm (¼ in) depth; a paste can be made using dextranomer and sterile glycerin (3:1) to apply to hard to reach areas; beads appear gray-yellow when saturated and should be removed by irrigating with sterile water

Nonocclusive/ Foams	Advantages	Disadvantages	Comments	Indications for Use	Method of Application
LYO Foam (LYO Foam C Acme United Corp, Fairfield, CT) (Made of a modified polyurethane; consists of a hydrophilic surface placed on wound bed and a modified hydrophobic surface)	Easy to shape and conform to body surfaces; soft and flexible; maintains a moist wound environment that encourages reepithelialization; nonadherent; gas permeability reduces possibility of anaerobic bacteria and odor they cause; impedes bacterial migration; Lyofoam C contains activated carbon to control odor		Expensive but can be reused until saturated; be sure to place smooth shiny side on wound bed, since foam side will stick to wound and is nonabsorbent	Useful for covering wounds surrounded by fragile or friable skin and draining or odorous wounds	Select or cut a piece that will give at least a 1-in (2.5-cm) margin around the wound; place smooth shiny side directly onto wound surface; secure with gauze, gauze wrapping, elastic bandage, or hypoallergenic tape
Exu-Dry (Frastec Wound Care Products, The Bronx, NY)	Highly absorbent; wicking action draws exudate away from wound; soft and pliable, conforms to body contours; easy to apply and remove	Nonadherent; may be difficult to obtain in retail stores	Available in a variety of sizes and absorbancies; frequency of dressing change depends on amount of wound drainage	Used for burns, skin ulcers, and draining chronic wounds	Dressing must be pressed firmly against wound to ensure absorption; must be secured in place with gauze roll, elastic bandage, or hypoallergenic tape; change dressing when saturated
Epithelial Stimulants	**Advantages**	**Disadvantages**	**Comments**	**Indications for Use**	**Method of Application**
Biolex Wound Gel (Catalina Biomedical, Duarte, CA) Carrington Wound Gel (Carrington Laboratories, Dallas, TX)	Creates and maintains moist wound environment, which promotes epithelialization	Not to be used in infected wounds	Recommend using Biolex and Cara-Klenz to cleanse wound before application; frequency of dressing changes will vary, but do not let wound bed "dry out"; dressings will adhere to wound bed; may be moistened with cleanser to aid removal	Maintain moist wound bed	Cleanse wound first; apply gel to all areas of wound bed and 1 in (2.5 cm) beyond wound bed, including healthy tissue; cover with nonocclusive dressing; change dressings three times a day

Source: Compiled by Kathleen Farley, RN, MS, and Ann McDonald-Lynch, RN, MS, Rush-Presbyterian St. Luke's Medical Center, Chicago, ILL.

Chapter 31

Oncologic Emergencies

Kathleen A. Dietz, RN, MA, MS
Anne Marie Flaherty, RN, MS

INTRODUCTION

Individuals with cancer often experience medical emergencies as a result of the disease process or the treatment protocol. As more effective and aggressive treatments are discovered, patients with cancer live longer and therefore have a greater likelihood of complications from either the treatment or the disease. Some oncologic emergencies, however, can be the presenting symptoms of the malignancy. Prompt diagnosis and treatment of an oncologic emergency can enable further treatment of the primary cancer and thus prolong life. This chapter highlights the most frequent oncologic emergencies that confront the nurses who care for these patients.

SEPTIC SHOCK

Introduction

Septicemia, a systemic invasion of the blood by microorganisms, can lead to the life-threatening syndrome known as septic shock. Septic shock is a profound syndrome characterized by hemodynamic instability, coagulopathies, and alterations in metabolism. Mortality rates are high (>75%) for cancer patients in whom septic shock develops. Rapid and aggressive therapy is needed.[1]

Pathophysiology

Microorganisms, bacterial or fungal, responsible for septic shock can enter the blood either by local invasion of a blood vessel or by entering the venous system via the lymphatic vessels. Endotoxins are produced by gram-negative bacteria, whereas gram-positive organisms produce exotoxins; both cause the release of chemical mediators and hormones and initiate the inflammatory response. Antigen-antibody complexes are formed, activating the complement protein system. The complement proteins directly destroy organisms, enhance phagocytosis, promote chemotaxis, release histamine, activate the kinin system, promote vasodilation, and increase capillary permeability.[2] Plasma leaks into interstitial tissues and causes depletion of intravascular volume, which leads to hypotension. Tissue perfusion is compromised secondary to fluid in the lungs, decreased circulating oxygen-carrying blood, and microemboli caused by the activation of factor XII and the clotting process.[3]

Septic shock is classified into two patterns: early hyperdynamic shock and late hypodynamic shock. In the early or hyperdynamic phase of shock, cardiac output increases and systemic vascular resistance decreases in an attempt to maintain adequate tissue perfusion. The blood pressure may be normal initally, but it soon falls as vasodilation persists and the respiratory rate increases in an attempt to provide oxygen. As hypoxemia develops, cells shift from aerobic to anaerobic metabolism, leading to metabolic acidosis. Pulmonary edema and adult respiratory distress syndrome can develop in the early phase of septic shock.[1] In the advanced or hypodynamic phase of shock, there is vasoconstriction of the splanchnic, pulmonary, and renal circulation, which produces ischemia of the abdominal organs, impaired alveolar gas exchange, and decreased urine output. This compensatory vasoconstriction actually decreases cardiac output, venous return, and blood pressure by trapping blood in vascular beds.[4] Progressive lactic acidosis results from the prolonged anaerobic metabolism. As septic shock progresses, respiratory and renal failure occur, poor cerebral perfusion leads to coma, and inadequate perfusion of heart muscle leads to ischemia, arrythmias, and death.

Etiology

Sepsis is the most common cause of shock in the cancer patient.[1] Cancer patients are at risk of infections that may lead to septic shock because of the local effects of tumor growth, immunologic effects of neoplastic disease or treatment, iatrogenic factors, and nosocomial sources.[5] Local tumor growth (ie, cancer of the skin, head and neck, and gastrointestinal tract) can disrupt normal mucocutaneous barriers, thus enabling invasion by endogenous or acquired pathogens.[3] Likewise, such tumors as head and neck or lung cancers, may obstruct natural passages causing retention or aspiration of secretions that result in pneumonia. Cellular immunity is impaired in Hodgkin's disease and also in persons receiving radiotherapy and chemotherapy. Cancers that involve B lymphocytes, such as multiple myeloma, chronic lymphocytic leukemia, and Waldenström's macroglobulinemia, may impair humoral immunity. Splenectomy for staging or treatment purposes (ie, in lymphoma and leukemia) can increase the risk of infection. Neutropenia may be caused by the cancer itself but is also a potential side effect of radiation and chemotherapy. Invasive procedures, such as placement of vascular access devices, chest tubes, stents, and urinary catheters, can alter the patient's barriers against infection. Hospital-acquired organisms may be transmitted by humidifiers, respirators, flowers, and most especially by hospital personnel. In patients who receive long-term antibiotic therapy resistant organisms often develop, or there may be overgrowth of normal endogenous bacteria or fungi.

Assessment

When caring for individuals with cancer, a high index of suspicion and close monitoring are essential to recognizing persons at high risk of septic shock.[6,7] The clinical picture varies from patient to patient. However, tachypnea, hyperventilation, and respiratory alkalosis are usually the earliest signs of developing sepsis.[1]

Clinical characteristics

Fever or shaking chills in the granulocytopenic and/or immunosuppressed patient may herald a life-threatening infection that can lead to septic shock if left untreated. Vital signs and level of consciousness are monitored closely. In hyperdynamic or "warm" shock, cardiac output increases, causing a rise in blood pressure, an increased heart rate, and a widened pulse pressure (Figure 31-1). The skin is warm as a result of vasodilation and respiratory rate increases because of capillary leakage in the lungs, causing hypoxia. Since there is a high incidence of associated adult respiratory distress syndrome, bilateral rales will be auscultated if pulmonary edema develops.[8,9] Mental status often deteriorates early, as evidenced by lethargy and confusion. Urine output may be normal to increased initially, but as blood flow to vital organs is reduced, oliguria develops. In the hypodynamic or "cold" shock phase, the patient is cool, clammy, and cyanotic, the pulse is rapid and thready, and the blood pressure begins to fall with a narrowing pulse pressure. Arterial blood gases will initially show respiratory alkalosis, but as an-

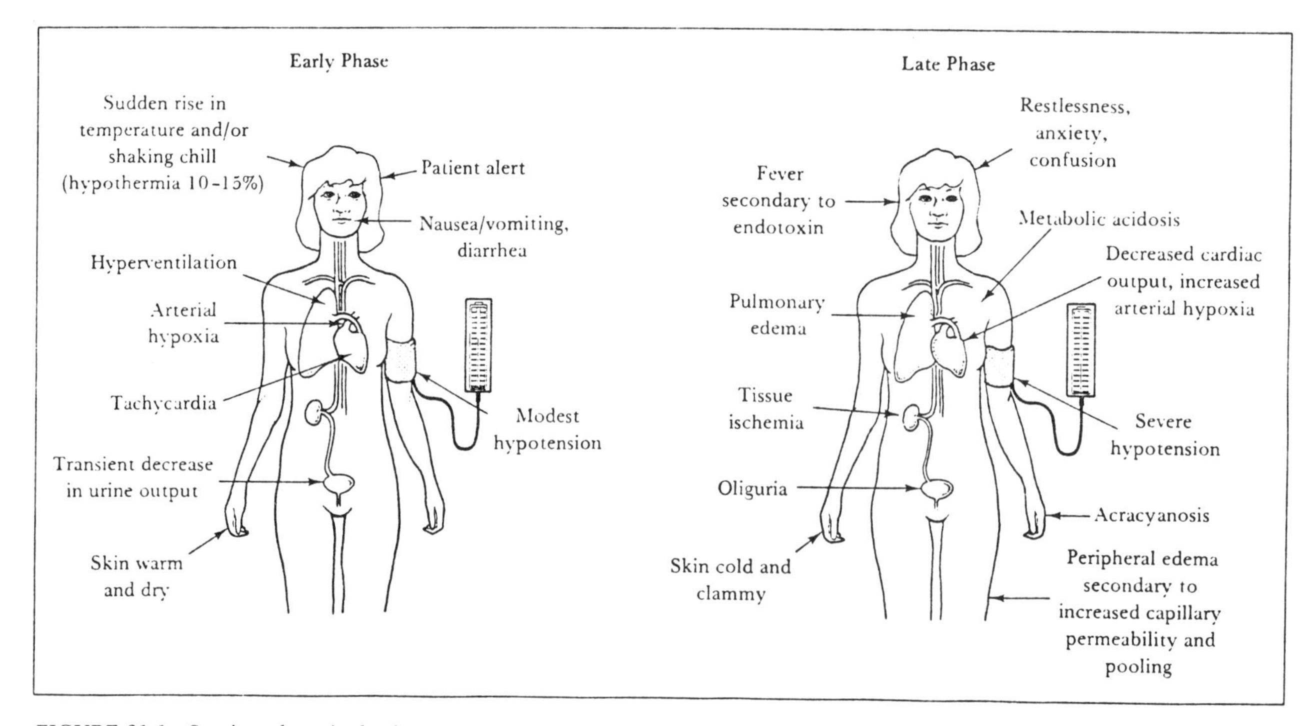

FIGURE 31-1 Sepsis and septic shock.

aerobic metabolism persists, a combination of metabolic and respiratory acidosis occurs. Decreased venous return leads to pulmonary edema, adult respiratory distress syndrome, coma, and death.

Diagnostic studies

Cancer patients at greatest risk of septic shock have granulocyte counts of less than $100/mm^3$.[1] During early sepsis a low $Paco_2$ indicates respiratory alkalosis, which in the later stage progresses to a metabolic acidosis and elevation of lactic acid levels to more than 1 to 2 mmol/L above normal.[1] In cancer patients, rapid muscle wasting, negative nitrogen balance, decreased intravascular volume, and renal dysfunction contribute to elevated blood urea nitrogen levels.[1] When disseminated intravascular coagulation occurs in association with sepsis, thrombocytopenia and coagulation abnormalities (eg, prolonged prothrombin and activated partial thromboplastin time and decreased fibrinogen) may be noted.

Treatment

Knowledge of the pathophysiology of the various cancers, treatment protocols, patient history, physical assessment, and results of laboratory tests provides the data base necessary to predict which individuals are at risk of septic shock. Early identification may prevent an episode of fever from becoming a critical event. Because death from septic shock can occur rapidly among cancer patients, immediate therapy is necessary. The primary therapeutic intervention is directed toward controlling sepsis. Administration of emperic broad-spectrum antibiotics is instituted immediately after appropriate microbiology cultures are obtained.[10] A recommended initial approach for neutropenic patients includes administration of an aminoglycoside, an extended-spectrum penicillin active against anaerobes and *Pseudomonas aeruginosa*, and a cephalosporin for staphylococcal and *Klebsiella* coverage. If *Staphylococcus epidermidis* is suspected or if *Corynebacterium* is identified, an agent such as vancomycin should be added to the regimen.[1,10] If shock develops in the presence of prolonged antibiotic therapy and persistent neutropenia, a fungal source is anticipated and treatment with amphotericin B is initiated. An infectious agent may not be identified in 30% of cancer patients with sepsis.[1] Antibiotic therapy must not be delayed, even in the absence of a positive blood culture.

Additional measures are taken in an effort to stabilize the patient and to gain time until the source of sepsis is controlled or eliminated. Vital signs, urine output, and level of consciousness are monitored frequently.[11] Venous access is maintained for the administration of fluids, crystalloids, colloids, and vasopressors. Fluid status is closely monitored. Vigorous fluid replacement is given to expand plasma volume that is depleted because of diffuse capillary leakage. Unless the patient exhibits signs of fluid overload, a fluid challenge of 500 mL within 20 to 30 minutes is infused.[12] Crystalloid solutions, such as normal saline or Ringer's lactate, or colloids, such as albumin, are administered to increase intravascular volume.[10] Fresh frozen plasma can be given in an infusion of 250 mL every 10 to 20 minutes until a mean arterial pressure of 80 mm Hg is reached.[1] Controversy exists over the use of crystalloids versus colloids for volume replacement.[1,10,12] Blood and colloid solutions expand the intravascular volume more rapidly and with less fluid. When crystalloids are given, peripheral edema often develops and may be mistaken for fluid overload. Central venous pressure or pulmonary artery pressures must be monitored to assure proper repletion of fluid and intravascular volume without complications of fluid overload.

When vital signs do not improve in response to fluids, vasopressors such as dopamine or levarterenol are given in an attempt to maintain cerebral, coronary, and renal perfusion. Although controversial, high-dose corticosteroids may be administered early in the course of shock to produce anti-inflammatory activity and enhance survival. However if steroids are given later in the course, they may delay death without effecting survival.[3] One commonly used approach is to give methylprednisolone, 30 mg/kg intravenously every 6 hours, during the initial 24 hours after septic shock is diagnosed.[1]

Airway patency is maintained and nasopharyngeal suctioning is instituted as necessary. Oxygen therapy is administered, and if respiratory status continues to decompensate, intubation and mechanical ventilatory assistance are indicated.[9] Arterial blood gases and electrolytes are monitored, and the physician is immediately notified of results. Since metabolic acidosis occurs as anaerobic metabolism develops, intravenous injections of sodium bicarbonate are given to maintain the blood pH within the normal range. An indwelling urinary catheter is used to assist in monitoring of renal perfusion. Hypotensive patients are placed in the Trendelenberg position to promote venous return, and skin is assessed for color, temperature, and moisture.

The effectiveness of the therapies administered is assessed by continuous monitoring of blood pressure, central venous or pulmonary artery pressure, apical rate, frequency and character of respirations, skin color and temperature, level of consciousness, and urinary output.[6,11] When therapy is effective, the vital signs should stabilize, pressure should reflect proper intravascular volume, and urine output should be adequate. Maintaining this high level of care is paramount to the resolution of septic shock.

Prognosis and Follow-Up Care

The mortality rate associated with septic shock is estimated at between 50% and 90%. The higher rates are observed among persons with hematologic malignancies.[3] The frequency of shock and the mortality rate increase if the patient does not mount an initial febrile response, as may occur in patients who are taking steroids or who are severely debilitated.[1]

DISSEMINATED INTRAVASCULAR COAGULATION

Introduction

Disseminated intravascular coagulation (DIC), an abnormality of the coagulation system, is characterized by widespread clotting within arterioles and capillaries and simultaneous hemorrhage. DIC can be acute or chronic. Acute DIC must be treated as a medical emergency, whereas chronic DIC produces coagulation abnormalities, with or without clinical manifestations, that can be medically managed.[13]

Pathophysiology

Normally, the body has a steady state between clot formation (thrombosis) and clot dissolution (fibrinolysis).[14] When a vessel is severed or ruptured, the wall of the vessel contracts to reduce blood flow. The endothelium loses its normal smoothness and becomes wet and sticky, thus allowing the endothelial surfaces to become glued together. On coming into contact with this sticky endothelial surface, platelets, which are usually round or oval disks, assume bizarre, irregular forms with irradiating processes that adhere to the endothelial surface and to other platelets, forming a plug. Since the platelet plug is relatively unstable, procoagulants from both the traumatized vascular wall and the adhering platelets act to form a stable clot.

For clotting to be effective, both platelets and the 13 different clotting factors are required. These clotting factors are proteins involved in a series of enzymatic reactions that have a cascading or domino effect. The clotting cascade is initiated either by the intrinsic mechanism (via factor XII) when the blood itself is traumatized or by the extrinsic mechanism (via factor VII) when there is tissue injury (Figure 31-2). Factor X is the common pathway for the intrinsic and extrinsic systems and converts prothrombin to thrombin in the presence of factor V, platelets, and calcium. Both calcium and lipid are essential for clotting; calcium is normally present in the body, and lipid is provided by platelet membranes. Prothrombin is an unstable plasma protein that is continually produced by the liver. Vitamin K, produced by the intestinal flora, is required by the liver for the normal function of prothrombin. Thrombin is the enzyme responsible for converting fibrinogen to a fibrin clot, which is stabilized by factor XIII. Once healing has occurred, the anticlotting system is activated and plasmin dissolves the clot, resulting in the release of fibrin split products (FSPs). These degradation products are normally cleared by the liver. The normal homeostatic balance between the procoagulant and anticoagulant systems prevents thrombosis and hemorrhage.

In DIC, both microvascular thrombosis and bleeding from numerous sites occur simultaneously. Disseminated coagulation takes place so rapidly that the liver is unable to clear the FSPs. When a large quantity of FSPs are circulating, they produce a feedback inhibition of clotting and have an anticoagulant effect. At the same time, the consumable factors I, II, V, and VIII and platelets are depleted by the extensive microvascular clotting.

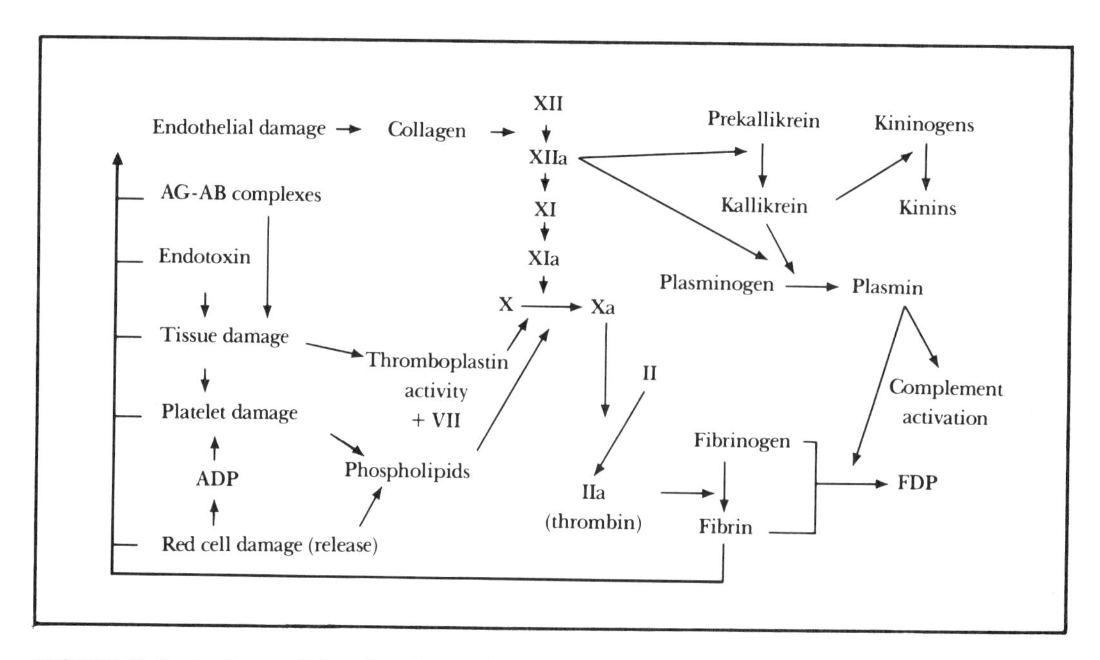

FIGURE 31-2 A schema of the triggering mechanisms in disseminated intravascular coagulation. (*AG-AB*, Antigen-antibody.) (Source: Bick RL: Disseminated intravascular coagulation and related syndromes: A clinical review, in *Seminars in Thrombosis and Hemostasis,* Volume 14, Number 4, New York, 1988, Thieme Medical Publishers, Inc. Reprinted by permission.)

TABLE 31-1 Conditions Associated with Acute Disseminated Intravascular Coagulation

Obstetric accidents
Amniotic fluid embolism
Placental abruption
Retained fetus syndrome
Eclampsia
Intravascular hemolysis
Hemolytic transfusion reactions
Minor hemolysis
Massive transfusions
Bacteremia
Gram-negative (endotoxin)
Gram-positive (mucopolysaccharides)
Viremias
Cytomegalovirus
Hepatitis
Varicella
Disseminated malignancy
Leukemia
Acute promyelocytic
Acute myelomonocytic
Many others
Burns
Crush injuries and tissue necrosis
Liver disease
Obstructive jaundice
Acute hepatic failure
Prosthetic devices
(LeVeen shunting and aortic balloon)
Vascular disorders

Source: Bick RL: Disseminated intravascular coagulation and related syndromes: A clinical review in *Seminars in Thrombosis and Hemostasis,* Volume 14, Number 4, New York, 1988, Thieme Medical Publishers, Inc. Reprinted by permission.

Etiology

DIC is not a primary disorder; it is always a reflection of another event that is occurring in the body (Table 31-1). The DIC syndrome is seen in fewer than 15% of persons with cancer and can be related to either the disease process or the treatment protocol.[15] Solid tumors develop new vasculature, which has an abnormal endothelial lining that may activate the procoagulant system. It is also thought that tumors may release into the circulation necrotic tissue or tumor enzymes that could activate the coagulation system.[13] Solid tumors associated with DIC include mucin-producing adenocarcinomas, such as gastric, lung, pancreas, and prostate tumors (Table 31-2).

Patients with solid tumors may have laboratory evidence of a low-grade, chronic DIC that does not produce clinical manifestations. Patients with cancer of the pancreas or prostate, however, will usually have overt signs of DIC. A study at the Mayo Clinic showed that a coagulation screening should be performed before prostate surgery, since there appears to be a direct correlation between preoperative laboratory findings of DIC and postprostatectomy blood loss. Patients with cancer of the body or tail of the pancreas may experience "migratory thrombophlebitis" as a result of ductal obstruction with subsequent release of trypsin into the systemic circulation. Trypsin acts like thrombin and activates the coagulation cascade, causing thrombosis.[13]

TABLE 31-2 Disseminated Intravascular Coagulation and Common Malignancies

Gastrointestinal	Ovary
Pancreas	Melanoma
Prostate	Acute leukemia
Lung	Myeloma
Breast	Myeloproliferative syndromes

Source: Bick RL: Disseminated intravascular coagulation and related syndromes: A clinical review in *Seminars in Thrombosis and Hemostasis,* Volume 14, Number 4, New York, 1988, Thieme Medical Publishers, Inc. Reprinted by permission.

Persons with acute promyelocytic leukemia (APL) have a high incidence of DIC (about 85%),[16] which can occur both before and in conjunction with chemotherapy.[17-19] Studies indicate that in persons with APL the tendency to bleed is associated with a white blood cell count of $\geq$ 10,000/mm^3 at diagnosis.[17,20] This bleeding diathesis is thought to be due to the release of procoagulant material from granules on the promyelocytes. Autopsy studies of individuals with APL have revealed diffuse thrombosis with fibrin deposition in 15% to 25% of cases.[21] Likewise, in patients with large tumor burdens, as occurs with some other leukemias and lymphomas, DIC may develop during treatment when cells are rapidly lysed.[22]

Complications of cancer therapy are also associated with DIC. *Meningococcus* and other gram-negative organisms causing sepsis may provide the triggering event that initiates the clotting cascade.[23] Endotoxins can activate factor XII, induce a platelet-release reaction, cause endothelial sloughing, and initiate a release of granulocytic procoagulant materials—all mechanisms capable of initiating the clotting cascade.[13] Gram-positive bacterial sepsis and acidosis associated with DIC occur in a similar fashion. Viremias, most commonly involving varicella, hepatitis and cytomegalovirus, are also associated with DIC, possibly because of an antigen-antibody activation of factor XII.

Intravascular hemolysis (eg, hemolytic transfusion reaction) can cause DIC by the release of red cell adenosine diphosphate or red cell phospholipoproteins, which may activate the procoagulant system.[13] Foreign surfaces in the circulatory system may cause the generation of microthrombi and subsequent fibrinolysis leading to DIC. This may be an obstacle to the use of prosthetic devices. The LeVeen shunt and other peritoneovenous shunts placed to alleviate intractable malignant ascites are also associated with both acute and chronic DIC. The DIC may be a result of both placement of a foreign device and the fact that ascitic fluid precipitates procoagulant activity.[13,24]

Assessment

Clinical characteristics

Persons with cancer who are considered at risk of DIC should be monitored closely.[25] Observation and reporting of early signs of bleeding will aid in the diagnosis of DIC. Patients with acute DIC will usually have clinical evidence of bleeding from at least three unrelated sites.[13] The organ systems most often compromised by bleeding include the skin, heart, lungs, gastrointestinal tract, and central nervous system.[26] Signs of internal bleeding include anxiety, restlessness, confusion, tachycardia, tachypnea, abdominal tenderness, and increased abdominal girth. The person may have headaches, change in mentation, epistaxis, conjunctival hemorrhage, periorbital petechiae, bleeding gums, hemoptysis, diffuse ecchymoses, joint pain, and oozing of blood from wounds, previous injection sites, or bone marrow aspiration sites.[14,25] Women should be asked whether menses has been unusually prolonged or heavy and whether there is midcycle spotting. Emesis, urine, and stool are tested for the presence of occult blood if frank bleeding is not apparent.

Patients with chronic DIC commonly have gingival bleeding, spontaneous, large cutaneous ecchymoses, and mild to moderate genitourinary or gastrointestinal bleeding. Pulmonary hemorrhage is an early and prominent sign of chronic DIC in the patient with cancer.[13]

Diagnostic studies

DIC has been defined as the presence of two or more of the following coagulation abnormalities: (a) prothrombin (PT), 3 or more seconds greater than control; (b) activated partial thromboplastin time (APTT), 5 or more seconds greater than the upper limit of the normal range; (c) thrombin time (TT) prolonged by 3 or more seconds more than control; (d) fibrinogen (Fib) greater than 150 mg/dL; and (e) fibrin split products (FSP) equal to or greater than 40 μg/mL.[16]

No single coagulation abnormality will definitely diagnose DIC. In acute DIC, the PT is prolonged in 75% of patients, and the APTT is prolonged in only 50% to 60%. Thrombin time is often normal in persons with DIC. Fibrin split products are elevated in 85% to 100% of patients with acute DIC.[13] Fibrinogen levels have been reported as normal in up to 57% of patients with acute DIC.[22] Fibrinogen is an acute-phase reactant in infection, causing the fibrinogen level to be normal in DIC associated with infection. Serial fibrinogen levels should be determined to ascertain whether there is a downward trend. Protamine sulfate or ethanol gelation tests will be positive in persons with acute DIC, and the platelet count will be decreased as a result of consumption. The degree of thrombocytopenia in DIC averages about 60,000 mm^3.[13] In patients with leukemia and DIC, thrombocytopenia is more severe because of decreased thrombopoiesis.

Red cell fragments called schistocytes can be seen on peripheral blood smears in all patients with chronic DIC but in only 50% of patients with acute DIC. Fibrin split products are usually elevated in chronic DIC and induce platelet dysfunction.[13]

Treatment

The major and only effective treatment for DIC is treatment of the underlying cause of the syndrome.[23] Aggressive management of the underlying cause (tumor- or therapy-related) must be undertaken immediately in cases of acute DIC. Concomitant interventions to control DIC include administration of platelets and fresh frozen plasma to replace consumable factors as well as cryoprecipitate to replace fibrinogen.[22,23] Fresh frozen plasma or antithrombin III concentrates neutralize excess thrombin and slow the DIC process.

Heparin, although controversial, may be given to inhibit factors IX and X, thereby halting the clotting cascade.[16,17,19,20,26,27] Heparin is given in a continuous intravenous infusion to avoid peaks in the effect that result from intermittent subcutaneous injections. The usual administration of heparin is a controlled infusion of 7.5 U/kg per hour with incremental increases of 2.5 U until the fibrinogen level reflects an upward trend.[17] Heparin therapy is contraindicated in patients in whom excessive bleeding occurs in a closed space so that it compromises vital function (eg, intracranial, intraspinal, pericardial, or paratracheal bleeding).[22] The heparin infusion should be stopped immediately if the person complains of headache, displays signs of intracranial bleeding, or has observable frank bleeding (for example, gastrointestinal bleeding). Epsilon-aminocaproic acid (EACA), 1 g/hr intravenously, has been given in conjunction with heparin therapy to maintain platelet and fibrinogen levels, but its use is controversial.[22,26,28] "EACA should not be used in the great majority of patients with DIC because inhibition of the fibrinolytic system may lead to widespread fibrin deposition in the microcirculation and result in ischemic organ dysfunction or failure."[22]

In patients with DIC caused by septicemia, anticoagulant therapy is usually not indicated since the DIC most often resolves after the initiation of antibiotic therapy and no difference in survival has been shown when heparin was given.[22] Anticoagulant therapy is initiated only if the patient with septicemia has evidence of fibrin deposition, acral or dermal ischemia, venous or arterial thromboembolism, or bleeding associated with thrombocytopenia and decreased fibrinogen level after a trial of antibiotic therapy.[13,22]

TABLE 31-3 Patient Information: Guidelines for Patients Who Have a Low Platelet Count

1. Protect yourself from injury when performing daily activities:
   a. Brush with a soft toothbrush and gently floss gums
   b. Wear gloves when gardening, cooking, and doing home repairs
   c. Use an electric razor when shaving
   d. Avoid unsafe conditions, contact sports, and activities such as riding a bicycle
   e. Avoid use of rectal suppositories, enemas, and vaginal tampons
2. Avoid aspirin and aspirin-containing products
3. Call your doctor if you have:
   a. Excessive bruising
   b. Faint red rash on trunk, arms, and legs
   c. Black bowel movements
   d. Blood in urine
   e. Headaches that persist
   f. Vaginal spotting
   g. Any bleeding that persists

Source: Division of Nursing, Memorial Sloan-Kettering Cancer Center, New York, 1984.

During acute DIC, the patient is assessed for signs of bleeding or increased bleeding. A quiet environment is maintained, and vital signs with neurologic checks are recorded every 2 to 4 hours. Medications are given to suppress symptoms that will increase intracranial pressure (for example, coughing or vomiting). Patients are assisted during ambulation after receiving medications that cause drowsiness or orthostatic changes. Medications that interfere with platelet function, such as aspirin-containing products or nonsteroidal anti-inflammatory drugs should be avoided.[23,29] Bleeding should be prevented and minimized by institution of bleeding precautions (Table 31-3).[30] An accurate record of blood loss should be kept by counting of wound dressings or vaginal pads and measurement of emesis, urine, or stool containing frank blood.[29,31] The patient should be monitored for signs of cardiogenic shock, including hypovolemia, hypoxia, hypotension, and oliguria.[32]

Clinically manifest chronic DIC associated with solid tumors can be effectively treated with subcutaneous injections of heparin or antiplatelet agents, such as aspirin or dipyridamole.[13] It should be noted that oral warfarin has been shown to be ineffective.[22]

Prognosis

Resolution of acute DIC will be accomplished only when the underlying cause of this medical emergency is successfully treated. Evaluation is accomplished by monitoring the coagulation screen and platelet count for an upward trend in fibrinogen and a decrease in fibrin split products. If the patient is not receiving chemotherapy, an increase in platelet count should also occur.

When the process that triggers an acute episode of DIC is removed, the intravascular clotting process is stopped, and blood component therapy is given as indicated, there is a 75% survival rate and low morbidity in patients with classic acute DIC.[13] The lowest incidences of hemorrhagic deaths in patients with APL and acute DIC, with or without heparin therapy, are 14% and 15%, respectively.[16,17]

SUPERIOR VENA CAVA SYNDROME

Introduction

Superior vena cava syndrome (SVCS) is a medical emergency that may also be the presenting sign of a malignancy. Ninety-seven percent of all cases of SVCS are due to cancer. This syndrome is the result of compression of the superior vena cava by tumor, which leads to a characteristic pattern of upper extremity manifestations. If untreated, SVCS can lead to airway obstruction.

Pathophysiology

The superior vena cava is a thin-walled vessel with relatively low intravascular pressure; it is surrounded by rigid structures, including the right mainstem bronchus, vertebral bodies, sternum, and lymph nodes.[33] It is the main vessel for venous return from the upper thorax. The presence of an expanding mass or lymphadenopathy in the mediastinum can compress the superior vena cava vessel. Compression produces markedly increased venous pressure in the upper part of the thorax. Three pathophysiologic states can cause an obstruction of the superior vena cava: (a) external compression of the vessel by tumor or lymph nodes, (b) direct invasion of the vessel wall by tumor, and (c) thrombosis of the vessel.

Etiology

Two malignancies—lung cancer and lymphoma—are most frequently the cause of SVCS. Small cell tumor is the most common histologic type of lung cancer.[34]

A benign source of SVCS observed in the oncology population is thrombus formation around a central venous catheter, such as those placed for long-term therapy. Fibrinolytic therapy directly into the vena cava and surgical removal of the catheter usually reverse this SVCS.

Assessment

Clinical characteristics

Superior vena cava obstruction causes elevated venous pressure and congestion, resulting in an array of signs and symptoms that are hallmarks of this syndrome. The severity of symptoms is related to the rapidity of onset, the degree and location of the obstruction, and the adequacy of collateral circulation.[33]

Clinical characteristics include shortness of breath, facial edema, trunk and upper extremity edema, neck and chest vein distention, cough, hoarseness, and stridor. The patient may be dyspneic, cyanotic, or plethoric. The conjunctiva may also be engorged. Neurologic symptoms are related to increased intracranial pressure and include headache, dizziness, visual disturbance, and occasionally alterations in mental status. A rapidly developing SVCS may be fatal, whereas gradual onset of SVCS allows the collateral circulation to shunt enough blood to minimize complications.[33] Airway obstruction can occur with rapidly developing SVCS, leading to respiratory failure.

Diagnostic studies

In addition to clinical evidence, a radiograph of the chest will usually reveal a mediastinal mass or adenopathy. Extensive diagnostic tests to establish SVCS are unnecessary. In the past, prompt treatment of SVCS with mediastinal irradiation was initiated, regardless of the type of underlying malignancy. Recently, however, oncologists believe that most cases of SVCS do not represent a life-threatening emergency and that invasive tests to establish the histopathologic diagnosis of the underlying malignancy are well tolerated.[35,36] Type of treatment, future therapy, and prognosis are dependent on a definitive tissue diagnosis. Therefore a tissue specimen should be obtained if the patient's clinical condition permits. Biopsy is performed if abnormal tissue, such as an enlarged supraclavicular lymph node, is readily accessible.[37]

Treatment

Patients with severe SVCS who are experiencing acute respiratory distress, massive edema, and markedly elevated venous pressure require immediate intervention to avoid respiratory arrest.[35] In an acute crisis with no tissue diagnosis, fractionated irradiation of the mediastinum is the treatment of choice. High doses of fractionation, 300 to 400 cGy per day are given initially, followed by 200-cGy doses to complete a cumulative 3000- to 3500-cGy dose to the obstructing tumor site.[38]

In slower progressing, less critical SVCS, tissue diagnosis is obtained and proper treatment for the underlying disease is initiated. For example, small cell lung cancer is very responsive to combination chemotherapy. When SVCS occurs in patients with small cell lung cancer, chemotherapy is initiated immediately. If there is a lack of tumor response or if SVCS continues to progress, mediastinal irradiation can be added to the treatment regimen.

Lymphomas are extremely radiosensitive. Therefore fractionated radiation for SVCS is reasonable. If the mass, however, is so large that a significant portion of lung tissue would be irradiated, combination chemotherapy may be preferred to reverse the SVCS.[34] Hodgkin's disease and diffuse histiocytic lymphoma are sensitive to combination chemotherapy. Chemotherapy is also the preferred treatment if the patient has undergone previous mediastinal radiation therapy.

The timing of systemic chemotherapy and/or mediastinal irradiation is crucial so that optimal therapy is administered with the least amount of normal tissue damage and maximal tumor destruction. Steroids and anticoagulant therapy are sometimes used in the treatment of SVCS. Although an inflammatory reaction is usually not associated with SVCS, steroids are probably indicated when respiratory distress is present.[39] Anticoagulants can prevent thrombosis in the presence of decreased circulatory time and decreased blood flow through the obstructed vessel, and fibrinolytic agents may reduce intramural thrombi.[40]

Nursing care of patients experiencing SVCS is directed toward maintaining adequate cardiopulmonary status, monitoring the progression of SVCS, assisting with medical intervention, and reducing the patient's anxiety.

Invasive or constrictive procedures are avoided in the upper extremities because of impaired venous return and the potential for hemorrhage. Blood pressure measures are taken on the thigh, using the popliteal pulse, and venipuncture is performed on the lower extremities. The administration of chemotherapeutic agents that are irritants or vesicants is of considerable concern. There is some controversy about the safety of administering vesicants and irritants via the peripheral veins of the lower extremities. Upper extremity administration is avoided since SVCS causes pooling of the irritant or vesicant in the upper thorax, with inadequate drug distribution and possible phlebitis or thrombosis.[34] Probably the safest route for administration of chemotherapy during the acute phase of SVCS is surgical cannulation of the femoral vein, either temporarily or with placement of a Silastic cuffed catheter, such as a Hickman or a Broviac catheter. Fluid management during and after administration of chemotherapy is also a challenge. Although kidney function needs to be preserved, care is taken to avoid overhydration and subsequent exacerbation of SVCS. The use of diuretic agents may be necessary to maintain an adequate fluid balance.

Patients require careful monitoring of respiratory, neurologic, and hemodynamic status during the acute phase of SVCS. Coagulation profiles are monitored routinely if anticoagulants are administered. Positioning the patient comfortably with the head elevated will help maximize breathing and allay anxiety. A calm environment with visible support will significantly reassure the patient who is experiencing this crisis. It is important to stress that the physical appearance is temporary and will subside once the SVCS is resolved.

Resolution of the clinical manifestations is adequate evidence of effective treatment. This may occur within 24 to 72 hours after the initiation of therapy. Thrombus is usually suspected if the syndrome does not respond rapidly. Fibrolytic therapy and surgery may then have to be pursued. If diagnostic evaluation of the underlying malignancy is incomplete, it can begin or proceed, once the clinical condition of SVCS improves.

Prognosis and Follow-Up Care

The prognosis following resolution of SVCS is favorable and depends on the prognosis of the underlying malignancy. More than 50% of patients with SVCS have either a complete (38%) or a partial (23%) response to treatment of the syndrome.[41] Recurrence of SVCS is infrequent in the lymphoma population but is rather common in patients with small cell lung cancer.

After the resolution of SVCS, rehabilitation is rather rapid, with disappearance of the physical effects. Thereafter, routine follow-up care provided for the oncology patient is sufficient.

Superior vena cava syndrome is a relatively rare entity; it is most often caused by an intrathoracic malignancy. An iatrogenic cause can be long-term indwelling central venous catheters. If respiratory distress is not present, tissue diagnosis should be obtained before the initiation of therapy, since the type of cancer will dictate the most effective therapy. Current literature is revealing low morbidity and mortality associated with invasive procedures in patients with SVCS.

CARDIAC TAMPONADE

Introduction

Cardiac tamponade is a life-threatening emergency in which excessive fluid accumulation in the pericardial space creates pressure of such magnitude that the heart's ability to fill and pump is severely compromised. Decreased cardiac output and impaired systemic perfusion result. The prognosis is dependent on the rapidity of this fluid accumulation, the pressure developed, and prompt diagnosis and treatment.

Pathophysiology

The pericardial space, a double-layered serous membrane between the visceral and parietal layers of the serous pericardium, normally holds 25 to 35 ml of lymphatic fluid. Intrapericardial pressure results from the amount of fluid in this space and the elasticity or flexibility of the pericardium. Increased fluid or fibrosis and thickening of the pericardium can raise the intrapericardial pressure to the point where the pressure interferes with the heart's function.

Intraventricular diastolic pressure rises as a result of higher intrapericardial pressure. This prevents adequate filling of the ventricle during diastole, causes venous congestion, and thereby decreases cardiac output. Multiple physiologic changes occur as other pressures are subsequently affected, including an elevated central venous pressure and a lowered left atrial pressure (Figure 31-3). The compensatory mechanisms that attempt to counteract these pressures and maintain cardiac output are an increase in heart rate (tachycardia) and peripheral vasoconstriction, which in turn help maintain arterial pressure and venous return. Peripheral vasoconstriction decreases renal blood flow, and this leads to water and sodium retention and an increase in blood volume.[42]

If these compensatory mechanisms fail and intervention does not reverse the syndrome of progressive pericardial effusion, then cardiac output falls and impedes coronary artery flow, leading to severe myocardial ischemia, further cardiac decline, and eventual circulatory collapse.[43]

Etiology

Cardiac tamponade is caused by either an abnormal accumulation of fluid in the pericardial space or, less commonly, constrictive fibrosis of the pericardium. Both cancer and cancer therapy can initiate these changes.

Pericardial effusion and constrictive pericarditis can be caused by metastatic tumors involving the pericardium through direct extension or hematogenous or lymphatic spread. Tumors that most commonly metastasize to the pericardium include lung cancer, breast cancer, leukemia, Hodgkin's disease, lymphoma, melanoma, gastrointestinal tumors, and sarcomas. Although rare, primary tumors of the heart, including mesothelioma and sarcoma, can also involve the pericardium.[42] Hemopericardium can occur in patients with thrombocytopenia or other coagulopathies.[44]

Radiation therapy, especially when it involves high doses to the mediastinum, can damage the pericardium, causing a constrictive pericarditis and/or pericardial effusion.[43] Doses ranging from 4000 to 6000 cGy, delivered to a large portion of the heart, may induce either acute or chronic pericarditis, which can progress to cardiac tamponade with or without an effusion.[45]

Assessment

Cardiac tamponade can lead to sudden death. Early diagnosis and intervention are dependent on the assessment skills and knowledge of the health professional who first encounters the patient. No single sign or symptom is definitively characteristic of cardiac tamponade. Many factors must be taken into consideration.

Clinical characteristics

The cancer patient with impending cardiac tamponade may complain of retrosternal chest pain and shortness of breath. The chest pain is relieved somewhat by leaning forward but is more severe when the patient is in the supine position.[43] The primary clinical signs of cardiac tamponade are venous distention, distant heart sounds, and paradoxical pulse.[46] Venous distention can mimic heart failure, with jugular neck vein distention, orthopnea, hepatic congestion, and possible bilateral pleural effusions.[42] Neck vein distention will usually increase during inspiration if the tamponade is significant. Hypotension

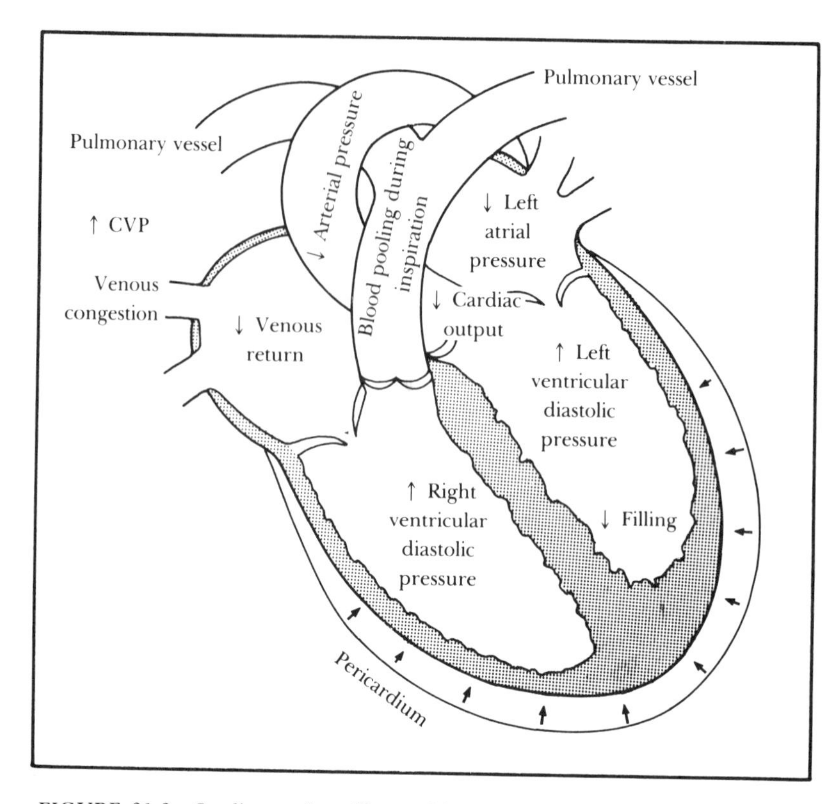

FIGURE 31-3 Cardiovascular effects of increased intrapleural pressure. Intraventricular diastolic pressure rises as a result of higher intrapericardial pressure. This prevents adequate filling of the ventricle, causing venous congestion, decreased cardiac output, lowered left atrial pressure, and elevated central venous pressure. ↑, Increased; ↓, decreased.

and tachycardia are usually present and reflect a decreased cardiac output. Distant heart sounds and dullness over the precordium occur when tamponade is caused by pericardial effusion. Conversely, heart sounds will be easily heard and a friction rub and atrial arrhythmia may be present if tamponade is caused by tumor encroachment and/or constrictive pericarditis.[47]

A paradoxical pulse is defined as a pulse that is significantly weaker during inspiration than during expiration.[48] Systolic blood pressure is normally 8 to 10 mm Hg lower during inspiration and is attributed to increased blood volume in the lungs, decreased venous return, and decreased stroke volume. Cardiac tamponade further decreases venous return and stroke volume, thereby causing a difference of more than 10 mm Hg in systolic blood pressure at inspiration and expiration.[44] If cardiac tamponade is severe, a palpated arterial pulse may also diminish during inspiration. Additional findings include dyspnea, cough, chest pain, narrowed pulse pressure, cyanosis, diaphoresis, confusion, and peripheral edema.

Diagnostic studies

If the clinical signs suggest cardiac tamponade, the echocardiogram is the easiest, most sensitive, and most accurate tool with which to determine the presence of pericardial effusion. Large or small (15 mL or less) accumulations of fluid can be observed easily. With tamponade, two echos rather than one are seen with a single heart beat and anterior mitral leaflet motion may be aberrant.[42] A computerized tomography scan can also be helpful in estimating the volume of the effusion. A radiograph of the chest will usually reveal a cardiac silhouette that is enlarged and globular in shape. An electrocardiogram (EKG) is not a sensitive diagnostic tool for cardiac tamponade, but it can show low voltage, nonspecific ST and T changes, and electrical alternans, where P waves and QRS complexes vary in size.

Treatment

In the face of life-threatening cardiac tamponade, immediate goals include hemodynamic stabilization and removal of the fluid by pericardiocentesis. Pericardiocentesis involves placement of a 16-gauge needle into the pericardial sac from a left parasternal or substernal paraxiphoid approach. The patient is supine, and the head of the bed is elevated 10° to 20°. With a syringe, pericardial fluid is withdrawn and sent for cytologic study and culture. False-negative cytologic findings in the face of a malignant effusion are quite common. Although pericardiocentesis will immediately reverse cardiac tamponade, more permanent resolution is sought through systemic therapy or local treatment. If effective systemic therapy is an option, it should be instituted as soon as the emergent tamponade is resolved.

For recurrent pericardial effusions and prolonged palliation, formation of a pericardial pleural window is recommended. Creation of a pericardial pleural window is a fairly successful surgical procedure with a greater than 90% reponse rate. It has limited risks, with adhesion formation as the major drawback.[49] Some oncologists prefer drainage and sclerosing by means of a catheter insertion similar to the approach for pleural effusions. Common sclerosing agents are tetracycline, quinacrine, thiotepa, nitrogen mustard, and 5-fluorouracil. Sclerosing is successful in about 50% of the attempts and causes transient chest pain, nausea, and fever.[42]

Recent advances in intracavitary therapy, the instillation of cytotoxic agents into a body cavity to destroy cancer cells rather than sclerose the cavity, have been applied to the treatment of malignant pericardial effusions. Markman and Howell[50] have effectively treated recurrent pericardial effusions with intrapericardial instillation of cisplatin, 10 mg in 50 mL normal saline solution administered daily for 5 days.

Successful treatment of cardiac tamponade is evident, with immediate clinical improvement seen, when as little as 50 mL of pericardial fluid is removed. Resolution of cardiac tamponade occurs rapidly after the effusion is drained. Vital signs return to normal and cardiopulmonary status stabilizes.

For patients with a favorable prognosis who are considered free of malignant disease, those with chronic pericarditis from mediastinal irradiation, or those with constrictive pericarditis, total pericardectomy by thoracotomy may be the treatment of choice. Total pericardectomy carries a high morbidity and should be chosen for a very limited population. Corticosteroids can help alleviate the inflammation of constrictive pericarditis as a short-term measure. Radiation therapy has also been used to prevent recurrent pericardial effusions but carries the risk of damage to the pericardium and myocardium. Long-term resolution is a challenge, since there is a significant rate of recurrence of pericardial effusions.

Nursing management of the patient with cardiac tamponade begins with early recognition and prompt diagnosis. Populations at risk, patients with cardiothoracic malignancies and widely disseminated disease, should be skillfully assessed, particularly if shortness of breath, fatigue, tachycardia, or hypotension is present. Right heart catheterization (Swan-Ganz) assists in diagnosis of cardiac tamponade and in monitoring of hemodynamic status during therapeutic reversal of tamponade. Right atrial, right ventricular diastolic, and pulmonary artery diastolic pressures are usually 10 mm Hg or higher in classic tamponade due to pericardial effusion.[44]

Once cardiac tamponade is suspected, supportive therapy is instituted to stabilize the patient while preparations are made for an emergency pericardiocentesis.[46] Supportive therapy includes volume expanders such as saline solution, 5% Plasmanate, or fresh frozen plasma, given to improve cardiac filling pressures and to compensate for a decreased cardiac output.[44,45] Cardiac output can be further maximized by infusions of positive inotropic agents such as isoproterenol or dobutamine.[44,46,51] Oxygen should be given as needed, but intubation with positive pressure breathing should be avoided since this would further decrease venous return and increase intrapleural and intrapericardial pressures.[46]

During pericardiocentesis, the patient's hemodynamic status and electrocardiogram are closely monitored. The nurse observes the patient for possible complications, which include puncture of the right atrium or ventricle, arrythmia, infection, injury to the lungs, laceration of a coronary artery, and inadvertent injection of air into the heart.[51] If catheters are kept in place for continuous drainage and/or instillation of either sclerosing or antineoplastic agents, asepsis and patency are maintained as well as accurate records of drainage output and vital signs.

Nurses can provide invaluable support to patients and their families during this life-threatening experience. Explaining the procedures and equipment can greatly reduce the patient's anxiety and foster hope and confidence in the outcome of the emergency interventions.

Prognosis and Follow-Up Care

Development of a pericardial effusion is a significant prognostic indicator. It usually occurs in the face of widely metastatic cancer or a rapidly progressing cardiothoracic malignancy. No studies have compared the prognosis of patients with or without pericardial effusion in various types of cancer.[46] In small trials of different treatment options available for pericardial effusions caused by a variety of cancers, overall average survival ranges from 3 to 17 months.[49,52,53] Death is most often attributed to the disseminated cancer and not to cardiac complications.

For patients who have an acute episode, tamponade is usually reversible and recovery is rapid, once effective treatment is initiated. Rehabilitation requirements are short term. The patient's status, however, is monitored through frequent office visits. Resolution of the effusion and/or cardiac tamponade is achieved by treatment of the underlying disease.

Chronic pericardial effusion, constrictive pericarditis, and unsuccessful treatment can severely debilitate the cancer patient, who already has a limited outlook for survival. Home care needs may include assistance with activities of daily living, assistive devices, oxygen therapy, and possible admission to an extended-care facility. Supportive care is critical during the terminal phase of the disease.

Since effective treatments for cancer have prolonged overall survival, the incidence of metastasis to the pericardium and of cardiac complications of cancer treatment are increasing. When recognized and treated early, pericardial effusion and cardiac tamponade are reversible emergency conditions. Tumor encroachment and invasion of the heart most often cause fatal cardiac tamponade.

HYPERCALCEMIA

Introduction

The two most common causes of hypercalcemia are primary hyperparathyroidism and cancer. This medical emergency will occur in 8% to 20% of cancer patients. Its occurrence often heralds a lack of control of the malignant disease process.[54] It is estimated that 150 cancer patients per million per year will have hypercalcemia.[55,56] The course of hypercalcemia associated with malignancy is steadily progressive. Death can occur from hypercalcemic crisis within 12 hours, but fewer than 5% of patients will require urgent lifesaving therapy.[56]

Pathophysiology

Hypercalcemia is a metabolic disorder that can occur in persons with cancer as a result of increased bone resorption caused by either bone destruction by tumor invasion or increased levels of parathyroid hormone (PTH), osteoclast-activating factor (OAF), or prostaglandin produced by the cancer.[57] If adequate renal clearance of calcium is not preserved, hypercalcemia can develop. Untreated or uncontrolled hypercalcemia can lead to life-threatening alterations in cardiac, neurologic, and renal function.

Normal serum calcium levels are maintained by absorption of calcium from the gastrointestinal tract, secretion of PTH and calcitonin, effects of vitamin D, deposition or resorption of calcium from bone, renal clearance of calcium, and binding of calcium to serum proteins, usually albumin.[54]

PTH, produced by the parathyroid gland, promotes the release of calcium from bone when the calcium level in the extracellular fluid surrounding the parathyroid is low. PTH stimulates osteoclasts to break down bone structure, thus liberating calcium phosphate crystals. PTH increases gastrointestinal absorption of calcium by stimulating the active-transport system to move calcium from the intestinal lumen to the blood. In addition, vitamin D stimulates calcium absorption from the intestine. PTH also stimulates increased renal tubular absorption of calcium while reducing reabsorption of phosphate to lower extracellular phosphate concentration.[58] Calcitonin, secreted by the thyroid, is part of a feedback mechanism to lower serum calcium by inhibiting bone resorption and opposing the effects of PTH. Ninety-nine percent of body calcium is bound in bone and teeth. The other 1% is present in the plasma as ionized (0.5%) and protein bound (0.5%) calcium. When serum albumin levels are reduced, there is a disproportionate increase of ionized (free) calcium in the blood. Ionized (free) calcium is the critical component in clinical hypercalcemia.

Etiology

Persons at greatest risk of hypercalcemia include those with bone metastases from primary tumors of the breast, lung, and kidney because of extensive bone destruction and release of calcium into the extracellular fluid. Hypercalcemia also occurs in persons with osteolytic bone lesions and with hematologic malignancies such as multiple myeloma and lymphomas, particularly HTLV-1 associated T-cell lymphoma or leukemia. Squamous cell lung cancer and carcinoma of the head and neck are thought to produce PTH, OAF, and prostaglandin, which stimulate bone resorption.

Other factors that contribute to the occurrence of hypercalcemia in cancer patients include hyperparathyroidism, immobilization, anorexia, nausea, vomiting, dehydration, and renal failure. Cancer patients have an increased incidence of primary hyperparathyroidism, which should be considered in the differential diagnosis.[57] Prolonged immobilization is associated with increased resorption of calcium from the bones.[59] Dehydration results in a decreased glomerular filtration rate (GFR) and an increased sodium reabsorption to conserve water, which then increases calcium reabsorption and decreases calcium excretion, respectively. An elevated serum calcium level causes a decrease in smooth muscle tone of the gastrointestinal tract, resulting in anorexia, nausea, vomiting, and constipation. Likewise, a renal tubular defect can cause an inability to conserve water as evidenced by polyuria and polydipsia, with worsening dehydration, and the vicious cycle of hypercalcemia persists. Decreased GFR may be a side effect of some chemotherapeutic or antibiotic medications and could contribute to hypercalcemia. Therapy with estrogen, androgen, progesterone, or tamoxifen has been associated with hypercalcemia in women with breast cancer.[54]

Assessment

Clinical characteristics

Knowledge of the specific cancers and factors that contribute to hypercalcemia is necessary for determination of who is at risk of this metabolic emergency.[60] Clinical characteristics are usually related to the effects of increased calcium on smooth, skeletal, and cardiac muscle. The main systems affected include gastrointestinal, neuromuscular, cardiac, and renal. The effects of hypercalcemia on the gastrointestinal tract can be manifested as anorexia, nausea, vomiting, constipation, abdominal pain, and dehydration.[60] Neuromuscular manifestations are lethargy, confusion, stupor, convulsions, and hyporeflexia.[61] Abnormalities in cardiac function may be bradycardia or tachycardia and electrocardiographic abnormalities reflecting an increased PR interval and a decreased QT interval. Signs of alterations in renal function are polyuria, polydipsia, decreased renal concentrating ability, progressive renal insufficiency, and eventually renal failure.[61] Dry mucous membranes, poor skin turgor, rapid thready pulse, and orthostatic hypotension may signify dehydration. Cancer patients who have hypercalcemia usually experience a progressive course with recurrent episodes.

Diagnostic studies

Mundy and Martin[56] have outlined three categories of patients with hypercalcemia and indications for treatment: (1) Patients with serum calcium levels of 10.5 to 12.0 mg/dL (2.62 to 3.0 mm/L) who are asymptomatic should be observed carefully and may be given chronic therapy as outpatients. (2) Patients with serum calcium levels of 12 to 13 mg/dL (3.0 to 3.25 mm/L) and who are asymptomatic require specific but nonurgent therapy. (3) Patients with serum calcium levels of 13 mg/dL (3.25 mm/L) or higher and any patients with symptoms require emergency treatment of hypercalcemia.

It is important to note that since calcium is bound to protein, the serum calcium level must be "corrected" for albumin less than 4 to obtain an accurate measure of the calcium level. The formula for this calculation is

"Corrected" total serum calcium (TSC) =
Measured TSC + (4.0 − Serum albumin) × 0.8.[56]

TABLE 31-4 Therapy of Malignancy-Associated Hypercalcemia

Tumor ablation
Rehydration/calciuresis
Saline infusion
Furosemide
Inhibition of bone resorption
Prostaglandin synthetase inhibitors
Calcitonin
Mithramycin
Diphosphonates
Galium nitrate
Miscellaneous
Oral phosphorus
Limitation of parenteral calcium intake
Mobilization
Dialysis
Glucocorticoids

Source: Adapted from Stewart AF: Therapy of malignancy-associated hypercalcemia: 1983. Am J Med 74:476, 1983.

Treatment

Tumor control or reduction of tumor burden is the only long-term measure that is effective for reversing hypercalcemia (Table 31-4).[62] Cancer therapy and emergency medical intervention must be instituted for patients who have symptoms or who have a serum calcium level of 13 mg/dL or more. For cancer patients, severe hypercalcemia is a medical emergency that requires vigorous hydration to restore the normal volume of extracellular compartment fluid, increase glomerular filtration, and promote urinary calcium excretion. Infusion of 4 to 6 liters of normal saline solution (0.9%) each day for 48 hours will raise the glomerular filtration rate and interfere with calcium reabsorption in the proximal tubule. Serum calcium will likely decrease by 2 to 3 mg/dL over 1 to 2 days.[62] Parenteral furosemide, 40 to 80 mg every 4 to 6 hours, can produce sodium diuresis, which in turn causes calcium diuresis while preventing heart failure from fluid overload and hypernatremia.[63] When hypercalcemia is emergent, fluid and electrolyte balance is monitored closely. Fluid balance is assessed by monitoring intake, output, and weight and observing for edema of lower extremities or sacrum, noting distended neck veins and shortness of breath, and auscultating the lungs for rales. Serum electrolytes are monitored closely since vigorous hydration can lead to hypokalemia, hyponatremia, hypocalcemia, and hypomagnesemia.[64] Likewise, blood urea nitrogen and creatinine are monitored to evaluate the adequacy of renal function.

Intravenous mithramycin, 15 to 25 μg/kg body weight, is given in a single dose to inhibit bone resorption of calcium; it usually decreases serum calcium within 12 hours, with a peak effect at 48 to 96 hours.[62] Intravenous mithramycin, initially developed as a cytotoxic agent, may cause nausea and vomiting, bone marrow suppression, clotting abnormalities, and hepatic and renal changes. Mithramycin is administered cautiously through an intravenous line since infiltration can cause tissue necrosis at the site. Antiemetic agents are administered, but they may cause increased lethargy, particularly if liver function is compromised. The limiting toxic effects associated with mithramycin are thrombocytopenia and bleeding diathesis despite a normal platelet count.[56] Prothrombin and partial thromboplastin levels are monitored and precautions are instituted to prevent bleeding, especially when other antineoplastic agents are given concomitantly. Mithramycin is nephrotoxic, eliminated by the kidneys, and cannot be used when renal function is impaired. Many cancer patients have impaired renal function as a result of previous antibiotic or cytotoxic therapy. Patients with multiple myeloma may have impaired renal function from Bence-Jones proteinuria.[56]

Calcitonin, 4 Medical Research Council units per kilogram of body weight subcutaneously every 12 hours, also can inhibit bone resorption, with a rapid effect, but the duration of the response is limited.[62] Serum calcium level is reduced by 2 to 3 mg/dL.[62] However, the effect is transient and limited to 24 to 72 hours, despite repeated administration. This phenomenon "may be due to down-regulation of calcitonin receptors on bone cells which occurs in the continued presence of calcitonin."[56] Glucocorticosteroids (eg, hydrocortisone, 100 mg intravenously every 6 hours) are often administered concomitantly to prevent this phenomenon. Since there is a risk of anaphylaxis with calcitonin injections, skin testing is done before administration. Epinephrine, antihistamines, and oxygen should be available for emergency use.

Phosphate, 75 mmol intravenously, although extremely toxic, may be administered as a single injection if other measures fail to promote the precipitation of inorganic calcium phosphate.[56] Intravenous phosphates act within minutes of administration; however, there is danger of hypotension, hypocalcemia, renal failure, and visceral calcification.[57]

Gallium nitrate, 200 mg/m^2 in continuous intravenous infusion for 5 days, has been shown to be an effective agent in decreasing serum calcium salts in the bone.[57,65] Diphosphates, such as etridonale plus ADP, are currently being studied for effectiveness.[62,66] When there is preexistent renal disease, or if renal failure occurs, dialysis will be necessary.

Oral phosphate, 1 to 3 g three times daily, may be given to control chronic, mild hypercalcemia when the serum phosphorus level is less than 3.7 mg/dL; however, diarrhea may be a dose-limiting side effect.[56] When oral phosphates are prescribed, the patient is taught that perianal care after defecation is necessary to prevent skin breakdown caused by the caustic effect of excreted phosphate. If perianal pain or excoriation develops, sitz baths are encouraged and anesthetic ointment is applied. Indomethacin and oral steroids may be prescribed for patients with hypercalcemia, but the effectiveness of these agents is controversial.[56] Patients who are taking steroids or indomethacin are taught that immunosuppressive agents may mask fever as an early sign of infection, and precautionary measures are reviewed.

Recognition of the early signs of hypercalcemia is an important nursing intervention to prevent further complications of hypercalcemia.[67] Patients and family members are taught to observe for these symptoms, and the importance of frequent ambulation or mobilization of extremities is stressed.[60,67,68] Analgesic agents are administered before mobility exercises if chronic pain is a problem. However, any new bone pain must be reported, since patients at risk of hypercalcemia may develop pathologic fractures.[68] Patients at risk of hypercalcemia are encouraged to drink 2 to 3 liters of fluid each day to prevent dehydration and promote urinary excretion of calcium.

Thiazide diuretics inhibit calcium excretion; therefore they are contraindicated in persons who are at risk of hypercalcemia. Likewise, the dosage of digitalis preparations may need to be lowered and digitalis toxicity carefully assessed, since the action of digitalis is potentiated in a hypercalcemic state.[69]

Prognosis

Emergent hypercalcemia can be reversed in 80% of episodes with aggressive, immediate intervention. However, the duration of normocalcemia may last only a few days to 3 weeks unless there is control of the underlying tumor that is causing the hypercalcemia. Oral steroids and indomethacin are only 20% to 30% effective in controlling chronic hypercalcemia.[56]

TUMOR LYSIS SYNDROME

Introduction

Acute tumor lysis syndrome (ATLS) is a complication of cancer therapy that occurs when a large number of rapidly proliferating tumor cells are lysed. Many chemotherapeutic agents destroy tumor cells while the cells are dividing; likewise, cells that are undergoing division are more sensitive to radiation therapy. Therefore cancer patients with massive tumor burdens that are rapidly dividing are at risk of acute tumor lysis syndrome, particularly as treatment is instituted.

Pathophysiology

Within the cell are the minerals potassium and phosphorus and nucleic acids that form DNA and RNA. When the cell membrane is ruptured, released nucleic acids are converted by the liver into uric acid while potassium and phosphorus are released into the bloodstream, causing abnormally high levels of these minerals and a decrease in calcium (Figure 31-4). An inverse relationship exists between phosphorus and calcium; increased serum phosphorus results in decreased serum calcium because serum phosphorus binds with circulating calcium. When a large number of cells are lysed within a short period of time, the result is acute tumor lysis syndrome characterized by acute hyperuricemia, hyperkalemia, hyperphosphatemia and hypocalcemia, and/or acute renal failure.[70] The degree of metabolic abnormality depends on the adequacy of renal

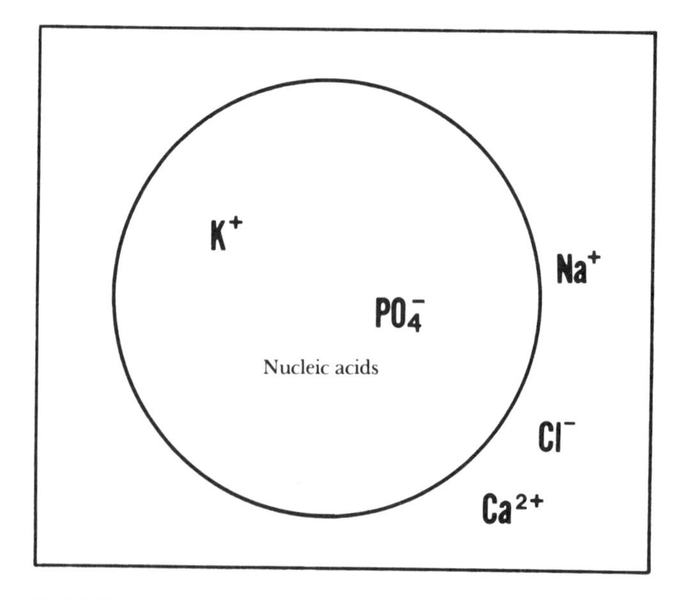

FIGURE 31-4 Normal intracellular components include potassium, phosphorus, and nucleic acids. When cell lysis occurs, the intracellular components are released, causing abnormally high levels of circulating minerals and uric acid production. Serum phosphorus binds with circulating calcium and this results in hypocalcemia.

function, since uric acid, potassium, and phosphorus are excreted in the urine.[71] These metabolic abnormalities can develop alone or in combination. Acute renal failure results from intratubular precipitation of uric acid or calcium phosphate crystallization.[71]

Etiology

Acute tumor lysis syndrome can occur when a cancer patient with a rapidly growing large tumor burden receives cytotoxic therapy. ATLS is most commonly seen in cancer patients with high-grade lymphoma or acute lymphoblastic leukemia, since these cancer cells are particularly sensitive to treatment and will rapidly lyse.[72] In addition, immature lymphoblasts contain an abnormally high level of phosphorus, which is released when the cells are lysed.[73] In untreated persons with cancer, acute tumor lysis syndrome can also develop when there is a rapidly growing large tumor mass that undergoes profound cell destruction.[71]

Assessment

When cancer patients with rapidly proliferating tumors are receiving cytotoxic therapy, acute tumor lysis syndrome should be anticipated. Patients with large tumor burdens in combination with high white blood cell count, lymphadenopathy, splenomegaly, and elevated lactate dehydrogenase are at particularly high risk. They will require close monitoring of metabolic parameters, including potassium, phosphorus, calcium, uric acid, blood urea nitrogen, and creatinine levels. For high-risk patients, baseline renal function is assessed before the initiation of aggressive antineoplastic therapy.

Clinical characteristics

Pretreatment serum potassium levels may be elevated because of dehydration, compromised renal function, acidosis resulting from sepsis, adrenal insufficiency as steroids are tapered, and medications such as indomethacin, potassium supplements, and potassium-sparing diuretics.[74] Signs of hyperkalemia include weakness, paresthesia, muscle cramps, ascending flaccid paralysis, bradycardia, EKG changes, diarrhea, and nausea.

Clinical indicators of hyperphosphatemia include oliguria, anuria, and renal insufficiency. Patients with hypocalcemia may exhibit muscle twitching, carpopedal spasm, tetany, laryngospasm, paresthesia, convulsions, hypotension, and EKG changes. Hypomagnesemia, acute pancreatitis, vitamin D deficiency, diarrhea, multiple blood transfusions, and anorexia are predisposing factors for hypocalcemia.[74] Medications that may potentiate hyperphosphatemia and hypocalcemia include phosphates, furosemide, mithramycin, gallium nitrate, and anticonvulsants.[74]

Signs of hyperuricemia and compromised renal function include nausea, vomiting, diarrhea, lethargy, edema, flank pain, hematuria, crystalluria, azotemia, oliguria, and anuria. Thiazide diuretics potentiate hyperuricemia.

Treatment

Knowledge of cancer patients who are at risk of acute tumor lysis syndrome and close monitoring for hyperuricemia, hyperkalemia, hyperphosphatemia, hypocalcemia, and impaired renal function is essential.[73,75] Adequate renal function must be preserved during treatment for cancers associated with acute tumor lysis syndrome. Uric acid crystallization in the renal tubules causing obstruction, decreased glomerular filtration, and/or acute renal failure is a major complication that can be prevented by prophylactic alkalinization of urine, thus increasing the solubility of uric acid. This is accomplished by maintaining the urine pH at a level greater than 7, with the use of sodium bicarbonate and vigorous intravenous hydration to decrease the uric acid concentration in the urine.[70,76] A recommended fluid regimen is D5W/0.45NS with sodium bicarbonate, 60 meg/L, at 150 mL/hr.

Potassium and magnesium may need to be replaced if deficits in these electrolytes appear.[71] Simultaneous hydration and diuresis promote the excretion of phosphorus and potassium. Urine output should be maintained at 3 liters or more per day.[71] Diuretics may be administered as adjunctive therapy, particularly when the person has a coexisting condition (eg, impaired cardiac function) that could potentiate the risk of fluid overload. If adequate urine output is not achieved, furosemide, 40 to 80 mg intravenously, or mannitol, 12.5 g intravenously, may be given to promote diuresis.[71] Fluid balance is assessed by monitoring of intake, output, and weight and observation for edema of lower extremities or sacrum. Distended neck veins or shortness of breath should be noted and the lungs should be auscultated for adventitious sounds (rales). Decreased urine output, hematuria, and urine pH <7 are reported immediately.

If acute tumor lysis syndrome is a potential complication of the cytotoxic therapy, allopurinol is generally given as a prophylactic measure.[70] Allopurinol decreases uric acid levels by interfering with purine metabolism. It may cause a skin rash within 7 days of initial dosage, requiring palliative relief measures with lotion or diphenhydramine hydrochloride.

Persons with cancer that infiltrates the kidney (eg, lymphoma or leukemia) may require radiation therapy to the kidney area before they receive chemotherapy, which should reduce the overall tumor burden.[71] Also, leukapheresis may be employed when the white blood cell count is extraordinarily elevated (eg, 100,000/mm^3) to reduce both the tumor burden and the risk of tumor lysis syndrome. If the aforementioned interventions fail to promote adequate renal function, dialysis may be necessary.

If hyperkalemia develops, an intravenous solution of 50% glucose (25 g) is administered to raise plasma insulin levels, thereby causing an intracellular shift of potassium. It is recommended that 1 unit of regular insulin be given with each 4 g of glucose administered.[71] An ion exchange resin, such as Kayexalate (Winthrop-Breon) may be given orally or rectally in conjunction with sorbitol to promote excretion of potassium in feces. Oral Kayexalate is given in a dose of 15 to 30 g with 50 mL of 20% sorbitol two to four times daily. If the patient is unable to tolerate oral medications, then a retention enema of 50 g in 200 mL of 20% sorbitol, held for 30 to 60 minutes, is recommended.[71] If cardiac or neuromuscular toxicity is exhibited, calcium gluconate is given to decrease these symptoms.

Hyperphosphatemia and hypocalcemia are treated by administration of calcium supplements and phosphate-binding antacids, such as Amphogel (Wyeth) or Basaljel (Wyeth). Pulse rate, rhythm, and EKG should be monitored frequently and changes should be reported. Serum potassium, phosphorus, calcium, uric acid, blood urea nitrogen, and creatinine levels should be monitored every 6 hours, or as ordered.

Prognosis

The occurrence and resolution of acute tumor lysis syndrome are dependent on the tumor's responsiveness to the radiation and/or chemotherapy administered. Since cytolysis occurs within 7 days following treatment, acute tumor lysis syndrome usually resolves during that time frame if adequate renal function has been maintained and metabolic parameters have been corrected. If a person who has a hematologic malignancy and a rapidly rising white blood cell count has a relapse, there is usually a recurrence of acute tumor lysis syndrome when therapy is instituted again.

SYNDROME OF INAPPROPRIATE ANTIDIURETIC HORMONE

Introduction

Syndrome of inappropriate antidiuretic hormone (SIADH) is a paraneoplastic disease that usually occurs as a result of the presence of a malignancy. It is often the presenting symptom in patients with small cell lung cancer.

Pathophysiology

Antidiuretic hormone (ADH) or arginine vasopressin is produced by the hypothalamus and stored in the posterior lobe of the pituitary. In response to either an increase in plasma concentration (serum osmolality) or a decrease in plasma volume, ADH is secreted. ADH increases the permeability of the distal tubules of the kidney, which then conserve water. As a result, plasma osmolality is lowered by the dilutional effect of additional water and plasma volume increases.[77] A feedback loop of osmoreceptors in the hypothalamus and pressoreceptors in the left atrium and carotid sinus monitor plasma osmolality and circulation volume to adjust ADH secretion appropriately.

The syndrome of inappropriate antidiuretic hormone (SIADH) is usually associated with an excess of ADH resulting from ectopic production or abnormal stimulation of the hypothalamus-pituitary network. SIADH may, however, occur as a result of direct effect on the renal tubules of external factors (ie, chemotherapy and analgesics) that mimic the action of ADH. The resulting pathophysiologic state is water intoxication. When excessive amounts of water are retained, plasma osmolality drops and dilutional hyponatremia occurs. In addition, urinary excretion of sodium increases, causing further hyponatremia, and urinary osmolality becomes inappropriately higher than plasma osmolality.[78]

Etiology

The tumors most frequently associated with ectopic ADH production are small cell tumors of the lung. ADH levels are elevated in approximately 50% of the cases of small-cell lung cancer, while only about 10% have clinically evident SIADH.[79,81] Other malignancies that produce inappropriate levels of ADH are gastrointestinal cancers, thymoma, lymphoma, Hodgkin's disease, bladder cancer, and some sarcomas.[78,82]

Certain antineoplastic agents, drugs, and chemicals (eg, cyclophosphamide, vincristine, chlorpropamide, morphine, nicotine, and ethanol) can induce SIADH.[78] Some agents directly stimulate ADH secretion, whereas others affect the renal tubules. Cisplatin administration has been associated with the development of SIADH, but whether it increases ADH secretion or affects the renal tubules has not been established.[83] Other medical conditions, such as pulmonary and central nervous system infections, neurologic trauma, and primary or metastatic brain tumors, can also cause SIADH. SIADH is most frequently associated with ectopic ADH production in small cell lung cancer.

Assessment

Identification of patients at risk of SIADH and its manifestations aids in recognition and treatment of this emergency. Initially, symptoms are vague and easily attributed to side effects of therapy or tumor. Assessment of blood and urine chemistries and physical manifestations will help develop the diagnosis of SIADH.

Clinical characteristics

The primary clinical characteristics are manifestations of water intoxication and the severity depends on the degree of abnormality of the serum sodium and plasma osmolality as well as the rapidity with which the syndrome develops. Symptoms are attributed to the effects of cerebral edema. In persons with mild hyponatremia (serum sodium levels ≤ 130 mEq/L), thirst, headache, anorexia, muscle cramps, and lethargy may be seen. As the serum sodium level falls below 125 mEq/L, nausea, vomiting, hyporeflexia, and confusion may ensue. Severe hypona-

TABLE 31-5 Laboratory Values in SIADH

Serum sodium	<130 mEq/L
Plasma osmolality	<280 mOsm/kg
Urine osmolality	>330 mOsm/kg
Urine sodium	>20 mEq/L

tremia (serum sodium < 120 mEq/L) can cause seizures, coma, and death.

Other clinical characteristics may include decreased urine output (less than 400 mL/24 hr) and unexplained weight gain without evidence of edema.[85]

Diagnostic studies

Hyponatremia (serum sodium level less than 130 mEq/L) is not solely diagnostic of SIADH. It may, in fact, be due to rigorous hydration or recent diuretic administration. Hyponatremia associated with a low serum osmolality, high urine sodium level, and high urine osmolality is indicative of SIADH. Table 31-5 lists the laboratory parameters used to diagnose SIADH. Adrenal and renal function are normal in SIADH. Blood urea nitrogen and serum uric acid levels may be low as a result of the expanded intravascular volume of SIADH.

Treatment

The management of SIADH depends on the severity of the hyponatremia, the patient's clinical condition, and the underlying cause of the syndrome. Initial therapy usually consists of water restriction to induce a net negative water balance. In the oncology population, most often the underlying malignancy and its ectopic hormone production are causing SIADH. If the cancer patient's condition permits, systemic chemotherapy should be instituted immediately, since no other medical intervention will effectively suppress tumor production of ADH. Most chemotherapy regimens require adequate hydration, so this situation demands critical assessment and monitoring skills to manage the patient's fluid and electrolyte status. In mild hyponatremia, the minimal amount of hydration during chemotherapy administration with normal saline solution and subsequent fluid restriction of 500 mL/24 hr will control the syndrome until the tumor regresses.

Moderate SIADH, when the serum sodium level is less than 125 mEq/L and the patient has symptoms, may require infusion of normal saline solution and electrolytes and diuresis with furosemide before initiation of systemic chemotherapy to treat the underlying tumor. Patients who are severely hyponatremic (serum sodium level less than 120 mEq/L) and experiencing profound neurologic changes may require 3% hypertonic saline infusions and furosemide diuresis.[86] Systemic chemotherapy may have to be delayed for several days until the patient's fluid and electrolyte balance and neurologic status are improved. When neurologic status is impaired, patient safety is a priority and a protective environment is provided.

Some of the systemic chemotherapy agents currently used to treat small cell lung cancer are vincristine, cyclophosphamide, and cisplatin. When managing patients with SIADH who are receiving these chemotherapeutic agents, one should consider the ADH effects and toxicities associated with each particular agent. Vincristine, cisplatin, and cyclophosphamide may exacerbate SIADH. Fluid restriction may promote hemorrhagic cystitis with cyclophosphamide, nephrotoxicity with cisplatin, and uric acid nephrolithiasis from tumor cell lysis. If hydration is critical to the administration of chemotherapy, normal saline solution is used with or without furosemide diuresis. Weight, neurologic status, intake and output, plasma and urine osmolality, and urine and serum sodium levels are carefully monitored and used as critical parameters for management. Any other medications that can induce SIADH must be withheld and possible substitutions made.

SIADH that is chronic or recurs despite systemic chemotherapy may require therapy with demeclocycline (900 to 1200 mg/24 hr). Demeclocycline can partially inhibit the action of ADH, but it induces a reversible diabetes insipidus.[87] Lithium may also be used to inhibit ADH effect on the kidney.

SIADH commonly occurs as a presenting symptom of small cell lung cancer. Nursing interventions are directed toward reversing SIADH, administering chemotherapy and managing its side effects, educating the patient and the family about the disease, treatment, side effects, and self-care measures, and also providing support to the patient and family during this crisis. Since most therapy for lung cancer is administered on an outpatient basis, education and home care instructions are essential. Patients are taught about fluid restrictions, measurement of intake and output, signs and symptoms of hyponatremia, and when a condition indicates the need to contact the physician.

Reversal of SIADH is evident when the serum sodium level approaches normal. When the permeability of the renal tubules to water normalizes, not only the serum sodium level but the urine and plasma osmolality and the urine sodium value also return to normal. Mental status improves and other symptoms resolve as fluid and electrolyte balance is restored. This balance must be restored slowly since rapid changes in serum sodium and water levels can cause shrinkage of neurons, leading to cerebral edema and seizures.[88]

Prognosis and Follow-up Care

The overall prognosis for the cancer patient with SIADH depends on the underlying cause. SIADH usually resolves as the tumor regresses, but it can persist despite tumor control. It may recur and suggest tumor progression, but recurrence is sometimes seen with stable disease during the maintenance phase of chemotherapy.[2] Neurologic impairment from water intoxication is usually reversible and does not require long-term rehabilitation. Frequent assessment of the patient and monitoring of the serum sodium level is needed in the initial period following SIADH.

Because of the increased incidence of small cell lung cancer and other tumors associated with ectopic production of ADH, the incidence of SIADH is increasing.[88] SIADH can progress to seizure, coma, and death. The insidious onset of SIADH can delay early diagnosis; therefore the nurse must be aware of the population at risk and of the predisposing factors. Involvement of the patient and the family is crucial in effective management, since compliance with fluid restriction, monitoring of symptoms, and reporting of changes is necessary to reverse SIADH.

SPINAL CORD COMPRESSION

Introduction

For the oncology patient, spinal cord compression is a neurologic emergency that requires prompt diagnosis and intervention so that neurologic function can be preserved and maintained. It is estimated that spinal cord compression develops in about 5% of patients with systemic cancer and that 95% of these cases are due to tumor in the epidural space or outside the spinal cord.[89]

Pathophysiology

Compression of the spinal cord can occur through one of four mechanisms: epidural metastases, intramedullary metastases, vertebral subluxation, and spinal subdural hematoma.[90] Metastatic tumor in the epidural space of the spine is the most common cause of cord compression. Tumor usually reaches the epidural space by first metastasizing to the vertebral body and then invading the anterior epidural space. Another pathway for epidural metastasis is direct extension through the intervertebral foramina by paravertebral tumors, such as tumors in retroperitoneal or mediastinal lymph nodes. A third (and rare) mechanism of epidural metastasis is hematogenous spread.[90]

Intramedullary metastasis is rare. Tumor cells reach the interior cord by hematogenous spread, growth along nerve roots by paravertebral tumors, or seeding from leptomeningeal metastases. Vertebral subluxation (dislocation) causing spinal cord compression is an infrequent occurrence that is most often associated with cervical spine metastasis. Metastasis to the cervical axis leads to pathologic fracture, dislocation of the atlas into or onto the axis, and cervical cord compression with possible respiratory arrest. Spinal subdural hematoma is a complication that has a rapid onset, usually associated with lumbar puncture in patients with thrombocytopenia.

Compression of the spinal cord in any circumstance leads to edema of the cord and ischemia, which mechanically distort and damage neural tissue. Further insult can occur from direct tumor infiltration that destroys cord tissue.[91,92] The rate and degree of compression and resulting cord damage are responsible for the array of clinical manifestations. The spinal cord has sensory, motor, and autonomic functions and the amount of damage can range from minor neurologic changes to complete paralysis (paraplegia).

Etiology

Although primary tumors of the spinal cord can cause compression, it is more likely to be metastatic disease that causes spinal cord compression. Epidural metastasis is most frequently associated with vertebral body metastasis. Therefore cancers that metastasize to bone can cause spinal cord compression. The most common cancers that metastasize to bone are those of the breast, lung, prostate, and kidney and myeloma. Lymphomas have a high correlation with spinal cord compression, but lymphomas invade the cord by direct extension through the intervertebral foramina.[90,93] In the past decade the incidence of lymphoma-induced spinal cord compression has declined because of the use of aggressive radiation early in the treatment of lymphoma.[90,94] Neuroblastomas also cause spinal cord compression via the direct extension route.

The site of epidural metastasis and compression is related to the origin of the primary cancer. In their classic study of cord compression, Gilbert and colleagues[94] concluded that lung and breast cancers most often cause thoracic spinal cord compression whereas gastrointestinal cancers most frequently metastasize to the lumbosacral spine. Breast cancer is also related to vertebral subluxation of the cervical spine. The relationship between primary tumors and epidural metastases is due to not only anatomic location but also to vascular supply and venous drainage.[93] Figure 31-5 illustrates the incidence of epidural metastasis by location on the spinal cord and primary cancer.[94]

Assessment

The importance of early recognition and diagnosis of spinal cord compression cannot be overemphasized. The single critical prognostic factor in spinal cord compression is the neurologic status before the initiation of therapy. The less extensive the injury to the cord before treatment, the greater the likelihood of full ambulation, sensation, and bowel and bladder control after treatment.[89,93] The converse is also true. Compromised neurologic status before treatment would indicate that posttreatment recovery will probably be limited.

Clinical characteristics

Four symptoms in particular are related to spinal cord compression: pain, weakness, autonomic dysfunction, and sensory loss. More than 90% of the patients with spinal cord compression have central back pain within one or two vertebrae of the actual compression. The pain may or

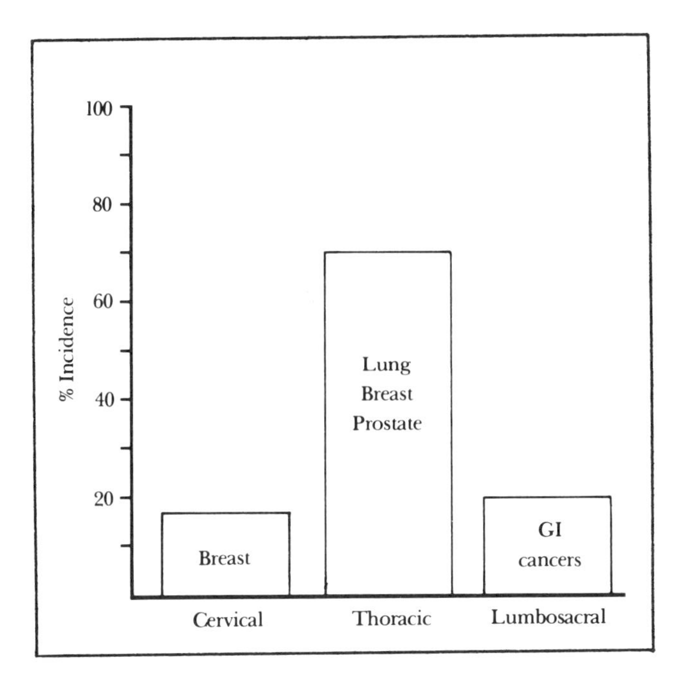

FIGURE 31-5 Primary cancers responsible for most cord compressions specific to location on spinal cord.

may not radiate. Pain related to lumbosacral and cervical compression tends to be radicular in nature. Pain is usually the presenting symptom and may be accentuated by percussion and, depending on the location, straight leg raising, neck flexion, or the valsalva maneuver. The pain differs from that of a herniated disk in that it is not relieved by lying down.

Motor weakness, although rarely a presenting symptom, is present in about three fourths of the patients at the time of diagnosis of spinal cord compression. Even more patients are found by neurologic examination to be paraparetic at the time of diagnosis. Sensory loss, autonomic dysfunction, and abnormal bowel and bladder sphincter control are seen in about half of the patients when cord compression is diagnosed.[94] These signs are less favorable in terms of full recovery after treatment. The extent of sensory and motor loss will depend on the level and degree of the compression.

Diagnostic studies

Even if back pain is the only symptom, spinal cord compression should be suspected in cancer patients. Radiographs of the spine will demonstrate vertebral body collapse, pedicle erosion, or vertebral lesions in more than 85% of the cases of epidural metastasis.[90,95] These films are an inexpensive and readily available diagnostic tool. A bone scan can also be helpful in the identification of vertebral body metastasis.

On the evidence of clinical manifestations, neurologic examination, and spine films/bone scan, myelography is performed to definitively diagnose spinal cord compression. Contrast media, such as Pantopaque or Metrizomide are injected via a lumbar puncture into the subarachnoid space, and flow is observed to identify any defects. These defects are measured in approximate percentages to describe the degree of tumor involvement in the epidural space. A complete block is present when no contrast flows above the level of the tumor. A cisternal puncture is performed to identify the upper level of the block. Cerebrospinal fluid (CSF) is withdrawn before the instillation of contrast medium and sent for cytologic study, cell count, and determination of glucose and protein levels. Examination of CSF also helps to diagnose leptomeningeal metastasis.

In contrast to epidural compression, an intramedullary lesion of the spine appears on the myelogram as an expanded spinal cord. Vertebral subluxation is evident on radiographs of the spine. On a myelogram, subdural hematoma appears similar to epidural tumor. Often myelography cannot be performed on the patient with thrombocytopenia or coagulopathy until multiple infusions of platelets and clotting factors have corrected the deficit.

Contrast dyes remain in the subarachnoid space after a myelogram, so that repeat films can be obtained to assess the efficacy of treatment. Computed tomography and magnetic resonance imaging may also be done at the time of myelography and after treatment to evaluate response. The side effects of a myelogram include nausea, vomiting, headache, and the associated risk of further neurologic injury.

Treatment

Equally important to the rapid diagnosis of spinal cord compression is timely treatment. Neurologic deficits can quickly progress and render the patient paraplegic if intervention is not initiated immediately. Controversy exists concerning the initial treatment of choice: radiation therapy, surgical decompression via laminectomy, or a combined approach of surgery followed by irradiation.

Radiation therapy is the treatment most often used for patients with epidural metastasis and spinal cord compression.[90] The radiation port extends one to two vertebral bodies above and below the compression. A total dose of 3000 to 4000 cGy is delivered in fractionated doses over a few weeks. The side effects of radiation to the involved area are minimal and relate to location on the spinal column. Overall, the radiation treatments are well tolerated.

Surgical decompression with laminectomy or vertebral body resection can promptly relieve spinal cord compression. In the past, a posterior approach was used and complete tumor resection was impossible since most epidural metastases are anterior to the spine. The major obstacle to an anterior surgical approach has been stabilization of the spine, but new acrylic materials and advances in surgical technique have made this approach more feasible.[96]

With the traditional posterior approach, surgery followed by radiation offered the same results as radiation alone.[94] Surgery is indicated in certain instances: when maximum radiation has been previously received, when tissue diagnosis is mandatory, when rapid neurologic deterioration ensues despite radiation, or when the cause of compression is unknown but there is a possibility of abscess or hematoma.[90,97] Clearly, the morbidity associated with surgery for patients with advanced cancer makes the surgical approach appropriate for only a highly select group. Further investigation is needed to identify specific criteria to help determine which treatment—radiation alone, surgery alone, or surgery with radiation—would benefit different groups of patients. Chemotherapy may be used with extremely chemosensitive cancers, such as lymphoma and Hodgkin's disease.

Regardless of type of treatment, steroids are included as part of the management of spinal cord compression. Steroids are initiated as soon as there is a high degree of suspicion, even before a definitive diagnosis is made. If myelography reveals compression, high-dose steroids are administered: usually a 100 mg bolus of dexamethasone given intravenously, followed by 24 mg orally every 6 hours for 2 days, and then rapidly tapered.[90,97] The purpose of steroids is to reduce spinal cord edema and pain. With certain tumors, steroids have an oncolytic effect.[98] Some disagreement exists, however, about the ideal dosage of steroids. Frequently, severe and sometimes fatal complications are associated with prolonged steroid use.[99] These include gastric ulceration and bleeding, hyperglycemia, osteoporosis, hypertension, psychosis, and immunosuppression.[100] Greenberg and his colleagues[99] compared high-dose steroids to more traditional dosages and found that higher doses relieved pain more effectively and had a low incidence of complications.

Nursing care of patients with spinal cord compression is directed by the rapidity of onset, level and degree of compression, presenting symptoms, type of treatment, and response to treatment. Patient assessment is crucial throughout this emergency for evaluation of neurologic status and preservation of maximal function. Assessment includes monitoring of sensory and motor function as well as urinary and bowel sphincter control. Intensive care may be needed if acute decompensation occurs, resulting in increased intracranial pressure or seizures.

The nurse assists the patient in the management of sensory and motor deficits. The patient needs to be able to perform activities of daily living as independently as possible while incorporating any deficits. This may require the use of assistive devices and collaboration with rehabilitation specialists. Detailed exercise regimens should be reinforced and facilitated by the nurse. Preservation and maximizing of function are a priority, since many patients have excellent rehabilitative potential after treatment is initiated.

Since more than 95% of patients with spinal cord compression have pain, knowledge of the principles of analgesia in the oncology population is essential. Effective analgesia is established early and adjusted as steroids and treatment reduce pain. The variety of analgesic agents and the types of administration techniques available help health professionals provide adequate relief for patients.

Sphincter disturbances include bowel and bladder incontinence and retention. Establishment of a daily elimination regimen will help manage incontinence and retention. Urinary disturbances can be reversed by institution of a schedule of hydration, intermittent catheterization, and perineal hygiene. Bowel control can be established with the appropriate use of diet, laxatives, and suppositories.

Patients need instruction about the schedule of the steroid taper, side effects, and conditions requiring medical care. Patients also need support and reassurance during this stressful time. If the patient requires surgery, the nurse provides routine postlaminectomy care that includes turning, positioning, skin care, pain management, wound care, and rehabilitation. Newer anterior approaches require post-thoracotomy care. During radiation therapy, the nurse instructs the patient concerning side effects and measures to alleviate them, inspects skin, and assesses response to therapy.

Comparison of response rates shows that the type of tumor determines the response rate and that the various treatments currently yield similar results for that tumor type. Bruckman and Bloomer[89] pooled data from several studies to analyze satisfactory response rates of patients with various types of tumor who were treated for spinal cord compression. Satisfactory response rates were defined as ambulation and sphincter control for more than 3 months after treatment. The percentages of patients who had a satisfactory response to treatment, according to primary cancer, are as follows: lymphoma and myeloma, 50%; breast and prostate, 30%; and lung and kidney, 10%.[89]

General criteria for evaluation of treatment response are measured through neurologic examination and include pain, sphincter control, and motor function. Further evaluation includes myelography, CT scan, or magnetic resonance imaging to visualize and measure tumor response to treatment.

Prognosis and Follow-up Care

Effective treatment of spinal cord compression is related to prolonged survival.[97] The most important prognostic factor in spinal cord compression is pretreatment neurologic status. Approximately 80% of ambulatory patients remain ambulatory after treatment, whereas only 30% to 40% of patients with significant pretreatment motor dysfunction are ambulatory after treatment.[90,94,99] Other prognostic factors include the rate of onset of symptoms and the type of malignancy. A rapidly progressing syndrome has a poor recovery rate. In the earlier discussion of response rates, patients with lymphoma and myeloma did much better than those with lung, prostate, or renal cancers.

Rehabilitative potential is dependent on pretreatment status and response to treatment. Although some patients will regain lost function, the vast majority will not. Several weeks after radiation therapy, maximum benefit is evident. Further rehabilitation beyond this time is usually not possible and the goal is to preserve existing function. If surgical decompression is successful, rapid rehabilitation is expected after postoperative recovery.

After treatment is completed, intensive follow-up care is required to assess response to treatment, assist with the adjustment to any motor or autonomic dysfunction, and monitor existing neurologic status. Home care services, such as physical therapy or home health aid, may have to be obtained and coordinated. Additional follow-up care related to the primary disease and its systemic treatment and monitoring is also needed.

Spinal cord compression can produce devastating sequelae for a patient who is already physically and emotionally compromised by the diagnosis of cancer and its treatment. Nurses play a vital role in early recognition of spinal cord compression. Prompt diagnosis and treatment help ensure neurologic preservation and a higher quality of life for the patient. Symptom management and rehabilitation are the primary goals that direct nursing care in this population. A newer surgical approach to spinal cord compression—anterior resection and spine stabilization—may reduce neurologic deficits in the future, especially in those patients who are paraparetic or paraplegic at the time of diagnosis.

CONCLUSION

Radiation therapy, chemotherapeutic agents that affect bone marrow function, and primary malignancies of the bone marrow (ie, leukemia) predispose the patient to prolonged periods of neutropenia. Sepsis is the most common cause of septic shock in patients with cancer. Appropriate nursing diagnoses and interventions may prevent an episode of neutropenic fever from progressing to septic shock.

Septic shock is one process that can initiate disseminated intravascular coagulation (DIC), an abnormality of the clotting process that results in massive clotting and simultaneous hemorrhage. Patients with gastric, prostate, and pancreatic cancers as well as those with acute promyelocytic leukemia (APL) are also prone to DIC. Successful treatment of DIC is dependent on treatment of the underlying cause.

Intrathoracic malignancies are most often associated with superior vena cava syndrome (SVCS) and cardiac tamponade secondary to pericardial effusion. SVCS is a rare emergency resulting from compression of the superior vena cava and associated with upper body edema, venous congestion, and possible respiratory distress. In the past, treatment of SVCS often precluded diagnosis of the underlying malignancy. Current practitioners prefer definitive diagnosis before initiation of treatment. The prognosis of SVCS is dependent on treating the underlying malignancy.

Pericardial effusion, with or without cardiac tamponade, is easily reversible, provided it is recognized early. Unfortunately, early symptoms, fatigue, shortness of breath, and chest discomfort can be attributed to the effects of disease or treatment. Cardiac tamponade is usually caused by fluid accumulation and increased intrapericardial pressure but can also be caused by inflammation and inelasticity of the pericardium. The outcomes of SVCS and cardiac tamponade depend on the speed with which the emergency develops and on prompt diagnosis and treatment.

Various metabolic abnormalities are associated with cancer, its treatment, and necessary supportive therapy. Three of the most common metabolic emergencies in the oncology population are hypercalcemia, tumor lysis syndrome, and syndrome of inappropriate antidiuretic hormone (SIADH). When cancer infiltrates bony structures, life-threatening problems associated with the release of calcium into the blood arise. Hypercalcemia can also result from inappropriate production of PTH, OAF, and prostaglandin by tumors. Successful long-term treatment of hypercalcemia is dependent on tumor control and regression, but vigorous hydration and calcium-inhibiting agents can reverse an emergent episode of hypercalcemia.

Individuals with massive tumor burden, such as Burkitt's lymphoma, lymphoblastic leukemia, or any rapidly growing cancer, are at risk of tumor lysis syndrome. This syndrome is characterized by hyperkalemia, hyperphosphatemia, hyperuricemia, and hypocalcemia, and if not recognized early may cause renal failure as large numbers of sensitive tumor cells are destroyed. Tumor lysis syndrome is most successfully treated when it is anticipated and adequate renal function is maintained.

Syndrome of inappropriate antidiuretic hormone is a paraneoplastic syndrome characterized by ectopic tumor production of this hormone. It is most frequently associated with small cell lung cancer but can also be initiated by various medications, including those used to treat small-cell lung cancer. Again, this syndrome is most successfully reversed by removal of the underlying cause, but anticipation and planning can greatly reduce the degree of morbidity.

Spinal cord compression is one of the most common neurologic emergencies facing the patient with cancer. Prompt recognition and treatment preserve neurologic function and prevent permanent deficits, such as paraplegia and bowel and bladder incontinence or retention. Although radiation therapy has been the primary treatment modality, new techniques are making surgical treatment a more feasible option for a select group of patients.

Since cancer is not one disease with one treatment, the oncology nurse must be familiar with the various cancers, treatment protocols, and associated medical emergencies. This knowledge, along with the patient's history, physical assessment, and results of laboratory tests, provide the nurse with the data base necessary to predict which individuals are at risk and allow for the planning and nursing interventions required to prevent a critical event.

REFERENCES

1. Groeger JS: Shock states and cancer, in Howland WS, Carlon GC (eds): Critical Care of the Cancer Patient. Chicago, Yearbook Medical Publishers, 1985, pp 296-317.
2. Vander AJ, Sherman JH, Luciano DS (eds): Human Physiology—The Mechanisms of Body Function (ed 2). New York, McGraw-Hill, 1975.
3. Cunnion RE, Parrillo JE: Cardiovascular disease, in Parrillo JE, Masur H: The Critically Ill Immunosuppressed Patient. Rockville, Md, Aspen Publishers, 1987, pp 3-38.
4. Clowes GH: Stresses, mediators and responses of survival, in Clowes GH (ed): Trauma, Sepsis and Shock: The Physiological Basis of Therapy. New York, Marcel Dekker, 1988, pp 11-54.
5. Gucalp R, Dutcher JP: Fever and infection, in Dutcher JP, Wiernik PH (eds): Handbook of Hematologic and Oncologic Emergencies. New York, Plenum, 1987, pp 153-184.
6. Fromme L, Mesa D, Outlaw E: Septic shock, in Brown MH, Kiss ME, Outlaw EM, et al (eds): Standards of Oncology Nursing Practice. New York, John Wiley & Sons, 1986, pp 469-472.
7. Mason CA: Septic shock. J Assoc Pediatr Oncol Nurses 4(3-4):25-31, 1988.
8. Perry AG: Shock complications: Recognition and management. Crit Care Nurs Q 11:1-8, 1988.
9. Littleton MT: Pathophysiology and assessment of sepsis and septic shock. Crit Care Nurs Q 11:30-47, 1988.
10. Karakusis PH: Considerations in the therapy of septic shock. Med Clin North Am 70:933-944, 1986.
11. Barry SA: Septic shock: Special needs of patients with cancer. Oncol Nurs Forum 16:31-35, 1989.
12. Peters JI, Utset OM: Shock in the ICU: When to suspect, how to determine its cause. J Crit Illness 4(7):77-93, 1989.
13. Bick RL: Disseminated intravascular coagulation and related syndromes: A clinical review. Semin Thromb Hemost 14:229-338, 1988.
14. O'Brian BS, Woods S: The paradox of DIC. Am J Nurs 78(11):1878-1880, 1978.
15. Wolfe W: Hematologic complications of malignancy. Top Emerg Med 8(2):18-24, 1986.
16. Goldberg MA, Girsburg D, Mayer RM, et al: Is heparin administration necessary during induction chemotherapy for patients with acute promyelocytic leukemia? Blood 69(1):187-191, 1987.
17. Cunningham I, Gee TS, Reich LM, et al: Acute promyelocytic leukemia: Treatment results during a decade at Memorial Hospital. Blood 73:1116-1122, 1989.
18. Happ M: Life threatening hemorrhage in children with cancer. J Assoc Pediatr Oncol Nurses 4(3-4):36-40, 1988.
19. Drapkin RL, Gee TS, Dowling MD, et al: Prophylactic heparin therapy in acute promyelocytic leukemia. Cancer 41:2484-2490, 1978.
20. Kantarjian HM, Keating MJ, Walters RS, et al: Acute promyelocytic leukemia. Am J Med 80:789, 1986.
21. Lisiewicz J: Disseminated intravascular coagulation in acute leukemia. Semin Thromb Hemost 14:339-348, 1988.
22. Feinstein DI: Treatment of disseminated intravascular coagulation. Sem Thromb Hemost 14:351-362, 1988.
23. Fruchtman S, Aledort LM: Disseminated intravascular coagulation. J Am Coll Cardiol 8:159B-167B, 1986.
24. Tempero MA, Davis RB, Reed E, et al: Thrombocytopenia and laboratory evidence of disseminated intravascular coagulation after shunts for ascites in malignant disease. Cancer 55:2718-2721, 1985.
25. Rooney A, Haviley C: Nursing management of disseminated intravascular coagulation. Oncol Nurs Forum 12:15-22, 1985.
26. Rosen N, Kaufman D, Young RC: Medical emergencies in patients with solid tumors, in Parrillo JE, Masur H (eds): The Critically Ill Immunosuppressed Patient. Rockville, Md, Aspen Publishers, 1987, pp 481-498.
27. Kingsley EC, Durie BG, Gareival HS: Acute promyelocytic leukemia. West J Med 146:322-327, 1987.
28. Schwartz BS, Williams EC, Conlon MG, et al: Epsilonaminocaproic acid in the treatment of promyelocytic leukemia and acquired alpha$_2$-plasma inhibitor deficiency. Ann Intern Med 105:873-877, 1986.
29. Pilapil F: Disseminated intravascular coagulation (DIC), in Brown MH, Kiss ME, Outlaw EM, et al (eds): Standards of Oncology Nursing Practice. New York, John Wiley & Sons, 1986, pp 459-463.
30. Division of Nursing, Memorial Sloan-Kettering Cancer Center, New York, 1984.
31. Siegrist CW, Jones JA: Disseminated intravascular coagulopathy and nursing implications. Semin Oncol Nurs 1:237-243, 1985.
32. Bavier AR: Alterations in hemostasis, in Johnson BL, Gross J (eds): Handbook of Oncology Nursing. Bethany, Conn, Flescher, 1985, pp 506-516.
33. Simpson JR, Perez CA, Presant CA, et al: Superior vena cava syndrome, in Yarbro JW, Bornstein RS (eds): Oncologic Emergencies. New York, Grune & Stratton, 1981, pp 43-72.
34. Carabell SC, Goodman RL: Oncologic emergencies: Superior vena cava syndrome, in DeVita VT, Hellman S, Rosenberg SA (eds): Cancer Principles and Practice of Oncology. Philadelphia, JB Lippincott, 1985, pp 1855-1860.
35. Lopez MJ, Vincent RG: Malignant superior vena cava syndrome, in Kapoor AS (ed): Cancer and the Heart. New York, Springer-Verlag, 1986, pp 206-212.
36. Little AG, Golomb HM, Ferguson MK, et al: Malignant superior vena cava obstruction reconsidered: The role of diagnostic surgical intervention. Ann Thorac Surg 40:285-288, 1985.
37. Lokich JJ, Goodman RL: Superior vena cava syndrome. JAMA 231:58-61, 1975.
38. Perez CA, Presant CA, Amburg AL: Management of superior vena cava syndrome. Semin Oncol 5:123-134, 1978.
39. Varricchio C: Clinical management of superior vena cava syndrome. Heart Lung 14:411-416, 1985.
40. Adelstein DJ, Hines JD, Carter SG, et al: Thromboembolic events in patients with malignant superior vena cava syndrome and the role of anticoagulation. Cancer 62:2258-2262, 1988.
41. Lopez MJ, Sala JM: Malignant superior vena cava syndrome: A 15 year experience. Mo Med 79:810-815, 1982.
42. Mauch PM, Ullmann JE: Treatment of malignant pericardial effusions, in DeVita VT, Hellman S, Rosenberg SA (eds): Cancer Principles and Practice of Oncology. Philadelphia, JB Lippincott, 1985, pp 2141-2144.
43. Shabetai R: Diseases of the pericardium, in Wyngaarden JB, Smith LH (eds): Cecil's Textbook of Medicine. Philadelphia, WB Saunders, 1988, pp 362-367.
44. Groeger J. Shock states and cancer, in Carlon G, Howland W (eds): Critical Care of the Cancer Patient. Chicago, Yearbook Medical Publishers, 1985, pp 296-317.
45. Appelfeld MM, Cole JF, Pollock SH, et al: The late appearance of chronic pericardial disease in patients treated

by radiotherapy for Hodgkin's disease. Ann Intern Med 94:338-341, 1981.
46. Kapoor AS: Malignant pericardial effusion and cardiac tamponade, in Kapoor AS (ed): Cancer and the Heart. New York, Springer-Verlag, 1986, 216-231.
47. Hancock EW: Constrictive pericarditis: Clinical clues to diagnosis. JAMA 232:176, 1975.
48. Basmajian JV, Burke MD, Burnett GW, et al: Illustrated Stedman's Medical Dictionary (ed 24). Baltimore, Williams & Wilkins, 1982, p 1171.
49. Osuch JR, Khandikar JD, Fry WA: Emergency subxiphoid pericardial decompression for malignant pericardial effusion. Am Surg 51:298-300, 1985.
50. Markman M, Howell SB: Intrapericardial instillation of cisplatin in a patient with a large malignant effusion. Cancer Drug Deliv 2:49-52, 1985.
51. Concilus E, Bohachick P: Cancer: Pericardial effusion and tamponade. Cancer Nurs 7:391-398, 1984.
52. Shepherd FA, Morgan C, Evans WK, et al: Medical management of malignant pericardial effusion by tetracycline sclerosis. Am J Cardiol 60:1161-1166, 1987.
53. Woll PJ, Knight RK, Rubens RD: Pericardial effusion complicating breast cancer. J R Soc Med 80:490-491, 1987.
54. Deconti RC: Management of hypercalcemia of neoplastic disease. Curr Concepts Oncol (Spring):7-13, 1985.
55. Mundy GR, Ibbottson KJ, D'Souza SM, et al: The hypercalcemia of cancer. N Engl J Med 310:1718-1728, 1984.
56. Mundy GR, Martin TJ: The hypercalcemia of malignancy: Pathogenesis and management. Metabolism 31:1247-1277, 1982.
57. Borenstein M: Metabolic emergencies in cancer. Top Emerg Med 8(2):75-81, 1986.
58. Vander AJ, Sherman JH, Luciano DS: Human Physiology: The Mechanisms of Body Functions (ed 2). New York, McGraw-Hill, 1975.
59. Coward DD: Cancer-induced hypercalcemia. Cancer Nurs 9(3):125-132, 1986.
60. Mahon SM: Signs and symptoms associated with malignancy-induced hypercalcemia. Cancer Nurs 12:153-160, 1989.
61. Einzig AI: Hypercalcemia in malignancy, in Dutcher JP, Wiernik PH (eds): Handbook of Hematologic and Oncologic Emergencies. New York, Plenum, 1987, pp 17-27.
62. Stewart AF: Therapy of malignancy-associated hypercalcemia: 1983. Am J Med 74:475-480, 1983.
63. Singer FR, Fernandez M: Therapy of hypercalcemia of malignancy. Am J Med 82:34-41, 1987 (suppl 2A).
64. Poe CM, Radford AI: The challenge of hypercalcemia in cancer. Oncol Nurs Forum 12(6):29-34, 1985.
65. Warrel RP, Israel R, Frisone M: Gallium nitrate for acute treatment of cancer-related hypercalcemia. Ann Intern Med 108:669-674, 1988.
66. Hasling C, Charles P, Mosekilde L: Etidronate disodium in the management of malignancy-related hypercalcemia. Am J Med 82:51-54, 1987 (suppl 2A).
67. Moore JM: Metabolic emergencies, in Johnson BL, Gross J (eds): Handbook of Oncology Nursing. Bethany, Conn, Fleschner, 1985, pp 459-470.
68. Waters HF, Stuckey PA: Oncology alert for the home care nurse: Hypercalcemia. Home Health Care Nurse 6:32-36, 1988.
69. Henry P, Seery R, Outlaw E: Hypercalcemia, in Brown MH, Kiss ME (eds): Standards of Oncology Nursing Practice. New York, John Wiley & Sons, 1986, pp 488-493.
70. Marcus SL, Einzig AI: Acute tumor lysis syndrome, prevention and management, in Dutcher JP, Wiernik PH (eds): Handbook of Hematologic and Oncologic Emergencies. New York, Plenum, 1987, pp 9-16.
71. Flombaum C: Electrolyte and renal abnormalities in the cancer patient, in Howland WS, Carlon GC (eds): Critical Care of the Cancer Patient. Chicago, Yearbook Medical Publishers, 1985, pp 114-142.
72. Cohen LF, Balow JE, McGrath IT, et al: Acute tumor lysis syndrome: A review of 37 patients with Burkitt's lymphoma. Am J Med 68:486-491, 1980.
73. Moore JM: Tumor lysis syndrome, in Johnson BL, Gross J (eds): Handbook of Oncology Nursing. Bethany, Conn, Fleschner, 1985, pp 470-476.
74. Henry P, Seery R: Tumor lysis syndrome, in Brown MH, Kiss ME, et al (eds): Standards of Oncology Nursing Practice. New York, John Wiley & Sons, 1986, pp 473-479.
75. Patterson KL, Klopovich P: Metabolic emergencies in pediatric oncology: The acute tumor lysis syndrome. J Assoc Pediatr Oncol Nurses 4(3-4):19-24, 1988.
76. Nace CS, Nace GS: Acute tumor lysis syndrome: Pathophysiology and nursing management. Crit Care Nurse 5(3):26-34, 1985.
77. Burry M, Martens L: ADH: Antidiuretic hormone and its inappropriate secretion. Cancer Nurs 76(2):41-43, 1980.
78. Bunn PA, Ridgway EC: Paraneoplastic syndromes, in DeVita VT, Hellman S, Rosenberg SA (eds): Cancer Principles and Practice of Oncology, Philadelphia, JB Lippincott, 1989, pp 1902-1905.
79. Lokich JJ: The frequency and clinical biology of the ectopic hormone syndromes of small-cell carcinoma. Cancer 50:2111-2114, 1982.
80. Hansen M, Hansen HH, Hirsch FR, et al: Hormonal polypeptides and amine metabolites in small cell carcinoma of the lung with special reference to stage and subtypes. Cancer 45:1432-1437, 1980.
81. Hainsworth JD, Workman R, Greco FA: Management of the syndrome of inappropriate antidiuretic hormone secretion in small cell lung cancer. Cancer 51:161-165, 1983.
82. Moses AM, Blumenthal SA, Streeten DH, et al: Acid base and electrolyte disorders associated with endocrine disease, pituitary and thyroid, in Arieff AI, DeFronzo RA (eds): Fluid, Electrolyte and Acid-Base Disorders, vol II. New York, Churchill-Livingston, 1985, pp 872-877.
83. Ritch PS: Cis-dichlorodiammineplatinum II-induced syndrome of inappropriate antidiuretic hormone. Cancer 61:448-450, 1988.
84. Minna JD, Pass H, Glatstein EJ, et al: Cancer of the lung, in DeVita VT, Hellman S, Rosenberg SA (eds): Cancer Principles and Practice of Oncology, Philadelphia, JB Lippincott, 1989, pp 591-705.
85. Coleman P: Antidiuretic hormone: Physiology and pathophysiology—A review. J Neurosurg Nurs Dec 11, 1979, pp 199-204.
86. Hantman D, Rossier B, Zohlman R, et al: Rapid secretion correction of hyponatremia in the syndrome of inappropriate secretion of antidiuretic hormone, an alternative treatment to hypertonic saline. Ann Intern Med 78:870-875, 1973.
87. Kleger A, Lovett D: Electrolyte abnormalities in cancer patients, in Yarbro JW, Bornstein R (eds): Oncologic Emergencies, New York, Grune & Stratton, 1981, pp 215-246.
88. Poe CM, Taylor LM: Syndrome of inappropriate antidiuretic hormone: Assessment and nursing implications. Oncol Nurs Forum 16:373-381, 1989.
89. Bruckman JE, Bloomer WD: Management of spinal cord compression. Semin Oncol 5:135-140, 1978.
90. Cairncross JG, Posner JB: Neurological complications of

systemic cancer, in Yarbro JW, Bornstein RS (eds): Oncology Emergencies. New York, Grune & Stratton, 1981, pp 73-96.

91. Findley JP: Nursing management of common oncologic emergencies, in Ziegfeld CR (ed): Core Curriculum for Oncology Nursing. Philadelphia, WB Saunders, 1987, pp 321-332.
92. Klein PW: Neurologic emergencies in oncology. Semin Oncol Nurs 1:278-284, 1985.
93. Carabell SC: Central nervous system emergencies, in DeVita VT, Hellman S, Rosenberg SA (eds): Cancer Principles and Practice of Oncology. Philadelphia, JB Lippincott, 1985, pp 1860-1866.
94. Gilbert RW, Kim JH, Posner JB: Epidural spinal cord compression from metastatic tumor: Diagnosis and treatment. Ann Neurol 3:40-51, 1978.
95. Posner JB: Neurological complications of systemic cancer. Med Clin North Am 55:625-646, 1971.
96. Sundaresan N, Galicich JH, Lane JM, et al: Treatment of neoplastic epidural cord compression by vertebral body resecton and stabilization. J Neurosurg 63:676-684, 1985.
97. Marlenson JA, Evans RG, Lie MR, et al: Treatment outcome and complications in patients treated for malignant epidural spinal cord compression. J Neurooncol 3:77-84, 1985.
98. Posner JB, Howieson J, Cvitkovic E: Disappearing spinal cord compression: Oncolytic effects of glucocorticoids and other chemotherapeutic agents on epidural metastases. Ann Neurol 2:409-413, 1977.
99. Greenberg HS, Kim JH, Posner JB: Epidural spinal cord compression from metastatic tumor: Results with a new treatment protocol. Ann Neurol 8:361-366, 1980.
100. McEvoy GK: American Hospital Formulary Service Drug Information '88. Bethesda, American Society of Hospital Pharmacists, Inc. 1988.

Chapter 32

Late Effects of Cancer Treatment

Ida Marie (Ki) Moore, RN, DNSc

Kathy Ruccione, RN, MPH

INTRODUCTION

More than 5 million Americans with a history of cancer are alive today; 3 million of these cases were diagnosed 5 or more years ago. At least half these individuals can be considered biologically cured.[1] For children, in particular, 63% survive 5 years or more from the time of diagnosis, an improvement of 40% since the early 1970s. In fact, the current estimate is that by the year 2000, one in every 1000 young adults from 20 to 29 years of age will be a survivor of childhood cancer.[2]

Biologic cure refers to a patient who has no evidence of disease, has the same life expectancy as a person who never had cancer, and ultimately dies of unrelated causes.[3] Given the state of the art in cancer treatment, this cure is not without consequences. These consequences, or late effects, result from physiologic changes related to particular treatments or to the interactions among the treatment, the individual, and the disease. In contrast to the acute side effects of chemotherapy and radiation that are due to the death of proliferative cells in tissues with relatively rapid renewal, late biologic toxicity is believed to progress over time and by different mechanisms.

Late effects can appear months to years after treatment. They can be mild to severe to life threatening; they can be clinically obvious, clinically subtle, or subclinical. Their impact depends on the age and developmental stage of the patient. Young people may rebound from the acute toxicities of treatment better than adults, but the growing child may be more vulnerable to the effects of delayed toxicities. A great unknown is what will happen to individuals who received intensive treatment in their youth as they age. Although we may not be able to detect any obvious side effects soon after the completion of treatment, the effect of even subtle tissue damage on the process of aging is unknown. For adults, we do not know what will be the cumulative effect of mild, but permanent, treatment toxicity in hearts, lungs, and kidneys when combined with hereditary predisposition to particular health problems and environmental exposure to pollutants. This chapter summarizes what is currently known about the long-term consequences of treatment on organ systems and on the development of second malignancies. The treatments associated with specific late effects and individual risk factors are discussed. For many late toxicities the specific mechanisms of pathogenesis are not well understood. This content is included whenever possible.

CENTRAL NERVOUS SYSTEM

Neuropsychologic, neuroanatomic, and neurophysiologic changes can occur as a result of central nervous system (CNS) treatment. These late effects have been observed in children with acute lymphoblastic leukemia (ALL) and brain tumors and in adult small cell carcinoma of the lung (SCCL) patients, all of whom received CNS treatment for the primary tumor or as prophylaxis against meningeal disease.

Neuropsychologic Effects

The most frequently described neuropsychologic late effects of CNS treatment include significant decrements (10 to 20 points on the WIS-R) in general intellectual potential and academic achievement scores,[4-10] as well as specific deficits in visual-motor integration, attention, memory, and visuomotor skills.[6,11-19] Nonverbal, or performance, skills seem to be particularly vulnerable to the deleterious effects of CNS treatment,[15-17] and deficits in these areas may be among the first to appear.

An important hallmark of neuropsychologic late effects is that they do not become apparent until 24 to 36 months following treatment.[4,7,8] For example, Obetz et al[20] found that 48% of children with ALL who had received treatment that involved the CNS more than 2 years prior to the time of evaluation had neuropsychologic or neuroanatomic abnormalities. This latency between CNS treatment and the manifestation of neuropsychologic late effects also has been observed in other patient populations.[10,21]

To overcome the problem of obtaining reliable pretreatment measures of intellectual functioning, several studies of children treated with cranial radiation have used healthy siblings' scores as a baseline estimate because the intelligence scores of siblings show high correlation. The findings from these studies demonstrated that children whose treatment involved the CNS were functioning at a significantly lower level than their healthy brothers and sisters[22-26] and that the differences became more disparate over time.[22]

The type of CNS treatment that most closely has been associated with neuropsychologic deficits is cranial radiation alone or in combination with intrathecal (IT) chemotherapy. Numerous studies have compared children with ALL who received 2400 cGy of whole brain radiation in combination with IT methotrexate with those who received only IT methotrexate for CNS prophylaxis. The findings provide strong evidence that radiation is closely linked to long-term functional problems.[3,7,11,18,21,24,26-28] In contrast, cognitive deficits have not been associated with CNS prophylactic regimens in which only IT methotrexate was used.[27,29]

There may be a synergistic effect between cranial radiation and chemotherapy that increases the magnitude of the toxicity. Robison et al[5] found that longer duration of chemotherapy was closely associated with lower intelligence quotient (IQ) scores in children with ALL who were treated with 2400 cGy, and Duffner et al[10] reported that adjuvant chemotherapy was a significant risk factor associated with declines in IQ in patients with brain tumors who received radiation.

It is difficult to systematically determine if a radiation-dose response relationship exists for neuropsychologic sequelae. There is modest evidence that young children who received whole brain radiation doses of less than 1000 cGy in preparation for bone marrow transplantation are neurologically and intellectually normal.[30-32] Tameroff et al[33] reported that children who received either 1800 or 2400 cGy of whole brain radiation and IT methotrexate had significantly lower Full and Performance IQ and Visual Motor Integration test scores than those who received only IT methotrexate; however, there were no significant differences between the scores of children in the two radiation groups. In contrast, higher doses of radiation (eg, 2400 to 4800 cGy), which frequently are used in the treatment of brain tumors or micrometastasis in SCCL tend to result in more severe impairments.[26,34-37]

Age at the time of CNS treatment is an important risk factor for neurologic sequelae.[4-7,8,11,25] Children who receive at least 2400 cGy of cranial radiation before the age of 3,[10,25] 4,[38] or 5 [6,18] years are at greatest risk for neuropsychologic late effects. This age-at-time-of-treatment effect has been attributed to the deleterious effects of radiation and chemotherapy on the processes of brain development that occur during early childhood.[39,40] There are no reported studies of the significance of age at the time of CNS treatment with lower doses of radiation.

Neuroanatomic Effects

Computed tomography (CT) and magnetic resonance imaging (MRI) have been used to evaluate structural changes after CNS treatment. Brouwers et al[41] found that the CT scans of 13 of 23 (57%) long-term survivors of ALL who received 2400 cGy of whole brain radiation showed abnormalities. Similarly, there are reports that 73% of children with brain tumor[42] and from 70% to 100% of those with SCCL[12,21] treated with higher radiation doses have neuroanatomic changes that are unrelated to the tumor itself.

Atrophy and decreased subcortical white matter are the most frequently reported abnormalities. Atrophy usually is manifested as ventricular dilatation and widening of the subarachnoid spaces; it has been reported in 25% to 51% of patients treated with cranial radiation.[43-45] Periventricular hypodensity, believed to represent decreased white matter, has been documented in 26% of patients with brain tumors[42] and 45% of those with SCCL[21]; however, it has occurred less frequently in patients with ALL who received 1800 to 2400 cGy of radiation.[41,43,46]

Other less common neuroanatomic abnormalities include calcifications[26,34,43,45] and leukoencephalopathy.[12,34] As with neuropsychologic effects these neuroanatomic changes are associated most closely with cranial radiation, although mild indications of atrophy and white matter degeneration have been reported in up to 20% of children who received only IT methotrexate.[44,45]

These studies of neuroanatomic pathologic conditions suggest that higher radiation doses result in a greater incidence and severity of abnormalities. Age at the time of CNS treatment also may be important. Davis et al[42] reported that children with brain tumors who receive irradiation before the age of 3 years are at greatest risk for abnormalities, and Tsurada et al[47] found that the highest incidence of white matter degeneration in adult patients with brain tumor occurred in those older than 60 years of age. This finding is of interest because it suggests that the aging, as well as the developing, brain may be more vulnerable to the deleterious effects of cancer treatment involving the CNS.

Mechanisms of Pathogenesis

The pathogenesis of delayed injury to normal tissue after treatment of the CNS is not well understood. Sheline et al[48] suggest that demyelination may be important in the early stage of delayed injury, with ischemia becoming progressively significant over time. Oligodendroglia, the myelin-producing cells in the CNS, are proliferative during early childhood and therefore radiosensitive. Damage to or a reproductive loss of glial cells from radiation can disrupt the myelin membrane that insulates axons.

A synergistic relationship between radiation and methotrexate may account for progressive demyelination.[49,50] The reduction of dihydrofolate to tetrahydrofolate, which is necessary for 1-carbon transfers in phospholipid synthesis, is inhibited by methotrexate. Procarbazine, which frequently is used in combination with methotrexate in the treatment of SCCL, can further this neurotoxicity by potentiating the methotrexate-induced depletion of the 1-carbon pool.[21] The result is disruption and loss of integrity in phospholipid membranes, such as the myelin sheath. An interference with phospholipid synthesis has been hypothesized as the underlying mechanism of demyelination[49,50] and as a contributing factor to the pathogenesis of delayed tissue damage.[51-53] Degenerative changes of glial cells, disruption of myelin sheaths, thickened capillary walls, and necrotizing and sclerotic microangiopathy have been documented in children who died of leukoencephalopathy (progressive white matter destruction) and had been treated with a cumulative dose of 2000 cGy of cranial radiation and intravenous methotrexate.[53]

Myelin basic protein (MBP) has been used as a marker for the disruption in synthesis or increased breakdown of myelin following CNS treatment. Elevated MBP has been measured in the cerebral spinal fluid of patients with ALL who have clinical and neuroradiologic evidence of leukoencephalopathy.[54,55] In one study the persistent release of MBP correlated with the progression of neurotoxicity.[54] Patients with elevations in MBP had received CNS treatment involving either 2400 cGy of whole brain radiation in combination with IT methotrexate or triple IT therapy with methotrexate, hydrocortisone, and cytosine arabinoside. Children without evidence of leukoencephalopathy, however, did not have elevations in MBP. There is no evidence that links increased MBP in the cerebral spinal fluid with neuropsychologic and/or neuroanatomic sequelae in the absence of leukoencephalopathy.

Damage to the endothelial cells of the microvasculature is believed to play an important role in the pathogenesis of delayed injury following CNS treatment.[49,50,56,57] These cells may be particularly vulnerable to the damaging effects of radiation because of their replicating capacity.[56] The consequences of endothelial cell damage include increased synthesis and density of collagenous tissue and loss of the tight intracellular junctions that form the blood-brain barrier. These pathologic changes result in decreased perfusion, increased blood-brain barrier permeability, and disruption of active transport mechanisms. The net effect is inflammation, ischemia, and loss of parenchymal tissue function. Vascular changes have been documented in animals treated with low to moderate doses of radiation[58] and in human beings who received 1500 to 6000 cGy.[53,59]

Vision and Hearing

In addition to the long-term effects of CNS treatment that involves neuropsychologic function and neuroanatomy, visual deficits and hearing loss also can occur. Enucleation, which may be necessary in the treatment of ocular tumors such as retinoblastoma, is the most disabling visual deficit. Cataracts have been associated with cranial irradiation and long-term corticosteroid therapy.[60] They may be detected on a visual examination or require a slit-lamp examination.

Hearing loss in the high-tone range is most closely associated with cisplatin.[61] Recent evidence from a limited study of children with brain tumors suggests that treatment with high doses of cranial irradiation within 10 months of cisplatin administration increases the sensitivity to the ototoxic effects of this drug in young children. Profound hearing loss occurred in all frequency ranges.[62] The investigators postulated that postirradiation hyperemia may have increased the sensitivity of the cochlea to cisplatin damage. Recurrent otitis media, a common problem in young children receiving chemotherapy, as well as the use of antibiotics that are ototoxic, also can contribute to hearing loss.

ENDOCRINE SYSTEM

Cancer treatment can adversely affect a number of endocrine functions, including metabolism, growth, secondary sexual development, and reproduction. These late effects result from damage to the target organ (ie, thyroid, ovary, and testis), and/or the hypothalamic pituitary axis. Table 32-1 summarizes the major endocrine sequelae, related risk factors, and recommendations for evaluation and treatment.

Thyroid

Direct damage to the thyroid gland causes primary hypothyroidism with a decreased production of thyroxine (T_4) and triiodothyronine (T_3). These hormones have biologic effects on oxygen consumption, the central and peripheral nervous systems, skeletal and cardiac muscle, carbohydrate and cholesterol metabolism, and growth and development.[63] Primary hypothyroidism can be compensated when there is only partial organ damage and some function is preserved. The compensated state is maintained by an increased production of thyrotropin-releasing factor (TRF) and thyroid-stimulating hormone (TSH) from the hypothalamus and pituitary. This chronic overstimulation is of concern because it is believed to increase the risk of malignant transformation in previously damaged cells.

Overt or compensated primary hypothyroidism has been documented in 4% to 80% of patients who received radiation to the neck for Hodgkin's disease, other lymphomas, and carcinomas.[64-72] Damage to the thyroid gland usually occurs after radiation doses of more than 2000 cGy in multiple fractions. Sklar et al,[73] however, documented hypothyroidism in 47% of children who received a single dose of 750 cGy of whole body radiation in preparation for bone marrow transplantation. In general, the incidence and severity of thyroid dysfunction appear to increase with higher radiation doses and may be due to damage to thyroid follicular cells, thyroid vasculature, or connective tissue. There are no chemotherapeutic agents that have been associated with long-term thyroid damage.

The importance of age at time of irradiation has been difficult to access. Although hypothyroidism usually develops 3 to 4 years after treatment, it can occur as late as 7 to 14 years afterward.[70,74] A higher incidence of dysfunction in patients treated before the age of 20 years was reported by Glatstein et al,[64] which was attributed to an increased sensitivity of the thyroid in younger individuals or to an induced sensitivity from prolonged iodine release in the contrast used in lymphangiograms.[71] Others have found that age at time of irradiation is not a significant risk factor.[75,76]

When the hypothalamic pituitary axis is in the field of radiation to the nasopharynx or the CNS, secondary hypothyroidism can occur. Decreased levels of TRF, TSH, T_3, and T_4 have been reported in patients who received at least 5500 cGy of external beam radiation for nasopharyngeal, paranasal sinus, or brain tumors that did not involve the hypothalamus or pituitary.[77,78] These studies found no difference in the development of secondary hypothyroidism between children and adults; however, the majority of subjects were adults. As with primary thyroid dysfunction, secondary hypothyroidism may not develop until years after the completion of therapy.

Growth

Growth hormone deficiency with short stature is one of the most common long-term endocrine consequences of radiation to the CNS in children. Growth impairment with deficient growth hormone release and decreased linear growth rate has been found in 50% to 100% of children with brain tumor who received 2400 cGy or more of cranial or craniospinal radiation.[35,79-85] Children with ALL who received radiation for CNS prophylaxis have dem-

TABLE 32-1 Endocrine Late Effects and Associated Risk Factors

Organ	Chemotherapy	Radiation	High Risk	Evaluation	Treatment
Ovaries	Procarbazine Cyclophosphamide Nitrogen mustard Busulfan age-dependent	400-800 cGy Age-dependent	Older > younger age Abdominal and pelvic tumors Hodgkin's disease Spinal radiation (ALL, brain tumors)	LH FSH Estradiol	Oophoropexy before treatment Replacement hormones
Testes	Procarbazine Cyclophosphamide Nitrogen mustard Busulfan	≤400 cGy: Azospermia with recovery possible ≥600 cGy: Permanent azoospermia ≥2400 cGy: Leydig cell damage (↓ testosterone)	Pelvic tumors Testicular tumors Testicular leukemia Hodgkin's disease	LH FSH Testosterone	Sperm banking before treatment Transposition of testicles before treatment Replacement hormones
Thyroid	None currently identified	>2000 cGy: Overt or compensatory hypothyroidism; Graves' disease ≥750 cGy TBI for BMT: hypothyroidism	Younger > older age Hodgkin's disease Head and neck tumors Brain tumors Leukemia (cranial rad) Bone marrow transplantation	Free triiodothyronine Thyroxine Antithyroid and anticromosomal autoantibodies (follow-up to 15 yr)	Replacement hormones
Hypothalamic-pituitary axis	None currently identified	≥2400 cGy: Hypothalamic dysfunction ≥4000 cGy: Pituitary dysfunction	CNS tumors Head and neck tumors Leukemia with central nervous system irradiation	Growth chart Growth hormone Pulsatile test Stimulation test Somatomedin-C LH, FSH Prolactin	Replacement hormones Bromocriptine

All, Acute lymphocytic leukemia; *BMT*, bone marrow transplantation; *FSH*, follicle-stimulating hormone; *LH*, luteinizing hormone; *TBI*, total body irradiation.
Source: From Hobbie WL, Schwartz CL: Endocrine late effects among survivors of cancer. Semin Oncol Nurs 5:15, 1989.

onstrated a similar pattern of growth disturbances.[86-91] Pituitary dysfunction requires radiation doses of at least 4000 cGy, but damage to the hypothalamus occurs with lower doses.[92] Although the belief has been that growth disturbances as a result of hypothalamic damage require doses of at least 2400 cGy,[92,93] Starceski et al[94] observed a 25% decline in height percentile in children treated with 2400 cGy and 14% in children treated with 1800 cGy. In both groups, growth velocity decreased significantly over 3 years following treatment and did not recover. Sanders et al[95] observed partial growth hormone deficiency in 6 of 18 children who received total body irradiation in preparation for bone marrow transplantation. A dose-response relationship has been demonstrated, with higher doses resulting in more significant growth abnormalities[92]; similarly the fewer the number of fractionations for a given radiation dose, the greater the risk of long-term sequelae.[86] Children treated with cranial radiation before the age of 5 years are believed to be more susceptible to growth deficits,[89,96] which may become most apparent during periods of rapid growth.[96] Growth retardation may be more pronounced in children who receive cranial and spinal irradiation because of spinal shortening.[82]

Secondary Sexual Development and Reproduction

Chemotherapy, specifically alkylating agents (eg, cyclophosphamide, mechlorethamine, busulfan, and procarbazine) can cause permanent damage to the gonads. Primary ovarian failure, with amenorrhea, decreased estradiol, and elevated gonadotropins (luteinizing hormone and follicle-stimulating hormone), has been reported in women who received these agents for Hodgkin's disease,[97-99] breast cancer,[100,101] and ovarian germ cell tumors.[102] In younger patients, ovarian damage is manifested as failure to develop secondary sexual characteristics or as arrested pubertal development.[103] Shalet[104] observed ovarian dysfunction in 4 of 12 girls with ALL who received cyclophosphamide. In three patients normal pubertal development subsequently occurred, which suggests that both transient and permanent damage can occur.

Damage to the germinal epithelium of the testis with decreased or absent spermatogonia can occur in males treated with alkylating agents.[105] Leydig cell damage is unusual; thus testosterone production and pubertal development are not affected.[104] Testicular damage with azoospermia is most frequent in males with Hodgkin's disease who received MOPP (mechlorethamine, vincristine, procarbazine, and prednisone)[106-109] but also has been observed in males with ALL treated with cyclophosphamide and cytosine arabinoside.[110]

Age at time of treatment, sex, total drug dose, and the use of combinations of alkylating agents are important risk factors for gonadal failure. The quiescence of the prepubertal gonad provides some protection whereas the incidence of gonadal damage increases with age and stage of pubertal development. The testis appears to be more sensitive than the ovary to the damaging effects of therapy. Rivkees and Crawford[108] reported that the incidence of gonadal dysfunction increased from 0% in prepubertal girls and 14% in prepubertal boys to 71% in sexually mature women and 95% in mature men. Byrne et al[111] found that the fertility of men treated with alkylating agents was half that of the fertility of control subjects, whereas the fertility of women was unimpaired.

The risk of gonadal failure also increases with greater total doses of alkylating agents and the use of more than one drug, such as in MOPP therapy. For example, Koyama et al[100] found that the dose of cyclophosphamide that resulted in amenorrhea was 5.2 g in those women older than 40 years and 20.4 g in those 20 to 29 years of age. Similarly, 64% of men treated with less than three cycles of MOPP had recovery of spermatogenesis, whereas those treated with more than five cycles had persistent azoospermia.[112]

Radiation is another cause of gonadal dysfunction. Pathologic changes in women who receive radiation to the ovaries include reduced numbers of oocytes, inhibited follicle development, atrophic ovaries, and strong fibrohyalinization.[113-114] Older women are at greater risk for ovarian failure following radiation. The ovaries may be preserved in women who receive *800 cGy; however, ovarian failure has been reported in 100% of women older than 40 years of age treated with §400 cGy.[115,116]

The testis is extremely sensitive to the damaging effects of radiation. The threshold dose required to damage the germinal epithelium is as low as 300 to 900 cGy,[117] whereas the Leydig cells are more resistant, with permanent damage occurring following doses §2000 cGy.[118] Scatter to the ovaries and testes as a result of abdominal or craniospinal irradiation also can result in long-term damage.[119,120] In a large retrospective cohort study of 2283 survivors of childhood cancer, Byrne et al[111] found that radiation therapy directed below the diaphragm depressed fertility in men and women by approximately 25%, and combined therapy involving infradiaphragmatic radiation and alkylating agents reduced fertility to almost 50% of that in the control subjects.

Radiation to the cranium or nasopharynx can damage the hypothalamic pituitary axis, causing secondary gonadal failure. Subnormal levels of luteinizing hormone (LH), follicle-stimulating hormone (FSH), and prolactin-inhibiting factor (PIF) have been found in both sexes treated for head and neck tumors with 400 to 7800 cGy of radiation.[77,121] In addition to the effects of low LH and FSH levels on ovarian and testicular function, the decrease in PIF and resultant increase in prolactin caused irregular menses, anovulatory periods, low testosterone, reduced libido, and impotence.[77,122]

IMMUNE SYSTEM

Immunosuppression has long been recognized as one of the most serious acute toxic effects of chemotherapy and radiation. A more recent discovery is that certain aspects of immune function can be adversely affected for years after the completion of treatment. These immunologic late effects have been studied most thoroughly in patients treated for leukemia, Hodgkin's disease, and breast cancer.

The early studies of children who received combination chemotherapy for ALL measured immune system recovery by absolute lymphocyte, T-cell, and B-cell counts and by immunoglobulin production.[123,124] A rebound of these parameters within the first 12 months was observed and may have contributed to the assumption that immunocompetence is restored during this time period.

More recent studies provide compelling evidence for persistent immunologic impairments following radiation and chemotherapy. The lymphopenia that occurs immediately after radiation usually involves both cellular (T cell) and humoral (B cell) immunity.[125] The time required for recovery of these cell populations, however, is very different.[126-129] The B lymphocytes gradually repopulate within 12 months,[128,130] whereas T-lymphocyte depletion is much more prolonged. Of particular significance is the finding that suppressor T cells recover more rapidly than helper T cells, which seem to be particularly radiosensitive. The result is an inversion of the helper-to-suppressor ratio that can persist for as long as 10 years following local radiation for breast cancer,[128,129] nodal radiation for Hodgkin's disease,[130,131] and total body irradiation prior to bone marrow transplantation.[132] Decreased lymphocyte proliferative capacity, natural killer cells, and immunoglobulin production associated with defective suppressor-cell immunoregulation and an abnormal helper-to-suppressor cell ratio also have been observed in patients treated with multiagent chemotherapy for Hodgkin's disease[133] and leukemia.[134-136] In addition, a pronounced long-term effect on plasma cell and immunoglobulin production, with a possible effect on T-cell function, also has been observed in children with ALL.[134,135]

The immunosuppressive effects of specific chemotherapeutic agents are not well known. The use of radiation in conjunction with multiagent chemotherapy can result in more frequent and more severe immune system impairment.[137] Larger volumes of irradiated bone marrow and greater total radiation doses result in more severe hematopoietic depression and more prolonged recovery. In a study of 32 patients with lymphoma who received either mantle or mantle with inverted Y radiation, bone marrow recovery was observed following doses of 2000 cGy, but recovery was markedly limited after 4000 cGy.[138] Compensation by hyperactivity of the nonradiated marrow persisted for up to 10 years after radiation. Bone marrow regeneration also has been found to be slower and less extensive in older patients (20 years of age or older).[139]

The clinical significance of these long-term alterations in immune function is not well understood. There is no evidence that patients with persistent immunologic abnormalities are at greater risk for infections. One group of patients who are at increased risk of infections are those who have undergone splenectomy. Overwhelming bacterial infections, primarily pneumococcal, are a major concern to these individuals because of the protective role of the spleen against encapsulated organisms. Persistent immune defects have not been linked to the occurrence of second malignancies. This may change, however, as survival time increases for larger numbers of patients.

CARDIOVASCULAR SYSTEM

The use of anthracyclines, such as daunorubicin and doxorubicin, has improved survival in patients with acute leukemias, lymphomas, pediatric solid tumors, and other cancers. One of the most serious late effects of these drugs is cardiac toxicity which typically presents as cardiomyopathy, with clinical signs of congestive heart failure. Recent evidence, however, indicates that structural damage to the heart can occur in the absence of clinical signs. Steinherz et al[140,141] detected abnormalities of contractility and rhythm, apparently related to myocardial fibrosis, on echocardiograms obtained 4 to 20 years after anthracycline therapy. These investigators also have documented cardiac failure, dysrhythmias, and sudden deaths many years following completion of therapy. Some of the patients with these late complications had no early symptoms. Myocardial fibrosis was present on autopsy in all cases of sudden death.[140,141]

The risk of cardiotoxicity is related to cumulative dose,[140,141] schedule of administration (continuous versus intermittent), and presence of other factors such as mediastinal irradiation.[142] Cumulative doses §550 mg/m^2 have been associated with cardiac toxicity[143,144]; similar abnormalities can occur after lower doses in children.[145] Table 32-2 includes a summary of cardiotoxicity, methods of assessment, and suggestions for intervention.

Individuals who received radiation therapy to a field that includes the heart, such as mediastinal radiation for Hodgkin's disease or other lymphomas, also are at risk for cardiotoxicity. Radiation-induced cardiotoxicity is manifested primarily as congestive heart failure. An acceleration of coronary artery disease that results in angina and myocardial infarction may occur in some patients.[142] Pericardial damage secondary to mediastinal irradiation is another cardiovascular complication.[146] Patients may have overt symptoms and/or abnormalities that are visible on x-ray examination. Pericardial damage may be self-limiting, but life-threatening pericardial effusions also can occur.[147] In general, peripheral vascular disease is a rare cardiovascular late effect. However, approximately 50% of patients with germ cell tumors of the testes treated with cisplatin, vinblastine, and bleomycin report having Raynaud's phenomenon.[148] Vinblastine is the suspected cause, but there is no evidence of a dose effect.

PULMONARY SYSTEM

Pneumonitis and pulmonary fibrosis are the major biologic late effects of treatment to the pulmonary system (see Table 32-2). These problems can be caused by chemotherapy, radiation therapy, and recurrent respiratory infections in immunosuppressed patients.[149,150] Pulmonary fibrosis occurs in 1% to 5% of patients who receive bleomycin for treatment of Hodgkin's disease, non-Hodgkin's lymphoma, testicular cancer, and head and neck tumors.[151] The effect is dose related, and the incidence of fibrosis increases to at least 10% if the cumulative dose exceeds 450 U.[152] Other factors that contribute to the toxic effects of bleomycin on the pulmonary system are advanced age and concurrent radiation therapy to the lungs.

Alkylating agents, primarily busulfan, and the nitrosourea agents (eg, lomustine and carmustine) also have been associated with the development of pulmonary fibrosis. Busulfan currently is used as part of the preparative regimen for bone marrow transplantation in patients with leukemia. Although acute pulmonary toxicity appears to be less than that following total body irradiation, long-term follow-up is needed to determine the actual incidence and severity of late toxic effects of busulfan. Pulmonary fibrosis also has been observed in some patients treated with nitrosourea agents for brain tumors, lymphomas, and a variety of solid tumors. The risk is related to total cumulative dose, the patient's age, number of cycles of chemotherapy, and underlying disease.[153]

Pulmonary fibrosis is the most common type of chronic lung damage following radiation therapy. Obstructive lung disease also can occur. Pulmonary damage is more likely when higher radiation doses are used and when larger lung volumes are irradiated. Radiation therapy also can potentiate the long-term toxicity induced by other agents such as bleomycin and the nitrosureas.

GASTROINTESTINAL SYSTEM

Radiation and radiation-enhancing chemotherapeutic agents can have long-term effects on the gastrointestinal tract and the liver.[154] Although rare, vascular abnormalities and altered digestive system activity can result in malabsorption.[155] Late effects in the liver are more common and

TABLE 32-2 Biologic Late Effects on Selected Organ Systems

Body System	Health Problem	Associated Treatment Modality	Method of Assessment	Management and Nursing Considerations
Cardiovascular	Cardiomyopathy	Anthracycline chemotherapy Risk increased with lifetime cumulative dose >550 mg/m^2, mediastinal irradiation	Detection is difficult: ECG, echocardiogram, scans may be inadequate Monitor with clinical observation for shortness of breath, weight gain, edema	Careful monitoring of anthracycline dosage to limit lifetime dose If congestive heart failure develops, support care with digitalis, diuretics, sodium restriction, provision of adequate rest periods
	Pericardial damage	Mediastinal irradiation (eg, 4000-6000 cGy)	Clinical observation for chest pain, dyspnea, fever, paradoxic pulse, venous distention, friction rub, Kussmaul's sign Abnormalities visible on chest film	May be self-limiting If pericardial effusion occurs, treatment may include anti-inflammatory agents, pericardiectomy
	Peripheral vascular disease	Vinblastine	History of digital cold sensitivity	Avoidance of cold
Respiratory	Pulmonary fibrosis	Lung irradiation Some chemotherapeutic agents Risk increased with larger lung volume in radiation field, dose: 4000 cGy, radiation-sensitizing chemotherapeutic agents	Clinical observation for dyspnea, rales, cough, decreased exercise tolerance, pulmonary insufficiency Monitor with physical examination, chest film, pulmonary function tests	Health education for smoking prevention/cessation Supportive care with provision of adequate rest periods Vigilance re: development of pulmonary infection
Musculoskeletal	Scoliosis, kyphosis	Radiation therapy for intra-abdominal tumor in which vertebrae absorb radiation unevenly	Regular physical examination May not become apparent until adolescent growth spurt	Referral to orthopedist for rehabilitative measures Instruction regarding normal weight maintenance to make problem less noticeable
	Spinal shortening (decrease in sitting height)	Spinal irradiation (eg, for medulloblastoma); direct effect of radiation on growth centers of vertebral bodies	Serial measurements of sitting height (crown to rump)	Referral to orthopedist Anticipatory teaching regarding disproportion between shorter-than-usual trunk and normal leg length as full growth is attained; reassurance that disproportion probably will not be obvious to others but may be a problem in fitting clothing
	Increased susceptibility to fractures, poor healing, deformities, or shortening of extremities	Irradiation to lesions in long bones (eg, Ewing's sarcoma)	Regular physical examination	Referral to orthopedist Teaching about protective measures such as avoiding rough contact sports
	Facial asymmetry	Surgery plus irradiation to head and neck area (eg, for rhabdomyosarcoma) causing altered growth in facial bones	Physical examination Early evaluation by reconstructive surgeon	Anticipatory guidance regarding possible adjustment problems with visible deformity Referral to family counseling to manage or prevent adjustment and behavior problems

	Dental problems: gingival irritation and bleeding; tooth loosening, migration (can lead to peridontal disease); delayed/arrested tooth development	Radiation therapy to maxilla, mandible areas; chemotherapy	Clinical observation with dental examination	Many dental problems can be minimized or prevented with good oral hygiene with flossing/brushing, gingival massage, use of plaque-disclosing tablets/solutions; preradiation therapy fluoride prophylaxis; dental evaluation 2 wk postradiation; orthodontic treatment for malocclusion; extraction of damaged, nonfunctional teeth
Gastrointestinal	Chronic enteritis	Radiation therapy Risk increased with doses >5000 cGy, previous abdominal surgery, radiation-sensitizing chemotherapeutic agents	Clinical observation for pain, dysphagia, recurrent vomiting, obstipation/constipation, bloody or mucus-containing diarrhea, malabsorption syndrome	Nutritional consultation for diet plan to diminish symptoms while providing adequate nutrition for growth and development to fit family routine, ethnic or cultural customs; dietary modifications may include low-fat, low-residue, gluten-free, free of milk and milk products If enterostomy is performed, coordination with enterostomal therapist for patient family teaching about stoma care
	Hepatic fibrosis, cirrhosis	Radiation therapy Some chemotherapeutic agents	Clinical observation for pain, hepatomegaly, jaundice Monitoring with liver function tests and liver scans may be inconclusive; thus periodic liver biopsy may be necessary	Supportive care with nutritional consultation
Kidney and urinary tract	Chronic nephritis (may lead to renal failure, cardiovascular damage)	Radiation to renal structures Risk increased with concomitant chemotherapy	Clinical observation and monitoring with blood pressure readings, urinalysis, CBC, BUN	If progressive renal failure develops, supportive care (possibly dialysis and/or transplantation)
	Chronic hemorrhagic cystitis	Chemotherapy (cyclophosphamide) Risk increased with pelvic radiation, inadequate hydration before, during, and after chemotherapy	Clinical observation for dysuria, urinary frequency, hematuria Monitoring with urinalysis	Ensure adequate hydration before, during, and after chemotherapy (3000 mL/m^2/24 hr) Bladder hemorrhage may be treated with formalin instillation and/or fulguration of bleeding sites
	Unilateral kidney	Nephrectomy for Wilms' tumor	Clinical observation for dysuria, urinary frequency, flank pain, hematuria Monitoring with urinalysis	Health education to avoid injury to remaining kidney (eg, contact sports) If urinary tract infection develops: identification of causative organism, antibiotic treatment, repeat urinalysis Medic-Alert identification bracelet/tag

Source: Adapted from Ruccione K, Weinberg K: Late effects in multiple body systems. Semin Oncol Nurs 5:6-8, 1989.

include hepatic fibrosis, cirrhosis, and portal hypertension. Radiation therapy in combination with radiation-enhancing agents, such as actinomycin D and possibly vincristine, can result in hepatic fibrosis. Portal hypertension can occur if the fibrosis is severe.[156] Methotrexate also has been linked to hepatic fibrosis and cirrhosis (although the use of citrovorum factor may minimize or prevent these effects), and methotrexate in combination with 6-mercaptopurine can result in cirrhosis with portal hypertension.[157] Finally, the administration of blood products as part of the supportive care of myelosuppressed patients can cause chronic hepatitis. Table 32-2 includes a summary of late biologic toxic effects in the gastrointestinal tract.

RENAL SYSTEM

Nephritis and cystitis are the major long-term renal toxicities that result from cancer treatment (see Table 32-2). Damage to the nephrons and bladder has been documented in patients treated with cyclophosphamide, ifosfamide, and cisplatin. The hemorrhagic cystitis that can occur following cyclophosphamide therapy may persist, and the risk is increased by concurrent pelvic radiation.[158,159] Radiation also can damage the kidneys. Radiation doses of 2000 cGy or less may minimize the risk of renal toxicity, whereas concurrent administration of radiation-enhancing drugs increases the risk.[160,161] Clinical manifestations of nephritis include proteinuria, hypertension, anemia, and progressive renal failure, although early detection and intervention may prevent irreversible damage. The compensatory hypertrophy of the remaining kidney following nephrectomy for renal tumors such as Wilms' tumor has not been associated with any biologic consequences. However, urinary tract infections or trauma to the remaining kidney obviously can be a serious problem.

MUSCULOSKELETAL SYSTEM

The treatment most frequently associated with late effects in the musculoskeletal system is radiation. Age at time of irradiation, radiation dose, and volume of tissue irradiated are all risk factors. Children treated at an early age (younger than 6 years) and those undergoing puberty are at high risk because of rapid growth and development. Uneven irradiation to the vertebrae, soft tissue, and muscles (eg, radiation to one side of the body) for the treatment of intra-abdominal tumors frequently results in scoliosis or kyphosis, or both. Although more recent therapies have been modified to minimize these problems, skeletal abnormalities still occur in some children and tend to become most apparent during periods of rapid growth such as the adolescent growth spurt.[162]

Spinal shortening, which is another radiation-related effect, is caused by damage to the growth centers in the vertebral bodies.[163] Children who receive spinal radiation frequently do not achieve their full height potential; those who receive craniospinal irradiation are at great risk for growth retardation because of central (hypothalamic-pituitary), as well as direct (skeletal), effects.

The late effects on long bones include functional limitations, shortening of the extremity, osteonecrosis, increased susceptibility to fractures, and poor healing.[142] Radiation is the treatment most commonly associated with these problems; however, prolonged use of corticosteroids also can have degenerative effects. Finally, surgical procedures such as amputation or limb disarticulation have obvious immediate and lasting cosmetic, as well as physical, consequences.

Altered growth of facial bones following maxillofacial or orbital irradiation or surgery causes facial asymmetry. This is a difficult problem that frequently occurs in children treated for tumors such as rhabdomyosarcoma. Maxillofacial irradiation also can cause a number of dental problems such as foreshortening and blunting of the roots, incomplete calcification, delayed or arrested tooth development, caries, and loosening.[164,165] Recently, dental problems in patients who were treated with chemotherapy have been reported and include abnormal occlusion, hypoplasia, enamel opacities, and radiologic abnormalities.[166]

SECOND MALIGNANT NEOPLASMS

It has been clearly established that adults and children who have received chemotherapy or radiation therapy, or both, for a primary malignancy are at increased risk for the development of a second malignant neoplasm. For example, in patients with Hodgkin's disease there is a 77-fold increased risk of the development of leukemia within 4 years of initial treatment.[167] For children, the overall risk is estimated to be at least 10 times greater than the cancer incidence among age-matched children,[168] with a 20-year cumulative probability of 12%.[169] Malignant transformation of normal cells is due to nonlethal damage to the DNA that is not repaired. Alkylating agents and ionizing radiation are the treatments most closely linked to a second malignant neoplasm. In addition to the type and dose of treatment received, the risk of the development of a second cancer depends on several predisposing factors. Some tumors have a common underlying etiologic factor. For example, patients with bladder cancer are at greater risk for the development of lung cancer because both tumors are associated with smoking.[170] Genetic susceptibility is a second factor.[168] Children with the genetic form of retinoblastoma (which is usually bilateral) have a much higher incidence of sarcomas (as a second malignant neoplasm) than those with the nongenetic form of the disease.[171-173]

Second Malignancies Following Chemotherapy

Acute nonlymphocytic leukemia (ANL) following treatment with alkylating agents is the most common chemotherapy-related second malignant neoplasm. The disease usually is preceded by a period of prolonged pancytopenia and can occur as early as 1.3 years following the initiation of chemotherapy for the primary malignancy. The incidence of treatment-related ANL peaks at 5 years and plateaus at 10 years following treatment.[174]

ANL following Hodgkin's disease has been studied intensively in large cohorts of patients.[174-181] The overall cumulative risk has been reported to be 3.3% at 15 years post diagnosis but varies from 0.6% in patients who received only radiation therapy to 17% in those treated with combination chemotherapy.[174,182,183] Coleman[177] reported that the average length of survival after the diagnosis of ANL was 6 months. The treatment regimen with the greatest leukemogenic potential is MOPP, which is presumed to be due to the mechlorethamine and procarbazine.[174,176-183] A dose-response relationship between alkylating agents and the occurrence of a second malignant neoplasm has been reported[182,183]; Aisenberg[176] has suggested that leukemia is most likely to develop in patients who received more than six cycles of MOPP or similar drug regimens that contain alkylating agents. The addition of radiation to the MOPP regimen does not appear to significantly increase the risk of ANL,[174] whereas the recent use of ABVD (Adriamycin [doxorubicin], bleomycin, vinblastine, and dacarbazine) and a regimen involving procarbazine, melphalan, and vinblastine have not been found to carry an increased risk of acute leukemia, which is attributed to a lower total dose of alkylating agents.[174,182-184]

In patients with multiple myeloma the risk is unusually high, more than 200 times that of the incidence in the general population, for the development of ANL. In a study of 364 patients the cumulative risk of ANL reached 17.5% at 50 months of follow-up.[185] The drug most closely associated with ANL was melphalan, although multiple myeloma may also be associated with an increased risk of ANL that is unrelated to treatment.[181]

Although the incidence is not as great as with Hodgkin's disease or multiple myeloma, treatment-related acute leukemia has occurred in patients with non-Hodgkin's lymphoma,[186-188] breast cancer,[189-190] gastrointestinal cancer,[191,192] lung cancer,[193,194] germ cell tumors in men,[195] and ovarian cancer[196] and in survivors of childhood cancer.[197] In all these studies, alkylating agents, primarily cyclophosphamide and melphalan, have been linked to the occurrence of ANL. ANL was two to three times more likely to develop in women who received melphalan for the treatment of ovarian cancer than in those who received cyclophosphamide, which suggests that of the two drugs melphalan has the greater leukemogenic potential.[198]

Second Malignancies Following Radiation

Sarcomas of the bone and soft tissue are the most common second malignant neoplasm after radiation therapy. Although the latency period can be as short as 5 months,[199] it ranges from 10 to 20 years following radiation.[200] The incidence has been found to peak at 15 to 20 years after the initial diagnosis.[200,201] Malignant transformation can occur in doses ranging from 1000 to 8000 cGy. The relative risk increases from 8 following doses of 1000 to 2000 cGy to 40 following doses §6000 cGy.[200,201] It has been postulated that the decreased risk following doses §8000 cGy is due to the phenomenon of cell killing rather than nonlethal cell damage.

In a large study of 9170 survivors of childhood cancer, 48 cases of bone cancer occurred as opposed to the 0.4 expected (relative risk, 133).[200] The risk was highest among children treated for retinoblastoma (relative risk 999) and Ewing's sarcoma (relative risk 649) but also was increased significantly in patients treated for rhabdomyosarcoma, Wilms' tumor, and Hodgkin's disease. Of the patients with sarcoma 84% had received radiation, and 83% of the subsequent tumors occurred within the field of radiation.

ANL following radiation therapy is uncommon but has been reported in childhood cancer[182,201] and non-Hodgkin's lymphoma.[187] Women with breast cancer treated with postoperative radiation also have a slightly increased risk of ANL.[189] In addition to sarcomas and leukemia, a variety of other solid tumors have been linked to treatment with radiation. Carcinomas of the breast can occur in girls treated with pulmonary irradiation,[182] and a slightly excessive number of tumors of the bladder, rectum, uterus, bone, and connective tissue has been reported in women who received radiation for gynecologic cancer.[202,203] Brain tumors can occur after cranial irradiation for CNS prophylaxis in childhood ALL.[204,205] Finally, lung cancer following mantle radiation for Hodgkin's disease has been reported.[206] The average latency period was 7 years, and smoking was a contributing factor in only 53% of the patients. Table 32-3 summarizes the findings from selected studies on the risk of ANL in patients treated for various types of cancer.

CONCLUSION

This chapter has provided a comprehensive review of the biologic late effects that can be caused by curative cancer therapy. Long-term surveillance for these toxic affects is a recent and challenging area for oncology nurses and physicians. A long-range perspective is essential because the latency period for some late toxicities is many years after completion of treatment and the consequences of permanent tissue damage in terms of life span is unknown.

General recommendations for long-term follow-up include an annual physical examination with a complete

TABLE 32-3 Selected Studies of Risk of Acute Nonlymphocytic Leukemia in Patients Treated for Several Types of Cancer

Series	Total No. of Patients	No. of Leukemias Observed	Relative Risk	Cumulative Risk (No. yr Follow-Up)
Hodgkin's disease				
Tucker et al[174]	1507	28	66	3.3% ± 0.6% (15)
Valagussa et al[175]	1329	27		3.6% ± 0.9% (12)
Tucker et al[183]	1036	12	89	4.2% ± 1.9% (20)
Coleman et al[179]	730	8	86	
Blayney et al[180]	193	12*	96	10% ± 3% (15)
Multiple myeloma				
Bergsagel et al[185]	364	14	214	17% ± 4 (4)
Ovarian cancer				
Greene et al[196]	1399	12	67	4.7% ± 1.6% (7)
Greene et al[198]	3363	28	23.5	8.4% ± 1.6% (10)*,†
Non-Hodgkin's lymphoma				
Gomez et al[187]	117	4	341	NA
Greene et al[188]	517	9	105	7.9% ± 3.2% (10)
Child cancer				
Tucker et al[197]	9170	22	14	0.8% ± 0.2% (20)
Breast cancer				
Fisher et al[189]	8483	43*	NA	<2% (10)
Gastrointestinal cancer				
Boice et al[191]	1402	6	1.6‡	NA
Boice et al[192]	3633	17*		3.2% (7)
Lung cancer				
Chak et al[193]	158	3	316	25% ± 13% (3.1)
Ratain et al[194]	119	4	NA	44% ± 24% (2.5)

*Includes myelodysplastic disorders.
†Cumulative risk among women treated with chemotherapy only.
‡Risk not statistically significant.
NA, Data not available.
Source: Adapted from Fraser MC, Tucker MA: Second malignancies following cancer therapy. Semin Oncol Nurs 5:43-55, 1989.

blood cell count and urinanalysis. Evaluation of specific toxicity to organ systems and second malignancies depends on the initial diagnosis, type and amount of treatment received, and host risk factors. In some treatment centers surveillance guidelines have been established. Such guidelines, however, have not been standardized or adopted at all institutions. For example, the most efficient and cost-effective method for evaluating cardiotoxicity remains unclear. For all biologic late effects a careful balance must be struck between monitoring and the creation of needless anxiety that could hinder the patient's overall rehabilitation and emotional adjustment.

REFERENCES

1. Cancer Facts and Figures: 1989. Atlanta, American Cancer Society, 1989, p 3.
2. Meadows AT, Hobbie WL: The medical consequences of cure. Cancer 58:524-528, 1986.
3. van Eys J: Living beyond cure: Transcending survival. Am J Pediatr Hematol Oncol 9:114-118, 1987.
4. Meadows AT, Massari DJ, Fergusson J, et al: Declines in IQ scores and cognitive dysfunctions in children with acute lymphoblastic leukemia treated with cranial irradiation. Lancet 2:1015-1018, 1981.

5. Robison LL, Nesbit ME, Sather HN, et al: Factors associated with IQ scores in long-term survivors of childhood acute lymphoblastic leukemia. Am J Pediatr Hematol Oncol 6:115-121, 1984.
6. Moore IM, Kramer JH, Ablin AR: Late effects of central nervous system prophylactic leukemia therapy on cognitive functioning. Oncol Nurs Forum 13:45-51, 1986.
7. Lansky SB, Cairns NU, Lansky LL, et al: Central nervous system prophylaxis. Am J Pediatr Hematol Oncol 6:183-190, 1984.
8. Stebhens JA, Kisker CT: Intelligence and achievement testing in childhood cancer: Three years postdiagnosis. J Dev Behav Pediatr 5:184-188, 1984.
9. Moehle KA, Berg RA, Ch'ien LT, et al: Language-related skills in children with acute lymphocytic leukemia. J Dev Behav Pediatr 4:257-261, 1983.
10. Duffner PK, Cohen ME, Parker MS: Prospective intellectual testing in children with brain tumors. Ann Neurol 23:575-579, 1988.
11. Chak LK, Zatz IM, Wasserstein P, et al: Neurologic dysfunction in patients treated for small cell carcinoma of the lung: A clinical and radiological study. Int J Radiat Oncol Biol Phys 12:385-389, 1986.
12. Frytak S, Earnest F, O'Neill B, et al: Magnetic resonance imaging for neurotoxicity in long-term survivors of carcinoma. Mayo Clin Proc 60:803-813, 1985.
13. Pfefferbaum-Levine B, Copeland DR, Fletcher JM, et al: Neuropsychological assessment of long-term survivors of childhood leukemia. Am J Pediatr Hematol Oncol 6:123-128, 1984.
14. Fletcher JM: Neurobehavioral effects of central nervous system prophylactic treatment of cancer in children. J Clin Exp Neuropsychol 10:495-538, 1988.
15. Goff JR, Anderson HR, Cooper PF: Distractability and memory deficits in long-term survivors of acute lymphoblastic leukemia. J Dev Behav Pediatr 1:158-163, 1980.
16. Kramer JH, Moore IM: Verbal learning deficits in long-term survivors of acute lymphoblastic leukemia. Proceedings of the annual conference of the American Psychological Association 97:401, 1985 (abstr).
17. Kramer JH, Moore IM: Age at time of treatment effect on mnemestic functioning following CNS irradiation and intrathecal methotrexate. J Clin Exp Neuropsychol 7:627, 1985 (abstr).
18. Copeland DR, Fletcher JM, Pfefferbaum-Levine B, et al: Neuropsychological sequelae of childhood cancer in long-term survivors. Pediatrics 75:745-753, 1985.
19. Ellison N, Bernath A, Kane R, et al: Disturbing problems of success: Clinical status of long-term survivors of small cell lung cancer. Proc Am Soc Clin Oncol 1:149, 1982 (abstr).
20. Obetz SW, Smithson WA, Groover RV, et al: Neuropsychological follow-up of children with acute lymphoblastic leukemia. Am J Pediatr Hematol Oncol 1:207-213, 1979.
21. Lee JS, Unsawadsi T, Lee Y, et al: Neurotoxicity in long-term survivors of small cell lung cancer. Int J Radiat Oncol Biol Phys 12:313-321, 1986.
22. Twaddle V, Britton PG, Craft AC, et al: Intellectual function after treatment for leukaemia or solid tumors. Arch Dis Child 58:949-952, 1985.
23. Taylor HG: Postirradiation treatment outcomes for children with acute lymphoblastic leukemia: Clarification of risks. J Pediatr Psychol 12:395-411, 1987.
24. Moss HA, Nannis ED, Poplack DG: The effects of prophylactic treatment of the central nervous system on the intellectual functioning of children with acute lymphocytic leukemia. Am J Med 71:47-52, 1981.
25. Jannoun L: Are cognitive and educational development affected by age at which prophylactic therapy is given in acute lymphoblastic leukemia? Arch Dis Child 58:953-958, 1983.
26. Silverman CL, Palkes H, Talent B, et al: Late effects of radiotherapy on patients with cerebellar medulloblastoma. Cancer 54:825-829, 1984.
27. Rowland JH, Glidewell OJ, Sibley RF, et al: Effects of different forms of central nervous system prophylaxis on neuropsychological function in childhood leukemia. J Clin Oncol 2:1327-1335, 1984.
28. Pavlovsky S, Castano J, Leiguarda R, et al: Neuropsychological study in patients with ALL. Am J Pediatr Hematol Oncol 5:79-128, 1983.
29. Tamaroff M, Miller DR, Murphy ML: Immediate and long-term post-therapy neuropsychologic performance in children with acute lymphoblastic leukemia treated without central nervous system radiation. J Pediatr 101:524-529, 1982.
30. Kaleita T, Tesler A, Feig SA: Prospective neurodevelopmental studies of two children treated with total body irradiation and bone marrow transplantation for acute leukemia in infancy. Prog Bone Marrow Transplant 1:157-164, 1987.
31. Smedler AC, Bergman H, Bolme P, et al: Neuropsychological functioning in children treated with bone marrow transplantation. J Clin Exp Neuropsychol 10:325-326, 1988.
32. Halberg F, Wara W, Kramer JH, et al: Total body irradiation in infancy: Effect on growth and development after bone marrow transplant for SIDS. Int J Radiat Oncol Biol Phys 15:154, 1988 (abstr).
33. Tamaroff M, Salwen R, Miller D, et al: Neuropsychological sequelae in irradiated (1800 rads [r] and 2400 r) and non-irradiated children with acute lymphoblastic leukemia (ALL). Proc Amer Soc Clin Oncol 4:C-644, 1985 (abstr).
34. Duffner PK, Cohen ME, Thomas PR, et al: The long-term effects of cranial irradiation on the central nervous system. Cancer 56:1841-1846, 1985.
35. Berry MP, Jenkins DT, Green GW, et al: Radiation treatment for medulloblastoma. J Neurosurg 55:43-51, 1981.
36. Mulhern RK, Crisco JJ, Kun LE: Neuropsychological sequelae of childhood brain tumors: A review. J Child Clin Psychol 12:66-73, 1983.
37. Packer RJ, Zimmerman RA, Bilaniuk LT: Magnetic resonance imaging in the evaluation of treatment-related central nervous system damage. Cancer 58:635-640, 1986.
38. Chin HW, Maruyama Y: Age at treatment and long-term performance results in medulloblastoma. Cancer 53:1952-1958, 1984.
39. Dobbing J, Sands J: Quantitative growth and development of the human brain. Arch Dis Child 48:757-767, 1973.
40. Davison AN, Dobbing J: Myelination as a vulnerable period in brain development. Br Med J 22:40-44, 1966.
41. Brouwers P, Riccardi R, Fedio P, et al: Long-term neuropsychological sequelae of childhood leukemia: Correlation with CT brain scan abnormalities. J Pediatr 106:723-728, 1985.
42. Davis PC, Hoffman JC, Pearl GS, et al: CT evaluation of effects of cranial radiation therapy in children. Am J Neuroradiol 7:639-644, 1986.
43. Peylan-Ramu N, Poplack D, Pizzo D, et al: Abnormal CT scans of the brain in asymptomatic children with acute lymphoblastic leukemia after prophylactic treatment of the central nervous system with radiation and intrathecal chemotherapy. N Engl J Med 298:815-819, 1978.

44. Ochs JJ, Berger P, Brecher ML, et al: Computed tomography brain scans in children with acute lymphoblastic leukemia receiving methotrexate alone as central nervous system prophylaxis. Cancer 45:2274-2278, 1980.
45. Ochs JJ, Parvey LS, Whitaker JN, et al: Serial cranial computed tomography scans in children with leukemia given two different forms of central nervous system therapy. J Clin Oncol 1:793-798, 1983.
46. Kramer JH, Norman D, Brant-Zawadski M, et al: Absence of white matter changes on magnetic resonance imaging in children treated with CNS prophylaxis therapy for leukemia. Cancer 61:928-930, 1988.
47. Tsurada JS, Kortman KE, Bradley WG, et al: Radiation effects on cerebral white matter: MR evaluation. Am J Radiat 149:165-171, 1987.
48. Sheline GE, Wara WM, Smith V: Therapeutic irradiation and brain injury. Int J Radiat Oncol Biol Phys 6:1215-1228, 1980.
49. Cassarett G: Basic mechanisms of permanent and delayed radiation pathology. Cancer 37:1002-1010, 1976.
50. Committee for Radiation Oncology Studies: Normal tissue tolerance and damage. Cancer 37:2046-2055, 1976.
51. Allen JC: The effects of cancer therapy on the nervous system. J Pediatr 93:903-909, 1978.
52. Creasey W: Basic mechanisms of tissue injury by chemotherapy. Cancer 37:999-1002, 1976.
53. Price RA, Jamieson PA: The central nervous system in childhood leukemia. II. Subacute leukoencephalopathy. Cancer 35:306-318, 1975.
54. Mahoney DH, Fernbach DJ, Glaze DG, et al: Elevated myelin basic protein level in the cerebral spinal fluid of children with acute lymphoblastic leukemia. J Clin Oncol 2:58-61, 1984.
55. Gangji D, Reaman GH, Cohen SR, et al: Leukoencephalopathy and elevated levels of myelin basic protein in the cerebral spinal fluid of patients with acute lymphoblastic leukemia. Medical Intelligence 303:19-21, 1980.
56. Packer R, Meadows AT, Rorke L, et al: Long-term sequelae of cancer treatment on the central nervous system in childhood. Med Pediatr Oncol 15:241-253, 1987.
57. Hopewell JW: Late radiation damage to the central nervous system: A radiobiological interpretation. Neuropathol Appl Neurobiol 5:329-343, 1979.
58. Tiller-Boricich JK, Fike JR, Phillips TL, et al: Pathology of delayed radiation brain damage: An experimental canine model. Radiat Res 110:161-172, 1987.
59. Deck MD: Imaging techniques in the diagnosis of radiation damage to the central nervous system, in Gilbert HA, Kagen AR (eds): Radiation Damage to the Nervous System. New York, Raven Press, 1980, pp 107-127.
60. Wharam MD: Radiation therapy, in Altman AJ, Schwartz AD (eds): Malignant Diseases of Infancy, Childhood and Adolescence. Philadelphia, WB Saunders, 1983, p 103.
61. Piehl IJ, Meyer D, Perlia CP, et al: Effects of cixsdiammine dichloroplatinum (NSC-119875) on hearing function in man. Cancer Chemother Rep 58:871-875, 1974.
62. Walkwe DA, Pillov J, Waters KD, et al: Enhanced cisplatinum ototoxicity in children with brain tumors who have received simultaneous or prior cranial irradiation. Med Pediatr Oncol 17:48-52, 1989.
63. Ganong WF: The thyroid gland, in Ganong WF (ed): Review of Medical Physiology. Palo Alto, Calif, Appleton & Lange, 1987, pp 262-275.
64. Glatstein E, McHardy-Young S, Brast N, et al: Alterations in serum thyrotropin (TSH) and thyroid function following radiotherapy in patients with malignant lymphoma. J Clin Endocrinol Metab 32:838-841, 1971.
65. Shalet SM, Rosenstock JD, Beardwell CG, et al: Thyroid dysfunction following external irradiation to the neck for Hodgkin's disease in childhood. Radiology 28:511-515, 1977.
66. Smith RE, Adler RA, Clark P, et al: Thyroid function after mantle radiation in Hodgkin's disease. JAMA 245:46-49, 1981.
67. Donaldson SS, Glatstein E, Rosenberg SA, et al: Pediatric Hodgkin's disease. II. Results of therapy. Cancer 37:2436-2447, 1976.
68. Ramsay N, Kim T, Coccia P, et al: Thyroid dysfunction in pediatric patients after mantle field radiation therapy for Hodgkin's disease. Proc Am Soc Clin Oncol 19:331, 1978 (abstr).
69. Mortimer RH, Hill GE, Galligan JP, et al: Hypothyroidism and Graves' disease after mantle irradiation: A follow-up study. Aust N Z J Med 16:347-351, 1986.
70. Joensuu H, Viikari J: Thyroid function after postoperative radiation therapy in patients with breast cancer. Acta Radiol Oncol 25:167-170, 1986.
71. Fuks Z, Glatstein E, Marsa G, et al: Long-term effects of external radiation on the pituitary and thyroid glands. Cancer 37:1157-1161, 1979 (suppl).
72. Mauch PM, Weinstein H, Botnick L, et al: An evaluation of long-term survival and treatment complications in children with Hodgkin's disease. Cancer 51:925-932, 1983.
73. Sklar C, Kim T, Ramsay N: Thyroid dysfunction among long-term survivors of bone marrow transplantation. Am J Med 73:688-694, 1982.
74. Constine LS, Rubin P, Woolf PD: Hyperprolactinemia and hypothyroidism following cytotoxic therapy for central nervous system malignancies. J Clin Oncol 5:1841-1851, 1987.
75. Samaan N, Scholtz P, Yang KP: Endocrine complications after radiotherapy for tumors of the head and neck. J Lab Clin Med 109:364-372, 1987.
76. Nelson DF, Reddy KV, O'Mara RE, et al: Thyroid abnormalities following neck irradiation for Hodgkin's disease. Cancer 42:2553-2562, 1978.
77. Schimpff SC, Diggs CH, Wiswell JG, et al: Radiation-related thyroid dysfunction: Implications for the treatment of Hodgkin's disease. Ann Intern Med 92:91-98, 1980.
78. Samaan NA, Vieto R, Schultz PN, et al: Hypothalamic, pituitary and thyroid dysfunction after radiotherapy to the head and neck. Int J Radiat Oncol Biol Phys 8:1857-1867, 1982.
79. Richards GE, Wara WM, Grumbach MM, et al: Delayed onset of hypopituitarism: Sequelae of therapeutic irradiation of central nervous system, ear, and middle ear tumors. J Pediatr 89:553-559, 1976.
80. Shalet SM, Beardwell CG, Aarous BM, et al: Growth impairment of children treated for brain tumors. Arch Dis Child 53:491-494, 1978.
81. Bamford FN, Morris Jones PH, Pearson D, et al: Residual disabilities in children treated for intracranial space-occupying lesions. Cancer 37:1149-1151, 1976.
82. Brauner R, Rappaport R, Prevot C, et al: A prospective study of growth hormone deficiency in children given cranial irradiation, and its relation to statural growth. J Clin Endocrinol Metab 68:346-351, 1989.
83. Pasqualini T, Diez B, Domene H, et al: Long-term endocrine sequelae after surgery, radiation therapy and chemotherapy in younger children with medulloblastoma. Cancer 59:801-806, 1987.

84. Oberfield SE, Allen JC, Pollack J, et al: Long-term endocrine sequelae after treatment of medulloblastoma: Perspective study of growth and thyroid function. J Pediatr 108:219-223, 1986.
85. Ahmed SR, Shalet SM, Beardwell CG: The effects of cranial irradiation on growth hormone secretion. Acta Paediatr Scand 75:255-260, 1986.
86. Shalet SM, Beardwell CG, Morris Jones PH, et al: Growth hormone deficiency after treatment of acute leukemia in children. Arch Dis Child 51:489-493, 1971.
87. Wells RJ, Foster MB, D'Ercole JD, et al: The impact of cranial irradiation on growth of children with acute lymphoblastic leukemia. Am J Dis Child 137:37-39, 1983.
88. Blatt J, Bercu BB, Gillin C, et al: Reduced pulsatile growth hormone secretion in children after therapy for acute lymphoblastic leukemia. J Pediatr 104:182-186, 1984.
89. Berry DH, Elders MJ, Crist WM, et al: Growth in children with acute lymphoblastic leukemia: A Pediatric Oncology Group Study. Med Pediatr Oncol 11:39-45, 1983.
90. Hakami N, Mohammad A, Meyer J: Growth and growth hormone of children with acute lymphoblastic leukemia following central nervous system prophylaxis with and without cranial irradiation. Am J Pediatr Hematol Oncol 2:311-316, 1985.
91. Robison LL, Nesbit ME, Sather HN, et al: Height of children successfully treated for acute lymphoblastic leukemia: A report from the late effects study committee of Children's Cancer Study Group. Med Pediatr Oncol 13:13-21, 1985.
92. Shalet SM, Bearwell CG, Pearson D, et al: The effect of varying doses of cerebral irradiation on growth hormone production in childhood. Clin Endocrinol 5:287-290, 1976.
93. Cicognani A, Cacciari E, Veechi V, et al: Differential effects of 18- and 24-Gy cranial irradiation on growth rate and growth hormone release in children with prolonged survival after acute lymphoblastic leukemia. Am J Dis Child 142:1199-1202, 1988.
94. Starceski PJ, Lee PA, Blatt J, et al: Comparable effects of 1800- and 2400-rad cranial irradiation on height and weight in children treated for acute lymphoblastic leukemia. Am J Dis Child 141:550-552, 1987.
95. Sanders JE, Pritchard S, Mahoney P, et al: Growth and development following marrow transplantation for leukemia. Blood 68:1129-1135, 1986.
96. Brauner R, Czernichow P, Rappaport R: Greater susceptibility to hypothalamopituitary irradiation in younger children with acute lymphoblastic leukemia. J Pediatr 108:332, 1986.
97. Chapman R, Sutcliffe S, Malpas J: Cytotoxic-induced ovarian failure in Hodgkin's disease. II. Effects on sexual function. JAMA 242:1882-1884, 1979.
98. Chapman R, Sutcliffe S, Malpas J: Cytotoxic-induced ovarian failure in women with Hodgkin's disease. I. Hormone function. JAMA 242:1877-1881, 1979.
99. Andrieu J, Ochoa-Molina ME: Menstrual cycle, pregnancies and offspring before and after MOPP therapy for Hodgkin's disease. Cancer 52:435-438, 1983.
100. Koyama H, Wada T, Nishizawa Y, et al: Cyclophosphamide-induced ovarian failure and its therapeutic significance in patients with breast cancer. Cancer 39:1403-1409, 1977.
101. Jordan VC, Fritz NF, Tormey DC: Endocrine effects of adjuvant chemotherapy and long-term tamoxifen administration on node-positive patients with breast cancer. Cancer Res 47:624-630, 1987.
102. Gershenson DM: Menstrual and reproductive function after treatment with combination chemotherapy for malignant ovarian germ cell tumors. J Clin Oncol 6:270-275, 1988.
103. Hobbie WL, Schwartz CL: Endocrine late effects among survivors of cancer. Semin Oncol Nurs 5:14-21, 1989.
104. Shalet SM: The effects of cancer treatment on growth and sexual development. Clin Oncol 4:223-238, 1985.
105. Hensle T, Burbige K, Shepard B, et al: Chemotherapy and its effect on testicular morphology in children. J Urol 131:1142-1144, 1982.
106. Sherins RJ, Olweny CLM, Ziegler JL: Gynaecomastia and gonadal dysfunction in adolescent boys treated with combination chemotherapy for Hodgkin's disease. N Engl J Med 299:12-16, 1978.
107. Whilthead E, Shalet SM, Morris Jones PH, et al: Gonadal function after combination chemotherapy for Hodgkin's disease in childhood. Arch Dis Child 57:287-291, 1982.
108. Rivkees SA, Crawford JD: The relationship of gonadal activity and chemotherapy-induced gonadal damage. JAMA 259:2123-2125, 1988.
109. Green DM, Brecher BL, Lindsay AN, et al: Gonadal function in pediatric patients following treatment for Hodgkin's disease. Pediatr Oncol 9:235-244, 1981.
110. Shalet SM, Hann IM, Lendon M, et al: Testicular function after combination chemotherapy in childhood for acute lymphoblastic leukemia. J Pediatr 94:719-722, 1981.
111. Byrne J, Mulvihill JJ, Myers MH, et al: Effects of treatment on fertility in long-term survivors of childhood or adolescent cancer. N Engl J Med 317:1315-1321, 1987.
112. De Cunhna MF, Meistrich ML, Fuller IM, et al: Recovery of spermatogenesis after treatment for Hodgkin's disease: Limiting dose of MOPP chemotherapy. J Clin Oncol 2:571-577, 1984.
113. Nicosia S, Matus-Ridley M, Meadows AT: Gonadal effects of cancer therapy in girls. Cancer 55:2364-2372, 1985.
114. Himelstein-Braw R, Peters H, Faber M: Morphological study of the ovaries of leukemic children. Br J Cancer 38:82-87, 1978.
115. Ash P: The influence of radiation on fertility in man. Br J Radiol 53:271-278, 1980.
116. Fischer B, Cheung A: Delayed effect of radiation therapy with or without chemotherapy on ovarian function in women with Hodgkin's disease. Acta Radiol Oncol 23:43-48, 1984.
117. Shalet SM, Beardwell CG, Jacobs HG, et al: Testicular function following irradiation of the human prepubertal testis. Clin Endocrinol 9:483-490, 1978.
118. Shalet SM, Horner A, Ahmed SR, et al: Leydig cell damage and testicular function combination chemotherapy in childhood for acute lymphoblastic leukemia. Med Pediatr Oncol 13:65-68, 1985.
119. Hamre MR, Robison LL, Nesbit ME, et al: Effects of radiation on ovarian function in long-term survivors of childhood acute lymphoblastic leukemia: A report from the Children's Cancer Study Group. J Clin Oncol 5:1759-1765, 1987.
120. Shalet SM, Beardwell CG, Morris Jones PH, et al: Ovarian failure following abdominal irradiation in childhood. Br J Cancer 33:655-658, 1976.
121. Saman N, Vieto R, Schultz B, et al: Hypothalamic, pituitary and thyroid dysfunction after radiotherapy to the head and neck. Int J Radiat Oncol Biol Phys 8:1857-1867, 1982.
122. Buvat J, LeMarie A, Burat-Herbaut M, et al: Hyperprolactinemia and sexual function in men. Horm Res 22:196-203, 1985.
123. Hitzig WH, Pluss HJ, Joller P, et al: Studies on the immune status of children with acute lymphocytic leukemia. II. In remission with and without cytostatic treatment. Clin Exp Immunol 26:414-418, 1976.

124. Borella L, Green AA, Webster RG: Immunologic rebound after cessation of long-term chemotherapy in acute leukemia. Blood 40:42-51, 1972.
125. Hancock BW, Bruce L, Whitman MD, et al: The effects of radiotherapy on immunity in patients with cured localized carcinoma of the cervix uteri. Cancer 53:884-887, 1984.
126. Job G, Pfreundschuh M, Bauer M, et al: The influence of radiation therapy on T lymphocyte subpopulations defined by monoclonal antibodies. Int J Radiat Oncol Biol Phys 10:2077-2081, 1984.
127. Rotstein S, Blomgren H, Petrini B, et al: Long-term effects of the immune system following local radiation therapy for breast cancer. I. Cellular composition of peripheral blood lymphocyte population. Int J Radiat Oncol Biol Phys 11:921-925, 1985.
128. Rotstein S, Blomgren H, Petrini B, et al: Long-term effects on the immune system following local radiation therapy for breast cancer. IV. Proliferative responses and induction of suppressor activity of the blood lymphocyte population. Radiother Oncol 6:223-230, 1986.
129. Wasserman J, Blomgren H, Petrini B, et al: Effect of radiation therapy and in vitro x-ray exposure on lymphocyte subpopulations and their functions. Am J Clin Oncol 5:195-208, 1982.
130. Haas GS, Halperin E, Poseretz D, et al: Differential recovery of circulating T cell subsets after nodal irradiation for Hodgkin's disease. J Immunol 132:1026-1030, 1984.
131. Fuks Z, Strober S, Bobrove AM, et al: Long-term effects of radiation on peripheral blood of patients with Hodgkin's disease. J Clin Invest 58:803-814, 1976.
132. Ueda M, Harada N, Shiobara S, et al: T lymphocyte reconstitution in long-term survivors after allogeneic and autologous transplantation. Transplantation 3:552-556, 1984.
133. Van Rijswijk RE, Sybesma JPH, Kater L: A prospective study of the changes in the immune status before, during and after multiple agent chemotherapy for Hodgkin's disease. Cancer 51:637-644, 1983.
134. Layward L, Levinsky RJ, Butler M: Long-term abnormalities in T and B lymphocyte function in children following treatment for acute lymphoblastic leukemia. J Haematol 49:251-258, 1981.
135. Paolucci P, Layward L, Hayward AR, et al: Increase and inhibition of pre–B cell proliferation in culture by T cells. Clin Exp Immunol 43:336-341, 1979.
136. Katz J, Walter BN, Bennetts GA, et al: Abnormal cellular and humoral immunity in childhood acute lymphoblastic leukemia in long-term remission. West J Med 146:179-187, 1988.
137. Workman ML: Immunologic late effects in children and adults. Semin Oncol Nurs 5:36-42, 1989.
138. Parmentier L, Morardet N, Tubina M: Late effects on human bone marrow after extended field radiotherapy. Int J Radiat Oncol Biol Phys 9:1303-1311, 1983.
139. Sacks EL, Goris ML, Glatstein E: Bone marrow regeneration following large field radiation. Cancer 42:1057-1065, 1978.
140. Steinherz LJ, Steinherz P, Tan C, et al: Cardiac toxicity 4-20 years after completing anthracycline therapy. Proc Am Soc Clin Oncol 8:296, 1989 (abstr).
141. Steinherz LJ, Steinherz P, Tan C: Cardiac failure more than six years post anthracyclines. Proc Int Soc Paediatric Oncol, SIOP XIX Meeting, 1987, p 136 (abstr).
142. Ruccione K, Weinberg K: Late effects in multiple body systems. Semin Oncol Nurs 5:4-13, 1989.
143. Von Hoff DD, Layward MW, Basa P, et al: Risk factors for doxorubicin induced congestive heart failure. Ann Intern Med 91:710-717, 1979.
144. Von Hooff DD, Rozencweig M, Piccart M: The cardiotoxicity of anticancer agents. Semin Oncol 9:23-33, 1982.
145. Pratt CG, Ransom JL, Evans WE: Age-related Adriamycin cardiotoxicity in children. Cancer Treat Rep 62:1381-1384, 1978.
146. Muggia FM, Cassileth PA: Constrictive pericarditis following radiation therapy. Am J Med 44:116-123, 1968.
147. Martin RG, Ruckdeschel JC, Chang P, et al: Radiation-related pericarditis. Am J Cardiol 35:216-220, 1975.
148. Roth BJ, Greist A, Kubilis PS, et al: Cisplatin-based combination chemotherapy for disseminated germ cell tumors: Long-term follow-up. J Clin Oncol 6:1239-1247, 1988.
149. Libshitz JI, Southard ME: Complications of radiation therapy: The thorax. Semin Roentgenol 9:41-49, 1974.
150. Ginsberg AJ, Cormis RL: The pulmonary toxicity of antineoplastic agents. Semin Oncol 9:35-51, 1982.
151. DeLena M, Guzzon A, Monfardini S, et al: Clinical, radiologic and histopathologic studies on pulmonary toxicity induced by treatment with bleomycin (NSC-125066). Cancer Chemother Rep 56:343-356, 1972.
152. Blum RH, Carter SK, Agre K: A clinical review of bleomycin: A new antineoplastic agent. Cancer 31:903-913, 1973.
153. Aronin PA, Mahaley MS, Rudnick SA, et al: Prediction of BCNU pulmonary toxicity in patients with malignant gliomas. N Engl J Med 303:183-188, 1980.
154. Donaldson SS, Jundt S, Ricour C, et al: Radiation enteritis in children: A retrospective review, clinicopathologic correlation, and dietary management. Cancer 35:1167-1178, 1975.
155. Jaffe N: Biological consequences of cancer and its treatment and their relationship to current treatment planning. Am J Pediatr Hemat Oncol 9:62-67, 1987.
156. D'Angio GJ, Pearson D: Radiation therapy, in Bloom HGJ, et al (eds): Cancer in Children. Berlin, Springer-Verlag, 1975, pp 217-241.
157. Jaffe N: Late sequelae of cancer therapy, in Sutow SS, Fernbach DJ, Vietti TJ (eds): Clinical Pediatric Oncology. St Louis, CV Mosby, 1984, pp 810-832.
158. Aron BS, Schlesinger A: Complications of radiation therapy: The genitourinary tract. Semin Roentgenol 9:132-145, 1974.
159. Bennett AH: Cyclophosphamide and hemorrhagic cystitis. Urology 111:603-606, 1974.
160. D'Angio GJ, Farber S, Maddock CL: Potentiation of x-ray effects by actinomycin-D. Radiology 73:175-177, 1959.
161. Tefft M, Lattin PB, Jerab B, et al: Acute and late effects of normal tissues following combined chemo- and radiotherapy of childhood rhabdomyosarcoma and Ewing's sarcoma. Cancer 37:1202-1213, 1976.
162. Probert JC, Parker BR: The effects of radiation therapy on bone growth. Radiology 114:155-162, 1975.
163. Shalet SM, Gibson B, Swindell R, et al: Effect of spinal irradiation on growth. Arch Dis Child 62:461-464, 1987.
164. Jaffe N, Toth BB, Hoar RE, et al: Dental and maxillofacial abnormalities in long-term survivors of childhood cancer: Effects of treatment with chemotherapy and radiation to the head and neck. Pediatrics 73:816-823, 1984.
165. Hazra TA, Shipman B: Dental problems in pediatric patients with head and neck tumors undergoing multiple modality therapy. Med Pediatr Oncol 10:91-95, 1984.
166. Maguire A, Craft AW, Evans RGB, et al: The long-term effects of treatment on the dental conditions of children surviving malignant disease. Cancer 60:2570-2575, 1987.
167. Roller AC, Pembrook L, Plese L, et al: One-in-five Hodgkin's patients still at risk after 15 years. Oncol Nurs Update 2:13, 1987.

168. Meadows AT: Second malignant neoplasms in childhood cancer survivors. J Assoc Pediatr Oncol Nurs 6:7-11, 1989.
169. Li FP, Cassady R, Jaffe N: Risk of second tumors in survivors of childhood cancer. Cancer 35:1230-1235, 1975.
170. Fraser MC, Tucker MA: Second malignancies following cancer therapy. Semin Oncol Nurs 5:43-55, 1989.
171. Meadows AT: Second malignant neoplasms in children: An update from the Late Effects Study Group. J Clin Oncol 3:532-538, 1985.
172. Meadows AT, Strong LC, Li FP, et al: Bone sarcoma as a second malignant neoplasm in children: Influence of radiation and genetic predisposition. Cancer 46:2603-2606, 1980.
173. Tucker MA, D'Angio GI, Boice JD, et al: Bone sarcomas linked to radiotherapy and chemotherapy in children. N Engl J Med 317:588-593, 1987.
174. Tucker MH, Coleman CN, Cox RS, et al: Risk of second cancers after treatment for Hodgkin's disease. N Engl J Med 318:76-81, 1988.
175. Valagussa P, Santoro A, Fossati-Bellani F, et al: Second acute leukemia and other malignancies following treatment for Hodgkin's disease. J Clin Oncol 4:830-837, 1986.
176. Aisenberg AC: Acute nonlymphocytic leukemia after treatment for Hodgkin's disease. Am J Med 75:449-454, 1983.
177. Coleman CN: Secondary neoplasms in patients treated for cancer: Etiology and perspective. Radiat Res 92:188-200, 1982.
178. Coleman CN, Kaplan HS, Cox R, et al: Leukemia, non-Hodgkin's lymphoma and solid tumors in patients treated for Hodgkin's disease. Cancer Surv 1:733-744, 1982.
179. Coleman M, Easton DF, Horwich A, et al: Second malignancies and Hodgkin's disease—The Royal Marsden Hospital experience. Radiother Oncol 11:229-238, 1988.
180. Blayney DW, Longo DL, Young RC, et al: Decreasing risk of leukemia with prolonged follow-up after chemotherapy and radiation for Hodgkin's disease. N Engl J Med 316:710-714, 1987.
181. Greene MH: Epidemiologic studies of chemotherapy related acute leukemia, in Castellani A (ed): Epidemiology and Quantitation of Environmental Risk in Humans from Radiation and Other Agents. New York, Plenum, 1985, 499-514.
182. Meadows AT: Second malignant neoplasms. Clin Oncol 4:247-261, 1985.
183. Tucker MA, Meadows AT, Boice JD, et al: Cancer risk following treatment of childhood cancer, in Boice JD Jr, Fraumeni JF Jr (eds): Radiation Carcinogenesis: Epidemiology and Biological Significance. New York, Raven, 1984, pp 211-224.
184. Valagussa P, Santoro S, Kenda R, et al: Second malignancies in Hodgkin's disease: A complication of certain forms of treatment. Br Med J 280:216-219, 1980.
185. Bergasgel DE, Bailey AJ, Langley GR, et al: The chemotherapy of plasma cell myeloma and the incidence of acute leukemia. N Engl J Med 301:743-748, 1979.
186. Pedersen-Bjergaard J, Ersboll J, Sorensen HM, et al: Risk of acute nonlymphocytic leukemia and preleukemia in patients treated with cyclophosphamide for non-Hodgkin's lymphomas. Ann Intern Med 103:195-200, 1985.
187. Gomez GA, Aggarwal KK, Han R: Post-therapeutic acute malignant myeloproliferative syndrome and acute nonlymphocytic leukemia in non-Hodgkin's lymphoma: Correlation with intensity of treatment. Cancer 50:2285-2288, 1982.
188. Greene MH, Young RC, Merrill JM, et al: Evidence of a treatment dose response in acute nonlymphocytic leukemias which occur after therapy of non-Hodgkin's lymphoma. Cancer Res 43:1891-1898, 1983.
189. Fisher B, Rockette H, Fisher ER, et al: Leukemia in breast cancer patients following adjuvant chemotherapy or postoperative radiation: The NSABP experience. J Clin Oncol 3:1640-1658, 1985.
190. Lerner HJ: Acute myelogenous leukemia in patients receiving chorambucil as long-term adjuvant chemotherapy for stage II breast cancer. Cancer Treat Rep 62:1135-1138, 1979.
191. Boice JD, Greene MH, Killen JY, et al: Late effects of low dose adjuvant chemotherapy in colorectal cancer. J Natl Cancer Inst 64:501-511, 1980.
192. Boice JD, Greene MH, Killen JY, et al: Leukemia and preleukemia after adjuvant chemotherapy of gastrointestinal cancer with semustine (methyl-CCNU). N Engl J Med 309:1079-1084, 1983.
193. Chak LY, Sikic BL, Tucker MA, et al: Increased incidence of acute nonlymphocytic leukemia following therapy in patients with small cell carcinoma of the lung. J Clin Oncol 2:385-390, 1984.
194. Ratain MJ, Kaminer LS, Bitran JD, et al: Acute nonlymphocytic leukemia following etoposide and cisplatin combination chemotherapy for advanced non–small cell carcinoma of the lung. Blood 70:1412-1417, 1987.
195. Redman JR, Vugrin D, Arlin ZA, et al: Leukemia following treatment of germ cell tumors in men. J Clin Oncol 2:1080-1087, 1984.
196. Greene MH, Boice JD Jr, Greer GE, et al: Acute nonlymphocytic leukemia after therapy with alkylating agents for ovarian cancer. N Engl J Med 307:1416-1421, 1982.
197. Tucker MA, Meadows AT, Boice JD Jr, et al: Leukemia after therapy with alkylating agents for childhood cancer. J Natl Cancer Inst 78:459-464, 1987.
198. Greene MH, Harris EL, Gershenson DM, et al: Mephalan may be a more potent leukemogen than cyclophosphamide. Ann Intern Med 105:360-367, 1986.
199. Meadows AT, D'Angio GJ, Mike V, et al: Patterns of second malignant neoplasms in children. Cancer 40:1903-1911, 1977.
200. Tucker MA, D'Angio GJ, Boice JD, et al: Bone sarcomas linked to radiotherapy and chemotherapy in children. N Engl J Med 317:588-593, 1987.
201. Schwartz AD, Lee H, Baum ES: Leukemia in children with Wilms' tumor. J Pediatr 87:374-376, 1975.
202. Boice JD Jr, Blettner M, Kleinerman RA, et al: Radiation dose and second cancer risk in patients treated for cancer of the cervix. Radiat Res 116:3-55, 1988.
203. Storm HH: Secondary primary cancer after treatment for cervical cancer: Late effects of radiotherapy. Cancer 61:679-688, 1988.
204. Rimm IJ, Li FC, Tarbell NJ: Brain tumors after cranial irradiation for childhood acute lymphoblastic leukemia: A 13 year experience from the Dana Farber Cancer Institute and The Children's Hospital. Cancer 59:1506-1508, 1987.
205. Gilmann PA, Miller RW: Cancer after acute lymphocytic leukemia. Am J Dis Child 135:311-312, 1981.
206. List AF, Doll DC, Creco A: Lung cancer in Hodgkin's disease: Association with previous radiotherapy. J Clin Oncol 3:215-221, 1985.

PART VI

THE CARE OF INDIVIDUALS WITH CANCER

Chapter 33

AIDS-Related Malignancies

Theresa A. Moran, RN, MS

Gayling Gee, RN, MS

INTRODUCTION

For decades scientists and medical researchers have been attempting to prove or disprove the hypothesis of immune surveillance and the evolution of cancer. As the research in this area continues, it appears that human immunodeficiency virus (HIV) infection contributes yet another piece of evidence that supports this theory. The devastation wreaked by HIV on the immune system, particularly the cell-mediated arm, results in the diagnosis of a malignancy during some point of the illness in approximately 70% of those with acquired immunodeficiency syndrome.[1] Neoplasms of all organs and body systems also have been reported in patients whose serum is positive for HIV antibody. The three most common malignancies in AIDS are Kaposi's sarcoma (KS), non-Hodgkin's lymphoma (NHL), and primary central nervous system (CNS) lymphoma. These diseases have been referred to as *opportunistic* malignancies because they occur in patients with preexisting immunodeficiency, for example, in persons with primary immunodeficiency, in those who undergo therapeutic immunosuppression, and now in persons with HIV infection. Because these individuals are immunosuppressed, the aforementioned cancers proliferate rapidly.

KAPOSI'S SARCOMA

In 1872 Dr. Moritz Kaposi first described the lesions of Kaposi's sarcoma in seven men of Mediterranean or Jewish ancestry. In 1947 the literature indicated that only 500 cases had been reported, and by 1960 only 1200 total cases had been documented in the 100 years since the disease was first described. The incidence in the general population was estimated to be two to six cases per 100 million people; thus dermatologists and oncologists were not likely to diagnose this rare malignancy in the course of their professional careers. Beginning in the 1970s, however, the incidence of KS increased dramatically. As more sophisticated technologic advances brought on the era of organ transplantation, an increasing number of reports documented the occurrence of this malignancy in patients who were chemically immunosuppressed to prevent organ rejection.[1,2] With the development of new drugs, oncologists began seeing KS in patients treated with antineoplastic agents. Reports from Africa in the late 1970s revealed that KS was endemic in certain areas of the continent. In 1981 KS was reported in yet another population, that of previously healthy, young, homosexual men who were neither receiving chemotherapy nor undergoing organ transplantations.[3,4] This particular outbreak of what once was believed to be a rare skin cancer initially was considered an isolated anomaly, but as other cities in the United States began noting the increasing numbers of young men with KS, it became obvious that a new phenomenon was occurring. Although controversy exists over whether KS is a malignancy at all or a highly dysplastic phenomenon, the relationship of KS to AIDS is indisputable.[5] In addition to KS, other opportunistic infections, primarily *Pneumocystis carinii* pneumonia, were diagnosed in this same population.[3,4]

In an effort to determine the cause of this disease, researchers began examining the immune systems of these young homosexual men. All were found to have some degree of immunosuppression.[4] In 1982 these findings led to the clinical definition of a new disease, acquired immunodeficiency syndrome (AIDS), in which the underlying immunodeficiency resulted in the appearance of indicator diseases.[6] One of the indicator diseases included the diagnosis of KS in a person younger than 60 years of age. In 1987 the diagnosis of AIDS was expanded to include the advent of KS in a person of any age who is seropositive for HIV antibody.[7]

Epidemiology

Before the occurrence of HIV infection, KS was divided into the following categories: classic KS (non-African), African KS (endemic), and KS that occurred in transplant recipients. Cases of classic KS are found in the United States and Europe. Predominantly a disease that occurs in men, it has a male/female ratio of 10 to 15:1 and affects men of Mediterranean or Jewish ancestry in the fifth to eighth decades of life.[2] This malignancy is characterized as an indolent, slow-growing cutaneous nodule or plaque-like lesion. In 88% of those diagnosed, lesions will be confined to the lower extremities, distal to the knee, without invasive or disseminated disease. Treatment generally is not indicated because of its indolent nature. It is predictably a chronic, fairly benign malignancy that is rarely fatal.[2]

In contrast, African KS (endemic) is a malignant disease that affects persons of all ages, including children, and is found almost exclusively in black Africans. Cases of KS appear to cluster near the equator in the eastern half of the continent. African KS affects men twice as often as women, with a male/female ratio of 2.5:1.[8] Clinical presentations range from one similar to that observed in classic KS (nodular and indolent skin lesion) to a florid, infiltrative, and highly aggressive lymphadenopathic form that progresses rapidly and is frequently fatal.[8]

Transplant recipients experience an increased incidence of KS as high as 150 to 200 times the number of cases found in the general population.[9] KS affects men at a higher incidence than women (2 to 3:1), and presentations can range from localized skin lesions to disseminated visceral and mucocutaneous disease. A correlation seems to exist between the degree of immunosuppression and the incidence of KS. The more depressed the immune system, the greater the incidence of KS. Spontaneous remissions also have been documented in transplantation patients whose immunosuppression has been reversed.[9]

The fourth category, AIDS-related KS, was first described in 1981 and is distinctly different from the other categories of KS (Table 33-1).[10] Clinical presentation

TABLE 33-1 Clinical Features of Kaposi's Sarcoma

Group	Clinical Features	Response to Therapy
Classic: elderly men, especially of Jewish, Mediterranean ancestry	Indolent; cutaneous lesions of legs, feet; immunologic attrition of aging	Local radiation: good control; rarely fatal
Endemic: black Africans	Variable; children: aggressive, lymphadenopathic; adults: usually indolent, affects extremities; no underlying immunodeficiency	Systemic chemotherapy: poor response in lymphadenopathic form; excellent response in indolent, adult form
Renal transplant recipients	Aggressive, localized to visceral involvement; chemotherapy-induced immunosuppression	Controlled by stopping immunosuppressive medications
AIDS-related	Aggressive, disseminated disease with cutaneous, visceral, and lymphadenopathic involvement; virally induced immunodeficiency	Systemic chemotherapy: response rates of 25%-50% Radiation therapy: good response but recurrence common: palliative not curative Treatment selection is complex; need to control tumor without exacerbating immunodeficiency

Source: Adapted from Volberding PA: Kaposi's sarcoma in AIDS, in Levy JA (ed): AIDS, Pathogenesis and Treatment. New York, Marcel Dekker, 1989, p 349.

ranges from localized skin lesions to disseminated disease that involves multiple body organs. KS that occurs with AIDS tends to be a highly aggressive disease.[1] Despite the aggressive nature of AIDS-related KS, patients rarely die as a direct result of KS. Overall, the mortality rate in this group is approximately 41%, with more than 60% of all patients alive at 1 year and more than 50% alive at 22 months. This rate contrasts with the average survival rate of 18 months for all persons diagnosed with AIDS.[1] Patients with only KS and no opportunistic infections tend to live longer, and there are a number of anecdotal reports of persons with AIDS-related KS who have survived from 3 to 7 years.[9] The cause of death in patients with AIDS-related KS is usually from concomitant opportunistic infections or the pathologic effects of HIV itself.

Etiology

Although the link between immunosuppression and KS is established, it does not predict those persons in whom KS will develop. When KS was first reported, it was the initial indicator disease in 30% to 35% of all diagnosed AIDS cases. Recent reports reveal that KS is the initial AIDS diagnosis in only 23% of all AIDS cases.[11] Possible explanations for this reduction in incidence of initial diagnosis include medical advancements that enable opportunistic infections to be diagnosed earlier than KS and the elimination of a co-factor that promotes the development of KS. Some researchers link the decreased incidence of KS to the decreased use of "poppers," or amyl nitrite, believed to be a co-factor in the development of AIDS-related KS.[12] This connection was suggested in several studies; however, large enough cohorts have not been collected and studied to document a causal relationship. Another group of researchers believe that hereditary or genetic predisposition plays an important role in the development of KS in both immunocompetent and immunodeficient populations. These researchers postulate that men infected with HIV who carry the human leukocyte antigen (HLA)–DR5 allele may be at an increased risk of KS development. Again, a causal relationship has not been established and the postulate remains controversial.[13]

KS also seems to be a disease found predominantly in homosexual and bisexual men with AIDS. Other groups diagnosed with AIDS (women, children, or men who are heterosexual or intravenous drug users, or both) do not have as high an incidence of KS as homosexual men with AIDS.[14,15] One study found the DNA of cytomegalovirus (CMV) in the nucleus of cells of KS lesions, which suggests a viral cause of KS.[16] Serologic testing demonstrates that as many as 94% of all homosexual men have been infected by CMV, as evidenced by antibodies to CMV.[17] CMV also has been isolated from the blood, semen, gastrointestinal tract, central nervous system (CNS), and lungs of patients with AIDS, which suggests the possible role of latent CMV infection in AIDS-related KS. Together with high CMV antibody seroprevalence, this viral link may offer an explanation for the diagnosis of KS predominantly in homosexual men.

Detection

Detection of KS is typically by self-observation of cutaneous lesions. This makes patient education in lesion identification an important method of detection. Additionally, all health care providers should routinely perform a careful visual examination of cutaneous surfaces of all persons who are seropositive for HIV or who are in a high-risk group for AIDS. Visual inspection includes the skin of the head (including the sclera), neck, torso, extremities, perirectal area, palms of the hands, soles of the feet, and the oral cavity. Biopsy specimens of suspicious lesions are then examined. KS also may be a differential diagnosis in patients with enlarged lymph nodes or with pulmonary symptoms and a chest film with abnormal findings.

Pathophysiology

After histologic examination the pathologist has the responsibility of diagnosis. All types of KS (endemic, classic, transplantation-induced, and epidemic) are microscopically similar. Descriptions of lesions include interlacing bands of spindle cells, with vascular structures in a network of reticular and collagen fibers. As the integrity of this network is lost, clefts usually occur among the vascular structures, which allows the extravasation of red blood cells. Lymphatic and blood vessels are present throughout the lesion and on its periphery. The nucleus of the spindle cells are frequently pleomorphic. Hemosiderin, extravasated red cells, and red cells that phagocytose the hemosiderin may be found between spindle cells. An inflammatory response involving histiocytes, lymphocytes, and plasma cells also may be seen.

Diagnosis can be difficult, especially in the early or immature lesions. This stage has been referred to as the *macular stage*. Changes in this stage may be subtle and the pathologist may observe only abnormally dilated vessels surrounding normal superficial vasculature. There may be little or no inflammatory response at this stage. Nuclear pleomorphism may be seen in mitosis, with nuclear atypia. As the lesion matures and becomes a plaque, it demonstrates more extensive neoplastic involvement, with proliferation through many layers, including the dermis and occasionally the adipose layers. A marked inflammatory response occurs at this stage, with a corresponding increase in numbers of spindle cells and extravasation of red cells. The prominence of hemosiderin deposits also is noted at this time. As the lesion advances toward nodular formation, these effects become more exaggerated. Spindle cells are dense, with considerable reticulum deposition.[13,18-20]

Clinical Manifestations

The clinical presentation of AIDS-related KS resembles that of KS in transplant recipients. Multicentric skin lesions may be observed on any part of the body, and disseminated mucocutaneous and visceral disease frequently affects the lymphatic, pulmonary, gastrointestinal, cardiac, renal, biliary, and adrenal systems. There is no characteristic site of initial involvement as there is in the classic form of the disease. Lesions can be found on almost any skin surface, including the palms of the hands, soles of the feet, genitals, and head and neck. These lesions generally do not metastasize; instead they are multicentric (ie, each lesion is a primary lesion unto itself). The lesions range in pigmentation from brown, brown-red, purple, dark red, to violet; in rare cases they may appear to be deep blue-purple, resembling ecchymosis. They may be raised bullous nodules or flat plaquelike lesions. In either presentation they do not blanch when pressure is applied and are not painful unless they are responsible for structural damage or impinge on vital organs or nerves. Black persons commonly have nodular lesions, and white persons tend to have either nodular or plaquelike lesions. As with HIV infection the average age range for AIDS-related KS is from 20 to 40 years.

This tumor can involve not only the skin but also the mucocutaneous surface of the buccal mucosa, the hard and soft palate, and the gums, as well as the sclera of the eyes. In fact, at the time of initial diagnosis of KS, approximately 72% of patients will already have involvement of one or more organ systems.[1] Internal organs most frequently affected include lymph nodes (81%), gastrointestinal tract (33%), and the lungs (11%).[1,21] KS in these organ systems can cause severe morbidity. Lesions also have been found in the liver, pancreas, adrenal glands, spleen, testes, and heart. Symptoms caused by these lesions usually are minimal.[1,15]

As HIV infection progresses, the immune system becomes increasingly suppressed; with it the occurrence and severity of KS also increases. Increasing numbers of skin lesions may be found all over the body surface. The multicentric skin lesions continue to enlarge, frequently coalescing with each other to form one large confluent lesion, often encompassing as large an area as the thigh, shin, or forearm. Malignant cells may involve the lymph nodes, thus compromising lymphatic drainage and blood circulation, resulting in severe edema distal to the affected area and stasis ulcers from edematous tissue. The lymph node involvement may be so severe as to cause major shifts in body fluids, limiting the flow of vital protein from lymph to plasma. The patient may succumb to anasarca, which is due to internal coalesced lesions and a decreased total serum protein/albumin resulting from the shift of fluid.

Additionally, when the gastrointestinal tract is involved, the patient may have a protein-losing enteropathy.[22] In this instance protein is not absorbed from the gastrointestinal tract, which results in a decreased total serum protein/albumin level. In cases where progression of KS involves the lung, symptoms include dyspnea and shortness of breath, eventually culminating in fatal respiratory distress.[21,23,24]

Staging

The ability to classify patients with similar stages of the disease would enable researchers to compare data and patient outcomes. Although an official method of staging KS does not exist, Laubenstein[25] and Krigel et al,[26] and later Mitsuyasu,[11] proposed a staging system for AIDS-related KS (Table 33-2).[13,26]

There are some patients with KS whose prognosis is

TABLE 33-2 Staging of Epidemic Kaposi's Sarcoma

	NYU Staging System*	Mitsuyasu Staging System†
Stage		
I	Cutaneous, locally indolent	Limited cutaneous (*10 lesions or one anatomical area)
II	Cutaneous, locally aggressive with or without regional lymph nodes	Disseminated cutaneous (§10 lesions or more than one anatomical area)
III	Generalized mucocutaneous and/or lymph node involvement‡	Visceral only (GI, lymph node)
IV	Visceral	Cutaneous and visceral, or pulmonary KS
Subtype		
A	No systemic signs or symptoms	No systemic signs or symptoms
B	Systemic signs; weight loss (10%) or fever (§100BF orally, unrelated to an identifiable source of infection lasting §2 weeks)	Fevers §37.8BC unrelated to identifiable infection lasting §2 weeks, or weight loss §10% of body weight

*Krigel RL et al: Kaposi's sarcoma: A new staging classification. Cancer Treat Rep 67:531, 1983.

†Mitsuyasu RT, Groopman JE: Biology and therapy of Kaposi's sarcoma. Semin Oncol 11:53, 1984.

‡Generalized z more than upper or lower extremities alone; includes minimal GI disease defined as *5 lesions and *2 cm in combined diameters.

Source: From Groopman J, Broder S: Cancer in AIDS and other immunodeficiency states, in DeVita V, Hellman S, Rosenberg S (eds): Cancer Principles and Practice of Oncology. Philadelphia, JB Lippincott, 1989, p 1962.

better than others with KS. The reasons are not clear, nor have all the variables been examined. Some studies have correlated the relationship between the absolute T4 lymphocyte count and prognosis. For example, the lower the T4 value in a patient with KS, the poorer the prognosis. A person with a helper/suppressor (H:S) ratio of greater than 0.5 (>1:2) and a T4 lymphocyte count of greater than 300/mm^3 has a relatively good prognosis. A helper/suppressor ratio of less than 0.2 (<1:5) and a T4 lymphocyte count of less than 100/mm^3 indicates a very poor prognosis. The area inbetween these values is of unclear prognostic value.[27-29] Other data also indicate that patients with head and neck involvement,[30] patients with prior or concomitant opportunistic infections, and patients exhibiting "B" symptoms (weight loss, fevers, chills, night sweats, diarrhea) all have a shorter life expectancy than those without these factors. With the exception of the lung, organ involvement does not seem to influence prognosis, nor does tumor burden correlate with prognosis.[31]

Assessment

A complete history and physical examination is indicated, including the patient's past history of drug use, sexual practice, and ethnic ancestry, along with close examination of the sclera, oral cavity, and integumentary system. Suspicious lesions must be biopsied before a diagnosis can be established. Visual inspection of lesions alone is insufficient to establish a diagnosis. Experienced physicians who care for patients with AIDS reflect anecdotally on lesions that appeared to be symptomatic of KS but were not histologically confirmed; conversely, examination of tissue from lesions that did not resemble those of KS proved to be diagnostic of KS. A lesion that visually suggests KS may be an immature lesion and thus does not show the distinctive pathologic changes that are diagnostic of KS. Repeat biopsies of other suspicious lesions at a later date (eg, in 2 weeks) may in fact yield a diagnosis of KS.

Examination of preparations from a 3, 4, or 6 mm punch biopsy of skin lesions is the most common method of diagnosis. Patients with KS involvement of the oral cavity should be referred to an oral surgeon for a diagnostic biopsy. Suspicious lymph nodes are best evaluated by means of an open (excisional) biopsy. Suspected KS involvement of other organs requires more invasive diagnostic procedures. For example, documentation of lung involvement requires a bronchoscopic examination. Similarly, documentation of gastrointestinal lesions requires endoscopic examination of the upper or lower tract. Lesions visualized by means of bronchoscopy or endoscopy may be examined by biopsy, but because of the submucosal and highly vascular nature of the tumor, removal of tissue from these sites may cause bleeding and increased morbidity. For this reason, visual inspection and identification may be adequate for diagnosing lung or gastrointestinal involvement.

Documenting organ involvement by other means can be difficult. KS that involves the lung cannot be diagnosed or distinguished from other causes of respiratory distress by means of chest films. An upper gastrointestinal series may demonstrate lesions in the gut, but the cause remains unknown without tissue biopsy. Because it appears that the presence or absence of organ involvement, with the exception of the lung, does not affect survival, documentation of extent of disease is not useful in treatment decisions. If treatment of a specific site is to be initiated (eg, radiation therapy to treat enlarged lymph nodes), then tissue diagnosis must be determined.[29,30]

Patients with AIDS-related KS also may show laboratory abnormalities that probably are more related to HIV infection than to KS. These include elevated erythrocyte sedimentation rate (ESR), mild anemia, and leukopenia. Depressed test results with cosyntropin stimulation, elevated serum transaminase levels, and depressed platelet count may result from KS involvement of the adrenal glands, liver, or spleen respectively.

Treatment

Medical

Before the epidemic of AIDS and HIV infection, the KS seen in the United States was primarily classic KS (ie, indolent, slow growing, and chronic), which required little or no treatment. In the transplant recipient the reversal of immunosuppression by withdrawing immunosuppressive drugs generally resolved the problem. In AIDS-related KS, treatment of the malignancy provides only temporary remission or stabilization of disease and does not improve survival rate. The main goal of treatment is to lessen the morbidity associated with the disease.

As with other malignancies, three treatment options exist: surgery, radiation therapy, and chemotherapy. Other than enabling the provider to establish a diagnosis, surgery has almost no role in the treatment of KS. Radiation therapy is highly effective and plays a role in local control of lesions and in cosmetic effect. This treatment, however, is not free of side effects and affects patients with KS in the same manner as it does others who receive radiation therapy. Irradiation of a tonsillar or oral lesion, for example, may cause severe stomatitis because of a preexisting candidal infection. Chemotherapeutic agents are useful in the treatment of AIDS-related KS when a systemic effect is necessary and the benefits of treatment outweigh the risks to the patient. Guidelines for treatment of AIDS-related KS are outlined in Table 33-3.[10,11,32]

Patients with limited disease include those with a few localized, indolent lesions. Such patients may not require any treatment so long as the lesions remain stable. Careful observation may determine the natural history of the disease, and chemotherapeutic treatment can be initiated if the lesions begin to enlarge and multiply. Experimental antiviral agents may be considered as an alternative therapy if the patient is not comfortable with observation alone. If the localized lesions involve areas of the face, the patient could be offered radiation therapy.[10,11,32,33]

Patients with aggressive or extensive disease and who have an absolute neutrophil count greater than 1000/mm^3 may receive weekly single-agent chemotherapy. Those single agents include doxorubicin, 10 to 15 mg/m^2; vinblastine, 0.1 mg/kg; or vincristine, 2 mg. A patient with rapidly progressing disease, with disease unresponsive to single-agent therapy, or with lung involvement may be offered combination chemotherapy consisting of doxorubicin, bleomycin, and vincristine, administered every other week on the basis of the patient's complete blood cell count (CBC). Overall, lung involvement is a poor prognostic sign. Patients who are unable to tolerate aggressive chemotherapy because of low CBC receive a weekly course of either bleomycin or vincristine, alternating with vinblastine every other week.[10,11,32,33]

To minimize systemic side effects, investigators also have explored the use of intralesional recombinant tumor necrosis factor and intralesional vinblastine for local control. The results of these treatment options have not yet been reported.

The response of KS lesions to chemotherapy can be dramatic. The lesions frequently will decrease in size, flatten, and lose their pigmentation; however, they do not completely go away. The area remains pigmented, both after treatment with chemotherapy or radiation therapy, or both.

Nursing

Nursing care includes assessment of the patient in terms of the health-illness continuum. Consideration is given to the psychosocial aspects of the disease, as well as to the physical status of the patient. A determination of the patient's risk group and whether KS is the patient's first diagnosis or one in a long line of indicator diseases will help the nurse establish a plan of care.

Although great strides have been made to reduce phobia concerning AIDS and homosexual men, it is important to remember that the patient may be explaining his sexual preference to his family for the first time and informing them that he has a fatal disease. Emotional support is crucial. If the patient is an intravenous drug user, philosophic dilemmas may arise concerning the patient entering drug rehabilitation programs. Realistic goals are necessary in this patient population because of both drug-seeking and manipulative behavior.

The complications associated with the use of chemotherapeutic agents in patients with KS are similar to the complications experienced by other patient populations receiving the same agents. Nausea, vomiting, anorexia, stomatitis, and alopecia all occur with the same frequency as in other populations. What appears to differ in the AIDS population is the severity of the complications. For this reason nurses should be aggressive in the assessment of potential complications, should alert the physician promptly, and should implement appropriate nursing interventions. It also should be remembered that these patients have an underlying illness that predisposes them to other opportunistic infections and malignancies.

Patients with KS, on receiving the first dose of Vinca alkaloids, may experience severe jaw pain. Although this reaction is a reported side effect of treatment with the Vinca alkaloids, patients with AIDS and KS seem to have an increased incidence. Treatment with Vinca alkaloids should be discontinued in patients with this reaction because they may cause irreversible nerve damage.[34]

NON-HODGKIN'S LYMPHOMA

Epidemiology

Beginning in 1982 physicians in San Francisco, Los Angeles, and New York noted an increased incidence of NHL in homosexual patients. Because they believed that this incidence of NHL was somehow linked to the same im-

TABLE 33-3 Guidelines for Therapy in AIDS-Related Kaposi's Sarcoma

Group	Recommendations	Regimen
Minimal KS; <25 cutaneous lesions, stable disease, no history of opportunistic infections and/or "B" symptoms	No treatment with expectant observation for disease progression	No treatment
	or Experimental immunomodulators and/or antiviral drugs	Alpha interferon, 20-50 million units qd; SQ, IM, or IV or Azidothymidine, 200 mg q4h, PO
	or Vinblastine or other single-agent therapy	Vinblastine, 4-8 mg/wk, IV or Vincristine, 2 mg/wk or qowk, IV or Doxorubicin, 15-20 mg/m²/wk, IV or Vinblastine/vincristine, doses as above; each drug used individually on an alternating weekly basis
Minimal KS; <25 cutaneous lesions, stable disease, prior history of opportunistic infections and/or "B" symptoms	Vinblastine or other single-agent therapy	Vinblastine; doses as above or Vincristine; doses as above or Doxorubicin; doses as above or Vinblastine/vincristine; doses as above
	and Experimental immunomodulators and/or antiviral drugs if used in conjunction with cytotoxic agents	Alpha interferon or azidothymidine; doses as above
Advanced KS; extensive disease, prior history of opportunistic infection and/or "B" symptoms	Etoposide or doxorubicin as single agent therapy	Etoposide, 150 mg/m² qd × 3d, then q28d, IV doxorubicin; doses as above
	or Multiple agent chemotherapy with doxorubicin, bleomycin and vinblastine	Doxorubicin, 40 mg/m² q21-28d, IV; bleomycin, 15 units/m² q15d, IV; vinblastine, 6 mg/m² q21d, IV
KS with severe neutropenia or thrombocytopenia	Vincristine with or without bleomycin	Vincristine; doses as above with or without bleomycin, doses as above
Pulmonary KS	Etoposide or doxorubicin with or without radiation therapy	Etoposide; doses as above
Localized, bulky KS lesions of oral cavity, face, legs, or lymph nodes	Radiation therapy	Local therapy, 800-3000 cGy; fractionation or slow dose administration to oral cavity or oropharynx

Sources: Volberding PA: Kaposi's sarcoma in AIDS, in Levy JA (ed): AIDS, Pathogenesis and Treatment. New York, Marcel Dekker, 1989, pp 352-354. Mitsuyasu RT: Kaposi's sarcoma in the acquired immunodeficiency syndrome, in Sande MA, Volberding PA (eds): The Medical Management of AIDS. Philadelphia, WB Saunders, 1988, pp 296-302.

munodeficiency seen in AIDS, they began to prospectively collect blood for evaluation of the immune system. In fact, the immune deficiencies found in these patients with NHL were similar to those found in other patients with AIDS. Inasmuch as cancer in and of itself is immunosuppressive, this finding alone did not establish a diagnosis of AIDS. It did, however, initiate further investigation. When the HIV antibody test became available, these patients with NHL were found to be seropositive. Thus the link to HIV disease was found, and a new category of malignancy was added to the case definition of AIDS. NHL in a person who also is seropositive for HIV antibody or has positive culture results is considered to affirm a diagnosis of AIDS.[7,35-37]

It is difficult to determine the impact of HIV-related NHL on cancer statistics. Approximately 30,000 cases of NHL will be diagnosed in 1989[38]; however, the percentage of those cases that are HIV-related cannot be determined because statistics concerning tumors do not account for HIV status. Because the reporting of AIDS cases to the Centers for Disease Control (CDC) now is required by law, the incidence of HIV-related NHL eventually may become known. It has been estimated that NHL has been diagnosed in 4% to 10% of patients with AIDS. However, HIV antibody status is not determined in all patients with NHL; thus some underreporting may occur.

Etiology

The connection between cancers and virus has not been fully established; however, there are some malignancies in which a causative viral agent has been isolated. One such association exists between the malignancy known as African lymphoma, or Burkitt's lymphoma, which is a type of high-grade NHL, and Epstein-Barr virus (EBV). In 1962 Dr. Dennis Burkitt described a malignant lymphoma in African children that was typically extranodal in origin, with an affinity for facial bones. There appeared to be an increased incidence of this malignancy in regions of high temperature and rainfall. This suggested to Burkitt some type of insect vector as a method of infection (or transmission). Since then, serologic studies and tissue cultures have established a constant association with the DNA-containing herpes virus known as EBV and the development of Burkitt's lymphoma.[37] Although the significance of the geographic distribution remains unclear, it has been hypothesized that malaria or some other insect-borne infection results in a reticuloendothelial hyperplasia that may be a necessary co-factor for the oncogenic virus in the development of the malignancy. EBV also has been implicated as the causative agent in nasopharyngeal carcinoma and in the development of NHL in transplant recipients; it also has been suggested as an important etiologic agent in AIDS-NHL.[37]

Of interest is that similar research involving patients with AIDS could not causally link EBV to HIV-related NHL. Although the EBV genome has been isolated in the DNA of HIV-positive patients with NHL, a direct relationship is not apparent.[38] The role of EBV in the development of NHL remains unclear; however, even though the viral link cannot be causally established, it is strongly suspected. Ziegler[39] hypothesized that once infection with HIV occurs, EBV may trigger lymphocyte proliferation that remains unchecked as a result of immune dysfunction caused by HIV. This proliferation, in turn, may allow the expression of two oncogenes, resulting in a polyclonal or monoclonal NHL.[39]

It is now known that therapeutic immunosuppression increases the risk of lymphoma development. For example, the risk for transplant recipients has been estimated to be between 35 and 200 times greater than that for the general population.[40]

Pathophysiology

AIDS-associated NHLs are predominantly B-cell malignancies, typically intermediate to high grade. However, there have been a few isolated reports of lymphomas that are T cell in origin in men who show HIV seropositivity. The significance of these few cases is unclear inasmuch as the numbers are small and simply may represent the normal distribution of T-cell lymphoma in the general population. Only through an increase in the frequency of this type of lymphoma can significance be determined. Presently, it remains an interesting phenomenon.[41,42] Most cases of AIDS-NHL also have been associated with a previous history of persistent generalized lymphadenopathy. Benign follicular hyperplasia is a typical histologic finding upon biopsy, which suggests that this lymphoma may arise from a polyclonal B-cell activation. This polyclonal B-cell lymphoproliferation appears to be a complex result of EBV and HIV infection.[38,43-46] Current research is under way on the role of human T lymphotropic virus type I as a co-infecting retrovirus in the development of lymphomas in AIDS.[47]

If the process of AIDS-associated NHL begins in a lymph node, the growing tumor causes structural damage, including effacement of the normal node architecture, replacement of normal cellularity by uniform and/or grossly abnormal cells, and the random extension of cellular proliferations beyond the original structural confines of the node. Development of lymphoma, however, is not limited to lymph nodes or the spleen; all organs have lymphocytes within their boundaries that are capable of transforming and forming tumors.

Clinical Manifestations

In the general population the earliest sign of NHL unrelated to AIDS is usually a painless, enlarged, discrete lymph node located in the neck. Although most patients have no symptoms, approximately 20% may experience "B" symptoms, including fever, night sweats, and weight loss.[38] Patients who do not have AIDS frequently have a history of intermittent lymphadenopathy that has been present for several months. Although axillary or inguinal lymph nodes may be the first to enlarge, this enlargement is not common. Frequently, there is involvement of Waldeyer's ring, epitrochlear nodes, the testes, and the gastrointestinal tract. The liver and bone marrow may be involved. There is a higher incidence of CNS involvement in patients with NHL unrelated to AIDS who have bone marrow involvement. The disease will be localized in fewer than 10% of patients who do not have AIDS.[38] Because of the diffuse presentation of lymphoma, non-AIDS NHL should be included in the differential diagnosis of patients with superior vena cava syndrome, acute spinal cord compression, solitary thyroid nodules, isolated tumor nodules of the skin, bone tumors, unexplained anemias, testicular masses, or solitary brain lesions.

In contrast to the presentation just described, patients with HIV-related NHL have very advanced disease, which frequently involves extranodal sites. In one study[48] of 90 cases of AIDS-NHL, 19% were classified as intermediate-grade diffuse large cell, 28% as high-grade, large-cell immunoblastic, and 36% as high-grade, small, noncleaved lymphomas. Extranodal sites most commonly involved include the CNS, bone marrow, bowel, and anorectum; less commonly involved is the myocardium. In addition, these extranodal sites may be the only site of disease; that is, peripheral lymphadenopathy may be absent. If nodal sites are involved, there does not appear to be any predisposition to specific nodes.[45,46,48] In addition, these patients also may have underlying signs and symptoms of HIV infection, AIDS-related complex, or AIDS, including wasting, anorexia, nausea, vomiting, and fever, which confounds the work-up and makes diagnosis difficult.

Assessment

The diagnosis and classification of lymphoma can be made only by means of a biopsy specimen that is examined by a pathologist. Fine-needle aspirations may be helpful in differentiating a benign versus a malignant process, but, because of insufficient tissue yield, they are not useful in classifying the lymphoma. To fully assess HIV-related NHL, the patient's status must be staged and graded. Staging—that is, determining the extent of disease involvement—is accomplished by means of the Ann Arbor staging classification system (see Chapter 44). The staging work-up includes a careful history, which notes the presence or absence of "B" symptoms, and a complete physical examination with special attention to Waldeyer's ring, the liver, and the spleen. Laboratory tests include CBC, differential cell and platelet count, sedimentation rate, serum chemistries, and liver function tests. These laboratory tests are not specific to lymphoma; they can indicate the overall wellness of the patient and are helpful in screening for hypercalcemia, hyperphosphatemia, and hyperuricemia. A chest film and computed tomography (CT) scans of the chest, abdomen, and pelvis also are indicated. These usually are not indicated for patients with NHL in the general population, but because of the extensive extranodal involvement characteristic of HIV-related NHL, they are extremely important. A bilateral bone marrow biopsy and aspiration, as well as a lumbar puncture, should be performed. Once all the tests are complete, the patient is assigned a staging number that can help predict responsiveness to treatment.

If AIDS has not been previously diagnosed, then an HIV antibody test is indicated. It is important to note that not all swollen lymph nodes are malignant; benign reactive lymphadenopathy is a common finding in this HIV-seropositive population and is postulated to be an adaptive physiologic response to HIV insult. Abdominal masses or lymph nodes in a person who is HIV seropositive could be related to *Mycobacterium avium–intracellulare* infection; thus it is essential to obtain a biopsy specimen and compare it with normal tissue before a diagnosis is made. It is unusual for patients with HIV-related NHL to present at a stage lower than stage III.[49-51]

Treatment

Medical

Once the disease is staged and graded, treatment for NHL may begin. Treatment options can be determined on the basis of method (surgery, radiation therapy, and chemotherapy), as well as by grade of tumor. Low-grade tumors are uncommon in the population infected with HIV; in the general population the tumors are indolent and slow growing, requiring no treatment until they impinge on a vital structure or cause symptoms. At that time radiation therapy to the affected site usually is sufficient to treat the tumor, although chemotherapy may be used as well. Intermediate-grade tumors are more common in the population infected with HIV and may account for as much as 50% of HIV-related NHL. This grade of tumor in the general population can be treated with either chemotherapy or radiation therapy, depending on the stage at presentation.

The remaining HIV-related NHL occurs as high-grade, advanced stage disease. DiCarlo et al[49] found that 41% of patients with HIV-related NHL had high-grade disease. Ahmed et al[50] found that all patients with HIV-related NHL in their review had either intermediate or high-grade disease.

The treatment of choice for advanced intermediate/high-grade lymphoma is combination chemotherapy. The single most active and effective agent used in the treatment of NHL is cyclophosphamide. Other drugs that are also active and effective include doxorubicin, vincristine, vinblastine, methotrexate, prednisone, and cytosine arabinoside. Generally, these agents are used in some combination. The most common regimens include M-BACOD (methotrexate, bleomycin, doxorubicin cyclophosphamide, vincristine, dexamethasone), MACOP-B (methotrexate, doxorubicin, cyclophosphamide, vincristine, prednisone, bleomycin), and CHOP (cyclophosphamide, doxorubicin, vincristine, prednisone) (see Chapter 44 for a description of these regimens). Initial responses to chemotherapy usually are dramatic, with shrinkage of the tumor noted within 24 hours. The response, however, is not usually long-lived. Typically, patients remain disease-free while receiving chemotherapy, and relapse occurs within 4 to 6 weeks after the discontinuation of chemotherapy. Once chemotherapy is reinstituted, response rates are somewhat diminished. The neutropenia that results from treatment is severe (attributed to poor bone marrow reserve as a result of either HIV or *M. avium intracellulare*) and sometimes precipitates an opportunistic infection. It is important to remember that these patients have an underlying immune disorder and that whatever the outcome, they still have HIV infection and AIDS.

Radiation therapy may be useful for patients with limited bulky disease, for those who are unable to tolerate chemotherapy either because of poor health or low blood counts, for local control, or in some instances, for CNS prophylaxis. Surgery plays no role in the treatment of NHL other than to obtain a biopsy specimen.

Nursing

Nursing care of patients with AIDS-related NHL is no different from the care of those patients in the general population with non-AIDS-related NHL, with the exception of the emotional (psychosocial) aspect.

It should be noted that patients with big, bulky, high-grade disease are at high risk for tumor lysis syndrome. The exact numbers of patients with tumor lysis syndrome are unknown; some clinicians estimate that it may occur in as many as 10% of patients, whether or not their NHL is related to HIV. Anecdotally, it appears that patients with HIV-related NHL have a high incidence of this phenomena. Tumor lysis syndrome generally occurs when the patient is initially treated. It is the result of the lysing of rapidly growing tumor cells that spill their contents into the general circulation, causing a metabolic imbalance. This results in hypocalcemia, hyperkalemia, hyperphosphatemia, and hyperuricemia. If left uncorrected, this condition may result in renal failure and death. The treatment of choice is prevention. Therefore any patient suspected of being at high risk for tumor lysis should receive vigorous hydration (300 to 500 mL/hr) and may receive sodium bicarbonate to alkalinize the urine and prevent hyperuricemia nephropathy. In addition, allopurinol, a drug that blocks the conversion of metabolic wastes to uric acid, should be administered either intravenously or orally. The patient's urine output needs to be monitored every hour, and the physician should be alerted to any sign of urinary insufficiency. Serum chemistry levels are monitored every 6 hours in patients who are at high risk for tumor lysis, and in some cases the patient may need to be transferred to the intensive care unit. Dialysis may be necessary if the patient's electrolyte levels continue to rise and renal function deteriorates. Generally, there is less morbidity if the patient receives dialysis before renal failure occurs.

Although tumor lysis occurs in most patients 48 to 72 hours after the initiation of chemotherapy, some patients with HIV-related NHL may have this phenomenon sooner, usually within 24 hours.[51] However, all patients with HIV-related NHL should be observed for a full 72-hour period for any sign of tumor lysis syndrome. These signs and symptoms include a decreased urine output and increased lethargy. If the patient is being monitored by telemetry, arrhythmias may be noted.

It also should be noted that some patients with HIV-related NHL have some form of tumor lysis before they receive treatment. This may be due to the tumor cells replicating and dying at an extraordinary rate, spilling their cellular contents into the general circulation.[52] These patients also may have tumors that produce lactic acid, causing metabolic acidosis before treatment.[52]

The complications in this group are the same as those experienced by all patients with NHL: neutropenia-related sepsis, thrombocytopenia, and untreated tumor lysis syndrome.

PRIMARY CENTRAL NERVOUS SYSTEM LYMPHOMA

Epidemiology

Primary CNS lymphoma is a rare malignancy, which accounts for 0.3% to 2% of all newly diagnosed lymphomas.[53] Although it can affect immunocompetent hosts, most of those diagnosed with primary CNS lymphoma are immunocompromised. Therefore those with primary immunodeficiency, acquired immunodeficiency, and iatrogenic immunologic abnormalities (organ transplant recipients) are at increased risk of the development of primary CNS lymphoma.[54-56] In the case of organ transplant recipients, primary lymphoma involving the brain accounts for 50% of lymphomas that occur in this population; it is common enough to predict its occurrence 28 months after transplantation.[57] It is not surprising then that primary CNS lymphoma develops in those infected with HIV who have subsequent immune dysfunction. Before the AIDS epidemic, primary CNS lymphomas were noted in the 50- to 70-year-old age-group, with men at increased risk. Since the advent of AIDS the peak incidence has dropped to the 40- to 50-year-old age range.[58] In the general population the average time from onset of symptoms to disease is 1 to 2 months. Unfortunately, patients with AIDS are also at risk for the development of infectious CNS disease. Cryptococcosis and toxoplasmosis are AIDS-related opportunistic infections of the CNS. The differential evaluation of these diseases can prolong and complicate the diagnostic process; yet, in the setting of HIV infection, a complete evaluation of all possible pathologic causes is required.

The early medical literature reflects the confusion encountered in attempting to identify the cell of origin for primary CNS lymphoma. Perithelial sarcoma, reticulum cell sarcoma, and microglioma were a few of the names used to classify primary lymphoma involving the brain. It is now accepted that the cell of origin is the same as that causing NHL elsewhere in the body. The transformed cell, which multiplies in an area that does not allow expansion, is the cause of most presenting symptoms. In approximately 30% of all cases, this neoplasm will be multicentric, arising in several different areas of the brain at the same time.[54] This presentation is similar to that described in either spontaneously occurring tumors or in those tumors arising in immunodeficient states.

Clinical Manifestations

Two retrospective reviews[58,59] of a total of 26 patients revealed that the most frequently observed symptoms of HIV-associated CNS lymphomas included confusion, lethargy, and memory loss (12/26) and alterations in personality and behavior (5/26). Of the 26 patients, hemiparesis or aphasia was seen in 7, three patients had seizures, two had cranial nerve palsy, one had headache as the only symptom, one had headache associated with a lack of coordination, and one had no symptoms. Further review by So et al[58] revealed that although only three patients had seizures initially, seizures later developed in four additional patients. More than half the patients also reported more specific symptoms that consisted of focal seizures and progression of focal neurologic symptoms over days or weeks. In the review by Gill et al,[59] all six patients studied had disease within the cranium; four had disease in the frontoparietal region, and two had involvement of the pons cerebellum.

These clinical manifestations are typical of spontaneous primary CNS lymphoma. They also are typical symptoms caused by other mass lesions in the CNS. This similarity in symptomatology often makes it difficult to distinguish between CNS lymphoma and vascular and infectious disorders. The most common explanation for a mass lesion in the CNS is toxoplasmosis, which occurs in 10% of patients with AIDS.[60] Because of the morbidity associated with brain biopsy, primary CNS lymphoma is usually a diagnosis of exclusion. That is, the patient with CNS symptoms and a demonstrated brain mass will generally be treated empirically for toxoplasmosis for approximately 2 weeks. If the lesion fails to respond to treatment, the diagnosis of primary CNS lymphoma will then be considered. At this point, a brain biopsy could yield a definitive diagnosis; however, due to the invasiveness of the procedure for the patient in obtaining a biopsy and to the dismal response of primary CNS lymphoma to treatment, a presumptive diagnosis may be established.

In most patients, the radiographic findings from the CT and magnetic resonance imaging (MRI) examinations will reveal single or multiple discrete lesions. Prior to the use of a contrast medium on CT scanning, low-density lesions will appear, and a shift of midline structures also may be apparent. After the administration of contrast material, the lesion will characteristically appear enhanced. Reports differ on the type of enhancement; both uniform and patchy nodular enhancement with varying degrees of surrounding edema have been reported.[58,59] Primary CNS lymphoma usually appears as single or multiple discrete lesions and exhibits a characteristic pre- and postconstrast appearance. Some primary CNS lymphoma patients, however, have demonstrated ring-enhancing lesions on CT scan that are frequently indistinguishable from lesions seen in patients with cerebral toxoplasmosis. It is important to remember that a diagnosis of lymphoma cannot be determined by scans alone. In addition, MRI does not contribute to the differential diagnosis, although MRI may be useful in revealing lesions undetectable by the CT scan and may provide alternate biopsy sites.[58,59]

Examination of cerebral spinal fluid (CSF) may reveal some abnormalities; however, the results are nonspecific and useful only in that they indicate some abnormality in the CNS. Tests ordered on CSF include toxoplasmosis titers, the Veneral Disease Research Laboratory (VDRL) test, and cytologic examination. Cytologic findings will be positive in approximately 50% of patients who have CNS lymphoma.[61] This result, however, tends to depend on the volume of CSF obtained. Toxoplasmosis titers and VDRL results can help rule out toxoplasmosis and syphilis as causes for behavioral changes and altered mental status.

Treatment

Medical

It appears that whether or not patients with AIDS-associated CNS lymphoma are treated, the outcome remains the same. In a review by So et al[58] they noted that in one study six patients experienced a highly aggressive course and died within 2 weeks. In another, seven of 20 patients underwent treatment with radiation therapy.[58] Doses ranged from 3000 to 6000 cGy. Of the four patients who had CT scans after radiation therapy, three showed dramatic improvement. However, only two of seven patients were alive at 2 months. Most patients die of the concomitant opportunistic infections frequently experienced in AIDS. In a review by Gill et al[59] four patients were treated with subtotal resection of the tumor, followed by whole brain radiation and systemic chemotherapy. One patient remained alive at 28 months after diagnosis. It should be noted that the diagnosis of this particular patient was based on a pathologic finding of low-grade lymphoma. The other patients survived less than 2 months. An average survival time of 1.7 to 2.7 months has been reported.[59]

Nursing

Nursing responsibility in the care of these patients includes a thorough assessment, paying particular attention to any focal findings, motor incoordination, and cognitive deficits. Safety in the environment must be considered in both the acute care setting and the home. Provisions for activities of daily living also must be anticipated and a long-term plan developed. For example, if the patient cannot be maintained at home, plans should be made for transfer to a skilled nursing care facility. Providing emotional support to the patient and family is essential, whether this be through referrals to counselors or by the nurse. Ethical issues may be encountered when treatment is discussed. A determination should be made as to whether the patient is mentally competent to make decisions; if not, it should be determined who is the next of kin or whether someone has been authorized power of attorney. If the patient is deemed incompetent, has no next of kin, or has not transferred power of attorney, then a legal guardian will need to be appointed by a court of law to make decisions for that patient.

Complications

The most frequent complication in the treatment of AIDS-associated CNS lymphoma is the patient's mental deterioration to the point of becoming moribund and comatose. The reason for this downhill course associated with treatment is unclear. Unfortunately, there appears to be no preventive intervention. It may be a function of general debilitation caused by HIV, by HIV involvement of the brain, by the treatment itself, a combination of these, or another factor that has yet to be explored. Current research is not encouraging. Combining chemotherapy and radiation therapy in an attempt to control or eliminate the primary CNS lymphoma currently is being explored but is confounded by the low numbers of enrollable patients and their rapid deterioration. As a result the hope is for an effective antiviral agent that will control the HIV infection and for regeneration of the immune system through the use of immunomodulators.

OTHER MALIGNANCIES AND HUMAN IMMUNODEFICIENCY VIRUS

Kaposi's sarcoma, non-Hodgkin's lymphoma, and primary CNS lymphoma account for approximately 95% of all cancers diagnosed in patients with AIDS, but they are not the only malignancies seen in persons who are seropositive for HIV antibody.[62] Hodgkin's disease, squamous cell cancers of the rectum, nasopharyngeal cancers, malignant melanomas, and multiple myelomas have all been reported in patients infected with HIV. The difference between the indicator malignancies (KS, NHL, and primary CNS lymphoma) and other malignancies in individuals with HIV is the frequency with which they occur. There is a significantly greater incidence of the indicator malignancies in those who are seropositive for HIV. The same is not true for the other malignancies described in AIDS patients. Although these cancers may be seen in AIDS patients, no epidemiologic link or direct causal relationship has been established. HIV positivity does not prevent the development of any other cancer at the same rate seen in those who are seronegative. It is useful to know, however, the HIV status of a patient with a malignancy because response to therapy is typically poor in the person with HIV infection. It is reasonable to expect an increasing incidence of virally linked malignancies (eg, hepatomas and cervical cancer) as the incidence of AIDS and HIV infection continues to rise.[63]

CONCLUSION

The care of patients with a malignant disease who also are infected with HIV presents a demanding challenge for nurses. In addition to the already difficult task of managing the care of a patient receiving chemotherapy, infection with an immunosuppressive virus must be taken into account. The patient also may be receiving antiviral agents or immunomodulators, or both. Sorting out the side effects, as well as providing a comprehensive plan of care for these patients, presents an opportunity to participate in the nursing challenge of the 1990s.

REFERENCES

1. Longo DL, Seis RG, Lane HC, et al: Malignancies in the AIDS patient: Natural history, treatment strategies, and preliminary results. Ann NY Acad Sci 437:421-430, 1984.
2. Steis R, Broder S: AIDS: A general overview, in DeVita V, Hellman S, Rosenberg S (eds): AIDS Etiology, Diagnosis, Treatment and Prevention. Philadelphia, JB Lippincott, 1985, pp 299-338.
3. Centers for Disease Control: Kaposi's sarcoma and *Pneumocystis* pneumonia among homosexual men—New York City and California. MMWR 30:305-308, 1981.
4. Centers for Disease Control: Follow-up on Kaposi's sarcoma and *Pneumocystis* pneumonia. MMWR 30:409-410, 1981.
5. Brooks JJ: Kaposi's sarcoma: A reversible hyperplasia. Lancet 2:1309-1311, 1986.
6. Centers for Disease Control: Update on acquired immune deficiency syndrome (AIDS)—United States. MMWR 31:507-514, 1982.
7. Centers for Disease Control: Revision of the CDC surveillance case definition for acquired immunodeficiency syndrome. MMWR 35:3S-15S, 1987.
8. Rosenberg S, Suit H, Baker L, et al: Sarcomas of the soft tissue and bone, in DeVita V, Hellman S, Rosenberg S (eds): Cancer Principles and Practice of Oncology. Philadelphia, JB Lippincott, 1982, pp 1036-1093.
9. Krigel R, Friedman-Kien A: Kaposi's sarcoma in AIDS, in DeVita V, Hellman S, Rosenberg S (eds): AIDS Etiology, Diagnosis, Treatment and Prevention. Philadelphia, JB Lippincott, 1985, pp 185-212.
10. Volberding P: Kaposi's sarcoma in AIDS, in Levy J (ed): AIDS, Pathogenesis and Treatment. New York, Marcel Dekker, 1989, p 349.
11. Mitsuyasu RT: Kaposi's sarcoma in the acquired immunodeficiency syndrome. Infect Dis Clin North Am 2:511-523, 1988.
12. Haverdos HW, Pinsky PF, Drotman DP, et al: Disease manifestation and homosexual men with acquired immunodeficiency syndrome: A possible role of nitrites in Kaposi's sarcoma. Sex Transm Dis 23:203-208, 1985.
13. Groopman J, Broder S: Cancer in AIDS and other immunodeficiency states, in DeVita V, Hellman S, Rosenberg S (eds): Cancer Principles and Practice of Oncology. Philadelphia, JB Lippincott, 1989, pp 1953-1970.
14. Garrett T, Lange M, Ashford A, et al: Kaposi's sarcoma in heterosexual intravenous drug users. Cancer 55:1146-1158, 1985.
15. Nissenblatt M: Cancers and AIDS, in Gong V (ed): Understanding AIDS. New Brunswick, NJ, Rutgers University Press, 1985, pp 65-74.
16. Urmacher C, Myskowski P, Ochoa M, et al: Outbreak of KS with CMV infection in young homosexual men. Am J Med 74:569-575, 1982.
17. Drew L, Mintz L, Miner R: Prevalence of cytomegalovirus in homosexual men. J Infect Dis 143:188-192, 1981.
18. McNutt N: Kaposi's sarcoma, in Thiers B, Dobson R (eds): Pathogenesis of Skin Disease. New York, Churchill Livingstone, 1986, pp 459-474.
19. Caro W, Bronstein B: Tumors of the skin, in Moschella S, Hurley H (eds): Dermatology, vol 2 (ed 2). Philadelphia, WB Saunders, 1985, pp 1639-1671.
20. MacKie R: Tumors of the skin, in Rook A, Ebling F, Wilkinson E, et al (eds): Textbook of Dermatology, vol 3. London, Blackwell Scientific Publications, 1986, pp 2375-2478.
21. Meduri G, Stover D, Lee M, et al: Pulmonary Kaposi's sarcoma in the acquired immune deficiency syndrome: Clinical, radiographic and pathologic manifestations. Am J Med 81:11-18, 1986.
22. Laine L, Plitoske E, Pardash G: Protein-losing enteropathy in acquired immunodeficiency syndrome due to intestinal Kaposi's sarcoma. Arch Intern Med 147:1174-1175, 1988.
23. Kaplan L, Hopewell P, Jaffe H, et al: Kaposi's sarcoma involving the lung in patients with acquired immunodeficiency syndrome. J AIDS 1:25-31, 1988.
24. Brown R, Huberman R, Vanley G: Pulmonary features of KS. Am J Radiol 139:659-660, 1986.
25. Laubenstein L: Staging and treatment of Kaposi's sarcoma in patients with AIDS, in Friedman-Kien A, Laubenstein L

(eds): AIDS: The Epidemic of Kaposi's Sarcoma and Opportunistic Infections. New York, Masson, 1984, pp 51-56.
26. Krigel R, Laubenstein L, Muggia F: Kaposi's sarcoma: A new staging classification. Cancer Treat Rep 67:531-534, 1983.
27. Krigel R: Prognostic factors in Kaposi's sarcoma, in Friedman-Kien A, Laubenstein L (eds): AIDS: The Epidemic of Kaposi's Sarcoma and Opportunistic Infections. New York, Masson, 1984, pp 69-72.
28. Taylor J, Afrasia R, Fahey J, et al: Prognostically significant classification of immune changes in AIDS with Kaposi's sarcoma. Blood 76:666-671, 1986.
29. Afrasiabi A, Mitsuyasu R, Nishanian R, et al: Characteristics of a distinct subgroup of high-risk persons with KS and good prognosis who present with normal T4 cell number and T4:T8 ratio and negative HTLV/LAV serologic test results. Am J Med 81:969-973, 1986.
30. Gnepp D, Chandler W, Hyams V: Primary Kaposi's sarcoma of the head and neck. Ann Intern Med 100:107-114, 1984.
31. Saafai B, Sarngadharan M, Koziner B, et al: Spectrum of KS in the epidemic of AIDS. Cancer Res 45:6465-6485, 1985 (suppl 9).
32. Mitsuyasu R: Kaposi's sarcoma in the acquired immunodeficiency syndrome, in Sande M, Volberding P (eds): The Medical Management of AIDS. Philadelphia, WB Saunders, 1988, pp 296-302.
33. Safai B: Kaposi's sarcoma and other neoplasms in acquired immunodeficiency syndrome, in Gallin J, Fauci A (eds): Advances in Host Defense Mechanisms, vol 5, Acquired Immunodeficiency Syndrome (AIDS). New York, Raven Press, 1985, pp 59-73.
34. Luce J, MD: Personal communication, Aug 3, 1989.
35. Kaplan L, Wofsy C, Volberding PA: Treatment of patients with acquired immunodeficiency syndrome and associated manifestations. JAMA 257:1367-1373, 1987.
36. Diffuse, undifferentiated non-Hodgkin's lymphoma among homosexual males—United States. MMWR 31:277-279, 1982.
37. Aisenberg A: Malignant lymphoma. N Engl J Med 288:883-890, 1973.
38. DeVita V, Jaffe E, Mauch P, et al: Lymphocytic lymphomas, in DeVita V, Hellman S, Rosenberg S (eds): Cancer Principles and Practice of Oncology. Philadelphia, JB Lippincott, 1989, pp 1953-1970.
39. Ziegler J: AIDS and cancer. Ann Inst Pasteur Immunol 138:253-260, 1987.
40. Kaplan L: AIDS-associated lymphomas, in Sande M, Volberding P (eds): The Medical Management of AIDS. Philadelphia, WB Saunders, 1988, pp 307-315.
41. Nasr S, Brynes R, Garrison C, et al: Peripheral T-cell lymphoma in a patient with acquired immune deficiency disease. Cancer 61:947-951, 1988.
42. Presant C, et al: Human immunodeficiency virus associated with T-cell lymphoblastic lymphoma in AIDS. Cancer 60:1459-1461, 1987.
43. Yarchoan R, Redfield R, Broder S: Mechanisms of B-cell activation in patients with acquired immunodeficiency syndrome. J Clin Invest 78:439-447, 1986.
44. Ziegler J: Lymphomas and other neoplasms associated with AIDS, in Levy J (ed): AIDS, Pathogenesis and Treatment. New York, Marcel Dekker, 1989, pp 359-370.
45. Knowles D, Chamulak G, Subar M, et al: Lymphoid neoplasia associated with the acquired immunodeficiency syndrome (AIDS). The New York University Medical Center experience with 105 patients (1981-1986). Ann Intern Med 108:744-753, 1988.
46. Italian cooperative group for AIDS-related tumors, 1988. Malignant lymphomas in patients with or at risk for AIDS in Italy. JNCI 80:855-860, 1988.
47. McGrath M, MD: Personal communication, Aug 3, 1989.
48. Zeigler J, Beckstead J, Volberding P, et al: Non-Hodgkin's lymphoma in 90 homosexual men—relation to generalized lymphadenopathy and the acquired immunodeficiency syndrome. N Engl J Med 311:565-570, 1984.
49. DiCarlo E, Amberson J, Metroda C, et al: Malignant lymphomas and the acquired immunodeficiency syndrome. Arch Pathol Lab Med 110:1012-1016, 1986.
50. Ahmed S, Wormser G, Stahl R, et al: Malignant lymphomas in a population at risk for acquired immune deficiency syndrome. Cancer 60:719-723, 1987.
51. Kaplan L, MD: Personal communication, Aug 3, 1989.
52. Warrell R Jr, Bockman R: Oncologic emergencies, in DeVita V, Hellman S, Rosenberg S (eds): Cancer Principles and Practice of Oncology. Philadelphia, JB Lippincott, 1989, pp 1996-1997.
53. Henry J, Heffner R, Dillard S, et al: Primary malignant lymphomas of the central nervous system. Cancer 34:1293-1302, 1974.
54. Frizzera G, Rosai J, Dehner L, et al: Lymphoreticular disorders in primary immunodeficiency: New findings based on an up to date histologic classification of 35 cases. Cancer 46:692-699, 1980.
55. Good A, Russo R, Schnitzer B, et al: Intercranial histiocytic lymphoma with rheumatoid arthritis. J Rheumatol 5:75-78, 1978.
56. Frizzera G, Hanto D, Gaji-Peczalska K, et al: Polymorphic diffuse B-cell hyperplasia and lymphomas in renal transplant recipients. Cancer Res 41:4262-4279, 1981.
57. Levin V, Sheline G, Gutin P: Neoplasms of the central nervous system, in DeVita V, Hellman S, Rosenberg S (eds): Cancer Practice and Principles of Oncology. Philadelphia, JB Lippincott, 1989, pp 1557-1611.
58. So Y, Beckstead J, Davis R: Primary central nervous system lymphoma in acquired immunodeficiency syndrome: A clinical and pathological study. Ann Neurol 20:566-572, 1986.
59. Gill P, Levine A, Meyer P, et al: Primary central nervous system lymphoma in homosexual men. Am J Med 78:742-748, 1985.
60. Mills J: *Pneumocystis carinii* and *Toxoplasmosis gondii* infections in patients with AIDS. Rev Infect Dis 8:1001-1011, 1986.
61. Casciato D, Lowitz B: Neuromuscular complication, in Casciato D, Lowitz B (eds): Manual of Clinical Oncology, Boston, Little, Brown & Co, 1988, pp 468-483.
62. Levine A: Non-Hodgkin's lymphomas and other malignancies in the acquired immune deficiency syndrome. Semin Oncol 14:34-39, 1987 (suppl 3).
63. Friedman S: Gastrointestinal and hepatobiliary neoplasms in AIDS. Gastroenterol Clin North Am 17:465-486, 1988.

Chapter 34

Bone Cancer

Patricia A. Piasecki, RN, MS

INTRODUCTION

Bone malignancies are so uncommon that they are not listed among the five leading cancer sites. Diagnosis and treatment of these lesions are complex. Teamwork is essential. Key members of the health care team include the patient and family, the orthopedic surgeon, medical oncologist, roentgenologist, pathologist, radiation oncologist, thoracic surgeon, physical therapist, nurse, prosthetist, and social worker. Increased knowledge about bone cancer and a multidisciplinary approach to treatment have improved the results of bone tumor treatment in recent years.

EPIDEMIOLOGY

The incidence of primary malignant bone tumors is remarkably low. These tumors comprise only 0.2% of all malignant tumors diagnosed in the United States.[1] The American Cancer Society estimated in 1989 that 2100 new cases of bone cancer will be discovered annually. Incidence is slightly higher for men and white persons. The estimated number of deaths that occurred in 1989 from bone cancer is 1300, which represents a decrease over prior years.[2] Mortality statistics reveal that patterns of occurrence are bimodal, with peaks at the ages of 15 to 19 years and after 65 years.

ETIOLOGY

At present relatively little is known regarding the cause of primary bone tumors. Consequently, prevention and detection of bone cancer remain difficult because few risk factors have been identified. Cancer therapy in the form of high-dose irradiation has been linked to the development of bone cancer. Unlike other types of cancer, however, there is no increase in the incidence of bone neoplasms among survivors of the atomic bomb in Japan.[3] There is no evidence to demonstrate that other environmental factors are involved in the cause of human bone cancer.

Evidence of a familial tendency in bone cancer has been demonstrated by reports of siblings with osteosarcoma, Ewing's sarcoma, and chondrosarcoma. Bone sarcomas may be only part of a complex of different tumors that cluster in families.[4] These findings suggest that common susceptibility may be the critical factor in predisposition to diverse forms of cancer.

Malignant bone neoplasms have been associated with a number of preexisting bone conditions. Paget's disease primarily predisposes individuals to osteosarcoma but occasionally to fibrosarcoma, chondrosarcoma, and giant cell tumor. The incidence of sarcomas in patients with symptoms of Paget's disease is 0.8%.[5] It has been proposed that the mechanisms responsible for the relationship are prolonged growth or overstimulated metabolism, or both. These mechanisms also are implicated in the occurrence of bone tumors associated with hyperparathyroidism, chronic osteomyelitis, old bone infarct, and fracture callus.

Other factors such as syndromes of skeletal maldevelopment and skeletal growth patterns have been implicated in the etiology of bone cancer. These factors are discussed here in conjunction with the specific bone tumor type to which they apply.

PATHOPHYSIOLOGY

Primary malignant bone tumors are derived from the cells that have a common ancestry, namely the mesoderm. One group of bone tumors is produced by cells characterized by their ability to produce collagen. This group includes the osteogenic tumors arising from osteoblasts, the chondrogenic tumors arising from chondroblasts, and the fibrogenic tumors arising from fibroblasts. Another group of bone tumors originates in the bone marrow reticulum and includes round cell tumors such as Ewing's sarcoma and reticulum cell sarcoma. The third group of primary malignant bone tumors arises in blood vessels of the bone and includes the angiosarcomas.

Little can be said regarding the pathophysiology of bone tumors in general because of the individualized behavior demonstrated by the different types of tumors. Nearly every bone in the skeleton may be affected; however, individual tumors have a predilection for certain bones. Likewise, the segment of the bone involved usually varies according to the type of tumor. In addition, there are differences in cellular characteristics and in the progression of disease. In general, bone tumors tend to involve contiguous tissue and muscle aggressively and metastasize early to the lungs via the hematogenous route.

ASSESSMENT

Patient History

The evaluation of pain assumes a major focus in the patient interview. To begin obtaining information regarding the location, onset, and duration of the pain assists in the differential diagnosis. It is important to rule out a traumatic injury to the area, which could result in a condition such as hematoma or myositis ossificans that can resemble tumors. More commonly an injury merely brings a preexisting neoplasm to the attention of the individual. Bone tumor pain often has a gradual onset and may be present for a few months before the person seeks medical advice. The pain often is local but may be radiating if the tumor has spread and involves nerves. An abrupt onset of pain does not necessarily rule out the presence of bone tumor because a pathologic fracture may be the presenting symptom.

The character of the pain is investigated because it helps to differentiate the site of origin and extent of tumor growth. Bone pain usually is described as dull, deep, and having a quality of boring into the bone. Fracture pain usually is described as sharp. Muscle pain usually is described as crampy, and joint pain may be described with any number of adjectives because of the variety of tissues involved.

The evaluation of pain also includes a description of frequency and course. Pain resulting from a bone tumor often is constant and worse at night. The severity of pain steadily increases as the tumor enlarges. Finally, the relationship of pain characteristics to rest and activity also must be determined.

Other presenting symptoms such as a history of swelling need to be assessed during the patient interview. Attention is given to symptoms suggestive of pulmonary metastasis. A history of hemoptysis, chest pain, cough, fever, weight loss, malaise, exposure to toxic substances, radiation, or travel out of the country is noted.

To determine potential problems and needs a psychosocial assessment should be incorporated into the initial interview. The individual may have a life-threatening tumor that may require mutilating surgery. The nature of family, peer, love relationships, and other support systems is explored. It often is helpful to identify the person in whom the patient most frequently confides and the patient's usual coping strategies when confronting stress. To further delineate possible resources the significance of religion, work, and leisure activities is assessed.

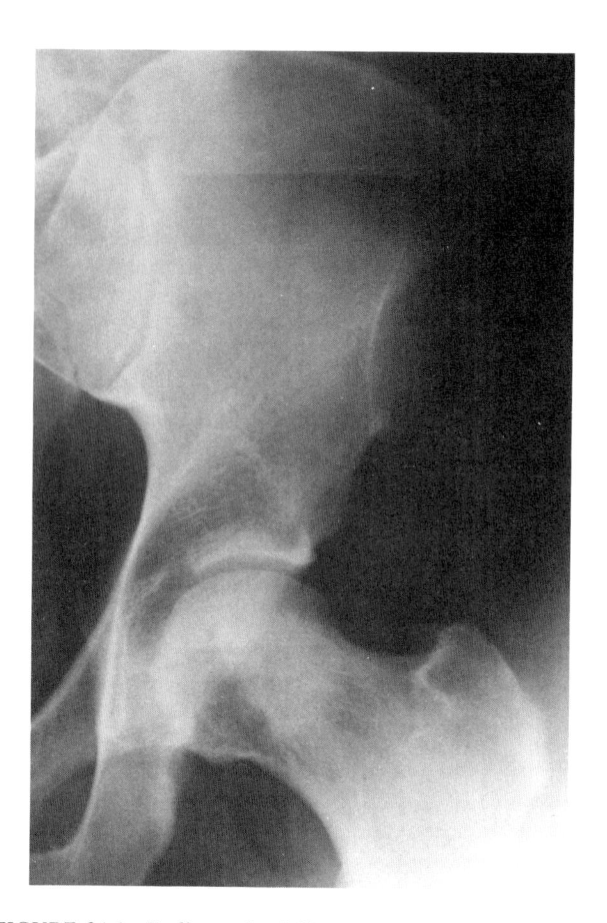

FIGURE 34-1 Radiograph of 67-year-old man with primary osteosarcoma of the femur.

Physical Examination

The physical examination of the individual with a suspected bone lesion involves inspection and palpation of the affected area. Inspection may reveal a visible mass or swelling. Dilated surface veins may be evident. A firm, nontender, warm enlargement may be palpated over the affected portions, although malignant bone tumors are not always visible or palpable. Evaluation for adenopathy and hepatomegaly also is performed. Limitations in movement or motion are noted.

Diagnostic Studies

Evaluation of the individual with symptoms suggestive of a bone tumor necessitates the collaboration of the radiologist, orthopedic surgeon, and pathologist. Before any diagnostic conclusions are made, the person's clinical history is reviewed, as well as the radiologic and histologic features of the lesion.

Radiographs, although they frequently do not yield a specific diagnosis, provide the opportunity to view the location and the anatomy of the lesion, as well as the status of surrounding tissue (Figure 34-1). In general, radiographic changes can be appreciated only when the tumor is far advanced. Three basic patterns of tumor destruction that may be viewed radiographically are described as geographic, moth-eaten, or permeative. These patterns (Figure 34-2) may be correlated with the pathologic aggressiveness or quiescence of the tumor and may occur alone or in combination with one or both of the other patterns.[6] The geographic pattern indicates that the tumor has a slow rate of growth. It is characterized by a large, well-defined hole in which the edge of completely destroyed bone interfaces with the edge of bone that is completely intact. The moth-eaten pattern indicates a moderately aggressive tumor. It is characterized by multiple holes that tend to coalesce. This pattern implies severe cortical destruction. Finally, the permeative pattern indicates an aggressive tumor with a strong capacity for infiltration. It is characterized by multiple tiny holes in cortical bone. These holes diminish in size and number in the peripheral areas of the lesion. The moth-eaten pattern indicates that the tumor has breached the cortex and has extended longitudinally within the bone.

Several other radiologic methods may be used in the evaluation of primary malignant bone cancer. These include bone scans, arteriography, computed tomography (CT), fluoroscopy, and magnetic resonance imaging (MRI). A bone scan is not helpful in distinguishing one bone condition from another but is useful in verifying the

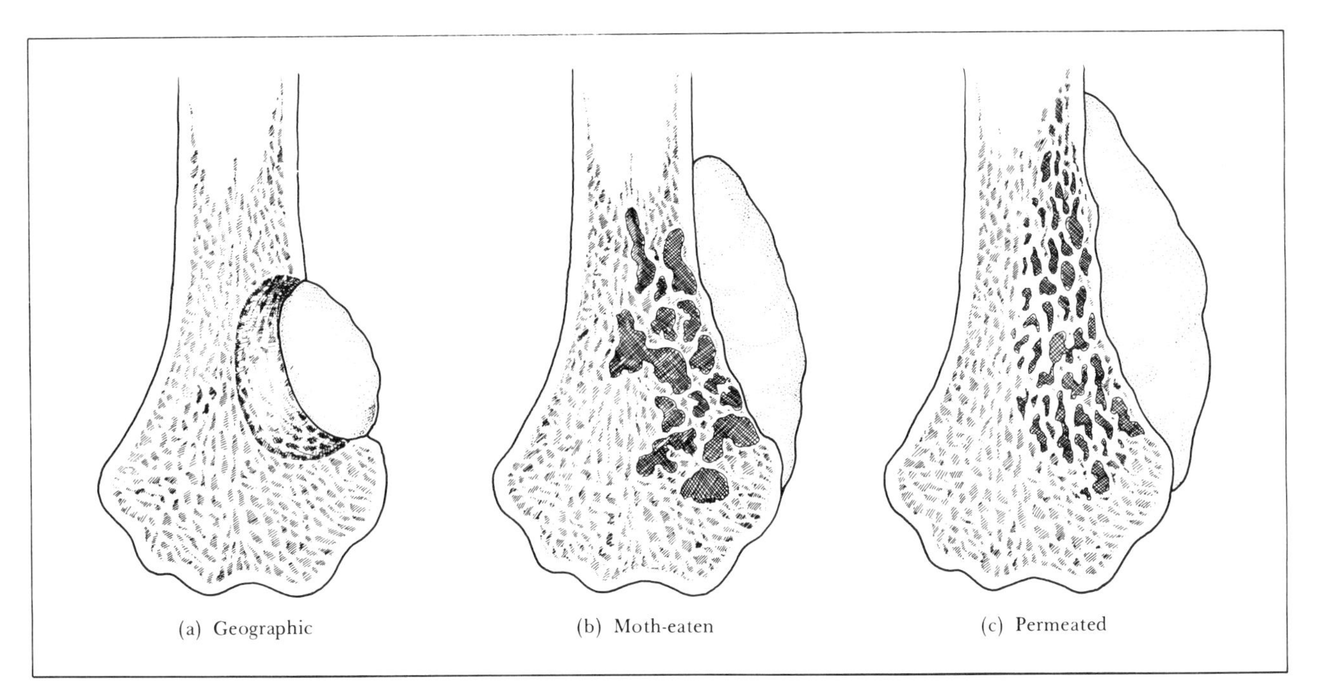

FIGURE 34-2 Radiographic patterns of tumor destruction. (a) Geographic pattern, indicating a slow rate of tumor growth. (b) Moth-eaten pattern, indicating moderately aggressive tumor growth. (c) Permeated pattern, indicating aggressive tumor growth. (Source: Lodwick GS: Solitary malignant tumors of the bone. Semin Roentgenol 1:293-313, 1966.)

presence of abnormal bone when plain radiographs show normal findings. A bone scan helps to detect or exclude the presence of additional lesions in the skeleton. Likewise, arteriography is not diagnostic but aids in the planning of surgical, radiation, and perfusion chemotherapy treatments by outlining tumor margins and mapping arterial blood supply to the tumor. CT provides an accurate evaluation of the true extent of the disease. Fluoroscopy is used in the operating room to document the location in the lesion from which the biopsy specimen is taken.

MRI uses a magnetic field to produce an image. The MRI is superior to a CT scan in demonstrating the tumor extent in marrow and soft tissue and in detecting recurrence in the presence of surgical clips and metallic prostheses.[7]

Biopsy not only is important for diagnosis but also contributes information necessary to determine the best treatment for a particular lesion. The biopsy should include the most representative section of the lesion as determined by the radiographs. Biopsy tissue may be obtained by use of a large needle or by open surgical methods.

Incisional biopsy is the most common type of biopsy used for bone lesions. With the patient under general anesthesia, an incision is made over the tumor mass and through to the soft tissue. Bone biopsies are more painful, weaken the bone, and need to be processed in the pathology department for a few days before diagnosis is made. Incisional biopsy yields a larger volume of tissue for examination.

The location and size of the incision are equally important to the surgeon and radiation oncologist. If hindquarter or forequarter amputation eventually is indicated, the biopsy scar must not compromise the skin flap. Therefore it is advisable for the orthopedic oncologist rather than the referring surgeon to perform the biopsy. If resection of the tumor is performed, the site of the biopsy incision is removed en bloc with the tumor. The radiation oncologist includes the incision site in the field of treatment. The patient has less tissue injury with a smaller field of radiation.

Frozen sections are done during incisional biopsy to ensure that representative material has been obtained. In circumstances in which clinical and radiologic findings are highly suggestive of a particular lesion, frozen sections are obtained with the intention of performing surgery while the patient is still anesthetized. For many bone tumors, however, it is advisable to await permanent paraffin sections.

Percutaneous needle biopsy has been recommended on the basis that it is technically simple, involves minimal patient risk, is cost and time effective, may be repeated without any ill effects, and makes it possible to extract material from different depths of the tumor. In addition, it is always possible to do incisional biopsy if the diagnosis remains unclear. Although positive results of biopsy nearly always are accurate, biopsy yields a 25% false-negative rate. For this reason needle biopsy generally is not the preferred method except in individuals with known metastatic disease.

In general, laboratory studies are not helpful in the diagnosis of bone tumors. There are a few exceptions, which will be addressed in conjunction with the specific tumor type to which they apply.

TABLE 34-1 Histologic Typing of Primary Bone Tumors and Tumorlike Lesions

Bone-forming tumors
- Benign
  - Osteoma
  - Osteoid osteoma and osteoblastoma (benign osteoblastoma)
- Malignant
  - Osteosarcoma (osteogenic sarcoma)
  - Juxtacortical osteosarcoma (parosteal osteosarcoma)

Cartilage-forming tumors
- Benign
  - Chondroma
  - Osteochondroma (osteocartilaginous exostosis)
  - Chondroblastoma (benign chondroblastoma; epiphyseal chondroblastoma)
  - Chondromyxoid fibroma
- Malignant
  - Chondrosarcoma
  - Juxtacortical chondrosarcoma
  - Mesenchymal chondrosarcoma

Giant cell tumor (osteoclastoma)

Marrow tumors
- Ewing's sarcoma
- Reticulosarcoma of bone
- Lymphosarcoma of bone
- Myeloma

Vascular tumors
- Benign
  - Hemangioma
  - Lymphangioma
  - Glomus tumor (glomangioma)
- Intermediate or indeterminate
  - Hemangioendothelioma
  - Hemangiopericytoma
- Malignant
  - Angiosarcoma

Other connective tissue tumors
- Benign
  - Desmoplastic fibroma
  - Lipoma
- Malignant
  - Fibrosarcoma
  - Liposarcoma
  - Malignant mesenchymoma
  - Undifferentiated sarcoma

Other tumors
- Chordoma
- "Adamantinoma" of long bones
- Neurilemmoma (schwannoma. neurinoma)
- Neurofibroma

Unclassified tumors

Tumorlike lesions
- Solitary bone cyst (simple or unicameral bone cyst)
- Aneurysmal bone cyst
- Juxta-articular bone cyst (intraosseous ganglion)
- Metaphyseal fibrous defect (nonossifying fibroma)
- Eosinophilic granuloma
- Fibrous dysplasia
- "Myositis ossificans"
- "Brown tumor" of hyperparathyroidism

Source: Schajowicz F, Ackerman LV, Sissions HA: International histological classification of tumours. Geneva, World Health Organization, monograph no. 6, 1972.

CLASSIFICATION AND STAGING

The classification of bone tumors currently is based on histologic patterns. These patterns correlate in general with the gross appearance, radiologic features, and biologic behavior of the tumor. Uncertainty with regard to the definition of terms used in pathologic nomenclature and classification cannot only complicate the treatment of bone tumors but also impedes research efforts aimed at the development of staging classification for primary malignant bone tumors. Consequently, the American Joint Committee on Cancer has recommended that *International Histological Classification of Tumors,* published by the World Health Organization, be used for specific definitions of histologic typing.[8]

The World Health Organization scheme of classification (Table 34-1) is based on the type of differentiation shown by the tumor cells and the type of intracellular material they produce.[9] The main types of primary bone tumors are listed according to whether they are bone-forming, cartilage-forming, or marrow-forming.

The surgical staging system for musculoskeletal sarcomas includes surgical grade, surgical site, and presence of metastases (Table 34-2).[10] Stage I includes low-grade lesions with low incidence of metastases, such as periosteal osteosarcoma and giant cell tumors. Stage II includes high-grade lesions with high incidence of metastases, such as classic osteosarcoma and angiosarcoma. The site is noted to be "A," which indicates an intracompartmental lesion, or "B," which indicates an extracompartmental lesion. Anatomic compartments have barriers to tumor extension. In bone, these barriers are cortical bone and articular cartilage; in joints, articular cartilage and joint capsule; and in soft tissue, the major fascial septa and the tendinous origins and insertions of muscle. Lesions that involve the

TABLE 34-2 Surgical Stages of Musculoskeletal Sarcomas

Stage	Grade	Site
IA	Low (G_1)	Intracompartmental (T_1)
IB	Low (G_1)	Extracompartmental (T_2)
IIA	High (G_2)	Intracompartmental (T_1)
IIB	High (G_2)	Extracompartmental (T_2)
III	Any (G) Regional or distant metastasis	Any (T)

Source: Enneking WF, Spanier S, Goodman M: A system for surgical staging of musculoskeletal sarcomas. Clin Orthop 153:106-119, 1980.

neurovascular bundle are extracompartmental. Stage III includes any site or grade lesion with metastases.

TREATMENT

The goals of treatment of primary malignant bone cancer include eradication of the tumor, avoidance of amputation when possible, and preservation of maximum function. The primary lesion is managed by surgery, radiotherapy, or chemotherapy, or a combination of these therapies. To a limited extent, immunotherapy is being evaluated for its usefulness as an adjuvant treatment. Treatment is highly individualized because an optimal treatment program has not been identified.

Surgery

Surgical management of primary neoplasia of the bone is strongly influenced by the histopathologic features of the lesion, the anatomic site of the lesion, and the physical size of the lesion. Clinical and radiographic data also are considered because they provide further information about the biologic behavior of a given lesion.

In the past 20 years, research indicated that no procedure short of ablation would control or eradicate aggressive forms of osteosarcoma, fibrosarcoma, and chondrosarcoma.[11] Historically, the amputation included the joint above the tumor. Tumors in inaccessible areas such as the pelvis, spine, or skull pose unique and difficult problems, with treatment frequently aimed at palliation.

In 1984 the National Institutes of Health held a conference to evaluate the efficacy of limb-sparing surgery. Experts reported their experiences with 2000 individuals diagnosed with sarcoma. The same disease-free survival rate was reported for individuals who underwent limb-sparing surgery as for those who underwent amputation.[12] The traditional contraindications for limb salvage are as follows: (1) inability to attain adequate surgical margin, (2) neurovascular bundle involved by tumor, and (3) age-group, that is, children younger than 10 years old, because of resultant limb length discrepancy.

An expandable prosthesis was developed in the early 1980s. The implantation of this prosthesis into the resected bone allows retention of the child's limb. Every 6 to 12 months surgery is performed to expand the prosthesis. The long-term outcome of these implants is unknown.[13]

Limb salvage is indicated for late metastasizing lesions such as periosteal osteosarcoma and locally aggressive chondrosarcomas or fibrosarcomas that have not invaded soft tissue.[14] Wide resection is necessary in limb surgery to ensure adequate tumor excision.

If the tumor extends to the incision surface at any point or cannot be removed entirely, amputation at a more proximal level may be indicated. Amputation also is indicated if a nonfunctional limb would result from a salvage procedure.

Radical resection with reconstruction

It is necessary to determine preoperatively what expectations the person has regarding postoperative management and rehabilitation of radical resection and reconstruction. The patient needs to be aware that revision surgery because of implant failure may occur at a later date.

Postoperative management in terms of levels of activity, mobilization, joint motion, weight bearing, the use of bracing devices, or external immobilization will vary according to the extensiveness of surgery, amount of bone and soft tissue resected, location, and stability of the implant or graft. The extensiveness of the surgery and subsequent effects on function cannot be predicted as readily as when an amputation is planned. It is important to clarify postoperatively if the planned procedure was carried out as anticipated.

Prevention of postoperative complications begins with adequate preoperative teaching in conjunction with conscientious follow-up after surgery. The extensive nature of most resections requires longer exposure to anesthesia, necessitating scrupulous attention to pulmonary hygiene. In the preoperative period the individual is familiarized with the pulmonary regimen and exercises to counteract venous stasis.

The nurse conducts a baseline assessment of neuromuscular function distal to the surgical site. Because nerve injury may occur during the surgical procedure, the assessment provides the opportunity to observe for changes in sensation and motor function that occur. In the immediate postoperative period the nurse observes for signs of hemorrhage and hematoma because of the vascularity of bone.

Nursing care also involves continuous attention to position and alignment of the involved extremity. Improper movement or positioning may impair healing. Postoper-

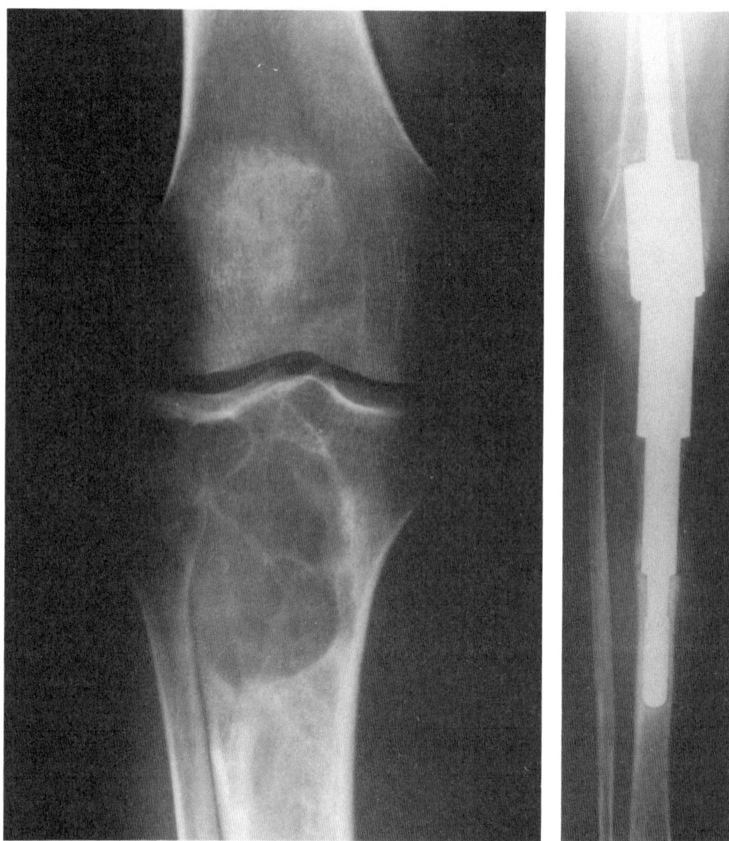

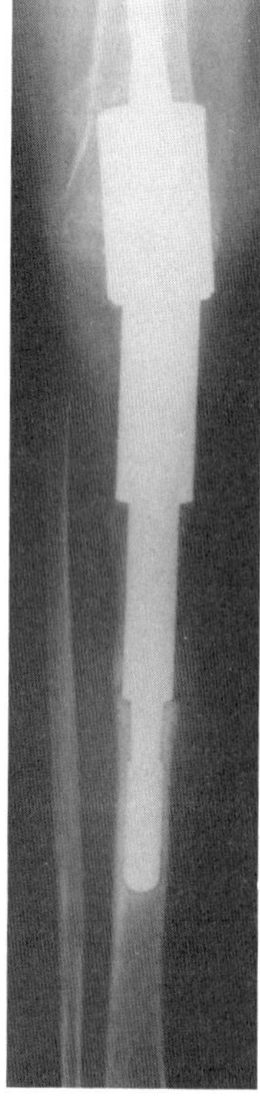

FIGURE 34-3 Radiograph of 30-year-old woman with fibrosarcoma of the proximal tibia, who underwent a wide excision of the tumor and received a segmental arthrodesis. She is disease-free after 6 years.

ative infection remains a significant concern because adjuvant therapies adversely affect patient immunity. Considerable bone damage can occur before detection. Once infection is identified, treatment involves removal of the graft or implant, insertion of drains, immobilization, intravenous antibiotic therapy for 6 weeks, and oral antibiotic therapy for 6 to 12 months. Amputation of the limb is a possibility if complications occur. Consequently, the nurse must be vigilant in observing for signs of infection. Assessment for pneumonia and deep vein thrombosis is done during the postoperative period.

Independence and an adapted body image are the goals of rehabilitation. Resection often involves muscle tissue; therefore physical therapy regimens often are indicated to improve and develop muscle tone. Assistive walking and brace devices may be needed if motor function is limited temporarily or permanently. For lower extremity resections, leg length discrepancies may necessitate gait retraining or may be managed simply through the use of shoe lifts. Finally, the importance of safety within the home environment cannot be overemphasized. Most patients who are discharged to their previous home environment are able to negotiate stairs. Life-long activity restrictions, such as no jogging, heavy lifting, or racquet sports, may be imposed and therefore alter the individual's career and recreation.

After wide resection, reconstruction to provide stability can be accomplished through the use of metal and synthetic materials; the use of bone autografts, which are those transplanted from one area to another in the same individual; or the use of bone allografts, which are those transferred between two genetically different members of the same species. The three most common methods of reconstruction after sarcoma resection are arthrodesis, arthroplasty with metallic or allograft implant, and intercalary allograft reconstruction. Careful consideration should be given to type of reconstruction, particularly in view of the patient's functional needs.[15]

Arthrodesis, or fusion, results in a stiff joint, which is a handicap for the individual. This form of reconstruction, however, is sturdy and permits activities such as running and jumping. There are a variety of surgical techniques for arthrodesis that use metallic implants, allograft implants, or autograft bone (Figure 34-3). Complications include infection and nonunion. In 1985 Otis and colleagues[16] found that patients who underwent segmental replacement have lower energy cost during gait than those with above-the-knee amputation, which could be a con-

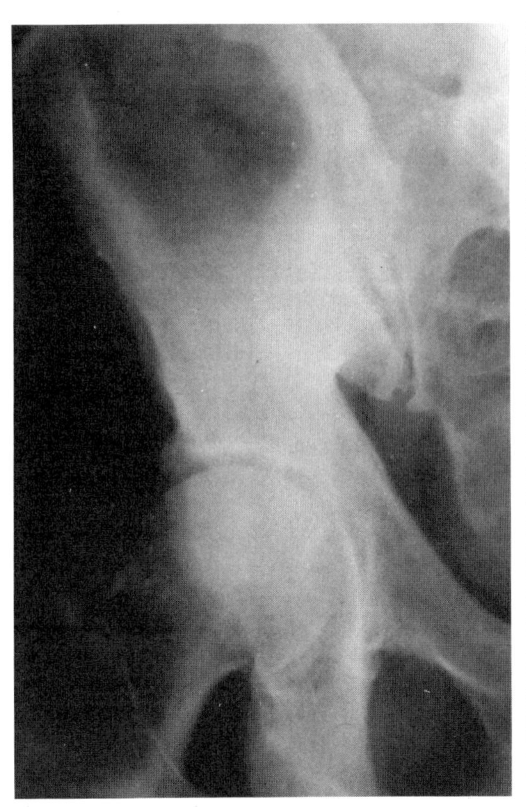
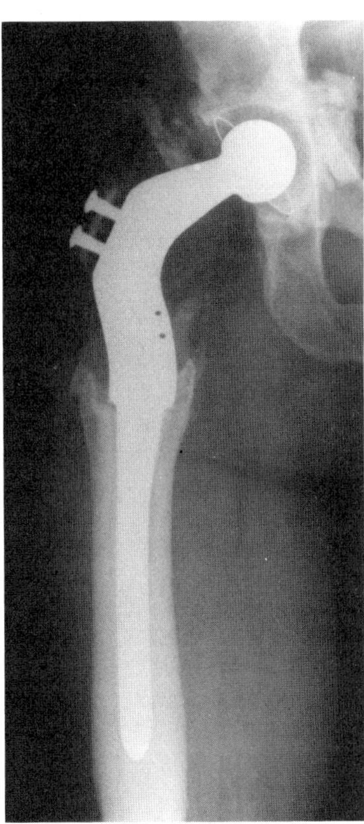

FIGURE 34-4 Radiograph of 25-year-old man with osteosarcoma of the proximal femur, who underwent a wide excision of the tumor with proximal one-third femur replacement with a metallic implant. He is disease-free after 10 years.

sideration in elderly patients who frequently have compromised cardiac status.

Arthroplasty with metallic or bone allograft implant or a combination of metal and allograft allows maintenance of joint function (Figure 34-4). The implant, however, is an artificial joint and will not tolerate percussive activities such as jogging and racquet sports or heavy lifting. Complications include infection, implant fracture, loosening of implant, and nonunion. In all these limb salvage surgeries, muscle flaps and skin graft may be necessary.

Osseous and osteochondral intercalary allografts provide a theoretically superior alternative to metallic implants because they provide joint mobility and are biologic materials.

In an intercalary allograft the allograft is placed between two segments of the host bone (Figure 34-5). The allograft actually heals to the host bone after being secured by metallic plates and screws. Research indicates successful results in the replacement of long bone tumors with fresh-frozen allografts.[17-19] Freezing diminishes the immunogenicity of bone. Currently, no immunosuppressive agents are given to these individuals.[20]

Long-term activity restrictions for individuals undergoing allografts are the same as for those receiving metallic implants. However, the individual needs to limit weight bearing and often must wear a cast or brace, sometimes for up to 6 to 12 months, until the allograft is healed to the host bone. Complications of this procedure include infection, allograft fracture, and nonunion. Chemotherapy retards allograft healing; postoperative chemotherapy increased complications from 44% to 51% in two series of studies.[21,22] The future of allograft reconstruction appears promising for individuals whose bone is destroyed by malignant tumors.

The role of surgery in the management of disseminated disease has gained support in recent years. Bone tumors frequently metastasize to the lung before involving other sites. If untreated, most patients with pulmonary metastases will die within 18 months. Individuals in whom lung metastases develop are good candidates for resection, provided the primary tumor is controlled, there is no indication of other visceral metastatic disease, and the pulmonary nodules are resectable. CT of the chest and chest roentgenogram are performed at the time of diagnosis and every 3 months to assess for extent of disease. Wedge excision is the preferred procedure for lung lesions. The nodule is adequately resected without compromising lung function. Patients generally recover rapidly after a thoracotomy. The 5-year actuarial survival cure is 40%.[23]

Amputation preparation

The psychologic needs of the individual who undergoes amputation should be considered during preopera-

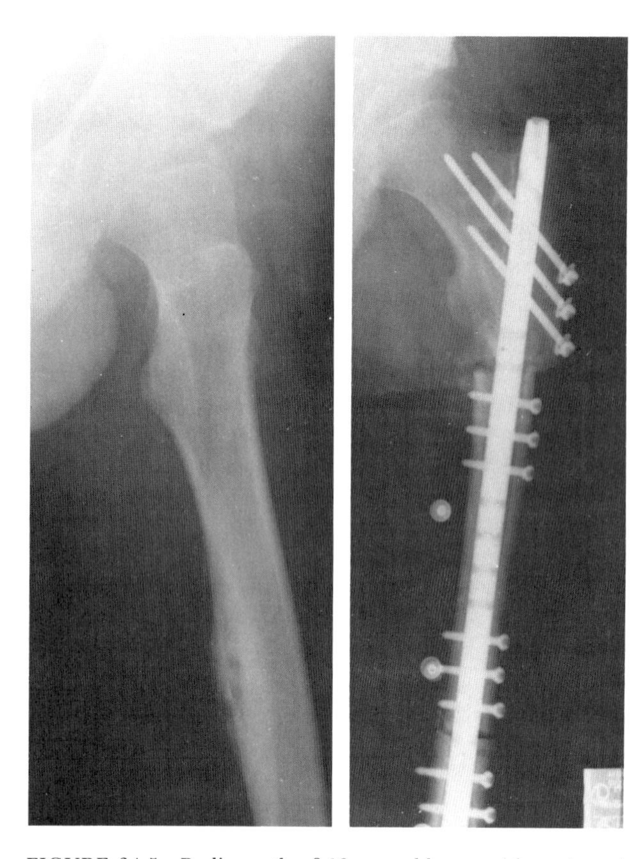

FIGURE 34-5 Radiograph of 18-year-old man with periosteal osteosarcoma of the diaphysis of the femur. He underwent a wide excision of the tumor with an intercalary allograft reconstruction. In the postoperative radiograph, it is difficult to detect the junction between the allograft and host bone. The individual is disease-free after 5 years.

tive preparation. It is reasonable to assume that the person facing an amputation has fears regarding death, disability, and deformity. In addition, the person may be concerned about the potential loss of social and economic self-sufficiency. These fears and concerns may lead to changes in self-esteem, which can be manifested by anxiety and depression. All these factors will affect the individual's readiness to learn and ability to participate in rehabilitation. Consequently, the plan of care includes interventions aimed at minimizing fear, decreasing anxiety, and promoting realistic optimism. The individual and family may wish to express their fears and doubts. Efforts are made to integrate their expectations with reality by providing accurate information from nursing and medical staff regarding the postoperative recovery period and future rehabilitation.

The individual having a hemipelvectomy may harbor fears concerning sexual adequacy. If appropriate a woman needs to be reassured that pregnancy and normal delivery are possible after surgery. A decision concerning future pregnancies, however, may be influenced by the fact that the prosthesis cannot be worn during pregnancy. Impotence in a man often is related to age. Loss of erectile power is due primarily to a decrease in blood supply; however, pelvic nerve function may be compromised. Most men recover potency over time. The younger the individual the more rapid recovery of potency.

To reduce anxiety it sometimes is helpful for the person undergoing surgery to meet preoperatively those individuals who will be involved in his or her postoperative care. Depending on the institution's program, this may include physical and occupational therapists, the prosthetist, the social worker, and the psychologist. Likewise, in some instances it may be helpful to arrange a preoperative visit from a person with an amputated limb who has mastered his or her prosthesis and achieved independence. Information regarding local organizations that train such volunteers can be obtained from the American Cancer Society. Care is taken in assessing which individuals could benefit by interaction with these resources. An overload of information and stimuli may serve only to increase the person's anxiety and fear.

The nurse consults social service personnel to inform the patient and family about financial resources and rehabilitation programs available in the state. There is underutilization of available resources for individuals with cancer. Other support is available through groups such as the American Cancer Society and American Handicapped Association.

It is important for the nurse to help establish realistic expectations regarding the patient's postamputation function. Many individuals who have lower extremity amputation can expect a return to full function and a relatively normal active life through the use of a lower limb prosthesis and occasionally walking aids. Amputees resume activities such as downhill skiing, swimming, and basketball. The person who has a hemicorporectomy is wheelchair bound. Hemipelvectomy prostheses will approximate only soft tissue, and the use of a walker or crutches will be necessary for additional stability. Because of the significantly increased energy expenditure required, it may be necessary for the person with a more proximal amputation to spend more time in a wheelchair. Elderly patients or those with cardiac conditions may find prosthetic use tiring and may need to use at least a cane.

Ideally, the goal for the individual is independent function with the use of prostheses. In evaluating rehabilitation potential, the nurse considers other factors such as age, effects of adjuvant therapy, the existence of unrelated disease, and the person's attitude. Prosthetic rehabilitation requires cooperation, coordination, and tremendous physical energy.

The nurse learns from the physician whether the patient will have an immediate postsurgical prosthetic fitting or a conventional delayed prosthetic fitting. This decision is made before surgery, which permits adequate preparation of the individual for the postoperative care regimen.

Phantom limb phenomenon Preoperative teaching includes a frank discussion of phantom limb sensation and pain. It is a frightening experience for an individual with a recent amputation to feel sensation or pain, or both, in a limb that no longer exists. Consequently, the person who is not adequately prepared may neglect to report the occurrence of the phantom limb phenomenon and may harbor doubts about his or her sanity.

All individuals who have an amputation can expect to feel some phantom limb sensation, whereas only 35% of those experience phantom limb pain.[24] Phantom limb sensation is described as an awareness of the position or existence of the limb. Itching, pressure, or tingling sensations may be described. Phantom limb pain is described as severe cramping, throbbing, or burning pain in various areas of the amputated limb. Phantom limb sensations usually are experienced shortly after surgery. Phantom limb pain usually does not occur until 1 to 4 weeks after surgery and may be triggered by fatigue, excitement, sickness, weather changes, stress, and other stimuli. Roth and Sugarbaker[25] demonstrated in a retrospective study of 63 individuals that the incidence and severity of phantom limb pain are greater when the amputation site is more proximal. For many individuals phantom limb pain resolves gradually in a few months. However, the pain becomes worse over the years for 5% to 10% of those who have amputations of limbs. It is suggested that increased severity of phantom limb pain after a few months may be a symptom of locally recurrent cancer in a stump, or it may be a sign of a neuroma.[26]

Phantom limb pain is poorly understood but seems to depend on a combination of physical and emotional factors. The physical component relates to the surgical interruption of neural reflex pathways, with resultant transmission of abnormal patterns of nerve impulses. Melzack noted a correlation between the length of time a person experiences limb pain before surgery and the incidence and duration of phantom limb pain.[24] Other factors that contribute to phantom pain include the maladaptive use of pain for secondary gain, the availability of support systems, and the ability to cope with loss.[27]

A variety of measures are used to alleviate phantom limb pain. Relief may be obtained simply by applying heat to the stump or by pressure, such as with elastic bandages. Distraction and diversion techniques may decrease the person's awareness of the pain. Tranquilizers, muscle relaxants, or local anesthesia are occasionally effective in managing the pain. Psychotherapy and behavioral therapy also may be useful. Procedures that are available for intractable pain include hypnosis, nerve blocks, sympathectomy, cordotomy, acupuncture, biofeedback, and transcutaneous nerve stimulation. In rare cases revision of the stump with reamputation at a higher level may be done.

Amputation of the lower extremity Preoperative preparation of the individual having a lower extremity amputation incorporates all considerations routinely given to any person undergoing general anesthesia. The individual who is to have a hemipelvectomy will need to know that a urethral catheter will be inserted and that preoperative cleansing enemas and antibiotics will be given to decrease the bacterial count of the intestinal tract.

General strengthening measures and mobility training should be initiated for all individuals undergoing amputation. In recent years insurance companies have restricted early admissions for surgery, making strengthening and mobility training difficult to achieve. A number of these exercises may be taught in the physician's office before surgery so that the individual can practice them at home. Pull-ups provide effective preparation for walking with crutches. Active and active-resistive exercises of the unaffected extremity maintain and increase muscle strength. The person also should be instructed in transfer maneuvers from bed to chair to commode. Finally, the person should be instructed to ambulate with the use of a walker or crutches. Control of weight bearing on the affected side should be emphasized.

The goals of postoperative care are to maintain the individual's general health status, to use modern prostheses, to achieve the highest level of function possible, and to minimize the negative psychosocial consequences of amputation. These goals remain the same for all individuals after an amputation; however, the actual postoperative care varies according to whether the individual has had an immediate prosthetic fitting or a conventional delayed prosthetic fitting.

Immediate postsurgical prosthetic fittings consist of a rigid dressing and cast that is applied to the stump at the time of surgery. A socket on the distal end of the cast is designed so that a pylon prosthetic unit may be attached to the cast (Figure 34-6). Restraining straps that go over the shoulder or attach to the waistband contribute to controlled pressure, improved stump shaping, and tissue support provided by the cast.

If a conventional delayed prosthesis fitting is planned, the patient will return from surgery with the stump covered with a dressing and an elastic bandage. During the second postoperative week the sutures or staples are removed. To shrink and shape the stump, elastic bandages or elastic stump shrinkers are used until the first fitting (Figure 34-7). The individual is fitted with a temporary or intermediate prosthesis at approximately 3 to 6 weeks, when acute swelling has decreased. An intermediate prosthesis, however, lacks a cosmetic covering. Ambulation with weight bearing is encouraged as tolerated. Approximately 3 months after surgery the individual is fitted with a permanent prosthesis.

The relative advantages and disadvantages for immediate and delayed prosthesis fitting are summarized in Table 34-3.

With the conventional delayed fitting, drains frequently are inserted during surgery to remove blood and serous drainage. The nurse observes for signs of hemorrhage such as excessive bleeding through the dressing or an increase in pain, tenderness, or swelling of the stump.

The stump usually is elevated for 24 hours after surgery to prevent edema and promote venous return. To prevent hip contractures the individual is assisted into the prone position three to four times a day for a minimum of 15 minutes and encouraged to assume that position for sleep. Exercises to maintain muscle tone and prevent edema, joint contractures, and muscle atrophy are initi-

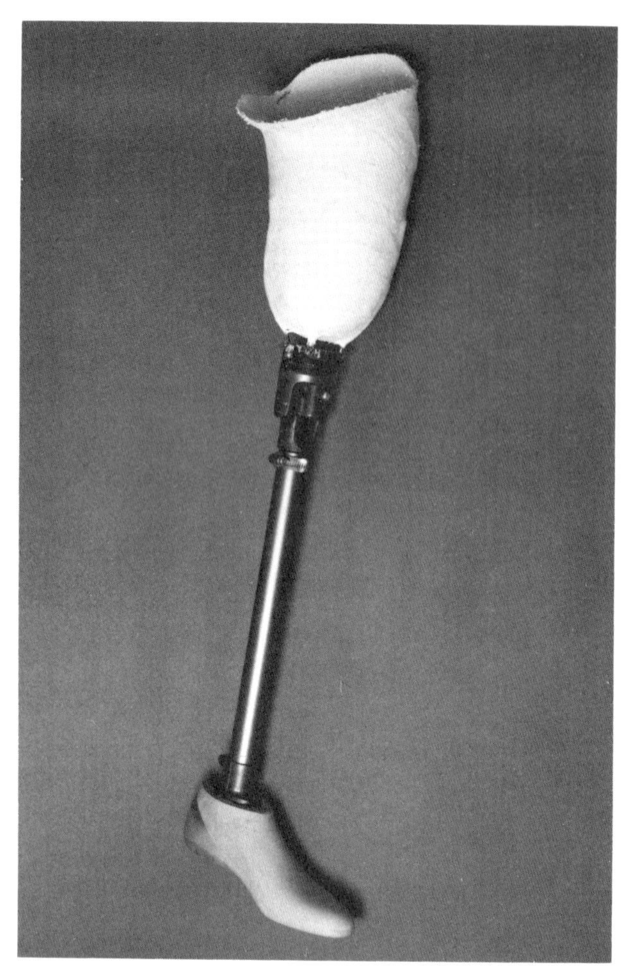

FIGURE 34-6 Immediate postsurgical prosthetic fitting with a pylon prosthetic unit attached to the cast.

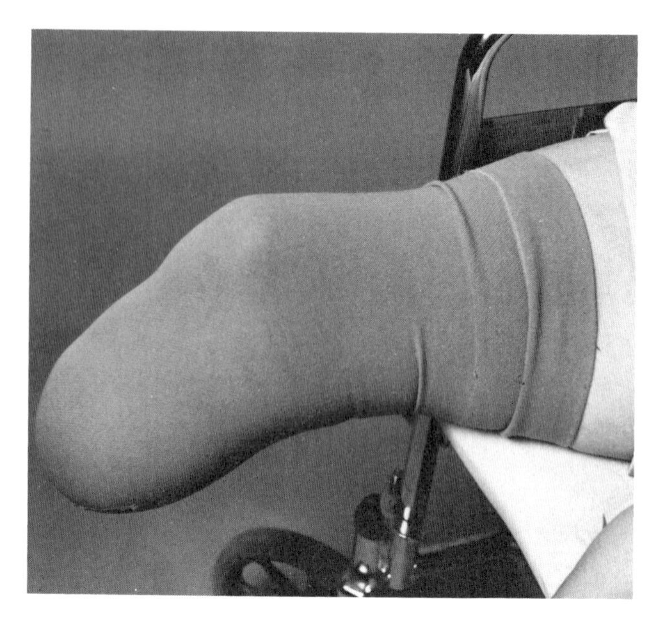

FIGURE 34-7 Elastic stump shrinker applied to shape stump.

ated on the first postoperative day. Exercises include active range of motion, strengthening exercises for the upper extremities, and hyperextension of the stump.

Stump care involves frequent wrapping with elastic bandages or stump shrinkers to facilitate stump shrinking. Dangling and transfer to a chair are encouraged on the first postoperative day. Crutch walking is started as soon as the person is strong enough. Sutures or staples are removed approximately 2 weeks after surgery. Temporary prosthetic fitting will occur at 3 to 6 weeks. For the individual having a hemipelvectomy, mobilization also is possible on the second or third postoperative day. The permanent prosthesis may be fitted within 12 weeks. A sitting or bucket prosthesis also is needed for an individual with a hemipelvectomy because of the absence of an ischium on which to sit. Until the bucket prosthesis is fabricated, a pillow is placed under the surgical site for balance.

With an immediate prosthetic fitting, hemorrhage is less likely because of the compression effects of the cast. However, evidence of blood staining on the cast should be noted. The rigid cast also minimizes acute swelling; however, the stump is routinely elevated for 24 hours. Care must be taken to prevent the cast from slipping off the stump, which would rapidly lead to edema and wound disruption. Should this occur, the stump should be wrapped with an elastic bandage and the surgeon notified. Because the wound cannot be visualized, it is important to monitor for signs of infection such as fever, increased white blood cell count, and significant stump pain. Such symptoms would necessitate immediate removal of the cast for wound inspection.

Nursing management includes cast care. The skin near the edges of the cast should be inspected for friction rubs, swelling, or discoloration. In addition, the cast should be inspected routinely for cracks. The rigid cast assists in the prevention of hip and joint contractures. However, maintenance of neutral alignment and frequent position changes remain important nursing measures. Exercises should not be overlooked, even though complications as a result of immobilization are significantly reduced because of early ambulation.

Ambulation with the pylon and crutches or walker is initiated on the first or second postoperative day. The length of time permitted for ambulation increases gradually. The individual advances to the use of parallel bars and to crutches while bearing touch-down weight on the pylon. The sutures are removed and the cast changed approximately 2 weeks after surgery. Temporary prosthetic fitting occurs at 3 to 6 weeks. After the swelling is diminished, fitting for a permanent prosthesis is undertaken at 12 weeks after surgery. Chemotherapy may increase stump swelling and delay fitting of the permanent prosthesis.

The primary nurse assumes the responsibility for coordinating the efforts of the health professionals involved in the care during hospitalization of a person undergoing amputation, as well as for making the appropriate referrals to those professionals in the community who will become involved in the person's total rehabilitation. This

TABLE 34-3 Relative Advantages and Disadvantages of Delayed Versus Immediate Prosthetic Fitting

	Delayed Fitting	Immediate Fitting
Advantages	Wound can be inspected for healing Skin can be conditioned	Better emotional adjustment with immediate substitute limb Motivation increased with early ambulation Decreased stump edema, pain, phantom limb pain, and contractures (caused by pressure of device)
Disadvantages	Edema delays shrinking and shaping of stump Continuous rewrapping with elastic bandages is required Attention must be given to prevention of contractures and other complications of immobility	Wound cannot be visualized Temporary prosthesis is heavy Poor gait pattern can develop because of heavy prosthesis and discomfort in early ambulation period Prosthetist must go to operating room to apply

may include a referral to a community nurse, community physical therapist, and local rehabilitation programs involved with vocational rehabilitation. Most individuals with amputated limbs are capable of returning to work with restrictions.

The primary nurse also contributes to improved health and the prevention of complications through patient and family education. Teaching the individual how to care for the stump is an essential element of the rehabilitation program. The person needs to be responsible for daily stump hygiene with the use of a mild soap and water. The person also should be instructed to avoid the use of skin creams, oils, and rubbing alcohol. Daily inspection for redness, blisters, or abrasions should be incorporated into the person's routine. The stump socks or elastic wraps should be fit properly and changed daily. When the wound has healed, the individual can prevent edema by putting on the prosthesis immediately after arising and keeping it on all day. The person with an immediate postsurgical prosthetic fitting also should be instructed regarding cast care and inspection for fit.

The individual also is taught how to put on and care for the prosthesis. The prosthesis socket is wiped out daily with a damp, soapy cloth. Care is taken to remove thoroughly the soap and to dry the socket to prevent a source of skin irritation and prosthesis rust. The individual is taught the importance of never attempting to make mechanical adjustments to the prosthesis. Discomfort or difficulties in use necessitate an immediate visit to the prosthetist.

The primary nurse and physical therapist review the exercises that contribute to achievement of the highest level of functioning with optimal grace and coordination. Exercises that contribute to balance and movement patterns include standing, weight shifting, heel and toe balance, rocking, hip hiking, and stair climbing. The individual is advised to practice these exercises after discharge from the hospital.

The physician and prosthetist collaborate in the planning of the prosthetic device to be constructed. The prosthetist ultimately is accountable for the construction and fit of the prosthesis and should be certified by the American Board for Certification of Prosthetists. Lower limb prostheses generally consist of a socket, suspension such as a waistband or suction or latex sleeve, knee joint, ankle joint, and foot (Figure 34-8). Many varieties of these

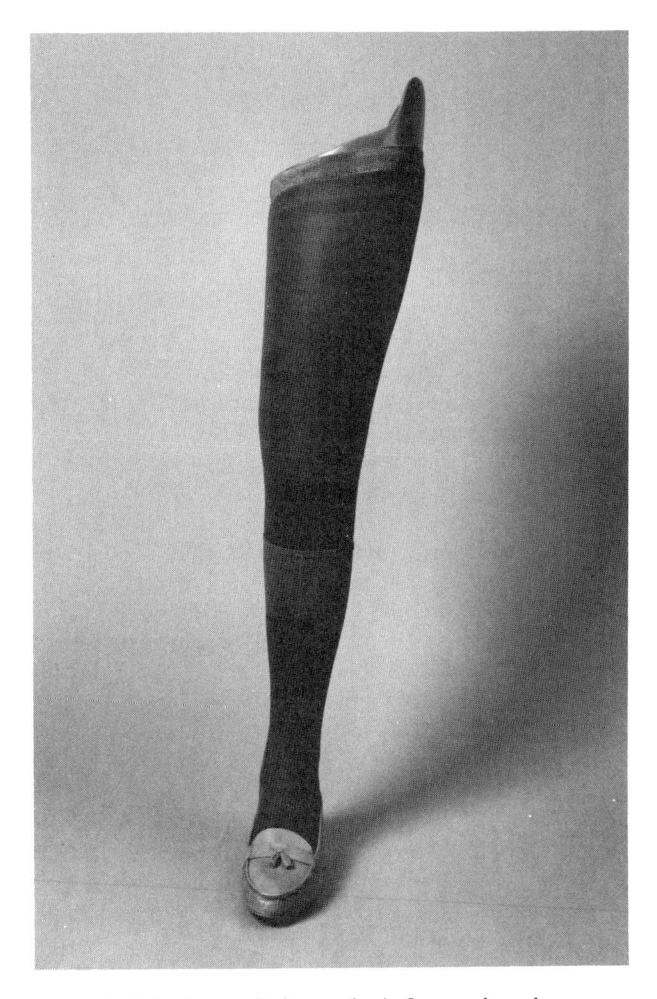

FIGURE 34-8 Lower limb prosthesis for an above-knee amputation showing the socket, waistband suspension, joints, foot, and ankle.

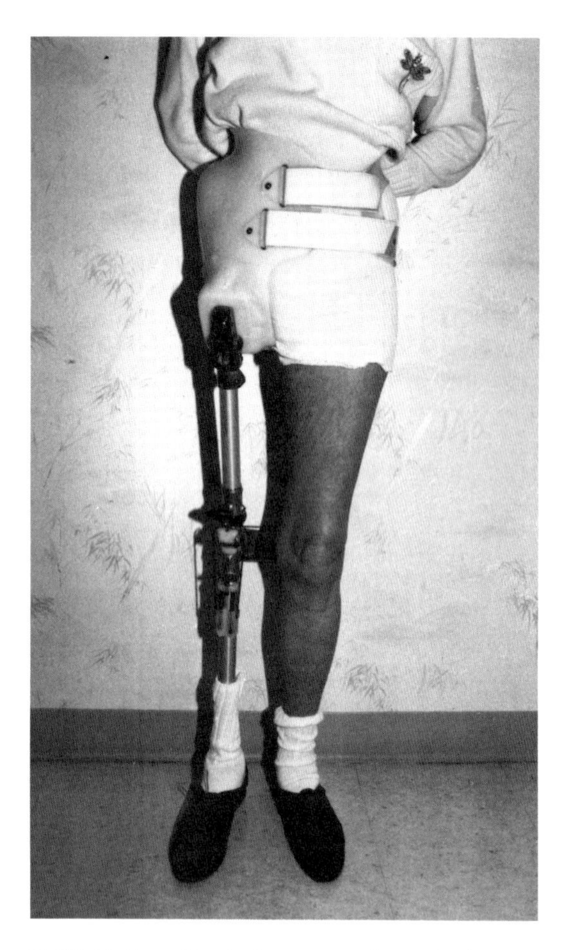

FIGURE 34-9 Hemipelvectomy endoprosthesis.

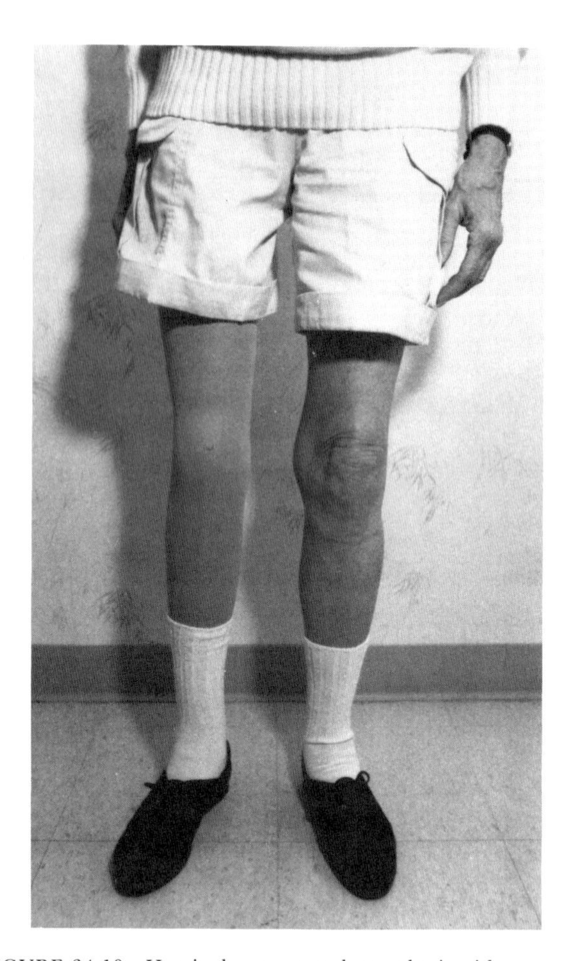

FIGURE 34-10 Hemipelvectomy endoprosthesis with cosmetic urethane foam cover.

components are available; consequently, numerous combinations can be developed to meet the needs of each individual. For example, knee joints are available that provide either mechanical or hydraulic assistance in controlling the swing phase of walking and provide increased stability during standing. These features, however, increase weight, cost, and maintenance. In designing the prosthesis, consideration is given to the person's age, ability, endurance, financial status, occupation goals, and motivation, as well as comfort, fit, alignment, safety, ease of application, and appearance. The primary nurse can assess these factors and communicate them to the prosthetist. Figure 34-9 shows an endoprosthesis for the individual with a hemipelvectomy before application of the cosmetic urethane foam cover pictured in Figure 34-10.

After discharge, the individual with an amputation should be seen by the prosthetist every 4 to 6 weeks for the first postoperative year. It is the responsibility of the community health nurse to observe for problems related to fit, comfort, physical stress, or psychologic maladjustment. These problems then should be explored with the individual and/or the prosthetist or physician. The rehabilitation process is complete when the individual has attained an optimal level of independence and successfully incorporated the prosthesis into his or her body image.

Amputation of the upper extremity Many of the considerations concerning preoperative, postoperative, and rehabilitative care that were discussed in the preceding section apply to individuals having a lower extremity amputation. There are, however, some significant differences.

Upper limb prostheses are far less satisfactory than those created for lower extremities in both appearance and function. The functional capabilities of the prosthesis for upper extremity amputation decrease as the level of amputation becomes more proximal. Power and motion are supplied in only a comparatively gross fashion. The most functional terminal (hand) device is a hook. The development of a substitute for the complex actions of the intricate muscles of the hand has thus far been impossible. Adequate cosmetic appearance can be obtained at the expense of function. Polyvinyl cosmetic gloves with realistic skin creases, veins, and hair are available. Skin tones are matched; shade changes that occur in the normal hand as a result of position and season cannot be reproduced. In addition, the glove must be replaced frequently because ink, newsprint, and other stains are impossible to remove.

Conventional prostheses for the upper extremities consist of a hand terminal device, a harness to supply force from the proximal muscles, appropriate segments between

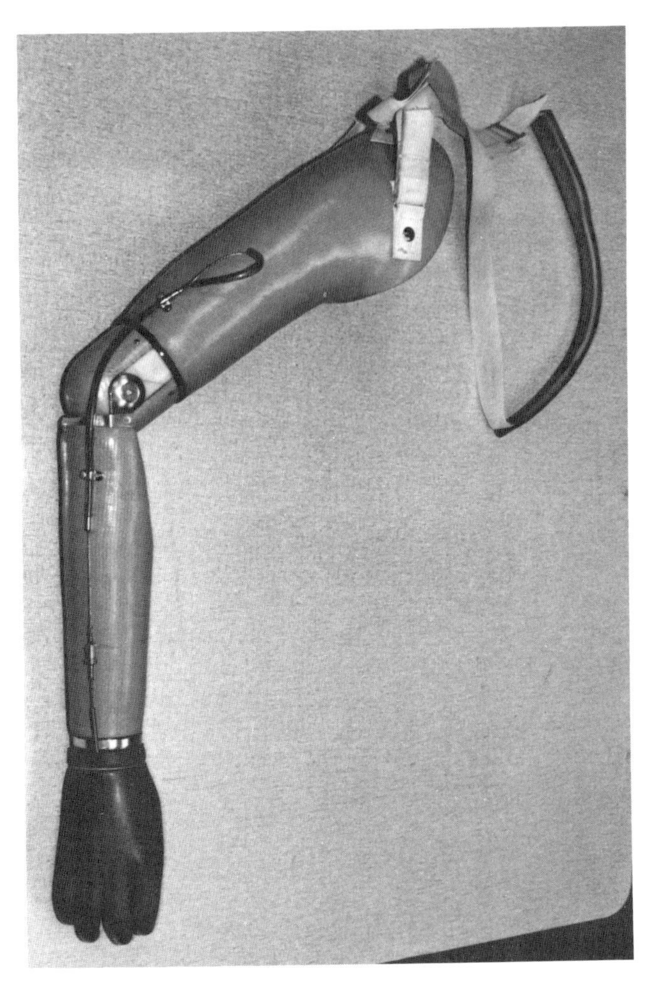

FIGURE 34-11 Upper extremity prosthetic device showing a cable system, elbow joint, and hand terminal device.

them, including a socket for the stumps, and cable system that provides motion at the terminal device and/or the elbow (Figure 34-11). Abduction of the scapula or flexion of the shoulder on the side of the prosthesis initiates movement. Flexion and extension of the wrist usually are omitted, although wrist units in flexed or extended positions are available. Pronation and supination are achieved by rotating the terminal device with the opposite hand. Likewise, opening and closing of the terminal device are accomplished through the use of the opposite hand.

Prostheses for interscapulothoracic amputations are fitted over the upper portion of the chest. Motion is severely limited because sources of power are unavailable. Some force can be initiated from the opposite shoulder and chest expansion. The primary function of the prosthesis, however, is cosmetic. Rejection of upper extremity prosthetic devices occurs more often than with prostheses of the lower extremity because of a combination of poor function, low cosmetic value, and lack of motivation.

Upper extremity prosthetic research has been directed at the development of myoelectric limb substitution. In this system electrical impulses from the contraction of extensor and flexor muscle in the stump are picked up by electrodes in the socket and are in turn amplified, switching on and off electrical motors in the prosthesis. An external battery pack may be worn to provide an additional electrical supply. Opening and closing of the terminal device, pronation and supination, and elbow flexion can be provided. The individual must be assessed first for the ability to elicit and control myoelectric signals.[28] The advantages include an increase in control with less energy expenditure and improved physical appearance. The disadvantages include electrical interference or inadvertent contraction of the muscles when the user coughs or stretches and the cost of the device.

The reality is that the inadequacy of available upper limb prostheses can be disappointing for the person with an upper limb amputation. The nurse, in conjunction with the physician, provides realistic information regarding the functional and cosmetic features of upper extremity prostheses. It is important to discuss with the individual the negative social stigma attached to the hook, as well as its functional capabilities. Equal emphasis should be placed on the functional limitations and cosmetic value of the glove. Some individuals are willing to sacrifice function to obtain the best cosmetic replacement.

As with lower extremity amputations, immediate or delayed postsurgical prosthesis fitting is possible. When delayed fitting is planned, the individual will return from surgery with a soft dressing and elastic bandages covering the stump. Compression of the traumatized area is to be avoided until healing takes place.

As with the lower extremity amputation, independence and an adapted body image can be facilitated through the provision of psychologic support, patient and family education, and appropriate referral to community resources. Rehabilitation goals emphasize use of the remaining arm for activities of daily living. The patient should be evaluated preoperatively by an occupational therapist for information on one-handedness. Vocational rehabilitation assumes particular importance for the individual with an upper extremity amputation because the ensuing disability could prevent the resumption of previous employment.

Radiotherapy

The use of radiotherapy in the management of primary or metastatic malignant bone tumors depends on the radiosensitivity of the particular tumor type. Most bone tumors are relatively unresponsive to radiation. Consequently, radiation is reserved for palliation and may be used in conjunction with chemotherapy for inoperable tumors or in conjunction with surgery to reduce the tumor load of partially resectable tumors. Conventional radiation doses for palliative treatment of primary bone tumors often result in fibrosis and contractures that lead to amputation even if the tumor is controlled. Neutron beam therapy, however, which is produced by heavy particle accelerators, can deliver higher doses with fewer complications. At the Fermilab Neutron Therapy Facility in Batavia, Illinois, 25 individuals were treated with neutron beam therapy for bone sarcoma in the axial skeleton or when surgery was refused for cosmetic or emotional reasons. The local control rate was 44% and the crude survival rate was 39%.[29] Neutron beam irradiation may be an effective option for nonresectable sarcoma.

In contrast, radiotherapy plays an integral role in the management of Ewing's sarcoma, a highly radiosensitive tumor. Complications of treatment include tendon contractures, edema of the involved extremity distal to the site of irradiation, cessation of growth of the extremity, and nonhealing fractures.

Chemotherapy and Immunotherapy

Since the addition of postoperative chemotherapy to the treatment of sarcomas in the early 1970s the survival rates have increased from 20% to more than 50%.[30] Currently chemotherapy is given preoperatively. The rationale for preoperative chemotherapy is to treat the micrometastasis, to decrease the primary tumor size, thereby increasing the likelihood of limb salvage surgery, and to assess the effectiveness of the chemotherapeutic agents for 2 to 3 months.[31] The route of the chemotherapy is either intravenous or intra-arterial. The duration of treatment ranges from 6 to 12 months.

OSTEOSARCOMA

Epidemiology and Etiology

Osteosarcoma is the most common osseous malignant bone tumor, accounting for an estimated 20% of such lesions.[11] Its incidence is greatest in individuals between 10 and 25 years of age, and it affects males twice as often as females. The incidence of osteosarcoma peaks again in older adults with Paget's disease.

The increased incidence of osteosarcoma during adolescence has been correlated with skeletal growth patterns, which in turn may account for the greater overall occurrence in males.

Pathophysiology

Osteosarcoma appears to arise from primitive bone-forming mesenchyma in the medullary cavity. Proliferating connective tissue generally gives rise to tumor osteoid and bone directly. The proliferating connective tissue also may form some tumor cartilage that undergoes rapid osseous transformation.

The duration, extent, and vascularity of the tumor, as well as the amount of bone production, are factors that affect the gross appearance of osteosarcoma. Sclerosing forms of osteosarcoma are characterized by abundant new bone formation. This form frequently involves the metaphysis of a long bone and extends outward through the periosteum, involving soft tissue and muscle. In addition, it usually extends upward into the epiphysis without involving the joint. This process gives the tumor a fan-shaped appearance.

In contrast, the osteolytic form of osteosarcoma is characterized by little bone formation but greater bone destruction. Large areas of hemorrhage and necrosis are seen with osteolytic osteosarcoma. Fragmentation and invasion of the periosteum occur early. The periosteum confines the tumor. Extension of the tumor occurs beneath the periosteum, with bone formation occurring at right angles to the shaft, forming a cuff that extends around part of the circumference of the bone. This process gives the tumor a spindle-shaped appearance.

Periosteal osteosarcoma, a variant of osteosarcoma, was originally described by Unni et al.[32] These tumors develop through slow but progressive proliferation of bone-forming periosteal connective tissue. They occur as a hard mass on the bone surface. The tumor is confined to the periosteum and cortex without a medullary component.

The histologic pattern of osteosarcoma is so variable that no two specimens are exactly alike. Specimens have varying mixtures of malignant bone, malignant cartilage, and malignant stroma. Consequently, the tumor may be described as osteoblastic, chondroblastic, or fibroblastic, depending on which component is dominant. Whatever the pattern, the essential criteria for the diagnosis of osteosarcoma are the presence of frankly sarcomatous stroma and the formation of tumor osteoid and bone by malignant connective tissue.

The most frequent sites of osteosarcoma include the distal end of the femur, the proximal end of the tibia, and the proximal end of the humerus. Osteosarcomas may be discovered in the iliac bone, vertebral column, mandible, and in rare cases the scapula, clavicle, or bones in the hands and feet.

Metastatic spread occurs primarily to the lungs by the hematogenous route. Radiologic evidence of pulmonary or bony metastases usually appears within 24 months of the definitive surgery. Late metastasis in one or more of the other bones occurs occasionally, often in the presence of pulmonary metastases.

Assessment

The individual with osteosarcoma typically has pain and a mass. The pain becomes more severe and, as the tumor progresses in size, usually is worse at night.

If the tumor is allowed to follow its natural course, the affected limb becomes swollen and its superficial veins significantly dilated. In individuals with rapidly growing tumors, weight loss and moderately severe anemia may be seen. This is especially true in children. In addition, pathologic fractures are not uncommon. The duration of symptoms varies from weeks to 6 months or more before medical advice and treatment are sought.

Half the individuals with osteosarcoma have an elevation in the serum alkaline phosphatase level. This level, which represents osteoblastic activity, tends to decline after removal of the tumor and to return to the initially high level in the presence of pulmonary metastasis. In the normal growing child the levels are elevated. Other laboratory data do not appear to be significant in the diagnosis of osteosarcoma.

The classic radiologic features of osteosarcoma include cortical bone destruction, extension of the tumor into soft tissues, and periosteal new bone formation that may appear in a perpendicular striated, or "sunburst," pattern. These findings can be diagnostic on plain radiographs.

Treatment

The 5-year survival rate for individuals treated with surgery alone or irradiation and surgery has been approximately 10% to 20%.[33] The high mortality rate is due principally to pulmonary metastasis, which is assumed to be present microscopically at time of presentation. Reports evaluating adjuvant chemotherapy after surgery for osteosarcoma indicate a significant prolongation of the disease-free interval. Reports from the 1970s show that the 5-year survival rate increased from 40% to 60% with the use of adjuvant chemotherapy.[34] These chemotherapy protocols have used doxorubicin, high-dose cyclophosphamide, or high-dose methotrexate with leucovorin rescue or combination chemotherapy incorporating both doxorubicin and/or high-dose methotrexate with other drugs. The drugs are given via an intravenous or intra-arterial route. Rosen and colleagues[35] and Lane and colleagues[36] demonstrated an 85% to 93% disease-free state at 2 years. When preoperative or neoadjuvant chemotherapy is used, effectiveness is assessed at the time of tumor resection. If there is 90% tumor necrosis, the high-dose methotrexate regimen is continued postoperatively for 9 to 12 months. The greater the necrosis, the greater the survival. If tumor necrosis is less, the chemotherapy is changed to cisplatin. This regimen allows an in vivo study of the tumor cells. During the 8 to 20 weeks of preoperative chemotherapy, physical examination of the tumor site is performed to assess for effectiveness of treatment by indices such as decreased pain and swelling.

Prospective randomized chemotherapy studies in osteosarcoma have shown improvement in overall survival (up to 60%) and disease-free intervals when adjuvant chemotherapy is given.[35-38]

The improved results of chemotherapy have sparked interest in limb salvage resections. The chemotherapy can result in decreased tumor size.[39] There is concern that if preoperative chemotherapy is not effective, the delay in surgery could allow tumor growth. The limb salvage criteria apply to these patients. Amputations are indicated for patients with large and invasive tumors. The occurrence of occult medullary extension or skip metastasis within a single bone or across joints is uncommon, which allows cross bone amputation with wide margins of normal tissue. Disarticulation, which results in greater disability and no greater overall survival, is performed as a last resort.[23] It is advisable to obtain a second opinion if an amputation is recommended. Local recurrence is as frequent in amputation surgery as in limb salvage surgeries (under 5%).[40] Resumption of chemotherapy after definitive surgery is delayed for 1 to 3 weeks.

Significant improvement of patient survival with metastatic disease has been demonstrated in the 1980s. Of patients with osteosarcoma who had thoracotomies for metastases 41% were free of disease more than 4 years after surgery.[30] No patients survived the development of pulmonary metastases unless they had surgical resection of gross disease. In these situations, chemotherapy is given after thoracotomy to eradicate microscopic disease.

Radiation currently is reserved for palliation or inoperable cases. Significant morbidity and mortality were reported when irradiation alone was used for treatment of the primary tumor.

CHONDROSARCOMA

Epidemiology and Etiology

Chondrosarcoma accounts for approximately 13% of malignant bone tumors. The incidence is greatest in individuals between 30 and 60 years of age and among males.

The occurrence of chondrosarcoma has been associated with syndromes of skeletal maldevelopment. Transformation of cartilaginous exostosis, enchondromas, or chondroplasia to chondrosarcoma has occurred. Chondrosarcoma also occurs in individuals with Ollier's disease, a syndrome of polyostotic benign cartilage tumors.

Pathophysiology

Chondrosarcoma arises from the cartilage. Large areas of the intracellular matrix of tumor cartilage may become heavily ossified (noncalcified bone-forming tissue); however, unlike osteosarcoma the osteoid tissue does not directly evolve out of sarcomatous stroma.

There are two forms of chondrosarcoma. The central form arises in the interior of the medullary cavity and may do so spontaneously or through malignant changes in a preexisting enchondroma. The peripheral form grows out from the bone through malignant changes in the cartilage cap of an osteochondroma, usually in individuals with multiple exostoses, which are benign cartilage tumors. In peripheral chondrosarcoma and central chondrosarcomas that have arisen from enchondromas, heavy calcification or ossification of larger parts of the intracellular matrix of the tumor cartilage occurs. In other chondrosarcomas the neoplastic tissue generally consists of compacted islands of cartilage with hyaline matrix. If the tumor is large and bulky, areas may exist in which the cartilage is softer, myxomatous, and necrotic.

The diagnosis of chondrosarcoma is based on cytologic changes of the cartilage cells. A cartilage tumor is considered malignant in the presence of many cells with plump nuclei, that is, more than a few cells with two such nuclei or clumps of chromatin.

The most frequent sites of chondrosarcoma include the pelvic bones, long bones, scapula, and ribs. Less frequent sites include bones of the hand and foot, the nose, the maxilla, and the base of the skull.

Most chondrosarcomas do not tend to metastasize early but rather remain slow growing and locally invasive. When advanced chondrosarcoma does become aggressive, it tends to metastasize via venous channels to the lungs and heart. Regional lymph nodes occasionally may be involved.

Assessment

Individuals with chondrosarcoma usually have a relatively long but unremarkable history. Medical advice often is sought for a slow-growing mass with intermittent dull, aching, pain at the tumor site. Physical examination can reveal a firm enlargement over the affected area. Joints may be swollen and exhibit restricted motion if they are near the affected area.

Radiographs of chondrosarcoma show a lobular pattern with or without calcification. If calcification is present, it usually is seen in a circular or semicircular pattern. Central chondrosarcomas in the long bones may show thickening of the cortex because of swelling of the shaft. The peripheral chondrosarcoma may demonstrate a vast, dense, blotchy appearance. Ragged, irregular, radiopaque streaks extending away from the central part of the lesion may be seen.

Treatment

When the diagnosis of chondrosarcoma has been established, surgery is indicated. If the tumor is of central origin and has not extended through the cortex, wide resection and reconstruction are considered. Limb salvage surgery or amputation are options.

At present, chondrosarcoma remains nearly totally refractory to chemotherapeutic efforts inasmuch as chondrosarcomas usually have a poor blood supply. Consequently, drugs given intravenously do not reach the tumor in concentrations that are high enough to be effective. The benefit of chemotherapy as an adjuvant to surgery has not been established.

Radiotherapy has limited effectiveness and is reserved for palliation of advanced or inoperable chondrosarcomas.

Individuals with a diagnosis of chondrosarcoma have a considerably better prognosis than those with osteosarcoma. The overall survival rate of individuals treated with wide resection or amputation has been reported to be 67% at 5 years and 50% at 10 years.[41] In this series survival correlated well with the designated histologic grade of the lesion. The estimated 10-year survival rate of individuals with grade 1 tumors is 87% and that of individuals with grade 2 tumors is 41%. For those with grade 3 lesions, the 5-year survival rate is 44%, and the 10-year survival rate is 27%.

FIBROSARCOMA

Epidemiology and Etiology

Fibrosarcoma is rare and accounts for fewer than 4% of primary malignant bone tumors.[20] This type of neoplasm may occur at any age but is rare in children. There is no evident sex predominance.

Paget's disease may be a predisposing factor in the development of fibrosarcoma. In addition, the tumor may develop as a sequel to therapeutic irradiation or may develop at the site of an old bone infarct. Chronic osteomyelitis or fibrous dysplasia also may be a predisposing factor in the development of fibrosarcoma.

Pathophysiology

Fibrosarcoma is a malignant fibroblastic tumor that fails to develop tumor osteoid or bone in its local invasive growth site or in its metastatic foci. Periosteal new bone may be laid down as a direct extension of the tumor.

Like osteosarcoma, fibrosarcoma usually originates within the medullary cavity. It eventually penetrates the overlying cortex and extends into the periosteum and muscle. Occasionally a fibrosarcoma may arise periosteally and extend into the interior of contiguous bone.

Histologic findings show that fibrosarcomas range from well differentiated to poorly differentiated. Rapidly growing tumors reflect cytologic changes such as moderate anaplasia, cell irregularity, and many mitotic figures, and they tend to metastasize early. Less aggressive fibrosarcomas develop more slowly, taking longer to penetrate the cortex of the bone. Some fibrosarcomas are surprisingly indolent in their growth patterns and may show very little change over a period of years.

The femur and the tibia are the most common sites of occurrence and account for 50% of all fibrosarcomas.[23] The neoplasm also may be observed in the humerus, radius, ulna, skull, and facial and pelvic bones. Metastasis occurs primarily to the lungs.

Assessment

The person with a fibrosarcoma, like those with other primary bone tumors, usually has initial pain and swelling of the affected area.

There are no radiologic features that distinguish fibrosarcoma from osteosarcoma. If the cortex is destroyed, extension into soft tissue frequently occurs. Periosteal bone reaction may be seen.

The diagnosis of fibrosarcoma is based on histologic study. The degree of differentiation of the malignant fibroblasts, the cellular pattern, and the amount of collagen produced vary. The poorly differentiated tumors are more aggressive.

Treatment

When the diagnosis of fibrosarcoma has been established, radical surgery is indicated. A radical resection may be considered for a well-differentiated tumor or low-grade tumor that is still confined to the cortex. Amputation is an option. Fibrosarcoma is considered to be radioresistant; consequently, the use of radiotherapy is reserved for inoperable tumors. Adjuvant chemotherapy programs after surgical treatment are being evaluated for reducing the incidence of microscopic residual metastatic disease.[23]

The prognosis for fibrosarcoma is guarded. The 5- and 10-year survival rates after radical surgery have been reported at 21.8% and 28%, respectively.[23] Individuals with poorly differentiated lesions have an extremely poor prognosis.

EWING'S SARCOMA

Epidemiology and Etiology

Ewing's sarcoma accounts for 5% of all malignant bone tumors.[23] Eighty percent of such tumors are diagnosed in individuals younger than 30 years of age, and 66% more males are affected than females. These patients are younger than any other patient affected by primary malignant bone tumors. The development of Ewing's sarcoma has not been strongly linked to any specific etiologic factor.

Pathophysiology

Ewing's sarcoma is a primitive, multicentric tumor that appears to be derived from the mesenchymal connective tissue framework of bone marrow. The tumor usually arises in the marrow spaces in the shaft of long bones and rarely involves the epiphysis.

The early stage of development is characterized by condensation of the shaft of the bone, followed by subperiosteal and endosteal formation of new bone in the cortex. The tumor itself does not give rise to bone directly. New bone is the result of periosteal reaction to the neoplastic tissue that has penetrated the cortex. The tumor proceeds to involve a greater portion of the shaft and finally extends through the periosteum, involving surrounding soft tissue.

On microscopic examination, Ewing's sarcoma is characterized by the presence of uniform cells with indistinct borders. These cells are packed closely together and contain prominent round or ovoid nuclei and have finely divided chromatin.

No one site seems to predominate in the development of Ewing's sarcoma. The tumor commonly is situated in the pelvis and the diaphyseal or metadiaphyseal regions of long bones. Ewing's sarcomas metastasize early and most frequently involve the lungs. The lymph nodes and the skull are other frequent sites of metastasis. On autopsy, a considerable portion of skeleton is affected. It is unclear whether these bone lesions represent metastatic spread or independent development of disease in multiple sites. Metastasis may be present in nearly 20% of individuals at the time of diagnosis.

The individual with Ewing's sarcoma frequently has a history of pain that has become increasingly severe and persistent. In addition to local pain, the person may complain of disability or stiffness in a corresponding joint. The physical examination usually reveals a palpable and tender mass. The temperature of the overlying skin is increased, and small superficial blood vessels may be seen.

Assessment

Many individuals have initial fever, anemia, high erythrocyte sedimentation rates, and sometimes leukocytosis. These symptoms can lead to an incorrect diagnosis of osteomyelitis. It has been observed that such findings result in a fulminating disease course that ends in death within a few months. Individuals who did not initially have such findings tended to survive longer. Glaubiger and colleagues[42] noted that normal lactic dehydrogenase, small distal primary lesion (8 cm), and absence of metastasis were better prognostic factors for the patient with Ewing's sarcoma.

Radiographs of Ewing's sarcoma show bone destruction that involves the shaft. Varying amounts of periosteal thickening may be present, with "onion skin" layers of laminated subperiosteal new bone. A large soft tissue mass frequently will be visualized as well. It is difficult to diagnose Ewing's sarcoma on the basis of radiographic findings.

Treatment

Integrated therapy with radiation and/or surgery in combination with chemotherapy is the treatment of choice for Ewing's sarcoma. The tumor is extremely radiosensitive and capable of being cured locally with 5000 cGy by means of shrinking fields. Improved techniques and the use of supervoltage radiation contribute to effective irradiation of the tumor without unacceptable damage to normal bone, skin, and subcutaneous tissue. The National Cancer Institute reports a 3% incidence of radiation-induced sarcoma after combined chemotherapy and radiation in Ewing's patients.[43] Physical therapy for gentle range of motion exercises during radiotherapy and for approximately 1 year after therapy has improved leg function.[44]

Surgery combined with radiotherapy improves the local control rate. Surgery can decrease the need for extremely high radiation doses.[45] Limb salvage and amputation are both options. The goal is to eradicate the tumor and maintain function. This goal is considered during the planning of treatment.

Surgery or radiation alone will not prevent the appearance of tumor foci elsewhere in the skeleton nor pulmonary metastasis. Consequently, neoadjuvant chemotherapy, as prophylactic therapy for micrometastases, is used as part of the initial treatment for all patients. Using actinomycin, doxorubicin, vincristine, and cyclophosphamide, Sim[23] reported an actuarial 5-year disease-free survival rate of 40% to 50%. Ifosfamide is a new agent with a response rate approaching 50%.[46] Treatment duration is usually 6 to 12 months. Local treatment (surgery and/or radiation) begins approximately 3 months after chemotherapy starts.

METASTATIC BONE TUMORS

The incidence of metastatic bone tumors has decreased because of the advent of multimodal treatment approaches to controlling local disease and distant metastases. When metastatic bone tumors do occur, they significantly affect musculoskeletal function and decrease life expectancy. Pain, functional limitation, and coping with the knowledge of recurrent disease place the individual under considerable stress. Metastasis to bone occurs by means of one of three mechanisms: direct extension of the tumor to adjacent bone, arterial embolization after passage through the right cardiopulmonary circulation, and direct venous spread through the pelvic and vertebral veins. A number of tumors have a predilection for metastasizing to bone. These include primary tumors of the lung, breast, prostate, kidney, and thyroid. Gastric, colonic, pancreatic, and testicular tumors also have been shown to metastasize to bone.

The individual with a metastatic bone lesion typically has initial dull, aching bone pain. Bone pain will increase steadily as the day progresses, peaking in the night hours and interfering with usual sleep patterns. If the lesion is permitted to progress, the pain may become so severe that weight bearing becomes intolerable. Fractures may occur if a sufficient amount of bone is involved. Tenderness and/or warmth over the lesion may be found on physical examination. In addition, loss of range of motion of involved joints may be noted.

Diagnostic evaluation includes conventional radiography and bone scanning techniques. Biopsy is not necessary if the appearance of the lesion is consistent with the known primary tumor. Biopsy is indicated in the absence of a known or suspected primary tumor. Alterations in the results of a number of laboratory studies may occur, depending on the nature of the primary lesion. For example, normocytic, normochromic anemia and a rapid erythrocyte sedimentation rate are characteristic of multiple myeloma. Hypercalcemia in the presence of a normal alkaline phosphatase level is associated with breast carcinoma. Elevations of serum acid phosphatase occur with prostatic cancer. Tumors of the lung may mimic a number of endocrinopathies.

Once the diagnosis of a metastatic bone lesion has been established, treatment may include surgery, chemotherapy, or radiotherapy. The goals of surgical interventions are augmenting the material strength of the bone, increasing resistance to fracture, improving functional use of the part, and resuming ambulatory status. This may be accomplished through prosthetic arthroplasty, including allograft arthroplasty or the use of an intramedullary stabilizing device.[47] Bone cement or methyl methacrylate is used to fill the cavity created by the tumor and to stabilize the implant. Individuals treated prophylactically for an impending pathologic hip fracture have fewer complications, a lower incidence of stabilization failure, and a high level of postoperative ambulation.[48]

Spinal lesions usually are managed by external bracing by means of collars and rigid braces. If the lesion is well advanced, however, more extensive procedures, such as use of the Harrington rod, may be necessary to provide stability and prevent paraplegia.

Amputation is indicated for tumors of the lower extremity that cannot be stabilized or that continue to fracture despite surgical intervention. Amputation also is an option for nonhealing lesions that do not respond to local care or radiotherapy.

Preoperative radiotherapy may be used to shrink the tumor to facilitate surgical intervention or for palliation of pain. In addition, it may be used postoperatively as adjuvant therapy or alone in cases in which surgical intervention would not provide any benefits. After internal fixation of involved bone, radiation is given to kill tumor cells and allow the surgical implant to maintain anatomic alignment. If the patient survives 6 months, near-normal bone structure may be restored.[49]

Chemotherapy also is used to reduce the tumor cell mass. Chemotherapy and its effect on normal cell function, however, interfere adversely with wound healing. If chemotherapy has been used before surgery, it is necessary to delay surgery until the leukocyte count is near normal. Similarly, institution of chemotherapy in the postoperative phase should be delayed until adequate collagen synthesis has occurred.

CONCLUSION

The treatment of bone malignancies is complex. The overall survival rates have improved since the late 1970s. Progress can be attributed to factors such as improved staging, adjuvant chemotherapy, and pulmonary resections. With the advent of limb salvage surgery, fewer patients are having amputations without altering their survival rates. It is hoped that ongoing studies will continue to show improved survival rates for bone cancer.

REFERENCES

1. Del Ragato JA, Spjut HJ: Cancer: Diagnosis, Treatment and Prognosis. St Louis, CV Mosby, 1985.
2. American Cancer Society: Cancer Facts and Figures, 1989. New York, American Cancer Society, 1989.

3. Yamamoto T, Wakabayshi T: Bone tumors among the atomic bomb survivors of Hiroshima and Nagasaki. Acta Pathol Jpn 19:201-202, 1969.
4. Miller RW: Deaths from childhood leukemia and solid tumors among twins and other sibs in the United States, 1960-67. NCI Monogr 46:203-209, 1971.
5. Uhthoff H: Current concept of diagnosis and treatment of bone and soft tissue tumor. Berlin, Springer-Verlag, 1984.
6. Lodwick G: Solitary malignant tumors of bone. Semin Roentgenol 1:293-313, 1966.
7. Zimmer W, Berquist T, McLeod R, et al: Bone tumor magnetic resonance imaging versus computed tomography. Radiology 155:709-718, 1985.
8. American Joint Committee on Cancer: Manual for Staging of Cancer (ed 3). New York, JB Lippincott, 1988.
9. Schajowicz I, Ackerman V, Sissions HA: International histological classification of tumours. Geneva, World Health Organization, monograph no. 6, 1972.
10. Enneking WF, Spanier S, Goodman M: A system for surgical staging of musculoskeletal sarcomas. Clin Orthop 153:106-119, 1980.
11. Dahlin DC, Unni K: Bone Tumors. Springfield, Ill, Charles C Thomas, 1986.
12. Consensus conference: Limb-sparing treatment of adult soft tissue sarcoma and osteosarcomas. JAMA 254:1791-1794, 1985.
13. Lewis M: The use of an expandable and adjustable prosthesis in the treatment of childhood malignant bone tumors of the extremity. Cancer 57:499-502, 1986.
14. Simon M, Aschliman M, Thomas N, et al: Limb-salvage treatment versus amputation for osteosarcoma of the distal end of femur. J Bone Joint Surg [AM] 68:1331-1337, 1986.
15. Sim FH, et al: Reconstruction of musculo-skeletal defects about the knee for tumor. Clin Orthop 221:188-201, 1987.
16. Otis J, et al: Energy cost during gait in osteosarcoma patients after resection and knee replacement and after above-the-knee amputation. J Bone Joint Surg [AM] 67:606-610, 1985.
17. Parrish FF: Allograft replacement of all or part of the end of a long bone following excision of a tumor: Report of twenty-one cases. J Bone Joint Surg [AM] 55:1-22, 1973.
18. Mankin HJ, Fogelson FS, Thrasber AZ: Massive resection and allograft transplantation in the treatment of malignant bone tumors. N Engl J Med 294:1247-1255, 1976.
19. Gitelis S, Heligman D, Quill G, et al: The use of large allograft for tumor reconstruction and salvage of the failed total hip arthroplasty. Clin Orthop 231:62-70, 1988.
20. Piasecki P, Rodts M: Bone banking: Its role in skeletal tumor reconstruction. Orthop Nurs 4(5):56-60, 1985.
21. Eilber FR, Morton DL, Eckardt J, et al: Limb salvage for skeletal and soft tissue sarcomas. Cancer 54:2579-2589, 1984.
22. Dick H, Malinin T, Mnaymneh W, et al: Massive allograft implantation following radical resection of high-grade tumor requiring adjuvant chemotherapy treatment. Clin Orthop 197:88-95, 1985.
23. Sim FH: Diagnosis and Treatment of Bone Tumors: A Team Approach. Thorofare, N J, Slack, 1983.
24. Melzack R: The Challenge of Pain. New York, Basic Books, 1983.
25. Roth Y, Sugarbaker P: Pains and sensations after amputation. Arch Phys Med Rehabil 61:490-493, 1980.
26. Sugarbaker P, Weiss C, Davidson D, et al: Increasing phantom limb pain as a symptom of cancer recurrence. Cancer 54:373-375, 1984.
27. Sherman R, Ernst J, Barja R, et al: Phantom pain: A lesson in the necessity for careful clinical research on chronic pain problems. J Rehabil Res Dev 25(2):7-10, 1988.
28. Kostuik J, Gillespie M: Amputation surgery and rehabilitation. New York, Churchill Livingstone, 1981.
29. Cohen L, Hendrickson J, Mansell J, et al: Response of sarcomas of bone and of soft tissue to neutron beam therapy. Int J Radiat Oncol Biol Phy 10:821-824, 1984.
30. Schaller R, Haas J, Schaller J, et al: Improved survival in children following resection of pulmonary metastases. J Pediatr Surg 17:546-555, 1987.
31. Malawer M: Impact of short course of neoadjuvant chemotherapy and the choice of surgical procedure for high grade sarcoma of extremities. Proc Am Soc Clin Oncol 8:320, 1989.
32. Unni KK, Dahlin DC, Baebout JW: Periosteal osteogenic sarcoma. Cancer 37:2476-2485, 1976.
33. Campanacci M, Bacci G, Gaetano S, et al: The treatment of osteosarcoma of the extremities. Cancer 48:1569-1581, 1981.
34. Sutow WW, Gehan E, Dyment P, et al: Multidrug adjuvant chemotherapy of osteosarcoma: Interim report of Southwest Oncology Group studies. Cancer Treat Rep 62:265-270, 1978.
35. Rosen G, Caparros B, Hovos A, et al: Preoperative chemotherapy for osteogenic sarcoma. Cancer 49:1221-1230, 1982.
36. Lane J: Surgical management of osteogenic sarcoma of lower limb. Bull N Y Acad Med 61:395-403, 1985.
37. Eilber F, Giulano A, Eckardt J, et al: Adjuvant chemotherapy for osteosarcoma: A prospective trial. J Clin Oncol 5:21-26, 1987.
38. Winkler W, Beron G, Kotz R, et al: Adjuvant chemotherapy of osteosarcoma. J Clin Oncol 6:329-337, 1988.
39. DeVita V, Hellman S, Rosenberg S, et al: Cancer (ed 3). Philadelphia, JB Lippincott, 1989.
40. Bacci G, Springfield D, Capanna R, et al: Neoadjuvant chemotherapy for osteosarcoma of the extremity. Clin Orthop 224:268-276, 1987.
41. Gitelis S, Bertoni S, Picci P, et al: Chondrosarcoma of bone. J Bone Joint Surg [Am] 63:1248-1257, 1981.
42. Glaubiger D, Makoch R, Schwarz J, et al: Determination of prognostic factors and their influence on therapeutic results of Ewing's sarcoma. Cancer 45:2213-2219, 1980.
43. Donaldson S: The value of adjuvant chemotherapy in the management of sarcomas in children. Cancer 55:2184-2197, 1985.
44. Jentzsch R, Binder H, Cramer H, et al: Leg function after radiotherapy for Ewing's sarcoma. Cancer 47:1267-1278, 1981.
45. Brown A, Fixsen J, Plowman P: Local control of Ewing's sarcoma: An analysis of 67 patients. Br J Radiol 60:261-268, 1987.
46. Magrath I, Sandlund J, Raynor A, et al: A phase II study of ifosfamide in treatment of recurrent sarcomas in young people. Cancer Chemother Pharmacol 18(2):25-28, 1986 (suppl).
47. Jaffe M, Goorin A, Link M, et al: Reconstruction for defects of the proximal part of the femur using allograft arthroplasty. J Bone Joint Surg [Am] 70:507-516, 1988.
48. Gitelis S, Hammerberg K, Sheinkop S, et al: Surgery in the management of metastic hip disease. Orthopedics 5:1004-1011, 1982.
49. Shocker J, Brady L: Radiation therapy for bone metastasis. Clin Orthop 169:38-43, 1982.

Chapter 35

Breast Cancer

Michelle Goodman, RN, MS

Nancy Harte, RN, MS

INTRODUCTION

Breast cancer is one of the leading causes of cancer death for women 35 to 54 years of age. The incidence of breast cancer increases rapidly with age until menopause, after which time it increases more slowly with advancing years. Over 70% of all breast cancer occurs in women who are older than 50, and less than 2% of all breast cancer occurs before the age of 30.[1] In 1963, the lifetime risk of the disease was about 5.5%, or 1 in every 18 women with an estimated general life span of 72 years.[2] The present statistics indicate that a woman in the general population has a 7% risk of developing breast cancer by the age of 70, or 1 in every 10 women.[3]

Despite improvements in therapeutic strategies, the death rate of breast cancer has remained unchanged over the past four decades. This may in part be related to the fact that there has been a relative increase in the incidence of breast cancer, especially among premenopausal women.[4] The average 32-year-old woman has an 8% risk of developing breast cancer. Of interest is the age-specific incidence rate for women between 35 and 39 years of age, which has increased more than 50% during the past 30 years. The incidence has increased in each of the 5-year age groups between 25 and 54 years of age.

Nearly 120,000 new cases of female breast cancer are diagnosed yearly. Of that number, approximately one third of women will die of their disease. Until screening methods become more sophisticated and available to detect preinvasive disease earlier, and until more is known about preventive measures (both endocrine and chemoprevention), the mortality rate is likely to remain unchanged.

The nurse caring for the woman with breast cancer must be acutely aware of the natural history of the disease, the known high-risk factors associated with breast cancer, and the controversies surrounding detection techniques and treatment choices.

ETIOLOGY

Experimental and clinical data indicate that the development of breast cancer is not a chance event. The genesis of breast cancer seems to be a multiphasic process involving many factors that are influential in the ongoing duel between tumor growth potential and host resistance.

Attempts are being made to reveal the etiology of breast cancer through an intense study of its epidemiology. As populations are identified in whom the incidence of the disease is increased, a genetic, hormonal, or biochemical factor may be identified that is considered significant in etiology. Epidemiologic features, when statistically correlated with incidence of disease, designate a particular factor as a "risk factor." Each risk factor merely serves as one piece of the puzzle because there are so many different factors that either increase or decrease a woman's risk of developing breast cancer. The highest incidence of breast cancer is in women 50 to 59 years of age. There is, however, a first-peak occurrence in premenopausal women or menopausal women between the ages of 45 and 49. The high incidence in this age group is thought to be related to ovarian estrogens. The second peak incidence occurs in women between 65 and 69 years of age and appears to be related to an imbalance of adrenal estrogens.

Hormonal Factors

Hormones have long been implicated in the genesis of breast cancer. The fact that women have much higher rates of breast cancer than men (100:1), the beneficial effect of hormonal manipulation by bilateral oophorectomy, and the therapeutic administration of pharmacologic doses of exogenous hormones substantiate the important role of hormones in certain human breast cancers. Women who have an adverse hormonal milieu are considered to be at high risk (eg, a woman who had a menarche before age 12 or a late natural menopause, with 40 or more years of ovarian function, has 2.5 times the normal risk of breast cancer). Women who have had an oophorectomy before 40 years of age without exogenous estrogen replacement have one-half the risk. Because lactation effectively inhibits ovarian function, it has been hypothesized, although not proved, that breast-feeding, like oophorectomy, reduces the risk of breast cancer.

The age at which a woman has her first full-term child appears to be strongly related to the subsequent risk of developing breast cancer. Women who have their first full-term pregnancy before age 20 have a relative risk of breast cancer that is only one third that of women who have had their first full-term pregnancy after age 35. Nulliparous women are at greater risk than most parous women, except for women who have their first full-term pregnancy after age 35, in whom the risk is greater.[1] The protective effect of early age at first birth is significant even among the elderly (age 70 to 80 years) and is of concern given the trend toward delay in having children together with an apparent rise in infertility.[5]

Hormones undoubtedly play a significant role in the etiology of breast cancer. Although these hormones are not mutagenic, it seems reasonable to assume that they act as cocarcinogens or promoters whereby they affect the rate of cellular proliferation, cellular atrophy, or differentiation of epithelial stem cells.[6]

In women three estrogens are normally found: estradiol, estrone, and estriol. Estriol has little if any estrogenic action and virtually no carcinogenic potential. When estriol and progesterone are present in adequate amounts, they are thought to have a biochemical antineoplastic effect that opposes estradiol, the strongest estrogen.

During pregnancy, estriol is increased tenfold over the other two more potent estrogens, especially in the last trimester. Estriol is thought to behave antagonistically to the carcinogenic actions of estradiol and estrone. The ratio of estriol to estradiol and estrone has been found to be lowered in women with a high risk of developing breast cancer. These hormone ratios may be genetically determined. Further research is needed before these findings can be applied to the detection or possible prevention of breast cancer.

The evidence that endogenous hormones are somehow related to the development of breast cancer suggests that exogenous hormones might increase a woman's risk of benign or malignant breast disease. There is evidence to suggest that high doses of exogenous estrogens are carcinogenic.[6] For instance, high doses of exogenous estrogens result in the development of mammary tumors in experimental animals and male transsexuals. The incidence of breast cancer is also increased in women who are given high doses of estrogens as treatment for infertility.[6] In women receiving low doses of conjugated estrogens (Premarin) for menopausal symptoms, the risk of breast cancer does not appear to be increased. However, when higher doses of estrogens are used for many years (more than 6) in the presence of additional risk factors such as nulliparity and family history, the risk of breast cancer is increased, particularly for perimenopausal women using estrogen (estradiol) and progestin in combination.[7] There is no firm evidence that the risk of breast cancer is either increased or decreased in women who use oral contraceptives, even for prolonged periods.[8,9] However, the significance of such issues as duration of oral contraceptive use, hormonal composition of the drug, reproductive age, and their relationship with other risk factors remains controversial.

Diet

Another epidemiologic finding related to endocrine factors is the greater incidence of breast cancer in postmenopausal women who are obese. A diet high in saturated fats increases the amount of biliary steroids needed to digest the fats, and androstenedione is converted to estrone in adipose tissue. These biliary steroids are converted to estrone and estradiol and are the primary sources of estrogen in postmenopausal women. However, despite the National Cancer Institute's recommendation to limit fat intake as a way to decrease the risk of developing breast cancer, it is important to note that there have been no prospective studies to demonstrate that dietary modification (decreased fat intake) in women will decrease the risk of developing breast cancer.[10] Although the epidemiologic data linking risk of developing breast cancer and high-fat diets are relatively strong, the major impact of high-fat diets may occur in children, especially at puberty, and influence risk by affecting endocrine function.[1,11]

It is reasonable to surmise that factors that determine tumor development may also affect the course of the disease. The influence of dietary fat consumption and obesity on breast cancer recurrence and survival has been documented.[12-14] Although not all studies support this relationship, overall findings seem to indicate that, whatever the reason for weight gain in the woman with breast cancer, the evidence of association between disease recurrence and decreased survival appears strong. Women who have breast cancer and who are obese are more likely to develop metastases and have a shorter survival than nonobese women.[13] Ingram et al[14] note that obese women are more likely to have menstrual irregularities and have been found to have elevated levels of non-protein-bound and total estrogens, thus providing a possible mechanism by which obesity may influence the development of breast disease.

Hereditary Factors

Evidence indicates that a woman whose family tree includes a first- or second-degree relative with breast cancer is herself at risk. A woman whose mother has breast cancer may expect a lifetime risk of between 9% and 23%, depending on the mother's age and menopausal status when the disease occurred and whether the mother had unilateral or bilateral disease.[15] The cumulative lifetime risk is nearly normal if the woman's mother was postmenopausal and had unilateral disease, whereas this risk increases to 18% if the mother was postmenopausal with bilateral cancer. If the woman was premenopausal with bilateral cancer, the cumulative lifetime risk rises to 53%.[16] If a woman has two female relatives with breast cancer, her risk ranges from 10% to 50%.[17] Women with a family history of breast cancer generally are found to have breast cancer at a younger age (20 to 44 years) and have bilateral breast cancer five times more often than do premenopausal women with no family history. Lynch et al[18] suggest that mothers with breast cancer may transmit a deleterious gene to 50% of their daughters that selectively predisposes breast and ovarian tissues to malignant transformation. Caution must be exercised in interpreting these findings, especially in terms of counseling women who have a family history of breast cancer. Not all family studies show familial aggregation. In fact, the majority (75% to 85%) of women with breast cancer have no known relative with the disease.[19]

The well-known differences in breast cancer throughout the world suggest a genetic influence. The most frequently noted difference is the extremely low risk of breast cancer in Japanese women in Japan. This low risk seems to hold also for Japanese women in the United States who maintain their low-fat dietary habits. Jewish women of European descent are at an increased risk of developing breast cancer compared with those of non-European descent. A study conducted by Rosen et al[20] reveals evidence that suggests that the incidence of breast cancer in premenopausal black women is increasing.

A woman who has breast cancer in one breast has approximately a 14% chance of developing cancer in the other breast, and about one third of these malignancies will be present at the same time as the original cancer.[19] Women with breast cancer are also at risk for subsequent development of cancer of the endometrium, ovary, and colon. Women with carcinoma of the uterine cervix are at a lower risk of developing breast cancer than the general population. The explanation for this negative correlation may be that the risk of cervical carcinoma is greater if sexual intercourse is begun at an earlier age, increasing the potential for full-term pregnancy at a young age, which decreases risk for breast cancer.

Fibrocystic Changes

The term *fibrocystic disease* is defined imprecisely in the literature and has been largely eliminated from medical terminology. The term *fibrocystic change* is preferable when describing simple proliferation of ductal epithelium and cystic changes in the breast. Although fibrocystic changes in the breast do occur, there is no correlation between these changes and the incidence of breast cancer. However, there is a four to five times greater risk of breast cancer in women who have atypical epithelial hyperplasia.[21,22] When other risk factors such as family history are also considered, risk for breast cancer can more than double.[21]

Noninvasive carcinoma in situ is rarely a palpable tumor and is usually diagnosed during a biopsy of a palpable lesion nearby. However, currently in situ cancers (intraductal, lobular, or intraepithelial carcinoma) may be detected on the basis of mammographic changes in the breast. In situ carcinoma, although it may be followed with frequent mammography, usually leads to mastectomy, since the goal is to eradicate potential foci of carcinoma in situ that are likely to become invasive carcinoma. This recommendation is complicated by the fact that according to Love et al[21] and others,[23] the risk of invasive carcinoma is usually equally distributed between both breasts and tends to be bilateral in 30% of cases.

Radiation

Women whose breast tissue has been exposed to repeated low doses of radiation are at higher risk of developing breast cancer. Specific examples would be women exposed to repeated fluoroscopic examinations to monitor pneumothorax therapy for tuberculosis,[24] women who received irradiation for the treatment of postpartum mastitis, women who received irradition for severe chest acne, and women exposed to ionizing radiation to the thymus in infancy.[25] Japanese women who were exposed to radiation following the atomic bombings of Hiroshima and Nagasaki continue to develop breast cancer at a higher rate than age-matched controls.

Nurses encounter many women who might be at risk of developing breast cancer. Nurses play an active role in detection and in instructing women in the community and the hospital about the technique of breast self-examination. Knowledge of the risk factors and a commitment to preventive health care practices will increase the nurse's ability to do casefinding and early detection.

TABLE 35-1 Risk Factors Related to the Development of Breast Cancer

Primary risk factors
Sex—female
Advanced age
Personal history of breast cancer
History of breast cancer in mother or sister
Secondary risk factors
History of breast cancer in a maternal or paternal grandmother or aunt
History of cystic breast disease
Birth of first infant after 30 years of age
Oral contraceptive use
Nulliparity
Early menarche and late menopause
Excessive exposure to ionizing radiation
History of cancer of the endometrium, ovary, or colon
Obesity or high intake of animal fat
Estrogen replacement therapy
Possible risk factors
Alcohol intake

PREVENTION AND DETECTION

Prevention

Prevention implies that one knows the cause of an event and can therefore intercede and stop the event from occurring. When addressing prevention of breast cancer, the exact causative factor is not known, so prevention is mainly limited to a discussion of risk reduction. Many of the risk factors for the development of breast cancer (Table 35-1) are not things that a woman has any direct control over, namely, her sex, her age, her past cancer history, her family history of cancer, or her menstrual factors.

Prophylactic Mastectomy

A prophylactic mastectomy, that is, the removal of all breast tissue, may be warranted in high-risk women; however, controversy exists over how much risk is enough to justify performing this procedure. Women for whom a prophylactic mastectomy may be indicated have been identified by Pennisi[26] as those with:

1. A strong family history of breast cancer and breasts exhibiting progressive nodularity.
2. A proven history of breast cancer in one breast and nodularity or cystic disease in the opposite breast. The incidence of a second breast cancer in the opposite breast is estimated to be 15% to 20%.

3. A suspicious mammogram and bilateral nodular breasts.
4. A breast biopsy that indicates moderate to severe microcystic or macrocystic disease, sclerosing adenosis, intraductal hyperplasia, papillomatosis, lobular neoplasia, or noninvasive forms of intraductal carcinoma.
5. Chronic cystic mastitis with repeated surgical biopsies and an overwhelming fear of breast cancer.

Two procedures are classified as a prophylactic mastectomy: a subcutaneous mastectomy or a total glandular mastectomy. A subcutaneous mastectomy removes a large portion of the breast tissue while retaining the skin and nipple-areola complex and is followed by implant reconstruction.[28] A total glandular mastectomy is the same procedure as a mastectomy for cancer except no axillary dissection is performed. Either procedure is only a means of risk reduction for the development of breast cancer because some residual breast tissue does remain.[29] Complications include hematoma formation, infection, flap necrosis, and problems with the implant.[30] Prophylactic mastectomy to prevent breast cancer may appear to be a drastic procedure, but it may be indicated for the young woman who has had a mastectomy for breast cancer in one breast or who has a strong family history and cystic nodular breasts.

Breast cancer may also be prevented if a woman reduces the risk factors within her control. Evidence suggests that avoiding obesity is one way to decrease the morbidity and mortality of breast cancer.[6] Similarly, reducing dietary fat and alcohol intake is also recommended. Studies regarding oral contraceptive use are suggestive but not yet conclusive. Women should consider these potential risks when making decisions about the use of these substances.

A new and developing area in cancer research is chemoprevention. The prophylactic use of the antiestrogen tamoxifen by women at high risk for the development of breast cancer has been proposed[31] and is currently being studied.

Detection and Screening

The majority of breast cancers (90%) are self-detected by women but are for the most part accidental findings. Even with the nationwide emphasis on early detection and instruction regarding breast self-examination, most lesions are quite large by the time a woman seeks medical attention. Larger tumors are associated with a higher incidence of nodal involvement, which can be directly related to survival. Likewise, data support the belief that survival of the woman with breast cancer is significantly increased when the disease is treated at an early stage (a reduction in mortality from 10% to 60%).[32]

The goal of screening and early detection is to decrease breast cancer mortality. Despite efforts at early detection, advancements in therapy, and various social and economic factors, the summary indicator of the seriousness of the breast cancer problem (ie, mortality from the disease) has been at a constant level for the past 55 years. This is partly attributable to underuse of the appropriate techniques of early detection.

In an attempt to determine the possible role of periodic screening in lowering breast cancer mortality, the American Cancer Society and the National Cancer Institute conducted a long-term randomized trial at the Health Insurance Plan of Greater New York (HIP) and the Breast Cancer Detection Demonstration Project (BCDDP). One of the major contributions of this nationwide effort was information about the diagnostic worth of mammography. Mammography was to be a major part of the screening effort and as such came under close scrutiny because of concern about radiation exposure. As a result, state radiation control boards examined radiation doses at various institutions, and, where doses were excessive, it was recommended that the total radiation exposure be 0.5 rad (cGy) for two views. At this dose a woman would need to undergo 13 mammograms per year to increase her lifetime inherent risk of breast cancer from 7% to 8%. The controversy regarding the risk of breast cancer's increasing as a result of mammography is for the most part resolved.[33]

The summary report of the BCDDP[34] suggests that mammography alone can detect 41.6% of the cancers discovered, compared with 33% in the HIP study. In addition, mammography can locate cancers that are nonpalpable (less than 1 cm) even to the most trained clinicians.

There are three established methods of early detection of breast cancer: physical examination, mammography, and breast self-examination. All three methods were used in the screening projects. The benefits of physical examination are well established in detecting breast cancer. In fact, 60% to 70% of the individuals in the HIP study had breast lumps first detected by this method. An important finding was that neither mammography nor physical examination alone is sufficient for early detection; rather, the two are complementary. This is especially true for younger women (under 40 years of age), whose breasts are more dense and in whom mammography is less effective in detecting small lesions that may be obvious on palpation.

The combination of mammography and physical examination was found to result in a higher percentage of negative axillary nodes in women diagnosed with breast cancer and the detection of a higher proportion of minimal noninvasive cancers. The prognosis for these women is assumed to be very good, which, loosely translated, means a decrease in mortality. However, the only screening program that has been found to decrease mortality was the HIP program. This detection and screening program used both mammography and physical examination and resulted in a 30% reduction in breast cancer mortality in women over 50 years of age. Regardless of how the data were analyzed, there was no benefit of screening in women 40 to 49 years of age. Routine screening was not recommended for women under 40 years of age for two reasons: (1) there is a lower incidence of breast cancer in this age group and (2) mammography is less diagnostic in this age group because of the increased density of the breast tissue. The recommendation of both the HIP and the BCDDP was that mass screening is not recommended on an ongoing basis. The cost is too high, and the yield is too low.

The current recommendations of the American Cancer Society and the National Cancer Institute for early detection of breast cancer in asymptomatic women include breast self-examination monthly for all women 20 years of age and older, physical examination by a trained clinician every 3 years for women 20 to 40 years of age, and physical examination every year for women over 40 years of age. Mammography is recommended for women 35 to 39 years of age to establish a baseline for comparison. In women 40 to 49 years of age, a mammogram is done yearly in women at high risk or according to the recommendation of each woman's personal physician. For women 50 years of age and older, a mammogram is recommended yearly.

For the majority of women, these guidelines seem appropriate and cost effective. However, women who have a higher risk of developing breast cancer need additional consideration. Woodward et al[25] found screening to be beneficial both in terms of cost effectiveness and detection of breast cancer in a cohort of women at increased risk for breast cancer because of prior irradiation for acute mastitis and a positive family history. In addition, the screening of asymptomatic women with a positive family history results in detection rates of 4.2 per 1000 in addition to the 5.9 to 9.4 per 1000, which is the prevalent rate in the general population.

Knowledge of a woman's risk factors for cancer should be incorporated into any educational session concerning breast self-examination. Based on these risk factors, a woman is given the current recommendations for early detection, including physical examination and mammography. Every woman is at risk for breast cancer, and health care professionals should depend less on obvious risk factors and more on the fact that breast cancer increases dramatically until menopause and continues thereafter at a steady rate.

Nurses can take an active role both in the community and in their work settings in teaching breast self-examination and in designing a comprehensive plan for early detection of breast cancer. The topic of breast self-examination and its role in early detection of breast cancer has come under close scrutiny over the past years.

At the National Breast Cancer Conference in New York in 1979, it was proposed that breast self-examination be evaluated scientifically to determine its overall worth and possible impact on survival. Unless there is good proof that breast self-examination is beneficial, promoting it would only lead to a false sense of security in some women and increased anxiety and frequent visits to a physician in other women.[35,36] These reasons for not promoting breast self-examination lack scientific rationale and imply that women are unable to discern an abnormality in their own breasts and that they would be frantically palpating their breasts and running to their physician with every complaint seeking reassurance. Another common argument against breast self-examination is that it would somehow replace the physician's examination. This has not been suggested by proponents of breast self-examination; rather, breast self-examination is only a part of the process of early detection, and a woman should be examined by a physician on a regular basis.

The important issues seem to be that breast self-examination is one early detection method that can aid in decreasing mortality, provided women have regular physical examinations, undergo mammography as recommended, and seek medical advice as soon as an abnormality is detected. It is a matter of great concern that most women know about the importance of breast self-examination but too few actually examine their breasts. Several surveys have been conducted to determine the knowledge base and attitudes women have toward breast self-examination as well as the actual performance of breast self-examination.[37-39] The findings are that 95% of women surveyed know about breast self-examination, 66% report practicing breast self-examination in a year's time, and 27% perform regular monthly examinations; however, only 13% do so correctly. The conclusion may be drawn that a significant number of women are aware of their risk of breast cancer and know how to perform breast self-examination, but these two factors are not enough to motivate a woman to examine her breasts regularly.

Recently a study was undertaken to examine breast self-examination compliance in women in light of the Health Belief Model.[40] There are two main constructs of this model: perceived threat of illness and perceived benefit of some health action in reducing the threat. Data were collected by questionnaire from 248 women, and several important findings were revealed that should be taken into account by the nurse when teaching breast self-examination. Embarassment, worry associated with breast self-examination, complexity of the procedure, effects of breast surgery on femininity, and lack of awareness of breast reconstruction were all related to poor breast self-examination compliance. Good compliance was associated with physician's practice of breast examination and interest in the patient's performing the task. In addition, providing patients with a reminder cue to facilitate the regular performance of the task was significant in increasing compliance.

One possible solution in the effort to motivate women to practice breast self-examination is to attempt to affect behavior when it is learned by incorporating early detection measures at a young age when health behaviors such as hygiene are first introduced. Theoretically, this would be far more effective than teaching a preventive health behavior at the adult level, when beliefs, fears, and mores are established. However, there will always be situations when the adult woman is the target of the teaching. Several authors[41,42] have recently written to address the needs of elderly women as they relate to breast self-examination instruction and practice, and the reader is referred to these for more detailed information.

PATHOPHYSIOLOGY

Recently clinicians have come to appreciate that breast cancer is not a homogeneous disease but rather protean, differing in histologic, biologic, and immunologic characteristics. Furthermore, breast cancer is often a systemic disease when first detected, as evidenced by the impressive failure rate following local therapy alone.[43] Therefore, attempts to treat the disease aggressively on a local level often fail to improve mortality.

The biologic nature of breast cancer provides for the existence of three populations of individuals with breast cancer:

1. Individuals whose tumors rarely metastasize and may even regress independent of therapy. The survival time of women with untreated breast cancer varies from 6 months to 19 years. Approximately 20% of women with untreated breast cancer survive 5 years or more.
2. Individuals whose disease metastasizes early to regional lymph nodes with only late systemic spread.
3. Individuals whose disease metastasizes early to adjacent lymph nodes and distant sites.

Cellular Characteristics

Each breast is composed of 15 to 20 glandular lobes that are arranged radially around the nipple. The lobes are drained by ducts that are slightly dilated just before opening into the nipple and are lined by columnar epithelium. There are a number of histopathologic types of breast cancer. The majority of primary breast cancers are adenocarcinomas, specifically infiltrating intraductal and infiltrating lobular carcinomas. Histologic and nuclear grading of tumor cells more completely define cellular characteristics. Histologic grading takes into account the growth pattern and cytologic features of differentiation, that is, the extent of tubule formation, nuclear characteristics, and mitotic rate. Nuclear grading involves the cytologic evaluation of the structural features of tumor nuclei. Histologic grades are recorded in a sequence that is the reverse of that used in nuclear grading.[44] Nuclear grade 3 refers to a well-differentiated tumor nuclei; a grade 2 implies intermediate changes; and grade 1, poorly differentiated tumor nuclei. Histologic grade I refers to well-differentiated cytologic features; grade II, intermediate changes; and grade III suggests poorly differentiated cytologic features and growth patterns. Patients with a high-grade, poorly differentiated invasive carcinoma have a significantly higher frequency of axillary node involvement, develop more recurrences, and are more likely to die of metastatic disease than women with low grade tumors.[44]

Epithelial tumors

The most common malignant tumor of the breast is an infiltrating intraductal carcinoma that may take various histologic forms, either well differentiated and slow growing, poorly differentiated and infiltrating, or highly malignant and undifferentiated with many mitoses and multinucleated giant cells. Infiltrating intraductal carcinoma comprises approximately 80% of carcinomas of the breast, may appear bilaterally, and unfortunately carries a poor prognosis. It primarily affects women in their early fifties. The overall 10-year survival rate is approximately 50%.

Colloid carcinoma, another type of epithelial carcinoma, is characterized by the presence of large pools of mucin interspersed with small islands of tumor cells. It constitutes about 2% of breast cancers and tends to metastasize late. Medullary carcinoma tends to be more circumscribed, which is a favorable prognostic sign. It is characterized by prominent lymphocytic infiltrate at the periphery.

Infiltrating lobular carcinoma occurs most frequently in women around 55 years of age and comprises about 7% of the carcinomas of the breast. Lobular carcinoma may be multifocal and is more frequently bilateral than intraductal carcinoma. Survival rates are similar to those noted for intraductal carcinoma.

Other malignant tumors

Cystosarcoma phyllodes is a bulky and usually circumscribed tumor with a low malignant potential that tends to be locally aggressive. More aggressive tumors may be difficult to distinguish from sarcomas and by nature tend to metastasize widely. Pure sarcomas of the breast are uncommon, as are lymphomas, but they have been reported.[44] Papillary carcinoma, metaplastic carcinoma, apocrine carcinoma, adenoid cystic carcinoma, and squamous cell carcinomas of the breast have also been reported.

Inflammatory carcinoma is characterized by a purplish color of the skin over the tumor. Because of subdermal lymphatic spread, prominent pores in the skin become congested, causing skin edema by lymph stasis. This peau d'orange (skin of the orange) appearance to the skin over the breast is characteristic of inflammatory carcinoma.[45]

In most situations, a palpable tumor is not present. There is usually invasion of the intramammary vascular spaces within the breast. Inflammatory breast cancer as a clinical entity occurs infrequently and is generally considered to be a grave prognostic sign.

Progression of Disease

Breast cancer metastasizes both by lymphatic and hematologic emboli. The primary lymphatic drainage is to the ipsilateral axillary nodes. These nodes may be bypassed, and the first nodes to be involved might be the supracla-

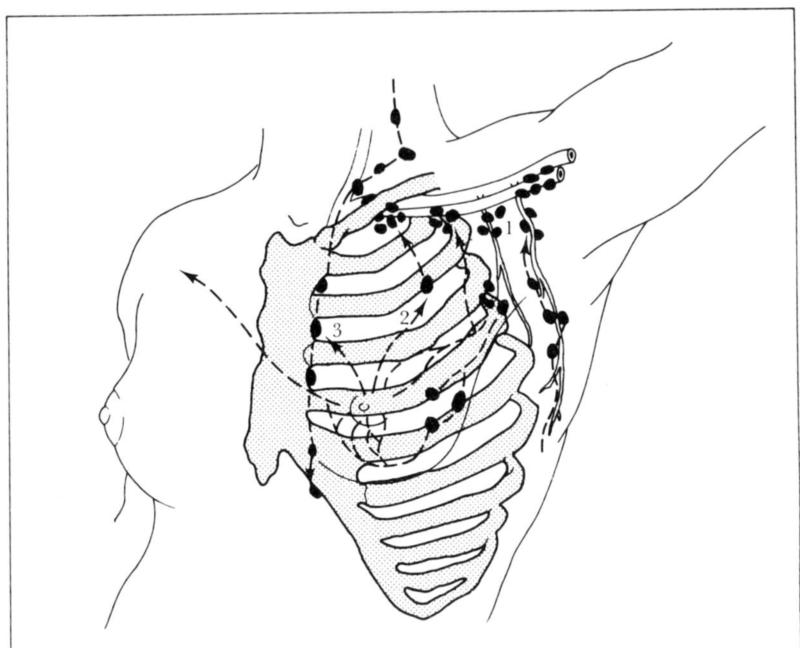

Lymphatics of the breast leading to (1) axillary nodes which are distributed over a large area from the lateral aspects of the breast proper to the axillary vessels; (2) interpectoral chain leading to interpectoral node (circle detail) and to high nodes in the axilla; (3) chain of the internal mammary leading frequently to node in second interspace and to supraclavicular and cervical nodes. The lymphatics of the breast may empty into the opposite axillary nodes.

FIGURE 35-1 Lymphatic drainage of the breast. (Source: Modified from Del Regato J, Spjut H (eds): Cancer: Diagnosis, Treatment, and Prognosis (ed 5). St Louis, CV Mosby, 1977.)

vicular and infraclavicular lymph nodes. Involvement of the supraclavicular nodes is routinely associated with distant spread. For lesions located more medially in the breast, the internal mammary nodes are involved as frequently as the axillary nodes, but there is an increased incidence of disease recurrence when medial nodes are involved compared with axillary node involvement. Approximately 50% of patients with breast cancer have axillary node involvement. The likelihood of axillary node involvement correlates directly with the size of the primary lesion. A 1-cm tumor is associated with a 25% risk, while a 3- to 4-cm tumor is associated with a 50% risk. The relationship between tumor size and metastases is fairly well established. Koscielny et al[47] found that metastases does not occur in half the cases until the tumor exceeds 3.56 cm in diameter. This finding lends optimism to the importance of early detection measures. With involvement of the internal mammary nodes, the cure rates drop precipitously because of the lack of local control and distant spread of the disease. Internal mammary node involvement occurs in about 20% of patients. When axillary nodes are positive, internal mammary node involvement rises to 30%. When axillary nodes are negative, internal mammary nodes are positive only 10% of the time.[47] Figure 35-1 depicts the major lymphatic drainage of the breast in order of occurrence. Each lymph node group may be involved singly or in combination with another group.

Breast cancer may metastasize widely and unpredictably either early in the course of the disease or late after a disease-free interval of many years. The time course to distant metastases depends on the size of the primary tumor, the number of positive nodes, and the histologic grade of the tumor. As a group, premenopausal women tend to have more widespread disease. The pulmonary system, bone, and liver are the most common sites of metastasis in breast cancer. Once pulmonary metastasis occurs, the tumor cells gain entrance into the arterial circulation, and brain as well as liver metastases are more common.

The areas of bone most commonly involved are the ribs, thoracic vertebrae, skull, pelvis, and upper femurs. Osseous metastases occur from hematologic emboli, disseminate through the vertebral vein, and may exist without pulmonary metastasis. Other metastatic sites of breast cancer include the pleura, kidneys, ovaries, pituitary gland, adrenal glands, and thyroid gland.

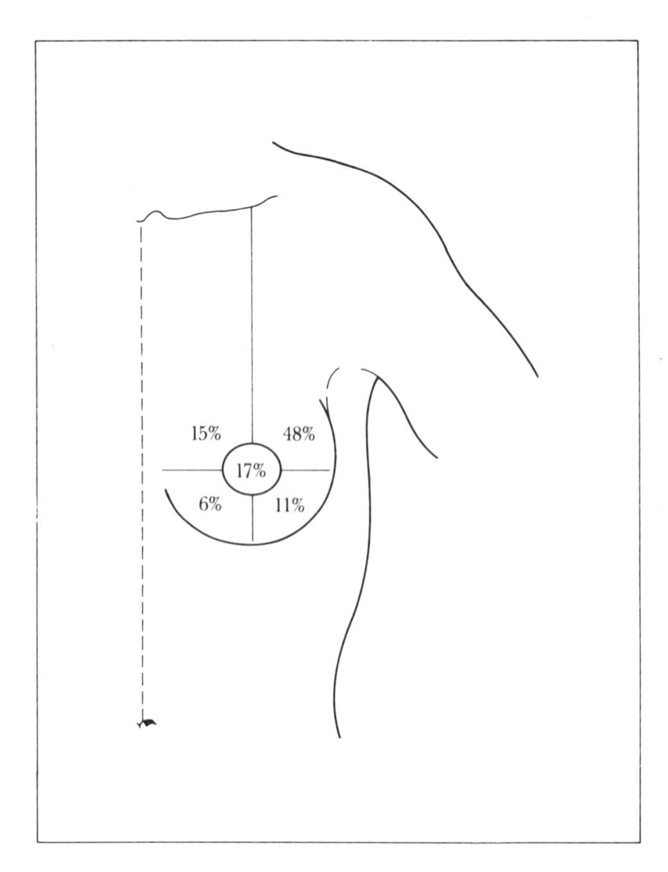

FIGURE 35-2 Incidence of breast cancer according to location.

CLINICAL MANIFESTATIONS

Carcinomas of the breast are most often located in the upper outer quadrant or beneath the nipple. The incidence of malignant disease is thought to be increased in these regions because a majority of breast tissue is found there (Figure 35-2). Breast carcinomas are more often located in the left breast than in the right breast.

Nearly eight of ten lumps that are biopsied are found to be benign. The clinical differences between benign and malignant disease are clear. The more obvious mobile mass that is encapsulated or circumscribed, with a distinct barrier from adjacent tissues, and found particularly in a premenopausal woman is most likely a fibroadenoma or a cyst. Malignant disease, on the other hand, usually has less distinct boundaries and lack of mobility because of tumor infiltration into adjacent tissues. A benign lesion is often soft and smooth with regular borders, whereas a malignant lesion is a firm, three-dimensional area with irregular borders.

Benign disease is frequently associated with bilateral, diffuse breast pain and tenderness that is more prominent at the time of the menstrual period. Often this pain radiates to the axilla. Pain is not a common symptom of breast carcinomas, but it may be present with more advanced local disease. The pain is characterized as focal, constant, and nonradiating and is not related to the menstrual period.

Benign disease is usually clear on transillumination, whereas malignant disease is opaque. Malignant disease is usually a solitary, unilateral lesion; benign disease may be multiple, bilateral lesions. Nipple discharge is most often a sign of benign disease but can indicate breast cancer if it is bloody, clear, or milky, spontaneous, and unilateral. Nipple ulceration or scaly skin at the nipple is suspicious of Paget's disease, an early form of breast carcinoma.

Clinical manifestations that are more suspicious of malignant disease are nipple retraction or elevation, which may be due to tumor fixation or infiltration into the underlying tissues. Skin dimpling or retraction also may be present and is possibly due to invasion of the suspensory ligaments and fixation to the chest wall. Heat and erythema of the breast skin may be related to inflammation, but they are also signs of inflammatory breast carcinoma. Skin edema, or peau d' orange (Figure 35-3), is characteristic of malignant disease. The edema is thought to be due to the invasion and obstruction of dermal lymphatics by tumor. Ulceration of the skin with secondary infection may be present. The presence of isolated skin nodules indicates invasion of blood vessels and lymphatics. This often results in implantation of tumor emboli in adjacent tissues and indicates that distant metastases are likely. Clinical presentation may also include, or be limited to, signs of local or distant metastatic disease.

Approximately 10% of women present with metastasis as the first indication of malignant disease. Firm, enlarged axillary lymph nodes that may be fixated are the result of tumor invasion into adjacent structures. This can result in obstruction of lymphatics and venous flow, with resultant edema of the arm. The most common complaint of women with distant metastatic disease is bone pain due to osseous metastasis. A pathologic fracture may be a presenting symptom as a result of metastatic disease to the bone. Parenchymal lung metastasis and pleural metastasis can present as a cough, pleuritic pain, shortness of breath, or vague chest discomfort; these, however, are not common presenting symptoms. Neurologic complaints suggest central nervous system (CNS) metastasis. Weight loss and anemia are signs of advancing disease and are rarely presenting symptoms.

ASSESSMENT AND DIAGNOSIS

The goal of the initial assessment of the woman with a breast mass is to determine the likelihood of a malignancy. A complete history of the patient is required, including a risk-factor profile, past history of breast disease, breast biopsies, and diagnostic studies of the breast as well as the chronology and character of the breast complaint according to the patient. Symptoms that might indicate distant metastasis may also be reviewed at this time. On completion of the history, a physical examination is performed. Careful inspection of both breasts, areolae, and nipples is

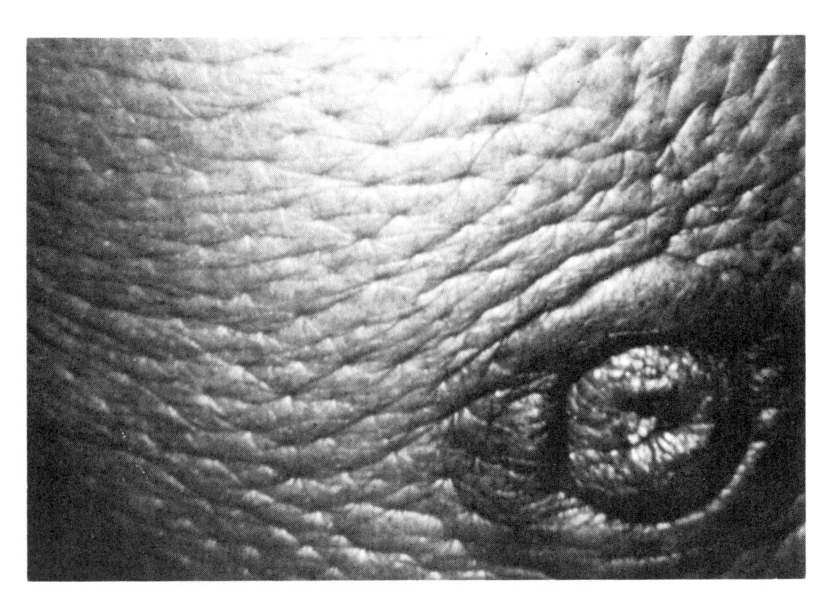

FIGURE 35-3 Peau d'orange.

followed by palpation of the breasts, nipples, suspicious masses, and supraclavicular and axillary lymph nodes.

Depending on the clinical evidence of disease, diagnostic studies may be indicated to evaluate one or both breasts. Mammography and ultrasonography are the most useful and routinely performed noninvasive tests. These tests should be obtained before proceeding with any invasive, diagnostic procedures. Thermography, computed tomography (CT), transillumination, and magnetic resonance imaging (MRI) are not standardly recommended in the diagnostic workup of a breast mass. This is due to their inability to diagnose small tumors, their inability to detect microcalcifications, their increased level of radiation exposure, and their expense.[49,50] Mammography is an adjunct to the physical examination and is not meant to replace it. Mammography is not solely done to evaluate a palpable mass but to detect an occult cancer in the same or other breast. According to Danforth et al,[51] "a negative mammogram should never be substituted for cytological or histological evaluation of a palpable mass and should never prevent the adequate evaluation of a mass seen as suspicious on physical exam."

The positive diagnosis of breast cancer can only be made by histologic examination following a closed or open biopsy. A closed biopsy is usually performed under local anesthesia in the physician's office by either a needle core biopsy or a fine needle aspiration (FNA). It should be noted that a FNA is only diagnostic if it is positive for malignant disease. Open biopsy techniques are either excisional or incisional and may be done under a general or local anesthetic. Excisional biopsies are usually indicated for masses smaller than 2 or 3 cm and allow for removal of the lump as well as a margin of normal tissue. For a larger mass, an incisional biopsy removes a part of the lesion only, from which histologic tests and estrogen-receptor status may be obtained to plan further treatment if necessary.

CLASSIFICATION AND STAGING

Women with breast cancer are grouped into various categories, or stages, according to characteristics of the tumor, nodal involvement, and the presence or absence of distant metastasis. Clinical staging of breast cancer is necessary because it indicates which therapeutic approaches may be advised and also assists in defining the prognosis. If surgery is indicated, a more accurate evaluation of the extent of the disease can be performed. Postsurgical staging affords the physician the opportunity to define the involvement of the nodes with greater precision and thereby predict the presence of occult metastasis and the advisability of adjuvant therapy.

Additional studies are indicated to determine the extent of disease and facilitate accurate clinical staging. The choice of these studies is based on the common sites for breast cancer to metastasize, which include lung, bone, liver, and adrenal glands. A chest film is obtained to evaluate the lungs for metastatic disease. A bone scan is done before treatment, especially if the woman is symptomatic and metastatic disease is suspected. A bone scan is a marginally sensitive test in that a lesion must be at least 1.5 to 2.0 cm to be detected. Unlike a radiograph, a bone scan permits bony metastases to be detected while the individual remains asymptomatic. A radiograph of a suspicious area found on bone scan will help differentiate a benign from a malignant lesion. Blood tests are done to evaluate blood chemistries, assess for anemia, and obtain baseline biologic markers (ie, carcinoembryonic antigen, human chorionic gonadotropin, and ferritin). An elevated alkaline phosphatase level may indicate liver or bony metastasis. A liver scan may be done if liver function tests are elevated, there is evidence of liver enlargement, or the woman complains of anorexia. Serum carcinoembryonic

TABLE 35-2 TNM Classification System for Breast Cancer

Clinical-Diagnostic Classification		Postsurgical Treatment Pathologic Classification	
Primary Tumor (T)			
TX	No tumor	Same	
T0	No evidence of primary tumor		
Tis	Carcinoma in situ/Paget's disease		
T1	Tumor [2 cm		
T1a	Tumor 0.5 cm or less		
T1b	Tumor > 0.5 cm but [1.0 cm		
T1c	Tumor > 1.0 cm but [2.0 cm		
T2	Tumor > 2.0 cm but [5.0 cm		
T3	Tumor > 5.0 cm		
T4	Tumor of any size with direct extension to chest wall or skin		
T4a	Extension to chest wall		
T4b	Edema, ulceration, or satellite nodules		
T4c	Both T4a and T4b		
T4d	Inflammatory carcinoma		
Nodal Involvement (N)			
NX	Regional lymph nodes cannot be assessed	pNX	Regional lymph nodes cannot be assessed
N0	No regional lymph node metastasis	pN0	No regional lymph node metastasis
N1	Metastasis to movable ipsilateral axillary lymph node(s)	pN1	Metastasis to movable ipsilateral axillary lymph node(s)
		pN1a	Only micrometastasis
		pN1b	Metastasis to lymph node(s) i Metastasis in one to three lymph nodes ii Metastasis to four or more lymph nodes iii Extension beyond the node capsule iv Any positive nodes 2 cm or more in dimension
N2	Metastasis to ipsilateral axillary lymph node(s) fixed to one another or to other structures	pN2	Metastasis to ipsilateral axillary lymph nodes that are fixed to one another or other structures
N3	Metastasis to ipsilateral internal mammary lymph node(s)	pN3	Metastasis to ipsilateral internal mammary lymph node(s)
Distant Metastasis (M)			
MX	Not assessed	Same	
M0	No known metastasis		
M1	Distant metastasis		

Stage Grouping

Stage	T	N	M
Stage 0	Tis	N0	M0
Stage I	T1	N0	M0
Stage 1A	T0	N1	M0
	T1	N1	M0
	T2	N0	M0
Stage IIB	T2	N1	M0
	T3	N0	M0
Stage IIIA	T0	N2	M0
	T1	N2	M0
	T2	N2	M0
	T3	N1,N2	M0
Stage IIIB	T4	Any N	M0
	Any T	N3	M0
Stage IV	Any T	Any N	M1

Source: Adapted from Beahrs OH, Henson DE, Hutter RV, et al (eds): Manual for Staging of Cancer (ed 3). Philadelphia, Lippincott, 1988, pp 145-150.

antigen is a frequently studied tumor marker in breast cancer and has been found to be elevated in 70% to 80% of patients with metastatic disease.[51,52]

The most widely used clinical staging system for breast cancer is the TNM (tumor-node-metastasis) system recommended by the American Joint Committee for Cancer Staging (1988) and the International Union Against Cancer (Table 35-2).

Regardless of the staging system used, women with stage I disease have approximately an 80% chance of 10-year survival with no evidence of disease (NED); stage II is associated with a 10-year survival rate of 60% (NED); stage III carries a 10-year survival rate of 40% (NED); and stage IV carries a 10-year survival rate of less than 10% (NED).[53]

PROGNOSIS

At diagnosis, the prognosis for the woman with breast cancer depends on many factors. The most important prognostic indicators include the degree of invasiveness of the tumor, tumor size, and axillary node status. Degree of invasiveness is determined by whether the tumor is attached to the overlying skin or the underlying chest wall. A direct correlation exists between tumor size and the likelihood of metastatic disease; conversely, there also exists a decrease in disease-free survival. It is estimated that 80% of women with tumors less than 1 cm in diameter, 55% of women with tumors 3 to 4 cm in diameter, and 45% of women with tumors 5 to 7.5 cm in diameter are alive after 10 years. The histologic presence of cancer in the axillary lymph nodes reduces the overall survival rate. Regardless of the absolute number of nodes removed, the actual number of nodes involved with tumor is the single most important prognosticator of survival and recurrence of breast cancer (Table 35-3).[54] It should be noted that the previously established practice of combining all patients with four or more positive nodes into one group gives misleading information regarding prognosis and benefits of treatment.[55]

TABLE 35-3 Survival of Patients with Breast Cancer in Relation to Axillary Nodal Involvement*

Number of Lymph Nodes	5-Year Survival (%)	10-Year Survival (%)
0	72	60
1-3	58	45
4-10	44	30
11-20	28	18
>20	18	16

*Percentages listed are approximate values within ± 2 percentage points.

Source: Adapted from Clark GM, McGuire WL: Steroid receptors and other prognostic factors in primary breast cancer. Semin Oncol 15:20-25, 1988 (suppl 1).

The histologic grade and the estrogen-receptor protein status of the tumor are prognostic factors that are also noted at diagnosis. A tumor with a high degree of anaplasia is considered poorly differentiated and is associated with a poor prognosis.[56,57] The assessment of cell proliferative potential may have important prognostic significance. Determination and evaluation of the cellular DNA content by flow cytometry can identify patients at risk for recurrence. Those patients with high S-phase fraction tumors are associated with a worse prognosis. Reports indicate that survival rates are significantly better in women whose tumors contain estrogen receptors than in those whose tumors do not. Increased survival rates are not correlated with a higher estrogen-receptor value. The prognostic value for positive estrogen-receptor status is more important for postmenopausal women than premenopausal women.[58] A controversial issue at present is the prognostic value of estrogen-receptor status in women without metastasis to the axillary lymph nodes; however, it is generally accepted that node-negative, estrogen-receptor-negative women have a worse prognosis than node-negative, estrogen-receptor-positive women.[57] For node-positive women, the absence of estrogen receptors is also associated with a poor prognosis.[59]

On the average, 40% to 45% of the women who have breast cancer will develop a recurrence. More than 50% of women who relapse with breast cancer do so after 3 years.[60] Fifty to 60% of the metastases will be clinically evident within 5 years of treatment, and 98% will have evidence of metastasis within 10 years of treatment.[61,62] At initial recurrence, the most important prognostic factors are the site(s) of recurrence and the number of recurrences.[56,63] Estrogen-receptor positive tumors more frequently recur in bone, while estrogen-receptor negative tumors tend to recur in visceral or soft tissue sites.

In 1942 Haagensen and Stout[64] identified the following clinical features of breast cancer that are generally related to a poor prognosis and high recurrence rates:

1. Extensive edema of the skin over the breast
2. Satellite tumor nodules in the skin over the breast
3. Inflammatory carcinoma
4. Supraclavicular node involvement
5. Large (>2.5 cm) or fixed axillary nodes
6. Intercostal or parasternal tumor nodules

These classic signs of unfavorable disease are still accepted today and are generally considered contraindications for mastectomy, unless it is done for cosmetic reasons.

TREATMENT ALTERNATIVES

Many diagnostic and therapeutic alternatives related to breast cancer are now available to women that were not

50 years ago. According to McKenna and Toghea,[65] "the combinations and permutations of treatment options available today for breast cancer number over 90." In addition, women are now more active health consumers who seek information regarding their options. This climate necessitates that the nurse working with these women be knowledgeable of the current options available to educate women regarding their options, to guide them in their decision making, and to make appropriate referrals.

The first alternative a woman may face is whether to have a biopsy done as a one- or two-step procedure. A one-step procedure is usually done under general anesthesia with immediate frozen section. If the biopsy is positive for malignancy, and it is appropriate, a mastectomy is then performed, thus avoiding the need for a second anesthesia. Today, the trend is toward biopsy under local anesthesia, followed by histologic examination and further discussion between the individual, family, and physician concerning possible therapy. This approach gives the woman time to prepare herself and her family for decisions regarding treatment and the possible loss of her breast, if indicated. That she is given a few days to consider her alternatives and participate in the decision-making process can possibly decrease the feeling of loss of control and can promote family cohesiveness and adaptation to changes in body image should a mastectomy be the treatment of choice. Undoubtedly, the treatment alternatives available to an individual woman are limited by the extent of disease at diagnosis.

Another option that may be discussed before cancer treatment is breast reconstruction. Immediate reconstruction takes place at mastectomy, whereas delayed reconstruction begins months to years after mastectomy. Although immediate reconstruction is being performed more frequently than before, delayed reconstruction allows a woman time to decide if she really wants reconstruction and to choose a plastic surgeon carefully.

Not all alternatives will be available to a woman at her present place of health care. Appropriate referrals should be made as requested or indicated. Comprehensive breast care centers, which are located in approximately 60 centers nationally, offer a woman with the diagnosis of breast cancer the opportunity to receive a formal, multidisciplinary team approach to her care.[66] The team consists of a surgeon, a radiation therapist, and a medical oncologist and may also include a plastic surgeon, pathologist, nurse, and social worker. Some women use this team approach for their definitive plan of therapy, while others use it for a second or a third opinion.

As members of the health care team, physicians and nurses are responsible for informing women with breast cancer of their rights and treatment alternatives. Since 1979, several states, including Michigan, Massachusetts, California, Hawaii, Kansas, Kentucky, Virginia, Georgia, and New York, have acknowledged these rights.[66] These states have passed laws regarding the management of breast cancer care. More specifically, the laws require the physician or the hospital to inform a breast cancer patient of all the therapeutic options available to her.

Surgical Interventions

For the woman found to have local minimal disease with no evidence of nodal metastasis or distant spread, cure is the goal of therapy. A modified radical mastectomy, also termed total mastectomy with axillary dissection, may be advocated for even minimal disease. This approach allows for surgical removal and pathologic examination of the breast and axillary lymph nodes, identifying women at risk for systemic recurrence.[67] Although more limited procedures such as lumpectomy or tylectomy have been proposed, the rationale for a modified radical mastectomy is that breast cancer can be multifocal, and lymph nodes felt to be negative at clinical staging may prove to be positive on pathologic examination. The incidence of multicentric breast cancer occurring in sites distant from the biopsy in mastectomy specimens varies from 9% to 75%.[67] The incidence of error in clinically staging lymph nodes is approximately 30%. Therefore, surgical evaluative staging of lymph nodes is the only dependable method of evaluating a woman's risk for distant spread and subsequent need for systemic therapy, which is the key element in breast cancer survival.

For women who have stage II or III disease, the modified radical mastectomy has been the treatment of choice. The procedure involves the en bloc removal of the breast, pectoralis minor muscles, intervening lymphatics (including the subpectoral and intrapectoral lymphatic chain), and a sampling of the axillary lymph nodes. The modified radical procedure usually leaves the woman with a relatively normal thickness of skin flaps because there is no evidence that thin skin flaps resulting from more radical procedures prevent recurrences.

The preservation of innervation to the pectoralis major muscles at the apex of the axilla allows for more shoulder mobility postoperatively. Maintenance of the pectoral fold gives a more normal feminine appearance to the shoulder, shoulder girdle, and infraclavicular area. When a horizontal incision is used and the skin flaps are healthy, the cosmetically superior results allow for the possibility of reconstructive breast surgery if the woman desires reconstruction. In addition to the more favorable cosmetic result, the modified radical procedure gained popularity as a result of various reports that indicate that 5- and 10-year survival rates of the modified radical mastectomy are essentially equal to those of the more extensive procedure. The Halsted radical mastectomy, once the mainstay of breast cancer treatment, has been abandoned in favor of more conservative procedures.

In 1971 the National Surgical Adjuvant Breast Project (NSABP) began protocol no. 4, which attempted to determine whether in women with clinical negative axillary nodes who subsequently develop positive nodes, a total mastectomy followed by axillary dissection is as effective a therapy as radical mastectomy. It also attempted to determine whether total mastectomy with postoperative regional irradiation is as effective a treatment as a radical mastectomy or total mastectomy with postponement of axillary dissection until positive nodes occur. In women with clinically positive nodes, the goal was to determine whether radical mastectomy and total mastectomy with postoperative regional irradiation are equivalent procedures. This study indicated that there is no significant difference in treatment failure or survival in women with clinically negative nodes who had a conventional radical mastectomy and those having a total mastectomy and axillary dissection only if positive axillary nodes subsequently occurred. Similarly, no significant difference in treatment failure or survival exists between women with clinically positive nodes who are treated by radical mastectomy or total mastectomy followed by irradiation. Following local therapy, disease may recur locally, regionally, or at distant sites. In general, if disease is detected beneath the scar or in the same area as the primary tumor, it is considered to be persistent cancer. However, a recurrence many years after primary treatment elsewhere in the breast is considered a new neoplasm.

Preoperative management

When biopsy and mastectomy are planned as a one-stage procedure, the woman has little opportunity to prepare herself for the loss and changes she will encounter postoperatively. For this reason, a woman may choose to have only a biopsy, after which she will make plans concerning treatment after considering the alternatives. There is no evidence that a brief delay (7 to 10 days) between biopsy and treatment is detrimental, although most physicians recommend that a woman have definitive treatment within 2 weeks of the biopsy if cure is the goal of therapy. As mentioned previously, the two-stage procedure also allows for pathologic analysis of the permanent sections of the breast tissue to ensure a thorough and accurate diagnosis.

The woman and her family must realize the individual nature of breast cancer and be able to discuss openly with the primary physician the alternatives of therapy. The need for such elucidation is extremely individual and is based on the woman's expressed needs. The nurse is often in a position to alert the physician of the individual's concerns regarding alternatives to therapy and can promote optimal communication between the patient and the physician. The nurse can help to clarify any misconceptions the woman may have regarding surgery and what to expect in the immediate postoperative period.

Before surgery, the basic issues that may be prominent in the minds of the woman and her family are (1) whether the surgeon will be able to remove all the cancer before it spreads and therefore improve her chances of being cured; (2) anticipatory grieving for the loss of the breast and consequent changes in body image; and (3) possible loss of self-esteem and sense of femininity. The woman may feel that she is paying a high price for the possibility of cure and may need to discuss these feelings before surgery. Conversely, she may be extremely relieved that an operation can be done that can potentially cure her of the cancer. Although it is not common practice at present in many institutions, these women may benefit from a visit by a volunteer from the American Cancer Society's "Reach to Recovery" program or by joining a support group of other women in similar circumstances before she has her mastectomy. This practice may become more widespread as women undergo outpatient aspiration biopsy and delayed mastectomy.

The question of the cost of two operations and double anesthesia is a valid one; however, the benefits a woman may gain by planning for this change in her life before it happens may be helpful in the adaptations she will make in her life after surgery.

Postoperative management

Immediate postoperative care involves preserving the integrity of the skin flaps overlying the chest wall, minimizing edema and loss of function of the arm, preventing infection of the surgical wound, pain management, and routine postoperative care with early ambulation and pulmonary hygiene.

Wound catheters are generally placed beneath the skin flap to prevent fluid collection and promote adherence of the skin flap to the chest wall to facilitate healing. Controlled suction is applied and maintained until the drainage is minimal. Any evidence of air (hissing), collapsed tubing, or excessive drainage should be reported to the physician. Air in the tubing can indicate that a leak exists and that the skin flaps are not adherent. The drainage tubes should be stripped to prevent blockage and subsequent collapse of the tubing. Excessive drainage (more than 200 mL in 8 hours) can indicate bleeding, which can lead to a hematoma or excessive blood loss. Hematoma formation beneath the flap can lead to necrosis of some portion of the skin flap. If the hematoma is evacuated promptly, healing usually occurs.

The woman may return from surgery with a bulky pressure dressing that must be observed for excessive drainage every 2 to 4 hours for the first 24 hours postoperatively. After the pressure dressing is removed, a sterile dressing is applied and should be monitored for drainage every 4 hours and changed as needed. The wound drains are removed 3 to 5 days after surgery, depending on the amount of drainage.

The affected arm should be in an adducted position to minimize tension on the suture line for the first couple of days after surgery. After the 2- to 3-day waiting period, the woman can usually begin limited range-of-motion exercises.

Because the lymphatics that traverse the pectoral muscles may not be resected by this modified operation, swelling of the arm is minimal. The woman's arm should, however, be positioned to promote adequate venous drainage and comfort. The arm should be adducted with the elbow even with the heart when the person is supine and sitting. To promote adequate drainage, the woman is encouraged from the first postoperative day to do isometric exercises with wrist and elbow flexion and extension. The use of a sling to support the arm seems to increase the incidence of frozen shoulder and less than optimal function and is generally not recommended.

Approximately 3 to 5 days after surgery, the woman is encouraged to do active range-of-motion exercises. These exercises should be designed specifically for each individual. The woman should be instructed to discontinue exercises if she feels pain and to resume exercising after resting. Transient edema may occur with increased use of the arm, but it subsides after about a month as collateral lymphatics develop.

Before the woman is discharged from the hospital, the nurse instructs her and her family on how she should protect her affected arm and hand from injury or trauma. These instructions are particularly important if the individual has had a more extensive axillary dissection than that of the standard modified radical mastectomy. The danger of infection is directly correlated with the degree of axillary dissection and whether the person is having adjuvant radiotherapy. Table 35-4 provides a list of "do's and don'ts" to help the woman prevent injury to her affected arm and hand. If the woman has not had an axillary dissection, there is no physiologic reason for not obtaining blood pressure readings on the affected side, and this may be done without harmful sequelae after complete healing has occurred.

Once the woman is discharged from the hospital, she should continue to monitor the status of her affected arm. If she has had an axillary dissection, she should be instructed to elevate the arm for 30 to 45 minutes every 2 hours for the first 2 to 3 weeks and then two to three times a day for an additional 6 weeks. The woman should be cautioned that just as lack of activity and favoring the arm can lead to edema and limited function, so too can excessive use of the arm. Overzealous use of the arm and excessive exercise can increase arterial flow beyond tissue tolerance and actually lead to edema. For the first 8 weeks after surgery, the woman should limit the use of the affected limb to 30 minutes at any one task. She also should continue sleeping with her forearm higher than her elbow and her elbow higher than or level with her heart. Lying on her affected side or arm will tend to decrease the efficiency of her lymph venous return and should be avoided. During the first 8 weeks after surgery, the woman should be instructed to measure the circumference of her arm 6 cm above and below the olecranon process once a week. If an increased circumference is noted over time, her physician should be notified, and an elastic stockinette may be indicated.

It is often beneficial for the woman who has had a mastectomy to have a Reach to Recovery volunteer visit in the early postoperative period. The volunteer can assist in instituting a rehabilitation program that includes the individual's physical, psychologic, and sociologic needs. With the physician's consent, the volunteer and nurse can design a program that best suits the woman's needs. The various exercises are usually demonstrated by the volunteer and reinforced by the nurse and physical therapists. The volunteer also may instruct the woman on the use of a temporary prosthesis and where she may obtain a more permanent prosthesis after complete wound healing has occurred. The volunteer also may discuss more intimate questions the woman may have regarding her sexuality and changes in body image.

TABLE 35-4 Hand and Arm Care*

Do's	Don'ts
Do wear your "Life Guard Medical Aid" tag engraved with "Caution—lymphedema arm—NO TESTS—NO HYPOS"	Do not allow injections of any kind on this arm
Do contact your physician if your arm gets red, warm, or unusually hard or swollen	Do not allow your blood to be drawn from this arm
Do wear a loose rubber glove on your hand when washing dishes	Do not carry your purse or anything heavy with this hand
Do protect your hand from pinpricks, scratches, or cuts of any kind	Do not hold a cigarette in this hand
Do apply a good lanolin hand cream several times daily	Do not cut or pick at the cuticles or nails on this hand
Do utilize cream cuticle remover for nail care	Do not wear constrictive clothing or jewelry on this arm
	Do not expose this hand or arm to excessive temperatures

*Guidelines apply to women who have had axillary lymph node dissections, axillary recurrence, or lymphedema.

Incision care is another important area of discharge teaching. The issue of whether the woman should be encouraged to look at her incision before discharge from the hospital is extremely individual. Viewing her chest before discharge does not imply that the woman will adjust more readily to her disfigurement. The goal of nursing is to remain available and be sensitive to the woman's reaction to her loss. If the woman must learn to apply a dressing or cleanse the incision, she should be encouraged to choose the time that she is ready to do this and the supportive person she wishes to assist her or be with her (ie, a loved one, physician, or nurse). She should be instructed to protect the incision from trauma or friction until complete healing has taken place, usually about 5 to 7 weeks after surgery. She should be encouraged to apply cocoa butter or lanolin cream to the incision to minimize drying and scar contracture. Cornstarch or talc powder can be applied to minimize itching and friction against clothing. It is not uncommon for women who have had a mastectomy to report "phantom breast" sensations. These sensations may be painful but generally range from twinges and itches to feelings of heaviness, coldness, and numbness. Discussing the possibility of these sensations before discharge is encouraged and may aid the woman in adapting to her loss.

Although such information is usually supplied by the Reach to Recovery volunteer, the nurse must be certain that the individual has information regarding the various prostheses that are available, their cost, and whether the woman's insurance will cover the cost. The nurse should

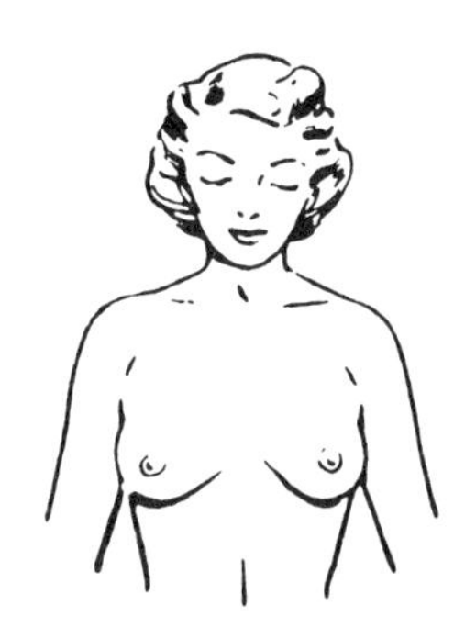

1. Careful examination of the breasts before a mirror for symmetry in size and shape, noting any puckering or dimpling of the skin or retraction of the nipple.

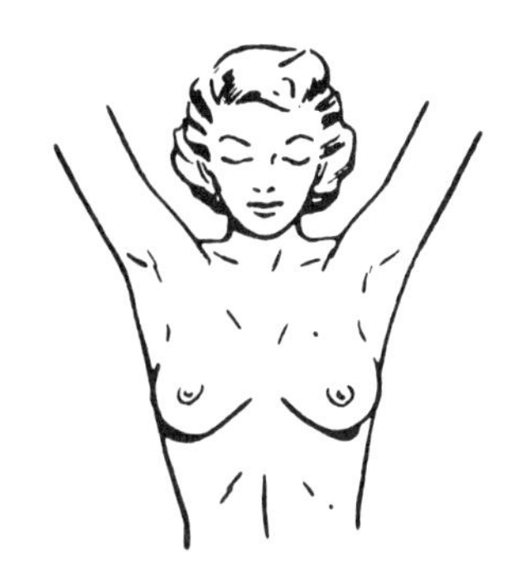

2. Arms raised over head, again studying the breasts in the mirror for the same signs.

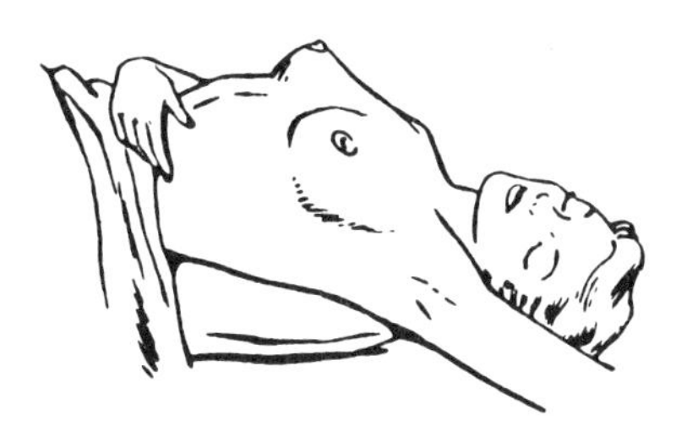

3. Reclining on bed with flat pillow or folded bath towel under the shoulder on the same side as breast to be examined.

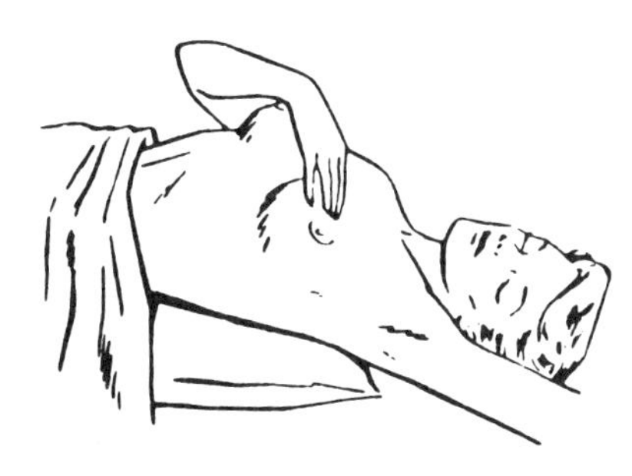

4. To examine the inner half of the breast the arm is raised over the head. Beginning at the breastbone and, in a series of steps, the inner half of the breast is palpated.

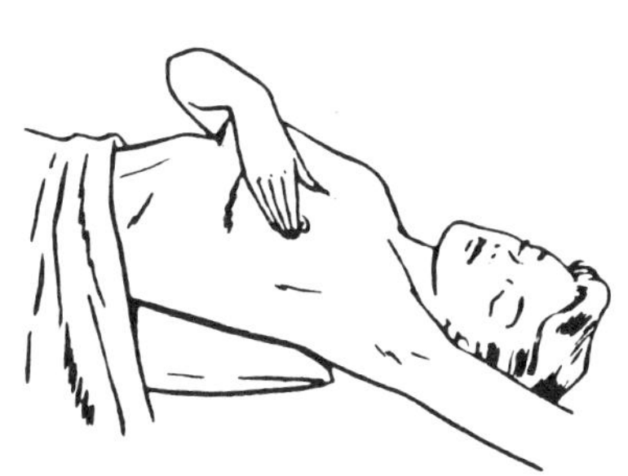

5. The area over the nipple is carefully palpated with the flat part of the fingers.

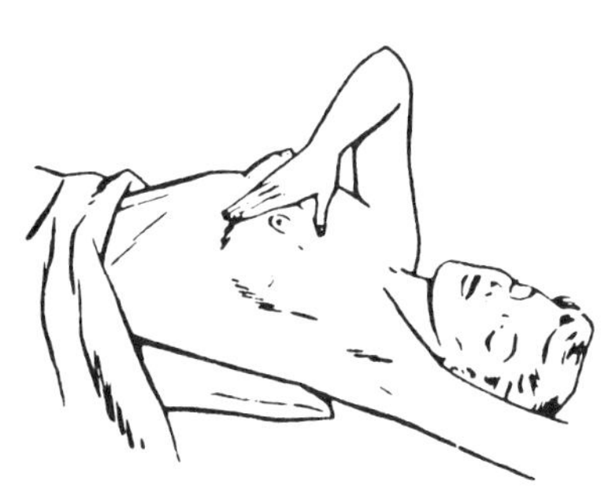

6. Examination of the lower inner half of the breast is completed.

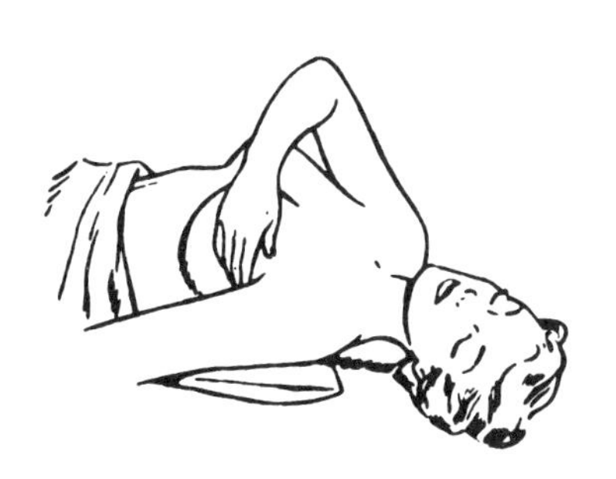

7. With arm down at side self examination of breasts continues by carefully feeling the tissues which extend to the armpit.

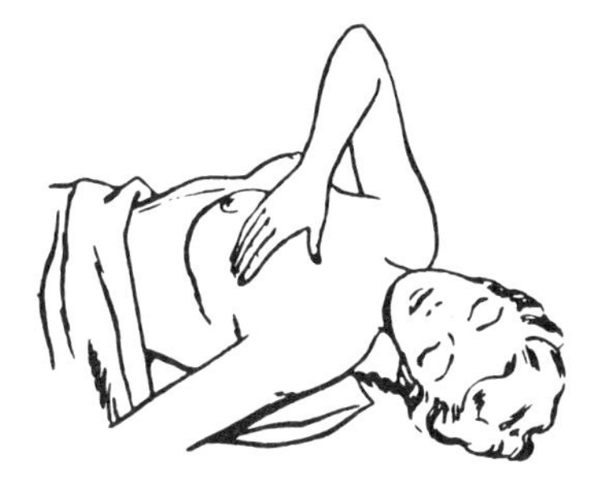

8. The upper outer quadrant of the breast is examined with the flat part of the fingers.

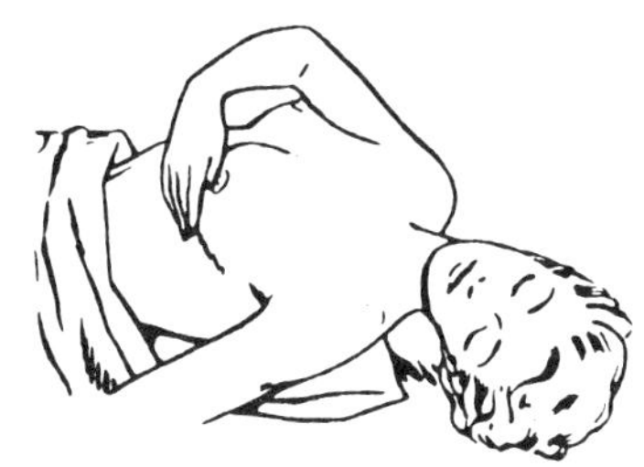

9. The lower outer quadrant of the breast is examined in successive stages with flat part of the fingers.

FIGURE 35-4 Technique of breast self-examination. (Courtesy American Cancer Society.)

be certain that the individual has the names of women who are responsible for the sale of breast prostheses at various department stores. A Reach to Recovery volunteer can supply such information, but if such a volunteer is not available, the nurse assumes this responsibility.

The rehabilitation program for the woman who has had a mastectomy is designed to promote functional use of the affected arm and shoulder and to facilitate psychological and emotional adaptation to the loss of the breast, the diagnosis of cancer, and the changes in body image and interpersonal relationships that she may experience.

It is not unusual for a woman to have misconceptions regarding breast cancer and its risk factors. She may be afraid that because she has breast cancer, her daughter will also have it, in which case the woman may feel guilty about "passing on" her disease. This myth should be dispelled with accurate information from the nurse and physician. Not infrequently a woman will request that her daughter or sister be present during any instruction of breast self-examination. This should be encouraged and the opportunity given to ask questions regarding breast examination and health maintenance. Figure 35-4 illustrates the technique of breast self-examination.

Follow-up

The woman who has a mastectomy for breast cancer, regardless of the type of surgical procedure, remains under the care of her physician for the rest of her life. The 5-year or 10-year disease-free gaps are encouraging milestones, but breast cancer can recur after many years.

Most women are scheduled to return for a checkup every 3 months for the first 2 years, every 6 months for 3 years, and then once a year after the 5-year mark. The timing of these visits serves to minimize the stress associated with the threat of recurrence without jeopardizing early detection of recurrence, metastasis, or a new carcinoma in the opposite breast.

A thorough physical examination is done routinely with each visit, and a chest radiograph is obtained every 3 to 6 months for the first 3 years. A yearly mammogram or xeroradiogram is usually recommended. Bone survey may be recommended every 12 months. Annual bone, liver, and brain scans are also appropriate, depending on the woman's individual case.

Along with the physical assessment, the physician and nurse must be particularly aware of the impact of illness on the individual and family, especially during the first year after the mastectomy. Maguire[68] has found that the incidence of psychiatric problems was higher among women who had undergone mastectomy than among controls who did not have a mastectomy. Twenty-five percent of the women examined required psychiatric intervention for depression or anxiety. Many complained of moderate or severe sexual difficulties. The woman's inability to cope with the changes brought about by the diagnosis and treatment of breast cancer may precipitate a crisis that requires the prompt attention of the interdisciplinary team. When lumpectomy is the treatment of choice, women report less of a loss of feelings of attractiveness and femininity, are less self-conscious, and are more open about their sexuality.[69]

BREAST RECONSTRUCTION

In the past 10 years, breast reconstruction has become an accepted and integral consideration in the management of breast cancer. There are a number of reasons for these advances. First, professionals are becoming increasingly aware of the changes in body image that the woman experiences and that deformity is not always accepted with equanimity, as was once thought. Rarely are the external breast prostheses incorporated into the woman's body image as a restored breast. These prostheses commonly are uncomfortable and easily displaced during normal activities of daily living, especially in the woman who exercises (swimming, aerobics, etc). Second, the mass media have publicized widely the procedure of breast reconstruction and in so doing have in essence assured the woman who has had a mastectomy that it is acceptable to inquire about or seek out the physicians who perform these procedures. The increasing public awareness serves to assure women that to inquire about reconstruction does not mean they have failed to adapt or are excessively vain. Physicians are approaching reconstruction as a planned part of the total treatment.

An additional reason for the advances in reconstructive breast surgery is that because of early detection and increasing awareness of the importance of breast self-examination, breast cancer may be detected at an earlier stage, thereby enabling less extensive curative procedures to be done.

Opponents of reconstruction may argue that the subsequent growth of implanted tumor cells could be concealed by the prosthesis, resulting in a treatment delay, or that the focus on local reconstruction might detract attention from systemic treatments designed to treat potential micrometastases. However, there is no scientific evidence to date that these arguments are valid or that reconstructive surgeries in any way hide local recurrence or affect the ultimate course of the illness adversely.

The best candidate for reconstruction is the woman who has a true stage I disease with no nodal involvement and no evidence of distant metastasis. Women with stage I disease have been found to exhibit a low incidence of local recurrence in the chest wall. Because the implant is usually placed submuscularly, any skin or subcutaneous recurrences are readily detected. Metastases occurring in the ribs or intercostal spaces under the implant are evidence of systemic disease, and reconstruction in such instance has little or no effect on the course of the disease.

A contraindication to reconstructive breast surgery would be the diagnosis of inflammatory carcinoma. In some instances high-dose radiotherapy may be a contraindication, depending on local damage. The presence of isolated distant metastasis is not necessarily a contraindication to breast reconstruction, particularly when local recurrence is absent. Another possible contraindication to breast reconstruction may be the woman's attitude and expectations regarding the cosmetic result. Before reconstruction, the woman and her family are made aware of the limitations of the surgery. Viewing "before" and "after" photographs of another woman in similar circumstances may be useful. The reconstructed breast may be far from perfect, perhaps only a mound that simulates a breast. This practice is useful because if the woman's hopes are unrealistically high, nothing short of perfection will be acceptable.

Current practice dictates that the woman wait 3 months to a year or until the completion of adjuvant chemotherapy or radiotherapy before beginning reconstruction, although it can be undertaken immediately after surgery. Immediate reconstruction is gaining acceptance, particularly for the woman who is not receiving adjuvant therapy. The use of the inflatable prosthesis allows for optimal healing. The rationale for delaying reconstruction until the completion of adjuvant therapy is to avoid interrupting therapy and possibly interfering with wound healing. The complications of immediate breast reconstruction following mastectomy are hematoma, seroma formation, skin necrosis, infection, and loss of the prosthesis. Delayed reconstruction allows for a more mature, supple scar and more pliable skin, which may accept a larger prosthesis. Also, a woman who has lived with a chest deformity for some time may be more accepting of the less-than-perfect results presently obtainable with reconstructive procedures. There is no maximum time after which reconstruction cannot be performed. A number of breast reconstruction techniques are possible, depending on the type of surgical deformity and the size of the remaining breast. The major challenges of breast reconstruction are to attain symmetry, correct the infraclavicular depression, and create the nipple-areolar complex. Depending on the degree of laxity of the overlying skin, an inflatable prosthesis or silicone gel implant is placed above or below the pectoralis muscle. Placement beneath the muscle helps to reduce capsular contracture, as does vigorous breast massage. If the tension on the skin is too great, necrosis or extrusion of the implant may result. Generally, the prosthesis is inflated gradually over 3 to 6 months to allow stretching of the skin. This is done once the prosthesis has settled into position on the chest wall. Currently, the use of a tissue expander, which is a silicone breast implant with a valve projecting from it, has gained popularity. This tissue expander is gradually filled with saline solution by a percutaneous injection into the fill valve.[4] The expander is later replaced by a permanent implant once the pocket has matured.

If sufficient skin and soft tissue are not present, as in the woman who has had a radical mastectomy, or if there has been skin grafting or excessive irradiation, then skin or muscle flaps or both obtained from the woman's chest, abdomen, or back may be used. The thoracoepigastric or the latissimus dorsi myocutaneous flap are most commonly used to ensure adequate blood supply and adequate tissue coverage to accommodate a prosthesis. The latissimus dorsi flap is preferred in many cases because it contains muscle and this appears to decrease fibrous capsule formation. The skin flap can be used to fill in the infraclavicular defect if one exists.

Except in women with micromastia, a reduction mammoplasty of the remaining breast is usually indicated if symmetry is to be obtained. In a high-risk individual, a subcutaneous mastectomy with immediate reconstruction may be indicated as a preventive measure.

If reconstructive breast surgery is a planned procedure, the surgeon may bank the nipple-areolar complex in the groin or abdominal area at the time of mastectomy. This is only done if thorough, multiple microscopic examinations are performed to ensure that the nipple-areolar complex is tumor-free. Involvement of the nipple is more likely if the primary tumor was found to be just below the nipple, the tumor was multicentric, or the primary tumor was greater than 4 cm. If such conditions exist, the nipple-areolar complex will be discarded.

If the nipple-areolar complex is not available to be transposed on the reconstructed breast mound, the plastic surgeon may create a nipple-areolar complex by sharing from the normal breast. If this is not possible, or if the woman is reluctant, the complex can be recreated by tattoos, by using local tissues, or by grafts from the labia minora or labia majora or both. The color match of such transplants is good, and complications are minimal.

Figure 35-5 depicts the cosmetic results of latissimus dorsi reconstruction following radical mastectomy.

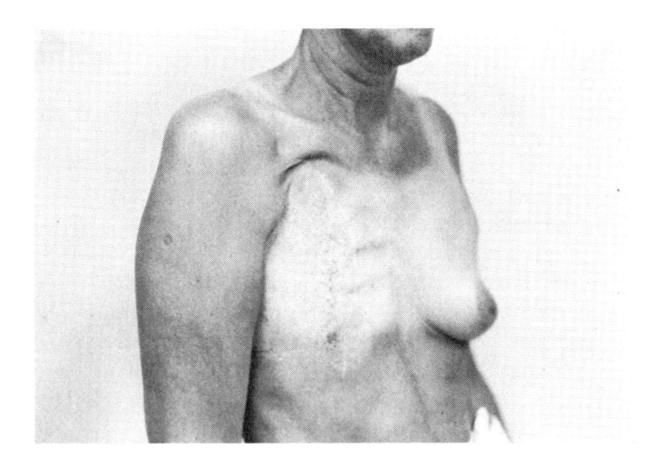

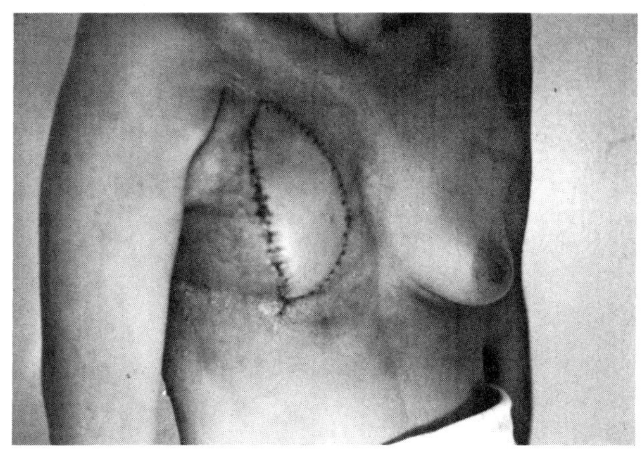

FIGURE 35-5 Lattisimus dorsi reconstruction following radical mastectomy.

ADJUVANT CHEMOTHERAPY IN OPERABLE BREAST CANCER

Failure of cure in breast cancer is related less to the type of primary treatment and more to the inability of local therapy to affect occult metastases that later become manifested to lung, bones, and viscera.

Because of the high incidence of treatment failures with local therapy alone, various clinical trials of adjuvant therapy continue to be conducted. The goals of these investigations are to examine therapeutic strategies for breast cancer and to attempt to identify those factors with a significant impact on overall survival.

When analyzing the results of studies involving the role of adjuvant chemotherapy, the important issues are the durability of the disease-free interval and the overall survival. These are balanced against the overall short- and long-term toxicities of the drugs and the impact on quality of life.

Most medical oncologists would agree on the general worth of adjuvant chemotherapy for all women with axillary nodes positive for cancer. While the true value for certain subgroups is as yet undefined, degree of nodal involvement remains an important predictor of breast cancer recurrence and heralds the need for adjuvant systemic therapy. Currently the benefit of adjuvant chemotherapy appears to be the greatest for premenopausal women with one to three nodes positive for cancer. Relapse-free survival has been found to be increased by adjuvant chemotherapy by as much as 15% to 25% in premenopausal women. There appears to be no significant survival advantage for postmenopausal women who receive adjuvant chemotherapy.[70]

Other significant findings are that combination chemotherapy is superior to single-agent treatment in improving relapse-free survival (RFS) as well as overall survival (OS). The greatest benefit of chemotherapy depends on the individual receiving the optimal dose at prescribed intervals; reduced dosages generally should be avoided. As demonstrated by Bonadonna and Valagussa,[71] the maximum cell kill in breast cancer appears to occur early in the treatment cycle; this is supported by the finding that individuals who receive six cycles of the cyclophosphamide-methotrexate-5-FU (CMF) regimen have the same response as those who receive twelve cycles.

Controversy exists over the optimal combination routine. Henderson[72] states that, at present, standard adjuvant chemotherapy for breast cancer is 6 months of CMF; others specify its use as standard therapy in premenopausal, node-positive women.[73,74] However, it is generally agreed that regimens containing doxorubicin are better than those that do not.[75] It appears that most authors[73,76,77] agree that there is no optimal combination as of yet; further randomized clinical trials are needed.

To pull together the available data on adjuvant chemotherapy and draw some basic conclusions about the matter, the National Institute for Health held a conference on Consensus Development on Adjuvant Chemotherapy for Breast Cancer in 1985. The following recommendations were produced from the meeting.[77]

1. Premenopausal, node-positive, estrogen-receptor-positive or -negative women should be treated with established combination chemotherapy.
2. Premenopausal, node-negative women are not recommended for chemotherapy unless they are at high risk.
3. Postmenopausal, node-positive, estrogen-receptor-positive women should be treated with tamoxifen.
4. Postmenopausal, node-positive, estrogen-receptor-negative women are not standardly treated with chemotherapy, but it may be considered.
5. Postmenopausal, node-negative, estrogen-receptor-positive or -negative women are not routinely given adjuvant chemotherapy.

These recommendations have been highlighted and supported by others[72,73]; however, others have questioned the clinical trials on which these conclusions have been based.[75] Recently, Glick[76] acknowledged that although the overall conclusions of the conference remain important and valid, the results of current trials will likely affect the validity of these recommendations in the future.

The most significant new finding regarding adjuvant chemotherapy are from four clinical trials conducted to evaluate the benefit of systemic therapy in node-negative women. Results of these trials (Table 35-5)[79-82] indicate the need for the medical community to reevaluate its recommendations for adjuvant therapy in this group of women. Results revealed improved disease-free survival for those women who were treated with either chemotherapy or hormonal therapy following primary treatment for breast cancer. To date, no change in overall survival rate has been noted owing to limited years of follow-up.

The overall results of postoperative adjuvant therapy for presumably local disease is less than optimal. Many trials have yet to show an improvement in crude survival. In the absence of new, more effective agents, efforts are being made to use drugs known to be effective in breast cancer in more creative ways. For instance, doxorubicin has routinely been reserved for women whose breast cancer recurs. Its use in adjuvant therapy has been investigated and currently is recommended by the National Surgical Adjuvant Breast Project (NSABP) for some patients

TABLE 35-5 Adjuvant Chemotherapy Studies with a Concomitant Control Group in Node-Negative Patients

First Author	No. of Patients	Adjuvant Treatment	Essential Findings
Fisher[79]	679	MF plus Leuco versus no treatment	4-year disease-free survival 80% versus 70%
Fisher[80]	2644	Tamoxifen versus placebo	4-year disease-free survival 83% versus 77%
Mansour[81]	406	CMFP versus no treatment	3-year median disease-free survival 84% versus 69%
Ludwig[82]	1275	CMF plus Leuco versus no treatment	4-year disease-free survival 77% versus 73%

M, methotrexate, *F,* 5-fluorouracil, *Leuco,* Leocovorin, *P,* prednisone, *C,* cyclophosphamide.

with stage II and most patients with stage III disease. The major question asked in these studies was whether disease-free intervals and survival rates in women with stage II breast cancer might be increased by adding doxorubicin to the standard PF (5-FU and phenylalanine mustard) regimen with or without tamoxifen based on age and hormone status.

In women at significant risk for recurrence of disease (stage III), doxorubicin is often used as a continuous infusion in combination with other drugs such as 5-FU or cyclophosphamide. It may also be given as a single monthly injection in combination with cyclophosphamide and 5-FU (CAF). Regimens that include doxorubicin are reported to be more toxic, causing myelosuppression, alopecia, and congestive heart failure. Although preliminary reports indicate that drug regimens containing doxorubicin may effectively reduce the incidence of early relapse and metastases in women with node-positive breast cancer, the impact on OS is yet to be determined.

Another approach to enhance survival in breast cancer is preoperative or induction chemotherapy. Administering chemotherapy at the earliest point possible after histologic diagnosis is thought to eliminate resistant cell lines at a time when they are most vulnerable. It is felt that the transition from a state of curability to a state of incurability can occur over a short period and that even a short delay in beginning therapy may decrease the chance of cure.[83,84] The use of preoperative chemotherapy requires further investigation but remains an encouraging possibility where discouraging survival rates persist.

If it is true that micrometastases increase in proliferative activity with resection of the primary disease, those malignant cells should be most vulnerable to chemotherapy in the operative period. Whatever the combination or scheduling used, use of adjuvant chemotherapy clearly is necessary with any evidence of nodal involvement. To improve survival rates, future trials likely will focus on newly designed drug combinations, testing different dose regimens, various schedules, and the use of effective non-cross-resistant combinations.

The long-term administration of cytotoxic agents may pose certain risks. Prolonged chemotherapy may be associated with second malignancies such as leukemia, and this risk is weighed against the benefits of treatment.

RADIOTHERAPY

Radiation is similar to surgical therapy in the management of breast cancer because both are essentially local forms of treatment. An analysis from the National Surgical Adjuvant Breast Project suggests that because a large percentage of women will have distant metastases at diagnosis, their survival is not likely to be affected by the choice of local therapy. The women who may be affected by the type of mastectomy or primary radiotherapy are those whose disease is limited to the breast and local lymph nodes. Current results from both prospective and retrospective trials suggest that primary radiotherapy for early breast cancer is an effective alternative to mastectomy. Primary radiation offers the possibility of both local tumor control and breast preservation.[85] Breast cancer has been shown to be a multicentric disease, and therefore any procedure less than a total mastectomy would seem inadequate. Currently, mammography helps to identify the woman with microcalcifications, which may indicate multicentric disease, and radiation may be deferred in these cases.

The basic principles of radiotherapy for breast cancer are outlined by Harris et al[86] as follows:

1. Large doses (6000 cGy) are generally required to control bulky lesions, and moderate doses (4500 to 5000 cGy) are sufficient to control subclinical or microscopic disease.
2. The effectiveness of radiotherapy in eradicating disease is increased if tumor bulk is reduced by gross removal of the tumor.
3. The tolerance of tissue to the radiation depends on dosage and fractionation of the radiation.
4. Local tumor eradication can be increased by combining external radiation with interstitial implantation either in residual sites or in sites where the risk of recurrent disease is increased.

Radiation has been used as the primary mode of therapy for stage I and II breast cancer. As previously mentioned, survival and local control rates do not differ for women treated locally with irradiation without mastectomy or for those who have had more conventional surgical treatment without irradiation.[87]

The findings of Fisher et al[88] support the use of lumpectomy and radiation in women with stage I and II disease (tumor $\leq$ 4 cm). At 8 years of follow-up, 90% of women (N = 1843) treated with radiation after lumpectomy remained free of ipsilateral breast tumor compared with 61% of those not treated with local radiation. Although there was no difference in rates of distant disease-free survival or survival among women who had lumpectomy with or without radiation, the radiation did serve to reduce the incidence of local recurrence. When local recurrence does occur, a salvage mastectomy results in a 5-year survival rate of 50%.

When irradiation is used as the primary mode of therapy without mastectomy, the individual undergoes a biopsy to confirm the diagnosis. This is generally an excisional biopsy (lumpectomy). Axillary nodes also may be sampled at this time to aid in determining the stage of disease and the need for adjuvant chemotherapy.

An external dose of 4500 to 6000 cGy may be delivered to the breast, ipsilateral mammary nodes, and supraclavicular and axillary nodes. If axillary nodes are found to be negative on surgical sampling, only the breast should be irradiated in women with outer quadrant lesions. If axillary nodes are negative in a woman with a medial/inner quadrant lesion, internal mammary and supraclavicular nodes are treated in addition to breast irradiation. A tangential field is used to minimize the volume of lung irradiated, and doses of 180 to 200 cGy per day are often delivered. The combination of the tangential field and low dose of radiation minimizes the incidence of rib fractures. The individual receives an additional 1000 to 2000 cGy by interstitial implantation of ^{192}Ir into and 2 cm around the area of the excisional biopsy. This implant remains in place for approximately 2 days.

The use of external irradiation plus implantation results in good cosmesis and a low incidence of radiation pneumonitis and radiation-induced rib fractures.

As mentioned previously, radiation is a form of local therapy, and adjuvant chemotherapy in women with stage II disease with nodal involvement is appropriate. An axillary dissection is usually done to determine the need for systemic therapy. However, drug doses may be compromised by prior radiation.

Radiotherapy to the chest wall and regional node-bearing areas enhances local and regional control in women with stage II and III breast cancer treated with radical or modified radical mastectomy. Stage III and regionally localized stage IV lesions indicate a poor prognosis. Surgery alone is inadequate. The best results probably can be achieved using a multimodal approach. This includes radiotherapy with or without surgery combined with systemic chemotherapy.

Skin reactions can be expected and depend on the dose of radiation delivered. Local skin changes vary from dry desquamation and hyperpigmentation to moist desquamation. These changes are transient and generally clear 1 to 3 weeks following cessation of therapy.

Late reactions to breast irradiation can occur several months or even years following therapy. Rib fractures may occur spontaneously or be precipitated by minor trauma. Such fractures may heal without treatment. Pulmonary manifestations such as transient chest wall discomfort, unproductive cough, tracheitis, and mild shortness of breath may occur. Radiation pneumonitis may occur 3 to 6 months after treatment and is characterized by a low-grade fever, malaise, and dry cough. Pleural effusions are uncommon, as is radiation-related pericarditis. If pericarditis occurs, surgical formation of a pericardial window may be needed to relieve cardiac tamponade.

Lymphedema of the arm may occur with higher doses of irradiation and is primarily due to progressive fibrosis of the lymphatic channels in and above the axilla. Management includes elevation of the arm and prevention of infection. With higher doses of radiation to the axilla and supraclavicular nodes, damage to the brachial plexus can occur because of radiation fibrosis. This may result in motor loss or intractable pain requiring analgesics.

TREATMENT FOR METASTATIC BREAST CANCER

Metastatic breast cancer is evident in approximately 50% of women who have breast cancer. It may be present at diagnosis or recur locally on the skin or soft tissue over or adjacent to the primary cancer site or in the regional lymphatics. It most commonly occurs at distant sites such as bone, liver, soft tissue, lung, or CNS. Although factors such as axillary node involvement and tumor size are predictive of risk for recurrence of disease, these factors have no bearing on prognosis once metastasis has occurred.[89]

When metastatic disease is suspected, an assessment of the extent of disease is made to determine response to therapy and help determine the most useful approach to management. Such clinical studies as chest film, liver scan, bone scan, CT brain scan, and cytologic analysis of the cerebrospinal fluid (CSF) may be indicated based on the woman's symptoms. The woman's performance status, peripheral blood counts, liver function tests, and serum calcium further define extent of disease, determine response, and predict to some degree the woman's ability to tolerate treatment. The carcinoembryonic antigen level may also be tested; it is elevated in up to 70% of women with metastatic cancer, especially those with liver involvement. A steady rise in this antigen during the disease-free interval may indicate the presence of metastatic disease as many as 3 months before clinical evidence of recurrence.

Although chemotherapy and hormonal therapy are very effective in relieving symptoms of metastatic disease, it is not firmly established that systemic therapy immediately, on evidence of recurrence, greatly alters overall survival. In the asymptomatic patient with a palpable node, a pulmonary nodule or bone lesion in a non-weight-bearing bone, it may be beneficial to assume a more conservative approach. Because treatment is palliative, it might be more judicious to offer a nontoxic therapy such as hormones or withhold therapy until the disease begins to affect the woman's quality of life. The patient can receive only a certain amount of radiation and chemotherapy (especially doxorubicin), and starting treatment later, when the patient has symptoms, rather than sooner permits treatment longevity when it is clearly needed. Additionally, the treatment generally is accompanied by side effects that outweigh the benefits in the asymptomatic patient.

In the symptomatic patient, especially one with lymphangitic pulmonary disease, hepatic involvement, asymptomatic brain metastases, bone marrow involvement, or lytic disease in bone, treatment is offered, especially when symptoms are likely to worsen in the near future.

The woman who is being evaluated for a possible metastasis is experiencing a great deal of fear and anxiety. Frequently the woman suspects recurrence even before it is proved. The nurse can be most helpful by knowing the history of the individual's disease, how the woman responded to the initial diagnosis and treatment, her past coping mechanisms, and what the interim time has been like for the woman and her family.

When diagnosis of recurrent disease is made, the woman and her family are often in a state of disbelief; feelings of anxiety and bitterness may surface. Anger and guilt may be directed toward the physician and nurse. The woman may have only recently begun to resume normal activities, and she may feel a sense of relief and pride in her ability to adapt to her mastectomy. Because of the actual work involved in adapting to the diagnosis of cancer and possible mastectomy, the woman's depression at learning that the cancer has recurred may be more severe than the depression she experienced with her initial diagnosis. The woman may now feel that her situation is hopeless. She also may feel defeated and have little personal strength with which to cope with this new crisis. She may have misconceptions regarding therapy for metastatic disease, which may be a source of additional stress. Her fears of dying are renewed, and denial may serve as an important coping mechanism at this time.

Nursing interventions are designed to encourage verbalization of fears and anxiety about the recurrence of disease and communicate an appreciation of the impact of illness on the individual and family. The family will require accurate information regarding the goals of therapy and measures that can be instituted to minimize the side effects of therapy.

There are many different combinations of therapy that can be offered to the woman with metastatic breast cancer; many are currently undergoing intense investigation. Systemic treatment usually includes chemotherapy, endocrine therapy, or a combination of the two.

Chemotherapy

Women who have hormone-receptor-negative tumors, are refractory to hormone therapy, or have aggressive disease in the liver or pulmonary system are candidates for chemotherapy. When chemotherapy is required, combination chemotherapy results in a higher response rate than does single-agent chemotherapy.

Combination chemotherapy often results in a response rate of 50% to 70% and can last for 9 to 12 months. However, the rate of complete response (percentage of individuals in whom all evidence of disease disappears) consistently has been seen in 10% to 20% of cases.[90]

Currently, CMF with or without prednisone and CAF are the two most commonly used treatment regimens for advanced or metastatic breast cancer. Whatever the combination used, it is important to note that none is clearly superior in response rates.

The majority of combination chemotherapy regimens are administered intermittently at 2- or 3-week intervals on an outpatient basis with infrequent clinic visits. Long-term responses are occasionally obtained, with complete relief of symptoms. Both individuals with slow-growing disease and those with rapidly progressing disease have a good response rate to chemotherapy. The response of individuals to cytotoxic agents is not significantly related to the predominant site of disease. Women with visceral metastasis, as well as those with bony involvement, will respond to chemotherapy. Although radiologic evidence of bone healing (the conversion of lytic to blastic lesions) may take as long as 6 months, subjective improvement occurs within a shorter time.

As a rule, premenopausal and especially perimenopausal women respond more often to chemotherapy than do postmenopausal women, whose disease is generally indolent. A possible explanation for this is that premenopausal and menopausal women typically have more aggressive disease than postmenopausal women. This faster growth rate increases the effectiveness of chemotherapeutic agents because more cells are undergoing cell division.

Newer approaches to treat metastatic and advanced breast cancer are currently being investigated. Mitoxantrone, bisantrene, vindesine, and platinum derivatives are chemotherapeutic agents currently undergoing clinical trials to test their efficacy in treating metastatic breast cancer. Based on the fact that there is a steep dose-response relationship for most cytotoxic agents used and that myelosuppression is the dose-limiting toxicity for most of these cytotoxic agents, the role of autologous bone marrow transplantation in this population is undergoing active study as well. Other new treatments include chemoimmunotherapy, chemohormonal therapy to induce cell synchronization, and hypothalamic hormone analogs such as buserelin and leuprolide.

Endocrine Therapy

Endocrine therapy is one of the major forms of treatment of the woman with metastatic breast disease. It is well known that the growth of normal mammary tissue is influenced by a variety of steroid hormones. Normal mammary cells contain cytoplasmic receptor sites for each of the hormones known to influence the growth and function of the mammary gland, specifically, estrogen, progesterone, and prolactin.

Steroid hormones can promote the growth of a breast cancer if the cells are hormonally dependent. In a woman who has a hormonally dependent tumor, estrogen enters the cell and binds to a specific cytoplasmic receptor protein called estrophillin or estrogen-receptor protein. The estrogen-receptor-hormone complex is then believed to undergo transformation and enter the cell nucleus to promote tumor growth. It is thought that if the source of estrogens is removed by surgical ablation or medical manipulation or if the hormone's access to the estrogen-receptor protein is blocked by antiestrogens, the chain of action is broken and the tumor regresses. Tumor cells that lack the cytoplasmic estrogen-receptor protein would not be expected to regress with hormonal or antiestrogen therapy. Knowledge of the individual's estrogen-receptor as well as progesterone-receptor status can help predict her response to endocrine therapy. Therefore, a large population of women can be identified who may be spared either unnecessary ablative surgical procedures or months of useless additive hormone therapy.

The amount of estrogen-receptor protein present in a tumor remains relatively constant throughout the course of a woman's disease, and its measurement provides information about the degree of hormone dependency of a tumor. Estrogen-receptor protein can be measured in a laboratory by assaying either the primary breast cancer at the time of surgery or a metastatic site such as a skin nodule[91] Approximately 100 mg of tumor tissue is required to perform the assay. Tumor specimens are reported as estrogen-receptor positive (ER+) or estrogen-receptor negative (ER−) based on the level of estrophillin present in the tumor specimen. Progesterone-receptor (PR) level information is also valuable in predicting response to hormone therapy and may be an indicator of estrogen-receptor protein activity. Progesterone receptors more than estrogen receptors correlate positively with disease-free interval in stage II breast cancer.[92]

Premenopausal women have a lower incidence of receptor-positive tumors (30%) than postmenopausal women (60%), and perimenopausal women have the lowest rate (10%).

Receptor-negative disease is usually associated with a short disease-free interval and more aggressive disease. Receptor-positive tumors are generally associated with a long disease-free interval between initial treatment and recurrence. These women often have slow-growing disease, usually in soft tissue or bone.

In summary, treatment with hormonal therapy, either additive or ablative, is indicated when there are metastases, the metastases are not amenable to treatment by surgery or radiotherapy, the disease is not life threatening, and the tumor is estrogen-receptor positive. If the disease is estrogen-receptor negative, aggressive, or both and life threatening, chemotherapy is indicated.

Estrogens

In women who are 5 or more years past menopause, the administration of pharmacologic doses of estrogens (diethylstilbestrol, 5 mg orally two or three times per day) can result in an objective remission in about 35% of the cases lasting several months to many years. The average duration of response is 1 year. Administration of high doses of exogenous estrogens suppresses pituitary follicle-stimulating hormone (FSH) and luteinizing hormone (LH) and therefore the production of endogenous estrogens.

At the initiation of therapy, nausea and occasional vomiting may occur for a few days. Nausea and vomiting accompanied by progressive lethargy or polyuria are symptoms of hypercalcemia, which may occur with the initiation of therapy. This is usually treated with fluids and mithramycin and is not necessarily an indication for discontinuing therapy. The woman taking estrogens should be instructed to limit sodium intake and be aware that she is likely to retain fluid and have decreased bladder tone as a result of estrogen administration. Diuretics are frequently needed to control fluid retention. Increased pigmentation of nipples and areolas and enlargement of the breasts are other side effects.

Objective evidence of tumor regression is seen most often in women with soft tissue disease. When the disease is reactivated, estrogen therapy is terminated. Estrogen withdrawal occasionally will result in a reinduction of a brief partial remission. Individuals may experience uterine bleeding with estrogen withdrawal. Women who respond to estrogen therapy and then experience a relapse may benefit from other forms of endocrine therapy.

Progestins

Megestrol acetate or high-dose medoxyprogesterone acetate have proved to be as effective as tamoxifen with a response rate of 33%. The standard dose of megestrol acetate is 40 mg, four times a day, while the dose of medroxyprogesterone acetate is 400 mg per day. These drugs are generally tolerated as well as tamoxifen. The most important side effect is weight gain, which occurs in up to 50% of patients. This weight gain is related both to increased food intake and fluid retention. Other side effects include hot flashes, hypercalcemia, and tumor flare as well as leukopenia and thrombocytopenia.

Androgens

Androgens may be employed in the treatment of all women with metastatic breast cancer, although oophorectomy, where feasible, is preferred in premenopausal women who are estrogen-receptor positive because remissions occur more frequently, are longer, and are of better quality than those obtained with androgens. Androgens exert their therapeutic effect by opposing endogenous estrogens. Androgen therapy may be added to oophorectomy in women under 35 years of age, but response rates are low. In the postmenopausal woman, androgens are indicated for the treatment of bone metastases. For soft tissue or pulmonary lesions, the response rate is less than that achieved with estrogens.[93]

Several androgens are available. The most widely accepted is fluoxymesterone (Halotestin), 20 mg per day orally. About 3 months of therapy with fluoxymesterone is needed before the maximum benefit is achieved. The systemic effects of fluoxymesterone include fluid retention, erythrocytosis, and masculinization. The woman may experience an increased libido and occasionally anorexia and nausea. In the woman who is premenopausal or early menopausal, there is the danger of precipitating hypercalcemia in the first few weeks of androgen therapy, and serum calcium levels should be monitored.

The androgenic hormones stimulate erythropoiesis and have therefore been employed to stimulate bone marrow function in women with chemotherapy-induced bone marrow suppression.

Corticosteroids

Pharmacologic doses of corticosteroids (prednisone, 30 mg orally every 8 hours, or dexamethasone, 6 mg orally every 8 hours) can result in a response in approximately 30% of women with metastatic breast disease that lasts about 3 months. Corticosteroids suppress pituitary adrenocorticotropic hormone (ACTH) estrogen-progesterone secretion from the adrenals. Corticosteroids are often used as adjuncts to radiotherapy of cerebral metastasis, in chemotherapy of advanced liver and lung metastasis, and in the management of hypercalcemia. The rate of response with steroids is not as great as with ablative procedures, nor is the duration of response as long. Because of their anti-inflammatory action, steroids can reduce peritumor edema, thereby relieving symptoms of cerebral and pulmonary metastasis. Steroids also increase the individual's appetite and feeling of well-being and can reduce pain from bone or visceral metastasis. The side effects and complications may be serious and include bleeding peptic ulcer, muscle weakness, hypertension, infection, edema, glucose intolerance, moon facies, and osteoporosis.

Antiestrogens

Potent nonsteroidal antiestrogens such as tamoxifen are indicated for the treatment of both primary and metastatic disease. These agents effectively compete with estrogen-receptor sites, thereby blocking the effect of estrogens on target tissues. Tamoxifen significantly increases survival rates when it is added to conventional adjuvant chemotherapy in metastatic disease. Tamoxifen can produce remissions similar to those obtained with other forms of endocrine therapy that last more than 10 months. Tamoxifen, 20 mg daily, has been shown to induce remission in women who have previously responded or failed to respond to adrenalectomy or oophorectomy. Currently, tamoxifen is the first-line hormone therapy in metastatic breast cancer in postmenopausal women with estrogen-receptor-positive tumors.[94]

Tamoxifen has some advantages over estrogens. It does not produce side effects such as nausea, urinary incontinence, breast tenderness, or fluid retention, which occur commonly with estrogen therapy. Furthermore, tamoxifen may be useful in some premenopausal and perimenopausal women. The best response from tamoxifen has been seen in postmenopausal women with soft tissue and lung metastasis rather than bone metastasis. The most common side effects of antiestrogens are hot flashes, mild nausea, and fluid retention with ankle swelling. Tumor flare of bone pain and hypercalcemia in patients with bone disease may occur transiently at the onset of therapy and is usually interpreted as a favorable antitumor response, although this is not well substantiated in the literature.

Oophorectomy

Surgical oophorectomy or ovarian radiation are equally effective in removing endogenous sources of estrogens in premenopausal and perimenopausal women and may be indicated in women with estrogen-receptor-positive tumor assays. Oophorectomy is not indicated in women with estrogen-receptor-negative tumors. The controversy over prophylactic versus therapeutic oophorectomy has for the most part been settled. Researchers have found that there is no therapeutic benefit to prophylactic oophorectomy in premenopausal women. Oophorectomy is therefore reserved for women with recurrent or metastatic disease, provided their disease at time of recurrence is not life threatening. Delaying oophorectomy is important to evaluate response and predict response to subsequent hormonal therapy.

About 32% of women who undergo oophorectomy obtain remission of disease, which may last for approximately 1 year.[94] Women who experience an objective response to oophorectomy are candidates for additional endocrine therapy.

Secondary ablative procedures

In the past, adrenalectomy or hypophysectomy resulted in objective remission in about 32% of women who responded to previous endocrine therapy. These procedures are no longer performed to treat women with disseminated breast cancer. The results of medical adrenalectomy with aminoglutethimide (Cytadren) therapy are equivalent to those of surgical ablation without the risks of surgery and permanent adrenal suppression. Aminoglutethimide effectively blocks the conversion of androstenedione to estrone in peripheral tissue and inhibits the conversion of cholesterol to pregnenolone, thus blocking all adrenal steroid synthesis. It also inhibits the peripheral conversion of androgens to estrogens. Hydrocortisone replacement is needed because of adrenal suppression. The side effects of aminoglutethimide administration include lethargy and skin rash occurring 7 to 10 days after initiation of therapy. If these reactions should occur, the aminoglutethimide is not discontinued, nor should the dose be decreased. The administration of increased doses of hydrocortisone for a week or more is effective in alleviating the rash.

MALE BREAST CANCER

Male breast cancer accounts for less than 1% of all breast cancers.[3] The anatomic structures of the male breast are the same as those of the female breast. It is the hormonal stimulation present in the female breast and absent in the male breast that accounts for the development and physiologic differences between the male and female breast. This lack of hormonal stimulation also may explain the comparatively low incidence of male breast cancer.

The incidence of breast cancer is increased in men who have undergone sex-change procedures. The administration of estrogens results in lobular development and enlargement of the male breast. Hormonal imbalance and gynecomastia are characteristic of Klinefelter's syndrome, and the incidence of breast cancer is increased in men with this chromosomal aberration.

The administration of diethylstilbestrol (DES) to men with carcinoma of the prostate has been associated with male breast cancer but is a rare occurrence. As pointed out by Buchanan-Davidson,[95] large numbers of men receiving DES for prostatic carcinoma do not exhibit an increased incidence of breast cancer. It is important to note that the life expectancy of these men is relatively short, and breast cancers may indeed be present but not yet manifested.

Breast cancer occurs most frequently in men 50 to 70 years old. It appears that after 40 years of age the Sertoli cells (elongated cells in the seminiferous tubules) secrete increasing amounts of estrogens. The majority of male breast cancers (75%) are known to be estrogen-receptor positive. They typically arise from ductal elements and present as infiltrating ductal carcinoma, which is commonly fixed to underlying fascia and skin. Nipple retraction and a bloody discharge may be present.

A painless, centrally located subareolar mass is usually the first symptom that brings the man to seek medical attention. Pectoral fixation, involvement of skin, nipple changes, and discharge are commonly present because of limited breast tissue. This factor may account for the increased frequency of widespread disease and early invasion of local and regional lymphatics. Ulceration may occur early in the course of the disease and carries a relatively poor prognosis.

Because of its relatively central location, male breast cancer can be expected to metastasize to the internal mammary nodes. The lungs and bony skeleton are the most common metastatic sites.

Because of the low incidence and relatively small number of patients, it is difficult to conduct controlled clinical trials to aid in establishing appropriate therapy. The treatment of male breast cancer is based in principle on the treatment of female breast cancer. The modified radical mastectomy has been the mainstay of therapy. The skin and underlying fascia are frequently involved, requiring skin grafting. Adjuvant radiotherapy, hormonal manipulation, and chemotherapy are the main methods of treatment.

With evidence of extensive disease, hormonal manipulation is indicated unless, as with female breast cancer, the disease is life threatening or aggressive, in which case chemotherapy would be indicated. The response rate to chemotherapy is about 44%.

Orchiectomy appears to remove the source of estrogen and androgen in recurrent male breast cancer and can result in a prompt remission. With recurrent disease, further hormonal manipulation, including tamoxifen, aminoglutethemide, progestin, and DES, may be beneficial.

COMPLICATIONS OF METASTATIC DISEASE

Bone Metastasis

Many individuals with breast cancer will, throughout the course of their illness, experience pain due to bony destruction by tumor. The individual may complain of pain over the rib cage, which is aggravated by a cough, or pain in the leg when rising from a sitting position. The person may also report feeling as if his or her back was strained while bending to pick something off the floor. In general, the pain is constant and grows progressively more severe. A radiograph of the area may demonstrate bony destruction and may be the first sign of metastasis or progression of disease. Bone pain may precede the development of skeletal radiographic changes by several weeks. Destructive bone lesions must be 1.0 to 1.5 cm in diameter and associated with a 30% to 50% loss of bone mineral content before they can be detected with conventional radiography. A bone scan is therefore indicated to determine the extent of disease. A more sensitive method than radiography for detecting metastatic disease, it should be obtained in all individuals with symptoms suggesting skeletal involvement.

In addition to radiography, examination of peripheral blood or serum chemistries may indicate metastatic disease. Anemia, thrombocytopenia, leukocytosis, and immature forms of circulating nucleated red blood cells may indicate metastasis to the bone marrow. Elevation of the serum alkaline phosphatase level may be observed with either bone or liver involvement. The serum calcium level also may be increased and indicates significant bone destruction. Individuals who complain of back pain should have a thorough neurologic examination as well as radiographic evaluation of the spine. A myelogram may be necessary to determine whether spinal cord compression is present or imminent.

For the individual who has had a long disease-free interval, a bone biopsy may be needed to document metastatic disease in bone. This is particularly true for the person who has no evidence of other metastatic deposits.

In addition to being painful, destructive lesions involving the femur or the humerus are highly susceptible to fracture. If fracture of the diseased bone should occur, severe vascular or neurologic damage may ensue, as well as immobility and severe pain. Irradiation in doses of 3000 to 4000 cGy to symptomatic areas often results in effective pain relief and recalcification of bone. If a fracture is pending or has occurred, surgery to stabilize the bone by internal fixation or replacement of the femoral head may be necessary. This is followed by 2500 to 3000 cGy of irradiation. This palliative surgery should allow the individual to remain ambulatory, thus decreasing the hazards of immobility such as hypercalcemia, deep vein thrombosis, and pneumonia. Physical therapy is instituted in the postoperative period and after discharge to ensure optimal rehabilitation.

In individuals with widespread bone involvement, radiation is given to areas that are painful and disabling. In cases where one or more fractures are pending, surgery is indicated and offers the least morbidity. Other forms of treatment for the individual with metastatic disease to bone include anti-inflammatory agents (such as prednisone), antiestrogens (such as tamoxifen), androgens, estrogens, or chemotherapy.

The nurse should be particularly aware of the vulnerability of the person with metastatic bone lesions. Simply turning the person improperly in bed can result in fracture of the affected area. The customary ways of repositioning patients in bed are contraindicated for the individual with disease in the clavicle. Lifting beneath the person's arms puts pressure on the clavicle and may cause a fracture. A pull sheet should be used to reposition the person with known disease in the hip, ribs, or vertebrae. At least two persons are needed to reposition these individuals properly so that correct body alignment is ensured. The nurse also should be aware of the intense pain often associated with metastatic bone disease, particularly if a fracture has occurred.

Spinal Cord Compression

Spinal cord compression constitutes an emergency because of the potential for developing paraplegia. Compression may be secondary to epidural tumor or altered bone alignment due to pathologic fracture. The initial signs and symptoms may be extremely subtle. Pain is usually present for several weeks before the development of additional neurologic symptoms. Imminent compression should be suspected in individuals who have progressive back pain associated with weakness, paresthesias, bowel or bladder dysfunction, or gait disturbances. A myelogram is performed as soon as the diagnosis is suspected to determine the exact level of the compression and identify other occult extradural lesions.

If the individual is found to have compression with an isolated extradural mass, radiotherapy combined with corticosteroids may produce optimal results and return of ambulation. The person is usually fitted with a brace or maintained on bed rest throughout the course of radiotherapy. Decompression laminectomy may be indicated for individuals who develop spinal cord compression and in whom the diagnosis of epidural metastasis is in doubt or whose neurologic deficits continue to worsen while they receive radiotherapy. Fewer than 50% of these individuals can be expected to regain ambulatory function.

Brain Metastasis and Leptomeningeal Carcinomatosis

Brain metastasis occurs in about 30% of individuals diagnosed with breast cancer and is often associated with devastating physical and emotional problems. The most frequent signs and symptoms of intracranial metastasis are headaches, seizures, visual defects, motor weakness, and mental changes. Therapy of brain or meningeal lesions requires accurate localization and adequate radiotherapy.

Most chemotherapeutic agents do not achieve a therapeutic concentration in the brain or CSF. This is why the CNS may be considered a potential sanctuary for tumor cells. Leptomeningeal metastases occur most likely by hematogenous spread through the capillary structure of the choroid plexis or by rupture of cerebral metastases that subsequently involve the subarachnoid space. The diagnosis of leptomeningeal metastases is made by lumbar puncture and analysis of the CSF. Headache and changes in mental status are the most common symptoms of meningeal carcinomatosis. Cranial nerve dysfunction also may be present. Ocular muscle parasis is common, as are facial weakness, hearing loss, and vision loss.

Treatment generally involves total brain irradiation (2400 to 3000 cGy in 8 to 10 fractions). This is commonly followed by intraventricular-intrathecal chemotherapy given through an Ommaya reservoir. Methotrexate, cytosine arabinoside, steroids, thiotepa, and derivatives of 5-FU may safely be given into the subarachnoid space. Treatment usually includes methotrexate and thiotepa given twice weekly initially, then once a week for life.

Chronic Lymphedema

With the recent trend in more conservative surgical resection with minimal axillary dissection for the individual undergoing mastectomy, the problem of massive lymphedema is less common. When axillary dissection is done, there may be transient edema initially while collateral vessels develop; however, it is unusual for edema to persist beyond 3 months after surgery.

The most common cause of chronic lymphedema is tumor recurrence or tumor enlargement in the axilla. When this occurs, there is an increased resistance to venous flow and a disturbance in oncotic pressure that develops in the affected arm. The longer the edema persists, the more difficult it is to manage. The individual is instructed to elevate the hand above the elbow and the forearm higher than or level with the heart whenever possible. If edema persists or worsens, the individual is instructed in the use of an elastic stockinette to aid in venous flow. The stockinette is measured precisely to ensure that it fits properly and does not constrict venous flow. The individual wears the stockinette when out of bed. While the individual is sleeping, the arm is positioned to aid venous flow. The individual is instructed to care for the skin and fingernails very carefully to avoid infection. Infection enhances lymphedema and slows regeneration of lymphatics. Individuals with chronic lymphedema are also instructed to control their weight and, in some situations, to lose weight.

For the individual who has massive edema without evidence of infection, a program of intermittent compression with a Jobst extremity pump may be necessary. The arm usually is treated daily as tolerated for 3 to 4 hours in the morning and 3 to 4 hours in the afternoon. When the arm reaches 1+ pitting edema, the treatment is discontinued and the arm is measured for a Jobst support. A compression pump is strictly contraindicated when there is evidence of acute phlebitis, perivascular lymphangitis, or cellulitis.

The lymphedematous arm is cosmetically unattractive and can be functionally useless. The arm can cause tremendous strain on the neck and shoulder muscles, which can result in pain. The woman may have difficulty adjusting her wardrobe to provide for the increasing size of her arm. Furthermore, the edematous arm can rarely be concealed adequately and can renew feelings of disfigurement and depression associated with the mastectomy that the woman may have resolved before the lymphedema occurred. When function of the arm is affected, the woman may not be able to work or perform activities of daily living. These limitations may not have been imposed on the woman following her mastectomy. Efforts should be made to discuss the goals and rationale of management with the woman, thereby enlisting her cooperation and participation in the planned treatment regimen.

PREGNANCY AND BREAST CANCER

The current literature reports the incidence of concurrent pregnancy or lactation and breast cancer to be 2% to 5%.[96] The diagnosis of breast cancer during pregnancy occurs in about 10% of eligible patients.[97] The average patient is in her fourth or early fifth decade of life, has had multiple pregnancies but relatively few deliveries, and has a long interval since a previous pregnancy or childbirth.[98]

The prognosis for women diagnosed with breast cancer during pregnancy has generally been poor, but today there is new optimism. It is now realized that the poor prognosis is more likely due to the increased incidence of delay in diagnosis in this population of women and subsequent discovery and treatment of advanced disease than it is due to the pregnancy itself. When compared with nonpregnant breast cancer patients of the same age, disease stage, and histologic grade, the prognosis for these patients is actually no worse.

Although the techniques of early detection and diagnosis in a pregnant patient can be difficult to perform because of the physiological changes in the breast, they are no less essential. Breast examinations should be performed as a regular part of prenatal care, and all women should be encouraged to practice breast self-examination throughout the duration of pregnancy. Any suspicious lump should receive a prompt workup as previously outlined. The effectiveness of mammography may be compromised by the increased density of the breast, and, if it is performed, the fetus should be shielded. The risk to the fetus in the event a breast biopsy is needed is minimal.

The treatment of breast cancer in this population of women is determined by the extent of the disease present and the term of pregnancy or lactation. In general, the same treatment principles apply. Early-stage disease should be surgically treated with little risk to the fetus. Radiation therapy is not recommended due to potential hazards to the fetus. Chemotherapy, if indicated, should not be administered during the first trimester but can be more safely used in the second and third. A therapeutic abortion at this stage is not necessary, nor has it been found to be therapeutically beneficial. A more advanced disease stage needs effective, urgent palliation and may indicate the need for termination of an early pregnancy to promptly begin treatment for the breast cancer. If the diagnosis is made in the third trimester, local therapy is carried out and adjuvant therapy is instituted once the child is born. When chemotherapy is deemed crucial because of more aggressive disease, cesarean section at the earliest opportunity may be recommended. Only a very small risk of metastasis to the fetus exists in these patients.

Advising a woman after treatment for breast cancer whether to become pregnant is based on several factors. Most important is considering if the woman is still fertile; some women are infertile as a result of chemotherapy. The next, and equally important consideration, is the woman's risk for recurrence as determined by the extent of nodal involvement at diagnosis and interval since completion of treatment. It is customary to advise a woman to wait 2 years after systemic therapy before becoming pregnant.

Data reveal that 7% to 10% of all premenopausal breast cancer patients become pregnant following treatment.[99] There are no data to support the belief that subsequent pregnancy activates quiescent micrometastases and triggers recurrent disease. However, if the woman has more advanced local disease (stage II or III), it is usually recommended that at least 3 or 4 years pass before she considers becoming pregnant, if at all. The issue in question is the woman's increased risk for recurrence and subsequent inability to raise her child. Despite prior thought, breast-feeding is not contraindicated in the woman who has been treated for breast cancer, although a radiated breast generally does not lactate.[100]

REFERENCES

1. Lynch HT, Watson P, Conway T, et al: Breast cancer family history as a risk factor for early onset breast cancer. Breast Cancer Res Treat 11:263-267, 1988.
2. Shimkin MB: Cancer of the breast. JAMA 183:358, 1963.
3. American Cancer Society: Cancer Facts and Figures. Atlanta, The Society, 1989.
4. Bostwick J: Breast reconstruction following mastectomy. CA 39:40-49, 1989.
5. Lippman ME: Epidemiology of breast cancer, in Lippman ME, Lichter AS, Danforth DN (eds): Diagnosis and Management of Breast Cancer. Philadelphia, WB Saunders, 1988, pp 1-9.
6. Thomas DB: Do hormones cause breast cancer? Cancer 53:595-604, 1984.
7. Bergkvist L, Adami HO, Persson I, et al: The risk of breast cancer after estrogen and estrogen-progestin replacement. N Engl J Med 321:293-297, 1989.
8. Center for Disease Control. Cancer and steroid hormone study. Long term oral contraceptive use and risk of breast cancer. JAMA 249:1591-1595, 1983.
9. Schlesselman JJ, Stadel BV, Murray P: Breast cancer in relation to early use of oral contraceptives: No evidence of latent effect. JAMA 259:1828-1833, 1988.
10. Hulka BS: Dietary fat and breast cancer: Case-control and cohort studies. Prevent Med 18:180-193, 1989.
11. Boyle P, Leake R: Progress in understanding breast cancer: Epidemiological and biological interactions. Breast Cancer Res Treat 11:91-112, 1988.
12. Rose DP, Boyar AP: Dietary fat and cancer risk: The rationale for intervention, in Reddy BS, Cohen LA (eds): Diet, Nutrition and Cancer: A Critical Evaluation. Boca Raton, Fla, CRC Press, 1986, pp 151-166.
13. Boyd NF: Body weight and prognosis in breast cancer. J Natl Cancer Inst 67:785-789, 1981
14. Ingram D, Nottage E, Ng S, et al: Obesity and breast cancer. Cancer 64:1049-1053, 1989.

15. Sattin RW, Rubin GL, Webster LA, et al: Family history and the risk of breast cancer. JAMA 253:1908-1913, 1985.
16. Petrakis NL: Genetic factors in the etiology of breast cancer. Cancer 39:2709-2715, 1977.
17. Anderson DE, Badzioch MD: Risk of familial breast cancer. Cancer 56:383-387, 1985.
18. Lynch HT, Albano WA, Danes BS, et al: Genetic predisposition to breast cancer. Cancer 53:612-622, 1984.
19. Dowden RV, Grundfest-Broniatowski S: Prophylactic mastectomy—when and how, in Grundfest-Broniatowski S, Esselstyn CB (eds): Controversies in Breast Disease: Diagnosis and Management. New York, Marcel Dekker, 1988, pp 219-231.
20. Rosen PP, Lesser ML, Senie RT, et al: Epidemiology of breast carcinoma. IV: Age and histologic tumor type. J Surg Oncol 19:44-51, 1982.
21. Love S, Schnitt SJ, Connolly JL, et al: Benign breast disorders, in Harris JR, Henderson IC, Hellman S, et al (eds): Breast Diseases. Philadelphia, JB Lippincott, 1987, pp 15-53.
22. Fisher ER: Relationship of fibrocystic disease to cancer of the breast, in Hoogstraten B, McDivitt RW (eds): Breast Cancer, Boca Raton, Fla, CRC Press, 1981, pp 119-135.
23. Page DL, Dupont WD, Rogers LW, et al: Atypical hyperplastic lesions of the female breast: A long-term follow-up study. Cancer 55:2698, 1985.
24. Miller AB, Howe GR, Sherman GJ: Mortality from breast cancer after irradiation during fluoroscopic examinations in patients being treated for tuberculosis. N Engl J Med 321:1285-1289, 1989.
25. Hildreth NG, Shore RE, Dvoretski PM: The risk of breast cancer after irradiation of the thymus in infancy. N Engl J Med 321:1281-1284, 1989.
26. Pennisi VR: The prevention of breast cancer by subcutaneous mastectomy. Surg Clin North Am 57:1023, 1987.
27. Synderman RK: Prophylactic mastectomy. Pros and cons. Cancer 53:803-808, 1984.
28. Bohmert HH: Subcutaneous mastectomy. Advantages and problems, in Grundfest-Broniatowski S, Esselstyn CB (eds): Controversies in Breast Disease. Diagnosis and Management. New York, Marcel Dekker, 1988, pp 235-259.
29. Woods JE: Prophylactic partial mastectomy. Surgery 101:120, 1987 (letter).
30. Dowden RV, Grundfest-Broniatowski S: Prophylactic mastectomy. When and how, in Grundfest-Broniatowski S, Esselstyn CB (ed): Controversies in Breast Disease. Diagnosis and Management. New York, Marcel Dekker, 1988, pp 219-231.
31. Cuzick J, Wang DY, Bulbrook RD: The prevention of breast cancer. Lancet 8472:83-86, 1986.
32. Eddy DM: Screening for breast cancer. Ann Intern Med 111:389-399, 1989.
33. Dodd GD: Screening for the early detection of breast cancer. Cancer 62:1781-1783, 1988.
34. Baker LH: Breast cancer detection demonstration project. Five-year summary report. CA 32:194-225, 1982.
35. Moore FD: Breast self-examination. N Engl J Med 299:304-305, 1978.
36. Venet L: Self-examination and clinical examination of the breast. Cancer 46:930-932, 1980.
37. American Cancer Society: Women's attitudes regarding breast cancer. Princeton NJ, Gallup Organization, 1973.
38. American Cancer Society: A basic study of public attitudes toward cancer and cancer tests. New York, Lieberman Research, 1978.
39. National Cancer Institute. Health education reports. J Natl Cancer Inst 3:1142-1146, 1981.
40. Rutledge DN, Davis GT: Breast self-examination compliance and the health belief model. Oncol Nurs Forum 15:175-179, 1988.
41. Welch-McCaffrey D, Dodge J: Planning breast self-examination programs for elderly women. Oncol Nurs Forum 15:811-814, 1988.
42. Williams RD: Factors affecting the practice of breast self-examination in older women. Oncol Nurs Forum 15:611-616, 1988.
43. Ahmann DL: A preliminary assessment of factors associated with recurrent disease in a surgical adjuvant clinical trial for patients with breast cancer with special emphasis on the aggressiveness of therapy. Am J Clin Oncol 5:371-381, 1982.
44. Nunez C: Fine needle aspiration biopsy of breast lesions, in Grundfest-Broniatowski S, Esselstyn CB (eds): Controversies in Breast Disease. New York, Marcel Dekker, 1988, pp 201-217.
45. Lee BJ, Tannenbaum E: Inflammatory carcinoma of the breast: A report of twenty eight cases from the breast clinic of the Memorial Hospital. Surg Gynecol Obstet 39:580, 1924.
46. Nemoto T, Vana J, Bedwani RN, et al: Management and survival of female breast cancer: Results of a national survey by the American College of Surgeons. Cancer 25:2917-2924, 1980.
47. Koscielny S, Tubiana L, Le MG, et al: Breast cancer: Relationship between the size of the primary tumor and the probability of metastatic dissemination. Br J Cancer 49:709, 1984.
48. Harris JR, Henderson IC: Natural history and staging of breast cancer, in Harris JR, Henderson IC, Hellman S, et al (eds): Breast Diseases. Philadelphia, JB Lippincott, 1987, pp 233-258.
49. Maisey MN: Imaging techniques in breast cancer. What is new. What is useful. A review. Eur J Cancer Clin Oncol 24:61-68, 1988.
50. Turner DA, Alcorn FS, Adler YT: Nuclear magnetic resonance in the diagnosis of breast cancer. Radiol Clin North Am 26:673-687, 1988.
51. Danforth DN, Lichter AS, Lippman ME: The diagnosis of breast cancer, in Lippman ME, Lichter AS, Danforth DN (eds): Diagnosis and Management of Breast Cancer. Philadelphia, WB Saunders, 1988, pp 50-94.
52. Smith RE: Biochemical detection of recurrent breast cancer. Cancer Detect Prev 11:303-309, 1988.
53. Henderson C, Canellos GP: Cancer of the breast. I and II. N Engl J Med 301:78-90, 1980.
54. Clark GM, McGuire WL: Steroid receptors and other prognostic factors in primary breast cancer. Semin Oncol 15:20-25, 1988 (suppl 1).
55. Fisher B, Bauer M, Wickerham DL, et al: Relation of number of positive axillary nodes to the prognosis of patients with primary breast cancer. Cancer 52:1551-1557, 1983.
56. Kamby C, Anderson J, Ejlertsen B, et al: Histological grade and steroid receptor content of primary breast cancer. Impact on prognosis and possible modes of action. Br J Cancer 58:480-486, 1988.
57. Fisher B, Redmond C, Fisher ER, et al: Relative worth of estrogen or progesterone receptor and pathologic characteristics of differentiation as indicators of prognosis in node negative breast cancer patients. Findings from National Surgical Adjuvant Breast and Bowel Project Protocol B-06. J Clin Oncol 6:1076-1087, 1988.

58. Chevallier B, Heintzmann F, Mosseri V, et al: Prognostic value of estrogen and progesterone receptors in operable breast cancer. Results of a univariate and multivariate analysis. Cancer 62:2517-2524, 1988.
59. Whitliff JL: Steroid hormone receptors in breast cancer. Cancer 53:630-643, 1984.
60. Obrist R: The significance and treatment of late distant metastasis in breast cancer. Helv Chir Acta 55:843-847, 1989.
61. Baker RR: Pre-operative assessment of the breast cancer patient. Surg Clin North Am 58:681-686, 1978.
62. Strax P: Evaluation and screening programs for the early diagnosis of breast cancer. Surg Clin North Am 58:667-679, 1978.
63. Clark GM, Sledge GW, Osborne CK, et al: Survival from first recurrence. Relative importance of prognostic factors in 1,015 breast cancer patients. J Clin Oncol 5:55-61, 1987.
64. Haagensen CC, Stout AP: Carcinoma of the breast. Ann Surg 116:801-815, 1942.
65. McKenna RJ, Toghia NJ: The law of informed consent and mastectomy, in Ariel I, Cleary J (ed): Breast Cancer. Diagnosis and Treatment. New York, McGraw-Hill, 1987, pp 544-556.
66. Harnes JK: Organizing for collaborative management. What are the options? In Harness J, Oberman H, Lichter A, et al (ed): Breast Cancer. Lewis, Mich, Collaborative Management, 1988, pp 3-9.
67. Kinne DW: Surgical management of clinically early breast cancer. Cancer 53:685-690, 1984.
68. Maguire GP: Psychiatric problems in the first year after mastectomy. Br Med J 1:963-965, 1978.
69. Steinbert MD, Juliano M, Wise L: Psychological outcome of lumpectomy versus mastectomy in the treatment of breast cancer. Am J Psychiatry 142:34-39, 1985.
70. Henderson CI: Adjuvant chemotherapy of breast cancer. A promising experiment or standard practice. J Clin Oncol 3:140-143, 1985.
71. Bonadonna G, Valagussa P: Adjuvant systemic therapy for resectable breast cancer. J Clin Oncol 3:259-275, 1985.
72. Henderson CI: Adjuvant systemic therapy for early breast cancer. Curr Probl Cancer 11:125-207, 1987.
73. Bonadonna G, Valagussa P: Current status of adjuvant chemotherapy for breast cancer. Semin Oncol 14:8-22, 1987.
74. Henderson CI, Harris JR, Kinne DW, et al: Cancer of the breast, in DeVita VT, Hellman S, Rosenberg SA (eds): Cancer Principles and Practice of Oncology. Philadelphia, JB Lippincott, 1989, pp 1197-1268.
75. Davidson NE, Lippman ME: Adjuvant therapy for breast cancer, in Lippman ME, Lichter AS, Danforth DN (eds): Diagnosis and Management of Breast Cancer. Philadelphia, WB Saunders, 1988, pp 348-374.
76. Glick JH: Meeting highlights. Adjuvant therapy for breast cancer. J Natl Cancer Inst 80:471-475, 1988.
77. Consensus Conference: Adjuvant chemotherapy for breast cancer. JAMA 254:3461-3463, 1985.
78. Levitt SH, Potish RA, Aeppli D, et al: The consensus statements on adjuvant chemotherapy in breast cancer. Fact or artifact. Am J Clin Oncol 11:73-76, 1988.
79. Fisher B, Redmond C, Dimitrov NV, et al: A randomized clinical trial evaluating sequential methotrexate and fluorouracil in the treatment of patients with node-negative breast cancer who have estrogen-receptor-negative tumors. N Engl J Med 320:473-478, 1989.
80. Fisher B, Constantino J, Redmond C, et al: A randomized clinical trial evaluating tamoxifen in the treatment of patients with node-negative breast cancer who have estrogen receptor-positive tumors. N Engl J Med 320:479-484,1989.
81. Mansour EG, Gray R, Shatila AH, et al: Efficacy of adjuvant chemotherapy in high-risk node-negative breast cancer. N Engl J Med 320:485-490, 1989.
82. Ludwig Breast Cancer Study Group: Prolonged disease-free survival after one course of perioperative adjuvant chemotherapy for node-negative breast cancer. N Engl J Med 320:491-496, 1989.
83. Goldie JH, Coldman AJ: A mathematic model for relating the drug sensitivity of tumors to their spontaneous mutation rate. Cancer Treat Rep 63:1727-1733, 1979.
84. Ragaz J, Baird R, Rebbeck P, et al: Neoadjuvant (preoperative) chemotherapy for breast cancer. Cancer 56:719-724, 1985.
85. Harris JR, Beadle GF: Clinical studies on the use of radiation therapy as primary treatment of early breast cancer. Cancer 53:705-711, 1984.
86. Harris JR, Levene MB, Hellman S: The role of radiation therapy in the primary treatment of carcinoma of the breast. Semin Oncol 5:403-416, 1978.
87. Danoff BF, Haller DG, Glick JH, et al: Conservative surgery and irradiation in the treatment of early breast cancer. Ann Intern Med 102:634-642, 1985.
88. Fisher B, Redmond C, Poisson R, et al: Eight year results of a randomized clinical trial comparing total mastectomy and lumpectomy with or without irradiation in the treatment of breast cancer. N Engl J Med 320:822-828, 1989.
89. Canellos GP: Treatment of metastases, in Harris JR, Henderson IC, Hellman S, et al (eds): Breast Diseases. Philadelphia, JB Lippincott, 1987, pp 385-398.
90. Canellos GP: Systemic therapy of breast cancer. Med J Aust 148:88-91, 1988.
91. Peetz ME: Multiple simultaneous and sequential estrogen receptor values in patients with breast cancer. Am J Surg 143:591-594, 1982.
92. Clark GM, McGuire WL: Steroid receptors and other prognostic factors in primary breast cancer. Semin Oncol 15:20-25, 1988 (suppl 1).
93. Ingle J: Additive hormonal therapy in women with advanced breast cancer. Cancer 53:766-777, 1984.
94. Wells SA: Ablative procedures in patients with metastatic breast carcinoma. Cancer 53:762-765, 1984.
95. Buchanan-Davidson DJ: Is breast cancer the same in men and women? Cancer Nurs 3:121-130, 1980.
96. Parente JT, Amsel M, Lerner R, et al: Breast cancer associated with pregnancy, Obstet Gynecol 71:861-864, 1988.
97. Ribiero G, Jones DA, Jones M: Carcinoma of the breast associated with pregnancy. Br J Surg 73:607-609, 1986.
98. Donegan WL: Mammary carcinoma and pregnancy, in Donegan WL, Spratt JS (eds): Cancer of the Breast. Philadelphia, WB Saunders, 1988, pp 679-688.
99. Deemarsky LJ, Semiglazov VF: Cancer of the breast and pregnancy, in Ariel IM, Cleary JB (eds): Breast Cancer. Diagnosis and Treatment. New York, McGraw-Hill, 1987, pp 475-488.
100. Hassey KM: Pregnancy and parenthood after treatment for breast cancer. Oncol Nurs Forum 15:439-444, 1988.

Chapter 36

Central Nervous System Cancers

Jo Ann Wegmann, RN, PhD

Patricia Hakius, RN, MSN

INTRODUCTION

The brain and spinal cord represent a closed system of intricately functioning organs. Tumor involvement within the central nervous system (CNS) is associated with a high degree of morbidity and mortality and occurs with some frequency. The CNS also is a common site for metastatic lesions; thus CNS tumor involvement often reflects advanced systemic disease.

ANATOMY AND PHYSIOLOGY

The intracranial cavity contains the cerebral hemispheres, the cerebellum, and brain stem. Each of the cerebral hemispheres has four lobes: frontal, temporal, parietal, and occipital (Figure 36-1). Below the cerebral hemisphere is the diencephalon, which contains the thalamus, basal ganglia, hypothalamus, and pineal gland. The midbrain, pons, and medulla make up the brain stem. The cerebellum is attached to the brain stem by three pairs of peduncles. The cerebellum has two hemispheres and a midline region called the vermis.

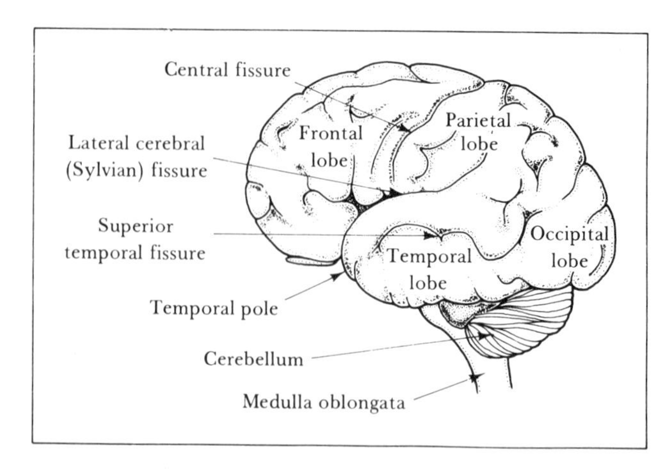

FIGURE 36-1 The four lobes of the cerebral hemispheres.

The cranial nerves have fiber pathways entering and exiting the brain and cranial cavity. The olfactory and optic nerves (I and II) are associated with cerebral hemispheres.

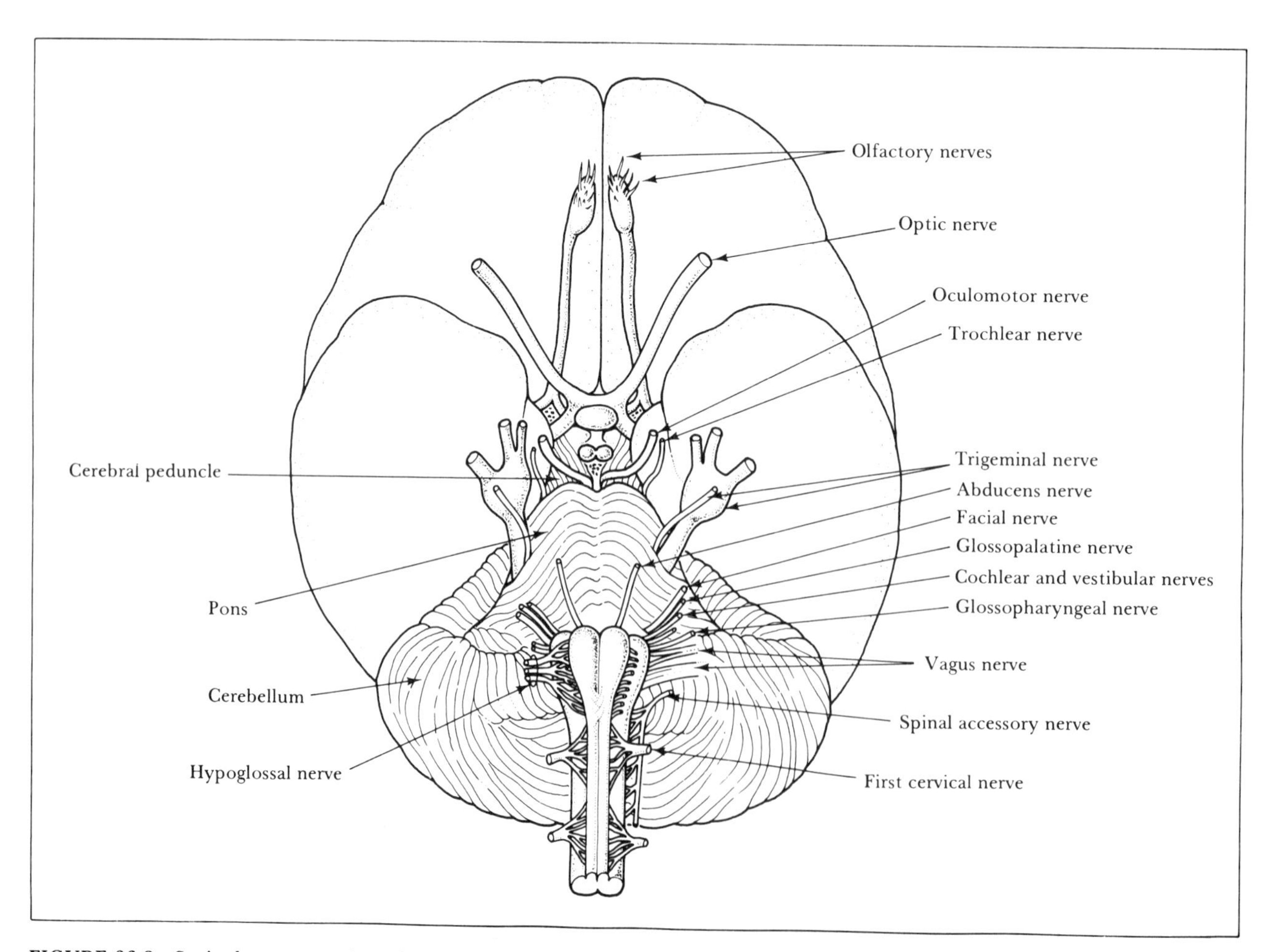

FIGURE 36-2 Sagittal representation of the brain.

The third and fourth cranial nerves, the occulomotor and trochlear, receive their fibers from the midbrain. The trigeminal nerve (V) is located between the midbrain and the pons; it has fibers running through the medulla, pons, and midbrain. The abducens and facial nerves (VI and VII) are located in the pons, with the abducens lying at the pontomedullary junction. The vestibulocochlear nerve (VIII) has fibers in the pons and in the medulla. The remaining central nerves—IX through XII (glossopharyngeal, vagus, spinal accessory, and hypoglossal)—are associated with the medulla (Figure 36-2). Symptoms of cranial nerve dysfunction provide valuable information for localizing an intracranial tumor.

The brain is supported and protected by the skull, meninges, and cerebrospinal fluid (CSF). The meninges consist of the tough dura mater below the skull, the arachnoid lining the dura, and the pia mater, which adheres directly to the surface of the brain. Cerebrospinal fluid circulates through the subarachnoid space, supporting and cushioning the brain and spinal cord (Figure 36-3).

The dura mater is a dense, tough layer of connective tissue. It is attached to the periosteum from which it receives small blood vessels. Two large partitions, or dural reflections, provide support for parts of the brain. These are the falx cerebri surrounding the cerebral hemispheres and the tentorium cerebelli, which wraps between the occipital lobes and the cerebellum. The edge of the tentorium runs along the midbrain. The space between the tentorial notch, or incisura, and the midbrain is small. This narrow space is the only passageway between the supratentorial and subtentorial regions (Figure 36-4).

Cerebrospinal fluid is formed in ventricles and circulates through the brain and spinal pathways. The choroid plexuses of the lateral, third, and fourth ventricles are responsible for the majority of CSF production. The flow of CSF is from the lateral ventricles through the intra-

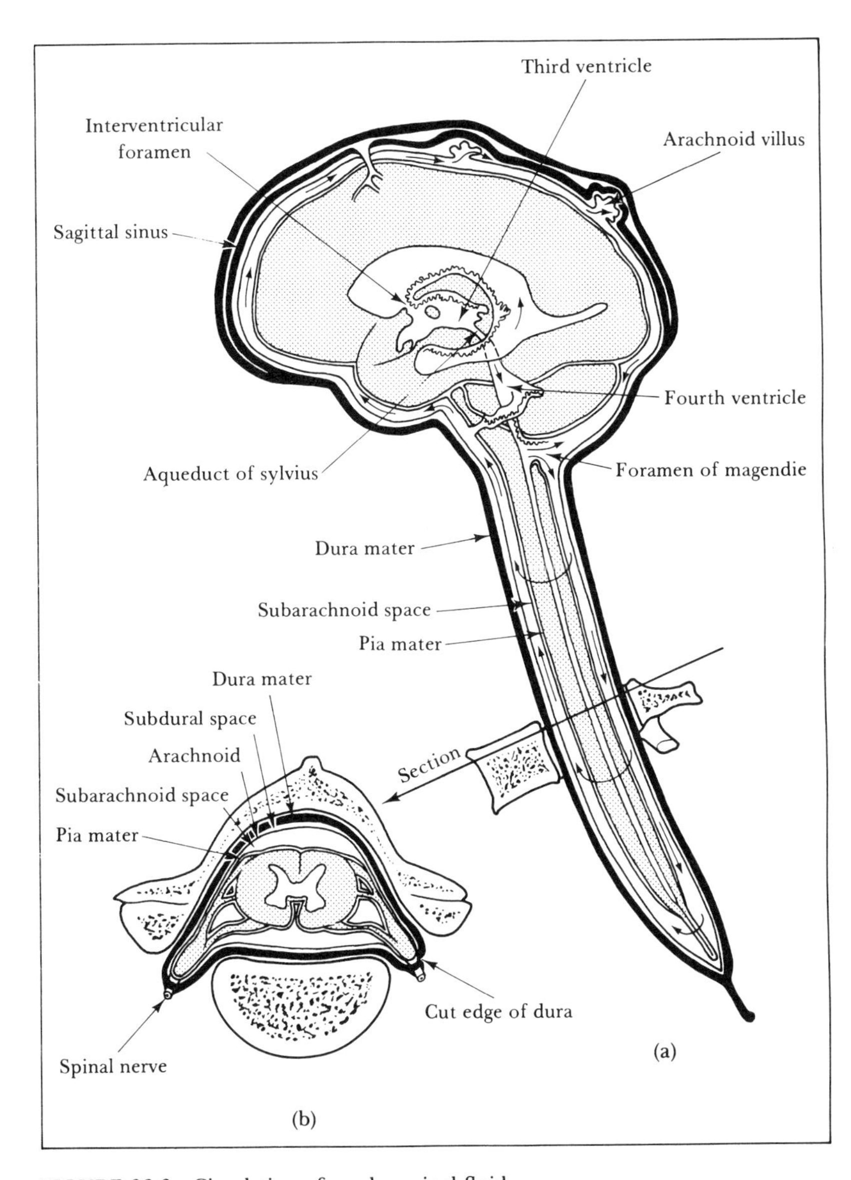

FIGURE 36-3 Circulation of cerebrospinal fluid.

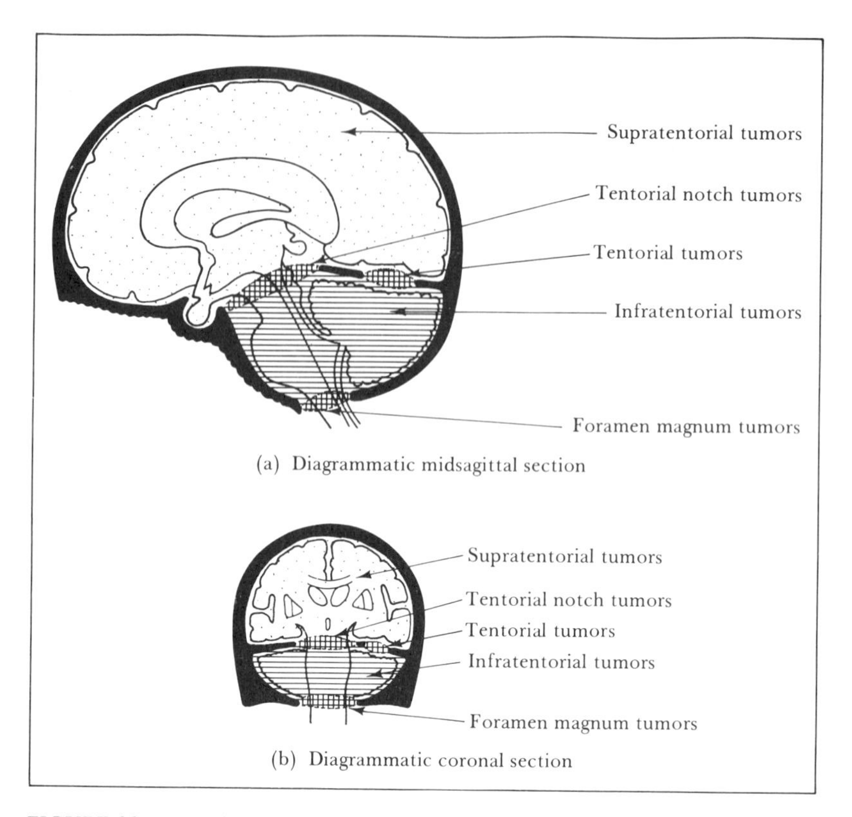

FIGURE 36-4 Localization of intracranial tumors.

ventricular foramen, into the third ventricle, through the aqueduct of Sylvius, and into the fourth ventricle. Cerebrospinal fluid exits from the ventricular system via the foramen of Magendie and the foramina of Luschka. Fluid circulates around the brain and the spinal cord. It is absorbed into the venous system by the arachnoid villi, which project into the dural venous sinuses. The sagittal sinus is an important site of reabsorption.

Blood flow to the brain is supplied by the two internal carotid arteries and the two vertebral arteries. The internal carotid arteries supply approximately 80% of this blood flow. The internal carotid bifurcates to form the anterior and middle cerebral arteries. These arteries supply blood to the frontal, temporal, and parietal lobes. The vertebral arteries enter the base of the skull and join to form the basilar artery. The cerebellum and the brain stem receive blood from the posterior cerebral artery. This artery supplies the occipital lobes and inferior and medial aspects of the temporal lobes.

Collateral circulation to the brain is provided by an intact circle of Willis (Figure 36-5). The posterior communicating arteries provide a connection between the internal carotid and posterior cerebral arteries. The two anterior cerebral arteries are connected by the anterior communicating artery. Blood can be shunted from one area of the brain to another in the event of sudden occlusion. This is possible only when the communicating arteries are present; these arteries are not present in all individuals.

Blood flow to the brain remains constant between systemic arterial pressures of 60 and 145 mm Hg. This regulatory mechanism is called autoregulation. Cerebral blood flow and blood volume in the brain are controlled through adjustments in the size of blood vessels. The cerebrovascular resistance (vasoconstriction or vasodilatation) regulates blood flow in accordance with metabolic needs. It also maintains a normal intracranial pressure despite fluctuations in arterial pressure and venous drainage.

Cerebral blood vessels dilate in response to decreased pH and increased Pa_{CO_2}. Decreased Pa_{CO_2} also will increase cerebral blood flow through vasodilatation. Declining Pa_{CO_2} causes a constriction of cerebral blood vessels and a decrease in blood flow. A decline in Pa_{CO_2} can occur as a result of decreased metabolic demand or hyperventilation.

Intracranial pressure (ICP) is maintained within the normal range by the autoregulatory mechanism. The two major determinants of ICP in normal and abnormal conditions are the arterial blood pressure and the intracranial venous pressure.[1] Arterial blood pressure increases with certain activities: sneezing, coughing, isometric muscle contraction, and performance of a Valsalva maneuver. Venous pressure is increased by obstruction of blood outflow. This is accomplished by jugular compression, flexion-extension of the neck, and rotation of the neck.[2] Because intracranial veins do not have valves, pressure in the venous system can be transmitted to the cranium. Increased intrathoracic or intraabdominal pressure can obstruct venous outflow. Activities that increase thoracic and abdom-

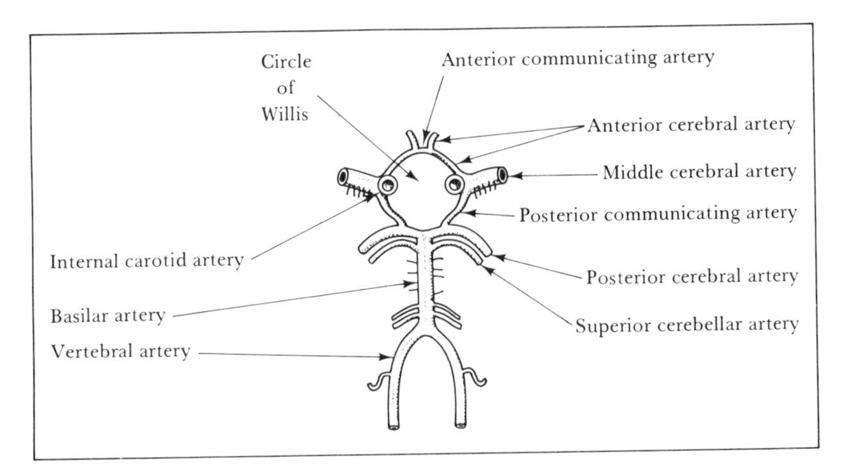

FIGURE 36-5 Circle of Willis.

inal cavity pressures include positive end-expiratory pressure (PEEP) treatments, hip flexion, Valsalva maneuvers, and lying on the abdomen. Elevating the head of the bed promotes venous drainage.

In the autoregulating brain, ICP remains constant despite changes in systemic arterial blood pressure and intracranial venous drainage. Loss of autoregulation means that cerebral blood flow and volume will fluctuate passively with systemic blood pressure. Activities that affect blood pressure and intracranial venous pressure will have significant effects on ICP.

EPIDEMIOLOGY

The most prevalent malignant CNS tumor is the tumor within the cranium, or the brain tumor. More than 50% of primary brain tumors are malignant and infiltrate the brain substance. Metastatic intracranial tumors occur predominantly in middle-aged individuals because the rate of metastasis increases with each decade of life, reaching a peak during the seventh decade in men and the sixth decade in women.

There are approximately 15,000 new cases of primary brain and CNS tumors and 11,000 deaths from CNS tumors each year in the United States.[3] Malignant brain tumors account for 1.4% of all cancer in the United States.[3] The death rate from brain and nervous system tumors is slightly higher for males than for females. Five-year survival rates for brain and nervous system cancer have been increasing slowly, with a 23% survival rate for white and a 31% survival rate for black persons.[3]

Most malignant CNS tumors are metastatic from a distant site. The most common primary sites include the lung, the breast, and the colon. Metastatic brain tumors occur with equal frequency in all races, and incidence rates are slightly higher for males.[4] The lung is considered the primary tumor site with the greatest propensity for brain metastasis; thus of the 28% of the total cancer deaths in the United States that were due to lung cancer, a significant number involved metastatic brain lesions.[3]

The incidence of primary malignant brain tumors is smaller, estimated at 5 per 100,000 individuals. At least 10% of all nontraumatic neurologic disease results from primary brain tumors.[5] A somewhat higher incidence of CNS cancer also has been found in persons with poor response to immunosuppressive agents, and a familial tendency is implicated for some brain tumors, particularly glioblastoma.[6]

ETIOLOGY

Specific causes of the various CNS tumors remain speculative. Prophylactic radiation therapy of the brain in children with other malignancies (eg, leukemia) has been linked with the subsequent appearance of malignant brain tumors.[7,8] Similarly, an increased incidence of both primary and metastatic brain tumors, including intracranial lymphoma, was found following immunosuppressive therapy.[9]

Evidence as yet is inconclusive, but several researchers suggest that certain occupational exposures may predispose an individual to the development of CNS tumors. These include exposure to vinyl chloride, plutonium, and petroleum.[10-12] Another area of occupational concern is that of electronics, where an increased risk of astrocytic brain tumors may exist.[11]

PATHOPHYSIOLOGY

Classification of primary CNS tumors is based on the presumed cell type of the tumor. The distinction between benign and malignant tumors is seldom made in epidemiologic studies of CNS tumors because of the similarity of symptoms, depending on locations. Yet there are several models for classification based on embryogenetics, grading systems, and other histologic classifications. A decade ago collaboration of various groups resulted in the universal histologic classification of CNS tumors.[13] This classification provided a uniform international nomenclature that considered both histologic type and degree of malignancy.[14] The histologic classification of CNS tumors is as follows:

- Tumors of neuroepithelial tissue
  Astrocytic tumors
  Oligodendroglial tumors
  Ependymal and choroid plexus tumors
  Pineal cell tumors
  Neuronal tumors
- Poorly differentiated and embryonal tumors
  Glioblastoma
  Medulloblastoma
  Medulloepithelioma
  Primitive polar spongioblastoma
  Gliomatosis cerebri
- Tumors of nerve sheath cells
  Neurilemmoma (schwannoma, neurinoma)
  Anaplastic (malignant) neurilemmoma (schwannoma, neurinoma)
  Neurofibroma
  Anaplastic (malignant) neurofibroma (neurofibrosarcoma, neurogenic sarcoma)
- Tumors of meningeal and related tissues
  Meningioma
  Meningeal sarcomas
  Xanthomatous tumors
  Primary melanotic tumors
- Tumors of blood vessel origin
  Hemangioblastoma (capillary hemangioblastoma)
  Monstrocellular sarcoma
- Germ cell tumors
  Germinoma
  Embryonal carcinoma
  Choriocarcinoma
  Teratoma

This classification represents the universally accepted histologic classifications of CNS tumors. Diagnostic classification and staging are discussed later in this chapter.

Primary brain tumors arise from neuroepithelial cells (glial cells) and are called gliomas. Glial cells are among the few neural cells that are capable of division. Gliomas include astrocytic tumors, oligodendroglial tumors, ependymal and choroid plexus tumors, pineal cell tumors, neuronal tumors, and poorly differentiated embryonal tumors. Those of astrocytic origin are the most common.[15]

Neuroepithelial tumor cells often are found diffusely in the perivascular spaces and subpial region of the cortex. Such tumors may appear to be multicentric. These tumors may spread via the CSF to distant parts of the nervous system. Metastases of primary neuroepithelial tumors outside the CNS are rare.[16] The most common primary CNS tumors of the adult are discussed in the sections that follow.

Astrocytoma

Astrocytomas make up the largest group of primary brain tumors of one cell type. In adults, astrocytomas are ranked third in frequency (10%), after glioblastomas and meningiomas.[6] Their incidence is greatest in individuals in the fifth and sixth decades of life and is somewhat higher in men than in women.[17]

Astrocytomas generally arise in the cerebral hemispheres of adults and develop in the central and subcortical white matter. Infrequently they may arise in the corpus striatum.[17] These tumors generally are solid but may appear as cystic lesions, such as cerebellar and spinal cord astrocytomas.[4] The histologic patterns of astrocytomas are varied. Grade I astrocytomas consist of well-differentiated astrocytes, whereas grade IV tumors demonstrate significant pleomorphism, cellularity, numerous mitoses, necrosis, and sometimes giant cells. Grades II and III are considered to be intermediate stages.

Astrocytoma grades III and IV (glioblastoma multiforme) may have multiple foci of origin. They are considered highly malignant because of their infiltrative character and lack of capsulation. Areas of necrosis and hemorrhage with frequent mitoses occur. Sloughing of tumor cells around necrotic foci is characteristic of these tumors. Vascular changes, such as endothelial proliferation, thrombosis, and fibroblastic proliferation, are features of these tumors.[4]

Oligodendroglioma

Fewer than 5% of all primary brain tumors are oligodendrogliomas. These tumors occur as typically circumscribed, spongy, and vascular masses, usually located in the frontal lobes. Calcification is a usual finding within the tumor and adjacent brain tissue.[4,6]

Cellular pleomorphism in the form of multinucleated giant cells of the Langhans type is a feature of the oligodendroglioma. Other anaplastic features include abundant necrotic zones and a proliferation of blood vessels. This is a slow-growing tumor, which is most commonly manifested as a seizure disorder. It has shown a unique chemosensitivity to procarbazine, CCNU, and vincristine, which has enhanced research interest in this rare tumor.[18]

Glioblastoma

Glioblastoma is the most common (60%) of the primary adult brain tumors.[6] Glioblastomas arise in the cerebral hemisphere of adults, with a somewhat higher incidence in men than in women. They occur typically during the fifth and sixth decades of life. Glioblastomas have a predilection for the frontal lobe.

Glioblastoma is characterized by necrosis, pseudopalisading, fistulous vessels, vascular endothelium proliferation, and areas of old and fresh hemorrhages.[13] This is typically a grade IV tumor. Thrombosis and fibroblastic proliferation are also present.

Primary Malignant Lymphomas

Primary central nervous system lymphoma is a rare form of neoplasm, formerly representing less than 1% of primary brain tumors. Since 1980, however, the number of cases has tripled. There is an increasing incidence of these tumors in the immunosuppressed patient (either inherited or acquired immunosuppression). Those populations at greatest risk include transplant recipients, patients with acquired immune deficiency syndrome (AIDS), and those with congenital immunodeficiencies. There also is a slightly higher incidence in men than in women. Approximately 3% of patients with AIDS will develop CNS lymphoma.[19]

This non-Hodgkin's lymphoma is mainly of B cell origin. Studies suggest that the Epstein-Barr virus plays a role in its development. This tumor may arise primarily in any part of the cerebrum, cerebellum, or brain stem and may be either monofocal or multifocal. Perivascular and meningeal spread results in shedding of cells into the CSF.[20]

CNS lymphoma appears in various ways, including neurologic dysfunction, apathy, confusion, or personality changes. Most of the AIDS-related primary brain lymphomas are reported to be of high or intermediate grade.[21]

Spinal Cord Tumors

CNS tumors include intraspinal tumors, which occur with considerably less frequency than intracranial tumors. Intraspinal tumors may be primary (approximately 15% of primary CNS tumors)[20] or metastatic. Regardless of pathophysiology, intraspinal tumors may result in spinal cord compression.

Cord compression is considered an oncologic emergency and is discussed in Chapter 31 of this text. Compression rapidly results in irreversible neurologic changes; therefore rapid surgical removal of the tumor is of utmost importance to relieve edema and related pressure.

Typically spinal cord tumors become clinically manifested in one of three ways.[20] Sensorimotor spinal tract syndromes compress the cord and cause destruction of cord tracts; initial asymmetric motor disturbance results. Radicular–spinal cord syndrome results in pain in the distribution of a sensory nerve root; the pain is intensified by straining and radiates in a distal direction, away from the spine. A syringomyelic syndrome results from an intramedullary tumor and produces a mixed sensorimotor tract syndrome.

Diagnosis of cord compression is established by spinal radiographs, CSF examination, and electromyography. Of particular importance to nursing are the ongoing assessment of neurologic status, prompt determination of a potential problem with compression, and immediate intervention to prevent irreversible neurologic damage and loss.

Metastatic Tumors

The incidence of metastatic brain tumors is estimated at 24% of the individuals who die of cancer.[22] Brain metastases are present at autopsy in 10% to 20% of individuals with systemic cancer.[5]

Intracranial metastases occur at three main sites: the skull and dura, the brain itself, and the meninges. The skull and dura are infiltrated by tumors that metastasize to the bone, particularly metastatic tumors of the breast and prostate. These metastases are believed to reach the skull via Batson's vertebral venous plexus, a valveless system of veins that runs the length of the vertebral column from the pelvic veins to the large venous sinuses of the skull, bypassing the systemic circulation.[20]

Metastases to the brain occur by hematogenous spread, with one third originating in the lung.[20] From the lungs, cancer cells may enter the pulmonary veins and reach the left atrium and ventricle. Tumor cells transported in this manner are widely dispersed and ultimately are deposited in the capillaries. Once within the arterial circulation, tumor cells readily travel to the brain and the liver. Tumor cells may return to the heart, enter the arterial circulation, and become generalized. Metastasis to the brain then occurs.

The most common site of metastasis in the brain is the cortex. Within the cortex is the terminal territory of the three main cerebral arteries: the middle, posterior, and anterior arteries. Because these arteries terminate so closely to one another, neoplastic emboli have a great tendency to develop there. In the majority of cases tumor cells spread to the brain via the arterial pathway described.

The individual at greatest risk of metastatic CNS involvement has widespread systemic disease when neurologic symptoms develop.[4] Tumors that metastasize to the brain are manifest in many ways and involve every portion of the brain. A metastatic brain tumor may mimic the presentation of any primary brain tumor. The major symptoms of metastatic brain tumors arise as a result of increased ICP. Early complaints include headache, nausea and vomiting, and personality changes. Destruction of neurologic structures, cerebral edema, and seizures lead to additional symptoms.

Meningeal carcinomatosis is rare and occurs with widespread dissemination of tumor cells throughout the meninges and ventricles. Adams and Victor[20] identify approximately 4% of neurologic metastases as meningeal carcinomatosis arising from adenocarcinoma of breast, lung, and gastrointestinal tract, melanoma, and childhood leukemia. Principal manifestations are headache, backache, radiculopathies, cranial nerve palsies, and dementia. Hydrocephalus may occur. Diagnosis is based partly on examination of the CSF, which shows elevated protein and low glucose levels. Treatment includes radiation therapy to symptomatic areas, followed by intraventricular administration of methotrexate. Reports of median survival range from 43 days to 5.8 months after diagnosis.[20]

CLINICAL MANIFESTATIONS

The signs and symptoms of brain tumors are variable. Clinical manifestations vary, depending on site, size, method of expansion, and other factors related to the nature of the tumor. The clinical manifestations can be classified into three major categories: generalized effects of increased ICP, secondary effects due to shifts or displacement of brain structures, and focal effects. Any one of these mechanisms may predominate throughout the course of an individual's illness. More often several of these mechanisms are producing effects simultaneously (Figure 36-6).

Increased Intracranial Pressure

In adults the skull acts as a rigid sphere. Its contents are fixed in total volume. The cranium encases the three normal components of the intracranial cavity: brain, cerebrospinal fluid, and blood. Each of these components is displaceable. To maintain normal ICP, an increase in the volume of one component must be accompanied by a proportional decrease in the volume of one or both of the other components. Compensatory mechanisms for accommodating a volume increase include decreased cerebral blood volume, decreased CSF production, increased CSF absorption, and brain fluid shifts from the head to the spinal cavity. The compensatory changes are limited, especially when a volume increase is too large or too sudden. Beyond, a certain point, additions of any further volume result in large increases in ICP. Once all the compensatory mechanisms are exhausted, relatively small increases in volume create large increases in ICP.

Brain tumors increase ICP by their size, cerebral edema, or obstruction of CSF pathways. A combination of tumor bulk and peritumoral edema usually is responsible for an increase in ICP. In the area of the third and fourth ventricles, a comparatively small tumor can block CSF flow. In contrast, extensive tumors can sometimes exist without causing an immediate increase in ICP. These are tumors in the frontal or temporal lobes (such as meningiomas) and diffusely infiltrative tumors (glioblastomas), which only partially damage structures during infiltration.

Clinical manifestations are produced by the effects of increasing ICP on nerve cells, blood vessels, and dura. Prolonged increase in ICP ultimately produces nerve cell damage and cell death. An expanding tumor mass can create a vicious cycle of intracranial hypertension (Figure 36-7). Once all the normal compensatory mechanisms have been used, increased ICP is compensated for by a decrease in cerebral blood flow (total blood volume in the brain). A decrease in the supply of oxygen and glucose to the brain leads to tissue hypoxia and a decreased blood supply impedes the removal of carbon dioxide and lactic acid. These two products of metabolism are potent vasodilatators. Vasodilatation of cerebral blood vessels creates further vasogenic edema. The total volume within the cranium is increased, intracranial pressure again rises, and the cycle repeats itself.

Cerebral blood flow is relatively constant in the healthy brain; blood flow to the brain is independent of changes in arterial blood pressure. This autoregulation of cerebral blood flow ensures a constant blood supply to the brain between the limits of mean systemic arterial pressures of 60 to 145 mm Hg.[1] In the normal autoregulating brain, changes in systemic blood pressure have no effect on ICP. When ICP rises to very high levels, however, the autoreg-

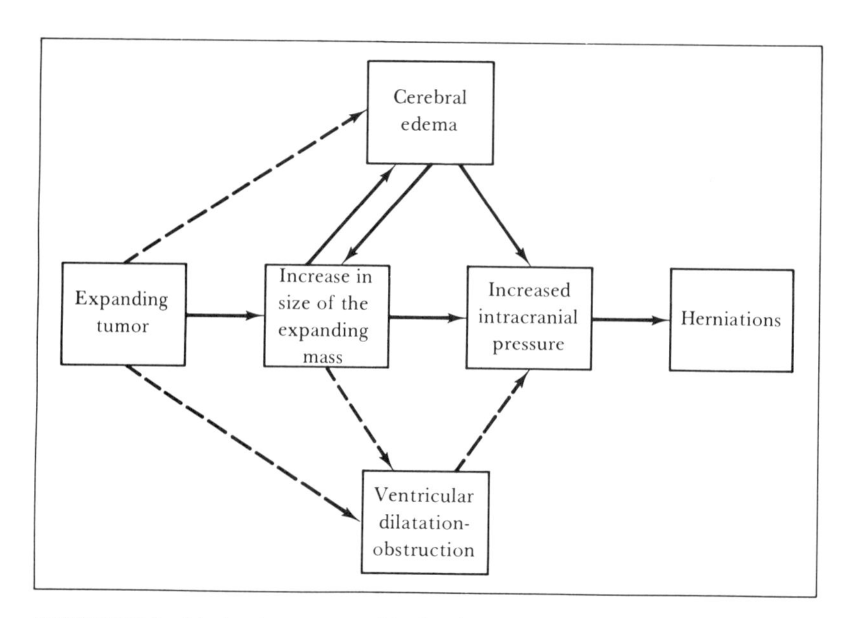

FIGURE 36-6 Mechanisms responsible for the clinical manifestations of intracranial tumors.

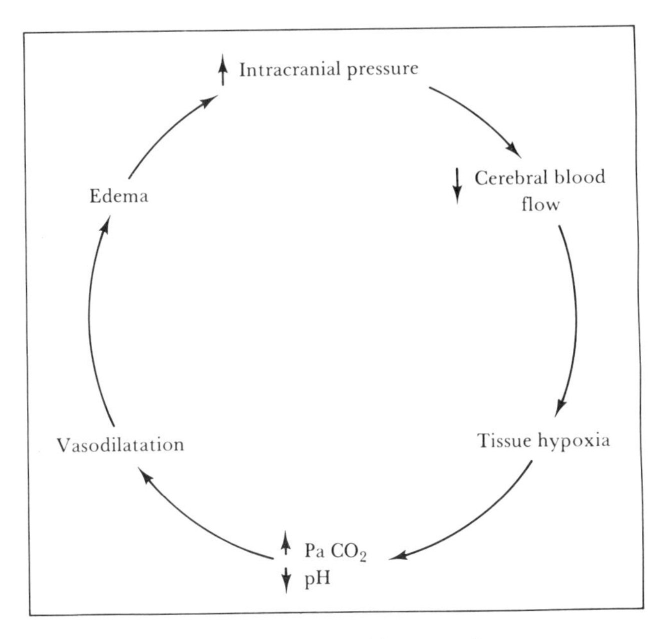

FIGURE 36-7 Cycle of intracranial hypertension.

ulatory system fails and the cerebral blood flow drops. The total blood supply to the brain is decreased. Lack of autoregulation means that cerebral blood flow fluctuates passively with the systemic arterial blood pressure. Increases in systemic blood pressure directly affect ICP. If the cycle of increasing pressure and decreasing cerebral blood flow continues, the brain tissue no longer receives an adequate blood supply and brain death occurs eventually.

The clinical manifestations of generalized increased ICP include mental changes, papilledema, headache, vomiting, and changes in vital signs. These signs and symptoms are nonspecific or nonlocalizing. Increased ICP can cause secondary effects by displacing brain tissue.

Changes in mental status include alterations in the level of consciousness, confusion, short-term memory loss, and personality changes. Each individual may show a wide variety of mental changes. These changes frequently are gradual in onset. Subtle initial changes may be evident only to the patient's family or to a skilled observer. In the early stages of increasing ICP, individuals may complain of drowsiness, a decreased attention span, and memory loss. Families may report changes in behavior and personality, mood changes, poor judgment, or blunting of intellectual functions. If the increased ICP is not treated, basic levels or states of consciousness are affected. The individual can go from a state of alertness (awake, fully aware of normal internal and external stimuli) to one of lethargy or somnolence. As ICP increases over time, the level of consciousness deteriorates from full alertness to somnolence, stupor, and finally coma.

Papilledema is considered a cardinal sign of increased ICP. An increase in CSF pressure around the optic nerve impairs the outflow of venous blood. Edema or swelling of the optic disk results. Blurred vision and visual field defects may accompany papilledema, especially in the presence of long-standing increased ICP. Papilledema may be an early or late finding, depending on the nature and location of the brain tumor.

Headaches are reported as an early symptom in approximately one third of the individuals with a brain tumor. These headaches are variable in nature and should be distinguished from other types of headache (eg, migraine, muscle contraction). It should be noted that some persons with elevated ICP never report headache. Because brain tissue itself does not contain pain sensors, headache pain is believed to be a result of pressure or traction on the pain-sensitive structures of the dura, venous sinuses, surface blood vessels, and cranial nerves.

The headache that accompanies a generalized increase in ICP usually is bilateral; it generally is located in the frontal or occipital regions. Individuals may give a history of early morning headache that subsides on arising. Bending over, coughing, or performing a Valsalva maneuver may aggravate or initiate a headache. Pain may be reported as dull, sharp, or throbbing. Over time the headaches increase in severity, frequency, and duration.

Vomiting is part of the classic triad of increased ICP (vomiting, papilledema, and headache). It appears unrelated to food ingestion. Vomiting may be preceded by nausea, or it may be sudden, unexpected, and forceful (projectile). Increased pressure on the vomiting center of the medulla is believed to precipitate this symptom.

Changes in vital signs are a late finding in cases of increased ICP. They result from increased pressure on the vasomotor centers of the medulla. As ICP increases, circulatory and respiratory responses to intracranial hypertension occur. Systolic blood pressure rises, diastolic blood pressure drops, and the pulse pressure widens. Bradycardia and slowed, irregular respirations are seen. The combination of hypertension, bradycardia, and respiratory slowing is called the Cushing triad and is not always seen in individuals with elevated ICP. When this response is seen, it is a late finding; usually the individual is already comatose.

Secondary Effects: Displacement of Brain Structures

The cranial cavity is divided into compartments by the rigid dura mater that surrounds the cerebral hemispheres (falx cerebri) and the cerebellum (tentorium cerebelli). Pressure normally is distributed equally throughout the compartments of the cranial cavity (Figure 36-8a). A growing tumor mass and the edema associated with it cause increased pressure within a cranial compartment. An increase in pressure in any one compartment can cause brain tissue to protrude from one compartment into another. Brain tissue shifts or herniates from the high-pressure compartment into a lower-pressure compartment. The resulting brain damage is life threatening.

Herniation is a neurologic emergency. Shifting brain tissue causes compression damage, cerebral edema, and ischemia. Blood vessels may be damaged by stretch and angulation pressures, which may produce an obstruction in blood flow or vessel rupture. Displaced brain tissue can obstruct CSF pathways, causing an obstructive hydrocephalus. These compressive, ischemic, vascular, and obstructive changes all add to and aggravate the original problem of increased ICP. The potentially reversible complications of an expanding tumor become irreversible.

An expanding tumor mass can displace tissue distant from the tumor site. The neurologic signs and symptoms that accompany these shifts may have true or false localizing value. There are two major classifications of herniation: supratentorial brain shifts and infratentorial brain shifts. The clinical manifestations of the two types differ. Supratentorial herniations cause changes in the level of consciousness and ocular, motor, and respiratory signs. Infratentorial herniations cause loss of consciousness and respiratory and cardiac changes. There is an orderly rostral-to-caudal progression of abnormal clinical signs. However, sudden changes in intracranial dynamics will rapidly precipitate medullary compression (as in hemorrhage or a lumbar puncture).

Supratentorial tumors, lesions above the tentorium cerebelli, displace brain structures in the anterior and middle fossae. An expanding tumor eventually takes up so much space that the supratentorial compartment can no longer tolerate the volume it displaces. The pressure of the tumor mass and its edema push the brain downward. The only outlet for this pressure is the opening at the tentorial notch (incisura). As pressure forces brain structures downward, the tissue becomes ischemic and edematous. Blood vessels may rupture. These reactions add to the problem of increasing ICP. Additional increases in pressure displace the swollen brain tissue farther downward.

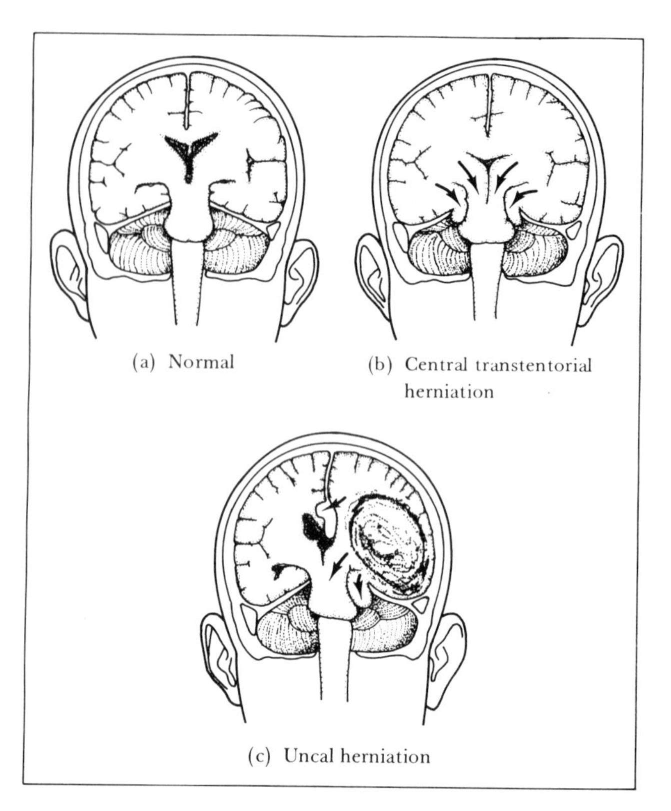

FIGURE 36-8 Intracranial shifts due to supratentorial lesions. (a) Normal. (b) Central transtentorial herniation. (c) Uncal herniation.

Central or transtentorial herniation occurs when the cerebral hemispheres, basal ganglia, diencephalon, and adjacent midbrain are displaced downward. The final result is a protrusion of the diencephalon and adjoining midbrain through the tentorial notch (Figure 36-8b). The first signs of impending central herniation are those of diencephalic dysfunction. A change in behavior or level of consciousness may signal early dysfunction. The individual may become agitated, drowsy, inattentive, or forgetful. As the tumor continues to displace tissue downward, the individual passes from alertness to stupor and then coma. Pupil size is reduced. Depending on the degree of diencephalic impairment, eye movements may be roving, conjugate, slightly disconjugate, or unmoving. Oculocephalic and oculovestibular responses may be impaired, and upward-gaze palsy may be seen. Motor signs include a bilateral Babinski's sign, contralateral hemiparesis, and ipsilateral paratonic resistance.

Uncal herniation occurs when the medial part of one of the temporal lobes is forced toward the midline and downward through the tentorial opening (Figure 36-8c). This characteristically occurs when the expanding tumor is in the temporal lobe. The pressure of the tumor shifts the medial aspect of the temporal lobe (the uncus) over the edge of the tentorial notch. The uncus compresses the midbrain laterally; the midbrain (cerebral peduncle) becomes compressed against the opposite tentorial notch. The herniated rim of the temporal lobe compresses the third cranial nerve, the cerebral peduncle, and the posterior cerebral artery. The downward pressure may also result in the stretching of blood vessels, which causes secondary brain stem hemorrhages.

In uncal herniation, the early signs of compression of the third nerve and lateral midbrain (cerebral peduncle) may precede changes in the level of consciousness. The third nerve passes through the tentorial notch on its way to the eye and is vulnerable to compression. The third nerve ipsilateral to the brain tumor is affected. Initially the pupil contracts sluggishly in response to direct light. With further compression on the third nerve, pupillary dilation results. With midbrain compression, the motor pathways of the cerebral peduncle are compromised. Compression of the cerebral peduncle produces a contralateral hemiparesis. Sometimes uncal herniation pushes the opposite cerebral peduncle against the tentorial notch opposite the side of herniation. This is referred to as Kernohan's notch. A hemiparesis ipsilateral to the third nerve palsy is produced; this may cause confusion in determination of the side on which a unilateral brain tumor is located. The important thing to remember is that the tumor is ipsilateral to the third nerve palsy.

Babinski's sign is seen with hemiparesis. Decerebrate or decorticate rigidity is a later finding. In the early stages, oculocephalic and oculovestibular responses are conjugate; later, they are dysconjugate because of impaired ipsilateral eye movement (third nerve). Third nerve function, motor signs, and changes in level of consciousness are early clinical manifestations of uncal herniation.

Both central and uncal herniations cause changes in the respiratory pattern. Irregular depth and rhythm often are more significant than changes in respiratory rate alone. In the initial stages respiration may be irregular with occasional pauses, sighs, or gasps. Later respiratory changes include Cheyne-Stokes breathing; sustained hyperventilation; slow, irregular (ataxic) breathing; apnea; and, finally, respiratory arrest.

The classic signs of Cushing's triad (rising systolic blood pressure, falling diastolic blood pressure, and bradycardia) do not occur with most supratentorial herniations. These changes in vital signs are seen during the terminal phase of herniation. The important clinical manifestations of supratentorial herniation are changes in level of consciousness, pupillary size and reaction to light, ocular movement, motor strength and response, and respiratory pattern.

Infratentorial herniations involve displacement of the cerebellum (Figure 36-9). Neurologic deficits are produced by the protrusion of the cerebellum either upward or downward. There are two exits from the infratentorial compartment: upward through the opening in the tentorium cerebelli and downward through the foramen magnum. When posterior fossa tumors expand, the cerebellum may be displaced upward, causing midbrain compression. More commonly, cerebellar herniation results in a downward protrusion of the cerebellar tonsils through the foramen magnum. This cerebellar pressure cone, or foramen magnum herniation, results in medullary compression. It is the most dangerous complication of intratentorial tumors, as medullary compression causes respiratory and circulatory arrest.

Upward transtentorial herniation compresses the midbrain. Vascular obstruction and blockage of CSF pathways can occur with the distortion of brain structures. It is not certain whether individuals with upward transtentorial herniation have a consistent syndrome of clinical manifestations. They often lose consciousness immediately. This is accompanied by altered respiratory, pupillary, ocular, and motor signs.

Downward cerebellar tonsillar herniation can be caused by generalized, increased intracranial pressure, midline tumor, or posterior fossa tumors. The outflow of the fourth ventricle is blocked by protrusion of the tonsils into the foramen magnum. The downward pressure also compresses the vasomotor centers of the medulla, causing respiratory changes. Sudden respiratory and circulatory arrest can occur. These may be precipitated by events that cause a sudden rise in intracranial pressure, such as sneezing, coughing, or performance of a Valsalva maneuver. Individuals with early signs of herniation may complain of a suboccipital headache and neck pain. The head may be held stiffly or to one side, or the neck may be arched. There may be vomiting and cranial nerve palsies (cranial nerves VII to XII). Altered consciousness with resulting coma is an early sign. Later signs of medullary dysfunction include respiratory irregularity (cluster breathing, gasping, ataxia), cardiac dysrhythmia, bradycardia or tachycardia, increased systolic blood pressure, and decreased diastolic blood pressure. Frequently, individuals with cerebellar–foramen magnum herniation have a sudden loss of consciousness followed by respiratory arrest.

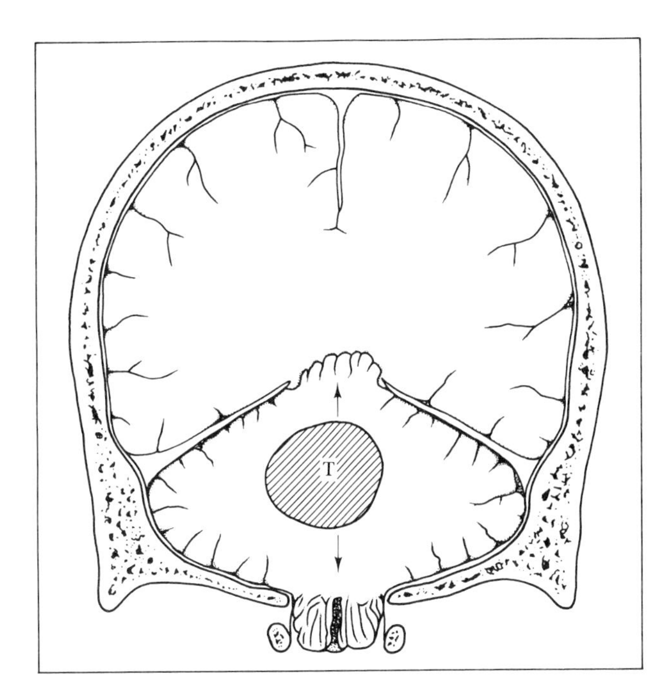

FIGURE 36-9 An infratentorial tumor causing an upward and downward shift of the cerebellum.

Focal Effects

Individual cranial nerves are associated with certain structures of the brain. Cranial nerve function may be affected by tumors that are located in intracranial compartments through which the cranial nerves pass. Neurologic deficits are related directly to the damaged area of the brain; the accompanying signs and symptoms therefore help one locate the tumor (Table 36-1). Intracranial tumors produce a wide variety of neurologic symptoms because of their direct focal effects on brain tissue. The focal effects of brain tumors are caused by direct compression of nerve tissue or destruction and invasion of brain tissue through infiltration.

Cerebral tumors of the motor and sensory strip cause deficits contralateral to the site of the tumor, whereas cerebellar tumors cause ipsilateral neurologic deficits. In the majority of individuals, the left side of the brain is the dominant hemisphere for speech representation. It is involved in the processing of information regarding language. The right hemisphere (nondominant in the majority of individuals) processes spatial-temporal information. A right-handed individual with a left hemisphere tumor may have problems with reading, arithmetic, writing, initiation of speech, or comprehension of speech in addition to some degree of motor loss. An individual with a tumor in the right hemisphere is more likely to have problems with right-left discrimination, body image (neglect of one side or part of the body), stereognosis, and other processing of sensory information.

TABLE 36-1 Clinical Manifestations of Intracranial Tumors

Location	Function	Abnormality
Frontal lobes	Intellect Personality Judgment Abstract thinking Mood and affect Memory Motor activity (contralateral) Expressive speech (left hemisphere)	Intellectual deterioration Personality changes Impaired judgment Bowel and bladder incontinence Emotional lability Memory loss Muscle weakness or paralysis Babinski's sign Decreased deep tendon reflexes Expressive aphasia
Parietal lobes	Sensory input (contralateral)	Decrease or loss of sensation (pain, temperature, pinprick, light touch, proprioception, vibration, two-point discrimination, double simultaneous stimulation, stereognosis, graphesthesia)
Occipital lobes	Sight Visual identification of objects	Visual field defects, hallucinations, inability to identify objects or symbols
Temporal lobes	Hearing Memory Receptive speech	Hearing changes, hallucinations Memory loss Receptive aphasia
Cerebellum	Coordination Balance (ipsilateral)	Ataxia, action tremor Nystagmus Loss of balance, wide-base gait Decreased deep, tendon reflexes

Seizures are a major manifestation of cerebral brain tumors, and in many adults they are the first clinical manifestation. Nerve tumor cells are abnormal, epileptogenic cells that are highly excitable and fire repetitively; focal or generalized seizures are the result. In some cases a generalized seizure is initiated focally and spreads rapidly to involve the entire brain. A careful description of the onset of the seizure, the seizure activity, and the postictal phase may have tumor-localizing value.

Patients with intracerebral metastases represent a subgroup of individuals with CNS tumors who may be at increased risk of late seizures. Yet, even in view of the known risk of postseizure sequelae, Cohen et al[23] recommend withholding of prophylactic anticonvulsant therapy until the first seizure.

ASSESSMENT

Patient assessment includes documentation of the presence and severity of both focal and generalized symptoms. The individual's response to the symptoms is identified, and a baseline measurement of neurologic dysfunction is made.

Posner[22] identifies the following symptoms of metastatic brain tumors in order of presentation: headache, focal weakness, mental disturbances, seizures, aphasia, and visual abnormalities. The evaluation of headache therefore assumes major importance in the interview with the patient. The assessment will ascertain information regarding the location, onset, and duration of headache. Episodic effects of headache also must be explored.

Other presenting symptoms, such as mental changes and sensory loss, are explored with the patient. Seizure represents an important area that warrants attention. The nurse determines whether the patient has had seizures or seizurelike activity, as well as the frequency and extent of such activity.

The physical examination includes a thorough neurologic examination, which involves an evaluation of the cranial nerves, the motor nervous system, the sensory nervous system, and cerebellar function and may also include extensive laboratory testing.

Testing of cranial nerve function is the most involved part of the neurologic examination. Table 36-2 lists the 12 cranial nerves, the methods of testing them, and the expected normal reactions.

TABLE 36-2 Examination of Cranial Nerves

Cranial Nerve	Method of Testing	Desired Response
I Olfactory	Inhalation of commonly recognized aromatic substance such as cloves; avoid the use of ammonia or alcohol because these stimulate the trigeminal nerve and evoke a pain response	Identification of the substance with each nostril
II Optic	Direct ophthalmoscopy; use finger movement and eye charts to test visual acuity and fields	Note the appearance of the optic disk, macula, vessels, and retina; correct eye movement and chart identification with each eye separately
III Oculomotor IV Trochlear VI Abducens	Individual follows the examiner's finger with the eyes to test eye movement; check pupil response to light; observe for ptosis of the eyelid, which indicates destruction of cranial nerve III	Movement of eyes should be equal in all six cardinal directions of gaze; pupils react to direct and consensual response to light; eyes are symmetric at rest and move conjugatively
V Trigeminal	Individual clamps the jaw, opens the mouth against resistance and masticates to check motor division of the nerve; touch both sides of the person's face, checking for pain, touch, and temperature response; gently touch the person's cornea with a cotton wisp to check the corneal reflex	Correct identification of sensations; rapid blinking
VII Facial	Observe for facial symmetry and the person's ability to contract muscles to check motor division; individual tastes sweet, sour, salty, and acidic flavors	Person smiles and frowns with symmetry; correct identification of tastes
VIII Acoustic	Test hearing ability with the use of whispered voice and tuning fork at various distances from the ear to check the cochlear nerve; check the vestibular nerve by having the person stand on one foot with eyes closed	Recognition of sound; maintain balance
IX Glossopharyngeal	Check the gag reflex by touching the pharynx with a tongue depressor	Gag response
X Vagus	Check the individual's swallowing ability; ask the person to cough and speak; glossopharyngeal and vagus nerves are easily examined together because of overlapping innervation of the pharynx	Speak without hoarseness or weakness
XI Spinal accessory	Ask the individual to elevate the shoulders, turn the head, and resist the examiner's attempts to pull the chin back to midline; check the symmetry of the trapezius and sternocleidomastoid muscles	Equal bilateral muscle strength; atrophy may indicate nerve dysfunction
XII Hypoglossal	Ask the individual to protrude the tongue	Absence of deviations, atrophy, or tremors

DIAGNOSTIC STUDIES

Numerous diagnostic measures have been designed to determine the presence of CNS tumors. All of these measures require direct nursing intervention to help the individual understand the procedures.

Pneumoencephalography, the study of the ventricular and cisternal systems, permits the observer to determine the shape and position of the ventricles and whether any abnormal masses exist in this area. The patient will experience a severe headache during and after this procedure and receives nothing to eat or drink before the procedure. If a brain tumor is present, the temporary increase of pressure within the cranium during pneumoencephalography may cause seizure activity. This is anticipated and proper precautions are taken. A permission form must be signed by the patient before the examination is conducted.

Many metastatic lesions are relatively avascular. They are demonstrable only by their mass effect in displacing normal cerebral arterial patterns. Cerebral arteriography allows the circle of Willis and the large blood vessels that penetrate the cerebrum to be visualized by serial imaging of the transit of a contrast medium through the brain's vascular bed. Cerebral arteriography is used most often to confirm metastatic tumor in the individual with a positive brain scan but with a doubtful diagnosis. This procedure can cause seizures, facial weakness, and decreased hand grip on the side opposite the injection of the contrast medium. The individual is observed for changes in pulse rate, blood pressure, and respiration after this procedure.

The diagnosis of brain tumors has been greatly facilitated by the development of computed tomography (CT) and magnetic resonance imaging (MRI). CT scanning measures the attenuation of x-ray beams passing through sections of the body from hundreds of different angles. On the basis of these measurements, a computer reconstructs pictures of the body's interior.[24] When used for the diagnosis of brain tumors, CT scanning views one plane of the cranium in circular fashion by a narrow x-ray beam over a period of seconds to minutes.[25] Lesions are seen as nodules of varying size, and photographs are produced for diagnostic purposes (Figures 36-10 and 36-11).

CT scanning offers advantages other than detection and diagnosis of brain tumors. It demonstrates the precise location of lytic metastases, as well as the extent of accompanying soft tissue masses, both intracranially and beneath the scalp. Edema surrounding a tumor also may be discerned by CT scanning.[26]

Because of its multiplanar capability, magnetic resonance imaging (MRI) reveals more about the chemistry of the tissue being examined than does a CT scan. MRI provides information about the chemical composition of tissue, whereas CT scanning provides a means of visualizing

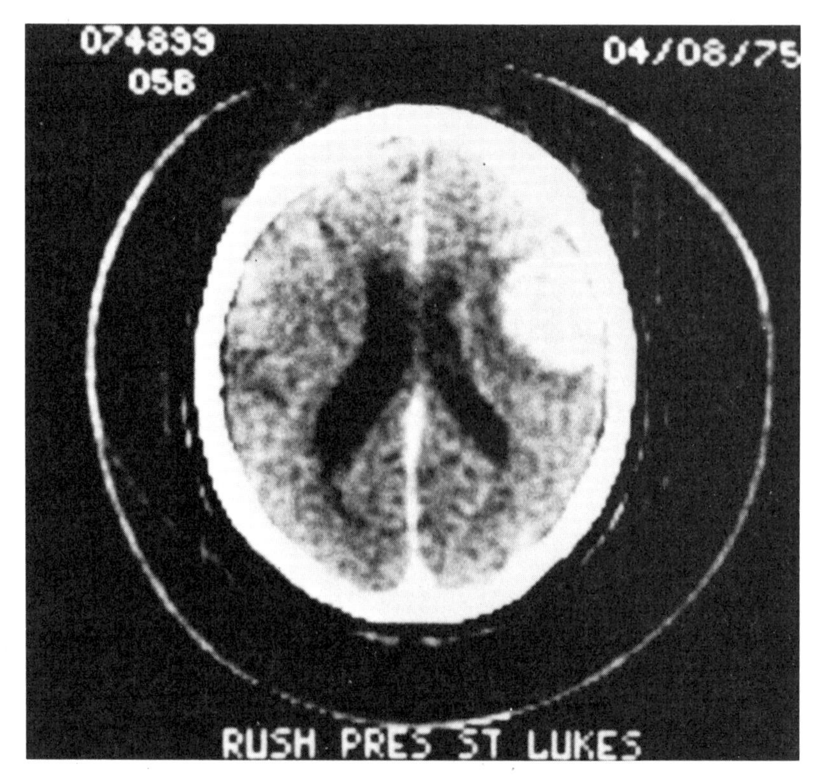

FIGURE 36-10 CT scan revealing a tumor of the right parietal lobe with some occlusion of the frontal horn of the ventricle. (Courtesy of Dr. M.S. Huckman, Chicago, Ill.)

the position and shape of the tissue. Various researchers have identified demonstrable advantages of MRI over CT scanning. Clarification of anatomic relationships and vessel patterns is greater with MRI, and diagnosis, staging, and follow-up are enhanced by MRI in children with neuroblastoma.[27,28] In some cases in which the CT scan is negative, MRI shows a tumor, because it has a higher soft tissue contrast.[29] Shuman et al[25] demonstrated that MRI identifies greater interface between tumor with edema and normal tissue. MRI is also effective in demonstrating secondary features of tumors, such as degree of edema, cyst formation, and presence of calcium aggregates. Particularly in the case of meningiomas, MRI can provide a clear histologic basis and offer crude predictions of pathologic subtype.[30]

Another noninvasive nuclear imaging technique being used for diagnostic purposes is positron-emission tomography (PET). This technique combines properties of conventional nuclear scanning with physical characteristics of positron-emitting radionuclides. Mathematical logarithms are applied that provide quantitative data to delineate the biochemistry in relation to the overall structure of the tissue in vivo.

While CT scanning is useful in discerning structures, the value of PET scanning is that metabolic processes may be quantified. "Time of flight" information is obtained by measuring the difference in arrival time of two annihilation photons after positron annihilation. This eliminates blurring in the final reconstructed image and improves the spatial resolution of an existing tumor.[31] PET also provides information on tumor metabolism through the study of blood flow and oxygen and glucose utilization.[32]

Francavilla et al[33] found that fluorodeoxygluconase (FDG) PET (with contrast) was helpful in the evaluation of malignant degeneration of low-grade gliomas. FDG-PET permits testing for ischemia and resulting tissue degeneration. Identification of degeneration helps the physician choose the appropriate treatment modality.

Further research with PET in patients with glioma demonstrates the ability to study glucose metabolism in hypometabolic and hypermetabolic tumors. Alavi et al[34] determined that PET distinguishes tumors with a good prognosis (hypometabolic) from tumors with a poor prognosis (hypermetabolic) and suggest that studies of glucose metabolism may provide an independent measure of the aggressiveness of a brain tumor, as well as supplement the pathologic grading.

The use of PET in diagnosis of brain tumor remains limited in comparison to CT and MRI. However, CT, MRI, and PET have produced a new era in the in vivo study of brain chemistry.[27]

Innovations in neuroradiology, including CT, PET, and MRI, have contributed greatly to the diagnosis and precise localization of brain tumors. The ultimate diagnosis and subsequent treatment arise from histopathologic findings.[34]

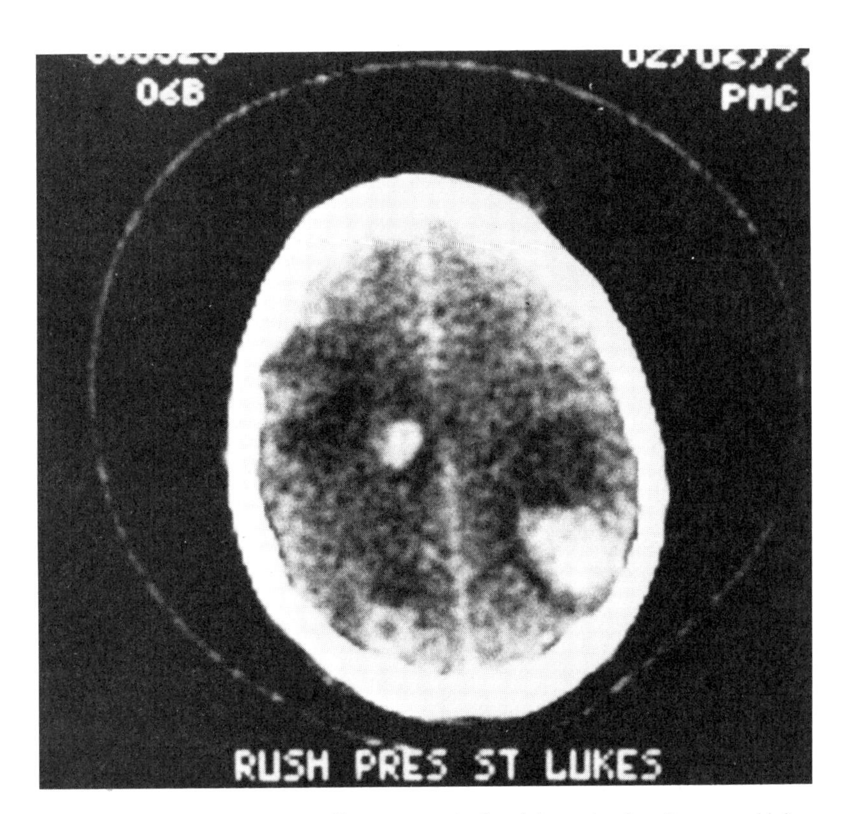

FIGURE 36-11 CT scan revealing a tumor in the right parietal and temporal lobes with surrounding edema and a smaller tumor in the left parietal lobe. (Courtesy of Dr. M.S. Huckman, Chicago, Ill.)

CLASSIFICATION AND STAGING

Beahrs et al[35] indicate that the most critical feature in the classification of CNS tumors is histopathology. Staging of such tumors, particularly intracranial tumors, has clinical and prognostic implications. Anatomic staging for tumors in general includes primary site, regional lymph nodes, and metastatic sites. There are no lymphatic structures draining the brain, but metastases from brain tumor may occur through seeding into the subarachnoid space.

Clinical staging of brain tumors is based on neurologic signs and symptoms, as well as on diagnostic tests. Pathologic staging is based on histopathology, grade, and microscopic evidence of completeness of removal of resected tumor. The histologic staging of brain tumors is found in Table 36-3.[35]

TABLE 36-3 Definition of TNM Classification of Brain Tumors

Primary tumor (T)

TX	Primary tumor cannot be assessed
TO	No evidence of primary tumor

Supratentorial tumor

T1	Tumor 5 cm or less in greatest dimension; limited to one side
T2	Tumor more than 5 cm in greatest dimension; limited to one side
T3	Tumor invades or encroaches upon the ventricular system
T4	Tumor crosses the midline, invades the opposite hemisphere, or invades infratentorially

Infratentorial tumor

T1	Tumor 3 cm or less in greatest dimension; limited to one side
T2	Tumor more than 3 cm in greatest dimension; limited to one side
T3	Tumor invades or encroaches upon the ventricular system
T4	Tumor crosses the midline, invades the opposite hemisphere, or invades supratentorially

Regional lymph nodes (N)

This category does not apply to this site.

Distant metastasis (M)

MX	Presence of distant metastasis cannot be assessed
MO	No distant metastasis
M1	Distant metastasis

Histopathologic grade (G)

GX	Grade cannot be assessed
G1	Well-differentiated
G2	Moderately well-differentiated
G3	Poorly differentiated
G4	Undifferentiated

Stage grouping

Stage IA	G1	T1	MO
Stage IB	G1	T2	MO
	G1	T3	MO
Stage IIA	G2	T1	MO
Stage IIB	G2	T2	MO
	G2	T3	MO
Stage IIIA	G3	T1	MO
Stage IIIB	G3	T2	MO
	G3	T3	MO
Stage IV	G1,2,3	T4	MO
	G4	Any T	MO
	Any G	Any T	M1

Source: Beahrs OH, Henson DE, Hutter R, et al: Manual for Staging of Cancer (ed 3). Philadelphia, JB Lippincott, 1988, pp 249-254.

TREATMENT

The treatment of CNS malignancies is determined by a number of factors, including primary site, tumor grade, and overall condition of the patient. Treatment is further defined by specific tumor types.[6] For purposes of this chapter, treatment is discussed in general terms that apply to any tumor of the CNS.

Surgery

The surgical treatment of brain tumors has improved with the use of the operating microscope and medical treatment to minimize cerebral edema. The individual with a primary brain tumor usually is a candidate for surgical excision as the initial treatment. Surgery may be performed on metastatic brain tumors as a palliative measure or to extend life. In rare cases cure can be achieved.

Several factors are considered in the evaluation of an individual for surgery: tumor location, size, method of spread, general condition of the individual, and the individual's neurologic status. For example, an encapsulated tumor that occupies a pole of the nondominant cerebral hemisphere lends itself to extensive resection. Complete excision of a rapidly growing glioblastoma in the center of the brain that has necrotic and hemorrhagic cysts may not be possible. Rather, internal decompression may be performed by removal of the main bulk of the tumor.

Fadul et al[36] explored factors that influence morbidity and mortality of craniotomy for excision of supratentorial gliomas. They found that patients with the highest morbidity and mortality were those with moderate to severe preoperative disabilities and deep midline lesions, persons over 55 years of age, and those receiving high doses of preoperative dexamethasone. These researchers also found that complete resection entailed no greater risks than biopsy or less extensive surgical procedures.

There are three approaches to the surgical management of the individual with a brain tumor: (1) surgery as the primary treatment, (2) surgery to facilitate nonsurgical therapy, and (3) no surgery at all. The aim of surgery as the primary treatment is complete removal of the tumor. The recent use of lasers and related approaches on eligible individuals permits more complete tumor excision. Partial tumor resection also may improve the individual's neurologic condition. Debulking the tumor may relieve symptoms by decreasing local compression and decreasing intracranial pressure. Small frontopolar, temporopolar, or occipitopolar tumors in the nondominant hemisphere are easier to resect. Resection is more difficult when the tumor is deep within the brain or in an area that controls vital human activities (brain stem, motor area). The surgical procedure must be technically possible and the projected quality of life for the individual worthwhile. The advantage of surgical therapy in carefully selected cases is increased survival time and an improved quality of survival.

Postoperative radiotherapy and/or chemotherapy is considered when tumor recurrence is likely. These treatments are indicated especially when excision is only partial. The aim of adjunctive therapy is to prevent or delay recurrence of the tumor.

Surgery may facilitate subsequent nonsurgical treatments, such as postoperative radiation. Surgery may be used to place radioactive substances within the tumor mass or to confirm the histologic or cytologic identification of a mass by biopsy. Stereotactic surgery was popular in the 1960s when it was used in the treatment of pain, movement disorders, epilepsy, and Parkinson's disease. More recently stereotactic surgery with computed tomography has been used in neurosurgery.[37] Coffey et al[38] propose stereotactic biopsy followed by radiation instead of surgical resection, especially for patients with malignant gliomas located in functionally important or inaccessible locations.

Surgical manipulation of a brain tumor may be inadvisable in individuals with invasive, rapidly growing tumors situated in critical areas of the brain who are in poor general health and have major neurologic deficits. Surgery or biopsy must be seriously evaluated and discussed with the patient and the family when the expected quality of survival is poor.

In the case of metastatic brain tumors, other factors should be considered. Factors favorable for surgery include a long interval between treatment of a primary extracranial neoplasm and diagnosis of an intracranial tumor, a single brain metastasis with no metastases to other parts of the body, an extracranial tumor that is responsive to therapy, a significant improvement in neurologic status with the administration of steroids, and minimal neurologic deficit, with increased intracranial pressure being the major problem. Tumors that are favorably situated and are not radiosensitive can be removed surgically. Good general health and neurologic status and a projected functional survival time of 6 months are strong indications for surgery.

Although there are many exceptions, depending on each individual's circumstances, factors considered unfavorable for surgical intervention include the presence of multiple small intracranial tumors, a major neurologic deficit that is unresponsive to steroid therapy, or a rapidly growing and disseminated tumor. Because of potential harm to future rehabilitation endeavors, it is more difficult to operate on tumors in the dominant hemisphere, basal ganglia, speech centers, or motor areas.

The most serious postoperative complications of neurosurgery are intracranial bleeding, cerebral edema, and water intoxication. The signs and symptoms of these complications may be the same: decreasing level of consciousness, increased ICP, progressive hemiparesis or other neurologic deficit, and possibly signs of herniation or seizures.

Hemorrhage into the operative cavity may take place within hours after surgery. Bleeding also may occur from traction on the bridging veins between the brain and the dura. Rupture of these vessels produces a subdural hematoma.

Postoperative cerebral edema frequently is severe after the excision of malignant tumors. In anticipation of brain swelling, the dura may be left open. Cerebral edema is treated with corticosteroids and osmotherapy. The effects of osmotic diuretic therapy on ICP are best determined by use of an intracranial pressure monitor. Other techniques for controlling intracranial hypertension include hyperventilation, hypothermia, and the use of anesthetic agents.

Other complications may follow a craniotomy. Wound infection, cerebral spinal fluid infection, or aseptic meningitis may develop within 3 or 4 days. Seizures may be an early or late postoperative problem and are controlled with anticonvulsant medication. Individuals undergoing neurosurgery also are susceptible to all of the systemic complications that can follow any period of immobility (ie, venous thrombosis and pulmonary embolism).

Surgery generally is the immediate treatment choice for tumors that cause spinal cord compression. Shaw, Mansfield, and Barges[39] discuss a one-stage posteriolateral decompression-stabilization procedure for patients with thoracolumbar intraspinal tumors. These authors demonstrated surgical success, with return to previous function, in their small (n = 9) sample. However, a rapid surgical approach was found to be less effective in the treatment of malignant astrocytomas of the spinal cord in the presence of hydrocephalus and dissemination of disease.[23]

Radiotherapy

The use of radiotherapy in the treatment of primary malignant brain tumors depends on the radiosensitivity of the particular tumor type. For example, glioblastoma is considered to have a negligible response to radiation. In contrast, medulloblastoma is considered to be highly radiosensitive, and radiotherapy may be initiated immediately after histologic confirmation of this tumor. Other primary brain tumors may be treated with radiation after surgical resection.

Radiotherapy also is used in the treatment of metastatic brain tumors. Typically, individuals have multiple cerebral metastases and are not considered to be candidates for surgical resection. When the presence of multiple intracranial tumors is documented, cranial radiotherapy is initiated. As with primary tumors, response rates vary with the histologic characteristics of the primary tumor. For example, metastases from breast and lung tumors respond better to irradiation than metastases from melanoma or sarcoma. Individuals with metastatic brain tumors also may undergo more than one course of cranial irradiation in conjunction with chemotherapy or in the presence of recurring metastases.

Radiation dosages to the brain vary according to tumor type and bulk and the individual's general condition. Initial irradiation may be delivered over a period of 2 to 4 weeks. West and Maor[40] suggest the delivery of 2000 rad (cGy) within 1 week or 300 cGy in 2 weeks for palliation of metastatic brain cancer. Higher doses of radiation delivered in shorter schedules are slightly superior in both promptness and duration of symptom relief.

Patients undergoing cranial radiotherapy may be given corticosteroids to promote more rapid improvement; however, this regimen does not contribute to overall survival or duration of improvement.[41]

Catterall[42] and others have identified the problem of decreased radiosensitivity of hypoxic malignant cells. Malignant brain tumors contain a large proportion of such cells, and hypoxia is believed to be a factor that limits the effectiveness of radiation. It is suggested that treatment with fast neutron therapy in addition to conventional megavoltage therapy may be advantageous in the treatment of hypoxic brain tumors.[43] Response to treatment is measured in part by the degree to which the individual is able to perform activities of daily living.

Irreversible radiation necrosis may develop after cranial radiotherapy.[44] This reaction is not common, but when it occurs, the necrosis is not distinguishable, clinically or on a CT scan, from a neoplastic lesion. This causes potential confusion in the diagnosis of tumor recurrence.

Radiation therapy also is used in conjunction with surgery for some tumors. Following surgical exposure of the tumor site, high-dose fractionated radiotherapy is delivered by means of a cone-shaped Lucite radiation applicator. This applicator protects healthy tissue from radiation while maintaining the integrity of the radiation fields, either during delivery of radiation in the operating room or during transport of the patient between the operating room and the radiation treatment room.[45] This combined modality remains experimental.

Another technique at use in only a few centers in the United States is stereotactic radiosurgery with the gamma knife that cross-fires an intracranial target with multiple beams of ionizing radiation.[46] Stereotactic radiosurgery with the gamma knife is a highly specialized radiation technique to treat focal neoplasms ranging in size from 5 to 40 mm. It is particularly useful for lesions that are deeply seated at the base of the brain or in areas where conventional surgical approaches could not be considered because of potential damage to brain tissue.

The role of stereotactic radiosurgery with the gamma knife is being assessed at centers throughout the United States. The procedure involves a precise radiation beam of cobalt 60 that is finely focused and administered with the aid of the stereotactic process. The procedure requires extensive collaboration among physicists and radiotherapists and involves specialized equipment. There are only a few centers in the United States where this treatment is currently available.

Chemotherapy and Related Drugs

An understanding of the blood-brain barrier is valuable for understanding the effect of chemotherapeutic agents on brain tumors. The blood-brain barrier (BBB) consists of a continuous lining of endothelial cells that are connected by tight junctions (Figure 36-12a). Transendothelial vesicular transport is not facilitated by the endothelial cells, and the junctions restrict intercellular diffusion.[47] This barrier limits blood-brain exchange of water-soluble drugs, ions, and proteins at the growing regions of a tumor

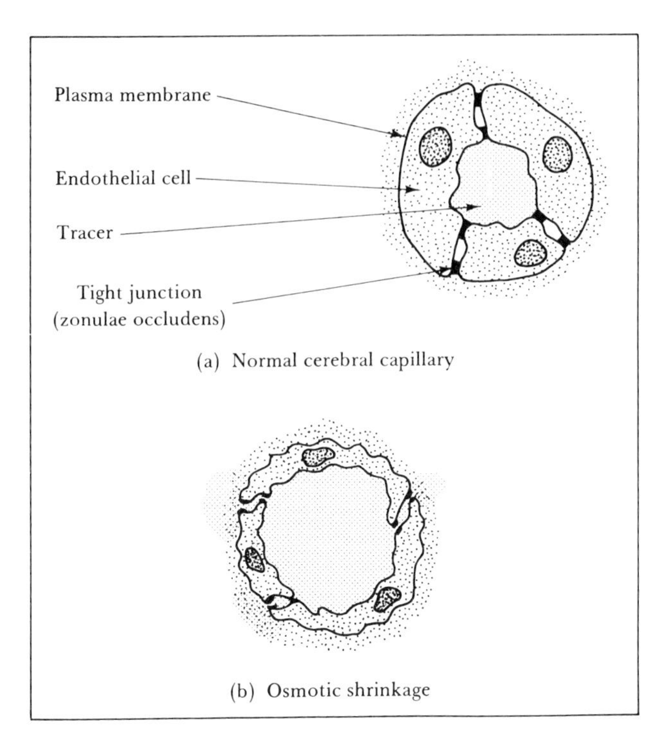

FIGURE 36-12 Schematic representation of the blood-brain barrier. (a) Normal cerebral capillary showing tight junctions. (b) Blood-brain barrier opening by widening of the interendothelial tight junctions. When the endothelial cells shrink in a hypertonic environment, the permeability of the junctions is increased.

edge but permits transport of lipid-soluble agents that can permeate the lipid membranes of the endothelial cells.[48] Furthermore, permeability of the BBB varies within the tumor and is believed to be greater in or near the central tumor bulk, where blood flow is reduced.[14]

The presence of openings between the vascular compartments of brain tumors and the parenchyma holds promise for chemotherapy.[47] Certain agents may have access to tumor tissue through bulk flow. Molecular size, lipid solubility, and degree of ionization are perhaps not the most crucial attributes of chemotherapeutic agents for brain tumors. Vick[47] suggests that agents be studied for their uptake and metabolic fat in tumor cells and for dosage and timing of delivery in relation to the kinetics of tumor cell growth.

Research suggests that malignant oligodendroglioma is a uniquely chemosensitive glial tumor.[18] Unfortunately, this is not true of other intracranial tumors, and within the accepted treatment methods for brain tumors chemotherapy represents a limited approach. Most chemotherapeutic agents do not cross the blood-brain barrier easily. However, the group of drugs classified as nitrosoureas are successful in penetrating the blood-brain barrier. These drugs include carmustine (BCNU), lomustine (CCNU), and semustine (methyl-CCNU), all of which are lipid soluble. Most commonly carmustine is used in combination with 5-fluorouracil. Chemotherapy is indicated for patients who have a histologic grade III or grade IV neoplasm.

Other means of delivering chemotherapy to brain tumors have been explored. For example, meningeal carcinomatosis either breaks down the blood-brain barrier or permits neovascularization and thereby circumvents the barrier. This has implications for the use of such agents as intravenous methotrexate, cisplatin, 5-fluorouracil, and interferon.

Hypertonic mannitol causes loss of fluid from the capillary endothelial cells, causing the endothelial cells to shrink and the tight junctions (zonulae occludens) to break, resulting in osmotic shrinkage (Figure 36-12, b). Materials of large molecular size may then diffuse through the junctions into the surrounding brain.

Transitory osmotic disruption of the blood-brain barrier by perfusion of the brain capillaries with a hypertonic solution of 25% mannitol opens the tight junctions for 15 to 30 minutes. Neuwalt[49] describes a protocol of combination chemotherapy, in conjunction with barrier disruption, at 28-day intervals. Intraarterial methotrexate with citrovorum rescue, followed by intravenous cyclophosphamide, is used. To date, the best results with this regimen have been achieved with primary CNS lymphomas.[49]

The sink effect also is of value in chemotherapy.[48] At the center of the tumor the blood-brain barrier is defective, but at the edge the vasculature may be partially intact. A drug that does enter can diffuse into the surrounding parenchyma (the sink effect).

The use of liposomes as drug carriers represents a recent approach in administration of chemotherapy. This permits penetration of the BBB with prolonged tissue concentrations of systemically administered drugs entrapped in liposomes such as cholesterol.[14]

Various other methods of drug administration have been described in an attempt to circumvent the BBB. These include intraarterial, intrathecal, and intratumoral administration.[14] Indeed, intratumoral injections of interleukin lymphoid effector cells have proved advantageous. However, these intracerebral injections are avoided in such areas of the brain as the thalamus, hypothalamus, and brain stem, where small amounts of edema may endanger the patient's life.[50]

Several other uses of chemotherapy are undergoing investigation. Autologous bone marrow transplantation in conjunction with high-dose etoposide (VP-16-213) has demonstrated activity in the treatment of malignant primary brain tumors and metastatic tumors from small-cell lung carcinoma.[51] Hidalgo et al[52] found enhanced responses to the treatment of brain metastases with weekly intravenous or intraarterial administration of cisplatin during whole-brain irradiation. Palliative and enhanced survival responses have been noted after osmotic BBB modification to enhance drug delivery to tumor and surrounding brain tissue.[53,54]

Intraarterial administration of chemotherapy has been used for regionally confined malignancies, including intracranial tumors. An intraarterial catheter is placed with fluoroscopic or angiographic visualization prior to infusion. A drug pump is used to deliver a high concentration of drug at the tumor site.

Floxuridine is one drug used successfully for intraarterial infusion for various tumors once considered incurable, such as certain metastatic and primary melanomas. Complications from such infusions include arterial aneurysm, arterial ischemia, arterial thrombosis, bleeding at catheter site, displaced or leaking catheter, infection at catheter site, and thrombophlebitis.[55]

The use of intraarterial chemotherapy for recurrent brain tumors remains experimental but continues to be an area of interest.[56] However, documentation of its benefits continues to be cloudy. Johnson et al[57] studied the use of intracarotid BCNU dissolved in 5% D5W and reported an 11% to 60% reduction of primary glioma in 8 of their 20 patients. Stewart et al[58] used intraarterial mitomycin C for treatment of recurrent brain metastases and reported a response in 6 of 13 patients. Both studies require clarification of the definition and significance of the response rates. Intraarterial administration of chemotherapy is not without problems. Of primary concern are the drugs' direct toxic effects to the ipsilateral eye and leukoencephalopathy.

The use of a combination of intraarterial and systemic chemotherapy was studied by Stewart et al.[59] It was found that a combination of systemic and regional drug therapy did not provide more effective therapy than the use of intraarterial drugs alone.

The final investigational drug therapy to be discussed is an antibody-toxin conjugate.[60] A genetically engineered toxin, CRM 107, is structurally similar to diphtheria toxin, with deviation in two amino acid chains. Intrathecal administration of CRM 107 has demonstrated selective destruction of human glioblastoma- and medulloblastoma-derived cell lines. This offers a wide therapeutic window, with extreme potency and general applicability against primary and metastatic tumors borne in cerebral spinal fluid, and warrants further clinical trial.

Hyperthermia

The use of hyperthermia in the treatment of malignant tumors has been under increased investigation during the 1980s. It is believed that normal cells have a higher thermal death point than malignant cells. This difference in cell death thermal points makes it possible for cancer cells to be destroyed while normal cells are spared. Tanaka et al[61] used hyperthermia by radiofrequency (RF) capacitive heating for sixteen malignant brain tumors and found that 6 of 10 evaluable tumors showed regression on CT scan. Hyperthermia also has been used successfully in conjunction with low-dose radiation on recurrent cancer cells in previously irradiated fields.[62]

Several clinical problems with the use of hyperthermia need to be solved, such as better control of heat to healthy brain and improved access to tumor during delivery. Tanaka et al suggest the use of hyperthermia along with other modes, such as chemotherapy and/or radiation therapy.[61] Studies in this area show promise, but long-term survival and side effects must be further evaluated.

GENERAL SUPPORTIVE MEASURES

The individual with a brain tumor may experience symptoms that drastically affect his or her ability to function normally. Furthermore, the prognosis for malignant CNS tumors has not changed greatly in the last 10 years, in spite of significant advances in therapeutic modalities.[14] Supportive nursing measures assume importance in all areas of patient care.

As mentioned previously, brain tumors increase ICP by their size, cerebral edema, or obstruction of CSF pathways. When CSF pathways are blocked, a hydrocephalus can develop, necessitating a shunting procedure. The tumor bulk and accompanying peritumoral edema usually are responsible for an increase in ICP. Therapeutic measures are aimed at controlling cerebral edema, cerebral blood flow, and other factors affecting ICP.

Chronic cerebral edema may be managed with corticosteroids. A reduction of peritumoral edema may occur over a period of hours or days. Corticosteroids are less helpful in the prompt reduction of acutely increased ICP. Osmotherapy is used to reduce the amount of fluid in the brain tissue. A hyperosmolar agent, such as mannitol, is administered intravenously. The drug creates an osmotic gradient across a semipermeable membrane. Fluid is drawn into the circulating bloodstream. Diuresis is achieved when the fluid is removed from the intravascular compartment by the kidneys. Osmotic diuretic agents remove fluid from normal brain cells (because they have an intact semipermeable cell membrane). The cerebral edema surrounding damaged cells is not directly removed by osmotherapy. Corticosteroids are administered concurrently because they are believed to have a direct effect on vasogenic brain edema. Fluid intake also is restricted to prevent intracellular swelling. Cellular edema adds to and aggravates increasing ICP.

Many activities affect cerebral blood flow and thus ICP. Suctioning reduces PaO_2, which creates a transient rise in ICP. Poor respiratory exchange also can elevate ICP. This is accomplished by an increased $PaCO_2$, which increases blood volume. Activities that increase systemic arterial blood pressure will also increase ICP. These include Valsalva maneuvers, isometric muscle contraction, coughing, and emotional arousal.

The venous outflow of blood from the cranial cavity affects ICP. A decrease in outflow increases the total blood volume in the cranium. Intracranial pressure rises when the total volume within the cranium is increased. The outflow of venous blood is impeded by jugular compression, head rotation, neck flexion, and neck extension. These head and neck positions should be avoided. Elevating the head of the patient's bed promotes venous drainage and is used as a therapeutic measure when increased ICP is present.

Intraabdominal and intrathoracic pressures affect ICP. This is due to the transmission of increased pressure along the venous system to the intracranial veins. Intracranial venous pressure is increased, and total blood volume increases with positive end-expiratory pressure (PEEP), sneezing, coughing, straining, and Valsalva maneuvers. Intraabdominal pressure increases with hip flexion and pressure on the abdomen (such as lying in the prone position). These activities should be avoided because they may produce dangerously high elevations in ICP.

Several nursing measures involve the performance of activities that affect ICP (turning, pulmonary hygiene, positioning, range-of-motion exercises, suctioning). Although certain activities cannot be avoided, it is recommended that activities be spread out over time. When individuals are turned in bed, the head and neck should be maintained in a neutral position. Alert patients are asked to permit themselves to be turned passively. Many individuals inadvertently perform a Valsalva maneuver or grab the side rails tightly (isometric muscle contraction) when they are being turned.

Intracranial hypertension may occasionally require special therapeutic measures. Levels of ICP must be determined by an intracranial pressure monitor. Intubation and hyperventilation may be used to control $Paco_2$ and Pao_2. The vasconstrictor effect of hyperventilation also reduces cerebral blood volume. Fluids are restricted and steroids and osmotic diuretics are used. The head of the bed is elevated to promote venous drainage. Anesthetic agents, such as barbiturates, may be used to decrease cerebral blood flow and metabolism. Hypothermia also may be used to reduce the cerebral metabolic rate.

Efforts to prevent seizures are important, since seizure activity may produce local brain tissue ischemia as well as alarm the individual and his or her family. Anticonvulsant agents may be used prophylactically because focal or generalized convulsions may lead to permanent neurologic disability. Diphenylhydantoin (phenytoin) is known to prevent convulsions without having a strong sedative effect and is therefore used most frequently.

A safe environment is essential for individuals with impaired intellect or those at risk of seizures. A defined daily schedule will help allay the patient's anxiety. The individual is encouraged to use his or her remaining cognitive functions as much as possible. If this can be accomplished through the use of safety shoes, a walker, and so on, such items are provided.

The use of steroids in the treatment of metastatic brain cancer has been discussed. Symptoms are ameliorated in 60% to 75% of individuals treated with adrenocorticosteroids. Dexamethasone (Decadron) is used frequently in neurologic settings to decrease cerebral edema. However, one of every six hospitalized individuals receiving corticosteroids experiences side effects, particularly individuals with low serum albumin levels and those who are receiving high doses of the drug.

Individuals receiving steroids should be observed for the following signs and symptoms:

1. Acute adrenal insufficiency, as evidenced by fatigue, muscular weakness, joint pain, fever, anorexia, nausea, and orthostatic hypotension.
2. Cardiovascular and renal problems, as evidenced by increased cardiac output and atrioventricular node conduction rate and sodium retention.
3. Gastrointestinal disturbances, as evidenced by induction or aggravation of peptic ulcers and melena with resulting anemia.
4. Metabolic problems, as evidenced by gluconeogenesis that leads to hyperglycemia and glucosuria, polydipsia, and polyuria.
5. Musculoskeletal problems, as evidenced by muscular atrophy and osteoporosis in immobilized individuals, petechiae, and decubitus ulcers.

Ongoing assessment of patients who are receiving steroids will alert the nurse to the development of steroid side effects. Steroid dosages are decreased immediately in the presence of side effects and are tapered slowly to prevent problems associated with hasty steroid withdrawal.

Individuals who are receiving phenobarbital or phenytoin may need higher dosages of corticosteroids, because these drugs stimulate hepatic corticosteroid metabolism. Individuals who receive high dosages for a prolonged period of time may develop a steroid psychosis. Such persons are observed for personality changes and paranoid behavior, which tend to develop suddenly and dramatically.

If the patient is unable to swallow, alternate routes for fluid and nutrient intake may be used. A nasogastric or gastrostomy tube may be used to prevent dehydration and malnutrition. Individuals with these tubes in place need to receive their liquid nutrition while in an upright position.

Planning for the hospital discharge of an individual who has been treated for a brain tumor encompasses an accurate assessment of existing limitations. Rehabilitation potential is always viewed with hope and optimism, and the attitude of realistic hope must be conveyed to the individual and the family. Discharge goals include helping the patient attain realistic goals and directing the family to appropriate resources.

Life expectancy at home is generally not of long duration. The patient may or may not be bedridden. A safe environment is required, regardless of activity level. Alterations in balance and confusion warrant housing the patient on the ground floor when possible. When ambulating, the patient uses sturdy footwear and obstacles are cleared from his or her pathway. Reality-orientation devices (clocks, calendars, etc.) should be readily available.

The patient with progressive CNS involvement generally is in a terminal state, and death at home may occur slowly, through progression of disease and complications of immobility. A resource available to patient and family is hospice care, which eases the terminal process and facilitates hope and integrity for all involved.

REFERENCES

1. Fishman RA: Cerebrospinal Fluid in the Diseases of the Nervous System. Philadelphia, WB Saunders, 1980, pp 1-15.
2. Mitchell PH, Mauss NK: Intercranial hypertension: Implications for research for nursing care. J Neurosurg Nurs 12:145-154, 1980.
3. Silverberg E, Lubera J: Cancer statistics. CA 39:3-21, 1989.
4. del Regato J, Spjut H, Cox JD: Cancer Diagnosis, Treatment and Prognosis (ed 6). St Louis, CV Mosby, 1985, pp 149-155.
5. Wilson CB, Fulton DS, Seager ML: Supportive management of the patient with malignant brain tumor. JAMA 244:1249-1251, 1980.
6. Kornblith PL, Walker MD, Cassady RR: Neurologic Oncology. Philadelphia, JB Lippincott, 1987.
7. Amendola B, Amendola M, McClatchey K: Radiation-induced malignant fibrous histiocytoma: A report of five cases including two occurring post whole brain irradiation. Cancer Invest 3:507-513, 1985.
8. Rimm I, Li F, Tabell N, et al: Brain tumors after cranial irradiation for childhood ALL. Cancer 59:1506-1508, 1987.
9. Penn I: Cancer is a complication of severe immunosuppression. Surg Gynecol Obstet 162:603-609, 1986.
10. Jones RD: Epidemiology of brain tumors in man and their relationship with chemical agents. Ed Chem Toxic 24:99-103, 1986.
11. Thomas T, Stewart P, Stemhagen A, et al: Risk of astrocytic brain tumors associated with occupational chemical exposure. Sc J Work, Env, Health 13:417-423, 1987.
12. Wilkinson G, Tietjen G, Wiggs L, et al: Mortality among plutonium and other radiation workers at a plutonium weapons facility. Am J Epidemiol 125:231-247, 1987.
13. Zulch KJ: Principles of the new World Health Organization (WHO) classification of brain tumors. Neuroradiology 19:59-66, 1980.
14. Jellinger K: Therapy of Malignant Brain Tumors. New York: Springer-Verlag, 1987.
15. Levin VA: Chemotherapy of primary brain tumors. Neurol Clin 3:855-865, 1985.
16. Schoenberg BS: The epidemiology of CNS tumors, in Walker MD (ed): Oncology of the Nervous System. Boston, Nijhoff, 1983, pp 1-311.
17. Popp JA, Horton J: Primary tumors of the brain. Curr Concepts Oncol 2:3-11, 1980.
18. Cairncross JG, MacDonald DR: Successful chemotherapy for recurrent malignant oligodendroglioma. Ann Neurol 23:360-364, 1988.
19. MacArthur JH, Palenicek JG: Human immunodeficiency virus and the nervous system. Nurs Clin North Am 23:823-841, 1988.
20. Adams RD, Victor M: Principles of Neurology (ed 3). New York, McGraw-Hill, 1985, pp 487-493.
21. Levin A: Non-Hodgkin's lymphomas and other malignancies in the acquired immune deficiency syndrome. Semin Oncol 14:34-39, 1987.
22. Posner JB: Brain metastases: A clinician's view, in Weiss L, Gilbert HA, Posner JB (eds): Brain Metastasis. Boston, Hall, 1980.
23. Cohen AR, Wisoff JH, Allan JC, et al: Malignant astrocytomas of the spinal cord. J Neurosurg 70:50-54, 1989.
24. Hounsfield GN: Computed medical imaging. Med Phys 7:283-290, 1980.
25. Shuman WP, Griffin BR, Haynar DR, et al: The utility of MR in planning the radiation therapy of oligodendroglioma. AJR 148:595-600, 1987.
26. Wagner HM: Images of the brain; past as prologue. J Nucl Med 27:1929-1937, 1987.
27. Mawhinney RR, Buckley JH, Holland IM, et al: The value of magnetic resonance imaging in the diagnosis of intracranial meningioma. Clin Radiol 37:429-439, 1986.
28. Dietrich RB, Kangarlov H, Lenarsky C, et al: The role of MR imaging. AJR 148:937-942, 1987.
29. Gado MH: MRI of the brain. Curr Probl Diagn Radiol 16:1-67, 1987.
30. Elster AD, Challa VR, Gilbert TH, et al: Mengiomas: MR and histological features. Radiology 170:857-862, 1989.
31. Phelps ME, Huang SC, Hoffman EJ, et al: An analysis of signal amplification using small detectors in positron emission tomography. J Comput Assist Tomogr 6:551-565, 1982.
32. Thomas D, Brooks D, Jones T: Metabolic studies of the brain tumors by P.E.T., in Chatel M, Darval F, Pecker J (eds): Brain Oncology. Boston, Kluwer Academic, 1987, pp 175-177.
33. Francavilla T, Miletich RS, Di Chiro G, et al: Positron emission tomography in the detection of malignant degeneration of low-grade gliomas. Neurosurgery 24:1-5, 1989.
34. Alavi JB, Alavi A, Chawluk J, et al: Positron emission tomography in patients with glioma. Cancer 62:1074-1078, 1988.
35. Beahrs OH, Henson DE, Hutter R, et al: Manual for Staging of Cancer (ed 3). Philadelphia, JB Lippincott, 1988, pp 249-254.
36. Fadul C, Wood J, Thaler H, et al: Morbidity and mortality of craniotomy for excision of supratentorial gliomas. Neuroradiology 38:1374-1379, 1988.
37. Glidenberg PL: Whatever happened to stereotactic surgery? Neurosurgery 20:983-987, 1987.
38. Coffey RJ, Lunsford LD, Taylor FH: Survival after steriotactic biopsy of malignant gliomas. Neurosurgery 22:465-471, 1988.
39. Shaw B, Mansfield FL, Borges L: One-stage posterolateral decompression and stabilization for primary and metastatic vertebral tumors in the thoracic and lumbar spine. J Neurosurg 70:405-410, 1989.
40. West J, Maor M: Intracranial metastases: Behavioral patterns related to primary site and results of treatment by whole brain irradiation. Int J Radiat Oncol Biol Phys 6:11-15, 1980.
41. Borget B: The palliation of brain metastases: Final results of the first two studies by the radiation therapy oncology group. Int J Radiat Oncol Biol Phys 6:1-9, 1980.
42. Catterall M: Fast neutrons compared with megavoltage x-rays in the treatment of patients with supratentorial glioblastoma; a controlled pilot study. Int J Radiat Oncol Biol Phys 6:262-266, 1980.
43. Batterman J: Fast neutron therapy for advanced brain tumors. Int J Radiat Oncol Biol Phys 6:333-335, 1980.
44. Shewmon DA, Mosdeu JC: Delayed radiation necrosis of the brain contralateral to original tumor. Arch Neurol 37:592-593, 1980.
45. Haibeck SV: Intraoperative radiation therapy. Oncol Nurs Forum 15:143-148, 1988.
46. Lunsford LD, Flickinger JC: Stereotactic Radiosurgery Using the Gamma Knife: An alternative to microsurgical removal. Proceedings of the 30th Annual Meeting of the American Society of Therapeutic Radiation Oncologists, January, 1989, New York, Abstract 78, p 156.
47. Vick NA: Brain tumor microvasculature, in Weiss L, Gilbert HA, Posner JB (eds): Brain Metastases. Boston, Hall, 1980.

48. Rapoport SI: Quantitative aspects of osmotic opening of the blood-brain barrier, in Weiss L, Gilbert HA, Posner JB (eds): Brain Metastasis. Boston, Hall, 1980.
49. Neuwalt ER: Implications of the Blood-Brain Barrier and Its Manipulation. New York, Plenum Press, 1989.
50. Merchant R, Grant A, Merchant P, et al: Adoptive immunotherapy for recurrent glioblastoma multiforme using LAK cells and RIL 2. Cancer 62:665-671, 1988.
51. Leff RS, Thompson JM, Daly MG, et al: Acute neurologic dysfunction after high-dose etoposide therapy for malignant glioma. Cancer 62:32-35, 1988.
52. Hidalgo V, Cy C, Fernandez-Hidalgo O, et al: Simultaneous radiotherapy and cis-platinum for the treatment of brain metastases: A pilot study. Am J Clin Oncol 10:205-209, 1987.
53. Neuwalt EA, Howieson J, Frenkel EP, et al: Therapeutic efficiency of multiagent chemotherapy with drug delivery enhancement by BBB modification in glioblastoma. Neurosurgery 19:573-580, 1986.
54. Rama B, Jansen J, Mennel HD, et al: Renaissance of intratumoral chemotherapy, in Chatel M, Darcel F, Pecker J (eds): Brain Oncology. Boston, Nijhoff, 1988, pp 433-434.
55. Frost DB, Patt YZ, Mavligit G, et al: Arterial infusion of dacarbazine and cisplatin for recurrent regionally confined melanoma. Arch Surg 120:478-480, 1985.
56. Morantz RA: Comments to intracarotid chemotherapy with 1, 3-BIS-(2-chloroethyl)-1-nitrosurea (BCNU) in 5% dextrose in water in the treatment of malignant glioma. Neurosurgery 20:583, 1987.
57. Johnson DW, Parkinson D, Wolpert SM, et al: Intraarterial Chemotherapy with 1, 3-Bis-(2-chloroethyl)-1-nitrosourea (BCNU) in 5% dextrose in water in the treatment of malignant glioma. Neurosurgery 20:577-582, 1987.
58. Stewart DJ, Grahovac Z, Hugenholtz H, et al: Intraarterial mitomycin-C for recurrent brain metastases. Am J Clin Oncol 10:432-436, 1987.
59. Stewart DJ, Grahovac Z, Hugenholtz H, et al: Combined intraarterial and systemic chemotherapy for intracerebral tumors. Neurosurgery 21:207-213, 1987.
60. Johnson VG, Wrobel C, Wilson D, et al: Improved tumor-specific immunotoxins in the treatment of CNS and leptomeningeal neoplasia. J Neurosurg 70:240-248, 1989.
61. Tanaka R, Kim CH, Yamada N, et al: Radiofrequency hyperthermia for malignant brain tumors: Preliminary results of clinical trails. Neurosurgery 21:478-483, 1987.
62. Knox SJ, Kapp DS, Hyperthermia and radiation therapy in the treatment of recurrent Merkel cell tumors. Cancer 62:1479-1486, 1988.

Chapter 37

Endocrine Cancer

Michele Girard Donehower, RN, MSN

INTRODUCTION

The endocrine system controls many of the body's most important physiologic functions through the release of hormones by endocrine glands. Hormones then initiate activities at the cellular level that permit target tissues to make the adaptive changes necessary to maintain homeostasis. When tumors arise in endocrine glands, the ability of these cells to perform their specific endocrine functions is altered. Although some endocrine tumors are not histologically malignant, in that they do not involve cellular changes characteristic of neoplastic transformation, they can, through hyperplasia and expansion, result in significant morbidity or death. With hyperplasia, the number of hormone-secreting cells increases. Because these cells are not subject to the normal regulatory feedback processes that control hormonal secretion, excessive secretion of hormones results. Depending on the location of the tumor, localized growth can cause compression of vital structures. The clinical presentation of these tumors depends on their anatomic location and their ability to produce excess hormone secretion. Tumors of the thyroid, parathyroid, adrenal, and pituitary glands will be discussed.

THYROID CANCER

Epidemiology

Although the incidence of thyroid cancer has risen slightly over the past 40 years, this neoplasm remains relatively rare.[1] It accounts for just over 1% of the total cancer incidence and approximately 0.2% of all cancer deaths.[2] Women are more than twice as likely as men to have a thyroid malignancy, with the majority of cases occurring between the ages of 25 and 65.[1] Thyroid tumors in childhood are relatively rare.[3]

Etiology

The only well-documented etiologic factor in the development of thyroid cancer is head and neck irradiation given during early childhood and adolescence.[4,5] Before the 1950s, radiotherapy was commonly used in the treatment of benign conditions, such as enlarged tonsils and adenoids, mastoiditis, sinusitis, hemangiomas, acne, tinea capitis, and eczema. The association between this widespread practice and the development of thyroid cancer was first reported by Duffy and Fitzgerald,[6] and later confirmed by other investigators.[4,5,7,8] The incidence of postirradiation thyroid cancer is a linear function of the dose received, with risk increasing up to 1200 rad (cGy).[1] The risk declines with doses over 2000 cGy because at those doses the thyroid gland becomes sterilized. Most cases of postirradiation thyroid cancer occur in patients who have received doses between 6.5 and 1200 cGy.[1,4,9] Usually there is a latency period of 5 to 10 years between radiation exposure and the development of thyroid cancer, but an increased risk of these malignancies persists for at least 35 years in exposed subjects.[4] For this reason, persons at risk of thyroid cancer as a result of childhood irradiation to the head and neck require lifelong follow-up.

Treatment of thyroid malignancies with radioactive isotopes does not appear to have the same carcinogenic effect as external irradiation. Isolated reports[10,11] of thyroid cancer after ^{131}I therapy for hyperthyroidism have not been substantiated by studies of larger populations of patients receiving ^{131}I therapy.[12,13]

The precise role of thyroid-stimulating hormone (TSH) in the development of thyroid cancer remains unclear. Under the influence of TSH, the thyroid gland forms two hormones: tetraiodothyronine (T_4) and triiodothyronine (T_3). The secretion of TSH by the pituitary gland is regulated by a negative-feedback mechanism. A decrease in T_3 or T_4 increases TSH secretion, while an increase has the opposite effect. Prolonged stimulation of the gland is known to occur with persistently low levels of thyroid hormones secondary to iodine deficiency or destruction or surgical removal of normal thyroid tissue.[14] Although thyroid cancer in animals can be induced by prolonged TSH stimulation, the role of TSH as a causative factor in humans is less well established.[14] It has been suggested that TSH does function as a growth factor for well-differentiated thyroid malignancies but may not actually induce neoplasia.[15]

The role of genetics in the etiology of thyroid cancers is not well defined except in the case of medullary thyroid cancer, where approximately 25% of cases occur as part of the genetically transmitted multiple endocrine neoplasia (MEN) syndromes.[16,17] In MEN syndromes, hyperplasia or neoplasia of endocrine cells occurs in more than one site, either synchronously or metachronously[18] (Table 37-1). Because these syndromes are transmitted genetically in an autosomal dominant fashion, it is recommended that the families of individuals with medullary carcinoma of the thyroid be screened. Such screening will increase the early detection of tumors and prevent the morbidity and mortality associated with MEN syndromes.[19]

Pathophysiology

Thyroid cancers demonstrate a wide range of biologic behavior, depending on the histologic characteristics of the tumor. There are four types of primary thyroid carcinoma that account for approximately 95% of all thyroid neoplasms: papillary, follicular, medullary, and anaplastic. These four major cancers and their clinical characteristics are outlined in Table 37-2.

The majority of thyroid tumors arise from the follicular and parafollicular cells (C cells) of the gland. Tumors arising from the follicular cells can be further divided into differentiated and undifferentiated types. Papillary and follicular carcinomas are well differentiated, in that they are histologically similar to their tissue of origin. Undif-

TABLE 37-1 Multiple Endocrine Neoplasia Syndromes

MEN Syndrome	Organs Involved	Affected (%)
I	Parathyroid adenomas	90
	Pancreatic islet adenomas	80
	Pituitary adenomas	65
	Adrenocortical adenomas	38
	Thyroid adenomas	18
IIa	Medullary thyroid carcinoma	80-100
	Pheochromocytoma	40-60
	Parathyroid adenoma or hyperplasia	40
IIb	Medullary thyroid carcinoma	90
	Pheochromocytoma	30
	Ganglioneuromatosis of tongue, lips, gastrointestinal tract	100
	Skeletal abnormalities (marfanoid habitus, pes cavus, scoliosis, and pectus excavatum)	70-80

Adapted from Kerr DJ, Burt AD, Anderson JR: Tumours of the diffuse neuroendocrine system. Eur J Surg Oncol 13:189-195, 1987.

ferentiated, or anaplastic, carcinomas bear little resemblance to their tissue of origin and lack the functional and histologic characteristics of normal thyroid tissue. Medullary carcinoma of the thyroid (MCT) is the only tumor of parafollicular, or C-cell, origin. Although MCT is generally well differentiated, poorly differentiated variants have been reported.[17] Thyroid tumors also vary in their ability to concentrate iodine. This has therapeutic implications, in that treatment with ^{131}I is effective only for tumors that are able to concentrate this radioisotope.

Papillary carcinoma

Papillary carcinoma generally follows a relatively indolent course and survival is measured in decades, even in patients with evidence of distant metastases.[20-25] It occurs in all age groups, but the biologic behavior and overall prognosis vary according to age. Older patients (more than 40 years of age) appear to have a more aggressive, rapidly growing form of the disease, with a significantly lower rate of survival. Other important prognostic factors include sex and extent of disease at the time of diagnosis. Men have a poorer prognosis than women, as do patients with extrathyroidal extension of their tumors. Symptoms indicative of advanced local disease (eg, dysphagia, dyspnea, dysphonia) have also been shown to confer a worse prognosis.[26]

Approximately 25% of papillary carcinomas are termed occult, in that they are small (<1.5 cm in diameter), nonpalpable lesions that are detected incidentally after thyroidectomy or during the search for a primary site of a nodal neck metastasis.[27] They are benign, even in the presence of nodal metastasis, and are highly curable when treated by conservative surgical means.

Cervical lymph node involvement occurs early in the course of papillary carcinoma and in approximately 24% to 32% of cases is present at the time of diagnosis; more than 50% of patients have involvement at some time in the course of their disease. Several studies have reported that lymph node involvement has no influence on long-term survival.[20,22,23] Tubiana et al[24] found the reverse to be true and suggest that the relatively good prognosis for patients with lymph node involvement may be due to the influence of age, since lymph node metastasis is more common in young patients.

The lung is the most common site of distant metastases, and lung involvement is present at diagnosis in approximately 6% of the cases. Bone involvement is present in approximately 3% of the cases. Pulmonary metastases can remain clinically dormant for years.

TABLE 37-2 Clinical Characteristics of Thyroid Carcinomas

Tumor Type (Cell of Origin)	Incidence[30]	Survival*	Metastatic Pattern
Papillary (follicular cells)	33%–73%	93%–20 years[22]‡	Cervical lymph nodes involved early in disease; metastasizes to lung and less frequently to bone
Follicular (follicular cells)	14%–33%	78%–10 years[28]†	More locally invasive than papillary, but less likely to have lymph node involvement; propensity for hematogenous spread to bone and, occasionally, lung
Anaplastic (follicular cells)	5%–10%	3.6%–5 years[34]‡	Rapid invasion and compression of adjacent structures early in disease; lung is most common site of metastases
Medullary (parafollicular or C-cells)	10%	61%–10 years[17]‡	50% have lymph node involvement at diagnosis; metastasizes to bone, liver, and lung

*With treatment.
†Disease-free survival.
‡Total survival.

Papillary carcinoma has a very slow doubling time, which accounts for the frequency of late relapses and the prolonged interval between relapse and death.[24] Death usually is due to recurrent or uncontrolled local disease, even in patients with distant metastases.

Follicular carcinomas

Follicular cancer tends to be more locally invasive than carcinoma of the papillary type. The average age at diagnosis is 45 to 50, and the tumor is rarely seen in children.[28-30] Compared with papillary carcinoma, follicular forms are less likely to metastasize to regional lymph nodes. When metastasis occurs, cervical involvement is more likely to be a result of direct extension of a locally invasive tumor. Bone metastases occur more frequently because of follicular carcinoma's propensity for hematogenous spread.[28,29] Unlike other forms of thyroid malignancies, follicular carcinomas are more likely to retain their ability to produce the thyroid hormones, T_3 and T_4, and occasionally to cause hyperthyroidism.[31]

Hürthle cell cancer of the thyroid is sometimes considered a distinct histologic entity. For practical purposes, however, it can be classified as a variant of follicular carcinoma since the clinical course and treatment recommendations are similar for both tumor types.[30]

Follicular tumors with capsular or vascular invasion are associated with a poorer prognosis.[28,29] Although most patients have metastatic disease at the time of death, death generally results from growth of local recurrent tumors.

Medullary carcinoma

In about 80% of cases medullary carcinoma of the thyroid (MCT) develops spontaneously, with the remaining 20% occurring as part of genetically transmitted multiple endocrine neoplasia syndromes.[30] MCT occurs equally in both sexes. The average age at occurrence of the sporadic form is 45 to 50 years, whereas the familial forms have been detected in patients ranging in age from 10 to 80 years.[30] MCT follows an indolent course in the majority of patients. Fifty percent of the patients have lymph node involvement at diagnosis. Hematogenous spread to lung, bone, and liver occurs later. Survival is highly variable, ranging from months to 30 years, and is significantly correlated with age, sex, and stage of disease. The best prognosis is for women younger than 40 years with an early stage of disease.[32] The familial form of MCT can occur as a component of MEN IIA or MEN IIB. Because the familial form that occurs as part of MEN IIB is particularly virulent, every effort should be made to screen family members of affected individuals for the presence of disease.[33] Identification of families at risk permits early detection of medullary thyroid cancer, with ultimate improvement of prognosis.

Anaplastic carcinoma

Anaplastic carcinomas of the thyroid are among the most rapidly growing, lethal neoplasms. Death usually occurs within months of diagnosis, regardless of therapy. The majority of patients are elderly individuals, with a mean age of 65 years, and females are affected more than males.[34,35] Eighty per cent of the patients have a history of goiter. The tumor rapidly invades surrounding structures and metastasizes early. Death usually occurs as a result of local invasion and tracheal encroachment.

There is some evidence that well-differentiated papillary thyroid cancers may evolve histologically to a more anaplastic variety.[20] This may reflect end-stage behavior in the natural history of papillary tumors, although previous irradiation may also be involved in the transformation process.

Clinical Manifestations

Clinical presentation may vary according to the type of thyroid malignancy. Incidental discovery of an otherwise asymptomatic thyroid mass on routine physical examination is frequently the first indication of disease in patients with papillary carcinoma. Cervical lymphadenopathy is also present in a large number of patients. Other symptoms occur with significantly less frequency and are related to compressive effects of the enlarging mass on adjacent structures. These complications are more commonly associated with the undifferentiated, anaplastic forms of the disease. Patients may experience a sensation of tightness or fullness in the neck that may progress to dyspnea or stridor when the trachea is compressed or infiltrated.[31] Compression of the esophagus can cause dysphagia. Hoarseness can result from malignant infiltration or destruction of the recurrent laryngeal or vagus nerves. Pain is uncommon and is usually indicative of advanced disease. It may be localized to the thyroid gland or reported as referred ear pain.

Osseous metastases are more likely in follicular carcinoma and patients may have signs of bone involvement. Approximately 20% to 30% of patients with medullary thyroid cancer experience persistent diarrhea, which may be related to production of prostaglandins, vasoactive intestinal peptide, and serotonin by the tumor.[16,17]

Diagnostic Evaluation

Assessment

Patient history/physical examination A comprehensive history of the patient may provide clues to the diagnosis. Information regarding growth rate of the tumor, associated symptoms, previous irradiation, and a family history of thyroid-related problems should be elicited.

On physical examination, the thyroid, adjacent neck structures, and surrounding lymph nodes are inspected for symmetry and palpated for masses. Diffusely enlarged thyroid glands can be attributed to a variety of nonmalignant causes and require further evaluation. The head and neck examination includes indirect laryngoscopy in all patients with a history of voice changes; this is done to assess the possibility of vocal cord paralysis and laryngeal nerve invasion.

Although altered hormonal secretion is unusual, pa-

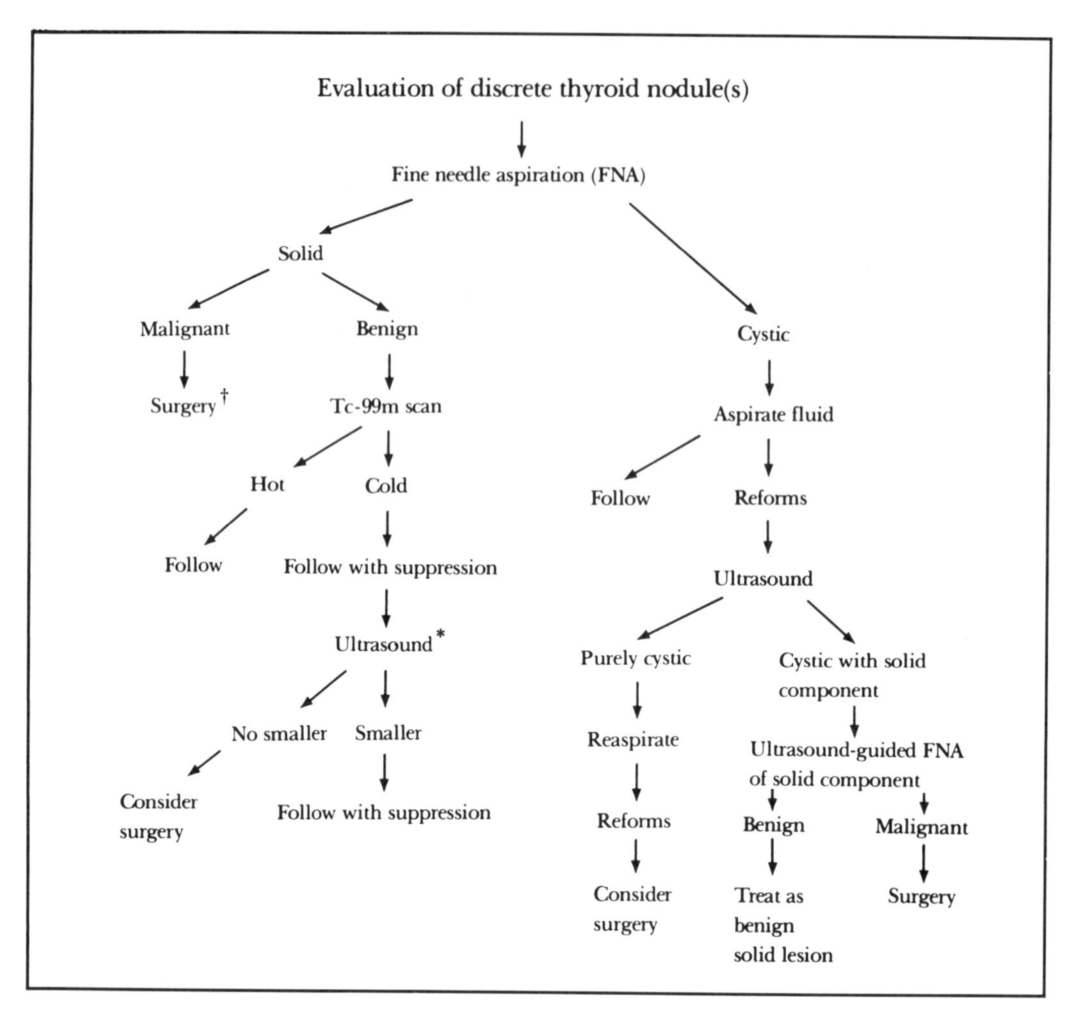

FIGURE 37-1 Evaluation of solitary thyroid nodules. Protocol for workup and management. Asterisk indicates one prominent nodule in a multinodular gland; dagger indicates ultrasonography only if the mass is difficult to palpate. *FNA*, Fine needle aspiration; *Tc-99m*, technitium-99m. (Source: From Friedman M, Toriumi DM, Mafee MF: Diagnostic imaging techniques in thyroid cancer. Am J Surg 155:215-223, 1988.)

tients may exhibit systemic manifestations of thyroid hormone excess or deficiency. Clinical symptoms of hyperthyroidism include fine tremors, lid lag, brisk tendon reflexes, increased appetite and weight loss, tachycardia, heat intolerance, proptosis, irritability, and muscle weakness. In thyroid hormone deficiency, patients may experience dry skin, hair loss, intolerance of cold, weight gain, slowed speech, bradycardia, decreased reflexes, and constipation. Individuals with thyroid nodules in whom thyroid cancer is suspected are systematically evaluated.

Fine-needle aspiration Fine-needle aspiration biopsy is widely used in the evaluation of nodular thyroid diseases, since it is the only diagnostic tool used in the workup of thyroid cancer that can differentiate benign from malignant nodules with a high degree of accuracy.[36] Hawkins et al[37] reported a false-negative rate of 2.4% and a false-positive rate of 6.5% in the interpretation of specimens categorized as suspicious. A suggested approach to the evaluation of thyroid nodules is depicted in Figure 37-1.[36] Patients with positive or suspicious aspirates generally require surgery.

TSH suppression Because of the influence of TSH on the growth of thyroid nodules, suppression of TSH is achieved by administration of exogenous thyroid hormone (thyroxine) to reduce the size of the nodules.[38] If, after several months of suppressive therapy, the size of the nodule increases or remains the same, surgery is indicated. There is a small possibility that nodules that respond to suppression may be malignant; therefore patients are observed for changes in the size of the nodule.[1,38]

Radionuclide imaging Thyroid scans provide useful information regarding the functional status of thyroid nodules. Normal thyroid tissue is functional, in that it concentrates iodine for use in the production of thyroid hormones. Radioactive isotopes are used to classify nodules according to their ability to concentrate iodine. Nodules may do this to the same, greater, or lesser extent than normal thyroid tissue.[39] Nonfunctioning nodules are "cold," normal thyroid tissue is "warm," and hyperfunctioning nodules are "hot." This classification technique is limited because it cannot distinguish benign from malignant nodules.[38]

TABLE 37-3 Staging Classification of Thyroid Carcinomas

DEFINITION OF TNM
Primary tumor (T)

Note: All categories may be subdivided: (a) solitary tumor, (b) multifocal tumor (the largest determines the classification).

TX Primary tumor cannot be assessed
T0 No evidence of primary tumor
T1 Tumor 1 cm or less in greatest dimension limited to the thyroid
T2 Tumor more than 1 cm but not more than 4 cm in greatest dimension limited to the thyroid
T3 Tumor more than 4 cm in greatest dimension limited to the thyroid
T4 Tumor of any size extending beyond the thyroid capsule

Regional lymph nodes (N)

Regional lymph nodes are the cervical and upper mediastinal lymph nodes.

NX Regional lymph nodes cannot be assessed
N0 No regional lymph node metastasis
N1 Regional lymph node metastasis
N1a Metastasis in ipsilateral cervical lymph node(s)
N1b Metastasis in bilateral, midline, or contralateral cervical or mediastinal lymph node(s)

Distant Metastasis (M)

MX Presence of distant metastasis cannot be assessed
M0 No distant metastasis
M1 Distant metastasis

STAGE GROUPING

Separate stage groupings are recommended for papillary and follicular, medullary, and undifferentiated.

Papillary or Follicular

	Under 45 years	45 Years and older
Stage I	Any T, Any N, M0	T1, N0, M0
Stage II	Any T, Any N, M1	T2, N0, M0
		T3, N0, M0
Stage III		T4, N0, M0
		Any T, N1, M0
Stage IV		Any T, Any N, M1

Medullary

Stage I	T1	N0	M0
Stage II	T2	N0	M0
	T3	N0	M0
	T4	N0	M0
Stage III	Any T	N1	M0
Stage IV	Any T	Any N	M1

Undifferentiated

All cases are stage IV.

Stage IV	Any T	Any N	Any M

Sources: Reprinted with permission from Beahrs OH, Henson DE, Hutter RVP, Myers (eds): Manual for Staging of Cancer (ed 3). Philadelphia, JB Lippincott, 1988, pp 57-59.

Laboratory tests If thyroid dysfunction is suggested by history or physical examination, routine thyroid function tests (RAI, T_3 uptake, total T_4, free T_4, and TSH) should be obtained, although these tests show nonspecifically elevated levels in all patients with nodular disease.[38]

Serum calcitonin is an important tumor marker for diagnosis and for evaluation of treatment response in patients with MCT. It is used routinely in screening for the familial forms of medullary thyroid cancer.[16]

Staging

The system proposed by the American Joint Committee of Cancer for staging thyroid cancer is widely used because it incorporates the important prognostic factors of age and histologic type into the classification (Table 37-3).[40]

TABLE 37-4 Guidelines for the Treatment of Thyroid Carcinomas

Age	Tumor Type	Extent of Disease	Treatment Recommendations
Any	Papillary Follicular	2 cm	Thyroid lobectomy or NTT with suppression[1]
45	Papillary Follicular	2-4 cm Confined to thyroid	NTT/TT with suppression[1]
45	Papillary Follicular	2-4 cm Confined to thyroid	NTT/TT with suppression and treatment with ^{131}I[1]
Any	Papillary Follicular	4 cm with extrathyroidal involvement or distant metastases	NTT/TT with suppression and treatment with ^{131}I ± external beam irradiation[1]
Any	Medullary	All patients	TT and modified neck dissection[17]
Any	Anaplastic	All patients	Thyroid lobectomy with excision of wide margins and isthmusectomy. Resection of clinically involved nodes[34]

TT, Total thyroidectomy; *NTT*, Near-total thyroidectomy.

Treatment

Early detection of disease before the occurrence of intraglandular or extraglandular invasion maximizes the potential for cure in patients with thyroid cancer. In well-differentiated carcinomas, an extended interval between initial therapy and recurrence and between recurrence and death necessitates prolonged follow-up. Because of the indolent nature of well-differentiated thyroid cancers and the lack of large prospective clinical trials, controversy continues regarding the best treatment for papillary and follicular carcinomas. General guidelines for the treatment of thyroid carcinomas are summarized in Table 37-4.

Surgery

The selection of type of surgical procedure depends on the histologic findings and the extent of disease. Near-total or total thyroidectomy is used widely as the initial treatment for all differentiated thyroid cancers. However, controversy regarding which procedure is superior continues.[20,22,23,41-47]

The advantages of total thyroidectomy are decreased local recurrences and increased effectiveness of treatment with ^{131}I because of total surgical ablation of the gland. Complications are higher with this approach but have decreased in recent years when the procedures were performed by skilled surgeons. In several studies, total thyroidectomy has been reserved for patients with adverse prognostic factors (age over 40 years, extracapsular extension of tumor, and follicular histology).[1,24,28]

Patients undergoing more conservative surgical procedures (near-total thyroidectomy, subtotal thyroidectomy) are less likely to experience postoperative complications. In this group, higher rates of recurrence have not been observed in patients followed up for up to 30 years after initial therapy, and survival rates have been comparable to those of patients undergoing total thyroidectomy.[1,23,45,47] Although ipsilateral total lobectomy may be performed in select cases where the lesion is less than 1.5 cm and is confined to one lobe, higher rates of recurrence have been observed with this approach.[20]

Total thyroidectomy is recommended for patients with medullary thyroid cancer because of the high incidence of bilateral involvement of the thyroid gland. Patients with anaplastic carcinoma who have resectable lesions generally are treated with lobectomy, because more radical surgery results in increased complications and does not alter the outcome of the disease.[34] In patients with unresectable lesions, palliative surgery is performed to debulk the tumor locally. Tracheostomy and gastrostomy also may be performed at this time.

Modified radical neck dissection is indicated when there is evidence of cervical node metastasis. Standard radical neck dissection can create residual cosmetic and functional deformities and is no longer warranted, since studies have shown that recurrences and survival are not influenced by the extent of lymph node surgery.

Postoperative complications Hemorrhage is possible because of the highly vascular nature of the gland. Since the patient is usually placed in a semi-Fowler's position, blood will flow to dependent areas. Bleeding is assessed by checking under the neck and shoulders as well as by inspecting the anterior dressing over the wound. Complaints of a sensation of pressure or tightness over the operative site may be indicative of hemorrhage.[48] A Penrose drain or other suction-type drain is used to prevent hematoma formation or accumulation of fluid at the operative site.[49] Individuals scheduled for surgery usually are given preoperative thyroid-suppressive therapy for several weeks to induce thyroid atrophy and reduce vascularity.[50]

The integrity of the parathyroid glands is threatened during resection of the thyroid because of their position on the posterior surface of the thyroid. Although every effort is made to preserve parathyroid tissue, the extent of surgery may not permit salvaging of these glands. If the parathyroid glands can be resected and are not involved with disease, they may be autotransplanted. The gland is minced at the time of surgery and then embedded into muscle tissue, usually the sternocleidomastoid muscle.[51] This process may permit the preservation of sufficient functioning parathyroid tissue to avert permanent hypoparathyroidism. Because the transplanted tissue does not become functional immediately, hypocalcemia resulting from loss of parathyroid hormone can occur. Patients are observed for signs of hypocalcemia and tetany in the immediate postoperative period. Symptoms include numbness, tingling, cramps in the extremities, stiffness, twitching, and a positive Chvostek's or Trousseau's sign. Serum calcium level is monitored daily, and calcium replacement is given until levels return to normal. If some parathyroid tissue has been preserved, normal function will gradually return. The duration of temporary hypoparathyroidism varies; periods ranging from 6 weeks to 1 year have been reported. Permanent hypoparathyroidism occurs in 1.2% to 11% of patients undergoing total thyroidectomy.[46]

Because the laryngeal nerves travel along the posterior surface of the thyroid, surgical resection of the thyroid may damage these nerves, resulting in temporary or permanent vocal cord paralysis. This can lead to respiratory obstruction if the vocal cords are closed, necessitating emergency tracheostomy. A tracheostomy set is kept at the patient's bedside at all times.[48] Transient nerve injury lasts from a few days to several months. The incidence of permanent recurrent laryngeal nerve injury has decreased in recent years, occurring in fewer than 1% of the cases when procedures are performed by surgeons skilled in thyroid surgery.[22,41,46]

Recurrent laryngeal nerve damage and postoperative local edema also contribute to alterations in vocal quality. With near-total thyroidectomy, the nerve on one side can be salvaged and patients will experience only hoarseness. Speech therapy may help the individual develop better vocal quality. If damage to both laryngeal nerves occurs, aphonia will result.[50]

In patients undergoing total or near-total thyroidectomy, postoperative administration of exogenous thyroid hormone is required to prevent clinical effects of hypothyroidism and suppress endogenous TSH that may serve as a growth factor for differentiated thyroid tumors. Patients are maintained permanently on suppressive therapy, with withdrawal only in preparation for ^{131}I therapy.

Radiotherapy

Use of ^{131}I is recommended for the treatment of residual and metastatic disease in certain patients with well-differentiated cancer after surgical resection of the thyroid. Well-differentiated cancers retain, to a variable extent, their ability to concentrate radioiodine. This characteristic makes them susceptible to treatment with ^{131}I after removal of normal thyroid tissue and the bulk of the primary tumor.[39] Anaplastic and medullary thyroid cancers are unable to concentrate this radioisotope, which precludes its effectiveness in treatment of these tumors.[17,34,35]

Before ^{131}I therapy is begun, administration of thyroid hormone is discontinued. Initiation of therapy is delayed for 4 to 6 weeks to permit blood levels of thyroid hormone to fall and previously suppressed TSH levels to rise. Radioiodine uptake depends on TSH levels. An increase in TSH levels augments uptake of ^{131}I into well-differentiated cancers. In patients with poor uptake, TSH stimulation may increase uptake and can be accomplished with injections of bovine TSH or administration of an antithyroid drug such as methimazole to induce endogenous TSH stimulation. The use of bovine TSH in repeated doses is controversial because it is associated with a high incidence of sensitivity reactions.[52] If TSH levels cannot be raised sufficiently, uptake of ^{131}I may be inadequate for the destruction of malignant tissue.[39]

^{131}I can be given for ablation and/or treatment after surgical resection. Ablation with ^{131}I is done before ^{131}I treatment for the purpose of totally eradicating any remaining normal thyroid tissue left in the neck after near-total thyroidectomy. Even after total thyroidectomy, residual functional thyroid tissue is detected on radionuclide scans. It optimizes the effectiveness of ^{131}I treatment so that the isotope will be concentrated in functional tumor tissue. Ablation is recommended for patients over the age of 40 and in patients whose tumors contain a follicular component.[44]

Two to 3 months after ablation, a whole-body scan is performed to detect metastatic disease or evidence of residual functioning tissue in the thyroid bed. Treatment with ^{131}I is not given less than 6 months after ablation because of residual radioactivity in the neck. Treatment with ^{131}I requires dosimetry calculations to determine the maximal dose to deliver to metastases of thyroid carcinoma while minimizing exposure of the blood. Therapy doses are given at 4- to 6-month intervals until whole-body imaging studies show no evidence of functioning tumor.[25]

Patients selected for ^{131}I therapy must be alert and capable of self-care activities. Inpatient admission in a private room for administration of ^{131}I treatment is required since radiation precautions are instituted. ^{131}I is administered orally and is present in all body secretions. No children or pregnant women are allowed in the patient's room after the isotope is administered. Patients may be discharged when radiation dose emission readings show less than 30 mCi ^{131}I—about 48 to 72 hours after 100 mCi is given. (Refer to Radiation Therapy chapter for other considerations for patients receiving brachytherapy.)

Complications of ^{131}I therapy include nausea and vomiting, fatigue, headache, sialadenitis (inflammation of the salivary glands), bone marrow suppression, and, rarely, pulmonary radiation fibrosis and leukemia.

Symptoms of fatigue, headache, and nausea and vomiting may be related to radiation sickness and can occur as early as 12 hours after ^{131}I administration. Premedication with antiemetics may be helpful.

Sialadenitis occurs within 24 hours after ^{131}I administration and may be due to the concentration of radioisotope in the salivary glands. Stimulation of salivary flow with hard candy may avert this problem.

Transient bone marrow suppression is seen in almost all patients receiving ^{131}I therapy. More severe aplasia may be seen in patients with extensive metastatic disease or in those who have had repeated doses of ^{131}I.

External-beam irradiation is used, either alone or in combination with ^{131}I, for patients with incompletely excised tumors. Tubiana et al[53] report that with high-dose external-beam therapy to the thyroid, neck, and superior mediastinum, they achieved local control of disease in approximately 90% of their patients with inoperable differentiated cancers.

Recent studies have shown that patients with MCT who were treated with postoperative irradiation had survival rates similar to those of patients treated with surgery alone, even though they had more advanced disease.[53,54]

Treatment of anaplastic carcinomas with ^{131}I and external irradiation has not been effective because of the radioresistance of this type of thyroid neoplasm, but Kim and Leeper[55] reported excellent results with local control obtained by combining external-beam radiation with low-dose doxorubicin as a radiosensitizer for hypoxic, radioresistant tumor cells. Because of the potentiation of bone marrow suppression and local toxicities affecting the oral mucosa and esophagus, dose reduction should be considered when chemotherapy and external radiation are administered concurrently.

External-beam irradiation may also be helpful in the palliation of painful bony metastases.

Chemotherapy

The role of chemotherapy in the treatment of advanced differentiated, medullary, and anaplastic thyroid cancer has been disappointing, with low response rates.[56] As a single agent, only doxorubicin has demonstrated any significant antitumor activity.[1] Shimaoka et al[57] report a 26% overall response rate when advanced differentiated and anaplastic thyroid carcinomas were treated with a combination of doxorubicin and cisplatin.

PITUITARY TUMORS

The diagnosis and management of patients with pituitary tumors have changed significantly over the past 20 years, with the refinement of microsurgical and radiotherapy techniques, advances in laboratory evaluation of hormonal activity, and pharmacologic developments for the management of tumor-related hormonal abnormalities.

Epidemiology

Pituitary tumors account for approximately 10% to 15% of all known intracranial neoplasms.[58] The great majority of these are benign pituitary adenomas that arise from the adenohypophyseal cells in the anterior portion of the gland. The other tumor types observed are craniopharyngiomas, which occur primarily in children, and pituitary carcinomas. Pituitary carcinoma is exceedingly rare.[59] This discussion will be limited to pituitary adenomas.

Although adenomas have been reported in all age groups, they are rarely seen before puberty and occur primarily in middle-aged and older patients.

Etiology

No definitive causative factors have been established, but changes in hormonal equilibrium within the pituitary may play a role in the development of pituitary adenomas.[60]

Hyperplasia of adenohypophyseal cells can result from prolonged stimulation of pituitary hormones. This generally occurs in clinical situations in which target glands of pituitary hormones are not secreting sufficient hormone to provide negative feedback to the pituitary gland. For example, hyperplasia of the cells that secrete TSH has been reported in patients with long-standing primary hypothyroidism.[61] This process can be reversed with administration of exogenous hormone, thereby inhibiting further stimulation of the pituitary gland. Although there is no conclusive evidence that hyperplastic cells are more susceptible to neoplastic transformation, the relationship between cellular proliferation and growth of adenomas requires further study.[58]

It also has been suggested that adenomas of the prolactin-secreting cells may result from disorders of dopamine synthesis and secretion. Because prolactin is inhibited by dopamine, disturbances in dopamine metabolism may result in an unopposed increase in prolactin secretion.[62]

There does not appear to be any genetic influence in the development of pituitary adenomas.[1]

Classification

Pituitary adenomas are categorized according to hormone secretion and size. The major hormones secreted by the anterior pituitary gland are prolactin, growth hormone (GH), adrenocorticotropin hormone (ACTH), TSH, follicle-stimulating hormone (FSH), and luteinizing hormone (LH). The hormonal classification of pituitary adenomas, their relative incidence, and associated clinical syndromes are listed in Table 37-5.[63]

Adenomas also are classified according to their size and extension outside the sella turcica.[64] Those smaller than 10 mm in diameter are classified as microadenomas. Microadenomas are associated with a better overall prognosis because they generally are confined to the sella turcica and are more easily resected.[65]

TABLE 37-5 Hormonal Classification of Pituitary Adenomas

Classification	Prevalence (approximate) (%)[63]	Hormone Secreted	Clinical Manifestations
Lactotroph	27	Prolactin	Women: amenorrhea, infertility, galactorrhea Men: decreased libido, impotence
Somatotroph	14	GH	Acromegaly, gigantism
Corticotroph	14	ACTH	Cushing's disease (approximately 6% have increased ACTH without endocrine symptoms)
Gonadotroph	6.5	FSH/LH	Frequently are clinically silent with only elevated blood hormone levels
Thyrotroph	1	TSH	Hyperthyroidism
Plurihormonal	10	Two or more adenohypophyseal hormones (GH, prolactin are most common)	Depends on type of hormone secreted
Null cell	25	None	Localized symptoms—headache, visual disturbances, dysfunction of cranial nerves

Pathophysiology

Although most pituitary adenomas do not exhibit the characteristic histologic changes indicative of malignant transformation, they are "malignant" by virtue of their ability to produce morbidity through growth in a confined space and mediation of hormonal dysfunction. Many adenomas are slow-growing, noninvasive tumors confined to the sella turcica. Others are more aggressive in their clinical behavior, exhibiting rapid growth rates, invading adjacent tissues, and causing symptoms indicative of compression of vital structures.[58,65,66] Invasion occurs more frequently with macroadenomas than with microadenomas.[65]

Adenohypophyseal carcinomas, although rare, are true malignant tumors in both their histologic appearance and their biologic behavior, and they uniformly result in distant metastases.[59]

The majority of pituitary tumors arising from adenohypophyseal cells are well differentiated and the cells retain their hormone-producing capabilities. The tumor cells are not subject to the normal regulatory mechanisms of the body and produce hormones, regardless of feedback from target organs.[58]

Clinical Presentation

The most common manifestations of pituitary adenoma are alterations in hormonal patterns and pressure symptoms from a growing tumor.

Patients with functional tumors will have symptoms of hormonal excess. Clinical effects of hypersecretion of the anterior pituitary hormones will be observed in these patients.

Infrequently, tumor expansion will cause destruction of normal adenohypophyseal cells, resulting in panhypopituitarism. The clinical picture generally reflects the degree of hormonal deficit, since abrupt cessation of all pituitary hormone secretion is rare.[64]

An expanding pituitary neoplasm can cause compression of surrounding critical structures, resulting in headache, visual disturbances, and functional impairment of cranial nerves (Figure 37-2).[67] Headache occurs when the expanding tumor distends the diaphragma sellae. Suprasellar extension may compress the optic nerves and chiasm. The most frequent ophthalmologic finding is a unilateral or bitemporal visual field defect. Lateral tumor extension also can involve oculomotor nerves, causing oculomotor paresis. Occasionally, penetration into the sphenoid sinus is associated with a spontaneous cerebral spinal fluid rhinorrhea.[64]

Diagnostic Evaluation

Although the histologic diagnosis of a pituitary adenoma cannot be confirmed before surgery, the anatomic extent of the pituitary mass and its functional status can be validated with appropriate endocrine and neuroradiologic studies.

Advances in radioimmunoassay techniques have made direct measurement of pituitary hormone secretion possible. Heretofore, assessment of pituitary hormones could be accomplished only indirectly by measurement of hormone secretion of target tissues.[68] Since hypersecretion of pituitary hormones can be caused by other pathologic pro-

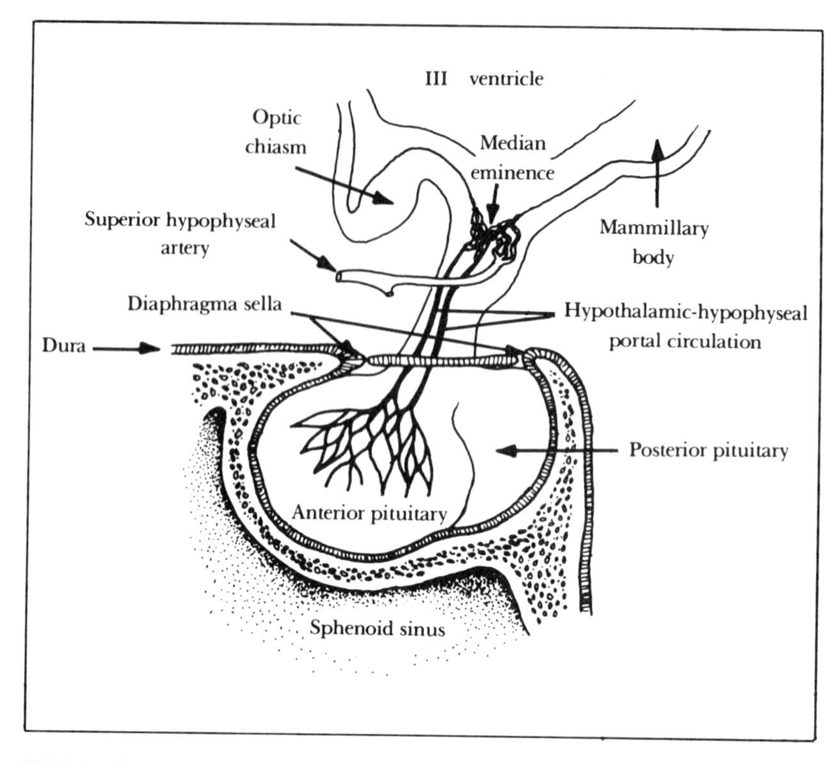

FIGURE 37-2 Anatomic relationship of pituitary gland to surrounding structures. (Source: From Boyd AE III, Jordan RM, Kohler PO: Disorders of the hypothalamus and anterior pituitary, in Kohler PO (ed): Clinical Endocrinology. New York, John Wiley & Sons, 1986, pp 11-51.)

cesses, documentation of elevated levels alone does not confirm the diagnosis of a pituitary adenoma.

Magnetic resonance imaging (MRI) and computed tomography (CT) are the imaging techniques most commonly used because they provide more precise information regarding tumor margins, effect of tumor on adjacent structures, location of vascular structures, the optic apparatus and cavernous sinus, consistency of the tumor, and presence of normal pituitary tissue.[69] Angiography defines the lumen of blood vessels and is indicated if there is a question of an aneurysm.

Information obtained during the diagnostic work-up may aid in the selection of a therapeutic approach, as well as provide baseline data for assessment of response to therapy. Diagnostic tests are repeated after initial therapy to assess adequacy of treatment and the need for additional management.

Treatment

The goals of treatment are removal or eradication of the tumor, restoration of normal hormonal function, and elimination of mass effects without residual morbidity.

Surgery

Prompt surgical intervention is indicated in patients with pituitary apoplexy (hemorrhage into the tumor and precipitous deterioration of neurologic status) and in patients with clinical manifestations of a progressive mass effect. Other indications for surgery remain controversial.

Surgical excision of hypersecreting pituitary microadenomas remains the most effective method of achieving rapid, durable responses in the treatment of these lesions.[70-73] In patients with hypersecreting macroadenomas, preoperative hormonal manipulation may be used to decrease the size of the tumor and increase resectability.[71,73]

Complete resection is not always possible in patients with macroadenomas, but subtotal resection followed by postoperative radiation can be curative in a large proportion of patients.[74,75]

Selection of the surgical technique depends on size of the tumor, extent of suprasellar extension, and involvement of the cavernous sinus. Approximately 96% of adenomas are resected by the transsphenoidal route,[70] with the remainder requiring craniotomy. The transsphenoidal approach permits selective removal of the tumor with preservation of normal pituitary tissue. Disadvantages of this technique are visual limitations in the surgical field, including inability to visualize the optic nerves. Craniotomy permits complete visualization of the pituitary gland and surrounding intracranial structures but is associated with higher morbidity. Whenever possible, normal pituitary tissue is preserved.

Diabetes insipidus, cerebrospinal fluid (CSF) leak, and meningitis are the most frequently reported complications that follow transsphenoidal surgery.

Transient diabetes insipidus is seen in 30% to 50% of patients and is managed with desmopressin.[76] This complication usually is transient, even in patients who have had complete hypophysectomy, since antidiuretic hormone (ADH) can be secreted directly from the hypothalamus without pituitary storage.

CSF rhinorrhea is managed with bed rest, elevation of the head of the bed, and fluid restrictions. Activities that increase intracranial pressure, such as sneezing, coughing, and blowing the nose, are avoided.[77]

Because of the increased risk of meningitis after surgery, patients frequently are given prophylactic antibiotics. Patients are monitored for symptoms of meningitis, including fever and stiff neck.[77]

Other possible surgical risks include damage to the hypothalamus, optic nerves, and carotid arteries. Additional nursing considerations during the immediate postoperative period pertain to the care of the operative site. It takes nasal mucosa approximately 1 month to heal after surgery. Sneezing and nose-blowing are contraindicated during this period to minimize pressure on the operative site. Because the surgical incision is located in the upper gingiva, oral inspection and meticulous mouth care are instituted to maintain integrity of the mucous membranes and to prevent infection.[77]

Postoperatively, measurement of pituitary hormone levels is done to assess the effectiveness of surgery in removing hypersecreting tumor tissue. As a result of surgery, normalization of hormonal levels occurs in 65% to 88% of patients with acromegaly[76] and 80% to 86% of patients with Cushing's disease.[78,79]

Radiotherapy

External-beam radiation is used in the management of patients with inoperable or incompletely resected tumors or those with persistent postoperative hyperfunctioning endocrinopathies.[50] Because of the recent advances in microsurgical techniques, irradiation seldom is used alone as a primary treatment of pituitary adenomas except in patients who are not optimal surgical candidates.[81] Ciric et al[72] report that, when combined with surgery, postoperative radiation can lower the recurrence rate of adenomas from 28% to 6%.

Radiation therapy is less effective in controlling endocrine hypersecretion than in controlling regrowth of pituitary adenomas.[75] Irradiation progressively lowers growth hormone level in approximately 80% of the patients with acromegaly and glucocorticoid level in 50% to 80% of the patients with Cushing's disease, but full effects may not be seen for months to years later. Because of the delay in radiation effect, this form of therapy alone is impractical for normalizing hormone levels in patients with hypersecreting tumors. The major complication of irradiation of pituitary adenomas is hypopituitarism, which may become evident years after treatment has been given.[81,82]

Pharmacotherapy

The focus of medical management of pituitary adenomas has been hormone manipulation of pituitary secretions.

Bromocriptine, a dopamine agonist, has been shown to be effective not only in reducing hormone levels in patients with prolactin-secreting tumors but in reducing tumor size as well.[83-85] This approach often is used as first-line therapy for patients with prolactinomas, but its use remains controversial. Bromocriptine as a single agent is not curative, and discontinuation results in rapid regrowth of tumor and hypersecretion of prolactin. It also has been suggested that preoperative treatment of prolactinomas with bromocriptine may adversely affect the outcome of surgery, since it can cause an increase in interstitial fibrosis. While it can make surgical resection technically more difficult, this fibrosis has not been found to affect the surgical outcome in patients receiving short-term (less than 6 weeks) preoperative therapy.[86]

A long-acting somatostatin analog, SMS 201-995 (Sandoz, Hanover, NJ), has been used in the preoperative treatment of GH-producing macroadenomas by suppressing GH hypersecretion as well as reducing tumor size.[87] Maximal tumor reduction occurs after 8 to 12 weeks of treatment and GH levels remain within the normal range in 80% of the patients postoperatively.

ADRENAL TUMORS

Adrenal tumors can arise from the cortical or medullary portions of the adrenal gland, with presentations differing significantly because of the physiologic diversity of these two types of tissue. The majority of cancers of the cortex are adenocarcinomas, while tumors of the adrenal medulla are either pheochromocytomas or neuroblastomas.[88]

Adrenocortical Carcinomas

Epidemiology

The incidence of adrenal neoplasms is rare, with adrenocortical tumors accounting for approximately 0.2% of all malignant tumors.[89] In several of the larger series of patients with adrenocortical carcinomas, the overall incidence was equal between sexes, although women had a much higher proportion of functional neoplasms.[90-93] Functional tumors are those that produce excess amounts of corticosteroids. Nonfunctional carcinomas occur most commonly in patients 40 to 70 years of age, with a 2:1

predominance in men. All series reported more frequent involvement of the left adrenal gland; bilateral occurrence was rarely seen.[93,94]

Pathophysiology

Adrenocortical carcinomas are aggressive malignancies, with 70% to 90% of the patients having either locally advanced or metastatic disease. The delay in detecting the disease is thought to be due to (1) difficulty in detecting retroperitoneal masses, (2) nonspecific symptoms in patients with nonfunctional tumors, and (3) gradual onset of symptoms in patients with functional tumors.[95]

The most common sites of metastasis are lung, liver, and lymph nodes. More than 50% of the patients in one series died of pulmonary insufficiency (from multiple lung metastases) and sepsis.[90] Sepsis was thought to be related to lack of immunocompetence in patients with disseminated cancer. Local tumor extension can involve the kidneys, liver, vena cava, pancreas, and diaphragm. Overall median survival with treatment ranges from 1 month to 5 years.[90-93]

Clinical presentation

Patients with nonfunctional tumors commonly have a palpable abdominal mass that may be associated with abdominal or back pain. Fever, weight loss, weakness, and lethargy are primarily seen in patients with advanced disease.[96]

Patients with functional tumors will have excessive production of one or more of the hormones secreted by the adrenal cortex. The five major steroid hormones are cortisol, aldosterone, progesterone, testosterone, and estradiol. The majority of functional tumors result in Cushing's disease, virilization and feminization syndromes, and hyperaldosteronism.[95]

Clinical features of Cushing's disease include weight gain, obesity of the trunk, face, and neck, hirsutism, hypertension, and muscle wasting.[96] In women, androgen-secreting tumors result in a virilization syndrome characterized by amenorrhea, hirsutism, increased muscle mass, and deepening of the voice.[97] In men, estrogen-secreting tumors result in gynecomastia, testicular atrophy, and impotence.[95] Estrogen-secreting tumors are difficult to detect until they are far advanced in premenopausal women. The occurrence of aldosterone-secreting tumors is rare. Hypersecretion of aldosterone leads to hypertension and hypokalemia.[98]

Diagnostic evaluation

Immunoassays of hormone precursors and mature hormones and their metabolites detect the presence of functional adrenal tumors. Patients with adrenocortical carcinoma commonly excrete large amounts of 17-ketosteroids if glucocorticoid or sex steroid production is excessive.[99]

CT is the most common means used to localize adrenal tumors[96] and provides information regarding hepatic, renal, and vena caval involvement. Widespread use of CT has resulted in increasing numbers of incidentally discovered adrenal masses.[100] These masses warrant careful evaluation to identify appropriate treatment interventions. Recent reports regarding the ability of MRI to distinguish benign adenomas from adrenocortical carcinomas and pheochromocytomas indicate that this is an invaluable diagnostic tool.[101,102] MRI may be particularly useful in the screening of asymptomatic masses. With earlier detection, the prognosis for patients with adrenocortical carcinomas may improve.[101]

Treatment

Surgery is the primary treatment for adrenocortical carcinoma, and it can be curative for patients with small localized tumors.[93] Unfortunately, many tumors are unresectable at the time of diagnosis because of local extension, lymphatic metastases, or distant metastases to the liver or lungs. In patients with locally advanced and invasive disease, maximal debulking should be undertaken before additional therapy is initiated. Results of treatment with conventional surgery, radiation therapy, and chemotherapy have been poor, with 5-year survival less than 30%.[90,103]

Because tumor hypersecretion may diffusely suppress adrenal hormone activity, causing atrophy of the uninvolved gland, glucocorticoids are administered before and after surgery until normal function of the unaffected gland returns. In patients with bilateral involvement, ablation of both adrenals necessitates permanent replacement therapy of the mineralocorticoids and glucocorticoids. Exogenous administration of catecholamines is not required, because of the ectopic sources at nerve endings and other ganglia in the sympathetic nervous system.[88]

The adrenocorticolytic drug, o,p'-DDD (mitotane), which causes selective necrosis of the adrenal cortex, has a limited role in the adjunctive management of adrenal cortical tumors after surgical debulking. In a large series of 60 patients who received o,p'-DDD, objective tumor regression was seen in 34% but the mean duration of response was approximately 10 months.[104] Treatment with o,p'-DDD is associated with disabling side effects that include nausea, vomiting, anorexia, diarrhea, lethargy, and profound depression that can alter a patient's quality of life. These toxic effects are seen with therapeutic doses of 8 to 10 grams per day. Patient tolerance has been improved with reduced doses.[105] Also, many of the side effects may be due to adrenal insufficiency and can be corrected by increased doses of replacement corticosteroids.[106]

Aminoglutethimide, which blocks corticosteroid secretion, can also be used for palliation of excess hormone production in patients with recurrent disease, but this drug does not inhibit further growth of the tumor.[88]

Evaluation of the efficacy of cytotoxic chemotherapy is limited because of the rarity of this neoplasm. Anecdotal reports of combination o,p'-DDD/streptozotocin and cisplatin/VP-16 have shown limited activity.[107,108]

Radiation therapy after surgical resection does not improve survival but can be effective in palliation of painful bone metastases.[92,93]

Phemochromocytoma

Epidemiology

Pheochromocytomas are rare catecholamine-secreting tumors that arise from chromaffin cells of the sympathoadrenal system. Chromaffin cells, found not only in the adrenals but in other ectopic sites along the sympathetic chain, have the enzymatic properties to synthesize amine hormones. Tumors that share these common biochemical characteristics for *a*mine *p*recursor *u*ptake and *d*ecarboxylation are referred to as APUD tumors.[109] APUD cells have been detected in the thyroid, adrenal medulla, sympathetic nervous system, and gastroenteropancreatic organs.

Pheochromocytomas are extremely rare, occurring in fewer than 0.1% to 1% of hypertensive patients.[110] Malignant pheochromocytomas occur in approximately 10% of patients with pheochromocytomas and can be differentiated from benign tumors only by their capacity for invasiveness and distant metastases.[110] Pheochromocytomas occasionally are associated with other endocrine tumors as part of a multiple endocrine neoplasia syndrome (Table 37-1). A genetic predisposition to development of pheochromocytomas in conjunction with other APUD-derived tumors is known to exist.[111]

Clinical presentation

Excess production of catecholamines accounts for most of the clinical manifestations of this tumor. Nearly all patients with symptoms of pheochromocytomas have sustained or paroxysmal diastolic hypertension, although in one study 35% of the patients with autopsy-proven pheochromocytomas had no previously documented hypertension.[112] Other symptoms include headache, sweating, nausea and vomiting, palpitations, and anxiety.

Diagnostic evaluation

Measurement of urinary and circulating catecholamines or their metabolites (metanephrine, normetanephrine, and vanillylmandelic acid) confirms the diagnosis of pheochromocytoma in 98% of cases.[113]

CT is used routinely to localize tumors before surgery in all patients with abnormal urinary test findings. The metaiodobenylguanidine scan (MIBG) also is helpful in localization of pheochromocytomas. MIBG is a noninvasive technique that uses an agent that mimics norepinephrine and is taken up by catecholamine-producing cells.[114]

Treatment

After biochemical confirmation of an existing pheochromocytoma, patients are pretreated with a-adrenergic blocking agents to minimize the possibility of uncontrolled catecholamine release during invasive localization procedures and surgery.

The goal of surgery is removal of all accessible disease and metastases, although resection of all functional catecholamine-secreting tissue may not be possible. Prolonged exposure to the b-adrenergic effect of circulating catecholamines may result in myocardial hypertrophy, thereby placing the patient at higher risk of cardiovascular complications during surgery.[115] Postoperatively, patients require rigorous monitoring for signs of shock related to the profound decrease in available catecholamines.

The role of cytotoxic therapy in the management of this tumor has not been fully ascertained. Averbuch et al[116] reported an overall response rate of 57% in 14 patients whose malignant pheochromocytoma was treated with combined cyclophosphamide, vincristine, and dacarbazine.

PARATHYROID TUMORS

Epidemiology

Malignant tumors of the parathyroid gland are extremely rare, accounting for only 1% to 4% of all cases of primary hyperparathyroidism.[117,118] The incidence is distributed equally between the sexes, with the majority of patients clustered between the ages of 30 and 60 years.[118] Carcinoma of the parathyroid causing hyperparathyroidism may occur as one entity of a multiple endocrine neoplasia syndrome.

Although no definitive causative factors have been identified, there is some evidence that irradiation of the head and neck may induce neoplastic transformation in hyperplastic glands.[119]

Pathophysiology

Generally, parathyroid carcinoma is an indolent, noninvasive tumor with the potential late in the course of the disease for metastases to regional nodes, liver, and lung.[118,120] Although the 5-year survival rate is only 50%,[118] prolonged survival has been observed, even when metastatic disease is present.[117,121]

Most parathyroid carcinomas are biochemically functional, causing clinical effects of hypercalcemia from hypersecretion of parathyroid hormone (PTH). Metabolic complications of hypercalcemia frequently are the cause of death.[117,120]

Clinical Presentation

Parathyroid tumors are most frequently detected by the finding of hypercalcemia during routine laboratory examination. On x-ray examination, approximately one half of the patients have evidence of bony disease caused by increased bone resorption, which occurs with elevations in PTH levels.[117] Only one third of the patients have palpable masses, and pain is rare.[121] Because parathyroid carcinoma presents a clinical and biochemical picture very similar to that of benign parathyroid disorders, it poses a difficult diagnostic problem.[117] To avoid unnecessary surgery, other disease processes that may cause hypercalcemia must be ruled out.

Treatment

Temporary control of hypercalcemia can be achieved with conservative medical therapy until adequate preoperative evaluation is completed.

Treatment consists of en bloc resection of the abnormal parathyroid tissue and ipsilateral neck dissection if cervical nodes are involved. Even after complete resection of macroscopic tumor, 30% to 65% of the patients will eventually have recurrent disease, either locally or at distant sites. Patients with recurrent disease are rarely cured, but since parathyroid carcinomas grow slowly, surgical resection of recurrent local tumors or functioning metastases is recommended because palliation can be achieved for prolonged periods of time.

Postoperative complications include hypoparathyroidism, recurrent laryngeal nerve damage, and hemorrhage. Residual normal parathyroid tissue may have atrophied as a result of suppressive effects of high circulating levels of PTH.[122] After removal of the hyperactive tissue, it may take 1 to 2 weeks for normal function to return. During this period of hypoparathyroidism, patients may experience tetany and require temporary administration of calcium replacement.[48] The postoperative nursing management of patients with parathyroid tumor is similar to that of individuals undergoing thyroidectomy.

Neither radiation therapy nor chemotherapy has been effective in the treatment of recurrent disease.

CONCLUSION

Progress in the treatment of endocrine tumors generally has been slow because of the lack of prospective, randomized clinical trials to evaluate new treatment approaches. This is due, in large part, to problems in accrual of patients because of the rarity of these tumors.

At this point, optimal management involves identification of high-risk groups, early detection of disease, and appropriate surgical intervention.

REFERENCES

1. Norton JA, Doppman JL, Jensen RT: Cancer of the endocrine system, in DeVita VT Jr, Hellman S, Rosenberg SA (eds): Cancer: Principles and Practice of Oncology. Philadelphia, JB Lippincott, 1989, pp 1269-1344.
2. Silverberg E, Lubera J: Cancer statistics, 1989. CA 39:3-20, 1989.
3. Schlumberger M, DeVathaire F, Travagli JP, et al: Differentiated thyroid carcinoma in childhood: Long term follow-up of 72 patients. J Clin Endocrinol Metab 65:1088-1094, 1987.
4. Favus MJ, Schneider AB, Stachura ME, et al: Thyroid cancer occurring as a late consequence of head and neck irradiation: Evaluation of 1056 patients. N Engl J Med 294:1019-25, 1975.
5. Refetoff S, Harrison J, Karanfilski BT, et al: Continuing occurrence of thyroid carcinoma after irradiation to the neck in infancy and childhood. N Engl J Med 292:171-175, 1975.
6. Duffy BJ, Fitzgerald PJ: Cancer of the thyroid in children: A report of 28 cases. J Clin Endocrinol 10:1296-1308, 1950.
7. Wilson SM, Platz C, Block GM: Thyroid carcinoma after irradiation: Characteristics and treatment. Arch Surg 100:330-337, 1970.
8. Hempleman LH, Pifer JW, Burke GJ, et al: Neoplasms in persons treated with x-rays in infancy for thymic enlargement; a report of the third follow-up survey. JNCI 38:317-341, 1967.
9. Schneider AB, Favus MJ, Stachura ME, et al: Incidence, prevalence and characteristics of radiation-induced thyroid tumors. Am J Med 64:243-52, 1978.
10. McDougall IR: Thyroid cancer after iodine-131 therapy. JAMA 227:438-440, 1974.
11. McDougall IR, Nelsen TS, Kempson RL: Papillary carcinoma of the thyroid seven years after I-131 therapy for Grave's disease. Clin Nucl Med 6:368-371, 1981.
12. Holm LE, Dahlquist I, Israelsson A, et al: Malignant thyroid tumors after iodine-131 therapy. N Engl J Med 303:188-191, 1980.
13. Spencer RP, Chapman CN, Rao H: Thyroid carcinoma after radioiodine therapy for hyperthyroidism: Analysis based on age, latency, and administered dose of I-131. Clin Nucl Med 8:216-220, 1983.
14. Williams ED: The aetiology of thyroid tumours. Clin Endocrinol Metab 8:193-207, 1979.
15. Clark OH: TSH suppression in the management of thyroid nodules and thyroid cancer. World J Surg 5:39-47, 1981.
16. Baylin SB, Wells SA: Management of hereditary medullary thyroid carcinoma. Clin Endocrinol Metab 10:367-377, 1981.
17. Saad MF, Ordonez NG, Rashid RK, et al: Medullary carcinoma of the thyroid: A study of the clinical features and prognostic factors in 161 patients. Medicine 63:319-342, 1984.
18. Kerr DJ, Burt AD, Anderson JR: Tumours of the diffuse neuroendocrine system. Eur J Surg Oncol 13:189-195, 1987.
19. Gagel RF, Tashjian AH, Cummings T, et al: The clinical outcome of prospective screening for multiple endocrine neoplasia type 2a: An 18-year experience. N Engl J Med 318:478-484, 1988.
20. Mazzaferri EL, Young RL, Oertel JE, et al: Papillary thyroid carcinoma: The impact of therapy in 576 patients. Medicine 56:171-196, 1977.
21. Schlumberger M, Tubiana M, deVathaire F, et al: Long-term results of treatment of 283 patients with lung and bone metastases from differentiated thyroid cancer. J Clin Endocrinol Metab 63:960-967, 1986.
22. McConahey WM, Hay ID, Woolner LB, et al: Papillary thyroid cancer treated at the Mayo Clinic, 1946 through 1970: Initial manifestations, pathologic findings, therapy, and outcome. Mayo Clin Proc 61:978-996, 1986.
23. Carcangiu ML, Giancarlo Z, Pupi A, et al: Papillary carcinoma of the thyroid: A clinicopathologic study of 241 cases treated at the University of Florence, Italy. Cancer 55:805-828, 1985.

24. Tubiana M, Schlumberger M, Rougier P, et al: Long-term results and prognostic factors in patients with differentiated thyroid cancer. Cancer 55:794-804, 1985.
25. Samaan NA, Schultz PN, Haynie TP, et al: Pulmonary metastasis of differentiated thyroid carcinoma: Treatment results in 101 patients. J Clin Endocrinol Metab 65:376-380, 1985.
26. Kerr DJ, Burt AD, Boyle P, et al: Prognostic factors in thyroid tumours. Br J Cancer 54:475-482, 1986.
27. Hubert JP, Kiernan PD, Beahrs OH, et al: Occult papillary carcinoma of the thyroid. Arch Surg 115:394-399, 1980.
28. Harness JK, Thompson NW, McLeod MK, et al: Follicular carcinoma of the thyroid gland: Trends and treatment. Surgery 96:972-978, 1984.
29. Schmidt RJ, Wang C: Encapsulated follicular carcinoma of the thyroid: Diagnosis, treatment, and results. Surgery 100:1068-1075, 1986.
30. Greenfield LD: Thyroid tumors, in Perez CA, Brady LW (eds): Principles and Practice of Radiation Oncology. Philadelphia, JB Lippincott, 1987, pp 1126-1156.
31. Leeper RD: Thyroid cancer. Med Clin North Am 69:1079-1096, 1985.
32. Schroder S, Bocker W, Baisch H, et al: Prognostic factors in medullary thyroid carcinomas. Cancer 61:806-816, 1988.
33. Kakudo K, Carney JA, Sizemore GW: Medullary carcinoma of thyroid: Biologic behavior of the sporadic and familial neoplasms. Cancer 55:2818-2821, 1985.
34. Nel CJC, VanHeerden JA, Goellner JR, et al: Anaplastic carcinoma of the thyroid: A clinicopathologic study of 82 cases. Mayo Clin Proc 60:51-58, 1985.
35. Carcangiu ML, Steeper T, Zampi G, et al: Anaplastic thyroid carcinoma: A study of 70 cases. Am J Clin Pathol 83:135-158, 1985.
36. Friedman M, Toriumi DM, Mafee MF: Diagnostic imaging techniques in thyroid cancer. Am J Surg 155:215-223, 1988.
37. Hawkins F, Gellido D, Bernal C, et al: Fine needle aspiration in the diagnosis of thyroid cancer and thyroid disease. Cancer 59:1206-1209, 1987.
38. Rojeski MT, Gharib H: Nodular thyroid disease: Evaluation and management. N Engl J Med 313:428-436, 1985.
39. Freitas JE, Gross MD, Ripley S, et al: Radionuclide diagnosis and therapy of thyroid cancer: Current status report. Semin Nucl Med 15:106-131, 1985.
40. Beahrs OH, Henson DE, Hutter RVP, et al (eds): Manual for Staging of Cancer (ed 3). Philadelphia, JB Lippincott, 1988, pp 57-59.
41. Clark OH, Levin K, Zeng Q, et al: Thyroid cancer: The case for total thyroidectomy. Eur J Cancer Clin Oncol 24:305-313, 1988.
42. Crile G Jr, Antunez AR, Esselstyn CB, et al: The advantages of subtotal thyroidectomy and suppression of TSH in the primary treatment of papillary carcinoma of the thyroid. Cancer 55:2691-2697, 1985.
43. Attie JN: Modified neck dissection in treatment of thyroid cancer: A safe procedure. Eur J Cancer Clin Oncol 24:315-324, 1988.
44. Goolden AWG: The use of radioactive iodine in thyroid carcinoma. Eur J Cancer Clin Oncol 24:339-343, 1988.
45. Schroder DM, Chambors A, France CJ: Operative strategy for thyroid cancer: Is total thyroidectomy worth the price? Cancer 58:2320-2328, 1986.
46. Harness JK, Fung L, Thompson NW, et al: Total thyroidectomy: Complications and technique. World J Surg 10:781-786, 1986.
47. Rossi RL, Cady B, Silverman ML, et al: Current results of conservative surgery for differentiated thyroid carcinoma. World J Surg 10:612-622, 1986.
48. Smeltzer SCO: Assessment and management of patients with endocrine disorders, in Brunner LS, Suddarth DS, Bare BG, et al (eds): Textbook of Medical-Surgical Nursing (ed 6). Philadelphia, JB Lippincott, 1988, pp 942-989.
49. Blahd WH: Treatment of thyroid cancer. Comp Ther 11(9):26-32, 1986.
50. Schreiber NW: Endocrine malignancies, in Groenwald S (ed): Cancer Nursing: Principles and Practice. Boston, Jones & Bartlett, 1987, pp 489-507.
51. Wells SA Jr, Ross AJ III, Dale JK, et al: Transplantation of the parathyroid glands: Current status. Surg Clin North Am 59:167-177, 1979.
52. Melmed S, Harada A, Hershman JM, et al: Neutralizing antibodies to bovine thyrotropin in immunized patients with cancer. J Clin Endocrinol Metab 51:358-363, 1980.
53. Tubiana M, Haddad E, Schlumberger M, et al: External radiotherapy in thyroid cancers. Cancer 55:2062-2071, 1985.
54. Rougier P, Parmentier C, Laplance A, et al: Medullary thyroid carcinoma: Prognostic factors and treatment. Int J Radiat Oncol Biol Phys 9:161-169, 1983.
55. Kim JH, Leeper RD: Treatment of anaplastic giant and spindle cell carcinoma of the thyroid gland with combination Adriamycin and radiation therapy: A new approach. Cancer 52:954-957, 1983.
56. Wells SA, Dilley WG, Farndon JA, et al: Early diagnosis and treatment of medullary thyroid carcinoma. Arch Intern Med 145:1248-1252, 1985.
57. Shimaoka K, Schoenfeld DA, DeWys WD, et al: A randomized trial of doxorubicin versus doxorubicin plus cisplatin in patients with advanced thyroid cancer. Cancer 56:2155-2158, 1985.
58. Kovacs K, Horvath E: Pathology of pituitary tumors. Endocrinol Metabol Clin 16:667-683, 1987.
59. Nudleman KL, Choi B, Kusske JA: Primary pituitary carcinoma: A clinical pathological study. Neurosurgery 16:90-95, 1985.
60. Molitch ME: Pathogenesis of pituitary tumors, Endocrinol Metab Clin 16:503-527, 1987.
61. Scheithauer BW, Kovacs K, Rangall RV, et al: Pituitary gland in hypothyroidism: Histologic and immunocytologic study. Arch Pathol Lab Med 109:499-508, 1985.
62. Camanni R, Ghigo E, Caccarelli, et al: Defective regulation of prolactin secretion after successful removal of prolactinomas. J Clin Endocrinol Metab 57:1270-1276, 1983.
63. Kovacs K, Horvath E: Tumors of the pituitary, in Atlas of Tumor Pathology, Fasc XXI, 2nd series, Washington DC, Armed Forces Institute of Pathology, 1986.
64. Ciric I: Pituitary tumors. Neurol Clin 3:751-766, 1985.
65. Scheithauer BW, Kovacs K, Laws ER Jr, et al: Pathology of invasive pituitary tumors with special reference to functional classification. J Neurosurg 65:733-744, 1986.
66. Landolt AM, Shibata T, Kleihues P: Growth rate of human pituitary adenomas. J Neurosurg 67:803-806, 1987.
67. Boyd AE III, Jordan RM, Kohler PO: Disorders of the hypothalamus and anterior pituitary, in Kohler PO (ed): Clinical Endocrinology. New York, John Wiley & Sons Inc, 1986, pp 11-51.
68. Earp HS, Ney RL: Pituitary tumors, in Holland JF, Frei E III (eds): Cancer Medicine (ed 2). Philadelphia, Lea & Febiger, 1982, pp 1634-1647.
69. Kaufman B, Kaufman BA, Arafah BM, et al: Large pituitary gland adenomas evaluated with magnetic resonance imaging. Neurosurgery 21:540-546, 1987.
70. Laws ER jr: Pituitary surgery. Endocrinol Metab Clin 16:647-665, 1987.

71. Ross DA, Wilson CB: Results of transsphenoidal microsurgery for growth hormone-secreting pituitary adenoma in a series of 214 patients. J Neurosurg 68:854-867, 1988.
72. Ciric I, Mikhael M, Stafford T, et al: Transsphenoidal microsurgery of pituitary macroadenomas with long-term follow-up results. J Neurosurg 59:395-401, 1983.
73. Bevan JS, Adams CBT, Burke CW, et al: Factors in the outcome of transsphenoidal surgery for prolactinoma and non-functioning pituitary tumour, including pre-operative bromocriptine therapy. Clin Endocrinol 26:541-556, 1987.
74. Ebersold MJ, Quast LM, Laws ER Jr, et al: Long-term results in transsphenoidal removal of nonfunctioning pituitary adenomas. J Neurosurg 64:713-719, 1986.
75. Levin VA, Sheline GE, Gutin PH: Neoplasms of the central nervous system, in DeVita VT Jr, Hellman S, Rosenberg SA (eds): Cancer: Principles and Practice of Oncology. Philadelphia, JB Lippincott, 1989, pp 1557-1611.
76. Laws ER Jr, Randall RV, Abboud CF: Surgical treatment of acromegaly: Results in 140 patients, in Givens J (ed): Hormone-Secreting Pituitary Tumors. Chicago, Year Book, 1982, pp 225-228.
77. Resio MJ: Nursing diagnosis: Alteration in oral/nasal mucous membranes related to trauma of transsphenoidal surgery. J Neurosci Nurs 18:112-115, 1986.
78. Wilson CB: A decade of pituitary microsurgery (The Herbert Olivecrona Lecture). J Neurosurg 61:814-833, 1984.
79. Zervas NT, Martin JB: Management of hormone-secreting pituitary adenomas. N Engl J Med 302:210-214, 1980.
80. Halberg FE, Sheline GE: Radiotherapy of pituitary tumors. Endocrinol Metab Clin 16:667-683, 1987.
81. Chun M, Masko GB, Hetelekisis S: Radiotherapy in the treatment of pituitary adenomas. Int J Radiat Oncol Biol Phys 15:305-309, 1988.
82. Snyder PJ, Fowble BF, Schatz NJ, et al: Hypopituitarism following radiation therapy of pituitary adenomas. Am J Med 81:457-462, 1986.
83. Molitch ME, Elton RL, Blackwell RE, et al: Bromocriptine as primary therapy for prolactin-secreting macroadenomas: Results of a prospective multicenter study. J Clin Endocrinol Metab 60:698-705, 1985.
84. Luizzi A, Dallabonzana D, Oppizzi G, et al: Low doses of dopamine agonists in the long-term treatment of macroprolactinomas. N Engl J Med 131:656-659, 1985.
85. Weiss MH, Wycoff RR, Yadley R, et al: Bromocriptine treatment of prolactin-secreting tumors: surgical implications. Neurosurgery 12:640-642, 1983.
86. Hubbard JL, Scheithauer BW, Abboud CF, et al: Prolactin-secreting adenomas: The preoperative response to bromocriptine treatment and surgical outcome. J Neurosurg 67:816-821, 1987.
87. Barkan AL, Lloyd RV, Chandler WF, et al: Preoperative treatment of acromegaly with long-acting somatostatin analog SMS-201-995: Shrinkage of invasive pituitary macroadenomas and improved surgical remission rate. J Clin Endocrinol Metab 67:1040-1048, 1988.
88. Geelhoed G: Adrenal tumors, in Pilch Y (ed): Surgical Oncology. New York, McGraw-Hill, 1984, pp 610-629.
89. Bradley L III: Primary and adjunctive therapy in carcinoma of the adrenal cortex. Surg Gynecol Obstet 141:507-511, 1975.
90. Didolkar MS, Besche RS, Elias EG, et al: Natural history of adrenocortical carcinoma: A clinicopathologic study of 42 patients. Cancer 47:2153-2161, 1981.
91. Schteingart DE, Matazedi A, Noonan RA, et al: Treatment of adrenal carcinomas. Arch Surg 117:1142-1146, 1982.
92. Karakousis CP, Rao U, Moore R: Adrenal adenocarcinomas: Histologic grading and survival. J Surg Oncol 29(2):105-111, 1985.
93. Cohn K, Gottesman L, Brennan M: Adrenocortical carcinoma. Surgery 100:1170-1177, 1986.
94. Hutter AM, Kayhoe DE: Adrenal cortical carcinoma: Clinical features of 138 patients. Am J Med 41:572-580, 1966.
95. Brennan MF: Adrenocortical cancer. CA 37:348-365, 1987.
96. Thompson NW, Cheung PSY: Diagnosis and treatment of functioning and nonfunctioning adrenocortical neoplasms including incidentalomas. Surg Clin North Am 67:423-36, 1987.
97. Loriaux DL, Cutler GB Jr: Diseases of the adrenal glands, in Kohler PO (ed): Clinical Endocrinology. New York, John Wiley & Sons, 1986, pp 167-238.
98. Alterman SL, Dominguez C, Lopez-Gomaz A, et al: Primary adrenocortical carcinoma causing aldosteronism. Cancer 24:602-609, 1969.
99. Samaan NA, Hickey RC: Adrenal cortical carcinoma. Semin Oncol 14:292-296, 1987.
100. Katz RL, Shirkhoda A: Diagnostic approach to incidental adrenal nodules in the cancer patients. Cancer 55:1995-2000, 1985.
101. Doppman JL, Reinig JW, Dwyer AJ, et al: Differentiation of adrenal masses by magnetic resonance imaging. Surgery 102:1018-1025, 1987.
102. Chang A, Glazer HS, Lee JKT, et al: Adrenal gland: MR imaging. Radiology 163:123-128, 1987.
103. Henley DJ, vanHeerden JA, Grant CS, et al: Adrenal cortical carcinoma—A continuing challenge. Surgery 94:926-31, 1983.
104. Plager JE: Carcinoma of the adrenal cortex: Clinical description, diagnosis and treatment. Int Adv Surg Oncol 7:329-353, 1984.
105. Jarabak J, Rice K: Metastatic adrenal cortical carcinoma: Prolonged regression with mitotane therapy. JAMA 246:1706-1707, 1981.
106. Robinson BG, Hales IB, Henniker K, et al: The effect of o,p'-DDD on adrenal steroid replacement therapy requirements. Clin Endocrinol 27:437-444, 1987.
107. Eriksson B, Oberg K, Curstedt T, et al: Treatment of hormone-producing adrenocortical cancer with o,p'DDD and streptozocin. Cancer 59:1398-1403, 1987.
108. Johnson DH, Greco FA: Treatment of metastatic adrenal cortical carcinoma with cisplatin and etoposide (VP-16). Cancer 58:2198-2202, 1986.
109. Pearse AGE: The diffuse neuroendocrine system and the APUD concept: Related endocrine peptides in brain, intestine, pituitary, placenta and anuran cutaneous glands. Med Biol 55:115-125, 1977.
110. Samaan NA, Hickey RC, Schutts PE: Diagnosis, localization and management of pheochromocytoma: Pitfalls and follow-up in 41 patients. Cancer 62:2451-2160, 1988.
111. Bravo EL, Gifford RW: Pheochromocytoma: Diagnosis, localization and management. N Engl J Med 311:1298-1303, 1984.
112. St John Sutton MG, Sheps SG, Lie JT: Prevalence of clinically unsuspected pheochromocytoma: A review of a 50-year autopsy series. Mayo Clin Proc 56:354-360, 1981.
113. Samaan NA, Hickey RC: Pheochromocytoma. Semin Oncol 14:297-305, 1987.
114. Sisson JC, Frager MS, Valk TW, et al: Scintigraphic localization of pheochromocytoma. N Engl J Med 305:12-17, 1981.
115. Hull CJ: Phaeochromocytoma: Diagnosis, preoperative

preparation and anesthetic management. Br J Anaesth 58:1453-1468, 1986.

116. Averbuch S, Steakley CS, Young RC, et al: Malignant pheochromocytoma: Effective treatment with a combination of cyclophosphamide, vincristine, and dacarbazine. Ann Intern Med 109:267-273, 1988.
117. Wang C, Gaz RD: Natural history of parathyroid carcinoma: diagnosis, treatment and results. Am J Surg 149:522-527, 1985.
118. Schantz A, Castleman B: Parathyroid carcinoma: A study of 70 cases. Cancer 31:600-605, 1973.
119. Ireland JP, Fleming SJ, Levison EA, et al: Parathyroid carcinoma associated with chronic renal failure and previous radiotherapy to the neck. J Clin Pathol 38:1114-1118, 1985.
120. McCance DR, Kenny BD, Sloan JM, et al: Parathyroid carcinoma: A review. J R Soc Med 80:505-509, 1987.
121. Shane E, Bilezidian JP: Parathyroid carcinoma: A review of 62 patients. Endocr Rev 3:218-226, 1982.
122. Flye MW, Brennen MF: Surgical resection of metastatic parathyroid carcinoma. Ann Surg 193:425-435, 1981.

Chapter 38

Gastrointestinal Cancer: Colon, Rectum, and Anus

Joy Boarini, RN, MSN, CETN

INTRODUCTION

Cancer of the large intestine is one of the most common cancers for both males and females in the United States. Colorectal cancer is second only to lung cancer for the greatest number of new cases and deaths, excluding common skin cancers. It was estimated in 1989 that there would be approximately 151,000 new cases detected and an estimated 61,300 individuals dying of colorectal cancer in the United States.[1] In males, only cancer of the lung and prostate show a higher incidence; in females, only breast cancer ranks higher.

An infant born today has a 5% chance of developing colorectal cancer in his or her lifetime. These figures serve to emphasize the magnitude of this disease and why the American Cancer Society declared colorectal cancer as the National Priority Program for 1985–1986.

EPIDEMIOLOGY

Trends in the prevalence of colorectal cancer have not shown drastic changes. Even with advances in treatment techniques, a stable 50% cure rate in persons undergoing resection of colon cancer has persisted.[2] The death rate for males with colorectal cancer over the past 30 years has shown no overall change. In contrast, the death rate for females has shown a noticeable decrease, coincident with a decline in deaths from uterine cancers although not as dramatic.[2,3]

Cancer of the large intestine can occur at any age, with one of the youngest documented cases in a 9-month-old infant.[4] However, a positive correlation does exist between advancing age and the occurrence of colorectal cancer, with the mean age at diagnosis occurring after 60 years of age. In the United States, most cases of colorectal cancers occur after age 40.[5]

Colorectal cancer shows no particular predilection for either sex, occurring essentially equally in males and females. This is a relatively uncommon relationship in the epidemiologic profile of other cancers. Generally, however, cancer of the colon is more common in women up to age 55, when it becomes slightly more common in men.[6] The occurrence of rectal cancer is essentially equal in both sexes to age 45, but it becomes twice as common in men after age 65.[6]

Studies of selected religious groups have yielded some interesting epidemiologic data. The Seventh-Day Adventists and Mormons have a cancer mortality below that of the general population.[5,7] The reason for the lower rates is speculated to be related to diet. Both these religious groups basically follow a vegetarian diet, abstaining to varying degrees from meat and meat products.

Similiarly, studies of migrant groups reveal environmental factors and again point to difference in dietary habits. Studies have demonstrated that as people move to new countries, they inherit the death rate of the new country rather than that of their original country.

ETIOLOGY

Diet

Peculiarities in the distribution of colorectal cancer support a multifactorial etiology.[6] Diet has long been suspected as a factor in the cause of colorectal cancer for two major reasons. First, food substances are obviously considered when one evaluates materials that would come in contact with the bowel surface. Second, wide variances in incidence rates between populations, rather than within them, suggest that the equally variable dietary habits of these groups play a role in etiology. One of the inherent difficulties with this type of investigation is the problem of obtaining accurate dietary histories in both study and control groups.

Although diet generally is accepted as a major etiologic agent, the action by which various substances are involved in the carcinogenic process is unclear. It is now thought that dietary factors affect the exposure of the gastrointestinal (GI) tract to promotors of carcinogenesis.[8] Some dietary agents are thought to increase exposure to promotor agents (fats), while other dietary factors (fiber, calcium) are thought to reduce exposure.

Fat

The substance currently receiving much attention as an etiologic factor in colorectal cancer is dietary fat. Fat itself is not thought to be the carcinogen but, rather, a promotor.[9,10]

The mechanism by which fat influences the development of colorectal cancer is uncertain. One theory is that a high-fat diet increases the level of fecal bile acids. Bile acids have also been implicated as another likely promotor.[11-13] Fat intake increases exposure of the GI tract to potentially mutagenic bile acids.[8] Therefore, diets high in fat, particularly unsaturated fat, may be a significant causative factor in colon cancer.[3,12]

Fiber

Citizens of underdeveloped countries with a lower incidence of colorectal cancer generally eat diets rich in fiber. Conversely, as civilizations become more westernized, fiber intake decreases and is replaced by a diet composed mostly of refined foods.

It is thought that low-fiber, high-fat foods work synergistically to increase the risk of colorectal cancer.[3,7,12] However, a diet high in fiber may actually protect against colorectal cancer even in the presence of a high-fat diet. This may be partially accomplished by limiting the time the colon is exposed to cancer promotors by decreasing intestinal transit time. It has also been suggested that fiber decreases fecal bile acid concentration.[8]

Although the American Cancer Society recommends a low-fat, high-fiber diet, the exact role of diet in colorectal cancer is a continued focus of ongoing clinical trials. Perhaps changes in dietary habits will serve to lower the cancer incidence in the United States in the future, but cultural adaptation is a slow process.[2] Other primary and secondary prevention techniques must be explored.

Calcium

Another interesting association has been suggested between calcium and colon cancer. In a number of studies, dairy product consumption has been demonstrated to decrease colon cancer risk.[14] The mechanism of this reduction has not been clearly identified but has been suggested to be related to dietary calcium's conversion of ionized fatty acids and bile acids to insoluble calcium compounds that reduce colonic epithelial proliferation.[15]

Predisposing Conditions

Knowledge of preexisting conditions that predispose an individual to develop cancer is important in identifying high-risk populations.

An increasing body of research supports the finding that most, if not all, colorectal cancers originate from a benign adenomatous polyp. As the polyp grows, so does its potential for malignant transformation.[12,16] Likewise, when multiple adenomas have been detected, the risk of cancer is greater.[17] Therefore, efforts must be made to redirect the focus from the cancer to the adenomatous polyp.[2]

Other predisposing conditions, some of them genetically linked, have also been associated with an increased risk of cancer of the colon and rectum. For example, there is general agreement that chronic ulcerative colitis is a true premalignant disease. However, all individuals with this condition are not believed to be at equal risk of developing colorectal cancer. Factors that have been identified in predicting the risk of subsequent cancer development include a total involvement of the colon and long duration of the colitis, with a significant increase after 7 to 10 years.[18]

Cancer associated with ulcerative colitis carries an unfavorable prognosis. It develops in relatively young individuals, and the tumors are usually infiltrative, multicentric, and highly anaplastic.[19,20] Diagnosis is often difficult because onset of symptoms suggesting cancer may be viewed as an exacerbation of the ulcerative colitis. For these reasons, a total proctocolectomy is eventually recommended to prevent the inevitable development of cancer. However, it is difficult for physicians to discuss and for the individual to consider a major, body-altering operation, especially when the ulcerative colitis has run a relatively mild course. One of the reasons physicians and patients often delayed surgical intervention in the past was that a total proctocolectomy necessitated a permanent ileostomy. This served as a significant deterrent to many, and many young people with ulcerative colitis developed and died of colon cancer.

Although conventional ileostomy remains the standard, other surgical options are available to people who might delay or avoid a curative resection that necessitates use of an ostomy appliance. Surgical options available to the person with chronic ulcerative colitis also include a continent ileostomy and an ileoanal reservoir.[21] These procedures eliminate the ulcerative colitis and thus the risk of colon cancer and do not require an ostomy pouch. A person with ulcerative colitis should make an informed decision based on surgical options plus risks and benefits.

Crohn's disease, which often only provides subtle diagnostic differences from chronic ulcerative colitis, also has been associated with an increased risk of colorectal cancer. Although this association is not as high as with ulcerative colitis, it is substantially higher than an age-matched control population.[20,22]

A number of GI-polyposis syndromes have been identified as precancerous. Familial polyposis is an inherited, autosomal dominant trait that affects both sexes equally. The disease is characterized by the presence of a hundred to several thousand adenomatous polyps in the large intestine. Without treatment, virtually 100% of afflicted individuals will develop cancer. Cancer usually occurs 10 to 15 years after the polyps appear and rarely occurs in individuals under 20 years of age. These people have the same curative options available as the person with ulcerative colitis.

Other groups have been reported to have a higher predisposition to colorectal cancer than the general population. These include individuals with a strong family history of colon cancer, familial colonic polyposis syndromes, and female genital and breast cancer.[20,23,24] Although this finding supports genetic factors, inheritance alone accounts for only a small percentage of colorectal cancers.

Other associations have been documented with individuals who have undergone ureterosigmoidostomy for urinary diversion and individuals with chronic, symptomatic, radiation-induced proctocolitis. Cholecystectomy has also recently been implicated as a possible precipitating factor, although this remains debatable.[25,26] Although information on these groups is somewhat limited, they deserve attention as high-risk groups for targeting detection and long-term follow-up.

PATHOPHYSIOLOGY

Cellular Characteristics

Cellular characteristics of large intestinal cancers vary according to tumor type. Adenocarcinoma is the most common of the colonic neoplasms, accounting for approximately 95% of the malignancies.

Histologically, colorectal tumors may be well differentiated, moderately differentiated, or poorly differentiated. Macroscopically, the tumor may display a number of forms, including scirrhous or infiltrating carcinomas, polypoid carcinomas, and ulcerating carcinomas.[7]

Evidence suggests that the development of colorectal cancer is a multistage process.[2,9] These tumors are relatively slow growing. Growth is rapid in the beginning but slows dramatically by the time the tumor is approximately 1 cm in diameter or 1 g in weight.[2] Symptoms typically occur early in the development of the tumor; metastasis occurs late.[7]

Carcinomas of the anus are relatively rare. They appear benign but are highly malignant. Anal cancer can occur at any age but is most likely in the fifth to seventh decades. Most studies show a higher frequency in women, although there has been a slight shift in the demographics. A new high-risk group has emerged to include males with admitted homosexuality, bisexuality, or a history of anal condylomata acuminata.[27] It is incumbent on the physician to regard with suspicion any anal lesion, especially if seen in a high-risk male patient.

Squamous cell carcinoma is rare and can be multifocal in the anal canal as well as the perianal skin, perineum, and vulvar areas.[28] On the perianal skin it presents as a slight thickening or a small, nodular elevation and may have a central ulceration. In the anal canal, patients may have symptoms of rectal bleeding, pruritis, mucus discharge, and tenesmus. These neoplasms originate in the stratified squamous epithelium and are usually well differentiated and slow growing; they may resemble fistulae, fissures, hemorrhoids, or other benign lesions.

Basal cell carcinomas, as the name implies, originate in the basal cell layer of the skin. They are very rare and occur at the anal verge or in the perianal region. The typical appearance is a chronic indurated growth with rolled edges and a central ulceration.[28] Patients usually report the sensation of a lump, bleeding, pain, pruritis, and discharge. Although they grow slowly and do not usually metastasize, they are highly malignant.

Malignant melanomas are ectodermal in origin and appear in the perianal region or anal canal. These lesions may be pigmented, are usually polypoid, and are firm. Patients may experience rectal bleeding, a change in bowel habits, and discomfort. The tumor may resemble thrombosed hemorrhoids, which may postpone diagnosis and appropriate treatment.

Other malignant neoplasms of the anal canal and perianal region include Bowen's disease, extramammary Paget's disease, and Kaposi's sarcoma.

Progression of Disease

The progression of colorectal cancer depends on a number of factors. Attempts have been made throughout the years to predict the prognosis more accurately. The classification of a tumor according to its degree of local and distant involvement is the best means of calculating survival rates.[29]

The earlier the malignancy is diagnosed, the better are the individual's chances for long-term survival and cure. Five-year survival rates based on Duke's classification show 67% to 81% for Duke's A, 51% to 64% for Duke's B, and 32% to 44% for Duke's C.[7] The 5-year survival nationally is about 50%.[1] Similarly, degree of differentiation of the neoplasm also affects the overall prognosis. These classification systems are discussed in detail in the section on classification and staging later in this chapter.

The duration of symptoms is not an effective means of predicting the degree of tumor advancement. However, the diagnosis of colorectal cancer in asymptomatic individuals has been shown to be related to improved survival.[12]

Individuals with obstructing or perforating carcinomas as well as those that develop in young people also carry a poor prognosis. Likewise, survival is about 10% poorer with tumors below the peritoneal reflection.[12]

Lymph node involvement in colorectal cancer is common, occurring in at least 50% of the patients reported in most series. Survival rates are closely linked to the degree of nodal involvement with an indirect relationship between prognosis and the number of positive nodes. Poorly differentiated lesions are associated with an increase in nodal involvement.

Venous invasion is a poor prognostic sign. The embolization of tumor cells through the vascular system leads to widespread dissemination of the disease. This type of metastasis does not lend itself to effective surgical resection, and the value of other adjuvant therapies such as chemotherapy or radiotherapy is still limited. The presence of intravascular involvement generally means visceral metastasis, usually to the liver. Hepatic metastasis is an ominous sign, usually indicating a greatly decreased survival time. Greater than 50% of deaths following surgery are secondary to hepatic metastasis.[30]

As a tumor grows, its chance to penetrate bowel wall layers increases. Once it invades the submucosal layer, it gains access to lymphatic and vascular channels, thereby increasing its potential for distant metastasis. These patients are at greater risk for local recurrence as well.[29] Direct extension of colon carcinomas usually involves neighboring structures and occurs in 10% to 20% of cases.[12] This local invasion is more common in the cecum and rectosigmoid areas because of the number of contiguous organs. An increase in the involvement of adjacent organs decreases survival rates and necessitates the need for more radical surgical intervention. The persistence or recurrence of a tumor locally is a major cause of therapeutic failure and mortality.

The liver is the most frequently reported site of metastatic involvement. The lungs may often be involved, but pulmonary involvement usually implies hepatic involvement as well because venous blood flow to the lungs is mainly by way of the liver. Other viscera also may be involved in venous spread. Other metastatic sites that are reported less often include the brain, bones, and adrenal glands.

Cancers of the perianal skin usually spread by direct invasion. Inguinal node involvement by anal cancers ranges from 20% to 25%. Anal canal carcinomas may involve the anal muscles and metastasize to the prostate, urethra, bladder, vagina, ischial tuberosity, and sacrum.[31]

CLINICAL MANIFESTATIONS

Tumors of the right colon typically are large, bulky growths that tend to ulcerate. Symptoms of tumors in this region usually include anemia, a palpable mass in the right lower quadrant, and pain. The pain is vague and dull and tends to persist for a long time. Because the pain is so nonspecific, right upper quadrant pain frequently is mistaken for gallbladder disease, whereas right lower quadrant pain may be misdiagnosed as appendicitis.

Obstruction is rare in the right colon for a number of reasons. First, tumors of this area typically grow in rather than around the bowel. Second, although the tumors are usually large and bulky, the lumen of the ascending colon is much larger in diameter than other areas of the colon. Therefore, the bowel can accommodate a larger mass without drastically compromising function. Third, the stool in this area is liquid, so even with a space-occupying neoplasm, the stool can pass through. Thus, obstructive symptoms usually do not occur despite the tumor's large size.

Cancer of the transverse colon commonly is manifested by a change in bowel habits and blood in the stool. Obstruction is more possible here than in the ascending colon because of a decrease in the bowel lumen, increase in the consistency of the stool, and narrowing of the lumen at the hepatic and splenic flexures.

Manifestation of malignancies in the descending and sigmoid colon again depends on the type of growth typical to this area. Tumors of this portion of the bowel are commonly the scirrhous, annular type. As a result, a change in bowel habits is a frequent symptom. Individuals usually describe increasing constipation or narrow, pencil-like stools. A history of increasing use of laxatives to counteract these persistent symptoms may be present. Blood will frequently be in or on the stool. As might be expected, symptoms of varying degrees of obstruction are common with neoplasms in this part of the colon. The obstructive phenomenon is a result of the type of tumors characteristic of this area, a decrease in the size of the bowel lumen, increase in the stool consistency, and decrease in peristaltic action.

Cancer of the rectum usually is manifested as bright red bleeding through the rectum. Unfortunately, this is often confused with bleeding from hemorrhoids, and therefore definitive diagnosis and treatment may be delayed unnecessarily. Sensations of incomplete evacuation and tenesmus also are prevalent signs. Some tumors characteristically produce a great amount of mucus, which leads to the complaint of mucus diarrhea. Pain is a late sign because this area is relatively insensitive, and the lesion is therefore quite large before it produces pain.

ASSESSMENT

The colon is a rather unusual internal organ in terms of assessment. It lends itself to direct visualization through the use of various scopes. It can be palpated directly to the length of the examiner's finger. Its entire length can be studied by radiologic techniques. Unfortunately, even with these diagnostic aids, less than half of all colorectal cancers are in a localized stage without lymph node involvement at diagnosis.

Physical Examination

A physical assessment is preceded by a careful history. The examiner proceeds with direct questioning regarding the presence of specific symptoms (eg, blood in the stool, change in bowel habits) as well as general complaints (eg, fatigue, weight loss). Careful note is made of any previous cancers, precancerous lesions (polyps), or a positive family history that would place the person in a high-risk group.

The abdomen is observed for distention or visible masses. In the event of portal obstruction, abdominal veins may be enlarged and visible. Inguinal and supraclavicular lymph nodes may show evidence of enlargement.

Auscultation follows inspection with an evaluation of peristaltic sound in all quadrants. Palpation and percussion of the abdomen will help to supplement the findings thus far obtained. In addition to any objective data collected, palpation also will reveal subjective information relating to pain. The presence of enlarged lymph nodes or organs can be assessed with more exactness at this time. Because the liver is the most frequent organ for metastasis, palpation and percussion of the liver may provide information regarding the extent of the disease.

Masses are palpated and described in terms of size, shape, location, tenderness, and mobility. Palpation of masses will be most successful in the right and transverse colon. Right-sided tumors typically are bulky, and a palpable mass frequently may be the first symptom. Because the transverse portion is the most anterior and movable part of the colon, tumors here are more accessible to detection by palpation.

The digital rectal examination is an essential part of every GI assessment. During the rectal examination, the anus and perianal region are inspected closely; highly malignant cacinomas may be present and mistaken for relatively benign lesions. The efficacy of this examination has been debated, since only 10% of the colorectal cancers are within the reach of the examiner's finger.[7] The examination is simple, cost effective, carries no risk, and has the potential benefit of detecting an early rectal or anal canal lesion. The American Cancer Society recommends a digital rectal examination every year after year 40.

Diagnostic Studies

Proctosigmoidoscopy, fiberoptic colonoscopy, radiographs, and fecal occult blood screening serve as valuable and necessary adjuncts in the diagnosis of colorectal cancer. Over the past 20 years, there has been a gradual shift in the site distribution of colorectal cancers. Studies have documented a decrease in rectal cancers with a progressive increase in more proximal tumors.[32] This phenomenon has led to an increase in the use of the flexible sigmoidoscope rather than the rigid sigmoidoscope to diagnose colorectal cancer.

The flexible fiberoptic sigmoidoscope detects more adenomatous polyps, provides a more proximal view of the colon (up to 60 cm), and generally is better tolerated than its rigid counterpart. With this instrument, approximately 60% of polyps and colorectal cancers are detectable.[16] The American Cancer Society recommends a proctosigmoidoscopy every 3 to 5 years after age 50 following two negative annual examinations.

Approximately one third of colorectal cancers are located in the right colon.[16] An experienced physician can visualize the entire length of the colon with the colonoscope. In addition to its diagnostic value, the colonoscope, like the sigmoidoscope, can be used therapeutically to remove suspicious polyps. Colonoscopy is not presently carried out on a routine basis and is not indicated for every person with a possible neoplasm.

The testing of stools for occult blood is a frequent screening procedure for colorectal cancer, but there are many false-positive and false-negative test results. The test appears to be more sensitive for cancers than for adenomas, but it can detect more adenomas if they are bleeding and larger than 2 cm.[33] Even though it has not been proved that when applied to a mass population it will actually alter the death rate, evidence suggests that stool testing for occult blood allows for earlier detection of colorectal cancers.[2,34,35]

The American Cancer Society recommends the fecal occult blood test every year after age 50. Many practitioners believe it is complementary to the proctosigmoidoscope examination.[2,20,33] An exhaustive review of fecal occult blood screening has been done by Simon.[36]

Determination of the individual's hemoglobin and hematocrit levels may be helpful in diagnosis. Anemia is a characteristic symptom in patients with tumors of the right side of the colon. Any individual who presents with unexplained anemia without other symptoms is evaluated further with one or more of the examinations discussed previously.

The possible role of carcinoembryonic antigen (CEA) in the evaluation of persons with colorectal cancer has been widely investigated.[37] Although it may be elevated in colorectal cancer, it is nonspecific and its use in mass screening and detection is limited. The value of CEA in the pretreatment phase is mainly as a prognostic tool. It is also used in evaluating the efficacy of various treatment regimens.

Computed tomography (CT) also has proved valuable in the detection or staging of pelvic abnormalities in individuals who have undergone resection for rectal or rectosigmoid cancers. Periodic postoperative CT evaluations may prolong survival by detecting early asymptomatic lesions.[30,38]

For anal cancer, physical examination and biopsy are the main diagnostic tools. In addition, these patients are tested for human immunodeficiency virus (HIV) antibodies because of the association of anal disease and acquired immune deficiency syndrome (AIDS).[39]

CLASSIFICATION AND STAGING

The first system for classifying rectal neoplasms was published by Dukes in 1932.[40] Since that time, the staging system for tumors of the colon and rectum has undergone many revisions, which has caused confusion when comparing data from various reports. A review of the various classification systems for colorectal cancer has been done by Zinkin.[41] There is no uniform or widely accepted staging system for anal carcinoma.[42]

TREATMENT

Surgery

The tumor's mode of spread dictates the type of surgical resection required. The surgeon will thus attempt to eliminate both the tumor and the established routes of metastasis. For example, cancer of the cecum or ascending colon usually requires a right hemicolectomy that includes the right colon as well as the related lymphatic and circulatory channels.

When a malignant lesion results in an obstruction, the surgeon may elect to do one of several procedures. The surgeon may resect the obstructing lesion and perform a primary anastomosis. A one-stage procedure is considered the standard and is possible in most instances.

A two-stage procedure involving a temporary colostomy or ileostomy may be necessary in some cases (eg, obstruction, perforation). This procedure carries with it the risks associated with two major operations.

In some instances, a three-stage procedure may be performed, which entails (1) a diverting colostomy, (2) a resection of the tumor, and (3) a takedown of the colostomy. Three operations are infrequently warranted, but the surgeon's experience and the patient's condition may influence the decision.

Carcinomas of the rectum present additional considerations for surgery. In the past, complete removal of the rectum was thought to be the best form of treatment. However, surgeons today are more selective in their approach, electing to do less radical procedures whenever possible.

Rectal cancer

The greatest distinction between procedures performed in this area of the large intestine is whether sphincter control can be maintained. However, preservation of anal continence is not an advantage if the person's survival is compromised as the result of a limited dissection. If the tumor is poorly differentiated, a sphincter-saving operation is not considered unless it is intended to be a palliative procedure.

For the surgeon trying to achieve a curative resection, a 2- to 5-cm distal margin (from the tumor to the anal verge) is important. This criterion is significant in the area of the rectum because the entire rectum is only 15 cm. This margin is probably the most critical variable in determining the type of surgical resection possible. Other factors that influence the surgeon's decision include the tumor's degree of differentiation, metastatic disease, and the patient's age, sex, and physical condition.[28] The final decision on the type of procedure may be reserved until surgery.

Lesions within the upper third of the rectum are best treated by a low anterior resection (LAR). The treatment of choice for lesions in the lower third of the rectum is an abdominoperineal resection. The greatest debate exists with those tumors that lie in the middle third—7 to 11 cm from the anal verge.

Low anterior resections As mentioned, LARs usually are carried out for lesions more than 10 cm from the anal verge. Because adequate exposure of the pelvis is critical, this procedure generally is easier in the female. However, with the advent of bowel-stapling instruments, the limits of the LAR have been extended. The stapling device provides a lower, safer bowel anastomosis than would be possible by the hand-sewn method.[43] The 2- to 5-cm distal margin must still be kept in mind with curative resections. Complications associated with LARs include hemorrhage, anastomotic leaks, stricture, abscess, irregular bowel function, and wound infection.

One of the greatest reservations with the LAR is the high incidence of tumor recurrence, particularly at the site of the suture line. Reported rates vary, but the survival rate for patients who have undergone the LAR or abdominoperineal resection is near 50%.[12] Recurrence usually develops within 2 years after the resection.[7] Once recurrence occurs, the prognosis is poor, since surgery is the most effective treatment.[2]

Abdominoperineal resection As its name implies, the abdominoperineal resection (APR) requires a combined surgical approach through the abdomen and perineum. It is a much more physically disruptive operative procedure that is associated with a relatively high morbidity rate[7] and requires major psychosocial adjustments. The wide excision results in a very high rate of impotency in males, and the removal of the rectum necessitates the creation of a permanent colostomy.

Complications reported following APR include ureteral injury, urinary dysfunction, urinary tract infections, sexual dysfunction, perineal and abdominal wound infections, and stomal complications.

Perineal wounds The perineal wound results after removal of the rectum, anus, muscle, and fatty tissue. Failure of this wound to heal properly can affect significantly the individual's postoperative adjustment and well-being as well as increase the length of hospitalization.

The time necessary for complete healing of the perineal wound varies greatly with each individual. Healing is often a slow process because of the large defect created, infections that occur frequently, and the fact that the blood supply to this area is not especially good.

There are several methods for closure of the perineal wound. The type of closure will determine the necessary postoperative care and teaching.

Leaving the wound open and packing it allows for healing by secondary intention. The packs usually are completely out within 2 to 3 days after surgery. Leaving the packing in for an extended period can lead to sepsis, a rigid wall, and delayed closure of the perineum.[44] After removal of the packing, meticulous hygiene is important in promoting granulation and healing. Irrigations or sitz baths are recommended until complete healing has occurred. In addition to its therapeutic effect, the sitz bath feels good. Patient education and close follow-up are necessary to avoid complications.

Another method of management is partial closure of the wound with an incisional drain. The suture line is examined for integrity and signs of infection. Dressings are used to contain the drainage.

Primary closure currently is advocated as the best method for closure of perineal wounds and is possible in most instances. Primary closure usually is more comfortable for the patient and easier to care for than an open wound. Primary closure is contraindicated when there is unsatisfactory hemostasis or fecal spillage.[43] Closed suction drains are placed in the perineal space and brought out anteriorly through a separate stab wound. Observation of the wound is important. Assessment is made of the wound and drain sites for evidence of infection and progression of healing. The amount and characteristics of the drainage from the drain sites are recorded. Drains are removed on the third to fifth postoperative day.

Sexual dysfunction Estimates of the percentage of sexual dysfunction in males following APR for cancer approaches 100%. The wide excision needed in an APR involves the dissection of areas responsible for sexual function in males. The sympathetic nerve fibers are particularly vulnerable when the rectosigmoid is dissected from the sacrum. Similarly, the nerves responsible for erection are intimately involved in the area between the rectum and the prostrate, which is dissected during a curative resection. Sexual dysfunction can range from partial to complete impotence.[45]

By contrast, female sexual response is controlled by the higher centers and peripheral sensory nerve stimuli that transverse the pudendal nerve fibers. These pudendal nerves run laterally in the pelvis and are not subject to dissection even if the whole rectum is removed.[45] Sexual dysfunction in females may occur secondary to scarring and contracture following surgery.

Sexual functioning is a multifaceted response involving more than the physical act of intercourse. Human sexuality encompasses an individual's self-identity and body image, feelings toward the other individual, and perceptions of the other person's acceptance. Therefore, sexual dysfunction may be the result of a negative emotional response to the surgery, the stoma, or the diagnosis of cancer and its concomitant treatment. The physician is responsible for discussing the possibility of sexual dysfunction with the patient preoperatively, regardless of the person's age. After surgery the individual receives guidance and counseling as needed.

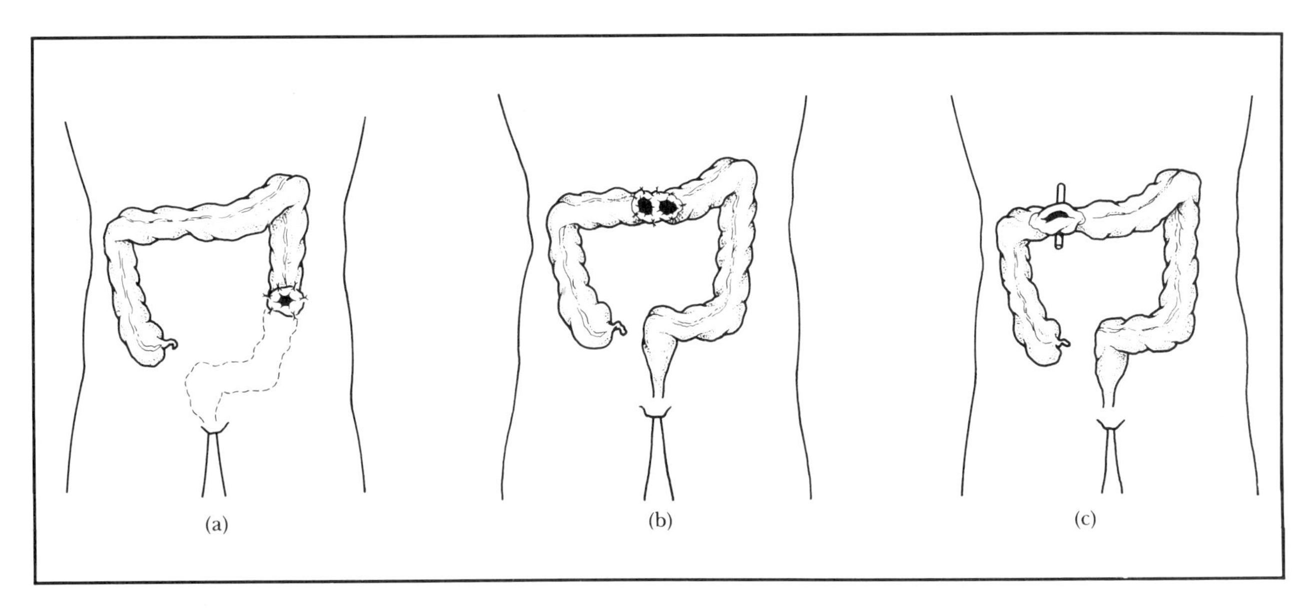

FIGURE 38-1 Colostomies identified according to structure. (a) End or single-barrel colostomy. Abdominoperineal resection has been performed. Sigmoid colon and rectum have been removed. (b) Double-barrel colostomy in transverse colon. (c) Loop colostomy in transverse colon.

Colon cancer

Colostomy There are three different types of colostomies according to surgical construction (Figure 38-1). An end or single-barrel colostomy is formed when the proximal portion of the colon is brought out and sutured to the abdominal wall. The distal segment of the bowel may be closed and placed back into the abdomen (Hartmann's pouch) or removed as in an APR. The removal of the rectum constitutes an irreversible procedure.

A double-barrel colostomy denotes the presence of two distinct stomas, which occurs when the defunctionalized section of the colon is not removed. The proximal portion of the bowel is sutured to the abdominal wall as an end stoma. The distal segment also is sutured to the abdominal wall as a stoma and is frequently called the mucus fistula. The two stomas will be in close proximity. Distinction between the functioning and nonfunctioning stoma is important in terms of pouching. If they are next to one another (see Figure 38-1), they may be incorporated into the same pouch. If they are located apart, a small dressing may be placed over the mucus fistula to absorb the bowel's normal secretion of mucus.

A loop colostomy is constructed by exteriorizing a loop of the colon and securing it over some device to prevent it from recessing back into the abdominal cavity. The device is left in place approximately 7 to 10 days until the bowel adheres to the abdominal wall.

A surgical technique that eliminates the need for any external supporting device is the fascial bridge. In this case, the surgeon brings out the loop of bowel and sutures the fascial layer of the abdomen under the loop to support it. This technique is preferred because special appliances are not required to accommodate the supporting device. A loop colostomy is seen most often in the transverse portion of the bowel. Frequently it is a temporary procedure to allow an anastomosis site or a diseased distal colon to heal, but it may serve as a palliative, diverting procedure to relieve an obstruction in an individual with terminal cancer.

Stoma marking Selection of an appliance that fits comfortably and securely depends on the construction of the stoma (eg, height, location of lumen), its location on the abdomen, and the characteristics of the surrounding skin surface (eg, integrity, wrinkles, bulges). Therefore, preoperative selection and marking of a stoma site is critical to postoperative management.

Proper selection of a stoma site involves the evaluation of many factors. It is important to have a smooth and adequate surface area around the stoma so that the appliance can adhere securely to the abdomen. This necessitates that it be placed away from skin folds, the suture line, bony prominences, scars, the umbilicus, and, preferably, the belt line. It is also crucial that the stoma be in a location that the individual can see without difficulty. To determine the ideal location of the stoma, the person's abdomen is observed in the sitting, standing, bending, and lying positions. The stoma site is located within the borders of the rectus muscle. Bringing the bowel through this muscle sheath prevents later complications of peristomal hernia and prolapse. The placement will also depend on the type of stoma to be created. For example, a sigmoid colostomy would usually be sited and marked in the left lower quadrant.

The individual who will actually select and mark the stoma site will vary in different institutions. Enterostomal therapy (ET) nurses are taught the principles of stoma site selection in their specialized education programs. If an ET nurse is not available, the physician or a nurse educated in this procedure may be responsible for this function. The marking of the stoma site is communicated to and approved by the surgeon so that the surgeon understands the intent of the preselected site.

Colostomy care An important postoperative nursing function is the assessment of stoma viability to identify early signs of compromised circulation to the stoma. In looking at an everted stoma, what is seen is the mucosal layer of the bowel wall. This innermost lining contains the vascular network that gives the stoma its normal, red appearance. This tissue is somewhat fragile and will bleed slightly when rubbed. A stoma that is dusky, gray, or black indicates an inadequate blood supply and is documented and brought to the surgeon's attention. A stoma that necroses will slough and generally leads to stomal stenosis.

When patients first view their stoma, they may be dismayed at its appearance. Stomas usually protrude and may be quite large postoperatively because of the trauma of surgery or the distention of the bowel due to an obstructive process. This initial edema will subside gradually over the next 6 to 8 weeks and even change remarkably before the patient is discharged from the hospital.

The time when the stoma will begin to function is somewhat variable. The degree to which the bowel was cleansed preoperatively will be a factor. As peristalsis returns and flatus is passed through the stoma, food will be introduced gradually and the nurse will see the initiation of or an increase in the amount of stool passed. Usually, the more proximal the stoma is in the bowel, the sooner it will begin to function.

Assessment of the skin surrounding the stoma is another important observation for which nurses are responsible. The peristomal skin should essentially look like any other skin on the abdomen. When an ostomy appliance is used, some erythema will be noted when the adhesive is removed, but this will disappear within a matter of minutes. Any other evidence of persistent redness or broken skin is abnormal and must be treated. A variety of skin care products are available to prevent skin breakdown and facilitate healing.

Considerations when selecting an appliance The selection of a stoma appliance is based on an evaluation of each individual. Stomal discharge, consistency and frequency of output, stoma profile, the condition of the peristomal skin, and the individual's abilities and activity level are some of the factors that influence the selection of an ostomy product.

Various products by different manufacturers offer numerous features that may be important to the person with a stoma. For example, some pouches have gas filters while others do not. Other variable features include odor-barrier pouch film, the pouch fabric or backing, color, closure clamps, skin barriers, convexity, belt tabs, adhesives, and the pouch size and shape. Some of these options may be desirable extras for one person and absolute necessities for another.

The cost of equipment varies. The individual with a stoma should not be burdened with unnecessary extras that are simply more costly. If money is not a concern, the nurse can mention various equipment options and allow

1. Assemble the necessary equipment: pouch, skin barrier, pattern or measuring guide, water, tissue or gauze, 1" paper tape, closure clip.
2. Prepare the pouch:
   - Trace the pattern onto the skin barrier. The skin barrier should be sized to fit around the base of the stoma(s).
   - Cut the skin barrier to the size of the pattern.
   - Cut the pouch ⅛" larger than the skin barrier.
   - Remove the protective backing from the pouch.
   - Apply the nonadhesive side of the skin barrier to the pouch, matching center openings.
   - Remove the protective backing from the skin barrier. Set aside.
3. Remove the used pouch and apply the new one:
   - Remove the used pouch, using one hand to gently push the skin away from the adhesive.
   - Discard the pouch, saving the closure clip.
   - Control any discharge with tissue or gauze.
   - Clean the skin with water. If soap is used, use a nonoily soap and rinse. Dry thoroughly.
   - Apply the clean pouch, centering the stoma in the opening.
   - Tape the edges of the pouch in a "picture frame" pattern with the paper tape.
   - Close the bottom of the pouch with the closure clip.
   - Empty the pouch when it is one-third full of flatus or stool.

FIGURE 38-2 Procedure for changing an ostomy pouch.

the patient to be involved in deciding what products to use.

Financial assistance is available from different agencies to help defer the cost of supplies. If a person qualifies, Medicaid will pay for the equipment. Medicare will reimburse the individual up to 80% for some supplies. However, many of the Medicare codes are outdated, and reimbursement may not be sufficient to offset the total cost of the supplies needed. Some private insurance carriers will cover all or part of the expenses. The nurse informs the person of the various sources of assistance or makes a referral to an ET nurse or social service agency. The person should not lack necessary equipment because of financial need.

For a discussion of the procedures for applying a pouch and irrigating a colostomy, see Figures 38-2 and 38-3.

Predischarge teaching A written checklist of tasks to be completed by and for the person with a stoma before discharge is useful. It helps to ensure that each person receives the same basic information and that nothing learned during this phase of hospitalization is forgotten. This information can be shared with the patient so that he or she knows what will be provided before discharge.

The individual with a new stoma should have at least two supervised opportunities to perform all the necessary steps of stoma care before discharge to increase his or her confidence in every aspect of care. It also provides time for the nurse and the patient to review objectives and evaluate the patient's level of competency. Patient teaching has become a greater challenge with shorter hospital stays as a result of the diagnosis-related groups (DRGs). Out-

1. Assemble the necessary equipment: colostomy irrigation set, cotton balls and water, IV pole or wall hook, clean pouch.
2. Prepare the equipment:
   - Close the water-control gauge on the irrigation bag.
   - Fill the water bag with 1000 cc of tepid tap water.
   - Hang the bag on a hook in the bathroom or on the IV pole, high enough to achieve adequate water pressure.
   - Open the water-control gauge and allow water to run through in order to remove air from the tubing, then close gauge.
   - Prepare the pouch to be worn after the irrigation procedure is completed. Set aside.
3. Procedure:
   - Remove the used pouch.
   - Put on the irrigation sleeve, centering the stoma in the middle of the ring. Fasten so that the belt is snug, creating a watertight seal against the abdomen.
   - Sit on the toilet or in a chair in front of the toilet, whichever is most comfortable.
   - Lubricate the cone tip.
   - Insert the tip gently into the stoma. Hold the cone firmly in order to prevent the water from escaping from the stoma.
   - Open the water-control gauge. It should take approximately 5 minutes to instill 1000 cc. If cramping occurs, slow down or stop the water flow temporarily.
   - Remain in the bathroom with the sleeve in the toilet for about 15 minutes.
   - After 15 minutes, you may choose to leave the bathroom. Rinse the sleeve with water, and bring the top and bottom of the sleeve together. Roll the sleeve two or three times and clamp.
   - During the next 45 minutes, some water and fecal matter will collect in the sleeve.
   - Remove the sleeve. Wash the skin around the stoma. Dry. Apply a clean pouch.
   - Rinse the irrigation sleeve and hang it to air dry. A mild soap can be used to clean the sleeve.
   - The entire procedure should take about 1 hour. Good control is established only if the procedure is repeated at about the same time each day.
   - The colostomy irrigation set is reusable. However, eventually the various parts wear out; at that time, they can be replaced individually.

FIGURE 38-3 Procedure for colostomy irrigation.

patient follow-up in the home or outpatient clinic is essential for successful rehabilitation.

The individual is provided with written information about everything he or she was taught, including the procedure for changing the pouch written out in a logical sequence. General instructions for the procedures commonly used can be printed and then individualized for each person.

Enough equipment is given to the patient to last at least 2 weeks after discharge. This gives the person an opportunity to get established at home without having to be concerned immediately with obtaining the necessary supplies.

A list of local vendors is provided so that when it is time to purchase new equipment, the individual will know where to get it. Most manufacturers also have dealer lists that are available without cost and can be obtained from their sales personnel or by writing to the company. It is helpful to have several of these lists on hand in the hospital. Local drug stores will sometimes order special equipment for their customers. Mail-order catalogs are also very popular and cost effective. Individuals should be encouraged to compare costs and services in selecting a vendor.

A number of referrals can be made to provide assistance to the person with a stoma after discharge from the hospital. Whenever possible, a visiting nurse is helpful in making the transition to the home environment. Any written instructions that have been provided for the person also are attached to the referral form. The United Ostomy Association (UOA) can provide many services for the individual with a stoma and his or her family. This association can put the family in contact with a local ostomy club and an ET nurse in the vicinity. In addition, the UOA publishes a number of audiovisual patient education aids, has a quarterly magazine, and has local support groups.

The American Cancer Society also offers assistance to the person with a stoma and the family through a variety of means including educational literature.

Anal cancer

Surgical treatment of anal cancer is used either alone or combined with other adjunct therapies. The choice depends on the stage of the tumor and depth of penetration.[7] Surgery may involve local excisions for carcinomas that are confined and well differentiated or an APR. As noted earlier, these more radical procedures are associated with a higher morbidity.

The inability of surgery alone to cure more than 55% of patients is due in part to the anatomy of the anal region, which makes it difficult to remove adequately the lateral and distal zones of the lymphatic spread.[31] If the anal margin is involved, a wider excision of perianal skin is required than in adenocarcinoma of the rectum.[28]

Radiotherapy

Despite advances in detection methods and surgical techniques, mortality from colorectal cancer has remained essentially unchanged throughout the past 20 years. The primary reason for failure after surgery alone is due to local or regional recurrence. Thus, researchers have proposed that better cure rates may be achieved by adjuvant therapy. Irradiation has been and is being investigated and tested as one means of improving survival rates for patients with colorectal cancer.

Studies have pointed to the potential value of irradiation before surgery. Evidence indicates that preoperative irradiation decreases the size of the tumor mass, thus transforming some unresectable lesions to resectable ones. The tumor actually may be downstaged, with substantially improved survival expectations.[46] It has also been demonstrated that preoperative irradiation does not adversely affect or limit subsequent surgical excision. Therefore, there has been no notable increase in morbidity and mortality in individuals treated with preoperative irradiation over those treated with surgery alone.

The time between the conclusion of the radiotherapy and the performance of surgery varies from immediately to 2 or 3 weeks. The dosage and amount of time over which the radiation is delivered also vary greatly. Despite these differences in protocol, the outcomes are quite similar.

Some authorities have advocated that the radiation be delivered after surgical excision. Although the value of postoperative irradiation is still being evaluated, it does seem to show some benefit in individuals at high risk of recurrence, but it is of limited value in individuals with Duke's C lesions because of the inability to control distant metastasis.[7] If it is used in these patients, the postoperative adjuvant therapy is initiated not sooner than 1 month following surgery to avoid problems with wound healing.

Some have suggested that a combined approach in which irradiation both precedes and follows surgery may provide a compromise. In theory this sandwich approach should include the advantages of both techniques. The disadvantage is that repopulation of residual malignant cells may occur with slow healing, which would further delay radiotherapy. Higher doses of radiation cannot subsequently be given to offset this phenomenon because of the preoperative irradiation already administered.

Radiation has been used as primary treatment in selected low-lying lesions.[47] However, the main advantage that can be obtained from radiation therapy at this time is an adjuvant to conservative or radical surgical excision.[48]

Local treatment of rectal lesions is advocated in selected cases. This may include endocavity direct-contact irradiation or electrocoagulation. When compared with the more radical surgical procedures, these techniques have a lower incidence of morbidity and mortality. Although they may in some instances be curative, they are better suited as palliative procedures to control symptoms in individuals who are poor surgical risks. These techniques are available in a limited number of medical centers.

Laser therapy is an exciting new tool available to the physician to be used in selected patients with inoperable tumors of the rectum and descending colon. The primary benefit is for symptomatic relief. Symptoms that are well controlled are bleeding, diarrhea, mucus discharge, tenesmus, and obstructive symptoms.[49] Fulguration by laser has a lower morbidity than electrocoagulation, is more widely available, has no mortality, can be done on an outpatient basis, and does not require anesthesia.[50]

The value of radiation therapy in anal cancer depends on tumor type, its location, and its degree of spread. For example, squamous cell carcinoma is a radiosensitive tumor, and radiotherapy thus may be used as a definitive treatment; its use with malignant melanoma, however, is of little value.[28] Complications associated with radiotherapy for anal cancer include proctitis, bleeding, cystitis and hematuria, anal radionecrosis, anal canal ulcers and strictures, and bleeding due to telangiectasia. The incidence of these complications is related to the dose delivered, size of the primary lesion, and type of radiotherapy used.[31]

Chemotherapy

The results of numerous trials with various antineoplastic drugs have been discouraging in the treatment of patients with colorectal cancer. Chemotherapy is used predominantly as an adjunct to surgical treatment. The primary patients to whom chemotherapy offers some hope are those with advanced resectable lesions and those with metastasis.

The one agent that has received the most attention as a potentially useful drug is 5-fluorouracil (5-FU). Since the initiation of its use in 1957, numerous intensive clinical studies have used 5-FU at different stages of the disease, in various dosage schedules, and by different routes of administration.[51,52] Unfortunately, the overall response rate is only 15% to 20%. As a single chemotherapeutic agent, 5-FU demonstrates a maximum 5-year survival benefit of only 5% to 10% greater than control groups, although it may improve patients' quality of life if they respond to the drug.[7,12]

Encouraging results have been obtained in more recent studies using (5-FU) in combination with other agents, specifically folinic acid, levamisole, interferon, methotrexate, MeCCNU, and cisplatin.[53-56] The combination of 5-FU and folinic acid (leukovorin, citrovorum factor) is especially useful in circumventing resistance through pharmacologic modulation. The enhancement of 5-FU antitumor activity by the coadministration of leukovorin has been well established.[57-59] The schedule and dosage of these agents varies. In general, 5-FU (300 to 750 mg/m^2 intravenous bolus) is given midway during a 2-hour infusion of leukovorin (200 to 500 mg/m^2). This treatment is repeated weekly for 6 weeks followed by a 2-week rest period. The 5-FU also may be given by single bolus injection or continuous infusion over 3 or 4 days every 4 weeks. When given by continuous infusion, patients tend to tolerate a higher dose of the 5-FU with minimal toxicity. Severe mucositis, diarrhea with or without nausea, and vomiting leading to dehydration have been reported.[60] Therefore, it is important to assess patients daily for toxicities. A complaint of diarrhea (3 or 4 times a day) on day 2 or 3 of treatment is usually sufficient to warrant cessation of therapy, especially if antidiarrheal agents are ineffective. To improve their ability as historians, patients are instructed to keep a diary of their intake and frequency and amount of diarrhea as well as daily weight.

A recent, as yet unpublished, study sponsored by the National Cancer Institute reports favorable results using 5-FU and levamisole in the treatment of 1300 patients with Duke's C colon cancer.[61] This study demonstrated increased survival rates in those patients treated with levamisole in combination with 5-FU. The drugs are initiated 3 to 5 weeks after surgery and continued for about 1 year. The levamisole is given by mouth three times a day for 3 days every 2 weeks and currently is available through the investigational drug branch of the National Cancer Institute. Other clinical trials evaluating the efficacy of 5-FU plus leukovorin with or without levamisole currently are underway. It is indeed encouraging that adjuvant chemotherapy has been shown not only to alter the natural history of colon and rectal carcinoma but to begin to demonstrate a prolongation of both disease-free survival and survival in patients with colorectal carcinoma.

Chemotherapy is used as an adjunct to radiotherapy and surgery in the management of anal cancers. This multimodality treatment approach has increased local control, improved cure rates, and decreased the number of patients who require more radical surgical procedures.[42] The most commonly used protocols include external radiation and 5-FU/mitomycin-C chemotherapy.[31] Side effects of chemoradiotherapy for anal cancer include leukopenia, thrombocytopenia, anemia, nausea, vomiting, diarrhea (40%), stomatitis, anal strictures or ulcers (13%), and radiation-induced dermatitis.[31]

CONCLUSION

It is well established that colorectal and anal cancers are a significant health concern. Some recent discoveries in the recognition of contributing factors and in treatment protocols have been encouraging; however, much work is yet to be done to improve the impact of this disease significantly.

The focus of future research efforts must be on prevention and education. Primary prevention (elimination of the cause) of colorectal cancer is preferrable to secondary prevention, which focuses on destroying the lesion once it has been detected.[2] Primary prevention would be directed at dietary alterations. This topic has drawn increased consumer awareness, mainly through the media. Many food advertisements are capitalizing not only on the nutritional value of their food products but also on their role (real or perceived) in the prevention of various health problems such as heart disease and colon cancer.[62]

Although this is a first step, it is not clear what quantities and types of dietary modifications are necessary to provide a measure of cancer prevention.[63] Additionally, cultural adaptation is a slow process that will probably take a couple of generations.[2]

Secondary prevention should focus on early detection and more effective therapy. This is best accomplished by monitoring high-risk groups and developing better diagnostic tools. Currently there is no cost-effective, easy, reliable, mass-screening tool available.

More effective adjuvant therapies also are needed to improve survival rates. Surgery has probably reached the limits of its effectiveness in the treatment of patients with colorectal cancer. Alternatives for patients who have advanced disease or who are not candidates for surgery as a primary mode of therapy are needed.

Overlying all the medical and scientific advancements researchers strive to achieve in the next decade is the need to remain cognizant of the moral, ethical, and financial issues. Helping people to live with dignity either with the disease or following radical therapy remains a concurrent goal.

REFERENCES

1. Silverberg E, Lubera JA: Cancer statistics, 1989. CA 39:3-20, 1989.
2. Finne CO III: Cancer of the colon—ruminations on the past and future. J Enterostom Ther 13:196-204, 1986.
3. American Cancer Society. Cancer Facts and Figures. New York, The Society, 1989.
4. Kern WH, White WC: Adenocarcinoma of the colon in a 9-month-old infant. Cancer 11:855-857, 1985.
5. Hedberg SE, Welch CE: The rectum and anus, in Nealon JF Jr (ed): Mangement of the Patient with Cancer. Philadelphia, WB Saunders, 1986, pp 389-417.
6. Boyle P, Zaridze DG, Smans M: Descriptive epidemiology of colorectal cancer. Int J Cancer 36:9-18, 1985.
7. Corman ML: Carcinoma of the colon, in Corman ML (ed): Colon and Rectal Surgery. Philadelphia, JB Lippincott, 1984, pp 268-328.
8. Foltz AT: Nutritional factors in the prevention of gastrointestinal cancer. Semin Oncol Nurs 4:239-245, 1988.
9. Zaridze DG: Environmental etiology of large-bowel cancer. J Nat Cancer Inst 70:d389-400, 1983.
10. Potter JD, McMichael AJ: Diet and cancer of the colon and rectum. A case-control study. J Nat Cancer Inst 76:557-569, 1986.
11. Willett WC, MacMahon B: Diet and cancer—an overview. N Engl J Med 310:697-703, 1984.
12. Sugarbaker PH, Gunderson LL, Wittes RE: Colorectal cancer, in DeVita VT Jr, Hellman S, Rosenberg SA, (eds): Cancer: Principles and Practice in Oncology. Philadelphia, JB Lippincott, 1985, pp 795-884.
13. Nigro ND, Bull AW: Experimental intestinal carcinogenesis. Br J Surg 72:S36-S37, 1985 (suppl).
14. Nelson RL, Tanure JC, Andrianopoulos G: The effect of dietary milk and calcium on experimental colorectal carcinogenesis. Dis Colon Rectum 30:947-949, 1987.
15. Liplein M, Newmark H: Effect of added dietary calcium on colonic epithelial cell proliferation in subjects at high risk for familial colonic cancer. N Engl J Med 313:1381-1384, 1985.
16. Swedberg K, Driggers DA, Deiss F: Screening for colorectal cancer. The role of the primary care physician. Postgrad Med 79:67-74, 1986.
17. Morson BC, Bussey HJR: Magnitude of risk for cancer patients with colorectal adenomas. Br J Surg 72:S23-S25, 1985 (suppl).
18. Ranshoff DF: Colon cancer in ulcerative colitis. Gastroenterology 94:1089-1091, 1988.
19. Slater G, Greenstein AJ, Gelernt I, et al: Distribution of colorectal cancer in patients with and without ulcerative colitis. Am J Surg 149:780-782, 1985.
20. Kahn AH: Colorectal carcinoma: Risk factors, screening and early detection. Geriatrics 39:42-47, 1984.
21. Buls JG, Goldberg SM: Surgical options in ulcerative colitis. Postgrad Med 74:175-178, 1983.
22. Hamilton SR: Colorectal carcinoma in patients with Crohn's disease. Gastroenterology 89:398-407, 1985.
23. Lynch HT, Kimberly WJ, Biscone KA, et al: Familial heterogeneity of colon cancer risk. Cancer 57:2212-2216, 1986.
24. Pietroiusti A, Caprilli R, Guiliano M, et al: Report of a family with hereditary site-specific colon cancer. Cancer 57:2438-2440, 1986.
25. Spitz M, Russell NC, Guinee VF, et al: Questionable relationship between cholecystectomy and colon cancer. J Surg Oncol 30:6-9, 1985.
26. Morrhead RJ, et al: Does cholecystectomy predispose to colorectal cancer? A case control study. Dis Colon Rectum 29:36-38, 1986.
27. Wexner SD, Milsom JW, Dailey TH: The demographics of anal cancers are changing: Identification of high-risk population. Dis Colon Rectum 30:942-946, 1987.
28. Corman ML: Malignant tumors of the anal canal, in Corman ML (ed): Colon and Rectal Surgery. Philadelphia, JB Lippincott, 1984, pp 217-223, 416-428.
29. Chapuis PH, Dent OF, Fisher R, et al: A multivariant analysis of clinical and pathological variables in prognosis after resection of large bowel cancer. Br J Surg 72:698-702, 1985.
30. Freeny PC, Marks WM, Ryan JA, et al: Colorectal carcinoma evaluation with CT: Preoperative staging and detection of postoperative occurrence. Radiology 158:347-353, 1986.
31. Hussain M, Al-Sarraf M: Anal carcinoma: New combined modality treatment approaches. Oncology 2:42-47, 1988.
32. Rosato FE, Marks G: Changing site distribution patterns of colorectal cancer at Thomas Jefferson University Hospital. Dis Colon Rectum 245:93-95, 1981.
33. Winawer SJ, Sherlock P: Surveillance for colorectal carcinoma: A critical review. Gastroenterology 88:820-837, 1982.
34. Gilbertson VA, McHugh R, Schuman L, et al: The earlier detection of colorectal cancers: A preliminary report of the results of the occult blood study. Cancer 45:2899-2901, 1980.
35. Fujita M, Nakano Y, Ohta J, et al: Mass screening for colorectal cancer by testing fecal occult blood. Cancer 57:2241-2245, 1986.
36. Simon JB: Occult blood screening for colorectal cancer. A critical review. Gastroenterology 88:820-837, 1985.
37. National Cancer Institute: Research Report: Cancer of the Colon and Rectum. Bethesda Md, National Institutes of Health, 1987, pp 1-11.
38. Thompson WM, Halvorson WM, Foster WL Jr, et al: Preoperative and postoperative CT staging of rectosigmoid carcinoma. Am J Radiol 146:703-710, 1986.
39. Sischy B: Review of anal carcinomas: New combined modality treatment approaches. Oncology 2:48, 1988.
40. Dukes CE: Classification of cancer of the rectum. J Pathol Bacteriol 35:323-332, 1932.
41. Zinkin LD: A critical review of the classification and staging of colorectal cancer. Dis Colon Rectum 26:37-43, 1983.
42. Cantril ST, Schoeppel P: Carcinoma of the anus: A review. Semin Oncol Nurs 4:293-299, 1988.

43. Goldberg SM, Gordon PH, Nivatvongs S: Malignant neoplasms of the rectum, in Goldberg SM, Gordon PH, Nivatvongs S (eds): Essentials of Anorectal Surgery. Philadelphia, JB Lippincott, 1980, pp 182-214.
44. Carson SM, Hawke GH: Nursing management of perineal wounds, in Broadwell DC, Jackson BS (eds): Principles of Ostomy Care. St. Louis, CV Mosby, 1982, pp 390-398.
45. Atkinson KG: Abdominoperineal resection of the rectum, in Broadwell DC, Jackson BS (eds): Principles of Ostomy Care, St. Louis, CV Mosby, 1982, pp 186-205.
46. Higgins GA: Current status of adjuvant therapy in the treatment of large bowel cancer. Surg Clin North Am 63:137-150, 1983.
47. Papillion J: Intracavity irradiation of early rectal cancer for cure. Cancer Treat Rep 69:1359-1363, 1975.
48. Minsky BD, Cohen AN: Conservative management of invasive rectal cancer: Alternative to abdominoperineal resection. Oncology 3:137-142, 1989.
49. McGowan I, Barr H, Krasner N: Palliative laser therapy for inoperable rectal cancer—does it work? A prospective study on quality of life. Cancer 63:967-969, 1989.
50. Russin DJ, Kaplan SR, Goldberg RI, et al: Neodymium-YAG laser: A new palliative tool in the treatment of colorectal cancer. Arch Surg 121:1399-1403, 1986.
51. Wolmarle N: Adjuvant chemotherapy in colorectal cancer. Can J Surg 28:416-419, 1985.
52. O'Connell MJ: Chemotherapy for colorectal carcinoma. CA 36:360-366, 1986.
53. Richards F II, Case D, White DR, et al: Combination chemotherapy (5-fluorouracil, methyl-CCNU, mitomycin-C) versus 5-fluorouracil alone for advanced previously untreated colorectal carcinoma. A phase III study of the Piedmont Oncology Association. J Clin Oncol 4:656-570, 1986.
54. Loehrer PJ, Einhorn LH, Williams SD, et al: Cisplatin plus 5-FU for the treatment of adenocarcinoma of the colon. Cancer Treat Rep 69:1359-1363, 1985.
55. Canobbio L, Nobile MT, Adrizzoni A, et al: Phase II study of sequential methotrexate and 5-FU combination in the treatment of advanced colorectal cancer. Cancer Treat Rep 70:419-420, 1986.
56. Leone BA, Romero A, Rabinovich MG, et al: Sequential therapy with methotrexate and 5-fluorouracil in the treatment of advanced colorectal carcinoma. J Clin Oncol 4:23-27, 1986.
57. Grem JL, Hoth DF, Hamilton TM, et al: Overview of current status and future direction of clinical trials with 5-fluorouracil in combination with folinic acid. Cancer Treat Rep 71:1249-1264, 1987.
58. Hines JD, Zakem MH, Adelstein DT, et al: Treatment of advanced stage colorectal adenocarcinoma with fluorouracil and high-dose leukovorin calcium: A pilot study. J Clin Oncol 6:142-146, 1988.
59. Berger SH, Hakala MT: Relationship of dUMP and free FdUMP pools to inhibition of thymidylaste synthetase by 5-fluorouracil. Mol Pharmacol 25:190-197, 1983.
60. Grem JL, Shoemaker DD, Petrelli NJ: Severe life-threatening toxicities observed in study using leukovorin with 5-fluorouracil. J Clin Oncol 5:1704, 1987.
61. AP News. 10/02/89.
62. Freundlich N, Cantrell W, Jereski L, et al: Where does the health end and the hype begin? Business Week October 9, 1989, pp 124-128.
63. Frogge MH: Future perspectives and nursing issues in gastrointestinal cancer. Semin Oncol Nurs 4:300-302, 1988.

Chapter 39

Gastrointestinal Cancer: Esophagus, Stomach, Liver, and Pancreas

Margaret Hansen Frogge, RN, MS

INTRODUCTION

Of all the organ systems in the body, the gastrointestinal tract accounts for the highest incidence of malignant tumors, more than 25% of cancer deaths annually in the United States. There are approximately 228,000 new cases of gastrointestinal cancer and 123,000 deaths from cancer of the gastrointestinal tract each year.[1] The colorectal area is the most frequent site of visceral cancer. Cancers of the pancreas and stomach follow next in incidence among gastrointestinal tumors. At one time gastric cancer was the most common type of gastrointestinal malignancy, but colon cancer has moved into the forefront, possibly as a result of the current techniques that aid in early detection and definitive diagnosis. Pancreatic cancer has been steadily increasing in incidence over the past 40 years, with a recent leveling off. Hepatobiliary and esophageal cancers rank next in the incidence of gastrointestinal tumors. Cancer of the small intestine is rare and comprises a small proportion of these tumors (about 1.0%).[1]

The incidence of cancer at different sites along the gastrointestinal tract presents an intriguing pattern when incidence among men is compared with that among women (Table 39-1). Incidence in men decreases from the esophagus to the large intestine, whereas the opposite is true for women. No clear explanations exist for this bidirectional pattern, but researchers are studying the question.

Tumors of the gastrointestinal tract often are insidious in onset and finally will present overt symptoms when the tumor is advanced. Early detection and diagnosis are difficult. Many etiologic risk factors linked to gastrointestinal tumors are nonspecific; therefore it is difficult to identify individuals at high risk. Persons considered to be at high risk are those with chronic diseases involving the gastrointestinal tract such as Crohn's disease, ulcerative colitis, or cirrhosis. Some hereditary conditions also are cited as possible links with gastrointestinal tumors, particularly Gardner's syndrome and familial polyposis. Nutritional factors have been the subject of great debate in recent years. Fiber, cholesterol, caffeine, fats, artificial ingredients, and preservatives are just a few of the food items with a controversial link to cancer, particularly gastrointestinal cancer. Although numerous animal studies demonstrate a correlation between certain nutritional factors and gastrointestinal tumors, insufficient data are available with human subjects to substantiate such claims. Securing data on humans is the epidemiologist's overwhelming challenge because nutrition histories are laborious and extend over lengthy periods of time; controlled nutrition studies are expensive, and compliance is a serious problem. Furthermore, the lag time between dietary intake and tumor development limits valid conclusion of cause and effect. Environmental factors, air and water quality, pollutants, soil composition, and disposal processes also have been questioned as carcinogenic factors.

Most tumors of the gastrointestinal tract are adenocarcinomas, with the exception of tumors of the esophagus and anus, in which squamous cell carcinomas predominate. Gastrointestinal tumors proliferate insidiously and extend locally, presenting signs and symptoms that can be misdiagnosed or self-treated for lengthy periods. As the tumor grows, it can exceed the distensible capacity of the gastrointestinal lumen and result in obstruction. The metastatic spread of gastrointestinal tumors typically occurs by local spread, blood vessel invasion, and dissemination via the lymphatic system. Prognosis depends on the tumor size, degree of cellular differentiation, extent of metastases, treatment efficacy, and the individual's general health status. The prognosis for persons with gastrointestinal tumors varies according to site. Tumors of the colon have a better prognosis than tumors of the esophagus or stomach; however, the prognosis for a person with any gastrointestinal tumor in the advanced stage is not optimistic.

Surgery plays the largest role in the treatment of gastrointestinal tumors. Poor survival and high mortality rates have caused oncologists to consider combinations of therapy to improve end results. Radiotherapy is used as adjuvant treatment, although it is limited by the highly radiosensitive gastrointestinal tract tissue and specific radioresistant adenocarcinomas. Esophageal and rectal tumors commonly are treated by irradiation. Chemotherapy has limited success in the treatment of gastrointestinal cancer, in part because of the large tumor burden of most cancers. The role of immunotherapy in the treatment of gastrointestinal tumors has not been established. New combinations of therapies and development of new technologies and drugs are considered to hold the greatest promise for effective treatment of gastrointestinal cancers.

TABLE 39-1 Gastrointestinal Tumors—Percentage Distribution by Sex

Site	Total Cases	Percentage of Males	Percentage of Females
Esophagus	10,100	71	29
Stomach	20,000	60	40
Pancreas	27,000	49	51
Liver	14,500	52	48
Small intestine	2,700	52	48
Colon-rectum	151,000	48	52

Source: Silverberg E, Lubera JA: Cancer statistics. CA 39:3-20, 1989.

ESOPHAGEAL TUMORS

Cancer of the esophagus occurs most often in persons 50 to 70 years of age. Many persons with esophageal cancer mistakenly attribute the signs and symptoms of esophageal cancer to more common disorders that affect older adults (eg, indigestion, heartburn, and decreased appetite).

If the person has delayed seeking medical attention for the presenting signs and symptoms, the tumor may be advanced and obstructing the esophageal lumen. The person can be dehydrated, malnourished, and debilitated as a result of inadequate nutrition and inappropriate self-treatment. Esophageal tumors that obstruct the lumen can cause a spillover of food, fluid, and saliva into the tracheobronchial tree, resulting in aspiration pneumonitis. The physician and nurse are faced with the challenge of several problems, principally a candidate at poor risk for aggressive therapy. Cancer of the esophagus grows rapidly, metastasizes early, and is diagnosed late; therefore survival rates are poor.

EPIDEMIOLOGY

Esophageal cancer is not common. It constitutes 1% of all forms of cancer and is responsible for 2% of all deaths from cancer. There are approximately 10,100 new cases and 9400 deaths from cancer of the esophagus in the United States annually.[1] The most alarming fact about esophageal cancer is that only 6% of those affected will be alive 5 years after diagnosis; this is one of the poorest survival rates among malignant diseases. In the United States the age-adjusted mortality rate from carcinoma of the esophagus per 100,000 persons is higher among white men (5.7) than among white women (1.5) and significantly increased among black men (16.4) and black women (4.1).[2] Carcinoma of the esophagus develops at a younger age in black persons than it does in white persons.[3] The overall average age of onset is 62 years. Most persons with this disease are 50 to 70 years of age.

A puzzling feature of esophageal cancer is the remarkable difference in incidence according to geographic location, sometimes varying by as much as 200 times.[4] No other tumor demonstrates such variation, which indicates possible environmental risk factors or carcinogens. There are countries in which the incidence of esophageal cancer is 400 to 500 times that of the United States.[5]

ETIOLOGY

Although a variety of relationships yield clues, the cause of esophageal cancer remains unknown. Incidence by geographic location points to nutritional and environmental factors. Individuals with esophageal cancer typically have a history of heavy alcohol intake, heavy tobacco use, and poor nutrition.[6] Cirrhosis, vitamin deficiency, anemia, and poor oral hygiene may be contributing etiologic factors. The use of maize husks in the brewing of beer has been associated with the high incidence of esophageal cancer in southern Africa.

Conditions of chronic irritation have been cited as possible etiologic agents: hiatus hernia, reflux esophagitis, and diverticula. In some cases esophageal cancer has developed in individuals who ingested lye or caustic agents. The cancer usually appeared 40 or more years after the agent was ingested.[7] Extremes of temperatures in food are suggested as a possible contributory factor, especially hot tea and coffee.

Persons with untreated achalasia have a sevenfold to eightfold greater risk of the development of esophageal cancer. Early treatment of achalasia would improve esophageal emptying and as a preventive measure could reduce the risk of cancer. Plummer-Vinson syndrome has been associated with esophageal cancer.[8]

A genetic factor is possibly involved as a risk factor with esophageal cancer. Tylosis, a syndrome characterized by hyperkeratosis of the palms or soles, has been reported in a few cases of persons with esophageal cancer. Tylosis develops during adolescence or later.[9] A routine examination of all family members of a person with hyperkeratosis for esophageal abnormalities or cancer would be worthwhile because of their risk for esophageal cancer.

Dietary deficiencies of certain mineral elements are considered risk factors for esophageal cancer. In areas with a high incidence of esophageal cancer, dietary deficiencies of selenium were correlated with esophageal cytologic changes. Because selenium potentially increases resistance to cancer, a deficiency may identify a high-risk person.[10]

PATHOPHYSIOLOGY

Cellular Characteristics

Squamous cell carcinoma (>90%) and adenocarcinoma (<8%) are the two major histologic types of esophageal cancer.[11] In an organ lined almost entirely with squamous epithelium, it follows that squamous cell carcinoma would dominate the area from the pharynx to within a few centimeters of the esophagogastric junction. In the distal few centimeters of the esophagus, adenocarcinomas and squamous cell carcinomas appear equally. However, tumors in the area of the esophagogastric junction are usually primary gastric adenocarcinomas that have extended from the stomach into the lower esophagus. The frequency of adenocarcinoma of the esophagus has increased in recent years.[11]

The site of esophageal tumors is an important factor in detection and prognosis. The following percentages represent the distribution of cancer according to site: cervical esophageal, 20%; upper thoracic esophagus, 37%; and lower thoracic esophagus, 43%.[12]

Carcinoma of the esophagus may be grossly classified as fungating, ulcerative, or infiltrating.[13] Most often the tumor is a fungating mass that projects into the esophageal lumen, producing significant pathophysiologic alterations. A compensatory dilation of the esophagus will occur at and proximal to the tumor mass. When tumor proportions exceed the distensible capacity of the esophageal wall, complete obstruction occurs. The ulcerative lesion with elevated, irregular, nodular edges is a common growth pattern. Elevation of the lesion is produced by tumor growth in the submucosa. Depending on the depth of ulceration the lesion can be elevated to such an extent that it obstructs the lumen. An infiltrating pattern of tumor growth can encircle and thicken the wall, both of which compromise the patency of the esophagus. Some lesions will remain localized, whereas others will extend over a wide area of the esophagus.

Squamous cell carcinomas and adenocarcinomas exhibit a range of cellular differentiation. Some lesions are so poorly differentiated that it is difficult to ascertain cellular origin. At present, studies are being conducted to determine if there is a correlation between the degree of differentiation and factors such as rapidity of growth, invasiveness, metastases, response to therapy, or prognosis. Flow cytometric analysis of DNA content,[14] epidermal growth factor receptors,[15] and karyometric measurements of cell contents[16] are some of the factors being studied as possible predictors of extent of disease and response to therapy.

Progression of Disease

Squamous cell carcinomas often extend beyond the lumen wall to invade contiguous structures. Tumors of the cervical esophagus may directly involve the carotid arteries, pleura, recurrent laryngeal nerves, trachea, or larynx. Tumors of the upper portion of the thoracic esophagus may involve the left main-stem bronchus, thoracic duct, aortic arch, or pleura. In the lower portion of the thoracic esophagus, tumors may invade pericardium, pleura, descending aorta, and diaphragm. If the phrenic nerve is involved, paralysis of the diaphragm can result. Tumor invasion of contiguous structures may be extensive enough to prevent separation during resection, thereby negating surgical cure and necessitating alternative therapies.

Tumors of the esophagus metastasize principally via the lymphatic system. The rich intramural plexus of lymphatic vessels and the lack of a serosal barrier permit early regional extension and dissemination of esophageal carcinoma before clinical signs appear. The lymph flow can be either cephalad or caudad. This unpredictable pattern of lymph drainage makes both staging and therapy difficult. Knowledge of the lymphatic flow is important for the nurse to perform adequate physical assessment. Lesions of the cervical and upper thoracic esophagus usually metastasize to the anterior jugular chain and high paratracheal nodes in the supraclavicular region. In the middle thoracic esophagus, tumor cells may metastasize to the mediastinum and subdiaphragmatic lymph nodes. Tumors in the lower part of the esophagus will disseminate to the abdominal lymph nodes and the gastric and celiac lymph channels.

Hematogenous spread of tumor cells or tumor emboli is another mode of metastases. Tumor emboli may dislodge into the caval system and become embedded in the lung or liver. Distant metastases to the lung, liver, adrenal glands, bone, brain, and kidney are common with advanced disease. Typically the natural history of the disease includes inability to swallow and subsequent malnutrition, which leads to anorexia, cachexia, muscle wasting, pneumonia, infection, and eventual death.

CLINICAL MANIFESTATIONS

Early symptoms of esophageal carcinoma may be nonspecific and cause little concern to the patient, nurse, or physician. The initial symptoms include a vague sense of pressure, fullness, indigestion, and occasional substernal distress. Symptoms may be present for only weeks or a few months; yet the esophageal carcinoma can be advanced.

As the disease advances, dysphagia becomes a dominant symptom in almost 90% of the cases. A significant characteristic of esophageal cancer is the progressive nature of the dysphagia. Because the esophagus initially will distend to allow liquid or food to pass the tumor, the individual unconsciously will masticate solid food more thoroughly and substitute soft and liquid foods to relieve the dysphagia. When tumor size exceeds a critical luminal circumference, saliva, food, and liquids may spill over into the lungs, causing aspiration pneumonitis. Pain on swallowing occurs in about 50% of the patients with esophageal cancer.[2]

Weight loss, which inevitably follows, is a symptom equaled in frequency only by pancreatic cancer. A loss of 40 to 50 pounds in 2 to 3 months is common. Anorexia, anemia, and dehydration may add to a debilitated state.

Substernal and epigastric pain often mimics heartburn. Coughing may indicate aspiration of food or a tracheoesophageal fistula. The person with a tracheoesophageal fistula has a characteristic swallow-cough sequence. Fever can signal pulmonary involvement by tumor or aspiration pneumonia. Superior vena cava obstruction, pleural effusion, and hepatomegaly may occur.

Tumor encroachment of the recurrent laryngeal nerve results in laryngeal paralysis and causes hoarseness. Phrenic nerve involvement can cause hiccups or paralysis of the arm or diaphragm. With invasion of the brachial plexus, paresthesia can occur.[17]

ASSESSMENT

The nurse's role in the prevention and detection of esophageal cancer can significantly influence early identification of this aggressive tumor. Any person with risk factors for esophageal cancer should be instructed both on the importance of adequate health care follow-up and on ways to reduce or eliminate risk factors. Counseling on nutrition, alcohol or smoking abuse, and good personal hygiene are important measures for prevention. Nurses should be acutely aware of chronic users of over-the-counter home medications for gastrointestinal upsets. Such persons should be encouraged to seek medical attention promptly. Industrial nurses have implemented screening programs aimed at cancer detection. In China mass screenings are conducted by means of an occult blood bead detector that is swallowed and then withdrawn to be evaluated for evidence of bleeding caused by tumor involvement.[18]

The diagnosis of esophageal cancer depends on a thorough patient history with particular attention to the sequelae of symptoms and nutritional alterations. The most definitive diagnostic procedures are routine and special radiologic examinations, endoscopic examinations, biopsy, cytologic examinations, and exploratory surgery.

Physical Examination

Physical examination reveals few findings definitive of the diagnosis, except in cases of advanced disease in which enlarged lymph nodes are palpable, organs are enlarged or displaced, dysphagia and weight loss are profound, and systemic manifestations such as aspiration pneumonia are present. Laboratory studies contribute little to the definitive diagnosis.

Diagnostic Studies

Radiologic examination

In addition to routine radiologic examination, barium studies are useful for diagnosis. The typical changes noted in a barium esophagram or swallow are irregularity, displacement, narrowing, and rigidity. Particular attention is directed toward tumor length, lumen caliber, marginal contour, peristalsis, mucosal pattern, displacement, and residue.[12] Small lesions are easily missed because of the subtle changes produced and the rapidity with which the barium passes. Large lesions may be detected by indirect evidence such as displacement of the trachea. Advanced lesions produce a characteristic cone-shaped dilation proximal to the tumor mass and area of stenosis. Ulceration is difficult to visualize but is indicated by irregularity, angulation, and distortion of the linear mucosal folds. Antispasmodic agents are used in cases of near complete obstruction to enhance visualization. Barium will leave the stomach within 2 to 6 hours. In consideration of the person's poor nutritional state, the nurse should be certain that laxatives or an enema are given after the test to prevent a barium impaction.

Computed tomography (CT) scan of the mediastinum and abdomen, bone scan, liver scan, and skeletal survey are indicated in most cases. Magnetic resonance imaging (MRI) does not offer a diagnostic advantage for detection of this disease.

Endoscopy and biopsy

Endoscopic visualization plays an important role in the differential diagnosis of esophageal tumors. The flexible instrument has the advantage of ease of placement, whereas the rigid esophagoscope permits a larger biopsy specimen to be obtained and often allows better visualization. Both instruments cause moderate irritation to the throat, which can be relieved with topical anesthetics.

Visualization of lesions by endoscopic examination has limitations and is therefore complemented by cytologic and microscopic examination. A diagnosis can be made by cytologic study with an accuracy rate of 90%.[4] Use of the fiberoptic esophagoscope makes it possible to obtain a sample for cytologic study by brushing the tumor directly. Washings for cytologic examination also have diagnostic value. In China cytologic examination is being used on a mass screening basis to detect early lesions and to monitor high-risk persons such as those with achalasia or tobacco and alcohol abuse.[19]

With all tumors of the cervical and upper portions of the thoracic esophagus, bronchoscopic examination is equally important to rule out invasion of the trachea or bronchus or incipient fistula.[20] A laryngoscopic examination may precede further studies if tumor involvement of the recurrent nerves and laryngeal paralysis is suspected. The carcinoma may appear elevated, irregular, friable, reddened, or as a patch of leukoplakia. The mucosa may appear normal in cases in which the submucosa is the involved area.

After instrumentation the individual will receive nothing to eat or drink and will remain with the head elevated until the effect of anesthesia dissipates. Nursing observations should be directed toward signs of esophageal perforation, fluid aspiration, and laryngospasm.

Biopsy of lymph nodes is a definitive diagnostic tool; however, nodes are not always accessible. If a laparotomy is performed as part of the therapeutic approach, extensive biopsy specimens of the entire area should be obtained because the rich network of lymph nodes often are metastatic sites.

CLASSIFICATION AND STAGING

Unlike more accessible cancers, clinical staging of esophageal cancer is difficult to accomplish without invasive measures. The extent of tumor growth (T) cannot be fully assessed by radiographic or endoscopic examination. The lymph node status (N) can be evaluated noninvasively only in cervical esophagus lesions. By the time a diagnosis is established, disease has frequently metastasized (M) to liver, lungs, or bone. The aggressiveness of the therapeutic approach is based on an evaluation of the individual and the extent to which the disease has progressed.

For purposes of classification and staging, the American Joint Committee for Cancer Staging and End-Results Reporting has developed a standardized classification system (Table 39-2).[21]

TREATMENT

Treatment Planning

Selection of the treatment plan

In view of the biologic nature and poor prognosis of esophageal carcinoma, the goal of interdisciplinary planning is to select the therapies most appropriate for the extent of the tumor and for the individual. Despite advances in surgery, radiotherapy, and chemotherapy, esophageal carcinoma has a poor outcome, with fewer than 6% of individuals surviving 5 years.[1] Careful interdisciplinary planning is needed to define the extent of the disease, to assess the individual's physiologic status, and to discuss alternatives completely with the individual before the course of treatment is selected. The nurse is in a

TABLE 39-2 TNM Classification System for Cancer of the Esophagus

Primary Tumor (T)

TX	Primary tumor cannot be assessed
T0	No evidence of primary tumor
Tis	Carcinoma *in situ*
T1	Tumor invades lamina propria or submucosa
T2	Tumor invades muscularis propria
T3	Tumor invades adventitia
T4	Tumor invades adjacent structures

Regional Lymph Nodes (N)

NX	Regional lymph nodes cannot be assessed
N0	No regional lymph node metastasis
N1	Regional lymph node metastasis

Distant Metastasis (M)

MX	Presence of distant metastasis cannot be assessed
M0	No distant metastasis
M1	Distant metastasis

Stage Grouping

Stage 0	Tis	N0	M0
Stage I	T1	N0	M0
Stage IIA	T2	N0	M0
	T3	N0	M0
Stage IIB	T1	N1	M0
	T2	N1	M0
Stage III	T3	N1	M0
	T4	Any N	M0
Stage IV	Any T	Any N	M1

Source: Beahrs OH, Henson DE, Hutter RV, et al (eds): American Joint Committee on Cancer: Manual for Staging of Cancer (ed 3). Philadelphia, JB Lippincott, 1988.

valuable position to evaluate the person's understanding and reaction to the anticipated therapy.

Surgical resection, radiotherapy, and chemotherapy are used to treat esophageal cancer, but it is a combination of these treatment methods that appears to offer the greatest hope of cure or control. The most effective combination or sequence of therapies has yet to be established. Preoperative irradiation and chemotherapy have been shown to improve resectability rates but not long-term survival rates. In the past, operative mortality rates were high (>50%) but are now decreasing to about 15%.[22] In light of the nature of this disease, aggressive efforts aimed at either cure or palliation are justifiable and constitute the only hope in many cases.

The optimal candidate for curative treatment should be free of concomitant renal, cardiac, and pulmonary diseases; relatively well nourished; and have a tumor that is localized, responsive, and accessible to treatment (ie, stage I or II). The interdisciplinary team will develop a plan that can include single or combined modalities of surgery, radiation, or chemotherapy.

The historical trend has been to treat lesions of the cervical esophagus initially with radiotherapy (4500 to 6000 cGy). Surgery is undertaken 3 to 4 weeks later.[2] Surgical resection is limited because of mortality risks associated with surgery and problems with reconstruction. Improvements in restoring the continuity of the cervical esophagus have been reported, but the outlook remains dismal.[23] The prognosis for tumors in the lower portion of the esophagus is somewhat better than for tumors in the other areas of the esophagus.

Certain findings usually preclude an individual from consideration for curative treatment (stage III disease):

1. Fixed lymph nodes (N3)
2. A fixed tumor mass (T3)
3. Extension of the tumor outside the esophagus (T3, M1)
4. Recurrent laryngeal nerve involvement (T3, M1)

In cases of advanced disease, restoration or maintenance of a patent alimentary tract is the aim of aggressive therapy. Treatment can be radiotherapy, surgical resection or bypass, prosthetic device implants, or systemic chemotherapy. Although long-term survival rarely is affected, aggressive therapy can be tolerated by many patients and results in an improvement in the individual's quality of life.

Preparation for treatment

If an aggressive treatment plan has been selected, ideally the patient will undergo supportive treatment to improve general health and nutrition before the course of therapy. If the disease is advanced and the symptoms and manifestations are severely debilitating, palliative therapy may need to be initiated immediately and supportive measures introduced whenever possible.

Progressive dysphagia affects about 90% of individuals with esophageal tumors.[2] Because of difficulty with swallowing, the individual's nutritional status usually is poor to severely compromised. Cachexia, muscle wasting, and negative nitrogen balance may be present. Intensive nutritional therapy that can include total parenteral nutrition, enteral tube feedings, or high-calorie, high-protein diets may be given, depending on the individual's intestinal patency. The degree of weight loss can be correlated with prognosis.[2]

Because of the high incidence of aspiration that occurs in individuals with esophageal cancer, pulmonary hygiene is a priority in pretreatment care. The person is taught to breathe deeply and cough, with careful attention to expectorating secretions. When an esophageal tumor hinders the ability to swallow, the nurse should instruct the individual to bend forward when coughing and expectorate into a tissue, cloth, or basin. Expectorants, antibiotics, or bronchodilators can be used to facilitate pulmonary hygiene. Esophageal lavage with a nasogastric tube placed above the obstruction may be necessary to prevent aspiration of accumulated food or secretions.

The individual with a large esophageal tumor usually cannot swallow saliva and will drool and spit frequently. The nurse must be acutely aware of the psychologic impact of this embarrassing problem and change in body image. The person should be assisted to establish an acceptable method for controlling drooling (eg, nearby basin, oral suction equipment, and abundant supply of tissues).

The period of treatment preparation is an excellent time to begin teaching the patient and family about the proposed therapy and anticipated course of the disease and to establish supportive relationships.

Radiotherapy

Esophageal squamous cell carcinoma is responsive to radiotherapy, which can result in rapid relief of an obstruction. Radiotherapy can be used alone, as preoperative or postoperative therapy, or as palliative therapy. Radiotherapy alone is not being employed as often now because newer methods of therapy that combine chemotherapy, radiation, and surgery are providing better results. Radiation alone, however, is an excellent therapeutic alternative for a person with advanced disease or for an elderly or severely debilitated person who cannot withstand the rigor of aggressive therapy.

Important factors in determining the selection of radiotherapy as treatment are the location and size of the tumor and the age and the general condition of the patient. Small lesions (*5 cm) can be treated for cure with radiotherapy alone or in combination. Tumoricidal doses of 5000 to 7000 cGy are administered over 6 to 8 weeks. Because esophageal cancer is a disease that results in a survival period of only a few months, radiation therapy can consume a significant portion of that time.

Radiotherapy is the treatment favored by many clinicians for stages I and II cervical esophageal lesions because surgical mortality rates are exceedingly high and the larynx can be preserved with irradiation. Unfortunately, few tumors are discovered early enough to be cured with radical radiotherapy alone. Tumors located in the cervical esophagus are complex to treat because of their proximity to the spinal cord. Tumors located in the upper thoracic esophagus respond well to radiotherapy. Lesions of the lower thoracic esophagus usually are treated with multimodal therapy.

Complications and side effects of radiotherapy relate to tissue tolerance, site and amount of radiation, and adjuvant therapy. Esophageal fistula, stricture, hemorrhage, radiation pneumonitis, and pericarditis are possible problems. Side effects expected during therapy are swallowing difficulties (burning, pain, dryness) and skin reactions. Nursing management should be aimed at anticipating and preventing complications of the radiation therapy and concomitant therapies, maintaining adequate nutritional intake, and minimizing the discomfort of esophageal and skin irritation. Nursing care of individuals who receive radiotherapy is discussed in detail in Chapter 12. The nurse or dietitian must plan an intensive dietary program based on the constraints of an obstructive tumor, the degree of nutritional deficit, and the person's preferences.

Preoperative radiotherapy

Preoperative radiotherapy can improve the outlook for persons with esophageal carcinomas. Because esophageal cancer is uncommon, individuals with such tumors should be treated in centers where cancer specialists combine their abilities. Preoperative radiotherapeutic doses of 3000 to 6000 cGy can reduce tumor bulk, enabling individuals with esophageal tumors to swallow, which leads to significantly improved nutritional status and less surgical risk. Preoperative radiation therapy potentially can eradicate local microscopic disease and reduce the risk of dissemination of tumor cells during surgery.

Prospective studies lend credibility to the effectiveness of the combination of preoperative radiation and surgery.[24,25] Increased resectability rates and decreased surgical mortality rates occur when combination therapy is used. The limitation to the aggressiveness of preoperative radiation or preoperative chemoradiation is toxicity.[25]

Postoperative radiotherapy

Postoperative radiotherapy is administered to eradicate residual tumor cells in the area of the surgical site. These cells may have been implanted during surgery or could be residual, that is, contained in the unresected tumor or adjacent tissue. If the tumor was an unresectable advanced esophageal cancer, postoperative radiotherapy can be effective for local control. The surgeon can mark the involved area with radiopaque clips, which enable more precise delivery of the radiation. If the tumor was resected and the stomach or colon used to restore intestinal continuity, a more limited radiation dose (4000 to 5000 cGy) will be required to avoid tissue injury.[2]

Postoperative radiotherapy does not affect surgical mortality, but it may not be as effective as chemoradiation before surgical resection. Further investigation is needed to determine the sequence of radiation therapy in the treatment pattern.

Surgery

Surgical intervention is employed selectively for lesions at all three levels of the esophagus.[26] The goal of surgery may be to cure or palliate, depending on the stage of the tumor and overall condition of the patient. Curative surgery attempts to eradicate the tumor and reestablish esophageal continuity, whereas palliative surgery may aim at maintaining esophageal patency.

Indications for curative surgery include a satisfactory nutritional state, a resectable tumor without evidence of invasion of contiguous structures (stages I and II), no distant metastases, and no serious concomitant disease. Age is not an issue, unless the person's general health is unsatisfactory. Curative surgery can be attempted if it is expected that the tumor will be removed completely and esophageal patency reestablished. If possible, blood, fluid, electrolyte, and nutritional balances should be established before aggressive surgical resection is done.[27] Impaired wound healing and increased incidence of infection are

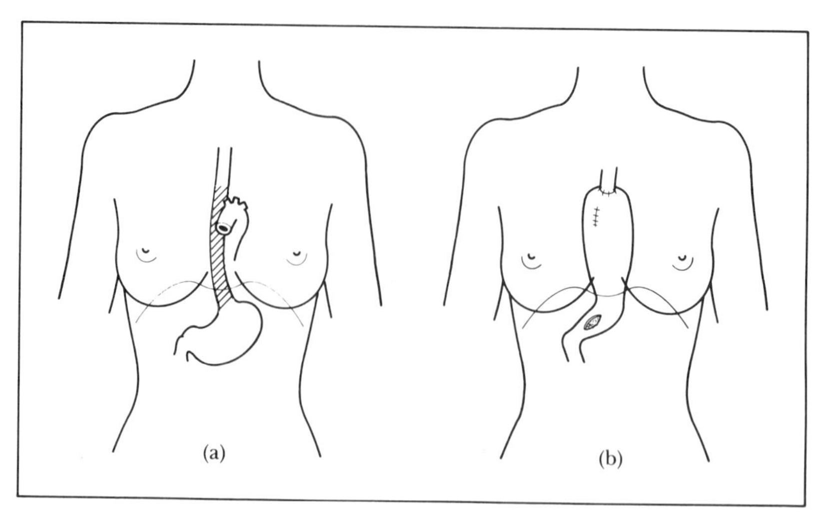

FIGURE 39-1 The technique of esophagectomy for cancers involving the mid-esophagus. (a) The extent of esophagus removed is shown by the darkened area. (b) The esophagogastrostomy above the aortic arch and pyloroplasty is illustrated.

associated with hypoalbuminemia.[28] Before surgery, chest physiotherapy includes respiratory exercise with intermittent positive pressure breathing and incentive spirometry. The patient is requested to refrain from smoking for 2 to 3 weeks before surgery.

Esophagectomy is the most widely accepted procedure for surgical resection aimed at potential cure. Because lymph node involvement can occur at a distance from the primary esophageal cancer, complete removal of the esophagus and adjacent lymph nodes is considered the procedure of choice. Included in the surgical resection are a margin of the lesser curvature of the stomach and adjacent lymph nodes from the immediate area and extending up to the cervical esophagus. Vital structures in the area (heart, aorta, main-stem bronchus) make complete resection of the esophagus and nodes difficult, hence the rationale for adjuvant therapies. Whenever there is evidence that cure is a strong possibility, a more extensive en bloc excision is performed. The en bloc continuous resection includes parietal pleura, pericardium, and all tissue between the esophagus and aorta.[29]

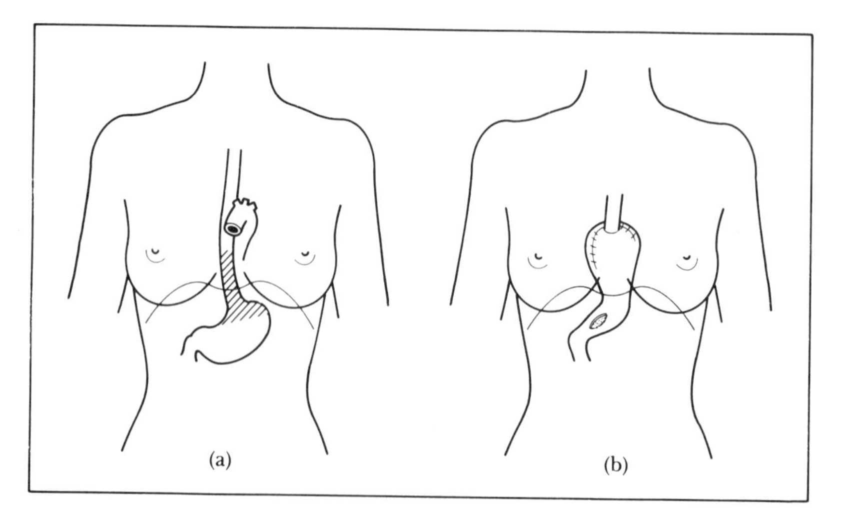

FIGURE 39-2 Esophagectomy for lesions of the lower esophagus. In most cases, the procedure can be performed through the left thoracic incision. The midline abdominal incision is used when the duodenum must be mobilized to permit the esophagogastrotomy to be performed. (a) The extent of esophagus and stomach removed is shown by the darkened area. The lymph nodes at the celiac axis are removed with the specimen. (b) The esophagogastrostomy is illustrated. A pyloroplasty is also done.

Surgical approaches

The actual approach to esophageal resection depends on the location of the tumor. Three surgical approaches currently are being used: left thoracotomy with a thoracoabdominal incision, right thoracotomy with laparotomy, or both a cervical and abdominal incision.[2] Right thoracotomy with laparotomy is the standard approach used by most surgeons. The laparotomy allows evaluation of the lower celiac nodes for tumor involvement. Left thoracotomy facilitates a higher intrathoracic resection of the esophagus and involved areas.[30]

Reconstruction after esophagectomy can be achieved by various procedures. Elevating the stomach to create an esophagogastrostomy is the most widely used reconstructive procedure (Figures 39-1 and 39-2). If a gastrectomy previously has been performed or the stomach is not suitable as a reconstructive organ, a colon interposition may be done (Figure 39-3). A gastric tube sometimes is created from the greater curvature of the stomach, reversed, and elevated to reconstruct the esophagus (Figure 39-4).

Special considerations: cervical esophagus

Resection of lesions of the cervical esophagus requires careful planning. Stage I tumors of the cervical esophagus can sometimes be resected completely without removing the larynx. The surgical procedure consists of a radical neck dissection and partial cervical esophagectomy. Stage I tumors are evaluated carefully to ensure that the involvement is localized. However, most squamous cell carcinomas of the cervical esophagus are first detected at a more advanced stage and require more extensive surgery. Usually resection of cervical esophagus lesions involves removing all or part of the pharynx, larynx, thyroid, and proximal esophagus.[2]

Reconstruction of intestinal patency is a major consideration, especially with irradiated tissue. Pharyngeal and esophageal reconstruction is necessary after this aggressive extirpation. The reconstructive procedure may be done at the time of the initial resection or later as a second-stage procedure. At present, cervical esophageal conti-

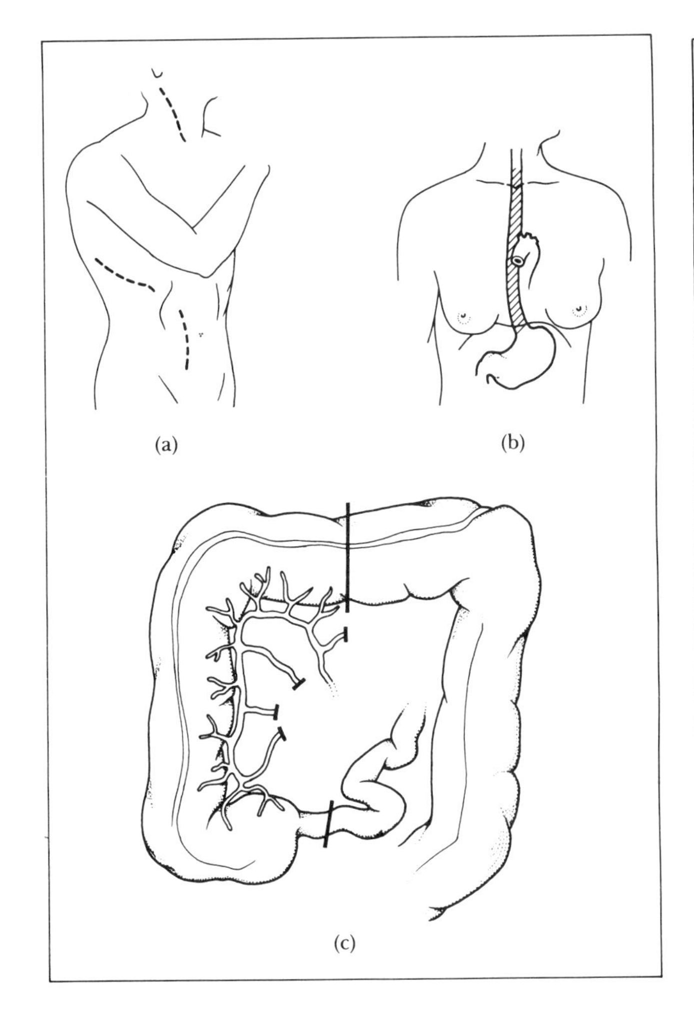

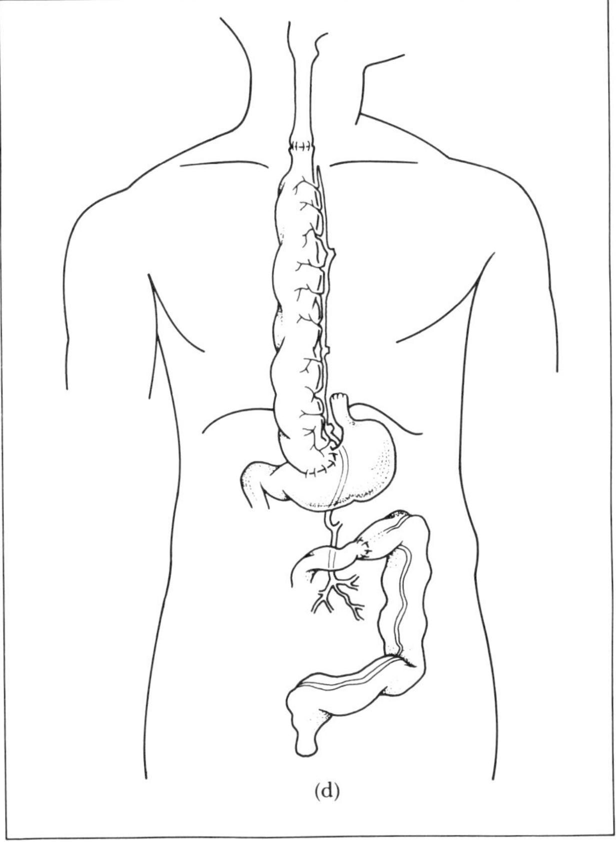

FIGURE 39-3 A right colon substernal transplant and total esophagectomy. (a) The cervical and abdominal incisions are made at the first stage of the operation. The right thoracic incision is used at the second stage to remove the esophagus. (b) The extent of esophageal resection is shown. (c) The right colon on a pedicle consisting of the midcolic artery and vein is illustrated. (d) The completed operation is shown.

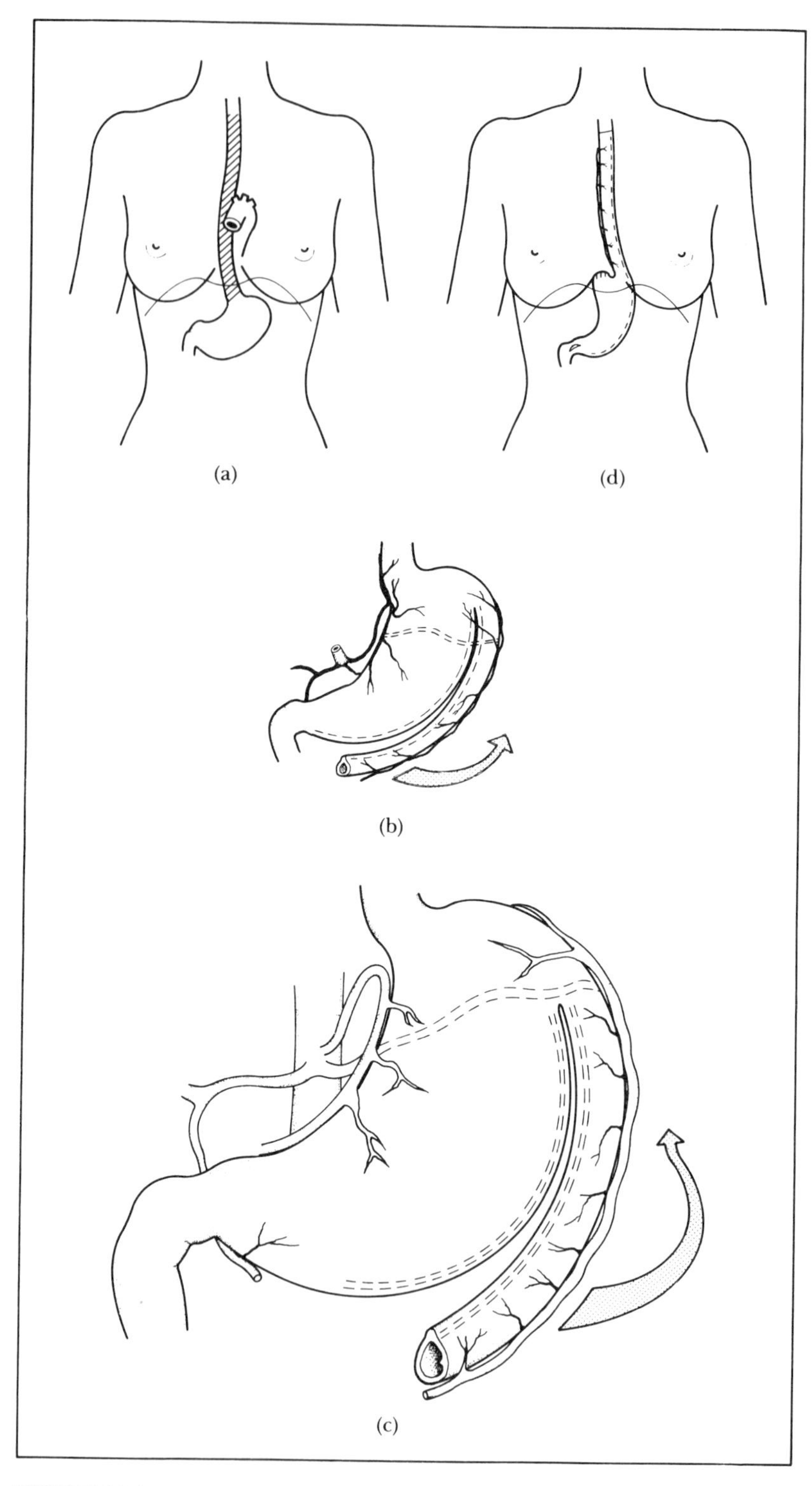

FIGURE 39-4 Reversed gastric tube and total esophagectomy. (a) The extent of esophageal resection is shown. (b) The reversed gastric tube created from two parallel rows of staples is shown. (c) The gastroepiploic vessels are carefully preserved and vascularize the gastric tube. (d) The completed operation, with gastrostomy and pyloroplasty, is shown.

nuity is reestablished by a variety of methods: pharyngogastrostomy, formation of a tube from the greater curvature of the stomach, use of skin tubes and skin grafts, or interposition of a segment of colon or jejunum. Pharyngogastrostomy is the reconstructive procedure of preference.

A satisfactory, functional result can be achieved with these procedures, but the postoperative period is plagued with complications of fistulas, anastomotic leaks, strictures, respiratory insufficiency, pulmonary embolism, obstruction, and infection.[2] Morbidity rates are high (25%),[20] and postoperative mortality ranges from 15% to 26%.[29,31] Particular attention should be directed toward preventing and anticipating the possible complications of each surgical procedure.

Postoperative care

Respiratory complications and anastomotic leaks comprise the bulk of complications after surgical resection for carcinoma of the esophagus. Severe atelectasis, pneumonia, respiratory failure, and pulmonary embolus are the major pulmonary complications that contribute to postoperative morbidity and mortality. Lengthy surgical procedures (5 to 8 hours) and a compromised preoperative pulmonary condition can precipitate problems. Because most individuals who undergo surgery for an esophageal tumor are in a precarious nutritional state, protein depletion and generalized muscle weakness are common. Ability to breathe deeply and cough is compromised by weakness and incisional pain. Aggressive respiratory care can include tracheal intubation, chest physical therapy, tracheobronchial aspiration, prevention of fluid overload, and antibiotic therapy. Early ambulation and mild exercise will improve respiratory status.

Because the esophagus is thin walled and drawn upward with each swallow, an anastomosis involving the esophagus has more of a tendency toward anastomotic leak than any other area of the gastrointestinal tract.[20,30,32] Decompression tubes, nasogastric or gastrostomy, must be patent at all times to prevent pressure or tension on the anastomotic site. Because the thoracoabdominal approach is used in many esophageal surgeries, chest tubes may be placed to facilitate full reexpansion of the lungs, extraesophageal drainage, and early identification of a disrupted anastomosis. Bloody, purulent, salivary, or excessive drainage from the chest tubes would indicate leakage. An anastomotic leak occasionally produces a pneumothorax or hydropneumothorax, which requires immediate drainage. The nurse routinely should auscultate the patient's chest to identify any changes in lung expansion or accumulation of fluid. Six or seven days after surgery a limited barium swallow is done to evaluate anastomotic healing. Small leaks usually close spontaneously, whereas large leaks require surgical approximation. Leaks at the cervical esophagogastric anastomosis may be opened, irrigated, and packed at the patient's bedside. Oral intake is stopped for 24 to 72 hours and replaced by enteral feedings. Once healing has occurred, a soft diet is initiated. Intrathoracic anastomotic leaks usually are managed with chest tube drainage, aggressive antibiotic therapy, cessation of oral intake, and open thoracotomy if the disruption is large.[33]

Infections are a serious threat to recovery. Virulent mouth organisms and overgrowth of pathogenic bacteria on ulcerating lesions may be the source of wound and intracavitary infections. If the individual has had previous radiotherapy, the risks of tissue breakdown, poor wound healing, and fistulas are greatly increased. Nursing assessments for signs of infection include inspection of incision lines; monitoring of vital signs, particularly temperature; pulmonary auscultation; and close attention to drainage, urinary output, and hematologic factors.

Meticulous suture line care and constant monitoring for signs of inflammation, drainage, and edema are necessary. Esophagocutaneous fistulas usually appear in raised, reddened, or necrotic areas along the suture line. The individual should be observed carefully during swallowing because a leak may occur at the suture line. Chylous fistulas produce a milky white secretion that gradually increases in amount. Systemic signs of fistula are fever, malaise, and increased respirations and pulse rate. The individual is maintained in proper body alignment to reduce tension on the anastomosis. Suction catheters are not introduced into the oropharyngeal cavity without knowledge of the location of the suture line because the suture line may be disrupted. The nasogastric tube should be advanced or manipulated only with the use of a fluoroscope.

If the individual had a cervical esophagectomy in conjunction with a laryngectomy, the nursing care needs are complex. The nursing care of the individual with a laryngectomy is discussed in detail in Chapter 41.

The postoperative nursing care of the individual with an esophagogastrectomy includes anticipation and prevention of reflux aspiration. The head of the bed should be elevated at all times. The individual may need assistance in developing a means of elevating the head of the bed at home. A foam rubber wedge or multiple pillows correctly aligned work well. Snacks or liquids after the evening meal should be avoided so that the stomach will be relatively empty at bedtime. The person should ingest all food and liquids in an upright position and remain upright for 20 to 30 minutes after eating.[33] Food and liquids should be swallowed in small amounts at all times. The person should be instructed to avoid bending over from the waist and especially any exercising or lifting that would increase intra-abdominal and thoracic pressure and cause reflux.[34] Squatting to lift objects will displace the stress to the legs rather than the abdomen.

When a segment of colon is used to reconstruct or bypass part of the esophagus, the individual will have complex nursing care needs in addition to those discussed previously for esophagectomy. Pulmonary hygiene, prevention of infection, prevention of reflux, control of odor, and nutrition are nursing priorities.

Before surgery for colon interposition, a regimen of antibiotics and sulfonamides is begun to suppress bacterial flora in the intestine. Despite efforts to sterilize and prepare the bowel for transposition, contamination of the peritoneal cavity and infection leading to fistula formation are common and serious complications. Gram-negative bacteria can produce endotoxic shock manifested by rapid pulse, decreased blood pressure, increased respirations and temperature, warm, dry skin, and confusion. The suture lines should be observed for signs of infection, vital signs monitored regularly, and careful lung assessments performed to detect an anastomotic leak or extraesophageal accumulation of fluid.

Foul-smelling breath is a distressing consequence of using a segment of bowel to reconstruct the esophagus. The extensive program of preoperative bowel preparation will reduce but not eliminate fecal odor. Frequent, meticulous oral care is necessary in the postoperative period and after discharge. The individual should be instructed to avoid foods that cause belching because the eructated air will have a fecal odor that could embarrass the person. The person can prepare a small, discreet travel kit that includes such items as a toothbrush, toothpaste, mouthwash, mint candies, and charcoal carbonate tablets. Some people find that commercially available breath sprays are useful. Charcoal carbonate tablets taken regularly help to control odor.

Chemotherapy

The role of chemotherapy in the treatment of esophageal tumors has not been clearly established, but it is known that esophageal cancers are chemosensitive. As more controlled research studies with chemotherapeutic agents are completed, the role of this treatment in the cure or control of esophageal tumors should become known. Single-agent and combination regimens have been studied but have not provided improved long-term disease-free intervals. Methotrexate, cisplatin, 5-fluorouracil (5-FU), mitomycin C, mitoguazone (MGBG), doxorubicin, and bleomycin have demonstrated cytotoxic activity with esophageal tumors.

Previously, chemotherapy was used only for palliation. As more was learned about the biologic nature of esophageal cancer and its metastatic characteristics, it became clear that esophageal cancer needs to be approached at the outset as though it were a systemic disease. The sequence of chemotherapy and its use in multimodal treatment approaches offer the most promising areas for exploration at this time.

Preoperative chemoradiation therapy, which allows an attack on local and metastatic disease simultaneously, is being investigated. Protocols include combination chemotherapy (usually cisplatin, 5-FU, and another agent) and fractionated radiation doses that total 3000 to 5000 cGy before surgery.[35-39] Tumor regression is effected in most cases. Cisplatin and 5-FU may act as radiosensitizers and improve the therapeutic effect. The toxicities associated with the extensive combination of chemotherapy, radiation therapy, and surgery are compounded and may be intolerable for some patients.[37] Severe mucositis and myelosuppression are the major toxic effects.[36,38] Surgical morbidity and mortality have not been increased.[37,39] Some chemotherapeutic agents (doxorubicin, actinomycin D, and daunorubicin) can produce radiation-recall esophagitis and skin reactions in individuals who have received previous irradiation.[40] Therefore, to reduce the severity of this effect, chemotherapy should not be initiated for several weeks after radiotherapy. Because few randomized trials have been completed, it is not yet known whether this approach to esophageal cancer will improve long-term disease-free intervals.

Chemoradiation alone without surgery has received attention.[41-43] Early results indicate that a better response is achieved with chemoradiation alone than with surgery or radiation alone. Optimal management of esophageal cancer is an unanswered question that requires further study.

Palliative Therapy

The objective of palliative therapy is to relieve the distressing symptoms of esophageal cancer, thereby improving the quality of the individual's life. Progressive dysphagia is probably the most debilitating of the symptoms, occurring in about 90% of the patients with advanced disease. Selection of a particular form of palliative therapy depends on the individual's preference, nutritional status, hematologic status, and ability to tolerate palliative therapy.

Palliative radiotherapy, although it cannot alter morbidity or survival rates, provides rapid symptomatic and objective relief. Usually 3000 to 5000 cGy will be given to decrease the size of the tumor or reduce bleeding, or both. Because of its noninvasive nature many oncologists select palliative radiotherapy over other forms of supportive treatment for the individual who can tolerate the therapy.

In selected individuals with advanced disease, palliative resection with reconstruction or surgical bypass of the esophagus is done to relieve severe symptoms of the disease or to reduce the size of the tumor. Radiotherapy, however, usually is the treatment of choice. Surgical mortality is high as a result of pulmonary complications, anastomotic leak, infection, and thromboembolism.[22] Limited resection or bypass of the tumor can be achieved by elevation of the stomach, substernal or subcutaneous colon interposition, or a tube formed from the greater curvature of the stomach.[2]

A number of synthetic endoesophageal prosthetic tubes have been designed to create an open passage for swallowing when the esophagus is obstructed by an inoperable tumor. The two methods most commonly used to place the tube are the push-through method and the pull-through method. With the push-through method the tube is placed blindly or through the esophagoscope. The pull-through method involves pulling the tube into place by means of a guidewire or gastrostomy. Radiologic dilation before tube placement can reduce complications of tube placement.[44] Esophageal perforation is a technical complication that occurs in about 5% to 10% of individuals.[45,46] Dislodgement and/or obstruction with food occurs frequently. Satisfactory palliative results achieved with either type of tube are limited; however, increased food intake occurs in about 80% of the patients after tube placement.[47]

Nursing care of the individual with an endoprosthesis is aimed at preventing complications and maintaining tube patency. Individuals need to understand the purpose, function, and care of the endoesophageal prosthesis. Aspiration pneumonia, which is the major cause of death in those with esophageal cancer, is a serious potential complication with the use of prosthesis. With the prosthesis in place, reflux of gastric contents can lead to aspiration pneumonia.[48]

Nursing care measures to prevent reflux include elevating the head of the bed at all times, ensuring patency of decompression tubes, and pursuing aggressive pulmonary hygiene. When the individual is able to begin eating, about 5 days after placement, the nurse must develop strategies to prevent reflux. The individual is instructed to take all meals and liquids in an upright position. The first attempts at swallowing may be uncomfortable, but encouragement by the nurse can greatly increase the person's confidence. Smaller amounts of liquid or food with each swallow may be necessary. If food should become lodged in the tube because it is too large or inadequately chewed, it usually can be dislodged carefully with a nasogastric tube. Predischarge teaching should include instructions to drink at least a half glass of water or a carbonated beverage at the end of a meal to clear the tube completely.

In addition to prosthetic tube placement to palliate an obstruction, high-dose photoirradiation and laser therapy are being used to reduce the obstructive mass.[49-52] Laser therapy is used to reduce esophageal stricture caused by tumor.

Gastrostomy and jejunostomy are alternative palliative procedures for individuals with esophageal cancer. Although they permit nutritional maintenance, they do not relieve the debilitating problem of inability to swallow solids, liquids, or saliva. Nursing measures to increase tolerance of tube feedings are discussed in Chapter 24. Nursing management of the individual with advanced esophageal cancer includes control of pain, nutritional support, and psychologic support. Esophageal cancer grows rapidly and disseminates early; therefore the nurse can be most helpful by anticipating problems and providing support to the individual and family.

CONCLUSION

In light of the dreary outlook on esophageal cancer, it is important to consider what the future may hold for persons with esophageal cancer. Early detection is the crux of all cancer control, and this area is receiving international attention.

Is it possible to identify biologic markers or definitive risk factors that would be helpful in detecting esophageal cancer at an early stage or even in predicting the onset of esophageal cancer? In China mass screening programs for esophageal cancer have proven successful in detecting early cases of esophageal carcinoma. Unfortunately, the present detection techniques are expensive, inefficient, and prohibitive for continued use on a large scale.

The role of multimodal therapy in the treatment of esophageal carcinoma is emerging. At present, a number of controlled studies are based on the use of multimodal therapy. It is hoped that these studies will lead to the development of a definitive set of guidelines for the treatment and management of esophageal tumors.

STOMACH TUMORS

INTRODUCTION

For reasons unknown at this time the incidence of gastric cancer is decreasing in some parts of the world and increasing steadily in others. In the United States the incidence has declined progressively since 1930 when it was the leading cause of cancer mortality.[1] On the other hand, gastric cancer continues to take a significant toll among inhabitants of Japan, Chile, Finland, Poland, Austria, Yugoslavia, and Costa Rica.[53]

If detected at an early stage and treated aggressively, cancer of the stomach can be cured.[54] As with all other forms of gastrointestinal cancer, stomach cancer is insidious in its onset and development. Cancer of the stomach usually infiltrates rapidly and can be disseminated throughout the body before overt signs of cancer are manifested. Overall 5-year survival rates are reported to range from about 8% to 16%.[1,53] Stomach cancer mimics several other gastrointestinal maladies and diseases such as polyps, ulcers, dyspepsia, and gastritis. Some of the most difficult aspects of prevention and early detection are informing and motivating people at risk for the development of gastric cancer to seek medical attention for chronic "stomach problems." Inappropriate use of home remedies, self-medication, and misdiagnosis are major hurdles to overcome.

ANATOMY

The stomach is a hollow, pouchlike reservoir that extends from the esophageal sphincter (cardiac) to the duodenal opening (pyloric sphincter). It is divided into three major areas: fundus, corpus or body, and antrum (Figure 39-5). The stomach wall is composed of four layers: serosa, muscle, submucosa, and mucosa. Liver, diaphragm, left suprarenal gland, kidney, pancreas, duodenum, and transverse colon are in contact with or in proximity to the stomach.

The stomach has a rich lymphatic network running through the mucosal, submucosal, muscular, and serosal layers. These lymphatic networks intercommunicate freely

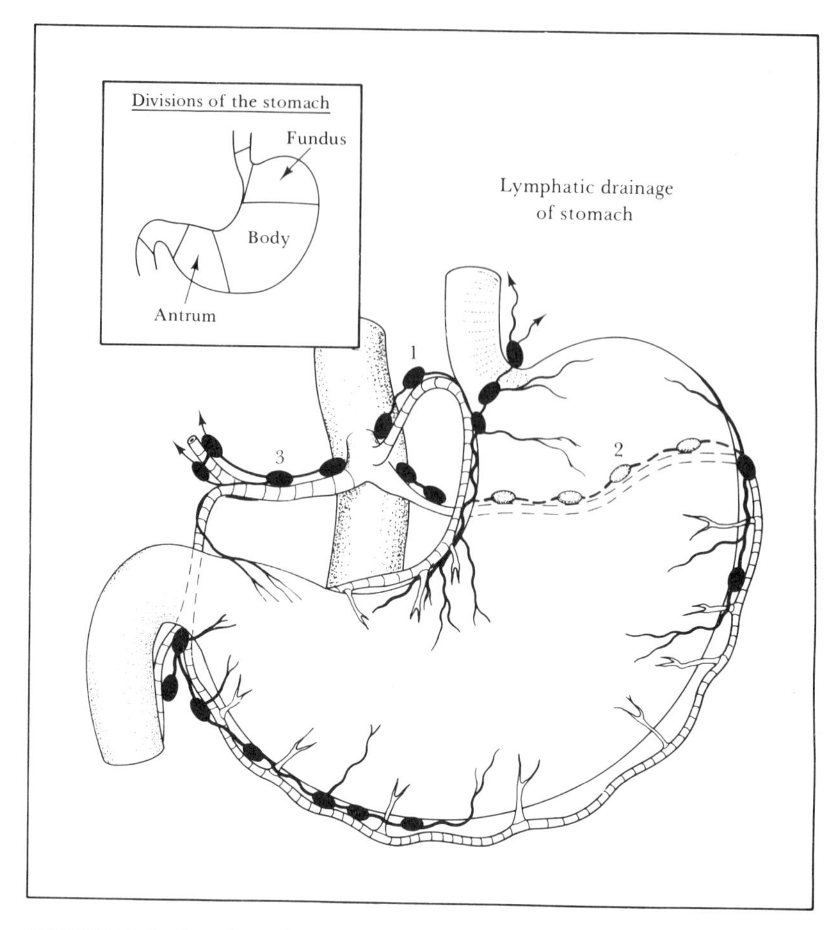

FIGURE 39-5 Lymphatic drainage of stomach showing (1) collecting trunks of left gastric artery, (2) splenic artery, and (3) hepatic artery. Inset: Divisions of the stomach: fundus, body, and antrum.

with each other and with the esophagus and duodenum, thereby serving as a conduit for tumor spread. Blood vessels approximate the course of the lymphatic vessels as shown in Figure 39-5.

EPIDEMIOLOGY

Gastric cancer is one of the few tumors that is decreasing in overall incidence. Japan has the highest incidence in the world of gastric cancer for both men and women, and stomach cancer is the major cause of death in Japan.[12,54] On the other hand, the incidence of gastric cancer is low in the United States.[1] The dramatic differences in geographic distribution throughout the world remain an enigma to epidemiologists.[55]

In the United States there are approximately 25,000 new cases and 14,500 deaths from gastric cancer each year.[1] This reflects a 50% decrease in incidence within the past 25 years, with the greatest decline occurring among white persons. Gastric cancer occurs among black men and women almost twice as often as among white persons. The reason for this is not clear. In the United States, black individuals, Japanese, Chinese, and native Hawaiians have a higher incidence and mortality rate than do white persons.[56] There also is great variation of incidence among the Indian, Hispanic white, and non-Hispanic white residents of New Mexico.[55]

ETIOLOGY

Factors that are believed to contribute to or that are associated with gastric cancer are largely environmental and genetic. The fact that immigrants exhibit incidence rates similar to those of their country of origin has led researchers to examine closely exogenous influences such as environment and diet. Mineral composition of the soil, especially nitroso compounds, is being questioned as a mutagenic and carcinogenic factor. Great controversy exists over the role of nitrites found in soil-grown foods, drinking water, and preserved foods. Because refrigeration and a high intake of ascorbic acid inhibit the formation of nitrites, it is postulated that the presence of these factors in modern American society may account for the decrease in gastric cancer in the United States.[57]

Those at greatest risk for the development of gastric cancer are older than 40 years of age and are at risk because of one or several of the following factors:

- Low socioeconomic status[58]
- Poor nutritional habits[59]
- Vitamin A deficiency[58]
- Food additives
- Pernicious anemia
- Achlorhydria
- Hypochlorhydria
- Gastric polyps
- Intestinal metaplasia
- Benign peptic ulcer disease[60]
- Smoking
- Alcohol consumption

Although gastric cancer in children is rare, it does occur. The highest incidence of gastric cancer occurs in men older than 70 years of age.[53]

PATHOPHYSIOLOGY

Cellular Characteristics

Almost all (95%) gastric cancers are epithelial tumors, predominantly adenocarcinomas.[61] Although uncommon, other types of gastric cancers are nonepithelial, carcinoid, hematopoietic, and lymphoid. Gastric tumors may be grossly classified as polypoid, scirrhous, ulcerative, or superficial. Most gastric cancers arise in the antrum, the lower third of the stomach. Tumor involves the lesser curvature of the stomach six times more often than it does the greater curvature.[27]

Adenocarcinomas that arise in the esophagocardia are considered to be a different disease than other gastric adenocarcinomas. Usually adenocarcinomas of the esophagocardia are primary cancers of the stomach that have extended to the esophagus. There are different male/female and ethnic distribution ratios.[62]

Progression of Disease

Because of the elusive nature of gastric disorders, gastric cancer usually is advanced when symptoms first appear. Gastric tumors can cause ulceration, obstruction, hemorrhage, or manifestations of metastatic involvement. There are several characteristic routes by which gastric carcinoma will progress and metastasize: (1) by extension and infiltration along the mucosal surface and stomach wall or lymphatic vessels, (2) via lymphatic or vascular embolism, probably to regional lymph nodes, (3) by direct extension into adjacent structures such as the pancreas, liver, or esophagus, and (4) by blood-borne spread. The pattern of metastatic spread of gastric cancer correlates with the size and the location of the tumor. Lesions of the distal portion of the stomach usually metastasize to infrapyloric, inferior gastric, and celiac lymph nodes. Tumors in the proximal portion often metastasize to pancreatic, pericardial, and gastric lymph nodes. With advanced gastric cancer, involvement of the left supraclavicular nodes may occur. Distant metastatic sites are the lung, adrenal glands, bone, liver, pancreas, and peritoneal cavity.

CLINICAL MANIFESTATIONS

Persons with gastric cancer have vague, poorly defined symptoms of variable duration. Individuals usually will delay several months between the onset of symptoms and initial medical consultation. The earliest symptoms are readily passed off as a "stomach upset." The individual with gastric cancer initially complains of a vague, uneasy sense of fullness, a feeling of heaviness, and moderate distention after meals. Home remedies and self-medication often are employed successfully for a while until more definitive signs and symptoms appear. As the disease advances, progressive weight loss can result from disturbances in appetite, nausea, and vomiting. Weakness, fatigue, and anemia are common findings. Dysphagia may occur with tumors of the proximal portion of the stomach. Pain in the epigastric, back, or retrosternal area often is cited as an early symptom that was ignored or that responded temporarily to symptomatic treatment. Hematemesis, melena, or a change in bowel habits sometimes is reported. Unfortunately, definitive clinical signs occur mostly with advanced disease. Common clinical signs of gastric carcinoma are weight loss, pain, vomiting, palpable abdominal mass, anorexia, and dysphagia.[61]

ASSESSMENT

The use of radiography, gastroscopy, and laparotomy may be necessary to establish a diagnosis of gastric carcinoma. Because the initial symptoms are vague, it is not unusual for misdiagnosis or treatment delay to occur. However, all individuals at risk for the development of gastric cancer should be examined periodically, have a complete assessment, and undergo radiologic, cytologic, and endoscopic examination.[63] Although the incidence of gastric cancer is decreasing, aggressive preventive health care in high-risk individuals is necessary to ensure that this decline continues.

Patient and Family History

To establish a clinical picture a complete assessment of the individual's nutritional status, physical examination, and social and family history should be done. An in-depth nutritional assessment and history aid in diagnosis and treatment planning by identifying subtle changes in dietary habits or contributory signs such as pain or bowel changes. Areas to include in a nutritional history/assessment are as follows:

1. Food and fluid intake patterns (types, amount, number, calories)
2. Symptoms associated with eating (pain, eructation, dysphagia, nausea, fullness, reflux)
3. Change in dietary habits or appetite (food intolerance, aversions, volume, types of food)
4. Weight (actual, usual, ideal)
5. Bowel patterns and habits (frequency, consistency, color, flatulence)
6. Medications (over-the-counter, home remedies, prescriptions)
7. Previous/concurrent illness (childhood, adult, transient maladies)

Physical Examination

The physical examination includes palpation of the abdomen and lymph nodes, particularly the supraclavicular and axillary lymph nodes because they are possible metastatic sites. An abdominal mass and/or hepatomegaly may be palpated. A rectal examination could reveal a shelf of metastatic deposits. If an obstruction exists in the pyloric area, peristaltic activity moving in a left-to-right direction may be detected. Advanced gastric cancer can result in anemia and jaundice.

Diagnostic Studies

Any signs and symptoms suggestive of gastric cancer should be investigated by diagnostic procedures to identify their source. Enlarged lymph nodes and hepatomegaly indicate the need for biopsy. Radiologic examinations are essential in diagnosis. An upper gastrointestinal series and double-contrast upper gastrointestinal series will reveal the mucosal pattern, character of mobility, distensibility, and flexibility of the walls. Filling defects and rigidity of walls suggest malignant involvement. CT scanning is useful in defining metastases and tumor extension. After radiologic examinations that involve the use of barium, care must be taken to administer laxatives to prevent barium impaction.

Accuracy of diagnosis is enhanced by endoscopic examination to view the lesion directly and to obtain washings for biopsy and cytologic examination.[27,61] Flexible fiberoptic scopes are more comfortable for the individual, less traumatic to the gastrointestinal tissue, and provide a diagnostic accuracy rate of greater than 90% when combined with biopsy and cytology.[61,64] Topical anesthetics, analgesics, or sedatives are administered to facilitate the endoscopic instrumentation and to make the patient comfortable. For 2 to 4 hours after the procedure, nursing measures should be employed to prevent aspiration or trauma. The patient receives nothing to eat or drink until a gag reflex returns; hoarseness from throat irritation can be relieved by lozenges or warm saline gargles after the effects of anesthesia dissipate; and the patient should be observed periodically for signs of perforation (ie, fever, abdominal pain or distention, dyspnea, cyanosis, and subcutaneous crepitus).

Laboratory analyses include hematologic profiles, which may reveal anemia resulting from gradual blood loss in both gastric cancer and chronic gastric ulcer. Differential diagnosis between gastric ulcer and gastric cancer is difficult. Malignancy is highly probable when there is a chronic unresponsive gastric ulcer, gastric ulcer on the greater curvature of the stomach, obstruction in the presence of ulcer, or achlorhydria and positive cytologic findings. Karyometric studies of DNA content have correlated high ploidy gastric tumors with a higher incidence of lymphatic and vascular invasion.[65]

CLASSIFICATION AND STAGING

Treatment planning ensues once a diagnosis is confirmed and the extent of involvement is delineated. The prognosis and treatment plan depend on the stage of the disease and general well-being of the individual. The American Joint Committee for Cancer Staging and End-Results Reporting has established and adopted the TNM classification system listed in Table 39-3.

TREATMENT

Before the initiation of a treatment plan the patient and family should receive a thorough explanation of the anticipated course and expected outcomes. The overall plan of therapy for gastric cancer depends on the stage of the disease and current advances in surgery, radiotherapy, and chemotherapy.

Localized gastric carcinomas are treated with curative intent with aggressive surgery alone or in combination with chemotherapy or radiotherapy. Approximately 50% of patients are candidates for curative resection.

Advanced tumors that are partially resectable, unresectable, or disseminated are treated with therapy combining surgery and chemotherapy, with or without radiotherapy, and palliative surgery. Palliative procedures such as esophagojejunostomy or partial gastric resection alleviate obstructive tumors and restore intestinal continuity. If the individual cannot withstand or elects not to have such a procedure, less traumatic palliative procedures may be done such as insertion of a synthetic tube or a gastro-

TABLE 39-3 TNM Classification for Gastric Carcinoma

Primary Tumor (T)

TX	Primary tumor cannot be assessed
T0	No evidence of primary tumor
Tis	Carcinoma *in situ:* intraepithelial tumor without invasion of the lamina propria
T1	Tumor invades lamina propria or submucosa
T2	Tumor invades the muscularis propria or the subserosa
T3	Tumor penetrates the serosa (visceral peritoneum) without invasion of adjacent structures
T4	Tumor invades adjacent structures

Regional Lymph Nodes (N)

NX	Regional lymph node(s) cannot be assessed
N0	No regional lymph node metastasis
N1	Metastasis in perigastric lymph node(s) within 3 cm of the edge of the primary tumor
N2	Metastasis in perigastric lymph node(s) more than 3 cm from the edge of the primary tumor, or in lymph nodes along the left gastric, common hepatic, splenic, or celiac arteries

Distant Metastasis (M)

MX	Presence of distant metastasis cannot be assessed
M0	No distant metastasis
M1	Distant metastasis

Stage Grouping

Stage 0	Tis	N0	M0
Stage IA	T1	N0	M0
Stage IB	T1	N1	M0
	T2	N0	M0
Stage II	T1	N2	M0
	T2	N1	M0
	T3	N0	M0
Stage IIIA	T2	N2	M0
	T3	N1	M0
	T4	N0	M0
Stage IIIB	T3	N2	M0
	T4	N1	M0
Stage IV	T4	N2	M0
	Any T	Any N	M1

Source: Beahrs Oh, Henson DE, Hutter RV, et al (eds): American Joint Committee on Cancer: Manual for Staging of Cancer (ed 3). Philadelphia, JB Lippincott, 1988.

jejunostomy. Combinations of chemotherapeutic agents have produced transient improvements with advanced tumors.[61]

Surgery

Total gastrectomy

If the lesion is resectable and located in the midportion or body of the stomach, a total gastrectomy usually is performed. The entire stomach is removed en bloc, along with supporting mesentery and lymph nodes. The esophagus is anastomosed to the jejunum. A thoracic approach sometimes is necessary to perform the esophagojejunostomy. Pneumonia, infection, anastomotic leak, hemorrhage, or reflux aspiration are frequent complications. Overall mortality rates are 10% to 15% for persons who undergo total gastrectomy.[66] In Japan extended lymph node dissection and extended regional resection that include the pancreas are common.[54,67]

Radical subtotal gastrectomy

Lesions located in the middle and distal half of the stomach are treated by subtotal gastrectomy. A Billroth I or Billroth II procedure will be done. A Billroth I, or gastroduodenostomy, involves resecting the first portion of the duodenum, the distal stomach, pylorus, and supporting circulatory and lymph vessels. The remaining stomach is anastomosed to the duodenum. Billroth I is the procedure of choice in elderly or debilitated individuals, when intraoperative time is of paramount importance. Because the procedure limits the scope of resection, the Billroth I is not as desirable as the Billroth II for gastric cancer.

The Billroth II is the surgery of choice for a person who requires and can tolerate a more radical procedure. A wider resection that includes about 75% of the stomach is possible, thereby decreasing the possibility of nodal or metastatic growth. A Billroth II involves removal of the antrum, pylorus, first portion of the duodenum, supporting circulatory structures, and all visible and palpable lymph nodes. With this procedure, the remaining stomach is anastomosed end-to-side to the jejunum. The duodenal stump is closed with sutures.

Gastric emptying is altered by the Billroth I and II procedures. The complications and resultant sequelae of the Billroth I and II procedures are the same as in all postgastrectomy syndromes. Steatorrhea, dumping syndrome, nausea, vomiting, weight loss, diarrhea, vitamin deficiency, and anastomotic leak may develop.

Subtotal esophagogastrectomy

If a resectable tumor is located in the proximal portion of the stomach, cardia, or fundus, a subtotal esophagogastrectomy is performed. This entails en bloc removal of the lower portion of the esophagus and supporting circulatory and lymphatic structures; removal of most of the greater and lesser omenta; and resection of the cardia, fundus, and body (sometimes a total gastrectomy). The esophagus is sutured to the duodenum or jejunum. A thoracoabdominal approach may be required. Potential complications include pneumonia, anastomotic leak, infection, reflux aspiration, and esophagitis.[68]

Postoperative care

Nursing measures for the person with gastric cancer who undergoes surgical resection do not differ from those for other individuals who undergo gastric surgery. The nurse must be acutely aware of the preoperative status of the individual and employ the nursing measures necessary to maintain or improve the person's preoperative condition. Pneumonia, infection, anastomotic leak, hemorrhage, and reflux aspiration are frequent complications after radical gastric surgery.

Dumping syndrome is a potential sequela of subtotal gastrectomy and total gastrectomy that affects many but not all individuals. The same nursing principles and care measures apply to the person with gastric cancer who experiences dumping syndrome as to the person with any other gastric disease that requires a total gastrectomy. Small, frequent feedings of low carbohydrate, high-fat, high-protein foods are recommended. It is important to restrict liquids for 30 to 40 minutes before and after a meal to avoid the effects of dumping syndrome.[69] Vitamin B_{12} deficiency will occur; thus monthly parenteral replacement therapy is necessary.

Radiation Therapy

Gastric adenocarcinomas generally are radiosensitive. In the abdomen there are dose-limited organs (ie, stomach, liver, kidney, and spinal cord) that restrict the use of radiotherapy. Radiation therapy usually is administered as adjuvant therapy in conjunction with chemotherapy or surgery. It is particularly useful for the treatment of locally advanced or recurrent disease. Patients seem to tolerate 4000 to 5000 cGy administered in fractionated doses over 4 to 5 weeks.[61] Transient effects on the rapidly proliferating epithelial cells of the gastrointestinal tract may lead to abdominal cramps, diarrhea, anorexia, nausea, or vomiting.

Radiotherapy is used to augment local regional control of residual or unresectable gastric cancer. Radiotherapy combined with surgical resection has been documented to increase 3- and 5-year survival rates, as compared with surgical intervention alone.[64] Multimodal therapy of radiation and chemotherapy for patients with unresectable disease have been documented to improve survival versus either radiotherapy or chemotherapy alone.[61,70-72] The sequence of administration of chemotherapy and radiotherapy is being studied to determine if there is any radiosensitization effect, diminished repopulation between treatments, or synergistic effect.[73]

Intraoperative radiotherapy is being used most extensively in Japan, where gastric cancer is a critical problem.[74] The advantage of delivering radiotherapy intraoperatively is the capability for direct visualization of the site to be irradiated and the opportunity to physically move dose-limited tissues out of the field during the radiation. A cancericidal dose of 2800 to 3500 cGy is delivered directly to the tumor bed.[74] The disadvantages of this treatment approach are the special equipment, operating rooms, and extensive professional collaboration that are required. Intraoperative radiotherapy is provided by only a few institutions in the United States. Its role in the management of gastric cancer has not been well studied in the United States; therefore it is too early to know the full impact of this approach.

Chemotherapy

No one specific chemotherapeutic regimen for gastric cancer has had a clear impact on patient survival. Single agents (5-fluorouracil and 5-fluorouracil deoxyribonucleoside [FUDR]) have been studied, but combination drug therapy appears to be superior. Single agents typically produce response rates in 20% of the cases, whereas combination chemotherapy can result in 30% to 50% response rates.[75]

The combination regimen used most commonly is FAM (5-fluorouracil, doxorubicin [Adriamycin], and mitomycin C). Other drugs used in combination regimens include cisplatin and the nitrosoureas.[76,77] Toxic effects depend on the drug and the dose. Alternative methods of delivery are being investigated, such as intraoperative, intra-arterial, and intraperitoneal administration.[75,78,79]

Survival time is increased somewhat when chemotherapy is used with surgical resection or radiotherapy. At present, objective response rates of gastric tumors treated with chemotherapy are low and have not substantiated the use of chemotherapy as a standard clinical treatment.

Supportive Therapy

Advanced gastric cancer can result in the individual's rapid deterioration. Medical and nursing management is aimed at controlling symptoms and maintaining optimal function. As gastric cancer advances, nutrition becomes a serious problem, either because of disruption of gastric continuity or gastric dysfunction. Lack of gastric secretory function leads to both enzymatic and nutrient deficiencies. The resulting malnutrition decreases the individual's ability to withstand therapy, fight infection, and perform self-care activities. Nutritional surveillance and aggressive approaches to maintaining a high level of nutrition are nursing priorities. (Chapter 10 presents suggestions for the management of nutritional problems.) From the time of diagnosis until death due to gastric cancer, nutrition presents one of the most challenging management problems.

When gastric cancer spreads to the most common metastatic sites (regional lymph nodes, intraperitoneal, liver, pancreas, lung, and bone), the manifestations of disease in those areas require the anticipatory and symptomatic nursing measures discussed in the chapters on specific manifestations of cancer. Individuals with gastric cancer commonly die of bronchopneumonia or lung abscess as a result of malnutrition or immobility. Other causes of death in those with gastric cancer are deep vein thrombosis, pulmonary emboli, anastomotic rupture, or a second primary tumor.[64]

Many patients and their families may feel a strong sense of guilt and negligence if the patient delayed seeking medical attention or opted for self-medication for any length of time. The nurse can support the individual and family by dispelling misconceptions and by promoting a realistic sense of hope.

LIVER TUMORS

INTRODUCTION

Liver cancer, despite its relative rarity, continues to be a serious problem in many areas of the world. In Africa and Asia it is one of the leading causes of death from cancer. In the United States, experience with liver tumors in children and adults is limited by the small number of cases. Many critical questions about this disease remain unanswered. Liver cancers have unusual clinical and pathologic features. At present no specific treatment effectively controls this aggressive malignancy. Liver cancer disseminates within the liver early and frequently is associated with cirrhosis. Early detection and diagnosis are critical factors.

ANATOMY

The liver is divided into two functional parts: a right and left lobe. It has a far-reaching lymphatic system that consists of superficial and deep lymphatic vessels. Superficial lymphatic vessels course from the superficial lobules of the liver to the periphery and extend beneath the peritoneum. Other superficial lymphatic vessels pass through the diaphragm and flow into the pericardial and mediastinal nodes, some follow the esophagus to the coronary chain nodes, and others follow the liver to end in the hepatic pedicle nodes and the inferior vena cava. The deep lymphatic vessels originate in the deep lobules of the liver to follow several courses: along the portal and suprahepatic veins; through the diaphragm to the supradiaphragmatic nodes; and along the portal vein branches to end in the hepatic pedicle, hepatic artery, or coronary chain nodes.

The liver has a complex and rich network of circulation. Afferent vessels are the hepatic artery and portal vein. The hepatic artery supplies most of the oxygen to the liver, whereas the portal vein carries about 75% of the total blood flow to the liver. Blood drains from the liver via the hepatic veins into the inferior vena cava. The liver contains a mass of branching blood vessels of varying sizes that extend to all areas of the liver.[80]

EPIDEMIOLOGY

Primary liver cancer accounts for about 2% of all cancers in the world.[81] In the United States there are approximately 14,500 new cases and 11,400 deaths from primary liver cancer each year.[1] In some areas of the world, liver cancer is up to 10 times more prevalent among men than among women.[81] The average age of onset is 60 to 70 years; however, liver tumors are encountered in persons of all ages. Liver cancer in children is rare.

An unusual epidemiologic aspect of liver cancer is its geographic distribution. Liver cancer is uncommon in North America, but it is a major problem in some of the more populous areas of the world, including South Africa, Asia, and the Pacific areas.

ETIOLOGY

Hepatocellular carcinomas are associated with alcohol-induced, nutritional, or posthepatitic cirrhosis of the liver. A rare form of cirrhosis called *hemochromatosis* (a genetic disorder of iron deposits in parenchymal cells) in combination with cirrhosis is associated with primary liver tumors. It is suggested that the chronic liver injury and subsequent continuous regeneration associated with cirrhosis may precipitate a loss of normal cellular controls and lead to liver neoplasia.[82]

A close relationship has been identified between liver cancer and chronic hepatitis B infection. Chronic hepatitis B infection causes liver damage and cirrhosis and appears to increase the risk of liver cancer development.[83,84]

Malnutrition has been cited as an etiologic factor because many of the geographic areas with a high incidence of liver cancer experience food shortages, poverty, and malnutrition.[84] No particular nutrient deficiency has been identified, although the incidence of kwashiorkor (a form of protein-calorie malnutrition) closely parallels that of liver cancer.[85] There also is a high incidence of liver cancer in tropical climates and areas where mold spoilage is significant.

Several naturally occurring substances have been found to produce malignant hepatomas in animals and thus have become suspect as etiologic agents in human beings. Aflatoxin B1, a mycotoxin derived from the fungus *Aspergillus flavus* is among these.[84,86,87] In Africa and Taiwan, researchers have found a correlation between the incidence of liver cancer and areas in which food sources are heavily contaminated by aflatoxin.[87]

Thorotrast, a drug formerly used for diagnostic purposes, may have produced chronic, progressive liver damage.[86] After a latent period of approximately 20 years, liver cancer may develop.[88] An increased incidence of liver damage and liver tumors has been reported among industrial employees who work with vinyl chloride.

The association between etiologic factors and the development of liver cancer is not strong at this time, mostly because of the limited number of cases of primary liver cancer. Environmental, clinical, and genetic factors all have been suggested. It is hoped that further investigation will provide definitive explanations.

Oral contraceptives have been reported to have an association with liver tumors; however, mostly benign tumors were involved.[89-92] Short-term use appears to have no association.[93] The relationship of oral contraceptives to liver tumors is unclear and the evidence scanty.

PATHOPHYSIOLOGY

Tumors in the liver may be primary cancer of the liver or secondary tumors that have metastasized from other sites. *Primary malignant hepatoma* and *hepatocellular carcinoma* are terms used interchangeably in the literature. One of the most critical issues in the diagnosis of liver cancer is to ascertain whether the cancer is a primary liver tumor or a metastatic growth in the liver.

Cellular Characteristics

Primary liver carcinoma

Most primary malignant tumors of the liver are adenocarcinomas of two major cell types: about 90% are hepatocellular carcinomas arising from liver cells and about 8% are cholangiocarcinomas arising from the bile duct cells. A very small proportion are hepatoblastomas, angiosarcomas, or sarcomas.[27,84] Only hepatocellular and cholangiocarcinomas are discussed in this chapter.

The macroscopic appearance of primary hepatocellular carcinoma is characterized by three forms: nodular, massive, or diffuse. The nodular type consists of multiple, similarly sized, widely dispersed clusters of cells. The massive type often has a single dominant large mass from which there are associated satellite nodules. The diffuse form is characterized by an extensive pattern of infiltration that may involve the entire liver.[27] All three forms of hepatocellular carcinoma originate mainly in the right lobe. The tumor may have a multicentric origin, commonly seen in cirrhotic livers, or it may start from a single focus to subsequent satellite lesions and then enlarge. Hepatocellular carcinomas generally are soft, highly vascular, and diffluent with stroma. Parts of the liver may be dull gray or green as a result of the presence of bile. There may be areas of necrosis, which can lead to intraperitoneal hemorrhage. Infiltration of the diaphragm and neighboring tissues or invasion of the portal and/or hepatic veins may be a feature. Regional lymph node metastasis is uncommon, which is a definitive characteristic of liver cancer. Cholangiocarcinomas also exhibit nodular or diffuse forms but usually appear as a solitary grayish-white mass. This type of tumor is firm and fibrous and may secrete mucin but does not form bile. Cholangiocarcinoma tends to invade surrounding parenchyma in a disorderly, irregular form and metastasize late.

Liver tumors often are well-differentiated lesions that resemble the tissue of origin. The cells are larger than normal parenchymal cells, with clearly defined margins. An uncommon histologic variant is clear cell carcinoma of the liver, characterized by a high content of glycogen, which results in marked vacuolation that causes a clear cytoplasm.[94] Tumor doubling time may be used as an indicator of survival. Longer doubling times are associated with a longer survival period.[95]

Secondary liver carcinoma

The liver is a repository for metastatic deposits from nearly all forms of malignancies. A tumor in the liver is 20 times more likely to be a metastatic deposit than a primary liver cancer.[96] Metastases to the liver usually are from the following high-incidence sites: lung, breast, kidney, and the intestinal tract (gallbladder, extrahepatic bile ducts, pancreas, stomach, colon, and rectum). Two patterns of secondary liver carcinoma predominate: (1) invasive growth from cancer of neighboring organs or structures (such as the stomach or colon) and (2) metastases through the portal veins.[97] Metastasis may occur as a single mass, but more often metastatic deposits are multiple masses in the liver. Once metastatic tumor cells are in the liver, spread within the rest of the liver is through the venous system. Metastatic tumors in the liver usually indicate that the primary carcinoma is incurable. However, if a localized metastasis in the liver can be resected or controlled with chemotherapy, then the primary tumor can be pursued aggressively. It is uncommon for a cancer to metastasize to a cirrhotic liver, possibly because the tissue damage precludes a favorable environment for metastases.[98]

Progression of Disease

Liver cancer tends to advance by direct extension within and around the liver and by direct invasion of venous and lymphatic channels within the liver. The tumor will enlarge within the lobules that have been weakened by pressure and derangement of the blood supply. Venous invasion commonly accounts for the multinodular appearance of hepatocellular carcinoma. The tumor grows along the veins as a solid mass to distal parts of the liver.[84,94] About 50% of individuals with liver cancer will have distant metastases to regional lymph nodes, lungs, bone, adrenal glands, and brain.[81,84,86]

Liver tumors typically alter the pattern of blood flow within the liver. Tumors receive their blood supply almost exclusively from the hepatic artery and drain via the hepatic vein.[99] Normal liver tissue receives its blood supply from both the hepatic artery and portal vein and drains via the hepatic vein. Within the liver the tumor may spread by emboli or by directly permeating the hepatic and portal veins, resulting in rapid spread of the tumor throughout the liver. Portal vein occlusion is common.[84,94]

As liver cancer advances, serious complications arise, and multiple body systems become affected. Hemorrhage has been cited as the cause of death of about 50% of individuals with liver cancer.[100] It is postulated that if the portal vein becomes obstructed rapidly, as occurs with tumor emboli, there is insufficient time for the collateral branches of the hepatic circulatory system to compensate. As a result the tamponade effect can lead to necrosis, rupture, and hemorrhage.[97] Esophageal varices and unrelenting ascites are common sequelae of either primary or secondary liver cancer.

Because of the late onset of definitive signs, liver cancer can be far advanced by the time of diagnosis. The prognosis is poor, with an overall 5-year survival rate of less than 2%.[1,101] If the disease is unresectable, death usually occurs within 6 months of diagnosis.[102] The cause of death from liver cancer most often is pneumonia, malnutrition, thromboemboli, hepatic failure, or hemorrhage.[86]

CLINICAL MANIFESTATIONS

The natural history of carcinoma of the liver is insidious and rapidly progressive, with characteristic clinical signs and symptoms. In adults the most common clinical manifestation is abdominal pain. Characteristically, the pain is not severe; rather it is dull, aching, and confined to the right upper quadrant of the abdomen. It may later radiate to the right scapula. The continuous pain may become more troublesome, prevent sleep, and be aggravated if the patient lies on the right side or experiences jolting movements. Profound, progressive weakness and fatigue are characteristic of liver cancer. Fullness in the epigastrium, especially after meals, and constipation or diarrhea are common manifestations. Anorexia and loss of weight are indicators of advanced disease.

Mild jaundice is present in some cases. Liver cancer should be suspected in all persons with cirrhosis who experience sudden or unexpected deterioration in health. Cirrhosis is found in 30% to 70% of persons with hepatocellular carcinoma.[86,103] On palpation, the liver is an enlarged, hard, nodular mass; a pedunculated tumor occasionally can be felt. Enlargement may be diffuse or limited to one lobe (usually the right).

Ascites and signs of portal hypertension that result from portal vein compression frequently accompany advanced disease. Hematemesis as a result of esophageal varices or tumor invasion of the stomach can occur. Paraneoplastic syndromes may occur, including hypercalcemia, hypoglycemia, polycythemia, carcinoid syndrome, gynecomastia, porphyria, and coagulation abnormalities.[27]

ASSESSMENT

Primary liver cancer is silent for a long period before it produces signs and symptoms that prompt the individual to seek medical attention. The person may be treated initially for a disorder that mimics liver cell cancer, such as gastritis. Systemic signs and symptoms appear late in the course of the disease and make it easier to establish a definitive diagnosis. The choice of therapy will be based on the location and extent of tumor involvement, whether extrahepatic spread has occurred, and the individual's general condition.

Physical Examination

A complete physical examination usually reveals a painful, enlarged liver and such manifestations as ascites, edema, circulatory disorders, esophageal varices, jaundice, or hematemesis.[86] Endocrine changes such as menstrual disorders, testicular atrophy, or gynecomastia may be observed.

Diagnostic Studies

Radiologic examinations

A simple radiograph of the abdomen may establish hepatomegaly and displacement or deformity of contiguous structures. An upper gastrointestinal series may evidence organ displacement. Ultrasound of the abdomen, CT of the abdomen and lungs, and MRI are noninvasive techniques used in the diagnostic evaluation of liver cancer.

Radioisotope scanning is an effective noninvasive technique for outlining primary and metastatic tumors of the liver. Small lesions less than 2.5 cm in diameter may be missed by the photoscanning device. The difference between a malignant and benign tumor cannot be discerned with a scan; therefore this technique should be correlated with the biopsy, laboratory studies, and hepatic arteriogram.

If a patient is considered to be a candidate for surgery, angiography is a useful diagnostic tool to provide information about the appearance, size, and number of lesions. Splenoportography demonstrates the extent of tumor spread into the portal vein. If the tumor has spread above the bifurcation of the portal vein, surgery is hazardous and alternate treatment must be selected. Assessment of the inferior vena cava can be accomplished by means of venacavography. Hepatic resection is not advisable if the vena cava is infiltrated. Selective hepatic arteriography is the single most useful procedure for identifying tumor vasculature and showing any abnormalities in the liver's blood supply. This information will serve as the "road map" for ligation of vessels during hepatic resection, chemotherapy administration, or therapeutic diversion of blood flow. The individual who undergoes arteriographic examination should be observed carefully for 24 hours after the procedure for signs of hemorrhage from a perforated or weakened vessel.

Laboratory studies

The hematologic profiles and liver function tests of most individuals with localized primary liver cancer who do not have cirrhosis show normal findings. In the absence of cirrhosis, tumor growth can extensively involve parenchyma before liver function is impaired. Liver function tests are not definitive diagnostic aids but can alert the clinician to a possible tumor and assist in selecting the appropriate therapy. Elevated levels of bilirubin, alkaline phosphatase, aspartate aminotransferase (SGOT), and

LDH (lactic dehydrogenase) alert the clinician to a possible liver tumor.

Alpha-fetoprotein is a tumor marker that is elevated in the serum of 30% to 90% of persons with primary hepatocellular carcinoma.[84,86] Because levels of alpha-fetoprotein are not specific for liver cancer, histologic diagnosis is required. The alpha-fetoprotein test gives negative results in cholangiocarcinoma and metastatic cancer of the liver. Alpha-fetoprotein disappears 1 to 2 weeks after a hepatocellular carcinoma is successfully resected. A reappearance of alpha-fetoprotein can indicate a recurrence. Serial monitoring of alpha-fetoprotein levels is being evaluated for definitive use as a measure of the effectiveness of therapy.

Elevated levels of carcinoembryonic antigen (CEA) are not indicative of primary liver cancer but may signify metastatic involvement. Colon cancer often metastasizes to the liver and will produce elevated CEA levels.

Biopsy

Biopsy is required to establish a histologically verified diagnosis. Needle biopsy should be done only in cooperative individuals with normal hemostatic function. Because most liver tumors are highly vascular, the individual must be monitored closely for intra-abdominal hemorrhage after needle biopsy. Potential complications after liver biopsy are hemorrhage, shock, peritonitis, and pneumothorax. If the tumor is localized, a definitive needle biopsy specimen could be difficult to obtain. Ultrasound-guided percutaneous needle biopsy is a rapid, safe procedure that is commonly used. As with any biopsy, absence of tumor cells in the biopsy specimen should not rule out the possibility of cancer. Many clinicians believe strongly that needle biopsy should be avoided at all cost if there is any chance for curative resection. They believe that the needle violates the tumor capsule, thereby potentially seeding and spreading the cancer.

CLASSIFICATION AND STAGING

A staging system has been developed for liver cancer that incorporates tumor size, location within the liver, extent of disease within and external to the liver, and metastatic sites.[21] The staging system has not been universally accepted but is available for use (Table 39-4).

TABLE 39-4 TNM Classification System for Liver Cancer

Primary Tumor (T)

TX Primary tumor cannot be assessed
T0 No evidence of primary tumor
T1 Solitary tumor 2 cm or less in greatest dimension without vascular invasion
T2 Solitary tumor 2 cm or less in greatest dimension with vascular invasion, *or*
Multiple tumors limited to one lobe, none more than 2 cm in greatest dimension without vascular invasion, *or*
A solitary tumor more than 2 cm in greatest dimension without vascular invasion
T3 Solitary tumor more than 2 cm in greatest dimension with vascular invasion, *or*
Multiple tumors limited to one lobe, none more than 2 cm in greatest dimension, with vascular invasion, *or*
Multiple tumors limited to one lobe, any more than 2 cm in greatest dimension, with or without vascular invasion
T4 Multiple tumors in more than one lobe *or*
Tumor(s) involve(s) a major branch of portal or hepatic vein(s)

Regional Lymph Nodes (N)

NX Regional lymph nodes cannot be assessed
N0 No regional lymph node metastasis
N1 Regional lymph node metastasis

Distant Metastasis (M)

MX Presence of distant metastasis cannot be assessed
M0 No distant metastasis
M1 Distant metastasis

Stage Grouping

Stage I	T1	N0	M0
Stage II	T2	N0	M0
Stage III	T1	N1	M0
	T2	N1	M0
	T3	N0, N1	M0
Stage IVA	T4	Any N	M0
Stage IVB	Any T	Any N	M1

Source: Beahrs OH, Henson DE, Hutter RV, et al (eds): American Joint Committee on Cancer: Manual of Staging of Cancer (ed 3). Philadelphia, JB Lippincott, 1988.

TREATMENT

Treatment Planning

Treatment of liver cancer provides a twofold challenge. First, the limited number of cases of primary liver cancer makes systematic investigation of therapy difficult. Second, the dismal outlook for persons with liver cancer has led to misconceptions about the effectiveness of various treatments, which have taken years to dispel. Surgery, radiotherapy, and chemotherapy play a significant role in the treatment of both primary and secondary liver cancer. At present, immunotherapy has a more limited clinical role.

The 5-year survival rate for persons with primary liver cancer is low, less than 2%.[86] The mean survival time has been estimated at 6 months from diagnosis.[102] For individuals with solitary localized liver cancer, however, advances in surgery, radiotherapy, and chemotherapy offer hope of cure or extended control. The choice of treatment depends on a number of factors: type and extent of the tumor, concomitant diseases, liver function and reserve, patient and family preference, hematologic status, nutritional status, age, and skill of the principal clinicians. Assessment of the patient's learning ability, coping mechanisms, and compliance potential are of great importance, especially if long-term therapy is anticipated.

Pretreatment therapy

Before the initiation of any therapeutic modality, physiologic factors are examined carefully. Most individuals with primary liver cancer have some degree of anemia; therefore complete blood profiles should be compiled and the anemia corrected. Efforts are made by the nurse and other health care workers to conserve the individual's energy and to begin instruction in the appropriate measures to help minimize the anemia.

Depending on the extent of liver dysfunction produced by tumor involvement, deficits in clotting mechanisms can exist. Vitamin K is administered, fluid and electrolyte imbalances corrected, and measures to prevent trauma or bleeding are taken.

Vitamins A, C, D, and B complex can be given to reduce the effect of jaundice, if present. Pruritus, which frequently accompanies jaundice, is precipitated by irritation of the cutaneous sensory nerve fibers by accumulated bile salts. Meticulous skin hygiene and efforts to reduce itching are instituted. The use of deodorant soaps should be avoided because they tend to dry the skin and make the pruritus more intense. Relief is sometimes obtained with oil-based lotions, antihistamines, or cholestyramine. Side effects of cholestyramine are nausea, vomiting, constipation, and bleeding tendencies.[17] The only effective measure for relief of pruritis is resolution of the jaundice.

Most individuals with liver cancer are in a poor nutritional state and benefit greatly from a diet high in proteins and carbohydrates and moderate in fats. If weight loss has been significant (more than 7 kg/mo), enteral feedings or total parenteral nutrition may be used to correct the nutritional imbalance. If the treatment is expected to affect nutritional status adversely, aggressive nutrition regimens must begin early.

Objectives of treatment

Primary liver cancer Cure is the objective of therapy if the primary liver tumor is a localized, solitary mass without evidence of regional lymph node involvement, distant metastases, or cirrhosis. Aggressive efforts toward eradicating the tumor and possible micrometastases will be planned. Surgical excision of the primary liver cancer is the only definitive treatment for cure. Only about 25% of patients with primary liver cancer are candidates for radical resection.[84,104] Adjuvant chemotherapy and radiotherapy usually are initiated to eliminate residual cancer cells or micrometastases.

If the tumor is multicentric, involves a large portion of the liver, or involves extrahepatic areas, control of tumor growth is the objective of therapy. Control can be achieved by surgical resection to remove or debulk the tumor, radiotherapy, or specific vascular ligation or cannulation followed by aggressive use of chemotherapeutic agents.

Palliation of the disabling effects of liver cancer may be the objective of treatment for advanced disease. Surgery, chemotherapy, and radiotherapy are used selectively to increase the individual's comfort and quality of life.

Secondary liver tumors When metastatic deposits occur in the liver, cure of the primary cancer is difficult. Aggressive therapy is employed if the metastatic deposit is a solitary or well-defined mass in a single lobe of the liver. Treatment of metastatic tumors to the liver may be surgical excision, arterial infusion of chemotherapeutic agents, ligation of the hepatic artery, or radiotherapy.[105] The aim of aggressive treatment of metastatic tumors in the liver is to control the tumor, increase survival time, and palliate debilitating symptoms (such as jaundice, anemia, and pain). Individuals with colorectal carcinoma that has metastasized to the liver are the most typical candidates for resection of the liver metastases because the liver usually is the first metastatic site for colorectal tumors. Subsequently, the primary colon tumor can be eradicated in some cases.

Surgery

Surgical excision is the most definitive treatment for primary liver tumors.[106] If cirrhosis is present, the surgical risk is directly proportional to the degree of cirrhosis. If the noncancerous lobe of the liver is macroscopically normal or only mildly cirrhotic, lobectomy can be undertaken safely. If cirrhosis is moderately advanced, left lobectomy can be considered; however, right hepatic lobectomy would be difficult and potentially life threatening. Local resection, cryosurgery, or laser surgery may be possible.[106,107] Those with severe cirrhosis are not candidates for surgery.

Extensive assessment must be done before hepatic resection to identify any possible contraindications. In addition to severe cirrhosis, contraindications to major hepatic resection include the following factors[86,102,108]:

1. Distant metastases in the lung, bone, or lymph nodes indicate a futile attempt at cure or control. Multiple discrete tumor nodules throughout both anatomic lobes would rule out surgery as the treatment of choice.

2. Jaundice, although not always the case, could indicate tumor extension or obstruction of the common bile duct. Palliative resection of the tumor can be done to relieve the progressive jaundice.

3. Ascites usually indicates liver failure and inability to tolerate any surgical procedure. The ascites may result from tumor cell seeding in the peritoneal cavity and/or cirrhosis. In either case it is preferable to control the ascites medically; although surgery could be considered, it is risky.

4. Poor visualization on angiographic studies jeopardizes the certainty with which the surgeon resects the tumor. Because the liver is a highly vascular organ, intraoperative hemorrhage is a great risk in all hepatic surgical procedures.

5. Biochemical changes that indicate poor liver function lower the probability of survival.

6. Involvement of the inferior vena cava or retrograde intraluminal growth within and to the portal vein bifurcation makes surgical excision hazardous.

Therefore, if the tumor is localized, solitary, and can be defined anatomically, a wide en bloc surgical excision is the initial treatment of choice for both primary and secondary liver tumors. From 80 to 85% of the noncirrhotic liver can be removed safely, unless the tumor is in the posterior segment of the right lobe where the hepatic vein is embedded. Hepatic lobectomy includes all the vessels involved with the lobe and requires extensive operative time. Partial resections (segmentectomy, wedge resection) are used in patients with mild cirrhosis.[109] Cryosurgery with liquid nitrogen has been employed for local excision of tumors in patients with nonresectable liver cancer.[110] (Several sources[82,88,97,111] present detailed information about the techniques of the surgical procedure.) Liver transplantation is still in the experimental stage and fraught with a high incidence of recurrent cancer in the transplanted liver.[112]

As a form of therapy, ligation or embolization of the principal hepatic vessels that supply the tumor has been used to necrose the tumor. Gelfoam cubes, metal coils, chemotherapy-laden microspheres, and surgical ligation are techniques for restricting blood flow.[84,86,113] The approaches are considered experimental and have not been proved superior to other treatment methods at this time.

Postoperative care

Overall surgical mortality (individuals who do not survive the hospitalization period) is less than 15% with hepatic resection.[84,86,114,115] Individuals who have had hepatic resection require intensive medical and nursing support until the liver regenerates adequately and postoperative recovery is complete. The principal concerns in the care of an individual who undergoes hepatic surgery are control of hemorrhage, prevention of infection and pneumonia, and appropriate supportive care. The individual with cirrhosis has greater difficulty in the postoperative period than the individual who is free of cirrhosis. Knowledge of the potential complications, expected reactions, and anticipatory nursing care will aid immeasurably in the postoperative period. The major complications after liver resection include hemorrhage, biliary fistula, infection, transient metabolic consequences, subphrenic abscess, pneumonia, atelectasis, portal hypertension, and clotting defects.

Hemorrhage The abundant vascularity of the liver cannot be overemphasized. Despite preventive measures to control bleeding, intra-abdominal hemorrhage must be recognized early before the condition is irreversible. Hemorrhage usually appears within the first 24 hours after surgery. Nursing observations and assessments should include frequent monitoring of vital signs; monitoring of central venous pressure; examination of the skin and extremities for perfusion; accurate measurement of abdominal girth; frequent checks for bleeding from incision sites, urine, and stool; and close attention to fluid and electrolyte levels and blood profiles. In addition, individuals with cirrhosis should be watched closely for overt and subclinical signs of bleeding disorders as a result of their predisposition to hematologic complications.

Biliary fistula In most individuals who undergo hepatic resection a T-tube is placed in the common bile duct for drainage. A subhepatic drain also may be placed in the area of the surgical resection. A small amount of bile is expected to drain through the subhepatic drain from the necrosis on the edge of the liver. An excessive drainage of bile through the subhepatic drain, however, could indicate a biliary fistula that is pouring large amounts of bile into the subhepatic space. The T-tube also can slip outside the common bile duct. The dislodged T-tube may continue to drain small amounts of bile, thus masking its malposition, but the properly positioned T-tube normally will drain about 400 mL of bile per day. Fever, pain, and altered vital signs accompany biliary fistula.

Subphrenic abscess Incomplete or insufficient drainage of the surgical defect can precipitate a subphrenic abscess. Close attention to vital signs and the function and output of the drainage tubes should continue for an extended period because the abscess will appear later in the postoperative course. Auscultation of the base of the lungs could signal the presence of the abscess and fluid accumulation. Development of sharp, piercing pain in the right upper quadrant of the abdomen later in the postoperative course and a low-grade fever are other warning signs.

Infection Individuals with cirrhosis are more prone to infection after hepatic resection than are individuals without cirrhosis. The mortality associated with serious infection is high. Frequent monitoring of vital signs and assessment of the wound and drainage provide early clues of impending infection. Constant, intermittent, or remittent hyperthermia or hypothermia as a result of infection requires aggressive intervention.

Pneumonia and atelectasis Nursing care directed toward prevention of respiratory complications is similar to that for any other person who has abdominal or thoracic surgery. Aggressive pulmonary hygiene is especially important. These individuals will be reluctant to comply because respiratory exercises cause significant incisional pain. Early ambulation, administration of analgesics before pulmonary exercise, incisional support, and avoidance of contact with persons with respiratory infections are important nursing care measures.

Transient metabolic consequences Jaundice is common during the first postoperative week. Jaundice may result from the temporary inability of the remaining liver to handle bile, but the condition usually subsides by the third week when the remaining liver regenerates. More often, however, jaundice results from the multiple transfusions and anoxia of the hepatocytes caused by vascular occlusion during surgery. If the jaundice in an individual without cirrhosis does not subside after 10 days, mechanical obstruction should be suspected. Nursing measures to relieve the discomforts of jaundice were discussed earlier, in the section on pretreatment planning.

Portal hypertension Another transient postoperative consequence of hepatic resection that the nurse should anticipate is portal hypertension. Portal hypertension is the result of the surgical rerouting of portal venous flow through a small remnant of liver, which leads to splanchnic circulatory sequestration.[116] Fortunately, the liver has a great potential for increasing blood flow if it is given adequate time to compensate. Central venous pressure monitoring is a good indicator of blood volume. Bleeding episodes from any cavity, wound, or puncture site require immediate intervention.

Clotting defects The prothrombin time may be delayed during the first week. Severe coagulopathies generally develop during the operative period and usually are not a concern after surgery. The nurse should take measures to prevent and/or detect complications from deficiencies in the clotting mechanisms, such as applying pressure to injection sites, monitoring abdominal girth, and testing urine and stool for blood.

Chemotherapy

The majority of individuals with primary liver cancer are not candidates for curative or palliative surgery; therefore chemotherapy may be the treatment of choice for unresectable primary tumors of the liver. Chemotherapy also is used as adjuvant therapy after surgical extirpation. Metastatic tumors to the liver also can be treated with chemotherapeutic agents, but surgical excision is the preferred therapy.

Chemotherapeutic agents can be administered by two approaches: systemic administration of single or combination drug regimens and regional infusion via hepatic artery or portal vein. Single-agent therapy has produced poor results; however, current trials of combination therapy are producing promising results.[86]

The premise on which regional therapy is based is the ability to provide a high concentration of the drug directly and continuously to the tumor with minimal systemic exposure.[117,118] Dose limitations are related to toxic effects to the liver and the upper gastrointestinal tract.[117,119,120] Continuous infusion pumps and the totally implantable pumps have renewed clinicians' interest in regional therapy.[121] In addition, advances in surgical technique for catheter placement have improved outcomes. Catheters are placed into the specifically defined vessels that have been identified as the major source of blood supply to the tumor. Development of selective angiography techniques has greatly aided the clinician in determining the pattern of blood flow to the tumor and normal liver tissue. Dual catheter placement may be needed in some cases to ensure adequate chemoperfusion of the liver.[119]

In general, regional infusion is considered superior to systemic chemotherapy.[119,122-124] A recent study by Safi et al[125] indicates that the combination of both regional infusion and systemic therapy actually may prolong survival. Regional infusions have been combined with radiotherapy. However, if more than 50% of the liver is involved with tumor or if the major vessels to the liver are narrowed or nonfunctional, systemic chemotherapy usually is the route of administration selected.

Chemotherapeutic agents used with primary and secondary liver cancer include doxorubicin, neocarzinostatin, mitomycin C, FUDR, 5-FU, carmustine, streptozocin, and VM-26. Intraperitoneal administration of 5-FU has been well tolerated by patients and produces results comparable to those with regional infusion therapy.[126] Further investigation is being conducted to explore the role of intraperitoneal chemotherapy in liver cancer.

Radiotherapy

To date, the role of radiation alone in liver cancer therapy is limited to palliation of primary and metastatic disease. Liver tissue is radiosensitive, but many questions still are unanswered regarding how high a dose of radiation the liver can tolerate. Relief of pain, improvements in strength, increased appetite, and increased liver function have been reported with doses ranging from 1900 to 3100 cGy over a period from 2 to 20 days.[86,127]

In conjunction with surgery or chemotherapy, radiotherapy is used to palliate symptoms or to eradicate micrometastases. Researchers are investigating the effectiveness of concurrent chemotherapy and radiotherapy and are finding that such regimens have been well tolerated.[128] The major side effects of radiotherapy to the liver are nausea, vomiting, anorexia, and fatigue. These effects usually are compounded when two modalities are combined.

Supportive Therapy

The prognosis for the person with liver cancer is dismal. Most individuals die within 6 months after diagnosis. The tumor proliferates rapidly, is difficult to detect, and is difficult to treat. Individuals in advanced stages of the disease will experience hepatic failure, severe ascites, infection, bleeding, diathesis, pain, weight loss, weakness, and pneumonia. The patient and family should be kept informed of the treatment plans and assured that efforts will be made to provide relief of symptoms.[129]

Pain is one of the most difficult problems to manage. In later stages the pain is severe, worsens at night, and often radiates to the right scapular or subscapular area. Position, activity, coughing, and deep breathing make the pain worse. Pulmonary hygiene can be attempted only when pain relief measures are most effective.

Ascites can become severe in advanced disease. Palliative measures to control ascites include fluid and sodium restriction, diuretic therapy, paracentesis, or albumin administration.

Anorexia and vomiting may be late-stage manifestations in liver cancer. Antiemetics, vitamin supplements, antidepressants, and tranquilizers have helped some individuals. Relief is sometimes afforded by manipulating the environment, food presentation, and distraction techniques.[130]

Significant weakness, muscle atrophy, and immobility eventually lead to pulmonary congestion, atelectasis, pneumonia, and death. Anticipatory management of the rapidly developing symptoms and patient and family support are the major goals of nursing care in advanced disease.

PANCREATIC CANCER

INTRODUCTION

Cancer of the pancreas is presently the fourth most frequent cause of death from cancer in the United States. It is seventh among all cancers in incidence, which is a remarkable change from a few years ago when pancreatic cancer was believed to be rare.[1] Within the past 40 years, reported cases of primary pancreatic cancer have increased 300%.[131] The rate of increase in incidence and mortality, however, has actually decreased in the past 10 years.[132] The National Cancer Institute established the National Pancreatic Cancer Project to determine the contributory factors, evaluate the effectiveness of present therapies, and establish guidelines for prevention, detection, and treatment.

Pancreatic cancer is one of the most difficult tumors to detect or diagnose because of the anatomic location and biologic nature of the tumor. Its onset is insidious, with signs and symptoms that occur late, are vague and misleading, and mimic other diseases. The person with pancreatic cancer typically will ignore or rely on self-treatment of the initial signs and symptoms for months or until intolerable signs begin to appear. As a result of late detection and relatively limited therapeutic experience with pancratic cancer, the prognosis is extremely poor and the outlook for the person with the disease miserable. Fewer than 4% of individuals with pancreatic cancer are alive at 3 years.[1]

Future improvements in detection, diagnosis, and treatment of pancreatic cancer depend on systematic investigation of traditional and innovative therapeutic approaches and a willingness of practitioners to treat the disease aggressively.

ANATOMY AND PHYSIOLOGY

The pancreas is a racemose gland located in the retroperitoneum. It is approximately 15 cm in length and 2 to 3 cm in thickness, and it weighs about 90 g. The pancreas is divided into a head, body, and tail. The head is positioned over the vena cava and is lodged within the first three portions of the duodenum. The body and tail occupy a position slightly above and behind the head, extending transversely behind the stomach to almost touch the spleen.

Both endocrine and exocrine functions are vested in the pancreas. Secretory cells, called *acini,* line the multiple small alveoli that together form the lobules of the exocrine pancreas. The lobules contain small ducts to receive secretions from the alveoli. These small ducts empty pancreatic secretions into the Wirsung's canal, which runs from the tail to the head and empties into the duodenum. A branch of the main duct, the duct of Santorini, is in the upper half of the head and empties into the duodenum.

Each day, 300 to 800 mL of pancreatic juice is secreted directly into the duodenum. The major exocrine components are electrolytes and the digestive enzymes trypsin, amylase, and lipase. These enzymes are responsible for the hydrolysis of protein, starch, glycogen, and fats. Endocrine products of insulin, gastrin, and glucagon are released directly into the blood stream. Most endocrine tissue is contained in the tail and distal body of the pancreas.

EPIDEMIOLOGY

Reported cases of cancer of the pancreas comprise approximately 3% of all cancers in American men and women and result in 5% of all cancer deaths.[1] Cancer of the pancreas occurs at all ages, but peak incidence occurs between the ages of 60 to 70 years. It is rare before the age of 40 years.[132] Although predominantly a disease that affects adults, rare cases of children with pancreatic cancer have been reported. Pancreatic carcinoma demonstrates a male dominance, with a male to female ratio of 1:1.5.[132]

Race and ethnicity may be factors in this disease. The incidence of pancreatic cancer is 1.5 to 2.0 times higher in black than in native white persons.[132] Japanese immigrants to the United States have a higher incidence of pancreatic cancer than do native white Americans.[132,133] In the United States extensive studies have been done to correlate incidence with geography. Findings demonstrated some clustering in parts of Louisiana, a higher incidence in urban areas, and a higher incidence in American counties with many residents of Scandinavian or Russian descent.[133,134]

ETIOLOGY

An analysis of reported cases of pancreatic cancer yields relatively few causal effects for this disease. Increased risks attributed to environmental factors have been suggested. The sharp increase of pancreatic cancer in urban areas and among Japanese immigrants compared with native Japanese seems to implicate environmental factors, such as diet and exposure to industrial pollutants. Persons who work in aluminum milling or with coal tar pitch derivative, naphthalene, and benzidine are considered to be at higher risk for pancreatic cancer.[135] High-fat diets, alcohol abuse, diabetes, chronic pancreatitis, and lower socioeconomic status have possible associations with pancreatic cancer.[132,133,136-138]

Blot[134] and Blot and Fraumeni[3] found that the geographic mortality pattern in the United States for lung cancer and pancreatic cancer correlated closely, which suggests that tobacco may be a contributing factor. Persons who smoke more than two packs of cigarettes per day are at much higher risk for pancreatic cancer than are nonsmokers.[136] It has been hypothesized that carcinogenic elements in tobacco or chemicals excreted by the liver may be refluxed into the pancreatic duct and result in cancer.[139] Knowledge of specific risk factors and carcinogens associated with pancreatic cancer is limited by accessibility of epidemiologic data.

PATHOPHYSIOLOGY

Tumors in the pancreas develop in both the exocrine and endocrine parenchyma. Approximately 95% of pancreatic tumors arise from the exocrine parenchyma.[133] Islet cell tumors are rare, constituting 5% of the cases of pancreatic cancer.[140] Islet cell tumors develop in any part of the pancreas as functioning insulinomas or nonfunctioning carcinomas. The predominant morphologic type is adenocarcinoma of ductal cell origin. Giant cell carcinomas, cystadenocarcinomas, microadenocarcinomas, and adenosquamous carcinomas are rare and will not be discussed in this chapter.

Cellular Characteristics

Carcinomas most commonly arise in the proximal area of the gland, which includes the head, neck and uncinate process. Adenocarcinoma of the pancreas usually is a hard, nodular, firm mass with a large amount of fibrosis. Adenocarcinomas commonly invade the entire pancreas, obliterate the lobulated tissue, and cause obstruction of the common bile duct and Wirsung's canal. Exocrine functions of the gland are interrupted. As tumor growth advances within the pancreas or in lymph nodes along the biliary tree, complete obstruction and compression of the bile duct can result. The gallbladder becomes distended and the liver enlarges.

Carcinomas eventually may infiltrate the duodenal musculature, stomach, transverse colon, portal vein, and superior mesenteric vein. Venous invasion or encirclement by tumor growth results in obstruction, thrombosis, ascites, and portal hypertension.

At the time of detection, large tumor masses may be fixed to the retropancreatic tissues or the vertebral column. The tumor may directly invade the spleen, kidney, or diaphragm. Invasion by the celiac nerve plexus may account for the unrelenting pain associated with carcinoma of the body and tail of the pancreas. Obstruction of the portal vein and tributaries can lead to esophageal varices.

Although uncommon (<5%), islet cell tumors can arise from the endocrine parenchyma. The tumors usually occur in any portion of the gland as small, well-circumscribed, reddish tissue. Islet cell tumors rarely extend beyond the pancreas. On microscopic examination islet cell tumors are well vascularized, encapsulated, and usually compress adjacent parenchyma. Fibrosis and calcification may be seen. Islet cell tumors are difficult to distinguish as malignant because they closely resemble normal islet cells and retain secretory or synthetic functions. This leads many to believe that metastasis is the most reliable criterion for establishing malignancy. (Chapter 37 presents a more detailed discussion of endocrine cancers.)

Progression of Disease

Characteristically, tumors of the pancreas grow rapidly, showing late signs or symptoms of pathology. At the time of diagnosis the cancer has invaded locally or metastasized in 90% of individuals.[141-143] Tumor growth frequently extends or spreads to the common bile duct and celiac nerve plexus. Metastatic spread initially involves regional and paraduodenal lymph nodes and later develops in mesocolic, peripancreatic, paraaortic, mesenteric, and posterior mediastinal nodes and the hilum of the liver as the disease progresses. Supraclavicular nodes may be involved with carcinoma of the body and tail more frequently than with tumors of the head of the pancreas. Metastatic deposits reach the liver through the blood stream in later stages of the disease. Peritoneal seeding by metastatic deposits can occur. Metastases to the lung, pleura, abdominal viscera, adrenal glands, and bone are common.[133]

Ascites can develop late in the course of the disease. Localized effects of the tumor may be the cause of rapid decline or death. Individuals with advanced pancreatic cancer usually die in a short time of cachexia, infection, or liver failure. Of those diagnosed with cancer of the pancreas 86% die within 1 year of diagnosis.[141]

CLINICAL MANIFESTATIONS

Cancer of the pancreas has an insidious onset. In nine of ten individuals, cure is impossible by the time the cancer is discovered.[142] The early signs and symptoms are vague and often referred to other organs or systems. Careful assessment and extensive inquiry into the character, onset, duration, and modulators of presenting signs and symptoms will greatly aid definitive diagnosis. Manifestations of disease differ according to the location of the tumor in the pancreas.

Head of Pancreas

When carcinoma involves the head of the pancreas, the signs and symptoms often will appear earlier than with a tumor in the body or tail of the pancreas. Clinical manifestations, however, usually occur after the tumor is large or has disseminated. A classic triad of symptoms is apparent with cancer of the head of the pancreas: pain, profound weight loss, and progressive jaundice.

Most individuals experience pain as an early symptom. The pain is initially in the epigastric region, dull and intermittent in nature, and shrugged off as indigestion or gaseous distention. The pain later becomes much more distinctive in nature, possibly as a result of celiac plexus and perineural invasion by tumor. The pain often is continuous and radiates to the right upper quadrant of the abdomen or to the dorsolumbar area. It may be colicky, dull, or vague in nature. The intensity of the pain is affected by activity, eating, and posture. The pain often is ameliorated if the person lies supine or sits up and bends forward.

Jaundice, which is precipitated by common bile duct obstruction, is the presenting symptom in 80% to 90% of cases of cancer of the head of the pancreas.[143] Regardless of whether jaundice is the initial symptom or follows the onset of pain or gastrointestinal distress, it is the symptom that inevitably leads individuals to seek medical assistance. Contrary to previously held beliefs, pain with jaundice is far more common than painless jaundice.[133,144] The evolution of jaundice in pancreatic cancer is distinctive. It appears first on the mucous membranes, then on the palms of the hands, and gradually becomes generalized. The face, genitals, and linea alba are more discolored than other areas. The jaundice is progressive and persistent and leads to severe pruritus, dark urine, and clay-colored stools. The belief that jaundice indicates extensive disease and unresectability is not always true.

Weight loss and clinical wasting are classic symptoms of cancer in the head of the pancreas. The weight loss initially may not cause concern and can be attributed to gastric maladies. As the disease advances, weight loss of 20 to 30 pounds in a few weeks is common and often is accelerated by pain, anorexia, flatulence, nausea, and vomiting. Tumor involvement of the pancreas or common bile duct prevents secretion of digestive enzymes and often diminishes insulin production. Malabsorption can lead to diarrhea, constipation, steatorrhea, and muscle weakness. Metabolic disturbances such as hyperglycemia, glycosuria, and hypoalbuminemia may occur.[145]

Individuals with pancreatic cancer complain of emotional disturbances such as irritability, depression, and personality changes. Considering the sudden onset of symptoms, severity of pain, and inability to eat or sleep, it is not surprising to find such emotional reactions.

With advanced cancer of the head of the pancreas, hemorrhage and bleeding disorders can result from liver damage and impaired vitamin K production. Portal hypertension, hepatomegaly, and gallbladder enlargement are found in a large number of patients.

Body of Pancreas

Tumors in the body of the pancreas produce signs and symptoms late in the disease process, rendering early detection virtually impossible. By the time it is brought to the attention of a physician, the tumor may be large enough to be palpated. Severe epigastric pain usually is the first and predominant symptom. The individual may experience intense epigastric pain 3 to 4 hours after a meal. The pain often is excruciating and accompanied by vomiting. Relief is brought about by sitting up, leaning forward, or lying on the right side with both knees drawn up to the chest. These episodes of pain are short in duration and are more severe at night. The individual commonly fears that death is imminent and can become extremely anxious.

Hepatomegaly and splenomegaly may be found on palpation. Unexplained thrombophlebitis may be a clinical manifestation of cancer in the distal portion of the pancreas.[133] Jaundice occurs rarely.

Tail of Pancreas

Carcinoma in the tail of the pancreas mimics several other diseases. Metastases to liver, bone, lungs, peritoneum, and other organs may cause the first symptoms of carcinoma in the tail of the pancreas. Individuals with cancer of the tail of the pancreas complain of generalized weakness, gripping upper abdominal pain, vague indigestion, anorexia, and unexplained weight loss. Jaundice is an unusual finding. Pain radiates to the back left hypochondrial area. Pain is not encountered as often with tumors of the tail as with the head and body of the pancreas. Upper gastrointestinal bleeding, splenomegaly, and signs of portal hypertension or ascites may result from thrombosis of the portal system or extensive liver damage. In a few individuals a bruit may be auscultated in the upper left quadrant of the abdomen because of splenic artery compression or involvement by tumor.

ASSESSMENT

Physical Examination

Physical examination of the pancreas itself is difficult because it is an inaccessible organ. In many persons with cancer of the head of the pancreas, however, physical examination may demonstrate an enlarged gallbladder and a palpable, smooth liver. With tumors of the body and tail of the pancreas, a hard and well-defined mass may be palpated in the subumbilical or left hypochondrial region. The mass can adhere to the vertebral column or large vessels and may produce a pulsation. An abdominal bruit may be heard on auscultation of the left hypochondrium if the tumor has compressed or involved the splenic artery.

Diagnostic Studies

A variety of diagnostic measures are available to assist in the identification of pancreatic carcinoma. If definitive diagnosis cannot be made with these studies, exploratory laparotomy and biopsy may be necessary.

Radiologic examination

When pancreatic cancer is suspected, abdominal ultrasonographic examination is used as an initial diagnostic test. It provides a good outline of any pancreatic mass, dilated biliary ducts, or liver metastases. CT scanning affords similar but more explicit detailing of the extent of disease. CT scan cannot be used alone, however, to determine resectability.[146] MRI is being evaluated as a diagnostic tool in pancreatic cancer. Liver and bone scans are done to determine metastatic involvement.

Endoscopic retrograde cholangiopancreatography is a useful diagnostic test. The sensitivity and specificity of the test are greater than 90%.[147] During this endoscopic procedure specimens for biopsy and cytologic analysis can be obtained. If the bile duct has been abruptly terminated by an obstruction, endoscopic retrograde cholangiopancreatography will demonstrate the alteration. Because this invasive procedure involves the risk of infection and rupture, it should be performed only by skilled clinicians.

Selective arteriography can define the vasculature of the pancreas and delineate involvement or deviation of major vessels. Percutaneous transhepatic cholangiography is useful in determining whether the distal common bile duct is obstructed. The nurse should thoroughly explain these procedures to the patient and family beforehand. After these invasive procedures, catheter insertion sites and vital signs are monitored carefully to detect bleeding, peritonitis, and infection.[148]

Gastrointestinal tract barium studies and intravenous pyelogram rarely are useful in the early stages of pancreatic cancer. As the carcinoma advances, however, displacement of organs or defects in mucosal lining may be detected.

Laboratory tests

The use of laboratory tests is limited because early disease produces few alterations that laboratory tests definitively demonstrate. In about one third of the cases of pancreatic cancer, an abnormal glucose tolerance will be found. Occult blood may be present in stool if the tumor has invaded the duodenum or stomach. Serum bilirubin and alkaline phosphatase levels will be high, particularly if jaundice is present. Transaminase levels may be elevated moderately. In the presence of pancreatitis as a result of obstructive tumor, serum and urine amylase concentrations will be elevated. The prothrombin time is prolonged in individuals with jaundice or liver involvement. Exfoliative cytologic examination of duodenal aspirates and duodenal secretion tests often are employed. Islet cell tumors are diagnosed by plasma insulin immunoassay and fasting blood glucose levels. In the presence of an islet cell tumor, serum insulin levels are markedly elevated after periods of fasting.

Tumor markers

Biologic markers are on the frontier of cancer research. CEA, the carbohydrate antigen CA19-9, and pancreatic oncofetal antigen (POA) are the tumor-associated antigens being most extensively studied in relation to pancreatic cancer. CEA levels are elevated in pancreatic cancer (>2.5 ng/mL). Unfortunately, CEA levels are not elevated in early pancreatic cancer and are not specific to pancreatic cancer; therefore the determination of the CEA level is not useful for a definitive diagnosis of pancreatic cancer.[133] For example, CEA levels are elevated in smokers. With the carbohydrate antigen CA19-9, approximately 80% of the pancreatic cancer cases have been correctly diagnosed with the use of this marker.[133,144] POA is significantly elevated in more than 50% of individuals with pancreatic cancer.[147] As with CEA, POA is not specific to pancreatic cancer. It also has been found to be elevated in persons with bronchogenic and breast cancer. POA levels will decrease after effective therapy and increase with tumor recurrence or progression. Because POA has a tendency to be elevated with well-differentiated pancreatic tumors, it is not a strict indicator of tumor bulk.[149] The limitations to serial monitoring of tumor markers pertain to cost, sensitivity, reliability, and overall risk versus benefit.

CLASSIFICATION AND STAGING

Treatment and prognosis of pancreatic cancer are greatly aided by careful definition of the tumor classification and staging. The specific stage and classification system for pancreatic cancer being used by the Cancer of the Pancreas Task Force of the American Joint Committee on Cancer is illustrated in Table 39-5.

TABLE 39-5 TNM Classification System for Cancer of the Pancreas

Primary Tumor (T)

TX	Primary tumor cannot be assessed
T0	No evidence of primary tumor
T1	Tumor limited to the pancreas
	T1a Tumor 2 cm or less in greatest dimension
	T1b Tumor more than 2 cm in greatest dimension
T2	Tumor extends directly to the duodenum, bile duct, or peripancreatic tissues
T3	Tumor extends directly to the stomach, spleen, colon, or adjacent large vessels

Regional Lymph Nodes (N)

NX	Regional lymph nodes cannot be assessed
N0	No regional lymph node metastasis
N1	Regional lymph node metastasis

Distant Metastasis (M)

MX	Presence of distant metastasis cannot be assessed
M0	No distant metastasis
M1	Distant metastasis

Stage Grouping

Stage I	T1	N0	M0
	T2	N0	M0
Stage II	T3	N0	M0
Stage III	Any T	N1	M0
Stage IV	Any T	Any N	M1

Source: Beahrs OH, Henson DE, Hutter RV, et al (eds): American Joint Committee on Cancer: Manual of Staging of Cancer (ed 3). Philadelphia, JB Lippincott, 1988.

TREATMENT

Treatment Planning

The poor prognosis for persons with pancreatic cancer indicates that the extent of the tumor and its effect on the host should be carefully evaluated before initiation of any therapy. If the disease is believed to be potentially curable, the therapy will be radical. Therefore the individual must be physically and psychologically capable of withstanding radical therapy. Considering that 99% of individuals with pancreatic cancer are beyond hope of cure when their disease is diagnosed, most clinicians have an extremely dismal outlook and are reluctant to treat the disease aggressively.[144]

Surgery, radiotherapy, and chemotherapy are the major treatment methods used for pancreatic cancer. Surgery offers the only hope for cure at this time. Multimodal therapy that combines surgery, radiation therapy, and chemotherapy is being extensively studied. Palliation can be achieved with surgery, radiotherapy, chemotherapy, or combined modalities.

Once a diagnosis has been made, the extent of tumor involvement established, and complete assessment of the person's physiologic status undertaken, the interdisciplinary team will decide on a treatment plan. A number of factors contribute to the choice of therapy, including age, nutritional status, hematologic status, liver function, concomitant disease, and skill of the principal clinicians.

If the tumor is localized and not fixed to other structures and if there is no evidence of regional or distant metastases (T1-T3, N0, M0), cure is the objective of therapy. Radical surgical extirpation of the tumor will be done.

If the tumor is large and not localized, is fixed to other structures, or has metastasized to regional or distant nodes (T4, N1-N4, M0-M1), control or palliation is the goal of therapy. Surgical resection or bypass will be initiated and followed by adjuvant chemotherapy or radiation therapy.

Approximately 40% to 70% of all cases of pancreatic carcinoma are diagnosed when the tumor is unresectable.[143,150,151] Surgical bypass procedures, radiotherapy, chemotherapy, or combined-modality treatment aimed at palliating devastating symptoms will be selected.

Despite the urgent nature of therapy initiation, the patient must be adequately prepared physiologically and psychologically. Pretreatment biliary decompression may be needed to relieve obstruction and pressure while also reducing operative risk.[144]

Baseline assessments of lung capacity, blood pressure, blood volume, hematologic status, and liver function are done before initiation of therapy. Bleeding and prolonged clotting time usually can be controlled with vitamin K administration and blood component replacement. Nutritional assessments, which include family patterns, will be helpful in planning nutritional interventions. Adequate total protein level and a sound nutritional status can decrease surgical risk.[144,152] At the outset it is important to understand patterns of family support, coping, and communication.

Surgery

Current surgical approaches for pancreatic cancer are plagued by high rates of surgical mortality, low rates of resectability, limited prospective research experience evaluating the surgical procedures, and a dismal overall 4% 5-year survival rate.[144,151,153] The crux of the problem is late detection of pancreatic tumors. Until such time as improvements in early detection and diagnosis are made, curative surgery will be limited to very few candidates, and palliative procedures will continue as the mainstay of therapy for cancer of the pancreas.

The surgical approaches most used for pancreatic cancer when cure is the objective are total pancreatectomy and pancreatoduodenectomy (Whipple procedure). Regional pancreatectomy and distal pancreatectomy also are done. Great controversy exists over the advantages, disadvantages, and long term results with each of these surgeries (Table 39-6[154]). Proponents of total pancreatectomy and regional pancreatectomy believe that, although the procedure invariably induces diabetes, the risk of leaving behind microscopic disease is greatly reduced by a more extensive procedure.[133,151] There have been good results in controlling the diabetes. Proponents of pancre-

TABLE 39-6 Comparison of Types of Pancreatic Resections for Malignancy

	Pancreatico-duodenectomy (Whipple)	Total Pancreatectomy	Regional Pancreatectomy	Distal Pancreatectomy
Indications	Periampullary or small carcinoma of head	Large carcinoma of head or diffuse carcinoma	Carcinoma involving portal system	Carcinoma localized to body or tail
Tissues removed	Head of pancreas Duodenum Gastric antrum Bile duct Gallbladder	Whole pancreas Duodenum Gastric antrum Bile duct Gallbladder Spleen Peripancreatic nodes	Whole pancreas Duodenum Gastric antrum Bile duct Gallbladder Spleen Peripancreatic, celiac, mesenteric nodes	Distal pancreas Spleen
Anastomoses	Choledochojejunostomy Gastrojejunostomy Pancreaticojejunostomy	Choledochojejunostomy Gastrojejunostomy	Choledochojejunostomy Gastrojejunostomy Portal vein	None
Potential advantages	Pancreatic remnant may prevent diabetes and malabsorption.	Excision of pancreas may remove multifocal tumor. Complete peripancreatic nodal dissection No pancreaticojejunostomy	Wide excision may remove microscopic residual tumor. Complete regional nodal dissection No pancreaticojejunostomy	Pancreatic remnant may prevent diabetes and malabsorption. No pancreaticojejunostomy
Potential disadvantages	Limited resection may leave residual tumor. Pancreaticojejunostomy may fail.	Diabetes and malabsorption result.	Diabetes and malabsorption result. Technically complex Venous anastomosis may fail.	Limited resection may leave residual tumor.

Source: Sindelar WF, Kinsella TJ, Mayer RJ: Cancer of the pancreas, in DeVita VT, Hellman S, Rosenberg SA (eds): Cancer: Principles and Practice of Oncology (ed 2). Philadelphia, JB Lippincott, 1985, pp 691-739.

atoduodenectomy (Whipple procedure) for periampullary or small carcinomas of the head of the pancreas believe that this procedure removes the cancer without creating another disease (diabetes) and that it is technically easier.[142] Overall surgical mortality rates range from 10% to 50%[142,144,153]; however, survival rates are somewhat higher with the regional pancreatectomy.[151] Whether this is due to the surgeon's expertise with each surgery, to the extent of resection, or to the tumor cell characteristics can be determined only after more cases are systematically evaluated.

Before any portion of the pancreas is resected during surgery, the pancreas and lymph nodes are inspected for resectability, and then biopsy specimens are obtained. To determine resectability the mesentery is examined and the mobility of the duodenum and pancreas assessed. The vena cava, portal vein, and mesenteric veins also are checked for possible tumor involvement.

Total pancreatectomy

A total pancreatectomy is an en bloc resection in which a large number of lymph nodes (about 50) are removed. The antrum, common duct, gallbladder (if involved), pancreas, spleen, duodenum, proximal jejunum, and regional lymph nodes are resected en bloc. The biliary tract is anastomosed to the remaining jejunum proximal to a gastrojejunostomy (Figure 39-6). A vagotomy is done to decrease the risk of peptic ulcer. Biliary drains and a gastrostomy tube are inserted for drainage.

Pancreatoduodenectomy

Pancreatoduodenectomy (Whipple procedure) entails removal of the distal portion of the stomach, pancreas to the right of the superior mesenteric vein, duodenum, proximal jejunum, distal portion of the common bile duct, and gallbladder (Figure 39-7). Gastrointestinal continuity is restored by anastomosing the common bile duct and the remaining pancreas to the jejunum proximal to the gastrojejunostomy. A gastrojejunostomy is formed to allow the alkaline bile and pancreatic juices to enter the jejunum before acidic gastric secretions. This decreases the potential of ulceration at the gastrojejunostomy. Some surgeons also perform a bilateral vagotomy to minimize ulceration. Postoperative complications are infection, anastomotic leakage, fistulas, thrombophlebitis, abscess, and pneumonia.

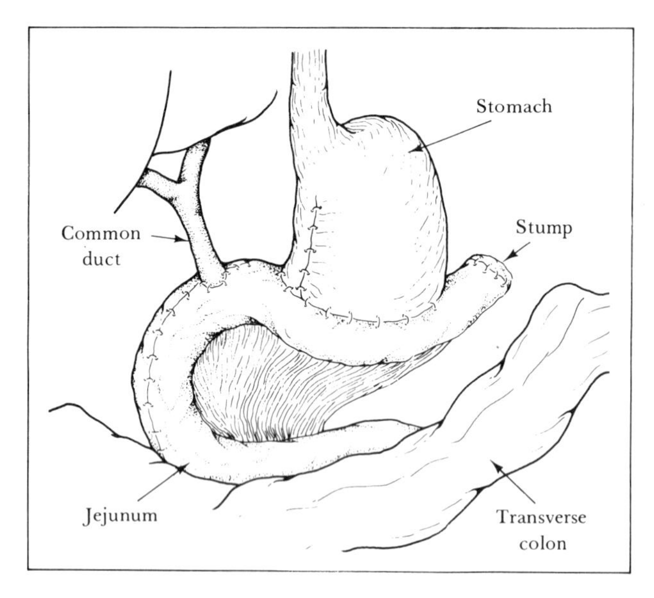

FIGURE 39-6 Total pancreatectomy. After resection of the pancreas, the biliary and gastrointestinal tracts are reconstructed by gastrojejunostomy and hepaticojejunostomy.

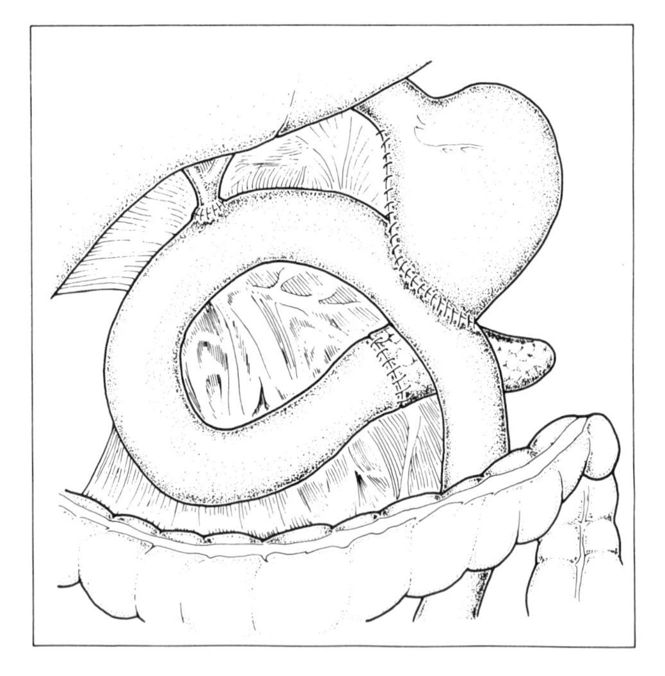

FIGURE 39-7 Whipple procedure. After resection of the head of the pancreas, reconstruction is achieved by pancreatojejunostomy, hepaticojejunostomy, and gastrojejunostomy. Vagotomy is performed to inhibit ulceration.

Regional pancreatectomy

Regional pancreatectomy is an extensive en bloc surgery that includes the entire pancreas, duodenum, gastric antrum, bile duct, gallbladder, spleen, the peripancreatic, celiac, and mesenteric nodes, and the sleeve resection of the portal vein.[142,151,155] Controversy regarding this surgical procedure relates to its technical complexity, higher surgical mortality rates, and limited experience to substantiate improved survival rates. Proponents believe that the high rate of failure in controlling pancreatic cancer supports the need to fully explore any promising methods to manage this lethal disease.

Distal pancreatectomy

In rare cases tumors of the body or tail of the pancreas are detected early enough to be considered curable. In such cases a distal pancreatectomy is performed. The entire tumor-bearing area plus a margin of safety is resected. The remaining pancreas is anastomosed to the duodenum and usually is capable of providing adequate exocrine and endocrine function.

Palliative surgical procedures

Palliative surgical procedures are used to remove tumor, relieve jaundice and obstruction, and decompress or bypass involved organs. Decompression procedures such as cholecystojejunostomy or choledochojejunostomy are used for biliary tract obstruction or pancreatojejunostomy for pancreatic duct obstruction.[143,156] If the duodenum has become obstructed or invaded by tumor, a bypass procedure (gastroenterostomy) will restore intestinal continuity. Delayed gastric emptying may be a serious postoperative problem for some patients.[157] Bypass procedures improve the quality of life and will relieve the debilitating symptoms of obstruction.[156,158]

Postoperative care

Intensive postoperative medical and nursing management of individuals who undergo pancreatic resection is critical for reducing the high overall surgical mortality rate of 15%.[142,159,160] Careful assessment, accurate observation, anticipatory management, appropriate interventions, and complete patient and family teaching will greatly enhance recovery and rehabilitation. In the immediate postoperative period, hemorrhage, hypovolemia, and hypotension pose the greatest threats. Fistula, infection, and anastomotic leak are potential problems.

Hemorrhage may occur from leakage at the surgical anastomosis or from generalized coagulopathy. Abdominal distention, shock, hematemesis, bloody stool, bloody drainage, or bleeding from the incision line warrant immediate attention. Retroperitoneal bleeding will manifest as a bluish-brown discoloration of either or both flanks. Prothrombin times should be monitored frequently and vitamin K and blood component therapy administered as needed. There have been reports of disseminated intravascular coagulation occurring in the postoperative period.

Hypovolemia can develop from fluids lost during extensive surgery, through drains, or from "third spacing" (the shift of fluid from the vascular space to the interstitial space). Malnutrition and hypoalbuminemia leading to low levels of circulating plasma proteins usually account for third spacing in the individual who has undergone surgery for pancreatic cancer. The first phase of fluid compartment shifting begins immediately after surgery and can last 48 to 72 hours. Signs of fluid shift are decreased blood pressure, increase pulse rate, low central venous pressure, decreased urine output, increased specific gravity, low levels of serum albumin, and hemoconcentration. When the plasma protein is replaced and levels return to normal, fluid reabsorption follows. Urine output will suddenly and dramatically increase, sometimes as much as 200 mL/hr. Urine output will greatly exceed intake. The individual is monitored closely for signs of circulatory overload such as central venous pressure above the normal range of 4 to 10 cm of water. The reabsorption phase will reach equilibrium within 24 to 48 hours.

Hypotension is a potential postoperative complication that is believed to result from severance of the sympathetic nerve fibers of the mesenteric complex.[17] Vital signs and urine output should be monitored frequently to detect alterations. Vasopressor drugs and liberal intravenous fluids may be administered.[17]

Pulmonary complications after surgery for pancreatic cancer are common, possibly as a result of immobility and inadequate lung expansion caused by pain and splinting. In addition, these individuals are highly susceptible to pneumonia because they are usually malnourished and protein-deficient before surgery. The importance of vigorous pulmonary hygiene and progressive ambulation cannot be overemphasized. Total parenteral nutrition often is needed to correct nutritional deficiencies.

After resection of the pancreas, exocrine and endocrine functions will be temporarily or permanently altered, depending on the amount of viable pancreatic tissue remaining. In the immediate postoperative period, laboratory tests will be useful in monitoring protein, fat, and glucose levels. Before discharge, the patient and family must become familiar with and able to recognize the signs of functional abnormalities such as hyperglycemia and hypoglycemia, steatorrhea, stupor, and lethargy.

Endocrine function (secretion of insulin and production of glucagon) most often is altered by resection involving the head of the pancreas. Serum and urine glucose levels are monitored at least every 6 hours and insulin therapy is initiated. Most individuals can be controlled with about 25 units of NPH insulin each morning[160] and a sliding scale of insulin dosages that maintain a mild hyperglycemia to prevent a precipitous drop in serum glucose.[148] Discharge teaching and home therapy programs are the same as those for individuals with diabetes. Inability to control glucose levels could indicate a recurrence of disease.

Alteration of exocrine function by removal of pancreatic tissue results in a malabsorption syndrome that is characterized by an inability to use ingested forms of fat and protein. The caloric requirement of an individual after surgery exceeds 3000 calories per day; adequate nutritional intake is essential to recovery. In the immediate postoperative period, nutritional maintenance is difficult. Parenteral hyperalimentation solutions contain approximately 1000 calories per liter; however, one of the major components is hypertonic dextrose. Serum and urine glucose levels are monitored at least every 6 hours and insulin administered as needed.

As soon as possible after pancreatectomy, the person is advanced to an oral diet. The aim of nutritional therapy is to replace calories lost as a result of the surgically induced inability to use ingested fats and proteins. Pancreatic enzymes are replaced with oral enzyme supplements. The two most reliable and frequently used forms are pancreatin (Viokase) and pancrelipase (Cotazym). Pancreatic enzyme supplements contain lipase, amylase, and trypsin.[17] Pancreatin and pancrelipase supplements are made from extracts of hog or beef pancreas enriched with bile salts and plant and fungal enzymes. The pancreas normally excretes 100,000 units of lipase per hour. Enzyme replacements contain about 4000 units of lipase per tablet. The usual therapeutic dose is eight tablets with each meal or 24 tablets (96,000 units) per day. It may require several approaches before the most appropriate dosage for each patient is determined because eating patterns and individual responses vary.[148] The individual should be informed that steatorrhea will decrease but may not be eliminated because oral pancreatic extracts are partially inactivated by acidic peptic fluids, whereas bile acids are activated by acidic duodenal contents.[161]

Most oral pancreatic enzyme supplements are enteric coated. There are conflicting reports regarding the efficacy of administering antacids with enzyme supplements. If diarrhea, steatorrhea, or weight loss persists with the administration of oral enzyme replacements, cimetidine, a potent gastric acid inhibitor, can be used.[162]

The second aim of nutritional therapy is to supply fats and proteins in a form that can be used. In most regular diets 98% of dietary fat consists of long-chain triglycerides that are difficult to break down into usable form. Administration of lipase is necessary so that the individual who has had a pancreatectomy can hydrolyze naturally occurring fats (ie, long-chain triglycerides). When lipase is administered in conjunction with pancreatic enzyme supplements, long-chain triglycerides can be broken down into medium-chain triglycerides. Food supplements that contain medium-chain triglycerides also can be ingested. These triglycerides are easily absorbed directly into the portal venous system, and bile salts or lipase are not required for absorption. Unfortunately, supplemental medium-chain triglycerides are unpalatable and expensive.

After a pancreatectomy, individuals are placed on a diet of bland, low-fat foods that are high in carbohydrate and protein. Several small feedings are tolerated better than large meals. Restrictions include overindulgence (which places a great demand on the pancreas), caffeine, and alcohol. It is advantageous for a clinical dietitian to consult with the individual and select the most agreeable diet plan on the basis of individual needs and life-style. The patient and family should be instructed on how to monitor the patient's tolerance to the diet and pancreatic enzyme replacement therapy. The stool should be examined daily for the characteristic signs of steatorrhea: frothy, floating, foul-smelling stool with fat particles floating in the water. If observed, this should be reported to the physician or nurse.

Chemotherapy

Chemotherapy as adjuvant treatment for pancreatic cancer is still being explored. A limited number of studies have been done because these individuals often cannot tolerate the drugs and toxic effects. The high rate of mortality associated with metastatic disease indicates that systemic therapy is needed; however, current applications of chemotherapy have failed to produce significant results. Perhaps new approaches in sequencing drugs and therapies or new drug combinations will improve the outcome.

Only a few agents have been determined to be effective as single agents: 5-FU, mitomycin C, streptozocin, methyl CCNU, and doxorubicin.[133,163] It is hoped that combinations of chemotherapeutic agents will produce high response rates, but few studies have substantiated this.[164,165] The combination regimens used most often are SMF (streptozocin, mitomycin C, and 5-FU) and FAM (5-FU, doxorubicin, [Adriamycin], and mitomycin C).

Chemotherapy alone has made no significant difference in survival periods, although it has provided palliation of pain in some cases. When both chemotherapy and radiation therapy are administered to individuals who have had pancreatic resection, the survival period may be increased slightly.[166-168]

Radiotherapy

External irradiation has been used for both palliative and curative therapy of pancreatic cancer. If the cancer is unresectable, many clinicians advocate the use of a combination of chemotherapy and radiotherapy. Local control of tumor growth and relief of debilitating symptoms are accomplished in about 50% of individuals.[169,170] Several specialized methods of radiotherapy have been used, such as interstitial implants, intraoperative radiotherapy, high linear energy transfer radiation, and charged-particle irradiation. These methods have resulted in a slight increase in short-term survival, but 5-year survival rates are unaffected.[169,171] None of these methods have had a significant impact on survival. The major limitation to radiotherapy appears to be the large volume of tumor that usually is present at diagnosis.

Combinations of radiotherapy and chemotherapy have resulted in significant increases in survival time as compared with patients treated with radiation or chemotherapy alone.[166-168] The average survival time with radiotherapy alone is 6 months, but with combination radiotherapy and chemotherapy is 11 months.[150,170,172] It is postulated that chemotherapeutic agents may reduce tumor burden and act as intrinsic radiation sensitizers, increasing the impact of radiotherapy.

Supportive Therapy

Cancer of the pancreas is an aggressive and unrelenting invasive disease in the advanced stages. The obstructive process will begin to fully manifest itself and can lead to hepatic failure, ascites, severe jaundice, hemorrhage, infection, and pain. The goal of therapy is palliative, intended to reduce the debilitating symptoms of the disease.

Relief of pain is a primary objective inasmuch as pancreatic tumors usually invade the celiac plexus and cause excruciating pain. The most effective approach to pain therapy is to prevent it from peaking by routinely administering the selected relief measures. Narcotics, sedatives, nerve blocks, relaxation therapy, and proper positioning may provide pain relief. Surgery, radiotherapy, or chemotherapy also have been used selectively to reduce pain.

As a result of the obstructive nature of advanced pancreatic cancer, nutritional support is a serious problem. Oral feedings should be maintained as long as caloric requirements can be met. Frequent small feedings and supplemental mixtures may be tolerated better than larger meals. Antiemetics before eating will assist in controlling nausea or vomiting. A feeding tube may be inserted below the point of obstruction if the individual can tolerate a surgical procedure. If exocrine function is disturbed, pancreatic enzyme replacements must be administered with oral or enteral feedings.

Jaundice as a result of ductal obstruction or liver damage can be a debilitating symptom that occurs in 40% to 70% of patients.[173] It causes severe pruritis and dry, friable skin. Cholestyramine, which combines with and promotes excretion of excess bile acids, may provide some relief of pruritus. The patient and family should be instructed to use soap sparingly, preferably mild soaps. Oil-based lotions, calamine lotion, cocoa butter, or bathing in sodium bicarbonate may help to relieve pruritus.[17]

Nonsurgical procedures are used to relieve obstructive jaundice in the patient with advanced cancer. Percutaneous transhepatic biliary drainage is performed under fluoroscopy with the patient receiving mild sedation and prophylactic antibiotics.[173] Endoscopic endoprosthesis placement can be done immediately after endoscopic retrograde cholangiopancreatography (ERCP). Successful placement of the endoprosthesis or biliary stent occurs in 90% of the cases attempted.[144,174] Palliative percutaneous transhepatic biliary drainage produces modest relief; however, care of the drainage apparatus is generally tedious for the family.

Liver damage may lead to ascites, hemorrhage, and confusion. Almost 90% of persons with pancreatic cancer die within a year of diagnosis. The course of the disease is rapid, and supporting the individual and family through the process is critical. It is important that the patient and family understand that some form of treatment or another medication always will be available to make the individual as comfortable as possible.

REFERENCES

1. Silverberg E, Lubera JA: Cancer statistics. CA 39:3-20, 1989.
2. Rosenberg JC, Lichter AS, Leichman LP: Cancer of the esophagus, in DeVita VT, Hellman S, Rosenberg SA (eds):

Cancer: Principles and Practice of Oncology (ed 3). Philadelphia, JB Lippincott, 1989, pp 725-764.
3. Blot WJ, Fraumeni JF: Trends in esophageal mortality among US blacks and whites. Am J Public Health 77:296-298, 1987.
4. Rosenberg JC, Roth JA, Lichter AS, et al: Cancer of the esophagus, in DeVita VT, Hellman S, Rosenberg SA (eds): Cancer: Principles and Practice of Oncology. Philadelphia, JB Lippincott, 1985, pp 622-657.
5. Qui S, Yang G: Precursor lesions of esophageal cancer in high risk populations in Henan Province, China. Cancer 62:551-557, 1988.
6. Ziegler RG: Alcohol-nutrient interactions in cancer etiology. Cancer 58:1942-1948, 1986.
7. Applequist P, Salmo M: Lye corrosion carcinoma of the esophagus. Cancer 45:2655-2658, 1980.
8. Mizroch S: Epidemiology of esophageal carcinoma. JAMA 239:2340, 1978.
9. Helm F: Cancer Dermatology. Philadelphia, Lea & Febiger, 1979, pp 48-49.
10. Jaskiewicz K, Marasas WF, Rossouw JE, et al: Selenium and other mineral elements in populations at risk for esophageal cancer. Cancer 62:2635-2639, 1988.
11. Hesketh PJ, Clapp RW, Doos WG, et al: The increasing frequency of adenocarcinoma of the esophagus. Cancer 64:526-530, 1989.
12. Morton JM, Poulter CA, Pandya KJ: Alimentary tract cancer, in Rubin P (ed): Clinical Oncology (ed 6). Philadelphia, WB Saunders, 1983, pp 154-177.
13. Sasajima K, Takai A, Taniguchi Y, et al: Polypoid squamous cell carcinoma of the esophagus. Cancer 64:94-97, 1989.
14. Jin-Ming Y, Li-Hua Y, Guo-Qian, et al: Flow cytometric analysis of DNA content in esophageal carcinoma. Cancer 64:80-82, 1989.
15. Ozawa S, Ueda M, Ando N, et al: Prognostic significance of epidermal growth factor receptor in esophageal squamous cell carcinomas. Cancer 63:2169-2173, 1989.
16. Stephens JK, Bibbo M, Dytch H, et al: Correlation between automated karyometric measurements of squamous cell carcinoma of the esophagus and histopathologic and clinical features. Cancer 64:83-87, 1989.
17. Given B, Simmons SJ: Gastroenterology in Nursing. St Louis, CV Mosby, 1979.
18. Qin D, Wang G, Yuan F, et al: Screening for upper digestive tract cancer with an occult blood bead detector. Cancer 62:1030-1034, 1988.
19. Huang CJ: Esophageal cancer. Jpn J Surg 11:399, 1981.
20. Postlethwait RW: Carcinoma of the esophagus. Curr Probl Cancer 2(8):1-43, 1978.
21. American Joint Committee on Cancer. Manual for staging of cancer ed 3, In Beahrs OH, Henson DE, Hutter RV, et al (eds). Philadelphia, JB Lippincott, 1988.
22. Postlethwait RW: Carcinoma of the thoracic esophagus. Surg Clin North Am 63:933-940, 1983.
23. Parker E: Carcinoma of the esophagus: Is there a role for surgery? Am J Digest Dis 23:730-734, 1978.
24. Wilson SE: Cancer of the distal esophagus and cardia: Preoperative irradiation prolongs survival. Am J Surg 150:114-121, 1985.
25. Gignoux M, Roussel A, Paillot B, et al: The value of preoperative radiotherapy in esophageal cancer: Results of a study of the E.O.R.T.C. World J Surg 11:426-432, 1987.
26. Austin JC, Postier RG, Elkins RC: Treatment of esophageal cancer: The continued need for surgical resection. Am J Surg 152:592-596, 1986.
27. Ramming KP, Haskell CM, Tesler AS: Neoplasms of the esophagus, in Haskell CM (ed): Cancer Treatment (ed 2). Philadelphia, WB Saunders, 1985, pp 231-246.
28. Naini AB, Dickerson JW, Brown MM: Preoperative and postoperative levels of plasma protein and amino acid in esophageal and lung cancer patients. Cancer 62:355-360, 1988.
29. Skinner DB, Ferguson MK, Soriano A, et al: Selection of operation for esophageal cancer based on staging. Ann Surg 204:391-401, 1986.
30. Mathisen DJ, Grillo HC, Wilkins EW, et al: Thoracic esophagectomy: A safe approach to carcinoma of the esophagus. Ann Thorac Surg 45:137-143, 1988.
31. Orringer MB: Transthoracic versus transhiatal esophagectomy: What difference does it make? Ann Thorac Surg 44:116-118, 1987.
32. Wong J: Esophageal resection for cancer: The rationale of current practice. Am J Surg 153:18-24, 1987 (suppl).
33. Medvec BR: Esophageal cancer: Treatment and nursing interventions. Semin Oncol Nurs 4:246-256, 1988.
34. Cameron M: What patients need most before and after thoracotomy. Nursing 8(5):28-36, 1978.
35. Campbell WR, Taylor SA, Pierce GE, et al: Therapeutic alternatives in patients with esophageal cancer. Am J Surg 150:665-668, 1985.
36. Poplin E, Fleming T, Leichman L, et al: Combined therapies for squamous-cell carcinoma of the esophagus, a Southwest Oncology Group study (SWOG-8037). J Clin Oncol 5:622-628, 1987.
37. Stewart FM, Harkins BJ, Hahn SS, et al: Cisplatin, 5-fluorouracil, mitomycin C, and concurrent radiation therapy with and without esophagectomy for esophageal carcinoma. Cancer 64:622-628, 1989.
38. Kies MS, Rosen ST, Tsang TK, et al: Cisplatin and 5-fluorouracil in the primary management of squamous esophageal cancer. Cancer 60:2156-2160, 1987.
39. Kelsen DP: Preoperative chemotherapy in esophageal carcinoma. World J Surg 11:433-438, 1987.
40. Dorr RT, Fritz WL: Cancer Chemotherapy Handbook. New York, Elsevier, 1981.
41. John MJ, Flam MS, Mowry PA, et al: Radiotherapy alone and chemoradiation for nonmetastatic esophageal carcinoma. Cancer 63:2397-2403, 1989.
42. Saika TK, Advani SH, Ramakrishnan G, et al: Intermediate-dose methotrexate and cisplatin in the treatment of advanced epidermoid esophageal carcinoma. Cancer 64:371-373, 1989.
43. Klaassen DJ, MacIntyre JM, Catton GE, et al: Treatment of locally unresectable cancer of the stomach and pancreas. J Clin Oncol 3:373-378, 1985.
44. Chisholm RJ, Stoller JL, Carpenter CM, et al: Radiologic dilatation preceding palliative surgical tube placement for esophageal cancer. Am J Surg 151:397-399, 1986.
45. Proctor DS: Esophageal intubation for carcinoma of the esophagus. World J Surg 4:451-455, 1980.
46. Tytgat GN, Bartelsman JF, Jager FC, et al: Upper intestinal and biliary tract endoprosthesis. Dig Dis Sci 31(9):57S-76S, 1986.
47. Chavy AL, Rougier M, Pieddeloup C, et al: Esophageal prosthesis for neoplastic stenosis. Cancer 57:1426-1431, 1986.
48. Mackety CJ: Caring for the cancer patient who has an esophageal endoprosthesis. RN 40:51-53, 1977.
49. Thomas RJ, Abbott M, Bhathal PS, et al: High-dose photoirradiation of esophageal cancer. Ann Surg 206:193-199, 1987.
50. Nava HR, Schuh ME, Nambisan R, et al: Endoscopic ablation of esophageal malignancies with the neodymium-YAG laser and electrofulgeration. Arch Surg 124:225-228, 1989.

51. Ahlquist DA, Gostout CJ, Viggiano TR, et al: Endoscopic laser palliation of malignant dysphagia: A prospective study. Mayo Clin Proc 62:867-874, 1987.
52. Jensen DM, Machicado G, Randall G, et al: Comparison of low-power YAG laser and BICAP tumor probe for palliation of esophageal cancer strictures. Gastroenterology 94:1263-1270, 1988.
53. Dupont BJ, Cohn I: Gastric adenocarcinoma. Curr Probl Cancer 4(8):1-35, 1980.
54. Maruyama K, Okabayashi K, Kinoshita T: Progress in gastric cancer surgery in Japan and its limits of radicality. World J Surg 11:418-425, 1987.
55. Wiggins CL, Becker TM, Key CR, et al: Stomach cancer among New Mexico's American Indians, Hispanic whites, and non-Hispanic whites. Cancer Res 49:1595-1599, 1989.
56. Horm JW, Asire AJ, Young JL, et al (eds): SEER Program: Cancer Incidence and Mortality in the United States 1973-1981, NIH Publication No. 85-1837. Bethesda, Md, National Cancer Institute, 1984.
57. Weisburger JH: Mechanism of action of diet as a carcinogen. Cancer 43:1987-1995, 1979.
58. Stehr PA, Gloninger MF, Kuller LH, et al: Dietary vitamin A deficiencies and stomach cancer. Am J Epidemiol 121:65-70, 1985.
59. Risch HA, Jain M, Choi NW, et al: Dietary factors and the incidence of cancer of the stomach. Am J Epidemiol 122:947-959, 1985.
60. Lundegardh G, Adami HO, Hellmick C, et al: Stomach cancer after partial gastrectomy for benign ulcer disease. N Engl J Med 319:195-200, 1988.
61. MacDonald JS, Steele G, Gunderson LL: Cancer of the stomach, in DeVita VT, Hellman S, Rosenberg SA (eds): Cancer Principles and Practice of Oncology (ed 3). Philadelphia, JB Lippincott, 1989, pp 765-799.
62. MacDonald WC, Mac Donald JB: Adenocarcinoma of the esophagus and/or gastric cardia. Cancer 60:1094-1098, 1987.
63. Seifert E, Butke H, Gail K, et al. Diagnosis of early gastric cancer. Am J Gastroenterol 71:563-567, 1979.
64. Olearchyk A: Gastric carcinoma. Am J Gastroenterol 70:25-45, 1978.
65. Baba H, Korenga D, Okamura T, et al: Prognostic significance of DNA content with special reference to age in gastric cancer. Cancer 63:1768-1772, 1989.
66. Adashek K: Cancer of the stomach. Ann Surg 189:6-10, 1979.
67. Mishima Y, Hirayama R: The role of lymph node surgery in gastric cancer. World J Surg 11:406-411, 1987.
68. Alfonso A: Adenocarcinoma of the proximal third of the stomach: Pitfalls in surgical management. Am J Surg 134:326-330, 1977.
69. Wang JF: Stomach cancer. Semin Oncol Nurs 4:257-264, 1988.
70. Gastrointestinal Tumor Study Group: Controlled trial of adjuvant chemotherapy following curative resection for gastric cancer. Cancer 49:1116-1122, 1982.
71. Moertel CG, Childs DS, O'Fallon JR, et al: Combined 5-fluorouracil and radiation therapy as surgical adjuvant for poor prognosis gastric carcinoma. J Clin Oncol 2:1249-1253, 1984.
72. Gunderson LL, Hoskins B, Cohen A, et al: Combined modality treatment of gastric cancer. Proc Am Soc Therapeutic Radiologists Int J Radiol Oncol 5:118, 1979.
73. O'Connell MJ, Gunderson LL, Moertel CG, et al: A pilot study to determine clinical tolerability of intensive combined therapy for locally unresectable gastric cancer. Int J Radiat Oncol Biol Phys 11:1827, 1985.
74. Abe M, Shibamoto Y, Takahashi, et al: Intraoperative radiotherapy in carcinoma of the stomach and pancreas. World J Surg 11:459-464, 1987.
75. MacDonald JS, Gohmann JJ: Chemotherapy of advanced gastric cancer: Present status, future prospects. Semin Oncol 15(3):42-49, 1988 (suppl).
76. Epelbaum R, Haim N, Stein M, et al: Treatment of advanced gastric cancer with DDP (cisplatin), Adriamycin, and 5-fluorouracil (DAF). Oncology 44:201-206, 1987.
77. Allum WH, Hallissey MT, Kelly KA: Adjuvant chemotherapy in operable gastric cancer. Lancet 1:571-574, 1989.
78. Schlag P: Adjuvant chemotherapy in gastric cancer. World J Surg 11:473-477, 1987.
79. Raab K: Intraperitoneal techniques offer daring alternative for abdominal cancer. Oncol Biotechnol News, August 1989, p 19.
80. Wright R: Liver and Biliary Disease. Philadelphia, WB Saunders, 1979.
81. Adams JT, Poulter CA, Pandya KJ: Cancer of the major digestive glands, in Rubin E (ed): Clinical Oncology (ed 6). New York, American Cancer Society, 1983, pp 178-189.
82. Foster JH, Berman MM: Solid Liver Tumors. Philadelphia, WB Saunders, 1977.
83. Blumberg BS, London WT: Hepatitis B virus and the prevention of primary hepatocellular carcinoma. N Engl J Med 304:732-735, 1981.
84. Wanebo HJ, Falkson G, Order SE: Cancer of the hepatobiliary system, in DeVita VT, Hellman S, Rosenberg SA (eds): Cancer: Principles and Practice of Oncology (ed 3). Philadelphia, JB Lippincott, 1989, pp 836-874.
85. Nealon T: Management of the patient with cancer. Philadelphia, WB Saunders, 1976.
86. Oberfield RA, Steele G, Gollan JL, et al: Liver cancer. CA 39:206-218, 1989.
87. Linsell A: Primary liver cancer: Epidemiology and etiology, in Wanebo JH (ed): Hepatic and Biliary Cancer. New York, Marcel Dekker, 1987, pp 3-15.
88. Okuda K, Peters R: Hepatocellular Carcinoma. New York, John Wiley & Sons, 1976.
89. Baum JK, et al: Possible association between benign hepatomas and oral contraceptives. Lancet 2:926-928, 1973.
90. Christopherson W: Hepatocellular carcinoma in young women on oral contraceptives. Lancet 2:38-39, 1978.
91. Jick H: Oral contraceptive induced benign liver tumors—The magnitude of the problem. JAMA 240:828-829, 1978.
92. Kent D: Effect of pregnancy on liver tumors associated with oral contraceptives. Obstet Gynecol 51:148-151, 1978.
93. World Health Organization: Collaborative study of neoplasia and steroid contraceptives. Int J Cancer 43:254-259, 1989.
94. Cameron HM, Linsell DA, Warwick GP: Liver Cell Cancer. New York, Elsevier, 1976.
95. Okazaki N, Yosshino M, Yoshida T, et al: Evaluation of the prognosis for small hepatocellular carcinoma based on tumor volume doubling time. Cancer 63:2207-2210, 1989.
96. Saddler D: Focus on the patient with metastic disease. Hepatic metastasis: A nursing perspective. Dimens Oncol Nurs 1(2):4-6, 1985.
97. Ong GB: Techniques and therapies for primary and metastatic liver cancer. Curr Probl Cancer 2(6):1-48, 1977.
98. Melato M, Laurino L, Mucli E, et al: Relationship between cirrhosis, liver cancer, and hepatic metastases. Cancer 64:455-459, 1989.

99. Bierman HR, Byron RL, Kelley KH, et al: Studies on blood supply of tumors in man. Vascular patterns of liver by hepatic arteriography in vivo. J NCI 12:107-131, 1951.
100. Case record of the Massachusetts General Hospital. N Engl J Med 302:1132, 1980.
101. Okuda K: Primary liver cancer in Japan. Cancer 45:2663-2667, 1980.
102. Lee YT: Nonsystemic treatment of metastatic tumors of the liver—A review. Med Pediatr Oncol 4:185-203, 1978.
103. Bengmark S, Hafstrom L: The natural course for liver cancer. Prog Clin Cancer 7:195-200, 1978.
104. Niederhuber JE, Ensminger WD: Surgical consideration in the management of hepatic neoplasia. Semin Oncol 10:135-147, 1983.
105. Adson MA: Resection of liver metastases—When is it worthwhile? World J Surg 11:511-529, 1987.
106. Zhuo X, Tang Z, Yu Y, et al: Long-term survivors after resection for primary liver cancer. Cancer 63:2201-2206, 1989.
107. Tang Z, Yu Y, Zhou X: The changing role of surgery in the treatment of primary liver cancer. Semin Surg Oncol 2:103-112, 1986.
108. Vitale GC, Heuser LS, Polk HC: Malignant tumors of the liver. Surg Clin North Am 66:723-741, 1986.
109. Li GH, Zhu SL, Li JQ, et al: Evaluation of partial hepatectomy for primary liver carcinoma. J Surg Oncol 41:5-8, 1989.
110. Zhou XD, Tang ZY, Yu YQ, et al: Clinical evaluation of cryosurgery in the treatment of primary liver cancer. Cancer 61:1889-1892, 1988.
111. Wanebo HJ: Hepatic and Biliary Cancer. New York, WB Saunders, 1987.
112. Flye MW, McCullough CS: Liver transplantation for malignant disease. PPO Updates 3(4):1-12, 1989.
113. Wollner IS, Walker-Andrews SC, Smith JE, et al: Phase II study of hepatic arterial degradable starch microspheres and mitomycin. Cancer Drug Delivery 3:279-284, 1986.
114. Fortner JG, Kim S, MacLean BJ: Major hepatic resection for neoplasia: Personal experience in 108 patients. Ann Surg 188:363-365, 1978.
115. Staryl T: Right trisegmentectomy for hepatic neoplasms. Surg Gynecol Obstetr 150:208-211, 1980.
116. Stone HH: Physiologic considerations in major hepatic resections. Am J Surg 117:78-83, 1969.
117. Niederhuber JE, Grochow LB: Status of infusion chemotherapy for the treatment of liver metastases. PPO Updates (3):1-9, 1989.
118. Albano WA, Durr M, Gutierrez AR, et al: Hepatic artery infusion: Surgical approach. Cancer Drug Delivery 1:213-226, 1984.
119. Sterchi JM, Richards F, White DR, et al: Chemoinfusion of the hepatic artery for metastases to the liver. Surg Obstetr Gynecol 168:291-295, 1989.
120. Balch CM, Levin B: Regional and systemic chemotherapy for colorectal metastases to the liver. World J Surg 11:521-526, 1987.
121. Ramming KP, O'Toole K: The use of the implantable chemoinfusion pump in the treatment of hepatic metastases of colorectal cancer. Arch Surg 121:1440-1444, 1986.
122. Kemeny N, Daly J, Reichman B, et al: Intrahepatic or systemic infusion of fluorodeoxyuridine in patients with liver metastases from colorectal carcinoma: A randomized trial. Ann Intern Med 107:459-465, 1987.
123. Chang AE, Schneider PD, Sugarbaker PH, et al: A prospective randomized trial of regional versus systemic continuous 5-fluorodeoxyuridine chemotherapy in the treatment of colorectal liver metastases. Ann Surg 206:685-693, 1987.
124. Schwemmle K, Link KH, Rieck B: Rationale and indications for perfusion in liver tumors: Current data. World J Surg 11:534-540, 1987.
125. Safi F, Bittner R, Roscher R, et al: Regional chemotherapy for hepatic metastases of colorectal carcinoma (continuous intraarterial versus continuous intraarterial/intravenous therapy). Cancer 64:379-387, 1989.
126. Ekberg H, Tranberg KG, Persson B, et al: Intraperitoneal infusion of 5-FU in liver metastases from colorectal cancer. J Surg Oncol 37:94-99, 1988.
127. Prasad B, Lee MS, Hendrickson FR: Irradiation of hepatic metastases. Int J Radiat Oncol Biol Phys 2:129-132, 1977.
128. Miller RL, Bukowski RM, Andersen S, et al: Phase II evaluation of sequential hepatic artery infusion of 5-fluorouracil and hepatic irradiation in metastatic colorectal carcinoma. J Surg Oncol 37:1-4, 1988.
129. O'Mary SS: Liver cancer: Primary and metastatic disease. Semin Oncol Nurs 4:265-273, 1988.
130. Welch D: Nursing the patient with advanced liver metastases. Cancer Nurs 2:297-303, 1979.
131. Mack TN: Pancreas, in Schottenfeld S, Fraumeni JL (eds): Cancer Epidemiology and Prevention. Philadelphia, WB Saunders, 1982.
132. Fontham ET, Correa P: Epidemiology of pancreatic cancer. Surg Clin North Am 69:551-567, 1989.
133. Brennan MF, Kinsella T, Friedman M: Cancer of the pancreas, in DeVita VT, Hellman S, Rosenberg SA (eds): Cancer Principles and Practice of Oncology (ed 3). Philadelphia, JB Lippincott, 1989, pp 800-835.
134. Blot W: Geographic correlates of pancreas cancer in the United States. Cancer 42:373-380, 1978.
135. Fraumeni JF: Cancers of the pancreas and biliary tract: Epidemiological considerations. Cancer Res 35:3437-3446, 1975.
136. Hiatt RA, Klatsky AL, Armstrong MA: Pancreatic cancer, blood glucose and beverage consumption. Int J Cancer 41:794-797, 1988.
137. Ishikawa O, Ohhigashi H, Wada A, et al: Morphologic characteristics of pancreatic carcinoma with diabetes mellitus. Cancer 64:1107-1112, 1989.
138. DiMagno EP: Early diagnosis of chronic pancreatitis and pancreatic cancer. Med Clin North Am 72:979-992, 1988.
139. Wynder EL, Mabuchi K, Maruchi N, et al: Epidemiology of cancer of the pancreas. J NCI 50:645-667, 1973.
140. Yamada T: Secretory tumors of the pancreas, in Sleisenger NH, Fordtran JS (eds): Gastrointestinal Disease (ed 3). Philadelphia, WB Saunders, 1983.
141. Brooks JR: Surgery of the Pancreas. Philadelphia, WB Saunders, 1983.
142. Sindelar WF: Clinical experience with regional pancreatectomy for adenocarcinoma of the pancreas. Arch Surg 124:127-132, 1989.
143. Singh SM, Reber HA: Surgical palliation for pancreatic cancer. Surg Clin North Am 69:599-611, 1989.
144. Warshaw AL, Swanson RS: Pancreatic cancer in 1988. Ann Surg 208:541-553, 1988.
145. Diamond DW, Fisler B: Pancreatic cancer. Surg Clin North Am 55(3):363-376, 1975.
146. Ross CR, Sharp KW, Kaufman AJ, et al: Efficacy of computerized tomography in the preoperative staging of pancreatic carcinoma. Am Surg 54:221-226, 1988.
147. Levin B: Panel: Cancer of the pancreas. Am J Surg 135:185-191, 1978.

148. Spross JA, Manalatos A, Thorpe M: Pancreatic cancer: Nursing challenges. Semin Oncol Nurs 4:274-284, 1988.
149. Moosa AR, Levin B: Collaborative studies in the diagnosis of pancreatic cancer. Semin Oncol 6:298-308, 1979.
150. Schein PS, Smith F, Wooley PV, et al (eds): Chemotherapy of pancreatic cancer, in Advances in Medical Oncology, Research and Education, vol 9. New York, Pergamon Press, 1978, pp 187-191.
151. Manabe T, Ohshio G, Baba N, et al: Radical pancreatectomy for ductal cell carcinoma of the head of the pancreas. Cancer 64:1132-1137, 1989.
152. Pedrazzoli S, Bonadimani B, Sperti C, et al: Forecast of surgical risk in pancreatic cancer. Am J Surg 153:374-377, 1987.
153. Beaszley RM, Cohn I: Update on pancreatic cancer. CA 38:310-318, 1988.
154. Sindelar WF, Kinsella TJ, Mayer RJ: Cancer of the pancreas, in DeVita VT, Hellman S, Rosenberg SA (eds): Cancer: Principles and Practice of Oncology (ed 2). Philadelphia, JB Lippincott, 1985, pp 691-739.
155. Lebow F: Regional pancreatectomy betters survival for pancreas cancer. Oncology Times (1):1, 1989.
156. McGrath PC, McNeill PM, Neifeld JP, et al: Management of biliary obstruction in patients with unresectable carcinoma of the pancreas. Ann Surg 209:284-288, 1989.
157. Doderneck RC, Berndt GA: Delayed gastric emptying after palliative gastrojejunostomy for carcinoma of the pancreas. Arch Surg 122:827-829, 1987.
158. Rosemurgy AS, Burnett CM, Wasselle JA: A comparison of choledochoenteric bypass and cholecystenteric bypass in patients with biliary obstruction due to pancreatic cancer. Am Surg 55:55-60, 1989.
159. Mannell A, Weiland LH, Heerden JA, et al: Factors influencing survival after resection for ductal adenocarcinoma of the pancreas. Ann Surg 203:403-407, 1986.
160. Brooks JR: Operative approach to pancreatic cancer. Semin Oncol 6:357-367, 1979.
161. Regan PT, DiMagno EP: The medical management of malabsorption. Mayo Clin Proc 54:267-274, 1979.
162. Moosa AR: Tumors of the Pancreas. Baltimore, Williams & Wilkins, 1980.
163. Bruckner HW, Crown J, McKenna A, et al: Leucovorin and 5-fluorouracil as a treatment for disseminated cancer of the pancreas and unknown primary tumors. Cancer Res 48:5570-5572, 1988.
164. Gastrointestinal Tumor Study Group: Phase II studies of drug combinations in advanced pancreatic carcinoma: Fluorouracil plus doxorubicin plus mitomycin-C plus fluorouracil. J Clin Oncol 4:1794-1798, 1986.
165. Cullinan SA, Moertel CG, Fleming TR, et al: A comparison of chemotherapeutic regimens in the treatment of advanced pancreatic and gastric carcinoma. JAMA 253:2061, 1985.
166. Douglass HO, Stablein DM, Thomas PR: An organized multiinstitutional interdisciplinary evaluation of role of radiation therapy alone or combined with chemotherapy in treatment of adenocarcinoma of the gastrointestinal tract. NCI Monogr 6:253-257, 1988.
167. Gastrointestinal Tumor Study Group: Treatment of locally unresectable carcinoma of the pancreas: Comparison of combined-modality therapy to chemotherapy alone. J Natl Cancer Inst 80:751-755, 1988.
168. Gastrointestinal Tumor Study Group: Further evidence of effective adjuvant combined radiation and chemotherapy following curative resection of pancreatic cancer. Cancer 59:2006-2010, 1987.
169. Roldan GE, Gunderson LL, Nagorney DM, et al: External beam versus intraoperative and external beam irradiation for locally advanced pancreatic cancer. Cancer 61:1110-1116, 1988.
170. Dobelbower RR: Pancreatic carcinoma treated with high dose, small volume irradiation. Cancer 42:1087-1092, 1978.
171. Bagne FR, Dobelbower RR, Milligan AJ, et al: Treatment of cancer of the pancreas by intraoperative electron beam therapy: Physical and biological aspects. Int J Radiat Oncol Biol Phys 16:231-242, 1989.
172. Borgelt BB: Betatron therapy for unresectable pancreatic cancer. Am J Surg 135:76-80, 1978.
173. Brandabur JJ, Kozarek RA, Ball TJ, et al: Nonoperative versus operative treatment of obstructive jaundice in pancreatic cancer: Cost and survival analysis. Am J Gastroenterol 83:1132-1139, 1988.
174. Cotton PB: Nonsurgical palliation of jaundice in pancreatic cancer. Surg Clin North Am 69:613-627, 1989.

Chapter 40

Gynecologic Cancers

Diane M. Otte, RN, MS, ET

INTRODUCTION

Approximately 71,900 new cases of invasive female genital cancer will be diagnosed in 1990 in the United States (Table 40-1).[1] This accounts for about 13% of cancers in women. Approximately 23,500 women will die of gynecologic malignancies in 1990.[1] This number has decreased dramatically since the introduction of the Papanicolaou (Pap) smear in 1941. This cytologic screening test allows most cervical cancer to be detected in the preneoplastic state. If every woman had an annual Pap smear, cervical cancer could be prevented or cured. Unfortunately, only 10% to 15% of women in the United States obtain a yearly Pap smear.[2]

Cervical cancer predominantly occurs during a woman's reproductive years, when women are more likely to receive regular gynecologic care. Endometrial cancer, on the other hand, is generally a postmenopausal disease. Regular gynecologic visits that include screening endometrial biopsy in postmenopausal women would increase the early detection of curable adenocarcinoma of the endometrium.

In contrast, ovarian cancer is usually widespread at diagnosis. Localized disease is asymptomatic in the vast majority of cases. Routine pelvic examinations frequently fail to detect ovarian tumors in asymptomatic women. Efforts to develop tools for early detection have been unsuccessful. Therefore, ovarian cancer is the fifth leading cause of cancer death in women, accounting for 12,400 deaths annually.[1]

TABLE 40-1 Gynecologic Cancer in the United States—1990

	Estimated New Cases	Estimated Deaths
Carcinoma of the cervix (invasive)	13,500	6,000
Carcinoma of the endometrium	33,000	4,000
Carcinoma of the ovary	20,500	12,400
Other gynecologic tumors	4,900	1,100

Source: Adapted from Silverberg E, Boring CC, Squires TS: Cancer Statistics, 1990. CA 40:9-26, 1990.

PREINVASIVE DISEASE

Cervical Intraepithelial Neoplasia

The cervix, the lower part of the uterus, extends from the isthmus into the vagina. The cervix is composed of two major parts: the endocervix and the exocervix. The endocervix is contiguous to the exocervix, which includes the external os and extends to the vaginal fornix. The squamocolumnar junction refers to the area in which the columnar epithelium of the endocervix joins the squamous epithelium of the exocervix at the os.[3]

Cancer of the cervix begins as a neoplastic alteration in the squamocolumnar junction. Over time, these abnormal cells will progress to involve the full thickness of this epithelium. These initial changes are considered preinvasive, premalignant, or cervical intraepithelial neoplasia (CIN).

CIN can be divided into three categories: CIN I, mild dysplasia; CIN II, moderate dysplasia; and CIN III, severe dysplasia or carcinoma in situ. Dysplasia actually means "abnormality of development" and is used to describe atypical changes in the cervical epithelium involving less than the full thickness of the epithelium. The term *carcinoma in situ* describes a lesion that has passed from dysplasia to one of neoplasia and involves full-thickness involvement.[4,5] There are no areas of invasion or metastases (Figure 40-1).[4]

All these lesions can regress, persist, or become invasive. CIN III is more likely to progress than the milder forms, which may regress spontaneously to normal. Because there is no way to predict which lesions will invade and which will not, all patients should be treated as soon as lesions are discovered.

Epidemiology

The incidence of carcinoma in situ has climbed dramatically since 1945. At the same time, the incidence of invasive cancer has decreased by nearly 50%. Instead of 23 cases per 100,000 women annually, there are now 12. During the same period, mortality has decreased from 15 to 6 deaths per 100,000 women. More than 50,000 new cases of carcinoma in situ will be diagnosed in 1990.[1] The mean age for women with carcinoma in situ is 15.6 years younger than women with invasive disease.[6] Women in their 20s are most often diagnosed with cervical dysplasia; those 30 to 39, with in situ cancer; and those over age 40, with invasive cancer.[7]

Etiology

Many personal risk factors have been shown to be associated with precancerous lesions of the cervix (Table 40-2).[8] A higher incidence of the disease occurs in lower socioeconomic groups. It is more common in blacks and Hispanics and in women who became sexually active at an early age, have many sexual partners, and are multiparous. Conversely, cervical carcinoma is infrequent in women who are nulliparous, those with inactive sex lives, and those who are lifetime celibates or lifetime monogamous.

The male's role in the epidemiology of cervical cancer has been reviewed. Kessler[9] discovered that women married to men whose previous spouses had cervical cancer were at a higher risk of developing cervical cancer. The cause for this apparent relationship has not yet been determined. The male partner's age at first coitus, smoking habits, visitation of prostitutes, and number of sexual partners also may affect relative risk.[8]

Females exposed to diethylstilbestrol (DES) in utero have a higher incidence of clear cell adenocarcinoma of the cervix and vagina.[10]

Certain sexually transmitted infectious oncogenes have been suggested as possible etiologic agents associated with cervical cancer. Herpes simplex virus type 2 has been shown to be carcinogenic in animals. Women with elevated herpes virus titers are at risk of developing cervical cancer.[11] Amstey[12] discovered that up to 25% of women with a Pap smear showing herpes developed cervical cancer, compared with only 2% of women in the control group. Despite these and other studies that show a correlation

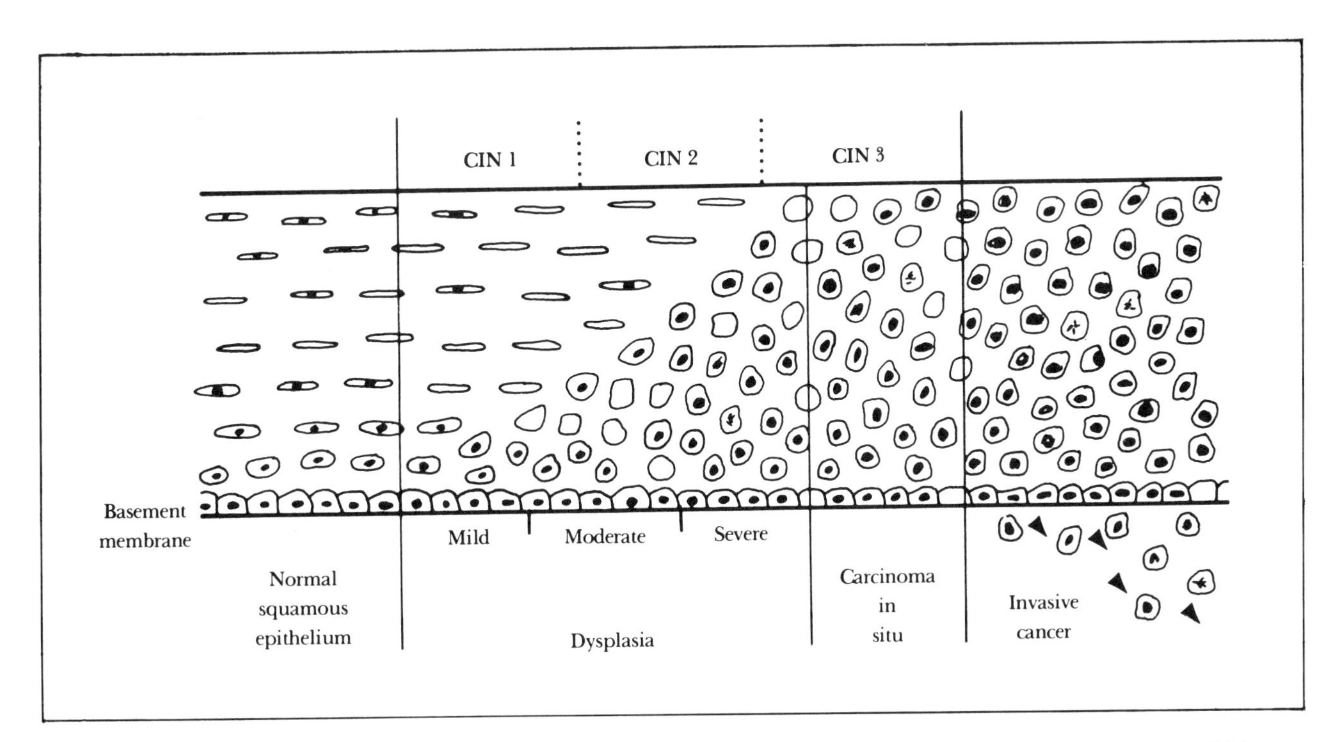

FIGURE 40-1 Schematic representation of precancerous cervical lesions. *CIN*,-cervical epithelial neoplasia. (Source: Jones HW, Jones GS: Novak's Textbook of Gynecology, Baltimore, Williams & Wilkins, 1981. © 1981, The Williams & Wilkins Co., Baltimore.)

TABLE 40-2 Risk Factors Associated with Precancerous Lesions in the Uterine Cervix

Risk factors
Strong association
Genital infections
Human papillomaviruses
Herpes simplex 2
Cigarette habit
Abnormal transformation zone
Immunosuppression
Chemotherapy
Multiple sexual partners
Tentative association
Genital schistosomiasis
Oral contraceptive use
Wine consumption
Coital factors
First, on the ground
No bathing before coitus
Douching after coitus
No abstinence during menses
Regular douching habit
Negative affect
Low socioeconomic status
Male factors
Smoking habit
Multiple sexual partners
Visitation of prostitutes
Occupational exposure to oncogenic agents
Penile warts or cancer
Previous wives with precancerous lesions or invasive cervical cancer

Source: Lovejoy NC: Precancerous lesions of the cervix: Personal risk factors. Cancer Nurs 10:2-14, 1987.

between herpetic infections and the development of cervical cancer, there is no absolute proof that the herpes virus causes cervical cancer.[13]

Human papillomaviruses (HPV) can cause a variety of warty infections. The female genital variety is called papilloma acuminata and is sexually transmitted. More than 46 distinct subtypes of the virus have been identified.[14] Kurman et al[15] studied 322 cases of CIN and carcinoma in situ. Twenty percent had associated papillomavirus structural protein.[15] Some types of HPV (6, 10, 11, 16, 18, 31, 33, 35, 39, 42, 43, and 44) are associated in precancerous lesions or invasive cervical carcinoma.[16-20] Both HPV 16 and 18 are associated with high-grade CIN or invasive cancer. HPV 18 is associated with 15% to 50% of invasive cervical cancer lesions.[21-23] The prevalence of HPV 16 appears to increase with the severity of the lesion.[22] Meanwell et al[18] suggest that this finding may be the effect of increasing age and that future reports on the association of HPV and cervical neoplasia should include details relating to the ages of patients under study. More studies must be done before a definite link can be established; however, there is strong evidence demonstrating a relationship of papillomavirus to intraepithelial neoplasia of the cervix.[16,24] The role of HPV and the need for practical clinical methods to identify which wart or lesion carries a risk of neoplasia must be clarified.[25]

Several factors may lower the risk of precancerous lesions of the cervix. These include barrier-type contraception, vasectomy, and recommended daily allowances of vitamin A, beta carotene, and vitamin C.[8]

Evaluation of an abnormal Pap smear

The Pap smear is one of the most effective, accurate, and economical techniques used to detect cervical neoplasia. Accuracy of the examination depends on the sampling method, staining, and microscopic examination.[13] Computerized microscope systems can prescreen Pap smears at a lower false-negative rate than human screeners. However, the cost-benefit relationship still remains a limiting factor with the automated method.[26]

The American Cancer Society has modified its recommendations regarding when Pap smears should be done. Previously it recommended that asymptomatic women 20 years of age and older and those under 20 who are sexually active have a Pap smear annually for two consecutive negative examinations and at least one every 3 years until 65 years of age and that women at high risk should have a yearly Pap smear. The American Cancer Society now recommends that all women who are or have been sexually active or who are 18 years or older should have an annual Pap test and pelvic examination. After a women has had three or more consecutive normal annual examinations, the Pap test may be performed less frequently at the discretion of her physician.[27] These guidelines are more in agreement with groups such as the American College of Obstetricians and Gynecologists, which recommends annual examinations to begin with the onset of sexual activity or at 18 years of age.

False-negative Pap smears occur and are thought to be due to sampling inefficiency.[28] Sexually active women should have annual Pap smears but should also have any pelvic pain, vaginal discharge, or abnormal bleeding evaluated by their physician promptly. A negative Pap smear offers no guarantee that the woman is free of cervical or uterine cancer.[28]

The correlation between cytologic diagnosis and subsequent histologic examination is over 90%.[29] A class II report (Table 40-3)[25] should be followed up in 2 weeks and any infection treated. If the findings persist, the woman should be followed every 6 months with repeat Pap smears; some physicians recommend colposcopy.

When the Pap smear report shows class III or IV, inspection should take place. This inspection is done by col-

TABLE 40-3 Cytologic Report Correlations

Class	Description
I	Smear normal, no abnormal cells
II	Atypical cells present below the level of cervical neoplasia
III	Smear contains abnormal cells consistent with dysplasia—mild: CIN I; moderate: CIN II
IV	Smear contains abnormal cells consistent with carcinoma in situ—severe: CIN III
V	Smear contains abnormal cells consistent with invasive carcinoma of squamous cell origin

CIN, Cervical intraepithelial neoplasia.
Source: Adapted from Nelson JH, Averette HE, Richart RM: Cervical intraepithelial neoplasia (dysplasia and carcinoma in situ) and early invasive cervical carcinoma. CA 39:157-178, 1989.

poscopy. A colposcope is a stereoscopic, binocular microscope that provides an eightfold to eighteenfold magnified view of the cervix. When colposcopy is done, the cervix is swabbed with 3% acetic acid solution, which accentuates the abnormalities and differentiates them from normal or metaplastic areas.[13] The epithelium of the cervix is visualized and the abnormal areas biopsied.

Treatment

It is critical that the extent of the disease be determined as accurately as possible before treatment begins. The Pap smear, colposcopy, and biopsy determine the extent and severity of the cervical lesion, differentiating between dysplasia and invasive carcinoma of the cervix. Treatment for CIN may be a direct cervical biopsy, cautery or cryosurgery, laser surgery, cone biopsy, or hysterectomy.[13] Electrocautery destroys the abnormal tissue by burning and is more widely used in Europe and Australia than in the United States. CIN can be successfully eradicated, with failure rates of only about 3% for all stages.[30] This procedure is painful, and general anesthesia is required to obtain adequate results. Extensive necrosis, tissue sloughing, and vascular injury result.

Cryosurgery, use of a portable cautery to induce freezing of cervical tissue, is a painless treatment that can be performed in the office. DiSaia and Creasman[5] report on six studies that show failure rates of 5%, 7%, and 12% after cryosurgery for CIN I, II, and III lesions, respectively. Patients complain of a watery discharge for 2 to 4 weeks after treatment.

Research is ongoing, but studies[31-33] show that approximately 80% to 90% of CIN of all grades can be eradicated by laser. The word *LASER* is an acronym for Light Amplification of Stimulated Emission of Radiation. The laser is mounted on the colposcope, and the laser beam is directed under colposcopic control. The advantage of using the laser is that significantly less disease-free tissue is removed along with the entire lesion. Patients experience a little more discomfort than with cryosurgery; however, after treatment there is less vaginal discharge, and the healing process is complete in 2 weeks. In 1983, Townsend and Richart[34] compared laser therapy with cryosurgery and found no significant difference in cure rates. They favor cryosurgery because it is less expensive. Ferenczy[35] suggests that laser should be used for lesions larger than 3 cm or for lesions extending into the external os that are still visible or that have not responded to two cryocautery or electrocautery treatments.

Conization involves removal of a cone-shaped piece of tissue from the exocervix and endocervix (Figure 40-2).[5] This procedure is done under general anesthesia and can be used as a diagnostic or therapeutic technique. The exact size of the cone depends on the colposcopic findings. Conization must be performed in specific situations: (1) when no lesion of the cervix is noted and an endocervical tumor is suspected, (2) when microinvasion is diagnosed on biopsy, (3) when the entire lesion cannot be seen with the colposcope, (4) when there are discrepancies between the cytologic report and the histologic appearance of the lesions, and (5) when the patient is not reliable for follow-up.[25] Major immediate complications of conization include hemorrhage, uterine perforation, and complications of anesthesia. Delayed complications are bleeding, cervical stenosis, infertility, cervical incompetence, and increased preterm (low birth weight) delivery. These are all functions of the amount of endocervix removed.[5]

Vaginal hysterectomy has been the treatment of choice for individuals with carcinoma in situ. Abdominal hysterectomy and oophorectomy are appropriate for individuals with CIN who have completed childbearing. These individuals must be followed as closely for recurrence as individuals treated with more conservative measures.[5]

Decisions regarding therapy are based on the extent of the disease, the patient's decision, and the physician's

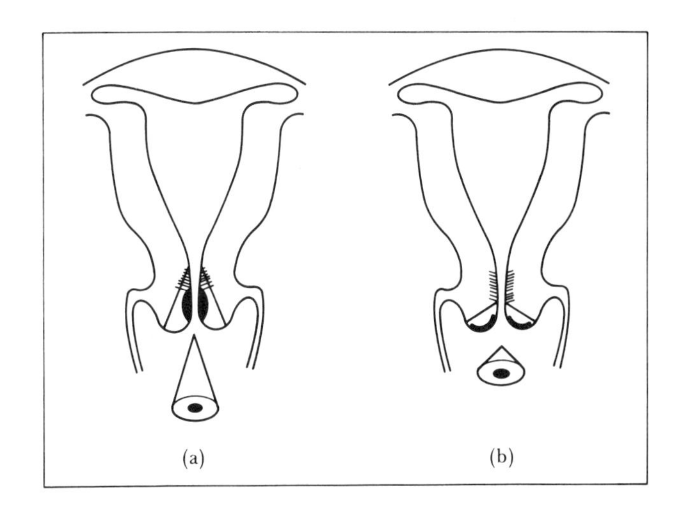

FIGURE 40-2 (a) Cone biopsy for endocervical disease. (b) Cone biopsy for CIN of the exocervix. *CIN,* Cervical epithelial neoplasia. (Source: DiSaia PJ, Creasman WT: Clinical Gynecologic Oncology. St Louis, CV Mosby, 1984.)

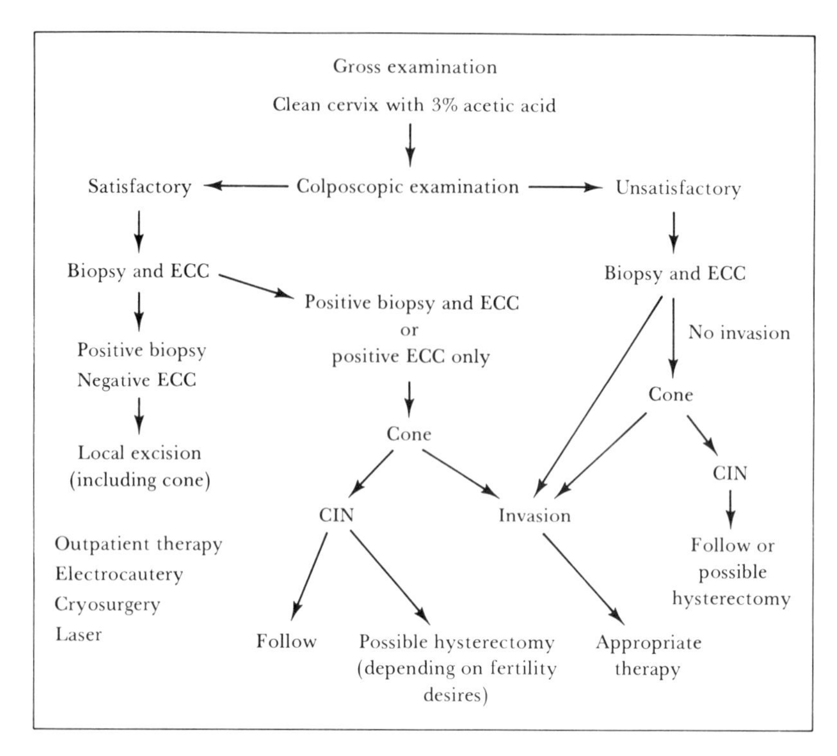

FIGURE 40-3 Evaluation and management schema for individual with abnormal pap smear. (Source: DiSaia PJ, Creasman WT: Clinical Gynecologic Oncology. St Louis, CV Mosby, 1984.)

experience. Women who wish to maintain optimum fertility and who have CIN I or II can be considered for electrocautery, laser therapy, or cryosurgery. CIN III also can be treated in this manner as long as the woman realizes that there is a slightly higher incidence of recurrence.[5]

Figure 40-3 summarizes the appropriate management of a patient with an abnormal Pap smear.[5] Regardless of the type of management used in CIN, frequent follow-up is essential.

Vulvar Intraepithelial Neoplasia

Epidemiology

Intraepithelial neoplasia of the vulva historically has been considered a disease of older women; however, it appears to be increasing in younger women.[36] Fifty percent of women are asymptomatic, whereas others may experience pruritus.

A variety of premalignant vulvar conditions can progress over time to intraepithelial carcinoma or carcinoma in situ. These lesions may vary clinically (eg, papules or macules, coalescent or discrete, single or multiple). Colors include white epithelium and pink, red, or brown hyperpigmented areas.[5]

Etiology

The etiology of intraepithelial neoplasia of the vulva is unclear. Some connection with venereal diseases, including herpes simplex virus type 2 and condylomata acuminatum, has been suggested.[37,38] The relationship between HPV and vulvar neoplasia remains unclear.[36]

Assessment

The most important diagnostic tool available is methodical inspection. Colposcopy is helpful in detecting multicentric lesions. A 1% toluidine blue solution can be used to stain suspicious areas but has a 20% false-positive rate.[38] To diagnose the underlying condition, vulvar biopsies should be employed liberally in the presence of any lesion.[5]

Treatment

Some controversy exists about the treatment of choice in patients with vulvar disease. Currently, wide local excision using either primary-closure skin flaps or skin graft is recommended with close follow-up.[38] For multicentric lesions, a skinning vulvectomy (Figure 40-4)[5] is performed. Rutledge and Sinclair[39] developed this procedure, which excises the vulvar skin, conserving the fat, muscle, and glands below the skin. A split-thickness skin graft is applied. This procedure produces excellent cosmetic and functional results. DiSaia and Creasman[5] report that of 35 women treated with skinning vulvectomy, none had complaints of dyspareunia or diminished sexual responsiveness.[5] A simple vulvectomy may be indicated in elderly women with chronic medical problems because healing of

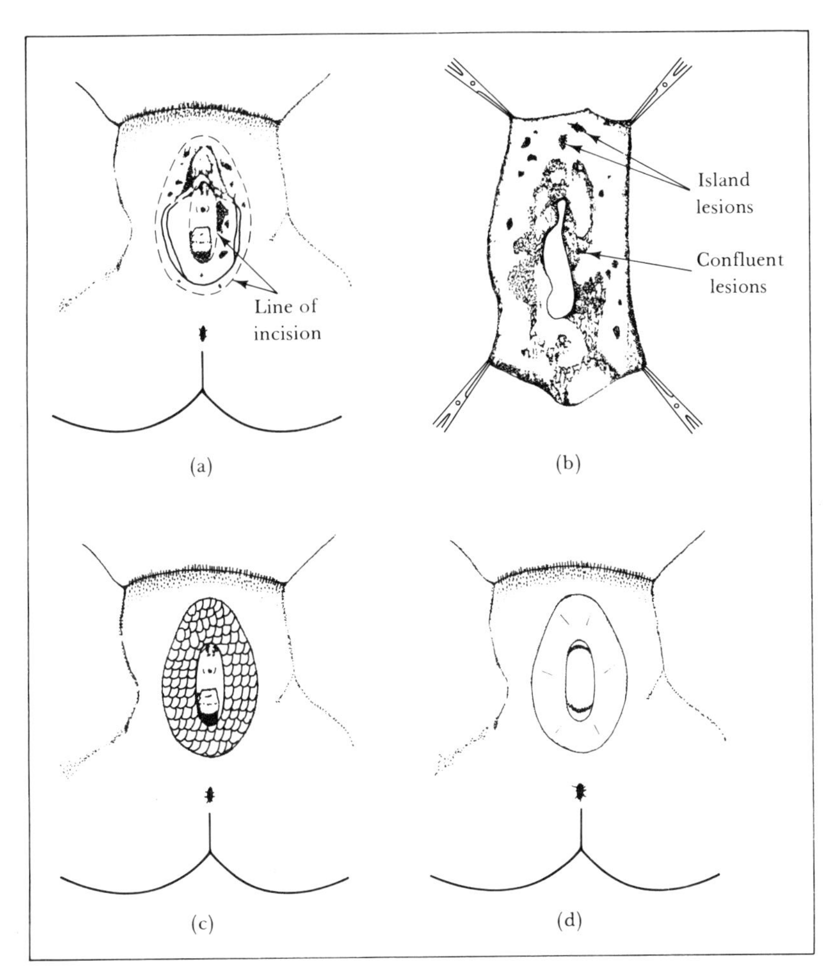

FIGURE 40-4 Skinning vulvectomy and skin graft. (a) Excise all areas of involvement en bloc. (b) Lesions may be isolated or confluent. (c) Preserve all subcutaneous tissue as the graft bed. (d) Suture to graft bed. (Source: DiSaia PJ, Creasman WT: Clinical Gynecologic Oncology. St Louis, CV Mosby, 1984.)

the skin graft after skinning vulvectomy requires prolonged bed rest.

Lesions also may be treated locally by electrocautery, cryosurgery, or laser. These treatments often result in painful ulcers that may take up to 3 months to heal.[40] Some authors support the use of the carbon dioxide laser rather than simple vulvectomy and split-graft skinning vulvectomy to treat patients with vulvar intraepithelial neoplasia. They feel this therapeutic approach is best because the majority of these women are young, with a mean age of 28.[41,42] Other local therapies that also result in painful, long-healing ulcers include topical 5% 5-fluorouracil (5-FU) and dinitrochlorobenzene (DNCB).[38,43]

Vaginal Intraepithelial Neoplasia

Carcinoma in situ of the vagina is much less common than that of the cervix or vulva. It is usually seen in women who have been treated for cervical CIN or after radiotherapy for invasive cervical cancer. The incidence of vaginal CIN after treatment of cervical CIN ranges from 0.7% to 6.6%.[44]

An abnormal Pap smear usually initiates the search for a definitive diagnosis because most lesions are asymptomatic. Colposcopic examination is done and biopsies taken.

Location of the lesion, the size of the lesion, and whether it is a single focus or multiple foci determine the treatment option.[38] Local excision is the treatment of choice for single lesions or several lesions in a single portion of the vagina.[38] Total vaginectomy with reconstruction should be reserved for the woman in whom more conservative therapy has failed. Varied results have been obtained using local application of 5-FU cream, but Cagler et al[45] indicated that this treatment can be effective. Laser therapy can cure approximately 80% of patients with vaginal intraepithelial lesions. Results are especially good for single lesions or multifocal lesions clustered in one area of the vagina.[35] Townsend et al[42] treated 36 patients with a 92% response rate. The use of intravaginal radium and cesium has been disappointing because of marked recurrences and vaginal stenosis.[44]

Nursing Care of Women with Preinvasive Disease

The primary nursing responsibilities for women with CIN focus on education. This educational process includes defining the disease, explaining treatment, and stressing the importance of close follow-up.

When the biopsies indicate CIN, the woman must understand that she does not have cancer. CIN is a premalignant condition that is easily treated provided the woman follows instructions carefully.

After biopsy, treatment is discussed. The nurse ensures that the woman understands the type of treatment the clinician is recommending. Outpatient treatment is usually cryosurgery or laser surgery. The nurse explains the purpose of treatment, which is to remove the abnormal cells on the cervix. Cryosurgery destroys the cells by freezing them, and laser surgery destroys cells using a light beam. The treatments take 10 to 20 minutes. The woman may feel a little discomfort but no severe pain. Electrocautery and conization are performed in an operating room under general anesthesia.

Following treatment, the nurse instructs the woman on how to care for herself at home. Minimal bleeding and vaginal discharge may be present for a week or longer after biopsy, cryosurgery, or laser. Minimal bleeding and vaginal discharge can continue for several weeks following conization. Douching, tampons, and sexual intercourse are prohibited for at least 2 to 4 weeks, depending on the treatment the woman received. A return visit must be arranged in 2 to 4 weeks, every 3 months for a year, and every 6 months thereafter. The importance of this follow-up must be stressed because these treatments are not always successful. There is a possibility of treatment failure or recurrence of the CIN.

Information concerning sexual functioning and fertility should be discussed by women undergoing treatment for CIN. Electrocautery, cryosurgery, laser therapy, and conization rarely cause physiologic sexual dysfunction.[46] Fertility is maintained, but, as previously mentioned, conization may cause cervical stenosis and cervical incompetence. If these conditions occur, there are potential fertility problems.

Sixty-four women were interviewed after conization about their sexual function, and they reported a significant decrease in dysmenorrhea and dyspareunia. There was no change in libido, experience of orgasm, coital frequency, or overall satisfaction of sex life.[47]

INVASIVE CERVICAL CANCER

According to the American Cancer Society, 13,500 new cases of invasive cervical cancer will be diagnosed in the United States in 1990, and approximately 6,000 women will die of the disease.[1] The incidence of invasive cervical cancer has steadily decreased as a result of the Pap smear, which has increased the ability to diagnose cervical cancer in a preinvasive state. However, cervical cancer is a significant health problem for elderly women, since 24% of new cases and 40% of deaths from cervical cancer occur in women age 65 years and older.[48]

Clinical Manifestations

There are no characteristic signs or symptoms of preinvasive disease. The first symptom of cancer may be a thin, watery, blood-tinged vaginal discharge that frequently goes unrecognized by the woman. The symptoms that may prompt the woman to seek medical attention are postcoital bleeding, intermenstrual bleeding, or heavy menstrual flow. If this bleeding is chronic, the woman may complain of symptoms related to anemia.

Late symptoms, which usually indicate advanced disease, include pain in the pelvis, hypogastrium, flank, or leg. This is secondary to involvement of the pelvic wall, ureters, lymph nodes, or sciatic nerve roots. Urinary and rectal symptoms may indicate invasion of these structures by tumor. End-stage disease may be characterized by edema of the lower extremities due to lymphatic and venous obstructon. Massive vaginal hemorrhage and development of renal failure may result from local invasion of blood vessels by tumor and bilateral ureteral obstruction by tumor.

Pathophysiology and Disease Progression

On gross examination, there are three types of lesions: exophytic, excavating or ulcerative, and endophytic. Exophytic lesions (Figure 40-5a)[49] are the most common and appear as cauliflowerlike, fungating cancers. These lesions are very friable and bleed easily. The lesions may be small, involving a small area of the cervix, or quite extensive, involving the entire cervix and upper vagina.

The excavating or ulcerative lesion (Figure 40-5b)[49] is a necrotic lesion that replaces the cervix and upper vagina with an ulcer or crater that bleeds easily. These lesions are often associated with local infection and purulent discharge.

The endophytic lesion (Figure 40-5c)[49] is located within the endocervical canal and shows no visible tumor or ulceration. The cervix appears normal but is hard to the touch. If there is parametrial involvement, the parametrium may also be hard and nodular.

Histologically, 80% to 90% of all tumors are squamous, 10% to 20% are adenocarcinomas, and a very small number are mixed (adenosquamous), verrucous carcinoma, melanoma, adenocystic carcinoma, or sarcoma. Adenocarcinomas generally are seen in higher percentages in younger women. Adenocarcinomas impose a greater risk because the tumor is within the cervix and can be quite bulky before it becomes clinically evident. The bulkiness makes it harder to treat, and this tumor thus has a high rate of local recurrence.[5,50] Adenocarcinomas appear to be increasing in prevalence.[50]

Cervical cancer spreads by three routes: direct extension, by way of the lymphatics, and by hematogenous

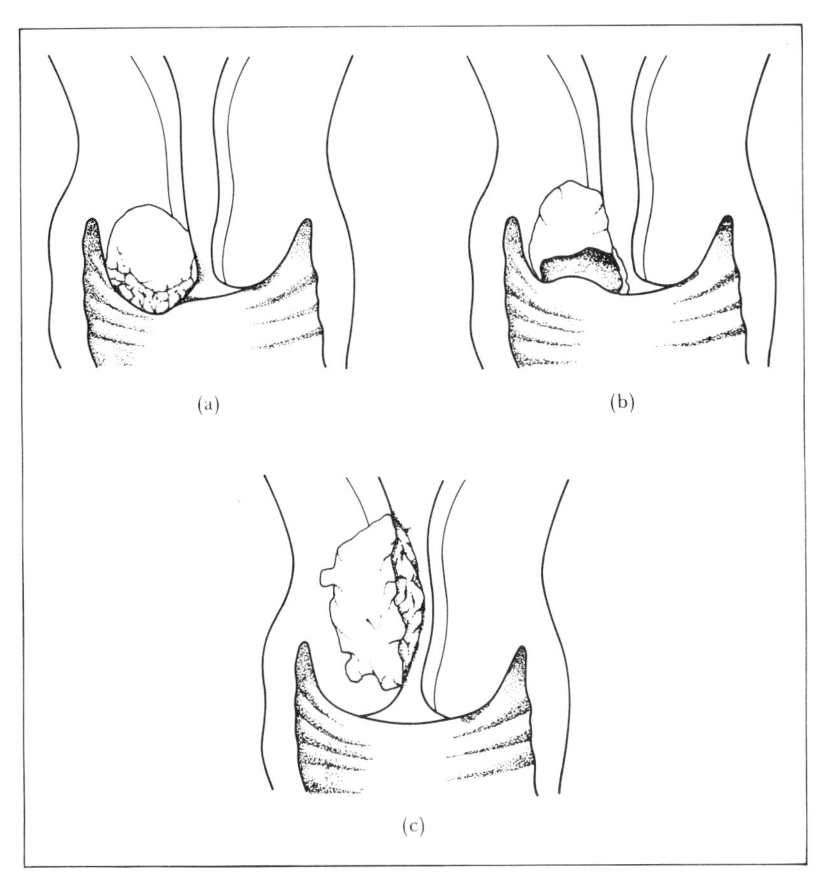

FIGURE 40-5 (a) Exophytic lesion. (b) Excavating or ulcerative lesion. (c) Endophytic lesion. (Source: Caputo TA: Uterine Cervical Cancer: The Current Approach to Diagnosis and Treatment. Syracuse, NY, Bristol Laboratories, 1979.)

spread. Direct extension is the most common route. The lesion starts on the endocervix and spreads throughout the entire cervix, the surrounding cervical tissue, into the parametrium, and through the vesicovaginal and rectovaginal septum into the bladder and rectum. The vagina and body of the uterus also may be involved.

Henricksen[51] studied lymphatic spread in cervical cancer extensively (Figure 40-6).[51] The primary nodes involved include parametrial, paracervical, obturator, hypogastric, external iliac, and sacral. The secondary group of lymph nodes involved are the common iliacs, inguinal, and para-aortic. Lymph node involvement can be correlated with stage of disease. The prevalence of positive nodes is 15% to 20% in stage 1, 25% to 40% in stage II, and at least 50% in stage III.[5]

Hematogenous spread through the venous plexus and the paracervical veins occurs less frequently than lymphatic spread but is relatively common in more advanced stages. Carlson et al[52] reviewed 2220 cases of squamous cell cervical cancer and found that only 15% of women developed distant metastases during the course of their disease. The majority of these individuals had stage III and IV disease. The most common sites of metastasis are the lungs, mediastinal and supraclavicular nodes, liver, and bone.

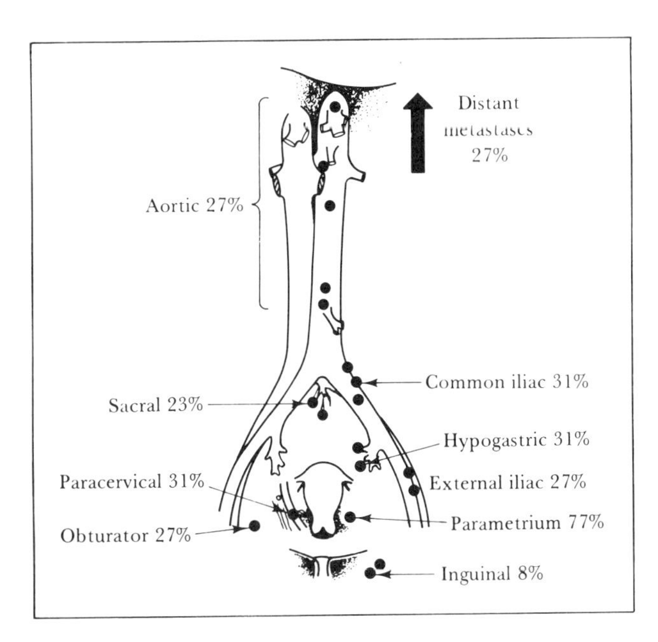

FIGURE 40-6 Lymph node involvement in cervical cancer. (Source: Hendriksen E: The lymphatic spread of carcinoma of the cervix and the body of the uterus. A study of 420 necropsies. Am J Obstet Gynecol. 1949, 58:924-942.)

Assessment and Staging

Cervical cancer is staged clinically, with confirmation obtained from examinations completed with the patient receiving anesthesia. The clinical stage is not changed at surgery or if the disease recurs. Staging is one of the best prognostic indicators. Approximate 5-year survival rates are: stage I, 80.5%; stage II, 59%; stage III, 33%; and stage IV, 7%.[14] Unfortunately there is a 30% to 40% understaging of cervical cancer when clinical and surgical stage are compared.[14,50]

A thorough clinical examination under anesthesia includes cervical biopsies, endocervical curettage, cystoscopy, and proctosigmoidoscopy. Additional diagnostic tests are chest radiograph, intravenous pyelogram (IVP), barium enema, complete blood count (CBC), and blood chemistries. If liver enzymes are elevated, a liver scan or computed tomographic (CT) scan is indicated.[5]

CT may also be used to determine the extent of pelvic disease and to define radiotherapy portals. It may be used in some institutions to evaluate lymph node status instead of lymphangiogram; however, there is no evidence that this is a reliable procedure to evaluate nodes for the initial staging of cervical cancer.[53] Magnetic resonance imaging (MRI) holds promise for determining tumor extent and tissue characterization more accurately than is presently available with CT and ultrasonography (US). It is hoped that MRI eventually will determine the presence of both pelvic and retroperitoneal nodes more accurately than CT. Unfortunately, at present, differentiation between benign versus malignant nodes cannot be determined by MRI.[54] Verification of tumor volume (the most important prognostic factor for survival of the patient with cervical cancer) by MRI may help the physician to determine the best treatment modality.[55]

Lymphangiogram may be indicated in selected individuals. The use of lymphangiography has been controversial owing to a high false-negative rate, with 21% of lymphangiograms interpreted as normal found to be histologically positive at laparotomy.[14] If enlarged nodes are seen on lymphangiogram, fine needle aspiration may be done. Tumor recurrence and radiation fibrosis may also be differentiated with fine needle CT-guided aspiration.[54] This may save the woman unnecessary surgery. Lymphangiogram may also be valuable in outlining abnormal lymph nodes to be included in radiotherapy ports.[38]

Clinical staging is not changed on the basis of surgical findings, but treatment may be altered. In selected cases where lymphangiogram is equivocal, a selected pelvic and periaortic lymphadenectomy may be performed. However, Wharton et al[56] have found that considerable morbidity and mortality result from this procedure when it is followed by radiotherapy. These researchers recommend evaluation of lymph nodes by lymphangiogram and percutaneous needle biopsy whenever possible.

Supraclavicular node biopsy is done if one of these nodes is palpable. The left node is usually positive because this is where the thoracic duct enters into the subclavian vein. Buchsbaum[57] has reported a 35% incidence of positive supraclavicular nodes with positive aortic nodes. He recommends a blind scalene node biopsy before therapy in any woman with positive aortic nodes. A positive scalene node biopsy indicates the need for therapy outside the pelvis. Following a thorough evaluation, the woman is clinically staged (Table 40-4).[58] This should be done jointly by the gynecologic oncologist and the radiation therapist. A team approach is essential because close cooperation is needed by these two disciplines in the treatment of patients with invasive cervical carcinoma.

Treatment

Once invasive cervical cancer is diagnosed and the stage established, treatment is based on the woman's age, general medical condition, extent of the cancer, and the presence of any complicating abnormalities. Either radical surgery or radiation therapy can be used equally effectively for patients with stages Ib and IIa cervical cancer. Comparable survival rates are generally obtained with both treatments in early-stage disease. Radiotherapy can be used for all individuals, whereas radical surgery is indicated only for women who are considered good surgical candidates.[5] A key component is that the patient be treated in an institution that has the appropriate personnel and equipment for either type of treatment and that all involved jointly decide what should be done.[38] In general, patients with stage IIb to IV are treated with radiotherapy.

Stage Ia

Stage Ia disease (microinvasion) has been divided into Ia1 and Ia2. Stage Ia1, microinvasive disease too small to be measured, should be treated by abdominal or vaginal hysterectomy if the patient is healthy and does not desire further childbearing. Conization can be done for those who are poor surgical risks or who wish to preserve fertility as long as the biopsy margins are free of disease and the patient is followed closely.[38]

Stage Ia2 disease is treated by abdominal or vaginal hysterectomy if invasion is less than 3 mm and there is no lymphovascular space involvement. If the invasion is greater than 3 mm or there is lymphovascular invasion, the disease is managed the same as a Stage Ib.[38] Intracavitary radiotherapy may also be used. Five-year survival in patients with properly staged Ia cervical cancer is close to 100%.[38]

Stage Ib and IIa

The choice of therapy for patients with Stage Ib and IIa disease remains controversial, and the preference of one treatment over another depends on the gynecologist and radiation oncologist involved as well as on the woman's condition and the lesion's characteristics.

Stage Ib disease and Stage IIa disease can be treated with radical hysterectomy and pelvic lymphadenectomy or with one or two intracavitary insertions (5000 to 8000 mgh). External radiotherapy to the pelvic sidewalls also may be included (2000 to 5000 rad [cGy]).[5]

TABLE 40-4 Staging Classification for Cervical Cancer

TNM	FIGO	Primary Tumor (T) Definition
TX		Primary tumor cannot be assessed
T0		No evidence of primary tumor
Tis	0	Carcinoma *in situ*
T1	I	Cervical carcinoma confined to uterus (extension to corpus should be disregarded)
T1a	Ia	Preclinical invasive carcinoma, diagnosed by microscopy only
T1a1	Iaa1	Minimal microscopic stromal invasion
T1a2	Ia2	Tumor with invasive component 5 mm or less in depth taken from the base of the epithelium and 7 mm or less in horizontal spread
T1b	Ib	Tumor larger than T1a2
T2	II	Cervical carcinoma invades beyond uterus but not to pelvic wall or to the lower third of vagina
T2a	IIa	Without parametrial invasion
T2b	IIb	With parametrial invasion
T3	III	Cervical carcinoma extends to the pelvic wall and/or involves lower third of vagina and/or causes hydronephrosis or nonfunctioning kidney
T3a	IIIa	Tumor involves lower third of the vagina, no extension to pelvic wall
T3b	IIIb	Tumor extends to pelvic wall and/or causes hydronephrosis or nonfunctioning kidney
T4	IVa	Tumor invades mucosa of bladder or rectum and/or extends beyond true pelvis
M1	IVb	Distant metastasis

Regional Lymph Nodes (N)

Regional lymph nodes include paracervical, parametrial, hypogastric (obturator), common, internal and external iliac, presacral and sacral.

NX	Regional lymph nodes cannot be assessed
N0	No regional lymph node metastasis
N1	Regional lymph node metastasis

Distant Metastasis (M)

MX		Presence of distant metastasis cannot be assessed
M0		No distant metastasis
M1	IVb	Distant metastasis

Stage Grouping

Stage 0	Tis	N0	M0
Stage IA	T1a	N0	M0
Stage IB	T1b	N0	M0
Stage IIA	T2a	N0	M0
Stage IIB	T2b	N0	M0
Stage IIIA	T3a	N0	M0
Stage IIIB	T1	N1	M0
	T2	N1	M0
	T3a	N1	M0
	T3b	Any N	M0
Stage IVA	T4	Any N	M0
Stage IVB	Any T	Any N	M1

Source: American Joint Committee on Cancer: Manual for Staging of Cancer (ed 3). Chicago, The Committee, 1988.

Surgery is preferred to radiotherapy by some oncologists, since ovarian function can be preserved, the vagina usually remains more pliable than with radiation, the overall treatment time is shorter, and long-term radiation complications to pelvic tissue can be avoided. Using radiation therapy has the advantages of avoiding major intraoperative and postoperative complications, and the patient can receive the therapy as an outpatient.[38]

Patients with bulky disease (barrel-shaped cervix) have a higher incidence of central recurrence, pelvic and para-aortic lymph node metastasis, and distant dissemination. An increased dose of radiation to the central pelvis or removal of the uterus, or both, have been advocated in patients with bulky disease.[38] The use of combined radical surgery followed by radiation remains controversial, and Barter et al[59] suggest use in a research setting only until the efficacy can truly be determined.[38]

Stage IIb, III, and IVa

Women with stage IIb, III, and IV cervical cancer are usually treated with high doses of external pelvic radiation, intracavitary radiation, and additional parametrial boosts or with a pelvic exenteration.[38] Radiation doses of 5500 cGy to 6000 cGy to the whole pelvis over 5 or 6 weeks are recommended.[14] Interstitial parametrial implants may also be used to supplement standard radiation techniques.[38] The 5-year survival rates of patients with stage IIb cancer are 60% to 65%, while those with stage IIIb cancer have survival rates of 25% to 48%.[38]

The role of surgery in the management of patients with advanced cervical cancer has increased. Pretreatment surgical staging of advanced cases is being advocated in an attempt to gain a more precise evaluation of the extent of the disease before definitive therapy.[60] Arguments for pretreatment laparotomy include the following: (1) the extent of the disease can be ascertained, (2) patients who have disease not curable by radiation can be offered palliative therapy, and (3) those patients most likely to benefit from extended field radiation can be identified. Arguments against pretreatment laparotomy are that (1) surgical staging can cause morbidity and mortality, (2) many patients with para-aortic nodal metastases also have systemic disease not detected by surgery, (3) there is only minimal improvement in net survival, and (4) surviving patients have high morbidity. This procedure warrants further study and is not recommended for routine use.[60]

At present, no chemotherapeutic agents have proved useful as adjuvant therapy for women who are at high risk.

Complications of surgery

Radical hysterectomy involves removal of the uterus, upper third of the vagina, entire uterosacral and uterovesical ligaments, all the parametrium on each side, and pelvic node dissection (ureteral, obturator, hypogastric, and iliac nodes). This is a complex procedure because the organs removed are proximal to many vital organs: the bladder, ureters, rectum, and great vessels of the pelvis.[5]

The major complications of radical hysterectomy include ureteral fistulas, bladder dysfunction, pulmonary embolus, lymphocysts, pelvic infection, bowel obstruction, rectovaginal fistulas, and hemorrhage. All these complications are becoming less common with improved surgical techniques.[5]

Complications of radiotherapy

Morbidity resulting from properly administered radiotherapy in cervical cancer is usually minimal. There are reported adverse reactions when poor technique is used, but these reactions generally do not occur in properly treated women. The higher the dose of radiation, the greater the rate of complications. Some morbidity attributed to radiation is secondary to uncontrolled tumor and not a direct result of the radiation. Major complications of radiotherapy for patients with stage I and IIa disease range from 3% to 5%, respectively, and are 10% to 15%, respectively, for patients with stage IIb and III disease.[61]

The most frequent major complications are rectovaginal fistulas, rectouterine fistulas, sigmoid perforation or stricture, rectal ulcer or proctitis, intestinal obstruction, vesicovaginal fistulas, ureteral stricture, severe cystitis, bladder ulcer, pulmonary embolus, pelvic hemorrhage, pelvic abscess, and sexual dysfunction secondary to vaginal stenosis.

Recurrent or persistent disease

Approximately 35% of women with invasive cervical cancer will have recurrent or persistent disease.[5] Therefore, intensive follow-up after treatment is essential and is the key to early detection of recurrence (Table 40-5).[5] Recurrent cervical cancer is difficult to diagnose. Clinical evaluation of an irradiated cervix is problematic because it is distorted from the radiation, and cytologic interpretation is difficult because the cells are altered by the radiation. Therefore, histologic confirmation of recurrence is essential.[5]

Most recurrences occur within 2 years after therapy; however, the signs and symptoms may be subtle and varied. They may include unexplained weight loss, leg edema (excessive and often unilateral), pelvic or thigh and buttock pain, serosanguinous vaginal discharge, progressive ureteral obstruction, supraclavicular lymph node enlargement (usually on the left side), cough, hemoptysis, or chest pain. If the woman presents with the triad of weight loss, leg edema, and pelvic pain, the outlook is grim. Evaluation after histologic confirmation will usually include chest radiograph, IVP, CBC, and blood chemistries. Some physicians will include a CT scan and lympangiography to evaluate the status of the regional lymph nodes, liver, and kidneys. Fluoroscopically directed needle biopsies have replaced more elaborate operative procedures to provide histologic confirmation of recurrence.[5]

Following surgery or radiotherapy as primary treatment for patients with cervical cancer, about 75% of all recurrences are local (cervix, uterus, vagina, parametrium, and regional lymph nodes). The remaining 25% of recurrences involve distant metastases to the lung, liver, bone, or mediastinal or supraclavicular lymph nodes.[51]

TABLE 40-5 Interval Evaluation of Cervical Cancer Following Radiotherapy (Asymptomatic Patient)*

Year	Frequency	Examination
1	3 months	Pelvic examination, Pap smear
	6 months	Chest radiograph, CBC, BUN, creatinine
	1 year	IVP
2	4 months	Pelvic examination, Pap smear
	1 year	Chest radiograph, CBC, BUN, creatinine, IVP
3	6 months	Pelvic examination, Pap smear
	1 year	Chest radiograph

*Symptomatic patients should have appropriate examinations where indicated.

CBC, Complete blood count; *BUN,* blood urea nitrogen; *IVP,* intravenous pyelogram.

Source: Adapted from DiSaia PJ, Creasman WT: Clinical Gynecologic Oncology. St Louis, CV Mosby, 1984.

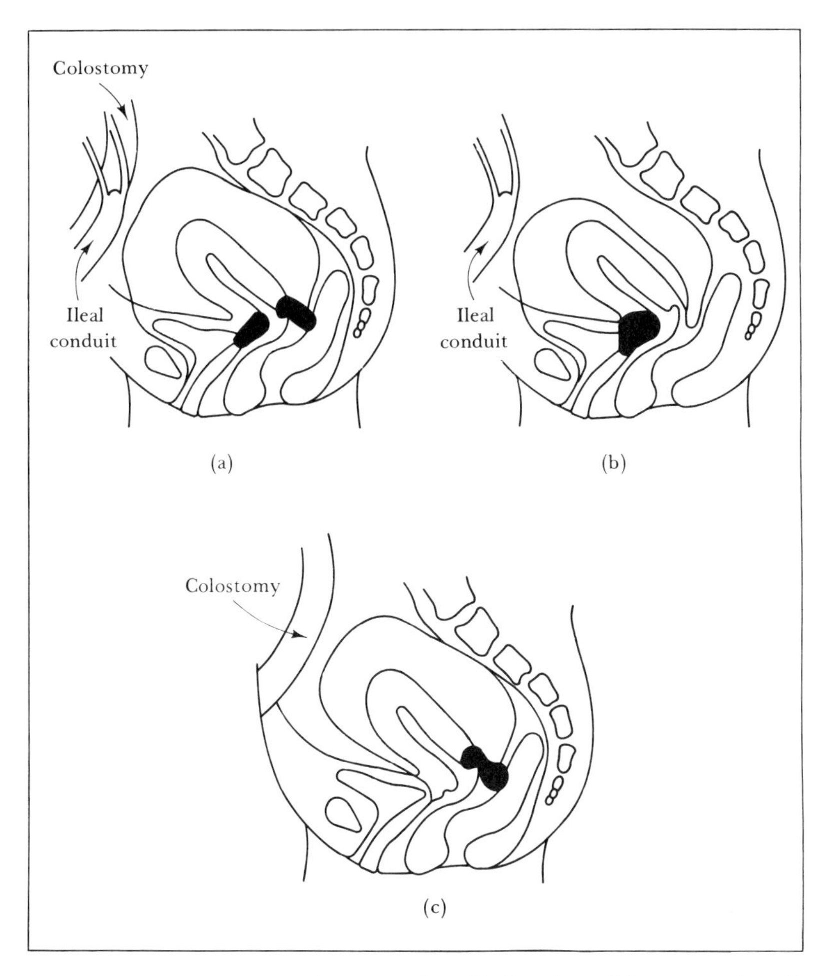

FIGURE 40-7 (a) Total pelvic exenteration. (b) Anterior pelvic exenteration. (c) Posterior pelvic exenteration. (Source: DiSaia PJ, Creasman WT: Clinical Gynecologic Oncology. St Louis, CV Mosby, 1984.)

The prognosis for patients with persistent or recurrent carcinoma of the cervix is dismal. One-year survival rates are 10% to 15%.[5] Survival averages 6 to 10 months once recurrent cervical cancer is diagnosed.[50] The aim of treatment in recurrent disease is palliation because control or cure is rare.

Surgery When cervical cancer recurs centrally following radiotherapy, pelvic exenteration may be considered. Total pelvic exenteration includes radical hysterectomy, pelvic lymph node dissection, and removal of the bladder and rectosigmoid colon. Occasionally, a posterior exenteration (which preserves the bladder) or anterior exenteration (which preserves the rectum) can be performed (Figure 40-7).[5] Partial pelvic exenterations are usually not done because the bladder and rectum have residual radiation effects and are prone to complications.

Only a small percentage of women are candidates for pelvic exenteration. This procedure is curative in intent. Women with disease outside the pelvis or with the triad of unilateral leg edema, sciatic pain, and ureteral obstruction are not candidates for pelvic exenteration. Obesity, severe medical problems, and advanced age may have a negative bearing on the advisability of the surgery.

Extensive preoperative evaluation must be done to ensure that there is not disease outside the pelvis and that renal function is adequate. Studies usually performed include chest radiography, IVP, blood chemistries, creatinine clearance, CT scan, bone scan, and liver-spleen scan. Some clinicians also do lymphangiography to evaluate the regional lymph nodes. If lymphadenopathy is present, a needle aspiration of the nodes may be done. If the aspirate is positive for malignancy, the woman can be spared an unnecessary laparotomy. A blind scalene node biopsy may be recommended to complete the evaluation.

At laparotomy, the entire abdomen and pelvis is explored for metastases. A selective para-aortic lymphadenectomy, bilateral pelvic lymphadenectomy, and biopsies of the pelvic sidewall are done and sent for frozen section. If any of these is positive, the exenteration is usually aborted because the disease is considered incurable.[5] However, some surgeons support doing pelvic exenterations in patients with recurrent disease complicated by pelvic lymph node metastases.[60]

The use of the end-to-end anastomotic (EEA) stapling device has resulted in patients' not needing a permanent colostomy after pelvic exenteration. Permanent colostomy can also be avoided by using a segment of sigmoid colon as a rectal substitute.[62,63]

Immediate postoperative problems include pulmonary embolism, pulmonary edema, cardiovascular accident, hemorrhage, myocardial infarction, sepsis, and small-bowel obstruction. Long-term problems include fistula formation, urinary obstruction and infection, and sepsis. Psychosexual and social rehabilitation of surviving patients is a major challenge.[60] Vaginal reconstruction at the time of exenteration and psychological support in the post-operative period can help patients adjust.

The use of pelvic exenteration has been limited to a highly select group of candidates, since reports indicate a 5-year survival of 23% and an operative mortality of approximately 9.8%.[38]

Radiotherapy In previously irradiated individuals, metastatic disease outside the initial radiation field may be treated cautiously with radiation to provide local control and relieve symptoms. In selected cases radiation within previously treated areas may be used.[5,38] For women treated initially with surgery, full-dose radiotherapy using a combination of external and intracavitary may afford excellent palliation or even cure.[38]

Because cervical cancer can be treated successfully with radiotherapy, research with hyperbaric oxygen, hypoxic sensitizers, and hyperthermia is being done to increase the benefits of traditional radiotherapy. The results using hyperbaric oxygen are mixed, with some studies showing improvement in survival for women below the age of 55, while others do not show any significant benefit. Complications are seen more with those patients treated in this fashion.[38] Use of misonidazole as a hypoxic cell sensitizer is being investigated by the Gynecologic Oncology Group in a protocol that compares misonidazole or hydroxyurea in combination with definitive radiation for patients with stages IIb, III, or IV cervical cancer.[38] Use of hyperthermia is limited because it is difficult to deliver heat to a large part of the body such as the pelvis.[38] Interstitial brachytherapy and the use of intraoperative radiation therapy with electron beam are innovative procedures that may help the patient with recurrent disease.[64] The use of accelerated hyperfractionation may also hold promise.[65]

Chemotherapy Chemotherapy for patients with cervical carcinoma is complicated because patients with cervical cancer frequently have decreased pelvic vascular perfusion, a limited bone marrow reserve, and poor renal function related to previous radiation, surgery, or ureteral obstruction from tumor or scarring.[14,66]

Response rates for patients with recurrent cervical cancer treated with single-agent chemotherapy (Tables 40-6 and 40-7)[38,67] range from 0% to 40%. In general, there is not long-term benefit, with responses lasting 4 to 6 months and variable lengths of survival. Single agent drugs showing significant activity include only 5-FU and cisplatin. Recently documented activity has been shown for dibromodulcitol, dianhydrogalactitol, ifosfamide, CHIP (iproplatin), and carboplatin.[38] Of the single agents, cisplatin remains the drug with the greatest antineoplastic activity.[38]

TABLE 40-6 Single-Agent Chemotherapy in Cervical Cancer

Drugs	Responders/ Total Treated	Overall Response (%)
Alkylating agents		
Cyclophosphamide	31/228	14
Chlorambucil	11/44	25
Dibromodulcitol	4/15	27
Dianhydrogalactitol	7/36	17
Ifosfamide	10/30	30
Antimetabolites		
5-Fluorouracil	68/348	20
Methotrexate	12/77	16
Mitotic inhibitors		
Vincristine	10/44	23
Antitumor antibiotics		
Doxorubicin (Adriamycin)	8/78	10
Bleomycin	17/172	10
Other agents		
Cisplatin	21/52	40
CHIP	7/36	21
Carboplatin	11/39	28
Piprazinedione	5/38	13

CHIP, iproplatin

Source: Hoskins WJ, Perez C, Young RC: Gynecologic tumors, in DeVita VT Jr, Hellman S, Rosenberg SA (eds): Cancer: Principles and Practice of Oncology (ed 3). Philadelphia, JB Lippincott, 1989, p 1133.

Combination chemotherapy (Table 40-8)[38] has not been definitely shown to be more effective than single agents. Complete response rates of 10% to 29% shown in several recent studies suggest some enhancement of effect using a combination of drugs. Rotmensch et al[68] used a combination of cisplatin and continuous-infusion 5-FU with a 50% response rate and feel this is a promising chemotherapy regimen for treating squamous cell carcinoma of the cervix. There is a necessity for larger, randomized trials before conclusions can be drawn about the most effective combination chemotherapy for patients with cervical carcinoma.[66]

Pelvic intra-arterial infusion of bleomycin, vincristine, and mitomycin-C has been studied in women with recurrent cervical cancer. Toxicity was significant, including pulmonary fibrosis from bleomycin and infectious or embolic complications from the catheterization. Response rates were low. More studies are needed to establish any benefits of this therapy.[38]

Chemotherapy as part of the initial treatment of patients with cervical cancer is also being investigated. Vogl[69] proposes its use in tumor debulking, spatial restoration,

TABLE 40-7 Cervical Carcinoma: Single-Agent Activity of Investigational Drugs in Patients with Squamous Cell Carcinoma

Drug	Patients	Responses No.	Responses (%)
AMSA	20	0	(0)
	25	1	(4)
Baker's antifol	32	5	(16)
Dianhydrogalactitol	36	7	(19)
Dibromodulcitol	47	7	(15)
ICRF-159	28	5	(18)
Maytansine	29	1	(2)
Mitotoxantrone	25	2	(8)
PALA	33	0	(0)
Piperazinedione	43	2	(5)
Spirogermanium	14	0	(0)
Vindesine	21	5	(24)
Yoshi 864	18	0	(0)

AMSA, Amsacrine; *PALA*, PALA disodium.

Source: Thigpen JT: Chemotherapy, in Morrow CP, Townsend DE (eds): Synopsis of Gynecologic Oncology (ed 3). New York, Wiley & Sons, 1987, pp 409-458. © John Wiley & Sons, Inc.

as a radiation sensitizer, and as adjuvant therapy. Because radiotherapy works better on a smaller tumor volume, induction chemotherapy may debulk the tumor before other therapies are started. This might reduce the incidence of pelvic failures. As a result of the debulking process, normal cervical size and architecture may be restored by chemotherapy before radiotherapy.[70] If the cervix is of normal size and configuration, intracavitary radiotherapy is more effective and less toxic.

Kim et al[71,72] used a regimen of vinblastine, bleomycin, and cisplatin initially in 54 patients (stages Ib and II with bulky tumors) followed by radical hysterectomy and found that it was effective in reducing tumor volume, the stage of the disease, and lymph node involvement and in improving the 2-year tumor-free survival rate.

Chemotherapy can be used as a radiation sensitizer, particularly hydroxyurea and cisplatin. Two studies have shown improved survival rates from the concurrent administration of radiation and hydroxyurea.[73,74] Several ongoing studies are using cisplatin concomitant with radiotherapy. Weekly low-dose cisplatin with radiation has been associated with a modest improvement in disease-free survival without any significant increases in toxicity.[38]

Chemotherapy might be studied for adjuvant use after definitive therapy in high-risk women. This could include women with positive nodes, bulky lesions, or adenocarcinomas. Weiner et al[75] suggest that a combination of mitomycin, vincristine, bleomycin, and cisplatin (MOBP) given before radiation therapy to patients with early disease and positive nodes may be beneficial.

Immunotherapy Recombinant alpha-2b-interferon for patients with disseminated cervical carcinoma is also being investigated in a phase II trial. Because cervical car-

TABLE 40-8 Combination Chemotherapy in Cervical Carcinoma

Regimen	Evaluable Patients	Number of Responses (%)	Complete Responses (%)
Doxorubicin (Adriamycin) and methotrexate	59	39 (66)	13 (22)
	24	7 (28)	0 (0)
Doxorubicin and methyl-CCNU	13	14 (45)	9 (29)
Doxorubicin and cisplatin	19	6 (31)	2 (10)
Mitomycin C and bleomycin	33	12 (36)	5 (15)
Mitomycin C, vincristine and bleomycin	91	46 (51)	14 (15)
Mitomycin C, vincristine, bleomycin and cisplatin	14	6 (43)	4 (29)
Cisplatin, bleomycin and velban	33	22 (66)	6 (18)
Cisplatin, bleomycin, vincristine and methotrexate	15	10 (66)	3 (20)

Source: Hoskins WJ, Perez C, Young RC: Gynecologic tumors, in DeVita VT Jr, Hellman S, Rosenberg SA (eds): Cancer: Principles and Practice of Oncology (ed 3). Philadelphia, JB Lippincott, 1989, p 1134.

cinoma is closely associated with HPV, and premalignant lesions of the female genital tract appear to be sensitive to interferon, it is hoped that this will be a helpful approach to the management of patients with this disease.[76]

ENDOMETRIAL CANCER

Epidemiology

Cancer of the endometrium is the most common malignancy of the female genital tract. Approximately 33,000 new cases of endometrial cancer will be diagnosed in the United States and approximately 4000 women will die of the disease in 1990.[1]

Endometrial cancer is primarily a postmenopausal disease. The median age at diagnosis is 61 years, with the largest number of women being between 50 and 59 years of age. Approximately 5% of women will be diagnosed before 40 years of age, and 20% to 25% will be diagnosed before menopause.[5]

Etiology

Multiple risk factors have been associated with the development of endometrial cancer. They include obesity, nulliparity, late menopause, diabetes, hypertension, infertility, irregular menses, failure of ovulation, a history of breast or ovarian cancer, adenomatous hyperplasia, and prolonged use of exogenous estrogen therapy. An obese, nulliparous woman who has menopause after 59 years of age appears to have a fivefold greater risk of developing endometrial cancer.[77]

An underlying derangement in endogenous estrogen metabolism or production has long been presumed to play a role in the development of endometrial cancer. Several hormonal aberrations can be linked to obesity. Fat is an excellent storage depot for estrogen. Chronic slow release of estrogen from fat cells may account for an increased risk of estrogen effects on the endometrium. In obese, postmenopausal women, secretion of serum sex hormone-binding globulin (SHBG) is depressed, leaving higher concentrations of free estradiol in the blood. Women above a certain body weight have endocrine malfunctions that cause anovulatory cycles with irregular menses. This results in failure of progesterone to oppose chronic estrogen effects on the endometrium. Another source of endogenous estrogen can be feminizing ovarian tumors (eg, granulosa cell tumors).[77]

Use of unopposed exogenous estrogens has been linked to an increased incidence of endometrial cancer. This problem could be virtually eliminated with regular gynecologic examinations that include endometrial evaluation and the use of cyclic estrogen. For example, oral estrogens could be given on days 1 through 25 of the menstrual cycle, with oral progesterone given on days 25 through 30.[5]

Either exogenous or endogenous estrogen may lead to endometrial hyperplasia. Adenomatous hyperplasia is the most worrisome because it is a precursor of endometrial carcinoma.

Clinical Manifestations

Postmenopausal bleeding should be considered a symptom of endometrial cancer until proven otherwise. Onset of irregular or heavy menstrual flow in a premenopausal woman also may be significant. Other more infrequent symptoms are yellow or serosanguineous vaginal discharge, pyometria, hematometria, and lumbosacral, hypogastric, or pelvic pain.[38]

Pathophysiology and Disease Progression

The uterine corpus is a muscular, hollow, pear-shaped organ that is lined by a mucous membrane called the endometrium. The endometrium is lined by ciliated surface epithelial cells. Throughout the epithelium are small, tubular glands that extend to the myometrium. The stroma is the connective tissue between the glands.[3]

Cancer usually starts in the fundus and may spread to involve the entire endometrium. It can infiltrate the myometrium and extend through the serosa. The tumor may extend into the endocervical canal and involve the entire cervix. It may expand into the parametrium, fallopian tubes, and ovaries.

Metastatic spread is usually to pelvic and para-aortic lymph nodes and has been correlated with tumor differentiation, stage of disease, and amount of myometrial invasion. Less common sites of metastases include the vagina, peritoneal cavity, omentum, and inguinal lymph nodes. Hematogenous spread, mostly seen in sarcomas, often involves the lung, liver, bone, and brain.

Over 90% of endometrial cancers are adenocarcinomas. The remainder are sarcoma, lymphoma, clear cell carcinoma, or epidermoid carcinoma. The following discussion focuses on adenocarcinomas.

Multiple factors have been identified for endometrial cancer that have prognostic significance. They include histologic type and differentiation, uterine size, stage of disease, myometrial invasion, peritoneal cytology, lymph node metastasis, and adnexal metastasis.

Histologic differentiation is one of the most sensitive prognostic indicators. The less differentiated the tumor, the poorer the prognosis. Grade 1 tumors are highly differentiated, grade 2 tumors are moderately differentiated, and grade 3 tumors are mostly solid or undifferentiated carcinomas.[38] Five-year survival rates are 92% for patients with grade I tumors, 74% for those with grade II tumors, and 48% for those with grade III tumors.[14] The less differentiated the tumor, the greater the chance of myometrial invasion.

The size of the uterus, measured by uterine sound, may affect survival. Large uterine size can be secondary to intercurrent disease, such as fibroids, so some authors disagree that size is a prognostic factor. The 5-year survival rate for women with a normal-sized uterus is 84%, whereas that for women with an enlarged uterus is 67%.[78]

Pretreatment staging helps to determine tumor size and extent. The majority of patients are first diagnosed with stage I disease.[14] Survival rates for endometrial cancer by stage are 76% for patients with stage I, 50% for those with stage II, 30% for those with stage III, and 9% for those with stage IV.[14]

The degree of myometrial invasion indicates how aggressive the tumor is. The extent of myometrial invasion is generally classified as endometrial (no muscular invasion), superficial (invasion into the first third), or deep (more than one third).[14] The greater the invasion, the poorer the prognosis. The grade of the tumor is combined with the degree of myometrial invasion to estimate survival. For example, a woman with deep myometrial invasion and a high-grade tumor has a poorer prognosis than one without myometrial invasion and a tumor of a lower grade.

During laparotomy, samples of peritoneal fluid or washings of the peritoneal cavity are obtained. This is for staging purposes, but the results also have prognostic significance. Women with positive washings are at a higher risk of pelvic recurrences. DiSaia and Creasman[5] report that 15% of their patients with stage I disease had positive washings. Recurrence developed in 34% of these individuals, compared with 10% in patients showing negative cytologic change.

Pelvic and para-aortic lymph node metastases may be present, even in women with stage I disease (Figure 40-8).[5] Less than 5% of patients with stage I disease have positive nodes, however. Of individuals with stage II disease, 36% have positive nodes.[79]

Endometrial cancer frequently metastasizes to the adnexa. If there are palpable adnexal masses, the woman is classified as having stage III disease. However, 10% of women with stage I disease have clinically undetected adnexal metastasis at surgery. Recurrences appear in 38% of women with adnexal metastasis versus 11% of those without adnexal involvement.[5]

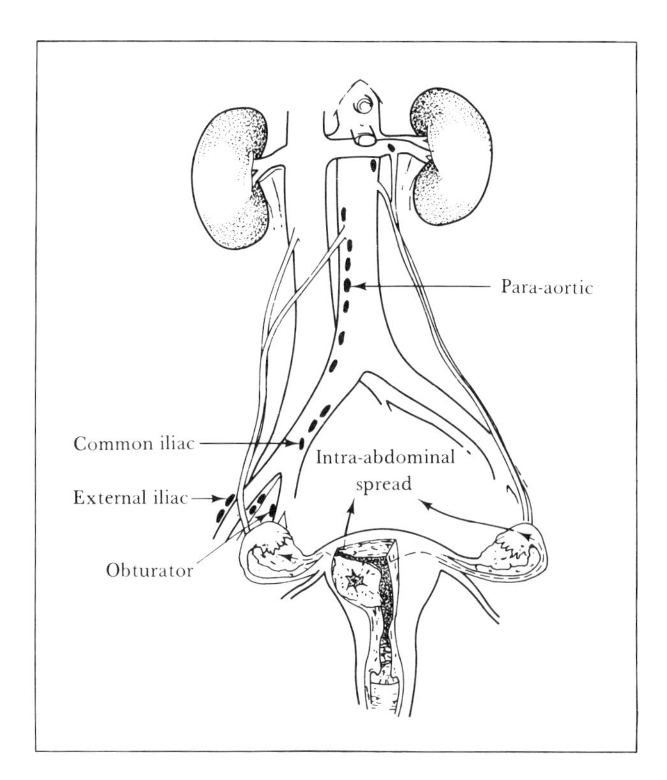

FIGURE 40-8 Spread pattern of endometrial cancer, with particular emphasis on potential lymph node spread. Pelvic and para-aortic nodes are at risk, even in stage I disease. (Source: DiSaia PJ, Creasman WT: Clinical Gynecologic Oncology. St Louis, CV Mosby, 1984.)

Assessment and Staging

In women suspected of having endometrial cancer, a thorough pelvic examination is performed, with particular attention to the vagina, since this is a frequent site of metastasis. A Pap smear may be performed but is not a reliable method of detecting endometrial cancer.[38] A more reliable technique is endometrial biopsy, which can be performed in the outpatient setting with local anesthesia. This procedure allows the woman to avoid hospitalization and is 90% effective in detecting endometrial cancer.[5] The American Cancer Society recommends endometrial sampling for women at high risk for the development of endometrial cancer at menopause.[80]

Fractional dilatation and curettage (D & C) is performed after biopsy-proven diagnosis or when persistent symptoms exist despite normal biopsy and cytology. In addition to dilating and curetting the endometrial cavity, it is imperative to obtain a separate endocervical curetting. This procedure helps to differentiate a cervical primary lesion from an endometrial primary tumor that has spread to the cervix.[5]

Other diagnostic tests include chest radiograph, IVP, CBC, and blood chemistry profiles. Cystoscopy, barium enema, and proctoscopy are performed if bladder or rectal involvement is suspected. Optional investigational studies include hysterography, hysteroscopy, lymphangiography, and CT scanning.[81]

Endometrial cancer is now staged surgically. Table 40-9[82] describes this method. Approximately 74% of tumors are stage I, 13% are stage II, 9% are stage III, and 3% are stage IV at diagnosis.[14]

Treatment

Primary

Many factors are considered by the radiation oncologist and gynecologist in planning therapy for women with endometrial cancer. The therapeutic approach is determined by tumor stage, histologic type and degree of differentiation, the size of the uterus, and the woman's medical condition.[38] Figure 40-9[5] summarizes the primary surgical treatment of patients with stage I endometrial cancer. The use of preoperative or postoperative irradia-

TABLE 40-9 Corpus Cancer Staging

Carcinoma of the uterine corpus

The Committee decided that corpus cancer should be surgically staged and as a result additional factors of prognostic importance are included in the staging. The Committee also decided to change the current definitions of tumour grading to coincide with the new recommendations of the International Society of Gynaecological Pathologists. The recommended staging is as follows:

Stage

IA	G123	Tumour limited to endometrium
IB	G123	Invasion to <1/2 myometrium
IC	G123	Invasion to >1/2 myometrium
IIA	G123	Endocervical glandular involvement only
IIB	G123	Cervical stromal invasion
IIIA	G123	Tumour invades serosa and/or adnexa and/or positive peritoneal cytology
IIIB	G123	Metastases to pelvic and/or para-aortic lymph nodes
IVA	G123	Tumour invasion of bladder and/or bowel mucosa
IVB		Distant metastases including intra-abdominal and/or inguinal lymph nodes

Histopathology: degree of differentiation

Cases of carcinoma of the corpus should be grouped with regard to the degree of differentiation of the adenocarcinoma as follows:

G1 5% or less of a non-squamous or non-morular solid growth pattern
G2 6%-50% of a non-squamous or non-morular solid growth pattern
G3 More than 50% of a non-squamous or nonmorular solid growth pattern

Notes on pathological grading

(1) Notable nuclear atypia, inappropriate for the architectural grade, raises the grade of a grade I or grade II tumour by one.
(2) In serous adenocarcinomas, clear-cell adenocarcinomas, and squamous-cell carcinomas, nuclear grading takes precedence.
(3) Adenocarcinomas with squamous differentiation are graded according to the nuclear grade of the glandular component.

Rules related to staging

(1) Since corpus cancer is now surgically staged, procedures used previously for the differentiation of stages are no longer applicable, such as using dilatation and curettage findings to differentiate between stage I and stage II. (It is appreciated that there may be a small number of patients with corpus cancer who will be treated primarily with radiation therapy. If that is the case, the clinical staging adopted by FIGO* in 1971 would still apply but designation of that staging system would be noted.)
(2) Ideally, the thickness of the myometrium should be measured along with the depth of tumour invasion.

* *FIGO*, International Federation of Gynecology & Obstetrics.

Source: Shepard JH: Revised FIGO staging for gynaecological cancer. Br J Obstet Gynaecol 96(8):889-892, 1989. Blackwell Scientific Publications Ltd.

tion has been extensively investigated with no evidence of a survival benefit.[14] Patients with tumors of poor histologic grade, deep myometrial invasion, or extensive involvement of the lower uterine segment or cervix may benefit from intracavitary or external-beam irradiation to reduce vaginal recurrence.[14]

Women with stage II endometrial carcinoma may be treated in the same manner as those with stage I, grade II and III disease if no visible disease is present on the cervix and no parametrial disease is present. If the disease is more extensive, preoperative radiotherapy may be used.

Stage III and IV disease is uncommon; therefore, treatment is highly individualized and is usually palliative.[83] Systemic therapy (hormonal therapy or chemotherapy) is usually given because of distant metastasis.[5]

Recurrent disease

Despite the fact that almost 75% of endometrial cancers are stage I, there are deaths due to this disease. Endometrial cancer is one of the most difficult cancers to treat when metastasis has occurred.[84] Local sites of metastases include the pelvis, vagina, and para-aortic lymph nodes.[38]

Patients with vaginal recurrences can be treated successfully with surgery or radiotherapy. These individuals do well and usually are long-term survivors.[5]

Women with recurrences outside the upper vagina (pelvis or distant) are not easily treated. Radiotherapy has a limited role in recurrent disease; therefore, hormonal therapy or chemotherapy is the treatment of choice.[5]

Hormonal therapy The most commonly used systemic therapy for recurrent endometrial cancer has been synthetic progestational agents. Response rates range from 30% to 37%. Response seems to be related to histologic grade of the tumor, length of the disease-free interval, the woman's age, and presence of areas of squamous metaplasia within the tumor.[38] Receptor status also appears to predict which tumors will respond to progestins. Positive

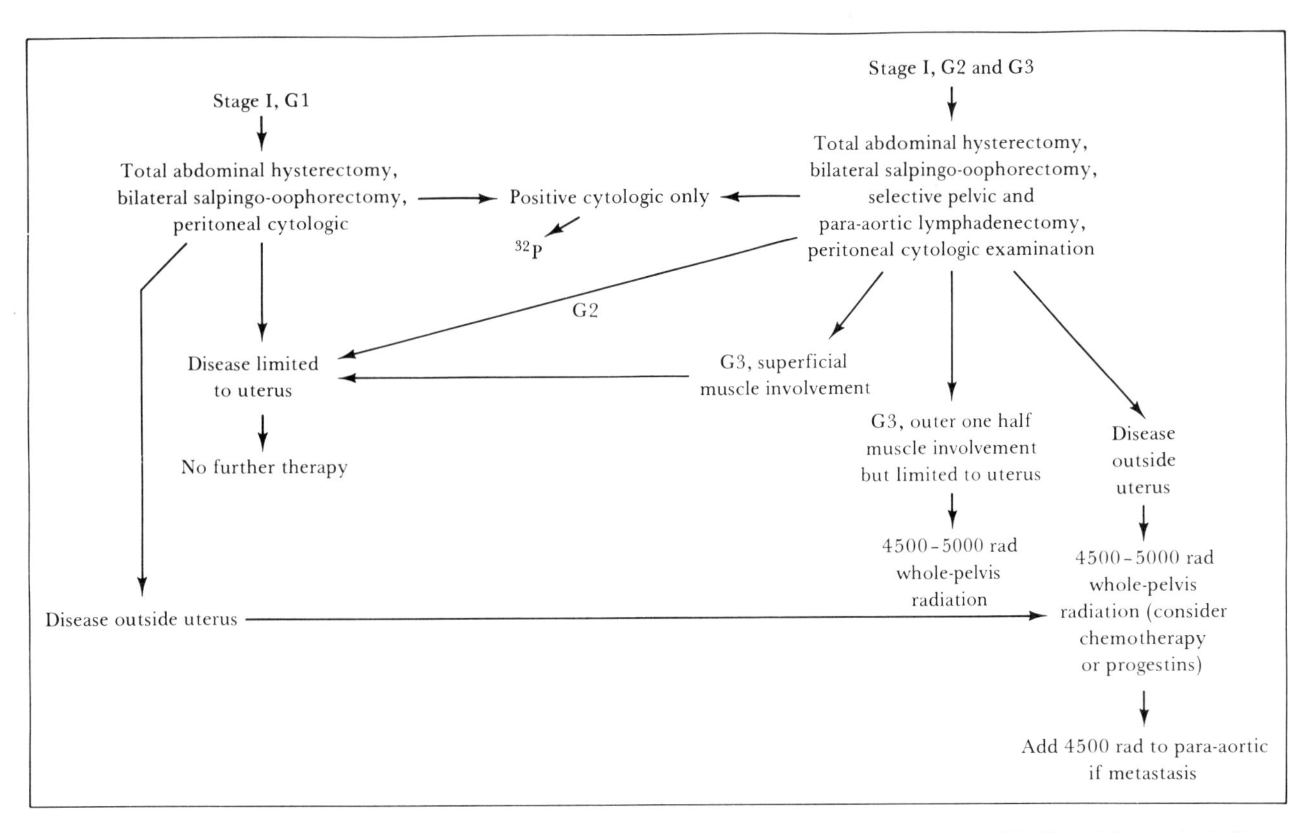

FIGURE 40-9 Primary surgical management of endometrial cancer. (Source: DiSaia PJ, Creasman WT: Clinical Gynecologic Oncology. St Louis, CV Mosby, 1984.)

receptor status correlates with a better chance to respond to progestins. Those positive for both receptors have a 77% response rate to progestins compared with only a 9% response rate among those who are negative for both receptors.[66]

Oral preparations of megestrol acetate (Megace) or intramuscular medroxyprogesterone acetate (Depo-Provera) are effective agents against endometrial cancer.[38] The progestins are continued until the disease progresses. At that time, chemotherapy is considered.

Kauppila et al[85] reported on over 1100 patients who received adjuvant progestin therapy for 2 years after primary treatment for endometrial cancer; recurrence occurred even in women with stage I disease. The effectiveness of adjuvant hormonal therapy in endometrial cancer is considered unproven and remains controversial.[38]

Considerable interest has been shown in the specific estrogen-progesterone receptors in malignant endometrial cells. With the availability of assays for receptors, more information can be collected on the response to hormonal therapy. Preliminary studies showed a positive correlation between the presence of progesterone receptors and clinical response to progestin therapy.[86] This information also might be correlated with prognostic factors to pinpoint even more specifically women who will respond. Theoretically, women with positive estrogen receptors should respond to antiestrogen therapy. If both estrogen receptors and progesterone receptors are positive, future trials may employ combination hormonal therapy. Utaaker et al[87] concluded from their study that steroid receptors were found in more than 85% of primary endometrial carcinomas. Highly differentiated tumors were more often estrogen receptor and progesterone receptor rich than poorly differentiated ones, but receptor status was not significantly associated with surgical stages.

Tamoxifen has been used in patients with advanced endometrial cancer in an attempt to induce progesterone receptor positivity. No improvement in length of response was seen, although the drug was shown to increase the number of receptors per tumor.[88] The use of tamoxifen is still experimental.[14] Quinn and Campbell[89] suggest using a combination of tamoxifen and a progestagen as the first choice of endocrine therapy.

Chemotherapy Because progestin therapy has been the mainstay of systemic therapy for endometrial cancer, few chemotherapy trials have been conducted. In single-agent trials, the most promising results were obtained by Thigpen et al[90] using 60 mg/m^2 of doxorubicin every 3 weeks. These researchers reported a 37% response rate, with 26% complete responses. Prognostic factors had no effect on the probability of response.

Administration of cisplatin has achieved response rates of 46% when used in high doses (100 mg/m^2) in women with no prior chemotherapy.[91] However, when cisplatin was used as second-line treatment, the results were not impressive (4% response rate).[92] Thigpen et al[93] studied 49 patients with advanced or recurrent endometrial carcinoma who had not received prior chemotherapy and who were no longer controllable with other treatment modalities. Patients were treated with cisplatin, 50 mg/m^2 intravenously, every 3 weeks; 45% exhibited stable disease for at least 2 months, while 35% progressed in less than 2 months after beginning chemotherapy.[93]

Combination therapy has been studied to a limited degree; however, cisplatin, doxorubicin, and cyclophosphamide resulted in an overall response rate of 45% in 209 patients.[94] Other studies have shown little improvement over response rates seen with single agents.

Thigpen et al[97] suggest that there is little evidence at present to support the use of combination chemotherapy in the management of endometrial carcinoma. Well-controlled clinical trials examining the role of combination chemotherapy in patients with advanced or recurrent endometrial carcinoma are needed.[14]

OVARIAN CANCER

Epidemiology

Approximately 27% of all gynecologic cancers are ovarian, with 52% of deaths from cancer of the female genital tract occuring as a result of ovarian cancer. It is the most common cause of death from gynecologic cancers in the United States.[95] There will be approximately 20,500 new cases diagnosed in the United States and over 12,400 deaths in 1990.[1]

It is estimated that one of every 70 women will develop ovarian cancer, with most cases seen in women between 55 and 59 years of age.[96,97] Only 7% to 8% of ovarian carcinoma occurs in women under 35 years of age.[98]

Ovarian cancers are common in modern or highly industrialized nations (Switzerland, United States, and Scandinavia) but occur less frequently in the Orient and Latin America.[81]

Etiology

Little is known regarding the etiology of ovarian cancer. Because the incidence is higher in industrialized countries (except Japan), environmental factors may play a role. Hormonal factors, such as nulliparity, infertility, and estrogen therapy, may play a role in epithelial ovarian cancer. Marked premenstrual tension, abnormal breast swelling, and marked dysmenorrhea are suspected of linkage to ovarian cancer. There is not good evidence that irradiation increases the frequency of ovarian cancer. Use of oral contraceptives and pregnancy may be protective factors.[99] Talc has been examined as a potential etiologic agent. It has been suggested that talc may act as a tumor-promotor by direct contact with the ovaries after passage through the vagina.[95,97] The relationship to diet is controversial, with some authors stating that there "seems to be no relationship between ovarian cancer and dietary practices"[95] and others stating that ovarian cancer is associated with a diet high in fats.[96,97]

Women with a family history of ovarian cancer are at an increased risk of developing the disease, but these situations are rare.[95,96] A history of breast cancer doubles the risk of ovarian cancer.[95] Cancer of the colon also places a woman at risk of ovarian cancer.[100] The overall 5-year survival rate for women with ovarian cancer is about 30% to 35%. This figure has not changed in the past 30 years. The poor survival rate is partially because ovarian neoplasms are difficult to diagnose early (60% to 70% of tumors are stage III or IV at diagnosis), treatment has not been perfected, a high-risk population has not been defined, and the etiology is essentially unknown.

Clinical Manifestations

Unfortunately, there are typically no early manifestations of ovarian cancer. Truly localized disease limited to the ovary is asymptomatic in the majority of women. As the mass enlarges, the woman may experience abdominal discomfort, dyspepsia, indigestion, flatulence, eructations, loss of appetite, pelvic pressure, or urinary frequency. These vague complaints are often not recognized as anything more than "middle-age indigestion" and may precede other symptoms by months.[97] A physician examining a 40- to 70-year-old woman with these persistent symptoms should include ovarian cancer in the differential diagnostic workup. Unfortunately, these nonspecific complaints are not disabling, so physicians may overlook the possibility of ovarian cancer. Not until the woman has a palpable mass or ascites does the appropriate evaluation begin.[5] At diagnosis, the cancer has spread beyond the ovary in 75% of patients.[99]

Pathophysiology and Disease Progression

Ovarian cancer is not one disease but rather is composed of several cell types that may occur in different age groups, exhibit different methods of spread, and respond to different therapeutic regimens. Epithelial, stromal, and germinal cells give rise to the four major subsets of ovarian cancer. Epithelial tumors constitute 80% to 90% of all malignant ovarian neoplasms.[95,96,99] The histologic categories of these tumors include serous, mucinous, endometroid, clear cell, Brenner, and undifferentiated carcinomas. Some ovarian tumors that are in the epithelial subset (10% to 20%) are characterized as "low malignant potential" (LMP) carcinomas. These tumors are intermediate between benign tumors and those with invasive characteristics.[96,97] Malignant germ cell tumors account for 4% of ovarian malignancies and are most often encountered in children and premenopausal women. The remaining 6% of ovarian malignancies are sex cord or stromal tumors. The following discussion focuses only on the epithelial ovarian cancers.

Histologic grade seems to be an important predictor of treatment response and survival.[99] Although important for all stages of disease, the grade seems to be prognostically significant in stage I and II disease. More differentiated tumors may respond better to treatment.[99]

Knowledge of the natural history of ovarian cancer is essential to appreciate the difficulties in staging and treatment. The most common mechanisms of spread are by direct extension and serosal seeding. Direct extension occurs when tumor cells penetrate the capsule of the ovary and invade adjacent structures. These structures include the fallopian tubes, uterus, bladder, and rectosigmoid and pelvic peritoneum. Peritoneal seeding can be microscopic or macroscopic and is the major route of dissemination. These tumor nodules or seeds are found on the peritoneal surfaces of the liver, diaphragm, bladder, and large and small bowel. This seeding is the basis for the formation of ascites in ovarian cancer. In addition, the diaphragmatic and substernal lymphatics that drain the peritoneal cavity can become obstructed, and peritoneal fluid subsequently accumulates.[99]

Although intraperitoneal spread is the most common method of dissemination, ovarian lymphatics are also an important pathway for dissemination. The ovary contains an extensive lymphatic network that flows cephalad toward the aortic nodes. Piver et al[101] found a 10% incidence of aortic and pelvic lymph node metastasis in stage I and II ovarian cancer. It is essential that these nodes be sampled during surgery to ensure proper staging.

Hematogenous spread of disease is the least common method of dissemination. The most frequently encountered distant sites are the liver, lung, pleura, kidney, bone, adrenal glands, bladder, and spleen.[99]

Death is usually due to intra-abdominal tumor dissemination. Bowel and mesentery are most commonly involved, producing multiple areas of malfunction, malabsorption, and varying degrees of alteration of peristalsis and obstruction. Women with intra-abdominal tumor dissemination gradually deteriorate and eventually die of electrolyte imbalance, sepsis, or cardiovascular collapse. Other contributing causes of death include toxicities of treatment, intercurrent medical problems, and pulmonary embolus.[100]

Assessment and Staging

Routine pelvic examinations will detect one ovarian carcinoma in 10,000 examinations of asymptomatic women. Despite this, pelvic examinations remain the most reliable method of detecting early disease. Pap smears are positive in a very small percentage of women. Any ovary that can be palpated in a woman 3 to 5 years or more after menopause should raise a high index of suspicion for an early ovarian neoplasm.[5] Barber[97] refers to this as "the postmenopausal palpable ovary syndrome" and states that it must be "investigated promptly for the presence or absence of an ovarian tumor."

Routine diagnostic tests are not of great value in the diagnosis of ovarian cancer. The major value of the tests is to rule out another primary tumor as the source of the pelvic mass. A complete physical examination is carried out, with careful attention to the pelvis, abdomen, and breasts. Barium enema is done to rule out primary rectosigmoid cancer, which can metastasize to ovaries. Proctosigmoidoscopy is valuable if the woman has lower intestinal symptoms. An upper gastrointestinal series can be individualized to the woman's symptoms. Chest radiography is done to look for pleural effusions and parenchymal metastases. IVP is done to rule out the kidney as the source of the pelvic mass. US and CT scans are often used to evaluate the potential size and location of the mass. MRI may be helpful for detecting lesions smaller than are possible with either US and CT but probably will be most helpful in monitoring therapy.[97] Paracentesis is avoided because it can rupture an encapsulated ovarian mass; malignant cells would then be spilled into the peritonteal cavity.[5] A laparotomy is necessary regardless of whether the fluid is malignant.

The staging of ovarian cancer is based on surgical evaluation (Table 40-10)[58] and is the cornerstone for all subsequent therapy. Approximately 15% to 20% of patients present as stage I, 10% to 15% as stage II, 60% to 70% as stage III, and 10% to 15% as stage IV.[14] Figure 40-10[102] summarizes the surgical approach in ovarian cancer. The purposes of the initial surgical exploration are precise diagnosis, accurate staging, and optimal debulking. Unfortunately, accurate surgical staging is obtained in a minority of patients presenting with early ovarian cancer.[95] Only about 25% of women operated on in the Untied States have a surgical incision adequate to allow evaluation of the entire pelvis and abdominal cavity. Understaging is common; 33% of patients thought to be free of disease at initial surgery have residual disease, and in 75% of women the disease has spread intra-abdominally.[103] Thorough cytoreductive surgery is paramount for effective postoperative adjuvant therapy. A major prognostic factor in ovarian cancer is the diameter of the largest residual tumor.[95,96,104]

Treatment

Ovarian cancer therapy is usually staged and surgically resected at the same time. Thorough evaluation and maximum tumor reduction are the goal of the initial operation. However, because the majority of cases of epithelial ovarian cancer are not diagnosed in the early stages, adjuvant therapy is usually indicated. Selection of the appropriate adjuvant therapy is based on stage, the size and location of residual tumor, the presence of ascites, or the discovery that the peritoneal fluid is contaminated with malignant cells.[105]

Stage I

Total abdominal hysterectomy with bilateral salpingo-oophorectomy (TAH-BSO) is the therapy of choice for patients with stage I disease. Omentectomy is essential, not only to look for microscopic disease but to facilitate the

TABLE 40-10 Staging Classification of Malignant Ovarian Tumors

Primary Tumor (T)

TNM	FIGO	Definition
TX		Primary tumor cannot be assessed
T0		No evidence of primary tumor
T1	I	Tumor limited to ovaries
T1a	Ia	Tumor limited to one ovary; capsule intact, no tumor on ovarian surface
T1b	Ib	Tumor limited to both ovaries; capsules intact, no tumor on ovarian surface
T1c	Ic	Tumor limited to one or both ovaries with any of the following: capsule ruptured, tumor on ovarian surface, malignant cells in ascites, or peritoneal washing
T2	II	Tumor involves one or both ovaries with pelvic extension
T2a	IIa	Extension and/or implants on uterus and/or tube(s)
T2b	IIb	Extension to other pelvic tissues
T2c	IIc	Pelvic extension (2a or 2b) with malignant cells in ascites or peritoneal washing
T3 and/or N1	III	Tumor involves one or both ovaries with microscopically confirmed peritoneal metastasis outside the pelvis and/or regional lymph node metastasis
T3a	IIIa	Microscopic peritoneal metastasis beyond pelvis
T3b	IIIb	Macroscopic peritoneal metastasis beyond pelvis 2 cm or less in greatest dimension
T3c and/or N1	IIIc	Peritoneal metastasis beyond pelvis more than 2 cm in greatest dimension and/or regional lymph node metastasis
M1	IV	Distant metastasis (excludes peritoneal metastasis)

Regional Lymph Nodes (N)

Regional lymph nodes include hypogastric (obturator), common iliac, external iliac, internal iliac, lateral sacral, para-aortic, and inguinal.

NX	Regional lymph nodes cannot be assessed
N0	No regional lymph node metastasis
N1	Regional lymph node metastasis

Distant Metastasis (M)

TNM	FIGO	Definition
MX		Presence of distant metastasis cannot be assessed
M0		No distant metastasis
M1	IV	Distant metastasis (excludes peritoneal metastasis)

Stage Grouping

Stage IA	T1a	N0	M0
Stage IB	T1b	N0	M0
Stage IC	T1c	N0	M0
Stage IIA	T2a	N0	M0
Stage IIB	T2b	N0	M0
Stage IIC	T2c	N0	M0
Stage IIIA	T3a	N0	M0
Stage IIIB	T3b	N0	M0
Stage IIIC	T3c	N0	M0
	Any T	N1	M0
Stage IV	Any T	Any N	M1

Source: American Joint Committee on Cancer; Manual For Staging of Cancer (ed 3). Chicago, The Committee, 1988.

use of intraperitoneal radioisotopes. Because 10% to 20% of women will have nodal involvement, lymphadenectomy may be done.[5]

Occasionally, disease may be of low histologic grade and confined to one ovary and therefore of favorable prognosis. In this situation, conservative surgical treatment may be acceptable.[5] If fertility is a concern, a unilateral salpingo-oophorectomy may be performed for select candidates.

No standard adjuvant therapy can be recommended for stage 1 ovarian cancer; therapies vary and are still under investigation. The therapies used are intraperitoneal radioisotopes, external radiotherapy, and systemic and intraperitoneal chemotherapy.

Radioactive chromic phosphate (^{32}P) and radioactive gold (^{198}Au) have been used as adjuvant therapy in women with stage I ovarian cancer (Figure 40-11).[5] Colloidal gold is not presently available for therapy. Complications can include small-bowel obstruction and stenosis.[99] Complications are slightly higher in women who have uneven distribution of the radioactive material in the peritoneal cavity.[99,106,107] Potter et al[108] treated 59 patients with intra-

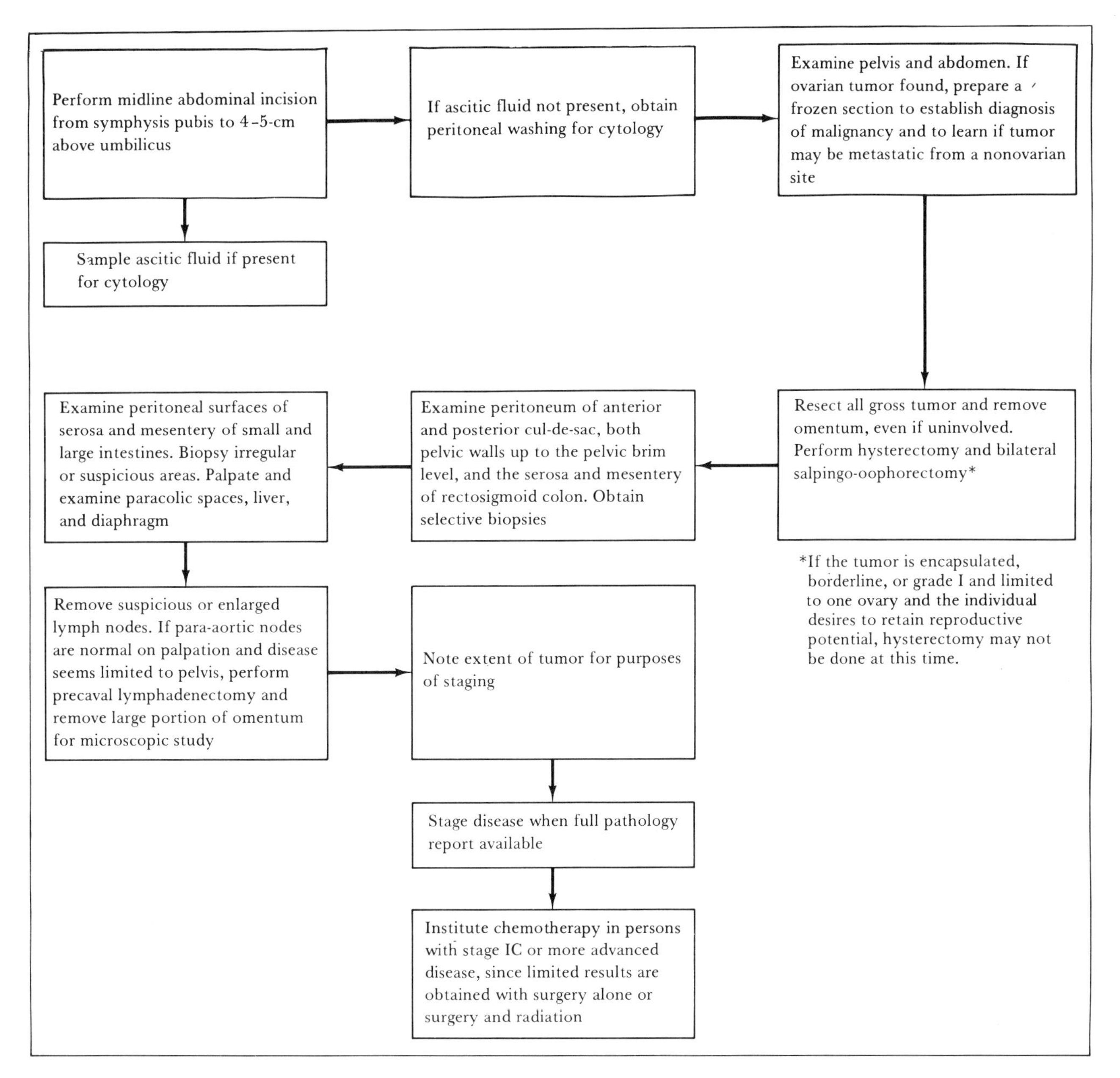

FIGURE 40-10 Surgery for ovarian carcinoma. (Source: Bristol Laboratories, Division of Bristol-Myers Co: Platinol: Effective palliation therapy in metastatic ovarian cancer. Syracuse, NY, Bristol Laboratories, 1982.)

peritoneal chromic phosphate and concluded that it is an alternative to chemotherapy or external radiation in the primary treatment of early stage ovarian lesions. It may also be useful for second-line therapy of early stage or low-grade ovarian lesions after a positive second-look surgery, but only if no gross residual disease remains. In general, reported cure rates for stage I tumors have been in the range of 90%, but there is not evidence that those results are better than what might have been achieved in the same patients without radiotherapy.[107]

Early studies of localized ovarian cancer did not include careful surgical staging and thus were not conclusive in determining optimum treatment for early-stage disease.[95] Generally patients received no additional therapy, pelvic irradiation, or intermittent oral melphalan after the initial surgery. Relapse after pelvic irradiation was 30%, compared with observation (17%) and intermittent oral melphalan (6%).[95] Carefully controlled studies are now being done to determine the best approach for treating stage I ovarian cancer patients, since approximately 20% of patients with early-stage disease still relapse and die.[14,109]

Stage II

The treatment of choice for women with stage II ovarian cancer is a TAH-BSO, omentectomy, and appendec-

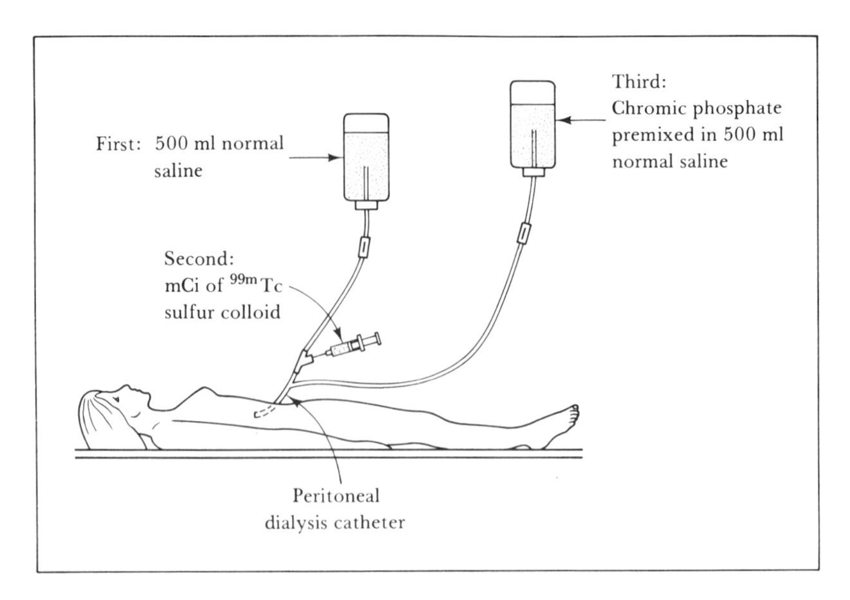

FIGURE 40-11 Method of administration of radioactive colloidal chromic phosphate into the peritoneal cavity. (Source: DiSaia PJ, Creasman WT: Clinical Gynecology Oncology. St Louis, CV Mosby, 1984.)

tomy; intraperitoneal ^{32}P instillation is optional.[97] Data on the therapy of stage II ovarian cancer is sparse because few women are diagnosed at this stage.

Stage III and IV

Advanced ovarian cancer is not curable by surgery alone. Controversy exists about the initial surgical approach to be used, the role of abdominal radiation therapy, and the choice of postoperative chemotherapy.[95] The unresolved issue related to use of cytoreductive surgery is whether the poor prognosis associated with bulky disease is due to increased tumor burden or if there is a difference in tumor biology associated with bulky disease or a decreased sensitivity to chemotherapeutic agents. It is also not clear when surgery is best performed (ie, before any chemotherapy, after one to three cycles of induction chemotherapy, or after completion of a full course of chemotherapy).[95]

Chemotherapy

Single agent therapy The mainstay of adjuvant therapy for stage III and IV epithelial ovarian cancer is chemotherapy. Historically, standard therapy has been single-alkylating agents: melphalan, chlorambucil, thiotepa, cyclophosphamide, and nitrosoureas. In the United States, the agent of choice was usually melphalan because it could be given orally and rarely caused alopecia or nausea.[110] Response rates seen with alkylating agents were 33% to 65%.[99] A small number of women (5% to 10%) are cured with single alkylating agent therapy.[99] Other single agents, including hexamethylmelamine, doxorubicin, and cisplatin, have response rates in the range of 20% to 35%. Cisplatin is considered to be one of the most active agents for treatment of ovarian cancer.[99] Other single agents that may have some activity in advanced ovarian cancer include ifosfamide, AZQ, VP-16 (etoposide), Peptichemio, and low-dose mitomycin C (Table 40-11).[99]

Combination chemotherapy Combination chemotherapy for advanced ovarian cancer has been studied extensively. It is difficult to compare the studies because of great variation in patient selection, prognostic factors, and response criteria. However, the studies generally compare

TABLE 40-11 Single Agents Active in Advanced Ovarian Adenocarcinoma

Alkylating agents	Plant alkaloids
Melphalan	Vinblastine
Chlorambucil	VP-16
Thiotepa	
Cyclophosphamide	Miscellaneous
Mechlorethamine	Hexamethylmelamine
Ifosfamide	Cisplatin
AZQ	Carboplatin
	Dianhydrogalacticol
Antimetabolites	Peptichemio
5-Fluorouracil	
Methotrexate	
Antitumor antibiotics	
Doxorubicin (Adriamycin)	
Mitomycin C	

AZQ, Aziridinyl benzoquinone; *VP-16*, etoposide.
Source: Adapted from Young R, Fuks Z, Hoskins WJ: Cancer of the ovary, in DeVita VT, Hellman S, Rosenberg SA (eds): Cancer: Principles and Practice of Oncology (ed 3). Philadelphia, JB Lippincott, 1989, p 1179.

single agents to combination chemotherapy and salvage chemotherapy regimens for those women who did not respond to previous therapy.[99]

The first study that demonstrated significantly improved survival using combination chemotherapy compared HexaCAF (hexamethylmelamine, cyclophosphamide, methotrexate, and 5-FU) with melphalan alone. The four-drug combination yielded better results, with an overall response rate of 75% versus 54%, a complete response rate of 33% versus 16%, and median survival of 29 months versus 17 months.[99,111] Several studies followed, showing that combination therapy is more beneficial than single-agent therapy in advanced ovarian cancer. It appears that a combination of full-dose chemotherapy offers the best chance for achieving a complete remission in women with advanced ovarian carcinoma.[99]

Table 40-12[99] summarizes results of studies using combination chemotherapy in advanced ovarian cancers. The overall response rate is 60% to 80%, with clinical complete remission seen in approximately 40% to 50% of women. Half the women who have complete clinical remission demonstrate residual disease at second-look laparotomy. About 25% to 30% of women will be disease-free at restaging and these women have prolonged disease-free survival.[99] The optimal combination regimen remains elusive.[112] The optimal duration of chemotherapy also is not clear. Gershenson et al[112] believe that maximum benefit from combination chemotherapy is achieved with six to nine cyles of therapy. There is substantial evidence to demonstrate that cisplatin is an important agent in any ovarian cancer chemotherapy regimen. Randomized comparisons of combination regimens indicate that there is not a com-

TABLE 40-12 Combination Chemotherapy in Advanced Ovarian Carcinoma

Regimen	Schedule	No. of Evaluable Patients	Complete and Partial Remissions (%)	No. of Clinical CR (%)	No. of Pathologic CR (%)
PAC		56	44/56 (79)	23/56 (41)	10/56 (18)
Cisplatin	20mg/m² IV day × 5 q 4 wk				
Adriamycin	50 mg/m² IV day 1 q 4 wk				
Cyclophosphamide	750 mg/m² IV day 1 q 4 wk				
A-C		41	35/41 (83)	20/41 (48)	12/41 (29)
Cyclophosphamide	500 mg/m² IV				
Adriamycin	40 mg/m²				
Hexa-CAF		40	30/40 (75)		13/40 (33)
Hexamethylmelamine	150 mg/m² PO qd × 14				
Cyclophosphamide	150 mg/m² PO qd × 14				
Methotrexate	40 mg/m² IV days 1,8				
5-Fluorouracil	600 mg/m² IV days 1,8				
CHAD		46	45/46 (98)	35/46 (76)	14/46 (30)
Cyclophosphamide	600 mg/m² IV day 1				
Hexamethylmelamine	200 mg/m² PO days 8–22				
Adriamycin	25 mg/m² IV day 1				
Cisplatin	50 mg/m² IV day 1				
CHEX-UP		62	43/62 (69)	29/62 (47)	12/62 (19)
Cyclophosphamide	150 mg/m² PO days 2–8 and 2–16				
Hexamethylmelamine	150 mg/m² PO days 2–8 and 9–16				
5-Fluorouracil	600 mg/m² IV days 1 and 8				
Cisplatin	30 mg/m² IV days 1 and 8				
CHAP-5		84	66/84 (79)	Not stated	25/84 (30)
Cyclophosphamide	100 mg/m² PO days 15–29				
Hexamethylmelamine	150 mg/m² PO days 15–29				
Adriamycin	35 mg/m² IV day 1				
Cisplatin	20 mg/m² IV days 1–5				
PC		52	Not stated	Not stated	12/52 (23)
Cisplatin	20 mg/m² IV days 1 5				
Cyclophosphamide	600 mg/m² IV day 4				

CR, complete remission.

Source: Young R, Fuks Z, Hoskins WJ: Cancer of the ovary, in DeVita VT, Hellman S, Rosenberg SA (eds): Cancer: Principles and Practice of Oncology (ed 3). Philadelphia, JB Lippincott, 1989, p 1181.

bination of drugs that produces better results than the CP (cyclophosphamide and cisplatin) regimen in full therapeutic doses.[99]

A number of studies have also demonstrated a clinically important dose relationship with cisplatin. Patients who were refractory to initial therapy or had recurrent disease and those patients not previously treated have received various schedules and ranges of high-dose cisplatin. The major dose-limiting toxicity of high-dose cisplatin is neurotoxicity.[95] Results of these studies are not clear in terms of survival, but it does appear that the high-dose chemotherapy regimen is markedly effective in rapidly debulking tumors in patients who present with advanced-stage disease and large abdominal tumors.[95] Cisplatin analogs, carboplatin and tetraplatin, are being investigated, as are pharmacologic techniques to decrease some of the toxicities associated with cisplatin and its analogs. A randomized trial comparing a CHAP-5 regimen (cisplatin, 20 mg/m^2 daily $\times 5$; doxorubicin, 35 mg/m^2 on day 1, hexamethylmelamine, 150 mg/m^2; cyclophosphamide, 100 mg/m^2 orally on days 14 to 28) with CHAC-1 (Carboplatin 350 mg/m^2 on day 1, all other drugs the same as CHAP-5) showed that antitumor activity did not appear to have any statistical differences between the two regimens but that the toxicity pattern observed in patients treated with CHAC-1 was much milder and more tolerable.[113] Diethyldithiocarbamate (DDTC) may protect against the myelosuppression of carboplatin and the dose-limiting neurotoxicity of cisplatin without changing the antitumor effect. If this is so, dose escalation could be achieved without increased toxicity.[95] Rothenberg et al[114] studied 21 patients with relapsed or refractory ovarian cancer who were treated with high-dose carboplatin followed 3 hours later with DDTC (4 g/m^2). The overall response rate was 19%; however, the regimen was associated with clinically significant hematologic and autonomic toxic effects.[114]

Unfortunately, the majority of patients suffer disease recurrence following response to initial chemotherapy. Second-line single agents have response rates ranging from 0% to 6% in those women who have received prior cisplatin therapy, and generally the responses are partial and of short duration.[115]

Alberts et al[115] studied 25 relapsed ovarian cancer patients who received mitomycin C, 10 mg/m^2 intravenously on day 1 every 6 weeks, and 5-FU, 500 mg/m^2 intravenously daily on days 1 to 3 every 3 weeks. The overall objective response rate was 40%, and the most prevalent toxicity was bone marrow suppression. They suggest further trials of this combination and possibly adding cisplatin to the regimen for first-line therapy in patients with clinically measurable diseases.[115]

Hormone therapy Hormone therapy for ovarian cancer has resulted in uneven responses.[116] Tamoxifen has been investigated as a second-line drug in individuals who have failed combination chemotherapy.[81,117] Belinson et al[118] randomly treated 33 patients with either megestrol acetate alone or megestrol acetate and tamoxifen. Doses were 160 mg/day of megestrol acetate and 20 mg/day of tamoxifen. No patients demonstrated tumor regression, but overall 39% showed stabilization of disease from 4 to 16+ months. Kavanagh et al[116] used leuprolide acetate (1 mg subcutaneously daily for a minimum of 8 weeks) for patients with refractory epithelial ovarian cancer and found better responses in patients with grade 1 disease. Further clinical trials are needed.

Drug resistance Tumors that develop multidrug resistance severely limit the effectiveness of chemotherapy in treating patients with ovarian cancer. Drug resistance is likely due to multiple factors, including (1) presence of the *MDR*-1 gene with its protein product, (2) the P-170 glycoprotein, (3) the elevation of intracellular glutathione (GSH), and (4) increased DNA repair.[99] It may be possible to pharmacologically reverse the drug resistance.[99,119] Clinical trials using verapamil and buthionine sulfoximine (BSO) are under study.[99]

It is clear that debulking surgery to reduce tumor burden to aggregates of 2 cm or less improves the response to postoperative chemotherapy.[99] Moreover, complete responses are associated with significant increase in survival as compared with partial responses or no responses. Chemotherapeutic combinations are associated with higher overall response rates and, more important, with an increase in complete responses. New combinations, alternate dosing schedules, and sequential and continuous infusion administration techniques continue to be investigated.[120,121]

Intraperitoneal chemotherapy One approach to chemotherapy administration is the intraperitoneal method. Because the primary spread of ovarian cancer is intraperitoneal, this is a logical approach. The aim of this method is to increase cytotoxic drug levels intraperitoneally while keeping systemic levels low. Patients with ovarian carcinoma who most likely will benefit from intraperitoneal therapy will be those with minimal residual disease following either surgery alone or surgery plus chemotherapy.[122] Other potential uses of intraperitoneal chemotherapy in ovarian cancer are (1) as an adjuvant to surgery in early-stage patients at high risk of relapse, (2) together with systemic therapy in patients with advanced disease and those not previously treated, and (3) as consolidation therapy in patients who achieve a complete remission with systemic therapy.[123] Intraperitoneal chemotherapy has been used for many years to control malignant ascites.[99] The current techniques differ from previous methods in the use of a semipermanent Tenckhoff dialysis catheter or implanted port system and the delivery of the agents in a large volume (2 liters of dialysate) instead of 50 to 100 mL of saline.

Researchers have used methotrexate,[124] doxorubicin,[125] 5-FU,[126] cisplatin with systemic thiosulfate protection,[127] mitomycin-c,[128] mitoxantrone,[129] cytarabine,[130] and recombinant alpha interferon.[131] Aclacinomycin, (an analog of adriamycin) and carboplatin (a cisplatin analog) are being evaluated to determine their efficacy as intraperitoneal drugs.[123] Intraperitoneal combination chemotherapy approaches are also being studied in clinical trials.[95,132] Intraperitoneal use of biologic agents being investigated in-

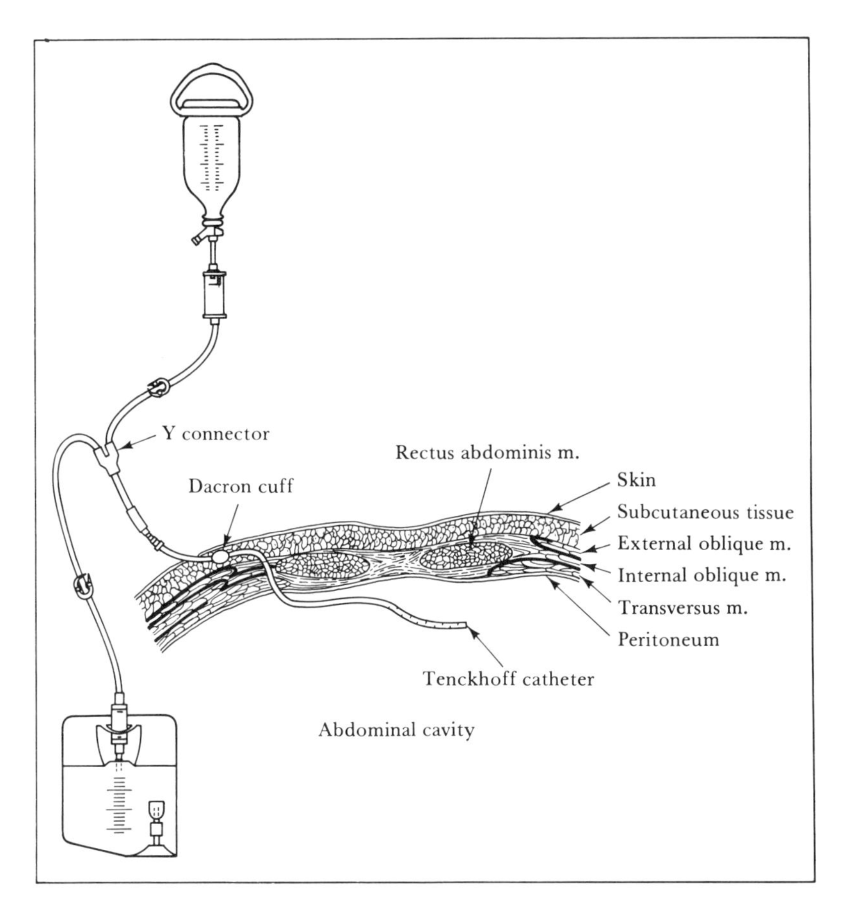

FIGURE 40-12 Tenckhoff dialysis catheter system for the delivery of intraperitoneal chemotherapy in ovarian cancer. (Source: Young R, Knapp RC, Fuks Z, et al: Cancer of the ovary, in DeVita VT, Hellman S, Rosenberg SA (eds): Cancer: Principles and Practice of Oncology (ed 3). Philadelphia, JB Lippincott, 1989.)

cludes gamma-interferon, tumor necrosis factor, interleukin-2, and monoclonal antibodies.[133-135] Intraperitoneal delivery of antineoplastic agents in 10% dimethyl sulfoxide (DMSO) may also be useful with certain ovarian cancers.[136]

Intraperitoneal chemotherapy is administered through a Tenckhoff dialysis catheter (Figure 40-12)[99] or an infusion port. The procedure is performed in a manner similar to peritoneal dialysis, except that the chemotherapeutic agent is mixed in the dialysate. There are problems associated with the Tenckhoff catheter. In approximately 20% of cases fluid will flow in readily but will not drain, most likely due to kinking of the catheter or adhesion development that leads to a one-way valve effect.[95,122,123] Use of the totally implanted system also presents similar problems.[132] A new catheter, specifically designed for patients with intraperitoneal tumors and adhesions, would be a great benefit.[125,137]

Concerns associated with intraperitoneal therapy include (1) no assurance that drugs instilled into the cavity will come into contact with the tumor, (2) establishing an effective method to deliver the drugs, (3) the potential for unique toxicities not observed with systemic chemotherapy, that is, infection secondary to bowel perforation or to the introduction of organisms from the skin into the peritoneal cavity, and (4) the risk of chronic and long-term consequences, that is, adhesion formation and bowel obstruction.[122] Ozols and Young[95] point out that there remain unresolved clinical issues related to intraperitoneal chemotherapy: (1) Can intraperitoneal chemotherapy produce a significant objective response rate? (2) In what clinical situations should it be used? (3) What is the optimum drug to use? (4) What role do drug combinations have? and (5) What is the optimum technique to deliver intraperitoneal drugs.[95]

Chemoimmunotherapy The role of chemoimmunotherapy has been investigated by two cooperative groups. The Gynecologic Oncology Group[138] compared melphalan with melphalan plus *Corynebacterium parvum*. The response rate with melphalan alone was 55%, whereas the response rate with melphalan plus *C parvum* was 65%. The Southwest Oncology Group[139] compared doxorubicin-cyclophosphamide alone and in combination with bacillus Calmette-Guerin (BCG). The response rates were 43% and 51%, respectively. In addition, Alberts et al[140] reported that the use of BCG did not add to the efficacy of a doxorubicin, cyclophosphamide, and cisplatin (DCP) regimen in patients with measurable stage III or IV disease. Adoptive cellular immunotherapy using intraperitoneal lymphokine-activated killer cells (LAK) and interleukin-2 (IL-2) is being examined in the treatment of women with minimal residual disease ovarian cancer.[14,95,133] Since immunotherapy is nonspecific, results are unpredictable. It is hoped that nonspecific immunotherapy will soon be replaced by specific vaccines.[97]

Radiotherapy

The role of radiotherapy has also been explored in managing advanced disease, and its effectiveness is directly related to the volume of disease at the time radiation is administered.[14,95] Patients who have less than 2 cm of disease have an approximately equivalent result with either combination chemotherapy or total abdominal radiation; however, only a small number of patients with advanced ovarian cancer have less than 2 cm of disease after initial laparotomy.[95] Whole abdominal radiation (WAR) appears to be effective therapy in those individuals with little or no gross residual disease.[141,142] The use of WAR as salvage therapy for patients with persistent or progressive disease after combination chemotherapy who have been explored and who have residual cancer [2 cm has also been studied.[141-143] Schray et al[143] found that patients with well- to moderately differentiated tumors or those with small-volume residual disease after the initial operation had a significantly better outcome from salvage radiation therapy. They suggest further randomized study to determine the best option for patients with poor prognostic factors. Simultaneous administration of WAR and chemotherapy (cisplatin and VP-16 [etoposide]) is also being evaluated.

Second-look surgery

A second-look operation is performed following the full course of chemotherapy (usually 6 to 12 cycles) to assess the patient's status and plan further therapy. This surgery is advocated for the following reasons: (1) to determine if therapy can be stopped and the patient has had a complete remission, (2) to assess the response and determine whether a change in the therapy is necessary, and (3) to perform secondary cytoreductive surgery to attempt to prolong survival. Controversy exists over whether there is real therapeutic value in doing second-look laparotomy and when it should be done.[95,96,142,144] Sonnendecker[145] challenges whether second-look laparotomy is justified, especially in patients with initial stage I disease, since 71.8% of patients in his study were found to have no gross or microscopic evidence of disease at the time of second-look surgery. He proposes that second-look surgery should be limited to clinical trials to define either optimum or minimum doses of chemotherapy or in the assessment of new single or combination chemotherapeutic agents.[145] Barber[97] feels that even though there are no prospective, randomized clinical studies demonstrating that second-look surgery adds to long-term survival, data suggest that patients live longer and more comfortably.[97] Lawton et al[144] did secondary surgical cytoreduction after only two or three cycles of intensive chemotherapy in patients with bulky disease remaining after primary laparotomy. They feel earlier intervention may have a role, especially if the primary surgical procedure was performed in a peripheral institution.[144]

A second-look operation is performed through a vertical incision. If gross tumor is found, it is resected. The surgeon evaluates whether there is more or less tumor than was present at the initial laparotomy. If no gross disease is present, a thorough staging evaluation is performed, including saline washings, biopsies of any irregularities or adhesions, multiple biopsies of areas where residual tumor was at the initial operation, precaval lymphadenectomy, and thorough evaluation of the intestine. TAH-BSO and omentectomy should be done if it was not done earlier. Overall, 26 to 30 biopsy specimens are secured.[105] Use of the Nd:YAG laser may be useful in resecting tumors that are fixed to the sacrum, pelvic side wall, or pubic symphysis.[146]

If the second-look operation yields negative results, the woman is followed regularly for signs of recurrence. If the second-look operation yields positive results, further therapy is needed. If the disease is microscopic, whole abdominal and pelvic irradiation may be considered. If gross disease remains, second-line chemotherapy or investigational treatment should be initiated. Additional controlled clinical trials may further delineate the role of second-look surgery. Peritoneoscopy may also be used in certain situations rather than second-look laparatomy.[99]

Tumor-associated antigens

If tumor-associated antigens specific for epithelial ovarian cancer could be detected in the bloodstream, they would provide a means for disease to be diagnosed at an early stage when patients could be cured. Tumor-associated antigens would also provide a means of monitoring disease regression during therapy and potentially allow discrimination between benign and malignant pelvic masses.[147] A monoclonal antibody that reacts with epithelial ovarian cancer cells has been developed and studied extensively.[148] It can detect an antigen (CA 125) in the blood of women with ovarian cancer. CA 125 has been elevated in serum in approximately 83% to 96% of ovarian cancer patients.[149] Elevations of CA 125 have preceeded clinical disease recurrence by 1 to 11 months.[148,150,151] A negative CA 125 value does not mean the patient is disease-free, since almost half will have residual disease.[95] CA 125 is being used to supplement standard methods of disease monitoring. If this method is perfected, second-look surgery might become unnecessary. Jager et al[152] propose that second-look surgery be done when serum CA-125 levels have fallen or returned to normal and that patients with rising serum CA-125 levels should not undergo second-look surgery. However, Potter et al[153] studied 45 women and found that a positive or negative CA 125 level was not predictive of the potential for reresection of disease at second-look.

CA 19-9 is another tumor marker used in combination with CA 125. It is a monosialoganglioside originally isolated from a colonic tumor cell.[154] Fioretti et al[155] studied CA 125 and CA 19-9 levels in 21 patients receiving both surgical and chemotherapeutic treatment for ovarian carcinoma. They found an 89.7% correlation of CA 125 levels with disease status and a 72.2% correlation with CA 19-9. Rising values may precede the clinical and ultrasonographic detection of recurrence by several months. They think that measuring CA 19-9 in addition to CA 125 could offer some benefit in monitoring patients. Neunteufel and Breitenbecker[149] also believe there is value in using more than one tumor marker. This will remain a controversial area that will only be resolved with further study.

Biologic therapy

Monoclonal antibodies, adoptive cellular immunotherapy, and interferon may soon become the fourth modality of therapy for ovarian cancer (in addition to surgery, radiation, and chemotherapy).[133] These agents are promising because they (1) have cytotoxic mechanisms that are probably unrelated to the other treatment modalities and most likely are different enough from each other not to exclude each other from sequential use, (2) can remain in the peritoneal cavity for prolonged periods when administered intraperitoneally, (3) are most likely not mutagenic, and (4) probably have manageable toxicities.[133]

A phase II study with human leukocyte interferon suggested possible activity in epithelial ovarian cancer.[156] Recombinant alpha-interferon has also shown some promise in patients with small-volume residual disease who were given intraperitoneally.[133] Combination therapy of alpha-interferon and doxorubicin produced complete and partial responses with acceptable toxicity in 29% of 24 recurring ovarian cancer patients.[157] Lichtenstein et al[158] conducted a phase I study using intraperitoneal recombinant alpha-interferon for 11 patients with persistent epithelial ovarian cancer at second-look surgery and found that 45% experienced a surgically documented antitumor response. A clinical trial using intraperitoneal human monocytes activated with recombinant gamma-interferon along with gamma-interferon is in progress.[133]

Mullerian inhibitory substance (MIS) is a biologic agent that may have potential as an anticancer agent. Radiolabeled antibodies may be able to demonstrate the presence of tumor, thus avoiding second-look laparotomy. Immunotoxins, antitumor antibodies conjugated to potent plant or bacterial toxins, are also under clinical trial. Antibodies conjugated to cytotoxic chemotherapeutic agents may improve the therapeutic index.[133] There remains a great deal still to be learned about these agents.

INVASIVE VAGINAL CANCER

Epidemiology and Etiology

Carcinoma of the vagina is a rare malignancy that accounts for 1% to 2% of gynecologic malignancies.[38,159-161] The peak incidence of squamous carcinoma of the vagina, the most common cell type, occurs in women between 50 and 70 years of age. In contrast, the peak incidence for clear cell adenocarcinoma occurs in women 18 to 19 years of age.

In 1970 Herbst and Scully[162] reported a series of seven adolescent women with adenocarcinoma arising in the vagina. This led to an intensive study that linked the maternal use of DES during pregnancy to the development of this malignancy in female offspring.

DES was used in the management of diabetic pregnancies, threatened abortion, habitual abortion, and other high-risk obstetric problems. The drug was taken during the first 18 weeks of pregnancy. The development of malignancy in the daughters of these women does not seem to be dose related. From the late 1940s to 1970, an estimated 2 million pregnant women received DES.[163]

Clinical Manifestations

The most frequent initial symptoms are abnormal vaginal bleeding, foul-smelling discharge, and dysuria. Urinary symptoms are more common with vaginal carcinoma than with cervical cancer because vaginal tumors are in close proximity to the bladder neck and can compress the urethra at an earlier stage of disease.[5]

Pathophysiology and Disease Progression

Squamous cell carcinoma comprises 75% to 95% of the cases seen.[161] Vaginal cancers occur most commonly on the posterior wall of the upper third of the vagina. The tumor may spread along the vaginal wall to involve the cervix or vulva. However, if the cervix is involved, the tumor is initially considered a primary cervical lesion. Anterior vaginal lesions penetrate into the vesicovaginal septum in an early stage. Posterior lesions can invade the rectum, but this is usually in the late stages. The tumor spreads by direct extension into the paracolpial and parametrial tissues, with extension into the obturator fossa, cardinal ligaments, lateral pelvic walls, and uterosacral ligament.[38]

The lymphatic drainage of the vagina consists of a vast, interconnecting network. Because of this complex arrangement, drainage may occur into any of the local nodal groups regardless of the location of the vaginal lesion. The incidence of lymph node metastasis is directly proportional to the stage of the vaginal cancer. The overall incidence of positive nodes is about 21%. Metastasis to the lungs or supraclavicular nodes in squamous cell carcinoma tends to occur in more advanced stages.[164] In clear cell carcinoma, metastasis to the lungs and supraclavicular nodes occurs more frequently than would be expected.[38]

Secondary carcinoma of the vagina occurs more frequently than primary cancer of the vagina. Extension of cervical cancer to the vagina is the most common secondary cancer. Cancers of the endometrium, ovary, urethra, bladder, rectum, and malignant trophoblastic disease also metastasize to the vaginal area.[5]

Assessment and Staging

Clinical diagnosis of vaginal cancer is made by careful visual examination and palpation of the vagina. Pap smear is helpful for squamous carcinoma but not for adenocarcinoma because it is often subepithelial. Colposcopy is particularly helpful for directed biopsies in abnormal vaginal areas.[38]

Women with invasive vaginal cancer should be investigated in the same manner as those with cervical cancer. All patients should have a history and physical examination, chest radiograph, biochemical profile, IVP, barium enema, cystoscopy, and proctosigmoidoscopy. Optional, but often helpful, are CT, MRI, and lymphangiogram.[38]

The disease is evaluated and staged under anesthesia by the gynecologist and the radiation therapist. Further vaginal biopsies and multiple cervical biopsies are performed. Negative biopsies of the cervix are necessary to diagnose primary vaginal carcinoma. Vaginal cancer is staged clinically using one of the staging classification systems shown in Table 40-13.[58]

Treatment

Radiotherapy is the treatment of choice for most invasive vaginal cancer (Table 40-14).[5] Intracavitary radiotherapy is accomplished with various types of devices: cylinders, intrauterine tandems with vaginal colpostats, needles, or Syed/Neblet applicators with perineal templates. The choice of devices is based on tumor location and extent. The use of hyperfractionated high-dose local radiotherapy concomitantly with chemotherapeutic drugs with both cytotoxic- and radiation-sensitizing properties is being explored.[165]

Surgery may be used in stage I adenocarcinoma. This surgery involves vaginectomy (total or partial), radical hysterectomy, and lymph node dissection. Lesions in the middle or lower vagina may require either anterior or posterior exenteration as the primary surgical therapy.[38]

The overall 5-year survival rate for all stages of squamous vaginal carcinoma is 51%. The survival rate is 65% for patients with stage I, 60% for those with stage II, 35% for those with stage III, and 39% for those with stage IV.

TABLE 40-13 Staging Classification for Carcinoma of the Vagina

Primary Tumor (T)

TNM	FIGO	Definition
TX		Primary tumor cannot be assessed
T0		No evidence of primary tumor
Tis	0	Carcinoma *in situ*
T1	I	Tumor confined to vagina
T2	II	Tumor invades paravaginal tissues but not to pelvic wall
T3	III	Tumor extends to pelvic wall
T4	IVa	Tumor invades *mucosa* of bladder or rectum and/or extends beyond the true pelvis
M1	IVb	Distant metastasis

Regional Lymph Nodes (N)

NX Regional lymph nodes cannot be assessed
N0 No regional lymph node metastasis

Upper two thirds of vagina:
N1 Pelvic lymph node metastasis

Lower one third of vagina:
N1 Unilateral inguinal lymph node metastasis
N2 Bilateral inguinal lymph node metastasis

Distant Metastasis (M)

TNM	FIGO	Definition
MX		Presence of distant metastasis cannot be assessed
M0		No distant metastasis
M1	IVb	Distant metastasis

Stage Grouping

Stage 0	Tis	No	M0
Stage I	T1	N0	M0
Stage II	T2	N0	M0
Stage III	T1	N1	M0
	T2	N1	M0
	T3	N0, N1	M0
Stage IVA	T1	N2	M0
	T2	N2	M0
	T3	N2	M0
	T4	Any N	M0
Stage IVB	Any T	Any N	M1

Source: American Joint Committee on Cancer; Manual For Staging of Cancer (ed 3). Chicago, The Committee, 1988.

TABLE 40-14 Radiotherapy of Vaginal Cancer

Stage	External Irradiation	Vaginal Therapy
Stage 0	Surgical excision preferred for localized disease	7000 rads surface dose
Stage I		
1–2 cm lesion	Omit	Interstitial irradiation, 6000–7000 rads
Larger lesions	4000–5000 rads whole pelvis	Interstitial implant delivering 3000–4000 rads
Stage II	4000–5000 rads whole pelvis	Same as above
Stage III	5000 rads whole pelvis optional (1000–2000 rads through reduced fields)	Interstitial implant, 2000–3000 rads (if tumor regression is optimal)
Stage IV (pelvis only)	Same as above	Same as above

Source: DiSaia PJ, Creasman WT: Clinical Gynecologic Oncology, St Louis, CV Mosby, 1984.

The 5-year survival rate in patients with adenocarcinoma is 80% because of early detection.[5]

Of women with recurrent disease, 80% have pelvic recurrences within 2 years of primary treatment.[5] Radiation failures can be treated effectively with surgery. Surgery for recurrence may range from wide local excision to total pelvic exenteration depending on extent of the disease.

Chemotherapy for squamous cell carcinoma of the vagina is the same as previously discussed for cervical squamous carcinoma.[5,38]

INVASIVE VULVAR CANCER

Epidemiology and Etiology

Invasive vulvar carcinoma is a disease of the elderly, with the peak incidence occurring in the seventh decade of life. It rarely occurs in women under 40 years of age. It accounts for only 3% to 4% of all gynecologic cancers.[159]

Clinical characteristics of the woman with vulvar carcinoma are described in Table 40-15.[166] Unlike cervical and endometrial malignancies, no definite precursor lesions exist for vulvar cancer. Vulvar dystrophies and CIN may occur in the presence of invasive vulvar cancer, but they rarely progress to vulvar cancer. Associated medical problems include hypertension, cardiovascular disease, obesity, and diabetes. These are probably related to the advanced age of most women who present with vulvar cancer. Chronic irritation and exposure to coal tar derivatives are also suspected.[159] Herpes simplex type 2 and HPV have been identifed in vulvar cancers.[14] Breast, cervical, and endometrial malignancies are associated with invasive vulvar carcinoma.[37]

TABLE 40-15 Clinical Features of the Patient with Vulvar Carcinoma

Feature	Percentage
Advanced age (>60 years)	68
Hypertension	41
Obesity	26
Nulliparity	22
Diabetes mellitus	13
Other malignancy	11
Positive serology (syphilis)	5

Source: Morrow CP, Townsend DE (eds): Synopsis of Gynecologic Oncology (ed 3). New York, John Wiley & Sons, 1987, pp 57-89. © John Wiley & Sons, Inc.

Clinical Manifestations

The symptoms of invasive vulvar carcinoma are variable and insidious. Twenty percent of women are asymptomatic, with lesions detected during routine pelvic examination. The most common complaint is the presence of a mass or growth in the vulvar area. Other symptoms include vulvar pruritus, bleeding, and pain.[38] Delay in treating the woman with vulvar cancer occurs for two reasons: the woman may have symptoms for 2 to 16 months before seeking medical attention, or medical treatment of vulvar lesions may continue for up to 12 months or longer without biopsy for definitive diagnosis.[5] Fortunately, vulvar cancer is commonly indolent, extends slowly, and metastasizes fairly late.

Pathophysiology and Disease Progression

The labia is the site of vulvar cancer in 70% of cases, with the labia majora involved three times more often than the labia minora. The clitoris, Bartholin's glands, and perineum may also be involved.[164] Squamous cancer accounts for 85% to 90% of all vulvar malignancies.[88] Less common malignancies include carcinoma of Bartholin's glands (adenocarcinoma and squamous), melanoma, sarcoma, basal cell carcinoma, Paget's disease, and verrucous carcinomas.[81]

The most common methods of metastatic spread are through direct extension and lymphatic dissemination. Squamous cancer may spread to involve the vagina, urethra, and anus. It spreads rapidly in the lymphatics, involving the inguinal, femoral, and pelvic nodes. The overall incidence of positive lymph nodes (both inguinal and pelvic) is 40%. For lesions smaller than 2 cm, the incidence of positive lymph nodes is 21%, and for lesions larger than 2 cm, the incidence of positive nodes is 45%.[167] The incidence of positive pelvic nodes is about 5% to 10%.[38]

Assessment and Staging

Diagnosis is usually established by local excisional biopsy of the lesions. Colposcopy is very useful in defining areas

TABLE 40-16 Staging Classification of Carcinoma of the Vulva

Primary Tumor (T)	
TX	Primary tumor cannot be assessed
T0	No evidence of primary tumor
Tis	Preinvasive carcinoma (carcinoma *in situ*)
T1	Tumor confined to the vulva, 2 cm or less in greatest dimension
T2	Tumor confined to the vulva, more than 2 cm in greatest dimension
T3	Tumor invades any of the following: urethra, vagina, perineum, or anus
T4	Tumor invades any of the following: bladder mucosa, upper part of the urethral mucosa, rectal mucosa, or tumor fixed to the bone
Regional Lymph Nodes (N)	
NX	Regional lymph nodes cannot be assessed
N0	No nodes palpable
N1	Nodes palpable in either groin, not enlarged, mobile (not clinically suspicious of neoplasm)
N2	Nodes palpable in either groin, enlarged, firm and mobile (clinically suspicious of neoplasm)
N3	Fixed or ulcerated nodes
Distant Metastasis (M)	
MX	Presence of distant metastasis cannot be assessed
M0	No clinical metastasis
M1a	Palpable deep pelvic lymph nodes
M1b	Other distant metastases

Stage Grouping: Definitions of the Clinical Stages in Carcinoma of the Vulva

(Correlation of the FIGO, UICC, and AJCC nomenclatures)

Stage	T	N	M	Description
Stage 0	Tis			Carcinoma *in situ*, intraepithelial carcinoma
Stage I	T1	N0	M0	Tumor confined to the vulva; 2 cm or less in greatest dimension. Nodes are not palpable or are palpable in either groin, not enlarged, mobile (not clinically suspicious of neoplasm)
	T1	N1	M0	
Stage II	T2	N0	M0	Tumor confined to the vulva; more than 2 cm in greatest dimension. Nodes are not palpable or are palpable in either groin, not enlarged, mobile (not clinically suspicious of neoplasm)
	T2	N1	M0	
Stage III	T3	N0	M0	Tumor of any size with (1) Adjacent spread to the lower urethra and/or the vagina, the perineum, or the anus, and/or (2) nodes palpable in either one or both groins (enlarged, firm, and mobile, not fixed but clinically suspicious of neoplasm)
	T3	N1	M0	
	T3	N2	M0	
	T1	N2	M0	
	T2	N2	M0	
Stage IV	T4	N0	M0	Tumor of any size (1) infiltrating the bladder mucosa and/or the upper part of the urethral mucosa and/or the rectal mucosa and/or
	T4	N1	M0	
	T4	N2	M0	
	Any T	Any N	M1a	(2) fixed to the bone or other distant metastases, and/or
	Any T	Any N	M1b	
	Any T	N3	M0	(3) fixed or ulcerated nodes either one or both groins

Source: American Joint Committee on Cancer: Manual for Staging of Cancer (ed 3). Chicago, The Committee, 1988.

to biopsy. Pap smear is essential because 10% of women with vulvar neoplasia have cervical CIN or invasive cancer. Examination under anesthesia may be needed to evaluate the cervix, vagina, and pelvis fully; dilatation and curettage should be performed at this time. Careful physical examination with attention to the inguinal lymph nodes is mandatory. Metastatic evaluation includes chest radiograph, proctosigmoidoscopy, cystoscopy, barium enema, IVP, and biochemical profile. CT or MRI of the pelvis may help to evaluate retroperitoneal nodal areas.[38] The classification system for vulvar cancer is clinical (Table 40-16).[58] This is limiting because 38% of women with clinically palpable nodes were free of tumor and 35% of women with clinically normal nodes showed microscopic invasion in a study by Plentl and Friedman.[164] There is some evidence to suggest that the depth of stromal invasion may relate to nodal positivity and therefore to prognosis, even though this is not currently part of the staging classification.[14]

Treatment

The traditional treatment for women with cancer of the vulva has been surgical: en bloc dissection of the tumor, contiguous skin, subcutaneous fat, and regional inguinal and femoral nodes. Some physicians recommend routine pelvic dissection; however, this procedure has essentially been reserved for women with positive groin nodes, very large lesions, melanomas, sarcomas, and adenocarcinomas.[168] Many surgeons have abandoned the en bloc approach and are now performing the nodal dissections through separate groin incisions.

Stage I lesions are generally treated with radical vulvectomy and bilateral groin dissection (Figure 40-13).[38,169] Early lesions under 2 cm in diameter with less than 5 mm of stromal invasion can be treated with a simple vulvectomy without groin dissection. A growing body of knowledge suggests that certain early lesions should be placed in a microinvasive category.[38] In a study by Wharton et al[170] no positive nodes, no recurrences, and no deaths were found in women with microinvasion. The term *microinvasion* remains controversial, as does the appropriate treatment for this stage of the disease.[38,171] Studies directed at defining microinvasive carcinoma and finding methods to reduce the radical extent of surgical procedures are especially important.[38]

Stage II and III lesions may require more extensive surgery than stage I tumors. If the lesion involves the urethra, vagina, or anus, resection of these organs may be necessary to remove adequate tissue to allow for tumor-free margins. The use of pelvic lymph node dissection is controversial because only 10% of women have positive

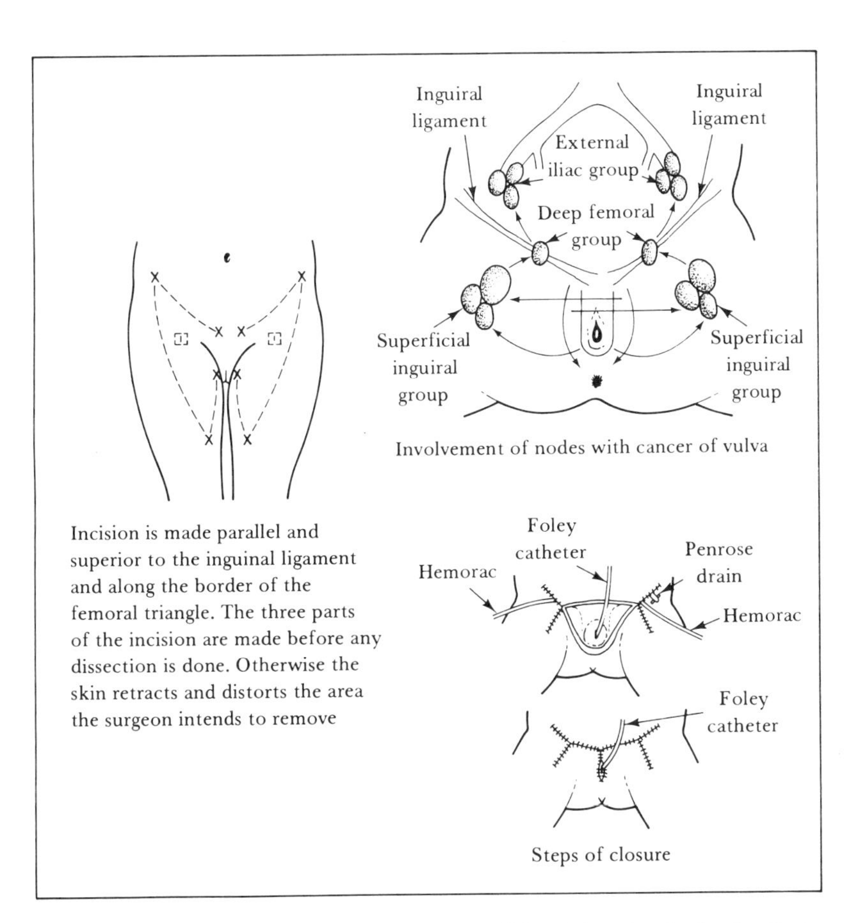

FIGURE 40-13 Radical vulvectomy. (Source: Ball B: Easing the shock of radical vulvectomy. Nursing, 5:27-31, 1975.

TABLE 40-17 Reported Complications After Radical Surgery for Vulvar Cancer

Complication	Percentage of All Cases
Wound breakdown or infection	54
Chronic leg edema	30
Lymphocyst	10
Genital prolapse	7
Stress incontinence	5
Thrombophlebitis	3.5
Grafting of skin flaps	1.7
Hernia (femoral, inguinal)	1.5
Pulmonary embolus	1.2
Ruptured femoral artery	1.9
Hospital deaths	3.3

Source: Adapted from Morrow CP, Townsend DE (eds): Synopsis of Gynecologic Oncology (ed 3). New York, John Wiley & Sons, 1987, pp 57-89. © John Wiley & Sons, Inc.

pelvic nodes, and the pelvic nodes usually will not be positive unless the inguinal nodes are positive.[37] Clinical trials comparing pelvic and inguinal irradiation versus inguinal lymphadenectomy in patients with stage I and II vulvar cancer are in progress.[38]

Patients with stage IV disease may require pelvic exenteration in addition to radical vulvectomy if the bladder or rectum is involved. If the disease is very advanced, conservative surgery and radiotherapy may be used. Operative mortality is only 1% to 2%. This figure is low considering the age of most women who develop vulvar cancer. Table 40-17 describes reported complications after radical surgery.[166] Wound breakdown occurs in about 54% of all patients. Varying degrees of lymphedema of the lower extremities occur in about 30% of patients. The use of elastic stockings is recommended for 12 months after surgery. Other infrequent complications include lymphocyst formation in the groin area, stress incontinence, and genital prolapse.

Radiotherapy has not generally been used as primary treatment in vulvar cancer because of the good results obtained with surgery. At present, the Gynecologic Oncology Group[38] is studying radiotherapy as an adjunct to groin dissection in women with positive nodes. Moderately high doses (4500 to 5500 cGy) of radiotherapy can be used preoperatively to increase the resectability rate.[38] Those patients who have undergone a resection of the primary lesion and are considered at high risk for recurrence due to inadequate resection margins are good candidates for postoperative irradiation of 4500 to 5000 cGy.[38] Radiotherapy also has a role in palliation of advanced disease.[172] In the future, radiation therapy may play a very important role in managing patients with vulvar carcinoma.[38]

The 5-year survival rate in vulvar cancer can be correlated with stage and nodal involvement. Beecham et al[81] collated data from several studies and found the overall 5-year survival rate to be 74% for all stages; the survival rate for women with stage I and II disease is 90%, and the survival rate for those with stage III disease is 44%. The survival rate for women with negative nodes is 90%, that for women with positive groin nodes is 30%, and that for women with positive pelvic nodes is 20%.

Over 80% of all recurrences will occur within the first 2 years after treatment. Over half the recurrences are local and near the site of the primary lesion. These recurrences can be treated with local excision or interstitial radiation. Distant recurrences or those in local lymph nodes are difficult to treat, and the salvage rate is poor.[5] Results with all chemotherapeutic agents studied have been very disappointing. Regimens have included methotrexate, vincristine, hydroxyurea, bleomycin, mitomycin-C, and cisplatin.[81] One study used preoperative mitomycin C and 5-FU followed by pelvic irradiation before surgery, which resulted in marked local tumor shrinkage to allow more definitive surgery.[173]

NURSING CARE OF THE WOMAN WITH GYNECOLOGIC CANCER

The nursing care of the woman with gynecologic cancer can be very complex and involves detailed assessment, planning, intervention, and evaluation. The following discussion focuses on the ten functional health patterns suggested by the National Group for Classification of Nursing Diagnosis. Individuals with gynecologic cancer are treated with multimodal therapy. Because the specific problems associated with chemotherapy, radiotherapy, and biologic therapy have been presented in other chapters, these discussions are omitted.

Moreland[174] has developed the Gynecology Initial Patient Assessment Record (GIPAR) to be used initially with women to provide a consistent and concise nursing assessment. A diagnosis of gynecologic cancer necessitates broad teaching about life-style changes for these women to achieve maximum rehabilitation.

Health Perception and Health Management Pattern

The nurse assumes a major role in prevention and detection of cervical dysplasia and cervical cancer by encouraging and educating women about PAP smears.[13] Stimulating an awareness of the potential threat of ovarian cancer to a woman's health and well-being is important, since ovarian cancer claims the greatest mortality of tumors of the female reproductive system.[175] In addition, every woman seen in a health care setting should be evaluated to determine her knowledge and practice of breast self-examination (BSE). This is particularly true for the woman with gynecologic cancer. A current or previous gynecologic malignancy (endometrial) places a woman at greater risk for breast cancer. Therefore, strict adherence to a monthly BSE schedule is essential. The nurse is responsible for ensuring that the woman is instructed on BSE and understands the importance of complying with this procedure.

Sandella[176] feels that vulvar self-examination should also be a health practice that is initiated early and continued throughout the life span. She has developed a brochure on vulvar self-examination that may be useful for cancer screenings or for the woman who has been treated for vulvar cancer to assess for recurrences.

Women having gynecologic surgical procedures are at risk of infections secondary to the presence of urinary catheters and surgical drains. The highest risk of infection occurs in women who have radical vulvectomy with bilateral groin dissections, since many are elderly, obese, diabetic, and may have other medical problems that make them susceptible to wound infections. Some 85% of groin wounds must be opened and healed by secondary intention.[177] Complete closure may take 2 or 3 months.

Wound care is initially a nursing activity. The wounds must be irrigated and packed, and the perineum must be kept dry. After cleaning the wound, a hair dryer is an ideal way of keeping the wound and the perineum dry. Bed cradles also may be effective in allowing air to reach the perineal area. Each surgical wound may require specialized care.

The patient should be encouraged from the outset to participate in wound care. She will be responsible for this after discharge and should be totally independent in this activity while still hospitalized. The nurse should begin teaching by encouraging the woman to look at the wound. Next the woman may feel comfortable touching the area. During this period of adjustment and learning, the nurse must reassure the woman that the wounds will heal completely with time. If the woman is unable to do the wound care herself, a family member, neighbor, relative, or other designated person must be taught how to do the care. Referral to a home health agency for frequent assessment and follow-up is essential.

Nutritional-Metabolic Pattern

Nutritional problems can occur in all stages of gynecologic cancers. Before major abdominopelvic surgery, these individuals will undergo a bowel preparation program. Because gynecologic cancers metastasize intraperitoneally, and the bowel may be involved, these women must always be prepared for possible bowel surgery. A bowel cleansing preparation program consists of a clear liquid diet (which has very little nutritional value), laxatives, enemas, and antibiotics. Fluid and electrolyte imbalances are possible, and the woman may be in a catabolic state before major surgery. Elemental diets (Vivonex, Flexical, etc) may be part of the preoperative care plan. These preparations can be taken orally and will ensure that the woman is in the best possible nutritional state before surgery. Before radical surgical procedures, some physicians will support patients preoperatively with total parenteral nutrition. An optimal nutritional state is imperative to ensure wound healing and decrease recovery time.

After surgery, fluid and electrolyte balance may be a problem due to ostomies, fistulas, and nasogastric tubes. If the woman must receive nothing to eat or drink by mouth for an extended period, total parenteral nutrition (TPN) may be indicated after surgery. TPN may be indicated on a long-term basis for patients with short-bowel syndrome secondary to an extensive small-bowel resection or a bowel obstruction.

In later stages of gynecologic cancer, nutritional problems always exist. These women have anorexia, cachexia, early satiety, bowel obstruction (intermittent or complete), nausea, and vomiting. Enteral feedings (either oral or by tube) may be used if the woman does not have an obstruction. The enteral route is usually contraindicated because the gastrointestinal tract is generally not intact. The woman may benefit from TPN if aggressive therapy is being pursued. If the woman is terminally ill, the physician may choose to maintain hydration with intravenous fluids only.

Discharge planning and teaching are necessary if the patient is to go home with tube feedings or parenteral fluids. The woman and her family must be taught how to administer these products and what to do if a problem arises at home. The home care nurse or the nurse from the company providing the supplies should be involved in discharge planning and teaching. Many times multiple community agencies and resources are involved in coordinating care of the woman in the home setting. This makes multiagency communication critical.

Lymphedema is a potential problem in all women with gynecologic cancer because these diseases tend to spread to lymph nodes. If a lymphadenectomy is performed as part of an abdominopelvic surgical procedure, pedal lymphedema can be a complication. This is especially true after radical vulvectomy with groin dissection.

In end-stage disease, lymphedema may develop secondary to lymphatic obstruction from tumor. This edema may progress to anasarca. The skin may actually break open and fluid seep out. This fluid loss may be so severe that towels must be wrapped around the woman's legs.

If the lymphedema is from lymphadenectomy, antiemboli leotards, leg elevation, salt restriction, and mild diuretics may be helpful. These measures rarely help if the edema is from obstruction. Palliative comfort measures should be employed.

After radical vulvectomy, the woman may be placed on bed rest for several days. Postoperatively, the woman should be placed on an air-fluidized or low-air-loss bed to prevent skin breakdown. Skin breakdown is always a potential problem if there are ostomies or draining fistulas. Ascites and pleural effusions are common problems in women with gynecologic cancer. Detailed nursing care measures for ascites and pleural effusions are discussed in Chapter 27.

Elimination Patterns

Aberrations in bowel and bladder function may include diarrhea, constipation, urinary tract infections, vesicovaginal or rectovaginal fistulas, incontinence, and altered routes of elimination (colostomy, ileostomy, nephrostomies, urinary catheters, and ileal-conduit).

Instruction for self-management of ostomies and catheters should begin preoperatively. The enterostomal therapist should be consulted to mark potential ostomy sites and begin patient teaching. This educational process will continue through the postoperative period.

If the woman is scheduled for radical hysterectomy, she probably will be discharged with a urinary drainage catheter. Detailed instructions for the care of the catheter, bladder training, and removal procedure must be given. Jusenius[178] has developed an excellent teaching aid for the woman undergoing radical hysterectomy that includes catheter care.

The use of intermittent catheterization for women who have undergone radical hysterectomy may become more commonplace. It can decrease infection, stimulate the normal voiding mechanism, and maintain the integrity of the urethrovesical junction.[179] This technique also requires a motivated woman who is receptive to learning the procedure. Follow-up after discharge from the hospital may be necessary.

Fistula formation and incontinence can be very distressing. Skin breakdown and odor are additional potential problems. Perineal pads or diapers may be necessary to absorb the drainage. Colostomies or urinary diversions are sometimes performed to correct fistulas. Constipation or diarrhea may result from narcotics, radiotherapy, chemotherapy, inactivity, or bowel obstruction. Routine nursing interventions for these problems should be employed. A colostomy or ileostomy may be necessary to relieve an obstruction.

Activity-Exercise Pattern

Women with gynecologic cancers may have extended hospital stays, especially after radical vulvectomy and pelvic exenteration. During the recovery phase, the patient could benefit from activities to occupy her time and provide constructive diversion. A consultation with the occupational therapist or recreational therapist may be indicated. Recovery time, psychological adjustment, and pain control can all be affected by distraction and diversion activities.

If the woman is weak or has ascites or lymphedema, there are potential mobility problems. A physical therapist may be able to help the woman attain her maximal level of independence. A music therapist may also be helpful to allow the woman an opportunity to express some of the feelings she may have about her diagnosis and treatment. The use of a video cassette recorder for women undergoing radiation implants may also be useful to pass time.

Until quite recently aggressive rehabilitation of the patient with cancer was not considered. Rehabilitation efforts can help maintain and improve function, but negative attitudes still persist and serve as barriers to rehabilitation. Increasing the awareness of cancer patients' rehabilitation needs and educating health care professionals and the public may be strategies to remove these barriers.[180]

Cognitive-Perceptual Pattern

Women with gynecologic cancer may experience pain from many sources: pressure from an enlarging pelvic mass, abdominal pain from recurring bowel obstruction, bone pain from metastases, and back or leg pain from encasement of nerve roots by tumor. For a thorough review of pain management, see Chapter 20.

Care of these women can be very complex, and knowledge deficits usually exist requiring nursing intervention, such as: pain management, ostomy care, catheter care, and wound care. Other areas for patient education are radiotherapy, surgery, chemotherapy, biotherapy, and sexuality.

Sleep-Rest Pattern

Potential alterations in sleep and rest are the same as those for any hospitalized individual diagnosed with cancer and may include pain, general inactivity, interrupted sleep, and anxiety.

Self-Perception–Self-Concept Pattern

Alterations in body image, decreased self-esteem, anxiety, and depression are all associated with the diagnosis of a gynecologic malignancy and the medical interventions used to treat them. A detailed discussion of these problems is included in the section on sexuality patterns.

Role Relationship Pattern

A particular concern of women who have gynecologic cancer is their sexual relationship. This is discussed in the section on sexuality-reproductive patterns.

A family relationship requiring careful assessment is that between the mother who took DES during pregnancy and her daughter who develops gynecologic cancer. Burke et al[181] describe the feelings of daughters of women who took DES during pregnancy: 80% of daughters displayed trust and a strong alliance with their mothers, only 10% expressed hostility toward their mothers, and 10% of daughters had an overwhelming preoccupation with sexual concerns and cancer.

Schwartz and Stewart[182] found that mothers suffered guilt and were more emotionally disturbed than their daughters. Feelings of rage, fear, despair, and helplessness were common. Mothers can minimize the trauma by sharing their feelings of resentment, disappointment, betrayal, and helplessness.

Konicki[183] states that the majority of daughters of women who took DES during pregnancy are asymptomatic but remain at risk for gynecologic abnormalities. Cancer phobia, fear of sexual inadequacy, and fear of fertility problems remain a constant source of anxiety for these women.

Sexuality-Reproductive Pattern

Alterations in sexuality and body image present major problems for most women with gynecologic cancer. Andersen[184] states that "30% to 90% of all women with gynecologic cancer will experience significant sexual problems." The disease itself, and the results of surgical treatment, chemotherapy, and radiotherapy, may greatly affect the quality of life of these women.[46,185-189] Reproductive abilities may be lost because of treatment modalities that result in irreversible changes.[190] A comprehensive counseling approach involving the patient, her family, and her sexual partner is recommended in the early stages of the disease process and before treatment.[46,188,191]

With invasive gynecologic cancers, women undergo at least simple hysterectomy or unilateral oophorectomy. Total pelvic exenteration and radical vulvectomy are the most extensive procedures. The most common surgical intervention is a TAH-BSO. If the uterus is removed, the woman loses her ability to reproduce. If both ovaries are removed, she not only loses her ability to reproduce but may also develop menopausal symptoms. These symptoms can include hot flashes, depression, facial hair growth, and decreased vaginal lubrication.

In addition to reproductive function, the uterus is involved in the sexual response cycle. During the excitement phase, it elevates from its usual position in the pelvis; during the orgasmic phase, it contracts rhythmically. The cervix contributes to orgasm but is not essential for climax.[192]

Radical pelvic surgery (exenteration, hysterectomy, or vulvectomy) means loss of sexually responsive tissue. Human sexual response is a total body vasocongestive neuromuscular response mediated through the autonomic nervous system. Loss of parasympathetic nerves and pelvic vasculature may delay physiologic response, but gynecologic surgery does not destroy sexual function.[193]

Although the uterus and ovaries are not external confirmation of sexuality, their loss can be devastating to a woman. Many women feel that their femininity is vested in procreation. They view menstruation as a badge of femininity. Following a hysterectomy, they feel defeminized and sexually inadequate. These feelings are heightened when more radical surgery is performed. Postoperative depression is the most common outward response to this perceived loss of femininity. This depression is significant even without oophorectomy. Glasgow et al[185] state that it is difficult to distinguish between the loss of sexual interest that is secondary to cancer and its treatment and the loss of interest that results from depression.

Much of the adverse response is predicated on myths and misconceptions about the role of the uterus and the effect of its removal. Some common myths about hysterectomy are that it brings about weight gain, cessation of sexual enjoyment, manifestations of old age, and mental deterioration. A common misconception of the woman with cancer is that sexual activity may spread the disease or that her partner may contract cancer.

Dennerstein et al[194] studied women who had hysterectomies with oophorectomies. Preoperatively the women were primarily worried about altered sexual function, weight gain, the surgery itself, cancer, loss of femininity, mental deterioration, and excessive hair growth. Women who worried about sexual alterations preoperatively had the greatest deterioration of sexual relationships postoperatively. Glasgow[185] supports open discussion with the patient regarding issues of sexuality before treatment so that misunderstandings are less likely.

Jenkins[187] studied 20 sexually active women following surgical and radiation treatment for endometrial and cervical cancer. Statistically significant negative changes were shown at a 95% level for indicators of sexual functioning, including frequency of intercourse and orgasm and feelings of desire and enjoyment. Some 59% of the women indicated that they received no information related to sexual changes, and no sexual counseling was given by nurses or physicians despite the fact that 88% wanted sexual discussions initiated by the physician or nurse. Jenkins[187] points out that "a patient cannot be expected to initiate a discussion she does not know is needed."

Hysterectomy for benign disease may significantly alter self-esteem and sexual performance. Problems are compounded if this procedure is coupled with the diagnosis of cancer, since the woman must cope with the biologic, psychological, and social factors that surround the diagnosis of cancer. Anxiety, depression, guilt, shame, and societal attitudes may all adversely affect her sexuality and sexual function. Harris et al[195] found that women newly diagnosed with gynecologic cancer felt the disease was punishment for previous sexual behaviors. They also experienced a significant decrease in sexual activity and satisfaction.

If bilateral oophorectomy is performed, the administration of estrogen can prevent the menopausal changes that follow. Dennerstein et al[194] found estrogen therapy to be unsuccessful for the treatment of decreased or absent libido. Atrophic changes in the vagina are prevented, but it has not been determined what effect, if any, estrogen has on human sexual behavior. Dennerstein et al[194] gave 89 women estrogen therapy, teaching, and counseling. Thirty-seven percent of the women reported a decrease in the frequency of sexual activity, 30% stated that sexual relations had improved, and 29% reported no change in sexual activity. There was no relationship between giving hormones and sexual dysfunction, desire for sex, ability to reach orgasm, and ease of vaginal lubrication. In gynecologic cancer (particularly adenocarcinoma), many physicians will not give supplemental estrogen therapy because of the association between exogenous estrogen therapy and cancer.

A negative preoperative expectation of the operation was significantly associated with a poor overall sexual outcome and loss of desire after surgery. These negative expectations may be related to lack of knowledge of the expected sexual outcome, negative comments by friends and relatives concerning the operation and its results, and change in treatment by the partner, even when positive.

Because some of the untoward reactions to hysterectomy stem from lack of information, the nurse must assess the woman's knowledge of anatomy, physiology, and sexual function. Other data that must be gathered preoperatively include support systems, sexual relationships, coping strategies, the woman's attitudes about herself, and whether she has completed her family. Glasgow et al[185] state that it is important to do a sexual history at the initial evaluation so that the patient feels free to bring up questions and be comfortable in later discussions. Specific questions that may be asked include, "Do you have any difficulty experiencing orgasm when you want to?" and "Many persons in your situation are concerned about how their illness will affect their sexuality or sexual relationships. To what extent have you had these concerns?"

Hogan[192] has determined five characteristics that place women at greatest risk of adverse psychosexual effects from surgery:

1. Women who regard the uterus and menstruation as a badge of femininity
2. Women who have had poor sexual activity before surgery with limited coital and orgasmic experience
3. Women who have not completed their families
4. Women who verbalize negative expectations of the sexual outcome of surgery
5. Women with a poor understanding of the reproductive tract and its function

The focus of preoperative counseling is education and giving the woman an opportunity to verbalize her feelings. The nurse functions as a listener, counselor, and support person. However, recent studies have identified that sexuality has not been a major concern of oncology nurses.[186,196] Wilson and Williams[186] conducted a survey of 937 oncology nurses and found that only 57.9% were comfortable initiating a discussion of sexuality with their patients. They also found that nurses with more years of experience and education reported more nursing practices related to sexuality. Increasing nurses' knowledge of alterations in sexuality, providing opportunities to discuss specific approaches with peers, and structured practice opportunities are all suggestions to change nurses' attitudes that may lead to increased nursing interventions. Fisher[197] also makes recommendations for education for nurses related to sexuality. First, nurses must be prepared to address the basic sexual health care needs of patients. Second, faculty who will be teaching these concepts to students must be prepared, possibly with the assistance of a nurse sex educator. Third, the concepts of sexual health care must be integrated into nursing practice so that it becomes a constant consideration in each nurse's care of patients. Jenkins[187] agrees that curricula designed to help nurses accept their own sexuality and that of others is necessary.

The nurse can increase the woman's self-esteem and self-worth by helping her redefine her self-concept in ways other than reproduction and help her to realize her intrinsic worth and dignity. This is also an opportunity to allow time for the woman to verbalize her feelings about cancer and what the diagnosis means to her.

As an educator, the nurse can teach the woman about reproduction and sexual function. This teaching should include drawings, diagrams, or models to explain anatomic and physiologic functions affected by the disease and its treatment.[185] The nurse can dispel any myths or misconceptions the woman may have about hysterectomy and cancer. The nurse discusses when sex may be resumed and the changes in sexual activity that may be needed if the vagina is shortened after surgery. These changes may include different coital positions and alternative forms of sexual expression. If the woman is discharged from the hospital while receiving hormone therapy, she must be instructed about the dosage, schedule, and possible side effects.

Hogan[197] has identified the following outcome criteria for the woman undergoing hysterectomy and her sexual partner:

1. Describe the function of the uterus in relation to the sexual response cycle and other female physiologic processes
2. State when sexual activity may be resumed
3. Describe alternate forms of sexual expression, if indicated, and positions for intercourse
4. Identify the importance of the medication that is prescribed and state the role of estrogen in preventing menopausal symptoms
5. State that she is still valued as a woman

In addition, the woman with gynecologic cancer may be receiving postoperative radiotherapy or chemotherapy. The woman should verbalize the rationale, side effects, and potential effects these therapies may have on her sexual function.

Sexual adjustment is a very real problem following hysterectomy. These problems are compounded after a pelvic exenteration. The woman has the stress of radical surgery, significant changes in body image as a result of the removal of genital organs and the formation of one or two stomas, and adjustment to changes in work, social, and sexual patterns.

Lamont et al[193] have found that women undergoing pelvic exenteration cannot accept that their partners see them as desirable, cannot see that they are inherently attractive as persons, cannot accept nudity in front of their partners, suffer from reactive depression, and lose their sexual appetite. Traditional societal attitudes linking normal sexuality, coitus, and reproduction present the woman who has undergone exenteration and her partner with particular problems they may never have discussed. Participation in autoeroticism, mutual masturbation, oral-genital sex, and fantasy may be impossible for the couple to consider without counseling.

Strong marital relationships are essential to sexual rehabilitation after surgical exenteration. If there are preexisting problems in the relationship, the exenteration may become the focus of all the problems. The surgery can arouse profound emotions in the man. He may be forced to confront his own emotions and evaluate the depth of his feelings for this woman and their relationship. He has to accept a shortened or reconstructed vagina, one or two stomas, and perhaps a complete change in the traditional coital experience he may be accustomed to. Several studies have found that the majority of women undergoing pelvic exenteration experience major, unresolved psychosexual problems after surgery.[193,198,199] This is significant because pelvic exenteration is usually performed with curative intent. These women have the rest of their lives ahead of them and deserve a satisfying sexual relationship. The woman's psychosexual adjustment begins before surgery. This requires a team approach. The team includes the physician, nurse, social worker, enterostomal therapist, dietician, and chaplain. Yarbrough[200] developed a teaching plan that incorporates objectives, content, teaching action, and outcome criteria for the members of the team. It is imperative that someone on this team be prepared to deal with the sexual problems that can follow exenterative surgery. The goal of rehabilitation is to return the woman to her home and occupation with the ability to deal with her altered body functions. Immediately after surgery the woman's physical needs take priority. As she begins to recover, the task of psychosexual adjustment becomes more obvious. Before optimum psychosexual adjustment can occur, it is imperative that hygienic needs are met. Femininity and attractiveness should be maintained and independence in physical care achieved. Only after these criteria are met can the woman proceed to more complex areas of concern.[198]

Women can be fully rehabilitated sexually following pelvic exenteration if proper attention is paid to the educational process and reassurance that they can be rehabilitated. Lamont et al[193] suggest that a psychosexual counselor see the woman before and after surgery, every 2 to 4 weeks after discharge for 6 months, and every 3 to 6 months thereafter. In their study, six of seven women were orgasmic within 6 months of surgery.

Crisis intervention counseling during initial hospitalization in women with gynecologic cancer has a significant effect in reducing sexual dysfunction and in enhancing the rate of return to pretreatment frequency of intercourse.[199] Springer[201] has described the physical, social, and sexual impact of radical vulvectomy. Disfigurement of the external genitals can result in distortions of body image and sexual functioning. The woman's vagina and clitoris may be mutilated or removed, which can make the woman feel sexually unattractive. When distal portions of the vagina are removed, the fine sensory perceptions so important to foreplay are lost. In addition, there are specific changes in sexual function due to the surgery. Introital stenosis can make intercourse painful or difficult.[201] Extensive counseling may be necessary to foster improved body image and self-esteem for postvulvectomy patients.[46]

Andersen and Hacker[202] interviewed 15 women who underwent surgery for vulvar cancer. The women exhibited similar psychologic distress to those who had undergone exenteration. These women had a decrease in sexual activity, low sexual arousal, sexual anxiety, limited sexual satisfaction, and disruption of body image. The interventions proposed for women undergoing pelvic exenteration also can be used for the woman undergoing radical vulvectomy.

Health care professionals often fail to consider the sexual consequences of gynecologic cancer for women who are elderly or in the later stages of their disease process.[185,203] Frank-Stromborg[203] suggests that advice to these women include (1) longer, slower, more direct stimulation (manual or oral), (2) the use of touch or perfume to enhance, (3) nontraditional sexual positions, and (4) not depending on simultaneous orgasm for sexual pleasure. These women may experience an even greater need for love and affection. The nurse can help the woman's partner and family understand and respond to these needs. Providing ample private time is imperative.[46]

Coping–Stress Tolerance Pattern

Adjustment to the diagnosis of cancer, subsequent treatment, recurrence, and death are a terrible burden for someone to face. For the woman with a gynecologic malignancy, it is compounded by the associated changes in body image and sexuality. Krouse[180] developed a four-stage model to describe the adjustment process that women with gynecologic cancer experience. This four-stage process includes (1) recognition-exploration, which involves the first awareness of disease symptoms and diagnosis; (2) crisis-climax, which is the period around the time of surgery and shortly after; (3) adaptation-maladaptation, during which the woman uses a number of mechanisms to allow her to adapt to the disease and treatment; and (4) resolution-disorganization, during which the woman is either able to return to a level of previous function or to a long period of disorganization. Implementing effective crisis intervention strategies can decrease the incidence of postsurgical psychologic dysfunction and increase the likelihood that the woman will adjust to her illness.[204] Psychological evaluation of the woman with gynecologic cancer and preparation of the family are essential.[205] The psychosocial aspects of the cancer diagnosis are discussed in detail in Chapters 16 to 19.

Value-Belief Pattern

The diagnosis of cancer creates feelings of anxiety, depression, body image destruction, guilt, shame, and dependency. Cancer of the genital tract may intensify these feelings. The hospital chaplain may be able to help relieve the guilt and shame associated with the disease.

CONCLUSION

Gynecologic cancer represents almost 15% of all cancers in women and results in 10% of all cancer deaths.[38] If women routinely had pelvic examinations and Pap smears, many more gynecologic cancers could be detected at an early stage when they may be curable. Treatment modalities for women with these malignancies are often very aggressive, regardless of whether the approach is surgery, radiotherapy, chemotherapy, or biologic therapy. Unfortunately, recurrences are not recognized early; therefore effective palliation for these patients remains a challenge for the health care professional. Gynecologic cancers have not only profound physical effects on the woman and her family but also have a major impact on body image and sexuality. Self-care is a necessity for many women with gynecologic cancer, although family support and involvement is also crucial. It is hoped that with earlier detection and improved treatment regimens, the incidence and mortality of gynecologic cancer will be reduced.

REFERENCES

1. Silverberg E, Boring CC, Squires TS: Cancer statistics, 1990. CA 40:9-26, 1990.
2. Guzick DS: Efficacy of screening for cervical cancer: A Review. Am J Publ Health 68:125-134, 1978.
3. Anthony CP: Textbook of Anatomy and Physiology. St Louis, CV Mosby, 1983.
4. Jones HW, Jones GS: Novak's Textbook of Gynecology. Baltimore, Williams & Wilkins, 1981.
5. DiSaia PJ, Creasman WT: Clinical Gynecologic Oncology. St Louis, CV Mosby, 1984.
6. Cramer DW, Cutler SJ: Incidence and histopathology of malignancies of the female genital organs in the United States. Am J Obstet Gynecol 118:443-460, 1974.
7. Brinton LA, Fraumeni JF Jr: Epidemiology of uterine cervical cancer. J Chron Dis 39:1051-1065, 1986.
8. Lovejoy NC: Precancerous lesions of the cervix: Personal risk factors. Cancer Nurs 10:2-14, 1987.
9. Kessler II: Cervical cancer epidemiology in historical perspective. J Reprod Med 12:173-185, 1974.
10. Herbst AL, Cole P, Norusis MJ, et al: Epidemiologic aspects and factors related to survival in 384 registry cases of clear cell adenocarcinoma of the vagina and cervix. Am J Obstet Gynecol 135:876-883, 1979.
11. Aurelian L, Strand B, Smith M: Immunodiagnostic potential of a virus-coded, tumor-associated antigen (AG-4) in cervical cancer. Cancer 39:1834-1849, 1977.
12. Amstey M: Relationship between herpes virus and cervical cancer. Contemp Ob Gyn 3:99-102, 1974.
13. Cashavelly BJ: Cervical dysplasia: An overview of current concepts in epidemiology, diagnosis, and treatments. Cancer Nurs 10:199-206, 1987.
14. Young RC: Gynecologic cancers, in Wittes RE (ed): Manual of Oncologic Therapeutics: 1989/1990. Philadelphia, JB Lippincott, 1989, pp 270-291.
15. Kurman RJ, Jenson AB, Lancaster MD: Papillomavirus infection of the cervix: Relationship to intraepithelial neoplasia based on the presence of specific viral structural proteins. Am J Surg Pathol 7:39-52, 1983.
16. Koss LG: Cytologic and histologic manifestations of human papillomavirus infection of the female genital tract and their clinical significance. Cancer 60:1942-1950, 1987.
17. Syrjanen K, Vayrynen M, Saarikoski S, et al: Natural history of cervical human papillomavirus (HPV) infections based on prospective follow-up. Br J Obstet Gynaecol 92:1086-1092, 1985.
18. Meanwell CA, Blackledge G, Cox MF, et al: HPV 16 DNA in normal and malignant cervical epithelium: Implications for the aetiology and behaviour of cervical neoplasia. Lancet 1:703-707, 1987.
19. Howley PM, Schlegel R: The human papillomaviruses. Am J Med 85:155-158, 1988 (suppl 2A).
20. Richart RM: Causes and management of cervical intraepithelial neoplasia. Cancer 60:1951-1959, 1987.
21. Boshart M, Gissmann L, Ikenberg H, et al: A new type of papillomavirus DNA, its presence in genital cancer biopsies and in cell lines derived from cervical cancer. EMBO J 3:1151-1157, 1984.
22. McCance DJ, Campion MJ, Clarkson PK, et al: Prevalence of human papillomavirus type 16 DNA sequences in cervical intraepithelial neoplasia and invasive carcinoma of the cervix. Br J Obstet Gynaecol 92:1101-1105, 1985.
23. Yoshikawa H, Matsukura T, Yamamoto E, et al: Occurrence of human papillomavirus types 16 and 18 DNA in cervical carcinomas from Japan: Age of patients and histologic type of carcinomas. Jpn J Cancer Res 76:667-671, 1985.
24. Munoz N, Bosch X, Kaldor JM: Does human papillomavirus cause cervical cancer? The state of the epidemiological evidence. Br J Cancer 57:1-5, 1988.
25. Nelson JH, Averette HE, Richart RM: Cervical intraepithelial neoplasia (dysplasia and carcinoma in situ) and early invasive cervical carcinoma. CA 39:157-178, 1989.
26. Stenkvist B, Bergstrom R, Brinne U, et al: Automatic analysis of Papanicolaou smears by digital image processing. Gynecol Oncol 27:1-14, 1987.
27. Fink DJ: Change in American Cancer Society checkup guidelines for detection of cervical cancer. CA 38:127-128, 1988.
28. Schwartz PE, Merino MJ, McCrea Curnen MG: Clinical management of patients with invasive cervical cancer following a negative Pap smear. Yale J Biol Med 61:327-338, 1988.
29. Kern WH, Zivolich MR: The accuracy and consistency of the cytologic classification of squamous lesions of the uterine cervix. Acta Cytol 21:519-523, 1977.
30. Chanen W, Rome RM: Electrocoagulation diathermy for cervical dysplasia and carcinoma-in-situ: A 15-year survey. Obstet Gynecol 61:673-679, 1983.
31. Masterson BJ, Krantz KE, Calkins JW, et al: The carbon dioxide laser in cervical epithelial neoplasia: A five-year experience in treating 230 patients. Am J Obstet Gynecol 139:565-567, 1981.
32. Burke L: The use of carbon dioxide laser in the therapy of cervical intraepithelial neoplasia. Am J Obstet Gynecol 144:337-340, 1982.
33. Anderson MC: Treatment of cervical intraepithelial neoplasia with the carbon dioxide laser: Report of 543 patients. Obstet Gynecol 59:720-725, 1982.
34. Townsend DE, Richart RM: Cryosurgery and carbon dioxide laser management of cervical intraepithelial neoplasia: A controlled comparison. Obstet Gynecol 61:75-81, 1983.

35. Ferenczy A: Laser treatment of patients with condylomata and squamous carcinoma precursors of the lower female genital tract. CA 37:334-347, 1987.
36. Husseinzadeh N, Newman NJ, Wesseler TA: Vulvar intraepithelial neoplasia: A clinicopathological study of carcinoma in situ of the vulva. Gynecol Oncol 33:157-163, 1989.
37. Green TH: Carcinoma of the vulva: A reassessment. Obstet Gynecol 50:462-468, 1978.
38. Hoskins WJ, Perez C, Young RC: Gynecologic tumors, in DeVita VT Jr, Hellman S, Rosenberg SA (eds): Cancer: Principles and Practice of Oncology (ed 3). Philadelphia, JB Lippincott, 1989, pp 1099-1161.
39. Rutledge F, Sinclair M: Treatment of intraepithelial carcinoma of the vulva by skin excision and graft. Am J Obstet Gynecol 102:806-815, 1968.
40. Baggish MS, Dorsey JH: CO_2 laser for the treatment of vulvar carcinoma-in-situ. Obstet Gynecol 57:371-375, 1981.
41. Ferenczy A: Using the laser to treat vulvar condylomata and intraepidermal neoplasia. Can Med Assoc J 128:135-137, 1983.
42. Townsend DE, Levine RU, Richart RM, et al: Management of vulvar intraepithelial neoplasia by carbon dioxide laser. Obstet Gynecol 60:49-52, 1982.
43. Raaf JH, Krown SE, Pinsky CM, et al: Treatment of Bowen's disease with topical dinitrochlorobenzene and 5-fluorouracil. Cancer 37:1633-1642, 1976.
44. Hernandez-Linares W, Puthawala A, Nolan JF, et al: Carcinoma in situ of the vagina: Past and present management. Obstet Gynecol 56:356-360, 1980.
45. Cagler H, Hurtzog RW, Hreshchyshyn MM: Topical 5-FU treatment of vaginal intraepithelial neoplasia. Obstet Gynecol 58:580-583, 1981.
46. Lamb MA: Sexual dysfunction in the gynecologic oncology patient. Semin Oncol Nurs 1:9-17, 1985.
47. Kilkku P, Gronroos M, Punnonen R: Sexual function after conization of the uterine cervix. Gynecol Oncol 14:209-212, 1982.
48. Celentano DD, Shapiro S, Weisman CS: Cancer: Preventive screening behavior among elderly women. Prev Med 11:454-463, 1982.
49. Caputo TA: Uterine cervical cancer: The current approach to diagnosis and treatment. Syracuse, NY, Bristol Laboratories, 1979.
50. Brand E, Berek JS, Hacker NF: Controversies in the management of cervical adenocarcinoma. Obstet Gynecol 71:261-269, 1988.
51. Henriksen E: The lymphatic spread of carcinoma of the cervix and the body of the uterus. Am J Obstet Gynecol 58:924-942, 1949.
52. Carlson V, Delclos L, Fletcher GH: Distant metastases in squamous-cell carcinoma of the uterine cervix. Radiology 88:961-966, 1967.
53. Walsh JW, Amendola MA, Konerding KF, et al: Computed tomographic detection of pelvic and inguinal lymph node metastases from primary and recurrent pelvic malignant diseases. Radiology 137:157-166, 1980.
54. Lewis E: The use and abuse of imaging in gynecologic cancer. Cancer 60:1993-2009, 1987.
55. Burghardt E, Hofmann HMH, Ebner F, et al: Magnetic resonance imaging in cervical cancer: A basis for objective classification. Gynecol Oncol 33:61-67, 1989.
56. Wharton JT, Jones HW, Day TG Jr, et al: Preirradiation celiotomy and extended-field irradiation for invasive carcinoma of the cervix. Obstet Gynecol 49:333-338, 1977.
57. Buchsbaum HJ: Extrapelvic lymph node metastases in cervical carcinoma. Am J Obstet Gynecol 133:814-824, 1979.
58. American Joint Committee On Cancer: Manual for Staging of Cancer (ed 3). Chicago, The Committee, 1988.
59. Barter JF, Soong SJ, Shingleton HM, et al: Complications of combined radical hysterectomy—postoperative radiation therapy in women with early stage cervical cancer. Gynecol Oncol 32:292-296, 1989.
60. Jones WB: Surgical approaches for advanced or recurrent cancer of the cervix. Cancer 60:2094-2103, 1987.
61. Perez CA, Breaux S, Bedwinek JM, et al: Radiation therapy alone in treatment of the uterine cervix. II. Analysis of complications. Cancer 54:235-246, 1984.
62. Lagasse LD, Johnson GH, Smith ML, et al: Use of sigmoid colon for rectal substitution following pelvic exenteration. Am J Obstet Gynecol 116:106-110, 1973.
63. Hatch KD, Shingleton HM, Potter ME, et al: Low rectal resection and anastomosis at the time of pelvic exenteration. Gynecol Oncol 31:262-267, 1988.
64. Brady LW, Markoe AM, DeEulis T, et al: Treatment of advanced and recurrent gynecologic cancer. Cancer 60: 2081-2093, 1987.
65. Wang CC: Altered fractionation radiation therapy for gynecologic cancers. Cancer 60:2064-2067, 1987.
66. Thigpen T, Vance R, Lambuth B, et al: Chemotherapy for advanced or recurrent gynecologic cancer. Cancer 60:2104-2116, 1987.
67. Thigpen JT: Chemotherapy, in Morrow CP, Townsend DE (eds): Synopsis of Gynecologic Oncology (ed 3). New York, Wiley & Sons, 1987, pp 409-458.
68. Rotmensch J, Senekjian EK, Javaheri G, et al: Evaluation of bolus cisplatinum and continuous 5-flourouracil infusion for metastatic and recurrent squamous cell carcinoma of the cervix. Gynecol Oncol 29:76-81, 1988.
69. Vogl SE: Chemotherapy of squamous cell carcinoma of the uterine cervix: Progress and potential. Curr Concepts Oncol 5:10-11, 15-17, 1983.
70. Stuart GCE, Robertson DI, Fedorkow DM, et al: Recurrent and persistent squamous cell cervical carcinoma in women under age 35. Gynecol Oncol 30:163-172, 1988.
71. Kim DS, Moon H, Kim KT, et al: Two-year survival: Preoperative adjuvant chemotherapy in the treatment of cervical cancer stages Ib and II with bulky tumor. Gynecol Oncol 33:225-230, 1989.
72. Kim DS, Moon H, Hwang YY, et al: Preoperative adjuvant chemotherapy in the treatment of cervical cancer stage Ib, IIa, and IIb with bulky tumor. Gynecol Oncol 29:321-332, 1988.
73. Hreshchyshyn MM, Aron BS, Boronow RC, et al: Hydroxyurea or placebo combined with radiation to treat stages IIIB and IV cervical cancer confined to the pelvis. Int J Radiat Oncol Biol Phys 5:317-322, 1979.
74. Piver MS, Barlow JJ, Vongtama V, et al: Hydroxyurea and radiation therapy in advanced cervical cancer. Am J Obstet Gynecol 120:969-972, 1974.
75. Weiner SA, Aristizabal S, Alberts DS, et al: A phase II trial of mitomycin, vincristine, bleomycin, and cisplatin (MOBP) as neoadjuvant therapy in high-risk cervical carcinoma. Gynecol Oncol 30:1-6, 1988.
76. Dutcher JP, Wadler S, Wiernik PH: Biologic response modifiers in gynecologic malignancies. Yale J Biol Med 61:367-378, 1988.
77. MacMahon B: Risk factors for endometrial cancer. Gynecol Oncol 2:122-129, 1974.
78. Jones HW: Treatment of adenocarcinoma of the endometrium. Obstet Gynecol Surg 30:147-169, 1975.
79. Morrow CP, DiSaia PJ, Townsend DE: Current management of endometrial carcinoma. Obstet Gynecol 42:399-406, 1973.

80. American Cancer Society: Summary of current guidelines for the cancer-related health check-up: Recommendations. New York, The Society, 1988.
81. Beecham JB, Helmkamp BF, Rubin P: Tumors of the female reproductive organs, in Rubin P (ed): Clinical Oncology: A Multidisciplinary Approach. New York, American Cancer Society, 1983, pp 428-480.
82. Shepherd JH: Revised FIGO staging for gynaecological cancer. Br J Obstet Gynaecol 96(8):889-892, 1989.
83. Shell JA, Carter J: The gynecological implant patient. Semin Oncol Nurs 3:54-66, 1987.
84. Edmonson JH, Krook JE, Hilton JF, et al: Randomized phase II studies of cisplatin and a combination of cyclophosphamide-doxorubicin-cisplatin (CAP) in patients with progestin-refractory advanced endometrial carcinoma. Gynecol Oncol 28:20-24, 1987.
85. Kauppila A, Gornroos N, Nieminen U: Clinical outcome in endometrial cancer. Obstet Gynecol 60:473-480, 1980.
86. Creasman WT, McCarty KS Sr, McCarty KS Jr: Clinical correlation of estrogen, progesterone binding proteins in human endometrial adenocarcinoma. Obstet Gynecol 55:363-370, 1980.
87. Utaaker E, Iversen OE, Skaarland E: The distribution and prognostic implications of steroid receptors in endometrial carcinomas. Gynecol Oncol 28:89-100, 1987.
88. Weintraub NT, Freedman ML: Gynecologic malignancies of the elderly. Clin Geriatr Med 3:669-694, 1987.
89. Quinn MA, Campbell JJ: Tamoxifen therapy in advanced/recurrent endometrial carcinoma. Gynecol Oncol 32:1-3, 1989.
90. Thigpen T, Buchsbaum HJ, Mangan C, et al: Phase II trial of adriamycin in treatment of advanced or recurrent endometrial carcinoma. Cancer Treat Rep 63:21-27, 1979.
91. Seski JC, Edwards CL, Herson J, et al: Cisplatin chemotherapy for disseminated endometrial cancer. Obstet Gynecol 59:225-228, 1982.
92. Thigpen T, Shingleton H, Homesley H, et al: Phase II trial of cisplatinum in the management of advanced or recurrent endometrial carcinoma. Proc Am Soc Clin Oncol 22:469, 1981.
93. Thigpen JT, Blessing JA, Homesley H, et al: Phase II trial of cisplatin as first-line chemotherapy in patients with advanced or recurrent endometrial carcinoma: A gynecologic oncology group study. Gynecol Oncol 33:68-70, 1989.
94. Turbow MM, Thornton J, Ballon S, et al: Chemotherapy of advanced endometrial cancer with platinum, adriamycin and cyclophosphamide. Proc Am Soc Clin Oncol 1:108, 1982.
95. Ozols RF, Young RC: Ovarian cancer. Curr Probl Cancer 11:57-122, 1987.
96. Runowicz CD: Ovarian cancer. Mediguide Oncol 7:1-5, 1987.
97. Barber HRK: Ovarian cancer. CA 36:149-184, 1986.
98. Hubbard SM: Ovarian carcinoma: An overview of current concepts in diagnosis and management. Cancer Nurs 1:115-128, 1978.
99. Young R, Fuks Z, Hoskins WJ: Cancer of the ovary, in DeVita VT, Hellman S, Rosenberg SA (eds): Cancer: Principles and Practice of Oncology (ed 3). Philadelphia, JB Lippincott Company, 1989, pp 1162-1196.
100. McGowan L: Ovarian cancer, in McGowan L (ed): Gynecologic Oncology. New York, Appleton-Century-Crofts, 1978.
101. Piver MS, Barlow JJ, Lele SB: Incidence of sub-clinical metastasis in stage I and II ovarian carcinoma. Obstet Gynecol 52:100-104, 1978.
102. Bristol Laboratories, Division of Bristol-Myers Co: Platinol: Effective palliation therapy in metastatic ovarian cancer. Syracuse, NY, Bristol Laboratories, 1982.
103. Young RC: Initial therapy for early ovarian carcinoma. Cancer 60:2042-2049, 1987.
104. Smith JP, Day TG: Review of ovarian cancer at the University of Texas Systems Cancer Center, M.D. Anderson Hospital and Tumor Institute. Am J Obstet Gynecology 135:984-993, 1979.
105. Stanhope CR, Smith JP: Ovarian cancer: The current approach to diagnosis and treatment. Syracuse, NY, Bristol Laboratories, 1981.
106. Pezner RD, Stevens KR Jr, Tong D, et al: Limited epithelial carcinoma of the ovary treated with curative intent by intraperitoneal instillation of radiocolloids. Cancer 42:2563-2671, 1978.
107. Richardson GS, Scully RE, Nikrui N, et al: Common epithelial cancer of the ovary. N Engl J Med 312:474-483, 1985.
108. Potter ME, Partridge EE, Shingleton HM, et al: Intraperitoneal chromic phosphate in ovarian cancer: Risks and benefits. Gynecol Oncol 32:314-318, 1989.
109. Gallion HH, van Nagell JR, Donaldson ES, et al: Adjuvant oral alkylating chemotherapy in patients with stage I epithelial ovarian cancer. Cancer 63:1070-1073, 1989.
110. Tobias JS, Griffiths CT: Management of ovarian carcinoma. N Engl J Med 294:818-823, 1976.
111. Young RC, Chabner BA, Hubbard SM: Prospective trial of melphalan (1-PAM) versus combination chemotherapy (Hexa-CAF) in ovarian adenocarcinoma. N Engl J Med 299:1261-1266, 1978.
112. Gershenson DM, Taylor Wharton J, Copeland LJ, et al: Treatment of advanced epithelial ovarian cancer with cisplatin and cyclophosphamide. Gynecol Oncol 32:336-341, 1989.
113. ten Bokkel Huinink WW, van der Burg MEL, van Oosterom AT, et al: Carboplatin in combination therapy for ovarian cancer. Cancer Treat Rev 15:9-15, 1988 (suppl B).
114. Rothenberg ML, Ostchega Y, Steinberg SM, et al: High-dose carboplatin with diethyldithiocarbamate chemoprotection in treatment of women with relapsed ovarian cancer. J Natl Cancer Inst 80:1488-1492, 1988.
115. Alberts DS, Garcia-Kendall D, Surwit EA: Phase II trial of mitomycin C plus 5-FU in the treatment of drug-refractory ovarian cancer. Semin Oncol 15:22-26, 1988 (suppl 4).
116. Kavanagh JJ, Roberts W, Townsend P, et al: Leuprolide acetate in the treatment of refractory or persistent epithelial ovarian cancer. J Clin Oncol 7:115-118, 1989.
117. Weiner SA, Alberts DS, Surwit EA, et al: Tamoxifen therapy in recurrent epithelial ovarian carcinoma. Gynecol Oncol 27:208-213, 1987.
118. Belinson JL, McClure M, Badger G: Randomized trial of megestrol acetate vs. megestrol acetate/tamoxifen for the management of progressive or recurrent epithelial ovarian carcinoma. Gynecol Oncol 28:151-155, 1987.
119. Fojo A, Hamilton TC, Young RC, et al: Multidrug resistance in ovarian cancer. Cancer 60:2075-2080, 1987.
120. Donehower RC, Rosenshein NB, Rotmensch J, et al: Sequential methotrexate and 5-fluorouracil in advanced ovarian carcinoma. Gynecol Oncol 27:90-96, 1987.
121. Goodman HM, Dottino PR, Kredenster D, et al: Continuous infusion fluoropyrimidines as salvage therapy for patients with advanced ovarian carcinoma. Gynecol Oncol 29:348-355, 1988.
122. Markman M: Intraperitoneal chemotherapy as treatment of ovarian carcinoma: Why, how and when? Obstet Gynecol Survey 42:533-539, 1987.

123. Ozols RF: Intraperitoneal chemotherapy. Mediguide Oncol 5:1-5, 1986.
124. Jones RB, Collins JM, Myers CE, et al: High volume intraperitoneal chemotherapy with methotrexate in patients with cancer. Cancer Res 41:55-59, 1981.
125. Ozols RF, Young RC, Speyer JL, et al: Phase I and pharmacological studies of adriamycin administered intraperitoneally to patients with ovarian cancer. Cancer Res 42:4265-4269, 1982.
126. Speyer J, Collins JM, Dedrick RL, et al: Phase I and pharmacological studies of 5-FU administered intraperitoneally. Cancer 40:567-572, 1980.
127. Howell SB, Pfeifle CL, Wung WE, et al: Intraperitoneal cisplatin with systemic thiosulfate protection. Ann Intern Med 97:845-851, 1982.
128. Monk BJ, Surwit EA, Alberts DS, et al: Intraperitoneal mitomycin C in the treatment of peritoneal carcinomatosis following second-look surgery. Semin Oncol 15:27-31, 1988 (suppl 4).
129. Loeffler T, Freund W: Pharmacokinetics of mitosantrone intraperitoneal. Proc Am Assoc Cancer Res 27:175, 1986.
130. King ME, Pfeifle CE, Howell SB: Intraperitoneal cytosine arabinoside in ovarian carcinoma. J Clin Oncol 2:662, 1984.
131. Berek JS, Hacker NF, Lichtenstein A, et al: Intraperitoneal recombinant alpha-interferon for "salvage" immunotherapy in stage III epithelial ovarian cancer: A gynecologic oncology group study. Cancer Res 45:4447-4453, 1985.
132. Piccart MJ, Abrams J, Dodion PF, et al: Intraperitoneal chemotherapy with cisplatin and melphalan. J Natl Cancer Inst 80:1118-1124, 1988.
133. Hamilton TC, Ozols RF, Longo DL: Biologic therapy for the treatment of malignant common epithelial tumors of the ovary. Cancer 60:2054-2063, 1987.
134. Chapman PB, Hakes T, Gabrilove JL, et al: A phase I pilot study of intraperitoneal rIL-2 in ovarian cancer. Proc Am Soc Clin Oncol 5:23, 1986.
135. Smith LH, Teng NNH: Clinical applications of monoclonal antibodies in gynecologic oncology. Cancer 60:2068-2074, 1987.
136. Pommier RF, Woltering EA, Milo G, et al: Synergistic cytotoxicity between dimethyl sulfoxide and antineoplastic agents against ovarian cancer in vitro. Am J Obstet Gynecol 159:848-852, 1988.
137. Rubin SC, Hoskins WJ, Markman M, et al: Long-term access to the peritoneal cavity in ovarian cancer patients. Gynecol Oncol 33:46-48, 1989.
138. Creasman WT, Yale SA, Blessing JA, et al: Chemoimmunotherapy in the management of primary stage III ovarian cancer: A Gynecologic Oncology Group study. Cancer Treat Rep 63:319-323, 1979.
139. Alberts DS, Moon TE, Stephens RA, et al: Randomized trial of chemoimmunotherapy for advanced ovarian carcinoma: A preliminary report of a Southwest Oncology Group Study. Cancer Treat Rep 63:325-331, 1979.
140. Alberts DS, Mason-Liddil N, O'Toole RV, et al: Randomized phase III trial of chemoimmunotherapy in patients with previously untreated stages III and IV suboptimal disease ovarian cancer: A Southwest Oncology Group study. Gynecol Oncol 32:8-15, 1989.
141. Weiser EB, Burke TW, Heller PB, et al: Determinants of survival of patients with epithelial ovarian carcinoma following whole abdomen irradiation (WAR). Gynecol Oncol 30:201-208, 1988.
142. Solomon HJ, Atkinson KH, Coppleson JVM, et al: Ovarian carcinoma: Abdominopelvic irradiation following reexploration. Gynecol Oncol 31:396-401, 1988.
143. Schray MF, Martinez A, Howes AE, et al: Advanced epithelial ovarian cancer: Salvage whole abdominal irradiation for patients with recurrent or persistent disease after combination chemotherapy. J Clin Oncol 6:1433-1439, 1988.
144. Lawton FG, Redman CW, Luesley DM, et al: Neoadjuvant (cytoreductive) chemotherapy combined with intervention debulking surgery in advanced, unresected epithelial ovarian cancer. Obstet Gynecol 73:61-65, 1989.
145. Sonnendecker EWW: Is routine second-look laparotomy for ovarian cancer justified? Gynecol Oncol 31:249-255, 1988.
146. Brand E, Wade ME, Lagasse LD: Resection of fixed pelvic tumors using the Nd:YAG laser. J Surg Oncol 37:246-251, 1988.
147. Bast RC Jr, Hunter V, Knapp RC: Pros and cons of gynecologic tumor markers. Cancer 60:1984-1992, 1987.
148. Bast RC, Klug TL, St. John E, et al: A radioimmunoassay using a monoclonal antibody to monitor the course of epithelial ovarian cancer. N Engl J Med 309:883-887, 1983.
149. Neunteufel W, Breitenbecker G: Tissue expression of CA 125 in benign and malignant lesions of ovary and fallopian tube: A comparison with CA 19-9 and CEA. Gynecol Oncol 33:297-302, 1989.
150. Niloff JM, Bast RC Jr, Schaetzl EM, et al: Predictive value of CA 125 antigen levels at second look procedures in ovarian cancer. Am J Obstet Gynecol 151:981-986, 1985.
151. Berek JS, Knapp PC, Malkasian GD, et al: CA 125 serum levels correlate with second-look operations among ovarian cancer patients: A prospective multi-institutional study. Obstet Gynecol 67:685-689, 1986.
152. Jager W, Adam R, Wildt L, et al: Serum CA-125 as a guideline for the timing of a second-look operation and second-line treatment in ovarian cancer. Arch Gynecol Obstet 243:91-99, 1988.
153. Potter ME, Moradi M, To ACW, et al: Value of serum 125 CA levels: Does the result preclude a second look? Gynecol Oncol 33:201-203, 1989.
154. MacDonald F, Bird R, Stokes H, et al: Expression of CEA, CA 125, CA 19-9 and human milk fat globule membrane antigen in ovarian tumours. J Clin Pathol 41:260-264, 1988.
155. Fioretti P, Gadducci A, Ferdeghini M, et al: Correlation of CA 125 and CA 19-9 serum levels with clinical course and second-look findings in patients with ovarian carcinoma. Gynecol Oncol 28:278-283, 1987.
156. Einhorn N, Cantell K, Einhorn S, et al: Human leukocyte interferon therapy for advanced ovarian cancer. Am J Clin Oncol 5:167-172, 1982.
157. Welander CE: Use of interferon in the treatment of ovarian cancer as a single agent and in combination with cytotoxic drugs. Cancer 59:617-619, 1987.
158. Lichtenstein A, Spina C, Berek JS, et al: Intraperitoneal administration of human recombinant interferon-alpha in patients with ovarian cancer: Effects on lymphocyte phenotype and cytotoxicity. Cancer Res 48:5853-5859, 1988.
159. Smith DB: Gynecological cancers: Etiology and pathophysiology. Semin Oncol Nurs 2:270-274, 1986.
160. Podczaski E, Herbst AL: Cancer of the vagina and fallopian tube, in Knapp RS, Berkowitz RS (eds): Gynecologic Oncology. New York, Macmillan, 1986, pp 339-424.
161. Sulak P, Barnhill D, Heller P, et al: Nonsquamous cancer of the vagina. Gynecol Oncol 29:309-320, 1988.
162. Herbst AL, Scully RE: Adenocarcinoma of the vagina in adolescents. Cancer 25:745-757, 1970.
163. Auclair CA: Consequences of prenatal exposure to diethylstilbestrol. J Gynecol Nurs 8:35-39, 1979.
164. Plentl AA, Friedman EA: Lymphatic System in the Female Genitalia. Philadelphia, WB Saunders, 1971.

165. Reddy S, Lee MS, Graham JE, et al: Radiation therapy in primary carcinoma of the vagina. Gynecol Oncol 26:19-24, 1987.
166. Morrow CP, Townsend DE (eds): Synopsis of Gynecologic Oncology (ed 3). New York, Wiley & Sons, 1987.
167. Morley GW: Infiltrative carcinoma of the vulva: Results of surgical treatment. Am J Obstet Gynecol 124:874-880, 1976.
168. Curry SL, Wharton JT, Rutledge F: Positive lymph nodes in vulvar squamous carcinoma. Gynecol Oncol 9:63-67, 1980.
169. Ball B: Easing the shock of radical vulvectomy. Nursing 5:27-31, 1975.
170. Wharton JT, Gallagher S, Rutledge FN: Microinvasive carcinoma of the vulva. Am J Obstet Gynecol 118:159-162, 1974.
171. Averette HE, Donato DM, Lovecchio JL, et al: Surgical staging of gynecologic malignancies. Cancer 60:2010-2020, 1987.
172. Robertson C: Treatment modalities for gynecological cancers. Semin Oncol Nurs 2:275-280, 1986.
173. Levin W, Rad FF, Goldberg G, et al: The use of concomitant chemotherapy and radiotherapy prior to surgery in advanced stage carcinoma of the vulva. Gynecol Oncol 25:20, 1986.
174. Moreland BJ: A nursing form for gynecology patient assessment. Oncol Nurs Forum 14:19-23, 1987.
175. Sargis NM: Detecting ovarian cancer: A challenge for nursing assessment. Oncol Nurs Forum 10:48-52, 1983.
176. Sandella J: Vulvar self examination (VSE). Oncol Nurs Forum 14:71-73, 1987.
177. Podratz KC, Symmonds RE, Taylor MF: Carcinoma of the vulva: Analysis of treatment failures. Am J Obstet Gynecol 143:340-351, 1982.
178. Jusenius K: A teaching aid for the radical hysterectomy patient. Oncol Nurs Forum 10:71-75, 1983.
179. McConnell EA, Zimmerman MF: Care of patients with urologic problems. Philadelphia, JB Lippincott, 1983.
180. Dudas S, Carlson CE: Cancer rehabilitation. Oncol Nurs Forum 15:183-188, 1988.
181. Burke L, Apfel RJ, Fisher S, et al: Observations on the psychological impact of diethylstilbestrol exposure and suggestions on management. J Reprod Med 24:99-102, 1980.
182. Schwartz R, Stewart N: Psychological effects of diethylstilbestrol exposure. J Am Med Assoc 237:257-260, 1977.
183. Konicki AM: Physical and psychological effects of DES on exposed offspring. Cancer Nurs 8:233-237, 1985.
184. Andersen BL: Sexual functioning morbidity among cancer survivors: Present status and future research directions. Cancer 57:1880-1886, 1985.
185. Glasgow M, Halfin V, Althausen AF: Sexual response and cancer. CA 37:322-333, 1987.
186. Wilson ME, Williams HA: Oncology nurses' attitudes and behaviors related to sexuality of patients with cancer. Oncol Nurs Forum 15:49-53, 1988.
187. Jenkins B: Patients' reports of sexual changes after treatment for gynecological cancer. Oncol Nurs Forum 15:349-354, 1988.
188. Grunberg KJ: Sexual rehabilitation of the cancer patient undergoing ostomy surgery. J Enterostom Ther 13:148-152, 1986.
189. McCartney CF, Larson DB: Quality of life in patients with gynecologic cancer. Cancer 60:2129-2136, 1987.
190. Kaempfer SH, Major P: Fertility considerations in the gynecologic oncology patient. Oncol Nurs Forum 13:23-27, 1986.
191. Andersen BL: Sexual functioning complications in women with gynecologic cancer: Outcomes and directions for prevention. Cancer 60:2123-2128, 1987.
192. Hogan R: Human Sexuality: A Nursing Perspective. New York, Appleton-Century-Crofts, 1980.
193. Lamont JA, DePetrillo AD, Sargeant EJ: Psychosexual rehabilitation and exenterative surgery. Gynecol Oncol 6:236-242, 1978.
194. Dennerstein L, Wood C, Burrows GD: Sexual response following hysterectomy and oophorectomy. Obstet Gynecol 49:84-96, 1977.
195. Harris R, Good R, Pollack L: Sexual behavior of gynecologic cancer patients. Arch Sex Behav 11:503-510, 1982.
196. Williams HA, Wilson ME, Hongladarom G, et al: Nurses' attitudes toward sexuality in cancer patients. Oncol Nurs Forum 13:39-43, 1986.
197. Fisher SG: The sexual knowledge and attitudes of oncology nurses: Implications for nursing education. Semin Oncol Nurs 1:63-68, 1985.
198. Fisher SG: Psychosexual adjustment following total pelvic exenteration. Cancer Nurs 2:219-225, 1979.
199. Capone MA, Good RS, Westie KS, et al: Psychosocial rehabilitation of gynecologic oncology patients. Arch Phys Med Rehab 61:128-132, 1980.
200. Yarbrough B: Teaching plan for patients undergoing total pelvic exenteration. Oncol Nurs Forum 8:36-40, 1981.
201. Springer MO: Radical vulvectomy: Physical, psychological, social and sexual implications. Oncol Nurs Forum 9:19-29, 1982.
202. Andersen B, Hacker N: Psychosexual adjustment after vulvar surgery. Obstet Gynecol 62:457-462, 1983.
203. Frank-Stromborg M: Sexuality and the elderly cancer patient. Semin Oncol Nurs 1:49-55, 1985.
204. Krouse HJ: A psychological model of adjustment in gynecologic cancer patients. Oncol Nurs Forum 12:45-49, 1985.
205. Holmes BC: Psychological evaluation and preparation of the patient and family. Cancer 60:2021-2024, 1987.

Chapter 41

Head and Neck Cancer

Michelle Goodman, RN, MS

INTRODUCTION

The concepts of infiltration and invasion can be aptly applied to carcinomas of the head and neck. Within this group of malignancies are imaginary lines that separate one primary tumor site from another. The infiltration and invasion of a tumor in this region can proceed unmarked by anatomic boundaries, silently destroying and disrupting the intricate and highly sophisticated structure and function of the head and neck region.

Through our knowledge of this organization of structure and function, we are able to detect carcinoma in the head and neck region and anticipate the structural and functional losses that will occur as a consequence of destruction by the tumor and by treatment regimens.

Treatment often involves major physiologic changes in the highly complex, interrelated functions of eating, swallowing, speech, and respiration. The organs of special senses also may be altered. In addition to these losses, the individual often experiences major alterations in body image as a result of the unavoidable changes in physical appearance. Each person responds differently to these losses, but the majority of individuals eventually adapt to these losses as a necessary price to pay for possible cure of the disease. The adaptations these people make are often extraordinary.

Because rehabilitation is in part defined by the functional diagnosis (ie, what functions have been lost and what compensatory functions need to be made), each discussion of the various head and neck carcinomas first defines the anatomic function of the part, the physiologic problems created by surgery, and the rehabilitative measures that serve to minimize the losses and assist in the adaptation process.

ANATOMY AND PHYSIOLOGY

Prior to a discussion of the functional rehabilitation problems an individual can encounter after resection of a portion of the head and neck region, an understanding of the anatomy and physiology in this area is imperative. The following is a brief overview of the anatomy of this region and the physiology of swallowing and airway protection, two functions that are often altered by surgery of the head and neck region.

Figure 41-1 depicts the six major anatomic subdivisions of the upper aerodigestive tract.

Nasal Cavity and Paranasal Sinuses

The nasal cavities are triangular spaces, one on each side of the nasal septum. Each cavity communicates exteriorly through the anterior nares and posteriorly with the nasopharynx through the posterior nares, laterally with the maxillary sinus, and superiorly with the sphenoid, ethmoid, and frontal sinuses. The upper nasal cavity is considered to be olfactory and the lower nasal cavity respiratory in function. The major functions of these areas are to cleanse, humidify, and warm the air one breathes, to serve as airway passages, and for olfaction.

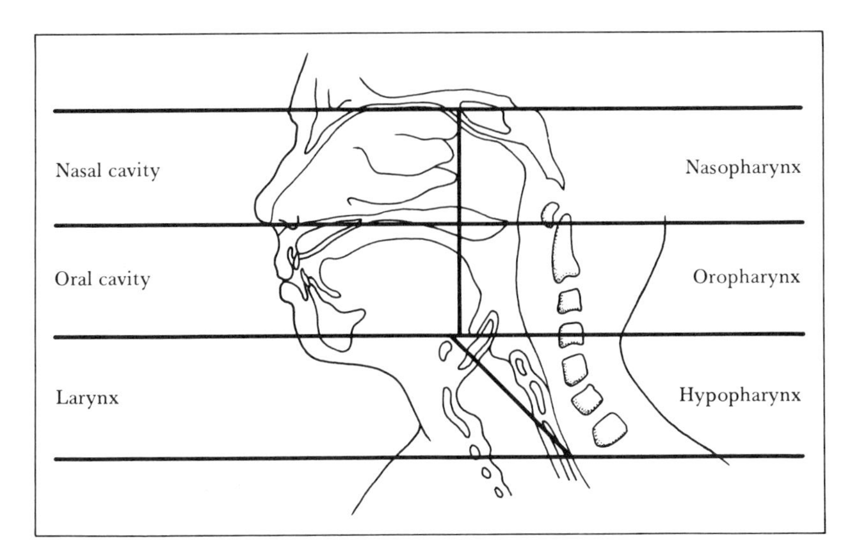

FIGURE 41-1 Major anatomic subdivisions of the upper aerodigestive tract.

Olfaction

The olfactory area is located high in the nasal vault, above the superior turbinate. The olfactory nerve (first cranial) innervates the nasal mucous membranes to mediate the sense of smell. When the sense of smell is poor or absent, the only immediate discomfort is a change in taste. The taste of food is recognized and enjoyed through simultaneous stimulation on the taste buds of the tongue and the olfactory cells of the nose. When odors cannot reach the olfactory area or when the sense of smell is absent (anosmia), food tastes flat and unpalatable. When the sense of smell is absent for a long time, as in persons who undergo laryngectomy, the sensitivity of the taste buds apparently increases, and the acuity of taste is increased in a compensatory fashion.

Humidification and temperature control

An important function of the nose is to condition the inspired air before it enters the trachea, bronchi, and lungs. The nose can add moisture to inspired air or remove it so that the air that reaches the pharynx is of almost constant relative humidity. The nose also cleanses particles and bacteria from air entering the nasal cavity. To control temperature, the capillaries of the nasal cavity enlarge or contract rapidly as necessary.

Nasopharynx

The nasopharynx is an open space situated just below the base of the skull and behind the nasal cavity. Anteriorly the nasopharynx communicates with the nasal cavity via the posterior nares, which are separated in the midline by the nasal septum. The inferior wall is bordered by the soft palate. The lateral walls contain the pharyngeal orifice of the eustachian tubes. The posterior and lateral walls of the nasopharynx are surrounded by fascia. This area is closely related to the gasserian ganglion and the cavernous sinus. The abducens nerve (VI) passes through the cavernous sinus, and the oculomotor nerve (III) and the trochlear nerve (IV) are found in its lateral wall. The optic nerve (II) lies medial to the cavernous sinus.

In front of the eustachian tube, the lateral wall of the nasopharynx is in proximity to the maxillopharyngeal space and the vertical ramus of the mandible. In this space is found the mandibular nerve as it descends from the foramen ovale. Behind the eustachian tube lies a space that contains the internal carotid artery, the internal jugular vein, and the glossopharyngeal, vagus, spinal accessory, and hypoglossal nerves (IX, X, XI, and XII), as well as the cervical sympathetic nerve, all of which emerge from the base of the skull through this space.

Oral Cavity

The oral cavity is composed of the anterior two thirds, or mobile portion, of the tongue, the floor of the mouth, the buccal mucosa, the hard palate, and the upper and lower alveolar ridges (gingivae).

The tongue is the chief organ of taste, speech, mastication, and deglutition. The articulators of speech are the lip, tongue, oral cavity, and jaw. The major function of the lips in speech is to produce a valving action that provides for the buildup of intraoral pressure, which is necessary for the production of plosive consonants such as *P* and *B*. The production sounds, such as *Y* and *F*, require good lip control and tension. An intact lower lip is most important for oral competence and mobility. The tongue plays a major role in articulation of sound for speech. The formation of many of the consonants and all of the vowels and diphthongs is related to tongue position and configuration. Extremely rapid changes in tongue position and shape are required for clear, concise articulation. Tongue-tip sounds of *N*, *T*, *D*, and *L* require elevation of the tip to the upper alveolus. The *TH* sounds require that the tongue tip be protruded beyond the incisor edges. The *R* sound is distinctive in that two curves are created in the tongue with the tip free of contact. The *S* and *Z* sounds are made with the tip against the palate and with a median opening for passage of turbulent air.

The sensory and motor innervation of the tongue is bilateral. This allows for the high degree of compensatory action that is accomplished with unilateral denervation after surgical ablation. Major sensory innervation is mediated via the lingual nerve from the mandibular branch of the fifth cranial nerve, which innervates the mucous membranes of the anterior tongue. Major motor innervation to the intrinsic and extrinsic muscles of the tongue is mediated via the hypoglossal (twelfth cranial) nerve. The major extrinsic muscles of the tongue are the genioglossus, which protrudes and depresses the tongue, the hypoglossus, which depresses and retracts the tongue, the styloglossus, which raises and retracts the tongue, and the palatoglossus, which elevates the tongue.

Oropharynx

The oropharynx is a posterior continuation of the oral cavity that includes the retromolar trigone and the anterior tonsillar pillar, the soft palate (or palatine arch), the base of the tongue, the pharyngeal walls, and the tonsils. For the purpose of this discussion, the major area of interest is the innervation of the base of the tongue and the soft palate. The major motor and sensory innervation to the pharynx and posterior third or base of the tongue is mediated by the glossopharyngeal, or ninth cranial, nerve. This nerve facilitates adequate swallowing and airway protection in that the glossopharyngeal is responsible for the gag reflex. The vagus, or tenth cranial, nerve innervates the soft palate and pharynx. Damage to this nerve results in palatal and pharyngeal paralysis, which can result in nasal regurgitation.

Laryngopharynx or Hypopharynx

The laryngopharyngeal region involves the lingual surface of the epiglottis, the vallecula (depression between the lateral and median glossoepiglottic folds), and the central portion of the posterior base of the tongue. It is formed by two elongated gutters (piriform sinuses), which extend on both sides of the larynx posteriorly from the pharyngoepiglottic fold to the mouth of the esophagus. The median wall of the piriform sinus is formed by the arytenoepiglottic fold above and by the muscles that form the mouth of the esophagus below.

The structures are intimately involved in swallowing and airway protection. The glossopharyngeal and vagus nerves innervate the pharyngeal constrictors, which constrict the upper, middle, and lower parts of the pharynx during the act of swallowing. During the act of swallowing the hypopharynx is separated and closed off from the endolarynx by the anterior elevation of the larynx.

Larnyx (Endolarynx)

The larynx is situated directly below the hypopharynx and is encased within three main cartilages that form the skeleton of the larynx: the epiglottis, the thyroid cartilage, and the cricoid cartilage, which are tightly interconnected by ligaments. The larynx is subdivided into three regions: the superglottic, glottic, and subglottic areas. The superglottic area extends from the free border of the epiglottis to and including the false cords, and the arytenoepiglottic folds form the boundary between the larynx and the piriform sinus. The glottis is formed by the true vocal cords, which extend from the thyroid cartilage anteriorly to the arytenoids posteriorly. The subglottic region includes the area directly below and continuous with the trachea; the subglottic region is surrounded entirely by the cricoid cartilage.

The major motor innervation of the larynx is via the external laryngeal branch of the superior laryngeal branch of the vagus nerve and the recurrent laryngeal nerve. The internal laryngeal branch of the superior larnygeal nerve from the vagus supplies the sensory innervation. During respiration, the framework of the larynx is ridged to maintain an adequate airway. To prevent substances from entering the trachea, the lateral cricoarytenoid and arytenoid muscles adduct the vocal cords. In forced respiration the glottis is opened by the action of the posterior cricoarytenoid muscle. During vocalization, pitch is changed through changes in the tension of the vocal cords. A higher pitch and increased tension are brought about by the cricothyroid muscles. Decreased tension, which shortens the vocal cords, is brought about through the action of the thyroarytenoid muscles.

Physiology of Swallowing

Swallowing is divided into four phases: the oral preparation phase, the oral phase, the pharyngeal phase, and the esophageal phase. The oral phase is voluntary, and both the pharyngeal and the esophageal phases are involuntary. Patients with head and neck cancer, especially those who are treated with surgery, often have disruption in the intricate motor actions characteristic of the various phases of swallowing.[1]

Oral preparation phase

Lip closure to prevent drooling and loss of food from the mouth and tongue movement to bring food together in a bolus are the two most important aspects of the oral preparation phase.

Oral phase

The oral phase of swallowing begins with the jaws closed and the lips together. The tongue is voluntarily raised against the hard palate. The entire tongue is lifted by the contraction of the mylohyoid, geniohyoid, and genioglossus muscles while the palatoglossus muscles relax; this removes the bolus to the level of the soft palate. The hypoglossal nerve supplies the innervation necessary to perform this action. At the same time, the base of the tongue is elevated and drawn back with a slight elevation of the larynx. As the dorsum of the tongue is pressed against the hard palate, the bolus is propelled into the pharynx. The styloglossus muscle is important in this function.

Pharyngeal phase

The pharyngeal phase is a reflex act and involves both propulsion of the bolus and protection of the airway. The pharynx, which is attached to the larynx, is raised and expanded to receive the bolus. Movement of the soft palate to the posterior nasopharyngeal wall is facilitated by contraction of the superior constrictor muscle. Simultaneously, the larynx is elevated against the base of the tongue. Next, the vocal cords close, and the base of the tongue is forcibly opposed to the posterior pharyngeal wall. This is followed immediately by contraction of the pharyngeal constrictors, creating a stripping wave to empty the pharynx.

Esophageal phase

The pharyngeal phase ends by the descent of the larynx and the contraction of the cricopharyngeal muscle, which presumably occurs to avoid regurgitation, and respiration is resumed. Respiration is inhibited during the oral and pharyngeal phases and is resumed during the esophageal phase.

Airway Protection

The epiglottis is relatively unimportant in the mechanism of airway protection and can be resected (epiglectomy) without danger of aspiration. It is the elevation and forward movement of the larynx against the base of the tongue that is the most important factor in prevention of aspiration and airway protection. The closing of the vocal cords constitutes an important secondary line of defense in the act of swallowing and the prevention of aspiration.

EPIDEMIOLOGY

Head and neck carcinomas (excluding cancers of the central nervous system, eye, skin, and thyroid) account for 4% of all malignancies in males and 2% in females and for about 13,375 deaths annually.[2] Although easily detected, the tumors are generally discovered late. When first seen by a physician, 80% to 90% of oral cancers are 2 cm or more in diameter. More than 60% of the 54,200 individuals in whom head and neck cancer is diagnosed each year in the United States have advanced disease when first seen. Diagnosis may be delayed because the lesions are generally painless and people procrastinate, partly out of fear and partly in the vain hope that the "sore" will go away. For these and other reasons, often metastasis to regional lymph nodes has occurred by the time these cancers are first detected. Tumor size and the presence of regional lymph node metastasis make treatment more complex and reconstructive procedures more complicated than they would be if the asymptomatic lesions were detected and treated earlier. These facts create special problems from the standpoint of rehabilitation and treatment. The incidence of head and neck carcinoma is high among lower socioeconomic groups, particularly males. The male/female ratio is 3:1, with the greatest incidence occurring during the fifth and seventh decades of life.

ETIOLOGY

The high incidence of head and neck cancer in lower socioeconomic groups has to do in part with personal and social habits. Heavy alcohol consumption combined with the use of tobacco (smoking and chewing) is highly correlated with the development of head and neck cancer. Tobacco is believed to be a physical and chemical carcinogen. The combination of alcohol and tobacco potentiates carcinogenesis and creates a significantly higher risk than does either one alone.[3] This finding is especially true for laryngeal and oropharyngeal carcinoma. Chewing tobacco has been linked to oral cancer. Snuff dipping, the placement and retention of tobacco in the cheek, is a common practice among women in rural areas and is becoming popular with young boys.

Poor dentition and poor oral hygiene in general are also risk facors, especially for carcinoma of the tongue, where constant irritation from a jagged carious tooth can set the stage for mucosal changes. Ill-fitting dentures have been suggested as causative agents in carcinoma of the gingiva and other sites. The inhalation of certain wood dusts, nickel compounds, nitrosamines, hydrocarbons, and asbestos is highly correlated with tumors of the oral cavity, nasal cavity, and paranasal sinuses. A close relationship has been documented between nasopharyngeal carcinoma, especially in younger persons, and the Epstein-Barr virus (EBV).[4] Henle and colleagues[5] report a decrease in EBV antibody titers in individuals being treated for nasopharyngeal carcinoma and an elevation in titers with increasing tumor burden in individuals with advancing disease. The high incidence of nasopharyngeal cancer among Cantonese populations and the presence of a specific HLA antigen profile in these persons suggests a genetic predisposition.[6]

A relatively high incidence of Plummer-Vinson syndrome is found among persons with carcinoma of the oral cavity and pharynx. This syndrome is characterized by generalized nutritional deficiencies (eg, iron and riboflavin), anemia, achlorhydria, chronic dysphagia, and splenic enlargement. There may be general signs of atrophy of the mucous membranes in the mouth and pharynx. Persons with Plummer-Vinson syndrome often have a history of loss of teeth early in life. A diet deficient in vitamin A and retinoids may play a role in the etiology of head and neck cancer, but the exact mechanism is not known.[7]

A review of the risk factors of head and neck carcinoma quickly alerts the nurse to the need for preventive teaching and to the population of persons who could best benefit from such an intervention.

To say that this group of cancers occurs only among indigent persons would be erroneous. Two distinct groups emerge in which the clinical presentation is quite different. The first includes individuals with early, relatively localized tumors, who may smoke and drink but rarely to excess. With early detection and prompt treatment, these persons can be cured or at least can expect long-term survival.[8] The second group, as previously mentioned, consists of individuals who pay little heed to their general health. In this group a tumor that is painful or growing large will not be brought to the atttention of a physician until the growth dramatically alters life-style (eg, causes difficulty in breathing or swallowing). The outlook for survival or long-term palliation is negligible in this group. These individuals usually return to previous patterns of self-abusive behavior and are, unless strictly followed (by telephone calls or visits from the visiting nurse), lost to follow-up. Early recognition of cases and general preventive health teaching are of paramount importance.

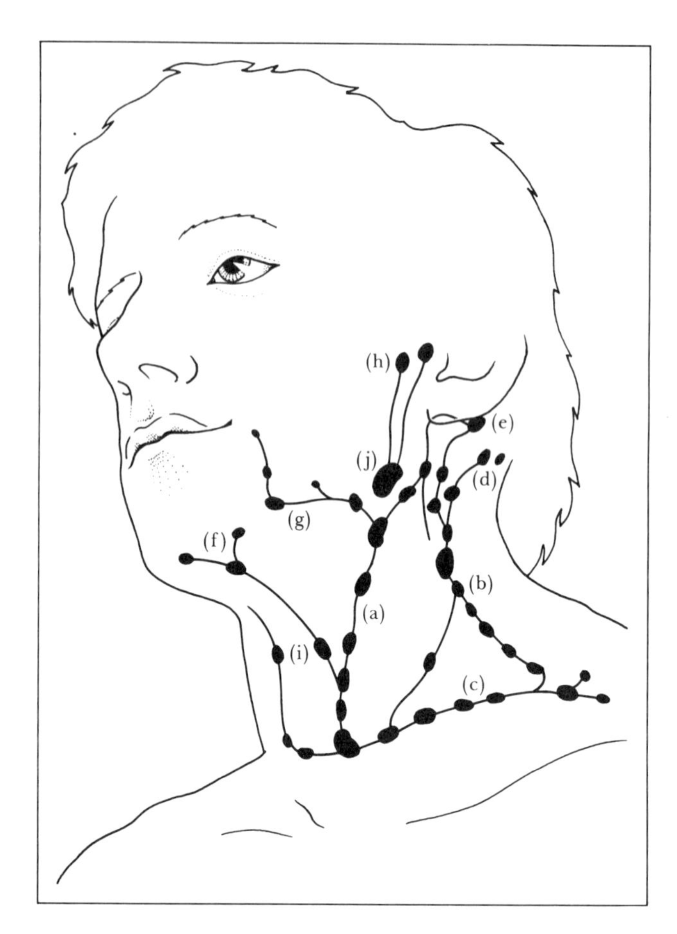

FIGURE 41-2 Lymphatic drainage of the head and neck. (a) Lateral cervical midjugular. (b) Midposterior cervical. (c) Supraclavicular. (d) Occipital. (e) Posterior auricular. (f) Submental. (g) Submandibular. (h) Preauricular. (i) Anterior cervical. (j) Subdigastric.

PATHOPHYSIOLOGY

Approximately 95% of all head and neck carcinomas are of squamous cell origin and arise from epithelium that lines the upper airways and the digestive tract. Leukoplakia or erythroplasia may or may not precede carcinoma but is considered to be a precancerous lesion, particularly in chronic users of alcohol or tobacco.

The majority of tumors of the head and neck region invade locally, deep into neighboring structures and along tissue planes far beyond the anatomic limits of the lesion. The perineural route is an important pathway for tumor spread. Intracranial spread may result from perineural extension of tumor along peripheral branches of cranial nerves.[9] Regional lymph node metastasis is predictable, depending on the site of the primary tumor and the degree of tumor cell differentiation. The more poorly differentiated tumors tend to metastasize early to regional lymph nodes and beyond. An enlarged lymph node may be the first sign that a tumor is present in the head and neck region. Lymphatic drainage of the head and neck area is depicted in Figure 41-2.

In the past it was believed that head and neck cancers as a group remained localized to the supraclavicular nodes and above and rarely metastasized. As local-regional control of disease is being achieved through advances in therapy, individuals are living longer and the incidence of clinically evident hematogenous metastases increases. For patients with tumors 2 to 4 cm in diameter, the incidence of microscopic or clinically evident lymph node metastasis is greater than 50%.[10] The incidence of distant metastasis, particularly to the lungs, bone, and liver, is approximately 12%. However, when a lymph node or distant metastasis is present in a patient with an early oral primary cancer, it is likely that a second primary upper aerodigestive or lung cancer is responsible.

The presence or absence of histologically proven lymph node metastasis plays an important role in determining the prognosis. As the number of nodes involved increases, the prognosis steadily decreases. Another factor that affects prognosis is the degree of lymph node involvement and the presence or absence of soft tissue spread after penetration of the lymph node capsule. As carcinoma spreads to lower nodes in the neck, there seems to be a corresponding reduction in the 5-year survival rate, at least in individuals with involvement in the lower third of the neck. The lowest survival rate is found in individuals with three or more positive nodes and involvement in the lower third of the neck.

Recurrence of disease locally and/or in the neck region after initial therapy presents special problems in terms of treatment and patient survival. Ninety percent of recurrences are detected within 18 months of therapy. Depending on previous therapy and the extent of recurrence, cure or long-term survival of the individual may still be possible.

The incidence of primary cancer and multiple primary cancer is high in this population of individuals and may be related to the unusually high degree of immunosuppression, even in the early stages of the disease.[11] These patients generally have suppressed T-cell function, and this suppression tends to be more pronounced with progression of the disease.

The greatest risk of a second primary tumor occurs within the initial 3-year period following treatment of the initial cancer. Approximately 30% of individuals with head and neck cancer will have a second primary cancer, which occurs predominantly in the upper aerodigestive tract.[12] It is believed that common contiguous tissues are subject to similar carcinogenic influences, and this is related to the idea that neoplastic induction of separate groups of cells by the same influences in an appropriate environment might occur in tissues with a common embryologic origin.

CLASSIFICATION AND STAGING

Cancers of the head and neck region may arise from any membranous lining of the upper aerodigestive tract. The T (tumor) classifications indicating the extent of the primary tumor are similar but differ in specific details for each site because of anatomic considerations. These differences are described in the subsequent sections, which discuss each region. The N (nodal) classification for cervical lymph node metastasis and the M (metastasis) classification for distant metastasis are uniform for all head and neck sites (Table 41-1).[13]

TABLE 41-1 TNM Classification System for Head and Neck Tumors: Nodal and Distant Sites

Nodal Involvement (N) Classification for All Head and Neck Malignant Neoplasms	
NX	Nodes cannot be assessed
N0	No clinically positive nodes
N1	Single clinically positive homolateral node 3 cm or less in diameter
N2	Single clinically positive homolateral node 3–6 cm in diameter
N2a	Single clinically positive homolateral node 3–6 cm in diameter
N2b	Multiple clinically positive homolateral nodes, none more than 6 cm in diameter
N3	Massive homolateral node(s), bilateral nodes, or contralateral node(s)
N3a	Clinically positive homolateral node(s), none more than 6 cm in diameter
N3b	Bilateral clinically positive nodes (each side of the neck is clinically staged separately)
N3c	Contralateral clinically positive node(s) only
Distant Metastasis (M) Classification for All Head and Neck Malignant Neoplasms	
MX	Not assessed
M0	No known distant metastasis
M1	Distant metastasis present; specify site and degree of organ impairment
Stage Grouping	
Stage I	T1, N0, M0
Stage II	T2, N0, M0
Stage III	T3, N0, M0 T1 or T2 or T3, N1, M0
Stage IV	T4, N0 or N1, M0 any T, N2 or N3, M0 any T, any N, M1

Source: Beahrs OH, Henson DE, Hutter RVP, et al (eds): Manual for Staging of Cancer (ed 3). Philadelphia, JB Lippencott, 1988.

TREATMENT

Treatment Planning

The anatomic location and the extent of the primary tumor will dictate the appropriate therapy. If, for example, the tumor is an isolated tongue lesion that is easily accessible, simple surgical excision with minimal or no functional loss is possible. If, however, the tumor is located in an area that is less accessible (eg, the nasopharynx), radiotherapy is most appropriate and affords the least structural change. Lesions that extend to neighboring tissues with nodal involvement will often require a combined therapeutic approach. No single modality of treatment has been universally successful in managing advanced (stages III and IV) head and neck cancers. While numerous combinations of surgery, radiation, chemotherapy, and immunotherapy have been tried, none have significantly improved survival in this population.[10]

Pretreatment planning includes joint consultation among surgeon, medical oncologist, radiotherapist, and prosthodontist. Computerized axial tomography, panendoscopy, barium swallow, and radiography of the chest will help to identify synchronous primary lesions. Photography and tattooing are used to determine the extent of disease before treatment and to objectively measure response to radiation and chemotherapy.

Assessment in the Pretreatment Phase

In the pretreatment period, the nurse has a unique opportunity to perform assessments that will help to minimize the complications of therapy. With the assistance of all members of the rehabilitation team, a plan of care is established on the basis of joint assessments and knowledge of the therapeutic plan.

Psychosocial assessment

The individual often has had previous surgical treatment, radiotherapy, or both for the tumor and may feel discouraged and depressed. Persons who can verbalize how their present condition is debilitating or unacceptable often are able to prepare themselves emotionally for treatment. For instance, perhaps the pain has been unbearable and constant for a period of time or eating has been nearly impossible, with resultant weight loss. The proposed treatment may cause anxiety but is preferable to the consequences of untreated disease.

The assistance of a psychiatric social worker or a chaplain in the pretreatment period can provide additional support to the individual. It is important that all members of the rehabilitation team who will be involved in the person's care after surgery become familiar to the patient and his or her family during the preoperative period. This is especially true if the individual is undergoing major surgery that involves temporary or permanent loss of speech or a major alteration of facial contour. This ensures not only a continuity of care but also spares the person the task of establishing new relationships in the immediate postoperative period when changes in body image are acute. It is important that in the preoperative period the individual and the family experience an overwhelming sense of acceptance and personalized care that will extend into the postoperative period.

Nutritional assessment

The individual with head and neck cancer often has nutritional deficiencies related to a variety of factors. The presence of a tumor in the oral cavity or pharyngeal area can obstruct normal deglutition. A tumor in the tongue can further interfere with the ability to eat, either by causing fixation and immobility or because of pain. If the tumor is exophytic and draining, with or without infection, esthetics can be a problem. These individuals are often edentulous which further complicates nutritional management.

Previous alcohol abuse, with or without liver dysfunction, leads to further nutritional deficits. Older individuals with financial limitations and restricted food preferences may have nutritional deficiencies. Pain and pain medications reduce appetite. Anorexia and resultant weight loss generate a vicious cycle: the weakness and lassitude they produce further decreases appetite.

Oral hygiene and dental care

The oral cavity is inspected carefully before treatment and a regimen of meticulous oral hygiene and peridontal care is established to minimize the risk of infection. An assessment of the teeth and gingival tissues is carried out by the prosthodontist or the nurse. These measures are particularly important if a mandibular prosthesis is being considered as part of the therapeutic plan.

If the individual has had prior irradiation, saliva production is usually reduced, acidic, or absent. Without the bacteriostatic properties of saliva, plaque builds up, leading to dental caries. In addition, infection is more likely in the presence of an ulcerative lesion. Bacteria often invade intraoral and pharyngeal suture lines postoperatively, causing infection and poor tissue healing.

Oral hygiene can be accomplished in a number of ways. Oxidizing agents, such as hydrogen peroxide (4:1 mixture) or baking soda (1/2 teaspoon in 8 ounces of water) adequately cleanse and free the oral cavity of debris. Oral gavaging with a drainage bag or a Water Pik irrigation device may be necessary to cleanse the oral cavity adequately. Commercial mouthwash should not be used because the majority of such agents contain an alcohol base and have a drying effect. Oral hygiene should be performed three to four times a day or when necessary. Fluoride treatments are recommended before irradiation and periodically to prevent decay.

Pulmonary hygiene

Because individuals with cancer of the head and neck are often moderate to heavy smokers, an aggressive program of pulmonary hygiene and rehabilitation is begun in the preoperative period; a trained pulmonary therapist usually is responsible for this program, but it also can be carried out adequately by a nurse. The person is instructed on proper lung-expansion techniques and breathing exercises that will be necessary in the postoperative period. This type of preventive mangement is important because the surgical procedures are often lengthy and the individual may have an alternate airway, either temporarily or permanently, after surgery. In addition, the major postoperative complications in the person with head and neck cancer are pneumonia and atelectasis.

Communication techniques

An appropriate method of communication to be used after surgery is established in the preoperative period. If the individual is to have a portion of the tongue or the larynx removed, the speech therapist will give instructions on methods of communicating. If swallowing will be altered, methods of muscle retraining may be instituted before surgery. The person is given a magic slate or a communication board to use after surgery. The individual's ability to write is assessed. If the writing is illegible or if the person speaks a foreign language, a picture board can be devised.

For the individual undergoing laryngectomy, a thorough speech and hearing evaluation is carried out before surgery. These individuals sometimes have hearing difficulties that will impede their progress in esophageal speech. If they cannot adequately hear the sounds they need to make, it is nearly impossible for them to learn esophageal speech successfully. Speech patterns are also assessed. The individual who has always been close-mouthed and reserved is not likely to verbalize a great deal with any form of speech therapy, and this could be wrongly interpreted as indicative of withdrawal or lack of motivation.

Surgery

Surgical intervention is often the treatment of choice for the majority of head and neck cancers. For localized superficial lesions, an excision with primary closure results in little or no functional loss to the individual. More extensive lesions may require a wide excision and a skin graft or local mucosal flap for closure. The intent of these major resections, commonly referred to as composite resection, monobloc, or commando procedures, is cure of the disease. A standard definition of a composition resection or monobloc procedure cannot be universal simply because the extent of the resection is defined by the extent of the tumor, which is sometimes unpredictable in dimension until actually visualized. A composite resection or monobloc procedure includes the resection of the tumor and a margin of regional lymphatic vessels. It may or may not include a portion of the mandible. This definition may be applied conceptually to any primary tumor in the head and neck region but is intended for resections that involve the oral cavity.

The more extensive the tumor involvement, the less the chance of cure; however, percentage probabilities of cure have little meaning when the tumor is obstructing and interfering with swallowing, speech, and respiration. Pain is a major symptom in individuals with extensive lesions. An acceptable quality of life may be obtainable only through surgery, although there are obvious trade-offs. The objective of aggressive surgical management is total resection of the primary tumor to provide cure. There must be adequate means of reconstructing the defect to provide compensatory function and an acceptable physical appearance. An accurate definition of the extent of the tumor in all its dimensions and a thorough assessment of potential losses and reconstructive procedures that are possible to compensate for these losses are required.

The definition of the tumor is accomplished by an examination of the head and neck region. Special radiologic techniques, such as nuclear magnetic resonance imaging (MRI), xeroradiography, or computed tomography (CT), are useful in the evaluation of bony invasion and areas that are difficult to assess, such as the sinuses and orbit.

Preoperative teaching

Depending on the therapeutic plan, the individual and the family are instructed about what they can expect and what will be expected of them in the immediate and extended postoperative period. The amount of information given depends on the person's needs, his or her desire to know, and the level of anxiety. The individual who knows what to expect will be less anxious and more in control of the situation. The individual's responsibilities in coughing, communicating, and early ambulation are all emphasized.

If a tracheostomy or a laryngectomy is to be performed, the individual can benefit from preoperative instruction on the use of the suctioning equipment, since tracheal suctioning often creates the most anxiety after surgery.

Postoperative complications

Special postoperative complications can occur after surgery in the head and neck region because of the complex anatomy of this area. Only the major complications peculiar to the area are addressed in this section.

The actual mortality rate of head and neck surgery is low (1% to 3%). However, the nurse should be familiar with possible complications and the interventions necessary to minimize their occurrence.

Hemorrhage Because of the length of the operative procedure, a blood loss of 500 mL is considered normal, but a loss of 1000 mL may occur if flap reconstruction is carried out. This volume is usually replaced during surgery without serious sequelae. Ligation or resection of the carotid artery involves a mortality rate of 25%, with central nervous system damage in about 50% of the survivors. Ophthalmoplethysmography may be carried out before surgery to assess whether there is adequate carotid crossover on the affected side. If tumor does not involve the carotid artery but the carotid is found to be a source of bleeding, an attempt is made to repair the vessel rather than ligate it. When a radical neck dissection is performed, an attempt usually is made to cover the carotid artery with a mucosal or muscle flap, such as the levator scapulae, for protection.

If the carotid artery is exposed after surgery as a result of skin flap necrosis or persistent tumor in the area, the individual is at risk of a carotid rupture, especially if the area is simultaneously infected. If there is a possibility that the carotid artery may rupture, the appropriate emergency supplies are placed at the bedside without unduly alarming the person.[14] (See Table 41-2.)

The first sign of an impending carotid artery rupture usually is a small trickle of blood from the area. This signal of impending blowout often calls for exploration and ligation of the vessel if necrosis of the carotid wall is evident. In the event that a carotid blowout occurs before the vessel can be ligated or repaired, the person nearest the patient must act without hesitation or the outcome may be fatal for the patient. A saline-soaked cotton dressing is wrapped around the two middle fingers, and constant digital pressure is applied directly in the wound over the carotid vessel. The person applying the pressure must not check to see whether the bleeding has stopped or attempt to apply a hemostat because this only results in further loss of blood. Meanwhile, a clot of blood is drawn and sent to the blood bank. The operating room is notified, and an intravenous line is started for administration of fluids. Only after the person is in the operating room and the arena is in readiness can the pressure be released and the vessel repaired. Hemiparesis remains a strong possibility,

TABLE 41-2 Carotid Precautions: Equipment

Sterile cotton dressings (6 packages 4 × 4s)
2 Cotton bath towels
Sterile bowl and normal saline solution
Ringer's lactate
Albumin
Type and crossmatch equipment (Vacutainer, holder, needle)
Completed requisitions for 2U of blood
Two 20 mL syringes
Alcohol swabs
1 Cuffed tracheostomy tube if indicated
Suction equipment

Adapted from Schwartz SS, Yuska CM: Common patient care issues following surgery for head and neck cancer. Semin Oncol Nurs 15(3):191-194, 1989.

but prevention of shock and fluid replacement for adequate perfusion of the brain via the opposite internal carotid artery help to decrease this risk.

This is a particularly frightening time for the patient. Patients need to be told what is being done to help them and what they can expect to happen. The person needs reassurance to remain calm and cooperative. If the individual has a tracheostomy or laryngectomy stoma, the cuff should be inflated to prevent blood from entering the trachea. Suctioning should be done as necessary to maintain the airway.

Hematoma may be a serious postoperative complication. Drainage tubes are usually placed beneath skin flaps to ensure adequate drainage and prevent the collection of fluid beneath the flaps. If there is excessive bleeding after surgery, as evidenced in the suction container, or if a hematoma develops beneath the flap, the patient may have to be returned to the operating room for evacuation of the hematoma or ligation of the vessel that is bleeding. In the first 24 hours after surgery the surgical incision should be assessed closely for bleeding and drainage tubes should be checked for patency. If the suction apparatus and drainage tubes are not functioning properly, skin flaps may fail to adhere and necrosis of the neck flap can be a serious problem, especially if it is located in the area of the carotid artery. Because of the excision of regional lymphatic vessels, venous drainage in the neck area must be accomplished by gravity. The head of the bed must be elevated to reduce swelling which, if persistent, can compromise blood flow to the skin flaps. Patients invariably complain of a headache for many days after surgery; this can be explained in part by irritation of the dura mater caused by a slight increase in cerebral pressure due to excision of regional lymphatic vessels and ligation of the internal jugular vein. The head of the bed should be elevated to between 30 and 45 degrees to make it easier for the person to swallow and to promote lymphatic and venous drainage.

Pain Pain is an uncommon problem in the postoperative period, mostly because sensory nerves that commonly transmit the pain are no longer present. If bone has been resected, the person will complain of a dull aching pain. A mild analgesic is usually sufficient to manage the discomfort.

Airway obstruction Airway obstruction is a complication that is usually prevented by a tracheostomy at the time of surgery, especially when a composite resection with radical neck dissection is performed. Tissue swelling, difficulty in clearing secretions from the tracheobronchial tree, and the danger of aspiration of secretions are all indications for a prophylactic tracheostomy. In the first 24 hours after surgery, the patient should be observed closely for any evidence of airway obstruction, especially if a tracheostomy has not been performed. Intrinsic laryngeal edema or hematoma, possibly triggered by increased anxiety or apprehension, can quickly cause airway obstruction. The possibility of airway obstruction should be assessed before the administration of narcotics or sedatives. A mucus plug or blood clot also can cause airway obstruction and requires prompt nursing action. The inner cannula of the tracheostomy tube should be removed and the airway suctioned. If the person is unable to cough out the obstructing agent, the tube may have to be removed by the physician and replaced. Trousseau dilators should be kept at the bedside, as well as another tracheostomy tube, in case the tracheostomy tube should become misplaced, coughed out, or need to be changed. Pulmonary atelectasis and bronchopneumonia are preventable by early ambulation, coughing, and clearing the airway of secretions. Antibiotics are usually administered if an infection is suspected.

Infection Infection of the incision line is an unfortunate occurrence because the person's hospital stay is usually lengthened and morbidity is increased. An infection with potential wound dehiscence is most likely to develop in a suture line in irradiated tissue. Tension on suture lines, either because of the intrinsic pressure of edema or malpositioning of the head, can predispose the suture line to breakdown and infection. An intraoral incision may heal poorly because of a previous intraoral infection since the mouth is not a sterile environment.

After surgery the incision lines should be cleansed thoroughly and gently with hydrogen peroxide and water to remove crusts, and a bactericidal ointment should be applied in a thin layer.

Oral hygiene is very important and should be done four times a day. However, oral hygiene should not be undertaken without knowledge of the location of intraoral sutures. A swab, Water Pik device, or toothbrush should be used carefully to avoid trauma to the incision line.

If a wound infection should occur, a culture is obtained and the appropriate antibiotics are administered. A wound infection commonly occurs in conjunction with the formation of a fistulous tract. A fistula can occur from the oral cavity through to the incision (orocutaneous) or from the pharyngeal area to the incision (pharyngocutaneous). A fistula becomes most obvious after the person begins to take fluids and the incision is noted to have increased drainage. The extent of the fistula may be assessed by a contrast study, such as a cine-esophogram. If a fistula exists, the person is allowed nothing to eat or drink by mouth until the area heals. Most fistulas close spontaneously in 10 to 12 days. Nasogastric or tube feedings are continued until complete healing occurs. If the fistula is large, with major skin flap necrosis, the area may have to be debrided of any nonviable tissue. This can be accomplished by packing the area loosely with wet saline dressings every 4 hours. This helps to debride the area, which may heal spontaneously. If healing does not occur, a surgical debridement with skin grafting or flap rotation may be necessary. If the skin flap breakdown has occurred in the area of the carotid artery, the patient must be observed closely and placed on a regimen of carotid precautions.

Thoracic duct leakage When surgery includes resection of lymphatic vessels in the neck, thoracic duct leakage may occur. The loss of fluid and protein may occur if a chyle leak exists, and the depletion of lymphocytes may be significant. A chyle leak appears as a milky white liquid that is often mixed with serous fluid as it exits the wound-drainage site through tubes in the inferior aspect of the wound. A chyle fistula usually will close spontaneously; if it does not, surgical closure may be necessary. The individual who has a major lymphatic leak following neck surgery requires fluid and protein replacement during convalescence.

Nerve injury During the course of radical neck dissection or other major head and neck surgery, nerves may be sacrificed as part of the surgical resection or they may be inadvertently severed.

Superior laryngeal nerve The superior laryngeal nerve is a branch of the vagus nerve that innervates a small portion of the base of the tongue. Severance of one superior laryngeal nerve produces some interference in the individual's ability to swallow, but the person usually compensates well for this loss over a month's time. Severance of both nerves results in a severe swallowing impairment, and laryngectomy may be necessary.

Vagus Resection of the vagus at a high level in the neck, including the main trunk with the pharyngeal and laryngeal branches, can cause unilateral palatal and pharyngeal paralysis, supraglottic anesthesia, and glottic incompetence due to unilateral vocal cord paralysis. These three conditions in combination can be crippling, and compensatory adaptation requires great concentration.

If the vagus is severed unilaterally and singly, an ipsilateral laryngeal paralysis results, which does not create serious problems unless the cord is paralyzed in the abducted (open) position. This results in a poor, raspy voice, frequent aspirations, and the inability to perform an adequate cough. When aspiration occurs as a result of vocal cord paralysis, a Teflon injection into the paralyzed cord adds bulk to the cord and improves closure during speech, swallowing, and coughing.

Recurrent laryngeal nerve The recurrent laryngeal nerve is included in the discussion of the vagus nerve. Bilateral paralysis, however, requires an immediate tracheostomy because the recurrent laryngeal nerve is responsible for adduction and abduction of the vocal cords.

Phrenic nerve The phrenic nerve, if severed on one side only, results in paralysis of the hemidiaphragm, which becomes a problem only if there are additional respiratory problems.

Hypoglossal nerve The hypoglossal nerve innervates the genioglossus muscle and is responsible for movement of the tongue. If it is severed, unilateral tongue paralysis results; this leads to speech impairment and masticatory difficulties.

Lingual nerve The lingual nerve is sensory, and numbness on the ipsilateral side of the tongue results if it is severed.

Glossopharyngeal nerve The glossopharyngeal nerve innervates the posterior third of the tongue. Damage to it causes difficulty in swallowing and altered taste sensation on the ipsilateral side, but the contralateral side generally compensates for this.

Sacrifice or resection of the superficial sensory nerves of the head and neck results in numbness over skin areas. The overlap of innervation of these nerves is such that sensation usually returns to large areas over time.

Damage to the facial nerve may occur because of the trauma of surgery, especially in the area of the parotid gland, in which case temporary paralysis may be noted. Facial nerve function usually returns to normal within 8 weeks. The mandibular branch of the facial nerve may be sectioned during a radical neck dissection or other major head and neck surgery. This results in paresthesia and drooling on the ipsilateral side.

Spinal accessory nerve The spinal accessory nerve innervates the trapezius muscle, which supports the shoulder and allows lateral abduction of the arm. It is often necessary to resect this nerve as part of the radical neck dissection. The postoperative result in approximately 50% of the cases is a painful shoulder droop with atrophy of the trapezius muscle, and individuals can no longer raise the arm above the shoulder. Once complete healing of tissues has occurred (10 to 12 days after surgery), the individual should begin an exercise program to support the shoulder while developing and strengthening the levator scapulae and the rhomboid muscles of the back (Figures 41-3 to 41-11). In addition, the exercises aid in stretching the trapezius muscle, which, if allowed to contract, causes pain in the neck and shoulder region.

These exercises also may be used for the individual who has had irradiation to the area of the spinal accessory nerve because radiation also can decrease innervation to the trapezius muscle.

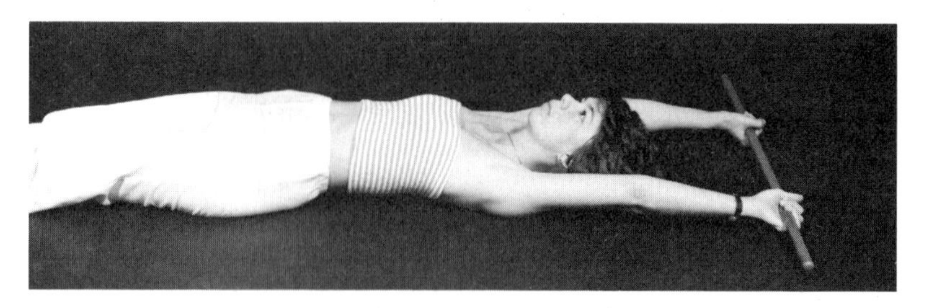

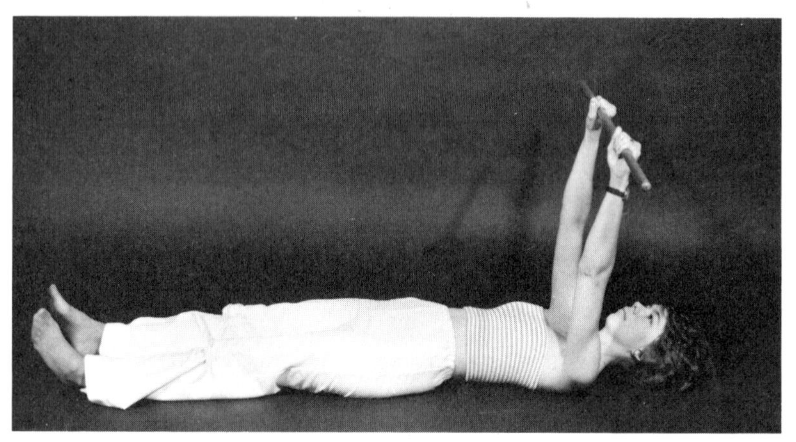

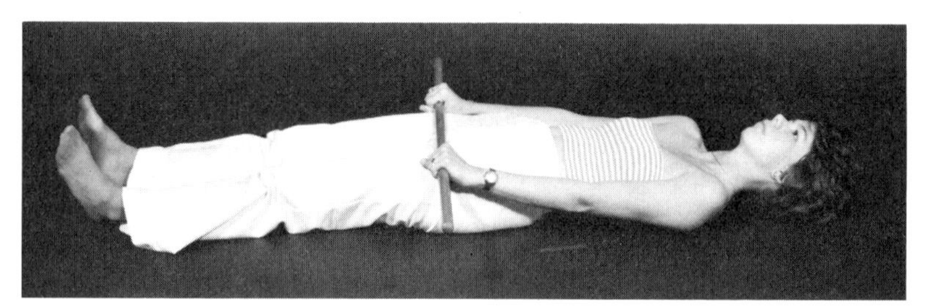

FIGURE 41-3 Shoulder flexion.

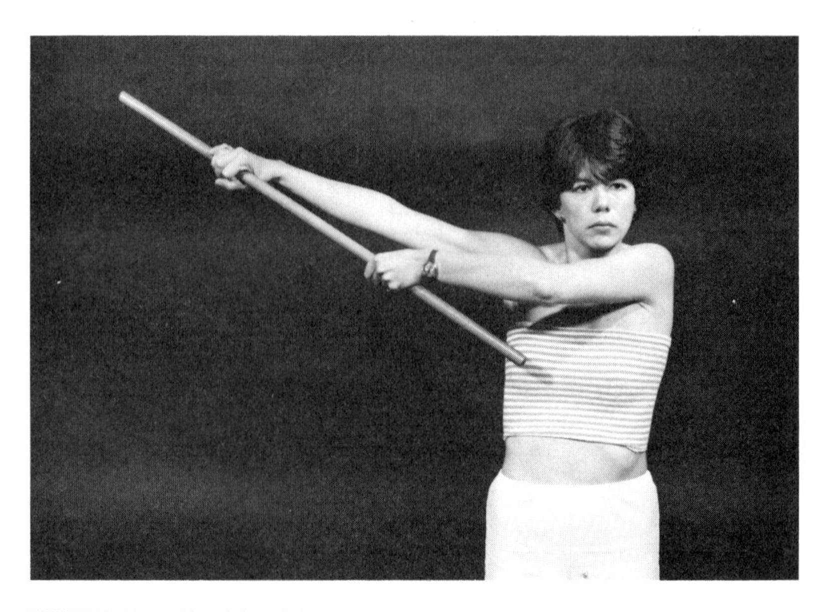

FIGURE 41-4 Shoulder abduction.

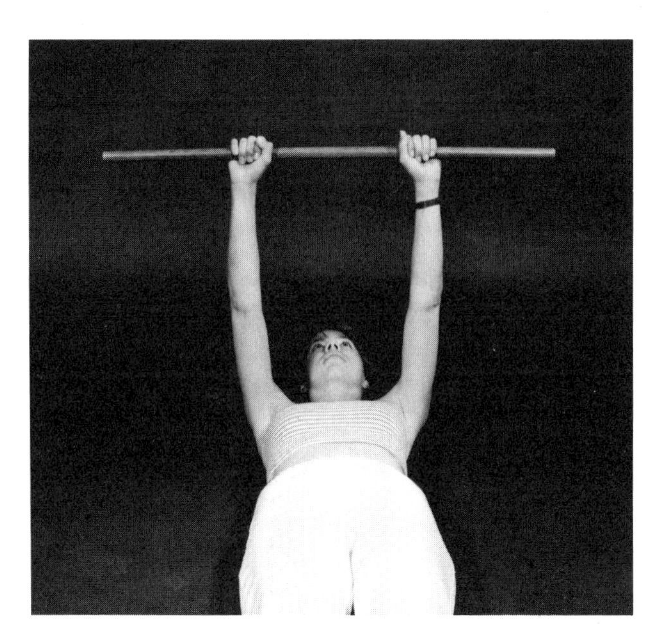

FIGURE 41-5 Shoulder horizontal abduction.

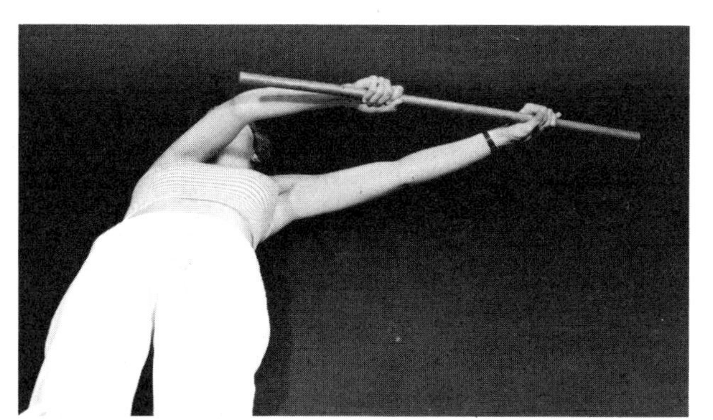

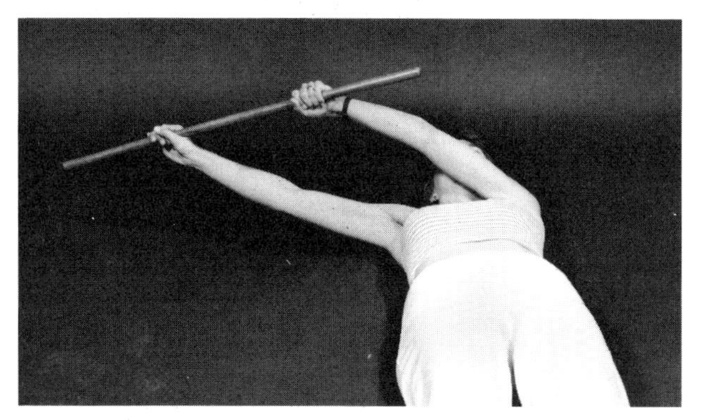

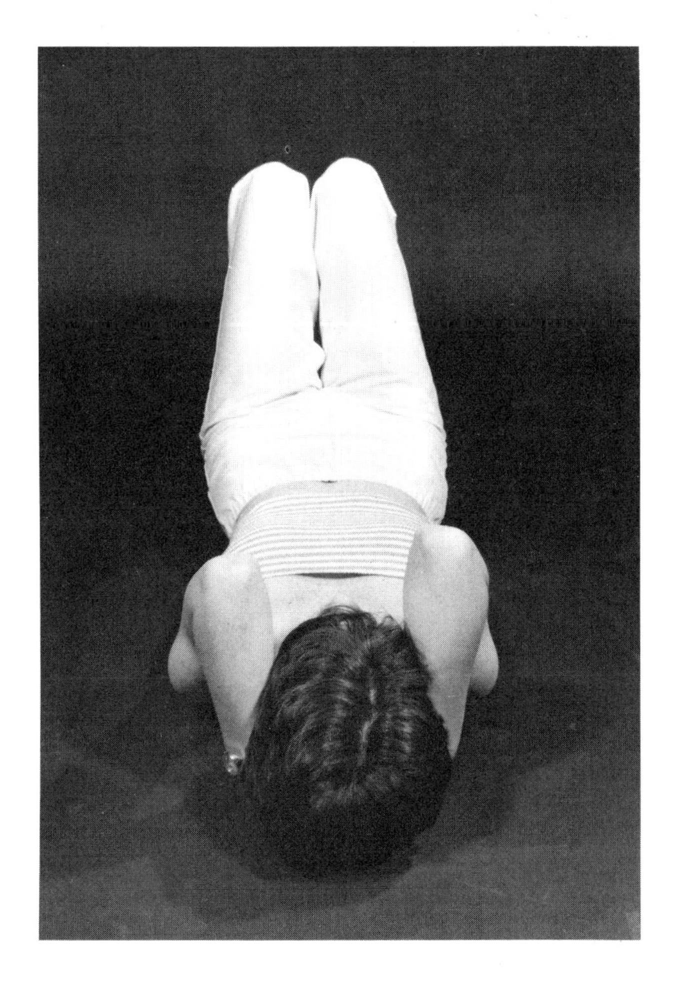

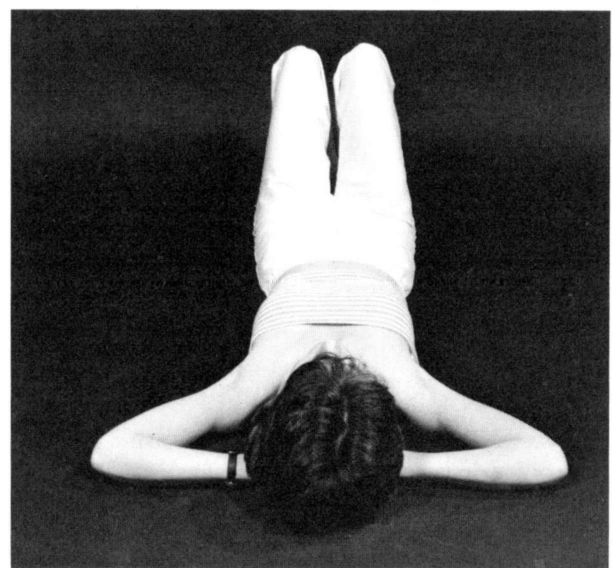

FIGURE 41-6 Shoulder external rotation.

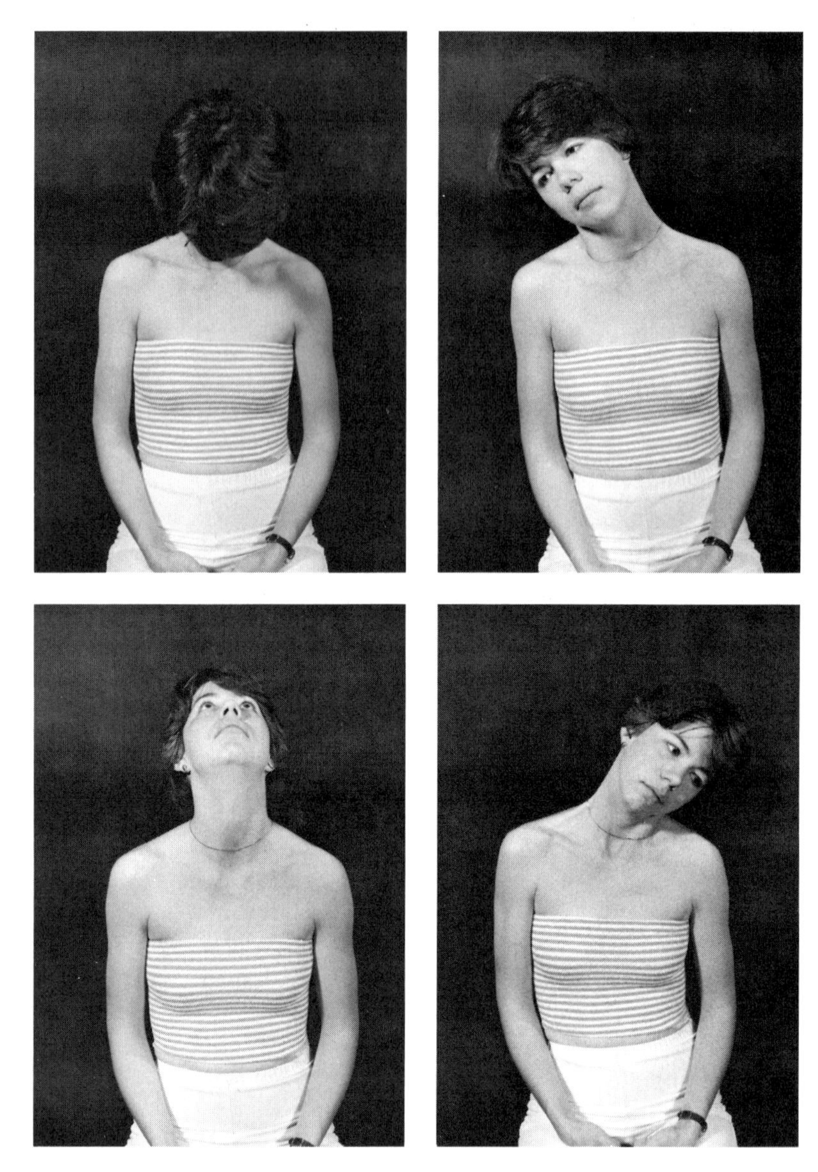

FIGURE 41-7 Neck circles.

Head and neck reconstruction

In no other area of the body is structure and function so intricately related as in the head and neck region. Only a superficial understanding of this interplay is needed to predict the varying array of disabilities that are associated with losses of structural integrity, which may be the consequence of surgical extirpation. These losses create deformities that are readily apparent visually. When the individual attempts to speak, he or she may not be understood. When trying to eat, the individual may drool and have little ability to control the direction of the food. The individual, realizing that others are uncomfortable and/or embarrassed, may withdraw from society.

In the past 30 years, extensive knowledge has been gained regarding the methods of head and neck reconstruction through the use of axial and random-patterned skin flaps and creative prosthetic devices. There is, however, little documentation or mention of the patient's acceptance or personal evaluation of reconstruction. It often is not realistic to expect that after reconstruction an individual will be able to regain his or her preoperative level of function. However, it is essential that the individual be able to achieve an appropriate level of rehabilitation, and this is possible only if the efforts in the areas of head and neck surgery are combined toward this end. That extensive head and neck surgery and reconstruction procedures are carried out in institutions without the coordinated efforts of physicians, prosthodontist, and supportive professionals documents the lack of understanding of the crippling impact of these surgically created defects.

Goals of reconstruction The goal of the surgeon is to maintain or secure adequate function after the surgical

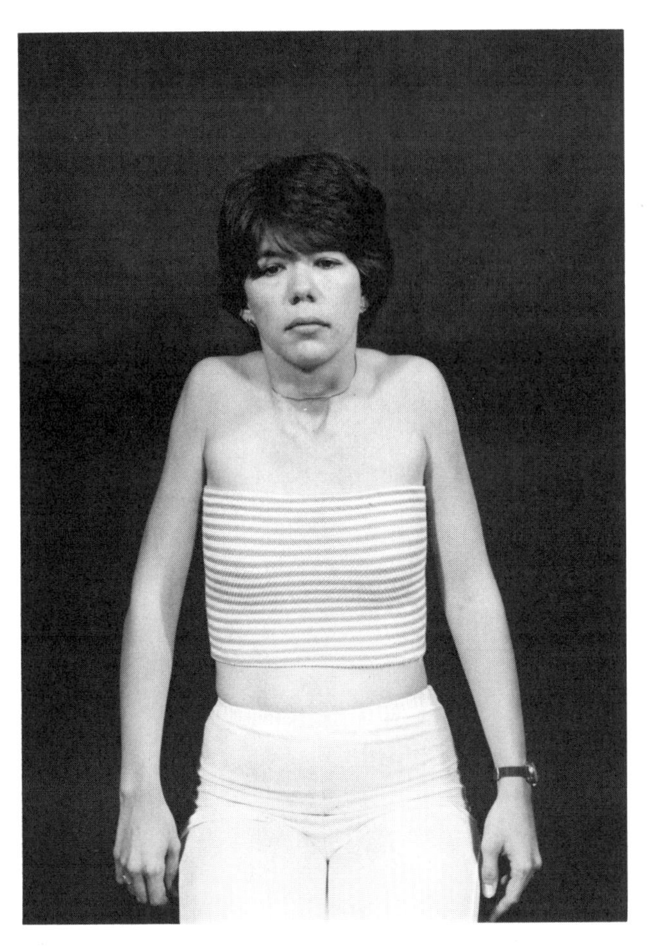

FIGURE 41-8 Levator strengthening.

removal of involved tissues. It is this functional result that is most important to the patient. Most persons can adapt to the physical disfigurement; however, the absence of the internal mechanisms of swallowing, articulation, and oral continence are most debilitating and crippling. That a reconstructive procedure can provide an acceptable cosmetic appearance documents the advances made in the surgical arena. Such accomplishments are recognized by the individual and his or her family only when the individual is able to resume an acceptable degree of function. The priority, then, for the individual and the family is primarily the restoration of functional capabilities and secondarily cosmesis. This fact clearly supports the emphasis on rehabilitation and the trend toward accomplishment of these goals. From a technical point of view, restoration of function is extremely difficult, especially when extensive ablative procedures are carried out. Such procedures often require mobilization of regional skin flaps into the oral cavity that cannot be trained to perform a function for which they were never intended.

Skin flap reconstruction Skin flaps allow for the maintenance of remaining structures and reconstructed parts in a more normal functional position. This prevents the forces of muscle imbalance and wound contracture from shifting areas, which could result in a functionally ineffective oral cavity. Structural support generally is maintained through skeletal support. When this support is lacking, various reconstructive procedures, such as intermaxillary fixation, extraoral appliances, implanted synthetic materials, or bone grafts, may be incorporated into the overall reconstructive plan.

Skin flaps may be used to cover full-thickness surface defects, such as those of the cheek or floor of the nasal cavity. They may be used to protect and cover the carotid

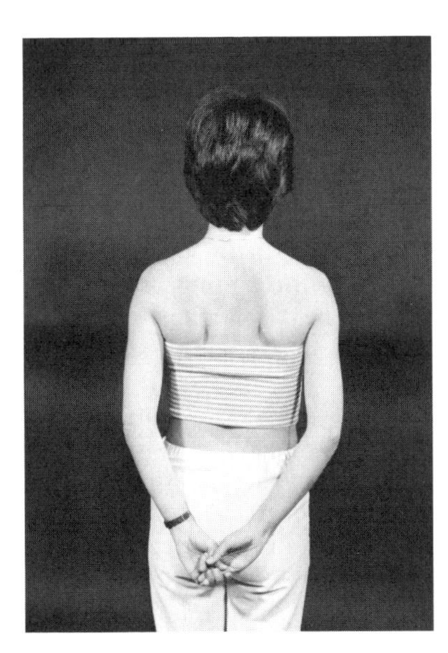

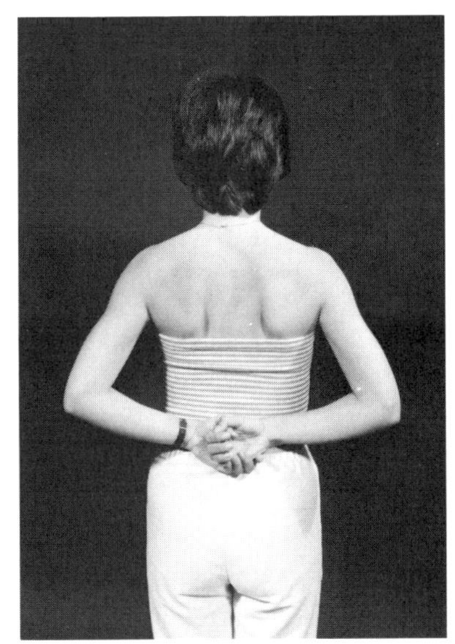

FIGURE 41-9 Shoulder internal rotation.

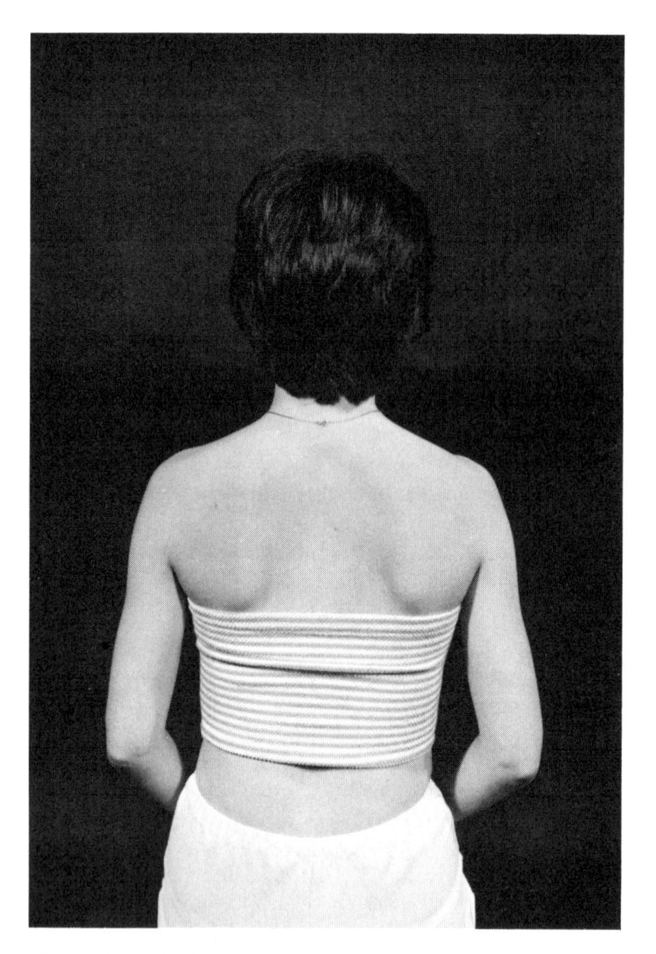

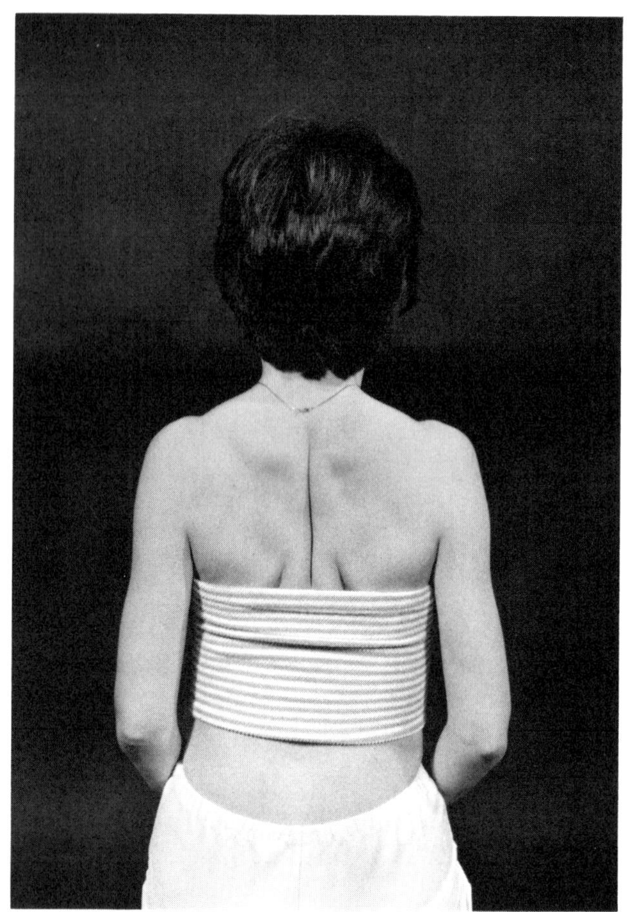

FIGURE 41-10 Rhomboid strengthening.

artery and nerves in the neck region after a radical neck dissection. Another role of the skin flap may be to line the oral mucosa or pharyngeal cavity or to replace the mucoperiosteum overlying the alveolar ridge or hard palate. When used to provide soft tissue stabilization, the flap aids in the prevention of wound contractures, which can significantly reduce functional capabilities. Functional support may be gained by use of a flap to fill in a defect that would otherwise create a gully for the entrapment and stagnation of food particles, a definite hindrance to swallowing. Flaps may be used to provide surface cover and line the oral cavity, as is needed when a full-thickness loss of buccal mucosa exists.

Mobility in the oral cavity is an important end result of head and neck reconstruction. Successful oral function (ie, continence, intelligible speech, efficient chewing, and swallowing) can be accomplished only when sufficient amounts of supple tissue are present to permit effective motion. This is particularly important for the tongue, cheeks, soft palate, and pharyngeal wall. Tissue lining is placed to give support and provide closure without presenting a physical impediment to the passage of food or the flow of saliva.

When tumor excision involves the removal of a significant portion of the structures that support the larynx, provisions must be made for replacement of this support; otherwise, aspiration will occur. At present, muscular function cannot be duplicated, but the provision of a skin flap for an anterior static apparatus allows for adequate laryngeal support.

The disadvantages of skin flap reconstruction are that the skin often undergoes desquamation and, because a skin flap does not produce mucus, the oral cavity may be dry, causing food to stick to the flap. This buildup of crusts results because the flap is not self-cleansing, as is the normal mucosa. A skin flap also lacks sensation, and the individual may complain of a feeling of anesthesia over the area of the flap.

A skin flap includes epidermis, dermis, and subcutaneous tissue. It characteristically maintains its vascular attachment at the base and, when rotated on that base, can be used to line the oral cavity, cover surface defects, and provide soft tissue stabilization. A distinct advantage to the use of regional skin flaps is that the flap has a functioning arterial and venous system that originates at its base. This property allows for the transfer of the flap into an area of compromised blood supply that would be inadequate to nourish a skin graft or provide for wound closure.

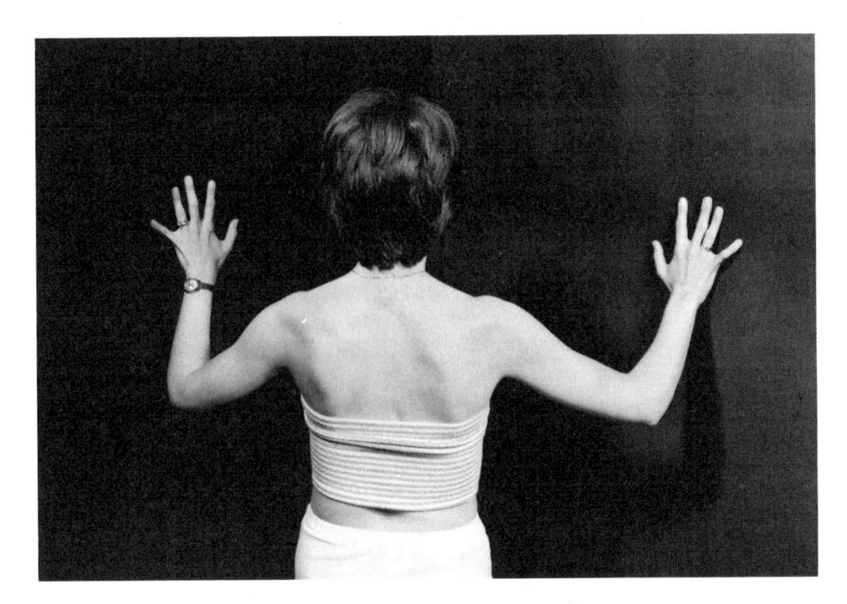

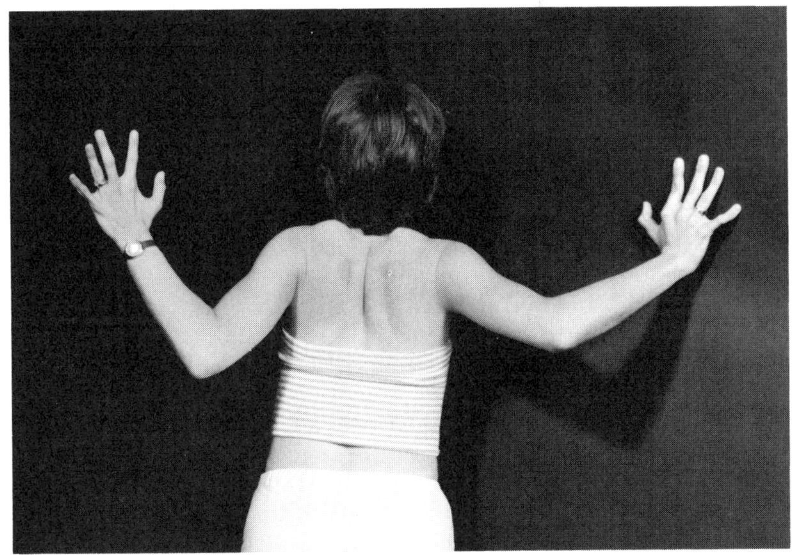

FIGURE 41-11 Pectoralis stretching.

Skin flaps are particularly useful for individuals who have had previous irradiation. Because the flap comes from an area that has not been exposed to the vascular sclerosing effects of radiation, the blood flow is technically uncompromised. The use of such flaps also allows for immediate reconstruction and restoration of physiologic function and cosmetic appearance.

Occasionally there is concern about the vascular supply to the flap or the region to which the flap is being transposed. The vascular supply may be compromised because of previous irradiation to the area or because of generalized disorders, such as diabetes or arteriosclerosis. In these cases the flap is tested and trained by the technique known as "delay." Superficial incisions down to the subcutaneous tissue are made precisely along the lines delineating the flap. Thus the flap is deprived of all vasculature except that at its base, on which it must depend at the time of its rotation. If the flap is viable at the end of the 7- to 10-day period, it is used in reconstruction.

The basic principles of reconstruction and nursing care are applicable regardless of the type of flap reconstruction an individual undergoes.

Mechanisms of flap failure The major factor in skin or myocutaneous flap survival is maintenance of vascular integrity. If the arterial or venous supply is hindered by a variety of mechanisms, all or a portion of a flap may necrose and eventually slough. Once a flap is transferred to its recipient bed, it should survive unless there is tension, kinking, pressure, hematoma, or infection in the flap.

When a flap or skin "paddle" is transposed, it is generally sutured in place with great caution to allow for the edema and swelling that are expected to occur. If edema is too great, however, tension can be placed on the suture line, resulting in a compromised blood supply. Tension also may occur if a flap is stretched too tightly in order to reach a distant wound. A confused or uncooperative patient may create tension at the suture line of the flap. Hyperextension of the neck can also produce tension on the suture line.

Kinking of a flap can be equally deleterious. Consider the individual who has a tubed pedicle. By bending the head to the operative side, the individual can create a crease that will directly affect the blood supply to the distal portion and at the same time prevent venous outflow. The increase in capillary permeability and the occlusion of lymphatic vessels and arterioles result in increased tissue turgor and vascular occlusion.

Pressure on a flap may be from an internal or an external source. An example of an external source would be a forehead flap tunneled beneath the right zygomatic arch. Another example would be the placement of circumferential tracheostomy ties across the base of a deltopectoral flap transposed to the neck. Whenever one of these patients requires a tracheostomy, the tracheostomy tube is generally sutured in place to prevent constricture and pressure from the ties that occlude the blood supply. Internal pressure is closely related to tension and is usually the result of edema due to surgical trauma and the resection of regional lymphatic vessels. For this reason, the individual should be positioned in such a way as to help the gravitational flow of the circulation from the tip to the base of the flap. Generally, the head of the bed is elevated to 45 degrees at all times during the day and night, especially when the deltopectoral flap is used following an extensive surgical procedure. Nighttime presents special problems because individuals have difficulty sleeping with the head of the bed elevated, and frequent repositioning is required throughout the night.

Hematoma formation is generally prevented by the placement of suction catheters superiorly and inferiorly in the wound. Suction catheters promote adherence of the flap to the recipient bed while eliminating dead space, where serosanguineous fluid could potentially accumulate. Rapid adhesion of the flap to the defect is desirable and necessary to achieve as fast a vascular linkup as possible. If drains become plugged or malfunction, or if there is excessive bleeding, vascular linkup is prevented and fluid collects, heralding the possibility of infection.

Infection occurs most often when a flap is placed in the oral cavity. For this reason, an aggressive program of oral hygiene and periodontal care is instituted in the preoperative period. Antibiotics may be given in the preoperative period and continued after surgery.

Because of its decreased blood flow, a recently elevated flap may be capable of supplying or supporting only its basic metabolic need and will not likely be able to provide the blood flow needed to overcome an inflammatory reaction. Assiduous care of the incision will aid in the prevention of infection.

It has been emphasized that flap viability depends closely on adequacy of circulation. A healthy flap is pink or slightly reddened. After blanching, this color reappears gradually. The surface skin is finely wrinkled. Early pallor suggests a lack of capillary filling. If this corrects itself within 24 hours, the flap may be expected to survive. If the whiteness persists, however, the flap will not survive. Early cyanosis occurs because of the presence of poorly oxygenated blood. Spontaneous correction within 24 to 48 hours means that the flap will probably survive. Persistence of this cyanosis usually results in necrosis within 12 days. An edematous flap with immediate color return after blanching suggests venous congestion. The skin is shiny, and blistering may occur. Such flaps fail, at least partially.

Partial flap failure may be recovered simply by careful cleansing and local debridement. Skin grafting occasionally may be performed to cover defects resulting from partial flap necrosis. Full-thickness failure necessitates a second flap, often from the cervical region.

Radiotherapy

When radiation alone is chosen as the primary mode of therapy, doses of 6000 to 7000 rad (cGy) are generally necessary to eradicate disease. Primary radiation therapy permits control of disease while preserving structure and function of the region. Radiation may be delivered by external ports, or external and internal radiation may be combined through the use of interstitial implantation. Radiation may be given preoperatively, postoperatively, or in combination with chemotherapy and/or hyperthermia.

The permanent damage that occurs in the irradiated tissues of the head and neck is a function of the radiobiologic effect. Lymphatic vessels, arteries, and veins are obliterated, which renders the skin and underlying structures virtually unable to withstand the insult of surgery. For the patient who received high-dose radiotherapy and then has a recurrence requiring surgical intervention, regional flaps may have to be rotated to cover the underlying structures and provide closure of the wound at the time of surgery. Wound infections, fistula formation, flap necrosis, and increased morbidity with longer hospitalization are common in the previously irradiated individual. Postoperative morbidity and complications are related to the radiation dosage, which is, in part, the rationale for a combined approach involving both radiation and surgery. Over time, the effects of radiation result in skin fibrosis, radiation caries, osteoradionecrosis, and trismus.[16]

Radiation and surgery

An important aspect of the combined use of radiation and surgery is the type of surgical procedure used. In general, radical resections are performed where indicated, but there is a trend toward more conservative surgical procedures that, when combined with radiation, would possibly yield the same cure rates with less anatomic deformity and physiologic deficit.

Preoperative irradiation Preoperative radiotherapy may be advocated because it is more effective when the circulation is intact. Individuals with large tumors may be more likely to have a recurrence after surgery, because of microextensions of disease that were not removed by surgery. For persons with localized disease, surgery alone may result in dissemination of viable tumor cells at the time of surgery. A further indication for preoperative radiotherapy is the presence of a large lesion that would be technically unresectable because of fixation to underlying structures. Irradiation can render these lesions resectable after partial regression. The preoperative radiation dosage ranges from 3000 to 4000 cGy in 3 to 4 weeks or 5000 cGy in 5 to 6 weeks, depending on the location of the primary tumor. Fractionation also allows for reoxygenation of hypoxic cells by reduction in the tumor bulk and revascularization. Before surgery is performed, the normal tissues are allowed to recover from the sublethal damage from irradiation.

The goal of combination therapy is not use of the maximum dose of radiation with the most extensive surgery to control the disease but, rather, the optimal application of both techniques to achieve higher cure rates with the least morbidity.

Postoperative radiation Arguments for radiotherapy in the postoperative period are that tissues do not heal as well, once irradiated, the extent of disease is known more accurately after surgical exploration, tumor removal and the tumor burden is substantially reduced, making the task of radiation cell kill easier. However, the radiation oncologist is careful to include the incision line and tumor bed in the radiation field. In addition, a planned rather than delayed surgical resection of the tumor can proceed without hindrances commonly associated with radiation fibrosis caused by preoperative radiotherapy.

Combined therapy for locally advanced disease

Randomized clinical trials have been conducted to determine whether adjuvant chemotherapy enhances local control, reduces distant metastasis, or improves survival in individuals with locally advanced head and neck cancer.[17] Neoadjuvant or induction chemotherapy is also useful because tumor responsiveness can be measured, indicating whether the chemotherapy is useful. Because the drugs are capable of shrinking ("medically debulking") the tumor, there is increased vascularization and subsequently increased oxygenation to the tumor. This increased oxygenation enhances the effectiveness of the radiation therapy, which is usually given concurrently. Also, synchronous chemotherapy may select patients who can receive less local therapy.[18] The use of chemotherapy early in the course of the disease would also seem beneficial because most individuals are nutritionally stable and may have small tumor burdens. For the most part, head and neck carcinoma also is difficult to control, once it has recurred locally. This speaks to the need for more definitive primary management.

Methotrexate, bleomycin, cisplatin, carboplatin, and 5-fluorouracil have been used, either singly or in combination, as adjuvant therapy before definitive surgery and/or radiotherapy or as treatment for advanced or recurrent disease. The use of cisplatin and 5-fluorouracil together with radiation results in significant tumor reduction. Chemotherapy produces a 75% response rate, with complete response ranging from 25% to 54%. Individuals who experience a complete response to induction chemotherapy or synchronous chemoradiotherapy have a high probability of local control and cure.[19] Cisplatin and 5-fluorouracil are known radiosensitizers and, when given simultaneously with radiation, are synergistic.[20,21] The radiation may be given twice daily (hyperfractionation) during chemotherapy infusion to maximize drug-radiation exposure time.

In general, previously treated individuals do not tolerate chemotherapy as well as untreated individuals. This is especially true among those who have received radiotherapy, in whom severe mucositis is the major dose-limiting problem. Previous irradiation appears to decrease tumor responsiveness and increase mucosal sensitivity to methotrexate and bleomycin. Furthermore, the nutritional status and general performance status of heavily pretreated patients are such that they are unable to tolerate adequate doses of chemotherapy over any length of time, making tumor control difficult. Too often, the individual who is a candidate for chemotherapy has experienced difficulty in swallowing, pain, and severe weight loss. The person who is malnourished according to weight loss and laboratory indices is more likely to experience dose-limiting toxicities, such as stomatitis, enteritis, and overwhelming infection. This is coupled with the added difficulty of improving the individual's nutritional status during chemotherapy and accounts for the generalized debilitation of these individuals, even in the presence of tumor regression. Aggressive nutritional management is instituted before and coincidental with the chemotherapy.

CARCINOMA OF THE NASAL CAVITY AND PARANASAL SINUSES

EPIDEMIOLOGY AND ETIOLOGY

All age groups may be affected by carcinoma of the nasal cavity and the paranasal cavities, but the highest incidence occurs in men 60 to 70 years of age. The majority of these tumors are of squamous cell origin, but adenocarcinoma is also seen. The incidence of nasal cavity carcinoma has increased among furniture workers and seems to be associated with the presence of wood dust or leather dust. A high rate of occurrence has also been noted among persons exposed to radium, nickel compounds, chromate compounds, hydrocarbons, nitrosamines, and dioxane. Others at risk include snuff users, workers in the shoe industry, and asbestos and textile workers. People who work with mustard gas, isopropyl alcohol, and petroleum are also at risk.

For the majority of individuals with carcinoma of the nasal or paranasal cavities, there is no history of exposure to any of these agents. Most individuals do relate the signs and symptoms of long-standing chronic sinusitis. Other possible signs of disease include a stuffy nose, a history of sinus headache and facial pain, excessive lacrimation, nasal swelling, bleeding, obstruction, discharge, diplopia, and cranial nerve palsies. It may be difficult to determine the primary site of origin of tumors throughout the nasal and paranasal cavities, since several sites are generally included because of the propensity for tumors in this region to remain undetected for prolonged periods.

CLINICAL MANIFESTATIONS

This area of the head and neck region is composed of a pair of nasal cavities that communicate with four pairs of sinus cavities—sphenoid, ethmoid, frontal, and maxillary (Figure 41-12). Nasal obstruction and bleeding occur as the tumor invades through the foramina and breaks into the nasal cavity. Maxillary sinus tumors generally appear as bumps on the hard palate. Swelling of the cheek and pain may be noted. Swelling of the gums may result in ill-fitting dentures and complaints of toothache. Encroachment of the tumor on the infraorbital nerve may cause numbness over the cheek, increased lacrimation, exophthalmos, and diplopia. If the maxillary tumor extends posteriorly into the pterygoid fossa, trismus may occur; this is a grave sign. Thus, in more advanced tumors, displacement of the eye, extraocular muscle palsy, hyperesthesia of the cheek, and inability to open the mouth are common signs.

Tumors of the frontal sinus often involve swelling and frontal pain and mimic a sinus headache. The pain is generally due to tumor invasion of bone and bony destruction. With invasion into the ethmoids and orbit, ocular displacement and double vision may be expected.

Individuals with carcinoma of the sphenoid sinus complain of ill-defined, steady, deep-seated temporoparietal headaches. The sphenoid sinus is in close proximity to the cavernous sinus, and tumor extension to this area can cause compression of the third, fourth, and sixth cranial nerves, resulting in diplopia. Pressure on the optic nerve can result in gradual loss of vision.

Manifestations of tumors arising in the ethmoid sinuses can include medial orbital swelling, puffiness, decreased vision, excessive tearing (epiphora), and olfactory complaints. Lymphatic drainage of these areas is to the retropharyngeal lymph nodes and deep nodes of the internal and anterior jugular chain. Distant metastasis from both nasal cavities and the paranasal sinuses may occur, but death is usually caused by direct extension of the tumor into vital areas of the brain.

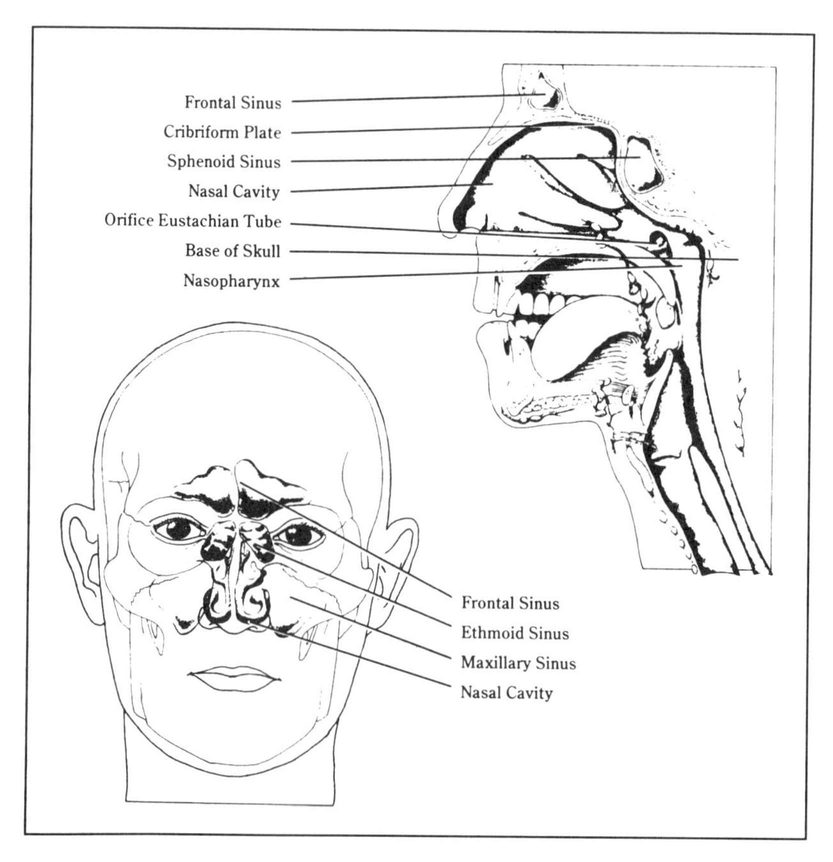

FIGURE 41-12 The nasal cavity and the paranasal sinuses. (Courtesy of Bristol Laboratories.)

ASSESSMENT

Diagnosis is difficult in the early stages of disease because early signs and symptoms are similar to those of common acute and chronic inflammatory diseases of the upper respiratory tract. Physical examination of the area includes evaluation of cranial nerve function and examination of facial contour and symmetry. A nasal speculum is used to examine the interior of the nose. Spraying the interior of the nose with a vasoconstrictor makes it easier to visualize the structures within the nose. Any unusual crusting, ulceration, inflammation, or tumor is noted.

Examination of the paranasal sinuses is not possible through the nose. These areas are studied by radiographic examination. The standard paranasal sinus radiographs offer information regarding both the nasal cavity and the paranasal sinuses. A biopsy of the external nose and nasal cavity is easily performed. Biopsy of the paranasal sinuses is carried out by lateral rhinotomy and the Caldwel-Luc operation.

One of the most important diagnostic findings is the presence or absence of bony destruction. Treatment is based on the stage of the disease and the general medical status of the patient (Table 41-3).

TABLE 41-3 TNM Classification System for Carcinoma of the Nasal and Paranasal Sinuses

Primary Tumor (T)

T0	No evidence of primary tumor
T1	Tumor confined to the antral mucosa of infrastructure with no bone erosion or bone destruction
T2	Tumor confined to the antral mucosa of infrastructure with no bone erosion or bone destruction
T3	Tumor with erosion or destruction of the infrastructure including the hard palate and/or the middle nasal meatus
T4	Massive tumor with invasion of cribriform plate, posterior ethmoids, sphenoid sinus, nasopharynx, pterygoid plates, or base of the skull

Source: American Joint Committee for Cancer Staging and End Results Reporting: 1988. Manual for Staging of Cancer. Philadelphia, JB Lippincott, 1988.

TREATMENT

The complex anatomy of this area, its close approximation to vital structures, and the usually advanced stage of the disease when the individual is first seen often result in failure to cure the patient. Because of the relative deformity that occurs as a result of surgical intervention, radiotherapy has been the treatment of choice, especially for stage I and stage II disease. Interstitial implants of radioactive material directly into tumors can be used to deliver higher doses of radiation to small tissue volumes. Additional doses of 2,000 to 4,000 cGy may be given through implants.[22] However, radiation results in severe morbidity, deformity, and dysfunction because of the high doses that are necessary for local control. The amount of radiation that can be safely given is limited by the radiobiologic effect of radiation to underlying bone. Implant needles may be used to deliver heat (hyperthermia) to the tumor before irradiation, which potentiates radiation and permits the use of lower-dose radiation with fewer complications.[23] Radiation salvage of patients in whom primary radiation therapy has failed is not encouraging and is associated with a significant degree of soft tissue necrosis. Likewise, the survival rates for persons with advanced disease treated with high-dose radiation are unsatisfactory (10% to 30%) and are associated with significant morbidity.

The feasibility of more radical surgical procedures with a curative intent has been influenced by the availability of superior prosthodontic techniques to restore the continuity of the oral cavity and to restore the facial contour with orbital and facial prostheses. Success cannot be complete without functional and cosmetic restoration.

It is difficult to obtain satisfactory repair of defects created in this area. The use of skin grafts and flaps can result in excessive tissue bulk and continuous downward displacement of tissue. Skin grafts are subject to crusting and require frequent lavaging. When the resection involves a part of the maxillary ridge or soft tissue without communication between the oral cavity and the nasal cavity, the disability is minimal and the prosthetic prognosis is excellent. The prosthetic design is modified to accommodate the altered anatomy and provide recontouring of the remaining soft tissues. If, however, the resection creates a communication between the oral cavity and the nasal cavity, sinuses, or nasopharynx, the disability can be severe. Speech is greatly impaired and unintelligible if the defect is not restored prosthetically. Oral competence is greatly compromised because nasal secretions drain into the oral cavity, often creating a fluid problem and an objectionable taste and odor. The individual also cannot drink liquids without their escaping through the nose. This can result in embarrassment and nutritional problems. In addition, food often will become trapped in the nasal cavity, predisposing the individual to infection.

Before surgical intervention, the prosthodontist often takes an impression of the hard and soft palate to create an obturator that will most accurately approximate the individual's normal contour. Restoration of any maxillary defect is greatly enhanced by the presence of natural teeth, which provide support and better stability of the prosthesis. After the surgical resection of the tumor, a skin graft is usually placed against the superior and lateral aspects of the wound to provide mucosal reconstruction. A surgical pack soaked in balsam of Peru or petroleum jelly is then placed to provide adherence of the graft and to occlude the defect. The patient's comfort is greatly enhanced if an obturator is placed at the time of surgery. The obturator helps to protect the wound from irritation and debris and also acts as a stent against which the postoperative tissue can heal and contour without contracture. The nasogastric tube can be removed earlier if a prosthesis is placed because the individual can eat without fear of damaging the surgical site or of getting fluid or liquid into the nasal area. The individual's morale is usually much better than it would be without the obturator.

Approximately 5 days is needed for the wound to heal and the skin grafts to adhere, after which the packing is changed. Once the obturator is removed, the pack generally is separated easily from within the defect. An interim obturator may then be placed to function as a hard palate. Minor adjustments in the prosthesis are generally necessary to maintain an adequate prosthesis-defect relationship during the postoperative period. Mucosal drying and atrophic changes will occur in the maxillectomy cavity as a result of surgical intervention. The protective-cleansing mechanism of mucociliary action is severely retarded and results in excessive crusting and drying. The skin grafts contribute to crusting, and superficial infection must be prevented. Problems of drying, crusting, and superficial infection are increased if the individual has had prior irradiation.

The patient is instructed about meticulous wound care before discharge from the hospital. The obturator can be difficult to remove because of its size, but with patience and encouragement, the individual will gain skill in removing and replacing it. An oral irrigating device that has a forceful jetting action is ideal for irrigation of these defects. The individual may complain that the jet stream causes piercing pain, which is a deterrent to meticulous oral hygiene. This problem is easily resolved by simply having the prosthodontist cut off the tip, thus increasing the caliber of the adapter and creating a larger outlet for fluid without decreasing the efficacy of the irrigation.

The most physiologically compatible irrigation solution has an alkaline base that increases ciliary action and prevents drying. An oxidizing agent may be used to free crusts and promote a clean wound. A solution of saline and baking soda provides adequate cleansing, does not burn (as does hydrogen peroxide), and is inexpensive. The individual should irrigate after each meal and at bedtime. To help minimize drying and irritation to the maxillary defect, the individual can irrigate the defect with a saline and viscous Xylocaine solution. After irrigation, the patient can instill a solution containing the following:

- 5 mL of mineral oil
- 2 drops of camphor
- 2 drops of eucalyptol
- 2 drops of menthol

This solution can be instilled with cotton-tipped applicators. A small portion also may be spread over the surface of the obturator, provided an adhesive is not needed. The individual who is receiving chemotherapy, radiotherapy, or both should be particularly aware of any mucositis and report this to both the oncologist and the prosthodontist.

The patient should not remove the obturator for prolonged periods, because atrophic changes may occur. A permanent obturator is usually constructed 6 months after the initial surgery to allow time for complete healing and consolidation of scar tissue.

Hyposomia and vocal changes should be expected as a result of extensive maxillectomy. Alteration in facial contour is minimal after partial or total maxillectomy because the incision along the nose is generally shaded and fades over time. However, when the tumor has extended through the roof of the antrum, the orbital contents must be resected with the maxilla. Maxillectomy with orbital exenteration may be performed if there is local recurrence of disease after partial maxillectomy or when disease is extensive. Such procedures are justified when one considers the natural history of this disease. It progresses slowly, it generally remains localized, and destructive invasion results in severe pain and inanition because of obstruction of the oropharynx. Erosion of major vessels and extension to the skull are predictable in uncontrolled disease. The future of the individual with uncontrolled local disease is bleak, and aggressive primary management is needed in an attempt to prevent recurrence and persistence of disease.

A maxillectomy with orbital exenteration may or may not include the skin of the cheek. A skin flap is generally used to close the wound and cover underlying structures. If skin should be included in the surgical specimen, the regional skin flaps are necessary to provide coverage and reconstruct the area. A deltopectoral, cervical, forehead, or scalp flap may be used to reconstruct the cheek after orbital exenteration. Skin grafts and packing are necessary for wound healing. An obturator may be placed at the time of surgery or after the packing is removed. General nursing management primarily includes preservation of the vascular integrity of the skin flaps and instructions on removal of the obturator and wound irrigation. If the orbit has been removed and the cheek is intact, the individual may choose to wear a patch or be fitted with an external orbit prosthesis, which is cosmetically acceptable, especially when worn with glasses.

CARCINOMA OF THE NASOPHARYNX

EPIDEMIOLOGY AND ETIOLOGY

The incidence of nasopharyngeal carcinoma is low (0.6 per 100,000 individuals). The incidence is higher in males, with a male/female ratio of 3:1. Nasopharyngeal carcinomas are largely of squamous cell origin and frequently are poorly differentiated or undifferentiated. Lymphoepithelioma, the predominant malignant nasopharyngeal tumor, occurs with unusually high frequency in southern Chinese and has been shown to have a close association with Epstein-Barr virus independent of geography.[24,25] The most probable factors accounting for the increased incidence of nasopharyngeal carcinoma among southern Chinese are the eating of salted fish and a deficiency of vitamin C in the diet early in life. Air pollutants also have been implicated.[24]

CLINICAL MANIFESTATIONS

Carcinoma of the nasopharynx is silent in the early stages. This is why most tumors in this area are discovered late and only after they have reached considerable size. In approximately 80% of the individuals with nasopharyngeal carcinoma, unilateral lymph node metastasis, usually to the cervical chain, is the initial presenting symptom. Metastasis occurs most often to the cervical triangle, the entire jugular chain, and the supraclavicular nodes. Extension is generally to the homolateral side, but contralateral metastasis is common because of the abundant interconnecting network of lymphatic vessels in the nasopharynx.

Symptoms of nasopharygeal carcinoma may include hearing impairment and tinnitus secondary to obstruction of the eustachian tube and persistent otitis media. Poorly localized headache in the frontal, temporal, or parietal region and facial pain are late symptoms caused by bony erosion and pressure on the fifth cranial nerve. Cranial nerve compression provides important diagnostic information (Table 41-4). Invasion through the base of the skull results in cranial nerve involvement.

Double vision occurs when the third, fourth, and sixth cranial nerves are involved. The presence of Horner's syndrome represents tumor invasion of the sympathetic nerve fibers accompanying the carotid artery as it passes intracranially. When sufficiently large, the tumor causes unilateral or bilateral nasal obstruction. Epistaxis may occur with necrosis of the tumor and vessel walls. A malignant tumor of the nasopharynx is one of the few tumors of the head and neck region that frequently metastasize widely. It spreads through the bloodstream to the lungs, liver, and bone (spine, pelvis, and femur).

TABLE 41-4 Symptoms of Cranial Nerve Compression from Nasopharyngeal Carcinoma

Nerve	Symptoms
Olfactory (I)	Seldom occurs; difficult to assess unilateral deficiency to olfaction
Optic (II)	Complete unilateral blindness
Oculomotor (III)	Paralysis of the upper, lower, and inner rectus muscle of the eye; complete fixation of the eye except for its lateral movement
Trochlear (IV)	Paralysis of the superior oblique muscles of the eye
Trigeminal (V)	Neurologic pain of the supraorbital and superior maxillary regions; painful anesthesia of half of the tongue, floor of the mouth, and buccal mucosa; compression of the mandibular branch results in paralysis of the temporal, internal pterygoid, and masseter muscles; lack of corneal reflex
Abducens (VI)	Paralysis of the external rectus muscle of the eye and diplopia
Facial (VII)	Peripheral facial paralysis; seldom occurs
Acoustic (VIII)	Loss of hearing and vertigo; seldom occurs
Glossopharyngeal (IX)	Difficulty swallowing, partial loss of taste, hoarseness, hemi-anesthesia of the soft palate
Vagus (X)	Anesthesia of the soft palate, pharynx, and larynx; tachycardia and tachypnea
Spinal accessory (XI)	Paralysis and atrophy of the trapezius and sternocleidomastoid muscles; hemiparesis of the soft palate and larynx
Hypoglossal (XII)	Rapid atrophy of the affected side of the tongue, which, when protracted, deviates toward the affected side
Cervical sympathetic nerve	Constriction of the pupil, retraction of the eye into the orbit, and narrowing of the palpebral fissure (Horner's syndrome)

ASSESSMENT

Diagnosis of nasopharyngeal carcinoma is made by careful examination and radiographic study of the area. The nasopharynx can be visualized with a head mirror, tongue depressor, and small mirror. A rubber catheter may be used to manually elevate the soft palate for easier viewing. A nasopharyngeal forceps is used to obtain a biopsy specimen. Radiographs and tomograms of the sinuses and base of the skull are often taken to depict bony destruction and extent of disease. The TNM classification system for nasopharyngeal carcinoma is presented in Table 41-5.

TREATMENT

Because of the anatomic location of the nasopharynx and its proximity to the base of the skull, it is virtually inaccessible to the surgeon, and radiotherapy is the primary treatment of choice.

Radiotherapy is designed to include all of the nasopharynx, the retropharyngeal nodes, and all lymph nodes on both sides of the neck. The usual dosage is 6000 to 7000 cGy delivered through lateral opposing fields over a 6- to 9-week period. Special care is taken to avoid exposing the spinal cord and medulla oblongata to doses of more than 5000 cGy. Radioactive implants may be used to augment the dosage. Most tumors of this area are relatively radiosensitive, and survival rates are good (25%), considering the advanced stages of the disease. Favorable results and better prognosis depend on diagnosis and treatment of the tumor at an earlier stage.

The individual with advanced disease often has severe pain and headaches as a result of bony invasion and erosion. Pain management is of the utmost importance. The individual often suffers from multiple cranial nerve palsies, visual problems, and sensory losses. Anorexia, severe weight loss, respiratory problems (secondary to vagal nerve paralysis), and laryngopharyngeal edema also occur. The individual often requires a tracheostomy and gastrostomy or esophagostomy as the disease progresses.

TABLE 41-5 TNM Classification System for Nasopharyngeal Carcinoma

Primary Tumor (T)	
TIS	Carcinoma in situ
T1	Tumor confined to one side of the nasopharynx or one subsite
T2	Tumor invades more than one subsite of nasopharynx
T3	Tumor invades nasal cavity and/or oropharynx
T4	Tumor invasion of the skull and/or cranial nerves

Source: American Joint Committee for Cancer Staging and End Results Reporting: Manual for Staging of Cancer. Philadelphia, JB Lippincott, 1988.

CARCINOMA OF THE ORAL CAVITY

EPIDEMIOLOGY AND ETIOLOGY

Age is a significant risk factor in oral cancer. The majority of oral cancers (75%) occur in persons over 60 years of age, and they occur twice as often in males as in females.

Malignant disease of the oral cavity has been associated with a number of etiologic agents, such as tobacco and alcohol use, riboflavin deficiencies, and trauma. Smokeless tobacco (chewing tobacco) has become popular recently and is associated with an increased risk of oral carcinoma.[26] In previous years an increased incidence of oral cancer, specifically carcinoma of the tongue, has been noted in persons with syphilis. It is not known whether this chronic infection leads to malignant changes in the mouth or whether persons exposed to spirochetal infections are also, because of socioeconomic factors, more susceptible to cancer of the oral cavity.[27] Persons who work with wool dust in the manufacture of textiles also have been known to have an increased incidence of oral cancer.

Two other infections are associated with oral cancer. Infection with *Candida albicans* often results in proliferative stomatitis and local epithelial hyperplasia and occurs with increased frequency in persons with leukoplakia. Herpes simplex virus (type 1) infection is also noted in the presence of leukoplakia.

Alcohol and tobacco have been noted to be cocarcinogens in head and neck cancer, especially oral carcinoma. Alcohol is thought to facilitate local absorption of carcinogens that pool in and are flushed through the mouth. The association of cirrhosis of the liver and cancer of the mouth is significant in that persons with both cirrhosis and cancer of the oral cavity have a much poorer survival rate than persons without cirrhosis.[28]

Long-standing malnutrition and anemia are related to mucosal changes and leukoplakia, which are often considered to be premalignant. Leukoplakia is associated with malignant change in up to 20% of the persons affected. The highest incidence occurs in persons with cancer of the buccal mucosa, mandibular mucosa, and mandibular sulcus. Poor oral hygiene, ill-fitting dentures, and trauma to mucous membranes have all been implicated in the etiology of oral carcinoma. The exact mechanisms are not known.

PATHOPHYSIOLOGY

Approximately 97% of the cancers that arise in the oral cavity are of squamous cell origin. Regardless of their origin, these cancers behave in a predictable manner, in that they tend to spread superficially to adjacent mucous membranes and thus commonly extend to neighboring structures (Figure 41-13).

Because of their tendency to extend deep into underlying structures, these cancers are often larger than they appear on the surface. Like other tumors in the head and neck region, cancers of the oral cavity metastasize to regional cervical nodes in a predictable manner. Lesions that approach the midline are likely to produce bilateral lymph node enlargement.

Of significance is the fact that more than 80% of the individuals with oral cancer who die of their disease die of uncontrolled local disease rather than distant metastasis. Metastasis below the clavicle does occur but generally late in the course of the disease.

When detected at an early stage, these cancers are highly curable. However, the majority of oral cancers are well advanced at the time of their diagnosis. An enlarged lymph node may be the first sign of a tumor in the oral cavity, and this indicates extensive disease. With the exception of skin cancer, probably no cancer is more easily detectable or accessible than cancers of the oral cavity. Dentists play a major role in the detection of early oral cancers, a factor that could significantly affect prognosis.

CLINICAL MANIFESTATIONS

The majority of oral cancers cause no symptoms in their early stages. An observant individual may note a white spot or sore, which is commonly attributed to dentures. Pain is seldom an early symptom. The most common complaint is that of a painless mass that has persisted for a prolonged period. Other complaints include persistent ulcerations, difficulty with dentures, and blood-tinged sputum. A complaint of difficulty in swallowing or in speech indicates more extensive disease.

ASSESSMENT

Adequate physical examination of the oral cavity requires good lighting, a tongue blade, and a finger cot to facilitate

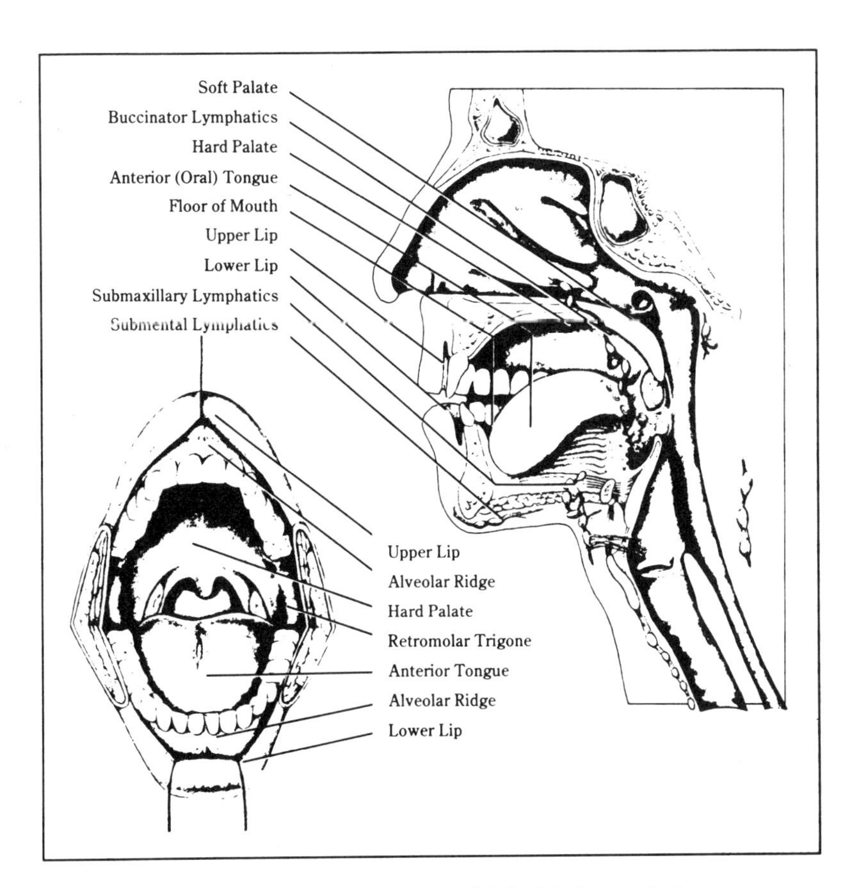

FIGURE 41-13 The oral cavity. (Courtesy of Bristol Laboratories.)

adequate bimanual palpation, which is an integral part of oral examination. Fissures, ulcers, or areas of induration in patches of leukoplakia may indicate malignant changes. However, erythroplasia or well-defined red patches with velvety consistency among tiny areas of ulceration are frequently the earliest evidence of malignant mucosal changes. Any ulcers, masses, or areas of pigmentation are considered suspicious.

Toluidine blue is a basic metachromatic dye which stains the nuclear material of malignant lesions. Topical application of the dye to suspicious lesions may indicate an area that has been missed by the clinician's subjective evaluation.[29] Biopsy specimens should be obtained from any areas of redness or inflammation that persist for longer than 2 weeks.

The neck is examined carefully for any cervical lymphadenopathy because an enlarged node may be the first indication of oral carcinoma.

Neurologic examination is also important. (For example, posterior tongue lesions may be suspected when there is hypoglossal nerve paralysis.) Numbness over the chin may indicate tumor invasion of the inferior alveolar ridge and compression of the mandibular nerve.

Because most lesions of the oral cavity are easily accessible, a simple biopsy can establish the diagnosis. When tumor is found adjacent to bone, such radiographs as a Panorex film of the mandible may be necessary for definition of the extent of the tumor and for proper staging (Table 41-6).

TABLE 41-6 TNM Classification System for Carcinoma of the Oral Cavity

Primary Tumor (T)	
TIS	Carcinoma in situ
T1	Primary tumor 2 cm or less in greatest diameter
T2	Primary tumor more than 2 cm but not more than 4 cm in greatest diameter
T3	Primary tumor more than 4 cm in greatest diameter
T4	Massive tumor more than 4 cm in diameter with deep invasion to the antrum, pterygoid muscles, maxillary sinus, base of the tongue, or skin of the neck

Source: American Joint Committee for Cancer Staging and End Results Reporting: Manual for Staging of Cancer. Philadelphia, JB Lippincott, 1988.

TREATMENT

The primary treatments for carcinoma of the oral cavity include radiotherapy and surgery. At present, it seems that in most cases either treatment may be equally successful in eradicating disease, particularly stage I and stage II disease. Combined therapy is also used and may include radiotherapy and chemotherapy before or after surgery. The treatment employed depends on the extent of the disease, the location of the primary tumor, the presence or absence of metastatic disease, the general health of the individual, and the personal preference of the physician and the patient.

In the past, surgery was often reserved for postradiation recurrences. This treatment plan has proven less than optimal because of poor healing and long-term morbidity associated with high-dose radiotherapy. In some cases (eg, small carcinomas of the tongue and leukoplakia) surgery, including CO_2 laser excision,[28] is curative and is found to be superior to radiation because it is more expedient. In cancers involving or adjacent to bone, surgery is often preferred because of the risk of radiation-induced mandibular necrosis. The deformity associated with resection of bone is a factor, however, and the individual may choose radiotherapy. The avoidance of severe physiologic, psychologic, and cosmetic defects with surgical procedures provides further impetus in the direction of radiotherapy. It should be noted, however, that approximately 50% of any part or organ in this complex anatomic area can be resected without serious functional disability. This is particulary important when one considers resection of the oral tongue.

The choice of initial therapy is critical in cancer of the oral cavity because the first therapeutic attempt is often decisive for cure. Treatment of recurrent disease, regardless of intial therapy, is associated with a high degree of failure. The difficulty inherent in the diagnosis of a recurrence and the biologic behavior of these tumors are important factors in early detection of a recurrence. At present, there is no way of determining biologic aggressiveness of a tumor at the initial diagnosis. Cancers of the tongue in individuals under 30 years of age tend to be more aggressive than cancers of the oral cavity in older persons. This suggests that more aggressive primary therapy may be indicated in this population.

Because each carcinoma that originates from the various sites of the oral cavity has distinct clinical features, course, and prognosis, the therapeutic approach is individualized. Each anatomic site in the oral cavity is discussed briefly, with emphasis on carcinoma of the tongue because this is the area most commonly involved.

Buccal Mucosa

The buccal mucosa forms the mucosal lining of the cheek and extends from the upper to the lower gingivobuccal gutters. Most neoplasms are encountered at the commissure of the mouth, along the occlusal plane of the teeth or at the retromolar area. Cancers in this region are common in geographic areas where people use snuff or chew tobacco.[27] Lesions related to cigars, pipes, and smokeless tobacco appear to develop in this region in response to direct contact with the oral mucosa.[29] Exophytic carcinoma is found most commonly and appears as a soft white outgrowth in an area of leukoplakia. These tumors may invade deep into the cheek and adjacent bone. Extension to the pharyngomaxillary fossa may occur in lesions that are situated posteriorly. Invasion of the anterior pillars of the soft palate, alveolar ridge, or pterygoid fossa is a grave sign.

Buccal carcinomas are usually insidious in their clinical behavior. Trismus produced by neoplastic infiltration of the masseter muscle or submaxillary lymphadenopathy may be the first clinical evidence of disease. Pain may be intense if the tumor is ulcerative.

For early T1 and T2 lesions, radiotherapy has resulted in a 50% 3-year recurrence-free rate of survival. A combination of external radiation and interstitial implants has been advocated.[30] Small lesions may be excised and covered with a skin graft of adjacent mucosa. Surgical resection with excision of the cheek may be indicated in lesions involving skin. Reconstruction often includes the use of the deltopectoral flap rotated in a tube fashion or rotation of the superiorly based cervical flap. After resection of a portion of the cheek and cheek muscles, individuals often have difficulty positioning food and controlling liquids for swallowing, and oral competence may be a problem initially. The loss of muscle will result in the inability of the cheek to stretch and store food. Jaw expansion also may be difficult.

Gingival Ridge (Gums)

Carcinoma of the gums generally occurs in the premolar and molar regions, with the lower jaw affected more often than the upper jaw. The clinical diagnosis may be difficult because of the similarity of signs and symptoms to those of benign inflammatory lesions, which are common in this area. Alveolar ridge carcinomas occur most often in edentulous areas. Interference with mastication or the fitting of a denture may be the first clinical sign. Leukoplakia also may be present. Invasion of underlying bone occurs early in the disease in approximately 50% of the cases and may account for the often observed loosening of teeth in the area.

Treatment depends on extent of the lesion, degree of bone involvement, and status of cervical lymph node involvement. When bone is involved, a partial mandibulectomy with radical neck dissection is often indicated.[30] Metastatic spread to regional lymphatic vessels is common with more advanced lesions, and radiotherapy is often given after resection to reduce the incidence of local recurrence of disease.

The alveolar ridge, particularly the lower ridge, is a common site for extension of carcinoma from the floor of the mouth and the tongue. Significant bone invasion can occur with tumor spread via the perineural lymphatic vessels of the inferior alveolar nerve. It is often necessary to resect a segment of the mandible, thus interrupting mandibular continuity. The disabilities incumbent in resection of a portion of the mandible depend on which part is resected and the extent of resection. Figures 41-14 to 41-17 illustrate the various types of mandibular resection that may be performed. Each type presents different functional problems and rehabilitation potentials.

Early efforts at mandibular reconstruction relied heavily on the use of stabilizing pins or autogenous bone grafts. Advances in technology have made possible the use of autogenous cancellous bone chips, homograft bone, complex prosthetic devices, and heterograft bone.

The use of autogenous bone grafts in mandibular reconstruction is based on the idea that these grafts contain viable marrow elements that provide a matrix to support revascularization with subsequent graft absorption and replacement with new bone. Bone grafts are usually constructed from ribs or ilium. The curvature of the ilium has been found to conform to the shape of the mandible and can be used to replace the angle of the mandible. Rib grafts have been found to be less stable and to fracture easily after trauma. Bone grafting has its drawbacks, in that failure may occur because of infection, nonunion, absorption, or sequestration.

Artificial implants may also be used to reconstruct the mandible. The material must be inert, durable, and well tolerated by the tissues. Vitallium and tantalum are two metals that have been used successfully. Unexplained pain or acute inflammation has been noted with these prostheses, necessitating removal in selected cases.

Kirschner wires and Steinmann pins have been used as temporary means of stabilizing the remaining mandibular segment and permit a more rapid return to normal function. The stabilizing device can be removed later and replaced by a permanent prosthesis. This method allows for healing and closure of the oral wound and ensures healing and viability of the lining flaps. Further dissection is minimal, and there is less threat of infection or hematoma and a greater likelihood of graft survival. The results of successful mandibular reconstruction are outstanding, both functionally and esthetically.

Not everyone who has a portion of the mandible resected requires reconstruction. When a minimal portion of the horizontal ramus is resected, excellent function and only minimal deformity are seen, and the individual may refuse reconstruction simply because he or she does not believe it is necessary.

The traumatic or surgical loss of a mandibular segment can potentially affect the total rehabilitation of an individual. Most important is the altered physiologic state of the oral cavity. This often involves the basic functions of mastication, deglutition, and phonation. Inadequate support of the oral cavity can result in aspiration. This disruption in mandibular continuity can result in facial disfigurement if a major portion is removed.

The following is a brief description of the types of mandibular resections and functional problems an individual may encounter.

Marginal mandibulectomy

Marginal mandibulectomy (Figure 41-14) is commonly performed when tumors are in continuity with the floor of the mouth. Rehabilitation is excellent because the con-

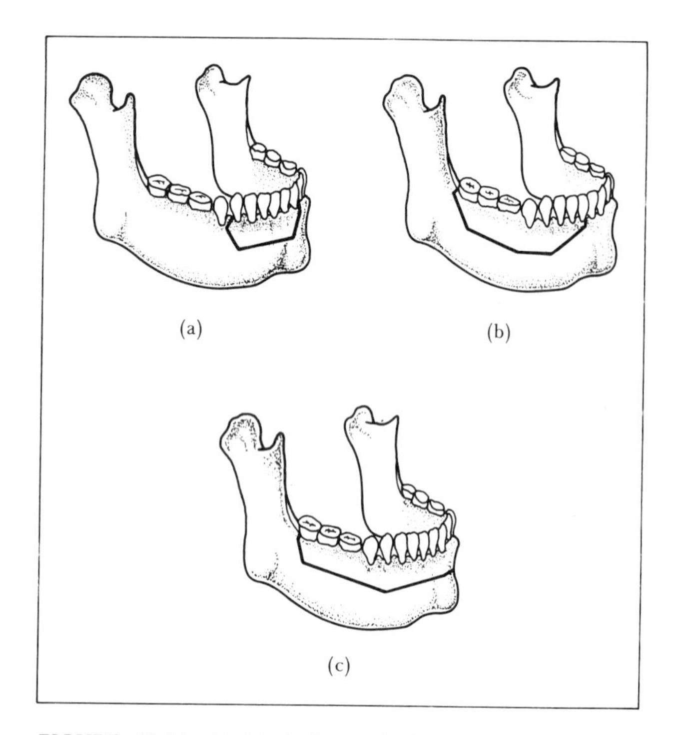

FIGURE 41-14 (a) Limited marginal mandibulectomy with teeth adjacent to defect. (b) More extensive marginal mandibulectomy with limited rehabilitation potential. (c) Total marginal mandibulectomy.

tinuity of the mandibular arch is maintained. The presence of teeth allows for anchorage of a dental prosthesis. In the normal edentulous mandible, a denture can be worn satisfactorily because the tongue and cheeks aid in stability. However, when the alveolar process and adjacent soft tissues are resected, scarring, loss of buccal and lingual sulci, and reduction in tongue and cheek mobility may occur. Secondary surgical procedures to rebuild denture-bearing bone may be necessary before a dental prosthesis is designed.

Lateral mandibulectomy

Lateral mandibulectomy (Figure 41-15) involves the body and ramus of the mandible posterior to the cuspid area. This procedure is commonly associated with resection of the floor of the mouth and tongue in a composite manner. Mandibular reconstruction may or may not be attempted, depending on whether the individual has had previous high-dose radiotherapy. Anterior facial contour is preserved with lateral mandibulectomy, but lateral facial contour is concave. The remaining mandible has a tendency to drift toward the resected side, causing malocclusion and difficulty with mastication. The remaining mandible may begin to tilt outward, causing pain and mucosal irritation. Pain also may occur at the temporomandibular joint because of the instability of the jaw. The individual is unable to wear a dental prosthesis, and nutritional maintenance is often a problem. Unilateral lip anesthesia occurs because of resection of the mandibular branch of the facial

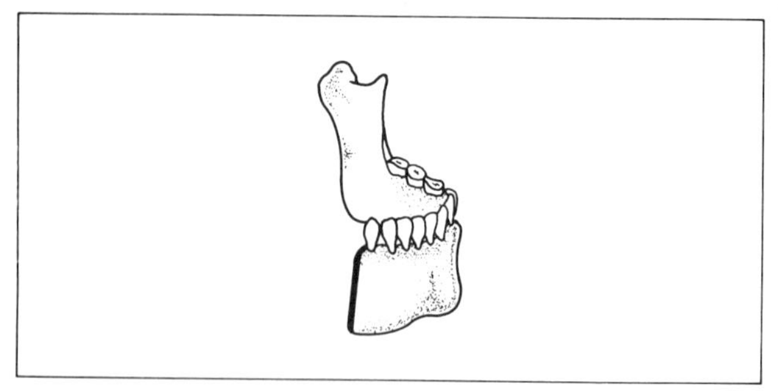

FIGURE 41-15 Lateral mandibulectomy.

nerve. Loss of normal buccal space with scar contracture further limits motion of the oral cavity. When this resection includes a portion of the tongue, function can be severely affected. These individuals should be evaluated for possible functional appliances that can facilitate retraining of remaining structures. A speech therapist can help evaluate the individual for muscle restrengthening and tongue mobility, as well as realignment exercises to maintain facial contour.

Hemimandibulectomy

The same problems exist for the individual who undergoes a hemimandibulectomy (Figure 41-16) as for the individual with a lateral mandibulectomy, only to a greater degree. Facial disfigurement is more marked, and speech, swallowing, and salivary control are compromised.

Anterior mandibulectomy

Anterior mandibulectomy (Figure 41-17) creates profound functional and cosmetic deformities. Functional loss of the hyomandibular complex impairs deglutition, articulation, salivary continence, mastication, and respiration. The lower lip lacks support and innervation; therefore oral continence and facial contour are severely affected. This resection is a major challenge to the reconstructive surgeon.

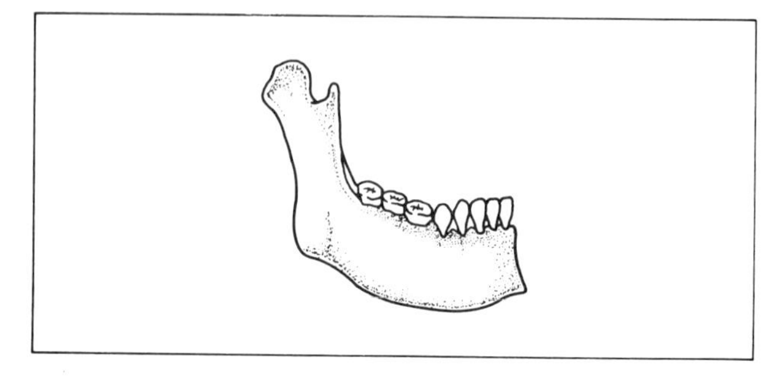

FIGURE 41-16 Hemimandibulectomy.

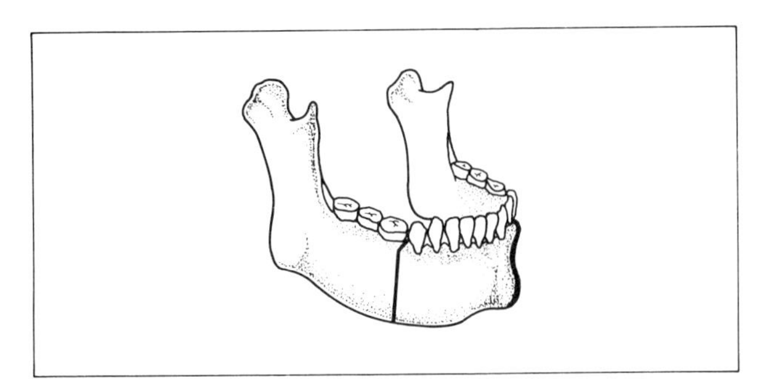

FIGURE 41-17 Anterior mandibulectomy.

Mobile Tongue

Cancer of the anterior tongue includes tumors arising from the mobile portion of the tongue anterior to the circumvallate palate and is the most common site of intraoral carcinoma. It is predominantly a disease of men between 40 and 70 years of age but is also seen in men under 30 years of age. The incidence in women is increasing, probably because of increasing alcohol and tobacco usage. Poor oral hygiene, excessive use of tobacco, including smokeless tobacco, and alcohol ingestion are important risk factors. The majority of cancers of the mobile tongue or anterior two thirds occur along the lateral border and may be etiologically related to dental trauma. The symptoms, clinical findings, and biologic behavior of carcinoma of the tongue vary considerably with the location of the neoplasm; the growth pattern is usually infiltrative, ulcerative, and/or exophytic. Neoplasms arising from the ventral surface tend to extend directly toward the floor of the mouth, and the extent of the disease can be difficult to assess. A painless superficial ulceration or focal thickening may be an early sign of disease. The deeply infiltrating types may manifest little or no surface ulceration until late in the disease. Metastasis to cervical lymph nodes occurs frequently and is often assumed, even if palpable lymph nodes are not present. Distant metastasis is not uncommon. The lungs and liver are most often the sites of metastasis.

The prognosis for individuals with carcinoma of the tongue is affected by many factors. The anteroposterior location is important, in that there is a marked decrease in 5-year survival as the primary site moves posteriorly toward the base of the tongue. The presence of positive lymph nodes adversely affects the prognosis, reducing 5-year survival rates by 50%.

As with other sites in the head and neck region, there is controversy regarding the most appropriate therapy. Early T1 and T2 lesions may be treated by either surgery or radiotherapy. When a tumor is easily accessible, surgical resection can be better tolerated by the individual than a prolonged course of radiotherapy. The combined use of radiation (4000 to 5000 cGy) and surgery is needed for more advanced lesions. The recurrence rate for carcinoma of the tongue is high, and therapy tends to be radical in the hope of preventing recurrence and establishing local control of the disease. In high-risk individuals, programs of combined chemotherapy and radiation for advanced disease are designed to induce remission and tumor shrinkage before surgery.

Transoral partial glossectomy is often the treatment of choice for limited lesions of the anterior tongue (Figure 41-18). The tongue itself may be used to close the wound, or a skin graft may be used if a large portion of the mucosal surface is resected. The functional result is usually good, with minimal scar contracture.

For larger lesions, a composite resection may be necessary. A composite resection is defined as the excision of an intraoral tumor (usually involving the tongue) in continuity with a radical neck dissection. The procedure may or may not include a portion of the mandible. When the individual has had previous irradiation, skin flaps may be necessary to reconstruct the defect.

Small marginal resections of the mandible and tongue do not create major problems in terms of function or cosmesis unless tongue mobility is impaired. Partial glossectomy of up to one third of the mobile tongue results in temporary difficulty in mobilization of a bolus but is usually compensated for in a few weeks. The major requirements for successful performance of bolus propulsion and speech articulation are sensation, freedom of motion, and motor control.

When a hemiglossectomy of the anterior two thirds of the tongue is performed as part of a composite resection, the functional goal is maximum mobility of the remaining tongue. The hypoglossal nerve on the ipsilateral side is sacrificed in this procedure, and function is compensated for by contralateral hypoglossal innervation. However, when extensive monobloc resections include one half or more of the tongue, floor of the mouth, adjacent lateral or hemimandible, and the ipsilateral side of the neck, moderate impairment of swallowing may result. Postoperative aspiration may occur, and adaptation may be slow, with retraining of the oral phase of swallowing requiring weeks to months. If the individual has had prior irradiation, there is the risk of fistula formation, which usually heals by secondary intention. This results in additional scarring, which contributes to functional disabilities.

If skin flaps are used to surface the tongue, function may be impaired because the flaps may serve to anchor the tongue and obstruct the flow of food from the anterior part of the mouth. These flaps lack sensation and muscle control, which further limits function of the remaining tongue.

Total glossectomy is the most debilitating of all oral cavity resections and virtually eliminates articulation and the oral phase of swallowing. The individual must evacuate the oral cavity by gravity, and inadequate reconstruction can result in oral incompetence and blockage of posterior flow. Skin flaps are often used to provide laryngeal support and protection. A cricopharyngeal myotomy can help to reduce aspiration by eliminating the normal delay in opening of the cricopharyngeal sphincter. Normal supraglottic sensation through intact superior laryngeal nerves is essential if aspiration is to be prevented. Chronic aspiration and recurrent pneumonia may necessitate laryngectomy.

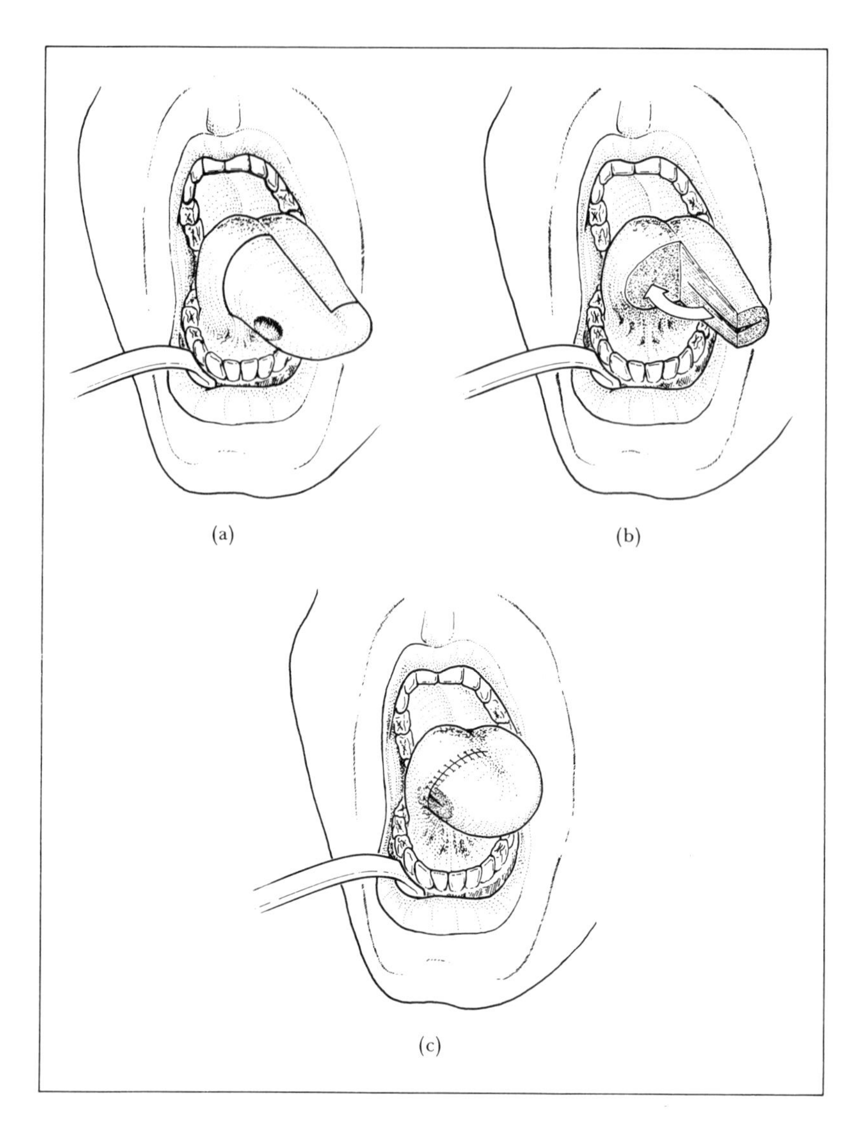

FIGURE 41-18 (a) Hemiglossectomy is recommended for small lesions of the anterior or middle third of the tongue. (b) A satisfactory closure can be obtained by removing a small portion and filleting the opposite tip. (c) The tip is then brought around and sutured to the posterior third.

Individuals who have undergone total glossectomy can eventually learn to swallow without aspiration. Some also are capable of reasonably intelligible speech. The sounds that are impossible to produce are *S*, *Z*, *T*, *D*, *H*, and *L*. The lips and buccal mucosa are the articulators, which, with much practice and energy, can enable the individual to produce intelligible speech.

Floor of the Mouth

The floor of the mouth is the second most common site for squamous cell carcinoma in the oral cavity and tumors at this site are often included in discussions of tongue lesions because the functional difficulties are similar. The most frequent site of origin is in the anterior segment of the floor of the mouth at the midline and lateral to or involving the frenulum. This area is considered a high-risk site for oral cancers because it is a dependent area where carcinogens remain in contact with the oral epithelium for extended periods of time. The larger proportion of these tumors are first detected at an advanced stage. They often are more extensive than they appear and may extend to the gums, tongue, and genioglossus muscle. Invasion of the root of the tongue is a grave prognostic sign. A significant number of individuals may have concurrent multiple primary tumors in the head and neck region.

Surgery and radiotherapy are the two major modes of therapy, although chemotherapy, cryotherapy, and CO_2 laser excision are also employed. Surgery is usually performed when small (T1) neoplasms are confined to the mucosa. Surgical excision and primary skin grafting generally present no functional difficulty. When larger portions of the floor of the mouth are resected, the posterior part of the tongue can be used as a lingual flap to resurface the lateral floor of the mouth and this does not routinely result in functional damage to the tongue. When tumor has invaded the mandible, surgical resection of the tumor in continuity with some portion of the mandible and radical neck dissection are performed. Composite resections, including the anterior portion of the mandible, floor of the mouth, and the anterior suprahyoid musculature, severely impair swallowing and present a challenge to reconstructive efforts. In addition to loss of lip sensation, salivary incontinence, and deficiencies in oral manipulation of ingested food, loss of laryngeal support and resultant aspiration are the most serious impairments. With loss of superior and anterior displacement during swallowing, the larynx is not protected sufficiently from aspiration. Functional reconstruction of the hyomandibular complex with regional skin flaps and laryngeal suspension can facilitate glottic protection. Cricopharyngeal myotomy helps to reduce salivary pooling and oral incompetence, as well as facilitate swallowing. The forehead flap, deltopectoral flap, or cervical flap may be used to reconstruct the floor of the mouth. The rotation of skin or myocutaneous flaps is usually done when the individual has had previous high-dose radiotherapy. The goal is to replace the postirradiation tissue that often deforms the tongue and to reconstruct the floor of the mouth with healthy tissue.

Radiation may be used to treat tumors of the floor of the mouth, either preoperatively or as the major mode of therapy. Proper radiation exposure may be accomplished by interstitial implant, by external therapy plus implant, or occasionally by a transoral cone. Radiotherapy in these lesions is possible only if the tumor has not infiltrated bone.

CARCINOMA OF THE OROPHARYNX

PATHOPHYSIOLOGY

The oropharynx is the posterior extension of the oral cavity and includes the soft palate, the posterior third or base of the tongue, the retromolar trigones, the anterior tonsillar pillar, the tonsil, the lateral and posterior pharyngeal wall, and the pharyngoepiglottic and glossoepiglottic folds, which bound the vallecula (Figure 41-19). Tumors arising from these regions are difficult to manage because often more than one anatomic site is involved. The biologic behavior of the carcinomas is predictable in

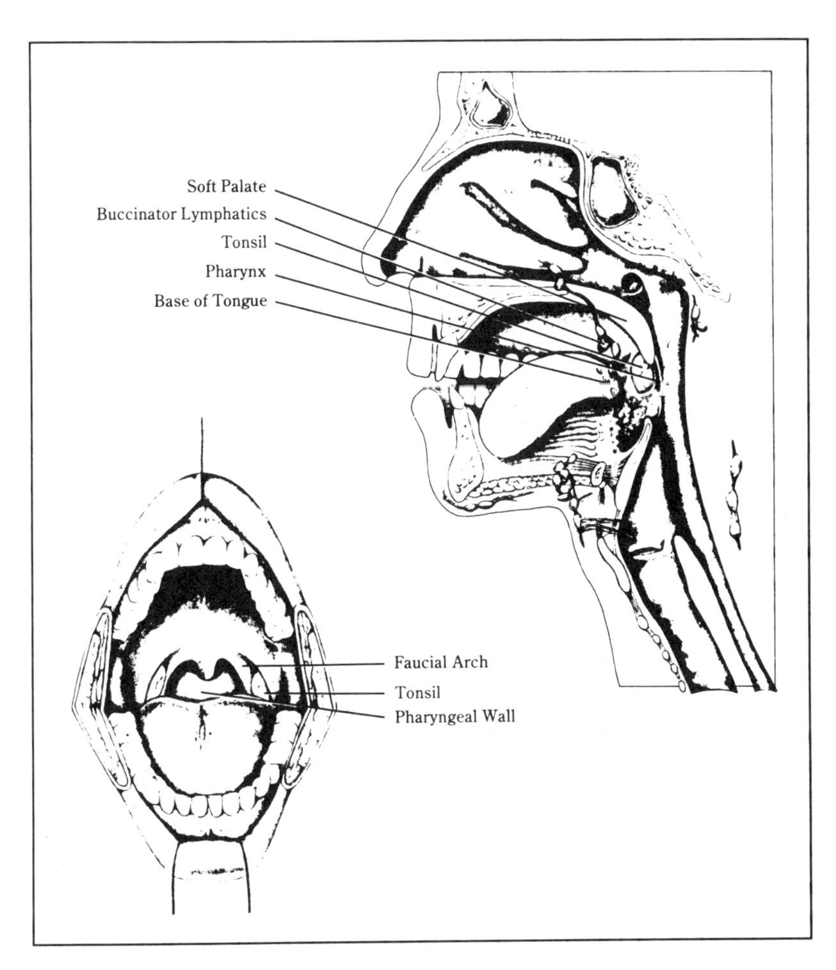

FIGURE 41-19 The oropharynx. (Courtesy of Bristol Laboratories.)

that they often extend to neighboring structures. For instance, primary carcinomas of the soft palate tend to involve the tonsillar pillars, the pterygoid plate, and the nasopharynx. Carcinomas of the tonsil and retromolar area advance toward the pharyngeal wall, the base of the tongue, the mandible, and the pterygoid muscle. The relatively poor prognosis for these individuals is influenced by the abundant lymphatic drainage of the area. The primary lymphatic connections of oropharyngeal lesions drain into the superior deep jugular lymph nodes and subdigastric lymph nodes. The incidence of nodal involvement at the time of diagnosis is greater than 60%, and the incidence of bilateral nodal involvement is high (23%) because of the relative midline location of these lesions. When metastasis does occur, it is usually to the lung, bone, and liver, in decreasing order of frequency. The incidence of metastasis increases with the more posterior lesions (base of the tongue and posterior tonsil).[31]

TABLE 41-7 TNM Classification System for Carcinoma of the Oropharynx

Primary Tumor (T)

TIS	Carcinoma in situ
T1	Tumor 2 cm or less in greatest diameter
T2	Tumor more than 2 cm but no more than 4 cm in greatest diameter
T4	Massive tumor more than 4 cm in diameter with invasion of bone, soft tissues of the neck, or deep (extrinsic) muscles of the tongue

Source: American Joint Committee for Cancer Staging and End Results Reporting: Manual for Staging of Cancer. Philadelphia, JB Lippincott, 1988.

CLINICAL MANIFESTATIONS

Squamous cell carcinoma in the oropharynx is more frequently found in individuals between 50 and 70 years of age; the male/female ratio is 5:1. A history of prolonged sore throat is probably the most common symptom of cancer in this area. If the tumor occurs in the palatine arch, ulceration and pain may be early symptoms because of the abundant nerve supply in this area. Tumors deep in the oropharynx (base of the tongue) ulcerate later, have fewer nerve fibers, and tend to be discovered later. A feeling of fullness, a lump in the throat, or a dull ache may be other presenting symptoms. A deep-seated earache (otalgia) is a common initial complaint. This represents referred pain to the ear along the ninth cranial nerve. Late symptoms include speech difficulties or nasal regurgitation from palatal obstruction. Fixation of the base of the tongue by tumor may cause difficulty in swallowing and aspiration. Trismus is an ominous sign and is common in advanced retromolar trigone and palatine arch lesions that have invaded the pterygoid muscle. In 25% of individuals, the first sign of oropharyngeal carcinoma is an asymptomatic mass in the neck.

ASSESSMENT

Examination and evaluation of the individual usually include direct visualization and palpation of the oropharynx. Mirror examination is necessary to evaluate the base of the tongue and periepiglottic lesions. A barium esophagogram may be valuable in determining the extent of the primary tumor or in detecting second primary tumors. Radiographic studies of the base of the skull may be indicated in individuals with trismus or neurologic symptoms. A metastatic survey, including bone and liver scans, is usually done only in individuals with advanced disease. Staging of disease is important in determining the appropriate therapy (Table 41-7).

TREATMENT

Therapeutic intervention depends on many factors and is controversial. Reports have shown that combined preoperative irradiation (5000 cGy) with surgery has produced higher survival rates and better control of distant metastasis than either treatment used alone.[31] An ipsilateral neck dissection is often done because there is a high frequency of metastasis to ipsilateral nodes. The anterior aspects of the anterior pillar or retromolar trigone are common sites for tumors of the oropharynx. The surgical resection of this region would involve a neck dissection in continuity with the tumor and regional tissues. A portion of the mandible (ascending ramus) may or may not be involved in the resection, depending on its actual involvement or proximity to the tumor. An osteotomy can be performed to gain access and provide for adequate closure of the wound. A typical resection would include the unilateral palatine arch, a portion of the retromolar trigone, the lateral aspect of the posterior tongue, and the lateral pharyngeal wall. The amount of pterygoid muscle resected depends on the extent of the tumor before radiotherapy. In most cases the defect is closed without the use of skin flaps, but such closure is more feasible when a portion of the mandible is resected. In some cases the ipsilateral remaining part of the anterior tongue may be used to reconstruct the base of the tongue and tonsillar region. The functional results are good, without further limitations for the individual. In larger tumors a forehead flap or a deltopectoral flap may be used to reconstruct the pharyngeal wall or soft palate. The objectives of reconstruction in this area are as follows:

1. To provide resurfacing of the palatine arch and lateral pharyngeal wall.
2. To close the wound and cover the carotid artery.
3. To maintain maximum motion of the remaining tongue.
4. To provide palatal competence.

Failure to accomplish these goals may result in dysphagia, poor speech, and nasal regurgitation.

Soft tissue reconstruction of the soft palate often provides less than optimal results. The construction of an upper jaw prosthesis with a posterior obturator provides better functional restoration, particularly in resections involving more than half of the soft palate.[32]

The individual's rehabilitation needs after surgery are congruent with the extent of the resection. The drains are generally removed on the fourth or fifth postoperative day. The tracheostomy may be plugged once edema has subsided and the individual is able to swallow without aspiration. The tube is later removed and the stoma is allowed to heal. The individual's nutritional status is maintained with a nasogastric tube or a gastrostomy tube, with or without parenteral hyperalimentation. The individual who has difficulty relearning the act of swallowing may need to be maintained on enteral feedings for an extended period of time. This is particularly true of individuals who have had a major resection of the base of the tongue and adjacent pharyngeal wall. The oral and pharyngeal phases of swallowing are impaired, and the remaining structures must compensate if swallowing is to be accomplished without aspiration. Such adaptation is aided by the remaining hypoglossal nerve and pharyngeal musculature on the contralateral side. A speech and swallowing therapist will often recommend that the individual be given soft food with the consistency of a peach. Such foods are easier to propel as a bolus, which aids in the oral and pharyngeal phase of swallowing. Liquids are most difficult to swallow because they are easily aspirated.

When the tumor extends to the supraglottic structures and the resection involves more than half of the base of the tongue and adjacent pharynx, the risk of aspiration is greatly increased. A total laryngectomy in continuity with the oropharyngeal lesion may be necessary, particularly if the individual is elderly and has chronic pulmonary disease.

Extensive surgical procedures are justified with this population of individuals regardless of age, because severe pain and great difficulty in swallowing and breathing accompany the expanding tumor. Surgery offers relief from these debilitating effects, and few people refuse. With creative rehabilitation nursing, these individuals will learn to compensate for and adapt to their structural and functional losses.

CARCINOMA OF THE HYPOPHARYNX

Because of its proximity to the larynx, the hypopharynx is also called the laryngopharynx. The hypopharynx is divided into (1) pyriform sinuses, (2) the posterior cricoid area, and (3) the posterior and lateral pharyngeal walls (Figure 41-20). The incidence of hypopharyngeal tumors is highest in men in the sixth and seventh decades of life. A history of Plummer-Vinson syndrome and alcohol and tobacco use are common predisposing factors.

PATHOPHYSIOLOGY

Most lesions in the hypopharynx are of squamous cell origin and are more undifferentiated than laryngeal tumors. The majority of individuals have a large lesion and a metastatic node, usually large and in the midportion of the jugular chain. Local extension by mucosal spread is common and results in the appearance of multifocal lesions. Direct extension may occur from the postcricoid region to the larynx or esophagus. Lesions of the posterior wall often extend to the posterior tonsillar pillar.

The overall survival figures of individuals with tumors of the hypopharynx have been uniformly poor, with a 5-year survival rate ranging from 23% to 29% when the currently available treatment methods are used.

CLINICAL MANIFESTATIONS

Like oropharyngeal tumors, lesions in the hypopharynx can have an insidious onset. The tumors may be large and still be asymptomatic. A lump in the neck may be the first sign of disease and the chief complaint. The individual may have had previous treatment for a persistent sore throat and complain of a burning sensation. The most common first symptom is the appearance of odynophagia, which is sometimes unilateral. Progressive dysphagia will be present and contribute to rapid weight loss. Otalgia on the same side of the lesion indicates tumor invasion of the superior laryngeal nerve. Hoarseness may be present if tumor has invaded the true cords or displaced the larynx, interfering with phonation. Foul, malodorous breath may be indicative of a tumor that is infected and necrotic.

ASSESSMENT

Tumors involve the pyriform sinus more frequently than other sites in the hypopharynx. Physical examination of

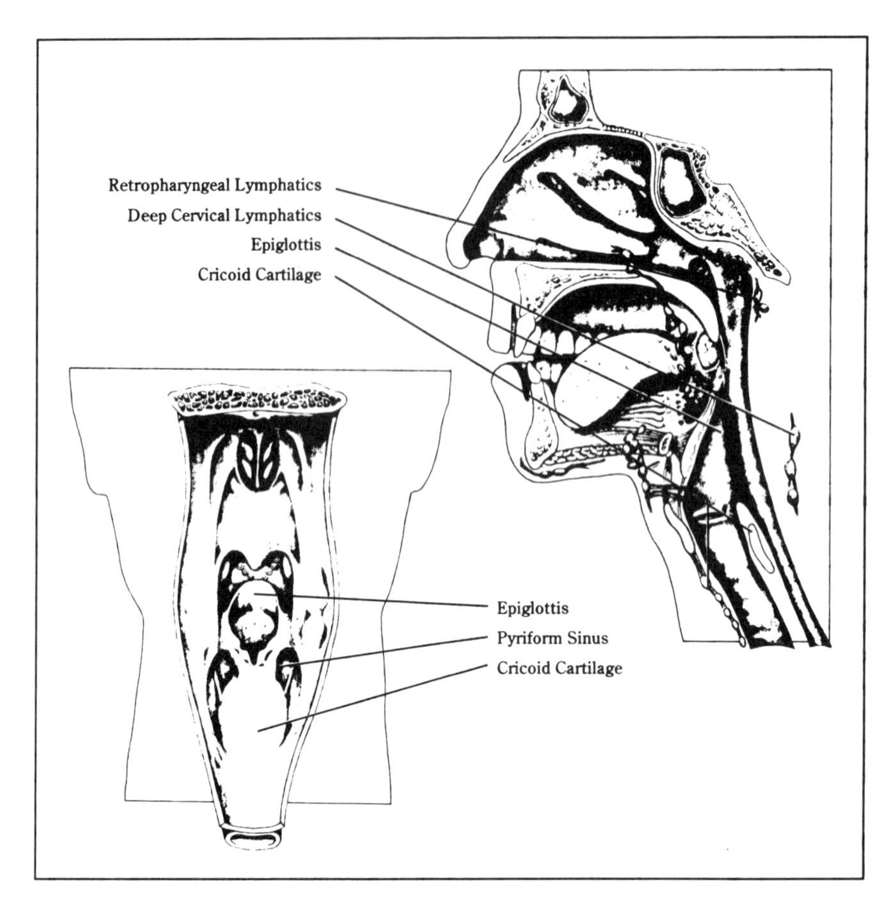

FIGURE 41-20 The hypopharynx. (Courtesy of Bristol Laboratories.)

the area can be carried out with a tongue depressor, a laryngeal mirror, and palpation. Mirror pharyngoscopy can yield clear visualization of the hypopharynx, excluding the postcricoid area. The pyriform sinuses are best visualized during phonation. When the mirror is angled against the soft palate, adequate viewing of the posterior and lateral pharyngeal wall is possible.

Diagnostic studies include soft tissue tomograms, contrast radiograms, and direct pharyngoscopy and/or laryngoscopy with biopsy. The propensity of pyriform sinus tumors to be necrotic often necessitates multiple deep biopsies to ensure an adequate tissue sample. Esophagoscopy with biopsy also may be necessary if posterior invasion of the esophagus appears evident on pharyngoscopy. Observations pertinent to treatment planning include the following:

1. *Presence or absence of laryngeal involvement by tumor.* If both cords are mobile, invasion by tumor has not occurred, and the lesion is exterior to the larynx. If one cord is fixed, the individual may be a candidate for a partial laryngectomy in continuity with the primary site.

2. *Tumor invasion and mucosal involvement of the posterior wall of the pharynx.* The posterior pharynx is often used to reconstruct the site after resection, but involvement by tumor would obviate its use for reconstruction, and alternate tissues would need to be used.

3. *Pooling of saliva in or around the pyriform sinus and pharynx.* This could indicate cervical esophageal extension or obstruction of the opening of the cervical esophagus, which would require aggressive treatment.

Treatment planning is based on the stage of disease (Table 41-8).

TREATMENT

Early exophytic tumors of the hypopharynx may be treated by either surgery or radiotherapy. Radiotherapy can potentially cure the individual when there is no evidence of metastasis. The more common event is an infiltrating tumor that involves neighboring tissues. Combined surgery, radiotherapy, and chemotherapy are often needed to control the disease.

Cancers of the pyriform sinus typically involve the laryngeal structures to some degree. With limited laryngeal involvement, the glottic sphincter can be preserved despite

TABLE 41-8 TNM Classification System for Carcinoma of the Hypopharynx

Primary Tumor (T)

TIS	Carcinoma in situ
T1	Tumor confined to the site of origin
T2	Extension of the tumor to the adjacent region without fixation of the hemilarynx
T3	Extension of the tumor to the adjacent region with fixation of the hemilarynx
T4	Massive tumor invading adjacent structures (eg, cartilage or soft tissues of neck)

Source: American Joint Committee for Cancer Staging and End Results Reporting. Manual for Staging of Cancer. Philadelphia, JB Lippincott, 1988.

resection of a portion of the larynx and the involved pharynx. Rehabilitation involves swallowing therapy to minimize aspiration. A nasogastric tube and tracheostomy tube may be necessary for extended periods of time until swallowing ability is restored and aspiration is reduced. However, difficulty in swallowing may be a long-term problem because extensive scarring often results in esophageal stricture. With involvement of the pyriform sinus, fixation of the cords, and invasion of the thyroid cartilage, more extensive procedures may be necessary. A total laryngectomy, pharyngectomy, and radical neck dissection are performed. The posterior pharyngeal wall is used to reconstruct a neogullet for swallowing. When the posterior pharyngeal wall cannot be used for reconstruction, cervical and regional flaps are necessary to close the defect. The reconstruction is usually done as a two- or three-stage procedure. The deltopectoral flap forms a tube that will provide an epithelial tissue source to reconstruct the oropharyngeal-esophageal area. The upper end of the tube is sutured at the level of the oropharynx, and the lower end is attached to the upper esophagus, with an opening on the external neck that acts as a temporary esophageal fistula. In approximately 3 weeks, the pedicle is divided, the esophagus is anastomosed, and wound closure is carried out. The result is that the individual has a reconstructed skin-lined conduit for food and saliva.

Surgical resections involving the pharyngeal constrictors interfere with the normal muscular contraction that controls a food bolus and delivers it into the esophagus during the act of swallowing. If more than half of the middle and lower constrictors are resected and reconstructed, scar contracture with impaired swallowing results but eventually becomes adequate as scar tissue softens. Complications after pharyngeal surgery are related to infection. Because any surgery in this area involves opening of the upper digestive tract and thus becomes a contaminated procedure, the individual receives antibiotic therapy. Meticulous wound care, nutritional support, and oral hygiene are major nursing interventions.

When the individual has had prior irradiation, wound healing is compromised and pharyngocutaneous fistula formation or infection of the anastomosis is common. If infection should occur, the integrity of the carotid artery is greatly threatened, and carotid rupture can be catastrophic.

Once healing has occurred, the individual can begin esophageal speech. The possibility of the person's gaining good speech through this method is less than optimal because of pharyngeal stricture, and success is rare. An electrical hand-held device is often needed for communication.

For the individual with an unresectable tumor, radiotherapy and chemotherapy are alternatives to local tumor control and palliation. High doses of radiation to the hypopharynx and bilateral neck are necessary for adequate control. Once three quarters of the dose is given, the spinal cord is shielded from the radiation source.

These individuals present major challenges to nursing management, particularly in terms of nutrition, side effects of surgery, radiotherapy, chemotherapy, and pain management. Many individuals will require permanent tracheostomy and gastrostomy tubes because of the obstructive nature of tumors in the hypopharynx. Every effort must be made to help the individual learn self-care while hospitalized. Major areas of patient and family teaching involve instruction on suctioning the trachea, cleansing and changing the entire tracheostomy tube, managing the gastrostomy tube, and nutritional counseling.

CARCINOMA OF THE LARYNX

EPIDEMIOLOGY AND ETIOLOGY

Laryngeal carcinoma accounts for 2% to 5% of all malignant tumors. Approximately 12,300 new cases are diagnosed annually in the United States, and in one third of these the individuals will die of uncontrolled local disease.[2] A higher incidence of cancer at any laryngeal location is found in males than in females (male/female ratio of 5:1). Approximately 80% of laryngeal carcinomas are found in persons over 50 years of age, with the highest incidence (40%) in the sixth decade of life. No single factor can be identified in the etiology of laryngeal carcinoma, although smoking and excessive alcohol intake have been implicated. The incidence of multiple primary tumors is 5% to 10%. The most common association is with bronchogenic carcinoma.

For practical purposes, cancer of the larynx cannot be considered as a single disease but, rather, as cancer involving the glottis, the space between the true cords, and cancer involving those structures above the glottis, or the

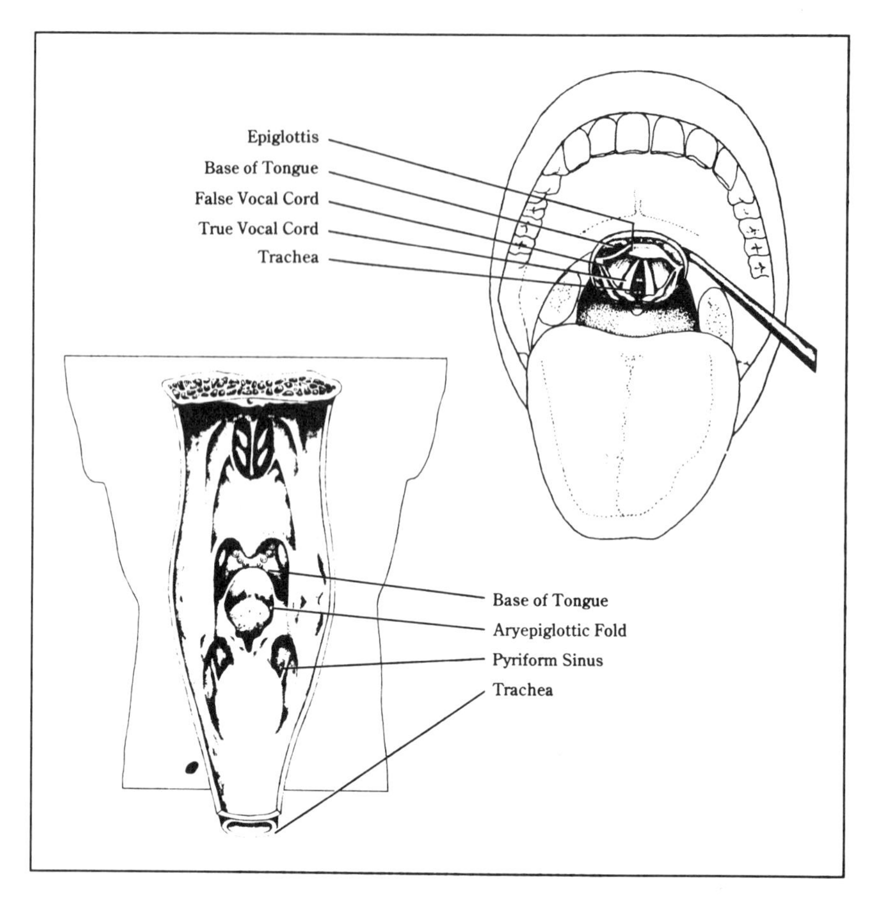

FIGURE 41-21 The larynx. (Courtesy of Bristol Laboratories.)

supraglottic region. (Figure 41-21 shows the structure of the larynx.) Cancer in each region involves distinct signs and symptoms, treatment regimens, and, most important, rehabilitation measures.

GLOTTIC CARCINOMA

Pathophysiology

Most glottic lesions begin on the anterior half of one cord and gradually extend to the anterior commissure, the opposite cord, or posteriorly to the arytenoid of the same cord. Fixation of one or both cords, either by infiltration of the cord or by nerve involvement, is common and indicative of more advanced disease. The lymphatic vessels are more abundant in the posterior larynx than in the anterior larynx; therefore, with arytenoid involvement, the likelihood of regional and distant metastasis is greater.

Glottic carcinoma is generally well differentiated, remains localized, and metastasizes high in the neck at the level of the carotid bifurcation (mid-digastric, midjugular). When a metastasis does occur, it is to regional nodes, is usually single, and remains movable until late.

When malignancy involves only one cord but not the arytenoid, the 5-year survival rate following proper treatment is 85% to 90%. If the posterior part of the larynx or any structures outside the larynx are involved, the 5-year survival rate drops precipitously to around 70%. If neck metastases are present, the prognosis is even worse.

Clinical Manifestations

Hoarseness is the cardinal symptom of glottic carcinoma. It is caused by any condition that interferes with the normal phonatory function of the true cords. As vocal cords approximate for phonation, they vibrate as air passes through the larynx. With cancer of the glottis, the vocal cords fail to perform properly because of vocal cord irregularities, occlusion or narrowing of the glottis, and invasion of the vocalis muscles or cricoarytenoid joints. Hoarseness alters the quality of the voice to one that is rough, grating, harsh, and of a lower pitch than normal. Pain and dysphagia occur in advanced disease. Any person who is hoarse for more than a 2-week period should have his or her larynx examined.

Assessment

A careful examination of the larynx is accomplished through indirect laryngoscopy. Tomograms of the larynx may be helpful. Laryngograms may be indicated to evaluate the epiglottis where it contracts the anterior commissure and the subglottic area for extension of disease. Laryngoscopy is done to define tumor extension and to obtain a biopsy specimen of the lesion, should one be found.

Important information that is obtained in the diagnostic phase includes the mobility of the cords, evidence of fixation of the cord, location of the lesion, involvement of the anterior commissure, and involvement of cervical lymphatic vessels. This information is important for staging the disease and determining the appropriate treatment (Table 41-9).

TABLE 41-9 TNM Classification System for Glottic Carcinoma

Primary Tumor (T)

TIS	Carcinoma in situ
T1	Tumor confined to the vocal cord(s) with normal mobility (includes involvement of anterior or posterior commissures)
T1a	Tumor limited to one vocal cord
T1b	Tumor involves both vocal cords
T2	Supraglottic and/or subglottic extension with normal or impaired cord mobility
T3	Tumor confined to the larynx with cord fixation
T4	Massive tumor with thyroid cartilage destruction and/or extends to other tissues beyond the larynx (eg, oropharynx, soft tissues of the neck)

Source: American Joint Committee for Cancer Staging and End Results Reporting: Manual for Staging of Cancer. Philadelphia, JB Lippincott, 1988.

Treatment

In recent years there has been a major emphasis on development of treatment techniques that will achieve cure of glottic carcinoma while simultaneously preserving the sphincteric, respiratory, and phonatory functions of the larynx. For early glottic carcinoma where there is no evidence of cord fixation, a conservative laryngeal resection is usually the treatment of choice. Conservative surgery for glottic cancer includes laryngofissure or partial laryngectomy and hemilaryngectomy. Aside from cord mobility, the major factor in the selection of a conservative surgical procedure is the age of the patient. Surgery, rather than radiation, is often preferred for younger individuals because it is advisable to reserve radiation until there is a recurrence of disease.

Early disease (T1 or T2)

A hemilaryngectomy is indicated when a glottic tumor extends beyond the membranous portion of the true cord or vocal process but does not extend more than 1 cm subglottically. The lesion may cross the anterior commissure to involve the anterior third of the contralateral cord. A hemilaryngectomy is usually not performed when the arytenoid and true cord are fixed. A hemilaryngectomy involves a tracheostomy, and after surgery the individual is fed through a nasogastric tube until there is complete healing and no evidence of aspiration. The individual will probably be decannulated between the tenth and fourteenth postoperative days. Voice is usually good and is accomplished by the adduction of the remaining cord against the scar tissue that eventually takes the place of the resected cord. Should the individual have difficulty with aspiration, a Teflon injection of the remaining redundant mucosa may serve to accomplish closure of the cords during swallowing. Damage to the superior and recurrent laryngeal nerves can lead to persistent aspiration in these individuals, in which case a total laryngectomy may be needed to prevent recurrent aspiration pneumonia.

Radiotherapy may be used in three basic treatment regimens for localized laryngeal carcinoma (T1 and T2 tumors with normal cord mobility). Because the intent is cure, the person usually receives 5500 to 7000 cGy over 6 to 7 weeks. Radiation may be employed as initial therapy to see how the tumor responds. If the tumor fails to respond after 4000 cGy, surgery may be indicated. If the individual responds, a full dose of radiation may be given. Surgery remains an option if the individual has persistent disease or a recurrence.

Because the biologic effect of radiation results in poor wound healing after laryngectomy, the combined sequential approach of surgery followed in 5 to 6 weeks by high-dose radiotherapy is gaining acceptance. Limited doses of radiation in the range of 4000 to 5000 cGy may be given before surgery, followed by surgery in 4 to 5 weeks.

Advanced disease (T3 to T4)

A total laryngectomy is reserved for individuals who have persistent or recurrent disease after radiotherapy for lesions involving one or both vocal cords with fixation of the cord, cancer of the cord with subglottic extension of more than 1 cm, extralaryngeal cancer, interarytenoid cancer, or layrngeal cartilage destruction. A total laryngectomy includes the removal of all laryngeal structures between and including the thyroid bone, thyroid cartilage, cricoid cartilage, and two to three tracheal rings. The procedure may or may not include a radical neck dissection. The chief alterations these individuals face are the loss of laryngeal tone and major airway alterations.

In the preoperative period, the person should be given the opportunity to verbalize fears and become an active member of the rehabilitation program. Preoperative and postoperative counseling by a speech therapist is imperative. During a speech and hearing evaluation, the speech therapist can assess whether the individual would benefit from a visit from someone who has had a laryngectomy and who has good esophageal speech. All individuals facing a laryngectomy should be given this unique opportunity to be assured that verbal communication is possible after surgery.

In the immediate postoperative period, the person will have moderate difficulty in managing secretions, which are often copious. Because the individual is unable to swallow because of postoperative edema, he or she should be instructed to suction the oral cavity as desired. Caution is used if the incision extends to the posterior oral cavity. About 6 to 7 days after surgery, oral secretions are no longer a problem because by then the person is generally able to swallow. Nasal secretions are a source of distress for the individual, because the cells in the nasal cavity continue to secrete mucus. Because of the altered airway, air no longer passes through the nose to dry the nasal cavity. Since these individuals cannot blow their noses, they have little control over nasal secretions, which for 7 to 10 days after surgery flow out the nares by gravity. The person should be assured that eventually the nasal cavity will secrete less mucus because of atrophy of mucus-secreting cells. Over time, the nasal cavity becomes dried, with frequent crusting. Nasal hygiene should include the removal of crusts and swabbing of the nares once daily with a mixture of eucalyptol in a mineral oil base.

Hyposmia occurs to some degree in every individual who has had a total laryngectomy. This loss is permanent and is known to the individual as soon as he or she is alert after surgery. Some limited odor detection and recognition will develop in the accessory olfactory areas over time. The exact mechanism of hyposmia in the person who has had a laryngectomy is not known but is thought to be related to motor denervation of the larynx or possibly to vascular changes that occur in the nasal mucous membranes. The ability to taste is closely related to stimulation of olfactory cells and is reduced significantly in the individual who has had a laryngectomy, especially if the person had previous irradiation that damaged taste buds and salivary gland secretion.

Weight loss is generally not a problem for the person who has had a laryngectomy. A nasogastric tube is placed during surgery to allow for alimentation until the suture lines have healed. Because the nasogastric tube rests on the incision line, it should not be manipulated in any way. If it should become dislodged or pulled out, the possibility of its being replaced without perforating the suture line is limited. This is particularly true in the individual who has had previous irradiation. The nasogastric tube remains in place for approximately 7 days in the nonirradiated person and for 10 days in the previously irradiated person. If the individual is able to swallow his or her own secretions without evidence of a fistula (that is, aspiration of secretions) the nasogastric tube is removed, and the person gradually progresses to a normal diet over a 3-day period. If a fistula does occur, the patient is maintained on nasogastric feedings until the fistula heals spontaneously, generally in 7 to 10 days.

The development of a fistula usually means an extended hospital stay and also increased scarring in the suture line, which can predispose the individual to esophageal stricture and dysphagia. Most strictures respond to periodic dilatation, although occasionally a secondary surgical procedure is necessary. Pseudodiverticuli at the base of the tongue and submucosal masses on the posterior pharyngeal wall caused by contraction of the detached constrictor muscles are common structural abnormalities found in individuals who have had laryngectomy. Dysphagia also can occur in the absence of stricture as a result of the uncoordinated contractions of the detached inferior constrictor muscles.

In the immediate postoperative period, it is routine for the individual to have a laryngectomy tube in place for 24 to 48 hours. The purpose of the tube is (1) to prevent trauma to the tracheal mucosa due to suctioning, (2) hemostasis, and (3) to ensure an adequate stoma. Once the laryngectomy tube is removed, the stoma should be kept free of crusting since crust formation can lead to infection and increased scar formation. The person who experiences stomal stricture over a period of months may need to wear a laryngectomy tube at night to help prevent further stricture.

Superficial infection of the trachea can occur as a result of the loss of humidification and protection afforded by the upper airway. If the person is without proper humidification, drying and infection can occur, leading to chronic bronchitis. The individual complains of a dry, hacking cough and secretions that are frequently tinged with blood. Instillation of saline solution with an atomizer, use of a room humidifier, and adequate fluid intake are generally satisfactory in preventing tracheitis. The oral administration of potassium iodine is helpful in increasing the volume and viscosity of secretions. Because the laryngeal sphincter is absent, intrabronchial pressure cannot be elevated, and therefore cough effectiveness is significantly reduced.

The absence of thoracic fixation after laryngectomy often limits the amount of lifting the person should attempt. The individual is instructed not to lift more than 10 pounds for 4 months after surgery. Heavy lifting and strenuous exercises may be performed gradually in spite of the lack of thoracic fixation; however, the person whose job has included repeated lifting of heavy objects may need another vocation. Most individuals who have had laryngectomy are able to resume their previous occupation, depending on the communication requirements and their level of vocal rehabilitation. Work that involves excessive exposure to water, harmful fumes, or dust should be avoided. The loss of the sphincteric action of the larynx results in loss of the ability to perform the Valsalva maneuver, which can lead to constipation and impaction. High-fiber foods and/or stool softeners may be necessary.

According to many surveys that have been conducted, between 60% and 75% of individuals who have laryngectomy develop usable esophageal speech.[33] Approximately 6% of these individuals achieve excellent esophageal speech. For those persons who are unable to achieve communication with esophageal speech, the major problems seem to be their inability to relax and control the upper esophageal sphincter secondary to excessive scarring.

Stricture formation or paralysis, limitations of tongue movement, hearing loss, advanced age, and lack of motivation all contribute to speech failure.

Esophageal tone is created by the person injecting air into the mouth and nose. The goal is to swallow the air, hold it in the upper esophagus, and release it in a controlled manner so that a tone is produced as the injected air vibrates against the cricopharyngeal musculature at the level of the esophageal sphincter. The tone that is produced by this method is generally lower than the normal tone, limited in range to one octave, and not as loud as conventional speech. Major articulators are not usually altered by a laryngectomy. Modification of esophageal tone occurs in the pharynx, nasopharynx, and oral cavity, where speech articulation is accomplished.

Complete air swallowing does occur to some degree in all esophageal speakers. This often results in upper abdominal distention and digestive disorders.

The hand-held artificial larynx, which is an electrical or mechanical instrument, may serve as an external tone source. Individuals can be understood in conversation and over the telephone.

There have been numerous creative attempts at surgical restoration of voice after total laryngectomy. A fistula tract is surgically created in the esophagus. The patient then learns to divert exhaled pulmonary air through this fistula, which causes the musculature at the top of the esophagus to vibrate. The patient learns to remove, clean, and replace a small prosthesis which fits into the fistula tract to prevent food from back-flowing into the trachea.

TABLE 41-10 TNM Classification System for Supraglottic Carcinoma

Primary Tumor (T)	
TIS	Carcinoma in situ
T1	Tumor confined to one subsite of supraglottis with normal cord mobility
T2	Tumor invades more than one subsite of supraglottis or glottis mobility with normal cord mobility
T3	Tumor limited to the larynx with vocal cord fixation and/or invades the postcricoid area, medial wall of the pyriform sinus, or preepiglottic space
T4	Tumor invades through thyroid cartilage and/or extends to other tissues beyond the larynx (eg, to oropharynx, soft tissues of the neck)

Source: American Joint Committee on Cancer Staging and End Results Reporting: Manual for Staging of Cancer. Philadelphia, JB Lippincott, 1988.

SUPRAGLOTTIC CARCINOMA

Pathophysiology

Cancers of the supraglottic larynx include those of the epiglottis, false cords, and aryepiglottic fold. Supraglottic carcinomas are generally more aggressive than glottic carcinomas, both in direct extension and in lymph node metastases. Because the predominant supraglottic structure, the epiglottis, is in the midline, both sides of the neck are threatened with metastasis. Approximately one third to one half of the individuals will have positive lymph nodes. The area is rich in lymphatic drainage, a factor that allows supraglottic lesions to metastasize more than glottic lesions. Lymphatic channels drain into the jugulodigastric, mid-jugular, and anterior jugular chain.

Clinical Manifestations

Supraglottic carcinoma is often advanced when first detected. Because of the location, there are few early symptoms of the disease. The patient may complain of pain and poorly defined throat and neck discomfort that occurs during swallowing. A few individuals may have severe pain when swallowing citrus juices; in short, the tumor has grown large and is exophytic. Others may have referred otalgia with throat pain. Glottic hoarseness may occur in advanced disease and usually means that vocal cord fixation has occurred from tumor extension. The presence or absence of vocal cord fixation is an important factor in deciding therapy, as it is in glottic carcinoma (Table 41-10).

Assessment

The diagnosis of supraglottic lesions is usually made by indirect laryngoscopy, with direct laryngoscopy used for obtaining a biopsy specimen. Lateral soft tissue radiographs, xerograms, tomograms, or contrast studies may be helpful in determining the inferior extent of disease.

Treatment

If the person's voice is near normal without hoarseness, the true cords and anterior commissure are generally not invaded by disease and a supraglottic laryngectomy, a surgical procedure that spares the true cords, may be contemplated. This conservative procedure is believed to be curative because supraglottic cancer remains localized above the ventricles and commonly does not invade the thyroid cartilage until late in the course of the disease. A block resection of the vallecula, epiglottis, hyoid bone, aryepiglottic folds, ventricular bands, upper third of the thyroid cartilage, and thyrohyoid membrane constitutes the classic supraglottic larnygectomy. A tracheostomy is performed to ensure an adequate airway during the postoperative period. With an uneventful postoperative course, voice and airway are essentially normal. For individuals with more extensive supraglottic tumors that extend to the base of the tongue or to the anterior commissure and true cords, a total laryngectomy is generally necessary to provide cure, rehabilitation, and quality of life.

The complications of a supraglottic laryngectomy include infection, wound breakdown, scarring, fistula formation, aspiration, and pneumonia. Resection of a portion of the structure responsible for the sphincteric action of the larynx automatically predisposes the person to aspiration unless the anatomic potential for glottic closure is surgically restored by reconstruction. The individual must then learn to swallow without aspirating. Because of the difficulties associated with aspiration, elderly individuals, especially those with chronic bronchitis or decreased lung compliance, may not be candidates for supraglottic laryngectomy. In many individuals, aspiration is relatively mild and of brief duration, allowing decannulation in 7 to 14 days after surgery. Other individuals may be sent home with a tracheostomy tube in place. Severe, prolonged aspiration may result in inanition and death. The person refuses to eat because every bite of food is aspirated. This quickly leads to weight loss and immobility. If pneumonia develops and is a persistent problem, a total laryngectomy will often be performed to save the person's life.

Paralysis of the internal branches of the superior laryngeal nerves is inherent in a supraglottic laryngectomy. This deficiency in sensory perception is generally well compensated for by residual structures, provided that damage to the external branches of the superior nerves and the recurrent laryngeal nerves is not incurred or the case is not complicated by other causes of aspiration, such as improper healing or postradiation fibrosis.

The prevention of aspiration after a supraglottic laryngectomy depends on good glottic closure, which can sometimes be augmented by a Teflon injection. The laryngeal remnant should closely approximate the base of the tongue during swallowing. If the elevation of the larynx against the base of the tongue is inadequate for protection of the glottis, aspiration will occur. Good tongue mobility is also mandatory for prevention of aspiration. Only limited resection of the base of the tongue can be tolerated without aspiration, and innervation of the tongue must be intact. If the person has had a neck dissection in conjunction with a supraglottic laryngectomy, a cricopharyngeal myotomy may be performed to eliminate delay and facilitate early transit of food into the esophagus.

A cineesophagogram and videofluoroscopy are usually obtained before decannulation to evaluate the person's ability to swallow without aspirating. Minimal aspiration is expected and, with proper instruction in swallowing techniques, the individual can overcome this complication.

Liquids are without question the most difficult for these people to swallow without aspiration. Attractive, textured foods with bulk should be used initially. Because adequate swallowing requires concentration, the person should be in a quiet environment without distractions. Swallowing is best accomplished with the person in the sitting position. The cuff of the tracheostomy tube should be deflated because an inflated cuff inhibits elevation of the laryngeal remnant against the base of the tongue. If the person cannot swallow without aspirating, the cuff should be inflated during meals only. Before swallowing food, the person should be familiar with the swallowing technique. The individual is instructed to take a breath and perform the Valsalva maneuver to assure glottic closure. The person then is instructed to swallow saliva while holding the breath and then immediately to cough. This is followed directly by another swallow and a cough. Once the person has learned the regimen, a bolus of food may be tried. The ideal food is one that will not fragment and will slip down easily, such as ice chips, gelatin, peaches, or custard.

The individual should be cautioned against tilting the head back, because this will surely result in aspiration. It is most important that the person not attempt to speak while eating and that a supportive professional be present during initial attempts at eating and at subsequent meals if necessary. Aspirating with every swallow of food is frightening and discouraging. The person requires frequent reassurance that success is possible and that occasional lack of concentration is not only acceptable but expected. The individual gradually progresses to solid foods, semisolids, and finally liquids.

Pulmonary hygiene is particularly important after a supraglottic laryngectomy. After each meal, a thorough tracheal toilet is mandatory. The individual is instructed to breathe deeply and cough every few hours. A high-humidity tracheostomy collar and adequate fluid intake aid in liquefying secretions. Should the person be found on videofluoroscopy to be aspirating more than 25% of what is swallowed, a nasogastric tube is generally reinserted and the person is sent home with a tracheostomy tube in place. The individual also may be instructed to pass an orogastric or nasogastric tube prior to each meal, depending on preference. With an extended healing time, scar tissue generally builds up and allows for adequate protection of the airway, and the person may be decannulated and swallow with only minimal or no aspiration.

CONCLUSION

In a number of treatment centers throughout the United States, efforts are being made to establish rehabilitation teams to manage the complex needs of the person with carcinoma of the head and neck region. This trend should continue, with special emphasis on the reconstruction of function and vocational rehabilitation of the individual. To date, there are few truly successful methods of vocal rehabilitation in these individuals. More research is needed and has implications for the individual's psychosocial and vocational adjustment.

With time, it is likely that more progress will be made in the use of microsurgery and island flap reconstruction in this area. Such advances can significantly affect the body image and functional adaptations these individuals are required to make.

REFERENCES

1. Logemann JA: Swallowing and communication rehabilitation. Semin Oncol Nurs 5:205-212, 1989.
2. Silverberg E, Lubera JA: Cancer statistics, 1989. CA 39:3-20, 1989.
3. Wynder EL, Mushinski M, Spivak J: Tobacco and alcohol consumption in relation to the development of multiple cancers. Cancer 40:1872-1878, 1977.
4. Sundar SK: Sera from patients with undifferentiated nasopharyngeal carcinoma contain a factor which abrogates specific Epstein-Barr antigen-induced lymphocyte response. Int J Cancer 29:407-412, 1982.
5. Henle W, et al: Nasopharyngeal carcinoma: Significance of changes in Epstein-Barr virus related antibody patterns following therapy. Int J Cancer 20:663-672, 1977.
6. Simons MJ, Chan SH, Wee GB, et al: Nasopharyngeal carcinoma and histocompatibility antigen, in de-The G, Ito Y (eds): Nasopharyngeal carcinoma: Etiology and control. Lyon, France, IARC Scientific Publications, 1978.
7. Ahlbom HE: Simple achlorhydric anemia, Plummer-Vinson syndrome, and carcinoma of the mouth, pharynx and esophagus in women. Br Med J 2:331-333, 1936.
8. Thomas LW: Head and neck cancer: Early detection. Semin Surg Oncol 5:168-175, 1989.
9. Lane M, Alford BR, Donovan DT: Neoplasms of the head and neck, in Calabresi P, Schein PS, Rosenberg SA (eds): Medical Oncology: Basic Principles and Clinical Management of Cancer, New York, Macmillan, 1985, pp 684-712.
10. Ervin TJ, Clark JR, Weichselbaum RR: Multidisciplinary treatment of advanced squamous carcinoma of the head and neck. Semin Oncol 12(4):71-78, 1985.
11. Perlin E: Chemotherapy for oral malignant disease. Otolaryngol Clin North Am 12:187-193, 1979.
12. Richardson MF: The problem of multiple primary tumors in patients with oral malignant disease. Otolaryngol Clin North Am 12:156-160, 1979.
13. Beahrs OH, Henson DE, Hutter RVP, et al (eds): Manual for Staging of Cancer (ed 3). Philadelphia, JB Lippincott, 1988, pp 27-51.
14. Schwartz SS, Yuska CM: Common patient care issues following surgery for head and neck cancer. Semin Oncol Nurs 15:191-194, 1989.
15. Stuart M: Skin flaps and grafts after head and neck surgery. Am J Nurs 78:1368-1374, 1978.
16. Strohl RA: Radiation therapy for head and neck cancers. Semin Oncol Nurs 15:166-173, 1989.
17. Adams GL: Treatment of head and neck cancer with combined modalities. Invest Radiol 24:562-567, 1989.
18. Clark JR, Fallon BG, Frei E III: Induction chemotherapy as initial treatment for advanced head and neck cancer: A model for the multidisciplinary treatment of solid tumors, in DeVita VT Jr, Hellman S, Rosenberg SA (eds): Important Advances in Oncology. Philadelphia, JB Lippincott, 1987, pp 175-195.
19. Ervine TJ, Clark JR, Weichselbaum R: Multidisciplinary treatment of advanced squamous carcinoma of the head and neck. Semin Oncol 12(4):71-78, 1985.
20. Taylor SG: Head and neck cancer, in Pinedo HM, Chabner BA (eds): Cancer Chemotherapy, New York, Elsevier, 1985.
21. Taylor SG: Combined simultaneous cisplatin/fluorouracil in multimodality therapy of head and neck cancer. J Clin Oncol 7:838-845, 1989.
22. Fontanesi J, Hetzler D, Ross J: Effect of dose rate on local control and complications in re-irradiation of head and neck tumors with interstitial irradium-192. Int J Radiat Oncol Biol Phys 17:365-369, 1989.
23. Manning MR, Cetas TC, Miller RC, et al: Clinical hyperthermia: Results of a phase I trail employing hyperthermia alone or in combination with external beam or interstitial radiotherapy. Cancer 49:205-216, 1982.
24. Ho JH: An epidemiologic and clinical study of nasopharyngeal carcinoma. Int J Radiat Oncol Biol Phys 4:183-197, 1978.
25. Coates HL, Pearson GR, Neel B: Epstein-Barr virus associated antigens in nasopharyngeal carcinoma. Arch Otolaryngol 104:427-430, 1978.
26. Squier CA: Introduction: Proceedings of a symposium on the health effects of smokeless tobacco, Washington DC, NCI-NIH 38:224-225, 1988.
27. Sellar SL: Epidemiology of oral cancer. Otolaryngol Clin North Am 12:45-55, 1979.
28. Chu FWK, Silverman S, Dedo HH: CO_2 laser treatment of oral leukoplakia. Laryngoscope 98:125-129, 1988.
29. Mashberg A, Samit AM: Early detection, diagnosis and management of oral and oropharyngeal cancer. CA 39(2):67-86, 1989.
30. Wang CC: Radiation therapy in the management of oral malignant disease. Otolaryngol Clin North Am 12:73-80, 1979.
31. Shumrick DA, Quenelle DJ: Malignant disease of the tonsillar region, retromolar trigone and buccal mucosa. Otolaryngol Clin North Am 12:115-124, 1979.
32. Hickey AJ, Drane JB: Prosthetic treatment and rehabilitation: Use in patients with cancer of the head and neck. Curr Probl Cancer 11(10):3-37, 1978.
33. Erskine MC: Treatment of the laryngectomy patients. Ear, Nose Throat J 58:53-54, 1979.

Chapter 42

Leukemia

Debra Wujcik, RN, MSN, OCN

INTRODUCTION

Leukemia is the name given to a group of hematologic malignancies that affect the bone marrow and lymph tissue. First described by the German pathologist Virchow in 1847 as simply "white blood," the term *leukemia* now includes abnormalities of proliferation and maturation in lymphocyte and nonlymphocyte cell lines. The acute leukemias are marked by an abnormal proliferation of immature blood cells with a short natural history (1 to 5 months) whereas the chronic leukemias are characterized by an excessive accumulation of more mature appearing, but still ineffective, cells and a slower, progressive course (2 to 5 years). The excessive proliferation of the leukemia cells results in an overcrowding of the bone marrow, which causes a decreased production and function of normal hematopoietic cells.

EPIDEMIOLOGY

Leukemia represents 3% of the cancer incidence with an estimated 27,800 new cases and 18,100 deaths expected in 1990.[1,2] Approximately one half of the cases are acute and the remaining cases are chronic, but the number of new cases per year is greater in adults (24,700) than in children (2,200). The most common types of leukemia in adults are acute myelogenous leukemia (AML) and chronic lymphocytic leukemia (CLL), whereas acute lymphocytic leukemia (ALL) accounts for 80% of all childhood leukemias.[3,4] The incidence of leukemia rose steeply from 1900 to the 1940s. Since then the incidence of AML has continued to increase steadily, both in the United States and developing countries, which suggests the influence of occupational and environmental exposure.[5]

ETIOLOGY

The cause of leukemia is not known. The etiologic factors most commonly considered are genetic predisposition, radiation, chemicals, drugs, and viruses.

Genetic Factors

The relationship of genetic factors to the incidence of leukemia has been suggested in terms of certain high-risk families and specific hereditary syndromes. There is evidence of familial clustering with a fourfold to sevenfold increased risk in individuals with a family member diagnosed with leukemia.[6,7] In addition, the disease develops in 10% to 20% of monozygous twins of individuals with leukemia.[6-8] Children with Down's syndrome (trisomy 21) have an 18-fold to 20-fold increased incidence of acute leukemia.[9,10] Other disorders with chromosome abnormalities or fragilities associated with acute leukemia are Bloom's syndrome, Fanconi's anemia, Klinefelter's syndrome, and Ellis-van Creveld syndrome.[3,11]

Diseases such as ataxia telangiectasia and congenital agammaglobulinemia also are prone to terminate in acute leukemia.[6] Although chromosomal abnormalities in these diseases are not detectable, deficiencies exist in humoral and cellular immunity. Whether congenital chromosomal defects cause or coexist with leukemia remains unclear; evidence of chromosomal abnormality and/or fragility appears to favor progression to a malignant state.

In addition to certain genetic factors being associated with the development of leukemia, new techniques in chromosome analysis allow investigators to correlate chromosomal aberrations with survival rates.[12] This should allow the modification of therapy to include intensive or investigational therapy to improve outcome for those with low response rates.

Radiation

Populations exposed to ionizing radiation have an increased incidence of leukemia, especially AML. Japanese survivors of the atomic bomb experienced a 20-fold increased incidence of AML and chronic myelogenous leukemia (CML). There appeared to be a direct relationship with the disease and the distance the individual was from the center of the explosion. The peak incidence was at 5 to 7 years following exposure, and increased risks continued for 20 years.[13,14] In addition, early radiologists exposed to excessive irradiation had a higher incidence of leukemia.[15] Also, patients who were diagnosed with ankylosing spondylitis and treated with 2000 rad (cGy) had a 14-fold increase of AML when compared with similar patients who did not receive irradiation.[16] Radiation remains the most conclusively identified leukemogenic factor in human beings.

Chemicals

Chronic exposure to certain chemicals has been associated with an increased incidence of pancytopenia and subsequent AML. Benzene, an aromatic hydrocarbon, is produced by natural processes and by industry. It was first implicated in the development of acute leukemia in Turkish cobblers in the early 1900s. Since then, other populations have been identified as being at risk, including workers with explosives, distillers, dye users, painters, and shoemakers.[17-21]

Drugs

Drugs that have demonstrated a causative relationship to acute leukemia include certain alkylating agents, the antibiotic chloramphenicol, and phenylbutazone. AML is the most frequently reported second cancer following ag-

TABLE 42-1 Characteristics of Treatment-Induced Acute Nonlymphocytic Leukemia (ANL) Compared to "Spontaneous" ANL

Treatment-Related ANL	"Spontaneous" ANL
Related to prior exposure to alkylating agents and/or radiotherapy	Etiology largely unknown; small % related to chemical exposure (eg, benzene)
Prolonged pancytopenia/preleukemia prior to onset	Approximately 30% present with preleukemia; rest have sudden onset
Latency period 2-5 years postexposure, with peak in incidence approximately 5 years	Latency period unknown
Dysplasia of one or more cell lines on marrow biopsy	May show dysplasia of cell lines
Specific cytogenetic abnormalities of chromosomes 3, 5, 7, 17. Approximately 90% have abnormalities of 5 and/or 7	Specific cytogenetic abnormalities of chromosomes 5, 7, 8, 11, 15, 16, 17, 21, (rarely 3, 4). Less than 5% have abnormalities of 5 and/or7
Refractory to treatment	Responsive to combination chemotherapy
Poor survival; almost uniformly fatal within a few months	Approximately 50% one year survival with some long-term survivors following bone marrow transplant
Peak age varies depending on primary tumor; age of onset about 5 years after treatment for first cancer	Peak age onset in 50s

Source: Fraser MC, Tucker MA: Late effects of cancer therapy: Chemotherapy related malignancies. Oncol Nurs Forum15:67-77,1988.

gressive chemotherapy and is associated with treatment for Hodgkin's disease, multiple myeloma, ovarian cancer, non-Hodgkin's lymphoma, and breast cancer.

Characteristics that distinguish therapy-related and de novo (arising without prior chemotherapy or radiation) leukemia are summarized in Table 42-1.[22] Therapy-related leukemia now represents 10% to 15% of all cases of AML,[23] and the overall median survival period is 4 to 8 months.[24,25] The time of greatest risk appears to be the first 10 years after treatment. Chloramphenicol and phenylbutazone are known to cause aplastic anemia and chromosomal breaks that eventually terminate in AML.[26-28]

Virus

The etiologic role of viruses in human leukemia is unclear. The enzyme reverse transcriptase is present primarily in C-type viruses, a group of RNA viruses that can cause leukemia in animals. This enzyme reverses the usual transcription of genetic information from DNA to RNA, allowing the RNA tumor virus to produce oncogenic DNA within the host cells.[29] There is evidence of horizontal transmission of this leukemogenic virus from cat to cat.[30] Reverse transcriptase has been detected in human leukemic blood cells but not in normal blood cells.

T-cell leukemia in Japan and the Caribbean is associated with the human T-cell lymphotrophic virus (HTLV-I). There is etiologic evidence for a role of HTLV-I in T-cell leukemia in the United States.[31] In addition, HTLV-II probably is involved in hairy cell leukemia, a rare chronic anemia.[32]

CLASSIFICATION

Leukemias are classified as either chronic or acute and as either myeloid or lymphoid. In chronic leukemia the predominant cell is mature-appearing although it does not function normally. The disease has a gradual onset, prolonged clinical course, and a relatively longer survival time. The predominant cell in acute leukemia is undifferentiated or immature, usually a "blast" cell. The abrupt onset and rapid disease progression result in a short survival time. However, as progress is made in the treatment of children with ALL and a longer survival period occurs, it may no longer be appropriate to describe acute leukemia in terms of short survival.

Figure 42-1 presents the major classification of leukemia according to the type of cell that predominates.[33] All cell lines arise from the same totipotent stem cell. From this cell, which has the potential to differentiate into a variety of cells, the myeloid and lymphocyte series are derived. The myeloid stem cell is pluripotent and gives rise to erythrocyte, thrombocyte, and granulocyte progenitors or committed cells. These are immature forms that mature into fully functional red blood cells, platelets, and white blood cells. The lymphoid stem cell matures in the thymus to form T-cell progenitors or in the bone marrow to form B-cell progenitors.

The type of leukemia is named according to the point at which cell maturation is arrested. Although the terms *lymphocytic* and *myelogenous* (nonlymphocytic) leukemia most commonly are used, further specification within each

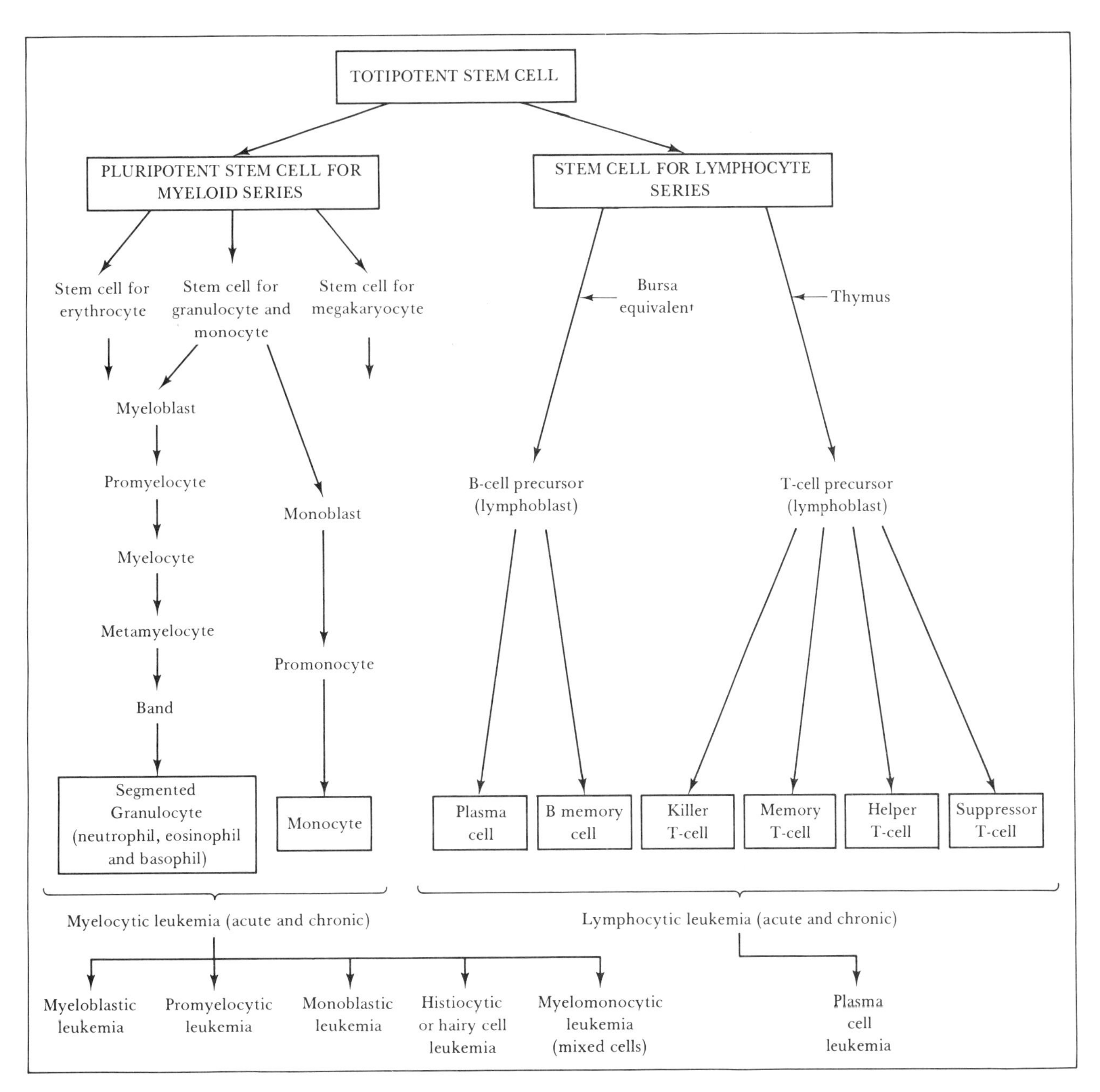

FIGURE 42-1 Hypothetical model of maturation of normal leukocytes and classification of leukemias. The two major classifications of leukemias are (1) the myelocytic leukemias, which arise from the myeloid series, and (2) the lymphocytic leukemias, which arise from the lymphocyte series. The two major classifications are further subdivided, and types of leukemias are named for their predominant cell type. The processes and terminology depicted are based on clinical data rather than on morphologic evidence and are therefore hypothetical.

class (eg, promyelocytic and myelocytic) describes the exact point at which arrest of maturation seems to occur.

In 1976 the French-American-British (FAB) Cooperative group developed criteria for the classification of the acute leukemias[34] (Table 42-2). The purpose was to provide a systematic, objective system that would be practical in most hematologic laboratories. The system, based on morphology and number of cells, has been revised and updated.[35,36] The additional information obtained through cytogenetics, identification of surface markers, and histochemical staining provides important therapeutic and prognostic information.

PATHOPHYSIOLOGY

In the normal bone marrow, efficient regulatory mechanisms ensure that cell proliferation and maturation are

TABLE 42-2 French-American-British (FAB) Classification of Acute Leukemia

Myeloid	Lymphocytic
M1, Undifferentiated myelocytic	L1, Childhood
M2, Myelocytic	L2, Adult
M3, Promyelocytic	L3, Resembles Burkitt's lymphoma
M4, Myelomonocytic	
M5, Monocytic	
M6, Erythroleukemia	
M7, Megakaryocytic	

Source: Data from Bennett et al.[34-36]

adequate for the needs of the individual. In leukemia control is missing or abnormal. The results are (1) arrest of the cell in an early phase of its maturation process, causing the accumulation of immature cells, (2) an abnormal proliferation of these immature cells, and (3) crowding of other marrow elements, resulting in inhibited growth or function of these elements and eventual replacement of the marrow by leukemic cells.

The pathologic defect in leukemia is an abnormal accumulation of immature leukocytes. Although it is often thought that the accumulation of leukocytes is due to a higher than normal mitotic rate, this is not the case. In fact, leukemia cells actually have a slower cell generation cycle than do their normal leukocyte counterparts. Control over their proliferation, however, is lost and more cells are capable of dividing; therefore they continue to divide and accumulate.

Manifestations of leukemia are related to three factors: (1) excessive proliferation of immature leukocytes within blood-forming organs such as the bone marrow, spleen, and lymph nodes, which results in destruction of tissue, (2) infiltration of proliferating leukocytes into various organs of the body, and (3) decrease in the number of normal leukocytes, erythrocytes, and thrombocytes as a result of crowding of the bone marrow by proliferating leukemic cells. Table 42-3 summarizes possible leukemic manifestations, although these vary considerably with each type of leukemia.[33] The presenting manifestations, complications, course of disease, and treatment for each major type are discussed separately (Table 42-4).[33]

Myelodysplastic Syndromes

Myelodysplastic syndromes (MDS) comprise a group of hematologic disorders with an increased risk of transformation to AML. They are characterized by a change in the quantity and quality of bone marrow products. Hematologic disorders that preceded acute leukemia were first reported in the late 1940s and referred to as *preleukemic anemia*.[37] Other terms used are preleukemia, hematopoietic dysplasia, refractory anemia with excess myeloblasts, subacute myeloid leukemia, oligoblastic leukemia, and dysmyelopoietic syndromes.[38]

Currently, myelodysplastic syndromes are divided into five subtypes according to the French-American-British (FAB) Cooperative Group Classification: refractory anemia (RA), refractory anemia with ringed sideroblasts (RARS), refractory anemia with excess blasts (RAEB), refractory anemia with excess blasts in transformation (RAEB-t), and chronic myelomonocytic leukemia (CMML).[39] Table 42-5 lists each type, along with diagnostic criteria, risk of evolution into acute leukemia, and average survival time.[38,39]

MDS are believed to occur as the result of an altered stem cell. The cause is unknown. Chromosome abnormalities are present at the level of the totipotent hematopoietic stem cell. Since MDS can progress to AML, ALL, or a mixed cell leukemia, it appears that both myeloid and lymphoid progenitors are involved.[40]

Approximately 30% of patients diagnosed with AML initially have a preleukemic syndrome.[10] MDS may be considered to be different stages of the same disease. Cases have been noted of transition from one type of MDS to another before transition to AML.[40] Even if the evolution to acute leukemia never occurs, life-threatening anemia, thrombocytopenia, and/or neutropenia invariably occurs. The defect usually is noted in the erythrocyte line first, then in the granulocytes and megakaryocytes.

Twenty percent of patients diagnosed with MDS are older than 50 years of age. The incidence is slightly higher in men than in women.[41] A bone marrow biopsy and aspirate usually reveal a hypercellular marrow with the predominant abnormality being morphologic changes in erythrocyte precursors. Poor prognostic indicators include excessive blast cells in the bone marrow, small clusters of immature myeloid precursors, pancytopenia, and complex chromosome abnormalities.[40] Death usually occurs within 2 years from complications related to bone marrow depression or transformation to acute leukemia.

Treatment for MDS is as aggressive as the course of the disease.[38] Serial bone marrow and peripheral blood examinations allow the physician to monitor the pace of the disease.[42] Supportive therapy includes replacement of red blood cells or platelets and antibiotics for infection. Continuous infusion of low-dose cytosine arabinoside (20 $mg/m^2/day$) is believed to induce differentiation of immature myeloid cells in 25% to 35% of patients with MDS.[40] Other differentiation inducers include retinoic acid, dimethylsulfoxide (DMSO) and vitamin D derivatives.[43] A synthetic androgen, danazol, sometimes is used to elevate platelet levels.[44] For the rare group of patients younger than 30 years of age with a donor matched for human leukocyte antigen (HLA), bone marrow transplantation is the treatment of choice.[38]

TABLE 42-3 Manifestations of Leukemia

	Organ	Manifestations
Primary Manifestations Result from the proliferation of leukocytes within blood-forming organs	Bone marrow	Hyperplasia of abnormal cells Hypoplasia of all normal cellular components Thrombocytopenia leads to bleeding Erythrocytopenia leads to anemia Leukocytopenia leads to infection
	Spleen and liver	Hepatosplenomegaly Changed consistency: Acute leukemia—soft Chronic leukemia—hard Infarction causes pain Hypersplenism leads to pancytopenia
	Lymph nodes	Lymphadenopathy May be painful Obstruction of adjacent organs or structures
Secondary Manifestations Result from the infiltration of leukemic cells into body tissues *or* consequences of bone marrow suppression	Liver	Hepatomegaly May be painful or tender
	Bones, joints, and muscle	Enlargement of the cortex of the long bones in children with acute lymphoblastic leukemia Osteolytic lesions Goutlike symptoms Pain Swelling
	Central nervous system	Thrombosis, Hemorrhage } paralysis Increased intracranial pressure Headache Vomiting
	Skin	Purpura Petechiae Ecchymoses Infection
	Gastrointestinal system	Ulceration Hemorrhage Infection
	Mouth, throat, and nose	Bleeding gums Epistaxis Ulceration Necrosis Infection
	Lungs	Infarction Infection Pleural effusion
	Eyes	Retinal hemorrhage Subconjunctival hemorrhage Papilledema Visual disturbances
	Kidneys	Bilateral asymmetric enlargement Hyperuricemia Rare pyelonephritis leads to renal failure

TABLE 42-4 Comparative Features of the Leukemias at Presentation

Description	Median Age	Initial Remission Rate*	Median Survival with Treatment	Splenomegaly	Infection	Adenopathy	Hemoglobin	White Blood Cell Count	Platelets
Acute myelogenous leukemia	20	50%	1 year	No	Yes	No	Low	Variable	Low
Acute lymphoblastic leukemia	4	Adult 70% Children 90%	2 years 5 years	Yes	Yes	Yes	Low	Variable	Low
Chronic myelogenous leukemia	49	90%	3 years	Yes	No	No	Low	100,000–300,000 granulocytes	Normal or low
Chronic lymphocytic leukemia	60	90%	4–6 years	Yes	Yes	Yes	Low	>20,000 lymphocytes	Low

* Remission is defined as <5% blasts appearing in the bone marrow.

TABLE 42-5 Classification of Myelodysplastic Syndrome with Percentage of Blast Cells, Leukemia Risk, and Average Survival

	Blasts (%)			
Category	Blood	Bone Marrow	Risk of Evolution to Acute Leukemia (%)	Survival (mo)
RA	<1	<5		
			0-25	40-71
RARS	<1	<5		
RAEB	<5	≥5	≤20	
RAEB-t	>5	20-30	27-60	5-20
CMML	<5	1-20		
	$>10^9$ monocytes			

RA, refractory anemia; *RARS*, refractory anemia with ringed sideroblasts; *RAEB*, refractory anemia with excess blasts; *RAEB-t*, refractory anemia with excess blasts in transmission; *CMML*, chronic myelomonocytic leukemia.

Source: Data from Buzaid et al[38] and Bennett et al.[39]

Acute Myelogenous Leukemia

AML, also referred to as *acute nonlymphocytic leukemia*, (ANLL), is a disease of the pluripotent myeloid stem cell. The malignant clone arises in the myeloid, monocytic, erythroid, or megakaryocytic lines. The exact event that triggers the malignant transformation is not known.

The leukemic cells have more abundant cytoplasm, and granulation in the cytoplasm is usually, but not always, present. Auer rods, which are abnormal lysosomal granules, are present in some patients with AML. Multiple nucleoli are present and tend to vary in size.

As previously stated, the type of leukemia is named for the predominant cell. The most common myelogenous leukemia is acute myelocytic leukemia (M1). Acute promyelocytic leukemia (M3) is associated with an increased risk of disseminated intravascular coagulation. This is due to the release of procoagulants from granules within the leukemic promyelocyte, especially during remission-induction therapy.[24] Patients with acute monocytic (M5) or myelomonocytic (M4) leukemia often exhibit extramedullary leukemic infiltration with gingival hypertrophy, cutaneouus leukemia, and liver, spleen, and lymph enlargement.[20] Cytogenetic abnormalities are present in most leukemias, and specific translocations are being increasingly recognized as associated with specific subtypes of leukemia and with prognosis.[45]

Erythroleukemia (M6), which was first described by DiGugliolmo, has both a chronic and an acute form.[3] As the erythroleukemia progresses, the morphologic picture resembles that of myelocytic or myelomonocytic leukemia. Megakaryocytic leukemia (M7), which occurs rarely, is less responsive to chemotherapy.[45]

By the time an individual is diagnosed with AML, the bone marrow and peripheral blood contain up to 10^{12} leukemic cells.[46] The accumulation within the bone marrow space results in inhibition and crowding out of normal marrow stem cells and infiltration of other organs by myeloblasts. Anemia, thrombocytopenia, and neutropenia result. If the disease is untreated, death occurs within a few months because of infection or uncontrolled bleeding.

Acute Lymphocytic Leukemia

ALL is a malignant disease of the lymphoid progenitors. The abnormal clone originates in the marrow, thymus, and lymph nodes, but the exact etiologic event is unknown. The leukemic lymphoblast is nongranular with little cytoplasm. The round nucleus resembles a normal lymphoblast. Although the defect does not involve the myeloid cell lines, the secondary effect of the high leukemic cell burden on the bone marrow interferes with normal hematopoietic activity.

The FAB classification for ALL is based on several cell properties: size; ratio of nucleus to cytoplasm; number, size, and shape of nucleoli; and amount and basophilia of the cytoplasm (Table 42-2).[34-36] In childhood ALL, 85% of cases have L1 morphology whereas the majority of adult cases have L2 morphology. L3 ALL, which resembles Burkitt's lymphoma, is rare.

Another classification system for ALL is based on immune features.[47,48] Four subtypes are identified by the presence of certain markers on the cell surface. Common ALL (C-ALL), which is the most frequent and least differentiated subtype,[49] is identified by the common ALL antigen (cALLa). T-cell markers such as sheep erythrocyte receptors and T-cell specific antigens identify T-cell ALL. Both cALLa and T-cell antigens contain another marker, terminal deoxynucleotidyl transferase (TdT). Other surface and cell immunoglobulins denote the rare B-cell ALL. Last, about one fourth are non-T, non-B, or null leukemias, which do not have any identifiable surface markers.

Lymphoblasts have a propensity for organ infiltration and may remain sequestered in sanctuary sites even after remission has been achieved. Leukemic cells infiltrate into the central nervous system (CNS) early in the disease.[50] Because drugs used for treatment penetrate poorly into the cerebrospinal fluid, the leukemic cells are sheltered from the cytotoxic effects of the drugs. Over time, the leukemic cells proliferate and cause relapse. Other cells can be harbored in the testes.[4] In addition, 80% of patients have lymphadenopathy or splenomegaly, or both, at the time of diagnosis as a result of the infiltration of these organs by leukemic cells.[10]

The prognosis for long-term survival is more favorable for individuals with ALL than with AML inasmuch as drugs are available that are uniquely effective against lymphocytes, for example, prednisone. CNS prophylaxis is used in ALL and has proved successful.

Chronic Myelogenous Leukemia

CML, also called *chronic granulocytic leukemia,* is a disorder of the myeloid stem cell and is characterized by marked splenomegaly and an increased production of granulocytes, especially neutrophils.[51] Approximately 90% of patients with CML have a diagnostic marker, the Philadelphia chromosome (Ph^1). The G group chromosome, number 22, is missing a portion of the long arm (q), which has been translocated to the long arm of number 9.[52,53] The significance of the marker is that a new gene is activated, and it is believed that this gene is related to the cause of CML. Patients with Ph^1-negative CML have been found to have activation of this same gene even though no visible chromosome change is present.[54] In addition, as long as the marker is present, the patient is not cured of the disease.

There is no specific cause for CML, except exposure to ionizing radiation.[53] The peak incidence is in the third and fourth decades, and both sexes are affected equally.[51]

The natural course of CML, is divided into a chronic and terminal phase. The initial chronic phase is characterized by excessive proliferation and accumulation of mature granulocytes and precursors. There is an absence of lymphadenopathy, but 90% of patients have palpable splenomegaly.[51] Within 30 to 40 months the disorder transforms into a terminal phase, which consists of accelerated and blastic phases. The accelerated phase includes progressive leukocytosis with increasing myeloid precursors (including blasts), increasing basophils, splenomegaly, weight loss, and weakness. There is increasing resistance to therapy, and serial cytogenetic studies indicate progressive chromosomal abnormalities.[53]

The blastic phase resembles AML in that 30% to 40% of the bone marrow cells are blasts or promyelocytes. A crisis occurs as blast cell counts rise rapidly, often exceeding 100,000/dL. Leukostatic lesions caused by the high cell count result in occlusion in the microvasculature of the CNS or lungs.[51] The majority have myeloblastic transformation, but some have lymphoblastic transformation evidenced by the presence of TdT or cALL-a. Median survival time after the onset of the terminal phase is 3 months.[52]

Chronic Lymphocytic Leukemia

A progressive accumulation of morphologically normal, but functionally inert, lymphocytes is found in CLL.[55] As the disease progresses, the abnormal lymphocytes accumulate in the bone marrow, spleen, liver, and lymph nodes. In 95% of the cases there is clonal (from a single cell) expansion of neoplastic B lymphocytes.[56] The median age at diagnosis is 60 years, and the majority of cases are in men.[53,57]

The diseased cells usually are small lymphocytes with markers of B lymphocytes and surface IgM or IgD.[46] Approximately one half of the individuals with CLL experience frequent viral and fungal infections caused by hypogammaglobulinemia.[56,57] For more than 25% of patients, the diagnosis is an incidental finding during routine examination. Anemia, lymphadenopathy, or infection may be present. Autoimmune hemolytic anemia, verified by positive results of Coombs' test, occurs in 25% of patients.[46]

The clinical course is variable, and as with the other hematologic malignancies, many attempts have been made to correlate a staging system with prognosis.[58-62] The two most commonly used systems are those of Rai and Binet. The Rai staging system has five levels based on the extent of tissue involvement and compromise of bone marrow function[55] whereas the Binet system identifies three groups, each with a subsequently worsening prognosis.[60] The International Workshop on CLL (IWCLL) attempted to combine the two systems (Table 42-6).[63] Binet et al reviewed numerous systems and concluded that all staging systems defined a high-risk group of patients with anemia and/or thrombocytopenia.[60] In general, treatment

TABLE 42-6 Three Systems for the Classification of Chronic Lymphocytic Leukemia

Rai	Binet	IWCLL	Prognosis
0	A	A(0), A(I), A(II)	Good: >10yr
II	B	B(I), B(II)	Intermediate: <7 yr
III	C	C(III), C(IV)	Poor: <2 yr
IV			

IWCLL, International Workshop on Chronic Lymphocytic Leukemia.

Source: Data from Binet JL, Cavotsky D, Chandra P, et al: Chronic lymphocytic leukemia: Proposals for a revised prognostic staging system. Br J Haematol 48:365-367, 1981.

is withheld until the patient shows evidence of hemolytic anemia, cytopenia, disfiguring or painful lymphadenopathy, symptomatic organomegaly, or marked systemic symptoms.[46]

Hairy Cell Leukemia

An unusual variant of the chronic leukemias is hairy cell leukemia (HCL), so named for the prominent cytoplasmic projections on circulating mononuclear cells. Golomb[64] suggested that these cells share a common stem cell origin with histocytes or monocytes and that the malignant cell is an immunoglobulin-bearing B lymphocyte. HCL also is called *leukemic reticuloendotheliosis.*

Clinically, HCL may be difficult to distinguish from CLL or malignant lymphoma. The distinguishing characteristics are massive splenomegaly and little or no adenopathy. The characteristic hairy cells stain positively for tartrate-resistant acid phosphatase.[46] Two thirds of individuals with HCL have pancytopenia, symptoms of anemia, bleeding, and infection.

The goal of therapy in HCL is palliation inasmuch as no curative therapy has yet been established. Patients without cytopenias require no immediate treatment. Because infection is the primary cause of death, however, patients with HCL should be monitored closely. Splenectomy, which is the treatment of choice for patients with marked pancytopenia, recurrent infections, massive splenomegaly, or rapid disease progression, may prolong survival for up to 15 years.[65] Low-dose daily chlorambucil and leukapheresis are two other treatments useful in HCL.[66] At present, recombinant interferon-alpha is considered the treatment of choice for those in whom disease progresses either before or after splenectomy.[67] Administered daily by intramuscular or subcutaneous injection, interferon-alpha decreases the need for transfusions, reduces risk of infection, and improves overall quality of life.

ACUTE LEUKEMIA

Assessment

Factors that influence symptoms and physical findings are (1) the type of leukemic cell, (2) the degree of leukemic cell burden (early stage or advanced disease), (3) the involvement of organs or systems outside the bone marrow or peripheral circulation, and (4) the depression of normal marrow elements by the leukemic process. For the purpose of this discussion the acute leukemias will be grouped together, and distinctions will be made according to specific subgroups. The chronic leukemias, CML and CLL, are discussed separately.

Patient history

Acute leukemia presents with a large and rapidly growing population of leukemic cells. Usually signs and symptoms have been present for less than 3 months and perhaps for only a few days. Although the diagnosis cannot be made by means of history alone, many of the findings are typical and essential in guiding the diagnostic work-up.

The most common complaints of the patient are nonspecific—that is, fatigue, malaise, weight loss, and fever. The presenting symptoms are the manifestations of the effects of leukemic cells on the normal marrow elements. Infections are recurrent in the common sites such as the skin, gingiva, perianal tissue, lung, and urinary tract. The patient may complain of sore throat and describe fever with or without signs of localized infection. Unexplained bleeding may occur with petechiae and ecchymoses noted in dependent areas. Gingival bleeding may result from a low platelet count or from hypertrophy. Midcycle menstrual flow or heavy bleeding with a period may occur. Symptoms of progressive anemia include fatigue, palpitations, shortness of breath, and anorexia. Pain may arise from several sources: bones such as the sternum, enlarged lymph nodes, and hepatosplenomegaly.

Neurologic complaints are frequent and may signal either leukemic infiltration (especially in ALL) or intracerebral hemorrhage. These include a history of headache, vomiting, visual disturbances, or seizures.

Review of the individual's past medical history may not be significant for diagnosis. It is, however, of etiologic importance to note a history of recurrent infections or bleeding tendencies as well as the type and time of any drug exposure, to attempt documentation of the approximate onset of leukemia. Similarly, the occupational (especially chemical and radiation exposure) and family history of genetic abnormalities or cancer contributes to the total epidemiologic picture.

An essential part of the initial history that serves as a baseline for understanding the individual and planning care is the psychosocial profile. Questions that elicit details concerning past and present coping strategies with illness or other crises should be asked. Determination of significant others may be made by asking such questions as, "Who can you talk to most easily about your illness?" Finally, the nurse must ascertain how the patient and family perceive the illness and what their previous experience with hospitalization has been.

Physical examination

The physical findings of acute leukemia usually relate directly to the effects of pancytopenia. Vital signs may reveal fever, tachycardia, and tachypena. The skin and mucous membranes generally appear pale, with readily apparent ecchymoses or petechiae. Generalized or localized adenopathy may be present as a result of leukemic infiltration or infection.

A comprehensive physical examination serves to validate findings elicited in a complete history and review of symptoms. Ophthalmoscopic examination may reveal retinal capillary hemorrhage or papilledema caused by leukostasis or thrombocytopenia-induced bleeding and/or increased intracranial pressure. An oral infection with *Candida albicans* may be present. Examination of the lungs and heart may reveal the effects of anemia (cardiac murmurs) or infection (abnormal lung sounds). Abdominal palpation may demonstrate hepatosplenomegaly or enlarged kidneys as a result of leukemic infiltration, especially in children with ALL. Perirectal tissue may be tender and swollen and the only evidence of an abscess or a fistula. Finally, gentle palpation of bones and joints may reveal swelling and elicit pain.

Diagnostic studies

Laboratory and radiographic studies are essential for proper diagnosis. It is important to distinguish AML from ALL because the treatment and prognosis differ markedly. An ongoing explanation to the patient and family of the plan and purpose of the exhaustive diagnostic workup will facilitate cooperation, decrease anxiety, and create an atmosphere of confidence and trust.

The diagnosis is suggested by the peripheral smear but requires a full examination of the bone marrow. The white blood cell count may be low, normal, or high, and 90% of patients have blast cells in the peripheral blood. Neutropenia (absolute granulocyte count <1000 cells/mm^3) is frequent, and thrombocytopenia is present in 40% of patients. Blood chemistry studies may reveal hyperuricemia and increased lactic dehydrogenase, as well as altered serum and urine muramidase levels (greatly increased with monocytic and myelomonocytic leukemia but normal to low with lymphoblastic leukemia). If acute promyelocytic leukemia (M3) is suspected, laboratory evaluation should include determinations of plasma fibrinogen, fibrin split products, and prothrombin time.

Bone marrow contents usually are hypercellular, with 60% to 90% blasts in the differential blood count. Auer rods are diagnostic of AML, as well as are special stains (Sudan black B fat stain and peroxidase).

Cytogenetic analysis demonstrates that 30% to 50% of patients have chromosomal abnormalities that disappear during remission and reappear with recurrence of the leukemia. Surface antigen markers can distinguish B-cell ALL and T-cell ALL and confirm the FAB categories of AML.

Treatment

The two major objectives for the therapeutic management of leukemia are (1) to reduce or eradicate the population of leukemic cells and (2) to support the patient's adaptation process throughout the course of illness. The degree to which these objectives will be met depends on the type of leukemia, the extent of the disease, the availability of sophisticated treatment resources, and the individual's state of health. Within this context the nursing care plan will reflect the nurse's understanding of the specific disease process as it affects each person. Appropriate management, which includes teaching, intervention, and evaluation, must be seen as a complex, interdisciplinary process that is carried out over a prolonged period of time. By setting realistic short- and long-term goals, the staff and patient can most successfully deal with a disease that offers periods of wellness, acute life-threatening events, and/or chronic debilitation that results in death.

The primary treatment for acute leukemia is chemotherapy. Immunotherapy remains controversial as an effective treatment method. Leukemic cells are relatively sensitive to radiotherapy, but the current use is for CNS prophylaxis. The current accepted treatments for AML and ALL are described in the following sections. Specific regimens may vary slightly from one institution to another.

Acute myelogenous leukemia

The goal of antileukemic treatment for AML is the eradication of the leukemic stem cell. Complete remission is defined as the restoration of normal peripheral counts and fewer than 5% blasts in the bone marrow.[68] Treatment regimens capable of inducing a complete remission are composed of several drugs, each of which is known to be effective against leukemic myeloblasts. The course of therapy is divided into two stages: induction and postremission therapy.

Induction therapy The goal of induction therapy is to cause severe bone marrow hypoplasia. At diagnosis the leukemic cells are proliferating more slowly than normal myeloid precursors. Therefore the myeloid stem cells repopulate the depleted marrow faster than leukemic cells. The cornerstone for remission induction is the cell cycle–specific antimetabolite cytosine arabinoside plus an anthracycline (daunorubicin, doxorubicin, mitoxantrone, amsacrine, or idarubicin).[69,70] It is theorized that a drug that is non-cycle-specific will have a synergistic effect when given sequentially with a cell cycle–specific drug by causing proliferating cells to enter the cell cycle concurrently.

Cytosine arabinoside is administered for 7 days, and the anthracycline is given for 3 days. This protocol is called "7 + 3",[71] but variations include 5-day or 10-day infusions of cytosine arabinoside. Gale and Foon,[72] in a review of the results of eight clinical studies, reported a complete response rate of 50% to 75%, with the best results in the protocols with 7 days of cytosine arabinoside.

The impact of the chemotherapy is assessed at 1 week after the completion of therapy, with a bone marrow biopsy and aspiration on day 14. If residual leukemia is present, a second course is begun. Bone marrow recovery usually takes 14 to 21 days after the end of the chemotherapy, with median time to complete recovery at 28 to 32 days. After extensive review of current studies, Mayer[73] concluded that complete response should now be observed in 65% to 70% of previously untreated adults with a complete remission rate in the 75% range if the patient is younger than 60 years of age. Unfortunately, in spite of improving remission rates, only 20% of patients remain in complete remission. Relapse occurs in the remaining cases within 1 to 2 years.[74,75] Thus postremission therapy is essential.

Postremission therapy By the addition of postremission therapy the median duration of remission can be increased from 4 to 8 months to 10 to 15 months.[73] Wolff et al[76] have used high-dose cytosine arabinoside to increase the continuing complete remission rate to 51%. The goal of further therapy is to prevent leukemic recurrence related to undetectable, resistant disease, also called *minimal residual disease*. Terms used to describe postremission therapies include *consolidation, intensification*, and *maintenance*.[77]

Consolidation therapy consists of one or two courses of very high doses of the same drugs used for induction. Up to 30 times the induction doses of cytosine arabinoside are used to consolidate the remission.[75] Although the patient is in a healthier state for this part of the treatment, the toxic effects are substantial, with extended myelosuppression, cerebellar dysfunction, dermatitis, hepatic dysfunction, and conjunctivitis. The longest remissions appear to occur after two or more courses of consolidation therapy, with a median remission of 1 to 2 years.[70]

Intensification may occur right after remission induction (early intensification) or several months later (late intensification), and different drugs are used with the hope that they will be noncross-resistant with the induction drugs. The terminology is somewhat confusing in various clinical investigations.

Maintenance therapy describes treatment with lower doses of the same or other drugs given monthly for a prolonged period of time. Maintenance therapy is not currently recommended in the treatment of AML.[73,77]

Because microscopic disease is being treated in postremission therapy, it is difficult to know how much treatment is enough. Investigation continues to determine the optimal curative treatment.

Patients who relapse after induction and postinduction chemotherapy have a 30% to 60% likelihood of achieving a second remission.[72,78,79] Leukemic cells acquire increasing resistance to chemotherapy. The cellular kinetics change because of an increased growth fraction and shortened generation time, resulting in a decreasing doubling time.[68] The second and subsequent remissions are influenced by prior treatment, length of remission, and the initial response to therapy. Patients whose relapses occur quickly or who have resistant leukemia should be considered for clinical trials or bone marrow transplantation.[79]

The role of bone marrow transplantation (BMT) in the treatment of AML remains controversial.[80,81] Approximately 40% of patients with AML are younger than 40 years of age. Of those, approximately 40% have an HLA-matched donor. Therefore only 16% or fewer of patients with AML are eligible for an allogeneic transplantation.[68] In patients younger than 30 years of age, bone marrow transplantation may offer a higher cure rate than does standard treatment. In patients in the fourth decade the results of chemotherapy versus BMT vary. Transplantation centers usually do not admit patients older than the age of 50 years. Because BMT carries the risk of graft-versus-host disease, interstitial pneumonia, and infection with cytomegalovirus, the decision for BMT is not easy. The question of optimal timing for transplantation remains unanswered. (See Chapter 15 for an in-depth discussion of bone marrow transplantation.)

A final consideration in the treatment of AML is the significance of prognostic factors. Prognostic indicators may be useful in determining the best course of therapy for AML (Table 42-7).[4,70,82,83] For example, patients with unfavorable factors such as older age or multiple chromosomal abnormalities may be treated with high-dose or investigational drugs. In a younger patient with an unfavorable morphologic subtype, bone marrow transplantation may be preferred to consolidation therapy.

Acute lymphocytic leukemia

As with AML, long-term survival and cure for individuals with ALL is possible only if complete remission is achieved. This is documented by a bone marrow aspirate containing fewer than 5% lymphoblasts and the disappearance of all peripheral manifestations of the disease.

In contrast to AML current chemotherapeutic regimens proven effective against ALL contain drugs that are selectively toxic to lymphoblasts and relatively sparing of normal hematopoietic stem cells. Therefore the patient experiences hypoplasia that is less severe and of shorter duration with greater leukemic cell kill. In addition, relapses may be more effectively treated because the marrow is better able to recover.

The focus of therapy for ALL is to eradicate all leukemic cells from the marrow and lymph tissue and eliminate any residual foci of disease within the CNS. Treatment is divided into three stages: induction, CNS prophylaxis, and maintenance.

Induction therapy Although it is possible to achieve complete remission in 93% of children with ALL by using a combination of vincristine, prednisone, and L-asparaginase,[84] the same drugs, even with the addition of an anthracycline, produce remission rates of only 70% to 75%

TABLE 42-7 Prognostic Factors in Acute Leukemia

	Poor Prognosis	Favorable Prognosis
Acute myelogenous leukemia	Age > 60 yr M4, M5, M6 Chromosome abnormalities: −5/5q −; −7/7q− t(6;9); t(4;11); t(9;22) Prior radiation/chemotherapy, prior MDS, infection at diagnosis	Age <60 yr M3 Chromosome abnormalities: t(15;17); t(8;21) inversion 16
Acute lymphocytic leukemia	Age > 60 yr L3 WBC >25,000/L T cell (children) Male Chromosome abnormalities: t(9;22); t(4;11); t(8;14) CNS involvement	Age <60 yr L1, L2 T cell (adults) Female

M3, Promyelocytic; M4, myelomonocytic; M5, monocytic; M6, erythroleukemia; MDS, myelodysplastic syndrome; L1, L2, L3, French-American-British classification of acute lymphocytic leukemia.

Source: Data from Maguire,[4] Clarkson et al,[50] Champlin,[70] Keating et al,[82] Priesler et al,[83] and Hoelzer and Gale.[85]

in adults with ALL.[44,84,85] Therapy usually begins in the hospital, but the duration of hypoplasia is shorter than with AML treatment. Once remission is documented, the therapy is completed on an outpatient basis.

CNS prophylaxis Meningeal leukemia is present at diagnosis in about 2% of patients and occurs in up to 50% of patients with ALL in the absence of CNS prophylaxis.[49,86] By comparison, in patients with AML the incidence is less than 5%. Leukemic lymphoblasts enter the leptomeninges either by direct extension from the blood of the meningeal vessels or by seeding from thrombocytopenic bleeding. The cells extend deeply into the cerebral sulci and nerve sheaths, causing a mechanical obstruction of the cerebrospinal fluid (CSF). If unchecked, hydrocephaly and death occur. Several factors may explain the increased incidence of CSF infiltration with ALL.[87] There is selective tendency for lymphoblasts rather than myeloblasts to enter the CNS. Drugs used in ALL enter the CSF slowly or in concentrations too low to be cytotoxic. The slower proliferation of lymphoblasts in the CSF may require longer drug exposure. Signs and symptoms of CNS leukemia include headache, blurred vision, nausea/vomiting, or cranial nerve palsies.[49]

CNS prophylaxis should start within a few weeks of the initiation of therapy. Treatment usually includes intracranial radiation and intrathecal methotrexate.[50,70,88,89] Cranial radiation delivered in fractionated doses of 200 cGy up to a total dose of 2400 cGy produces predictable penetration of leukemic cells regardless of CSF dynamics. This therapy also can kill or sterilize cells not undergoing cell division. However, there are now recognized side effects of this therapy, which include somnolence, chemical meningitis, paraparesis, and leukoencephalopathy.[49,89]

Maintenance therapy As in AML, even after complete remission patients with ALL harbor remaining leukemic cells. Relapse occurs in 2 to 3 months without continuing therapy. Prolonged chemotherapy may lead to a 40% overall cure rate, but the type and duration are not completely defined.[50] Methotrexate and 6-mercaptopurine may be added to the drug regimen used during induction,[4,89] and therapy often continues for 2 to 3 years.

The outlook for patients in whom relapse occurs during therapy is poor, and younger patients with an HLA-matched donor should be immediately referred for BMT.[88] If relapse occurs after the completion of therapy, treatment is continued with high-dose methotrexate, tenopiside, and cytarabine, or high-dose cytosine arabinoside with an anthracycline or amsacrine. Second remission can be achieved in up to 50% of cases.[85]

Prognostic factors also are important in planning treatment for ALL. They are summarized in Table 42-7.[50,70,85] Because patients treated with allogeneic BMT show a trend toward longer survival if the transplantation is performed during the first remission,[80] it is important to identify patients with unfavorable prognosis in the early stages of disease.

CHRONIC MYELOGENOUS LEUKEMIA

Assessment

CML may be diagnosed in the absence of any symptoms in up to 20% of individuals with the disease.[53] Most patients, however, have a history that reflects the gradual accumulation of a white blood cell mass that is 10 to 150 times the normal amount.

Patient history

The initial symptoms typically include those related to massive splenomegaly as a result of infiltration of the spleen by leukemic cells: pain in the upper left portion of the abdomen, early satiety, and vague abdominal fullness. Leukemic infiltration of joints also may cause bone and joint pain. A history of malaise, fatigue, weight loss, and fever caused by a gradually worsening hypercatabolic state may precede more acute symptoms of anemia.[90]

To a lesser extent than in acute leukemia, epidemiologic clues may be provided by a complete past medical and family history, such as a history of exposure to ionizing radiation or a family history of leukemia.

Physical examination

The vast majority of individuals are diagnosed during the chronic phase of their disease. The individual with anemia appears pale. Examination of the eyes, ears, nose, and throat may reveal leukemic infiltration. Splenomegaly and hepatomegaly are common.

The physical examination of the patient in blast crisis is similar to that for the patient with acute leukemia. In blast crisis, blastic transformation of the leukemic granulocytes has replaced the bone marrow, causing an acute illness and pancytopenia, infection, and hypercatabolism. Rapid diagnosis and treatment to reduce the number of proliferating blasts are essential.

Diagnostic studies

A complete blood cell count in the chronic phase reveals anemia and severe leukocytosis, that is, a white blood cell count (WBC) greater than 100,000 mm^3. The differential count of the leukocytes demonstrates white blood cells in every stage of maturation, with a predominance of more mature cells. The presence of functional, although leukemic granulocytes, accounts for the low incidence of infection during the chronic phase. There usually is moderate anemia and thrombocytosis. The anemia is normocytic and normochromic, with a median hemoglobin value of 9 to 10 g/dL.[53]

Other laboratory studies reveal high serum B_{12} levels and a low leukocyte alkaline phosphatase level.[52,91] Both may return to normal with successful therapy.[51] Bone marrow biopsy demonstrates hyperplasia with a myeloid to erythroid ratio of 15:1 and normal to increased megakaryocytes (platelet precursors). The abnormal Ph^1 chromosome is found in the granulocytic, erythrocytic, and megakaryocytic series of the marrow and confirms the diagnosis of CML.[92]

Treatment

The only chance for cure of CML is with ablation of the Ph^1 chromosome. Currently, this occurs after high-dose therapy followed by BMT. CML is a chronic disease and usually is suppressed by chemotherapy with hydroxyurea or busulfan. Late in the disease or at blastic crisis, investigational drugs are used. Recently, interferon has been found useful in early disease.[93]

Chronic phase

The standard therapy during the chronic phase is single-agent oral chemotherapy.[91,92] Busulfan, an alkylating agent, is active against primitive hematopoietic stem cells. The WBC begins to drop 10 to 14 days after therapy is begun. To prevent prolonged or severe myelosuppression, treatment is stopped if the WBC is less than 20,000/mm^3. Long-term side effects include skin hyperpigmentation and pulmonary or retroperitoneal fibrosis. Hydroxyurea is cytostatic to cycling cells and inhibits ribonucleotide reductase. It acts on late progenitor stem cells, which causes rapid disease control but requires frequent monitoring of blood levels. Because the toxic effects of hydroxyurea on pulmonary and bone marrow tissue are not long-term, it may be a better choice if future BMT is a consideration.[93] Although these drugs decrease the leukemic cell mass and improve the quality of life, the progression to a terminal, refractory stage is not altered.

Terminal phase

CML is a chronic neoplasm with a 100% incidence of blastic transformation.[94] This transformation, also described as a metamorphosis,[94] is a gradual failure of response to treatment and failure of production of erythrocytes and platelets. Serial cytogenetic analyses can reveal signs of blastic transformation by 3 to 4 months before clinical signs are evident. Bone marrow aspirations, however, are required, which are costly and uncomfortable for the patient.[52] The current trend is to treat the accelerated phase by continuing chronic phase therapy until evidence of the blastic phase appears. Because the transformation from benign to malignant state appears to be random in length, it is difficult to predict survival, although life expectancy is less than 1 year.[94]

Blast crisis requires intensive chemotherapy, similar to that used in the treatment of AML. If the transformation is myeloblastic, therapy includes cytosine arabinoside, an anthracycline, and thioguanine. If lymphoblastic transformation has occurred, vincristine and prednisone are added. Patients in whom lymphoblastic transformation develops are more responsive to treatment and live longer.[95]

In a review of 18 clinical investigaitons, Talpaz et al[93] concluded the median survival from diagnosis has increased from 19 months for untreated patients to a range of 30 to 45 months for those who receive conventional, single-agent therapy. The range for those treated with intensive therapy (during the chronic phase) is 50 to 65 months.

Although BMT remains the only chance for cure, it is an option for only 25% of patients.[91] The best results have been obtained in patients who receive allogeneic BMT during the chronic phase, with 55% to 70% being disease free at 3 to 5 years.[96] Both autologous and allogeneic transplantations are being performed. Other promising therapies include the use of interferon[93] and "differentiating" agents such as *cis*-retinoic acid or 5-azacytidine,[52] which induce differentiation of cells to more mature forms.

CHRONIC LYMPHOCYTIC LEUKEMIA

Assessment

Diagnosis of CLL is made in one fourth of individuals with CLL during a routine physical examination. Clues that alert the clinician early on, however, may be provided by a complete health history.

Patient history

Early CLL may produce no symptoms. Because CLL is a disease of immunoglobulin-secreting cells, however, a history of recurrent infections, especially of the skin and respiratory tract, may be elicited. The onset, location, duration, and response to treatment for infection should be documented.

Progressive infiltration and accumulation in nodal structures and the bone marrow gradually produce the symptoms that are typical of more advanced disease. Vague complaints of malaise, anorexia, and fatigue are common, as is noticeable and bothersome lymphadenopathy. Splenomegaly may cause early satiety and abdominal discomfort. The past medical history should focus on the documentation of any underlying autoimmune or immune-deficiency diseases, bleeding tendencies, and infectious episodes.

Physical examination

The individual with early CLL appears to be well. Splenomegaly may be the only clincal finding. In advanced disease there may be evidence of infection, fever and rashes. Lymphadenopathy occurs in 60% of patients, especially cervical, axillary, inguinal, and femoral nodes. The nodes are described as mobile, discrete and nontender.[56]

Diagnostic studies

Peripheral blood examination reveals lymphocytosis with normal or immature lymphocytes. The lymphocyte count is greater than 20,000/mm^3 in early disease and may be more than 100,000 cells/mm^3 in advanced disease. Protein electrophoresis documents the hypogammaglobulinemia that occurs in approximately 50% of patients.

Bone marrow aspirate reflects the lymphocytosis seen peripherally, with varying degrees of infiltration. The severity of infiltration depends on the severity of the disease. Although early CLL causes patchy or focal infiltrates of the mature-appearing lymphocytes, progressive disease leads to a "packed marrow" with few normal hematopoietic cells. Lymph node biopsy may be interpreted as well-differentiated lymphocytic lymphoma if the blood count and bone marrow findings are unknown to the pathologist.

Treatment

In general, treatment consists only of observation until the patient is symptomatic with cytopenia or organomegaly.[56] The rate of progressive lymphocytosis directs the frequency of observation and start of therapy. Patients may show a fluctuating moderate lymphocytosis for many years with no treatment at all.

Chlorambucil and cyclophosphamide are two alkylating agents used to treat CLL.[57,97] Chlorambucil is more effective in suppressing growth of well-differentiated, small lymphocytes. Cyclophosphamide suppresses growth of less mature lymphocytes, with relative sparing of neutrophils and platelets. These drugs provide a response rate of 60%, with complete remission in 10% to 20% of patients. There is a concern, however, that prolonged use of alkylating agents may cause development of AML.[97,98]

Corticosteroids are used to control leukocytosis and immunomediated cytopenias. When the patient no longer responds to steroid therapy, splenectomy may provide relief of symptoms.[97]

Radiation therapy may be used to treat lymphadenopathy or painful splenomegaly. Total body irradiation and extracorporeal irradiation of blood to reduce lymphocyte counts are being investigated at this time.[56]

For patients with advanced disease (stage III or IV) and anemia or thrombocytopenia, combination therapy is recommended.[60] This includes cyclophosphamide, vincristine, doxorubicin, and prednisone. Future studies include the use of interferon and monoclonal antibodies in the treatment of CLL[97,99]

SUPPORTIVE THERAPY

The increase in the length and quality of survival in leukemia is due not only to advances in antileukemic therapy but also to improved blood product and antimicrobial support and specialized nursing care. The complex means of providing effective supportive care includes medical management to maintain physiologic homeostasis and an interdisciplinary approach to the health care plan.

Effective nursing participation in the supportive care of any patient with leukemia depends on an understanding of the staging and natural history of each of the leukemias. From this base of knowledge the nurse contributes to the care of the patient with leukemia in each of the following areas: education, physical care, symptom management, and, psychosocial adaptation.

Education

Providing information related to the disease process and treatment is clearly a standard in oncology nursing.[100,101] The nurse caring for the patient with AML has the unique opportunity of providing information to the patient and family because the patient usually is hospitalized throughout the course of therapy. The teaching plan for all patients includes pertinent information related to the diagnosis, strategies for self-care in the prevention and treatment of side effects both in the hospital setting and at home, and methods to facilitate coping and adaptation to the illness.

For all patients with leukemia it is helpful to include the basic physiology of the bone marrow in the teaching plan. A hematologic malignancy is not as easy to understand as the concept of a solid tumor. Describing bone marrow as the center of the bone in which all blood prod-

White Blood Cells Fight Infection	Red Blood Cells Carry Oxygen	Platelets Control Bleeding
If bone marrow is not producing enough cells:		
1. may develop infection	1. anemia	1. may have nosebleeds
2. may develop sore mouth	2. feel out of breath	2. gums may bleed
	3. feel weak or tired	3. may notice bruises
		4. blood in urine or stool
Treatment:		
1. prevent infection	1. transfusions	1. prevent bleeding
		2. transfusions
Report to doctor or nurse:		
1. fever over 100°	1. feeling out of breath	1. nosebleed that will not stop
2. excess cough and sputum production	2. increasing weakness	2. blood in stool
3. burning with urination		3. cloudy urine

FIGURE 42-2 Blood cell production.

ucts are made is a simple start. Further explanation includes the type, function, and abnormalities of the blood cells (Figure 42-2). From this base, individualized instruction related to the specific leukemia is given. Educational materials can be obtained from the Leukemia Society, American Cancer Society, and the National Cancer Institute. Information for contacting these organizations is found in Yellow Pages: Cancer Nursing Resources at the end of this book.

Physical Care

The physical care needs of patients with leukemia require nurses who are skilled in physical assessment and experienced in the use of right atrial catheters (RACs) and vascular access devices (VADs). Patients with AML receive intensive therapy aimed at producing bone marrow aplasia for several weeks. Those with ALL who have defective lymphocytes that produce altered immunocompetence, are also receiving cytotoxic drugs. The hypogammaglobulinemia associated with CLL increases the patient's susceptibility to viral and fungal infections. In any type of leukemia the incidence of infection is high, but the usual signs and symptoms of infection are diminished or absent. Therefore the nurse must regularly conduct a thorough physical examination to detect any evidence of infection during each shift. Subtle changes in vital signs and mentation may indicate early sepsis. Oozing of blood from gums and intravenous sites may be the first signs of disseminated intravascular coagulation. Toxic effects related to chemotherapy to the cerebellum may be manifested as slightly altered responses in the neurologic examination. Each of these situations may be life threatening, and the skills of the experienced nurse may be the crucial factor in initiating appropriate treatment.

A double- or triple-lumen RAC often is placed before aggressive induction therapy is begun in hospitalized patients. These are used for blood sampling and for the infusion of fluids, chemotherapy, antibiotics, total parenteral nutrition, and blood products.[102] Patients who require ongoing treatment but less frequent blood sampling and no simultaneous infusion of multiple fluids may have a VAD placed subcutaneously.[103] The advantages, disadvantages, and nursing procedures associated with RAC and VAD are beyond the scope of this chapter. However, inasmuch as one of these devices is used in most patients with acute leukemia, it is important for the nurse to become familiar with them.

Symptom Management

Certain side effects associated with antileukemic therapy and disease-related complications can best be ameliorated if detected early and treated promptly. Knowing which side effects are expected and when they may occur allows the nurse to focus care appropriately.

Bone marrow depression

The desired effect of cytotoxic therapy is bone marrow hypoplasia. The duration of pancytopenia is variable, depending on the type of therapy and the person's ability to recover. However, acute leukemia in the induction phase or CML in blast crisis may cause severe hypoplasia for weeks at a time.

Neutropenia It takes 9 to 10 days for immature cells formed in the bone marrow to become mature granulocytes. Because granulocytes circulate for only 6 to 10 hours, any interruption in their production quickly places the patient at risk for infection. Infection is the major complication for patients with leukemia, with a 20% to 30% mortality rate.[74] Neutropenia commonly is defined as an absolute neutrophil count lower than 1000/mm^3. Because the neutrophils are responsible for phagocytosis, neutropenia eliminates one of the body's first lines of defense against infection. The patient with leukemia is particularly at risk as a result of a rapid drop in WBCs with the initiation of therapy, a continuing decrease until the nadir (lowest point) is reached, and a prolonged recovery time.[104]

Infection develops in approximately 60% of individuals with neutropenia. One third have documented bacteremia, another third have documented infection without bacteremia, and the final third have apparent infection with no microbiologically documented pathogen. The risk of infection rises as the neutrophil count decreases, with 100% incidence of infection if the neutrophil count remains lower than 100/mm^3 for 3 weeks.[105] Other factors that add to the risk of infection are corticosteroids, hospital environment, antibiotic agents that lead to increased colonization, and mucosal alteration.[106]

Adrenal corticosteroids frequently are used as part of the chemotherapeutic regimen or as supportive therapy. Steroids cause lysis of lymphocytes, suppression of antibody production, protein malnutrition, and suppression of inflammatory responses. As a result, the use of corticosteroids predisposes the patient to infection.

Most infections are due to organisms endogenous to the host or present in the environment.[107] The most common sites of infection are the alimentary tract (pharynx, esophagus, anorectum), sinuses, lungs, and skin.[104,108] The alimentary mucosa is directly damaged by the chemotherapy, and neutropenia allows colonization with yeasts and/or gram-negative bacilli. Perianal infection occurs in 25% of patients with AML, and the only signs may be induration, erythema, and pain on defecation. Pneumonia can be caused by gram-negative organisms such as *Pseudomonas aeruginosa*, *Klebsiella pneumoniae*, and *Escherichia coli*. The most common gram-positive organism that causes infection is *Staphylococcus epidermidis*.[104,108]

More serious infections associated with prolonged neutropenia are fungal infections with *Candida* species or *Aspergillus* or protozoa such as *Pneumocystis carinii*. When these infections occur during severe aplasia and immunodepression, recovery of the blood counts is the best hope for survival.[3]

Empiric antibiotic therapy is used to treat patients at high risk (those with neutropenia and fever) until an infecting organism is identified. Early empiric antibiotic therapy includes drugs to cover both gram-negative and gram-positive organisms. The usual combinations include an aminoglycoside plus an extended-spectrum cephalosporin or a broad-spectrum antipseudomonal penicillin.[104,106,109] There currently is a trend toward initial broad-spectrum monotherapy.[110]

Amphotericin B is used to treat life-threatening fungal infections in myelosuppressed, immunosuppressed individuals. It is indicated if fever continues for 5 to 7 days after the start of antibiotic therapy, if there is no identified source of infection, and if continued neutropenia is expected.[106] Side effects of this toxic therapy include fever, chills, and rigors (80% to 90%), nephrotoxicity (90%), headache (45%), anorexia (50%), vomiting (20%), and anemia.[111,112] Because anaphylaxis is a risk, a test dose of 1 mg is administered over 30 minutes. If cardiopulmonary or mental changes do not occur, the starting dose is given. Fever is not a contraindication when the patient has recurrent fevers before therapy. The dose is escalated daily until the desired dose is reached and therapy continues for weeks to months, depending on the organism being treated and the patient's response.

Symptom managment includes the following interventions to prevent or treat fever, chills, or rigors: premedication with corticosteroids, acetaminophen, diphenhydramine, and the addition of 10 to 15 mg hydrocortisone sodium succinate to the infusion. Intravenous meperidine, 25 to 50 mg, is given at the onset of chills or as a premedication.[111,112] Increasing room temperature, adding extra covers, and using relaxation, hypnosis, and isometric leg and arm movements are other suggested comfort measures.[113] Potential nephrotoxicity as a result of a decreased glomerular filtration rate requires close monitoring of blood urea nitrogen, creatinine, potassium, and magnesium levels, as well as evaluation of fluid balance. Peripheral phlebitis can be avoided by adding heparin to the solution. The anemia associated with amphotericin B is reversible and a problem only in that it compounds the existing myelosuppression.

Because the patient with neutropenia does not produce an adequate inflammatory response to infection, the usual signs and symptoms are absent. Fever usually is the first sign of infection, which then leads to closer inspection of high-risk areas (perirectal area, oral mucosa, sites of intravenous lines). Patients often are unable to produce sputum; thus the early indications of pneumonia are shortness of breath or cough. Vital signs are assessed every 4 hours. At the onset of fever higher than 100°F in the patient with neutropenia, blood, urine, and sputum cultures are obtained and empiric antibiotic therapy is initated. The importance of prompt reporting of fever and initiation of therapy cannot be overemphasized because delay of only a few hours can allow the patient to go into septic shock.

Prevention of infection focuses on restoring host defenses, decreasing invasive procedures, and decreasing colonization of organisms. Treatment and remission induction will restore normal defenses against infection. Decreasing invasive procedures includes avoiding the use of Foley catheters. If catheterization is necessary, the smallest possible lumen should be used and the catheter should be anchored. Other measures are meticulous care of intravenous sites or RAC exit sites and aseptic technique for any invasive procedure.

To decrease the number of gram-negative organisms, uncooked fruits and vegetables are avoided, especially salads. *P. aeruginosa* can be decreased by removing aerators from faucets, using ice machines in which the ice falls directly into the cup, and frequent changing of stagnant water sources such as oxygen humidifiers. Proper handwashing techniques by everyone in contact with the patient can eliminate the main source of gram-positive organisms. Fungi that are found in food or the air also can be decreased by cooking foods and eliminating live plants or flowers from the patient's room. A private room is necessary and visitors are restricted. All these measures are to be practiced by the health care team and taught to the patient and family.[114-116] Further information is provided in Chapter 21.

In certain circumstances such as BMT, total reverse isolation may be used. The patient is kept in a sterile laminar air flow room. Nonabsorbable antibiotics are used to sterilize the alimentary canal. Normal skin flora is decreased by frequent cleansing with hexachlorophene or an iodine-base soap.[3,74]

Granulocyte transfusions may be indicated for patients with profound neutropenia and documented infections unresponsive to antibiotics.[108,117] However, the hazards of this therapy (increased alloimmunization and refractoriness to platelet transfusions) and the high cost make it a controversial therapy.

Erythrocytopenia Tolerance for chronic low-grade anemia develops in individuals undergoing intensive chemotherapy. However, in severe cases of hypoplasia, sudden blood loss due to bleeding, or symptomatic anemia, support with transfusions of red blood cells is required. Premedication with acetaminophen and diphenhydramine can decrease the febrile response to antibodies to white cells that occurs after multiple transfusions. Leukocyte-poor red blood cells may be used to decrease the antibody production against antigens on the leukocytes.[118]

Thrombocytopenia Thrombocytopenia is the abnormal decrease in the number of circulating platelets. The potential for bleeding occurs when levels reach ≤50,000 platelets/mm^3 and spontaneous bleeding occurs at levels of ≤20,000 platelets/mm^3.[116] The first evidence of bleeding may be petechiae or ecchymoses on the skin of dependent limbs or mucous membranes or oozing from gums, nose, or intravenous sites.

Random donor platelets are given to keep the platelet count greater than 20,000/mm^3.[74] Once antibodies to the platelets develop, refractoriness to random donor platelets occurs. When blood counts 1 hour after transfusion reveal poor increments, the patient may require HLA-matched single-donor platelets.[108] Because chills and fever can destroy circulating platelets, the patient is premedicated with acetaminophen and diphenhydramine.[109] Additional measures used to prevent bleeding include maintaining skin integrity, preventing trauma, and avoiding medications that have the potential to induce or prolong bleeding. Stool softeners will prevent the Valsalva maneuver and rectal tears. (See Chapter 22.)

Complications

Certain complications of the specific leukemic process or therapy may be singled out as untoward, but not unexpected, side effects. Knowledge of these occurrences assists the nurse in anticipating problems in individuals at high risk. These complications include leukostasis, disseminated intravascular coagulation, oral complications, and cerebellar toxicity.

Leukostasis

Individuals with extremely high numbers of circulating blasts are at risk of leukostatic-induced hemorrhage. This occurs most often in patients with ALL. Leukostasis occurs as leukemic blasts accumulate and invade vessel walls, causing rupture and bleeding. Because of the extensive capillary network and the limited vasculature space of the brain, intracerebral hemorrhage is the most common and the most lethal manifestation of this complication. Therefore early detection of patients at risk (WBC >50,000 cells/mm^3) and immediate efforts to reduce the number of circulating cells are imperative. Treatment consists of high doses of cytotoxic drugs to reduce the burden of circulating cells. Leukapheresis and cranial irradiation may be used to provide immediate treatment.[3]

Disseminated intravascular coagulation

Disseminated intravascular coagulation (DIC) most frequently is associated with acute promyelocytic leukemia although it may occur with any acute leukemia.[24] During induction therapy there is excessive release of procoagulants from granules within the leukemic promyelocyte.[3] (See Chapters 22 and 31 for a discussion of DIC.)

Correction of the coagulopathy in DIC depends on the successful treatment of the leukemia. Therapy usually includes heparin and replacement of plasma factors and platelets.[3] Nursing care focuses on the prevention of injury, administration of prescribed therapy, and monitoring of the appropriate laboratory results.[120]

Oral complications

The oral complications of leukemia may be the result of the disease or the therapy. Gingival hypertrophy as a result of massive infiltration by leukemic cells is associated with acute myelomonocytic and monocytic leukemia.[10] The gingiva may be swollen, necrotic, and/or superinfected. The most effective treatment is therapy for the leukemia.

Stomatitis caused by the direct toxicity of chemotherpeutic agents such as the anthracyclines or methotrexate, combined with prolonged neutropenia and antibiotic therapy, renders the patient at high risk for oral infection. Oral care consists of regular cleansing with a solution of one quart of water with one teaspoon each of salt and sodium bicarbonate, treatment of infection with nystatin mouth rinses, and appropriate analgesia as needed.[121]

Cerebellar toxicity

The CNS can react to the toxicity of a drug and affect the cerebellum, for example, the toxicity associated with the administration of high-dose cytosine arabinoside (HDARAC). Conventional dosages are 100 to 200 mg/m^2 whereas HDARAC is $\geq$3 g/m^2. The incidence of neurotoxicity is 11% to 28% at dosages of 3 g/m^2 and as high as 67% in dosages up to 4.5 g/m^2.[122,123] This toxic effect also is age-related, with an increased risk in patients older than 50 years.[124] The syndrome may begin with signs of ataxia and nystagmus and progress to dysarthria (difficulty in articulating words) and adiadochokinesia (inability to perform rapid alternating movements). This toxic reaction may be irreversible if not detected early. Therefore it is essential that prior to each dose of HDARAC, the nurse completes a full neurologic assessment.[125] Any changes are reported, and the dosage is held until the physician evaluates the patient's condition.

PSYCHOSOCIAL SUPPORT

Individuals and their significant others are at risk for ineffective coping during the diagnostic work-up for malignancy and subsequent treatments.[126] A primary objective of supportive care must be to facilitate the most effective coping mechanisms for the individual and family and to enable the patient to live as full and normal a life as possible. Several factors should be taken into consideration as the nurse coordinates the care plan for psychologic and physical rehabilitation.

The age of the individual at the time of diagnosis may vary from infancy to old age. Issues may range from concern about fertility or the risk of a second malignancy in the young adult to fear of job stigma in the middle-aged individual. The elderly patient may be dealing with increasing physical decline in addition to the debilitating effects of cancer. Assessment of the individual's needs and degree of stress will facilitate the planning of suitable intervention.[127]

The stage and "curability" of the disease are other factors to be considered. It is imperative that the nurse understand the implications of the planned therapy and assist the patient in making appropriate decisions. For example, a young mother undergoing intensive chemotherapy for AML may need to make the necessary arrangements for child care and housekeeping for 6 to 8 weeks. A patient undergoing BMT may need to discuss with an employer the need for extended sick leave. The emotional ups and downs related to multiple remission inductions and relapses are exhausting to the patient and family.[128] Education and reassurance by consistent nursing staff members can help the individual regain a sense of control and hopefulness.

CONCLUSION

The care of the individual with a diagnosis of leukemia requires a multidisciplinary approach that considers many factors. The classification of acute or chronic and myeloid or lymphoid determines diverse plans and prognoses that are quite variable. The age of the patient and the stage of the disease determine the aggressiveness of therapy. Newer diagnostic studies allow the identification of both favorable and high-risk subsets of patients. As research continues, so it is hoped will the progress in achieving more durable cure rates.

The role of the nurse who provides direct care for patients with leukemia includes provision of education, physical care, symptom management, and psychosocial support. In addition, contributions to research studies are essential. Although the nurse has an indirect impact on the prognosis through correct administration of therapy and managment of side effects, the direct result of continuous support and education is an improved quality of life.

REFERENCES

1. Cancer Facts and Figures 1988. New York, American Cancer Society, 1988, p 14.
2. Cancer statistics, 1990. CA 40.9-26, 1990.
3. Henderson ES: Acute leukemia: General considerations, in Williams WJ, Beutler E, Erslev AJ, et al (eds): Hematology. New York, McGraw-Hill, 1983, pp 221-253.
4. Maguire ME: Leukemia, in Ziegfeld C (ed): Core Curriculum for Oncology Nursing. Philadelphia, WB Saunders, 1987, pp 173-192.
5. Sandler OP: Epidemiology of acute myelogenous leukemia. Semin Oncol 14:359-364, 1987.
6. Miller RW: Relation between cancer and congenital defects: An epidemiological evaluation. J Natl Cancer Inst 40:1079, 1968.
7. Keating MJ, Freireich EJ, McCredie KB, et al: Acute leukemia in adults, 1977. CA 27:2-25, 1977.
8. Gunz FW, Gunz JP, Veale AMO, et al: Familial leukemia: A study of 909 families. Scand J Haematol 15:117-131, 1975.
9. Rosner F, Lee SL: Down's syndrome and acute leukemia: Myeloblastic or lymphoblastic? Am J Med 53:203-218, 1972.
10. Wiernik PH: Acute leukemias of adults, in DeVita VT, Hellman S, Rosenberg SA (eds): Cancer: Principles and Practice of Oncology. Philadelphia, JB Lippincott, 1982, pp 1640-1657.
11. Zuelzer WW, Cox DE: Genetic aspects of leukemia. Semin Hematol 6:228, 1969.

12. Bloomfield CD, de la Chapelle A: Chromosome abnormalities in acute nonlymphocytic leukemia: Clinical and biological significance. Semin Oncol 14:372-383, 1987.
13. Brill AB, Tomonaga M, Heyssell RM: Leukemia in man following exposure to ionizing radiation: Summary of findings in Hiroshima and Nagasaki and a comparison with other human experience. Ann Intern Med 56:590-609, 1962.
14. Bizzozero OJ, Johnson KG, Crocco A: Radiation-related leukemia in Hiroshima and Nagasaki. N Engl J Med 274:1095-1097, 1966.
15. Matanowski GM, Seltser R, Sartwell PE: The current mortality rates of radiologists and other physician specialists: Specific causes of death. Am J Epidemiol 101:199-210, 1975.
16. Court-Brown WM, Doll R: Leukemia and aplastic anemia in patients irradiated for ankylosing spondylitis. Medical Research Council Special Report Series No 295, London, Her Majesty's Stationary Office, 1957.
17. Vigliani EC, Sarta G: Benzene and leukemia. N Engl J Med 271:872-875, 1964.
18. Thorpe JJ: Epidemiologic survey of leukemia in persons potentially exposed to benzene. J Occup Med 16:375-382, 1974.
19. Aksoy M: Malignancies due to occupational exposure to benzene. Am J Ind Med 7:395-402, 1985.
20. Cronkite EP: Chemical leukemogenesis: Benzene as a model. Semin Hematol 24:2-11, 1978.
21. Yin SN, Li G, Tain FD, et al: Leukemia in benzene workers: A retrospective cohort study. Br J Ind Med 44:124-128, 1987.
22. Fraser MC, Tucker MA: Late effects of cancer therapy: Chemotherapy related malignancies. Oncol Nurs Forum 15:67-77, 1988.
23. Keating M, Cork A, Broach Y, et al: Towards a clinically relevant cytogenetic classification of acute myelogenous leukemia. Leuk Res 11:119-133, 1987.
24. Foon KA, Gale RP: Controversies in the therapy of acute myelogenous leukemia. Am J Med 72:963-978, 1982.
25. Kantarjian HM, Keating M: Therapy related leukemia and myelodysplastic syndrome. Semin Oncol 14:435-443, 1987.
26. Dougan L, Woodleff AJ: Acute leukemia associated with phenylbutazone treatment. Med J Aust 1:217-219, 1965.
27. Brauer MJ, Dameshek W: Hypoplastic anemia and myeloblastic leukemia following chloramphenicol therapy. N Engl J Med 277:1003-1005, 1967.
28. Cohen T, Creger WB: Acute myeloid leukemia following seven years of aplastic anemia induced by chloramphenicol. Am J Med 43:762-770, 1967.
29. Gallagher RE, Gallo RC: Type of C RNA tumor virus isolated from cultured human acute myelogenous leukemia cells. Science 187:350-353, 1975.
30. Jarrett W, Essex M, Mackey L, et al: Horizontal transmission of leukemia virus and leukemia in the cat. J Natl Cancer Inst 51:833-841, 1973.
31. Heath CW: Epidemiology and hereditary aspects of acute leukemia, in Wiernick PH (ed): Neoplastic Diseases of the Blood, (vol 1). New York, Churchill Livingstone, 1985, pp 183-200.
32. Kalyanaraman VS, Sarngadharan MG, Robert-Guroff M, et al: A new subtype of human T-cell leukemia virus (HTLV-II) associated with a T-cell variant of hairy cell leukemia. Science 218:571-573, 1982.
33. Johnson BL: Leukemias, in Groenwald S (ed): Cancer Nursing: Principles and Practice. Boston, Jones & Bartlett, 1987, pp 654-670.
34. Bennett JM, Catovsky D, Daniel MT, et al: Proposals for the classification of the acute leukemias. Br J Haematol 33:451-458, 1976.
35. Bennett JM, Catovsky D, Daniel MT, et al: Criteria for the diagnosis of acute leukemia of megakaryocyte lineage (M7). Ann Intern Med 103:406-462, 1985.
36. Bennett JM, Catovsky D, Daniel MT, et al: Proposed revised criteria for the classification of acute myeloid leukemia. Ann Intern Med 103:626-629, 1985.
37. Hamilton-Paterson JL: Pre-leukemia anemia. Acta Haematol 2:309-316, 1949.
38. Buzaid AC, Garewal HS, Greenberg BR: Management of myelodysplastic syndromes. Am J Med 80:1149-1157, 1986.
39. Bennett JM, Catovsky D, Daniel MT, et al: The French-American-British (FAB) Co-operative Group: Proposals for the classification of the myelodysplastic syndromes. Br J Haematol 51:189-199, 1982.
40. Tricot GJ, Lauer RC, Appelbaum FR, et al: Management of the myelodysplastic syndromes. Semin Oncol 14:444-453, 1987.
41. Greenberg PL: The smoldering myeloid leukemic states: Clinical and biologic features. Blood 61:1035-1044, 1983.
42. Koeffler HP: Myelodysplastic syndromes (preleukemia). Semin Hematol 23:284-299, 1986.
43. Yoemans AC: Myelodysplastic syndromes: A preleukemic disorder. Cancer Nurs 10:32-40, 1987.
44. Cines DB, Cassileth PA, Kiss JE: Danazol therapy in myelodysplasia. Ann Intern Med 103:58-60, 1985.
45. Peterson BA, Ellis EG: Uncommon subtypes of acute nonlymphocytic leukemia: Clinical features and management of FAB M5, M6 and M7. Semin Oncol 14:425-434, 1987.
46. Champlin R, Golde DW: The leukemias, in Braunwald E, Isselbacher KJ, Pettersdorf RG, et al (eds): Harrison's Principles of Internal Medicine (ed 11). New York, McGraw-Hill, 1987, pp 1541-1550.
47. Foon KA, Todd RF: Immunologic classification of leukemia and lymphoma. Blood 68:1-31, 1986.
48. Foon KA, Gale RP, Todd RF: Recent advances in the immunologic classification of leukemia and lymphoma. Semin Hematol 23:257-283, 1986.
49. Henderson ES: Acute lymphocytic leukemia, in Williams WJ, Beutler E, Erslev AJ, et al (eds): Hematology, New York, McGraw-Hill, 1983, pp 970-978.
50. Clarkson B, Elles S, Little C, et al: Acute lymphoblastic leukemia in adults. Semin Oncol 12:160-179, 1985.
51. Adamson JW: The myeloproliferative diseases, in Braunwald E, Isselbacher KJ, Petersdorf RG, et al (eds): Harrison's Principles of Internal Medicine (ed 11). New York, McGraw-Hill, 1987, pp 1527-1533.
52. Coleman M, Allen SL: Chronic myelogenous leukemia: Evolving concepts in diagnosis and treatment. Mediguide to Oncology 3(4):1-5, 1983.
53. Canellos GP: Chronic leukemias, in Williams WJ, Beutler E, Erslev AJ, et al (eds): Hematology. New York, McGraw-Hill, 1983, pp 221-253.
54. Canellos GP: Chronic leukemias, in DeVita VT, Hellman S, Rosenberg SA (eds): Cancer: Principles and Practice of Oncology (ed 2). Philadelphia, JB Lippincott, 1985, pp 1739-1752.
55. Rai KR, Montserat E: Prognostic factors in chronic lymphocytic leukemia. Semin Hematol 24:252-256, 1987.
56. Rai KR, Sawitsky A, Jagathambal K, et al: Chronic lymphocytic leukemia. Med Clin North Am 68:697-711, 1984.
57. Rundles WR: Chronic lymphocytic leukemia. In Williams WJ, Beutler E, Erslev AJ, et al (eds): Hematology. New York, McGraw-Hill, 1983, pp 981-994.

58. Rundles RW, Moore JO: Chronic lymphocytic leukemia. Cancer 42:941-945, 1978.
59. Lipshutz MD, Mu R, Rai KR, et al: Bone marrow biopsy and clinical staging in chronic lymphocytic leukemia. Cancer 46:1422-1427, 1980.
60. Binet JL, Chastang C, Dighiero G, et al: Prognostic and therapeutic advances in CLL managment: The experience of the French Cooperative Group. Semin Hematol 24:275-290, 1987.
61. Lee JS, Dixon DO, Kantarjian HM, et al: Prognosis of chronic lymphocytic leukemia: A multivariate regression analysis of 325 untreated patients. Blood 69:929-936, 1987.
62. Mandelli F, De Rossi G, Mancini P, et al: Prognosis in chronic lymphocytic leukemia: A retrospective multicenter study from the GIMEMA Group. J Clin Oncol 5:398-406, 1987.
63. Binet JL, Cavotsky D, Chandra P, et al: Chronic lymphocytic leukemia: Proposals for a revised prognostic staging system. Br J Haematol 48:365-367, 1981.
64. Golomb HM: Hairy cell leukemia: An unusual lymphoproliferative disease. Cancer 42:946-956, 1978.
65. Steis RG, Longs DL: Update on the treatment of hairy cell leukemia, in DeVita VT, Hellman S, Rosenberg SA (eds): Cancer: Principles and Practice of Oncology. Philadelphia, JB Lippincott, 1982 (suppl), pp 1-12.
66. Portlock CS: Therapeutic approaches to the treatment of hairy cell leukemia. Semin Oncol 13:55-59, 1986 (suppl).
67. Portlock CS: Surgery, chemotherapy or biotherapy for hairy cell leukemia. Clin Oncol 1:1-4, 1988. (Quiz No 2.)
68. Cassileth PA: Adult acute nonlymphocytic leukemia. Med Clin North Am 68:675-695, 1984.
69. Larson RA, Daly KM, Choi KE, et al: A clinical and pharmacokinetic study of mitoxantrone in acute nonlymphocytic leukemia. J Clin Oncol 5:391-397, 1987.
70. Champlin R: Acute myelogenous leukemia: Biology and treatment. Mediguide to Oncology 8:1-9, 1988.
71. Preisler H, Davis RB, Kirshner J, et al: Comparison of three remission induction regimens and two postinduction strategies for the treatment of acute nonlymphocytic leukemia: A cancer and leukemia group B study. Blood 69:1441-1449, 1987.
72. Gale RP, Foon KA: Therapy of acute myelogenous leukemia. Semin Hematol 24:40-54, 1987.
73. Mayer RJ: Current chemotherapeutic treatment approaches to the management of previously untreated adults with de novo acute myelogenous leukemia. Semin Oncol 14:384-396, 1987.
74. Foon KA, Gale RP: Controversies in the therapy of acute myelogenous leukemia. Am J Med 72:963-978, 1982.
75. Wolff SN, Marion J, Stern RS, et al: High dose cytosine arabinoside and daunorubicin as consolidation therapy for acute nonlymphocytic leukemia in first remission: A pilot study. Blood 65:1407-1411, 1985.
76. Wolff SN, Herzig RH, Phillips CL, et al: High dose cytosine arabinoside and daunorubicin as consolidation therapy for acute nonlymphocytic leukemia in first remission: An update. Semin Oncol 14:12-17, 1987 (suppl).
77. Bloomfield CD: Post remission therapy in acute myeloid leukemia. J Clin Oncol 3:1570-1572, 1985 (editorial).
78. Cassileth PA, Begg CB, Bennett JM, et al: A randomized study of the efficacy of consolidation therapy in adult acute nonlymphocytic leukemia. Blood 63:843-847, 1984.
79. Grever MR: Treatment of patients with acute nonlymphocytic leukemia not in remission. Semin Oncol 14:416-424, 1987.
80. Champlin R, Gale RP: Bone marrow transplantation for acute leukemia: Recent advances and comparison with alternative therapies. Semin Hematol 24:55-67, 1987.
81. Applebaum FR, Fisher LD, Thomas ED, et al: Chemotherapy versus marrow transplantation for adults with acute nonlymphocytic leukemia: A five year follow-up. Blood 72:179-184, 1988.
82. Keating MJ, Gehan EA, Smith TL, et al: A strategy for evaluation of new treatments in untreated patients: Application to a clinical trial of AMSA for acute leukemia. J Clin Oncol 5:710-721, 1987.
83. Priesler HD, Raza A, Barcos M, et al: High dose cytosine arabinoside as the initial treatment of poor risk patients with acute nonlymphocytic leukemia: A leukemia intergroup study. J Clin Oncol 5:75-82, 1987.
84. Ortega JA, Nesbit ME, Donaldson MH, et al: L-Asparaginase, vincristine and prednisone for induction of first remission in acute lymphocytic leukemia. Cancer Res 37:535-540, 1977.
85. Hoelzer D, Gale RP: Acute lymphoblastic leukemia in adults: Recent progress, future directions. Semin Hematol 24:27-39, 1987.
86. Law IP, Blom J: Adult acute leukemia—Frequency of CNS involvement in long-term survivors. Cancer 40:1304-1306, 1977.
87. Kuo AH, Yataganas X, Galicich YY, et al: Proliferative kinetics of central nervous system leukemia. Cancer 36:232-239, 1975.
88. Chessells JM: Acute lymphoblastic leukemia. Semin Hematol 19:155-171, 1982.
89. Skeel RT: Leukemias, in Skeel RT (ed): Manual of Cancer Chemotherapy. Boston, Little, Brown, 1987, pp 209-221.
90. Spiers AS: Chronic granulocytic leukemia. Med Clin North Am 68:713-727, 1984.
91. Griffin JD: Managment of chronic myelogenous leukemia. Semin Hematol 23:20-26, 1986 (suppl 1).
92. Haines ME, Goldman JM, Worlsey AM, et al: Chemotherapy and autografting for chronic granulocytic leukemia in transformation: Probable prolongation of survival for some patients. Br J Haematol 58:711-721, 1984.
93. Talpaz M, Kantarjian HM, Kurzrock R, et al: Therapy of chronic myelogenous leukemia: Chemotherapy and interferons. Semin Hematol 25:62-73, 1988.
94. Sokal JE, Baccaran M, Russo D, et al: Staging and prognosis in chronic myelogenous leukemia. Semin Hematol 25:49-61, 1988.
95. Kantarjian HM, Smith TL, McCredie KB, et al: Chronic myelogenous leukemia: A multivariate analysis of the associations of patient characteristics and therapy with survival. Blood 66:1326-1335, 1985.
96. Champlin RE, Goldman JM, Gale RP: Bone marrow transplantation in chronic myelogenous leukemia. Semin Hematol 25:74-80, 1988.
97. Foon KA, Gale RT: Staging and therapy of chronic lymphocytic leukemia. Semin Hematol 24:264-274, 1987.
98. Pape LH: Therapy related acute leukemia: An overview. Cancer Nurs 11:295-302, 1988.
99. Foon KA, Bunn PA: Interferon treatment of cutaneous T cell lymphoma and chronic lymphocytic leukemia. Semin Oncol 13:35-39, 1986 (suppl 5).
100. Fanslow J: Knowledge deficit related to disease process, in McNally JC, Stair JC, Somerville ET (eds): Guidelines for Cancer Nursing Practice. Orlando, Fla, Grune & Stratton, 1985, pp 34-35.
101. Somerville ET: Knowledge deficit related to chemotherapy, in McNally JC, Stair JC, Somerville ET (eds): Guidelines for Cancer Nursing Practice. Orlando, Fla, Grune & Stratton, 1985, pp 36-39.
102. Wilson JM: Right atrial catheters (Broviac and Hickman): Indications for insertion, maintenance, and protocol for home care. Natl Int Ther Assoc J 6:23-27, 1983.

103. Goodman MS, Wickham R: Venous access devices: An overview. Oncol Nurs Forum 11(5):16-23, 1984.
104. Newman KA: The leukemias. Nurs Clin North Am 20:227-234, 1985.
105. Bodey GP: Infection in cancer patients. Cancer Treat Rev 2:89-129, 1975.
106. Carlson AC: Infection prophylaxis in the patient with cancer. Oncol Nurs Forum 12:56-64, 1985.
107. Reheis CE: Neutropenia: Causes, complications, treatment and resulting nursing care. Nurs Clin North Am 20:219-225, 1985.
108. Scheffer CA, Wade JC: Supportive care: Issues in the use of blood products and treatment of infection. Semin Oncol 14:454-467, 1987.
109. Young LS: Management of infections in leukemia and lymphoma, in Ruben RH, Young LS (eds): Clinical Approach to Infection in the Compromised Host. New York, Plenum Medicare Book Co, 1981, pp 461-497.
110. Hathorn JW, Ruben M, Pizzo PA: Empirical antibiotic therapy in the febrile neutropenic cancer patient: Clinical efficacy and impact of monotherapy. Antimicrob Agents Chemother 31:971-977, 1987.
111. Bodey CP: Topical and systemic antifungal agents. Med Clin North Am 72:637-659, 1988.
112. Mahon SM: Taking the terror out of amphotericin B. Am J Nurs 88:961-966, 1988.
113. Rutledge DN, Holtzclaw BJ: Amphotericin B–induced shivering in patients with cancer: A nursing approach. Heart Lung 17:432-440, 1988.
114. Nunnally C, Yasko JM: Infection, in Yasko JM (ed): Guidelines for Cancer Care: Symptom Management. Reston, Va, Reston Publishing, 1983, pp 38-62.
115. Brandt B: A nursing protocol for the client with neutropenia. Oncol Nurs Forum 11(2):24-28, 1984.
116. Spross JA: Protective mechanisms, in Johnson BL, Gross J: Handbook of Oncology Nursing. New York, John Wiley & Sons, 1985, pp 229-302.
117. Nusbacher J: Preservation and clinical use of leukocytes, in Williams WJ, Beutler EJ, Erslev AJ, et al (eds): Hematology. New York, McGraw-Hill, 1983, pp 1549-1555.
118. Masauredis SP: Preservation and clinical use of erythrocytes and whole blood, in Williams WJ, Beutler EJ, Erslev AJ, et al (eds): Hematology. New York, McGraw-Hill, 1983, pp 1529-1549.
119. Gannon CT: Bleeding due to thrombocytopenia, in Yasko JM (ed): Guidelines for Cancer Care: Symptom Management. Reston, Va, Reston Publishing, 1983, pp 25-32.
120. Rooney A, Hawley C: Nursing managment of disseminated intravascular coagulation. Oncol Nurs Forum 12(1):15-22, 1985.
121. Ziga SE: Stomatitis/mucositis, in Yasko JM (ed): Guidelines for Cancer Care: Symptom Management. Reston, Va, Reston Publishing, 1983, pp 212-229.
122. Sylvester RK, Fisher AJ, Lobell M: Cytarabine-induced cerebellar syndrome, case report and literature review. Drug Intell Clin Pharm 21:177-179, 1987.
123. Herzig RH, Lazarus GP, Herzig PF, et al: Central nervous system toxicity with high dose cytosine arabinoside. Semin Oncol 12:233-236, 1985 (suppl).
124. Herzig RH, Hines JD, Herzig GP, et al: Cerebellar toxicity with high dose cytosine arabinoside. J Clin Oncol 5:927-932, 1987.
125. Conrad KJ: Cerebellar toxicities associated with cytosine arabinoside: A nursing perspective. Oncol Nurs Forum 13(5):57-59, 1986.
126. Doublsky J: Ineffective individual coping, in McNally JC, Stair JC, Somerville ET (eds): Guidelines for Cancer Nursing Practice. Orlando, Fla, Grune & Stratton, 1985, pp 66-72.
127. Smith K, Lesko LM: Psychosocial problems in cancer survivors. Oncology 2:33-40, 1988.
128. Scott DW, Goode WL, Arlin ZA: The psychodynamics of multiple remissions in a patient with nonlymphoblastic leukemia. Cancer Nurs 6:201-206, 1983.

Chapter 43

Lung Cancer

Ellen Heid Elpern, RN, MSN

INTRODUCTION

Lung cancer has a devastating impact on our nation's health. Lung cancer is our most serious cancer problem and has become our most common cancer killer. In recent years improvements have been made in diagnostic and staging techniques, but without consistent advances in therapies. Five-year outcomes for individuals with bronchogenic cancer remain poor. Ironically, it has been estimated that 85% of lung cancers are preventable if cigarette smoking could be eliminated. Clearly, our best hope in controlling this disease lies in its prevention.

EPIDEMIOLOGY

Examination of epidemiologic studies related to lung cancer reveals alarming trends. In 1912, only 374 cases of lung cancer were reported worldwide. Today, lung cancer is the most frequent cause of death in people who die of malignant disease. The peak incidence is in males 50 to 60 years of age. Although lung cancer occurs predominantly in males, the incidence in females is rising dramatically and more quickly than in males. As a result, the sex ratio (ratio of the number of male cases to the number of female cases) has steadily decreased in the United States and is likely to continue to decline. Already the source of most male cancer deaths (Figure 43-1), in 1986 lung cancer became the leading cause of cancer death in women (Figure 43-2). In the United States, mortality due to lung cancer in both males and females is increasing almost twice as fast for nonwhites as for whites.

The highly virulent and rapidly fatal nature of lung cancer is obvious when data on incidence and mortality are examined. There is a close relationship between incidence and death rates, indicating that most individuals diagnosed with lung cancer die of the disease. Both incidence and death rates from lung cancer are highest in large industrial cities, emphasizing the environmental factors implicated in this disease. In the United States, 155,000 new cases of lung cancer and 142,000 deaths from lung cancer were estimated for 1989. The 5-year survival rate for individuals diagnosed with lung cancer is 13% for whites and 11% for blacks.[1]

ETIOLOGY

Lung cancers most commonly occur following repeated exposure to substances that cause tissue irritation and inflammation. Lung tissues are exposed to these substances primarily as they are inhaled with ambient air. Tobacco smoke, air pollutants, and exposure to certain metals, fibers, and gases are major risk factors in the development of lung cancer. For many single agents, a direct cause-and-effect relationship has not been firmly established. The interactive and synergistic effects of exposure to more than one carcinogenic agent have been recognized and must be emphasized in a discussion of the etiologies of lung cancer. A future challenge lies in determining the degree to which multiple factor interactions can be identified and ultimately prevented.

Tobacco Smoke

Europeans were introduced to tobacco smoking in the 1600s by the American Indians and quickly popularized the practice in their native countries. The automatic roller, patented in 1880, allowed for the mass production of cigarettes. In the past century changes in tobacco growing and curing methods altered the quality of tobacco smoke so that it became less caustic and more "inhalable." The mass production and marketing of cigarettes, along with the practice of repetitive inhalation of cigarette smoke, has had a devastating impact on the incidence of lung cancer. There is a strong and irrefutable causal relationship between smoking and lung cancer. This conclusion has been confirmed by an abundance of epidemiologic studies beginning in the 1950s and continuing to the present. In addition to a strong statistical relationship between lung cancer and smoking, Spencer[2] summarized further evidence for this association:

1. The finding of benzopyrene and other carcinogens in combusted tobacco.
2. The finding of precarcinomatous histologic changes in the bronchial epithelium of heavy smokers.
3. The increased incidence of other diseases associated with smoking in individuals with lung cancer.
4. The experimental production of tumors in animals following the internal and cutaneous application of tobacco condensates.

Accumulated evidence suggests that the relationship of smoking to lung cancer has a dose-response nature, where the relative risk of lung cancer increases with the quantity of cigarettes smoked. Fortunately, there is also a reduced risk of lung cancer over time for former smokers, eventually approaching that for lifetime nonsmokers. Although improvements begin shortly after the cessation of smoking, it appears to take approximately 15 years for a former smoker's risk of lung cancer to approximate that of a lifetime nonsmoker.[3] In determining risk, the number of pack years (packs of cigarettes consumed per day times the number of years of smoking) appears to be a crucial factor. Age at onset of smoking is also an influential factor. Individuals who start smoking at an early age (15 years) have a greater risk than do individuals who start smoking later (25 years or older). Other factors that influence cancer risk are smoking practices (size of puff, depth of inhalation, time of breath holding, amount of cigarette smoked) and type of cigarette smoked (tar content, filtered vs. nonfiltered).

Although it is true that the incidence of lung cancer corresponds to smoking habits, how tobacco smoke causes cancer is less clear. Cigarette smoke contains 3600 chemicals, many of which are carcinogens or mutagens. The potential interactive effects of inhalation of these chemicals with environmental or genetic factors in the causation of lung cancer are unclear. The correlation between cigarette smoking and lung cancer differs among the specific tumor cell types. Squamous and small cell cancers occur almost exclusively in smokers and are generally dose related.

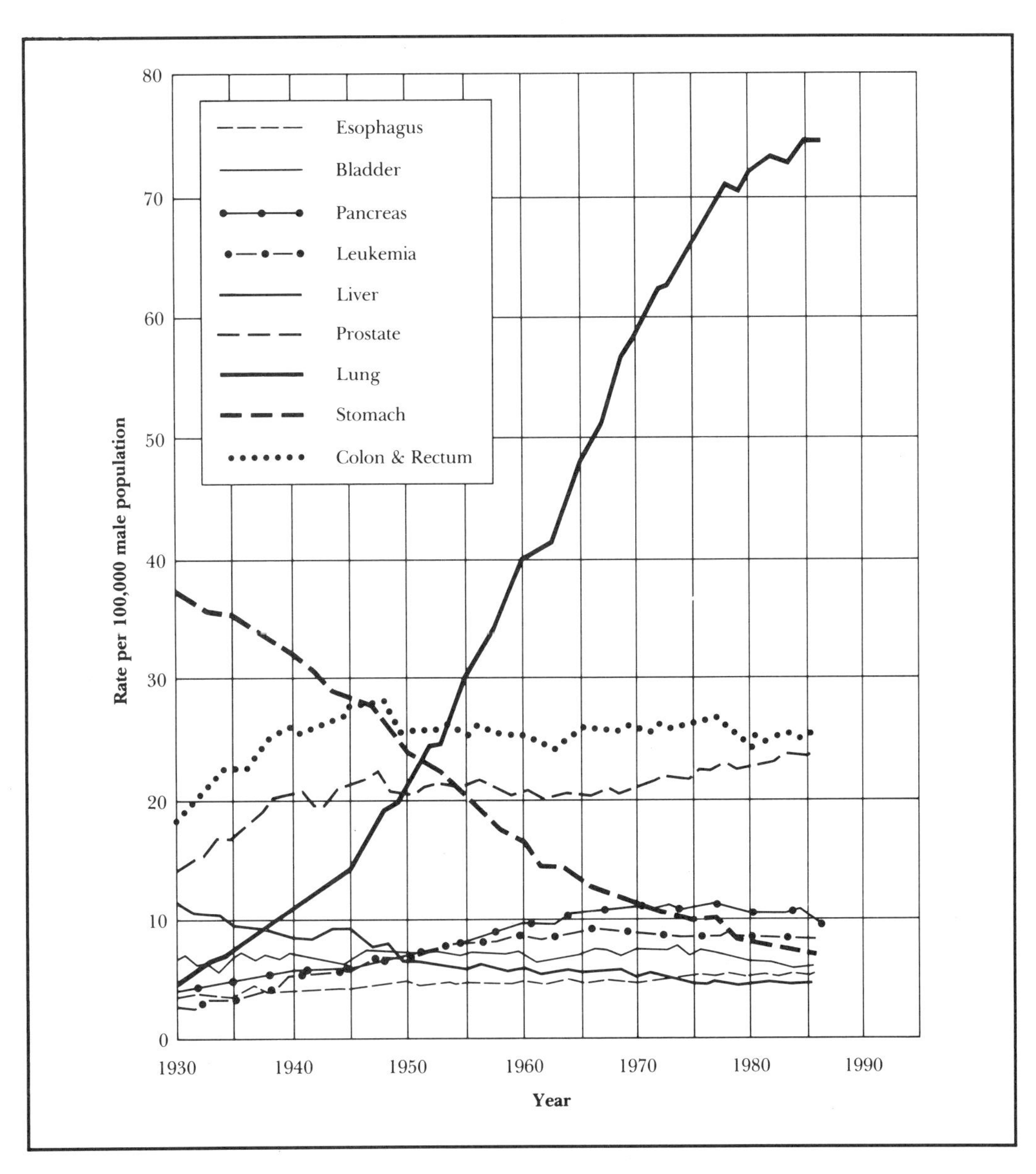

FIGURE 43-1 Age-adjusted (to the age distribution of the 1970 US Census population) cancer death rates for selected sites, males, United States, 1930-1986. (Source: Silverberg E, Boring CC, Squires TS: Cancer Statistics, 1990. CA 40:9-26, 1990.)

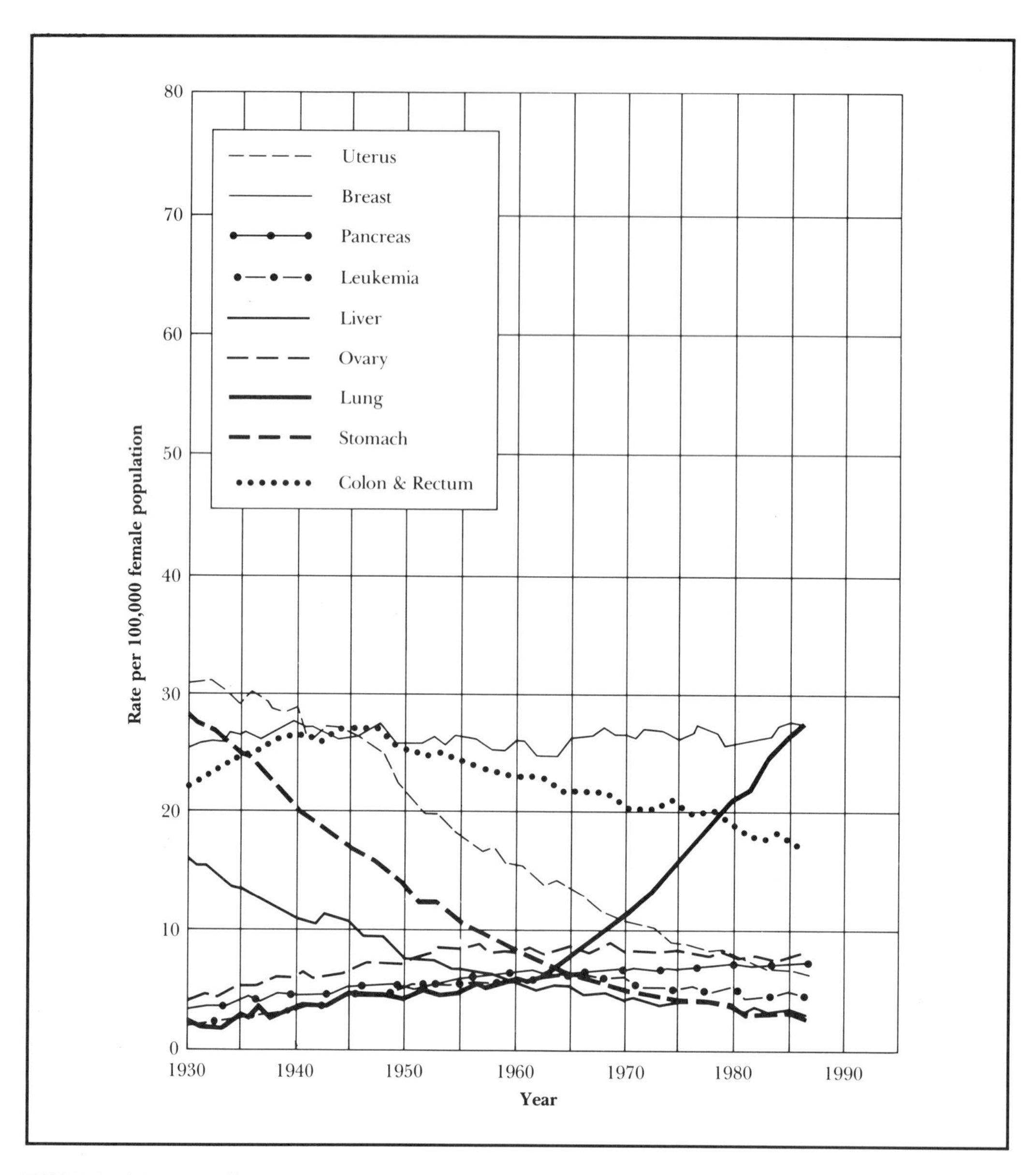

FIGURE 43-2 Age-adjusted cancer death rates (to the age distribution of the 1970 US Census population) for selected sites, females, United States, 1930-1986. (Source: Silverberg E, Boring CC, Squires TS: Cancer Statistics, 1990. CA 40:9-26, 1990.)

Passive Smoking

Passive smoking refers to the involuntary exposure of nonsmokers to tobacco combustion products in the indoor environment. Oleske[4] has summarized the evidence for an increased risk for lung cancer among nonsmokers with spouses who smoke. The 1986 Report of the Surgeon General[5] presented evidence that sidestream smoke is qualitatively similar to mainstream smoke inhaled by the smoker and that both act as carcinogens. The report concluded that involuntary smoking can cause lung cancer in nonsmokers. The number of lung cancers due to passive smoking is much less than those due to active smoking. The magnitude of increased lung cancer risk that results from passive smoking has yet to be clearly determined, but a dose-response relationship between exposure and risk is expected. One of the most important methodologic issues to be addressed in this emerging field of research relates to quantification of tobacco smoke exposure in passive smokers.

Air Pollution

There are three major sources and types of air pollution: (1) the sulfur oxide–particulate complex arising from the combustion of sulfur-containing fuels, (2) photochemical oxidants related to motor vehicle emissions, and (3) miscellaneous pollutants from localized sources such as refineries and manufacturing plants.[6] Known carcinogens have been identified in atmospheric pollution, and it has been hypothesized that repeated exposure to these pollutants causes lung cancer. At this time, this hypothesis remains neither proved nor disproved. There is evidence that the incidence of lung cancer increases in polluted urban areas, but the separate or interactive contributions of cigarette smoking, occupational exposure, and indoor air pollution to the development of lung cancer confuse the relationship. Some inhaled irritants may be more important as tumor promoters than as direct carcinogenic agents. Air pollutants most probably contribute little risk in themselves but exert a powerful effect in determining lung cancer occurrences in smokers.

Occupational Factors

A substantial number of chemicals are associated with lung cancer in humans. These chemicals and the occupations that result in exposure are listed in Table 43-1. Occupational exposure to such substances offers opportunities for tumor induction, usually after a long latency period. About 12% of the overall annual lung cancer deaths result from chronic exposure to industrial carcinogens. The interactive effects of smoking and occupational exposure must again be stressed. For example, smoking clearly compounds the risk of lung cancer for asbestos and uranium workers. Asbestos workers who smoke are up to 50 times more likely to develop lung cancer than are nonexposed nonsmokers. This illustrates the point that the carcinogenic potential of a single agent may be magnified and enhanced by interaction with another agent.

TABLE 43-1 Occupational Risk Factors to the Development of Lung Cancer

Cancer-Causing Substance	Occupations
Arsenic	Oil refining; copper smelting; mining; using pesticides; tanning; working in the chemical industry
Asbestos	Asbestos milling and manufacture; working with insulation; shipyard work; brake and clutch repair; asbestos mining
Bischloromethyl ether and mustard gas	Working in the chemical industry; making ion exchange resins
Chromates	Glassmaking; potting; acetylene and aniline manufacturing; bleaching; battery making; spray painting
Coke oven fumes	Steel mill, foundry, and petroleum workers
Nickel	Nickel refining
Petroleum products and oils	Working with lubricating oils, paraffins, or wax oils or coke and rubber filler
Radiation	Working in the atomic energy industry; medicine; radiology; uranium mining

Radon

Radon from uranium ore has long been recognized as a cause of lung cancer in uranium miners. Radon is now recognized as a cause of lung cancer in the general population as well. Radon is a naturally occurring radioactive gas that is colorless, odorless, and tasteless. It is found in variable concentrations in soil and rocks, formed by the natural decay of uranium and thorium. Radon can migrate up through porous soils and enter homes through basement or foundation cracks, sumps, drains, or deep private wells. Radon levels vary by geographic location, climate, season, and type of heating and ventilation system. It has been estimated that indoor radon may be responsible for 5,000 to 20,000 lung cancer deaths per year.[7,8] A synergistic effect exists between radon exposure and cigarette smoking. The longer the period of exposure, the greater the risk. Cancer risk decreases with time after cessation of exposure. Radon is measured in picocuries per liter (pCi/L). The Environmental Protection Agency (EPA) has set 4 pCi/L as the level at which action to lower radon levels is recommended. Detection devices are available for home monitoring.

Vitamin A

Studies compiled in the last 20 years suggest an inverse relationship between lung cancer and dietary intake of vitamin A.[9] These studies demonstrated that patients with lung cancer consumed smaller quantities of foods rich in Vitamin A or had lower blood levels of retinol or beta carotene than did matched controls. Although not all studies controlled for cigarette smoking, the association between low vitamin A levels and lung cancer held when smoking history was considered. This association may be stronger in males than in females. It is not yet clear whether or how dietary interventions can modify lung cancer risk, but the available epidemiologic evidence points to dietary intervention as an encouraging area for further study.

Constitutional Factors

Some researchers[10,11] claim that an individual's genetic makeup may predispose him or her to lung cancer. The finding of multiple cases of lung cancer in some families is used as supportive data. Strong evidence to confirm this hypothesis is lacking, and no conclusions can be drawn from available data.

Several studies[12,13] suggested that the presence of

chronic obstructive pulmonary disease is a risk factor for the development of lung cancer independent of smoking history. The mechanisms for this risk are not known but may relate to impaired mucociliary transport with enhanced deposition of carcinogens, chronic inflammation and scarring, and genetic predisposition to mucosal injury.

An association between progressive systemic sclerosis (PSS) and lung cancer has also been suggested.[14] The increased incidence of lung cancer with PSS may be associated more with the presence of pulmonary fibrosis in these patients than with cigarette smoking.

Both focal lung scars and more diffuse parenchymal fibrosis can become sites of lung malignancies. The "scar cancers" of the lung probably occur when regenerative hyperplasia becomes excessive and develops into malignant changes. Scar cancers are usually adenocarcinomas.

PREVENTION

Smoking Related

Lung cancer is a common and particularly lethal disease. Ironically, it is also a condition that could be readily controlled with the elimination of its major causative factor—cigarette smoking. Efforts aimed at lung cancer prevention must focus on changing smoking behaviors.

In 1985, 30% of adult Americans smoked cigarettes. The number of adult smokers peaked at 40% in the early 1960s and has declined since publication of the first Surgeon General's Report on Smoking and Health in 1964. Likewise, the per capita consumption of cigarettes has declined by 20% in the past 20 years. Despite these encouraging overall statistics, smoking remains a major health concern generally and for certain populations in particular. About 15% of adolescents from 12 to 17 years of age smoke cigarettes. In the past 10 years, the prevalence of adolescent smokers has been higher for females than for males. In the adult population, there are more black than white smokers. Blacks are also less likely to quit smoking than are whites.

Research increasingly supports the conclusion that multiple factors influence the initiation and maintenance of smoking. Generally, the reasons why an individual starts to smoke are entirely different from those that lead him or her to continue smoking. It seems clear, therefore, that activities aimed at reducing the development of smoking behaviors will be different from those designed to assist smokers to quit. The social and pyschological factors that influence the initiation or maintenance of smoking must be considered in such programs.

Horn[15] has concluded that smoking behaviors are usually initiated at a fairly young age and in response to opportunity, curiosity, and a need for self-expression. Several steps to reduce the development of smoking behavior have been proposed:

1. Reduce the easy availability of cigarettes to young people.
2. Encourage parents and important role models to set the example of not smoking.
3. Reduce the intensity of emotionally charged proscriptions against smoking, which serve to stimulate contrary action.
4. Stress the costs associated with smoking without denying the benefits. Encourage the achievement of these benefits in less damaging ways.
5. Avoid stereotyping smoking and smokers in ways that turn youth away from antismoking "do-gooders."
6. Help young people develop insight into their perception of smoking as attractive. Encourage them to seek alternate means of satisfying this need.

Past efforts to influence young people not to smoke have not been effective. The number of preadolescent and teenage smokers has steadily increased, particularly among females. Programs aimed at preventing youngsters from starting to smoke are of particular importance to lung cancer control and should be initiated as early as the first grade.

Whereas initiation of smoking is largely socially determined, maintenance of smoking involves others factors. The regular use of cigarettes leads to behavioral and pharmacologic dependence. Smoking becomes not only a habitual, conditioned response, but one necessary to satisfy a chemical dependence on nicotine. Nicotine is a drug with powerful physiologic and psychoactive effects that lead to its compulsive use. Changing smoking habits is an admittedly complex and difficult task. Despite the growing awareness of the serious health hazard that cigarette smoking represents, about one third of the U.S. population continues to smoke. Although the majority of these people indicate a desire to quit smoking, the long-term successful quit rate (abstinent 1 year after quiting) is about 30% at best. Ninety-five percent of those who quit smoking do so without the aid of an organized program.[16] Success at quitting increases with the number of attempts made. Clearly, successful self-help programs require attention to techniques first to achieve and then to maintain abstinence. Many program formats are available, including self-help manuals and broadcast media programs. Intensive individual programs using therapists or antismoking specialists are also available. A nicotine resin chewing gum is available to help control symptoms of nicotine withdrawal.

Nurses may play a prominent role in reducing smoking and lung cancer risk. Risser[17] has suggested strategies that include example setting, limiting smoking in the workplace, identification of high-risk individuals, counseling or referral of smokers motivated to quit, and reinforcement of cessation attempts. Colleagues as well as patients may benefit from such efforts. Between 10% and 15% of physicians smoke, and 20% to 25% of registered nurses are active smokers.[18,19]

It is likely that a large number of individuals will take up smoking or continue to smoke despite all contrary efforts. To reduce the risk of lung cancer in smokers, an additional research thrust has been the development of less harmful cigarettes. Such cigarettes would have to contain considerably less particulate matter and lower levels of those components known to be carcinogenic or tumor promoters. There is evidence that reducing the levels of tar and nicotine in cigarettes, as has been done in the last 15 years, can favorably affect lung histopathology in smokers. Smokers who died in the 1970s had less metaplasia and atypia on autopsy than did smokers who died in the 1950s, when tar content of cigarettes was twice as great.[20] Although it is now possible to manufacture cigarettes that are less hazardous than those currently available, their tastelessness makes them unacceptable to most smokers. It is also possible that smokers offset the potential benefits of switching to lower tar and nicotine cigarettes by adjusting their smoking habits (smoke more cigarettes, alter puffing characteristics) to maintain a certain intake of nicotine.

Legislative approaches to smoking control include taxation of cigarettes, warning label requirements, restrictions on advertising, and restrictions on smoking in public places. Numerous antismoking activist groups are available for concerned citizens. Some are more politically oriented than others, and the thrusts of the groups vary considerably. In addition to such groups, health care professionals should be aware of the resources and involvement the professional societies may have in relation to antismoking efforts.

In recent years a growing concern has arisen regarding the hazards of "passive" or involuntary smoking, that is, the exposure of nonsmokers to tobacco combustion products in the indoor environment. Health risks include increased incidence of lung cancer in nonsmoking women whose husbands smoke and increased frequency of respiratory infections and symptoms in children whose parents smoke. Concern over the effect of passive smoking is reflected in ongoing studies to ascertain its health consequences and in the proposal of laws and regulations restricting smoking in public places. Many cities have passed legislation requiring employers to regulate or, if necessary, ban smoking in the workplace. In 1988 a federal bill was passed banning smoking on commercial airline flights of 120 minutes or less.

Occupation Related

The prevention of occupational lung disease depends on eliminating or reducing lung exposure to toxic substances. Although the number of cases of lung cancer caused by occupational exposure alone is relatively small, job-related lung cancer is potentially entirely preventable. The risk of lung cancer from occupational exposure is multiplied greatly if the worker also smokes cigarettes.

As summarized by Landrigan and Selikoff,[21] prevention of occupational lung cancer may be achieved by a combination of techniques including premarket toxicologic testing of new chemical compounds, application of industrial hygiene techniques, legal and regulatory approaches, and epidemiologic surveillance. The federal government has taken some steps to ensure safer working conditions (Occupational Safety and Health Act [OSHA], Federal Mine Safety and Health Act, Toxic Substances Control Act), but the response of industry has been generally slow and often controversial. Special interest groups continue to debate the degree of carcinogenic risk for workers exposed to certain substances as well as the potential economic hardships imposed by stringent regulations. Governmental commitment to the control of job-related hazardous exposure has also been variable. An increased awareness of the health hazards of certain occupations on the part of labor, management, and government and voluntary compliance with exposure-reduction methods, although potentially costly and difficult to effect, would substantially reduce job-related lung cancer.

Dietary Related

In light of epidemiologic data suggesting a relation between vitamin A deficiency and lung cancer incidence, the National Cancer Institute has undertaken study of preventative research in nutrition and lung cancer. Vitamin A and its precursor, beta carotene, are among the agents to be tested. The potential benefits of chemoprevention are conceptually exciting but await confirmation by intervention trials.

EARLY DETECTION

The natural history of lung cancer usually includes years of tumor growth prior to clinical presentation. The potential benefits of the earliest possible detection of a lung malignancy seem straightforward. The earlier the disease is detected, the more probable it is that the cancer is localized and the better the chances for cure. Unfortunately, the diagnosis of an occult or localized lung cancer is a relatively infrequent occurrence. It is probable that this frequency could be significantly increased through mass screening programs.

The only screening tests currently available for the diagnosis of asymptomatic lung cancers are sputum cytologies and chest radiographs. These screening tests are generally used in combination. Cancerous lesions may be radiographically undetectable because of their small size or because their presence is obscured by other chest structures or abnormalities. The necessity of sputum cytologies for the detection of such lesions is obvious. Chest radiographs are more accurate in detecting peripherally located lung tumors, and sputum cytologies more often detect central lung tumors. Sputum cytologies are sensitive detectors of lung cancer only if multiple specimens are evaluated. Both sputum studies and chest radiographs are costly and require special facilities and personnel. The cost of performing these screening measures on the general adult population is considered excessive, and mass screening for lung cancer is considered unwarranted. Screening programs do exist but are applied only to individuals considered at high risk for lung cancer.

In the early 1970s the National Cancer Institute initiated a cooperative program of lung cancer screening at three sites. The objectives of this screening program were to determine (1) whether detection of lung cancer can be improved by adding modern sputum cytologic screening techniques to the examination at regular intervals by chest radiography and (2) whether the mortality from lung cancer can be reduced significantly with this type of screening program followed by newer localizing methods and appropriate treatment.[22] Enrollment was limited to individuals considered at risk: males, age 45 years or older, who chronically smoked at least one package of cigarettes per day. Approximately 10,000 men have been enrolled at each of the three centers. Analysis of results to date[23] demonstrate that the two screening modalities are effective and complementary in the detection of lung cancer. More tumors are detected by chest x-ray study than by sputum cytology. However, sputum cytology is the most effective detector of early resectable tumors. Unfortunately, although screening programs achieved earlier diagnoses and longer survival, no significant reduction in lung cancer mortality was demonstrated. Earlier detection appears to lengthen the interval between diagnosis and death without increasing total life span.

In light of the cost of even selective radiographic screening, many authorities have revised their recommendations in this regard. In 1980, the American Cancer Society advised against screening even in high-risk groups unless symptoms were present.

It has been repeatedly demonstrated that substances not produced by normal cells can be elaborated by cancer cells. If such ectopic substances could be identified and detected in human tissues, important new methods for screening for cancer and measuring the effects of therapy would become available. It has been demonstrated that the majority of individuals with lung cancer have increased concentrations of carcinoembryonic antigen (CEA) in their blood. The effective use of CEA as a tumor marker is limited, however, by the finding of increased levels of CEA in the blood of some smokers and individuals with chronic obstructive lung disease who do not have lung cancer. CEA levels may be used to evaluate treatment response.

Studies of individuals diagnosed with lung cancer using assays for adrenocorticotropic hormone (ACTH) or hormone precursors have suggested that ectopic production of ACTH by lung tumor cells may be much more universal than clinically evidenced. A biologically inactive precursor, proACTH, has been found in the blood of almost all individuals with untreated lung cancer. The usefulness of proACTH is compromised by similar elevations in some individuals with chronic obstructive lung disease who are not known to have lung cancer. The potential use of these and other substances as tumor markers is receiving intensive study, and future developments could have significant clinical implications.

HISTOGENESIS

Bronchogenic tumor cells differ in appearance and behavior from normal bronchial epithelial cells. Carcinogenic-induced alterations in chromosomes cause the aberrancies seen in cancer cells. It is believed that early tumor cells retain many of the morphologic and metabolic features of the tissue of origin and are classified as well differentiated. With rapid multiplication and growth, tumor cells may become dedifferentiated and less recognizable in morphology and arrangement from normal bronchial epithelial cells. Over 90% of all primary lung tumors arise from the bronchial epithelium.

Normal bronchial epithelial cells serve as a lining and protective function. They are derived from the endodermal cell layer of the human embryo. Pseudostratified columnar epithelial cells line the tracheobronchial tree from the trachea to the terminal bronchioles. The columnar cells rest on a basement membrane. Some of these columnar cells are ciliated, while others are mucus-secreting cells (goblet cells).

Interspersed between the columnar cells, but not reaching the bronchial lumen, are the smaller, shorter basal cells. Some of these basal cells are the reserve or stem cells that can differentiate to become mature columnar lining cells. Other basal cells (called Kulchitsky's cells) contain secretory granules. It is speculated that these basal cells have a neurosecretory or endocrine function of some kind.

As a protective layer between the body and the outer environment, the bronchial epithelium is continually damaged, shed, and replaced. Inhaled irritant substances are most commonly deposited in the airways at points of major bronchial bifurcation. Short-term exposure to cigarette smoke may change ciliary structure or reduce ciliary beating but is principally associated with mucous cell hyperplasia and hypersecretion of mucus. With continued years of smoking, ciliated cells are repeatedly damaged and shed from the basement membrane. More rapid loss of these cells stimulates an increase in the cell turnover rate in the basal cell layer (basal cell hyperplasia). With basal hyperplasia the epithelium appears more stratified, or layered. With repeated insult, the rapidly proliferating basal cells have less energy available for differentiation, and the cells assume the more primitive, flattened, and rounded appearance of squamous cells.

The protective ciliated and mucus-producing cells are replaced by these dysplastic cells, allowing easier access of irritants and carcinogens. Even at this point of squamous metaplasia, epithelial injury is not irreversible if the cause is removed. If heavy smoking continues, however, atypia of the epithelial cells progresses to nuclear enlargement, nuclear variability, hyperchromatism, and mitotic activity. Several sites of fully developed intraepithelial carcinomas that do not invade the basement membrane (carcinoma in situ) can develop, located in the bronchi of both lungs. Apparently, not all foci of carcinoma in situ will progress to become invasive tumors. Over time, invasion through the basement membrane may occur with downgrowth of the tumor. Figure 43-3 illustrates the response of the bronchial epithelium to chronic irritants.

The transformations of the bronchial epithelium that are described above occur over extended periods, usually several decades. The developmental period probably depends on the duration and degree of exposure to lung irritants or carcinogens.

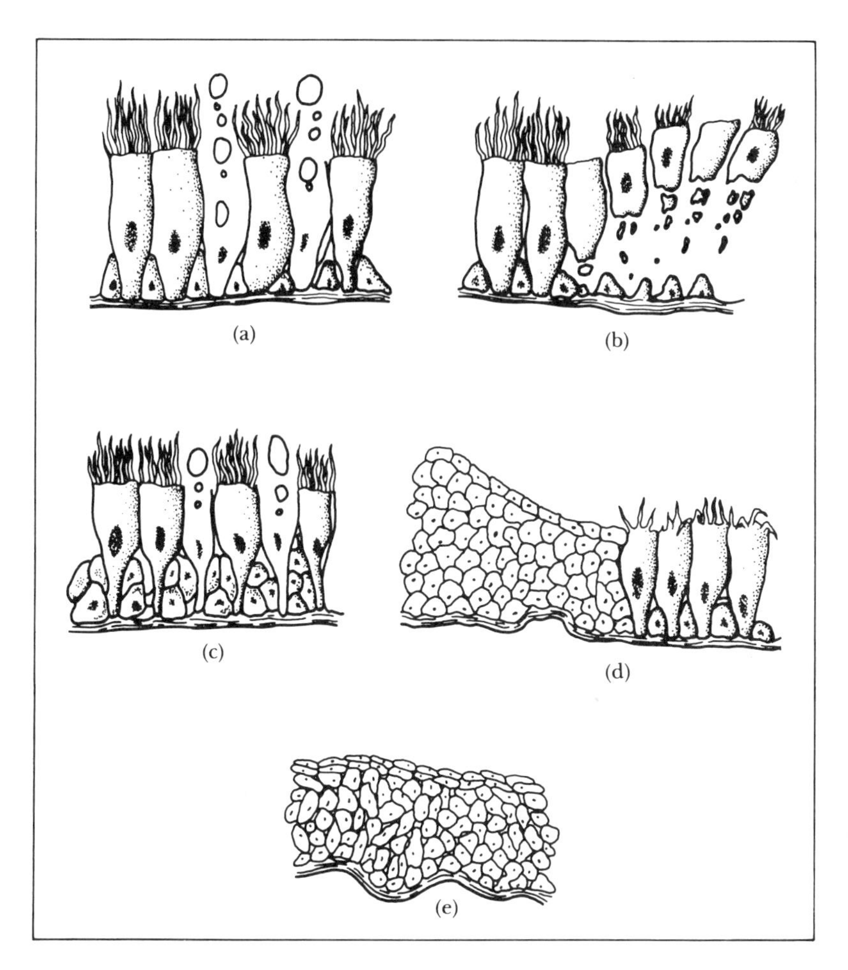

FIGURE 43-3 Response of bronchial epithelium to chronic irritation. (a) Normal bronchial epithelium; (b) ciliated airway cells are continuously shed and replaced in response to irritant exposure; (c) ciliated cells regenerate from basal cells; (d) chronic irritation results in an increased turnover of cells, damaged cilia, and basal cell proliferation; (e) continuation or irritation may produce bronchial epithelial dysplasia and carcinoma in situ. (Source: Adapted from Kotin P: Carcinogenesis of the lung, in Liebow AA, Smith DE (eds): The Lung. Baltimore, Williams & Wilkins, 1968.)

HISTOLOGY

Bronchogenic tumors are classified according to recognized variations in histology as squamous cell carcinomas, adenocarcinomas, large cell carcinomas, and small cell carcinomas. Histologic classifications are important to the organization of data on incidence, natural history, etiology, and treatment. Because of significant differences in presentation, natural history, and treatment response, lung tumors are usually referred to as small cell lung cancer (SCLC) or non-small cell lung cancer (NSCLC).

Histologic classification depends on identification of the distinct morphology of tumor cells. Unfortunately, many lung tumors contain more than one cellular element, or the cell type identified at diagnosis may evolve to a different type with treatment. The presence of multiple cell types in a single tumor mass, as well as the possibility of conversion to other cell types, suggests a common progenitor cell for all lung carcinomas. This unitary theory of histogenesis is a relatively new concept, since small cell tumors were thought historically to originate from a cell line different from other lung tumors. All tumors probably arise not from mature epithelial cell types but from proliferating simple pleuropotential reserve cells and differ only in their degree of differentiation. Yesner and Carter[25] suggest a spectrum of lung cancer ranging from poorly differentiated SCLC that evolves into more differentiated adeno and squamous tumors, with large cell undifferentiated tumors as intermediate (Figure 43-4). Characteristics of the various cell types of lung tumors are discussed below.

Non-Small Cell Lung Cancers

Squamous cell carcinomas

Squamous cancers show a very strong association with cigarette smoking that is of a dose-response nature; that is, the greater the quantity of cigarettes smoked, the higher the incidence of squamous cancer. Currently, squamous

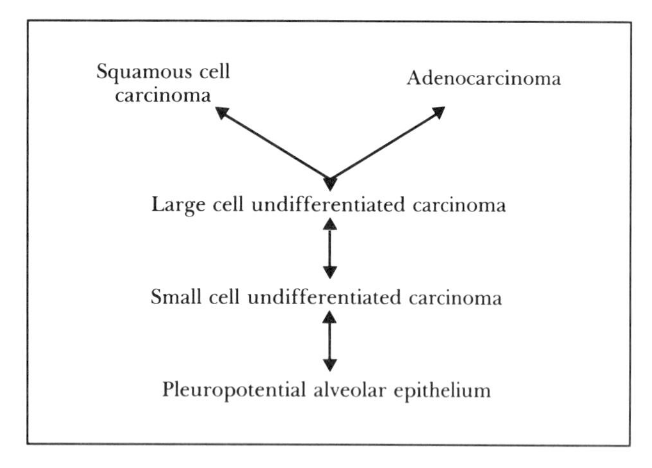

FIGURE 43-4 Proposed histological schema of lung cancer. (Source: Adapted from Yesner R, Carter D: Pathology of carcinoma of the lung. Clin Chest Med 3:257-289, 1982.)

cancers are more common in males than females, probably as a function of sex differences in relation to smoking history. This sex ratio is changing as the incidence of female smokers increases. Squamous tumors comprise about 30% of all bronchogenic cancers.

Histologically, these tumor cells can be elongated, spindle shaped, tadpole shaped, oval, or round. Well-differentiated cells can produce keratin. Tumor cells are often arranged in a whorling pattern. If intracellular bridges are seen, another criterion for designation to this group of tumors is satisfied.

Squamous tumors most often occur in the major bronchi or their primary divisions. Grossly, these tumors appear as gray, white, or yellowish masses. A tumor that arises in the central airways may invade, encircle, and compress the bronchus from which it originates. Others may grow into the bronchial lumen. In both instances, signs and symptoms of bronchial obstruction result. Other lesions may be seen as tumor plaques extending along the airway surface. Central necrosis and cavitation are not uncommon. Squamous tumors remain more localized than other cell types. Metastases to structures within the thorax commonly occur. Patients with squamous cancer survive longer than those with other cell types, probably as a function of slower growth rate, the possibility of surgical resection, and late metastasis.

Adenocarcinomas

Adenocarcinomas are the most common of the lung cancers (30% to 35% incidence). This is the most frequent type of lung cancer found in women (with as many female as male cases), nonsmokers, and young people.

Adenocarcinoma cells are characteristically found in a glandular formation. Prominent macronucleoli are seen within the cell nucleus. Vacuoles are seen in the cytoplasm, indicating secretory capabilities. Mucin production is frequently evident. The pathogenesis of adenocarcinoma is not well understood. Unlike other cell types, the adenocarcinoma shows poor dose-response correlation with cigarette smoking. Although no causal relationship can be concluded, adenocarcinomas have been known to develop after long-standing parenchymal irritation, scarring, or fibrosis. These tumors generally present as slow-growing peripheral masses. Hematogenous spread occurs frequently and relatively early in the course of the disease. Adenocarcinomas demonstrate a particular predilection to metastasize to the brain.

A variant of the adenocarcinoma classification is the bronchioloalveolar tumor. As with other adenocarcinomas, these tumors usually present in the periphery of the lung and are characteristically slow growing. Bronchioloalveolar tumors may vary widely in presentation from solitary nodules to diffuse interstitial infiltrates. The appearance of the more well-differentiated bronchioloalveolar tumor cells resembles that of the peripheral respiratory epithelial cells.

Large cell carcinomas

Large cell carcinomas are a heterogenous group of lung cancers, constituting 10% to 15% of all bronchogenic malignancies. Tumors of this type often show almost no differentiated histologic features. Some clinicians refer to this category as a "wastebasket" for all lesions that do not clearly fit into the other three categories. Large cell carcinomas show prominent macronucleoli and are usually mucin negative, with no glandular pattern to the cytoplasm. Peripheral lesions are more common than central ones. Patterns of metastasis are similar to those of adenocarcinomas, with an additional tendency to metastasize to the gastrointestinal tract. Survival rates are generally poor.

Small Cell Lung Cancer

SCLC is strongly associated with cigarette smoking, with an increasing incidence of small cell tumors associated with increased amount of smoking. About 25% of lung cancers are of the small cell variety. Small cell carcinomas are histologically identified as cells containing large nuclei and very little cytoplasm. Cells are often oval and described as resembling lymphocytes even though they are two or three times larger than lymphocytes. Tumors are usually located in central regions of the lung, often at the hilum. Tumors typically grow submucosally with early intralymphatic invasion. Because of their central location and early lymphatic metastases, small cell tumors often present as hilar or perihilar masses. Rapidly growing central tumors can cause bronchial obstruction and pneumonia.

In past years small cell cancers were believed to be derived from Kulchitsky's cells, which have neurosecretory capabilities. The finding of neurosecretory granules in small cell tumor cells and the frequent production of ectopic hormones by these tumors were considered supportive evidence. Such occurrences are now recognized as not exclusive to small cell cancers, and these tumors are thought not to have a unique histogenesis.

Patients with SCLC have a poor prognosis because of the tumors' high growth rate and tendency to metastasize early and widely. Although these tumors are the most sensitive of the histologic types to radiation and chemotherapy, short-term relapses are common.

METASTATIC PATTERN

As with any solid tumor, lung cancers spread by direct extension, lymphatic invasion, and blood-borne metastases. Tumors can spread within the bronchus of origin by direct invasion. Growth can occur in such a manner that the lumen is partially or completely filled and occluded. Other tumors extend in a flattened, plaquelike fashion along the inside of the lumen. Others may invade the bronchial wall and encircle and obstruct the airway. Intrapulmonary spread may lead to compression of lung structures other than airways such as blood or lymph vessels, alveoli, and nerves. Direct extension through the pleura can result in spread over the surface of the lung, chest wall, or diaphragm.

Most centrally located tumors spread to the hilar lymph structures, either by direct extension or lymphatic spread. When lymphatic structures are invaded by tumor, the pattern of subsequent spread depends on the tumor cell type and anatomic location. The central hilar, mediastinal, and paratracheal glands are most commonly affected by lung tumors, although supraclavicular, cervical, and abdominal channels may be invaded. Tumors in the lower lobes tend to spread more widely by lymph channels than do those located elsewhere in the lung.

The widespread pattern of hematogenous metastases in lung cancer is due to the invasion of the pulmonary vascular system and is associated with a poor prognosis. Once tumor cells enter the pulmonary venous system, they can be carried through the heart and disseminated systemically. Tumor emboli can become lodged in areas of organ systems where vessels become too narrow for their passage or where blood flow is reduced. Invasion of branches of the pulmonary arteries occurs less commonly, but this is not infrequent with small cell carcinomas and adenocarcinomas. Metastatic lesions outside the thorax frequently involve the liver, adrenal glands, bone, and brain.

PROGRESSION OF DISEASE

Cures in patients with lung cancer are very rare. Even with the slower-growing types of lung cancer, three out of four individuals will not be alive 5 years after diagnosis, with or without intensive therapy. The 5-year survival rate for patients with all types of bronchogenic cancer is about 11%. At diagnosis, most tumors have probably progressed through the majority of their life spans. As mentioned previously, metastatic spread occurs through the lymph and vascular routes, often before the primary site is detectable. Survival time can be extended by surgical, chemotherapeutic, and radiotherapeutic intervention. These and other forms of therapy are also critical in palliation. The prognosis and selection of appropriate treatment protocols are generally based on the anatomic extent or stage of the cancer at diagnosis.

CLINICAL MANIFESTATIONS

The presence and nature of symptoms in lung cancer depend on the location and extent of the tumor. Systemic symptoms such as anorexia, weight loss and fatigue may suggest cancer. Presenting pulmonary symptoms may include cough, chest pain, hemoptysis, dyspnea, and wheezing. Because most of these symptoms are also associated with cigarette smoking and chronic obstructive pulmonary disease, their significance as indicators of an oncologic process may be unappreciated initially. Symptoms of local metastases may include hoarseness (recurrent laryngeal nerve involvement), chest or shoulder pain (chest wall, pleural, or brachial plexus involvement), dysphagia (esophageal compression or invasion), or head and neck swelling (superior vena caval obstruction). Tumors of the superior sulcus or the apical cap of the lung may invade the brachial plexus, causing shoulder and arm pain. If the cervical nerves are involved, unilateral ptosis, pupillary constriction, and lack of perspiration (Horner's syndrome) may also be seen. Extrathoracic symptoms appear with tumor metastasis and depend on the site and extent of metastatic tumor growth.

Symptoms related to the systemic syndromes that can be associated with lung cancers are numerous and diverse. The ectopic hormone syndromes described in Chapter 26 are one set of syndromes that may occur. Numerous paraneoplastic syndromes are also associated with lung cancer.[26] These phenomena represent the release by tumor cells of hormones or other biologically active substances. Although ectopic hormone syndromes may occur with other carcinomas, they are seen most frequently with lung cancer. SCLCs are more often associated with paraneoplastic syndromes than are the NSCLCs. Exceptions to this are the hypercalcemic and ectopic parathyroid hormone syndromes that are seen with squamous cell tumors. Hypertrophic pulmonary osteoarthropathy and dermatomyositis are also more common in NSCLC. The appearance of these syndromes may precede any other symptoms of lung cancer and may provide the impetus for establishing the diagnosis. Treatment of the lung tumor may result in the remission of symptoms.

CLASSIFICATION AND STAGING

Non-Small Cell Lung Cancer

The staging of lung cancer is based on the TNM system recommended by the American Joint Committee on Cancer. This system provides standardized descriptors of the anatomic extent of disease, which is the crucial determinant of treatment and ultimate survival. Numerical suffixes under T describe increasing size or involvement of the primary tumor. N suffixes describe regional lymph node metastases. M suffixes describe the presence or absence of metastases to distant sites (Table 43-2).

Subsets of the TNM categories have been combined into stages that describe growth, dissemination, and prognosis for tumors in each stage. The International Staging System for Lung Cancer illustrated in Table 43-3 describes levels of tumor progression that are related to therapeutic options and to estimates of prognosis for NSCLC. Survival according to cell type and clinical staging criteria is illustrated in Figures 43-5 to 43-7.

Small Cell Lung Cancer

In SCLC the TNM staging system has little prognostic significance, as illustrated in Figure 43-5. SCLCs are aggressive tumors that disseminate rapidly and widely and carry a poor prognosis regardless of stage classification. The anatomic extent of disease in SCLC is most often described as "limited" or "extensive" using stages proposed by the Veterans Administration Lung Cancer Study Group (VALG). Limited disease can be treated within a single radiotherapy portal and is generally defined as tumor confined to one hemithorax and regional lymph nodes without pleural effusion. Extensive disease refers to spread beyond this area. This two-stage system does provide significant prognostic information. Long-term survival (>3 yrs) in SCLC occurs almost exclusively in the limited disease category.

Although extent of disease is the most important prognostic factor in SCLC, other variables have been shown to affect survival. Although patients with limited disease usually have a better initial performance status than those with extensive disease, performance status at diagnosis has been shown to be an important independent determinant of treatment response and survival. Similarly, weight loss, independent of performance status, has been shown to have prognostic significance. Poor response to chemotherapy, defined as either poor initial response or relapse after treatment, is an additional adverse prognostic sign. Factors known to have prognostic significance in SCLC are:

- Extent of disease (limited vs extensive)
- Performance status
- Weight loss
- Complete response to therapy

TABLE 43-2 TNM Definitions

Primary Tumor (T)	
TX	Tumor proven by the presence of malignant cells in bronchopulmonary secretions but not visualized by imaging or bronchoscopy
T0	No evidence of primary tumor
TIS	Carcinoma in situ
T1	A tumor 3 cm or less in greatest dimension, surrounded by lung or visceral pleura, and without evidence of invasion proximal to a lobar bronchus at bronchoscopy
T2	A tumor more than 3 cm in greatest dimension, or a tumor of any size that either invades the visceral pleura or has associated atelectasis or obstructive pneumonitis extending to the hilar region. At bronchoscopy, the proximal extent of demonstrable tumor must be within a lobar bronchus or at least 2 cm distal to the carina. Any associated atelectasis or obstructive pneumonitis must involve less than an entire lung
T3	A tumor of any size that directly invades into the chest wall (including superior sulcus tumors), diaphragm, or the mediastinal pleura or pericardium without involving the heart, great vessels, trachea, esophagus or vertebral body, or a tumor in the main bronchus within 2 cm of the carina without involving the carina, or associated atelectasis or obstructive pneumonitis of entire lung
T4	A tumor of any size that invades the mediastinum, heart, great vessels, trachea, esophagus, vertebral body or carina or presence of malignant pleural effusion
Nodal Involvement (N)	
N0	No demonstrable metastasis to regional lymph nodes
N1	Metastasis in the peribronchial or the ipsilateral hilar lymph nodes, or both, including direct extension
N2	Metastasis in ipsilateral mediastinal lymph nodes and/or subcarinal lymph nodes
N3	Metastasis in contralateral mediastinal, contralateral hilar, ipsilateral or contralateral scalene or supraclavicular lymph nodes
Distant Metastasis (M)	
M0	No distant metastasis
M1	Distant metastasis

DIAGNOSTIC AND STAGING TESTS

When an individual presents with symptoms that might indicate a lung malignancy, a battery of examinations are scheduled for diagnosis, staging, and treatment planning. Some individuals may be asymptomatic when first seen, with a lesion on a chest radiograph suspicious of a lung

TABLE 43-3 Stage Grouping

Occult Carcinoma	TX	N0	M0
Stage 0	TIS Carcinoma in situ		
Stage I	T1	N0	M0
	T2	N0	M0
Stage II	T1	N1	M0
	T2	N1	M0
Stage III-a	T3	N0	M0
	T3	N1	M0
	T1-3	N2	M0
Stage III-b	Any T	N3	M0
	T4	Any N	M0
Stage IV	Any T	Any N	M1

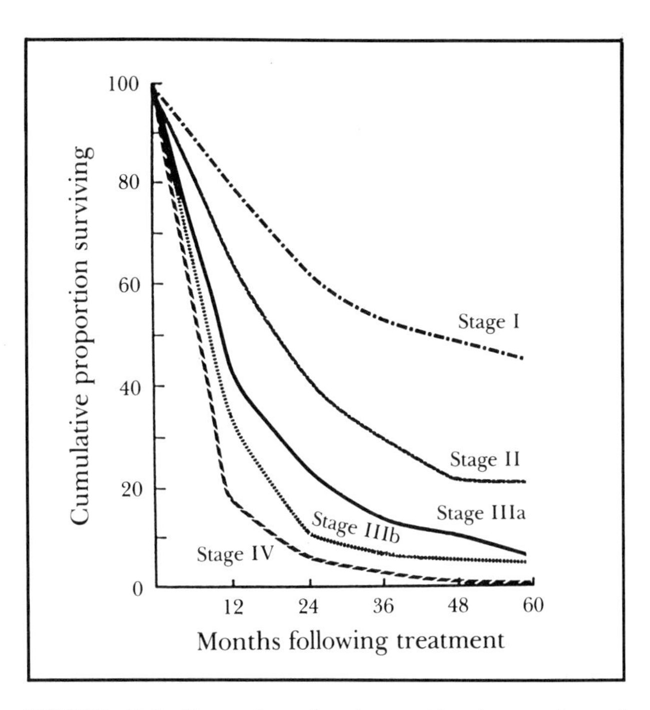

FIGURE 43-6 Proportion of patients with adenocarcinoma/large cell lung cancer expected to survive 5 years according to clinical stage of disease. (Source: Mountain CF: Prognostic implications of the International Staging System for Lung Cancer. Semin Oncol 15:236-245, 1988.)

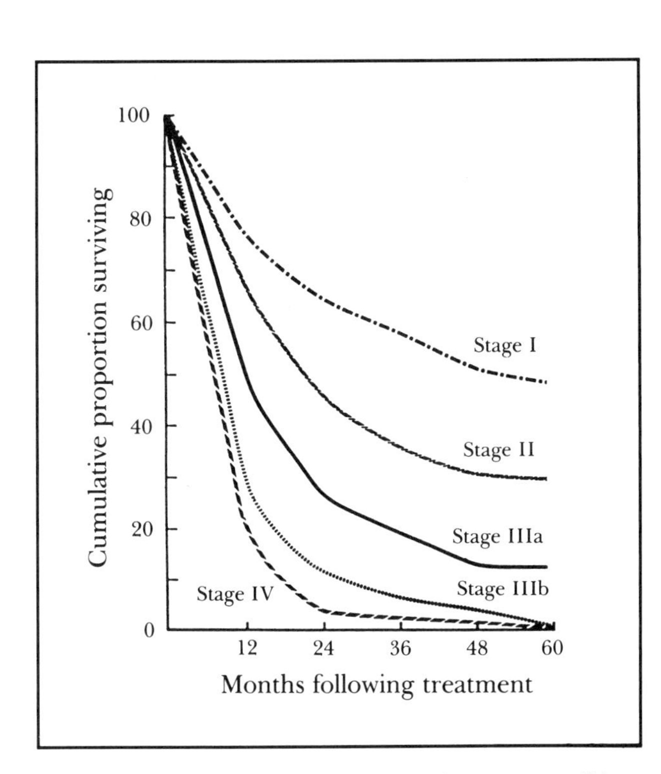

FIGURE 43-5 Proportion of patients with squamous cell lung cancer expected to survive 5 years according to clinical stage of disease. (Source: Mountain CF: Prognostic implications of the International Staging System for Lung Cancer. Semin Oncol 15:236-245, 1988.)

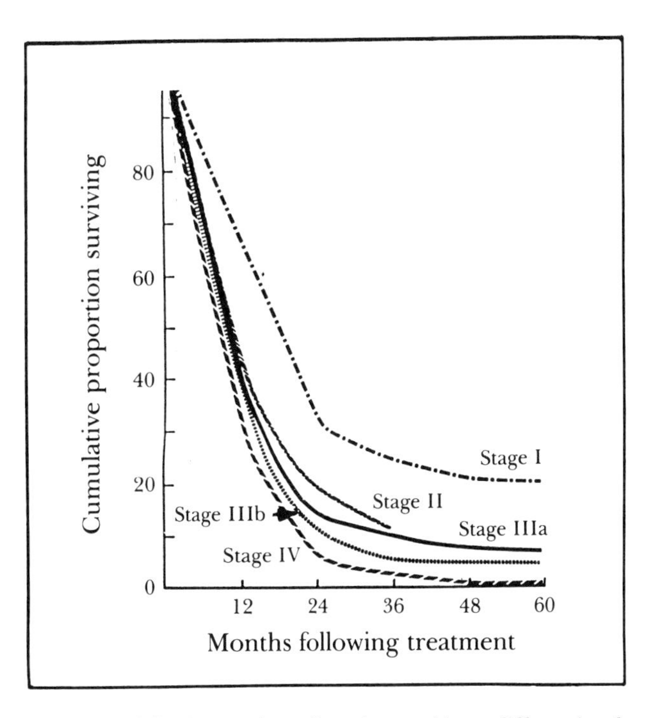

FIGURE 43-7 Proportion of patients with undifferentiated small cell lung cancer expected to survive 5 years according to clinical stage of disease. (Source: Mountain CF: Prognostic implications of the International Staging System for Lung Cancer. Semin Oncol 15:236-245, 1988.)

malignancy or, more rarely, positive sputum cytologic findings.

The initial evaluation includes an assessment of the presence, duration, and severity of pulmonary and extrapulmonary symptoms. The history includes questions regarding prolonged exposure to and inhalation of carcinogenic substances. A past medical history of tuberculosis or pulmonary inflammatory processes may suggest the development of tumors from pulmonary scars. Also of significance would be any apparent familial clustering of lung cancer, suggesting the possibility of an inherited susceptibility to bronchogenic carcinoma.

A number of procedures are available for investigating a possible lung tumor and for staging purposes. The following discussion of applications of the available techniques is organized according to the TNM system.

T (Tumor) Sites

Lesions present on plain chest radiographs may be visualized further by lung tomograms. Computed tomography (CT) scans may better define the characteristics of a suspected tumor, such as size, shape, cavitation, borders, and extent of involvement of surrounding tissue structures.

A diagnosis of lung cancer is ultimately established by cytologic examination of secretions or biopsied tissue. The method of choice for obtaining tissue depends on the location of the suspected tumor. Centrally located endobronchial tumors are most likely to yield positive sputum cytologies. The recommended procedure for the outpatient collection of pooled sputum specimens for cytologic examination is as follows:

1. The individual is given three to five containers, each containing 2 oz of fixative. Each container is labelled to indicate consecutive days of collection. The probability of detecting malignant cells is approximately 75% with three daily specimens and 90% with five consecutive daily specimens.
2. The person is instructed to cough and expectorate into one of these containers according to the following procedure:
   a. Specimens should be obtained on arising in the morning. This provides the best specimen for secretions from deep in the lungs.
   b. No mouth care, eating, or drinking of fluids other than water should be done prior to obtaining the specimen.
   c. The person should breathe deeply and cough to raise sputum. Saliva specimens have no benefit in cancer detection. Heated hypertonic aerosol, ultrasonic mist, and postural drainage may be used to assist in sputum induction.
   d. The person should expectorate directly into the specimen container.
3. Additional sputum raised by the individual should be added to the same container during the day.
4. A separate container is used for each day's sputum.

Nurses usually are responsible for instructing and assisting in sputum collection and can increase the efficiency of this method of cancer detection by collecting and handling the specimen appropriately.

Centrally located tumors are also accessible for bronchoscopic visualization and washing, brushing, and biopsy. The more peripherally located tumors may be reached by percutaneous needle biopsy. Pleural effusions may result from tumor extension to the pleural surface. Examination of pleural fluid and biopsied pleura may confirm the diagnosis of lung cancer. The presence of malignant cells in pleural fluid is usually considered a contraindication to surgical resection.

N (Node) Status

Approximately half of all individuals with lung cancer have mediastinal involvement at diagnosis. The evaluation of the presence and extent of regional lymph node metastases is critical to determining surgical resectability and prognosis. Individuals with mediastinal node metastases are usually considered to have unresectable disease, although this depends on the tumor cell type and location of the affected nodes.

A noninvasive method for evaluating thoracic lymph nodes is CT scanning, which is useful for distinguishing small differences in tissue density and detecting nodal enlargement. CT scanning is more sensitive than conventional tomography in detecting mediastinal adenopathy; unfortunately, neither method can distinguish malignant from nonmalignant adenopathy, nor can micrometastases be detected.

Regional nodes can be sampled by transbronchial needle aspiration, mediastinoscopy, and mediastinotomy. Transbronchial needle aspiration is accomplished through a flexible bronchoscope and allows tissue from the paratracheal, hilar, and subcarinal regions to be obtained. Mediastinoscopy is a more invasive procedure and is done under general anesthesia because of the coughing and pain that result from manipulation of the trachea. Some clinicians routinely employ mediastinoscopy in all cases of bronchogenic tumor without distant metastases to assess operability. Others continue to rely on CT scanning to define nodal involvement. A left anterior mediastinotomy through the left second intercostal space can be used to evaluate preaortic and subaortic mediastinal nodes, a common site of tumor spread from the left upper lobe and left hilum.

M (Metastasis) Status

A careful history and physical examination, along with routine blood chemistries, are the most useful techniques in evaluating metastatic spread. In the absence of signs or symptoms of specific organ involvement, organ scanning is of limited value in detecting unsuspected disease. Metastatic disease not detectable by physical examination or biochemical screening is rarely encountered. Also, the incidence of false-positive scans can be significant. Organ scans and biopsies may be employed to assess stage or operability.

TREATMENT

Non-Small Cell Lung Cancer

Surgery

With rare exceptions, complete surgical resection of a lung tumor offers the only chance for cure. Only 20% to 25% of patients with lung cancer qualify for curative resectional surgery. Patients who are considered surgical candidates are those with NSCLCs with occult, stage I or II disease. Occasionally, some patients with localized stage IIIa disease may be considered for surgery.

Occult and stage I cancer If the individual has an occult cancer or a tumor that is not detectable on chest radiograph, it is necessary to locate the source of the malignant cells seen in the sputum prior to surgery. Localization may be achieved by searching the tracheobronchial tree with fiberoptic bronchoscopy. The flexible fiberoptic bronchoscope allows visualization and biopsy down to the fourth or fifth branchings of the bronchial tree. Cancerous lesions may not appear as discrete and easily recognizable from surrounding mucosa, and any suspicious site is brushed and biopsied. This procedure may be repeated at frequent intervals (3 to 6 months) if localization is initially unsuccessful.

An alternative method has recently been developed for locating occult malignancies that arise from the trachea or central bronchi. This technique, bronchoscopic laser photoirradiation, depends on the use during bronchoscopy of the chemical hematoporphyrin derivative (HpD) as a tumor marker. HpD selectively accumulates in malignant tissue and produces a red fluorescence when photoirradiated with a laser light source. Laser photoirradiation may establish a diagnosis of lung cancer in individuals whose tumors have not been diagnosed by radiography or conventional fiberoptic bronchoscopy.

The nurse is in a position to provide information and support during the process of localizing the tumor. It is likely to be a difficult time for the individual and family. The person must adjust to the fact that he or she has a serious disease despite being entirely or largely asymptomatic. There is a realistic basis for optimism, however, in light of the improved survival statistics following surgical treatment of localized lung cancer. Accurate information presented in realistically optimistic terms is recommended in dealing with individuals with occult or stage I cancer and their families.

Several surgical procedures may be considered for resection of localized cancer, including wedge resection, segmentectomy, lobectomy, or pneumonectomy. Figure 43-8 illustrates three of the more common surgical procedures. Opinions on the most appropriate procedure differ, but in general the most conservative procedure that will encompass all the known tumor is selected. The anatomic location and extent of the tumor are crucial factors in the selection of the surgical approach. In all instances the risks of surgery are weighed against the purposes and realistic outcomes of the procedure.

The results of surgery vary by TNM category and cell type. The 5-year survival rate for patients with stage I disease is 50% or more.[29] Survival statistics for patients with squamous tumors are better than those for patients with adenocarcinomas or large cell cancers.

Thorough discussions of the nursing care of individuals before and after thoracotomy are available and will not be reiterated here. Several of the most important considerations are highlighted in the discussion that follows.

Preoperatively, all individuals scheduled for resectional surgery will undergo testing to evaluate operative risk and tolerance for the loss of lung tissue. The surgical decision may be a particularly complex one because individuals often present with two diseases related to cigarette smoking—lung cancer and chronic obstructive lung disease. General screening tests prior to lung resection include chest radiography, spirometry, and arterial blood gas analysis. Individuals with spirometric limitations or evidence of ventilatory failure are always at higher risk than those with normal pulmonary functions, and the greater the decline, the greater the risk. Measurement of the forced expiratory volume in 1 second (FEV_1) has been particularly relied on as a predictor of postoperative pulmonary impairment. A predicted postoperative FEV_1 of 0.8 to 1 liter has been defined as the lower limit of acceptable pulmonary function, below which there is great risk of ventilatory insufficiency and intolerance of exertion. Additional guidelines are available to assist in determining a specific individual's operability, but morbidity and mortality vary greatly. Individual recommendations must be formulated with consideration of such factors as age, overall constitutional status, the type of surgery contemplated, and the type of anesthesia to be used. In individuals with marginal pulmonary functions, more extensive tests may be ordered to assess tolerance for the degree of anticipated resection. Radioisotopic lung scanning techniques to ascertain regional lung function and predict postoperative values may be indicated. In individuals with pulmonary hypertension, pulmonary arterial pressures may be recorded during balloon occlusion of either the right or left pulmonary artery. This maneuver is used to help determine the adequacy of the pulmonary vasculature remaining after resection.

To maximize ventilatory capacities, particularly in individuals identified as at risk before surgery, airway clearance measures are employed. These include postural drainage, inhalation of aerosol solutions, and deep breathing and coughing techniques. Bronchodilators are indicated in instances of reversible airway obstruction. Pathogens identified by sputum culture are treated with appropriate antibiotics.

Cigarette smoking, which predisposes to oxygen de-

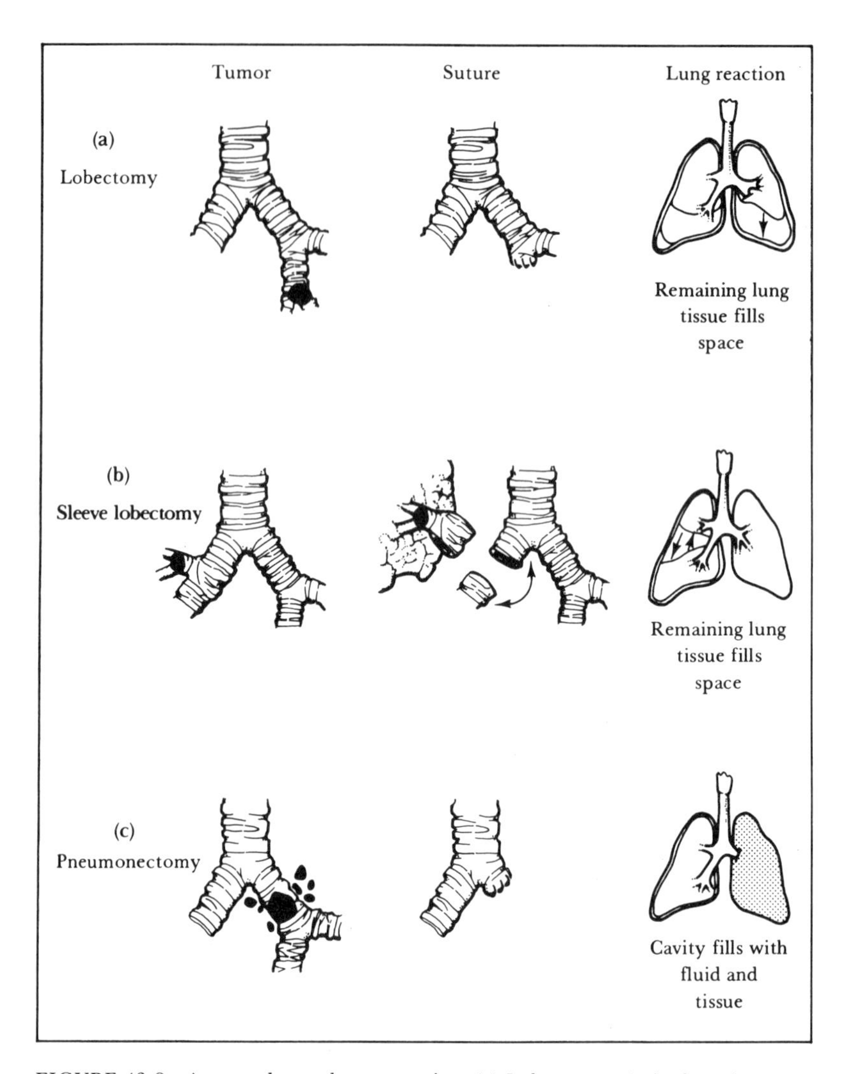

FIGURE 43-8 Approaches to lung resection. (a) Lobectomy: A single pulmonary lobe is resected. (b) Sleeve lobectomy: The tumor-bearing lobe is resected together with a segment of the main bronchus, followed by an end-to-end anastomosis. Classic indication is a carcinoma of the right upper lobe bronchus. (c) Pneumonectomy: The lung alone is removed (simple pneumonectomy) or the lung and involved adjacent nodes are removed (radical pneumonectomy).

saturation, excessive secretions, and pulmonary infection, should be curtailed before surgery. This prescription may be difficult for the individual to follow. In caring for such individuals, the nurse would do well to examine his or her feelings about smoking and lung cancer. For the most part, cancer is considered to be a disease that "attacks" unsuspecting victims. Lung cancer is notably at odds with this portrayal. The causal relationship between smoking and lung cancer has been much publicized. Smokers who develop lung cancer may be seen less as innocent victims than as active participants in the causation of their cancer. Although blaming the person serves no purpose, it is difficult to avoid ambivalence in dealing with such individuals, particularly if they continue to smoke after diagnosis. A judgmental approach by the nurse can increase the person's anxiety, discourage an open and therapeutic relationship, and deter cooperation toward important goals. It should be remembered that compulsive cigarette smoking is an addictive behavior, not one that results from a lack of willpower.

After surgery, individuals generally undergo mechanical ventilatory assistance for a brief period. In resective lung surgery, it is desirable to discontinue positive pressure ventilation as soon as feasible to minimize potential barotrauma to the sutured airway. Analgesics will be necessary to control incisional pain. After extubation, deep breathing and coughing exercises are crucial to mobilize secretions and prevent atelectasis and should be coordinated with times of analgesia administration to minimize the person's discomfort. The incision line should be splinted during deep breathing and coughing exercises. It is important to realize that many individuals forget their preoperative instructions regarding coughing and deep breathing. It may be necessary to repeat instructions from session to session because carryover of teaching may be poor. Other postoperative nursing care is specific to the operative procedure performed and is outlined in Tables 43-4 to 43-6.

Stage II cancer Surgical resection is usually the treatment of choice for stage II bronchogenic carcinomas other than those of the small cell variety. The goal is cure, although the incidence of cure in patients with stage II disease is low. The probability of residual tumor after resection is great, as is the probability of occult distant metastasis. Accordingly, some type of adjuvant therapy or combination of therapies are being used and studied. Most protocols involve the use of preoperative radiation and/or chemotherapy to improve resectability and survival. Such additions to the surgical procedure have not been impressive in influencing survival. Preoperative radiotherapy may be employed to debulk the primary tumor, control lymph node metastasis not accessible for removal, and reduce local and systemic dissemination of viable tumor cells during the operative procedure. If preoperative irradiation is employed, surgery may be postponed for 4 to 6 weeks. Postoperative irradiation is designed to kill any cancer cells not resected. Postoperative systemic chemotherapy may be employed to control occult metastasis and cancer recurrence. To date, survival rates have not been significantly affected by these adjuncts to the surgical regimen.

TABLE 43-4 Nursing Care of Individuals After Lobectomy

Discussion	Nursing Implications
Ventilation—perfusion relationships are disrupted by lobe removal	Gas exchange status must be monitored carefully, particularly through arterial blood gas analysis; supplemental oxygen is usually administered
After lobe removal, the remaining lobe(s) expand to fill the space created by removal	Position the person to foster expansion; avoid leaving the individual lying on the operative side for prolonged periods of time
The bronchus leading to the resected lobe is stapled or sutured closed	Suction only as necessary; suction returns should be carefully inspected for evidence of bleeding, necrosis, or infection of the stump
Closed chest-tube drainage is employed to remove air and fluid from the pleural space	The water seal must be maintained at all times; drainage collection devices must be below chest level at all times; chest tubes must be kept patent and free of leaks

Radiation therapy

In instances where curative resection is impossible either because of tumor extent or other disease, radiation therapy may be applied. Guidelines for radiation therapy have been summarized as follows[30]:

1. Radiation for cure in patients with intrathoracic but inoperable NSCLC is appropriate in those who are in good physical condition without extrathoracic metastases.

2. Curative radiation in clinically operable patients who are at increased risk because of advanced age or medical illness is an appropriate therapeutic approach.

3. Preoperative radiation can sterilize tumor and make inoperable patients operable, but overall survival is not improved and may be worse than with operation alone.

4. Postoperative irradiation is indicated in patients with mediastinal nodes removed at operation. In such circumstances, irradiation may prolong survival, although results of large-scale trials are not available.

5. Poor general condition, distant metastases, inadequate pulmonary reserve, malignant pleural effusion, and tumor size greater than 6 cm are contraindications to curative radiation. Palliative radiation can improve symptoms, often dramatically. Tumor shrinkage with relief of pressure on adjacent structures may help relieve dyspnea, cough, hemoptysis, and symptoms associated with superior vena caval obstruction, airway compression, paralysis of the recurrent laryngeal nerve, or pleural effusion. Bone and brain metastases are also managed by irradiation.

Most NSCLCs demonstrate poor radiosensitivity, and high doses of radiation (5000 to 6000 rad [cGy]) are necessary for cure. These doses of radiation therapy exceed normal lung tissue tolerance levels, and some degree of damage to the airways and parenchyma is inevitable. The occurrence and severity of the resulting inflammatory reaction depends on the dose of radiation received and the size of the treatment field. Acute radiation pneumonitis usually produces symptoms within 1 to 3 months after treatment. Symptoms include dyspnea, fever, night sweats, and thick sputum.[31] Pulmonary infections are an associated risk. Radiation fibrosis may develop 6 months after completion of radiation therapy and is discussed subsequently as a late complication of treatment.

Other structures in the irradiated field may also evidence tissue destruction. Radiation-induced pharyngitis and esophagitis with dysphagia are particularly common. During treatment, individuals may need to be placed on a high-protein, soft diet and monitored for signs of gastrointestinal bleeding. More serious complications such as radiation carditis, radiation myelitis, and bronchoesophageal fistulae occur in less than 3% of patients.

TABLE 43-5 Nursing Care of Individuals After Pneumonectomy

Discussion	Nursing Implications
All pulmonary volumes and capacities are reduced by approximately one-half as compared with the preoperative state	Volume and pressure settings on the mechanical ventilator must be determined accordingly; supplemental oxygen is usually administered; avoid positions that compress the remaining lung (Trendelenburg, lying on the unoperated side)
Blood flow to the remaining lung is increased	Carefully monitor individual for signs of pulmonary hypertension; fluid intake and output must be calculated carefully to avoid fluid overload; use of a volumetric pump for the administration of intravenous fluids is recommended
The thoracic cavity left after lung removal must be filled to prevent mediastinal shift of the heart and remaining lung	Chest tubes are not inserted or placed, but clamped; clamps should be left in place and labeled to prevent removal; the position of the trachea should be monitored closely and the physician notified immediately of a shift from the midline position; a shift toward the unoperated side may indicate hemorrhage or a bronchopleural fistula
The bronchial stump is stapled or sutured after lung removal	Intermittent positive-pressure breathing and blow bottles are generally not used postoperatively; vigorous, deep suctioning should be avoided to prevent suture line trauma or perforation; at the physician's discretion, suctioning may be contraindicated and secretions removed via a flexible bronchoscope; positioning the person on the unoperated side may be initially restricted to prevent fluid from leaking through the stump and into the remaining lung
If intrapericardial node dissection is done during pneumonectomy, herniation of the heart through the pericardial sac is a rare but lethal complication	Individuals must be monitored closely for the development of hypotension, tachycardia and central venous obstruction; immediate thoracotomy is essential to reposition the heart and correct the defect

Prophylactic brain irradiation has been given to patients with NSCLC, particularly those with adenocarcinoma, where brain metastases are frequent. Prophylactic brain irradiation has been given as part of curative therapy to prevent having the central nervous system (CNS) be a potential site of relapse. However, this has not been shown to improve survival.

The use of radiotherapy to improve the prognosis for individuals diagnosed with lung cancer has not yielded encouraging results. Several techniques to improve the response of lung tumors to radiotherapy have been suggested and are under investigation. It is hoped that dosage and fractionation schedules may be adjusted to be optimally effective in relation to the various cell types and stage groups of lung cancer. Hyperfractionation, short-course, and split-dose techniques are being studied for their effects on various tumors at various stages. Also, methods to increase the sensitivity of lung tumor cells to radiation using such agents as oxygen and vitamin K are being tested. Some clinicians have attempted to provide concentrated localized postoperative radiotherapy by implanting radioactive seeds in the bed of any unresectable tumor during the operative procedure. The role of elective irradiation of common relapse sites after "curative" surgery, radiotherapy, or chemotherapy also requires further investigation.

Chemotherapy

The role of chemotherapy in patients with nonresectable NSCLC has been seriously debated. With combination chemotherapy, tumor shrinkage may occur, but a consistent improvement in prognosis has not been produced. Chemotherapy is generally not considered as standard treatment for patients with disseminated NSCLC but may be undertaken in a research setting. Clinical investigation in NSCLC includes evaluation of drug regimens composed of doxorubicin, methotrexate, cyclophosphamide, vindesine, cisplatin, mitomycin C, etoposide, and carboplatin. Toxicity of treatment regimens is considerable. Since response rates are linked to pretreatment performance status, only patients who evidence good performance status should be selected for chemotherapy. To avoid needless toxicity, treatment should be discontinued if tumor shrinkage is not evident.

The limited benefits of chemotherapy in NSCLC have provided impetus to researchers seeking to improve tumor response. Strategies have included the use of lung cancer

TABLE 43-6 Discharge Planning of Individuals After Thoracotomy

Discussion	Nursing Implications
Painful or fatiguing coughing can occur following exposure to bronchial irritants	The importance of smoking cessation should be emphasized; the person should be instructed to avoid situations where exposure is likely (air pollution alerts, crowded or smoke-filled rooms); vocational counseling may be necessary
After resectional surgery, individuals are at risk for the development of pulmonary hypertension	Individual should be monitored for the development of right-sided heart failure
The development of pulmonary infection can threaten gas exchange status	Individual should be assessed to ensure that he or she is free of pulmonary congestion prior to discharge; instruct the person to avoid contact with persons with known infections; provide the person with information to monitor for the development of symptoms of a respiratory tract infection; the person may be vaccinated against influenza at the physician's discretion
Easy fatigability may persist after thoracotomy	A progressive activity regimen may be prescribed
Individuals with a previous lung cancer are at risk of cancer recurrence	Postdischarge follow-up will generally include semiannual chest radiographs and sputum cytologies; any new symptoms should be reported immediately to the physician

cell lines to identify new chemotherapy agents that are active specifically against lung tumors. A related approach has been the use of in vitro drug sensitivity testing using fresh tumor specimens to select agents for use in vivo. The laboratory techniques necessary for the success of these drug screening efforts are under development.

Small Cell Lung Cancer

Regardless of the findings at diagnosis, small cell cancer is considered a systemic disease. As such, the mainstay of treatment is combination chemotherapy with or without radiotherapy. SCLC is a highly responsive neoplasm and the most sensitive of all lung tumors to both chemotherapy and radiotherapy.

The role of surgery as an adjunctive treatment in SCLC is not clear. Surgical resection combined with preoperative or postoperative chemotherapy may be considered in the rare patient with a small peripheral tumor without apparent nodal involvement.

Chemotherapy

Combination chemotherapeutic regimens can dramatically influence survival. Major advances in chemotherapy in SCLC occurred in the 1970s, with only limited gains since then. The results of clinical trials have demonstrated several principles that guide current therapy:

1. Multiple simultaneously administered chemotherapeutic agents are preferable to single agents in both limited and extensive disease. Drugs that are particularly effective include cyclophosphamide, doxorubicin, vincristine, etoposide, and cisplatin. Regimens that combine three of the above agents are usually recommended.

2. Maximum results require high-dose therapy sufficient to produce serious toxicity. To a point, more intensive regimens appear to produce higher response rates. However, there is a limit to this dose response, above which increased toxicity occurs without increased benefit.

3. Tumor regression in response to chemotherapy often occurs quickly. Unfortunately, most responders relapse, frequently at the initial intrathoracic site. The optimal duration of chemotherapy is undetermined.

4. The development of drug resistance is a common problem. Alternating chemotherapy regimens to prevent the development of drug resistance is a proposed but not confirmed strategy.

5. Less than 20% of patients achieve long-term (>2 years) survival after initiation of treatment. Typically, these are patients with limited disease who achieve a complete response to therapy. Relapses in long-term survivors are often related to the appearance of NSCLC.[32]

It may be possible to improve significantly the prognosis of patients with SCLC if synergistic drugs could be combined in therapy, more effective modes of administration and schedules of administration developed, and appropriate combinations of multimodal approaches to therapy established. Several centers are attempting to achieve cures in patients with SCLC by using autologous bone marrow transplantation to individuals after megadose chemotherapy and total body irradiation.

Radiation therapy

The role of localized radiotherapy in the treatment of patients with SCLC is still being formulated. Chest irradiation has been combined with chemotherapy to reduce the frequency of intrathoracic relapses after chemotherapy alone. Although the frequency of tumor recurrence can be reduced with the addition of radiotherapy, it is premature to conclude that a clear survival advantage results from combined modality therapy. Combination therapy causes increased toxicity, particularly to the skin, esophagus, and lung parenchyma. Combined therapy is reserved for patients with limited disease, since patients with extensive disease have not been shown to benefit from the addition of radiotherapy.

Many patients with SCLC have brain metastasis at diagnosis or develop signs of brain metastasis sometime before death. The longer the patient with SCLC survives, the greater is the likelihood of detectable cerebral metastases. Prophylactic brain irradiation has been recommended for patients who have achieved a complete response to chemotherapy to eliminate the CNS as the site of early relapse. To date, no great survival advantage has resulted from prophylactic cranial irradiation, although the small numbers of patients studied may account in part for the lack of significant results.

Smoking Cessation

Smokers who develop lung cancer may believe that, since the worst danger of smoking has been realized, there is no compelling reason to quit smoking. There is evidence that cigarette smoking adversely affects prognosis in individuals with lung cancer. Investigations of patients with SCLC demonstrated that patients who discontinued smoking either prior to or at diagnosis survived longer than individuals who continued to smoke. The reasons underlying the relationship between cigarette smoking and survival were hypothesized to relate to impaired host defenses against tumor growth associated with smoking.[33] Additionally, patients who continue to smoke during therapy for SCLC had a greater risk of developing NSCLCs than did those who discontinued smoking. These findings illustrate the probable immunodepressive effects of cigarette smoking in terms of tumor development and growth. The potential benefits of smoking cessation after lung cancer is diagnosed should be recognized and efforts directed toward assisting patients to stop smoking.

Phototherapy

Phototherapy using a neodynium-yttrium-aluminum-garnet (YAG) laser has been applied as palliation in individuals with far-advanced obstructing airway tumors. Applied through a bronchoscope, the neodynium-YAG laser can produce thermal necrosis and shrinkage of the tumor, allowing pieces of the tumor to be removed through biopsy forceps. Heating also reduces blood supply and may help control bleeding, although hemorrhage is a recognized complication of neodynium-YAG laser therapy.

LATE COMPLICATIONS OF TREATMENT

The discussion of treatments rendered to patients with lung cancers, particularly SCLCs, has emphasized the intensity of therapy and the liklihood of serious side effects. Toxicities associated with radiation therapy and chemotherapy are discussed below.

Radiation Therapy

Pulmonary fibrosis is a common late effect of chest irradiation. The severity of this condition is related to the dose of radiation and the size of the treatment portal. Injury to lung tissue is markedly enhanced when chemotherapy and radiation are combined in treatment. Clinical manifestations include dry cough, dyspnea, weakness, hypoxemia, and perhaps cor pulmonale.

Pericarditis and myelitis can follow curative-dose radiotherapy to the heart or spinal cord. The frequency of occurrence increases with increasing doses. Because of the poor survival rate generally seen in lung cancer, patients may die of their cancer before these complications develop.

In cases of cranial irradiation, particularly when combined with chemotherapy, a "CNS syndrome" of unusual neurologic abnormalities has been seen. Memory loss, tremor, slurred speech, and somnolence can be acute. A similar syndrome with abnormalities on CT scan has been described in long-term survivors who received prophylactic cranial irradiation.

Chemotherapy

The aggressive multiagent chemotherapy regimens often used in lung cancer, particularly when combined with chest irradiation, can cause serious toxicities. An increased incidence of preleukemia and leukemia posttherapy has been seen and indicates long-term bone marrow toxicity. Patients aggressively treated with cytotoxic agents, particularly with alkylating agents, are at high risk of this hazard.

Many pharmacologic agents are associated with pulmonary parenchymal damage. Risks of pulmonary toxicity from cytotoxic drugs may increase with cumulative drug dose, age, use of chest radiotherapy, and concurrent oxygen therapy.[34] The agents that can cause lung injury are listed below:

Bleomycin	Azathioprine
Mitomycin	Mercaptopurine
Busulfan	Cytosine arabinoside
Cyclophosphamide	Procarbazine
Chlorambucil	VM-26
Melphalan	Vinblastine
BCNU	Vindasine
CCNU	Chlorozotocin
Methotrexate	

Lung injury in the form of pneumonitis and fibrosis most commonly occurs. Treatment involves withdrawing the offending agent and administering corticosteroids. Some syndromes of injury are self-limited, but progressive disease is more often encountered.

SYMPTOMATIC MANAGEMENT

Cough

A chronic cough may result from stimulation of irritant receptors in the bronchial mucosa through tumor infiltration. Hypersecretion of mucus also may cause coughing. The dry, irritating cough must be distinguished from the productive cough. Although it may be appropriate to suppress a dry, persistent, and debilitating cough, this should not be attempted at the expense of secretion retention. Narcotic medications, specifically codeine preparations, are generally used for cough suppression. In addition, inspired air should be warmed and humidified and cigarette smoking discouraged. Deep breathing and effective coughing techniques should be taught and reinforced as necessary. Tracheal suctioning should be used only if the person's cough is ineffective in removing secretions.

Pain

Chest pain due to a bronchogenic tumor is usually dull, poorly localized, and described as an ache. The mechanism of pain production is not clear, but the pain itself is seldom severe. A more sharp and severe type of chest pain can occur with tumor involvement of the bony thorax or parietal pleura. Radiotherapy is often effective in controlling pain. If standard cancer therapies fail to relieve or control pain, pharmacologic agents are usually ordered. If agents such as hydromorphone hydrochloride (Dilaudid), meperidine hydrochloride (Demerol), or morphine are ultimately necessary to control pain, such drugs should not be withheld because of fear of addiction. Individuals in pain generally have significant disease and a short life expectancy. They should be made as comfortable as possible in their remaining days.

Dyspnea

Dyspnea is a complex reaction that involves physiologic and psychologic processes. Dyspnea is a common presenting symptom in individuals with lung cancer and develops in others after diagnosis. The presence and severity of dyspnea may relate to multiple factors including airways obstruction, fibrosis, edema, tumor infiltration, pleural effusion, inspiratory muscle fatigue, anxiety, and depression. In patients with lung cancer the presence of dyspnea is often associated with fatigue and decreased energy.[35] Emotional stress may contribute to the production of dyspnea and may also result from the experience of dyspnea.

Nurses should assess the events that appear to stimulate dyspnea, the individual's description and interpretation of the experience, and individual management strategies. Such evaluation may suggest possible interventions to limit the frequency or severity of dyspneic episodes or to increase tolerance of this symptom. Depending on the cause, dyspnea may improve following thoracentesis, irradiation, chemotherapy, diuretics, steroids, or supplemental oxygen. Activity limitation, bronchial hygiene measures, appropriate positioning, and systematic relaxation training may help control persistent dyspnea. Although it is sometimes useful in controlling dyspnea in individuals with chronic airways obstruction, breathing retraining should not be automatically prescribed for lung cancer patients with dyspnea. Diaphragmatic breathing with slow exhalation through pursed lips may not be appropriate for patients whose dyspnea relates to restrictive pulmonary disorders and may, in fact, cause greater distress. In patients with intractable dyspnea, narcotics or anxiolytics may be of benefit in symptom reduction. The potential side effects, including hypoventilation, are considered acceptable risks in selected patients.

Hemoptysis

Hemoptysis is caused by tumor erosion into pulmonary blood vessels. Bleeding may appear as streaks or dots or as gross blood loss. Although infrequent, frank bleeding with significant blood loss requires immediate attention if shock and fatal hemorrhage are to be avoided. As soon as bleeding is encountered, the patient should be positioned on one side so that the lung most probably containing the bleeding site is dependent. Such positioning is undertaken to prevent spillover of blood into the unaffected lung. The bleeding site must be located and treated, usually through bronchoscopy. Radiotherapy may be effective in controlling hemorrhage. Less severe bleeding episodes are still likely to be frightening, and the individual should be reassured if the blood loss is not significant. Individuals with hemoptysis must be monitored carefully for increased blood loss, changes in blood pressure and pulse, and respiratory distress. Because blood provides an excellent medium for bacterial growth, antibiotics may be prescribed for the person with hemoptysis.

Wheezing

Unilateral persistent wheezing occurs if a tumor partially obstructs the bronchus. This troublesome symptom can generally be relieved by tumor shrinkage through irradiation. Wheezing may be more severe when the individual lies on one side, and positioning should be undertaken to protect bronchial patency.

PSYCHOSOCIAL ISSUES

Psychosocial issues and concerns of individuals with malignancies have been discussed elsewhere in this text. In caring for individuals with lung cancer, certain responses or dilemmas that may relate to this particular illness are discussed below.

Social Isolation

Individuals with lung cancer are usually symptomatic when they present for diagnosis. Presenting symptoms commonly include dyspnea, cough, weight loss, and fatigue. These symptoms may worsen as a result of treatment and/or disease progression. Social isolation is a coping strategy frequently used to deal with distressing symptoms, particularly dyspnea and fatigue.[35] Patients may find it necessary to curtail previously important social contact to prevent physical decompensation.

Individuals who continue to smoke beyond diagnosis may feel vulnerable to criticism and consequently avoid or limit contact with others. This behavior may prove to be an additional stressor for the patient or the family who feels isolated from social supports at a time when they are especially needed. To the extent possible, patients should be assisted to balance their need to avoid disabling emotional and physical activation against the reduced quality of life associated with psychosocial isolation.

Limited Prognosis

Individuals with cancer have indicated their need for caregivers to deal with them honestly and with hope. This need can be of greater importance than the need to discuss issues related to death and dying.[36] Given the typically limited prognosis of most patients with lung cancer, this may seem to pose a dilemma of how to balance optimism with realism. To prevent undue distress, it is important to keep several factors in mind. First, hope and honesty are not incompatible. Patients hope not only for a cure or an extension of life but to preserve the quality of their life. Second, patients' needs may vary in importance according to changing phases of illness. Fortunately, most patients provide cues, some overt and some subtle, regarding when and how much information they are prepared to handle. Nurses who are sensitive to such cues can help provide timely information and support. Although it is not helpful to give early and frequent reminders to a patient that his or her days may be limited, it is also a disservice to ignore disease progression and impending death. Patients with respiratory illness often express fear of a "smothering" type of death and are relieved to hear that such an experience is unlikely. Patients should also be given the opportunity to discuss the use of life-sustaining technologies and to describe their desires regarding the use of these supports. This discussion should take place well before a medical crisis necessitates decisions about the use of such supports. To commit hopelessly ill patients to mechanical ventilation and other resuscitative measures simply because no one has ascertained their preferences is unsupportable morally, ethically, and economically.

CONCLUSION

The challenges to those involved in the care of individuals with lung cancer are significant. Given the high potential for prevention and the low probabilities for cure, the oncology nurse's role assumes special prominence. Nurses may have particular opportunities and competencies in supporting individual efforts to avoid or cease smoking. In individuals with lung cancer for whom curative measures are impossible or unsuccessful, the nurse often becomes a principal coordinator and practitioner of interventions aimed at palliation. Practice in these areas is as much art as science. There is much to be learned from scientists, clinical colleagues, patients, and families. We know of many interventions that do not benefit patients; the challenge of the future is to develop and perfect more that do. Nurses who are willing to be educated and guided by experience and who remain open to investigating innovative and creative approaches are essential to all such efforts.

REFERENCES

1. Silverberg E, Lubera GA: Cancer statistics, 1989. CA 39:3-20, 1989.
2. Spencer H: Pathology of the Lung (vol 2, ed 4). Oxford, Pergamon Press, 1985.
3. Wynder EL, Stellman SD: Impact of long term filter cigarette usage on lung and laryngeal cancer risk. J Natl Cancer Inst 62:471-477, 1979.
4. Oleske DM: Epidemiology of lung cancer. Semin Oncol Nurs 3:165-173, 1987.
5. Report of the Surgeon General: The health consequences of involuntary smoking. Washington, DC, US Dept of Health and Human Services, 1986.
6. American Thoracic Society Scientific Assembling on Occupational and Environmental Health: Health effects of air pollution. ATS News 4:22-63, 1978.
7. American Lung Association: Facts about radon. New York, The Association, 1988.
8. Samet JM, Nero AV: Indoor radon and lung cancer. N Engl J Med 320:591-593, 1989.
9. Colditz GA, Stampfer MJ, Willett WC: Diet and lung cancer. Arch Intern Med 147:157-160, 1987.
10. Birrer MJ, Minna JD: Molecular genetics of lung cancer. Semin Oncol 15:226-235, 1988.
11. Mulvihill JJ, Bale AE: Ecogenetics of lung cancer, in Mizell M, Correa P (eds): Lung Cancer: Causes and Prevention. Deerfield Beach: Verlag Chemie International, 1984, pp 141-152.

12. Skillrud DM, Offord KP, Miller RD: Higher risk of lung cancer in chronic obstructive pulmonary disease. Ann Intern Med 105:503-507, 1986.
13. Filderman AE, Carter DC, Baue AE, et al: Lung cancer, in Matthay RA, Matthay MA, Wiedemann HP (eds): Annual Review of Pulmonary and Critical Care Medicine. Philadelphia, Hanley & Belfur, 1988, pp 53-75.
14. Baumm AD, Medsger TA: Cancer and systemic sclerosis: An epidemiologic study. Arthritis Rheum 28:1336-1340, 1985.
15. Horn D: Social and psychologic aspects of starting smoking, in Neiburgs HE (ed): Prevention and Detection of Cancer (vol 1). New York, Marcel Dekker, 1977, pp 739-746.
16. Report of the Surgeon General: The health consequences of smoking. Washington, DC, US Dept of Health and Human Services, 1982.
17. Risser NL: The key to prevention of lung cancer. Semin Oncol Nurs 3:228-236, 1987.
18. Garfinkel L, Stellman SD: Cigarette smoking among physicians, dentists and nurses. CA 36:2-8, 1986.
19. Gritz ER, Kanim L: Do fewer oncology nurses smoke? Oncol Nurs Forum 13:61-64, 1986.
20. Auerbach O, Hammond EC, Garfinkel L: Changes in bronchial epithelium in relation to cigarette smoking, 1955–1960 vs. 1970–1977. N Engl J Med 300:381-386, 1979.
21. Landrigan PJ, Selikoff IJ: Primary prevention against occupational carcinogens, in Bannasch P (ed): Cancer Risks, New York, Springer-Verlag, 1986, pp 94-100.
22. Berlin NI, Buncher CR, Fontana RS, et al: The National Cancer Institute cooperative early lung cancer detection program. Am Rev Respir Dis 130:545-549, 1984.
23. Early Lung Cancer Cooperative Study: Early lung cancer detection. Am Rev Respir Des 130:565-570, 1984.
24. Kotin P: Carcinogenesis of the lung, in Liebow AA, Smith DE (eds): The Lung. Baltimore, Williams & Wilkins, 1968.
25. Yesner R, Carter D: Pathology of carcinoma of the lung. Clin Chest Med 3:257-289, 1982.
26. Doyle LA, Aisner J: Clinical presentation of lung cancer, in Roth HA, Ruckdeschel JC, Weisenburger TH (eds): Thoracic Oncology. Philadelphia, WB Saunders, 1989, pp 52-76.
27. Mountain CF: Prognostic implications of the International Staging System for Lung Cancer. Semin Oncol 15:236-245, 1988.
28. Abrams J, Dole LA, Aisner J: Staging, prognostic factors and special considerations in small cell lung cancer. Semin Oncol 15:261-277, 1988.
29. Johnson MR: Selecting patients with lung cancer for surgical therapy. Semin Oncol 15:246-254, 1988.
30. Hande KR, Des Prez RM: Chemotherapy and radiation therapy for non-small cell lung carcinoma. Clin Chest Med 3:399-414, 1982.
31. McNaull FW: Radiation therapy for lung cancer. Semin Oncol Nurs 3:194-201, 1987.
32. Johnson BE, Ihde DC, Matthews MJ: Nonsmall cell lung cancer: Major cause of late mortality in patients with small cell lung cancer. Am J Med 80:1103-1110, 1986.
33. Johnston-Early A, Cohen MH, Minna JD, et al: Smoking abstinence and small cell lung cancer survival. JAMA 244:2175-2179, 1980.
34. Cooper JA, White DA, Matthay RA: Drug induced pulmonary disease: Cytotoxic drugs. Am Rev Respir Dis 133:321-340, 1986.
35. Brown ML, Carrieri V, Janson-Bjerklie S, et al: Lung cancer and dyspnea. Oncol Nurs Forum 13:19-24, 1986.
36. Young-Brockopp D: Cancer patients' perception of five psychosocial needs. Oncol Nurs Forum 9:31-35, 1982.

Chapter 44

Lymphomas

Connie Henke Yarbro, RN, BSN

INTRODUCTION

In 1832, in England, Thomas Hodgkin[1] described seven patients with a relentlessly progressive, ultimately fatal enlargement of the lymph nodes. The disease was later named after him.[2] Prior to that time the lymphomas had probably been mistaken for tuberculosis of the lymph nodes, which was once a very common infectious disease. A review of the original tissues many years later demonstrated that Hodgkin's cases actually represented examples of what we would now call Hodgkin's disease as well as non-Hodgkin's lymphoma. All lymphomas were called Hodgkin's disease until many years later, when Reed[3] and Sternberg[4] described the multinucleated (Reed-Sternberg) giant cell in some forms of lymphoma but not in others. Subsequently, those lymphomas demonstrating the Reed-Sternberg cell were classified as Hodgkin's disease (HD) and those in which this cell was absent were called lymphosarcoma or reticulum cell sarcoma and later non-Hodgkin's lymphoma (NHL).

The distinction between HD and NHL is important because the clinical course, prognosis, and treatment of these conditions are substantially different, although there are numerous superficial similarities. The nature and origin of the Reed-Sternberg cell remain uncertain, but it is clear that this cell is useful in prognosis since lymphocytic malignancies that are similar in pathologic appearance behave differently according to the presence or absence of this cell.

Even before treatment became available, it was clear that the behavior of the malignant lymphomas was highly variable. Some patients followed a rapidly downhill course, with progressive generalized adenopathy, fever, night sweats, splenomegaly, and infiltration of the liver, bone marrow, lung, and other organs by proliferating cells of malignant origin. Death resulted, usually in 1 to 2 years, from infection or hemorrhage due to bone marrow destruction by invading tumor cells or from failure of some vital organ due to infiltration. Other individuals followed a more indolent course in which the disease was limited to lymph nodes for many years, although ultimately the character of the disease usually became more aggressive with invasion of extranodal organs. These less aggressive forms of the disease sometimes were given separate names because of their behavior.

Because some individuals with lymphomas did well and others did poorly, numerous attempts were made to identify histologic characteristics useful in predicting the behavior of the disease and in selection of the best therapy. The resulting classification systems have become complex and confusing. There have been several histologic classifications for HD. At present there are several competing systems of classification for NHL. This often results in the same type of lymphoma having two or three different pathologic names attached to it. It is important, therefore, for the nurse to be aware of which classification scheme a pathologist is using in reporting the biopsy findings in order to understand the probable course the patient will follow and the basis for the choice of therapy.

At present the system of Lukes and Butler[5] is generally accepted for HD. Recently an international group has developed what is hoped will become a standard system of nomenclature, the so-called Working Formulation.[6]

This confusing welter of nomenclature is best understood from the perspective of the origin and development of the lymphocyte.[7] The lymphomas are preeminently a malignancy of the lymphocyte and represent a unique example in which there seems to be a separate malignancy for each sequential stage in the developmental sequence from primitive to mature lymphocyte. That is, at each stage of development, the potential exists for the normal maturing lymphocyte to be transformed into a cancer cell; once transformed, the new clone of malignant cells follows the behavior pattern of the stage of the lymphocyte at which the transformation took place. Thus, if the function of the maturing lymphocyte at the time it is transformed to a malignant cell is secretion of an antibody protein, the tumor cells will continue to secrete that normal protein in abnormal quantities. If the function at the time of transformation is for the lymphocyte to form maturing nodules in lymph nodes, the disease will be seen as a nodular lymphoma. As the maturation of the lymphocyte is described in the following section, the reader should consider the nature of the tumor that might result at each step if malignant transformation took place.

MATURATION OF THE LYMPHOCYTE

The origin of the lymphocyte can be traced to a stem cell in the bone marrow that has the potential to develop into any of the cells that normally circulate in the blood. At each step along the path of differentiation, the cell loses the capacity to proceed along an alternate route. In the first step, the stem cell matures so that it is either the precursor of the lymphocyte series or of all the other series of the blood (erythrocyte, megakaryocyte, polymorphonuclear leukocyte, or monocyte). The lymphocyte precursor then develops to become one of a number of types of mature lymphocytes. Figure 44-1 demonstrates the maturation sequence of the lymphocyte.

Lymphocytes are responsible for the two arms of the immunological defense system: the humoral arm, which consists of plasma cells that produce circulating antibodies against foreign antigens, and the cellular arm, which consists of circulating lymphocytes that have developed specificity against foreign antigens. These two arms of the immune process are distinct and function jointly in defending the host against foreign proteins. An early step in the differentiation of the maturing lymphocyte occurs when the cell is programmed either by the thymus or by the bone marrow (bursa equivalent), after which it becomes either a T lymphocyte or a B lymphocyte and functions in either the cellular immune arm or the humoral arm, respectively. Those lymphocytes that are programmed as B lymphocytes, when exposed to an appropriate foreign antigen, mature into plasma cells and pro-

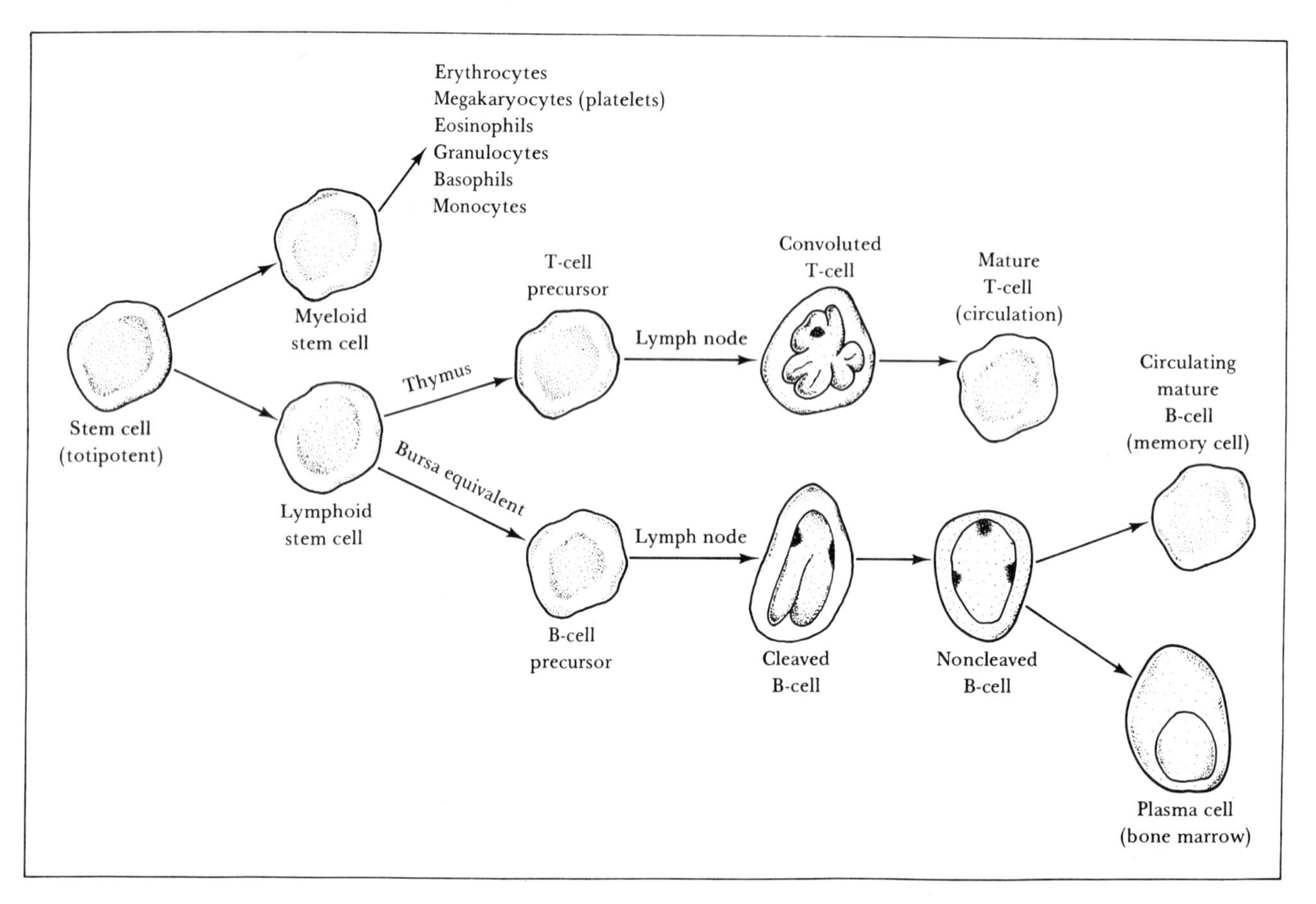

FIGURE 44-1 Maturation sequence of the lymphocyte.

duce antibodies against that antigen. Those lymphocytes programmed as T lymphocytes, when similarly exposed to a foreign antigen, develop into killer lymphocytes that will attack and destroy the foreign antigen without benefit of an antibody intermediary. In addition, some lymphocytes develop specific regulator roles in which they either suppress or stimulate immune functions (suppressor cells and helper cells).

In the course of this development, lymphocytes pass through a series of distinct phases, during which time they are characterized by specific and unique behavior; for example, during one phase of the development of the B lymphocyte, the cells are localized in follicles or nodules of normal lymph nodes. Lymphomas can be classified immunologically as malignancies of either T lymphocytes or B lymphocytes, and the malignant cells behave somewhat differently according to the cell of origin. For example, nodular lymphomas are almost exclusively diseases of the B lymphocytes and tend to follow a more indolent course than the lymphomas produced by transformation of T lymphocytes. Lymphomas of T lymphocytes tend to localize in the mediastinum in the region of the thymus.

EPIDEMIOLOGY

There are approximately 7400 new cases of HD in the United States each year.[8] This represents fewer than 1% of all cancers. Approximately 1500 people die of HD each year. Non-Hodgkin's lymphoma is almost four times as common as HD, and almost 17,300 die of non-Hodgkin's lymphoma annually.

Lymphoma is slightly more common in males than in females (4:3 for HD and 5:3 for NHL), and males may have a poorer prognosis. The incidence of NHL rises steadily, starting in the fourth or fifth decade. The age incidence curve for HD demonstrates a unique and unexplained phenomenon in developed countries, in that there is a double peak in the curve. The first peak occurs early in life, during the second and third decades, and the second peak occurs late in life, during the sixth and seventh decades. The second peak of the HD incidence curve is similar to that of NHL and is concentrated in the older age group, much like other forms of cancer. The early peak in HD is not understood but is thought to be related to the etiology of the nodular sclerosing type of HD, the tissue type that is observed commonly in young persons.

It has been suggested that HD is really two separate diseases and that the first incidence peak may represent a disease of viral etiology, more common in middle-class than in lower-class families and more common in developed than in underdeveloped countries.[9] These characteristics are consistent with a virus that is widely disseminated under conditions of poor hygiene and which, if contracted early, rarely leads to a severe illness. Such a pattern favors the development of subclinical or asymptomatic disease in low socioeconomic groups and underdeveloped countries because these children are exposed at a very early age, when they are resistant and able to develop immunity. In middle-class families and developed nations, however, improved hygiene delays exposure until adolescence or young adulthood. There is no proof to support this hypothesis, but it remains an interesting matter of speculation at the present time, increasingly so as there are suggestions of a possible relationship between the Epstein-Barr virus and nodular sclerosing HD.

NHL has an equally interesting epidemiologic characteristic, in that this disease seems to be predominant in individuals who have a defective immune system, either iatrogenically induced (for example, in a patient receiving immunosuppressive therapy in conjunction with a renal transplant), as a result of a hereditary deficiency of the immune system, or as a result of AIDS. The relationship between NHL and immune deficiency remains unexplained, but it is suggested that NHL may result from an abortive attempt on the part of the lymphocyte to respond to an antigenic stimulation.

ETIOLOGY

As noted above, the etiology of both HD and NHL remains obscure at the present time. The epidemiologic clues suggest either a viral origin or some aberration of the immune system.

One form of NHL, Burkitt's lymphoma, provides very strong evidence of the involvement of a virus.[10] A herpes virus, originally described by Epstein and Barr (usually referred to as Epstein-Barr virus or EBV), is the most likely etiologic agent of Burkitt's lymphoma. Burkitt's lymphoma is confined almost exclusively to Africa and is a disease of children who live in certain endemic areas. This disease is histologically distinct but similar to the lymphomas seen in the United States, although there are some unique differences (such as a predilection for involvement of the mandible). EBV is the etiologic agent of infectious mononucleosis in the United States, and there are suggestions of a relationship to HD, but the mechanism by which it produces Burkitt's lymphoma in Africa is incompletely understood, although it is generally assumed that some additional factor must be involved in Africa to promote the development of a malignancy rather than the self-limiting disease of infectious mononucleosis. Chronic malaria has been suggested as a factor interacting with the immune system to predispose one to EBV-induced lymphoma.[10]

PATHOPHYSIOLOGY

The malignant cell in NHL is obviously a lymphocyte that has been transformed at some stage of its development. The malignant cell in HD is less certain; indeed, it has not even been established whether the Reed-Sternberg cell is a neoplastic cell. The Reed-Sternberg cell may, in fact, represent an attempt at host reaction against the malignancy, because such cells are seen in a number of other diseases where they are part of the host defense mechanism.

In some lymphomas there are rather specific cytogenetic changes that provide a clue to the pathogenesis. Burkitt's lymphoma shows a characteristic transposition of a portion of chromosome No. 8 to chromosome No. 14 (or sometimes 2 or 22). This results in the juxtaposition of the *myc* gene, an oncogene associated with cellular proliferation, with one of the genes associated with antibody production.[10] This suggests that continued stimulation of antibody production might in some fashion activate cell proliferation. In NHL there are characteristic cytogenetic changes associated with certain histologic types that may be useful in prognosis.

The relentless proliferation of lymphocytes, however, is the major anatomic characteristic of both HD and NHL, and these proliferating cells invade and compromise the function of various organs, especially bone marrow. Most patients with HD exhibit evidence of immune deficiency early in the disease, even before treatment has been given. However, the treatment of both HD and NHL is immunosuppressive, rendering patients unusually susceptible to various infections with common pathogens and also with several uncommon pathogens, including herpes zoster and *Pneumocystis carinii*. In untreated individuals or those who have become resistant to further treatment, death usually results from infection or hemorrhage due to a compromise of bone marrow function.

CLINICAL MANIFESTATIONS

Most patients with lymphoma seek medical assistance because they have discovered one or more enlarged lymph nodes. Such nodes are characteristically painless, firm, rubbery in consistency, freely movable, and of variable size (from 1 cm to several centimeters). Three fourths of the patients present with enlargement of cervical lymph nodes, but enlarged axillary or inguinal nodes may be the presenting symptoms. Occasionally enlarged hilar nodes may be noted on routine chest radiograph. Less common presentations include gastric complaints from NHL in the gastrointestinal tract, bone tumors due to NHL, abdominal HD with malabsorption, autoimmune hemolytic anemia, and in rare cases a febrile illness simulating a systemic disease such as tuberculosis. Weakness, fatigue, and general malaise may be a part of the presenting picture.

Approximately one third of the individuals with lymphoma have an associated fever, night sweats, or weight loss. Such symptoms connote a poor prognosis because they often indicate generalized rather than localized disease. Patients with HD may have pruritus. They may also complain of pain in enlarged nodes after the ingestion of alcohol. Neither of these characteristic symptoms has a clear-cut pathophysiologic explanation.

ASSESSMENT

The diagnosis of lymphoma can be established only by biopsy of involved tissue, usually a lymph node. However, there are many causes of lymphadenopathy, especially in younger individuals. These include upper respiratory infection (bacterial or viral), infectious mononucleosis, allergic reactions, and other, often nonspecific, causes. Older persons with cancer of the head and neck may initially present with enlarged cervical lymph nodes.

When an enlarged node is detected on routine physical examination or when the patient reports such a complaint, a careful history and physical examination are essential to determine whether a biopsy should be performed. When there is evidence of a recent infection or other nonmalignant process, the physician may choose to delay biopsy and to observe the clinical course. In most cases, lymphadenopathy of infectious origin will resolve in a few days to a few weeks. For persistent lymphadenopathy or when the etiology is not apparent, a biopsy is usually indicated. Since a family history of HD increases the risk to other siblings, this may also be a factor in the decision to perform a biopsy. In older persons, the detection of an enlarged lymph node in the neck in the absence of fever or systemic complaints is an indication that a careful search of the mouth, pharynx, and larynx for the presence of a malignant process should be made.

Once the diagnosis is established on the basis of lymph node biopsy, it is necessary to obtain an accurate histologic typing and staging of the disease to determine the precise prognosis and selection of therapy.

HISTOPATHOLOGY

Lukes and Butler[5] developed a histopathologic system for HD which serves as the current standard for histologic classification (Table 44-1). Nodular sclerosis (NS), with its unique age incidence (the young) and its different sex incidence (females more commonly than males), has a unique histologic makeup that does not fit into the spectrum presented by the other three types. In NS-HD the lymph node is divided into nodules by sclerosing bands of collagen. The lymphocytes in the collagen-bound nodules may be of various types, from predominantly small lymphocytes to the large "histiocytic" forms. Such variation in cell types may influence prognosis in NS-HD.

The other three histologic types of HD form a spectrum of prognoses from good to poor. The lymphocyte-predominant (LP) is characterized by sheets of mature-appearing small lymphocytes with few Reed-Sternberg cells and carries a good prognosis. The lymphocyte-depleted (LD) type is characterized by a paucity of small lymphocytes, a large number of Reed-Sternberg cells, and a predominance of "histiocytes" (which are in reality large activated lymphocytes) and carries a poor prognosis. Mixed-cell (MC) HD is intermediate between LP and LD in terms of histology and prognosis. All three of these forms of HD are more common in males than in females and more common in the elderly than in the young, in contrast to NS-HD. Histologic variants have been defined that may influence the prognosis; for example, in LP-HD the diffuse variant has been reported by some to have a better prognosis for cure than the nodular subtype,[11] although this has not been confirmed in another study.[12]

Although the Reed-Sternberg cell is essential to the diagnosis, it is not absolute proof of HD because on rare occasions it may be seen in other conditions, infectious mononucleosis, lymph nodes receiving drainage from some infections, lymphadenopathy associated with an idio-

TABLE 44-1 Histologic Classification of Hodgkin's Disease and Relationship to Prognosis*

Histology	Frequency	Approximate 5-Year Survival	Comment
Nodular sclerosis (NS)	30–50%	70%	Young females especially
Lymphocyte predominant (LP)	5–15%	90%	Usually stage I or IIa
Mixed cellularity (MC)	30–40%	40%	Intermediate prognosis
Lymphocyte depleted (LD)	5–15%	40%	Usually stage III or IVb

*According to Lukes and Butler.[5]

TABLE 44-2 Histopathologic Classification of Malignant Lymphomas: Comparison of Working Formulation With Rappaport and Lukes-Collins Systems of Nomenclature

Working Formulation	Rappaport System	Lukes-Collins System
Low Grade		
A Small lymphocytic	Diffuse well-differentiated lymphocytic	Small lymphocytic B-cell or T-cell
B Follicular, small cleaved	Nodular poorly differentiated lymphocytic	Follicular, small cleaved FCC*
C Follicular, mixed small cleaved and large-cell	Nodular, mixed lymphocytic and histiocytic	Follicular, mixed small cleaved and large FCC
Intermediate Grade		
D Follicular, large-cell	Nodular histiocytic	Follicular, large cleaved and/or non-cleaved FCC
E Diffuse, small cleaved	Diffuse poorly differentiated lymphocytic	Diffuse small cleaved FCC
F Diffuse, mixed small and large	Diffuse mixed lymphocytic and histiocytic	Diffuse mixed small and large cleaved or noncleaved FCC
G Diffuse, large-cell	Diffuse histiocytic	Diffuse large cleaved or noncleaved FCC
High Grade		
H Immunoblastic, large-cell	Diffuse histiocytic	Immunoblastic sarcoma, B-cell or T-cell
I Lymphoblastic	Lymphoblastic	Convoluted T-cell
J Small, noncleaved	Undifferentiated, Burkitt and non-Burkitt	Small noncleaved FCC

* *FCC*, Follicular center cell.

syncratic reaction to diphenylhydantoin (phenytoin), and some other conditions. Therefore, it is the total histologic picture that characterizes HD.

Rappaport[13] described the histopathologic classification that until recently was most commonly used for NHL. This scheme separates NHL into types based on the predominant cell (well-differentiated lymphocyte, poorly differentiated lymphocyte, large "histiocytic" lymphocyte) and designates each cell type as either nodular or diffuse, depending on the macrostructure of the lymph node. This system is easily reproduced and correlates well with clinical observations, but it gives little insight into the pathophysiology involved.

Lukes and Collins[14] proposed an immunologic classification system that provides important correlations with the pathophysiology of the immune system. This approach is to separate NHL into either T-cell or B-cell lymphomas. Since B-lymphocytes normally mature in the nodular regions (follicular centers) of lymph nodes, they classify the B-cell lymphomas along the pattern of the presumed maturation sequence of the B-lymphocyte (small lymphocyte, small and large cleaved and noncleaved lymphocyte, and B-immunoblast). The T-cell lymphomas are classified as convoluted lymphocyte type, T-immunoblastic, mycosis fungoides, and Sézary syndrome (see Figure 44-1).

Additional classifications of NHL have been developed by Lennert (the Kiel classification), by the World Health Organization, and by Dorfman (see Magrath[7]). Recently an international working group has developed what is hoped will become an international standard histologic classification, currently referred to as the Working Formulation. This is shown in Table 44-2 and compared to the Rappaport and Lukes-Collins classifications.

STAGING

After the diagnosis of HD or NHL has been established on the basis of lymph node biopsy and the histologic type has been determined in accordance with the criteria outlined, the next step in patient management is the careful determination of the extent of disease involvement. This process is referred to as staging, and the object is to determine the extent of disease in accordance with the definitions developed at the Ann Arbor Conference on Staging[15] (Table 44-3). As noted previously, both HD and NHL almost always develop in a lymph node, usually a cervical node, and progress to involve other lymph nodes and subsequently nonlymphatic tissues. Therefore, the stage describes the degree of advancement and the extent of treatment that probably will be required; it also permits

TABLE 44-3 Ann Arbor Modification of the Rye Staging System for Lymphoma

Stage	Extent of Involvement
I	Involvement of a single lymph node region (I) or of a single extralymphatic organ or site (I_E)
II	Involvement of two or more lymph node regions on the same side of the diaphragm (II) or localized involvement of an extralymphatic organ or site and of one or more lymph node regions on the same side of the diaphragm (II_E).
III	Involvement of lymph node regions on both sides of the diaphragm (III), which may also be accompanied by localized involvement of an extralymphatic organ or site (III_E), involvement of the spleen (III_S), or both (III_{SE})
IV	Diffuse or disseminated involvement of one or more extralymphatic organs or tissues with or without associated lymph node enlargement

For Hodgkin's disease, the presence or absence of systemic manifestations should be indicated by adding either the letter A or B (A = asymptomatic and B = fever, sweats, and weight loss of more than 10% of body weight).

the clinician to draw an inference with regard to the aggressiveness of the disease process.

Several general principles will help one understand the importance of staging and the use of the information revealed during this work-up. In general, HD spreads from one lymph node group to an immediately adjacent lymph node group, whereas NHL has a propensity for skipping to noncontiguous lymph node groups. These relationships are illustrated in Figure 44-2. The histologic type provides some clue as to the probability of widespread involvement, in that the more aggressive histologic types such as LD-HD tend to be either stage III or IV at the time of presentation, whereas the less aggressive histologic types such as NS-HD and LP-HD tend to be stages I and II at the time of presentation. NHL, whether of the aggressive or the indolent variety, rarely presents as stage I.

Determination of the stage of disease in HD is important because it influences which treatment option (radiation therapy or combination chemotherapy) will be used. Radiotherapy is very effective for localized HD and has been, historically, the treatment of choice.[16-18] When delivered in a full therapeutic dose, radiation can be expected to eradicate disease from a given lymph node group in well over 90% of the cases.[19] On the other hand, as the number of involved lymph node groups increases, the proportion of patients cured by radiotherapy diminishes. Thus, radiotherapy is most effective in early-stage disease, whereas chemotherapy is the treatment of choice for late-stage disease. Chemotherapy in the appropriate combination is curative in HD.[20] Recently, as noted below, it has been shown that chemotherapy is as effective in early stage HD as is radiation.

NHL, on the other hand, is almost always treated with chemotherapy because it usually presents at an advanced stage. In a small number of cases the large-cell, or aggressive, form of NHL may present as localized disease and radiation therapy, usually followed by chemotherapy, may prove useful.

The following list outlines the sequential staging workup for lymphoma in the most frequently encountered clinical presentation, namely, cervical adenopathy:

1. History and physical examination.
2. Chest radiography.
3. Complete blood count and platelet count.
4. Blood chemistries, including liver and kidney function tests.
5. CT scan of the chest and abdomen.
6. Bone marrow biopsy. (*Note:* If the marrow biopsy is positive for lymphoma, the patient has stage IV disease and requires only minimal further evaluation.)
7. Percutaneous liver biopsy if liver function tests or scans are abnormal or the liver is enlarged. (*Note:* If the liver biopsy is positive for lymphoma, the patient has stage IV disease and requires only minimal further evaluation.)
8. Lower limb lymphangiography if not contraindicated by impaired pulmonary function. (*Note:* At this point a careful assessment of all data available should be made, with particular reference to histologic type of lymphoma. Additional tests, such as bone scan, mediastinal CT scan, and laparoscopy, may be ordered to clarify the situation.)
9. In selected individuals an exploratory laparotomy with multiple node biopsies, splenectomy, and liver and bone biopsies may be necessary for final determination of stage. This is necessary in some cases of HD, rarely in NHL.

History and physical examination findings, complete blood count, chest radiograph, and blood chemistries will usually be normal in the typical case but on occasion may provide evidence of lymph node involvement below the diaphragm, hepatomegaly or abnormal liver function, extension of the lymphoma to mediastinal lymph nodes, or splenomegaly. CT scan may reveal mediastinal or paraaortic adenopathy. If the bone marrow biopsy is positive, the patient has a stage IV lymphoma. In general, if the liver is enlarged or if tests indicate abnormal liver function, a percutaneous liver biopsy is indicated. If this biopsy is positive, the patient has stage IV disease and further work-up is not required.

On the basis of history and physical findings, the HD patient will be substaged as either A or B, depending on the presence or absence of fever, night sweats, or weight loss greater than 10% of body weight. The A and B staging system is rarely used for NHL.

If the initial assessment fails to allow a definitive staging, the next step is the performance of a bilateral lym-

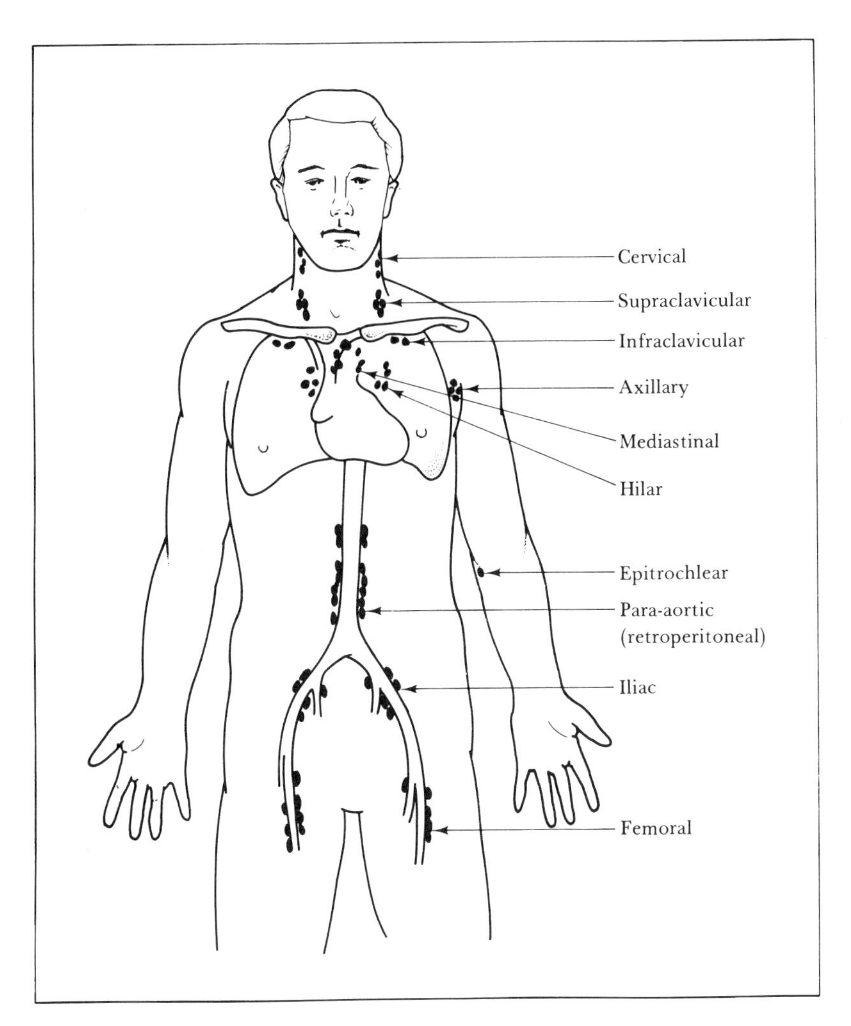

FIGURE 44-2 Major lymph node groups.

phangiogram (LAG). This study will permit a determination of involvement of the retroperitoneal lymph nodes and is often the first clue that the patient has at least clinical stage III disease. Unfortunately, in NHL the mesenteric lymph nodes are more often positive than the retroperitoneal lymph nodes, and mesenteric lymph nodes are not visualized by LAG; thus, unlike the person with HD, an individual with NHL often has abdominal lymph node involvement but a normal LAG. For this reason, an LAG is rarely performed in cases of NHL.

History and physical examination, blood chemistries, chest radiograph, bone marrow biopsy, liver biopsy (if tests indicate abnormal function), and LAG represent the generally accepted data base for determining the clinical stage in a patient with HD or NHL. In the majority of cases, an accurate staging can be made and treatment determined on the basis of such information. For some patients, however, additional information will be necessary, and this is usually obtained by an exploratory laparotomy for biopsy of multiple lymph node groups, removal of the spleen for pathologic study, and multiple biopsies of the liver.[21] In general, most individuals with lymphoma will not require explorative laparatomy. For example, almost 90% of the individuals with NHL will be found to have disease below the diaphragm at the time of exploratory laparotomy, regardless of the presence or absence of other clinical signs of advanced disease.[22] Thus, with a few exceptions, laparotomy is not routinely used for patients with NHL. Similarly, patients with NS-HD without mediastinal involvement usually do not have abdominal involvement, and in this group of individuals the procedure may be safely omitted. In other histologic types, however, the situation is less clear.

For HD, prognosis is most closely related to stage. For NHL, it is the histologic type that is important. The prognosis gradually worsens (in the absence of treatment) as one proceeds down the Working Formulation list of types from histologic type A to type J. The response to therapy, on the other hand, improves as the aggressiveness of the disease increases. Thus high-grade lymphomas are often cured by intensive chemotherapy, whereas the low-grade ones are not considered curable, although they often demonstrate a long survival without therapy.

It is customary to specify whether a stage is determined on the basis of clinical signs alone (eg, an abnormal lymphangiogram) or on the basis of pathologic examination of a biopsy specimen. Thus, a patient may be referred to as having "clinical" stage III (abbreviated CS III) or "pathologic" stage III (abbreviated PS III), depending on the strength of the evidence. The nurse should be familiar with these diagnostic procedures and terms in order to help the lymphoma patient follow the sequence and understand the significance of the staging work-up.

TREATMENT

Since both HD and high-grade NHL may be cured in a high percentage of cases, and since initial treatment failure substantially reduces the chance of cure with subsequent treatment, it is imperative that great care be exercised in the selection and delivery of the first therapeutic intervention. This requires input from a variety of disciplines (radiology, surgery, pathology, medical oncology) working together as an interdisciplinary team.

Contact with multiple physicians and the complexity of the staging procedures may cause the patient with a diagnosis of lymphoma to feel confused and "lost in the system." In some cases the nurse may be the only constant contact the patient has with the diagnostic and treatment team. It is essential that support be provided as the patient adjusts to a diagnosis of malignant disease. The complex and therapeutic procedures to which the patient will be subjected may require clarification and repeated explanation. These explanations must be given with understanding, empathy, compassion, and tact.[23]

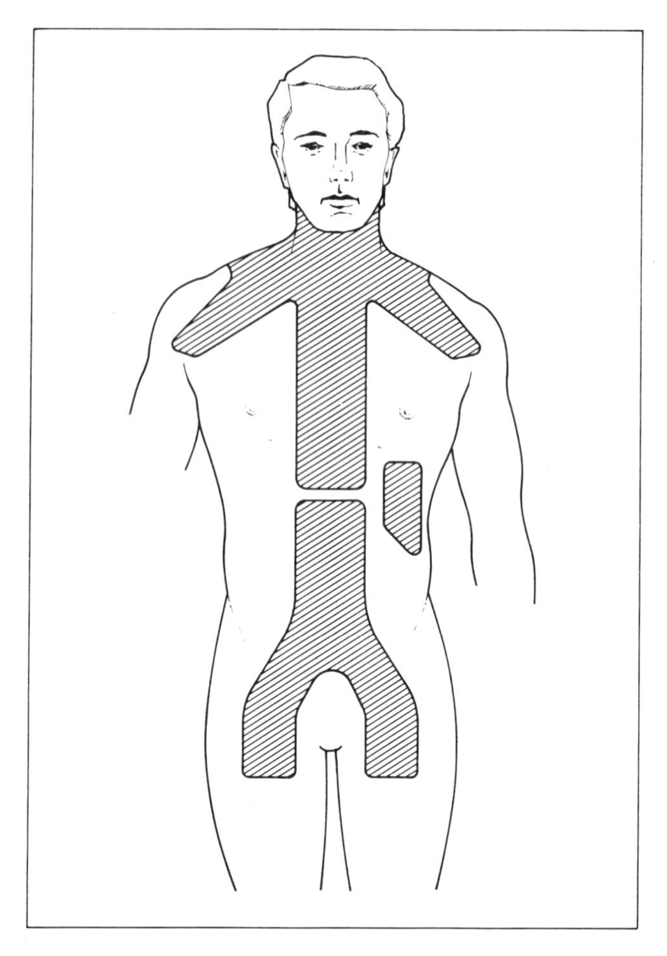

FIGURE 44-3 Ports used for total nodal irradiation. The upper port, called a mantle, extends from the mandible to the diaphragm and includes cervical, axillary, supraclavicular, infraclavicular, and mediastinal node chains. The heart and lungs are protected in part by lead shields. The lower port, called an inverted Y, extends from the diaphragm to the lower border of the pelvis and includes periaortic, iliac, inguinal, and femoral node chains. The small left lateral port, called the splenic port, includes the spleen and splenic hilar nodes.

Hodgkin's Disease

Current recommendations for treatment of HD are relatively noncontroversial.[24] For stage IA and IIA Hodgkin's disease above the diaphragm, without bulky mediastinal disease, patients should receive mantle irradiation to a total dose of 3500 to 4400 rad (cGy) over a period of 4 to 6 weeks. Usually paraaortic lymph nodes will be included, except in patients without mediastinal involvement or those with LP-HD (Figure 44-3). When bulky mediastinal disease is present, patients do not undergo laparotomy because it would not change the treatment they receive and combined radiation and chemotherapy are used. Stage IIIA patients with only splenic involvement may be treated with total or subtotal nodal radiation. Generally total nodal radiation is considered inappropriate for other stage IIIA patients.[25] Patients with IIIB and IV disease receive chemotherapy. Patients with stage IIB disease may receive total or subtotal nodal radiotherapy if careful laparotomy staging has been conducted, but otherwise they should receive chemotherapy.

There are several curative chemotherapy regimens. The MOPP regimen (Table 44-4) or the ABVD regimen (Table 44-5) can be expected to produce complete remissions in more than 80% of previously untreated patïeints, and 68% of the patients who achieve complete remissions will be alive with no evidence of disease at 10 years and presumably cured. No relapses have been seen beyond 42 months after induction of a complete remission with MOPP.[26] Results with ABVD are equal to or superior to MOPP.[27,28] It is important to note that either MOPP or ABVD can be expected to produce a complete remission in more than half of the patients who have recurrent disease after treatment with the other combination. At present, there is no evidence that maintenance chemotherapy for patients in complete remission adds to cure or control rates. The combination of MOPP and ABVD, three alternating cycles of each, may be superior to either alone.[28] Other curative regimens are reported.[29]

Recently the National Cancer Institute reported a randomized trial showing that chemotherapy is as effective in early-stage HD as radiotherapy.[30] This had been suspected on the basis of uncontrolled studies in Africa.[31] It

TABLE 44-4 The MOPP Regimen for Hodgkin's Disease

Drug	Dosage
Nitrogen mustard (Mustargen)	6 mg/m² IV on days 1 and 8
Vincristine (Oncovin)	1.4 mg/m² IV on days 1 and 8
Procarbazine	100 mg/m² PO daily × 14 days
Prednisone (first and fourth cycle only)	40 mg/m² PO daily × 14 days

Repeat the cycle starting on day 29 and continue through six cycles or for two cycles after induction of a complete remission, whichever is longer.

TABLE 44-5 The ABVD Regimen for Hodgkin's Disease

Drug	Dosage
Doxorubicin	25 mg/m² IV on days 1 and 15
Bleomycin	10 U/m² IV on days 1 and 15
Vinblastine	6 mg/m² IV on days 1 and 15
DTIC (dacarbazine)	375 mg/m² IV on days 1 and 15

Repeat the cycle starting on day 29 and continue through six cycles.

is generally accepted that chemotherapy is more toxic than radiotherapy, so the results of this trial will not substantially alter the pattern of treatment, except that in cases where the stage is in doubt there will be a tendency to err on the side of caution and use chemotherapy.

Some patients present with what has been called "bulky" disease, usually defined as mediastinal adenopathy greater than one third the width of the chest on x-ray examination. This pattern of disease has a high recurrence rate after radiotherapy alone[32,33] and poses some risk for exploratory laparotomy because the mediastinal mass may complicate anesthesia.[34] It is probably best to use chemotherapy as an adjuvant after radiotherapy in such patients.[35]

Age is a prognostic factor in HD,[36] as is the total number of node groups involved (independent of stage).[37] Subdiaphragmatic presentation, which is uncommon, also has a poorer prognosis than the usual cervical presentation; most of the recurrences are seen above the diaphragm, suggesting that the disease is often more advanced than suspected.[38]

Non-Hodgkin's Lymphoma

Since most NHL is disseminated at diagnosis, treatment is based on cell type. The spectrum of clinical behavior is wider for NHL, extending from the aggressive, rapidly fatal diffuse histiocytic lymphoma to the indolent nodular varieties. There is no evidence that treatment of the indolent forms of NHL improves survival; thus treatment is used largely to control symptoms in histologic types A and B of the Working Formulation.

Patients with types A and B NHL do well without therapy or with minimal symptomatic therapy, such as palliative radiation to a symptomatic area or alkylating agent therapy for anemia. Because such patients often show histologic changes in their tumors to one of the more aggressive forms after an indolent course of years, it has been suggested that perhaps the potent combination chemotherapy regimens should be withheld until the disease is likely to be more responsive to intensive treatment.

At present, NHL is considered far less curable by radiotherapy than is HD, except in the earliest stages. Unfortunately, less than 10% of NHL is truly stage I disease. Diffuse histiocytic lymphoma occasionally appears as true stage I disease, and in such cases cure rates of 90% have been reported.[39] When NHL occurs as a primary lesion in bone or stomach, radiotherapy has been reported to produce 50% cure rates in the past. Early-stage cases of NHL are the exception, however. Increasingly, even in localized NHL, chemotherapy is being added to radiotherapy for the high-grade malignancies.[40]

Type A NHL is the lymph node form of chronic lymphocytic leukemia (CLL). On occasion CLL presents with a relatively normal peripheral blood count but with lymphadenopathy. In such cases the lymph node biopsy will be interpreted as type A in the Working Formulation or as well-differentiated lymphocytic lymphoma in the Rappaport scheme. Management of this condition is discussed in the chapter on chronic leukemia. Generally, treatment is not given until symptoms develop, since prognosis is good without therapy and there is no evidence that treatment improves survival.

One of the most common forms of NHL is type B, called nodular poorly differentiated lymphocytic lymphoma in the Rappaport scheme. It has an excellent prognosis with no therapy. Most centers withhold treatment unless the patient becomes symptomatic or is entered in a clinical trial. There are no convincing trials indicating that aggressive therapy improves survival in comparison to symptomatic care. Attempts have been made to improve prognosis by immunologic studies,[41] but histology remains the best prognostic factor.[42]

Most individuals with intermediate and high-grade NHL will receive chemotherapy as their initial treatment. However, controversy exists as to the regimen of choice. The controversy relates to which regimen is best and whether very aggressive therapy, with its high complication rate, is more effective than moderately aggressive

TABLE 44-6 The CHOP Regimen for Intermediate and High-Grade Non-Hodgkin's Lymphoma

Cyclophosphamide	750 mg/m² IV push, day 1
Doxorubicin	50 mg/m² IV push, day 1
Vincristine	1.4 mg/m² (maximum 2 mg) IV push, day 1
Prednisone	100 mg PO, days 1-5 Repeated every 3 weeks for 8 courses (with dose adjustments for toxicity)

TABLE 44-7 The BACOP Regimen for Intermediate and High-Grade Non-Hodgkin's Lymphoma

Bleomycin	5 U/m² IV push, days 15, 22
Doxorubicin	25 mg/m² IV push, days 1, 8
Cyclophosphamide	650 mg/m² IV push, days 1, 8
Vincristine	1.2 mg/m² (maximum 2 mg) IV push, days 1, 8
Prednisone	60 mg/m² PO, days 15-28 Repeated every 4 weeks for 6 courses (with dose adjustments for toxicity)

therapy. There are also questions as to comparability of studies with regard to age, dose intensity, and histologic type. Multiple histologic types (by the Working Formulation) are contained in studies of "diffuse large cell lymphoma" (DLCL), which is the usual description of patients under study. There are very few randomized trials. Armitage and Cheson[43] have recently reviewed these data. One of the most frequently used regimens is CHOP (Table 44-6). This regimen will produce long-term survival in about half of the treated DLCL patients. CHOP was one of the first regimens that convincingly produced a high cure rate in DLCL. A second commonly used regimen is BACOP,[44] shown in Table 44-7. Subsequently a number of other regimens, more intensive and more toxic, have been developed. One of the most intensive and toxic regimens reported is the MACOP-B regimen[45] shown in Table 44-8. Many investigators believe that more aggressive treatment regimens will increase the cure rate, and uncontrolled trials with impressive results from intensive therapy continue to be reported.[46] DeVita et al[47] have reviewed the evidence of an increased cure rate with an increase in dose intensity and with an increase in the number of drugs used. However, there are too few randomized comparisons to provide convincing data to confirm the superiority of any one regimen.[43] A study by the Southwest Oncology Group (SWOG) is presently comparing CHOP with two more aggressive regimens in intermediate and high-grade lymphoma, and there are no data as yet to dispute the conclusion that CHOP remains the current standard treatment of choice.[48]

Despite the new histologic classification of NHL, prognosis remains difficult and the search continues for a more reliable prognostic scheme. Age is clearly important.[49] Stage remains an important prognostic factor.[50] The presence of a large tumor burden and/or an elevated lactic dehydrogenase level adversely affects survival.[51] There are cytogenetic changes that influence prognosis as well.[52] Research continues on prognostic models containing multiple variables.[53] Finally, high-grade NHL is being seen with increased frequency in persons with AIDS and the prognosis in this subset of patients is extremely poor. (See Chapter 33, AIDS-Related Malignancies.)

Adult T-cell lymphoma/leukemia[54] is a special consideration and will not be discussed in detail here. It represents a tumor induced by the HTLV 1 virus, which is common in Japan, the Caribbean, and the southeastern United States. The pathogenesis of this rare tumor is discussed further in Chapter 2.

Supportive Therapy

Supportive care of the patient with a lymphoma begins at diagnosis with an explanation of the disease, a description of the steps that will be taken for staging and treatment, and generation in the patient of a feeling of confidence in the multidisciplinary team responsible for care. Regardless of whether the primary treatment is radiotherapy or chemotherapy, it is certain that it will be lengthy and highly toxic, and the individual must be prepared to cope with this.

TABLE 44-8 The MACOP-B Regimen for Intermediate and High-Grade Non-Hodgkin's Lymphoma

Methotrexate with leucovorin rescue	100 mg/m² IV push, then 300 mg/m² IV over 4 hr, then in 24 hr leucovorin 15 mg PO q 6 hr × 6 doses; weeks 2, 6, 10
Doxorubicin	50 mg/m² IV push, weeks 1, 3, 5, 7, 9, 11
Cyclophosphamide	350 mg/m² IV push, weeks 1, 3, 5, 7, 9, 11
Vincristine	1.4 mg/m² IV push, weeks 2, 4, 6, 8, 10, 12
Prednisone	75 mg PO daily, tapered last 2 weeks
Bleomycin	10 U/m² IV push, weeks 4, 8, 12
Cotrimoxazole	2 tablets PO daily throughout

The person who presents with constitutional symptoms and receives several courses of chemotherapy often becomes completely asymptomatic. Because symptoms are relieved, the patient might question why he or she should proceed with treatment that causes adverse side effects. This follow-up period is crucial for the completion of the course of therapy. The nurse can play a major role by providing the understanding and emotional support the patient needs and by making sure that the patient understands that small foci of disease cause no symptoms but will, if untreated, lead to recurrence.

After the primary treatment, there will be a prolonged period (months to years) during which the patient will be observed for a recurrence of disease. This is a particularly trying period because the individual has, in his or her own mind, been very close to death by virtue of having to deal with the diagnosis of cancer. The treatment has (as a rule) produced complete remission, but each visit to the clinic now carries with it the threat that the disease may have recurred and the nightmare must begin all over again. The nurse must be aware that whereas the treatment team views this as a "routine" visit of a patient who has responded very well to therapy, the individual perceives every word or facial expression as a potential clue that the cancer has returned.

Complications of radiotherapy

Radiotherapy often causes complications during treatment (acute) or following the completion of treatment (subacute or late). The most common reactions associated with mantle irradiation are loss of taste, dry mouth, redness of skin, dysphagia, loss of hair at the nape of the neck, nausea, and vomiting. Because the amount of saliva is decreased, these individuals are at increased risk of dental caries. Instructions in proper dental hygiene, which includes routine dental examination and cleaning every 4 to 6 months, should be given.

Irradiation of the inverted-Y port usually results in nausea, vomiting, anorexia, diarrhea, and malaise. Bone marrow depression may occur and must be monitored by frequent complete blood counts. Total nodal irradiation leads to all the side effects noted previously and particularly to severe bone marrow depression.

Late reactions to irradiation may include radiation pneumonitis. Men will experience transient aspermia, but recovery of spermatogenesis with careful testicular shielding has been documented. Women who have not had an oophoropexy or shielding of the ovaries may undergo artificial menopause. At the time of exploratory laparotomy, surgical fixation of the ovaries to the uterus is often performed in the young female patient to preserve ovarian function. Young male and female patients must be informed of these potential effects on the reproductive system so that they will understand the implications on their present status, as well as those for the future. (See Chapter 12 for a detailed discussion of nursing care of the individual receiving radiotherapy.)

Complications of chemotherapy

The various combinations of chemotherapy used in the treatment of HD and NHL will invariably result in acute and chronic side effects. The nature of these side effects depend on the drugs used, but many are common to most drugs. The most frequent side effect is nausea and vomiting. Although this reaction varies from one individual to another, it is generally transient and can often be controlled with the use of antiemetics. Other reactions that can occur include alopecia, myalgia, chills, fever, euphoria, fluid retention, stomatitis, gastrointestinal disturbances, hemorrhagic cystitis, and mental depression, depending on the specific drug regimen used. Specific aspects of nursing care related to these side effects are covered elsewhere in this text. The most important side effect produced by all combination regimens is bone marrow depression, which renders the individual susceptible to infection and hemorrhage. Late reactions that result from cumulative toxicity may occur with doxorubicin (cardiotoxicity) and bleomycin (pulmonary fibrosis).

Transient and sometimes permanent male sterility is a recognized complication of induction chemotherapy for individuals with lymphoma. As a group, the alkylating agents are the most toxic to the testicular germ cells, with reversible changes occurring up to a threshold level and irreversible germinal aplasia occurring after the threshold has been exceeded. Individuals with Hodgkin's disease treated with MOPP have a greater than 80% likelihood of developing germinal aplasia, azoospermia, and testicular atrophy with elevated serum follicle-stimulating hormone levels.[55] Chapman and colleagues[56] reported 100% infertility during the first 12 months after therapy in 74 men with HD who were treated with MOPP. Return of active spermatogenesis was seen in only 4 of 64 men 15 to 51 months after therapy was stopped. An alternative chemotherapy program for Hodgkin's disease, ABVD, may be as effective as MOPP but is less toxic to germinal epithelium.[27] The use of combination chemotherapy in women also produces ovarian dysfunction, with women older than 35 to 40 years of age being the most susceptible. In the case of MOPP therapy, only 40% to 50% of the women experienced ovarian failure. Clearly, the complication of gonadal dysfunction may result in considerable psychosocial problems in men and women being treated for cure. Chapter 28 provides a detailed discussion of sexual and reproductive dysfunction in the cancer patient.

Infections

Because both chemotherapy and radiotherapy are immunosuppressive, bacterial infections as well as other unusual infections may occur. The most common gram-negative bacteria causing infections in individuals with lymphoma are *Escherichia coli, Pseudomonas aeruginosa*, and *Klebsiella*. Various species of *Staphylococcus* are increasingly common infectious agents in these patients. Although fever may be a presenting complaint attributable to the lymphoma itself, fever in a patient who has been treated (especially one who is neutropenic) must always be considered a sign of potentially life-threatening infection until proven otherwise. Appropriate cultures should be obtained and empiric antibiotic therapy should be started immediately.

The two most common fungal infections in lymphoma patients are candidiasis and aspergillosis. *Pneumocystis carinii* is a rare protozoal infestation in immunologically normal individuals but is frequent in lymphoma patients.

Herpes zoster is a troublesome complication that is often seen in individuals with lymphoma. It results from the reactivation of latent foci of chickenpox virus, presumably secondary to the immunosuppression caused by the lymphoma and/or the treatment. This is usually localized, but on occasion a life-threatening generalized infection may occur.

The nurse who is caring for the patient undergoing aggressive radiotherapy or chemotherapy must be familiar with the common manifestations of these infections and the appropriate therapy used to manage them. Supportive care is vital to these individuals and is discussed in more detail in Chapter 21.

Recurrent Disease

Fortunately, the lymphomas are sufficiently responsive to treatment that complications during the primary therapy are relatively mild in comparison with those associated with some other malignancies. It is the individual whose lymphoma has recurred and requires additional treatment for whom most problems arise. Such persons have a reduced bone marrow reserve as a result of the primary therapy (whether radiotherapy or chemotherapy) and tolerate secondary therapy poorly. They need a great deal of psychologic support because it rarely escapes their attention that recurrent lymphoma is much less likely to be cured than the initial disease.

For the patient with HD, it is possible to obtain a cure with intensive therapy after the first recurrence of disease following a complete remission. Third-line chemotherapy that is potentially curative and wide-field radiotherapy with curative intent have also been described.[57] Cure is rarely possible with recurrent NHL. These patients require platelet transfusions as the chemotherapy drives their platelet counts into the danger zone below 20,000/mm^3. Some institutions use granulocyte transfusions for bacterial infection or fever of unknown origin in the presence of a significantly reduced granulocyte count. Sepsis is a major cause of death in such individuals. Some treatment centers use protected environments, whereas others have found careful attention to isolation technique to be equally effective.

Bone marrow transplantation has recently been proposed as a means of salvaging patients with recurrent lymphoma when no curative regimen exists.[58] The availability of stored bone marrow, collected during a time of remission, may allow autologous bone marrow transplantation (ABMT) after very high doses of chemotherapeutic agents with complete remission, or even cure, of recurrent or refractory lymphoma.[59] It has been suggested that in especially poor-risk lymphoma, ABMT might be used early in the course of treatment.[60] There are as yet only preliminary results from the use of these approaches to treatment. However, there is a new technology for collecting stem cells from peripheral blood, and this may make ABMT easier in the future.[61,62]

Individuals with recurrent disease often require palliative radiotherapy to control a symptomatic lesion. Such therapy can safely be administered, even in a person with compromised bone marrow reserve because, in comparison with curative radiotherapy, the port sizes and the doses used are substantially reduced. In like manner, more generalized disease may be palliated with a single- (or double-) drug chemotherapy regimen selected on the basis of the patient's drug history or based on a phase 2 clinical trial and used in dosages tolerated by the individual's diminished marrow reserve. The goal is to improve the quality of the patient's remaining life, and it is essential to keep this in perspective so that excessive rigidity of treatment scheduling does not interfere with activities that are, in fact, more important. For example, it may be highly desirable to discontinue or reschedule palliative treatment to permit travel to attend a grandchild's graduation. For such individuals, control of pain is a primary responsibility of the management team.

SPECIAL CONSIDERATIONS

Superior Vena Cava Syndrome

Tumors of the superior mediastinum on the right side have the potential to obstruct the return of blood to the heart by the superior vena cava and produce a characteristic syndrome of edema of the upper half of the body associated with prominent collateral circulation. Lung cancer, especially the oat cell variety, is the most common cause of this complication, but the lymphomas represent the second most common cause. This is an oncologic emergency that necessitates prompt therapy aimed at relieving the pressure on the superior vena cava, and radiotherapy has been the traditional approach.[63] However, as chemotherapy has become more effective, it is clear that chemotherapy, alone or combined with radiotherapy if the tumor is large, represents the optimal approach.[64] Treatment should be designed so that the management of this emergency does not compromise the curative management of the lymphoma.

Spinal Cord Compression

Rare as a presenting symptom but commonly seen in progressive lymphoma, compression of the spinal cord represents a complication that is dreaded because of its potential to cripple with paraplegia a person who might otherwise have many productive years remaining. This oncologic emergency develops swiftly, with weakness of the lower extremities, increased tendon reflexes, positive Babinski signs, and the development of a sensory "level" below which sensation is lost. Precise localization of the compression by myelogram is essential. Recently magnetic resonance imaging has offered the promise of a noninvasive diagnostic technique, but myelography remains the standard diagnostic method.

Early diagnosis is critical to prevention of neurologic impairment. Patients who have already developed compromised neurologic function usually do not have a return of function after treatment.[65] The nurse should be sensitive to complaints of leg weakness or bowel and bladder dysfunction, especially in patients with back pain.

In the past, laminectomy has been the standard treatment, but radiotherapy has been compared in a randomized fashion to surgery plus radiation and no significant difference was seen.[66] The surgical approach has improved with the use of vertebral body resection for anterior tumors.[67] Primary chemotherapy has also been shown to be effective in children[68] and more recently in adults with epidural cord compression due to lymphoma.[69] Dexamethasone has been widely used to reduce edema associated with the tumor itself and with treatment. Delaney and Oldfield[70] have made treatment recommendations for spinal cord compression: radiation for radiosensitive tumors if the spine is stable; surgery followed by radiation for radioresistant tumors or if the spine is unstable as a result of pathologic fracture; surgery only for relapse at the site of prior radiation; and chemotherapy for responsive pediatric tumors, as an adjuvant in responsive adult tumors, and for relapse at the site of prior surgery and radiotherapy. Application of these recommendations to lymphoma would lead to radiotherapy plus chemotherapy as the usual treatment of choice in the absence of spinal instability, although primary chemotherapy may be increasingly used.

Hypothyroidism

The radiation ports used for the curative therapy of HD allow sufficient dosages to be delivered to the thyroid gland to produce hypofunction in later years. Most often such hypofunction is compensated by an increase in thyroid-stimulating hormone and escapes clinical detection unless searched for. When the hypofunction becomes overt, therapy is required with replacement doses of an appropriate thyroid hormone preparation, and it is likely that such therapy is also indicated for subclinical hypofunction manifested only by increased thyroid-stimulating hormone levels.[71]

Second Malignancies After Cure of Lymphoma

Second malignancies may develop after cure of a lymphoma.[72] Acute nonlymphocytic leukemia is the most common and well-recognized long-range complication of exposure to radiation or to alkylating anticancer drugs. Cumulative risk varies according to the intensity and nature of the treatment and the period of observation and may range from less than 1% to well over 10%.[72]

If both radiation and chemotherapy are used, the risk of subsequent leukemia is greatest. It is generally believed that the alkylating agents are more leukemogenic than other anticancer drugs; thus a regimen such as ABVD might be followed by a lower rate of leukemia than an alkylating regimen such as MOPP. Non-Hodgkin's lymphoma has been reported in patients cured of Hodgkin's disease.[73] Radiotherapy seems to selectively increase the risk for tumors of bones and soft tissues that are in the field of radiation.[74]

Employability

Because individuals with lymphoma are frequently cured of their disease, subsequent questions may be raised regarding their eligibility for employment. Many companies are reluctant to accept employees with a past history of cancer, even though the probability of cure may be very high (80% to 90%). This is a particularly difficult problem for the young person who has been in complete remission for several years (for example, after treatment of NS-HD) and who may be applying for graduate school or beginning a new career. Opportunities for such individuals may be severely curtailed when a prospective employer or graduate school admissions committee becomes aware of their past medical history. This may present a problem in some situations and cause painful difficulties for a person who has so recently survived a life-threatening cancer. Counseling, understanding, and support may be helpful, but the ultimate solution is societal rather than medical.

CONCLUSION

The lymphomas comprise more than a dozen separate clinical entities with a widely variable spectrum of disease ranging from slow, indolent growth to rapidly fatal progression. Some lymphomas are highly curable with appropriate therapy, others show no increase in survival following treatment. These different clinical entities are separated from each other on the basis of subtle clinical and histologic differences requiring expert pathologic interpretation and staging for accurate prognosis and selection of therapy. Megavoltage radiotherapy and combination chemotherapy have provided curative management techniques, leading to the expectation of cure in well over 50% of all individuals with lymphoma. However, not all varieties of lymphoma are equally curable. Thus, the skillful application of the complex and toxic treatments requires a precise delineation of histologic type and extent of disease in accordance with rigorously established principles of staging.

Although the etiology of the lymphomas remains elusive, tantalizing hints are provided by the strong suggestion of Epstein-Barr virus–induced Burkitt's lymphoma in Africa, the viruslike epidemiologic pattern of nodular sclerosing Hodgkin's disease, and the clear association between malfunction of the immune defense system and the development of non-Hodgkin's lymphoma.

Effective diagnosis, staging, and multimodal management of the lymphomas require the collaborative efforts of multiple health care disciplines. The nurse is an essential member of this team. The nurse has the opportunity not only to provide medical and nursing care but also to respond to an even greater challenge. It is the nurse who, to a greater extent than most others on the team, must respond to the patient's most desperate need for support and understanding; it is the nurse who must meet the patient's need for careful explanation of the complex diagnostic and therapeutic methods designed to deal with a life-threatening malignancy; it is the nurse who must be constantly alert to the possible complications of both the disease and its treatment.

In our haste to exercise our newfound curative therapeutic methods, we must be constantly aware of the impact of the disease and its treatment on a person's future quality of life. When cure was unknown, sterility, employability, and the difficulty of living with a cured cancer were unknown problems. Our progress has, as is so often the case, given us not a respite but a new set of challenges.

REFERENCES

1. Hodgkin T: On some morbid appearances of the absorbent glands and spleen. Med Chir Trans 17:68-114, 1832.
2. Wilks S: Cases of enlargement of the lymphatic glands and spleen, or, Hodgkin's disease. Guy's Hosp Rep 11:56-67, 1865.
3. Reed DM: On the pathological changes in Hodgkin's disease, with especial reference to tuberculosis. Johns Hopkins Rep 10:133-196, 1902.
4. Sternberg C: Über eine eigenartige unter dem Bilde der Pseukoleukamie verlaufende: Tuberculose des lymphatischen apparates. Z Heilkd 19:21-90, 1898.
5. Lukes RJ, Butler JJ: The pathology and nomenclature of Hodgkin's disease. Cancer Res 26:1063-1081, 1966.
6. Rosenberg SA, Berard CW, Brown BW, et al: National Cancer Institute study of classification of non-Hodgkin's lymphomas: Summary and description of a working formulation for clinical usage. Cancer 49:2112-2135, 1982.
7. Magrath IT: Lymphocyte differentiation: An essential basis for the comprehension of lymphoid neoplasia. JNCI 67:501-514, 1981.
8. Silverberg E, Lubera JA: Cancer statistics, 1989. CA 39:3-20, 1989.
9. Cole P, MacMahon B, Aisenberg A: Mortality from Hodgkin's disease in the United States: Evidence for the multiple etiology hypothesis. Lancet 2:1371-1376, 1968.
10. Poplack DG, Kun LE, Cassady JR, et al: Leukemias and lymphomas of childhood, in DeVita VT Jr, Hellman S, Rosenberg SA (eds): Cancer: Principles and Practice of Oncology. Philadelphia, JB Lippincott, 1989, pp 1671-1695.
11. Regula DP, Hoppe RT, Weiss LM: Nodular and diffuse types of lymphocyte predominance in Hodgkin's disease. N Engl J Med 318:214-219, 1988.
12. Borg-Grech A, Radford AJ, Crowther D, et al: A compar-
13. Rappaport H: Tumors of the hematopoietic system, in Atlas of Tumor Pathology, Section 3, Fascicle 8. Washington, DC, Armed Forces Institute of Pathology, 1966.
14. Lukes RJ, Collins RD: Immunological characterization of human malignant lymphomas. Cancer 34:1488-1503, 1974.
15. Carbonne PP, Kaplan HS, Musshoff K, et al: Report of the committee on Hodgkin's disease staging. Cancer Res 31:1860-1861, 1971.
16. Gilbert R: Radiotherapy of Hodgkin's disease: Anatomic and clinical foundations. AJR 41:198-241, 1939.
17. Peters MV: A study of survivals in Hodgkin's disease treated radiologically. AJR 63:299-311, 1950.
18. Hoppe RT: Radiation therapy in the treatment of Hodgkin's disease. Semin Oncol 7:136-143, 1980.
19. Kaplan H: Evidence for a tumoricidal dose level in the radiotherapy of Hodgkin's disease. Cancer Res 26:1221-1224, 1966.
20. DeVita VT, Serpick A, Carbone PP: Combination chemotherapy in the treatment of advanced Hodgkin's disease. Ann Intern Med 73:881-895, 1970.
21. Glatein R, Trueblood HW, Enright LP, et al: Surgical staging of abdominal involvement in unselected patients with Hodgkin's disease. Radiology 97:425-432, 1970.
22. Chabner BA, Johnson RE, Young RC, et al: Sequential nonsurgical and surgical staging of non-Hodgkin's lymphoma. Ann Intern Med 85:149-154, 1976.
23. Yarbro CH: Lymphomas, in Groenwald S (ed): Cancer Nursing: Principles and Practice. Boston, Jones & Bartlett, 1987, pp 671-683.
24. Hellman S, Jaffe ES, DeVita VT: Hodgkin's disease, in DeVita VT Jr, Hellman S, Rosenberg SA (eds): Cancer: Principles and Practice of Oncology. Philadelphia, JB Lippincott, 1989, pp 1696-1740.
25. Lister TA, Dorreen MS, Faux M, et al: The treatment of stage IIIA Hodgkin's disease. J Clin Oncol 1:745, 1983.
26. DeVita VT, Simon RM, Hubbard SM, et al: Curability of advanced Hodgkin's disease with chemotherapy: Long term follow-up of MOPP treated patients at the National Cancer Institute. Ann Intern Med 92:587-595, 1980.
27. Santoro A, Bonadonna G, Valagussa P, et al: Long-term results of combined chemotherapy-radiotherapy approach in Hodgkin's disease: Superiority of ABVD plus radiotherapy versus MOPP plus radiotherapy. J Clin Oncol 5:27-37, 1987.
28. Bonnadonna G, Valagussa P, Santoro A: Alternating non-cross-resistant combination chemotherapy or MOPP in stage IV Hodgkin's disease. Ann Intern Med 104:739-746, 1986.
29. Bakemeier RF, Anderson JR, Costello W, et al: BCVPP chemotherapy for advanced Hodgkin's disease: Evidence for greater duration of complete remission, greater survival, and less toxicity than with a MOPP regimen. Ann Intern Med 101:447-456, 1984.
30. Longo D, Glatstein E, Young R, et al: Randomized trial of MOPP chemotherapy vs. subtotal nodal radiation therapy in patients with laparotomy-documented early stage Hodgkin's disease. Proc Am Soc Clin Oncol 6:206, 1987 (abstr).
31. Olwney CLM, Katongole-Mbidda E, Kiire C, et al: Childhood Hodgkin's disease in Uganda: A ten-year experience. Cancer 42:787-792, 1978.
32. Schomberg PJ, Evans RG, O'Connell MJ, et al: Prognostic significance of mediastinal mass in adult Hodgkin's disease. Cancer 53:324-328, 1984.
33. Lee CK, Bloomfield CD, Goldman AL, et al: Prognostic significance of mediastinal involvement in Hodgkin's disease treated with curative radiotherapy. Cancer 46:2403-2409, 1980.
34. Prakash U, Abel MD: Mediastinal mass and tracheal obstruction during general anesthesia. Mayo Clin Proc 63:1004-1011, 1988.
35. Leopold KA, Canellos GP, Rosenthal D, et al: Stage IA-IIB

Hodgkin's disease: Staging and treatment of patients with large mediastinal adenopathy. J Clin Oncol 7:1059-1065, 1989.
36. Austin-Seymour MM, Hoppe RT, Cox RS, et al: Hodgkin's disease in patients over sixty years old. Ann Intern Med 100:13-18, 1984.
37. Tubiana M, Henry-Amar M, Hayat M, et al: Prognostic significance of the number of involved areas in the early stages of Hodgkin's disease. Cancer 54:885-894, 1984.
38. Leibenhaut MH, Hoppe RT, Varghese A, et al: Subdiaphragmatic Hodgkin's disease: Laparotomy and treatment results in 49 patients. J Clin Oncol 5:1050-1055, 1987.
39. Sweet DL and Golomb HM: The non-Hodgkin's lymphomas. Curr Probl Cancer 4(7):3-35, 1980.
40. Longo DL, Glatstein E, Duffey PL, et al: Treatment of localized aggressive lymphomas with combination chemotherapy followed by involved-field radiation therapy. J Clin Oncol 7:1295-1302, 1989.
41. Medeiros LJ, Picker LJ, Gelb AB, et al: Numbers of host "helper" T cells and proliferating cells predict survival in diffuse small-cell lymphomas. J Clin Oncol 7:1009-1017, 1989.
42. Fisher RI: Picking winners and losers in diffuse small-cell lymphomas. J Clin Oncol 7:991-992, 1989 (editorial).
43. Armitage JO, Cheson BD: Interpretation of clinical trials in diffuse large-cell lymphoma. J Clin Oncol 6:1335-1347, 1988.
44. Schein PS, DeVita VT, Hubbard S, et al: Bleomycin, adriamycin, cyclophosphamide, vincristine, and prednisone (BACOP) combination chemotherapy in the treatment of advanced diffuse histiocytic lymphoma. Ann Intern Med 85:417-422, 1976.
45. Conners JM, Klima P: MACOP-B chemotherapy for malignant lymphomas and related conditions: 1987 update and additional observations. Semin Hematol 25:41-46, 1988 (suppl 2).
46. Coiffier B, Gisselbrecht C, Herbrecht R, et al: LNH-84 regimen: A multicenter study of intensive chemotherapy in 737 patients with aggressive malignant lymphoma. J Clin Oncol 7:1018-1026, 1989.
47. DeVita VT Jr, Jaffe ES, Mauch P, et al: Lymphocytic lymphomas, in DeVita VT Jr, Hellman S, Rosenberg SA (eds): Cancer: Principles and Practice of Oncology. Philadelphia, JB Lippincott, 1989, pp 1741-1798.
48. Miller TP, Dana BW, Weick JK, et al: Southwest Oncology Group clinical trials for intermediate- and high-grade non-Hodgkin's lymphomas. Semin Hematol 25:17-22, 1988 (suppl 2).
49. Vose JM, Armitage JO, Weisenburger DD, et al: The importance of age in survival of patients treated with chemotherapy for aggressive non-Hodgkin's lymphoma. J Clin Oncol 6:1838-1844, 1988.
50. Jones SE, Miller TP, Connors JM: Long-term follow-up and analysis for prognostic factors for patients with limited-stage diffuse large-cell lymphoma treated with initial chemotherapy with or without adjuvant radiotherapy. J Clin Oncol 7:1186-1191, 1989.
51. Coiffer B, Lepage E: Prognosis of aggressive lymphomas: A study of five prognostic models with patients included in the LNH-84 regimen. Blood 74:558-564, 1989.
52. Yunis JJ, Okien MM, Kaplan ME, et al: Distinctive chromosomal abnormalities in histologic subtypes of non-Hodgkin's lymphoma. N Engl J Med 307:1231-1236, 1982.
53. Velasquez WS, Jagannath S, Tucker SL, et al: Risk classification as the basis for clinical staging of diffuse large-cell lymphoma derived from 10-year survival data. Blood 74:551-557, 1989.
54. Gibbs WN, Lofters WS, Campbell M, et al: Non-Hodgkin's lymphoma in Jamaica and its relation to adult T-cell leukemia-lymphoma. Ann Intern Med 106:361-368, 1987.
55. Sherins RJ, DeVita VT: Effects of drug treatment of lymphoma on male reproductive capacity. Ann Intern Med 79:216-220, 1973.
56. Chapman R, Rees L, Sutcliffe SB, et al: Cyclical combination chemotherapy and gonadal function: Retrospective study in males. Lancet 1:285-289, 1979.
57. Bergsagel DE: Salvage treatment for Hodgkin's disease in relapse. J Clin Oncol 5:525-526, 1987 (editorial).
58. Reece DE, Barnet MJ, Connors JW, et al: Allogeneic marrow transplantation for refractory Hodgkin's disease. J Clin Oncol 7:1039-1045, 1989.
59. Philip T, Armitage JO, Spitzer G, et al: High-dose therapy and autologous bone marrow transplantation after failure of conventional chemotherapy in adults with intermediate grade or high-grade non-Hodgkin's lymphoma. N Engl J Med 316:1493-1498, 1987.
60. Gulati SC, Shank B, Black P, et al: Autologous bone marrow transplantation for patients with poor-prognosis lymphoma. J Clin Oncol 6:1303-1313, 1988.
61. Takaue Y, Watanabe T, Kawano Y, et al: Isolation and storage of peripheral blood hematopoietic stem cells for autotransplantation into children with cancer. Blood 74:1245-1251, 1989.
62. Kessinger A, Armitage JO, Smith DM, et al: High-dose therapy and autologous peripheral blood stem cell transplantation for patients with lymphoma. Blood 74:1260-1265, 1989.
63. Perez C, Presant C, VanAmburg AL: Management of superior vena cava syndrome. Semin Oncol 5:123-133, 1978.
64. Perez-Soler R, McLaughlin P, Valasquez WS, et al: Clinical features and results of management of superior vena cava syndrome secondary to lymphoma. J Clin Oncol 2:260-266, 1984.
65. Bruckman JE, Bloomer WD: Management of spinal cord compression. Semin Oncol 5:135-140, 1978.
66. Young RF, Post EM, King GA: Treatment of spinal epidural metastases. Randomized prospective comparison of laminectomy and radiotherapy. J Neurosurg 53:741-748, 1980.
67. Siegal T, Siegal T: Surgical decompression of anterior and posterior malignant epidural tumors compressing the spinal cord: A prospective study. Neurosurgery 17:424-432, 1985.
68. Hayes FA, Thompson EL, Hvizdala E, et al: Chemotherapy as an alternative to laminectomy and radiation in management of epidural tumor. J Pediatr 104:221-224, 1984.
69. Burch PA, Grossman SA: Treatment of epidural cord compressions from Hodgkin's disease with chemotherapy: A report of two cases and a review of the literature. Am J Med 84:555-558, 1988.
70. Delaney TF, Oldfield EH: Spinal cord compression, in DeVita VT Jr, Hellman S, Rosenberg SA (eds): Cancer: Principles and Practice of Oncology. Philadelphia, JB Lippincott, 1989, pp 1978-1986.
71. Schimpff SC, Diggs CH, Wiswell JG, et al: Radiation-related thyroid dysfunction: Implications for the treatment of Hodgkin's disease. Ann Intern Med 92:91-98, 1980.
72. Fraser MC, Tucker MA: Second malignancies following cancer therapy. Semin Oncol Nurs 5:43-55, 1989.
73. Jacquillat C, Khayat D, Desprez-Curely JP, et al: Occurrence of non-Hodgkin's lymphoma after therapy for Hodgkin's disease. Cancer 53:459-462, 1984.
74. Boivin JF, O'Brien K: Solid cancer risk after treatment of Hodgkin's disease. Cancer 61:2541-2546, 1988.

Chapter 45

Multiple Myeloma

Mary Barton Cook, RN, BSN, OCN

INTRODUCTION

Multiple myeloma is a neoplastic proliferation of plasma cells. These cells are derived from one type, or clone, of plasma cell and produce a homogeneous immunoglobulin without any apparent antigenic stimulation. The disease is characterized by bone destruction, bone marrow involvement, and the presence of a homogeneous immunoglobulin in the urine or serum.

EPIDEMIOLOGY

Multiple myeloma is primarily a disease of late-middle-aged to elderly persons. The median age at diagnosis is 68 years; fewer than 2% of affected individuals are under 40 years of age.[1] The incidence among white men and women is 4.3 per 100,000 and 3.0 per 100,000, respectively. The incidence among black men (9.6 per 100,000) and women (6.7 per 100,000) is higher.[1]

There are approximately 11,600 new cases and almost 8600 deaths from multiple myeloma each year.[2] The reported death rate for multiple myeloma is 3 per 100,000 individuals per year. Multiple myeloma accounts for about 1% of all cancer deaths and 10% of deaths from hematologic malignancies.[2] The incidence and mortality of multiple myeloma have risen sharply in the last 40 years. However it is believed that this rise reflects previous underdiagnoses rather than a recent increase.

ETIOLOGY

The etiology of multiple myeloma is unknown. A variety of factors have been suggested in the pathogenesis of the disease. Genetic factors may play a role, particularly in light of the increased incidence among blacks. Genetic marker studies have yielded little information to date.

Environmental influences may be etiologic factors also. Some individuals with multiple myeloma have a history of chronic infections, but common environmental factors have not been identified.[3] Multiple myeloma has been linked with chronic low-level exposure to various types of occupational, diagnostic, or therapeutic radiation.[4] There is an increased incidence of multiple myeloma among Japanese who survived the atomic bomb explosions at Hiroshima and Nagasaki and among first-degree relatives of affected survivors. In a 6-year period, multiple myeloma was found in 8 of 440 siblings of individuals with multiple myeloma.[3]

PATHOPHYSIOLOGY

Normal Physiology of Plasma Cells

Figure 45-1 shows the development of plasma cells from lymphocytes. The function of plasma cells is the production of immunoglobulins, the basic units from which antibodies are formed. Each clone of plasma cells is thought to be responsible for the production of one specific type of immunoglobulin. There are five types of immunoglobulin: IgG, IgA, IgM, IgD, and IgE. IgG is responsible for major antibacterial and antiviral activity. IgA is the body's first line of defense against pathogens in the respiratory and gastrointestinal tracts and is present in external secretions, such as tears, gastrointestinal secretions, and mucus. IgM is responsible for the initial formation of antibodies after the administration of an antigen. The function of IgD is unknown. IgE is associated with allergic diseases, such as hay fever, asthma, and urticaria.

Pathologic Characteristics

In multiple myeloma, there is uncontrolled proliferation of plasma cells that have undergone malignant transformation. Typically, one specific clone of the plasma cells is transformed, resulting in the excessive production of one homogeneous immunoglobulin. The aberrant immunoglobulin differs from the normal immunoglobulin in two ways: increased level of production and homogeneity. In a healthy individual, the immunoglobulins that are produced are heterogeneous in nature because they are produced by many types of plasma cells. With multiple myeloma, however, the immunoglobulin is produced by a single clone of plasma cell, making it homogeneous. The abnormally increased production of a specific homogeneous immunoglobulin can be demonstrated by serum electrophoresis of blood from an individual with multiple myeloma (Figure 45-2).

The abnormal immunoglobulin produced by the malignant transformed plasma cell is called the M-protein, the *M* referring to monoclonal, myeloma, and/or malignant. This M-protein is produced in excessive amounts and is incapable of effective antibody production. M-protein is found in nearly all individuals with multiple myeloma and is responsible for many of the clinical manifestations of the disease. Nonsecreting myeloma, in which urine or serum proteins cannot be detected, occurs in about 1% of individuals.[5] The diagnosis must then be made on the basis of other clinical manifestations of the disease.

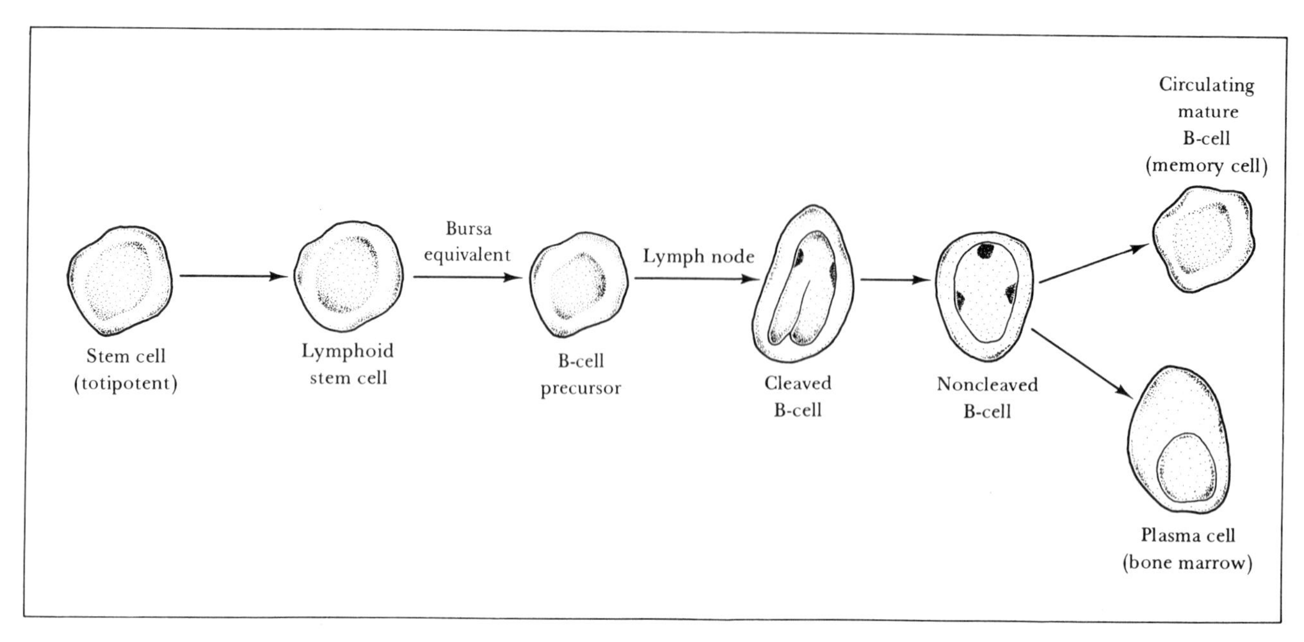

FIGURE 45-1 Development of plasma cells from lymphocytes.

CLINICAL MANIFESTATIONS AND ASSESSMENTS

The clinical manifestations of multiple myeloma result from the total body tumor burden of excessive malignant cell proliferation within the bone and the indirect effects of the secreted products of the abnormal proteins throughout the body. Multiple myeloma is a slow-growing neoplasm characterized by a long prodromal period during which the individual may be asymptomatic. It is usually during the more advanced stages that symptoms appear and the diagnosis is made. The common laboratory and radiographic studies performed to diagnose multiple myeloma are bone marrow aspiration and biopsy; skeletal x-ray survey; urine or serum electrophoresis; quantitative immunoglobulins; immunoelectrophoresis; determination of serum calcium, blood urea nitrogen, creatinine, albumin, uric acid, electrolyte, and Bence-Jones urine protein levels; complete blood cell counts; and urinalysis. In selected cases, magnetic resonance imaging (MRI) can be used to provide great detail of the vertebral involvement; however, MRI is expensive and requires several hours to complete.[6]

Bone Involvement

The most common presenting symptom of multiple myeloma is bone pain due to the excessive accumulation of abnormal plasma cells in the bone marrow. The myeloma cells produce osteoclast activating factor (OAF), a lymphokine that stimulates osteoclast proliferation and activ-

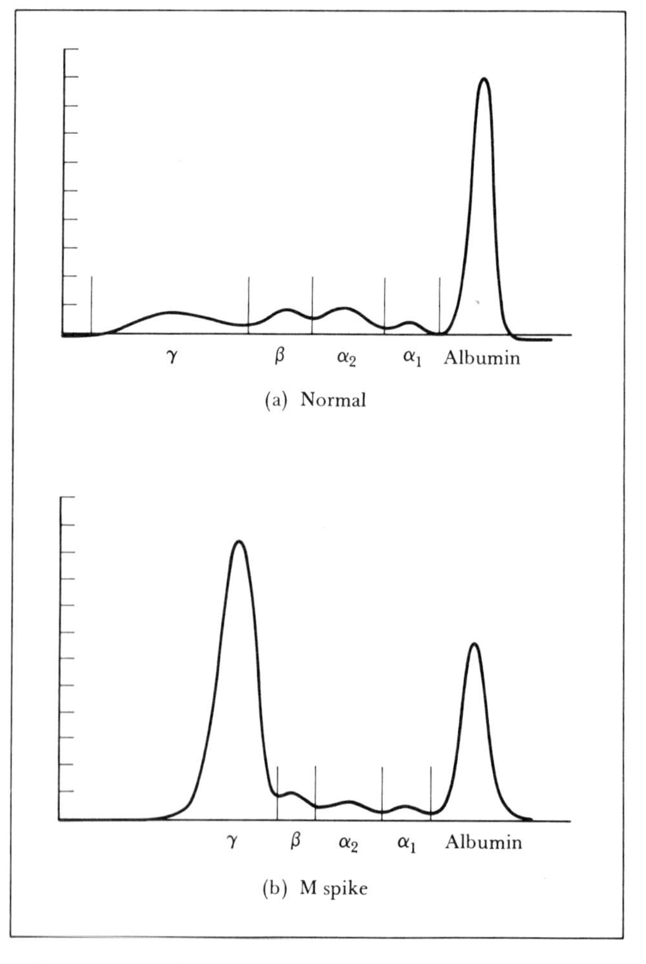

FIGURE 45-2 Abnormal electrophoresis in individuals with myeloma. Gamma globulin is elevated in individuals with myeloma, giving the so-called M spike.

ity, leading to extensive osteolysis, severe bone pain, and pathologic fractures.[5] Levels of osteoclast activating factor correlate with the extent of skeletal involvement.[7] The thoracic and lumbar vertebrae are most commonly involved, resulting in pain on movement or weight bearing. Compression fractures in the thoracic and lumbar spine area are sequelae of myeloma. The ribs, skull, pelvis, and proximal long bones are also frequently involved. Many individuals will initially have pathologic fractures and hypercalcemia. Radiographically, there are multiple "punched-out" osteolytic lesions and/or diffuse osteoporosis (Figure 45-3).

Bone Marrow Involvement

In individuals with multiple myeloma, 10% to 95% of the nucleated cells in the bone marrow are plasma cells with varying degrees of maturation.[8] Normally, plasma cells account for fewer than 3.5% of the nucleated cells in bone marrow.[8]

Anemia

Individuals with multiple myeloma commonly present with mild to moderate normochromic, normocytic anemia caused by crowding of the marrow by plasma cells. This

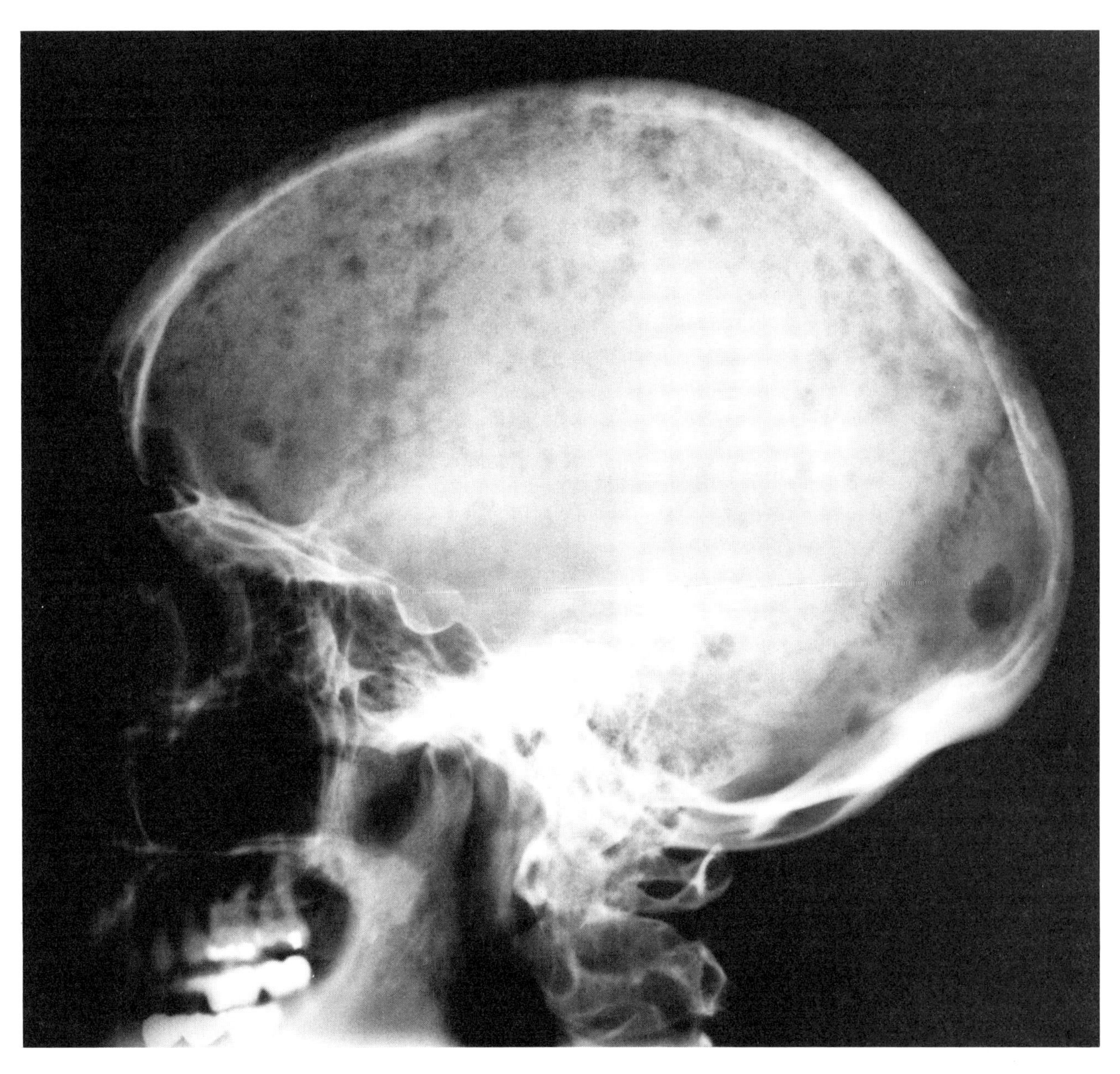

FIGURE 45-3 Skull radiograph of 68-year-old woman with multiple myeloma, showing characteristic picture of multiple, sharply circumscribed osteolytic (punched-out) lesions. (Courtesy Valley Radiology Group, Inc., San Jose, Calif.)

is classically manifest as fatigue and weakness. The degree of anemia is related to the percentage of plasma cells in the marrow. Other factors that contribute to anemia in individuals with multiple myeloma are reduced production of red blood cells and increased red cell destruction. Serum M-protein produces a coating that causes red cells to line up like rolls of coins, which is referred to as rouleau formation. Hemolysis and sludging result.

Thrombocytopenia

There is a predisposition to bleeding as a result of M-protein coating the platelets. The platelet count may be within normal limits, but tests show that platelet function (eg, bleeding time) is abnormal. The most common sites of bleeding are mucosal surfaces such as the nose and the gastrointestinal tract.

Renal Insufficiency

Renal insufficiency at the time of clinical presentation indicates a poor prognosis. Proteinuria is present in about 70% of the persons who have multiple myeloma. Bence-Jones proteins, the light chains of immunoglobulin molecules, are present initially, and it is these proteins that damage the renal tubular cells.[8] The presence of Bence-Jones proteins in the urine may lead to the formation of precipitates in the tubules, where the glomerular filtrate is concentrated. This may result in tubular obstruction, foreign body reaction, and tubular degeneration. There also may be an increased loss of amino acids, glucose, phosphorus, and potassium because of impaired reabsorption.

The serum uric acid is elevated in approximately two thirds of the individuals who have multiple myeloma.[8] The elevation is caused by an increased rate of cell death and the by-products of protein synthesis by tumor cells. Renal insufficiency contributes to the impaired renal clearance of uric acid. If left untreated, the elevated uric acid will add to further kidney damage. Hypercalcemia is present as a result of the bone destruction characteristic of multiple myeloma and may further impair renal function.

Pyelonephritis frequently occurs in persons with multiple myeloma. It is due to tubular obstruction and the resulting decrease in kidney function, as well as decreased immunity caused by the lack of normal immunoglobulins from the multiple myeloma and later by the myelosuppressive effects of the chemotherapy.

Another problem leading to decreased renal function is myeloma kidney, which is a result of the toxic effects of the Bence-Jones proteins on the renal tubules. A characteristic finding of myeloma kidney is the precipitation of dense tubular casts of light chains. Other conditions that interfere with renal function include deposits of calcium or amyloid within the parenchyma. The amyloid deposits cause renal glomerular damage and are the result of a reaction between the M-protein and tissue polysaccharides, which causes precipitation of starchy material. Amyloid deposits may also occur in the heart, blood vessels, and gastrointestinal tract.

Immune System

Infection is a common cause of death, with pneumonia specifically being responsible for 50% of the deaths.[8] The most common sites of infection are the respiratory tract, the urinary tract, skin, sinuses, and blood. In individuals with multiple myeloma, the normal serum antibody immunoglobulin levels are usually depressed. An acquired hyporesponsiveness to antigen stimulation that results in deficient antibody production is the primary reason for decreased immunity. This depression of normal serum antibody immunoglobulin production may be the result of a feedback mechanism involving the increased production of abnormal immunoglobulins.

Another factor that contributes to increased susceptibility to infection is impaired granulocyte function, which interferes with normal phagocytosis. Decreased granulocyte production results from infiltration of the bone marrow by abnormal plasma cells and later is exacerbated by the myelosuppressive and immunosuppressive effects of chemotherapy.

Hyperviscosity Syndrome

In about 5% of the individuals who have multiple myeloma (most commonly those with IgM myeloma and occasionally those with IgA and IgG myeloma), the presence of high concentrations of M-protein in the blood increases the serum viscosity, leading to a variety of problems.[1] Usually some degree of hyperviscosity is present in individuals with multiple myeloma, but symptoms generally do not appear until the serum viscosity exceeds 4.0 centipaise units.[1] The first problems encountered as a result of hyperviscosity are related to circulatory impairment caused by occlusion of small blood vessels with M-protein. The person may experience intermittent claudication because of the decreased circulation or, if the impairment is severe, may even develop gangrene in the distal extremities. The M-protein also interferes with circulation in the retinal vessels, leading to visual disturbances, retinal hemorrhages, and papilledema. Neurologic symptoms resulting from the circulatory impairment include irritability, headache, drowsiness, confusion, and in some cases even coma.

As the amount of M-protein increases, the high molecular mass of M-proteins produces increased osmotic pressure, leading to hypervolemia. Problems related to hypervolemia include anemia (normochromic, normocytic) due to hemodilution and congestive heart failure resulting from circulatory overload.

CLINICAL STAGING

A staging system that is universally accepted and used has not been developed. Several staging criteria models have been published but none has gained widespread acceptance. The Durie-Salmon myeloma staging system is frequently used as a basis for comparing survival by stages in clinical studies. Tumor burden is the pivotal criterion in this particular staging system (Table 45-1).[1]

As an alternative to a traditional staging system, some clinicians are using serum levels of B_2-microglobulin (B-2M) as a definitive prognostic factor. B_2-microglobulin is a protein synthesized by all nucleated cells. It can be measured by radioimmunoassay. Serum levels of B-2M correlate strongly with renal function and myeloma cell tumor burden.[9] It has been suggested that B-2M levels are an objective parameter to consider for prediction of survival and as a pretreatment prognostic indicator.

TABLE 45-1 Myeloma Staging System

Criteria	Measured Myeloma Cell Mass (Cells × $10^{12}/m^2$)
Stage I	
All of the following:	
Hemoglobin value >10 g/dL	
Serum calcium value normal (<12 mg/dL)	
On roentgenogram, normal bone structure (scale 0) or solitary bone plasmacytoma only	
Low M-component production rates	<0.6 (low)
IgG value <5 g/dL	
IgA value < 3g/dL	
Urine light chain M-component on electrophoresis <4g/24 hr	
Stage II	
Overall data not as minimally abnormal as shown for stage I and no single value as abnormal as defined for stage III	0.6-1.20 (intermediate)
Stage III	
One or more of the following	
Hemoglobin value <8.5 g/dL	
Serum calcium value >12 mg/dL	
Advanced lytic bone lesions (scale 3)	
High M-component production rates	>1.20 (high)
IgG value >7g/dL	
IgA value >5 g/dL	
Urine light chain M-component on electrophoresis >12 g/24 hr	
Subclassification	
A = relatively normal renal function (serum creatinine value >2.0 mg/dL)	
B = abnormal renal function (serum creatinine value ≥2.0 mg/dL)	
Examples	
Stage IA = low cell mass with normal renal function	
Stage IIIB = high cell mass with abnormal renal function	

IgA, Immunoglobulin A; *IgG*, immunoglobulin G.

Source: Salmon SE, Cassady JR: Plasma cell neoplasms, in DeVita VT, Hellman S, Rosenberg SA (eds): Cancer: Principles and Practice (ed 3). Philadelphia, JB Lippincott, 1989.

TREATMENT

Systemic antineoplastic therapy is the treatment of choice for multiple myeloma. Individuals diagnosed with asymptomatic stage I myeloma are not given chemotherapy until there are signs that the disease is progressing. The administration of chemotherapy for stage I disease has failed to demonstrate improved survival rates; therefore it is considered inappropriate to expose these individuals to the risks associated with chemotherapy.[1,10] Serial monitoring of M-protein levels may be useful to detect increasing disease activity in the asymptomatic patient. Clinical signs of disease progression that would indicate the need for systemic therapy include bone pain, hypercalcemia, renal failure, or bone marrow suppression. Pathologic fractures and serious infections are usually treated and controlled before initiation of systemic therapy. Others who should not be treated are those with benign monoclonal gammopathy (a condition that is initially not malignant but in some will later develop into multiple myeloma) and "smoldering myeloma," in which the disease remains stable without treatment.[1]

Most individuals with newly diagnosed stage II or III myeloma respond favorably to systemic therapy. Multiple myeloma treated with systemic therapy appears to respond in phases that include the following[1]:

1. An initial phase of drug sensitivity (usually 2 to 3 years)
2. A plateau phase when the disease appears stable
3. A drug-resistant phase of altered growth kinetics and resistance to chemotherapy

Median overall survival for persons with myeloma is about 3 to 4 years. Some persons will experience lengthy periods of drug sensitivity lasting 5 to 10 years.[1]

Cycle-nonspecific cytotoxic drugs, usually in combination with prednisone, are the agents of choice for treatment of multiple myeloma. Alkylating agents, alone or in combination with prednisone, are the mainstay of treatment. The most commonly used drug is phenylalanine mustard (L-PAM, melphalan) given on a high-dose intermittent or low-dose continuous schedule of administration. Intermittent dosing is thought to be superior because it allows the person to recover from the myelosuppressive and immunosuppressive effects of the chemotherapy[5,8,10] and potentially to avoid cumulative toxic reactions. During induction chemotherapy, if individuals do not experience significant myelosuppression, they should receive escalating doses of oral melphalan to assure maximum adsorption and avoid underdosing. Cyclophosphamide is the other alkylating agent used to treat myeloma, usually given on an intermittent schedule. In some individuals, responses may be obtained with cyclophosphamide after the person has developed resistance to phenylalanine mustard. The objective response rates to alkylating agents alone or in combination with prednisone range from 20% to 70%.[1]

Glucocorticoids, especially prednisone, are used in the treatment of multiple myeloma. Glucocorticoids may potentiate the activity of other chemotherapeutic drugs and are useful in reducing bone resorption; reducing hypercalcemia; decreasing serum M-protein concentrations, including that of the monoclonal protein; decreasing proteinuria; and producing a rise in the hematocrit level.[3,5,8,11]

Other chemotherapeutic agents that are being used in multiagent protocols in combination with melphalan and cyclophosphamide are doxorubicin, BCNU, prednisone, and vincristine. Because of difficulties in comparing results of the different protocols and evaluating responses, the choice of initial treatment is somewhat controversial; yet phenylalanine mustard and prednisone remain the most commonly used chemotherapeutic agents. Drugs under investigation include interferon and interleukin II. Studies using α-interferon have shown promising antitumor activity in the treatment of multiple myeloma.[12] The overall response rate in individuals with resistant disease ranges from 15% to 30%, depending on the prognostic subgroup.[13] The effects of α-interferon in combination with chemotherapy is being evaluated.[14]

The criteria for objective response to chemotherapy include sustained decrease in M-protein level in the serum, urine, or both, normal serum calcium value, and normal hemoglobin and hematocrit levels. Lytic lesions generally do not appear to heal, but the absence of new lesions on skeletal radiographs is considered a significant indicator of response. Criteria for subjective response include an increased sense of well-being, increased appetite, and decreased pain.[1]

Persons who do not respond to induction therapy are considered resistant to drugs and overall prognosis is poor. Individuals who have responded to induction therapy and later relapse, will more likely respond to alternate second-line therapy. Glucocorticoids have proved useful for a single-agent approach to the drug-resistant or relapsed person. Multiagent combination chemotherapy is being explored for second-line treatment.

Plasmapheresis, a procedure similar to hemodialysis, removes the excessive M-protein from the blood and returns the white blood cells and red blood cells to the individual. This procedure, in conjunction with chemotherapy, is used to treat individuals with hyperviscosity syndrome or myeloma kidney and those who are at risk of bleeding.

Radiation therapy has traditionally been used for palliation of bone pain in individuals with multiple myeloma. Advances in the application of radiotherapy have led to such approaches as hemibody irradiation and systemic radiotherapy, particularly for the person who has chemoresistant disease.

Multiple myeloma is highly radioresponsive. Therefore debilitating bone pain can be rapidly relieved with radiotherapy. Fractionated doses of 2000 to 2400 rad (cGy) over a period of 1 to 2 weeks will usually relieve pain, eradicate tumor growth at the site, and often prevent impending pathologic fractures.[15] Individuals who receive palliative radiotherapy to alleviate these disabling complications of myeloma experience a welcome improvement, albeit temporary, in the quality of their lives. Careful evaluation and treatment planning are needed if additional courses of radiotherapy are considered for recurrence of complications.

When a person with myeloma exhibits primary chemoresistance or relapses after induction therapy, systemic radiotherapy or hemibody irradiation have been employed as alternative treatment strategies.[16,17] In most cases 750 to 850 cGy are given at a low-dose rate (25 cGy/min) to the hemibody.[17] Pretreatment preparation for hemibody irradiation includes administration of corticosteroids and antiemetics. This therapeutic approach has resulted in a prolonged plateau phase, arrest of disease progression, and reduction in analgesia requirements. Attempts are being made to determine the effectiveness and appropriateness of systemic radiotherapy.

Goals and Interventions

The challenge in caring for the person with multiple myeloma lies in preventing or delaying the inevitable life-threatening complications. There is no known cure for multiple myeloma; therefore the goals shared by the physician and the nurse are to prolong survival and improve the quality of life.

Management of pain

Severe bone pain is a common manifestation of myeloma. Persons with multiple myeloma require the judicious use of analgesics to manage pain. The nurse plays an important role in helping to determine the effective dose and schedule to maximize comfort and avoid unacceptable side effects. Opiates and nonsteroidal anti-inflammatory agents are often used. The nonsteroidal anti-inflammatory agents, although useful, have been associated with renal failure.[18] A back brace, especially the lightweight type with Velcro fasteners, may be helpful for the debilitated person who has lesions of the lumbar spine. Radiotherapy for localized areas of bone disease may be useful to control pain.

Prevention of pathologic fractures

Individuals with multiple myeloma should avoid bed rest and should be encouraged to ambulate, thereby decreasing calcium resorption from the bone and increasing skeletal strength. Adequate pain control will facilitate ambulation. It is important to provide a safe environment by removing any obstacles that might interfere with ambulation. The use of a cane or walker provides a wider base of support and is helpful for some persons. Proper body mechanics reduce stress on involved bones. Radiotherapy may be necessary not only to control severe bone pain but also to stabilize lytic areas that are likely to fracture. In the event of a fracture involving a diseased area of bone, internal fixation is indicated because bone involved with myeloma will not heal. Internal fixation may also be done prophylactically in some instances to prevent a fracture from occurring. Because hypercalcemia is common with bone involvement, it is also important that the patient and the family know its signs and symptoms so that early intervention can minimize complications. (See Chapter 25.)

Maintenance of adequate renal function

Renal failure occurs in about 20% of all individuals with multiple myeloma.[1] Every effort should be taken to ensure an adequate fluid intake. Persons with multiple myeloma should be encouraged to drink at least 2 to 3 liters of fluid per day. Fluid intake and output should be carefully monitored, particularly if renal insufficiency is already present. High fluid intake can potentially prevent kidney damage from elevated levels of uric acid, calcium, and Bence-Jones proteins and other excretory products. Oral intake must never be withheld from individuals with multiple myeloma who are to undergo diagnostic testing or therapy unless they are receiving intravenous fluids, because this may precipitate renal failure. Intravenous pyelogram (IVP) contrast material may lead to renal failure because of the associated increase in osmotic load after administration of these agents. Allopurinol may be administered to protect the kidneys from high uric acid levels and the breakdown products of tumor cells lysed by chemotherapy. Hemodialysis, peritoneal dialysis, or plasmapheresis can be used to treat renal failure in the person who is undergoing intensive therapy. Aggressive dialysis measures are not indicated if there is progressive disease that is unresponsive to therapy.

Prevention of infection

Persons with multiple myeloma should not receive vaccinations with live organisms because these individuals are unable to form antibodies effectively. Adequate fluid intake, a diet high in calories and protein, and the maintenance of a safe environment are key factors to prevent infection. Vigorous chest physiotherapy may be indicated to prevent pneumonia. Any sign of infection, such as fever, sore throat, cough, rash, dysuria, or malaise, should be reported immediately. If signs of infection are present, appropriate cultures are taken and antibiotic therapy is initiated. Because of the risk that resistant strains of bacteria and secondary infections may develop, prophylactic antibiotics are generally not given.

Prevention of cardiovascular problems

Anemia is a common manifestation of myeloma. The severity of the anemia is usually correlated with the extent of the disease. The individual and the family are taught the signs and symptoms of anemia and assisted in the planning of activities to allow for adequate rest and to minimize fatigue. Transfusion of blood components may be necessary. Careful observation is required during blood transfusions, since there may be difficulty in accurately crossmatching blood because of the M-protein. The blood bank should be made aware of the diagnosis of multiple myeloma when transfusions are ordered.

Hyperviscosity syndrome occurs in fewer than 5% of myeloma patients. The signs and symptoms of hyperviscosity syndrome include hypervolemia, edema, congestive heart failure, hemorrhage, retinopathy, and neurologic changes. Plasmapheresis is the initial therapy for hyperviscosity syndrome. Persons undergoing plasmapheresis will require careful teaching before beginning these treatments.

Individuals with multiple myeloma must also be alert for signs of bleeding, such as bruising, petechiae, epistaxis, hematuria, melena, and hematochezia.

Provision of emotional support

The person with multiple myeloma may have many fears that involve death, dependency, disability, weakness, adverse reactions to treatment, the loss of role in the family or in professional life, or financial difficulties. Such a person will require emotional support and open and honest communication. A hopeful atmosphere is maintained, even though the individual is faced with an incurable chronic illness, the emphasis being placed on improving the quality of his or her life. Individuals should be encouraged to maintain as much independence and control over life as possible. The nurse assists the person to cope with changes as they occur and to plan activities around those changes. The individual and the family should be made aware of support groups, social services, the American Cancer Society, and home nursing services available in the community.

CONCLUSION

The prognosis in multiple myeloma has improved from an average length of survival of several months for untreated individuals to as long as 10 years with chemotherapy and aggressive management of complications.[5] Even when resistance to chemotherapy has occurred and the disease progresses, many individuals can be maintained in relative comfort for several years.

The hope for future success in improving survival in individuals with multiple myeloma will depend on further research into the etiology of the disease so that new and more effective treatment measures may be developed. A greater awareness of the subtle signs and symptoms of multiple myeloma, as well as availability of improved screening and detection measures, may facilitate early detection, thereby making treatment available as soon as it is appropriate.

Until the time when either of these is attained, nurses will need to be creative with interventions to promote comfort and optimal living for the individual with multiple myeloma. Further research into effective pain-control measures, techniques to prevent calcium resorption from bone, and more effective means of patient teaching will add to the ability of nurses to assist in improving the quality of life for individuals with multiple myeloma.

REFERENCES

1. Salmon SE, Cassady JR: Plasma cell neoplasms, in DeVita VT, Hellman S, Rosenberg SA (eds): Cancer: Principles and Practice (ed 3). Philadelphia, JB Lippincott, 1989.
2. Silverberg E, Lubera J: Cancer statistics, 1989. CA 39:3-20, 1989.
3. Bersagel D: Plasma cell neoplasms—General considerations, in Williams WJ, Beutler E, Erslev AJ, et al (eds): Hematology (ed 3). New York, McGraw-Hill, 1983.
4. McIntyre OR: Myeloma, in Calabresi P, Schein P, Rosenberg SA (eds): Medical Oncology: Basic Principles and Clinical Management of Cancer. New York, Macmillan, 1985.
5. Bersagel D: Plasma cell myeloma, in Williams WJ, Beutler E, Erslev AJ, et al (eds): Hematology (ed 3). New York, McGraw-Hill, 1983.
6. Ludwig M, Tscholakoff D, Neuhold A, et al: Magnetic resonance imaging of the spine in multiple myeloma. Lancet 2:364-366, 1987.
7. Durie BGM, Salmon SE, Mundy GR: Relation of osteoclast activating factor production to the extent of bone disease in multiple myeloma. Br J Haematol 47:21-30, 1981.
8. Bersagel D: Plasma cell neoplasms, in Holland J, Frei E (eds): Cancer Medicine (ed 2). Philadelphia, Lea & Febiger, 1982.
9. Bataille R, Grenier J: Serum beta-2 microglobulin in multiple myeloma—A critical review. Eur J Cancer 23:1829-1832, 1987.
10. Bersagel D, Rider W: Plasma cell neoplasms, in DeVita VT, Hellman S, Rosenberg SA (eds): Cancer: Principles and Practice of Oncology (ed 1). Philadelphia, JB Lippincott, 1982.
11. Dorr RT, Fritz WL: Cancer Chemotherapy Handbook. New York, Elsevier, 1980.
12. Mitsuyasu RT: The role of alpha interferon in the biotherapy of hematologic malignancies and AIDS-related Kaposi's sarcoma. Oncol Nurs Forum 15:7-12, 1989 (suppl).
13. Cooper MR: Interferons in the management of multiple myeloma. Semin Oncol 15:21-25, 1988 (suppl 5).
14. Cooper MR, Fefer A, Thompson I, et al: Alpha-2-interferon/melphalan/prednisone in previously untreated patients with multiple myeloma: A Phase I-II trial. Cancer Treat Rep 70:473-476, 1986.
15. Mill WB, Griffith R: The role of radiation therapy in the management of plasma cell tumors. Cancer 45: 647-652, 1980.
16. Rider WB: Half-body radiotherapy, an update. Int J Radiat Oncol Biol Phys 4:69-70, 1978 (suppl 2).
17. Singer CR, Tobias JS, Giles F, et al: Hemibody irradiation. Cancer 63:2446-2451, 1989.
18. Rota S, Moungenot B, Baudouin B, et al: Multiple myeloma and severe renal failure: A clinicopathologic study of outcome and prognosis in 34 patients. Medicine 66:126-137, 1987.

Chapter 46

Skin Cancer

Lois J. Loescher, RN, MS

Ann Booth, RN, BS

INTRODUCTION

Cancers of the skin consist of basal cell epithelioma (BCE), squamous cell carcinoma (SCC), and malignant melanoma. BCE (also known as basal cell carcinoma) and SCC are often grouped together and referred to as nonmelanoma skin cancers. Most melanomas are cutaneous (CM); others rarely originate in the eye or viscera. Although these cutaneous cancers share common etiologic factors, they vary in other respects. Nonmelanoma skin cancers have a higher incidence, but they have a low metastatic potential and mortality rate. The associated morbidity is of concern, since nonmelanoma skin cancers often require costly, extensive, and repeated treatments that may result in cosmetic and functional damage. Conversely, melanoma has a much lower incidence but a mortality rate that is triple that of the nonmelanoma skin cancers. The increased mortality is directly related to its high potential for metastasis. For oncology nurses to recognize the subtle and major differences among these skin cancers, the associated epidemiologic, etiologic, and pathophysiologic factors must be understood. Knowledge of assessment, treatment, and prevention of nonmelanoma and melanoma skin cancers enables nurses to provide quality care both for individuals with the disease and for those at high risk.

EPIDEMIOLOGY

More than 500,000 new skin cancers are reported annually, with most of those being BCE or SCC.[1] The incidence of nonmelanoma skin cancer among white persons in the United States is about 165 per 100,000 persons. BCE is the most common form of skin cancer, comprising at least 75% of the cases in the southern United States, and more than 90% of those in the northern United States.[2] BCE occurs twice as often in men as in women; similarly, SCC occurs two to three times more often in men.[3] BCE and SCC are associated with an overall 5-year survival rate of 95%, but they still account for an estimated 2,000 deaths per year.[1]

Approximately 27,000 cases of melanoma are reported annually.[1] Statistics reflecting the yearly incidence of CM since 1973 indicate that it is the most rapidly increasing cancer among white males and the fourth most rapidly increasing cancer among white females.[4] The nationwide incidence of CM appears to double about every 10 years. CM rates among white males are higher than those for white females, being approximately 11.9 and 8.9 per 100,000, respectively.[4]

Although CM represents only about 3% of all skin cancers, its malignant potential must not be underestimated, as it accounts for an estimated 6,000 cancer deaths annually and for 65% of all deaths from skin cancer.[1,5] In the age-adjusted cancer mortality rates reported by the SEER (*S*urveillance, *E*pidemiology, and *E*nd *R*esults) program in 1988, the percent increase in mortality for both sexes and for white and black races from 1973 to 1985 was 25.9%.[4] Early detection and treatment, however, increased the overall relative 5-year survival rate for white persons from 60% to 68% during 1960 to 1973 to 78% to 80% from 1974 to 1984. The relative 5-year survival rate for blacks was approximately 60% from 1974 to 1984.[6]

Skin cancers of any type are rare in children. Although the incidence rate increases with each decade of age, skin cancers generally occur in adults between 30 and 60 years of age.[5]

ETIOLOGY

Multiple etiologic and risk factors are associated with skin cancers (Table 46-1). Most individuals have many pigmented lesions (moles, freckles, birthmarks) on their bodies, and the average white adult averages 10 to 40 lesions.[7] A few of these lesions may be present at birth, whereas others develop throughout life. Almost all are normal, but a change in any pigmented area can be indicative of skin cancer.[8,9]

A persistently changed or changing mole or the presence of irregular pigmented precursor lesions (dysplastic nevi, congenital nevi, lentigo maligna) represents a major high-risk situation for CM. Dysplastic nevi are cutaneous markers that identify family members who are at extremely high risk for CM. Individuals with familial dysplastic nevi are several hundred times more likely to de-

TABLE 46-1 Risk Factors for Cutaneous Nonmelanoma and Melanoma Cancers

Risk Factor	Skin Cancer Type
Presence of precursor lesions	CM
Family history of melanoma	CM
History of primary skin cancer	BCE, CM
Ultraviolet light exposure	BCE, SCC, CM
Red hair, fair complexion	CM
Skin easily sunburned	BCE, SCC, CM
Occupational exposure	BCE, SCC
Ionizing radiation exposure	BCE, SCC
Immunologic changes	BCE, SCC, CM
Hormonal changes	CM
Congenital moles	CM
Scars, chronic inflammation	BCE, SCC

BCE, Basal cell epithelioma; *CM*, cutaneous melanoma; *SCC*, squamous cell carcinoma.

velop melanoma than control persons in the general population.[7] Dysplastic nevi are discussed in more detail in the "Cutaneous Melanoma" section of this chapter.

Ultraviolet (UV) radiation is a frequent cause of nonmelanoma skin cancers, which are commonly found on sun-exposed areas of the body, such as the head and neck, arms, upper back, and legs. Types of UV radiation harmful to the skin are UV-B and UV-A. UV-B rays have short wavelengths and are absorbed by the skin, causing sunburn. UV-A rays have long wavelengths and can penetrate deep into the lower levels of the skin. The incidence of both CM and nonmelanoma skin cancers is higher in latitudes close to the equator, which receive more UV radiation, and lower in latitudes farther from the equator.[2,10] However, the direct association of CM with UV radiation is controversial, as CM can also develop in areas that are not exposed to the sun.[10]

Skin pigmentation is clearly important in the etiology of skin cancers, in that American blacks and persons of African, Asian, or Mediterranean descent are known to have a lower incidence of skin cancer.[4] When these individuals do develop CM, it usually originates on the less densely pigmented areas of the body such as the palms, soles, and fingernails.[10] White persons with red hair and fair complexions, who tend to sunburn or freckle easily, have higher relative risks (RR) for all skin cancers (1.4 to 3.0 RR).[9,11]

Other possible risk factors for CM include age, hormonal factors, immunosuppression, and a previous history of melanoma.[5,9] A family history of CM increases its relative risk in the range of two to eight times.[12,13] There is no conclusive evidence regarding the use of oral contraceptives and the increased risk of CM.[14-16] However, some physicians recommend that women with a history of melanoma use a nonhormonal contraceptive.

NONMELANOMA SKIN CANCERS

Basal Cell Epithelioma

Pathophysiology

Basal cell epithelioma is the least aggressive type of skin cancer. This is an epithelial tumor with a disputed site of origin. It is believed to arise either from cells in the basal layer of the epidermis that have impaired ability to mature and keratinize or from cells in the surrounding dermal structures.[2,17] BCE usually grows slowly by direct extension and has the capacity to cause major local destruction. Although metastasis is rare, the most common metastatic sites are the regional lymph nodes.[2] Other rare sites of metastasis are bones, lungs, liver, brain, dura, kidneys, and, even less frequently, skin.[18]

Assessment

There are as many as ten types of BCE. However, only four types (nodular, superficial, pigmented, and morphea-like) will be described. Nodular BCE is the most common type. Histologically, nodular BCE consists of masses of tumor cells that have large oval nuclei, are uniform in appearance, and resemble basal cells of the epidermis. These cells descend from the epidermis and fill the dermis, with the peripheral cells resembling a picket fence pattern.[17,19] Clinically, nodular BCE begins as a small, firm, well-demarcated, dome-shaped papule. The color can be pearly white, pink, or skin-colored, with telangiectases often evident on the surface. As the lesion enlarges, it ulcerates peripherally or centrally and develops raised, pearly, well-circumscribed borders. Nodular BCE most commonly occurs on the face, head, and neck[2,19-21] (Color plate 8).

Superficial BCE is the second most common type, histologically exhibiting a bud of irregular proliferating tumor tissue attached to the undersurface of the epidermis. Clinically, it is flat and has erythematous or pink scaling plaques or papules with well-defined margins and occasional shallow erosions or crusts.[19-21] Superficial BCE usually develops on the trunk and extremities.

Pigmented BCE is less common and may be nodular or superficial. It has a melanin pigment concentrated in the center of a nest of BCE cells, causing a brown, black, or blue color. Also present is a shiny, pearly, papular border with well-defined margins and telangiectases.[19,20] Biologically, the behavior of pigmented BCE is similar to nodular BCE.[19] Pigmented BCE most commonly occurs on the head, neck, and face.

Morphea-like BCE is the most rare type. Histologically, this tumor has many roots with branching strands embedded in dense fibrous stroma of collagen and elastic fibers.[19-21] Clinically, it is flat, ivory-colored or colorless, resembles a scar, lacks translucency, and has ill-defined margins. This lesion is more aggressive than nodular BCE, having increased invasiveness and destructiveness of surrounding tissues, particularly muscle, nerve, and bone. Morphea-like BCE develops primarily on the head and neck.

Squamous Cell Carcinoma

Pathophysiology

Squamous cell carcinoma is a tumor that may arise in any epithelium. Its behavior in the skin is similar to that of neoplasms that arise from stratified squamous epithelium in other organ sites. The cells of SCC vary from well-differentiated to completely anaplastic. The well-differentiated tumor cell has a histologic appearance similar to that seen in normal squamous epithelium in that it is a large polygonal cell with intracellular bridges and round nuclei. Some individual cell keratinization exists, and formation of keratin pearls is common. Keratinization and keratin pearl formation diminish as the tumor becomes less well differentiated and disappears with high-grade tumors. As the tumor cells become more anaplastic, the nuclei become distorted in shape, mitoses become more numerous, cell shapes become more bizarre, and cell numbers increase.[2,22] SCC is more aggressive than BCE, as it has a faster growth rate, less well-demarcated margins, and a greater metastatic potential.[2,20,23] In addition, the metastatic potential of SCC is increased in patients who are receiving immunosuppressive agents.[2,20,22-24] Metastatic disease is usually first noted in the regional lymph nodes.

Assessment

SCC appears as a flesh-colored or erythematous, raised, firm papule. It may be crusted with keratin products and, in its early or late stages, may ulcerate and bleed, becoming tender and painful. Infiltration of the tumor into normal surrounding skin produces induration around the nodule (Color plate 9). SCC is usually confined to areas exposed to UV radiation. The most highly exposed areas of skin, such as the top of the nose, the forehead, the helices of the ear, the backs of the hands, and the lower lip tend to be more affected. With the exception of the lower lip site, SCC on these areas is less likely to metastasize than lesions located on areas that are not exposed to UV radiation.[20,25] SCC can also arise in old areas of radiation, in scars from thermal or chemical burns, in areas of chronic inflammation or increased cell proliferation, and in mucous membranes. Tumors that originate in these areas are more aggressive and have a high frequency of metastasis.

Several preexisting conditions may lead to invasive SCC. Intraepidermal SCC, also called carcinoma in situ, may develop in existing cutaneous lesions, such as scar tissue, solar keratoses, radiation keratoses, and Bowen's disease. Intraepidermal SCC remains in the epidermis for an extended time but unpredictably passes through the basement membrane and extends into the dermis. These lesions appear as slightly raised erythematous plaques with varying amounts of scaling and well-defined margins. Other conditions include keratoacanthomas, which are hyperkeratotic lesions morphologically similar to SCC, and epidermodysplasia verruciformis, characterized by multiple flat, wartlike lesions containing oncogenic type 5 human papillomavirus.[26]

Treatment of Nonmelanoma Skin Cancers

Standard treatment for nonmelanoma skin cancers includes surgical excision, chemosurgery, curettage and electrodesiccation, radiation, and cryotherapy. Factors to consider when choosing a treatment are tumor type, location, size, growth pattern, and whether the tumor is primary or secondary. The patient's age and general health also should be considered. No single therapy is applicable to all tumors. However, the primary goals of treatment are cure, preservation of tissue and function, minimal operative risk, and optimal cosmetic results.

An excisional biopsy is the preferred initial step of any treatment. This biopsy is indicated for small lesions located in areas where primary closure is not a problem and offers the advantage of complete tumor excision and a complete specimen for histology.[2] In unusual circumstances, such as large lesions or lesions located on the face, an incisional biopsy may be performed.

Surgical excision

Surgical excision can be performed for any nonmelanoma skin cancer and may be simple or complex, depending on tumor size and location. An elliptical excision, with suture closure, of a small to moderate lesion usually can be performed on an outpatient basis with the use of a local anesthetic. Surgical excision facilitates healing of large carcinoma sites where thin layers of subcutaneous tissue overlie bony areas, such as the forehead, scalp, and distal extremities. Surgical excision also is beneficial in the treatment of residual tumor and large carcinomas that occur in conjunction with late radiation dermatitis and those that arise in scars and ulcers, as these areas cannot tolerate radiation therapy. In addition, excision of large carcinomas of the eyelid and lip preserves function and allows reconstruction by graft or flap.[22]

A skin graft or flap may be performed as an adjunct to surgical excision. A graft or flap is indicated when a lesion is large or located in an area where insufficient tissue for primary closure would result in deformity. A skin flap consists of skin and subcutaneous tissue which is transferred from one area of the body to another. A flap contains its own blood supply, whereas a graft is avascular and depends on the blood supply of the recipient site for its survival. Skin grafting or flapping requires hospitalization, and possible complications include graft failure, hematoma, scarring, and infection.

The advantages of surgical excision are rapid healing, the availability of an entire specimen for histologic examination, and favorable cosmetic results. Disadvantages are related to the time-consuming aspect of the procedure and the need for a skilled physician to judge the exact extent of the tumor and the risk of infection.[19-21,25]

Chemosurgery

Another type of surgical treatment available for select tumors is Mohs' micrographic surgery, or chemosurgery. This procedure involves horizontal shaving and staining of tissue in thin layers, with careful histologic mapping of all specimen margins. This is the most accurate technique of assessing the actual extent of nonmelanoma skin cancers. Mohs' microsurgery is most often used as a first line of treatment for cancers in high-risk areas, such as the nose and nasolabial folds, the medial canthus, and pre- and postauricular locations.[27] It is also used for lesions with unclear margins, recurrent lesions, aggressive tumors, and extensive lesions (usually larger than 2 cm). Skin grafting may also have to accompany this treatment. The advantages of Mohs' microsurgery include preservation of the maximum amount of tissue for easier reconstruction, the ability to map tumor margins histologically, and the fact that the procedure can be performed on an outpatient basis with the use of a local anesthetic.[19,25,27,28] The disadvantages are the requirement of specialized training and equipment, the time-consuming aspects of the procedure, the need for daily wound care postoperatively, and the possibility of graft rejection and wound dehiscence.[27-29]

Curettage and electrodesiccation

Because of poor margin control, curettage and electrodesiccation is used only for BCE skin cancers that are small, superficial, or recurrent. The tumor is destroyed by scraping out the tumor mass through curettage and treating the tumor base with electrodesiccation or a low-voltage electrode. The physician uses the curettage to determine the tumor edges. As tumor tissue is softer and more friable than normal tissue, electrodesiccation maintains hemostasis and softens normal tissue so that a safe margin can be removed by curettage.[2,20-22] Advantages of this treatment are its rapidity, good cosmetic results, preservation of normal tissue, and the ability to obtain a tissue specimen for histopathologic study. Disadvantages include no margin control, prolonged healing, and the need for physician skill in seeking out the tumor tissue by "feel."[2,19]

Radiotherapy

Radiotherapy generally is recommended only for lesions that are inoperable, lesions located in sites such as the corner of the nose, eyelid, lip, and canthus, and lesions greater than 1 cm but less than 10 cm in diameter. Patients who are poor surgical candidates may benefit from radiotherapy, but the treatment is not recommended for young patients, since the irradiated area becomes more atrophic, erythematous, and irregular over the years.[2,19-21,25,30] Radiation is administered in fractional doses because increased skin tolerance may enhance its effectiveness.[22] Advantages of radiotherapy are painless treatment, preservation of normal anatomic contours, and the ability to extend treatment into areas surrounding the tumor if desired. Disadvantages include lack of histologic tissue for margin control, long treatment periods (3 to 4 weeks), the fact that treatment itself may lead to BCE or SCC, and the need for clinical facilities with persons trained in radiotherapy.

Cryotherapy

Cryotherapy involves tumor destruction by the use of liquid nitrogen to freeze and thaw tumor tissue. Liquid nitrogen is applied to the lesion by open spray, causing a quick, intense freezing of the tissue, which is then allowed to thaw slowly. This cycle is repeated, and tumor necrosis and erosion ensue. Healing time depends on the tumor location, with tumors of the face healing in 3 to 4 weeks, and lesions on the back or previously treated sites taking significantly longer.[2]

Cryotherapy can be used for small to large primary tumors, for certain recurrent lesions such as those in areas of previous radiation, for multiple superficial BCE, and for lesions that need palliative treatment. Only lesions with well-defined margins (both lateral and depth) benefit from this treatment.[21,29] Cryotherapy is not recommended for the medial canthal area and the rim of the ears, since frozen cartilage buckles during healing and recurrence rates are high.[21,25] Advantages of this treatment include minimal discomfort (a burning or hot sensation is usually experienced), performance on an outpatient basis, and speed of performance with good cosmetic results. Disadvantages include the need for wound care, prolonged healing time, possible temporary nerve damage, and bleeding.[29,31]

MELANOMA

Cutaneous Melanoma

Pathophysiology

CM arises from melanocytes, which are cells that specialize in the biosynthesis and transport of melanin. These pigment-producing cells migrate from the neural crest to the skin, uveal tract, meninges, and ectodermal mucosa by the third month of gestation.[5,32] Melanocytes are found throughout the skin but are most common in the basal layers of the epidermis. Melanocytes contain a melanosome, the specific granule that synthesizes the melanin pigment. When the melanosome-melanin package is transferred through the dendritic cytoplasm of the melanocyte, it is phagocytized by keratinocytes.[5] These then migrate upward from the basal layer through the epidermis and may be visible in the skin as pigmented melanin granules[5,32] (Color plate 10). In melanomas, the melanosomes may be abnormal or even absent in amelanotic clones.[32]

Precursor lesions Three specific precursor lesions of CM include dysplastic nevi, congenital nevi, and lentigo maligna. *Dysplastic nevi* (DN) may be familial (also known as B-K moles) or nonfamilial (sporadic dysplastic nevi). In melanoma-prone families, the risk of CM in a family member with DN approaches 100%, and 69% of familial melanomas show histologic evidence of DN contiguous with the melanoma.[33] Although an estimated 5% to 10% of all CM occurs in persons with a family history of DN, it has been reported that 50% of CM evolve from some form of DN.[7] DN are absent at birth; however, an early clinical indication may be the presence of an increased number of histologically normal nevi between the ages of 5 and 8 years, with dysplastic changes occurring after puberty.[7]

DN are often larger than 5 mm and they can number from one to 100 or more; most affected persons have 25 to 75 abnormal nevi.[7] Individuals with this syndrome also have normal moles. DN appear on the face, trunk, and arms but also may be seen on the buttocks, groin, scalp, and female breast. Pigmentation is irregular, with mixtures of tan, brown, and black or of red and pink. A distinctive feature is a "fried egg" appearance with a deeply pigmented papular area surrounded by an area of lighter pigmentation. The surface is pebbly, and the border is indistinct and irregular[5,9,34-36] (Color plate 11). Individuals should be thoroughly questioned about family or personal history of melanoma, atypical pigmented lesions, and previous excisions of lesions of any kind. Results of any previous skin biopsies should be obtained if possible. The entire skin surface, including the scalp, axilla, genitalia, and the area between the toes and fingers, should be examined. The first line of treatment is excisional biopsy of the most atypical-looking lesions to document the presence of histologic dysplasia and to rule out melanoma.[35,37,38] Once a diagnosis of DN has been established, the individual should have periodic skin examinations by a dermatologist, with accompanying photographs, every 3 to 6 months. Changing or new lesions suggestive of melanoma should be removed and a biopsy performed. Every individual with dysplastic nevi, as well as their first-degree relatives, should be taught to examine the entire body every 1 to 2 months and should be educated about melanoma risk factors and preventive behaviors.[9,35,39]

Congenital nevi are present at birth or appear shortly thereafter. They are classified as large or small and range in size from 1.5 to 3.0 cm to large lesions covering extensive body surfaces such as the trunk, an arm, or a hand. The color of a congenital nevus ranges from brown to black; lesions may be slightly raised, with an irregular surface and a fairly regular border. Larger lesions may contain areas of nodularity. A careful history and examination of congenital nevi are essential to management and should include dates of first appearance and subsequent changes. A biopsy should be done on any abnormal-appearing lesion to confirm its exact histology. Treatment consists primarily of surgical excision. There is some debate over whether smaller congenital nevi should be removed surgically as a preventive measure.[5,34] Removal of larger lesions may require several surgical procedures, which can be disfiguring depending on their location and size. After treatment, regular follow-up examinations are essential.

Lentigo maligna is detailed in the section that describes its very similar counterpart, lentigo maligna melanoma. Treatment of this precursor lesion is discussed in the section on treatment of melanoma.

Assessment

A thorough patient history and physical examination are essential for identification of individuals at high risk and for early detection of CM and suspicious lesions. Comments and complaints about a preexisting nevus or a new lesion should be investigated. Important questions to ask patients include the following: (1) When was the lesion first noted? (2) Is the lesion new or preexisting? How long has it been there? (3) What caused you to notice the lesion: change in color, size, or texture; bleeding; a different sensation such as burning, itching, tingling, etc.? (4) How long has the lesion been changing and over what time period? (5) Do you have a history of frequent or intense sun exposure, chemical or thermal injury, or trauma? (6) Do you have a family history of dysplastic nevus syndrome or melanoma?

The initial step of the physical examination includes a complete visual examination of the cutaneous surface, the questionable lesion(s), and the area surrounding the lesion to determine the presence of satellite lesions or in-transit metastases. All accessible lymph nodes, particularly those in the regional drainage sites, are palpated. A review of systems is obtained. The skin assessment is described in detail in the "Nursing Management" section of this chapter.

Melanoma can metastasize to virtually every organ in the body, and those with the diagnosis should undergo the recommended examinations for metastatic disease. Initially, a radiograph of the chest, a complete blood cell count, and serum chemistry determinations with liver function tests are performed after the diagnosis has been made. Liver function tests have proved to be most useful in determining liver metastasis.[40-42] The combination of elevated LDH, SGOT, and alkaline phosphatase levels is more specific for liver involvement and indicates that a computed tomography (CT) scan of the liver is necessary.[40]

If clinical findings indicate possible involvement of other common metastatic sites, such as skin, subcutaneous tissue, lymph nodes, lung, brain, and bone, a more extensive metastatic work-up is performed. This may include skin or lymph node biopsy for new lesions; a radiograph of the chest for increased shortness of breath, new cough, or hemoptysis; a CT scan of the brain for neurologic abnormality, headaches, mental deficits, or seizures; and a bone scan for undetermined bone pain.[43] Magnetic resonance imaging (MRI) scans offer clearer images and detect different characteristics of lesions than a CT scan. Since the cost of MRI is high, it may be reserved for special situations.

Classification

Melanoma has been classified into several types: lentigo maligna (LMM), superficial spreading (SSM), nodular, acral lentiginous (mucocutaneous), those in which the radial growth phase is not characteristic of SSM or LMM, those arising from congenital nevi, those arising from blue nevi, and visceral and ocular lesions. The four major types of CM described here include lentigo maligna, superficial spreading, nodular, and acral lentiginous (Table 46-2). Each of these is characterized by a radial and/or vertical growth phase. In the radial growth phase, tumor growth is parallel to the surface of the skin and may last for several years. During this phase, the propensity for the tumor to metastasize is very small, and surgical excision may be curative. In the vertical growth phase, however, there is focal deep penetration of atypical melanocytes into the dermis and subcutaneous tissue. This penetration occurs rapidly, increasing the risk of metastasis.[5,37,44-46]

Lentigo maligna melanoma constitutes 4% to 15% of all CMs and is the least serious type. It occurs on body areas that are heavily exposed to solar radiation, such as

TABLE 46-2 Comparisons of the Four Major Types of Cutaneous Melanoma

Type	Site	Radial Growth Phase	Vertical Growth Phase	Characteristics
Lentigo maligna melanoma	Face, neck, dorsal hands, lower legs	Yes (10-25 yr)	Yes (less aggressive)	Size: Large (10 cm) Color: Tan/brown Radial phase: Irregular mottling with regression Vertical phase: Raised nodules on surface
Superficial spreading	Men: trunk Women: legs	Yes (1-5 yr)	Yes (aggressive)	Radial phase: Flat with fine crust/scaly surface; tan/brown color Vertical phase: Shiny surface; tan/brown/black to red/white/blue color; borders irregular; raised nodules; ulceration
Nodular	Head, neck, trunk	No	Yes (aggressive)	Vertical phase: Raised, dome-shaped; blue-black/red color; ulcerations/bleeding may be present
Acral lentiginous	Palms, soles, nailbeds, mucous membranes	Yes	Yes (aggressive)	Radial phase: Flat, tan/brown/black color similar to lentigo maligna Nailbed: Tan/brown stain/streaking Vertical phase: Elevated, areas of nodularity

the face, neck, and occasionally the backs of the hands and the lower legs. Early premalignant in situ lesions often precede lentigo maligna melanoma and are termed lentigo maligna. Both lentigo maligna and lentigo maligna melanoma are large in size and are primarily tan in color with different shades of brown throughout (Color plate 12). The predominant histologic feature of lentigo maligna is proliferation of atypical melanocytes along the basal layer of the epidermis. This early radial growth phase usually lasts between 10 and 25 years, with the lesion growing as large as 10 cm. As soon as these melanocytes invade the dermis, the lesion becomes malignant. With increased growth of the lentigo maligna melanoma, irregular mottling or freckling may occur along with regression in some areas. A portion of the lesion may begin a vertical growth phase with accompanying raised nodules over the surface.[5,11,37,39,44,46] There is a 25% chance of a metastasis in the vertical phase.[5]

Superficial spreading melanoma accounts for approximately 50% to 75% of CM. This lesion is most commonly seen on the trunk in men and on the legs in women. Superficial spreading melanoma usually arises in a preexisting nevus. Early lesions are generally flat, with a fine crust or scaly surface. The radial growth phase lasts from 1 to 5 or more years. As the lesion enters the vertical phase, a rapid increase in growth occurs with a change in color ranging from a mixture of tan, brown, and black to a characteristic red, white, and blue appearance. As the lesion continues to grow, the borders become irregular and notched and the surface becomes shiny and irregular, with raised nodules and ulceration[5,39,44,46,47] (Color plate 13). A 35% to 85% chance of metastasis exists in the vertical growth phase.[5]

Nodular melanoma constitutes 12% to 30% of all CMs. This lesion appears as a raised, dome-shaped blue-black or red nodule on areas of the head, neck, and trunk that may or may not be exposed to the sun. Ulcerations and bleeding may be present (Color plate 14). Nodular melanoma has only a vertically invasive component, making early diagnosis difficult. It is more aggressive than the other types of melanoma and has a shorter clinical onset. Commonly, these lesions begin de novo in uninvolved skin rather than from a preexisting lesion. Because this lesion lacks a radial phase and is difficult to detect in its early stages, there is an increased chance of metastasis being present at diagnosis.[11,46,47]

Acral lentiginous or mucocutaneous melanoma is found in 35% to 60% of dark-skinned persons, particularly blacks, Orientals, and Hispanics, and only 2% to 10% of white persons.[11,39] This lesion occurs on the palms, soles, nailbeds, and mucous membranes. Acral lentiginous melanoma exhibits both a radial and a vertical growth phase. The radial growth phase may last for years and resembles an early lentigo maligna. In this phase the lesion is flat, with nonpalpable margins and is haphazardly pigmented with tan, brown, and black colors. In subungal areas, the radial growth phase appears as an irregular tan-brown stain of streaking in the nailbed (Color plate 15). Acral lentiginous melanomas in the vertical phase become elevated with areas of nodularity. A small percentage are flesh-colored. In the vertical phase, acral lentiginous melanomas are more aggressive and can metastasize.

Staging and prognostic factors

Microstaging is a term used to describe the level of invasion of the CM and maximum tumor thickness. Two parameters are used in assessing the depth of invasion of melanoma (Figure 46-1). The first is the anatomic level of invasion or the Clark level, and the second is the thickness of tumor tissue or the Breslow level. Clark categorized CM into five histologic levels based on vertical depth of tumor invasion, with the deeper lesions having the worst prognosis for metastases and survival. When the Clark system is used, there may be subjective difficulties in classifying certain melanomas, such as those located in thin-skinned areas (ie, the elbow, under the eye). As a result, Breslow modified the Clark system by using an ocular micrometer to measure, in millimeters, the maximum vertical tumor thickness. This measurement is made from the top of the granular cell layer of the tumor to the deepest level of invasion of the melanoma.

Controversy exists over which staging system should be used for CM. Several systems are currently in use; among them are the original clinicopathologic staging system for melanoma (the three-stage system), the modified three-stage system, the M.D. Anderson Hospital Staging System, and the International Union Against Cancer (UICC) staging system. The three-stage system (Table 46-3) is the most widely used; yet it does not include important disease criteria, such as tumor thickness. The American Joint Committee on Cancer now has a four-stage system for CM that they believe will be broadly applicable to different centers throughout the world and allow more consistent exchange of information (Table 46-4).[48]

TABLE 46-3 The Original Three-Stage System for Cutaneous Melanoma

Stage	Extent of Disease
I	Localized primary melanoma
IA	Local recurrence (satellite lesions)
II	Regional lymph node involvement or in-transit metastases
III	Distant metastases

Source: Adapted from Ketcham AS, Balch CM: Classification and staging systems, in Balch CM, Milton GW, Shaw HM, et al (eds): Cutaneous Melanoma. Philadelphia, JB Lippincott, 1985.

The prognosis for patients with metastatic disease at the time of diagnosis is poor, as most die within 5 years. The most extensive data about histologic and clinical prognostic factors are available for localized CM, clinical stage I (Table 46-5). It is well-documented that as CM thickness increases, survival rates decrease. Thus, the Breslow level has consistently proved to be a significant prognostic variable in stage I CM.[44,45,49-51]

Treatment

Surgery The initial surgical procedure for suspected CM is a biopsy. An excisional biopsy that entails removal

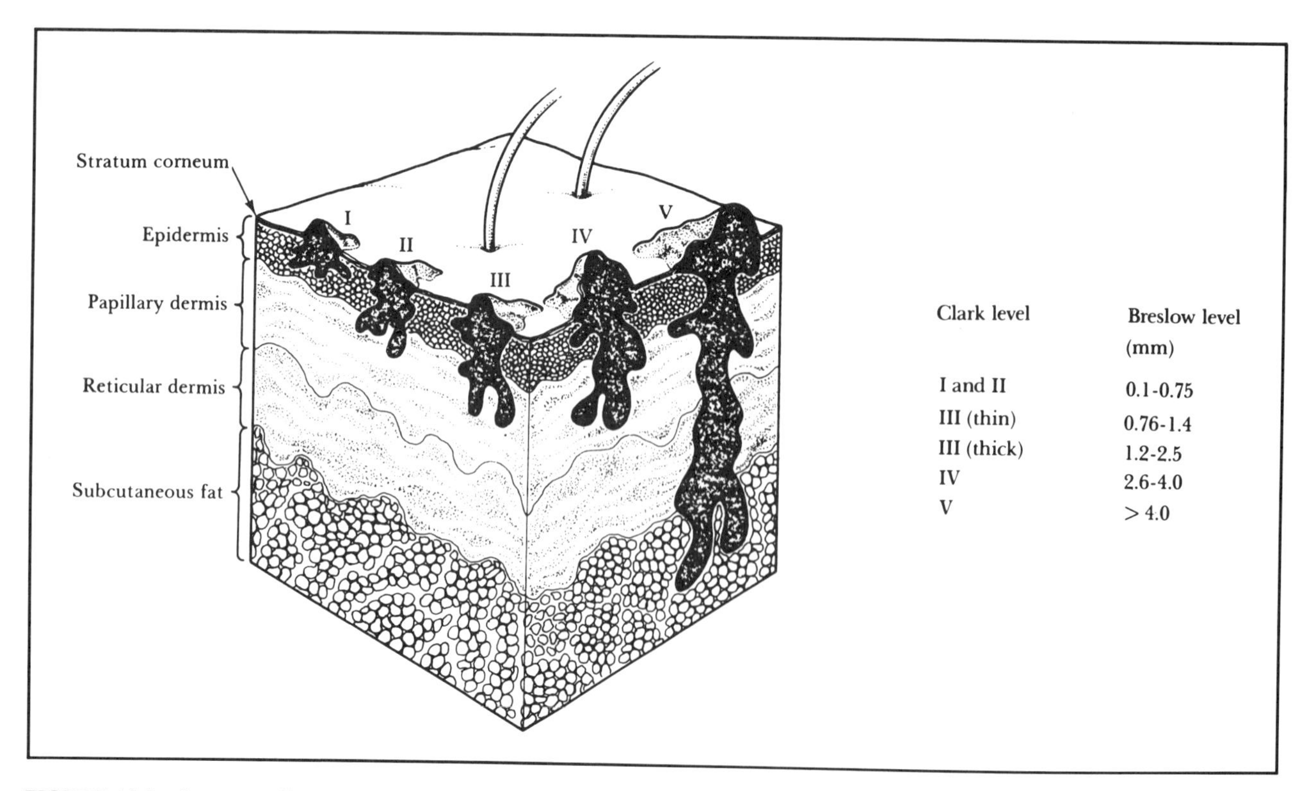

FIGURE 46-1 Corresponding thickness of Clark and Breslow levels.

TABLE 46-4 Four-Stage System for Cutaneous Melanoma

Clinical Stage	Breslow Level (mm)*	Clark Level*	TNM†
I	<0.75	II	T1, N0, M0 (localized)
II	>0.75-≤1.5	III	T2, N0, M0 (localized)
III	>1.5-≥4.0	IV	T3, N0, M0 (localized)
IIIA	(Can involve any T [T = any level above or 4.0 mm and level 5, and/or presence of satellite lesions], N1 [N1 = metastasis ≤3 cm greatest dimension in any regional lymph node(s)], M0)		
IV	Any T, any N [includes N1; N2 = nodal metastasis >3 cm greatest dimension and/or in-transit metastasis), M1 (distant metastasis in skin or subcutaneous tissue or distant lymph nodes or viscera)		

*When the thickness and the level-of-invasion criteria do not coincide within a T classification, thickness should take precedence.

† *T*, Tumor (for melanoma staging, tumor is designated by Breslow and Clark levels); *N*, node; *M*, metastasis.

Source: Adapted from Ketcham AS, Balch CM: Classification and staging systems, in Balch CM, Milton GW, Shaw HM, et al (eds): Cutaneous Melanoma. Philadelphia, JB Lippincott, 1985.

of a few millimeters of normal tissue surrounding the lesion is preferable, since it provides a definitive diagnosis along with microstaging information. An incisional biopsy can be used for lesions located in cosmetically sensitive areas or for large lesions. The incisional site should include any area of change, particularly suspicious raised or nodular-appearing areas. Both techniques should remove the full thickness of the skin and some underlying subcutaneous fat.[5,52,53] Electrocoagulation, curettage, shaving, and burning should never be used to remove a suspicious mole.

For stage I CM, the standard treatment is a wide excision. There has been some debate concerning the extent of the excision needed to achieve optimal control.[5,39,52-55] The common margin standard has been 3 to 5 cm of normal skin, but increasing evidence has shown that the risk of local recurrence correlates with the thickness of the lesion and that margin size does not influence survival.[52-54] Since a minimal risk of local recurrence exists for thin melanomas (<0.76 mm), only a 1 cm margin of normal skin around the lesion is required.[46,52,54] An excision margin 1 cm wide is also suitable for lentigo maligna melanoma, which has a low metastatic potential. Thicker lesions require a 3 to 5 cm margin of normal skin with a split-thickness graft.[5,52] For lesions in areas of sensitivity or where cosmesis is an issue, the surgeon determines the safest wide excision margin. Subungal lesions are treated by amputation.

There is controversy over the use of elective lymph node dissection (ELND) in the treatment of stage I disease. ELND has a high degree of morbidity, and use of this procedure is debatable when no clinical evidence of nodal involvement exists. There is agreement that a primary CM lesion of less than 0.76 mm and a lentigo maligna melanoma do not require an ELND. In addition, patients with large lesions (>4 mm) do not benefit from ELND because they most likely have microscopic metastases.[53,56,57] Proponents of ELND argue that 20% to 30% of the clinically normal nodes contain malignant cells, and that managing these nodes while the tumor burden is low will decrease the incidence of distant metastases. Opponents maintain that since nodal metastases are rare in patients with thinner melanomas, 70% to 80% of these individuals will undergo unnecessary surgery.[53,56,57] Reviews of some nonrandomized, prospective studies have demonstrated improved survival when patients with extremity lesions of intermediate thickness were treated with ELND.[54,57-59] Prospective randomized studies, however, have shown no benefit in terms of survival.[56-58] No prospective randomized trials have addressed the use of ELND for CM of the trunk, head, and neck.[57,58] Retrospective studies are also inconclusive, but there are some that suggest some patients with stage I CM of intermediate thickness (1 to 3.99 mm) may benefit from ELND.[5,53,59]

Standard surgical therapy of clinical stage II (clinical, but not histologic, evidence of draining lymph node involvement) disease includes a wide excision with full regional lymph node dissection.[5] In cases in which the index of suspicion is low for metastatic disease, a palpable node may be biopsied by either the open or the fine-needle approach.[60]

Surgery is also useful for palliation of disease and symptomatic involvement. Surgical removal of a solitary metastatic lesion is recommended if the lesion is easily accessible and if its removal will enhance quality and duration of survival. For example, craniotomy is indicated

TABLE 46-5 Factors Associated With Poor Prognosis of Stage I Cutaneous Melanoma

Histologic	Clinical
Tumor thickness (>3 mm)	Age (>50 yrs)
Level of invasion (>IV/V)	Sex (males)
Presence of microscopic satellites	Nodular type
Mitotic index (>6/mm²)	Presence of ulceration
Regression (original depth unknown)	Anatomic site (trunk)
Lack of lymphocytic infiltrate	Anatomic sub-site (BANS, HF)

BANS: *B*, interscapular area of upper back; *A*, posterior upper arms; *N*, posterior and lateral neck; *S*, scalp.
HF: *H*, hands; *F*, feet.

for removal of a solitary brain metastasis and thoracotomy for removal of an isolated lung lesion.[61]

Chemotherapy Metastatic malignant melanoma is highly resistant to systemic chemotherapeutic agents currently available, indicating the need for further research in this area. Dacarbazine (DTIC) is the most active agent, with an overall response rate of 15% to 28%.[5,39,44,62,63] The nitrosoureas (BCNU, CCNU, methyl-CCNU, and chlorozotocin) have shown some activity, with response rates of 10% to 18%.[5] Drug combinations that show some promise for treatment of metastatic disease are BCNU, hydroxyurea, and dacarbazine (response rate, 30%), and bleomycin, vincristine, CCNU, and dacarbazine (response rate, 39% to 48%).[44,63] In these regimens, toxicities are a dose-limiting factor. Cis-platinum, another single agent that demonstrates some antimelanoma activity, is being tested in combination with vinblastine and bleomycin, with mixed results.[5,63] The toxicities of the most frequently used chemotherapeutic agents are discussed in detail elsewhere in this text.

Isolated limb perfusion is a controversial adjuvant therapy for advanced melanoma confined to a limb or for disease involving melanoma satellites, in-transit metastasis, and poor-prognosis lesions of the extremities. The treatment consists of hyperthermia plus vascular perfusion of chemotherapy through an isolated region; this enables high concentrations of chemotherapeutic agents to be administered with minimal systemic toxicities. The agent most commonly used for this procedure is melphalan. Others, used alone and in combination, include thiotepa, dacarbazine, carmustine, cisplatin, and doxorubicin.[62,64-66] Complications of treatment include tissue necrosis, transient or persistent edema of the treated extremity, neurologic disorders, wound infection, pain, and deep-vein thrombosis.[64,65,67] Although isolated limb perfusion has been used since 1957, it remains expensive, investigational, and extremely controversial, since a limited number of control groups have been used in reported studies.[5,44,64,67,68]

Radiotherapy Recurrent or metastatic melanoma has a history of being radioresistant. New evidence, however, suggests that melanoma may be a radioresponsive tumor but that not all the tumor cells are sensitive. Radiotherapy is most effective when tumor volume is low and when a high dose per fewer fractions radiation level is used. The optimal radiation dose remains to be established. Radiotherapy is often used for palliation in patients who have subcutaneous, cutaneous, and nodal metastases that are inaccessible for surgical removal.[69-71] Palliative radiation to the brain in conjunction with steroids offers considerable relief of neurologic symptoms. Impending bone fractures and bone pain can also be reduced with the use of radiotherapy. Radiotherapy cannot be used to treat liver or lung metastases because of the resultant loss of function.[71]

Hormonal therapy A hormonal influence on proliferation of melanocytes and melanoma cells has been suggested by the usual occurrence of CM after puberty, increased incidence during menopause, and increased or decreased CM growth during pregnancy or after parturition.[15,72,73] Hormonal effects are also evidenced by the presence of estrogen and progesterone receptor sites on some CM cells, suggesting that endocrine therapy may be beneficial. Clinically, steroid hormones may directly affect CM growth or may be mediated indirectly by gonadotropins or other pituitary or hypothalamic factors modulated by steroids.[72] A high incidence of steroid binding in melanoma tissue has led to clinical trials demonstrating some tumor response with tamoxifen, diethylstilbestrol, estramustine phosphate, progesterone, and antiandrogens.[72] However, trials with endocrine therapy remain inconclusive.[5,63]

Biotherapy Biotherapy is a recent form of melanoma treatment; the rationale for use parallels the natural history of CM, indicating that immunologic intervention by the host may alter the growth pattern of CM. This immunologic interaction is demonstrated by the occurrence of more spontaneous remissions in CM than in other adult tumors. In addition, specific tumor antigen antibodies have been found in melanoma patients. Patients in whom there are lymphocytic infiltrates at the tumor site have a more favorable prognosis.[74]

Biotherapy is currently being investigated in the context of adjuvant therapy and as treatment for metastatic disease. Such agents as interferons, interleukins, tumor necrosis factors, monoclonal antibodies, and retinoids are being studied, either singly, in combination with each other, or in combination with chemotherapy. At present, no drug or combination of drugs is effective. In the past, injections of bacillus of Calmette-Guerin (BCG) were standard adjuvant treatments; however, this treatment is now considered to have little effect.[75]

Uveal Melanoma

Uveal melanoma affects the iris, ciliary body, and choroid portions of the eye and arises from uveal melanocytes that have a common embryologic origin with melanocytes of the conjunctiva and skin. The frequency of uveal melanomas in the right and left eyes is equal, but bilateral incidence is rare. Only one in 5 million white persons develop a choroidal melanoma each year.[76] Most melanomas of the choroid and ciliary body are diagnosed after the age of 50; iris melanomas can be diagnosed earlier. Uveal melanomas exhibit no familial tendency, although there is some controversy as to whether they have an association with dysplastic nevi.[76-78] Predisposing factors for uveal melanomas include ocular melanocytosis (congenital hyperpigmentation of the sclera and uvea), ocular nevi, and neurofibromatosis. Intermittent, intense exposure to ultraviolet (UV) radiation may be an important risk factor.[79] The role of chemicals and endocrine factors in the development of uveal melanoma is still unknown.[76]

Choroidal melanoma is the most common type of uveal

melanoma in adults. Large lesions that are left untreated can extend into surrounding tissues, metastasize, and inevitably become fatal. Metastasis is primarily to the liver or lung.[76] The treatment of small melanomas, particularly those that affect the choroid, may consist merely of observation, as these lesions have little potential to produce local tissue damage or to metastasize.[76] Tumors that affect the iris and ciliary body may be removed surgically. Small choroidal melanomas may also be treated with xenon arc light photocoagulation or laser photocoagulation. Treatment of larger choroidal melanomas remains controversial. For many years, standard therapy has been enucleation. However, some investigators have hypothesized that intraoperative manipulation leads to tumor cell dissemination and metastases.[80] Others, however, believe that the high postenucleation mortality is due to preexisting dormant or subclinical metastases.[81,82]

Radiotherapy is the most widely used nonenucleation therapy and has the potential advantage of preserving both life and vision. Radiotherapy is most commonly administered by means of radioactive cobalt or iodine plaques sutured onto the sclera. Tumor regression and survival rates (40% survival at 10 years) following radiotherapy are comparable to those for enucleation; however, more prospective research should be done in this area.[80,83,84] With severe extrascleral involvement, exenteration involving removal of the eye and orbital contents or structures may be performed.[76]

PREVENTION

Primary Prevention

Many skin cancers can be prevented by reduction of exposure to avoidable risk factors. Primary prevention of skin cancers involves the avoidance of excessive exposure to UV radiation. The harmful effects of this exposure begin in childhood, and because UV-induced damage is cumulative, severe effects may be seen by the time a person reaches young adulthood.[3] Thus, prevention measures for reducing exposure must start early in life. Specific behaviors recommended by the Skin Cancer Foundation[85] and the Arizona Sun Awareness Project[86] include the following:

1. Minimize sun exposure during the hours of 10 AM to 3 PM, when UV radiation is the strongest.
2. When in the sun, wear a hat, a long-sleeved shirt and long pants (both made of tightly woven material), and protective sunglasses.
3. Use sunscreen. Apply a sunscreen with a sun protection factor (SPF) of 15 or more before every exposure to the sun and reapply at least every 2 hours thereafter. Use waterproof sunscreen when perspiring heavily or swimming. Sunscreen should also be applied on overcast days because 70% to 80% of UV radiation can penetrate cloud cover. Individuals with any risk factors for skin cancer should get into the habit of applying sunscreen on a daily basis. If there is an allergic reaction to a particular product, another brand with different active ingredients can be tried. Sunscreens can be used on children as young as 6 months of age, but a "patch test" should be performed to determine whether the child's skin is sensitive to the product.
4. Be aware of photosensitivity caused by certain medications (ie, tetracycline, oral contraceptives) and cosmetics.
5. Be aware of such surfaces as sand, snow, concrete, or water, which can reflect more than one half of the UV radiation onto the skin. Sitting under a shade tree or a beach umbrella near these surfaces does not guarantee any added protection from UV radiation.
6. Avoid tanning parlors, as UV-A emitted by tanning booths damages the deep skin layers.
7. Keep infants out of the sun.

Other primary prevention behaviors, such as the avoidance of unnecessary radiographs, will reduce exposure to ionizing radiation. Furthermore, individuals who work with substances known to cause skin cancer should wear protective clothing and use protective equipment to reduce their exposure.

Secondary Prevention

Secondary prevention of skin cancers involves reduction of morbidity and mortality through early detection, diagnosis, and treatment in high-risk individuals with a changing or changed pigmented lesion, a precursor lesion, a previous history of skin cancer, and a family history of CM.[9] These persons should have periodic skin examinations by a qualified dermatologist. Ophthalmic examinations should also be performed for those at risk for uveal melanomas.

Early detection and diagnosis of skin cancers is of the utmost importance. Most changes on the skin are easily visible and can be detected early, thereby improving chances for cure. Both the general public and health care professionals must be made aware of the need for early evaluation of an unusual skin lesion. Figure 46-2 shows an example of a patient-education poster that describes these early changes.

Recently, randomized controlled clinical trials have been initiated; these involve treatment of individuals with precursor lesions for cutaneous cancers. Retinoids (vitamin A and its derivatives) used as biologic treatment agents have shown some effect as chemopreventive agents in persons with BCE, actinic keratosis, keratoacanthoma, epidermodysplasia verruciformis, and dysplastic nevi.[26,87] Retinoids used as dietary agents also exhibit potential anticancer effects.[88] The mineral selenium may have some protective benefit against skin cancers,[87] but definitive results from these and other chemoprevention studies will take several years.

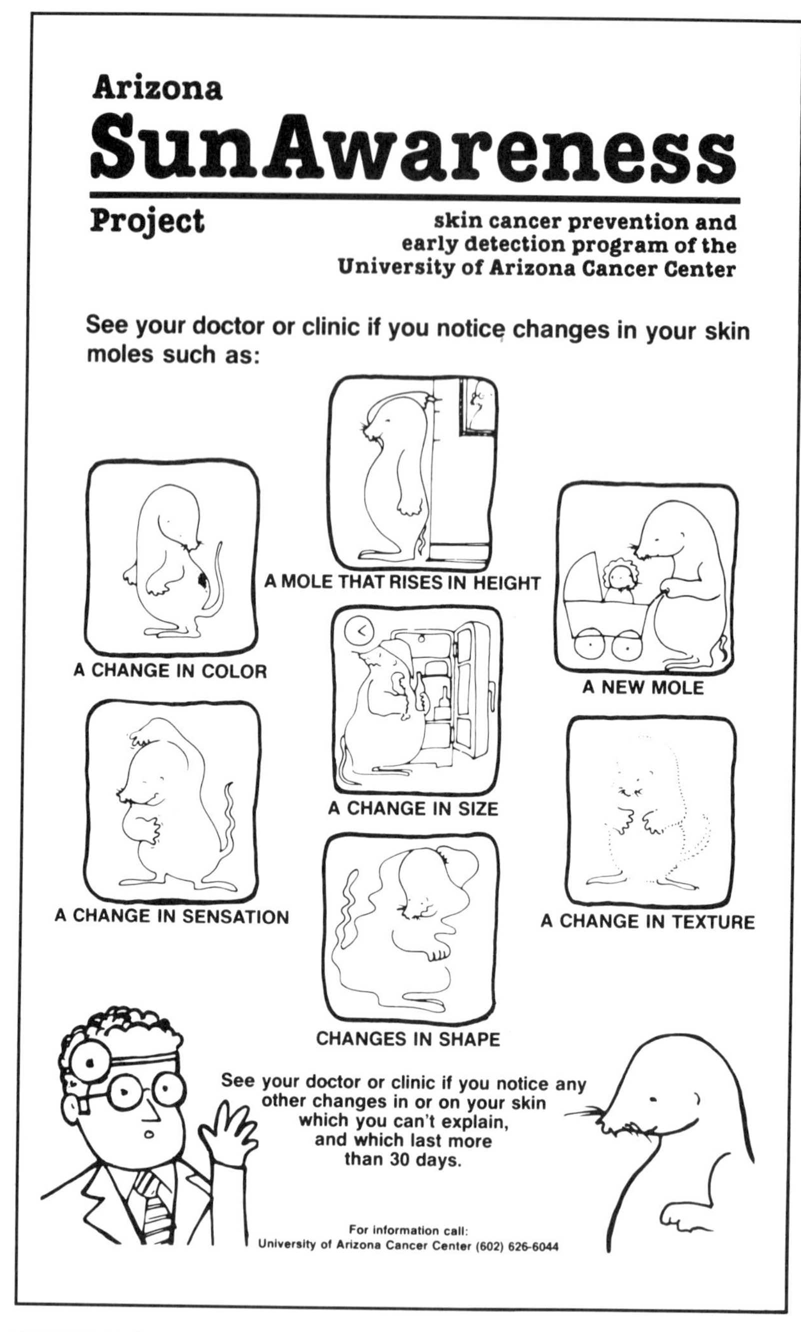

FIGURE 46-2 Patient-education poster describing mole changes that should be reported to a physician.

NURSING MANAGEMENT

Management of skin cancers presents a special challenge to the oncology nurse. Nursing involvement ranges from participation in prevention and early-detection education and screening of the general population to posttreatment management of patients with skin cancers. Important components of nursing management include interview, skin assessment, education, and posttreatment management.

Interview

All individuals with skin cancer or those at risk should be questioned about their knowledge of skin cancers, past medical history, and exposure to risk factors. Familiarity with the etiologic factors and clinical manifestations described throughout this chapter are an essential prerequisite for prevention and early-detection education and screening. The diagnosis of skin cancer can be frightening for the patient and the family members, and the interview elicits information about their knowledge and attitudes, potential fears, and coping mechanisms. Because attitudes toward the disease can influence health practices, the patient and family are given the opportunity to discuss any concerns or issues and are given appropriate information and reassurance.[89,90] Information about environmental factors, such as exposure to ultraviolet light, chemicals, and ionizing radiation, is routinely collected during the interview. A review of systems may reveal an overlooked cancer-related symptom.[91] Finally, a family pedigree is completed to ascertain family history of skin cancers. The history and exposure to risk factors will determine how detailed a skin assessment should be.[92]

Skin Assessment

A thorough nursing skin assessment can initially identify suspicious lesions. Persons with these lesions should then be referred to a qualified dermatologist for further review and diagnosis. Good lighting, preferably bright, natural light, is essential for the examination. Formal skin assessment is performed with the individual seated, although any opportunity such as bathing, dressing changes, or back rubs can be used to check a hospitalized patient's skin. Skin assessment consists of inspection and palpation to identify obvious lesions, visible swellings, adenopathy, alterations in normal borders and contour of nevi, discoloration in skin or mucosa, and areas of ulceration, scaling, crusting, and erosion. A magnifying glass may be used if necessary. The examination begins with the head and neck, including the entire scalp, eyelids, external ear and auditory canal, external and interior surfaces of the nose, the oral cavity, and the parotid, submaxillary, and sublingual glands. If the nurse has been trained to do indirect ophthalmoscopy, an eye examination should also be performed. Next, the thyroid is palpated, along with the regional lymph nodes of the neck. The examination then progresses to the chest, abdomen, back, and extremities, with special attention to intertriginous areas, such as under pendulous breasts, between the buttocks, the chin, an obese abdomen, hairy areas, axillae, nail beds, webs between fingers and toes, and soles of the feet. External genitalia are also examined. The location and descriptive characteristics of suspicious lesions should be recorded on an anatomic chart.[91,92] Warts, moles, scars, vascularities, and birthmarks should also be documented.

Education

Education about primary and secondary prevention behaviors and activities is of utmost importance. Numerous educational brochures describing various aspects of skin cancers and prevention are available from the American Cancer Society, the National Cancer Institute, the Skin Cancer Foundation, pharmaceutical companies that manufacture sunscreens, and other agencies.

Education for those who have or are at high risk of having skin cancers begins with an initial assessment of their knowledge deficit as related to skin cancers. Educational background, readiness to learn, and patient/family response to education are assessed. Clear and accurate information related to the diagnosis is then given to each patient and repeated several times, if necessary. Photographs of normal moles and birthmarks compared with photographs of skin cancers can be used as teaching aids. Patients are taught systematic self-assessment and are encouraged to examine their skin monthly.[89] Family members may assist in checking hard-to-see areas, such as the scalp, back, ears, and soles. Examinations should be performed at least twice yearly by a dermatologist or an oncologist who specializes in skin cancers. It is important for the nurse to emphasize that, with attentive self-care and medical management, most patients can lead relatively normal lives.[89] At the conclusion of any educational session, the nurse documents patient/family response to instruction, including comprehension and ability to perform skin self-examination.

Posttreatment Management

Surgical excision is still the most common treatment for skin cancers, and postoperative nursing management is determined by the extent of the procedure. Those patients who have had surgical excision only should be instructed to limit environmental insults to the surgical site and to protect the site against exposure to irritants and mechanical trauma. Patients who have undergone skin grafting or flapping require careful and frequent observation for signs of infection and hemorrhage in both donor and recipient sites. The recipient site should be immobilized to prevent separation, and involved limbs should be elevated to minimize edema. Some sloughing of a graft site may occur, but this can be controlled with the use of mineral oil or lanolin.[93]

Nursing management of patients who are undergoing chemotherapy, radiotherapy, or biotherapy is determined by the specific treatment regimen administered. General nursing care for patients receiving these therapies is described elsewhere in this text.

All patients with a diagnosis of melanoma should be evaluated at regular intervals for recurrence or metastatic disease. This evaluation should occur every 3 to 4 months for the first 2 years, every 6 months up to 5 years, and yearly thereafter. These intervals should be adjusted according to the risk of metastatic disease in any individual patient.[39,40] It is imperative that patients understand the importance of these follow-up visits and inform the physician or nurse of any physical or mental changes that occur.

CONCLUSION

This chapter has described three primary forms of skin cancer: basal cell epithelioma, squamous cell carcinoma, and cutaneous malignant melanoma. Uveal melanoma was also summarized. Since the best known treatment to date for most skin cancers is prevention, oncology nurses are in an ideal position to educate the public and other professionals about primary and secondary preventive behaviors. By practicing early detection, screening, and preventive behaviors themselves, oncology nurses can better serve as role models for the general population and for those at high risk.

REFERENCES

1. American Cancer Society: Cancer Facts and Figures. Atlanta, 1989.
2. Haynes HA, Mead KW, Goldwyn RM: Cancers of the skin, in DeVita VT, Hellman S, Rosenberg SA (eds): Cancer: Principles and Practice of Oncology (ed 2). Philadelphia, JB Lippincott, 1985, pp 1343-1369.
3. National Cancer Institute: Nonmelanoma Skin Cancers: Research Report. Bethesda, Md, NIH publication no. 88-2977, May, 1988.
4. National Cancer Institute: Annual Cancer Statistics Review Including Cancer Trends: 1950-1985. Bethesda, Md, January, 1988.
5. Mastrangelo MJ, Baker AR, Katz HR: Cutaneous melanoma, in DeVita VT, Hellman S, Rosenberg SA (eds): Cancer: Principles and Practice of Oncology (ed 2). Philadelphia, JB Lippincott, 1985, pp 1371-1422.
6. Silverberg E, Lubera J: Cancer statistics, 1989. CA 39:3-20, 1989.
7. Greene MH, Clark WH, Tucker MA, et al: Acquired precursors of cutaneous malignant melanoma: The familial dysplastic nevus syndrome. N Engl J Med 312:91-97, 1986.
8. Friedman RJ, Rigel DS, Kopf AW: The ABCD's of moles and melanomas. New York, The Skin Cancer Foundation, 1985.
9. Rhodes AR, Weinstock MA, Fitzpatrick TB, et al: Risk factors for cutaneous melanoma. JAMA 258:3146-3154, 1987.
10. Lee JAH: The causation of melanoma, in Balch CM, Milton GW, Shaw HM, et al (eds): Cutaneous Melanoma. Philadelphia, JB Lippincott, 1985, pp 303-311.
11. Milton GW, Balch CM, Shaw HM: Clinical characteristics, in Balch CM, Milton GW, Shaw HM, et al (eds): Cutaneous Melanoma. Philadelphia, JB Lippincott, 1985, pp 13-28.
12. Holman CDJ, Armstrong BK: Pigmentary traits, ethnic origin, benign nevi, and familial history as risk factors for cutaneous malignant melanoma. JNCI 72:257-266, 1984.
13. Green A, MacLennon R, Siskind V: Common acquired nevi and the risk of malignant melanoma. Int J Cancer 35:297-300, 1985.
14. Rampen FHJ: Sex differences in survival from cutaneous melanoma. Int J Dermatol 23:444-452, 1984.
15. Holly EA: Melanoma in pregnancy, in Gallagher RP (ed): Recent Results in Cancer Research: Epidemiology of Malignant Melanoma. New York, Springer-Verlag, 1986, pp 118-125.
16. Schwartz BK, Zashin SJ, Spencer SK, et al: Pregnancy and hormonal influences on malignant melanoma. J Dermatol Surg Oncol 13:276-281, 1987.
17. Grimwood RE, Siegle RJ, Ferris CF, et al: The biology of basal cell carcinomas: A revisit and recent developments. J Dermatol Surg Oncol 12:805-808, 1986.
18. Howat AJ, Levick PL: Metastatic basal cell carcinoma. Dermatologica 174:132-134, 1987.
19. McKinney P, Robinson JK: Basic principles in management of basal cell epithelioma. IMJ 173:105-111, 1988.
20. Edwards L, Levine N: Skin cancer: The best route to early diagnosis. Mod Med 54:42-54, 1986.
21. Tobinick EL: Basal cell carcinoma. Am Fam Physician 36:219-224, 1987.
22. Stoll HL, Scwartz RA: Squamous cell carcinoma, in Fitzpatrick TB, Eisen AZ, Wolff K, et al (eds): Dermatology in General Medicine. New York, McGraw-Hill, 1987, pp 746-758.
23. Marks R: Squamous cell carcinoma. Aust Fam Physician 15:937-938, 1986.
24. Friedman HI, Cooper PH, Wanebo HJ: Prognostic and therapeutic use of microstaging of cutaneous squamous cell carcinoma of the trunk and extremities. Cancer 56:1099-1105, 1985.
25. Stegman SJ: Basal cell carcinoma and squamous cell carcinoma: Recognition and treatment. Med Clin North Am 70:95-107, 1986.
26. Lippman SM, Kessler JF, Meyskens FL: Retinoids as preventive and therapeutic anticancer agents (parts 1 and 2). Cancer Treat Rep 71:391-405, 493-515, 1987.
27. Roenigk RK: Subspecialty clinics: Dermatology Mohs' micrographic surgery. Mayo Clin Proc 63:175-183, 1988.
28. Crawfort E, Girouard M, Johnson S, et al: Mohs' chemosurgery: Day surgery for cutaneous malignancies. AORN J 43:464-468, 1986.
29. Torre D: Cryosurgery of basal cell carcinoma. J Am Acad Dermatol 15:917-929, 1986.
30. Levine HL, Ratz JL, Bailin P: Squamous cell carcinoma of the head and neck: Selective management according to site and stage-skin. Otolaryngol Clin North Am 18:499-503, 1985.
31. Wheeland RG, Bailin PL, Ratz JL, et al: Carbon-dioxide laser vaporization and curettage in the treatment of multiple superficial basal cell carcinomas. J Dermatol Surg Oncol 13:119-125, 1987.
32. Worth AJ: Growth patterns in melanoma and its precursor lesions, in Gallagher RP (ed): Epidemiology of Malignant Melanoma. Berlin, Springer-Verlag, 1986, pp 1-7.
33. Greene MH, Clark WH, Tucker MA, et al: High risk of malignant melanoma in melanoma-prone families with dysplastic nevi. Ann Intern Med 102:458-465, 1985.
34. Rhodes AR: Benign neoplasias, hyperplasias and dysplasias of melanocytes, in Fitzpatrick TB, Eisen AZ, Wolff K, et al (eds): Dermatology in General Medicine. New York, McGraw-Hill, 1987, pp 877-946.
35. Barnhill RL, Hurwitz S, Duray PH: The dysplastic nevus: Recognition and management. Plast Reconstr Surg 81:280-288, 1988.
36. Landow KR: Differential diagnosis and treatment of pigmented skin lesions. Compr Ther 14:25-32, 1988.
37. Wade TR, White CR: The history of malignant melanoma. Med Clin North Am 70:57-69, 1986.
38. Bergman W, Ruiter DJ, Scheffer E, et al: Melanocytic atypia in dysplastic nevi. Cancer 61:1660-1666, 1988.
39. Kibbi AG, Mihm MC, Sober AJ, et al: Diagnosis and management of malignant melanoma. Compr Ther 12:23-31, 1986.
40. Berdeaux DH, Moon TE, Meyskens FL: Management of stage I cutaneous melanoma. Ariz Med 40:768-772, 1983.
41. Finck SJ, Giuliano AE, Morton DL: LDH and melanoma. Cancer 51:840-843, 1983.
42. Balch CM: Cutaneous melanoma: A review of clinical management. Texas Med 83:70-78, 1987.
43. Balch CM, Milton GW: Diagnosis of metastatic melanoma at distant sites, in Balch CM, Milton GW, Shaw HM, et al (eds):

Cutaneous Melanoma. Philadelphia, JB Lippincott, 1985, pp 221-250.
44. MacKie RM, Young D: Human malignant melanoma. Int J Dermatol 23:433-443, 1984.
45. Chanda JJ: The clinical recognition and prognostic factors of primary cutaneous malignant melanoma. Med Clin North Am 70:39-53, 1986.
46. Stal S, Loeb T, Spira M: Melanoma of the head and neck. Otolaryngol Clin North Am 19:549-564, 1986.
47. Briele HA, Walker MJ, Das G, et al: Melanoma of the head and neck: Update and perspective. Clin Plast Surg 12:495-502, 1985.
48. Beahrs OH, Henson DE, Hutter RP, et al (eds): Manual for Staging of Cancer: American Joint Committee on Cancer. Philadelphia, JB Lippincott, 1988, pp 139-140.
49. Balch CM, Soong SJ, Shaw HM, et al: An analysis of prognostic factors in 4000 patients with cutaneous melanoma, in Balch CM, Milton GW, Shaw HM, et al (eds): Cutaneous Melanoma. Philadelphia, JB Lippincott, 1985, pp 321-352.
50. Ketcham A, Balch CM: Classification and staging systems, in Balch CM, Milton GW, Shaw HM, et al (eds): Cutaneous Melanoma. Philadelphia, JB Lippincott, 1985, pp 55-62.
51. Kopf AW, Welkovich B, Frankel RE, et al: Thickness of malignant melanoma: Global analysis of related factors. J Dermatol Surg Oncol 13:345-420, 1987.
52. Urist MM, Balch CM, Milton GW: Surgical management of the primary melanoma, in Balch CM, Milton GW, Shaw HM, et al (eds): Cutaneous Melanoma. Philadelphia, JB Lippincott, 1985, pp 71-90.
53. Meyer KL, Kenady DE, Childers SJ: The surgical approach to primary malignant melanoma. Surg Gynecol Obstet 160:379-386, 1985.
54. Roses DF, Harris MN, Gumport SL: Surgery for primary cutaneous malignant melanoma. Dermatol Clin 3:315-326, 1985.
55. Veronesi U, Cascinelli N: How wide and deep is wide and deep enough? Am J Dermatopathol 7:123-126, 1985.
56. Sim FH, Taylor WF, Pritchard DJ, et al: Lymphadenectomy in the management of stage I malignant melanoma: A prospective randomized study. Mayo Clin Proc 61:697-705, 1986.
57. Veronesi U: Delayed node dissection in stage I malignant melanoma: Justification and advantages. Cancer Invest 5:47-53, 1987.
58. Balch CM: The role of elective lymph node dissection in melanoma: Rationale, results, and controversies. J Clin Oncol 6:163-172, 1988.
59. Day CL, Lew RA: Malignant melanoma prognostic factors: Elective lymph node dissection. J Dermatol Surg Oncol 11:233-239, 1985.
60. Balch CM, Urist MM, Maddox WM, et al: Management of regional metastatic melanoma, in Balch CM, Milton GW, Shaw HM, et al (eds): Cutaneous Melanoma. Philadelphia, JB Lippincott, 1985, pp 93-130.
61. Wornon IL, Smith JW, Soong SJ, et al: Surgery as palliative treatment for distant metastases of melanoma. Ann Surg 204:181-185, 1986.
62. Golumb FM: Chemotherapy of melanoma. Dermatol Clin 3:335-340, 1985.
63. Coates AS, Durant JR: Chemotherapy for metastatic malignant melanoma, in Balch CM, Milton GW, Shaw HM, et al (eds): Cutaneous Melanoma. Philadelphia, JB Lippincott, 1985, pp 275-282.
64. Klein ES, Ben-Ari GY: Isolation perfusion with cisplatin for malignant melanoma of the limbs. Cancer 59:1068-1071, 1987.
65. Krementz ET, Ryan RF, Carter RD, et al: Hyperthermic regional perfusion for melanoma of the limbs, in Balch CM, Milton GW, Shaw HM, et al (eds): Cutaneous Melanoma. Philadelphia, JB Lippincott, 1985, pp 171-195.
66. Muchmore JH, Carter RD, Krementz ET: Regional perfusion for malignant melanoma and soft tissue sarcoma: A review. Cancer Invest 3:129-143, 1985.
67. Ghussen F, Kruger I, Groth W, et al: The role of regional hyperthermia cytostatic perfusion in the treatment of extremity melanoma. Cancer 61:654-659, 1988.
68. Franklin HR, Koops HS, Oldhoff J, et al: To perfuse or not to perfuse? A retrospective comparative study to evaluate the effect of adjuvant isolated regional perfusion in patients with stage I extremity melanoma with a thickness of 1.5 mm or greater. J Clin Oncol 16:701-708, 1988.
69. Rofstad EK: Radiation biology of malignant melanoma. Acta Radiol 25:1-10, 1986.
70. Overgaard J: The role of radiotherapy in recurrent and metastatic malignant melanoma: A clinical radiobiological study. Int J Radiat Oncol 12:867-872, 1986.
71. Brascho DJ: Radiotherapy for metastatic melanoma, in Balch CM, Milton GW, Shaw HM, et al (eds): Cutaneous Melanoma. Philadelphia, JB Lippincott, 1985, pp 283-293.
72. Meyskens FL: The endocrinology of malignant melanoma. Rev Endocrine-Related Cancer 9:5-13, 1981.
73. Reintgen DS, McCarty KS, Vollmer R, et al: Malignant melanoma and pregnancy. Cancer 55:1340-1344, 1985.
74. Johnson BL: Malignant melanoma, in Groenwald SL (ed): Cancer Nursing: Principles and Practice. Boston, Jones & Bartlett, 1987. pp 684-692.
75. Meyskens FL, Loescher L, Serokman R, et al: Potential uses of biological response modifiers (BRM) in the adjuvant treatment of melanoma and results from a trial of BCG +/− vitamin A, in Salmon SE, Jones SE (eds): Proceedings of IV Adjuvant Conference. New York, Grune & Stratton, 1984, pp 583-590.
76. Shields JA: Diagnosis and Management of Intraocular Tumors. St Louis, CV Mosby, 1983.
77. Bellet RE, Shields JA, Soll DB, et al: Primary choroidal and cutaneous melanomas occurring in a patient with the B-K mole syndrome phenotype. Am J Ophthalmol 89:567-570, 1980.
78. Greene MH, Sanders RJ, Chu FC, et al: The familial occurrence of cutaneous melanoma, intraocular melanoma, and the dysplastic nevus syndrome. Am J Ophthalmol 96:238-245, 1983.
79. Tucker MA, Shields JA, Hartge P, et al: Sunlight exposure as a risk factor for intraocular malignant melanoma. N Engl J Med 313:789-792, 1985.
80. Zimmerman LE, McLean IW: Do growth and onset of symptoms of uveal melanomas indicate subclinical metastasis? Ophthalmology 91:685-691, 1984.
81. Shammas HF, Blodi FC: Prognostic factors in choroidal and ciliary body melanomas. Arch Ophthalmol 95:63-69, 1977.
82. Wilhelm JL, Zakov AN: Choroidal melanoma with liver metastasis before enucleation. Ann Ophthalmol 14:789-796, 1982.
83. Packer S, Rotman M, Salanitro P: Iodine-125 irradiation of choroidal melanoma: Clinical experience. Ophthalmology 91:1700-1708, 1984.
84. Augsburger JJ, Gamel JW, Sardi VF, et al: Enucleation vs cobalt plaque radiotherapy for malignant melanomas of the choroid and ciliary body. Arch Ophthalmol 104:655-661, 1986.

85. Simple Guidelines to Help Protect You From the Damaging Rays of the Sun. New York, Skin Cancer Foundation, 1988.
86. Arizona Sun Awareness Project: Sun Awareness. Arizona Cancer Center, 1985.
87. Bertram JS, Kolonel LN, Meyskens FL: Rationale and strategies for chemoprevention of cancer in humans. Cancer Res 47:3012-3031, 1987.
88. Ritenbaugh CK, Meyskens FL: Analysis of dietary associations of vitamin A with cancer, in Bland J (ed): The Year in Nutritional Medicine. New Canaan, Conn, Keats, 1986, pp 263-291.
89. Fraser MC: The nurse's role and malignant melanoma. Cancer Nurs 5:351-360, 1982.
90. Fraser MC, McGuire DB: Skin cancer's early warning system. Am J Nurs 84:1232-1236, 1984.
91. White LN, Cornelius JL, Judkins AF, et al: Screening of cancer by nurses. Cancer Nurs 1:15-20, 1978.
92. Schulmeister L: Screening for skin cancer: A necessary part of your assessment routine. Nursing 11:42-45, 1981.
93. Stern C: Melanoma: The most lethal skin cancer. RN 50:53-57, 1987.

Chapter 47

Soft Tissue Sarcomas

Shirley M. Gullo, RN, BSN, OCN

INTRODUCTION

Soft tissue sarcoma refers to a heterogeneous group of more than 50 types of cancers. Soft tissue sarcomas represent approximately 1% of all malignancies in men and 0.6% of those in women.[1] They affect all age groups, although some histologic types are more common in the younger or the older patient population. There are no identified populations that have either increased or decreased overall risks; sarcomas are found in all races.[2]

Soft tissue sarcomas are uncommon neoplasms that arise from supportive (connective) tissue other than bone. Soft tissue sarcomas may affect fibrous tissue (fibrosarcoma and fibrous histiocytoma), tendosynovial tissue (monophasic tendosynovial sarcoma), adipose tissue (liposarcoma), the muscles (rhabdomyosarcoma and leiomyosarcoma), vessels (lymphangiosarcoma, hemangiosarcoma), peripheral nerves, extraskeletal bone (chondrosarcoma), and miscellaneous tissue or combinations of tissue involvement (plasmacytoma, malignant mesenchymoma) (Table 47-1).[3] They are characterized by some common morphology and clinical behavior, although they vary in their potential to metastasize. Biologic and clinical data on sarcomas are limited because of the infrequent occurrence of these tumors. Further, soft tissue sarcomas lack sufficient homogeneous characteristics to aid in epidemiologic research. In spite of these hindrances, the prognosis for persons with soft tissue sarcoma appears to be improving with the increased use of combined-modality therapy.[2]

TABLE 47-1 Histogenic Classification of Sarcomas

Tissue of Origin	Type of Sarcoma
Fibrous tissue	Fibrous histiocytoma Fibrosarcoma
Tendosynovial tissue	Tendosynovial sarcoma
Adipose tissue	Liposarcoma
Muscle	Leiomyosarcoma Rhabdomyosarcoma
Vessels	Lymphangiosarcoma Hemangiosarcoma Kaposi's sarcoma
Peripheral nerve	Malignant peripheral nerve tumor
Bone	Osteogenic sarcoma Chondrosarcoma Ewing's sarcoma Chordoma
Miscellaneous tissue	Malignant granular cell tumor Alveolar soft-part sarcoma Malignant mesenchymoma

Source: Adapted from Hajdu SI: Pathology of Soft Tissue Tumors. Philadelphia, Lea & Febiger, 1979.

EPIDEMIOLOGY

In the United States an estimated 5600 new cases and 3000 deaths from soft tissue sarcomas are reported annually.[4] They are more common in children than in adults. Although soft tissue sarcomas are rare, they are responsible for about 6% of the malignant tumors that occur before the age of 25, and they account for nearly 2% of all deaths from malignancy. Only 0.7% of all cancers are sarcomas, with an age-adjusted incidence rate of 2 per 100,000. A composite of incidence reported by several researchers indicates that liposarcomas, rhabdomyosarcomas, fibrosarcomas, and synoviomas are the most common histologic types of soft tissue sarcoma.[1,4]

ETIOLOGY

The cause of soft tissue sarcoma is not known. The majority of the sarcomas appear to be malignant from the beginning, and very few develop in benign precursor tumors. Some possible exceptions are liposarcomas that infrequently develop from lipomas and neurofibrosarcoma that develops in approximately 10% of patients with neurofibromatosis (von Recklinghausen's disease). High-dose radiation therapy, usually greater than 10,000 rad (cGy), has been associated with an increased frequency of sarcomas. Angiosarcomas may arise in benign angiomas after radiation therapy, and fibrosarcomas have developed after intensive radiation for benign conditions such as tuberculosis of the skin or thyroid disease.[5]

Although sarcomas occasionally have developed in old scars, trauma has never been established as a causative factor. Granulation tissue sarcoma may originate in burn, surgical, or other scars. Lymphangiosarcoma may develop as a complication of prolonged, massive postmastectomy edema.[2,5]

Exposure to asbestos has been associated with mesothelioma. The relationship of other possible chemical and physical carcinogens and the development of sarcomas remains to be determined. Genetically linked diseases, such as tuberous sclerosis, Werner's syndrome, intestinal polyposis, Gardner's syndrome, and basal cell nevus syndrome, have been associated with soft tissue sarcomas.[6] Several animal viruses have been associated with sarcomas in animals, but a human sarcoma virus has not been unequivocally defined.[5,6]

PATHOPHYSIOLOGY OF SOFT TISSUE SARCOMAS

Fibrosarcomas

Malignant tumors of fibrous tissue constitute the most common sarcomas. There is a slight predominance in males and 70% of these tumors are seen between the ages of 20 and 50 years. The most common site is the thigh, followed by the trunk, buttock, arm, and miscellaneous sites.[7] Metastases can occur by direct extension of the connective tissue or nerve sheaths from which they originate and also by hematogenous routes.

Fibrosarcomas appear as single, firm, rounded, or slightly lobulated masses of grayish white, soft lesions with areas of necrosis. The size varies considerably, with many large tumors reported.

Treatment consists of wide excision, since these tumors have a high incidence of recurrence and are relatively resistant to radiotherapy as a single treatment modality. The ultimate therapeutic aim is eradication of the sarcoma with the least risk of local tumor recurrence consistent with minimal loss of tissue and function. Limb salvage is not always the best treatment, and amputation is often indicated in cases involving poorly differentiated fibrosarcomas. Although fibrosarcomas are not usually controlled by radiation therapy alone, postoperative radiation often is recommended. Clinical trials of adjuvant chemotherapy regimens are currently under investigation.[8]

Liposarcomas

Liposarcomas represent a more common form of soft tissue sarcoma. They usually are deep-seated neoplasms with an indolent course. They can occur almost anywhere that fat is present, but they most frequently arise in the trunk and extremities and rarely arise from lipomas. These tumors are frequently large, with multiple convolutions, and may be yellowish and gelatinous. Some of the largest sarcomas reported in man are liposarcomas. They are most common in persons 40 to 60 years of age and are extremely rare in children.

In general, all liposarcomas are prone to local recurrence. Studies of these neoplasms show that 67% recurred after surgical excision and more than 50% of the patients died of metastatic disease less than 5 years after the initial diagnosis.[3] Distant metastases are chiefly hematogenous, with the lung being the most common site.

Treatment consists of wide surgical excision with postoperative radiation therapy. This tumor is among the most radioresponsive of the soft tissue types. Overall 5-year survival is about 32%; however, survival rates vary with different classifications of liposarcoma.[9]

Synovial Sarcomas

Synovial sarcomas usually arise in or near tendinous sheaths, bursae, joints, and ligaments. Despite their name, they rarely involve the joint synovia. The tumor has a predilection for the extremities. About 60% of the cases occur in males. It has been reported to occur at all ages but has a predilection for individuals under 40 years of age. The usual presenting symptoms are tenderness, warmth, and a swelling or a palpable mass. Pain may precede a detectable mass by 1 to 18 months.[10] During physical assessment of individuals in this age group, the nurse should be suspicious of unexplained swellings and/or pain, especially near joints.

Synovial sarcomas are firm and gray, with hemorrhage, necrosis, and calcification present. The stippled appearance evident on microscopy can be seen by x-ray examination in about 30% of the patients.[11]

There is local recurrence in 60% to 90% of the cases after local excision. Postoperative radiation has been reported to control these tumors.[7] In some cases wide surgical excision may necessitate amputation, including hip disarticulation. Chemotherapy may be used in the palliation of these tumors.

Metastasis to lung occurs in 75% of cases and metastasis to bone is not uncommon. Most metastases and local recurrences occur within the first 2 years of diagnosis, but occasionally may occur even beyond 10 years.[13]

Malignant Tumors of Muscle

Rhabdomyosarcomas

Rhabdomyosarcomas occur more frequently in children than in adults. They are divided histologically into three separate entities: embyronal botryoid, embryonal alveolar, and adult pleomorphic. Embryonal botryoid rhabdomyosarcomas are named for their grapelike appearance. These are tumors of infancy and early childhood, and they usually occur in children under the age of 5 years. Occasionally cases occur after the age of 12, and there is a higher incidence in boys.[13] Common sites are the head and neck, especially the orbit and nasopharynx, and, more rarely, the genitourinary tract. Metastases are frequent in lymph nodes, lung, bone, and serous membranes. Combined-modality treatments have improved survival, but the 5-year prognosis remains grave.[1] Classically, embryonal alveolar rhabdomyosarcoma is a tumor of children and young adults and is found chiefly in the extremities. The tumor is aggressive, and many cases are well advanced at the time of diagnosis. The patients commonly have severe or intermittent pain in the affected area. Metastases to lymph nodes, lung, bone, and pancreas are common.[13] Total excision of the tumor with postoperative radiation and/or chemotherapy has improved the survival rates for this group of patients.[1] Adult pleomorphic rhabdomyosarcomas occur most frequently in the extremities, especially the thigh. The typical patient with this tumor is in his or her late 50s and tends to experience repeated local recurrences with ultimate metastases. Wide excision remains the treatment of choice. Local recurrence rates vary from 27% to 60% and 5-year survival ranges from 10% to 37%.[10]

Leiomyosarcomas

Leiomyosarcomas may be found along the distribution of smooth muscle, more frequently arising in specific visceral sites (ie, the uterus and the gastrointestinal tract). These tumors occur at all ages, with a peak incidence after the age of 60 years. They are aggressive tumors that frequently recur and metastasize, most often to the liver and lungs. For these reasons, radical resection is the primary treatment of choice.[1,13]

Malignant Tumors of Vessels

Malignant tumors of vessels include Kaposi's sarcoma, now most commonly associated with acquired immunodeficiency syndrome (AIDS) (see Chapter 33), angiosarcomas, lymphangiosarcomas, and hemangiosarcomas.

Angiosarcomas

The most common sites of angiosarcomas are the scalp, breast, and liver. They most often occur in elderly men except for breast angiosarcomas, which are more common in younger men and women. They are poorly defined lesions that resemble bruises or contusions, or they may be nodular with the appearance of a "blood blister." In general, growth is slow but persistent. They are somewhat responsive to radiation.[13]

Lymphangiosarcomas

Lymphangiosarcomas usually occur on the arms and in areas of lymph stasis. These tumors may occur from 1 to 27 years after radical mastectomy, often beginning as red and hemorrhagic macular skin lesions. Recurrence on the chest wall and metastasis to the lung are common. Even with multimodality therapy, the 5-year survival rate is poor.[14]

Hemangiosarcoma

Hemangiosarcomas have been reported at all ages, including infancy. These tumors affect men and women equally and occur in the lower and upper extremities, trunk, and head and neck area. They appear as painless, rather deep-seated masses. Surgery and chemotherapy are the treatments of choice.[13,14]

Malignant Tumors of Peripheral Nerves

These tumors are complex, and therapy is based on whether the tumor is small or large, solitary or multifocal. The tumors may occur at any age, the average age being in the early 40s. In general, the most common sites are those associated with sizeable nerves, such as the sciatic nerve, the medial nerve, the spinal nerve roots, and the brachial plexus. As a group they are aggressive, and the prognosis is generally worse if the tumor is associated with a history of neurofibromatosis. Malignant peripheral nerve neoplasms that occur in combination with neurofibromatosis or have a histologically high grade are usually treated by surgical resection and chemotherapy.[14]

Extraskeletal Malignant Bone Tumors

The thigh is the most common site of extraskeletal malignant bone tumors. Other locations include the popliteal area, leg, and foot. They usually appear as deep, circumscribed, gelatinous lesions, ranging from 4 to 7 cm in size. Generally, they are slow-growing tumors with a fairly high rate of recurrence following a lengthy disease-free interval. Wide surgical excision is the primary treatment of choice.[13] Ewing's sarcoma is the most common type of extraskeletal bone tumor, occurring most commonly in the midshaft of a long bone. Complete surgical resection or amputation of the primary lesion is recommended for most patients with Ewing's sarcomas. Whenever feasible, preoperative radiation is given in combination with chemotherapy.[16]

Miscellaneous Malignant Soft Tissue Tumors

Malignant granular cell tumors, alveolar soft-part sarcomas, granulocytic sarcomas, plasmacytomas, malignant mesenchymomas, and undifferentiated soft tissue sarcomas are rare tumors, and there is a paucity of information concerning them. Malignant granular cell tumors and alveolar soft-part sarcomas affect women more commonly than men. Multimodality treatment usually is designed on the basis of tumor size, location, cellularity, and duration of the neoplasm.[14]

CLINICAL MANIFESTATIONS

As a group, soft tissue sarcomas usually begin as painless masses or lumps. They often develop a hard consistency. About 40% occur in the lower extremities, 20% in the upper extremities, 20% in the trunk, and the rest in the head, neck, or retroperineum (Table 47-2).[15] Peripheral neuralgia (often characterized by stabbing pain), paralysis, or ischemia can occur because of pressure on nerve or vascular supply. The tumors also may interfere with visceral functions, resulting in obstruction of the bowel, ureters, or mediastinal structures. General malaise, fever, and weight loss may occur with more extensive disease. Endocrine disorders, such as goiter, pituitary dysfunction, and episodic hypoglycemia, also may occur with some large retroperitoneal or extrapleural sarcomas.

TABLE 47-2 Classification and Natural History of Soft Tissue Sarcomas

	Average Age	Sex Prevalence	Most Common Site	Most Common Presentation	Average Size (cm)	Histologic Pattern of Growth	Histologic Grade	Most Common Stage	Average 5-year Survival (%)
Malignant tumors of fibrous tissue									
Malignant fibroblastic fibrous histiocytoma	45	Male	Trunk	Superficial	10	Arranged	Low	I	85
Malignant histiocytic fibrous histiocytoma	50	Male	Knee	Deep	15	Epithelioid	—	II	55
Malignant pleomorphic fibrous histiocytoma	50	Male	Buttock and arm	Deep	5	Disarranged	—	III	50
Desmoid tumor	25	Male	Arm and thigh	Deep	5	Spreading	Low	I	95
Fibroblastic fibrosarcoma	45	Male	Thigh	Deep	10	Arranged	High	III	40
Pleomorphic fibrosarcoma	50	Male	Thigh	Deep	15	Disarranged	High	III	35
Malignant tumors of tendosynovial tissue									
Biphasic tendosynovial sarcoma	35	Male	Knee	Deep	10	Alveolar	—	II	55
Monophasic tendosynovial sarcoma	24	Male	Thigh	Deep	15	Spreading	High	III	30
Epithelioid sarcoma	25	Male	Forearm	Superficial	2	Epithelioid	—	II	65
Clear cell sarcoma	30	Male	Leg	Deep	5	Epithelioid	High	II	55
Chordoid sarcoma	40	Male	Hand	Superficial	2	Lacy	Low	0	75
Malignant tumors of adipose tissue									
Well-differentiated liposarcoma	55	Male	Trunk	—	5	Lacy	Low	I	95
Myxoid liposarcoma	40	Male	Thigh	Deep	10	Lacy	Low	II	95
Lipoblastic liposarcoma	45	Male	Thigh	Deep	10	Epithelioid	High	III	50
Fibroblastic liposarcoma	45	Male	Thigh	Deep	10	Arranged	High	III	60
Pleomorphic liposarcoma	55	Male	Thigh	Deep	20	Disarranged	High	III	45
Malignant tumors of muscle									
Leiomyosarcoma	55	Female	Leg	—	5	Spreading	—	II	60
Leiomyoblastoma	50	Female	—	Deep	5	Epithelioid	—	II	60
Embryonal rhabdomyosarcoma	10	Male	Thigh	Deep	15	Epithelioid	High	III	65
Rhabdomyoblastoma	20	Male	—	Deep	5	Epithelioid	High	II	40
Pleomorphic rhabdomyosarcoma	50	Male	Thigh	Deep	20	Disarranged	High	III	25

TABLE 47-2 Classification and Natural History of Soft Tissue Sarcomas (continued)

	Average Age	Sex Prevalence	Most Common Site	Most Common Presentation	Average Size (cm)	Histologic Pattern of Growth	Histologic Grade	Most Common Stage	Average 5-year Survival (%)
Malignant tumors of vessels									
Hemangiosarcoma	45	Male	Trunk	—	5	Alveolar	High	III	30
Hemangiopericytoma	40	Male	—	Deep	10	Alveolar	—	II	60
Kaposi's sarcoma	55	Male	Leg	Superficial	2	Alveolar	Low	0	90
Lymphangiosarcoma	50	Female	Arm	—	5	Alveolar	High	III	10
Malignant tumors of peripheral nerves									
Malignant peripheral nerve tumor	40	Female	Thigh	Deep	15	Spreading	—	II	60
Primitive neuroectodermal tumor	25	Male	Trunk	Deep	5	Epithelioid	High	III	30
Miscellaneous malignant soft tissue tumors									
Malignant granular cell tumor	45	Female	—	Superficial	5	Epithelioid	—	II	75
Alveolar soft-part sarcoma	35	Female	Thigh	Deep	15	Epithelioid	—	III	50
Malignant lymphoma	—	—	Thigh	Deep	10	—	—	—	—
Granulocytic sarcoma	20	Male	—	Deep	5	Epithelioid	High	III	5
Plasmacytoma	50	—	—	Deep	10	—	High	III	45
Malignant mesenchymoma	45	—	—	Deep	10	—	—	—	—
Postirradiation sarcoma	—	—	—	Deep	10	—	High	III	75
Undifferentiated soft tissue sarcoma	—	—	—	Deep	—	—	High	—	—

Source: Hajdu SI: Soft tissue sarcomas: Classification and natural history. CA 31:271-293, 1981.

Early detection is dependent on a high index of suspicion, particularly in specific age groups. Because of the rarity of the tumors, soft tissue masses often are assumed to be benign or are treated inadequately. All unexplained tumor masses require early biopsy or excision. Diagnosis involves careful evaluation of the mass, especially if size changes rapidly or if symptoms develop. Early detection is difficult since these tumors grow insidiously, are often in inaccessible sites, and are poorly encapsulated.[17]

DIAGNOSIS

The extent of the tumor is evaluated as accurately and quickly as possible to assure prompt treatment. The lesion is palpated gently and measured, and any regions of draining lymphatic sites are evaluated.[17]

The major focus of the diagnostic work-up for soft tissue sarcoma is to define the location, nature, and extent of disease. An individualized treatment plan to eradicate the neoplasm with preservation of maximum function is the primary goal. Routine admission tests in combination with a variety of radiologic techniques and other procedures are useful. A radiograph of the chest is obtained routinely to rule out pulmonary metastases. Tomograms of the lungs enhance efforts to locate early pulmonary metastases.

The area in question is scanned by computerized tomography (CT) in two places simultaneously at various angles. In the retroperitoneum, CT can detect the mass, the relationship of adjacent viscera, vessels, and lymph nodes, and abdominal and hepatic metastases. The CT scan more accurately defines the extent of the tumor because it adds a three-dimensional aspect to conventional radiographic examination and xeroradiography.[18]

Angiography is useful if the tumor has an identifiable blood supply. It displays the relationship of the tumor to the large vessels, reveals shunting, shows the size of the tumor mass and, in the late phase, delineates the major venous drainage that requires early control to limit embolization.

Bone scanning is useful to determine the proximity of the tumor to the bone or whether there is bone involvement. This is especially important in those cases that may require bone resection to assure sufficient surgical intervention.

Percutaneous needle biopsy provides histologic confirmation of the nature of the tumor. The biopsy site selected is the most invasive area as evidenced by radiographic evaluation of the size and position of the tumor. Areas of necrosis usually are avoided because the tissue specimen often is devoid of tumor cells. Aspiration cytology has a limited role in the primary diagnosis of soft tissue and bone sarcomas because of limited sampling and the marked cytologic resemblance of reactive, benign neoplastic, and malignant neoplastic lesions.[15]

Ultrasonography evaluates the deep structures of the body by measuring and recording the reflection of pulsed or continuous high-frequency sound waves. The examination can be completed in 5 minutes, and the exact size and shape of the tumor can be delineated. The liver, spleen, and kidneys usually are assessed accurately, with limitations of size and detectable lesions at 1.5 to 2.0 cm in diameter. Ultrasonography also has the advantage of imaging in two planes (longitudinal and transverse), which provides a better definition of acoustical interfaces.[18]

Metastases to the lungs develop in 30% to 50% of patients with tumors of high histologic grade. Lung metastases usually are defined by chest radiography and tomography. CT may be used if any question remains.[19]

Hepatic metastases have been reported in 21% of all sarcomas. Since the vascularity of these tumors determines the resolution of computed tomography, ultrasonography, and scintigraphy, these tests may not provide sufficient information to warrant their use. Angiography may be used for preoperative assessment of hepatic metastases confined to a resectable segment.[18]

The incidence of regional lymph node metastases is low (about 5%) but is more common in rhabdomyosarcoma, malignant fibrous histiocytoma, and epithelioid sarcoma. Lymphangiography is used when there is clinical evidence of lymph node involvement. Computed tomography may be used for diagnosis of large lymph nodes that may not necessarily indicate metastases.

Percutaneous biopsies of metastases to the lung, lymph nodes, and bones may be performed when the histologic information will influence management.

CLASSIFICATION AND STAGING

Histogenetically, sarcomas arise from diverse connective tissue elements and are named according to the tissues they most resemble. Because of the great variation in subtypes of soft tissue sarcomas, there is no clear consensus among pathologists as to the predominant cell type and grade. Differences in terminology and changes in histologic classification have added to the confusion in evaluation of the pathologic and clinical behavior of these tumors. For example, some sarcomas with the same histologic name exhibit different characteristics and behavior. This variability has limited the reproducibility of studies of pathology, physiology, classification, and treatment of sarcoma.[2] Yet the pathologic identification of tumor type is the most important factor in determining the choice of treatment and the prognosis.[18]

The grade of sarcoma also is a major consideration in determining the most appropriate therapy. It is the grade of sarcoma, not the anatomic extent of the tumor, that influences the stage determination. The grade of the sarcoma is based primarily on the number of mitoses present, necrosis, degree of cellularity, nuclear pleomorphism, capsulation, and neovascularity.[17]

Histologically, sarcomas are divided into two major groups: low- and high-grade tumors. The tumor grades are defined as G1, G2, or G3 in anatomic staging. G1, or low grade, represents a well-differentiated tumor; G2, or moderate grade, is moderately differentiated; and G3, or high grade, is poorly differentiated. Tumor size and nodal involvement are other considerations in anatomic staging (Table 47-3).[20] A recurrent or metastatic sarcoma may have a tendency to be less differentiated than the primary lesion and have a different histologic appearance. Therefore grading and staging should, if possible, be based on the appearance of the primary tumor.

TREATMENT

Surgery

Surgical removal is the principal method of treating soft tissue sarcoma, provided there is no evidence of local invasion or metastases. Wide excision of soft tissue sarcomas,

TABLE 47-3 Anatomic Staging

Rules for Classification

Clinical Staging. Clinical staging includes physical examination, clinical laboratory tests, and biopsy of the sarcoma for microscopic diagnosis and grading.

Pathologic Staging. Pathologic staging consists of the removal of the primary tumor, nodes, or suspected metastases.

Primary Tumors (T)

TX	Primary tumor cannot be assessed
T0	No evidence of primary tumor
T1	Tumor 5 cm or less in greatest dimension
T2	Tumor more than 5 cm in greatest dimension

Regional Lymph Nodes (N)

NX	Regional lymph nodes cannot be assessed
N0	No regional lymph node metastasis
N1	Regional lymph node metastasis

Distant Metastasis (M)

MX	Presence of distant metastasis cannot be assessed
M0	No distant metastasis
M1	Distant metastasis

Tumor Grade (G)

GX	Grade cannot be assessed
G1	Well differentiated
G2	Moderately well differentiated
G3-4	Poorly differentiated; undifferentiated

Stage Grouping

Stage IA	G1	T1	N0	M0
Stage IB	G1	T2	N0	M0
Stage IIA	G2	T1	N0	M0
Stage IIB	G2	T2	N0	M0
Stage IIIA	G3-4	T1	N0	M0
Stage IIIB	G3-4	T2	N0	M0
Stage IVA	Any G	Any T	N1	M0
Stage IVB	Any G	Any T	Any N	M1

Source: American Joint Committee on Cancer: Manual for Staging of Cancer. Philadelphia, JB Lippincott, 1988.

even with a margin of several centimeters of normal tissue surrounding a lesion in all directions, is associated with a local recurrence rate of 50%,[19,21] primarily because soft tissue sarcomas typically spread by local extension along the tissue planes, often far from the palpable tumor.[14] Surgical procedures vary from radical resection to marginal excision, depending on the location and size of the tumor, the age of the patient, and the stage of the disease.

The local anatomic and histopathologic features of a tumor often dictate the method of surgical treatment. In the past, amputation was regarded as the best treatment for sarcomas. In spite of the low risk of local recurrence, amputation did not offer a significant improvement in length of survival. Today amputation is used only when the tumor cannot be removed by less mutilating, function-saving surgical techniques. The ultimate aim of treatment is eradication of the sarcoma with the least risk of local recurrence consistent with minimal loss of tissue and function.[14,21]

Limb-sparing surgery is a procedure that removes a soft tissue sarcoma while preserving function and cosmesis. It is the preferred surgical approach when local disease can be resected completely. The muscles that surround the sarcoma are removed. Deeply situated sarcomas lying between or within muscle groups require the removal of all muscle bundles within that particular fascial compartment, all surrounding or adjacent fascia, periosteum, vessels, nerves, and connective tissues, and all skin adjacent to the lesions. These procedures are necessary because soft tissue sarcomas tend to infiltrate along the fascial and muscle planes beyond the palpable limits of the tumor. However, because of the high risk of local recurrence, adjuvant treatment modalities are required.

Limb-sparing surgery may not be indicated for primary lesions that involve major vessels and nerves, either at the proximal extremity or in a site that will critically compromise function, or for lesions of the extremities when it is impossible to achieve adequate surgical margins and when radiotherapy cannot be given without major complications.[5]

Generally, lymph node dissection is indicated only when the lesion is contiguous with the major node-bearing areas, the nodes are involved, or the lesion appears to have a predisposition for nodal spread.[22]

Radiotherapy

Radiotherapy plays an integral role in the management of soft tissue sarcomas. However, it is less effective than surgery or radiation combined with surgery. Radiation is recommended as the sole treatment only in those situations in which surgery is not feasible for technical or medical reasons. When radiation is combined with surgery, the radiation is used to clear the tissue of microscopic disease.

Radiation therapy alone can be considered in patients who are medically inoperable or who refuse surgery. Following high-dose irradiation of up to 7000 cGy, the 2-year disease-free survival in such patients is about 15%.[23] Unresectable lesions treated with radiotherapy alone have a local recurrence rate of approximately 60% when conventional fractionations are used.[23]

Radiation therapy may be given preoperatively, postoperatively, or intraoperatively. Unresectable soft tissue sarcomas of the extremities can be treated with a course of preoperative radiotherapy delivering 6000 cGY over a period of 6 weeks. After a rest period of 5 to 6 weeks, curative limb-salvage surgery often is performed. The advantages of preoperative radiotherapy are as follows: (1) Most cells in the surgical field are killed by the high doses of radiation, reducing the risk of intraoperative contamination of vascular spaces by viable tumor cells, and (2) reduction of tumor bulk may allow an easier surgical procedure.[24]

Postoperative radiation therapy is used to control microscopic disease. The advantages of employing postoperative radiation are as follows: (1) There is no delay in surgery (this is a psychologic advantage for some patients); (2) there is no radiation-induced delay in wound healing; (3) the entire specimen is available for histopathologic study to determine histologic type and grade; and (4) the exact size and pattern of extension of the tumor are defined. The goal of combining radiation with relatively conservative surgery is to preserve function and anatomy of the treated limb.

Preoperative and postoperative irradiation doses for retroperitoneal or thoracic soft tissue sarcomas are limited by the large volumes that must be treated and the tolerance of normal tissue, such as kidney and small intestine.[25]

Another technical approach to the management of soft tissue sarcomas is the use of conservative excision and intraoperative implantation of radioactive sources. Iodine 125 seed implantation has accomplished local control and improved survival in patients with residual tumor at surgery. Intraoperative electron beam therapy also is being investigated.[24,25]

Chemotherapy

Adjuvant chemotherapy is indicated whenever there is a possibility of metastasis in the patient with potentially curable disease. Chemotherapy also is indicated in cases of metastatic disease if there are disseminated lesions that are not amenable to other modes of treatment. Surgery or radiation therapy is preferred for solitary or small numbers of easily accessible metastases.

Although there are numerous types of soft tissue sarcoma, there are few differences regarding responsiveness to chemotherapeutic agents. Chondrosarcomas and leiomyosarcomas of gastrointestinal origin respond less frequently than other soft tissue sarcomas. Ewing's sarcoma and rhabdomyosarcoma are responsive in a fraction of cases to dactinomycin, vincristine, or both.[26,27] Chemotherapy may be employed preoperatively in an effort to shrink inoperable sarcomas so they may become operable. Preoperative induction chemotherapy also may eradicate microscopic disease that usually is present in highly malignant sarcomas. The problem of delay of chemotherapy because of postoperative complications is thus eliminated.

Chemotherapy may be given before radiation therapy to shrink the tumor and spare normal tissue from side effects of radiation. Shrinking a large tumor also may eliminate hypoxic necrotic areas within the tumor and make it more responsive to local radiation therapy.[14]

The most effective chemotherapeutic agent in the treatment of adult soft tissue sarcomas is doxorubicin. Dacarbazine is relatively ineffective when used as a single agent. When it is used in combination with doxorubicin, however, the duration of remission is prolonged and survival is improved.[27] Cyclophosphamide is included in many regimens, inspite of the fact that it has marginal efficacy when used alone. Activity of ifosfamide, an analogue of cyclophosphamide, has been documented in patients who are refractory to combinations containing cyclophosphamide. Clinical evidence that there is no cross-resistance between ifosfamide and cyclophosphamide was demonstrated when responses were obtained in patients who had progressive disease while receiving cyclophosphamide.[28] The role of ifosfamide and doxorubicin in combination currently is being evaluated.

A dose-response relationship exists for doxorubicin in the treatment of soft tissue sarcomas. At a dose of 45 mg/m^2, the response rate is less than 20%, compared with a 37% response rate at a dose of 75 mg/m^2. A similar dose-response relationship exists when doxorubicin is combined with other agents. The regimens with the best results are those that involve the highest doses of doxorubicin.[27]

The most effective chemotherapy regimen for soft tissue sarcomas consists of the combination of cyclophosphamide, doxorubicin, and dacarbazine, which is known as CyADIC. When vincristine is added to the regimen, the combination is referred to by the acronym CYVADIC.[27]

Research in the treatment of soft tissue sarcomas includes the use of epirubicin and ifosfamide as induction (neoadjuvant) chemotherapy. Epirubicin is used in place of doxorubicin, since it has less cardiotoxicity and myelotoxicity.[29] One study concludes that the combination of cyclophosphamide, doxorubicin, and dacarbazine, given by continuous infusion, is an effective treatment approach for patients with advanced soft tissue sarcoma.[30] Further studies are under way to determine the maximal dose intensity that can be achieved with longer infusion times (continuous infusion over 4 days) with this drug combination.

In soft tissue sarcomas of the extremities, infusion of intraarterial cisplatinum over 4 hours and bolus injection of doxorubucin before surgical resection had a demonstrable antitumor effect.[31]

Combined Modalities

The use of combined modalities in the treatment of most soft tissue sarcomas is of recognized value. The main problems of management of soft tissue sarcomas of the extremities are local tumor recurrence and the ever-present risk of distant metastases. Recent emphasis on preservation of affected limbs in patients with soft tissue sarcomas of the extremities has led to a careful exploration of the possible roles of adjuvant radiation therapy and chemotherapy in the treatment of these patients.[5-7] The role of each treatment modality is considered in the overall treatment plan.

Radiation therapy given as a postoperative adjuvant to surgery may be useful in reducing local recurrence rates. Knowledge of the ability of radiation therapy to sterilize microscopic disease is evolving from ongoing clinical investigations and prospective randomized protocols.[19]

Intraarterial preoperative infusion of doxorubicin through the femoral artery in conjunction with radiation therapy has been effective as a multimodality treatment approach for soft tissue sarcomas of the extremity.[32,33] Postoperative doxorubicin and high-dose methotrexate, known to be effective for established metastases, also may delay or prevent distant metastases.[5,6]

Therapy by tourniquet infusion may be considered in attempts to preserve affected extremities. Tourniquet infusion is a method of regional chemotherapy that consists of placing a catheter in the major artery of the diseased extremity, applying a pneumatic tourniquet above the tip of the catheter, inflating it, and then injecting a drug bolus through the catheter. Local skin reactions manifesting as pain, edema, discoloration, hyperpigmentation, and subcutaneous induration in the region of the tip of the catheter occurred in 90% of reported cases.[34] These reactions did not preclude planned surgical procedures. Since only a small number of soft tissue sarcomas were treated in this manner, additional studies appear justified.[32,34,35]

Locally advanced and recurrent, bulky sarcomas are usually unresponsive to surgical, chemotherapeutic, or radiation procedures. Some of these tumors have responded to hyperthermia because tumor blood flow is comparatively poor and sluggish and tumor neovascularity appears to be incapable of augmenting the flow in response to heat, in contrast with normal tissues.[5] Noninvasive radiofrequency instrumentation that produces uniform heat to any depth without injury to superficial tissues has allowed investigation of heating capacity and effects of hyperthermia in advanced sarcomas. Its role in multimodality treatment may be enhanced because hyperthermia causes vascular thrombosis, making tumors more operable. Hyperthermia also seems to intensify the effects of radiation therapy and chemotherapy, and the in situ destruction may augment host-immune responses.[36]

Immunotherapy, including the use of interferon, combined with chemotherapy, currently is under investigation.[33] Randomized comparative clinical studies against standard treatments will be necessary to establish the role of α-interferon in future treatment protocols for soft tissue sarcomas.

REFERENCES

1. Pories WJ, Murinson DS, Rubin P: Soft tissue sarcoma, in Rubin P: Clinical Oncology: A Multidisciplinary Approach (ed 6). New York, American Cancer Society, 1983, pp 308-326.
2. Sears H: Soft tissue sarcoma: A historical overview. Semin Oncol 8:129-132, 1981.
3. Hajdu SI: Differential Diagnosis of Soft Tissue and Bone Tumors. Philadelphia, Lea & Febiger, 1985.
4. American Cancer Society: Cancer Facts and Figures—1989. Atlanta, American Cancer Society, 1989, p 8.
5. Storm FK, Morton DL, Eiber FR, et al: Sarcoma: Etiology and advances in therapy with immunotherapy, limb salvage surgery, and hyperthermia. Semin Oncol 8:229-237, 1981.
6. Rosenberg SA, Suit H, Baker LH, et al: Sarcomas of the soft tissue and bone, in DeVita VT, Hellman S, Rosenberg SA (eds): Cancer: Principles and Practice of Oncology. Philadelphia, JB Lippincott, 1982, pp 1036-1068.
7. Stout AP, Lattes R: Tumors of the Soft Tissues: Atlas of Tumor Pathology, 2nd Series, Fasc 1. Washington, DC, Armed Forces Institute of Pathology, 1967.
8. Suit HD, Proppe KH, Mankin HJ, et al: Preoperative radiation therapy for sarcoma of soft tissue. Cancer 47:2267-2274, 1981.
9. Russell WO, Cohen J, Edmonson JH, et al: Staging system for soft tissue sarcoma. Semin Oncol 8:156-159, 1981.
10. del Regato JA, Spjut HJ, Cox JD: Sarcomas of the Soft Tissues, in Cancer: Diagnosis, Treatment, and Prognosis (ed 6). St Louis, CV Mosby, 1985, pp 945-963.
11. Cadman NL, Soule EH, Kelley P: Synovial sarcoma—An analysis of 134 tumors. Cancer 18:613-627, 1965.
12. Hajdu SI, Shiu MH, Fortner JG: Tendosynovial sarcoma—A clinicopathological study of 136 cases. Cancer 39:1201-1217, 1977.
13. Enterline HT: Histopathology of sarcomas. Semin Oncol 8:133-155, 1981.
14. Hajdu SI, Rosen G: Sarcomas, in Calabresis P (ed): Medical Oncology: Basic Principles and Clinical Management. New York, Macmillan, 1985, pp 1193-1225.
15. Hajdu SI: Soft tissue sarcomas: Classification and natural history. CA 31:271-293, 1981.
16. Rosen G, Juergens H, Caparros B, et al: Combination chemotherapy (T-6) in the multidisciplinary treatment of Ewing's sarcoma. Natl Cancer Inst Monogr 56:213-220, 1981.
17. Suit HD, Proppe KH: Multidisciplinary Decisions in Oncology: Soft Tissue Sarcoma. New York, Pergamon Press, 1982.
18. Lindell MM, Wallace S, de Santos LA, et al: Diagnostic technique for the evaluation of soft tissue sarcoma. Semin Oncol 8:160-171, 1981.
19. Rosenberg SA, Glatstein EJ: Perspectives on the role of surgery and radiation therapy in the treatment of soft tissue sarcomas of the extremities. Semin Oncol 8:190-200, 1981.
20. American Joint Committee for Cancer Staging: Manual for Staging of Cancer. Philadelphia, JB Lippincott, 1988.
21. Potter DA, Glenn J, Kinsella T, et al: Patterns of recurrence in patients with high grade soft tissue sarcomas. J Clin Oncol 3:353-359, 1985.
22. Shiu MH, Hajdu SI: Management of soft tissue sarcoma of the extremity. Semin Oncol 8:172-179, 1981.

23. Coia LR, Moylan DJ: Soft tissue sarcomas, in Coia, LR, Moylan DJ (eds): Therapeutic Radiology for the House Officer. Baltimore, Williams and Wilkins, 1984, pp 200-207.
24. Enneking WF, McAuliffe JA: Adjunctive preoperative radiation therapy in treatment of soft tissue sarcomas: a preliminary report. Cancer Treat Symp 3:37-47, 1985.
25. Carabell SC, Goodman RL: Radiation therapy for soft tissue sarcoma. Semin Oncol 8:201-206, 1981.
26. Rosenberg SA, Suit HD, Baker LH: Sarcomas of soft tissue, in DeVita VT Jr, Hellman S, Rosenberg SA (eds): Cancer: Principles and Practice of Oncology (ed 2). Philadelphia, JB Lippincott, 1986, pp 1264-1283.
27. Benjamin RS: Soft tissue sarcomas, in Skeel RT: Handbook of Cancer Chemotherapy (ed 2). Boston, Little, Brown, 1987, pp 198-203.
28. Higgs D, Nagy C, Einhorn L: Ifosfamide: A clinical review. Semin Oncol Nurs 5:72-73, 1989.
29. Frustaci S, Foladore G, LoRe V, et al: Full doses of ifosfamide and epirubicin in advanced soft tissue sarcomas. Proc Am Soc Clin Oncol 8:319, 1989 (abstr).
30. Savage PD, Skubitz KM: Continuous infusion chemotherapy for soft tissue sarcomas. Proc Am Soc Clin Oncol 8:321, 1989 (abstr).
31. Benedetto P, Mnaymneh W, Ghandur-Mnaymneh L, et al: Neoadjuvant chemotherapy for extremity soft tissue sarcomas. Proc Am Soc Clin Oncol 8:323, 1989 (abstr).
32. Morton DL, Eilber FR, Townsend CM Jr, et al: Limb salvage from a multidisciplinary treatment approach for skeletal and soft tissue sarcomas of the extremity. Ann Surg 184:268-278, 1976.
33. Morton DL, Eilber FR, Grant T, et al: Multimodality therapy of malignant melanoma, skeletal and soft tissue sarcomas using immunotherapy, chemotherapy, and radiation therapy, in Jones SE, Salmon SE (eds): Adjuvant Therapy of Cancer II. New York, Grune & Stratton, 1979, pp 497-506.
34. Jaffe N, Cangir A, Lee Y, et al: Treatment of pediatric bone and soft tissue sarcoma with intraarterial cis-diamminedichloroplatinum-II, in Aigner KR, Patt YZ, Link KH, et al (eds): Regional Cancer Treatment. New York, Karger, 1988, pp 292-303.
35. Karakousis CP, Kanter PM, Park HC, et al: Tourniquet infusion versus hyperthermic perfusion. Cancer 49:850-858, 1982.
36. Storm FK, Morton DL, Elliot RS, et al: Radiofrequency hyperthermia of advanced human sarcomas. J Surg Oncol 17:91-98, 1981.

Chapter 48

Urologic and Male Genital Cancers

Julena M. Lind, RN, MN

Susie Lee Nakao, RN, MN

INTRODUCTION

Cancers of the prostate gland, bladder, and kidney are common in adult men and women. Testicular tumors, although rare, are important because they are the most common solid tumors in men between 29 and 35 years of age. Tumors of the urethra, penis, scrotum, epididymis, and seminal vesicles are rare and are not discussed in this chapter.

Figure 48-1 gives an overview of the sites of genitourinary tumors and metastases in men. Figure 48-2 represents the sites and routes of genitourinary tumor metastases in women.

PROSTATIC CANCER

Anatomy and Physiology

The prostate is a small, firm organ that is shaped like an inverted and flattened pyramid. It is made up of glands and musculature enclosed in a fibrous capsule. In the adult male, the prostate is usually about the size of a walnut (4 to 6 cm long). It lies posterior to the symphysis pubis, just inferior to the bladder, and in front of the rectum (Figure 48-3). The prostate gland is inverted so that its base is at the neck of the bladder. A segment of the urethra runs through the prostate and is known as the prostatic urethra.

Epidemiology

There are approximately 103,000 new cases of prostate cancer and 28,500 deaths from the disease in the United States each year.[1] Prostate cancer accounts for approximately 18% of all cancer in men in the United States and 10% of cancer deaths. It is the second most common cancer in American men.

The highest rate of prostatic cancer in the world is among black Americans. The disease is reportedly less common in African blacks, which suggests more than a genetic basis to the disease. Japan has the lowest prostatic cancer rate among countries with reliable reporting. When Japanese men migrate to the United States, the incidence of prostate cancer rises but remains only about half that of American whites.[2]

The other important demographic variable is age. Prostatic cancer is rare in men under 40 years of age, and the risk increases with age. The peak incidence is in men between 60 and 70 years of age. The higher incidence in blacks appears not to be associated with social class, since the age-adjusted rates in blacks to whites is the same across all social classes.[2]

There has been a significant relative rise in the incidence of prostatic cancer in asymptomatic American males ranging in age from 55 to 70.[3]

Etiology

Age, infectious agents, and endocrine factors are the three main etiologic factors hypothesized to be related to prostatic cancer.

Infectious agents, transmitted through sexual activity, have been suggested as possible etiologic factors in prostate cancer. In reviewing the results of several epidemiologic studies, it was recently concluded that measures of sexual activity, including number of sex partners, frequency of intercourse, early age at first intercourse, and particularly a history of venereal disease are associated with a high risk of prostatic cancer.[2]

The sexual transmission hypothesis was tested by the University of Southern California Cancer Surveillance Program. This study examined death rates and cancer death rates in celibate men (Catholic priests in the Archdiocese of Los Angeles) and compared those rates with the expected number of cancer deaths in white males in the United States for the same years. They found that cancer mortality was 79% of that expected in celibate men, but the incidence of prostatic cancer deaths was higher in these men than would be expected. The relatively high cancer mortality among celibate men argues against the theory of sexual transmission of this disease.[2]

The prostate's growth and function are controlled by hormones. Adenocarcinoma of the prostate appears difficult to induce in animal models. But testosterone alone, given subcutaneously, can produce this cancer in rats,[4] thus lending support to the theory that prostatic cancer has a hormonal basis. A few human epidemiologic studies focus on this hypothesis. One study of 77 subjects showed that individuals with prostatic cancer had higher levels of serum testosterone than healthy controls of the same age.[5] Another study, looking at the circulating steroid hormone levels in white and black college students, found that the mean testosterone level in blacks was 15% higher than that of whites, which might explain the twofold increased risk of prostatic cancer in American blacks.[6]

Certain case-controlled studies have looked at the consumption of dietary fat and its association with the incidence of prostatic cancer and have found that persons whose fat intake was above the median were at higher risk for prostate cancer.[7] The hypothesis is that the conversion of dietary fat to steroids in some way changes the hormonal environment.

Pathophysiology

Cellular characteristics

Prostatic cancers are almost always adenocarcinomas that vary in appearance and differentiation. They arise most commonly in the posterior lobe and are usually multifocal.[8]

Progression of disease

Prostatic tumors grow and spread locally to the seminal vesicles, bladder, and peritoneum. Despite the fact that

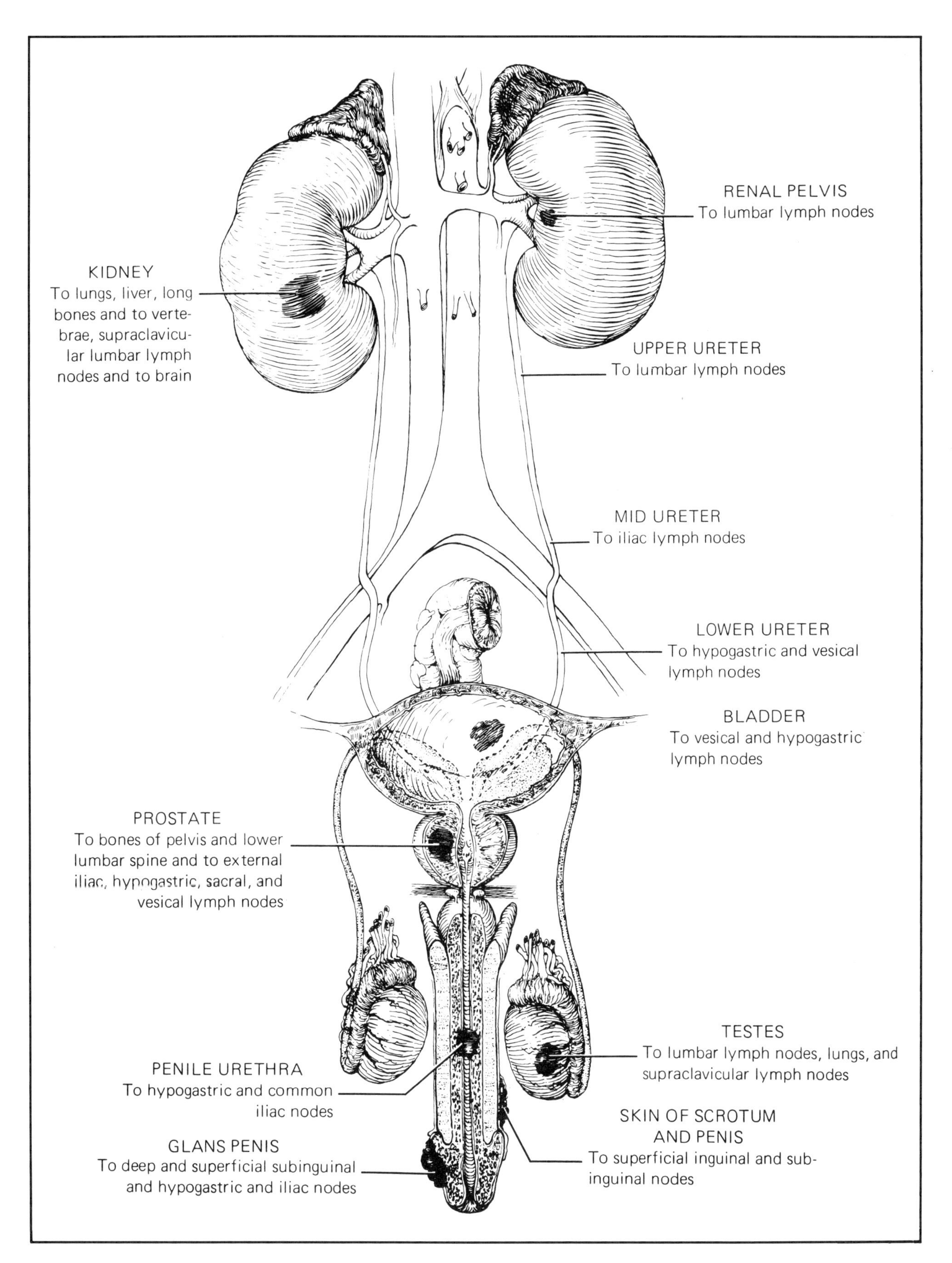

FIGURE 48-1 Sites of tumor origin and metastases in the male. (Source: Adapted from Johnson DE, Swanson DA, von Eschenbach AC: Tumors of the genitourinary tract, in Tanagho EA, McAninch, JW (eds) Smith's General Urology (ed 12). San Mateo, Calif, Appleton & Lange, 1987, p 332.)

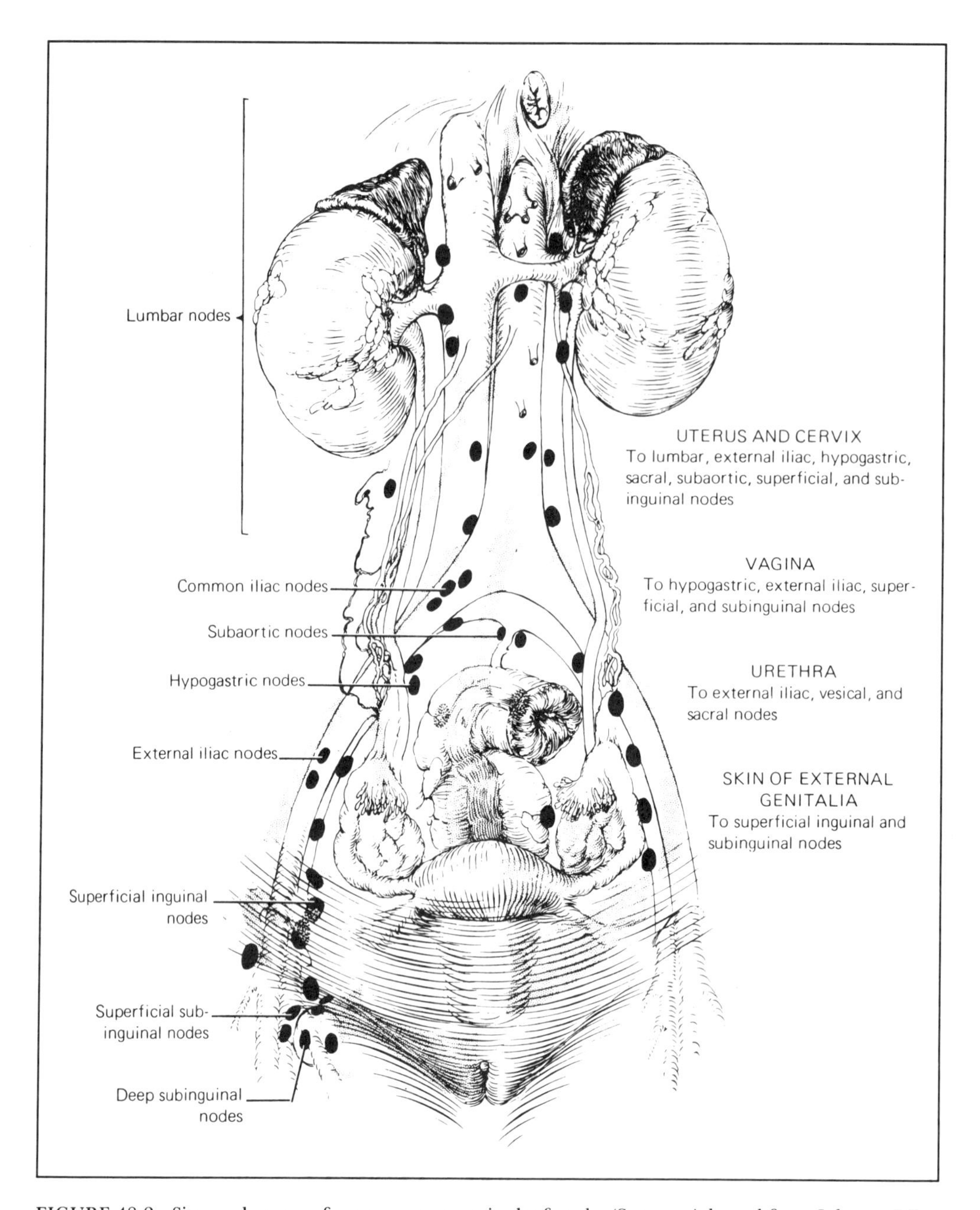

FIGURE 48-2 Sites and routes of tumor metastases in the female. (Source: Adapted from Johnson DE, Swanson DA, von Eschenbach AC: Tumors of the genitourinary tract, in Tanagho EA, McAninch JW (eds): Smith's General Urology (ed 12). San Mateo, Calif, Appleton & Lange, 1987, p 333.)

many prostatic tumors are extremely slow growing and indolent, it appears that there is an unusually wide range of biologic malignancy. Some prostatic tumors are rapidly progressive and fatal, some have intermediate behavior, and others are detected only accidentally and remain quiescent.

Adenocarcinoma of the prostate spreads by way of the blood vessels and lymphatic system. It spreads in the perineural lymphatics, involving the seminal vesicles and the sacral, external iliac, and lumbar lymph nodes. One third of men with early cancer have evidence of metastases to the pelvic lymph nodes.[9] From the pelvis the lymphatic fluids travel to the thoracic duct and enter the venous system at the junction of the left internal jugular and the left subclavian veins. Because the supraclavicular nodes lie adjacent to the veins that communicate with the thoracic duct, patients with widespread cancer often have scalene or supraclavicular node involvement.

Hematogenous spread of prostatic cancer typically involves the lungs, liver, kidneys, and bones. Nearly half the men who die of prostate cancer have lung metastases on autopsy, and 66% have bone metastases.[9] The vertebrae, pelvis, femur, and ribs are often involved.

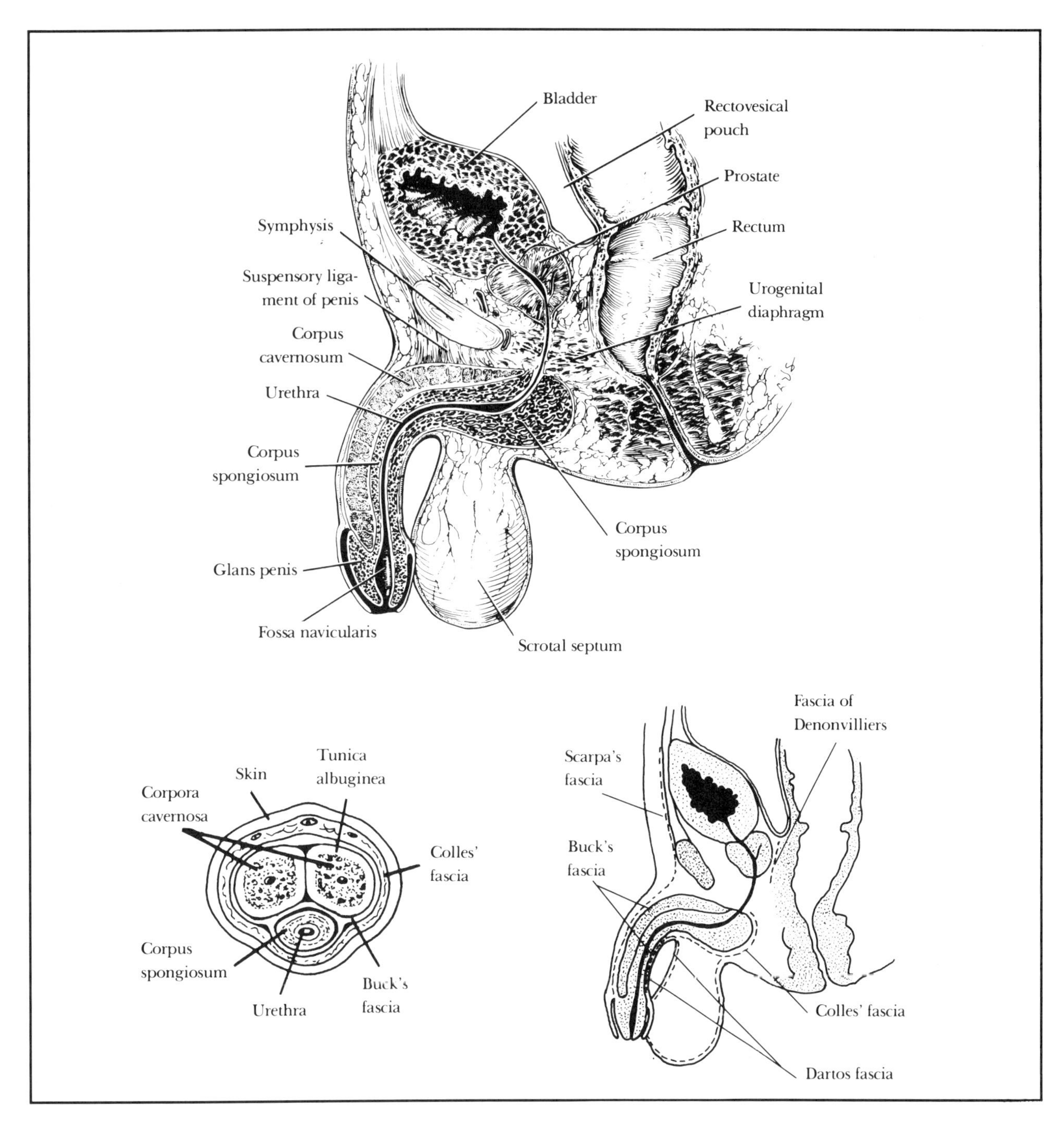

FIGURE 48-3 Relation of the bladder, prostate, seminal vesicles, penis, urethra, and scrotal contents. (Source: Tanagho EA: Anatomony of the genitourinary tract, in Tanagho EA, McAninch JW (eds): Smith's General Urology (ed 12). San Mateo, Calif, Appleton & Lange, 1987, p 10.)

Clinical Manifestations

Prostatic cancer is usually asymptomatic in its early stages. Detection occurs as a result of routine rectal examination that reveals a nodule or mass. Because the posterior surface of the prostate is in close contact with the rectum, it is the only portion that may be palpated. Tumors also may be discovered during examination of transurethral resection specimens.

A common presenting picture is an elderly man with weight loss, back pain, and prostatism. Other symptoms include urinary frequency and nocturia, dysuria, slow urinary stream, or hematuria. Unfortunately, many of these symptoms are similar to other disorders, particularly benign prostatic hypertrophy. About 5% of men with prostatic cancer will have their first symptoms from metastases. Signs related to spread of the disease are anemia and weight loss, lumbosacral pain (which may radiate to the hips or down the legs), and hematuria if the bladder or urethra has been invaded.

Assessment

Screening

Of the many prostatic cancer controversies, screening techniques and their value are among the most controversial. Screening of asymptomatic males for prostatic cancer by any means has not shown true benefit to date.[10] There are, however, several areas of disagreement. Three mechanisms currently exist to aid in early detection of prostatic cancer: digital rectal examination; transrectal ultrasonography; and biochemical markers, particularly prostatic acid phosphatase and prostate-specific antigen (PSA). An optimal screening test should be safe, inexpensive, widely available, accurate, and have a reasonable specificity for the disease. The goal of effective screening in prostatic cancer should be to diagnose more stage A and B1 lesions and to improve survival. There has been no satisfactory study of a true high-risk group of asymptomatic men that has met all the preceding requirements and detected more early cancers.[10]

Rectal palpation has been the most important step in detecting carcinoma of the prostate, and there is an increased incidence of early detection when digital rectal examination is done routinely.[11,12] However, the value of the rectal examination in screening an asymptomatic population is debatable. First, optimal age to begin screening has not been determined; second, many hard nodules are benign disorders, and several studies have shown that there is little correlation between the clinical impression during rectal examination and the biopsy results. It is currently estimated that the positive predictive value of an abnormal rectal examination ranges from 11% to 26%.[11]

Transrectal ultrasound was initially thought to be a very useful screening modality. Today, evaluation of this technique is being weighed in light of (1) the expense of the equipment, (2) the steep learning curves for both the imager and the clinicians, (3) the fact that the positive predictive value of a transrectal ultrasound is in the range of 30% to 35%, and (4) the fact that studies indicate the false-positive and false-negative rates are unacceptably high.[11] Others argue that the future of early detection and improved survival depends on finding those 70% of cancers that lie in the peripheral zone and that can be visualized by this procedure.[10,13] A recent study by Lee et al[14] concludes that transrectal ultrasound is more sensitive than digital rectal examination in detecting prostate cancer, and they advocate its broader implementation. Others counter that the study supports the concept of "case finding" and not screening in the true sense.[13]

Various markers including serum acid phosphatase, prostatic acid phosphatase, and serum and bone alkaline phosphatase have been used in the diagnosis and staging of prostatic cancer. However, none of these markers has been reliable in detecting early cancer.[15] A new serum marker, PSA, has recently been identified. This antigen is made exclusively by prostatic tissue, and it is immunologically distinct from prostatic acid phosphatase. Although PSA appears to be useful in monitoring patients with advanced disease, its use as a screening study has yet to be proved. It does, however, appear much more promising than the other markers, which all have high false-positive rates.[11,15]

In conclusion, to date there is no single, effective screening test for prostatic cancer. Several factors contribute to this lack:

1. Because of the puzzling natural history of prostate cancer, no test currently in use can reliably separate potentially aggressive tumors from those that will remain indolent.
2. The wide variations in applying screening techniques from digital rectal examinations to transrectal ultrasound prohibit accurate comparisons of results.
3. Two important biases confound the interpretation of screening study findings. Lead time bias happens when earlier diagnosis results in a greater duration of life (after diagnosis and treatment) without extending survival. The other bias is length bias, in which cancers that are not progressing or are progressing very slowly are included in statistical calculations. This automatically improves survival rates but actually dilutes the real impact of screening techniques.[16]

Although controversy surrounds screening for prostatic cancer, early detection is probably best done with routine yearly digital examination beginning at age 50. When an abnormality is found, other studies including biopsy, ultrasonography and serum prostatic acid phosphatase would be of benefit.[11]

Diagnosis

Common procedures used to diagnose prostatic cancer include rectal examination, biopsy, chemical studies, cytologic examination of urine and prostatic fluid, excretory urogram, bone scans, computed tomography (CT) and magnetic resonance imaging (MRI).

On rectal examination the consistency of the prostate normally feels rather rubbery. Early cancer presents as a nonraised, firm lesion that often has a sharp edge. Advanced cancer is hard and stonelike. The difficulty is in differentiating the firm areas of the prostate that might be cancer from infection, tuberculosis, and prostatic calculi.

Every suspected prostatic mass should be biopsied.[17] Various techniques are used. Transrectal or transperineal needle biopsy is most commonly used in the United States. Needle aspiration consists of inserting a fine needle into the prostate and aspirating cells with a syringe. Open biopsy is probably the most accurate technique, but a high degree of morbidity is associated with this procedure.

Because of the difficulty in diagnosing prostate cancer, some researchers have argued for the use of flow cytometry to help in confirming a cytopathologic diagnosis.[18] Flow cytometry can examine prostatic needle biopsy aspirate for DNA content and help to predict the biologic potential of the disease based on changes in the DNA.

Serum prostatic acid phosphatase can now be distinguished with a radioimmunologic technique. Eighty percent of men with stage D cancer have an increased serum prostatic acid phosphatase level.[17] An elevation of this enzyme is considered to indicate advanced disease regardless of whether the metastatic sites are obvious. The use of this test is generally inexpensive; although it is fairly accurate when in the high range, it is difficult to interpret when the acid phosphatase is in the normal or near normal range.[19]

As mentioned previously, PSA, has also been shown to be a good tumor marker. In fact, some researchers feel that serial serum PSAs are the most sensitive marker of localized and metastatic disease.[19]

Other serum factors also may be elevated. The isoenzyme of lactic dehydrogenase have been elevated in men with prostatic cancer. An increase in serum creatinine and urea nitrogen values occurs if the cancer is causing an obstruction associated with renal back pressure or ureteral occlusion.

Additional studies may include cytologic examination of urine and expressed prostatic fluid, which is positive in as many as 85% of men with prostate cancer. An excretory urogram may be done to demonstrate hydroureteronephrosis as a result of obstruction (caused by metastases to the pelvic lymph nodes) or direct invasion by the primary tumor. Bone scans have demonstrated metastases in 75% of patients with advanced disease.[17] CT scans can help to diagnose pelvic lymph node involvement, and MRI can demonstrate involvement of the seminal vesicles and changes in the contour of the prostate.[17,20]

Classification and Staging

The stages of prostatic cancer commonly used in the United States are as follows[21]:

Stage A	Tumor not clinically palpable but detectable in microscopic sections by biopsy or transurethral resection
Stage A1	Clinically occult carcinoma, well differentiated, focal
Stage A2	Clinically occult carcinoma, poorly differentiated, multifocal
Stage B	Palpable tumor confined to the prostate, with no distant metastases
Stage B1	Palpable tumor involving less than one lobe
Stage B2	Palpable tumor involving more than one lobe
Stage C	Tumor extending beyond the prostatic capsule (including the seminal vesicles), with or without invasion of contiguous organs but with no distant metastases
Stage D1	Metastases confined to the pelvis (including positive pelvic nodes)
Stage D2	Distant metastases

TABLE 48-1 TNM System of Staging Prostate Cancer

Primary Tumor (T)		
TX		Minimum requirements to assess the primary tumor cannot be met.
T0		No tumor present
	T1a	No palpable tumor; on histologic sections no more than three high-power fields of carcinoma found
	T1b	No palpable tumor; histologic sections revealing more than three high-power fields of prostatic carcinoma
	T2a	Palpable nodule less than 1.5 cm in diameter with compressible, normal-feeling tissue on at least three sides
	T2b	Palpable nodule more than 1.5 cm in diameter or nodule or induration in both lobes
T3		Palpable tumor extending into or beyond the prostatic capsule
	T3a	Palpable tumor extending into the periprostatic tissues or involving one seminal vesicle
	T3b	Palpable tumor extending into the periprostatic tissues, involving one or both seminal vesicles; tumor size more than 6 cm in diameter
T4		Tumor fixed or involving neighboring structures
Nodal Involvement (N)		
NX		Minimum requirements to assess the regional nodes cannot be met.
N0		No involvement of regional lymph nodes
N1		Involvement of a single homolateral regional lymph node
N2		Involvement of contralateral, bilateral, or multiple regional lymph nodes
N3		A fixed mass present on the pelvic wall with a free space between this and the tumor
Distant Metastasis (M)		
MX		Minimum requirements to assess the presence of distant metastasis cannot be met.
M0		No (known) distant metastasis
M1		Distant metastasis present

Source: American Joint Committee for Cancer Staging and End Results Reporting: Manual for Staging of Cancer. Chicago, The Committee, 1983.

Table 48-1 shows the TNM classification system for prostatic cancer, and Figure 48-4 illustrates staging according to the clinical and radiologic estimates of tumor involvement.

A staging workup to determine the presence of metastases should be done. The tests that might be included are chest radiography to show hilar nodes and involvement of lungs and ribs; plain radiograph of the abdomen to show typical osteoblastic metastases; bone scans to show areas of bony metastases; and pelvic CT scans to show extraprostatic extension, including enlarged lymph nodes.

In some centers staging pelvic lymphadenectomies have been advocated to aid in treatment selection. The rationale is that the pelvic lymphadenectomy will more

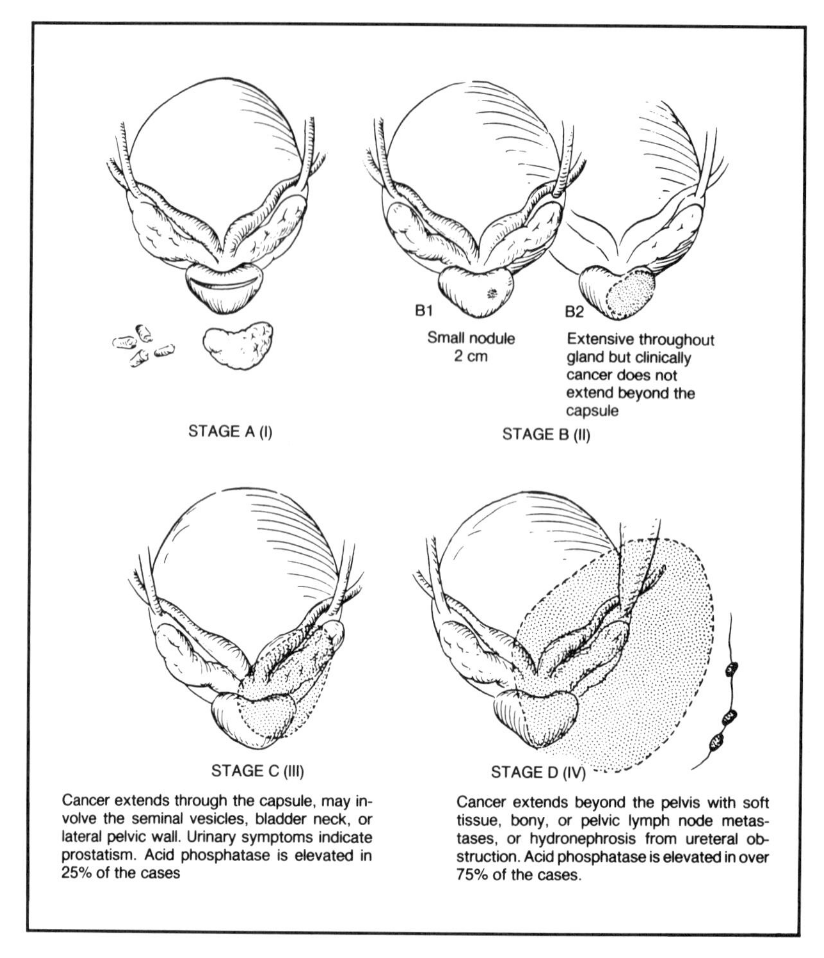

FIGURE 48-4 Staging according to clinical and radiologic involvement. (Source: From Skinner DG: Current concepts concerning carcinoma of the prostate, in Nyhus L (ed): Surgery Annual. New York, Appleton-Century-Crofts, 1973, p 393.)

accurately define the anatomic extent of spread. In men who are free of bony disease and have a negative acid phosphatase level and no other signs of metastases, it is important to define accurately whether there is nodal involvement.[17] Treatment will differ and will be less surgically aggressive if nodal involvement is present.

The Gleason classification system is also widely incorporated into today's staging profiles.[22] This is a system of histopathologic grading based on the glandular pattern of the tumor at relatively low magnification.[23] Combining clinical staging and histopathologic grading helps predict the biologic potential of prostate cancer.

Treatment

The treatment of prostatic cancer remains controversial. Four methods have been applied alone or in combination: surgery, radiotherapy, endocrine manipulation, and chemotherapy.

Surgery

Radical prostatectomy The term *radical prostatectomy* refers to the surgical removal of the entire prostate, including the true prostatic capsule, the seminal vesicles, and a portion of the bladder neck. Total prostatectomy may involve taking only a portion of the attached seminal vesicles. In the radical prostatectomy, removal is from the bladder neck to just beyond the apex of the prostate gland (Figure 48-5). The remaining portion of the bladder neck is then reanastomosed to the urethra.

Radical perineal prostatectomy is a common surgical method of choice.[24,25] Although this approach prohibits simultaneous pelvic lymphadenectomy, many authorities feel that it permits better visualization and better vesicle neck reconstruction and reanastomosis of the bladder to the urethra.[25] The individual is placed in an exaggerated lithotomy position for this surgery. Possible complications include infection and fecal incontinence from sphincter injury.

Radical retropubic prostatectomy provides for a simultaneous pelvic lymphadenectomy and may make a

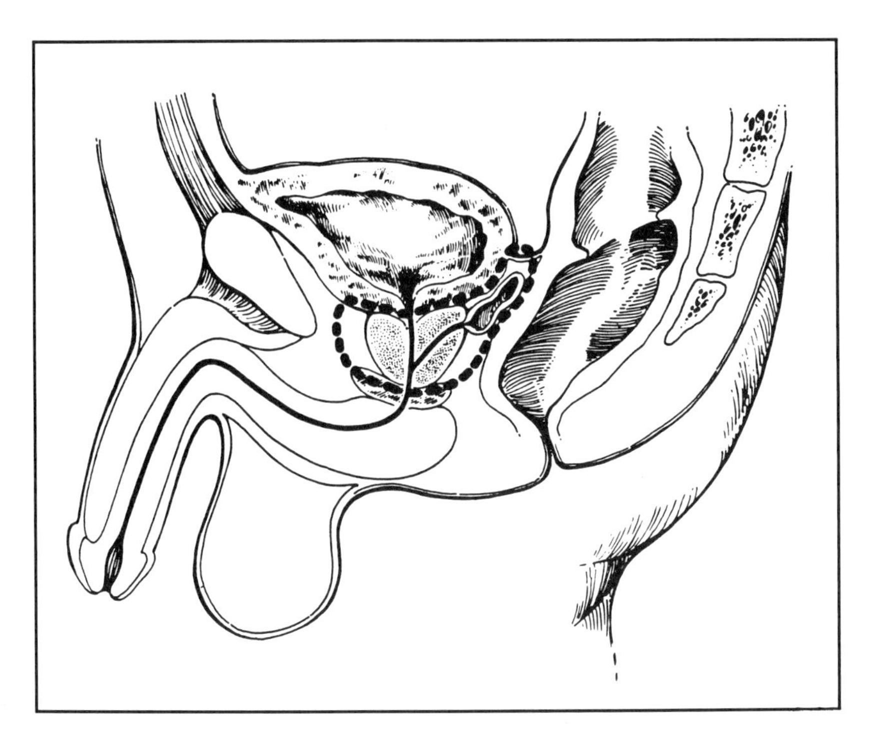

FIGURE 48-5 Surgical boundaries of a radical prostatectomy. The specimen includes the prostate with the true prostatic capsule and the seminal vesicles. (Source: Swanson D: Cancer of the bladder and prostate. The impact of therapy on sexual function, in von Eschenbach AC, Rodriguez D (eds): Sexual Rehabilitation of the Urologic Cancer Patient. Boston, GK Hall, 1981, p 93.)

high-riding prostate gland more accessible. The retropubic approach is preferred by some authorities, who feel that it provides more urinary control and less stricture formation.[26] Complications of this approach include thromboembolism (which can be prevented by administering anticoagulants postoperatively); infection (the risk of which is greater if a penile prosthesis is implanted at surgery); and rarely lymphedema.[26]

Sexual dysfunction is a common sequela of radical prostatectomy. All men undergoing radical prostatectomy will have absence of emission and ejaculation because of removal of the seminal vesicles and transection of the vas deferens. Loss of the ability to achieve an erection also occurs. An impotency rate of 90% has been reported following radical prostatectomy.[27] Erectile potency, however, does not depend on ejaculatory potency but rather on a combination of other factors. Psychologic aspects, blood supply, and nerve supply all work together to determine erectile potency. In a radical prostatectomy, it is not exactly clear why impotence should happen, and in fact up to 10% of men are still able to achieve an erection after this surgery.[27]

The internal pudendal artery is the major blood supply for the erectile tissue and should not be significantly damaged during surgery.[28] The nerves responsible for potency are much more at risk. The autonomic nerve fibers that supply the area are susceptible to damage during dissection of the prostate, prostatic capsule, and seminal vesicles. If a pelvic lymph node dissection is included, the risk of damage is even greater. Patients undergoing a radical retropubic prostatectomy with limited pelvic lymph node dissection will almost certainly experience erectile impotence.[26] Anatomic differences may influence which men retain erectile potency. In some men some nerves may simply escape surgical damage.

In 1982, it was suggested by Walsh and Donker[29] that postprostatectomy impotence was caused by damage to the pelvic nerve plexus that innervate the corpora cavernosa. Subsequently Walsh modified the technique for radical retropubic prostatectomy to avoid injury to the pelvic nerves by visualizing and preserving the nerve bundles intraoperatively. This approach has saved sexual function in a large majority of patients, up to 72% potency in some reports.[30] It has also shown fewer problems with incontinence.[31]

Subtotal prostatectomy Subtotal prostatectomy can be either an open enucleative approach or a TUR. In a TUR, a resectoscope is inserted through the urethra and the prostatic tissue is scraped out with a movable loop of metal that cuts tissue with a high-frequency current, which is turned on by a foot pedal. A resectoscope has an insulated sheath that protects the urethra from damage. This approach is not used as a curative surgical technique for prostatic cancer.

In the transurethral process, the bladder neck is altered anatomically. This virtually destroys the competence of the internal bladder sphincter. The closure of this physiologic sphincter is necessary for the ejaculation of seminal fluid. Thus the destruction of the sphincter allows the seminal fluid to pass retrograde (back into the bladder) rather than antegrade (out through the penis). This is known as retrograde ejaculation and almost always happens after TUR. Some men equate ejaculation with normal sexual functioning. The loss of the sensation of ejaculation may be confused with the loss of sexual interest or potency.

Reports about the incidence of actual erectile dysfunction after transurethral prostatectomy (TURP) are conflicting. Psychologic factors probably play a large part in this type of impotence.

Radiotherapy

External beam radiotherapy Radiotherapy as a cure for prostatic cancer is relatively new. The usual dose is 6000 to 7000 rad (cGy) for cure and 4000 to 5000 cGy for palliation. One example of a curative radiotherapy treatment regimen includes local and extended field irradiation of both the primary tumor and the first-echelon lymphatic drainage.[32] A four-field technique is used for anterior, posterior, left lateral, and right lateral fields (Figure 48-6). A dose of 7000 cGy is delivered in 7 weeks to the prostate at 200 cGy/day. A dose of 5000 cGy in 7 weeks is delivered to the pelvic lymph nodes at 200 cGy/day. This is accomplished by giving 2600 cGy (at 200 cGy/day) through the four-field technique. Another 2000 cGy is given to the prostate and the periprostatic tissue over a 2-week period, and then the four-field technique is reinstituted for another 2400 cGy.[32]

Common side effects of radiotherapy to the prostate are proctitis, diarrhea, and urinary frequency. These side effects usually develop toward the end of treatment, and complications requiring hospitalization are infrequent (only 6% of all men treated with curative radiotherapy).[33] Impotency rates following external beam radiotherapy vary from 20% to 40%.[32,33] The reason for the erectile dysfunction is unknown, but in most series age is a critical variable, and the higher potency rates usually apply to men under 60 years of age.[32]

Internal radiotherapy Interstitial radioactive gold (^{198}Au) and radioactive iodine implantation (^{125}I) have both been used as treatment methods in prostatic cancer. The radioactive gold grains have a half-life of 2.7 days

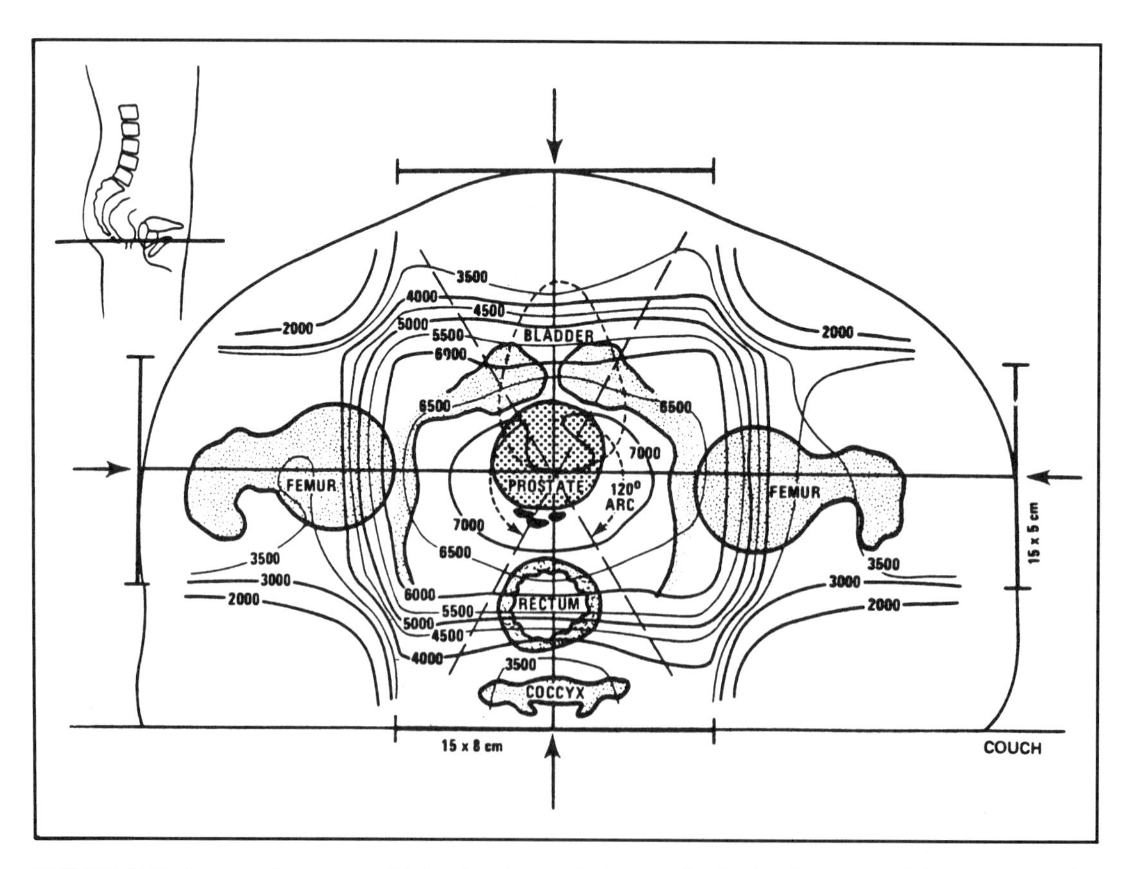

FIGURE 48-6 A composite pattern of full-pelvic-dose radiotherapy distribution for cancer of the prostate. Shows the four-field box technique integrated with the left and right 120-degree lateral arc for the prostatic boost. (Source: Bagshaw M: Radiation therapy for cancer of the prostate, in Skinner DG, deKernion J (eds): Genitourinary Cancer. Philadelphia, WB Saunders, 1978, p 367.)

and are inserted through a needle implanter after the prostate is surgically exposed. After implantation, the wound is irrigated and closed without drainage. This method delivers approximately 3000 to 3500 cGy directly to the prostate, thereby sparing normal local tissue. After 2 weeks, a course of external beam radiotherapy is begun, with 4000 to 5000 cGy delivered to the prostate and the periprostatic area.[34]

Radioactive iodine has a half-life of 60 days and is implanted under anesthesia with the patient in a modified lithotomy position. Hollow 17-gauge needles 15 cm long are placed in the prostate, parallel to one another about 1 cm apart in an anterioposterior direction. The radioactive iodine seeds, which are 4.5 mm long, are inserted through these hollow needles at intervals of 0.5 to 1.0 cm, and the needle is then withdrawn. The crossing of the prostatic urethra or bladder neck by the hollow needles is inevitable but does not seem to present later complications.[35]

The most common problem associated with ^{125}I implantation is delayed irritative voiding symptoms. Proctitis, rectal ulceration, or fistula has also occurred.[34] Complications of gold seed implantation are similar to ^{125}I. In both these methods, sexual function is preserved in 70% to 90% of individuals potent before treatment.[34]

Endocrine manipulation

About 85% of prostatic cancers are androgen dependent. Approximately 50% of patients have metastases at diagnosis, and the mainstay of treatment of advanced prostate cancer is to decrease the circulating androgens. Androgen-dependent tissues get androgen from the testes, the adrenal glands, or both. The testes produce 90% to 95% of the circulating testosterone, which is the most powerful androgen. Normally, a low level of testosterone signals the hypothalamus, through a negative feedback mechanism, to secrete gonadotropin-releasing hormone (GnRH), which stimulates the pituitary to release luteinizing hormone (LH). The LH stimulates Leydig's cells in the testes to synthesize testosterone. The testosterone secreted by Leydig's cells enables spermatogenesis at Sertoli's cells in the testicular seminiferous tubules. The adrenal glands also produce the weak androgens, androstenedione and dehydroepiandrosterone, which account for 5% of all androgens. By the same negative feedback mechanism, the hypothalamus signals the pituitary gland to release adrenocorticotropic hormone, (ACTH), which stimulates the adrenal glands to secrete androstenedione and dihydroepiandrosterone. If testosterone production through the testes has been inhibited for any reason, the adrenal glands will also produce testosterone.

The most common intracellular androgen is dihydrotestosterone. For the hormone to have an effect within the cell, it must bind with a receptor protein.

If the prostatic cancer cell depends on androgens for its growth, it seems logical to block androgen formation or use at some point in the cycle. The major methods of endocrine manipulation in the treatment of patients with prostate cancer are as follows:

1. Bilateral orchiectomy, which removes the organs that primarily produce androgens, and rapidly and directly lowers plasma testosterone levels
2. Administration of estrogen (in the form of diethylstilbestrol [DES]), which is the most common form of therapy and has been used for over 40 years to block the release of LH
3. Adrenalectomy, which removes the secondary source of androgen production either surgically or "medically" through the use of drugs
4. Administration of antiandrogen drugs, which interfere with intracellular androgen activity
5. Administration of GnRH analogs, which if given in large doses over time disrupt the pulsatile release of GnRH and cause a paradoxical suppression of gonadotropins and testosterone levels
6. Total androgen ablation, which simultaneously blocks both adrenal and testicular androgens

Orchiectomy, or removal of the testes, is a brief surgical procedure with little morbidity or mortality that immediately stops the production of testicular androgens. Bilateral orchiectomy will reduce plasma testosterone levels by 90%. Advantages of orchiectomy over a medical approach include immediate response, elimination of cardiac complications, and no problems with patient compliance.[36]

DES, 1 to 3 mg/day orally, is the estrogen most commonly used and is the least expensive. Examples include Premarin, estradiol, Stilphostrol (given intravenously in high doses), and estramustine phosphate, which is a combination of nitrogen mustard and estrogen. Major complications of DES are cardiogenic and include cardiac failure and edema. Other side effects are gynecomastia, loss of libido, and impotency. Individuals are also at increased risk of thrombophlebitis, especially if the dosages are high.[37]

Adrenalectomy (either surgical or medical with aminoglutethimide or other drugs) blocks adrenal androgens and has been proposed for those individuals who originally responded to hormonal therapy but have since relapsed. Surgical adrenalectomy is associated with significant mortality and is not commonly used today.[37] Aminoglutethimide may help one third of those who have relapsed after primary endocrine therapy (with orchiectomy or estrogen).[38] Side effects of aminoglutethimide therapy include lethargy, ataxia, hypotension, nausea, and hypothyroidism.[36] Other drugs that produce a medical adrenalectomy are ketoconazole, spironolactone, and glucocorticoids. Ketoconazole is an antifungal agent that, if given in high doses, will inhibit androgen production. Decreased libido, weakness, and lethargy are side effects of this drug.[38] Spironolactone inhibits adrenal and testicular precursors. Glucocorticoids suppress ACTH and provide only rare responses with significant side effects.[36]

Antiandrogens peripherally inhibit the action of dihydrotestosterone, usually by interfering with receptor steroid binding at the intracellular level. Cyproterone acetate, flutamide, and megesterol acetate are antiandrogen drugs that have been used.

Cyproterone acetate has fewer cardiac complications

than DES or megesterol acetate. Side effects include mild gynecomastia and peripheral edema. Flutamide is a potent antiandrogen without estrogenic activity and without cardiopulmonary complications. It seems to be more effective in patients who have received no prior endocrine therapy. Potency is retained in 33% to 80% of the patients who were potent before treatment.[36] Megesterol acetate decreases LH release, but studies show that there is an "escape" phenomenon after 6 months of treatment, where the androgen production is no longer totally blocked.[38]

Administration of GnRH analogs is one of the latest attempts at managing advanced prostate cancer through endocrine manipulation. The literature often confusingly describes specific drugs as luteinizing-hormone-releasing hormones (LHRH) rather than the broader, more generic term GnRH. For this text, the term GnRH will be used to refer to all gonadotropin-releasing hormone analogs.

Normally, GnRH is released in a pulselike manner from the hypothalamus and stimulates the pituitary gland to release LH in men. LH subsequently controls the release of testosterone. Administration of GnRH initially causes an abrupt *increase* in LH release and subsequent testosterone release. However, after the acute "flare" period, testosterone levels paradoxically fall to castration level.[38] The exact mechanism is not clear, but it probably involves changes and confusion in the central feedback control of LH release or desensitization of the gonad to high levels of LH by reducing the number of gonadal LH receptor sites.[38] Ultimately the biologic effect is that of chemical castration with fewer toxic side effects than estrogen therapy.

Three drugs have been studied in clinical trials: LHRH (Lupron, Leuporlide), Buserelin, and Zoladex. LHRH has been tested the most extensively in the United States. In trials, responses were equal to DES or orchiectomy in patients previously untreated by endocrine therapy. Side effects include loss of libido and hot flashes.[36]

Buserelin is a compound that can be given intranasally or subcutaneously with results similar to LHRH. One study reported a high frequency of durable objective and subjective responses in patients with advanced prostate cancer. Side effects consist of hot flashes, loss of libido, and impotence.[39]

Zoladex has been studied in Britain with clinical improvement demonstrated. Zoladex is given subcutaneously, with some irritation reported at the injection site.[36]

Total androgen ablation has been proposed for first-line endocrine treatment as an alternative to testicular androgen ablation alone. This can take various forms: antiandrogen drugs, such as flutamide combined with estrogen; orchiectomy plus adrenalectomy; or GnRH plus antiandrogens. It is not yet clear whether this type of treatment has any survival benefit over conventional endocrine therapy.[38]

In general, 70% to 85% of patients with advanced prostatic tumors respond to hormonal manipulation. This response is demonstrated by a definite regression in tumor size, lessening of the degree of urinary obstruction, disappearance of or decrease in bone pain, and weight gain. The duration of response is from 1 to 3 years. Only 10% survive 10 years after the start of endocrine therapy. The palliative role of hormonal therapy therefore is significant. It has not been possible, however, to establish whether orchiectomy and/or estrogen therapy can increase overall survival.[36]

Chemotherapy

There is a limited role for chemotherapy in the treatment of patients with advanced, hormonally unresponsive prostatic cancer. Both single agents and combination protocols have been attempted.

Chemotherapy appears to have a palliative benefit in men with hormone-resistant cancers. Single agents appear to be as effective as combination chemotherapy.[40] Active single agents include cyclophosphamide, methotrexate, doxorubicin, 5-fluorouracil (5-FU), cisplatin, mitomycin C and dacarbazine (DTIC). Drugs that have been used in combinations include doxorubicin, 5-FU, and mitomycin C. Other agents that combine a hormonal agent with an antineoplastic agent such as estramustine phosphate have been combined in protocols with cyclophosphamide.[41]

The results of a recent animal study argue for combining surgery and adjuvant cyclophosphamide chemotherapy in the treatment of patients with metastatic prostate cancer to minimize the total tumor burden and try to improve the cure rate.[42]

Numerous clinical studies have shown that chemotherapy has an acceptable risk-benefit ratio in the treatment of patients with advanced prostatic cancer.[41]

Treatment according to stage

Stage A In stage A disease, clinically occult cancer is detected incidentally. The tissue is described according to the degree of differentiation present. If the tumor is well differentiated, follow-up may be the only treatment recommendation, since most tumors have a slow growth potential. However, this approach may cause difficulties because it is common for prostatic tumors to have multiple foci, and the single needle biopsy might have missed the more aggressive cells in the neoplastic clone.

The common treatment approach for stage A tumors that are not well differentiated is radical perineal or retropubic prostatectomy. Some centers also recommend pelvic lymph node dissection.[26]

Stage B Stage B is defined as a palpable tumor in one or more lobes that has not extended through the prostatic capsule. Although radical prostatectomy is the standard treatment for these tumors, characteristics of the individual are important. A younger man or one who is more physically capable of tolerating surgery, with no evidence of metastases by bone scan and no increased level of prostatic acid phosphatase, is a much more likely surgical candidate. Pelvic lymphadenectomy might be included for those men at higher risk for metastases (ie, those with more than one lobe involved or with diffuse involvement of the prostate). The problems associated with this procedure are pulmonary embolus, sepsis, wound infection, and hematoma.

Radiotherapy for patients with stage B prostatic cancer is becoming increasingly popular. In the few studies available on stage B cancer, the long-term outcome for radical prostatectomy and radiation therapy is similar. For the 10% of prostate cancers detected at this stage, it appears that either radiation therapy or surgery has equally curative results, with fewer complications reported for radiation therapy.[33]

Stage C Between 40% and 50% of men present clinically with stage C disease, which extends through the prostatic capsule or involves the bladder neck or seminal vesicles. Many men with this stage of disease have occult bone or pelvic lymph node metastases. However, a well-differentiated tumor of this stage is less likely to have occult metastases. The acid phosphatase level may be elevated, but there should be no evidence of metastases on bone scan.[17]

A variety of treatment options have been recommended for patients with stage C prostatic cancer: (1) radical prostatectomy with or without pelvic lymph node dissection; (2) preoperative radiotherapy (to convert stage C to stage B) followed by radical prostatectomy and lymph node dissection; (3) external beam radiotherapy alone; (4) internal implants (^{125}I or ^{198}Au) with lymphadenectomy; and (5) hormonal therapy as a postsurgical or postradiotherapy adjunct. There are conflicting studies about whether lymph node dissection added to radical prostatectomy improves long-term survival.

Reports on external beam radiotherapy (as an alternative to radical surgery) also have interpretation problems. There are inconsistencies in the grading and staging of stage C tumors, making it difficult to compare survival statistics. Aggressive external beam radiotherapy of the prostate and potential regional adenopathy is recommended by some as the best hope for cure with the fewest side effects for men with stage C prostatic cancer.[32]

The results of interstitial implant treatment may well be comparable with external beam radiotherapy and offer fewer side effects.[34,35]

The addition of hormonal therapy to either surgery or radiotherapy has not been proved to add years to survival time.[32,36]

The choice of therapy depends on the person's physical condition, actual spread of cancer, degree of differentiation or grade of the tumor, and the person's preference.

Stage D Stage D disease involves metastases, either confined to the pelvis (including pelvic lymph nodes), D1, or distant metastases, D2. Stage D is the most common presenting clinical stage. There is no surgical cure for patients with this stage. Men with D1 lesions who have only limited nodal involvement might benefit from pelvic lymph dissection, but in individuals with extensive nodal disease, a biopsy is probably enough. Treatment options for men with advanced prostatic cancer include hormonal manipulation, interstitial or external beam radiotherapy, or chemotherapy. A common treatment plan for patients with stage D disease might include interstitial or external beam radiotherapy followed by hormonal therapy and possibly chemotherapy and then second-line hormonal manipulation followed by chemotherapy if the hormonal therapy fails.

Results and Prognosis

Survival rates from prostatic cancer have increased significantly for both whites and blacks.[1] Approximate survival rates after prostatectomy are shown in Table 48-2. Clearly, the survival rates for stage D disease are less encouraging.

Nursing Care

Nursing role in early detection

The American Cancer Society recommends an annual rectal examination for all men over 40 years of age. Even though other evaluation procedures such as transrectal ultrasound are being used in the initial evaluation, the digital examination is still the most efficient means for detecting early prostate cancer.[43] It is important to impress on men that regular rectal prostatic examination is the best way to detect prostatic cancer early enough for effective treatment.

As mentioned previously, black males in the United States have the highest incidence of prostate cancer in the world. American Cancer Society statistics revealed a significantly poorer outcome for blacks with prostate cancer. Limited cancer awareness has been cited as a major cause of poorer survival and higher mortality rates in this population. Minimal awareness leads to limited outcomes, probably because persons present themselves to the medical care system when their cancer is already at a later stage. Health care providers for the black community will want to target prostatic cancer patient education and early detection programs to meet that population's special needs.

Nursing care of patients undergoing rectal prostatic examination Having a rectal prostatic examination may be uncomfortable for the patient. The nurse can minimize the patient's discomfort by informing him about the procedure. Immediately before the rectal prostatic examination, the man should empty his bladder. This will make

TABLE 48-2 Approximate Survival Rates After Prostatectomy

Stage	5 Years	10 Years
A	88%	57%
B	73%	53%
C	62%	28%

the examination more accurate and comfortable. The nurse should also inform the patient that the examiner will ask him to "bear down" during insertion of the examining finger. Reassure the patient that it is normal to experience sensations of having to urinate or defecate during the procedure. Inform him that there are two possible positions that he may be asked to take during the examination: (1) knee-chest position with buttocks elevated or (2) bending from the hips with elbows either on the knees or on the examining table.[44]

Nursing care of patients undergoing treatment for prostate cancer

The major treatments for prostate cancer include surgery, radiotherapy, endocrine therapy, and cytotoxic chemotherapy. The nurse should be aware that these treatments may produce loss of libido, impotence, loss of fertility, or urinary incontinence. These possibilities and suggestions for management should be presented and discussed by the physician with the patient and his family before any treatment. The discussion should include alternate ways to achieve sexual gratification. Many individuals and their spouses are unprepared for the loss of sexual function that occurs after cancer treatment. Nurses should take a more active role in patient teaching in this area. Nurses usually spend more time with the patient and his family than any other caregiver. The nurse will want to assess fully the individual's areas of concern and act accordingly.

Preoperative nursing care Surgical approaches to removing the prostate include retropubic, perineal, and transurethral. (See the section on Treatment for indications for each approach.) The person undergoing prostate surgery is usually extremely anxious. The emotional implications of this surgery involve both the patient and his mate. The major concerns usually focus on sexual competence and urinary control. The nurse must encourage expressions of concern, assess the individual's needs and knowledge, and give information accordingly.

The preoperative regimen is very similar to that for other abdominal surgery. Preoperative bowel preparation consists of cathartics, enemas, antibiotics, and a low-residue diet. The person should be taught how to deep breathe, cough, and turn properly to minimize postoperative pulmonary complications. Leg exercises should be taught, and antiembolic stockings should be applied to avoid thrombophlebitis. A general description of what may be expected after surgery should be given. The person's fluid, electrolyte, and nutritional status should be optimum. If the individual has renal problems such as urinary retention or urinary obstruction, insertion of an indwelling urinary catheter may be necessary. Because the average age of the person diagnosed with prostate cancer is over 50, other coexisting diseases such as hypertension, cardiovascular disease, diabetes, and pulmonary disease may be present. Concurrent drug therapy for the coexisting diseases should not be overlooked.

Postoperative nursing care

Radical prostatectomy The person who has had a radical prostatectomy usually returns from surgery with a three-way indwelling urethral catheter. Monitoring the type and amount of urinary output and maintaining catheter patency are major nursing responsibilities. During the first 24 hours after surgery, frank bleeding rarely occurs. Hematuria is common during the first 3 or 4 days after surgery. The nurse must be alert for signs and symptoms of hemorrhage and shock. Vital signs must be monitored accurately and as frequently as indicated by the patient's clinical status. A normal blood pressure reading may be a significant drop for a person with hypertension. Thus baseline data must be available for assessment. The amount and color of the urinary drainage should be observed.

Bladder irrigation after radical prostatectomy is common. The irrigation can be continuous or intermittent according to the patient's need and the physician's choice. The purpose of irrigation is to avoid clot formation and promote adequate drainage of the bladder. Obstruction of urinary flow must be prevented because it can cause secondary hemorrhage by stretching the coagulated vessels. Catheter obstruction can be caused by kinked tubing, mucus plugs, or blood clots and can lead to uncomfortable bladder distention and painful bladder spasms.

Other nursing responsibilities include preventing infection and maintaining placement of the catheter. Urinary catheter, drainage tubing, and collecting bag must remain as a closed system to avoid urinary tract infection. Catheter care must be carried out diligently using aseptic technique to prevent the instillation of bacteria. Precautions should be taken to prevent accidental removal of the catheter. The individual should be encouraged to refrain from pulling on the catheter. Premature removal of the catheter can interfere with the patient's recovery, and surgical replacement may be required. Taping the drainage tubing to the inner thigh can prevent traction to the bladder and keep the tubing secure. With a radical prostatectomy, the urethral catheter serves as a splint for urethral anastomosis as well as for urinary drainage.

Bladder spasms may occur after prostatectomy. They can be caused by the presence of the urethral catheter or by bladder distention. These spasms have a rapid onset and usually subside in a few minutes. They can be quite painful, and antispasmodics may be required. The nurse should keep in mind that antispasmodics should not be given to individuals with cardiac problems or glaucoma because these drugs can increase heart rate and intraocular presence. If antispasmodics are used, stool softeners should be administered concurrently to avoid constipation.

The urethral catheter usually stays in place for 2 to 3 weeks after radical prostatectomy depending on the person's progress. After the urethral catheter is removed, the nurse should record the amount and frequency of voiding. There may be some dribbling and urgency for several weeks. For most individuals, this is transient and will gradually improve. Urinary incontinence is common after any type of prostate surgery, occurring in up to 15% of patients. Strengthening of the perineal muscles can usually help to return control. The nurse can instruct the person in the following exercises[45]:

1. Tense the perineal muscles by pressing the buttocks together. Hold this position as long as possible and then relax. Do this exercise 10 to 20 times per hour until full urinary control is gained.
2. When starting to void, shut off the stream for a few seconds, then continue with full voiding. This exercise should be done with each urination until urinary control is improved.
3. Urinate as soon as the desire is felt. Do not wait.

The person should be informed that his urine may be cloudy for several weeks after surgery and that it will clear up as the wound heals.

Individuals who have a radical prostatectomy also may have a suprapubic cystotomy catheter inserted to provide additional security against catheter obstruction. It is inserted directly into the bladder and may have some drainage around the tube, even though it is connected to gravity drainage. If the drainage is copious, the position of the tube should be checked for patency and displacement. This catheter may be removed 2 or 3 days after surgery and a simple dry dressing applied.

Wound care for the person who has had a radical prostatectomy depends on the surgical approach used during surgery. For retropubic prostatectomy, a Penrose-type rubber drain is inserted deep into the incision, advanced gradually, and removed in about 5 days. Because drainage is common, sterile dressing changes should be carried out every 4 to 8 hours and as needed. Individuals who have had perineal prostatectomy are prone to wound infection because of the location of the incision. About 1 to 2 days after surgery, the perineal area should be meticulously cleansed and a heat lamp treatment applied to promote healing. These individuals usually have had a Penrose drain inserted. To preserve skin integrity, it is advisable to use a T-binder rather than tape to hold the dressing in place. Sitz baths usually begin after the drain is removed. A low-residue diet is ordered to minimize bowel activity. Rectal tubes, rectal thermometers, and enemas should be avoided until the wound is healed.

Sexuality The incidence of sexual impotence following radical prostatectomy is about 90%.[27] The sexual dysfunction is usually caused by damage done during surgery to the nerves and muscular tissue surrounding the prostate capsule. Sexual dysfunction includes the loss of erectile potency and absence of emission and ejaculation. Recently the insertion of a penile prosthesis has made it possible for some men who are unable to achieve erection to have penile-vaginal intercourse. The nurse's important role in daily patient care affords an excellent opportunity to provide sexual counseling to the patient and his mate. Some useful guidelines in providing sexual counseling are[46]:

1. Wait until the person is ready.
2. Gauge your responses to the person's questions.
3. Emphasize the mind, not the body.
4. Help the person recognize his limitations.
5. Encourage the person to discuss sex openly with his partner.
6. Inform the person about his sexual alternatives.
7. Encourage the person to experiment with his partner.

It is vital that the nurse thoroughly assess the individual and his partner regarding their feelings about sexual activities after surgery. A brief sexual assessment may include such questions as: (1) Has being ill interfered with your being a husband? (2) Has your surgery changed the way you see yourself as a man? (3) Has your disability affected your sexual function?[47] Assessment should include learning about the couple's physical and emotional states, what they want to know, and what they need to know.[48] Nursing intervention depends on the person's level of need. The nurse may suggest to the individual alternative ways to achieve sexual gratification such as touching and caressing or masturbation. However, the nurse must recognize that some of the alternative sexual behaviors may not be acceptable to the individual or his significant other for personal or religious reasons. The individual and his partner must be reminded that there is no right or wrong way to achieve sexual gratification. Only they can determine what is fulfilling for them. Referral to a qualified therapist may be beneficial to those who desire it.

Transurethral resection TUR requires no incision. The tumor is removed transurethrally with a resectoscope. When the patient returns from the operating room, he will have a three-way indwelling urethral catheter present in his bladder with continuous irrigation. The purpose of the irrigation is to reduce blood clot formation and promote drainage. The most important nursing responsibilities after TUR are to watch carefully for any hemorrhage and to maintain catheter patency. Catheter care is similar to that described for individuals who have had a radical prostatectomy. The urethral catheter is usually removed 3 to 5 days after surgery, at which time the urine should be clear. After the catheter is removed, the nurse should monitor the person's ability to void and to observe any signs of bladder distention. Patients may be unable to void because of urethral edema, which may necessitate reinsertion of the urinary catheter. If the external sphincter has been injured during surgery, the person may experience urinary incontinence. Straining, dysuria, or a decrease in the size of the urinary stream may indicate urethral stricture. The physician should be notified of these symptoms, and the discharge teaching plan should include instructions to report these symptoms.

Nursing care of patients receiving radiotherapy

In recent years the curative potential of radiotherapy for prostatic cancer has been recognized. The incidence of impotence following radiation treatment is about 20%

to 40%, roughly half that associated with radical prostatectomy, and incontinence rarely occurs.[32,33]

Radiotherapy may be a frightening experience. Occasionally people mistakenly believe that the person receiving external radiation is radioactive and can cause harm to others. Answering questions and correcting any misconceptions is the first step in planning nursing care.

External radiotherapy Some of the common complications of external radiotherapy are cystitis, proctitis, skin reaction, and radiation syndrome.

Cystitis usually occurs during the first 1 to 3 weeks of therapy. The use of antispasmodics and analgesics can alleviate some of the symptoms. The patient should be encouraged to drink at least 2 quarts of fluid per day.

Proctitis is mainly due to damage of the intestinal lining. Antidiarrheal medication may decrease this symptom. Patients should eat a low-residue diet. The use of steroid enemas or suppositories also may alleviate the symptoms.

Skin reaction is one of the most common acute effects of radiation, although it is much less common now than it was 20 years ago. Radiodermatitis usually begins about 2 weeks after the beginning of treatment and reaches its peak during the fifth or sixth week. Skin reactions include epilation, erythema, or dry or wet desquamation. Patients must be educated about proper skin care to maintain skin integrity. The irradiated area should be kept clean and dry. Direct sun exposure to the irradiated area should be avoided, and the skin should not be exposed to extreme heat or cold. Commercial skin creams or lotions should be avoided because some contain metal bases, which can cause further burning. Some of the water-based lotions, such as Aquaphor, may be used with approval from the radiologist. Treatment of skin side effects differs. The nurse should assess the skin and report changes to the physician. See Chapter 20 for detailed information on care of the person receiving radiotherapy.

Internal radiotherapy Interstitial implants can deliver radiation doses that are relatively high to the diseased area with minimal damage to the surrounding tissues. Nursing care of the individual with interstitial implants is based on the penetration energy level of the radioactive substance and its half-life.[49] For those few individuals receiving ^{198}Au implants, the length of time the nurse spends with each patient should be determined by a physicist. Nursing care must be done quickly and efficiently, but the patient should not be made to feel abandoned. The allotted time for patient contact does not need to be used all at once. The nurse can divide the time, over the entire shift and use the principles of distance, time, and shielding to dictate care. Some of the person's feelings of rejection may be alleviated by explaining the need for shortened contact. The person also must be reminded that he is no longer radioactive after the radiation substance has decayed. The person who has had ^{125}I implants should have his urine and bed linen monitored. Nursing care of individuals with radioactive implants is discussed further in Chapter 20.

Nursing care of patients receiving hormonal therapy

DES is a drug commonly used for hormonal treatment of patients with prostatic cancer. One major side effect of DES is sodium retention, which can adversely affect a person with cardiovascular disease and may induce pulmonary edema and congestive heart failure. The concurrent use of diuretics may be necessary. Serious hypercalcemia may occur during the initial period of therapy, manifested by polyuria, general weakness, and mental disorientation. Other side effects of DES include nausea, hypertension, feminization, gynecomastia, loss of libido, and impotency. These individuals are also at higher risk for thromboembolic complications such as pulmonary embolus and strokes. Nurses should be aware of the potential side effects of estrogen therapy and pay special attention to individuals with a history of cardiopulmonary disease.

GnRH agonists are used in hormonal treatment of advanced prostatic cancer. These drugs do not cause gynecomastia. The patient may experience frequent high-intensity hot flashes, decreased libido, and erectile impotency. GnRH does not produce the metabolic side effects of estrogen.[50]

For patients with hormonally refractive metastatic prostate cancer, ketoconazole has been used combined with orchiectomy, estrogens, or GnRH agonists to achieve total androgen ablation. Because of ketoconazole's short duration of action, it is imperative that the nurse administer this drug on a strict 8-hour schedule. Hepatotoxicity has been reported in about 50% of patients.[51]

Nursing care of patients undergoing orchiectomy

Bilateral orchiectomy is another method of hormonal manipulation. Orchiectomy can provoke a high degree of anxiety for many men because of its connotation of castration. Some men mistakenly believe that removal of the testes will leave them with feminine voices and enlarged breasts. Having the testicles removed during adulthood has no impact on masculinity. Discussion of these side effects with patients is critical.

The immediate postorchiectomy nursing care plan includes pain management with analgesics, prevention of wound infection through aseptic care of the incision site, and maintenance of overall physiologic functions.

Nursing care of patients receiving chemotherapy

Patients with disseminated prostatic cancer have demonstrated various responses to cisplatin, cyclophosphamide, methotrexate, doxorubicin, 5-FU, and DTIC used singly and in combination. The nurse should be aware of the major toxicities of these drugs. Nephrotoxicity, severe nausea and vomiting, ototoxicity and peripheral neuropathies are the major side effects of cisplatin. Cyclophosphamide can cause hemorrhagic cystitis and myelosuppression. Methotrexate induces myelosuppression, stomatitis, and nephrotoxicity. Doxorubicin can cause alopecia, myelosuppression and cardiotoxicity. 5-FU induces myelosuppression, stomatitis, and diarrhea. DTIC causes severe nausea and vomiting and myelosuppression. Estramustine has no hematologic toxicity but causes gastrointestinal disturbances such as nausea and vomiting, which can be alleviated by antiemetics. Specific interventions for each drug are discussed in detail in Chapter 14.

BLADDER CANCER

Epidemiology

Bladder cancer is the second most common genitourinary cancer after prostate cancer. It accounts for 4% to 5% of cancers in the United States.

The four major variables related to bladder cancer incidence are race, gender, age, and geographic location. In the United States the most outstanding epidemiologic feature is the high incidence among white men. The age-adjusted bladder cancer rate in white men is twice the rate in black men.[52] In whites the bladder cancer ratio of men to women is 4:1.[52] Most of these cancers occur in men over 50 years of age. There is a high incidence of squamous cell carcinoma of the bladder in certain areas of the world, notably Egypt. This is linked to the parasite *Schistosoma haemotobium.*

Etiology

There are four etiologic hypotheses related to bladder cancer: cigarette smoking, occupational exposure to industrial chemicals, ingestion of other physical agents, and exposure to *Schistosoma haemotobium.*

Cigarette smoking was first associated with bladder cancer in 1956.[53] Since that time most case-controlled studies report a twofold relative risk for cigarette smokers compared with nonsmokers.[54,55] However, there are apparent inconsistencies between the case-controlled studies and supporting demographic evidence. For example, the incidence of smoking in women is increasing, while the incidence of bladder cancer in women is decreasing. Certain populations that have been studied for bladder cancer incidence, such as Polynesian men and American blacks, have a very high rate of cigarette smoking and a low incidence of bladder cancer.[52] Despite the inconsistencies, the overwhelming statistical evidence points to cigarette smoking as a prime epidemiologic factor, accounting for as much as 50% of all bladder cancer in American men.[52] The effect of cigarette smoking on bladder tissue seems to be different from that on lung cancer and is likely to be influenced by metabolic and genetic factors.

Among occupational exposure agents, arylamine(s), used in the synthetic textile dye industry, in the rubber industry, in hair dyes, and as paint pigment, is the class of chemicals most strongly related to bladder cancer.[52] Beta-naphthylamine and benzidine are two examples of this chemical class. Occupations known to be at risk for bladder cancer of two or greater include janitors and cleaners, mechanics, miners, and printers.[55]

Ingestion of other physical agents, such as coffee, alcohol, saccharin, and phenacetin, have been weakly linked to bladder cancer. None of these agents has consistently been related to bladder cancer incidence in humans.

The results of studies looking at coffee drinking as a possible etiologic factor in bladder cancer have generally been inconsistent, and the associated increases in risk are generally small.[52]

Although some recent reports have suggested bladder cancer association with alcohol consumption,[56,57] a recent study of 823 men and 2469 age-matched controls showed no association with bladder cancer.[55]

Animal studies have shown that saccharin may cause bladder cancer in rodents.[52] However, if the dose-incidence curve in rodents is extrapolated to humans, it has been calculated that saccharin users would experience only a 4% increase in bladder cancer occurrence. That level is not detectable by epidemiologic studies. Furthermore, diabetics (who consume a large quantity of artificial sweeteners) do not have a high incidence of bladder cancer.[52]

Heavy regular use of phenacetin has also been suggested as an etiologic link; however, the results of various studies have beeen confusing.[52]

Schistosomiasis is rare in the United States but common in many African countries and especially in Egypt. In areas where schistosomiasis is endemic, the incidence of squamous cell carcinoma of the bladder is much higher. In these areas a high percentage of individuals with squamous cell bladder cancer are found to have *S. haemotobium* ova in the bladder wall.[58]

Pathophysiology

Cellular characteristics

The urinary bladder is lined by transitional epithelium, often called the urothelium. About 90% to 95% of bladder tumors in North America are transitional cell carcinomas. Approximately 7% are squamous cell (associated with *S. haemotobium*), and 2% are adenocarcinomas.[59]

Transitional cell tumors arise in the epithelial layer of the bladder, which rests on the basement membrane. If the basement membrane remains intact, there is little chance of metastases to the vascular or lymphatic system.

Bladder cancer is a multifaceted problem. Within the transitional cell classification, the tumors may be subdivided into carcinoma in situ, papillary noninfiltrating or papillary infiltrating, and solid carcinomas. Figure 48-7 depicts the natural history of bladder cancer.

Grading of bladder tumors is commonly done to predict the speed of recurrence and the progression to invasion and metastases. The more well-differentiated bladder tumors (low grade) generally have a slower growth rate, and therefore these patients have a better prognosis.

Papillary tumors, although they may have a low cytologic grade and be noninvasive, tend to recur. Transitional

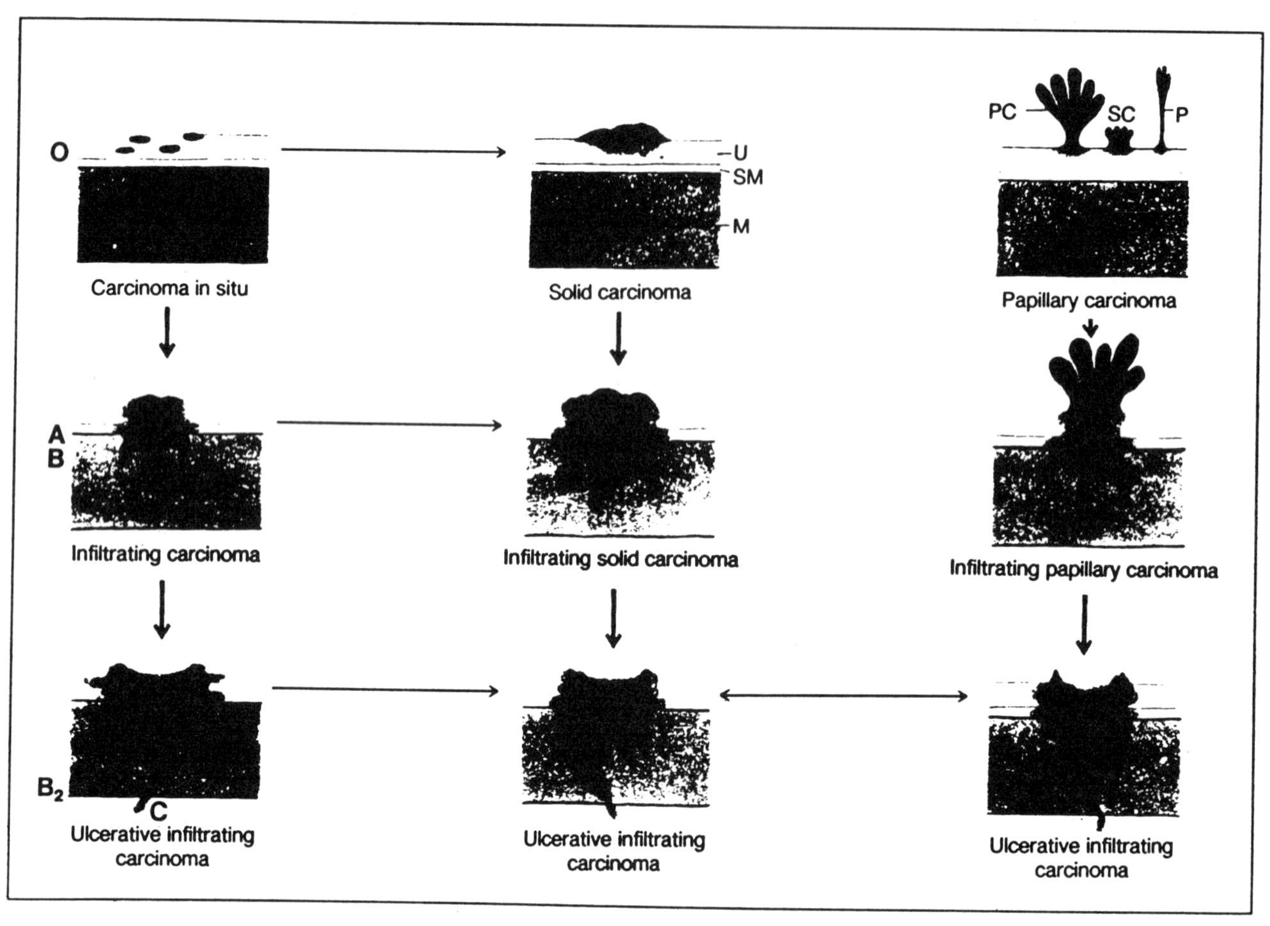

FIGURE 48-7 The natural history of bladder tumors. (Source: Melicow MM: Tumors of the bladder: A multifaceted problem. J Urol 112:468, 1974.)

cell carcinoma in situ is usually multifocal. This high recurrence rate and multicentricity necessitate aggressive follow-up after initial diagnosis and treatment.[59]

Progression of disease

Many of these tumors arise on the floor of the bladder and may involve one or both of the ureteral orifices.[60] The growth rate varies depending on the histologic type and grade of the tumor. The most important growth feature is the depth of penetration into the bladder wall.

Some tumors spread rapidly to the regional lymph nodes, which are the pelvic nodes just below the bifurcation of the common iliac arteries. Others grow more slowly and spread directly into pelvic tissues.

Growth occurs inward into the hollow aspect of bladder (in papillary tumors) and outward from the urothelial mucosa to the submucosa and to the detrusor muscle.

Metastasis takes place through direct extension out of the muscle of the bladder into the perivesicle fat (or serosa). Depending on the location of the tumor, it may obstruct the ureters or bladder neck and prostatic urethra. It can also spread by direct extension to involve other adjacent structures, particularly the sigmoid colon, the rectum, or the prostate as well as the uterus and vagina. Hematogenous spread occasionally occurs to the bones, liver, and lungs.[59]

Clinical Manifestations

Gross hematuria is the most common presenting symptom of bladder cancer. Painless hematuria is usually present through the entire stream of urine. This bleeding is rarely profuse and is often microscopic. Hematuria is usually intermittent.

Another symptom is irritability of the bladder. This manifests itself as dysuria, urinary frequency, and urgency and burning on urination if infection is present.

Symptoms associated with large tumor growth or metastasis also may be present. If the tumor is pushing on the internal urethral orifice, symptoms of bladder neck obstruction may be present including urinary hesitancy and decrease in the force and caliber of the stream. Obstruction of the ureters can cause flank pain and results in hydronephrosis.

Pain in the suprapubic region, rectum, or back as well as symptoms of lung, bone, or liver metastasis occur occasionally in individuals with advanced disease.

Assessment

Physical examination

There are no early signs of bladder cancer on physical examination. An invasive mass in the trigonal area occasionally may be revealed by rectal examination.

Diagnostic studies

Cytology Exfoliative urinary cytology is a relatively simple diagnostic tool in the assessment of bladder cancer. Many experts recommend the collection of a total voided specimen obtained late in the morning or early afternoon and sent immediately for cytologic examination to reduce the chance of obscuring the results.[60] Bladder washings produce even more reliable results.[61]

Flow cytometry In superficial transitional cell bladder cancer, the identification of those patients who might experience recurrent disease and those whose disease will progress to a higher stage are both important to assessment. Flow cytometry, which is a technique used to examine the DNA content of urine cells, has been useful in providing prognostic information beyond grading and staging. In this technique, automated machines are able to analyze large numbers of urine samples, sort the urine cells by size, and indirectly measure the DNA content. Aneuploidy, or large numbers of DNA per cell, indicates high-grade, high-stage transitional cell tumors.[18]

Excretory urogram (intravenous pyelogram) Excretory urogram (intravenous urogram) should be done before cystoscopy to help in evaluating the upper tracts at the same time.[61] Although it is not a conclusive diagnostic tool, excretory urography can help evaluate a suspected bladder tumor by possibly showing the tumor itself or by showing evidence of ureteral obstruction (hydronephrosis). Urethral obstruction also may be demonstrated with excretory urography.

Cystoscopy Cystoscopic examination can serve several purposes: tumor visualization, an opportunity for biopsy, and an opportunity for bimanual examination of the bladder.

Once the tumor is visualized, a deep biopsy specimen is taken from the center of the tumor and its outside border. The goal of these biopsies is to assess the presence or absence of muscle invasion. Multiple biopsy specimens of the rest of the bladder wall, the bladder neck, and the trigone also may be taken to diagnose carcinoma in situ or atypia. Selected mucosal biopsy can also be an effective adjunct to the management of superficial bladder cancer.[61]

Bimanual palpation performed under anesthesia may detect a palpable tumor or induration that could indicate deep muscle invasion, inflammation at the tumor site, or extension of the tumor into the serosa.

Tumor markers Serum carcinoembryonic antigen (CEA) levels are moderately elevated in 50% of late stage (T3 and T4) bladder cancer patients.[63] A greater CEA elevation is seen in tumors that are widely metastatic.

Cell locomotion is known to be an essential requirement for invasion and metastasis of cancer cells. Recent research has found that human bladder cancer elaborates an autocrine motility factor (AMF) and that tumor cell motility may be a major marker of metastasis.[64]

Computed tomography, ultrasound, magnetic resonance imaging Advocates of using CT scans in staging bladder cancer feel that it aids in defining the extent of the local tumor and in identifying pelvic lymph node metastasis.

Transurethral ultrasound has recently been used to define the local extension and degree of involvement of the bladder wall.[65] The exact role of both ultrasound and CT scanning remains to be determined.[61]

MRI has been successful in distinguishing cancer from the normal bladder wall because the tumor generates a higher signal intensity.[66] It has also been used to identify the presence of pelvic lymph node involvement.[67]

Classification and Staging

Several attempts have been made to develop a universal staging system for bladder cancer, but the most common systems used in the United States are the Jewett-Strong system (modified by Marshall) and the TNM system developed by the American Joint Committee for Cancer Staging and End Results Reporting.[61] A compilation of these systems is depicted in Figure 48-8.

Another factor sometimes considered in treatment but not included in the staging systems is the grade of the tumor, or its degree of cell differentiation. A grading system for cancer of the bladder is usually referred to as grade I, II, III, or IV, with IV designating the least well differentiated.

Treatment

Carcinoma in situ

Electrofulguration and thiotepa or radical cystectomy with urinary diversion are two common treatment options for patients with carcinoma in situ of the bladder. Radiotherapy has no proven value in the treatment of patients with carcinoma in situ.

Superficial, low-grade tumors

Superficial tumors of the bladder remain in the epithelium and lamina propria. Standard treatment is by transurethral surgery with resection and fulguration (if there are multiple small lesions). The overall 5-year survival rate of patients with superficial bladder cancer treated with TUR alone is approximately 70%.[68] Because the chance of recurrence is so great, intravesical chemotherapy following surgery has been investigated.

Several agents have shown some effectiveness in bladder cancer, including thiotepa, mitomycin C, Epodyl (triethylene glycol diglycerol ether), doxorubicin, VM-26 (epi-

1946 Jewett-Strong	1952 Jewett	1952 Marshall		1978, TNM Clinical	1978, TNM Pathologic
		0	No tumor, definitive specimen	T0	P0
			Carcinoma in situ	TIS	PIS
A	A		Papillary tumor s̄ invasion	Ta	Pa
		A	Invasion of the lamina propria	T1	P1
B	B1	B1	Superficial } Muscle invasion	T2	P2
	B2	B2	Deep	T3	P3A
C	C	C	Invasion of perivesical fat		P3B
			Invasion of prostate, vagina, or uterus	T4	P4A
		D1	Fixed to pelvic or abdominal wall		P4B
			Pelvic nodes		N1-3
		D2	Distant metastases		M1
			Nodes above the aortic bifurcation		N4

FIGURE 48-8 Staging systems for bladder cancer. (Source: Lieskovsky G, Ahlering T, Skinner DG: Diagnosis and staging of bladder cancer, in Skinner DG, Lieskovsky G (eds): Diagnosis and Management of Genitourinary Cancer. Philadelphia, WB Saunders, 1988, p 267.)

podophyllotoxin), and bacillus Calmette-Guérin (BCG). The most widely used drug for this purpose in the United States is thiotepa. Dosages vary from 30 to 60 mg diluted in equal amounts of sterile water. It is generally instilled and retained for 1 or 2 hours every week for 6 to 8 weeks and in some instances at monthly intervals for 2 years thereafter. The drug's side effects include severe bladder irritability, myelosuppression, and renal failure if there is reflux.[68]

Mitomycin C also has been used to treat patients with superficial disease. Because it has limited intravesical absorption, myelosuppression is rare, and the major side effects are chemical cystitis and skin reactions from contact with the drug.[68] If, as some believe, the benefits of mitomycin C and thiotepa are comparable, the deciding factor might be the greater expense of using mitomycin C.

The use of BCG intravesically has gained renewed attention. Complete responses of up to 79% and prolonged disease-free survival have been reported.[69-71] This treatment is considered both safe and effective in reducing transitional cell recurrences. Side effects include transient hematuria, dysuria, frequency of urination, and occasional influenza like symptoms.

Small superficial bladder tumors have also been treated by laser beams. One of the most useful lasers is the neodymium ytrium-aluminum-garnet laser (Nd:YAG). Laser therapy can be done through a small cystoscope without causing bleeding or stimulating the obturator nerve while the patient is under local anesthesia.[68]

Partial (or segmental) cystectomy is advocated by some authorities but only for individuals with diffuse unresectable tumors or tumors that have not responded to intravesical therapy.[68] The success of partial cystectomy is much higher with stage A, grade I or II lesions. The greatest disadvantage of partial cystectomy is a high tumor recurrence rate.

High-stage, high-grade tumors

Because of invasion of the bladder muscle, high-stage, high-grade tumors have dramatically altered prognoses. Common treatment options for these bladder tumors include definitive irradiation (ie, radiation alone with intent to cure), radical cystectomy with urinary diversion with or without pelvic lymph node dissection, or a combination of preoperative irradiation followed by surgical excision.

Definitive radiotherapy Historically, definitive radiotherapy involved approximately 7000 cGy delivered to the pelvis in 7 to 8 weeks, along with 5000 cGy delivered to the pelvic lymph nodes and was thought to have results comparable to radical surgery, with lesser morbidity. Today, however, many believe that definitive radiotherapy can cure no more than 16% to 30% of patients with invasive bladder cancer and that these figures are no longer comparable with the results achieved by protocols that include cystectomy.[72]

Preoperative irradiation A more typical use of radiotherapy for high-grade, high-stage bladder tumors is as a preoperative treatment in an effort to decrease both pelvic recurrence and dissemination during surgery. One protocol recommends 1600 cGy or preoperative radiation delivered over a 4-day period, followed by an immediate radical cystectomy and urinary diversion.[73]

A variety of other regimens are used: 2000 cGy in 1 week, 4000 cGy in 4 weeks, 4500 cGy in 4½ weeks, and 5000 cGy in 5 weeks. The radiation is delivered to the pelvis, sometimes with an extra radiation boost to the bladder alone. Fractionation of the radiation dose is most often used to decrease the side effects.

Radical cystectomy The term *radical cystectomy* in men is usually synonymous with prostatocystectomy. The pro-

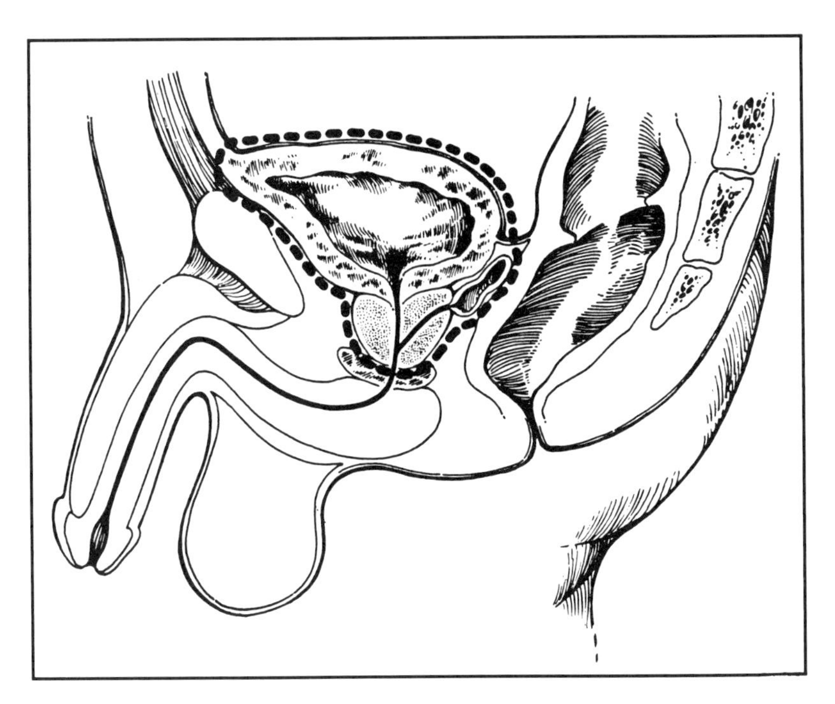

FIGURE 48-9 Surgical boundaries of radical cystectomy in a man. The specimen includes the bladder, the prostate, and the seminal vesicles. (Source: Swanson D: Cancer of the bladder and prostate. The impact of therapy on sexual function, in von Eschenbach AC, Rodriguez D, (eds): Sexual Rehabilitation of the Urologic Cancer Patient. Boston, GK Hall, 1981, p 102.)

cedure includes excision of the bladder with the pericystic fat, the attached peritoneum, and the entire prostate and seminal vesicles (Figure 48-9).

In women radical cystectomy includes removal of the bladder and entire urethra, uterus, ovaries, fallopian tubes, and anterior wall of the vagina (Figure 48-10).

Including pelvic lymphadenectomy with this surgery is controversial. The evidence that it improves survival is sparse and inconclusive. Some surgeons have demonstrated that adding a meticulous lymph node dissection has resulted in a low incidence of pelvic recurrence compared with results for simple total cystectomy without dissection or preoperative radiation therapy.[72]

Complications of this surgical procedure include ureterocutaneous fistula, wound dehiscence, partial small-bowel obstruction, wound infection, and small-bowel fistula.

Urinary diversion

Ileal conduit Since the early 1950s the Bricker ileal conduit has been a popular method of diverting urinary flow in the absence of bladder function. This procedure involves isolating a piece of terminal ileum, closing the proximal end, bringing the distal end out through a hole in the abdominal wall at a previously marked site, and suturing it to the skin, creating a stoma. For proper functioning the segment must reach from the retroperitoneum to the skin comfortably and without tension on the distal (stoma) end. The ureters are implanted into the ileal segment, urine flows into the conduit, and peristalsis propels it out through the stoma (Figure 48-11). Urinary stints may occasionally be threaded into the ureters to prevent ureteral anastomosis and to allow for free-flowing urine in the early postoperative period. Urinary stints are usually left in place for 7 to 10 days. Minimal electrolyte absorption occurs at the ileal conduit because it does not act as a reservoir.

Other portions of the bowel also have been used to divert the urine. A higher segment (the jejunum) will occasionally be used because of difficulties at the ileum. Portions of the sigmoid colon are used infrequently as conduits in urinary diversions associated with bladder cancer. Construction of any of these conduits necessitates that the person continually wear some sort of collection appliance.

Complications are related to stoma construction and placement and to the possibility of long-term kidney damage.

Stomas placed in skin creases, scars, or bony prominences make adherence of an appliance difficult to achieve. Stomas that are flush with the skin and recessed make the proper fit.

Other complications include stomal stenosis, which has a host of sequelae, including pain, stones, and potential pyelonephritis. Recent studies have indicated a high incidence of ureteral reflux and ascending infection that results in late kidney deterioration.

Loop stoma The Turnbull loop stoma has been used in an attempt to decrease the problems of stoma placement and stomal stenosis. In this technique,[75] an ileal or jejunal conduit is constructed, and both the distal and proximal ends are sutured closed. A loop of the conduit is pulled out through the abdominal wall, and the ureters are im-

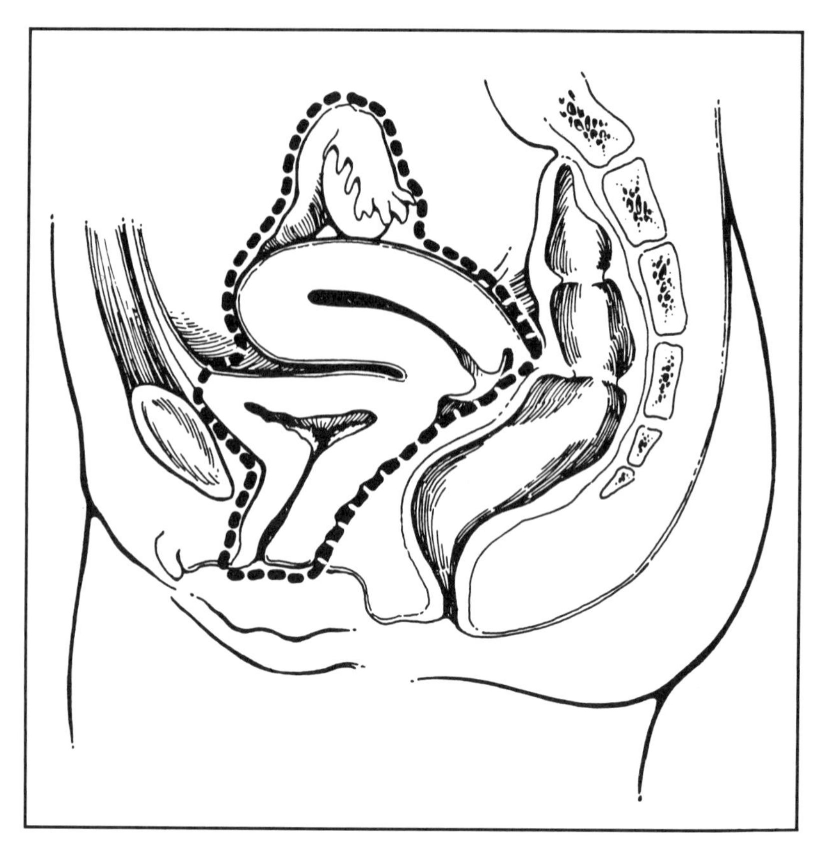

FIGURE 48-10 Surgical boundaries of a radical cystectomy in a woman. The specimen includes the bladder and entire urethra, uterus, ovaries, fallopian tubes, and the anterior wall of the vagina. (Source: Swanson D: Cancer of the bladder and prostate. The impact of therapy on sexual function, in von Eschenbach AC, Rodriguez D (eds): Sexual Rehabilitation of the Urologic Cancer Patient. Boston, GK Hall, 1981, p 103.)

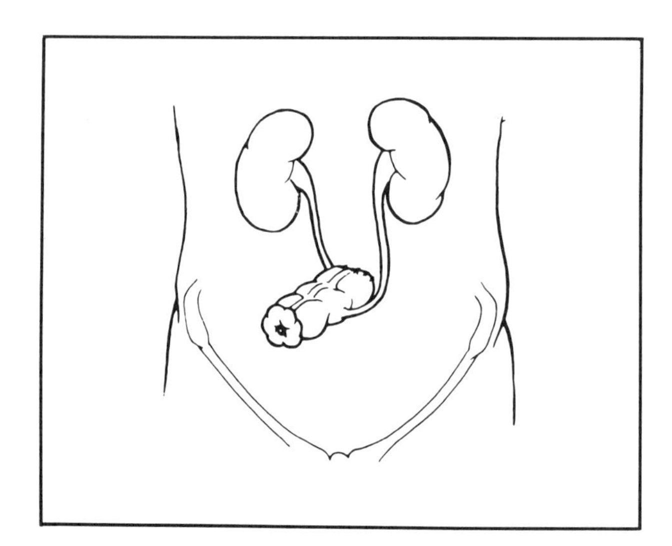

FIGURE 48-11 Ileal conduit. (Source: Bouchard R, Owens H: Nursing care of the cancer patient (ed 4). St Louis, CV Mosby, 1981, p 397.)

planted into the proximal portion (Figure 48-12). The loop is anchored to the skin, and the conduit is opened, creating a mucous fistula at the distal end of the conduit and a urinary diversion at the proximal end. The major complication is parastomal hernia.

Ureterosigmoidostomy A ureterosigmoidostomy involves implanting the ureters into the sigmoid colon using an antirefluxing anastomosis. The urine is then excreted through the rectum. The early and late complications include metabolic acidosis because of the absorptive quality of the sigmoid colon, potassium depletion, anastomotic stenosis, and ascending infection, particularly in individuals with impaired renal function.

Continent ileal reservoir for urinary diversion A new technique of urinary diversion attempts to substitute more effectively for the functions of the lower urinary tract. Ideally, voiding of urine would be under voluntary control at convenient intervals, and the upper renal tract would be protected from both obstruction and urine reflux.

The continent ileal reservoir for urinary diversion fulfills those criteria. Figure 48-13 illustrates one type of continent reservoir technique originated by Nils Kock[16] in Sweden and described by Gerber[74] and by Skinner et al.[77] Urinary diversion through a continent ileal reservoir pro-

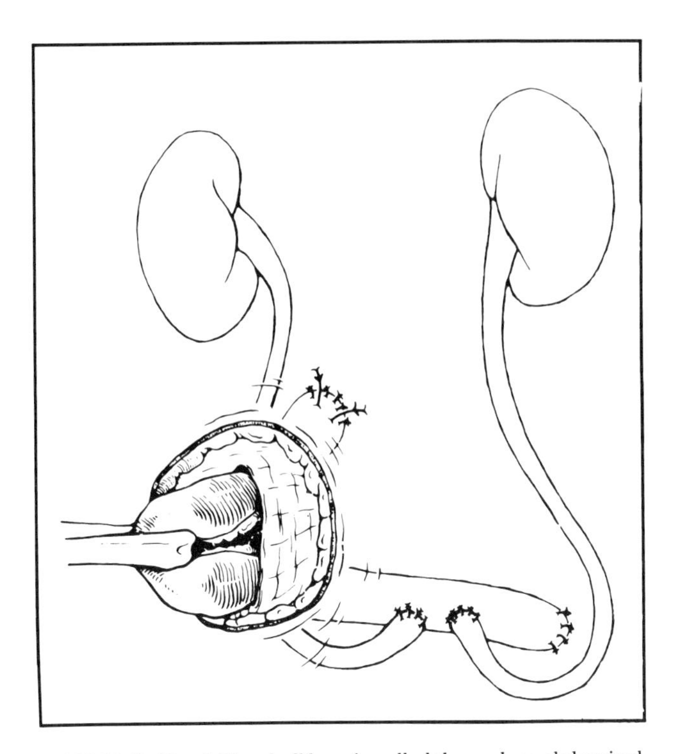

FIGURE 48-12 A Turnbull loop is pulled through an abdominal wall defect using a small Penrose drain as a tractor. (Source: Bloom DA, Lieskovsky G, Rainwater G, et al: The Turnbull loop stoma. J Urol 129:1983, 716.)

vides an intra-abdominal pouch for storage of urine and two nipple valves that maintain continence and prevent ureteral reflux. One procedure for constructing the urinary pouch describes using a 60- to 70-cm segment of ileum, isolated approximately 50 cm from the ileocecal valve. The ureters are anastomosed to a short segment of the ileum that leads into an ileal nipple, which prevents reflux of the urine to the kidneys. Proximal to this segment, two 22-cm segments are used to create the reservoir pouch itself. The remaining segment is used for the continence nipple and the stoma.[77]

When the lengthy surgical procedure is almost complete, a number 30 Medina tube is passed into the pouch and positioned so that the drainage holes are several centimeters beyond the efferent nipple. This tube is sutured in place to secure it for 3 weeks. A 1-inch Penrose drain is passed through a separate stab incision and sutured to the muscle or peritoneum to keep it from moving into the pouch.

To prevent mucus obstruction postoperatively, the Medina tube should be irrigated at least every 4 hours with 30 to 60 mL of normal saline. Three weeks following surgery the Medina tube is removed and the pouch is checked radiographically for any signs of leakage. If the pouch is patent, the patient is taught self-catheterization technique, beginning at 2- to 3-hour intervals.

Late complications usually involve problems with continence or catheterization such as urinary leakage at the

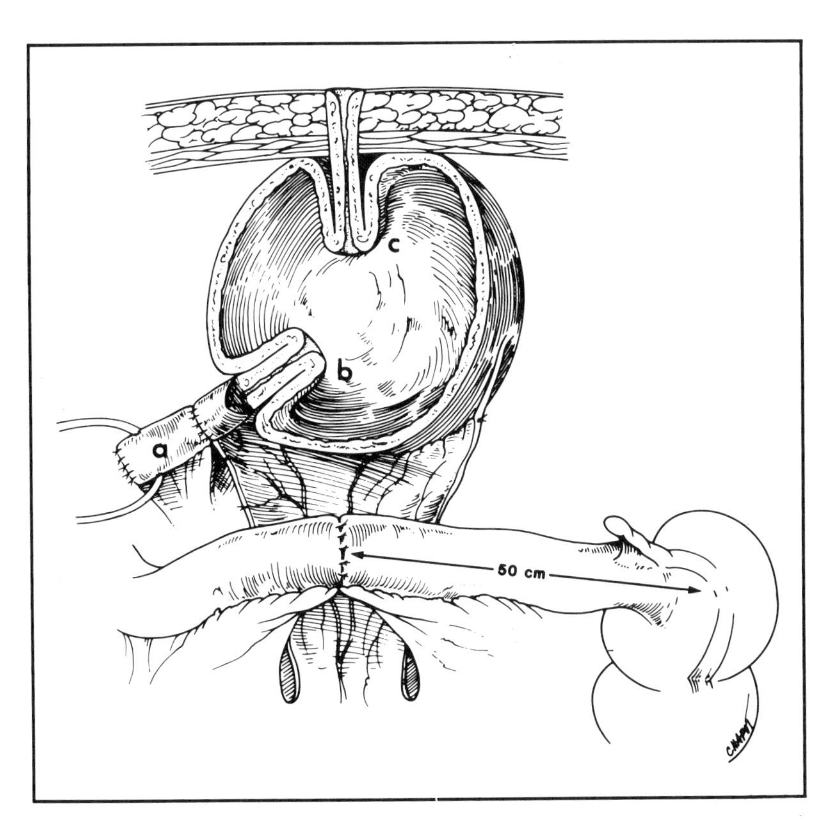

FIGURE 48-13 The continuent ileal reservoir. (a) The original ileal conduit with implanted ureters. (b) The reflux-preventing nipple valve. (c) The continence-maintaining nipple valve. (Source: Gerber A: The Kock continent ileal reservoir for supravesicle urinary diversion. Am J Surg 146:16, 1983.)

stoma, difficult catheterization, electrolyte abnormalities, pyelonephritis, hydronephrosis, and stone formation.

Sexuality A radical cystectomy with urinary diversion, particularly if accompanied by a lymphadenectomy, can affect many aspects of sexual functioning. The etiology of physiologic sexual dysfunction in men is similar to that associated with treatment for prostatic cancer. In addition, the psychologic impact of a stoma and external appliance may contribute to changes in body image and libido.[78]

The erectile impotence that results after radical cystectomy (or radical prostatectomy) may be helped by the insertion of a penile prosthesis. Three categories of devices are currently used. The Jonas prosthesis is an example of a malleable, semirigid, plastic rod that is inserted into the bodies of the corpora cavernosa (Figure 48-14). The result is a permanent semierection that is not painful and does not interfere with daily activities.

The Scott prosthesis, an example of various types of inflatable prostheses (Figure 48-15), makes it possible to control erectile function. When the man wishes to have an erection, he squeezes and repeatedly releases the pump bulb in the scrotum to pump fluid from the reservoir into both of the penile cylinders until an erection is achieved. To deflate the erection, finger pressure is exerted on the valve that holds the fluid under pressure.[79] The third and newest type of prosthesis consists of a self-contained inflatable cylinder.[80]

In women removal of the ovaries and uterus will result in sexuality changes similar to those following hysterectomy and oophorectomy for gynecologic malignancies. Psychologic problems may occur as a result of the external

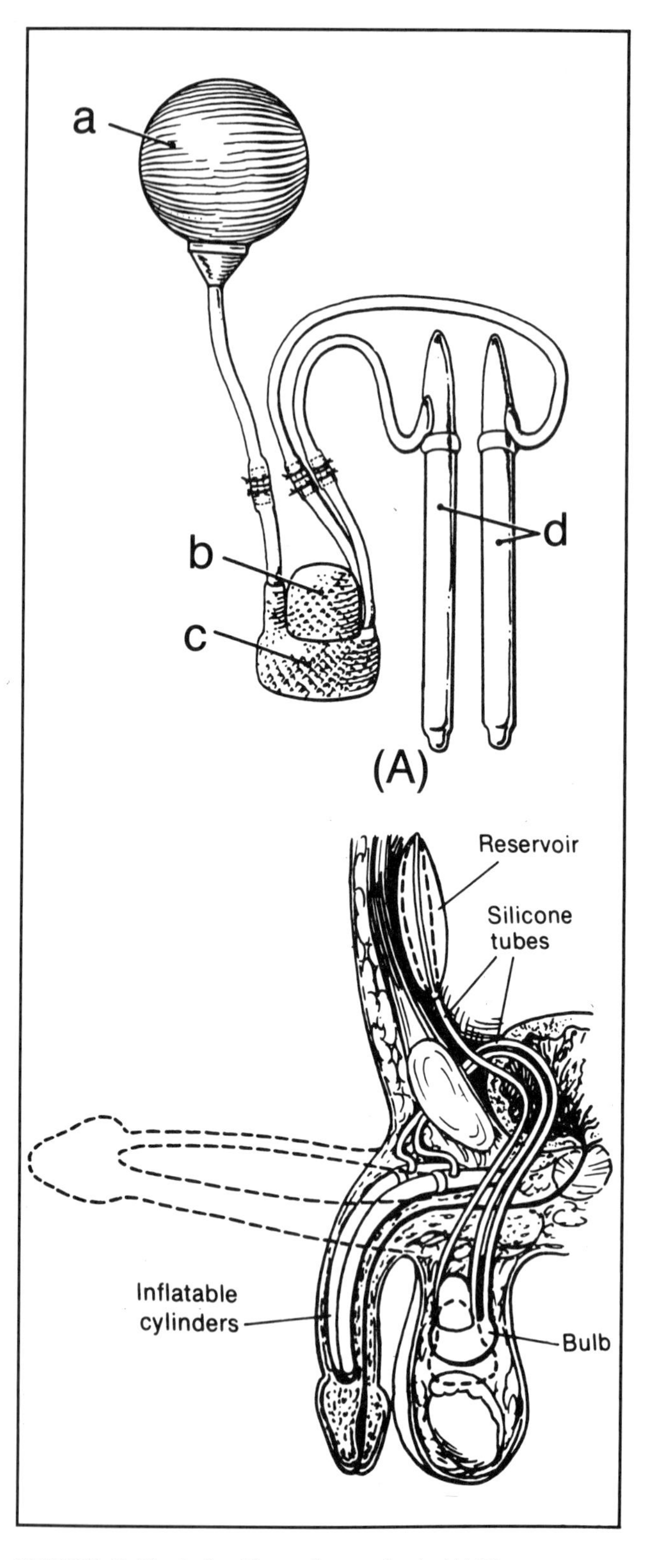

FIGURE 48-15 Inflatable penile prosthesis. (A) The apparatus: (a) spherical reservoir, (b) pump, (c) release valve, and (d) penile cylinders. (B) Prosthesis in place. (Source: Adapted from Scott FB, Kantzavelos D: Erectile impotence after urologic cancer surgery treated with the inflatable penile prosthesis, in von Eschenbach AC, Rodriguez D (eds): Sexual Rehabilitation of the Urologic Cancer Patient. Boston, GK Hall, 1981, p 243.)

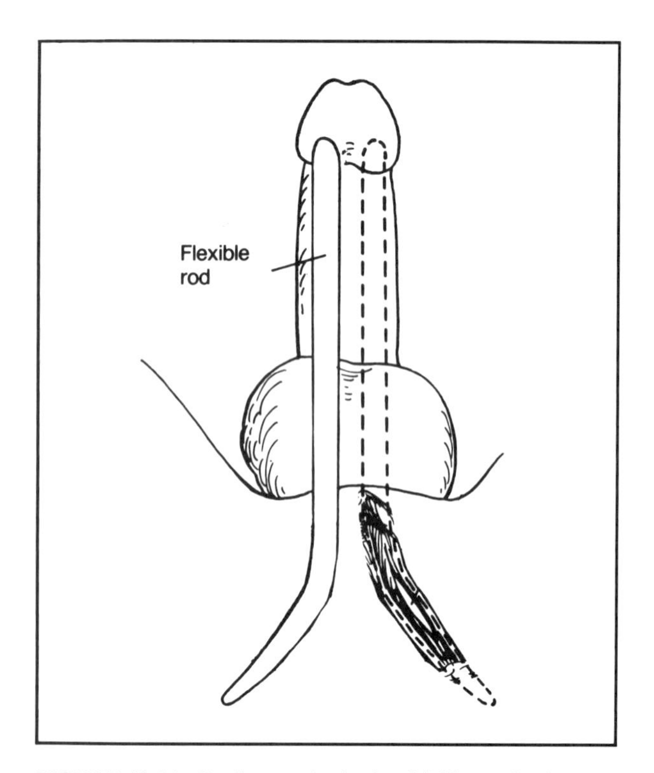

FIGURE 48-14 Penile prosthesis. Semirigid prosthesis consisting of flexible rods. (Source: Adapted from Luckmann J, Sorenson K: Medical-Surgical Nursing—A Psychophysiologic Approach. Philadelphia, WB Saunders, 1978, p 1843.)

urinary stoma or perceived losses related to hysterectomy and oophorectomy or may result from hormonal changes that occur as a result of surgery. A more direct physiologic effect, however, involves removal of the anterior wall of the vagina. The vagina is closed after surgery and therefore retains its original shape. However, if more than the anterior third of the vaginal wall is removed, the diameter of the introitus and the vaginal barrel can be severely compromised, and intercourse may be restricted. In addition, because of its close proximity to the urethral meatus, the clitoris may be injured or have compromised function because of subsequent scarring and fibrosis after surgery.[78] The physiologic changes can result in an alteration in sensation and potential for orgasm and impairment of the ability to permit insertion of the penis into the vagina.

Summary Optimal therapy for patients with high-stage, high-grade bladder tumors appears to be preoperative irradiation followed by radical cystectomy with urinary diversion or pelvic lymphadenectomy and radical cystectomy with urinary diversion. Definitive irradiation should be reserved only for those individuals who are not candidates for surgery.[72] Because of the high incidence of lymph node involvement, the nodes should be treated either by radiotherapy or lymphadenectomy. Short-course preoperative radiotherapy (eg, 2000 cGy in 4 to 5 days) followed by immediate radical cystectomy with pelvic lymph node dissection produces results that are as good as standard fractionation radiation therapy of 4000 to 5000 cGy over 4 to 6 weeks, followed by cystectomy 4 to 6 weeks later with or without pelvic node dissection.[72]

Advanced bladder cancer

Despite improvements in the diagnosis and treatment of bladder cancer, 50% of individuals with high-stage, high-grade tumors will eventually relapse.[81] Relapse is most likely related to the fact that many of these patients have undetectable micrometastases at the time of diagnosis. The use of chemotherapy early in the course of treatment may prove useful in lengthening the disease-free interval and overall survival. Complete responses have been seen in 40% to 50% of patients, with a 1-year median duration of response.[81] Single-agent and combination regimens have been attempted.

Table 48-3 represents most of the single agents tried in advanced bladder cancer. A review of the results of those studies indicates that in general, single agents produce only partial responses of short duration and that cisplatin and methotrexate demonstrate significant activity.

The following is a list of some of the combinations of chemotherapeutic drugs that have been studied in bladder cancer:

- Doxorubicin plus cyclophosphamide
- Doxorubicin plus cisplatin
- Doxorubicin plus 5-FU
- Cyclophosphamide plus cisplatin
- Doxorubicin plus cyclophosphamide plus cisplatin
- VM-26 plus cisplatin
- Methotrexate plus vinblastine

Reviewing the results of those studies indicates that (1) a good comparative assessment is difficult but that (2) intensive combination chemotherapy that includes cisplatin seems to produce a higher complete response rate than single-agent chemotherapy. Surgical treatment is seldom used to palliate symptoms of advanced bladder cancer. An individual with severe irritative symptoms due to a bladder tumor occasionally may have an improved quality of life if urinary diversion alone is performed.[81]

Radiotherapy can improve the problem of hemorrhage in the person with advanced bladder cancer and certainly plays an important role in treating bony metastases, but local irritative symptoms can be made worse by radiotherapy.

Results and Prognosis

The American Cancer Society reports 5-year survival rates (adjusted for normal life expectancy) to vary between American whites and blacks (Table 48-4).[1] Five-year survivals of over 80% have been reported for patients with stage A bladder cancer after treatment by radiotherapy, cystectomy, and node dissection.[72]

Nursing Care*

Preoperative nursing care

When a diagnosis of bladder cancer has been confirmed and the treatment of choice includes urinary diversion, the type of diversion best suited for the individual must be chosen. The decision is based on each person's needs, anatomy, history, and prognosis. Most urinary diversions that will use a segment of the bowel and require an external stoma for the excretion of urine have similar preoperative nursing considerations.

A low-residue diet is given 2 days before surgery, followed by a clear liquid diet on the day before surgery. Bowel preparation using antibiotics, cathartics, and low-residue and liquid diets is necessary, as before any intestinal bowel surgery. (See the section on colon and rectum cancer in Chapter 40.)

Emotional support is extremely important. The procedure to be performed should be explained to the person. It is important if possible to involve another family member or significant other. If indicated, the nurse can arrange for a preoperative visit by someone who has had similar surgery and has adjusted well.

Selection of a stoma site is an important preoperative

*The authors wish to acknowledge Gladys Frey, RN, MS, Director, USC Department of Nursing, Cosler Enterostomal Therapy Option, for her contribution to this section.

TABLE 48-3 Single Agent Regimens Used in Advanced Bladder Cancer

Drug	Dose
Adriamycin	25 to 75 mg/m^2 every 3 weeks
Bleomycin	5 units/m^2 biweekly
Etoposide	100 mg/m^2 every 3 weeks
Methotrexate	0.5 to 250 mg/m^2 every 1 to 2 weeks
Cisplatin	50 to 70 mg/m^2 every 3 or 4 weeks
Vinblastine	0.1 to 0.15 mg/m^2 every week

Source: Data from Daniels JR, Skinner DG, Lieskovsky G: Chemotherapy of cancer of the bladder, in Skinner D, Lieskovsky G (eds): Diagnosis and Management of Genitourinary Cancer. Philadelphia, WB Saunders, 1988, pp 313-321.

consideration, and the type of urinary diversion to be performed will dictate to some extent the stoma site selected. Any diversion that requires the wearing of an external appliance for the collection of urine must have an adequate surface for the appliance to adhere to properly.

The stoma site is selected and marked the day before surgery. It is crucial that an appropriate site be chosen only after discussing with the person his or her personal habits pertaining to work and recreational activities. The abdomen is examined and the individual observed while standing, sitting, and reclining. This is done to find an area at least 3 inches in diameter that is free of wrinkles and slightly convex. The site chosen should be visible to the individual and away from bony prominences, old scars or creases, and belt lines.

The Kock pouch, or continent ileal reservoir, needs no external collecting device, but the stoma must be placed for easy access by the person.

There are several methods of marking the site selected. After cleansing the site with alcohol, an insoluble dye such as gentian violet or methylene blue can be applied subdermally, or the dye can be tattooed into the midpoint of the selected site. Any method of marking the site that will remain visible after the surgical scrub is acceptable.

TABLE 48-4 Approximate 5-year Survival Rates for Bladder Cancer

Stage	Whites (%)	Blacks (%)
Localized	88	80
Disseminated	41	25
All Stages	79	56

Source: Data from Silverberg E, Lubera J: Cancer Statistics, 1989. CA 39:3-20, 1989.

Nursing care for patients undergoing ureterosigmoidostomy

Before Bricker described the ileal conduit in 1950, the ureterosigmoidostomy was the most popular form of urinary diversion. Diversion of urine from the bladder was accomplished by implanting the ureters into the sigmoid colon. Urine and feces were then excreted through the rectum and anal sphincter. Although it is not widely used today, a brief description of nursing care follows.

Preoperative bowel preparation is similar to that of any intestinal bowel surgery. Before surgery, the competency of the rectum and anal sphincter will be assessed by asking the individual to retain 200 to 300 mL of saline solution by enema as long as possible. Enemas may be given in increasing amounts to develop sphincter control and to acquaint the person with the rectal sensations he will feel after surgery.[82]

Following surgery, a large rectal tube will be inserted to drain urine and provide a means to measure urine accurately. Anuria in the early postoperative period may result from obstruction of the rectal tube with feces or mucus and may require irrigation with 20 to 30 mL of saline solution. If the tube must be changed within the first 4 or 5 days after surgery, care must be taken to avoid tissue perforation at the site of anastomosis and should not be reinserted more than 4 inches. Careful observation of intake and output is necessary to detect oliguria and anuria and reveal leakage, edema, obstruction, or stenosis at the site of anastomosis. Symptoms of abdominal distention with ileus, abdominal pain, a rising serum creatinine level, and poor urinary output after surgery indicate leakage of urine at the anastomosis between the ureter and the colon. Minor leaks may heal, but major leaks require immediate surgery.

When accurate urine measurement is no longer essential, the rectal tube may be removed during the day, and the individual instructed to empty the rectum every 2 to 3 hours. The rectal tube can be reinserted at night to allow for uninterrupted sleep, or the person can be instructed to awaken once or twice a night to empty the rectum. Until the rectal tube is removed, the individual is kept on a low-residue diet.

Initially, the stool will be diarrhea-like until the bowel adjusts to the presence of urine. Meticulous perianal skin care must be maintained to prevent irritation and breakdown. The skin should be kept clean and dry. Protective ointments may be necessary.

A high rate of complications has been recorded from this type of diversion. Reflux of urine and fecal reflux into the ureters and kidney pelvis, which can lead to pyelonephritis and possible uremia, result from a higher colonic pressure gradient.

A syndrome of hyperchloremic acidosis and hypokalemia occurs in about 50% of individuals undergoing urinary diversion, according to Skinner and Richie.[83] Symptoms of hyperchloremic acidosis include nausea, vomiting, irregular pulse, fever, muscle weakness, tachypnea, lethargy, and diarrhea. Urea reabsorption will result in dehydration, thirst, headache, and increased urinary output secondary to osmotic changes. Alkali therapy and potassium supplements may be helpful. Salt intake should be decreased and foods high in potassium such as orange or grapefruit juice, bananas, fresh apricots, cantaloupe, and potatoes should be included in the diet.

Foods that have a laxative effect or cause flatus, such as prunes, raisins, brussel sprouts, lentils, and cauliflower, should be avoided. Flatus can lead to incontinence of both urine and stool. Fluid intake should be increased to 2 to 3 liters/day to provide a natural irrigation of the urinary tract.

General nursing care following urinary diversion with an ileal conduit or continent reservoir

Unlike a fecal diversion that is subject to an adynamic ileus, the urinary diversion should produce urine from the time of surgery. As mentioned in the treatment section, the continent ileal reservoir will be intubated with a Medina Silastic catheter, which has been sutured to the skin line and connected to low-suction or gravity drainage. An ileoconduit may have stints threaded through the ureteral ileoanastomosis to provide for adequate urinary drainage while the anastomosis heals. The urinary flow should be rather continuous, and, in the case of an ileal conduit, a urinary appliance is needed to contain the drainage and to provide for accurate measurement. The appliance will prevent urine contamination of the new incisional site and protect the peristomal area from contact with the urine. The appliance is then connected to the bedside gravity drainage.

Nursing care following an ileal conduit

Stoma characteristics The intestinal stomal tissue can be compared with the mucosal lining of the mouth. The stoma may bleed when rubbed because of the capillaries in the area. A small amount of bleeding from the stoma is not serious, but it must be determined that the blood is from the stoma and not from the urine.

Ideally, a urinary stoma should protrude ½ to ¾ inches above the skin to allow the urine to drain into the aperture of an appliance. Flush stomas allow the urine to drain at skin level. This frequently is the cause of leakage and skin breakdown. The ileoconduit stoma is usually placed in the lower right quadrant. If a suitable area is not available to support an appliance there, it can be placed on the right side (within the confines of the rectus muscle to support the stoma).

Viability of the stoma is assessed by its color. This should be checked regularly, especially in the early postoperative period. Normal color of the stoma is deep pink to dark red. A dusky appearance ranging from purple to black may develop if circulation is seriously impaired. The appearance of a necrotic stoma may occur immediately after surgery or as late as 5 to 7 days after surgery.[82] The dusky appearance of the stoma immediately after surgery may change in a few hours and appear viable. Sustained color change of the stoma should be reported to the surgeon.

A necrotic stoma may develop from abdominal distention causing tension on the mesentery, from twisting of the conduit at surgery, or from arterial or venous insufficiency.[75] To determine the depth of the necrosis, a clear test tube can be inserted into the stoma with a small flashlight directed into the tube. The viable bowel will transilluminate the level of the necrosis. If the tissue at skin level is viable, surgical revision may be unnecessary. However, if necrotic, the tissue will slough, leaving a flush, retracted, or stenotic stoma. This leads to difficult management problems.

Stoma edema is normal in the early postoperative period as a result of surgical manipulation. This should not interfere with stoma functioning, but a larger opening will need to be cut in the appliance to prevent pressure or constriction of the stoma. The edema of the stoma should resolve in the first week or two after surgery. Most stomas continue to shrink over the next several months, and some will continue to decrease in size slightly for a year. Teaching the individual to continue to measure the stoma with a weekly change of appliance should alleviate the problem of the person's wearing an appliance with an aperture too large for the stoma. The stoma needs only ⅛ to ¹⁄₁₆ inch to allow for expansion during peristalsis.

Mucus production The intestine normally produces mucus, and mucus will be present in all diversions using segments of the bowel for a conduit or continent pouch. The amount of mucus produced varies with individuals and will cause the urine to appear cloudy. Excessive mucus also may be produced by an inflamed mucosa if infection is present. Excessive mucus can clog the urinary appliance outlet. Some agents on the market are designed to disperse mucus plugs but must be injected into the pouch each time it is emptied. Some urinary appliances provide larger outlets to assist with the free flow of urine. Increasing fluid intake to 3 liters/day also will help by acting as a natural irrigant.

Pouching a urinary stoma The fairly continuous flow of urine from a conduit requires the person to wear an appliance at all times. In the early postoperative period, any one of the many clear, disposable urinary pouches may be used. The selection of a particular type of pouch may be governed by the availability of supply in the facility or the surgeon's choice. The important element is the application of the appliance. Before removing the protective paper from the adhesive portion of the pouch, the stoma should be measured and the opening for the stoma cut to allow for a ⅛-inch space around the base of the stoma. If the pouch being used is a two-piece appliance with a skin barrier attached, it is not necessary to use an additional skin barrier. In the early postoperative period, it is imperative to protect the skin from direct contact with adhesives. Both shaving of the abdomen and the surgical scrub before surgery can irritate the abdominal skin. Appliances adhered without applied skin protection may further irritate the skin.

The skin around the stoma should be clean and thoroughly dry before positioning the appliance over the stoma. The pouch should initially be positioned to the person's side so that it can be attached to bedside drainage without placing stress on the seal. The flange can then be picture framed with microporous tape to enhance the seal.

Many of the urinary pouches today are manufactured with an antireflux valve. This is double thickness of the pouch, which prevents the urine from returning to the stoma. If stints are used to maintain patency, it may be necessary to thread them through the antireflux valve. The stoma should be clearly visible through the pouch.

Although not always possible, an effective urinary pouch should adhere for at least 3 days. If no leakage occurs, the same pouch can remain adhered to the skin for 5 days. It should then be changed for hygienic reasons and to observe the peristomal area.

Patient teaching for continuing care of a conduit The initial care rendered to the person with a new conduit is extremely important both physiologically and psychologically. Before the individual is able to actively participate in self-care, the nurse or enterostomal therapist can teach by example. Procedures are "talked" through as they are being performed. Applied pouches should remain in place without leakage for 3 to 5 days. Peristomal skin should remain intact without irritation. This reinforces the attitude that a normal life is possible with a conduit. As the individual's condition improves, he or she should be encouraged to verbalize concerns and fears. A visit from a person who has been rehabilitated with a similar diversion may be arranged to give reassurance. The patient should be given the opportunity to handle the equipment and do as much of the needed care as possible. All the procedures necessary for continuing care of the stoma should be written down. Names and addresses of where future supplies may be purchased also should be included. Names and telephone numbers of resource people to call if emergencies arise are a source of reassurance to the person.

Nursing care of the individual with a continent ileal reservoir for urinary diversion Three weeks after surgery, the individual will be readmitted to the hospital. The Medina tube and ureteral stints will be removed and a radiographic picture of the pouch (called a "loopogram") will be taken to confirm that there is no extravasation of urine from the pouch. The Medina tube should be intubated/catheterized every 2 hours during the day and every 3 hours at night during the first week after it is removed. This is increased gradually (by 1 hour each week) until the pouch is being intubated and drained approximately three or four times in 24 hours. The method of draining the pouch is simple, there is no need to wear an external appliance, and the time intervals between emptying the pouch can duplicate normal bladder function.

Follow-up nursing care Many complications of a urinary diversion can be averted by a periodic reevaluation of both the stoma and the function of the conduit. The stoma may continue to decrease in size for several months or more. The size of the appliance opening should reflect this change. An opening too large for the stoma will permit peristomal skin to be exposed to urine, causing maceration and denudation of the skin. Openings that are too large also can permit the formation of hypertrophic lesions, which are referred to as epitheliomatous hyperplasia. Epitheliomatous hyperplasia can appear as smooth epithelium that extends onto the stoma mucosa or as a rough keratosis that appears warty.[84] It can be painful to the individual and lead to poor adherance of the appliance because of the weeping or oozing, which in turn will cause continued leakage.

Alkaline encrustations around the stoma can lead to stoma stenosis as a result of skin contact with alkaline urine. Because bacteria thrive in an alkaline environment, infections can develop more readily when the pH of urine is allowed to become alkaline and is accompanied by serous weeping of the skin.

Stenosis, or narrowing, can occur in the stoma at the level of the skin, muscle, or fascia or at any level of the ileal segment. Stenosis interferes with drainage and can lead to stasis, dilatation of the intestine, and infection.

The urinary component of a conduit is formed by the kidneys and their collecting systems, the renal pelvis and ureters. Ureteral angulation, stenosis, obstruction, or lithiasis leads to hydronephrosis, or irreparable renal damage. Periodic evaluation by excretory pyelography or loopography can detect this before irreparable damage occurs.

The kidneys can be checked by the usual laboratory tests. The evaluations of the urea nitrogen, serum creatinine, urinary pH, and specific gravity or osmolality are the most useful tests of renal function. If urine is to be tested for culture, a sterile specimen must be obtained. Urine for analysis and culture should not be collected from the external appliance because the specimen collected will show bacteria and will not reflect the true conditions in the conduit.

Laboratory tests for the continent ileal reservoir are identical to those used to demonstrate kidney function. Urography is used to test the competence of the nipple valves and to ensure complete emptying of the reservoir.

Patient teaching accompanied by written instruction and periodic reevaluation of all components of the urinary diversion should facilitate the rehabilitation of the individual with minimal complications.

KIDNEY CANCER

Epidemiology

There are two major types of kidney cancer. Renal cell cancer is the most common form. It occurs in the parenchyma of the kidney and also has been known as renal cell carcinoma, renal adenocarcinoma, cancer of the kidney, and hypernephroma. The second major type is cancer of the renal pelvis.

Kidney cancer is not a common cancer in the United States, accounting for only about 3% of all cancers. Renal cell carcinoma accounts for about 75% of kidney cancers.[85] The American Cancer Society reports a slight steady increase in kidney cancer in men.[1]

There is a 2:1 male predominance in kidney cancer, especially in renal cell cancer.[86] There seem to be striking geographic differences, with the rate of kidney cancer being quite high in Scandinavian countries (about 11% of all cancers).[87] Japan has a low incidence, and the United States and most western European countries appear to have an intermediate risk. Interestingly enough, Scandinavians who migrate to Los Angeles do not have higher than expected rates of either cancer of the kidney or cancer of the renal pelvis.[85]

One of the most important demographic risk factors for both renal cell cancer and cancer of the renal pelvis is age. Both are rare in people under 35 years of age, and thereafter the incidence increases with age. The average age at diagnosis is 55 to 60 years.[86]

Etiology

Cigarette smoking

The causes of kidney cancer remain obscure. The only risk factor that has been linked persistently to kidney cancer by both cohort studies[88-90] and epidemiologic case-controlled studies[91-93] is cigarette smoking. For renal cell cancer, a consistent relationship between the number of cigarettes consumed and the risk of cancer has not been established. For cancer of the renal pelvis, however, there does appear to be a strong association between the number of cigarettes smoked and the risk for cancer.[85] It is not clear in what way cigarette smoking might induce kidney cancer, but studies have shown numerous mutagenic chemicals in the urine of cigarette smokers.[90]

Occupation

Kidney cancer seems to be associated with certain occupational exposures. Exposures to cadmium,[91] asbestos,[94] and lead (pigment in colored printing ink)[95] have each demonstrated a slightly increased risk for renal cell cancer than might otherwise be expected. But currently, occupational exposure is associated with only a very small proportion of all renal cancers.[85]

Analgesic use

Heavy use of analgesics, specifically aspirin, phenacetin, or acetaminophen-containing products, has been shown to increase the risk of cancer of the renal pelvis. A possible association between analgesics and renal cell cancer has been reported but not conclusively substantiated.[92]

Other factors

A strong association between renal cell cancer and obesity in women was first identified in 1974.[93] Others have found similar associations,[92] but there remains the question of whether the increased incidence in women is related to obesity or to hormonal (estrogen) influences.[86]

Although it is often mentioned speculatively, studies have failed to establish a uniform association between coffee drinking and kidney cancer.[85]

Pathophysiology

Cellular characteristics

There are two primary types of kidney cancer: renal cell carcinoma (also called renal cell cancer, renal adenocarcinoma, cancer of the kidney, adenocarcinoma of the renal parenchyma, and hypernephroma) and cancer of the renal pelvis.

Renal cell carcinoma is the most common form and accounts for about 75% to 85% of kidney cancers. Although the histology is diverse from tumor to tumor, renal cell carcinoma can be separated into two broad groups: clear cell tumors and granular cell tumors.

Cancer of the renal pelvis accounts for about 5% to 9% of all kidney cancers. The two major cell types in tumors of the renal pelvis are transitional cell cancer (most common) and squamous cell cancer.

Renal cell carcinoma arises from tubular epithelial cells that are found in the kidney parenchyma. Tumors of the renal pelvis generally arise from epithelial tissue anywhere in the renal pelvis and are often papillary.[63] These tumors often have independent, multifocal origins.[96]

Progression of disease

Renal cell cancers tend to grow toward the medullary portion of the kidney, whereas tumors of the renal pelvis often grow at the ureteropelvic junction and invade the underlying submucosa and muscular coats.

Cancer of the renal pelvis and renal cell carcinoma spread through the venous and lymphatic routes. Hematogenous spread most often involves the lungs, bones, and liver. Lymphatic drainage of the kidneys is to the nodes in the ipsilateral renal hilus. These nodes then drain into the regional lymph nodes.

Renal cell carcinoma also spreads by direct extension to the renal vein and sometimes farther into the vena cava. It can also extend by growing up through the renal capsule into the perinephric fat or the adjacent visceral structures.[97] Cancer of the renal pelvis grows by extension as mentioned, down into the ureter and out through the muscular coats.

Exact numbers vary, but somewhere between 30% and 50% of individuals with kidney cancer have metastasis at diagnosis.[98,99]

Paraneoplasia and Renal Cell Carcinoma

Renal cell carcinoma has a considerable association with certain paraneoplastic syndromes. The term *paraneoplastic syndrome* is used to describe systemic effects of a tumor on the host. The effects are not directly related to the tumor presence (such as compression or obstruction from a solid tumor) or to a particular metastatic lesion (eg, brain or bone metastasis). Rather, paraneoplastic syndromes are thought to be associated with compounds that the malignant cells synthesize that are not normally synthesized by cells of that type (see Chapter 28). Although uncommon in general, renal cell carcinomas seem to have a higher association with paraneoplasia, particularly that related to the endocrine system.[100] Some of the ectopic (or inappropriately secreted) hormones that have been ascribed to tumors of renal origin are parathyroid hormone, erythropoietin, renin, gonadotropins, and adrenocorticotropic hormone.[97,100,101]

Clinical Manifestations

Renal cell carcinoma

In 40% of individuals diagnosed with renal cell carcinoma, the initial symptom is gross hematuria. The hematuria appears uniform throughout the urinary stream, and lower tract discomfort is not present. Pain (which is usually dull and aching) is also a common presenting symptom, as is a palpable abdominal mass.[101] These three symptoms—hematuria, pain, and a palpable abdominal mass—represent the classic triad of symptoms of renal cell carcinoma. However, their simultaneous appearance on presentation is infrequent. Because of the well-protected anatomic position of the kidney, the presence of a tumor is unfortunately often concealed until advanced stages. Other, more generalized symptoms also have been described with cancer of the kidney, including fever, weight loss, an elevated erythrocyte sedimentation rate (ESR), or anemia.

Cancer of the renal pelvis

Only a few individuals with cancer of the renal pelvis present with the classic triad of symptoms. Most patients with tumors of the renal pelvis originally present with hematuria (gross or microscopic). Some individuals may have both hematuria and flank pain, which is probably caused by the passage of blood clots or by obstruction of the ureteropelvic junction.[96] A palpable mass in a tumor of the renal pelvis is almost always either because the tumor has extended outside the kidney or because of massive hydronephrosis (resulting from a ureteropelvic junction obstruction).

Techniques for early detection have not been identified for either renal cell carcinoma or cancer of renal pelvis.

Assessment

Renal cell carcinoma

Tests used in the diagnosis and staging of renal cell carcinoma include kidney, ureter, and bladder (KUB) radiographs, nephrotomograms, excretory urogram, retrograde urogram, renal ultrasound, renal CT, and renal angiography (Table 48-5). MRI examinations help to identify renal cysts more readily, and solid renal masses can be distinguished from normal renal parenchyma on MRI. Although some claim that the diagnosis of renal cancer has not been improved by MRI,[67] others believe it to be similar or slightly greater in accuracy than CT and maintain that its role in the systematic evaluation of kidney cancer is still evolving.[102]

Excretory urograms have traditionally been known as intravenous pyelograms. The prefix *pyelo* implies, however, that only the renal pelvis is shown. Excretory urogram is probably a more apt name because the test does show the entire urinary tract. Excretory urogram and renal tomography are considered by most to be the screening tests of choice for suspected renal mass lesions, although they are only 70% to 75% accurate in differentiating benign cysts from malignant lesions.[102]

The next test that might be employed is renal ultrasound. The apparent advantage of this test is that it is easy to do, noninvasive, relatively inexpensive, and requires a minimal physical expenditure on the person's part. It can generally differentiate solid from cystic masses. Individuals who have solid or questionable masses should undergo further tests.[103]

Renal ultrasound, which is generally the next step in the assessment of a renal mass, coupled with CT, makes it possible to diagnose small tumors suggestive of malignancy. A CT scan can accurately evaluate a questionable lesion, determine the local extent of the cancer, identify the presence of enlarged regional lymph nodes, and describe the presence of tumor within the main renal vein and the inferior vena cava.[104,105] A CT scan of the abdomen, chest, and brain also can aid in detecting distant metastases.

The value of renal angiography has decreased with the advent of ultrasound and CT. In most cases, the superiority of a technically adequate CT scan with ultrasound make diagnostic angiography a last resort.[102]

Recently, DNA flow cytometry has added information in predicting the prognosis of patients with renal cell cancer. Aneuploid tumors were found to be more likely to develop to invasive lesions than diploid tumors.[62]

Cancer of the renal pelvis

Excretory urogram, retrograde urogram, and urinary cytology are the most useful techniques for establishing a diagnosis of cancer of the renal pelvis. Angiography has been unsuccessful with these tumors. Routine use of ultrasound and CT scanning does not appear to have the same major impact on cancer of the renal pelvis as on renal cell cancer.[106] However, ultrasound may show a mass density in the central region of the kidney, and a CT scan might detect the presence of a soft tissue mass in the renal hilum.

Urinary cytology can be done on a freshly voided urine specimen or on washings from the renal pelvis obtained during a retrograde urogram. Cytology is helpful when findings are positive, but voided specimens are of questionable value because of the possible confusion with the presence of bladder cancer and because low-grade renal pelvis tumors often do not show positive findings.[106] Unfortunately, false-positive results have been reported in as many as 10% of cases, and false-negative results are common.[96]

Classification and Staging

Renal cell carcinoma

Staging for renal cell carcinoma, as with all cancers, is founded on those aspects that influence survival, including regional lymph node involvement, invasion through the renal capsule, extension to contiguous organs, and distant metastases.[107] Extension into the renal veins or the inferior vena cava is thought by some authorities to have no influence on prognosis if properly managed.[101] Likewise, the size of the primary tumor is not strongly correlated with survival and may not be a significant factor in staging.

The system that is used most often for classifying renal cell carcinoma is a modification of the system of Flocks and Kadesky[108] (Table 48-6). There are problems with this

TABLE 48-5 Diagnostic Evaluation of Renal Cell Carcinoma and Cancer of the Renal Pelvis

Test Name	Indications	Anatomic Features	Visualization Technique	Special Preparation	Side Effects/ Comments
KUB (kidney, ureter, bladder)	General initial study (sensitivity low)	Shows renal outlines for kidney size, shape, and position	X-ray film (plain film of abdomen)	None—patient will lie flat on x-ray table	Bowel content may obliterate renal shadow KUB should *not* follow barium studies
Nephrotomogram	Helps to differentiate between cysts and neoplasms and may reveal extrarenal masses	Enhances outlines, clarifies size, shape, and position of kidney	X-ray film of kidneys before and after opacification of renal arterial network and parenchyma with contrast medium	Nothing by mouth for 8 hours before test, injection of iodine-based contrast medium through antecubital vein (during test)	Possible allergic reaction to contrast medium Possible hematoma at antecubital fossa
Excretory urogram (intravenous pyelogram—IVP)	To evaluate structure and excretory function of the kidneys ureters and bladder	Allows visualization of the renal parenchyma, calyces and pelvis as well as the ureters and bladder	KUB x-ray first, then intravenous injection of contrast medium x-ray films at 1 minute, 5 minutes, 10 minutes and 15 or 20 minutes Ureteral compression may be done after 5 minutes through 10 minutes if needed to help visualize upper urinary tract; x-ray film of bladder after voiding	Good hydration, then nothing by mouth for 6 to 8 hours before test Laxative will decrease amount of gas and feces that might obscure delineation of the urinary tract	Possible allergic reaction to contrast medium, specific gravity of urine = 1.040 to 1.060 for 2 hours after test
Retrograde urograms (retrograde IVP, retrograde ureteropyelography)	Inadequate excretory urograms, assessment of degree of ureteral obstruction (tumors of renal pelvis) or sensitivity to intravenous contrast medium	Permits visualization of the renal collecting system (calyces, renal pelvis and ureters)	X-ray film of renal collecting system after injection of contrast medium through ureteral catheter during cystoscopy	Patient may be given a barbiturate or narcotic analgesic before the procedure; sometimes general anesthesia is indicated Laxatives the night before will cleanse the bowel	Instrumentation is always uncomfortable and can be painful; hematuria and dysuria and occasional voiding difficulty may occur after the procedure

TABLE 48-5 Diagnostic Evaluation of Renal Cell Carcinoma and Cancer of the Renal Pelvis (continued)

Test Name	Indications	Anatomic Features	Visualization Technique	Special Preparation	Side Effects/ Comments
Renal ultrasound	Differential diagnosis of renal cysts vs. neoplasms	Test not dependent on renal function, helps determine size, shape, position of kidneys, internal structures and perirenal tissues, including detecting differences in density of a mass	High-frequency sound waves transmitted through the kidneys and perirenal structures; the resulting echoes are converted into an anatomic image	None	Relatively inexpensive, safe, and painless
Renal computed tomography (CT scan)	Inadequate ultrasound, indeterminate cyst vs. tumor lesions, preoperative staging (extent of lymph node involvement, involvement of renal vein or inferior vena cava), assessing recurrence of renal cancer	Shows a series of cross sectioned slices of the whole urinary tract (kidney, perinephric space, renal hilum, inferior vena cava, and adjacent organs)	X-ray pictures of 10-mm contiguous transverse slices through both kidneys	Nothing by mouth for 4 hours before test if contrast enhancement performed. Prepare patient for large, possibly noisy machinery	If contrast medium used may experience transient flushing, headache or metallic taste in mouth
CT scans of brain, abdomen, chest	To evaluate distant metastasis	Series of cross-sectional (transverse) slices of body part being examined	Computerized x-ray technique	Same as above	Same as above
Renal angiography	May assist in detecting perinephric extension, lymph node involvement, renal vein and inferior vena caval involvement (plays a lesser role if CT scan employed)	Demonstrates the caliber of the great vessels and shows the renal arterial circulation	Usually a femoral catheter is passed into one of the renal arteries under fluoroscopy, and then radiopaque contrast medium is given intravenously	Nothing by mouth for 8 hours before test. Patient may be given a sedative or narcotic analgesic before the test; all metallic objects that may interfere with test results should be removed	May react to contast medium; bleeding or hematoma at injection site may occur; patient should be flat in bed for 8 to 12 hours after test Keep a pressure dressing in place and monitor popliteal and pedal pulses

staging system, primarily involving stage II and III. Stage III grouping includes tumors involving the renal vein or regional lymph nodes, with or without involvement of the vena cava or perinephric fat. Grouping renal vein, vena cava, and lymph node involvement into this stage causes the survival rate to be higher than in stage II because simple renal vein extension is not a dire prognostic factor.[107] Figure 48-16 demonstrates long-term survival by stage.

The TNM system (Table 48-7) solves that particular problem but is detailed and difficult to use.

Cancer of the renal pelvis

Because of the difficulty in establishing a diagnosis and the limited accuracy of available staging procedures, there is no official staging system for cancer of the renal pelvis.

Treatment of Renal Cell Carcinoma

Surgery

Patients with renal cell carcinoma are treated by surgical removal. A radical nephrectomy routinely includes

TABLE 48-6 Staging of Renal Cell Cancer

Stage	Description
Stage I	Tumor is confined to the kidney; perinephric fat, renal vein, and regional nodes show no evidence of malignancy
Stage II	Tumor involves the perinephric fat but is confined within Gerota's fascia; renal vein and regional nodes show no evidence of malignancy
Stage III	Tumor involves the renal vein or regional nodes, with or without involvement of the vena cava or perinephric fat
Stage IV	Distant metastases secondary to renal cell carcinoma present on admission or histologic involvement by tumor of contiguous visceral structures

removal of the lymph nodes in the renal hilar area.

Two surgical approaches have been used for radical nephrectomy. The abdominotransperitoneal approach is often performed with a midline or subcostal abdominal incision. Some authorities feel the use of this approach is limited because of the difficulty in dissecting the retroperitoneal region above and around the renal pedicles.[97] The thoracoabdominal approach may also be used.

Some experts suggest in the surgical management of renal cell carcinoma that the tumor must not be manipulated before the renal artery and vein are exposed and occluded. The origin of the right renal artery is directly behind the left renal vein, and it is felt that the right renal artery should be ligated at its origin from the aorta before the right kidney is mobilized or manipulated.[97]

Vena caval involvement

Only about 5% to 9% of individuals with renal cell carcinoma have varying degrees of tumor thrombus extending into the vena cava.[109] Because of the shorter right renal vein, tumor thrombus occurs more often on the right side. A tumor thrombus in the vena cava is removed in continuity with the renal tumor to prevent tumor embolization. Tumor invasion of the wall of the vena cava is no longer thought to be an unanimously incurable situation, and while the surgical treatment is complicated, recent published experience indicates a positive outcome for many of these patients if they are free of distant metastases.[110]

Classically, individuals with vena cava tumor thrombus have been classified as having stage III renal cell carcinoma and have been grouped along with individuals who have regional lymph node metastasis. This may be an inappropriate staging. Individuals who have vena caval extension (without capsular invasion, perinephric fat invasion, or regional lymph node metastases) have a prognosis comparable to individuals with stage I tumors.[111]

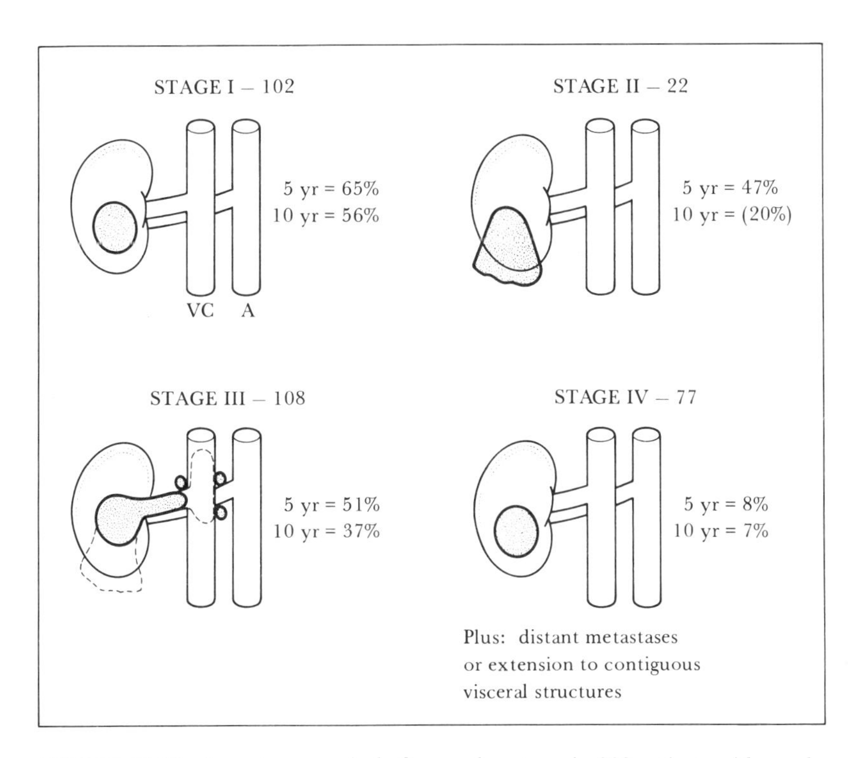

FIGURE 48-16 Long-term survival after nephrectomy in 309 patients with renal cell carcinoma. Results are grouped according to pathologic stage of the lesion. (Source: Skinner DG: The surgical management of renal cell carcinoma. J Urol 107:707, 1972.)

TABLE 48-7 TNM Classification System for Renal Cell Carcinoma

Primary Tumor (T)	
Tx	Minimum requirements cannot be met
T0	No evidence of primary tumor
T1	Small tumor, minimal renal and caliceal distortion or deformity. Circumscribed neovasculature surrounded by normal parenchyma
T2	Large tumor with deformity and/or enlargement of the kidney and/or collecting system
T3a	Tumor involving perinephric tissues
T3b	Tumor involving renal vein
T3c	Tumor involving renal vein and infradiaphragmatic vena cava
Note: Under T3, tumor may extend into perinephric tissues, into renal vein, and into vena cava as shown on cavography. In these instances, the T classification may be shown as T3a, b, and c, or some appropriate combination, depending on extension—for example, T3a,b is tumor in perinephric fat and extending into the renal vein	
T4a	Tumor invasion of neighboring structures (e.g., muscle, bowel)
T4b	Tumor involving supradiaphragmatic vena cava
Nodal Involvement (N)	
The regional lymph nodes are the para-aortic and paracaval nodes. The juxtaregional lymph nodes are the pelvic nodes and the mediastinal nodes.	
NX	Minimum requirements cannot be met
N0	No evidence of involvement of regional nodes
N1	Single, homolateral regional nodal involvement
N2	Involvement of multiple regional or contralateral or bilateral nodes
N3	Fixed regional nodes (assessable only at surgical exploration)
N4	Involvement of juxtaregional nodes
Note: If lymphography is source of staging, add "l" between "N" and designator number; if histologic proof is provided, "+" if positive, and "−" if negative. Thus, NI2 indicates multiple positive nodes seen on lymphography and proved at operation by biopsy	
Distant Metastasis (M)	
MX	Not assessed
M0	No (known) distant metastasis
M1	Distant metastasis present; specify sites according to the following notations:
	PUL—Pulmonary; MAR—Bone marrow
	OSS—Osseous; PLE—Pleura
	HEP—Hepatic; SKI—Skin
	BRA—Brain; EYE—Eye
	LYM—Lymph nodes; OTH—Other
Add "+" to the abbreviated notation to indicate that the pathology (p) is proven	

Source: American Joint Committee for Cancer Staging and End Results Reporting, Manual for Staging of Cancer. Chicago, The Committee, 1983.

Lymphadenectomy

Regional lymphadenectomy remains a controversial subject.[112] Lymphatic metastases has been found (by lymph node dissection) in 8% to 22% of individuals without other evidence of metastasis.[98] Those who argue against lymphadenectomy feel that (1) it does not improve survival, (2) its staging value in terms of predicting survival is limited because the cancer can spread through the venous system alone, and (3) because there is as yet no effective adjuvant therapy, identification of lymph node metastases is not important.[98,113]

Those who favor lymphadenectomy feel that it would add to a more comprehensive and meaningful staging using the TNM system.[114] Some settings routinely perform lymphadenectomy on all patients with stage I, II, or III disease; that is, it is argued that this offers the best chance of survival to those for whom radical nephrectomy is potentially curative.[115]

Bilateral tumors or tumors in a solitary kidney

In the unusual case of bilateral tumors or cancer in a solitary kidney, two treatment options are available. In bilateral tumors where there is a larger tumor in one kidney than in the other, partial nephrectomy is performed on the kidney with the smaller tumor, and several weeks later radical nephrectomy is carried out on the kidney with the larger tumor. In cases where there is a tumor in a solitary kidney with no evidence of metastasis, partial nephrectomy or radical nephrectomy with subsequent chronic hemodialysis are treatment alternatives.

Radiotherapy and chemotherapy

Renal cell carcinomas and their metastases are usually radioresistant, and the treatment role of radiotherapy is controversial. Some authors have reported that radiotherapy made surgery technically easier.[116] Metastatic bone pain can be palliated by irradiating the area involved with significant doses, up to 4000 to 5000 cGy.[117]

Adjuvant chemotherapy has not demonstrated any improvement in survival rates over those accomplished without chemotherapy.[101]

Treatment of Advanced Renal Cell Carcinoma

About 30% of individuals with renal cell carcinoma present with metastases at diagnosis. Another 50% will develop metastases after radical nephrectomy.[99] The mean survival rate in patients with metastases at diagnosis is approximately 4 months, and only about 10% survive 1 year.[118] Surgery, chemotherapy, hormonal therapy, and immunotherapy have all been suggested as means of managing the disease.

Surgery

Adjunctive or palliative nephrectomies have been described as approaches for individuals with metastatic renal cell carcinoma. Adjunctive nephrectomy is done to improve survival, whereas palliative nephrectomy is done to relieve symptoms of the primary renal tumor.

Individuals whose survival is improved by adjunctive nephrectomy are those who have the best performance status and least amount of tumor before surgery.[99]

Palliative nephrectomy may be justifiable for individuals who have severe disabling symptoms such as local pain, bleeding, or endocrinopathy but who otherwise have a reasonable life expectancy of greater than 6 months.[99] Radiotherapy might relieve these symptoms equally well.

Angioinfarction of the primary tumor with a subsequent radical nephrectomy has been used in an aggressive but unsuccessful attempt to improve survival.[119]

Chemotherapy

Chemotherapy has had no great impact on metastatic renal cell carcinoma.[98] Some clinicians, however, feel that chemotherapeutic trials might be appropriate for certain individuals because metastatic renal cell carcinoma presents so few options. Vinblastine (Velban) is one chemotherapeutic agent that has demonstrated some success in achieving tumor responses.[99]

Several clinical trials have tested chemotherapy combinations that include vinblastine. Better responses have been achieved than with vinblastine alone, but the response duration is short and the toxicity significant.[101]

Hormonal therapy

Because progestational agents have proved useful in DES-induced renal tumors in hamsters, several clinical trials in humans have been conducted in the last 20 years. Response rates vary from 2% to 15%. Drugs most often used have been progesterones such as medroxyprogesterone acetate (Depo-Provera) or megesterol acetate (Megace), testosterone, and antiestrogens such as tamoxifen. The infrequent responses to hormonal therapy have not significantly improved survival. A few individuals, however, may be helped by this relatively benign therapy.[101]

Immunotherapy

Although renal cell cancer has been resistant to chemotherapy and hormonal therapy, in 1985 Rosenberg et al[120] first demonstrated antitumor responses after adoptive immunotherapy with high doses of interleukin-2 (IL-2) and large numbers of lymphokine activated killer (LAK) cells in metastatic renal cancer. IL-2 has been used alone in patients with advanced disseminated disease, but complete and partial responses have been much higher when IL-2 is combined with LAK cells.[121]

The treatment is complicated, toxic, and expensive.[122] At this time, several phase II clinical studies are underway to confirm treatment effectiveness and to determine whether the complicated technology required can be transferred outside a pure research setting.[123] One current protocol requires a 16-day treatment cycle with patients initially being primed with 5 days of IL-2 to stimulate LAK cell precursors. After a 2-day rest, patients have 5 consecutive daily leukaphereses. The lymphocytes are incubated with IL-2 for three to four days. After the last leukapheresis, patient cells are reinfused along with additional IL-2 during the last 4 days of the cycle.[123]

This treatment is given in an intensive care unit because of the toxicity of IL-2, including fever, gastrointestinal bleeding, rash and pruritus, hepatic dysfunction, thrombocytopenia, somnolence, disorientation, and pulmonary edema.[123]

Alpha interferon has shown modest activity in the treatment of patients with advanced renal cancer. The side effects reported have been tolerable.[124]

Treatment of Cancer of the Renal Pelvis

Radical nephrectomy, including the kidney, all perinephric tissue, regional lymph nodes, the ureter, and the periureteral portion (or cuff) of the bladder is standard treatment for cancer of the renal pelvis. Proponents of this radical procedure feel it is necessary to treat the secondary ureteral and vesical tumors that may be present.[106] Others who argue for more conservative, kidney-sparing approaches to surgical treatment of this cancer stress the poor prognosis associated with advanced lesions and the mortality risks of radical procedures.[106]

Radiation therapy has not been proved an effective adjunct for the control of residual tumor, local recurrence, or unresectable disease.[106] Chemotherapeutic agents that have been used with limited results include doxorubicin, cisplatin, methotrexate, and vinblastine.[125]

TABLE 48-8 The 5- and 10-year Survival Rates for Patients with Renal Cell Cancer after Nephrectomy

Stage	5 Year (%)	10 Year (%)
I	65	56
II	47	20
III	51	37
IV	8	7

Source: Skinner DG: The surgical management of renal cell carcinoma. Urology 107:707, 1972.

Results and Prognosis

Survival rates for patients with renal cell carcinoma are shown in Table 48-8. Although the database for these figures is dated, in general the survival statistics have not changed.[101] There are, however, limitations in the previously described staging system in predicting the survival of patients with Stage III disease.

The prognosis for cancer of the renal pelvis is relatively poor and is closely correlated with the degree of differentiation and extent of the tumor. Although the overall survival rates are approximately 40%, the reported 5-year survival rate for individuals with differentiated transitional cell carcinoma of the renal pelvis is approximately 60%; for those with undifferentiated carcinomas, it is only 14%.[106] Extension outside the kidney indicates a very poor prognosis.

Nursing Care

Individuals who are undergoing diagnostic procedures or treatments for kidney malignancy are extremely anxious. Some individuals equate the loss of a kidney with imminent death. Others worry that the remaining kidney will not be able to meet the body's total need for complete urine elimination. The nurse can help by providing correct information to the individual and family. The nurse should assess the individual's knowledge and feelings about the disease and its treatment to help the patient set realistic goals for dealing with the malignancy.

Nursing care of patients undergoing surgery

In general, patients with primary renal carcinoma undergo surgical excision. Radical nephrectomy is performed on all resectable lesions in stage I to III and is sometimes done palliatively for symptoms such as pain and bleeding for individuals with advanced disease. The preoperative and postoperative nursing management of the person undergoing radical nephrectomy is similar to that of the individual undergoing laparotomy.

Preoperative nursing care A renal infarction may be done 2 or 3 days before surgery in an attempt to decrease surgical hemorrhage by decreasing tumor vascularity. Following this procedure, the individual may experience considerable pain, fever, nausea, and vomiting. Those symptoms may persist for up to 36 hours. Analgesic and antiemetic medications should be administered for symptomatic control. Intravenous fluid supplement may be necessary if the individual has a severe fluid loss. Emotional support and reassurance during this time can be comforting to the patient and family.

Postoperative nursing care

Pain relief The primary objectives during the postoperative period are the management of pain and the prevention of postoperative complications. Pain can be quite severe after nephrectomy. For lower pole renal tumors, the flank incision (retroperitoneal) approach is generally used, and the individual is placed in a hyperextended side-lying position. The thoracoabdominal incision approach is generally used for larger and upper pole lesions. In this approach the person is placed in an oblique position with rolled towels situated to elevate the flank.

As a result of the position on the operating table, the individual undergoing nephrectomy experiences not only incision pain but also muscular aches and pains. The nurse should administer analgesic medication on a regular schedule for the first 48 hours after surgery and then gradually decrease the frequency and strength of analgesics according to the person's needs per the physician's order. The use of moist heat, massage, and pillows to support the back while the person is on the side also can provide relief. The individual should be turned from side to side at least every 2 hours or whenever desired.

Prevention of atelectasis and pneumonia Because the incision is close to the diaphragm, deep breathing and coughing can be extremely uncomfortable. The person must be taught how to splint the incision while coughing. Use of analgesics at proper intervals will help the person perform deep breathing and coughing more effectively. The nurse should instruct the individual to take at least 10 deep breaths each hour while awake. The use of an incentive spirometer and intermittent positive-pressure breathing also may be beneficial.

Monitoring renal function If an indwelling catheter is in place, urine output should be monitored every hour immediately after surgery. The urine will be slightly blood-tinged for the first few hours after surgery. Urine output should be greater than 30 mL/hour. If the individual does not have a urinary catheter and has not voided within 8 to 10 hours after surgery, catheterization must be done to determine renal status. Accurate recording of fluid intake and output and weight should be done daily to determine the person's overall fluid balance.

Paralytic ileus is fairly common following renal surgery. It is thought to be due to a reflex paralysis of intestinal peristalsis. The individual is usually allowed nothing to eat or drink by mouth for the first 24 to 48 hours after surgery. Oral food and fluids are avoided until bowel sounds are heard and gas is passed. The symptoms of paralytic ileus are abdominal distension, pain, and absence of bowel sounds. Nothing is given by mouth, and a nasogastric or rectal tube is used to relieve abdominal distention. Other measures such as ambulation, turning the person, and use of a heating pad on the abdomen may also assist the individual in expelling flatus.

Hemorrhage Although not a frequent complication, postnephrectomy hemorrhage is a danger, because the kidney is a highly vascular organ. Acute massive hemorrhage manifests itself by profuse drainage and distension at the suture line or internally. It can be reflected by an elevation of pulse rate and a drop in blood pressure. However, slow bleeding may not manifest itself in such obvious changes in vital signs. The nurse should observe the individual closely for symptoms of hemorrhage and shock. The person should be turned and the underlying sheet examined for blood when the nephrectomy dressing is checked.

Wound care Wound care after nephrectomy is fairly routine. Frequently no drain is inserted. The frequency of dressing changes depends on the condition of the incision and the amount of drainage.

When the thoracoabdominal incision approach has been used for nephrectomy, pneumothorax may develop. The individual will have a chest tube placed during surgery to remove air and fluid from the thoracic cavity and to reexpand the lung. The nurse must maintain the chest tube under water drainage and keep it free of kinks. (See the section on chest tube care in Chapter 43.)

Discharge planning Discharge planning begins as soon as the individual is admitted to the hospital and is frequently updated. At discharge, the nurse must discuss with the individual the importance of continued liberal oral intake of fluids (at least 2500 mL/day) and the need to avoid any fad diets, which may result in excess protein catabolism. Individuals who are prone to hypertension should be encouraged to have frequent blood pressure checks because the nephrotic pressure gradient may change when only one kidney is present. Individuals who have had surgery to remove a renal tumor should be advised to have a complete physical examination and chest radiograph annually to rule out lung metastasis and to have an intravenous pyelogram yearly to check for contralateral tumors. The person also should be educated to report any symptoms of respiratory distress, hemoptysis, pain, or fracture of an extremity. These symptoms may signify metastasis. Last but not least, the person should be reassured that life with one kidney can be normal.

Nursing care of patients receiving chemotherapy

Antineoplastic agents have generally not had a significant effect on metastatic renal carcinoma. Vinblastine is the most effective single agent at present. The major toxicity of vinblastine is dose-related myelosuppression. Other infrequent side effects are alopecia, nausea, vomiting, stomatitis, neurotoxicity, and paralytic ileus. This drug is administered intravenously. The nurse must ensure vein patency before drug administration because extravasation can cause local skin and tissue necrosis.

Methyl-GAG, an investigational chemotherapeutic agent, has demonstrated some activity in renal carcinoma. This drug must be given as an intravenous infusion over at least 30 minutes to avoid possible orthostatic hypotension. Its major side effects are severe stomatitis, vasculitis, hyperglycemia, nausea, vomiting, and diarrhea. Other infrequent side effects are neuropathy, myopathy, and paralytic ileus.

The general nursing responsibilities regarding chemotherapy include familiarity with the normal dosage ranges and routes of administration, and potential acute and delay side effects. Patients should be educated accordingly. (See Chapter 14, Chemotherapy.)

Nursing care of patients receiving hormonal therapy

Progesterone and testosterone agents (eg, Depo-Provera and Megace) have been used in hormonal therapy to treat patients with metastatic renal cell carcinoma. They are generally well tolerated except for mild fluid retention and body weight gain. Testosterone (androgens) such as fluoxymesterone (Halotestin) and testolactone (Teslac) are also well tolerated. Acute side effects may include some nausea, vomiting, and edema.

Nursing care of patients receiving biologic response modifiers

Numerous clinical trials using a variety of biologic response modifiers (BRMs) such as interferon (INF), interleukin-2 (IL-2), and lymphokine activated killer cells (LAK) are being conducted in patients with metastatic renal cell carcinoma. Among the BRMs, interferons have had the broadest therapeutic experience in clinical oncology.[126] There are three distinct antigenic species, identified as alpha, beta, and gamma interferons. The alpha interferons have demonstrated positive response in metastatic renal cell carcinoma, while gamma interferon showed minimal activity in this disease.[126] Alpha interferon is usually administered by intramuscular or subcutaneous injection. In contrast, gamma interferon must be given intravenously.[127] Some of the common side effects of alpha interferon are malaise, weakness, fever, chills, pancytopenia, nausea, vomiting, and diarrhea.

IL-2 can be administered by various routes, including intravenous bolus, continuous infusion, subcutaneous injection, and peritoneal infusion. The optimal administration route and dosing schedule have not been established.[128] Some of the major toxicities are fluid retention, hypotension, confusion, oliguria, nausea, vomiting, diarrhea, hepatoxicity, skin rash, chills, fever, and malaise. The major dose-limiting toxicity of IL-2 is the fluid imbalance caused by capillary permeability; leaks allow intravascular fluids to shift into extravascular space. This is manifested as peripheral edema, abdominal ascites, or pulmonary infiltrates.[129] The nurse must monitor the patient's cardiovascular and pulmonary status carefully. Management of hypotension may require colloid solutions such as 5% human albumin. Fluid replacement must be carefully monitored to avoid fluid overload.

LAK is generally given as a part of IL-2 treatment. LAK is given intravenously using a tubing without filter over about 30 minutes after a test dose is given.[129] The patient may experience shaking chills, fever, nausea, vomiting, and other toxicities induced by IL-2.

In caring for patients undergoing BRM therapy, the nurse must assess the patient's anxiety and expectation and attempt to maintain a balance between hope and the possibility of negative clinical response. The nurse also must manage the many side effects of the BRMs, which at times may not be amenable to conventional nursing intervention. Severe toxicities may require reduction of the dose or discontinuation of the treatment. Patient and family should be educated about the potential side effects and when to seek help. Working with the patient receiving BRM treatment is indeed a nursing challenge.

TESTICULAR CANCER

Epidemiology

Testicular cancer is an uncommon cancer, accounting for only 1% to 2% of all cancer in men and less than 0.5% of all cancer deaths in men.[130] It is a striking type of cancer, however, for three reasons. First, it is the most common solid tumor in men between 29 and 35 years of age. Second, its incidence has been increasing over the last 50 years in whites, whereas the incidence in young black males is low. Third, the dramatic improvement in the management of this disease has been one of cancer's real success stories.

Age, race, and geographic location are all significant in the epidemiology of testicular cancer. The peak age is between 20 and 40 years of age. From 40 to 60 years of age the incidence declines, and then the incidence increases slightly. The rate in blacks is less than one third the rate in whites. Scandinavian countries have the highest incidence of testicular cancer; in Denmark it accounts for 6.7% of all cancers. However, there is an increase in incidence among young white males in all of Europe and North America. Asian and African countries have the lowest rate; Japan's testicular cancer incidence is 0.8%.[130]

The other epidemiologic factor of note is that the incidence of testis cancer is highest in men of the highest socioeconomic classes, regardless of ethnicity; that is, there is an association between higher incidence and higher economic status.

Etiology

Two factors have been associated with an increased incidence of testicular cancer: cryptorchidism and exogenous estrogens. Patients with cryptorchidism (undescended testicle) have a relative threefold to 14-fold risk for testicular cancer.[131,132] Normal descent of the testicle is under hormonal control. White persons have a three times greater risk of undescended testes than blacks do.[130]

Exogenous estrogens given to women as birth control pills or as DES (to prevent spontaneous abortion) have been hypothesized to influence the incidence of testicular cancer in subsequent male children. Case-controlled studies have examined the relationship between risk of testicular cancer of the testis and exogenous estrogen administration during pregnancy and found an increased risk of testicular cancer in the male children of women exposed to DES, estrogen, or estrogen-progestin combinations.[130]

Henderson et al[130] propose a unifying etiologic hypothesis that describes the initial carcinogenic event occurring in utero in response to free estrogen. Factors then combine throughout the boy's development and culminate in "abnormal" primitive germ cells, producing a neoplastic cell line.[130]

Pathophysiology

Cellular characteristics

Cell types of testicular cancer are classified in terms of embryonal tissue. Almost all these tumors arise from the primordial germ cell, a multipotent cell in the yolk sac of the embryo.[133] "Multipotent" refers to a cell that will have many varieties of cell types as its "offspring." This can explain why one primary testicular tumor may have a wide variety of cell types. It also explains why there are so many different types of primary testicular tumors. Several classification systems have been proposed for germ cell tumors. The following is a common grouping of the various histologic types of testicular cancer that separates the various types as seminomas or nonseminomas:

- Arising from germ tissue (germinal) (97%)
  - Seminoma (also called germinoma)
    - Typical (most common testicular tumor)
    - Anaplastic
    - Spermocytic
  - Nonseminomatous germ cell tumors (NSGCT)
    - Embryonal (including yolk sac)
    - Teratocarcinoma
    - Teratoma
    - Choriocarcinoma
- Arising from stromal tissue (3%)
  - Interstitial cell tumors (Leydig's cell tumors)
  - Gonadal-stromal tumors

This chapter focuses only on germinal tumors, that is, the seminomas and nonseminomas.

Most testicular tumors arise from germ tissue. They can arise either focally from a single cell or multifocally.[133] Malignant growth is fairly rapid. This cancer usually appears in only one testis.

Progression of disease

Metastases of germinal testicular cancers occur either by extension or through the lymphatics. Testicular germ cell tumors almost always spread lymphatically first and hematogenously later. Choriocarcinoma is the exception and spreads primarily by the hematogenous route. Lymphatic spread occurs in a step-wise fashion in the retroperitoneal lymph nodes. It spreads from the right testis to the interaortocaval, precaval, preaortic, paracaval, right common iliac, and right external iliac lymph nodes in that order and from the left testis to the para-aortic, preaortic, left common iliac and left external iliac lymph nodes.[134] Because of the complicated lymphatic network that surrounds the testes, metastasis can occur while the primary tumor is still small. Seminomas can spread to the mediastinal or supraclavicular nodes, but this usually occurs later. Lymph node invasion may cause displacement of the ureters or kidneys and occasionally may obstruct the ureters.

Testicular cancer also spreads by direct extension. The tumor may invade the epididymis, extend up the spermatic cord, or extend through the tunica vaginalis to the scrotum.

Germinal tumors of the testes ordinarily do not metastasize by hematogenous spread. Metastatic spread to the lung, liver, adrenal gland, or bone occasionally may occur as a late manifestation of the disease.

Clinical Manifestations

Painless enlargement of the testicle is the most common presenting symptom of testicular cancer. This can be discovered accidentally, or a dragging sensation, sometimes described as a "heaviness" in the scrotum (caused by the weight of the tumor), may call attention to the tumor's presence.

Lumbar pain, abdominal or supraclavicular masses, pain from obstruction, or a cough could all be symptoms related to metastases.

Trauma, which is often associated with the discovery of a lump, is not an etiologic factor but rather calls attention to an already present problem. Local signs of testicular cancer include a firm, diffuse enlargement, an inability to transilluminate the testis, and a lack of pain on palpation.[134] Any painless lump in the testis that does not respond promptly to antibiotics should be thought of as cancer until proved otherwise.

Assessment

The following is a list of the diagnostic procedures used for testicular cancer:

- Radical inguinal orchiectomy (as biopsy)
- Radiologic techniques
  - Chest radiograph
  - Full lung tomograms or chest CT scan
  - Lymphangiogram or abdominal CT scan (to detect retroperitoneal nodes)
  - Intravenous pyelogram
  - Testicular ultrasound (to help distinguish between epididymitis and tumor)
- Laboratory studies
  - Serum alpha-fetoprotein (AFP)
  - Serum beta human chorionic gonadotropin (HCG)

Physical examination includes palpation of the testes, abdominal palpation to exclude bulky abdominal disease, and supraclavicular lymph node palpation.

A high inguinal orchiectomy (with removal of the entire specimen) is done for biopsy purposes. A transscrotal testicular biopsy or exploration should not be done because of the risk of tumor seeding.[135]

Radiologic techniques include chest radiographs with full lung tomograms or chest CT scan to detect the presence of pulmonary metastases. Excretory urograms (intravenous pyelograms) are needed to determine any displacement by tumor of the ureters or kidneys, and they also indicate ureteral stenosis or obstruction.

Lymphangiograms or abdominal CT scans are important to demonstrate whether and to what extent the retroperitoneal lymph nodes are invloved. These procedures, when used in individuals with later-stage disease, can not only help assess response to therapy but also can help health care professionals plan for retroperitoneal lymphadenectomy.

Laboratory studies in testicular cancer have become important diagnostic aids in the last few years. Two radioimmunologic assays, alpha-fetoprotein (AFP) and beta human chorionic gonadotropin (HCG), have helped contribute to improved survival in individuals with testicular cancer.[134] These two tumor markers aid in detecting whether a germ cell tumor is present, marking the response to treatment, detecting the presence of residual tumor, and perhaps in differentiating between seminomas and nonseminomas.

Alpha-fetoprotein is a glycoprotein produced in the liver, yolk sac, and gastrointestinal tract of the fetus. Normal adult levels are less than 16 to 30 ng/ml. AFP is not elevated in patients with pure seminoma but is elevated in approximately 75% of those with nonseminomatous germ cell tumors.[136] High levels of AFP may indicate an aggressive biologic tumor.

Human chorionic gonadotropin is also a glycoprotein and is normally only produced in pregnant women. There are two subunits, alpha and beta. The beta subunit has more specifically been associated with testicular tumors. At present, 50% to 60% of individuals with nonseminomatous germ cell tumors will have an elevated level of beta HCG.[137] With a short half-life of less than 24 hours, the HCG falls rapidly after successful treatment and is thus an excellent tumor marker. One study reported that up to 30% of men with pure seminoma also will have an elevated beta HCG level.[138]

The clinical significance of AFP and HCG is to (1) corroborate initially the presence of a germinal testicular tumor, (2) determine whether treatment is effective (if the markers go down, the treatment is theoretically working), and (3) predict the prognosis and thereby aid in the choice of treatment by helping to differentiate between seminomas and nonseminomas and by possibly indicating the tumor's biologic aggressiveness.

Classification and Staging

Numerous classification systems have been developed, and many are in use today. A common staging system described by Skinner and Smith in 1980 is presented in Table 48-9. Table 48-10 describes a precise classification for patients with stage III or greater disease. This is typically applied to NSGCT. Table 48-11 outlines the TNM classification system as described by the American Joint Committee for Cancer Staging and End Results Reporting.

Treatment

Surgery

Surgical treatment for patients with testicular cancer includes high radical inguinal orchiectomy, which is considered a diagnostic step as well as the first phase of treatment, and possibly a radical retroperitoneal lymphadenectomy. Radical inguinal orchiectomy removes the testis, epididymis, a portion of the vas deferens, and portions of the gonadal lymphatics and blood supply. The remaining organ undergoes hyperplasia and produces enough testosterone to maintain sexual capacity, sexual characteristics, and libido.[139] After orchiectomy alone the potential for fertility theoretically remains the same. Some studies have shown, however, that a large percentage of men with testicular cancer had a low sperm count or reduced sperm motility after unilateral orchiectomy and before any other treatment.[140] The reason for the poor semen quality after orchiectomy is unclear. For many a low sperm count existed prior to orchiectomy as a baseline. On the other hand, it may be attributed to the stress of surgery or abnormality of the remaining testis. Clinical experience has shown that semen with a sperm count below 40 million/mL and sperm motility under 60% has only a remote chance of inducing pregnancy by artificial insemination. As a result, banking sperm or preserving semen after surgery may be of no benefit. The individual should be informed about the limitations of sperm preservation. Pretreatment fertility evaluation should be done for the person who wishes to father a child at a later time.

TABLE 48-9 Staging System for Testicular Carcinoma

Stage	Description
Stage A	Tumor is confined to the testicle; there is no evidence of spread beyond the confines of the scrotum
Stage B1	Evidence of *minimal* retroperitoneal lymph node metastases, determined either by retroperitoneal lymph node dissection or lymphangiogram (less than six positive nodes, well encapsulated)
Stage B2	Evidence of moderate retroperitoneal lymph node spread (more than six nodes)
Stage B3	Massive retroperitoneal lymph node involvement, usually a palpable mass on physical examination but without evidence of spread above the diaphragm (may directly invade contiguous structures)
Stage C	Metastatic tumor noted above the diaphragm or to solid visceral organs (liver, brain, or bone)

Source: Smith RB: Testicular cancer, in Haskell C (ed): Cancer Treatment (ed 2). Philadelphia, WB Saunders, 1985, p 397.

TABLE 48-10 TNM Classification System for Testicular Cancer

Primary Tumor (T)	
TX	Minimal requirements cannot be met (in the absence of orchiectomy, TX must be used)
T0	No evidence of primary tumor
T1	Tumor limited to body testis
T2	Tumor extends beyond the tunica albuginea
T3	Involvement of the rete testis or epididymis
T4a	Invasion of the spermatic cord
T4b	Invasion of the scrotal wall
Nodal Involvement (N)	
NX	Minimum requirements cannot be met
N0	No evidence of involvement of regional lymph nodes
N1	Involvement of a single homolateral regional lymph node which, if inguinal, is mobile
N2	Involvement of contralateral or bilateral or multiple regional lymph nodes which, if inguinal, are mobile
N3	Palpable abdominal mass present or fixed inguinal lymph nodes
N4	Involvement of juxtaregional nodes
Distant Metastasis (M)	
MX	Not assessed
M0	No (known) distant metastasis
M1	Distant metastasis present

Source: American Joint Committee for Cancer Staging and End Results Reporting. Manual for Staging of Cancer. Chicago, The Committee, 1983.

Lymphadenectomy

Retroperitoneal lymphadenectomy removes all perivascular tissue from the anatomic area that is bounded superiorally by the renal arteries and veins, laterally by both ureters, and inferiorally by the common iliac arteries to their bifurcation. This procedure is usually unilateral unless there is a large mass. Many autonomic nerves necessary for erectile potency and for ejaculation are located in this area, and surgery may damage the nerve supply to the prostate, seminal vesicles, vasa, and bladder neck. Therefore, ejaculatory ability may be altered even if

TABLE 48-11 Staging System for Later-Stage Testicular Cancer

Stage IIIA	Disease in superclavicular lymph nodes
Stage IIIB-1	Gynecomastia, either unilateral or bilateral, with or without elevated levels of human chorionic gonadotropin (HCG); no detectable gross disease
Stage IIIB-2	Minimal pulmonary disease; up to 5 metastatic masses in each lung, the largest no greater than 2 cm in diameter
Stage IIIB-3	Advanced pulmonary disease; any mediastinal or hilar mass, neoplastic pleural effusion, or intrapulmonary mass greater than 2 cm in diameter

Source: Johnson DE, Swanson DA, von Eschenbach AC: Tumors of the genitourinary tract, in Tanagho EA, McAninch JW (eds): Smith's General Urology (ed 12). San Mateo, Calif, Appleton & Lange, 1987, p 387.

erectile potency is maintained. Bracken[139] reported that 90% of men who had undergone postretroperitoneal lymphadenectomy had a reduction in or total loss of ejaculate.

Radiotherapy

External beam radiotherapy is aimed at the lymph node areas. In the pelvic (retroperitoneal) region, the ipsilateral inguinal, iliac, and bilateral para-aortic nodes are irradiated. In the chest the mediastinal or supraclavicular nodes, or both, are irradiated. The amount of radiation ranges from 2000 to 3500 cGy. (See the section below on treatment according to histologic type and stage for a discussion of how and when each of these two techniques is employed.)

Complications of radiotherapy are related to the port and dose of irradiation and vary from individual to individual. Side effects of radiation to the pelvic region may be fatigue, bone marrow suppression, and diarrhea. Even with testicular retraction and shielding, there may be radiation "scatter" to the remaining testicle. Rowley et al[141] have determined that the degree of damage to sperm production depends on the amount of radiation exposure. A single testicular dose of 8 to 50 cGy could induce oligospermia (scant numbers of sperm), and 80 to 300 cGy can cause azoospermia (no sperm production). The recovery of spermatogenesis is also dose related. At doses up to 100 cGy, sperm recovery requires 9 to 18 months; patients who received doses of 200 cGy require 30 months for sperm recovery; and patients who received doses of 600 cGy require 5 years or more to bring the sperm count back to preradiation levels.[139]

Chemotherapy

Chemotherapy has been used as an adjunct to other treatments, for disseminated disease, and for recurrences. Adjuvant chemotherapy has been attempted with both seminomas and nonseminomas. However, the experience with chemotherapy in the treatment of patients with seminomas has more typically been limited to recurrent disease.[142] Adjuvant chemotherapy as an adjunct to retroperitoneal lymphadenectomy for those patients with stage B NSGCT is recommended by some. These experts feel that even though recurrent disease can be cured with an appropriate cisplatin combination regimen, prophylactic use of less toxic outpatient chemotherapy can substantially reduce the recurrence rate and spare the patient the toxicities of a more agressive regimen.[143]

The major role of chemotherapy in patients with testicular cancer is in treatment of disseminated disease. In August 1974, early studies were begun at Indiana University on men with disseminated testicular cancer combining cisplatin, vinblastine, and bleomycin (PVB).[144] An example of this original regimen includes cisplatin, 20 mg/m2/day for 5 days every three weeks; bleomycin, 30 units on days 2, 9, and 16; and vinblastine, 0.2 mg/kg on days 1 and 2 every 3 weeks. This cycle is repeated three to four times.[144]

The result of this chemotherapy combination on nonseminomatous tumors has been remarkable. Einhorn[144] reports a regularly achieved 80% disease-free status; a relapse rate of approximately 10% with approximately 70% long-term survivors. This chemotherapeutic regimen has essentially revolutionized the treatment of patients with disseminated testicular cancer.

The toxicity of the PVB regimen, however, is considerable. The incidence of leukopenia and sepsis is high in these individuals. Other side effects reported include nausea, vomiting, and cisplatin-induced nephrotoxicity and neurotoxicity. Pulmonary fibrosis is an uncommon complication, but one associated with bleomycin. Myalgias, constipation, and paralytic ileus are all side effects associated with vinblastine.

Chemotherapy also has been used in those approximately 30% of men who have relapsed or who were refractory to chemotherapy initially. A variety of treatment programs have been tried, as follows:

- Cisplatin plus doxorubicin
- Cisplatin plus doxorubicin plus vincristine plus bleomycin
- Cisplatin plus vincristine plus bleomycin (PVB)
- PVB plus actinomycin D plus cyclophosphamide
- Cisplatin plus VP-16 (etoposide) plus bleomycin (BEP)
- Cisplatin plus VP-16 plus ifosfamide

Newer studies have looked at comparing three courses of BEP with four cycles of BEP; or comparing the standard BEP with a BEP regimen that has twice as much cisplatin.[144]

Treatment According to Histologic Type and Stage

Seminomas

Stage A, B1, and B2 seminomas are very radiosensitive. If there is no evidence of metastases and if retroperitoneal node involvement is not bulky, radical orchiectomy followed by radiotherapy of 2500 cGy over 3 weeks is the primary treatment. Men with evidence of retroperitoneal disease may receive additional 1000 cGy to the involved nodal areas.

In case of massive metastases to the retroperitoneal nodes or to other organs (stage B3 and C), preradiation chemotherapy typically using cisplatin, vinblastine, and bleomycin with or without doxorubicin is commonly used.[142]

Nonseminomas

With the revolutionary changes in management, Stage A, B1, and B2 tumors now have the highest cure rate of any solid tumor. Historically men with NSGCT had been treated with radiotherapy, retroperitoneal lymphadenectomy, and chemotherapy after orchiectomy. Today the most common approach to men with early-stage NSGCT is retroperitoneal lymphadenectomy and chemotherapy.[134,143] Postoperative radiotherapy, which before 1973 was used routinely, has now been replaced for the most part by postoperative chemotherapy.

Einhorn[144] describes cisplatin plus VP-16 (100 mg/m^2 × 5) plus bleomycin as standard therapy. The VP-16 protocol results in less neurotoxicity. Others recommend postoperative chemotherapy that is less toxic.[143] A "mini-VAB" combination is used that includes vinblastine, actinomycin D, and bleomycin. There is no cisplatin in this regimen.

Stage B3 and C testicular cancer generates the most treatment controversy. Aggressive primary chemotherapy using a cisplatin-based combination protocol is generally accepted as standard therapy. The controversy is usually over what drugs to combine with the cisplatin and whether retroperitoneal lymph node dissection should be done. Most centers advocate lymph node dissection for any residual disease after chemotherapy.[144] In other settings, surgery is only recommended in men who do not achieve a complete response from chemotherapy and in whom persistent retroperitoneal disease is suspected.[145]

Results and Prognosis

The survival rate for individuals with testicular cancer has improved significantly, especially for the nonseminomas. The advent of tumor markers and the use of sophisticated chemotherapy accounts for this improvement. For men with nonseminomatous testicular tumors treated by orchiectomy plus retroperitoneal lymph node dissection, or radiotherapy plus chemotherapy for bulky disease, the average reported 5-year survival rates are approximately 90% to 100% for stage A, 90% for stage B, and 80% to 85% for stage C.[134]

For men with seminomatous testicular cancers treated by radiotherapy, the reported 5-year survival rates are 98% for stage A, 75% to 94% for stage B1 and B2, and approximately 71% for stage B3 and C. The overall survival rate in this series was 92%.[134]

Nursing Role in Early Detection

The only routinely recommended screening methods for early detection of testicular cancer are monthly testicular self-examination (TSE) and the annual physical examination by a physician. Various research studies have revealed that very few men practice TSE. Blesch[146] studied 233 professional men and found that only 9.5% practiced TSE. Cummings et al[147] studied 266 male college students and found that only 16% had heard about TSE before the survey. Many men stated that vague discomfort and heaviness of the testicles alone would not seem serious enough for them to seek medical attention. This delay in consulting a physician probably accounts for the fact that 25% of seminomas[142] and 66% of nonseminomatous[143] testicular cancer has metastasized by the time it is diagnosed. There is a need for physicians and nurses to provide information on testicular cancer and on the benefits of practicing TSE. The technique and importance of TSE should be taught to young men so that they can practice this health behavior regularly.

Nursing Care

Surgery, radiation, and chemotherapy are all important components of testicular cancer treatment and play significant roles in the curative or palliative treatment of men with this disease.

Orchiectomy is usually the first diagnostic and curative step for all primary testicular tumors. Further treatment is based on the type of cells found in the tumor.

Orchiectomy has tremendous psychologic impact on many individuals. The nurse has a responsibility to provide psychologic support for these men and to teach them the implications of the diagnostic procedures and the phases of treatment.

Several diagnostic procedures (previously discussed in the section on assessment) assist in determining disease type and extent. To minimize the man's anxiety and fear, the nurse should provide easily understandable information about each test. Orchiectomy is a relatively minor operation, but it may present great emotional trauma for the man and his family. Before surgery, the nurse should assess the patient's knowledge and encourage the expression of fears and concerns. Preoperative patient teaching should include such matters as the location of the incision, intravenous infusions, coughing and deep breathing, and the availability of analgesics to control pain. Because of the location of the disease, patients may need a basic review of the anatomy and physiology of the surgical site and how the treatment will affect them.

Postoperative nursing care

For orchiectomy, the individual generally has a high inguinal incision. The nursing emphasis during the immediate postoperative period is primarily on alleviating pain. Drainage tubes are uncommon for this type of surgery. A simple dry, sterile dressing is applied to the incision. The nurse should watch for excessive bleeding and should use aseptic technique in wound care. Perhaps the greatest postoperative complication is altered body image. Although a unilateral orchiectomy will not alter a man's potency, some individuals may feel that they are less than whole with only one testis. These men should be assured that clinical experience has shown that men have normal sexual function after unilateral orchiectomy. The potential for fertility after unilateral orchiectomy is presumably unchanged if the remaining testis is normal. The actual fertility of these men may be eventually threatened by the treatments that follow orchiectomy, such as lymphadenectomy, radiotherapy, or chemotherapy.

Retroperitoneal lymphadenectomy, if indicated, is generally performed a few weeks following orchiectomy. A transabdominal approach is commonly used. No drainage tube is necessary for the wound. A nasogastric tube is usually placed for stomach decompression the first few days after surgery. Because the abdominal organs are handled during this surgery, bowel inertia may result. The man receives nothing to eat or drink by mouth until bowel sounds are noted. The person also may have a indwelling urinary catheter to monitor urinary output. Hemorrhage is a major (but uncommon) complication after retroperitoneal lymphadenectomy because many of the lymph nodes resected are located around the large abdominal vessels. Accurate monitoring of vital signs will detect any signs of hemorrhage and shock. The incisional dressing should be checked often to assess any excessive drainage. Pain and nutritional status also should be assessed. Nutritional status is important for wound healing and for preparing the individual for further therapy. About 10 days after surgery, the man may start radiotherapy or chemotherapy.

Another major and more common side effect of retroperitoneal lymphadenectomy is the loss of ejaculatory ability. It is important to assure the man that his ability to have an erection and experience orgasm is usually not permanently impaired by the surgery.

Nursing care of patients receiving radiotherapy

External beam radiotherapy is frequently the treatment of choice following orchiectomy for seminoma. Overall, individuals generally tolerate radiotherapy to the retroperitoneal regions very well. Some of the common side effects are mild nausea and vomiting, diarrhea, myelosuppression, and azoospermia. The transient nausea and vomiting may be controlled with antiemetics. Bone marrow suppression is usually mild unless the mediastinal and supraclavicular regions are also included in the treatment field. Azoospermia may result from inadvertent radiation scatter to the testis. To avoid unnecessary radiation exposure, a lead cup can be used to shield the remaining testis.

Nursing care of patients receiving chemotherapy

Testicular tumors have responded to a variety of cytotoxic agents, including cisplatin, vinblastine, and bleomycin. This drug combination is commonly known as PVB. If the patient does not respond to the PVB combination chemotherapy, the physician may initiate a salvage chemotherapy strategy that combines cisplatin with other active agents not previously used, such as VP-16 or ifosfamide.[148]

Since severe nausea and vomiting and nephrotoxicity are associated with cisplatin, antiemetics should be given before the infusion, on a regular basis or as needed during drug infusion to control nausea. Before drug administration, the nurse must be certain that the patient has been well hydrated and has adequate renal function. Mannitol and furosemide are commonly given with cisplatin to maintain adequate urinary output. The nurse must administer this drug with needles and intravenous sets free of aluminum because aluminum causes drug precipitation and subsequent loss of drug potency.

The major side effects of vinblastine are dose-related myelosuppression, neurotoxicity (constipation and paralytic ileus), mild nausea and vomiting, alopecia, and stomatitis. Because this drug is a vesicant, the nurse must ensure vein patency before drug administration. Prophylactic stool softeners may help prevent constipation.

The third agent in the PVB regimen is bleomycin. The nurse should be aware that bleomycin may precipitate an anaphylactoid reaction. A test dose should be given to individuals who have not previously received this agent. Emergency medications such as epinephrine, hydrocortisone, and diphenhydramine should be available at the bedside. The person may experience a fever 4 to 6 hours after receiving bleomycin. The nurse should obtain a baseline temperature before drug administration and monitor the temperature every 4 hours during the 24-hour period after chemotherapy. Diphenhydramine 50 mg and Tylenol 650 mg by mouth before bleomycin administration and repeated 4 to 6 hours later can prevent these unpleasant symptoms. The other side effects of bleomycin are stomatitis, alopecia, and delayed pulmonary toxicity. Maximum cumulative lifetime dose of bleomycin is 450 IU. Pulmonary fibrosis is by far the most serious side effect of bleomycin. Some of the manifestations are dry cough, dyspnea, rales, and pulmonary infiltrate.

Etoposide is incompatible with D5W; it should be diluted in at least 20 equivalent volumes of sodium chloride injection. It is given intravenously over at least 30 minutes. Hypotension may occur if the drug is administered too fast. Myelosuppression and alopecia are also considered common side effects of etoposide.

Ifosfamide is administered as a slow intravenous infusion lasting a minimum of 30 minutes each day for 5 days. The patient should be well hydrated during the therapy to minimize the potential for urotoxicity (eg, dysuria, urinary frequency and hemorrhagic cystitis). The uroprotectant mesna is useful in preventing these symptoms and is administered as an intravenous bolus equal to 20% of the usual dose of ifosamide 15 minutes before and 4 and 8 hours after administration of ifosamide. A daily urinalysis is done during ifosamide therapy to assess for hematuria. The patient may experience nausea, vomiting, central nervous system toxicity (lethargy), and a mild degree of leukopenia.

In general, treatment of testicular tumors can be lengthy and require surgery, radiation, and chemotherapy. The major nursing concern with this type of cancer is to anticipate the anxiety these young men will probably experience. There is a perceived and sometimes real threat to their sexual potency and fertility. Education, encouragement, and emotional support are essential nursing functions if these men are to cope fully with testicular cancer and its treatment.

REFERENCES

1. Silverberg E, Lubera JA: Cancer statistics, 1989. CA 39:3-32, 1989.
2. Ross RK, Paganini-Hill A, Henderson BE: Epidemiology of prostatic cancer, in Skinner D, Lieskovsky G (ed): Diagnosis and Management of Genitourinary Cancer. Philadelphia, WB Saunders, 1988, pp 40-45.
3. Fowler JE Jr, Mills SE: Operable prostatic carcinoma: Correlations among clinical stage, pathological stage, Gleason histological score and early disease-free survival. J Urol 133:40-42, 1985.
4. Noble RL: Production of Nb rat carcinoma of the dorsal prostate and response of estrogen-dependent transplants to sex hormones and tamoxifen. Cancer 40:3574-50, 1980.
5. Ghanadian R, Puah CM, O'Donoghue EPN: Serum testosterone and dihydrotestosterone in carcinoma of the prostate. Br J Cancer 39:P 696-699, 1979.
6. Ross RK, Bernstein L, Judd H, et al: Serum testosterone levels in healthy young black and white men. J Natl Cancer Inst 76:45-48, 1986.
7. Graham S, Haughey B, Marshall J, et al: Diet in the epidemiology of carcinoma of the prostate gland. J Natl Cancer Inst 70:687-692, 1983.
8. Waisman J, Mott LJM: Pathology of neoplasms of the prostate gland, in Skinner DG, deKernion J (eds): Genitourinary Cancer. Philadelphia, WB Saunders, 1978, pp 310-343.
9. Waisman J: Pathology of neoplasms of the prostate gland, in Skinner D, Lieskovsky G (ed): Diagnosis and Management of Genitourinary Cancer. Philadelphia, WB Saunders, 1988, pp 150-194.
10. Murphy GP: Screening for prostatic carcinoma—useful or not? EORTC Genitourinary Group Monograph 5: Progress and Controversies in Oncological Urology II. New York, Alan R Liss, 1988, pp 131-137.
11. Resnick MI: Background for screening—epidemiology and cost effectiveness. EORTC Genitourinary Group Monograph 5:Progress and Controversies in Oncological Urology II. New York, Alan R Liss, 1988, pp 111-120.
12. Thompson IM, Rounder JB, Teague JL, et al: Impact of routine screening for adenocarcinoma of the prostate on stage distribution. J Urol 137:424-426, 1987.
13. McClennan BL: Transrectal US of the prostate: Is the technology leading the science? Radiology 168:571-575, 1988.
14. Lee F, Littrup PJ, Torp-Pedersen ST, et al: Prostate cancer: Comparison of transrectal US and digital rectal examination for screening. Radiology 168:389-394, 1988.
15. Oesterling JE, Chan DW, Epstein JI, et al: Prostate specific antigen in the preoperative and postoperative evaluation of localized prostatic cancer treated with radical prostatectomy. J Urol 139:766-772, 1988.
16. Whitmore WF Jr: Background for screening: Natural history and treatment. EORTC Genitourinary Group Monograph 5:Progress and Controversies in Oncological Urology II. New York, Alan R Liss, 1988, pp 123-130.
17. McCullough DL: Diagnosis and staging of prostatic cancer, in Skinner D, Lieskovsky G (ed): Diagnosis and Management of Genitourinary Cancer. Philadelphia, WB Saunders, 1988, pp 405-416.
18. deVere White RW, Deitch AD: Flow cytometry in urologic cancer, in Williams RD (ed): Advances in Urologic Oncology (vol 1). New York, Macmillan, 1987, pp 25-42.
19. Cooper EH, Siddall JK, Newling DWW, et al: Acid phosphatase, alkaline phosphatase and prostate specific antigen: Which markers should we choose?, in EORTC Genitourinary Group Monograph 5: Progress and Controversies in Oncological Urology. New York, Alan R Liss, 1988, pp 43-53.
20. Poon PY, McCollum RW, Henkelinan MM: Magnetic resonance imaging of the prostate. Radiology 154:1985, 143-150.
21. deKernion JB: Cancer of the prostate, in Haskell C (ed): Cancer Treatment (ed 2). Philadelphia, WB Saunders, 1985, pp 352-366.
22. Kramer SA, Spahr J, Brendler C, et al: Experience with Gleasón's histopathologic grading in prostatic cancer. J Urol 124:223-225, 1980.
23. Gleason DF, Mellinger GT, et al: Prediction of prognosis for prostatic adenocarcinoma by combined histological grading and staging. J Urol 111:58-64, 1974.
24. Glenn J: Surgical therapy of cancer of the prostate, in Skinner DG, deKernion J (eds): Genitourinary Cancer. Philadelphia, WB Saunders, 1978, pp 344-354.
25. Paulson DF: Technique of radical perineal prostatectomy, in Skinner D, Lieskovsky G (ed): Diagnosis and Management of Genitourinary Cancer. Philadelphia, WB Saunders, 1988, pp 721-734.
26. Lieskovsky G: Technique of radical retropubic prostatectomy (Campbell's procedure) with limited pelvic lymph node dissection, in Skinner D, Lieskovsky G (eds): Diagnosis and Management of Genitourinary Cancer. Philadelphia, WB Saunders, 1988, pp 735-752.
27. Jewett HJ: Treatment of early cancer of the prostate. JAMA 183:373-375, 1963.
28. Lue TF: Male sexual dysfunction, in Tanagho EA, McAninch JW (eds): Smith's General Urology. San Mateo, Calif, Appleton & Lange, 1987, pp 663-678.
29. Walsh PC, Donker PJ: Impotence following radical prostatectomy: Insight into etiology and prevention. J Urol 128:492-497, 1982.
30. Walsh PC: Technique of radical retropubic prostatectomy with preservation of sexual function—an anatomic approach, in Skinner D, Lieskovsky G (eds): Diagnosis and Management of Genitourinary Cancer. Philadelphia, WB Saunders, 1988, pp 753-778.
31. Walsh PC, Mostwin JC: Radical prostatectomy and cystoprostatectomy with preservation of potency. Results using a new nerve-sparing technique. Br J Urol 56: 694-699, 1984.

32. Bagshaw MA: Radiation therapy for cancer of the prostate, in Skinner D, Lieskovsky G (ed): Diagnosis and Management of Genitourinary Cancer. Philadelphia, WB Saunders, 1988, pp 425-445.
33. Hanks GE: Radical prostatectomy or radiation therapy for early prostate cancer. Cancer 61:2153-2160, 1988.
34. Carlton CE: Radioactive isotope implantation for cancer of the prostate, in Skinner D, Lieskovsky G (eds): Diagnosis and Management of Genitourinary Cancer. Philadelphia, WB Saunders, 1988, pp 446-453.
35. Whitmore WF Jr: Experience with 125 iodine implantation in the treatment of prostate cancer, in Skinner DG (ed): Urological Cancer. New York, Grune & Stratton, 1983, pp 37-52.
36. Sogani PC, Fair WR: Treatment of advanced prostatic cancer. Urol Clin North Am 14:353-371, 1987.
37. Paulson DF: Role of endocrine therapy in the management of prostatic cancer, in Skinner D, Lieskovsky G (eds): Diagnosis and Management of Genitourinary Cancer. Philadelphia, WB Saunders, 1988, pp 464-472.
38. Trachtenberg J: Hormonal management of stage D carcinoma of the prostate. Urol Clin North Am 14:685-694, 1987.
39. Presant CA, Soloway MS, Klioze SS, et al: Buserelin treatment of advanced prostatic carcinoma: Long-term follow-up of antitumor responses and improved quality of life. Cancer 59:1713-1716, 1987.
40. Einhorn LH: An overview of chemotherapeutic trials in advanced cancer of the prostate, in Skinner DG (ed): Urological Cancers. New York, Grune & Stratton, 1983.
41. Huben RP, Murphy GP: Management of advanced cancer of the prostate, in Skinner D, Lieskovsky G (eds): Diagnosis and Management of Genitourinary Cancer. Philadelphia, WB Saunders, 1988, pp 473-482.
42. Henry JM, Isaacs JT: Relationship between tumor size and the curability of metastatic prostatic cancer by surgery alone or in combination with adjuvant chemotherapy. J Urol 139:1119-1128, 1988.
43. Chodak G, Eisenberger M, Scardino P, et al: Detecting prostate cancer early. Patient Care 4:69-73, 1987.
44. Luckmann J, Sorenson K: Medical-Surgical Nursing—A Psychophysiologic Approach (ed 3). Philadelphia, WB Saunders, 1987, p 1703.
45. Brunner LS, Suddarth D: The Lippincott Manual of Nursing Practice (ed 3). Philadelphia, JB Lippincott, 1982.
46. Baxter RT, Linn A: Sex counseling and the SCI patient . . . spinal cord injury. Nursing 78 8:46, 1978.
47. Lamb M, Woods N: Sexuality and the cancer patient. Cancer Nurs 4:137, 1981.
48. Shipes E, Lehr S: Sexuality of the male cancer patient. Cancer Nurs:375-381, 1982.
49. Sarna L: Concepts of nursing care for patients receiving radiation therapy, in Vredevoe D, et al (eds): Concepts of Oncology Nursing. Englewood Cliffs, NJ, Prentice-Hall, 1981, pp 154-205.
50. Lukkarinen O, Kontturi M: Treatment of advanced prostatic carcinoma with a slow release depot LHRH analogue (Zoladax depot r). Scand J Urol Nephrol 110:109-112, 1988.
51. Johnson D, Babaian R, von Eschenbach A, et al: Ketoconazole therapy for hormonally refractive metastatic prostate cancer. Urology 31:132-134, 1988.
52. Ross RK, Paganini-Hill A, Henderson BE: Epidemiology of bladder cancer, in Skinner D, Lieskovsky G (eds): Diagnosis and Management of Genitourinary Cancer. Philadelphia, WB Saunders, 1988, pp 23-31.
53. Lillienfeld AM, Levin ML, Moore GE: The association of smoking with cancer of the urinary bladder in humans. Arch Intern Med 98:129-135, 1956.
54. Wynder EL, Goldsmith R: The epidemiology of bladder cancer, a second look. Cancer 40:1246-1268, 1977.
55. Brownson RC, Chang JC, Davis JR: Occupation, smoking, and alcohol in the epidemiology of bladder cancer. Am J Public Health 77:1298-1300, 1987.
56. Claude J, Kunze E, Frentzel-Beyme R, et al: Life-style and occupational risk factors in cancer of the lower urinary tract. Am J Epidemiology 124:578-589, 1986.
57. Mommsen S, Aagaard J, Sell A: An epidemiological case-control study of bladder cancer in males from a predominantly rural district. Eur J Cancer Clin Oncol 18:1205-1210, 1982.
58. deKernion JB, Skinner DG: Epidemiology, diagnosis and staging of bladder cancer, in deKernion JB, Skinner DG (eds): Genitorurinary Cancer. Philadelphia, WB Saunders, 1978, pp 213-231.
59. Mostofi FK: Markers of bladder cancer. J Natl Cancer Inst 80:1184, 1988.
60. Tannenbaum M, Romas N: The pathobiology of early urothelial cancer, in Skinner DG, deKernion J (eds): Genitourinary Cancer. Philadelphia, WB Saunders, 1978, pp 232-255.
61. Lieskovsky G, Ahlering T, Skinner DG: Diagnosis and staging of bladder cancer, in Skinner D, Lieskovsky G (eds): Diagnosis and Management of Genitourinary Cancer. Philadelphia, WB Saunders, 1988, pp 264-280.
62. deVere White RW, Deitch AD, West B, et al: The predictive value of flow cytometric information in the clinical management of stage 0 (Ta) bladder cancer. J Urol 139:279-282, 1988.
63. Kern W: Bladder cancer: Flow cytometry, ABO predictors, and tumor markers, in Skinner DG (ed): Urological Cancer. New York, Grune & Stratton, 1983, pp 137-148.
64. Guirguis R, Schiffmann E, Liu B, et al: Detection of autocrine motility factor in urine as a marker of bladder cancer. J Natl Cancer Inst 80:1203-1211, 1988.
65. Marini F, Signori GB, Valente R: The relationship between transurethral ultrasound and pathological findings in 16 cases of tumor of the bladder. Prog Clin Biol Res 260:271-274, 1988.
66. Javadpour N, Lalehzarian M: Magnetic resonance imaging (MRI) in bladder cancer. Prog Clin Biol Res 260:265-270, 1988.
67. Williams RD: Magnetic resonance in the diagnosis and staging of urologic cancer, in Williams RD (ed): Advances in Urologic Oncology (vol 1). New York, Macmillan, 1987, pp 69-88.
68. Catalona WJ, Dresner SM, Haaff EO: Management of superficial bladder cancer, in Skinner D, Lieskovsky G (eds): Diagnosis and Management of Genitourinary Cancer. Philadelphia, WB Saunders, 1988, pp 281-294.
69. Lamm DL, Thor DE, Harris SC, et al: Bacillus Calmette-Guérin immunotherapy of superficial bladder cancer. J Urol 124:38-40, 1980.
70. Morales A, Ottenhof P, Emerson L: Treatment of residual non-infiltrating bladder cancer with bacillus Calmette-Guérin. J Urol 125:649-654, 1981.
71. Torrence RJ, Kavoussi LR, Catalona WJ, et al: Prognostic factors in patients treated with intravesical bacillus Calmette-Guérin for superficial bladder cancer. J Urol 139:941-944, 1988.
72. Skinner DG, Lieskovsky G: Management of invasive and high-grade bladder cancer, in Skinner D, Lieskovsky G

(eds): Diagnosis and Management of Genitourinary Cancer. Philadelphia, WB Saunders, 1988, pp 295-312.

73. Skinner DG, Tift JP, Kaufman JJ: High dose, short course preoperative radition therapy and immediate single stage radical cystectomy with pelvic node dissection in the management of bladder cancer. J Urol 127:671-674, 1982.
74. Gerber A: The Kock continent ileal reservoir for supravesical urinary diversion. Am J Surg 146:15-20, 1983.
75. Bloom DA, Lieskovsky G, Rainwater G, et al: The Turnbull loop stoma. J Urol 129:715-718, 1983.
76. Kock NG, Nilson AE, Nilsson LO, et al: Urinary diversion via a continent ileal reservoir: Clinical results in 12 patients. J Urol 128:469-475, 1982.
77. Skinner DG, Boyd SD, Lieskovsky G: Creation of the continent Kock ileal reservoir as an alternative to cutaneous urinary diversion, in Skinner D, Lieskovsky G (eds): Diagnosis and Management of Genitourinary Cancer. Philadelphia, WB Saunders, 1988, pp 653-674.
78. Swanson D: Cancer of the bladder and prostate: The impact of therapy on sexual function, in von Eschenbach A, Rodriguez D (eds): Sexual Rehabilitation of the Urologic Cancer Patient. Boston, GK Hall, 1981, pp 88-109.
79. Scott FB, Kantzavelos D: Erectile impotence after urologic cancer surgery treated with the inflatable penile prosthesis, in von Eschenbach A, Rodriguez D (eds): Sexual Rehabilitation of the Urologic Cancer Patient. Boston, GK Hall, 1981, pp 240-249.
80. Boyd SD: Management of male impotency, including technique of penile prosthesis placement, in Skinner D, Lieskovsky G (eds): Diagnosis and Management of Genitourinary Cancer. Philadelphia, WB Saunders, 1988, pp 675-683.
81. Daniels JR, Skinner DG, Lieskovsky G: Chemotherapy of carcinoma of bladder, in Skinner D, Lieskovsky G (eds): Diagnosis and Management of Genitourinary Cancer. Philadelphia, WB Saunders, 1988, pp 313-322.
82. Phipps WJ, Long BC, Woods NF: Medical Surgical Nursing: Concepts and Clinical Practice. St Louis, CV Mosby, 1987, pp 212-230.
83. Skinner DG, Richie JR: Ureterointestinal diversion, in Harrison JH, Gittes RF, Pearlmutter AD, et al (eds): Campbell's Urology (ed 4). Philadelphia, WB Saunders, 1979.
84. King A: Nursing management of stomas of the genitourinary system, in Broadwell D, Jackson B (eds): Principles of Ostomy Care. St Louis, CV Mosby, 1982.
85. Paganini-Hill A, Ross RK, Henderson BE: Epidemiology of renal cancer, in Skinner D, Lieskovsky G (eds): Diagnosis and Management of Genitourinary Cancer. Philadelphia, WB Saunders, 1988, pp 32-39.
86. FingerKantor AL, Meigs JW, Heston JF, et al: Epidemiology of renal cell cancer in Connecticut. J Natl Cancer Inst 57:495-500, 1976.
87. Waterhouse J, Muir C, Shanmugaratnom K, et al: Cancer incidence in five continents (vol 4). Lyon, France, IARC Scientific Publications, 42:1-807, 1982.
88. Hammond EC: Smoking in relation to death rates of 1 million men and women, in Epidemiological Approaches to the Study of Cancer and Other Chronic Diseases. Natl Cancer Inst Monograph 19. Washington, DC, US Government Printing Office, 1966.
89. Weir JM, Dunn JE: Smoking and mortality. A prospective study. Cancer 25:105-112, 1970.
90. Doll R, Peto R: Mortality in relation to smoking: 20 years' observations on male British doctors. Br Med J 2:1525-1536, 1976.
91. Kolonel LN: Association of cadmium with renal cancer. Cancer 37:1782-1787, 1976.
92. McLaughlin JK, Mandel JS, Blot WJ, et al: A population-based case-control study of renal cell carcinoma. J Natl Cancer Inst 72:275-284, 1984.
93. Wynder EL, Mabuchi K, Whitmore W: Epidemiology of adenocarcinoma of the kidney. J Natl Cancer Inst 53:1619-1634, 1974.
94. Selikoff IJ, Hammond EC, Seidman HP: Mortality experience of insulation workers in the United States and Canada, 1943-1976. Ann NY Acad Sci 330:91-116, 1979.
95. Paganini-Hill A, Glazer E, Henderson BE, et al: Cause-specific mortality among newspaper web pressmen. J Occup Med 22:542-544, 1980.
96. Fraley E: Cancer of the renal pelvis, in Skinner DG, deKernion J (eds): Genitourinary Cancer. Philadelphia, WB Saunders, 1978, pp 134-149.
97. Skinner DG, deKernion J: Clinical manifestations and treatment of renal parenchymal tumors, in Skinner DG, deKernion J (eds): Genitourinary Cancer. Philadelphia, WB Saunders, 1978, pp 107-133.
98. McDonald M: Current therapy for renal cell carcinoma. J Urol 127:211-217, 1982.
99. deKernion JB: Treatment of advanced renal cell cancer: Traditional methods and innovative approaches. J Urol 130:2-7, 1983.
100. Altaffer LF, 3rd, Chanault OW Jr: Paraneoplastic endocrinopathies associated with renal tumors. J Urol 122:573-577, 1979.
101. Pritchett TR, Lieskovsky G, Skinner DG: Clinical manifestations and treatment of renal parenchymal tumors, in Skinner D, Lieskovsky G (eds): Diagnosis and Management of Genitourinary Cancer. Philadelphia, WB Saunders, 1988, pp 337-361.
102. Boswell WD: Diagnostic imaging in genitourinary cancer, in Skinner D, Lieskovsky G (eds): Diagnosis and Management of Genitourinary Cancer. Philadelphia, WB Saunders, 1988, pp 237-263.
103. Lang E: Diagnosis of renal parenchymal tumors, in Skinner DG, deKernion J (eds): Genitourinary Cancer. Philadelphia, WB Saunders, 1978, pp 40-83.
104. Marks W, Korobkin M, Callen PW, et al: CT diagnosis of tumor of the renal vein and inferior vena cava. Am J Roentgenol 131:843-845, 1978.
105. Love L, Churchill R, Reynes C: Computed tomography staging of renal cancer. Urol Rad 1:35, 1979.
106. Richie JP: Carcinoma of renal pelvis and ureter, in Skinner D, Lieskovsky G (ed): Diagnosis and Management of Genitourinary Cancer. Philadelphia, WB Saunders, 1988, pp 323-336.
107. deKernion JB: Renal cell carcinoma, in Haskell C (ed): Cancer Treatment (ed 2). Philadelphia, WB Saunders, 1985, pp 382-393.
108. Flocks RH, Kadesky MC: Malignant neoplasms of the kidney; an analysis of 353 patients followed 5 years or more. J Urol 79:196, 1958.
109. Schefft P, Novick AC, Straffon RA, et al: Surgery for renal cell carcinoma extending into the inferior vena cava. J Urol 120:28-31, 1978.
110. Skinner DG, Lieskovsky G, Pritchett TR: Management of renal cell carcinoma involving the vena cava, in Skinner D, Lieskovsky G (eds): Diagnosis and Management of Genitourinary Cancer. Philadelphia, WB Saunders, 1988, pp 694-703.
111. Cherrie RJ, Goldman DG, Lindner A, et al: Prognostic implications of venal caval extension of renal cell carcinoma. J Urol 128:910-912, 1982.
112. Waters W, Richie JP: Aggressive surgical approach to renal

cell cancer: Review of 130 cases. J Urol 122:306-309, 1979.
113. deKernion JB: Lymphadenectomy for renal cell cancer: Therapeutic implications. Urol Clin North Am 7:697-703, 1980.
114. Marshall F, Powell K: Lymphadenectomy for renal cell cancer: Anatomical and therapeutic considerations. J Urol 128:677-681, 1982.
115. Skinner DG, Lieskovsky G, Pritchett TR: Technique of radical nephrectomy, in Skinner D, Lieskovsky G (eds): Diagnosis and Management of Genitourinary Cancer. Philadelphia, WB Saunders, 1988, pp 684-693.
116. Rost A, Brosig W: Preoperative irradiation of renal cell cancer. Urology 10:414-417, 1977.
117. Brady LW Jr: Carcinoma of the kidney: The role for radiation therapy. Semin Oncol 10:417-421, 1983.
118. deKernion JB, Ramming K, Smith R: The natural history of metastic renal cell cancer: A computer analysis. J Urol 120:148-152, 1978.
119. Swanson DA, Johnson DE, von Eschenbach AC, et al: Angioinfarction plus nephrectomy for metastatic renal cell carcinoma—an update. J Urol 130:449-452, 1983.
120. Rosenberg SA, Klotze MT, Muul LM, et al: Observations on the systematic administration of autologous lymphokine-activated killer cells and recombinant interleukin-2 with metastatic cancer. N Engl J Med 313:1485-1492, 1985.
121. Belldegrun A, Uppenkamp I, Rosenberg SA: Anti-tumor reactivity of human lymphokine activated killer (LAK) cells against fresh and cultured preparations of renal cell cancer. J Urol 139:150-155, 1988.
122. Fowler JE Jr.: Adoptive immunotherapy using lymphokine-activated killer cells. J Urol 139:148-149, 1988.
123. Fisher RI, Coltman CA, Doroshow JH, et al: Metastic renal cancer treated with interlukin-2 and lymphokine-activated killer cells. A phase II clinical trail. Ann Intern Med 108:518-523, 1988.
124. Sarna G, Figlin R, deKernion J: Interferon in renal cell carcinoma—the UCLA experience. Cancer 59:610-612, 1987.
125. Yagoda A: Chemotherapy for advanced urothelial cancer. Semin Urol 1:60-74, 1983.
126. Figlin RA: Biotherapy with interferon in solid tumors. Oncol Nurs Forum 14:23-26, 1987.
127. Irwin MM: Patients receiving biological response modifiers: Overview of nursing care. Oncol Nurs Forum 14:32-37, 1987.
128. Jassak PF, Sticklin LA: Interleukin 2: An overview. Oncol Nurs Forum 13:17-22, 1986.
129. Seipp C, Simpson C, Rosenberg S: Clinical trials with IL-2. Oncol Nurs Forum 13:25-29, 1986.
130. Henderson BE, Ross RK, Pike MC: Epidemiology of testicular cancer, in Skinner D, Lieskovsky G (eds): Diagnosis and Management of Genitourinary Cancer. Philadelphia, WB Saunders, 1988, pp 46-52.
131. Mostofi FK: Testicular tumors. Epidemiological, etiologic and pathologic features. Cancer 32:1186, 1978.
132. Henderson BE, Benton B, Jing J, et al: Risk factors for cancer of the testis in young men. Intl J Cancer 23:598-602, 1979.
133. Friedman NB: Pathology of testicular tumors, in Skinner D, Lieskovsky G (eds): Diagnosis and Management of Genitourinary Cancer. Philadelphia, WB Saunders, 1988, pp 215-234.
134. Johnson D, Swanson D, von Eschenbach A: Tumors of the genitourinary tract, in Smith's General Urology. San Mateo, Calif, Appleton & Lange, 1987, pp 330-434.
135. Smith R: Testicular carcinoma, in Haskell C (ed): Cancer Treatment (ed 2). Philadelphia, WB Saunders, 1985, pp 394-408.
136. Messing EM: Tumor antigens in the diagnosis, staging, and prognosis of urologic cancer, in Williams RD (ed): Advances in Urologic Oncology (vol 1). New York, Macmillan, 1987, pp 43-68.
137. Richie JP: Diagnosis and staging of testicular tumors, in Skinner D, Lieskovsky G (eds): Diagnosis and Management of Genitourinary Cancer. Philadelphia, WB Saunders, 1988, pp 498-507.
138. Lange PH, Nochomovitz LE, Rosai J, et al: Serum alpha fetoprotein and human chorionic gonadotropin in patients with seminoma. J Urol 124:472, 1980.
139. Bracken RB: Cancer of the testis, penis and urethra: The impact of therapy on sexual function, in von Eschenbach A, Rodriguez D (eds): Sexual Rehabilitation of the Urologic Cancer Patient. Boston, GK Hall, 1981, pp 108-127.
140. Bracken RB, Smith KD: Is semen cryopreservation helpful for the patient with testicular cancer? Urology 15:581-583, 1980.
141. Rowley MJ, Leach DR, Warner GA, et al: Effect of graded doses of ionizing radiation in the human testes. Rad Res 59:665-678, 1974.
142. Smith RB: Testicular seminoma, in Skinner D, Lieskovsky G (eds): Diagnosis and Management of Genitourinary Cancer. Philadelphia, WB Saunders, 1988, pp 508-515.
143. Skinner DG, Lieskovsky G: Management of early stage nonseminomatous germ cell tumors of testis, in Skinner D, Lieskovsky G (eds): Diagnosis and Management of Genitourinary Cancer. Philadelphia, WB Saunders, 1988, pp 516-525.
144. Einhorn LH: Chemotherapy of disseminated testicular cancer, in Skinner D, Lieskovsky G (eds): Diagnosis and Management of Genitourinary Cancer. Philadelphia, WB Saunders, 1988, pp 526-531.
145. Einhorn LH, Williams SD: Chemotherapy of disseminated testicular cancer—a random perspective study. Cancer 46:1339, 1980.
146. Blesch KS: Health beliefs about testicular cancer and self-examination among professional men. Oncol Nurs Forum 13:1986.
147. Cummings KB, Taylor WJ, Correa RJ, et al: Observations on definitive cobalt-60 radiation for cure in bladder carcinoma: 15 year follow-up. J Urol 115:152, 1976.
148. Einhorn LG: Complicated problems in testicular cancer. Semin Oncol 15:9-15, 1988.

PART VII

DELIVERY SYSTEMS FOR CANCER CARE

Chapter 49

Continuity of Care

Betty R. Ferrell, PhD, FAAN

Edith O'Neil-Page, RN, BS

INTRODUCTION

The Standards of Oncology Nursing Practice[1] emphasizes the importance of providing continuity of care throughout the span of diagnosis, treatment, rehabilitation, and terminal illness for the person with cancer. Part VIII of this book addresses the major delivery systems for cancer care. This chapter discusses the concept of continuity of care, care setting alternatives and issues, selecting and recommending settings, and the transition from hospital to the community. The three chapters that follow focus on the major delivery systems in the community: ambulatory care, home care, and hospice care.

CONTINUITY OF CARE—AN OVERVIEW

The eighties (1980-1990) will be known as the decade of drastic health care reforms and major alterations in systems of care. Although the full impact of these changes is yet to be realized, on the positive end of the continuum are alternative delivery systems that provide improved care. On the negative extreme is the potential for fragmentation of care and compromised outcomes for the patient. Interestingly, this same decade witnessed significant advancement in the specialty of oncology nursing. Oncology nurses will maintain the standards of oncology nursing practice within this rapidly changing environment by understanding the meaning and process of continuity of care.

Definition

While there is general agreement that *continuity of care* is a desirable goal,[2,3] few people have a clear definition of the term. The concept of continuity of care is often used interchangeably with the terms *discharge planning* or *continuing care*. Discharge planning can be considered the process of preparing the patient for transfer from one system and entry into the next phase of care.[2] Because patients' needs exist after discharge, there is generally continuing care, whether it is provided by the patient, the family, or another organized health care system. Continuity of care, however, implies a standard of care in which there is planned coordination of care that results in improved outcomes for the patient, irrespective of care setting or provider.

Several social and health care factors have stimulated increased emphasis on the concept of continuity of care. The most significant factor has been the implementation of diagnostic related groupings (DRGs), resulting in restricted use of acute care settings and reliance on alternative care systems. Shortened hospital stays, combined with more complex "high-tech" care, have also precipitated the concern and attention given to continuity of care. Cancer patients and their families are asked to assume nursing procedures at home that only a few years ago were limited to intensive care settings.

Another influence has been the evolution of cancer care delivered in multiple health care settings. Over the course of diagnosis and treatment, the cancer patient may experience a number of systems, including diagnostic clinics, physicians' offices, community hospitals, major cancer centers, ambulatory care centers, rehabilitation programs, home care, and hospice or nursing home care. The patient's experience will not be a linear progression from one system to another but, rather, a trajectory with multiple transitions between systems.

Therefore, continuity of care is much more than an empty phrase; it is a standard of care to be achieved. The outcome of continuity of care is efficient, optimum care over time. Studies have documented benefits of continuity of care that include decreased hospital stays, fewer hospital admissions, and increased patient satisfaction.[4,5] Figure 49-1 presents a model of continuity of care that illustrates the relationship of the patient and health care settings.

Principles Underlying Effective Continuity of Care

Since continuity of care has come to be uniformly valued, many health care agencies blindly assume that their settings are providing continuity. However, evaluation of the care in many instances would indicate that the concept is more idealistic than realistic. Table 49-1 lists the major characteristics of continuity of care. These characteristics are cited in the literature as referents of continuity of care.[2,6] This table can be used as a checklist by nurse managers or clinicians to evaluate their own settings.

Organizational philosophy is considered to be a prerequisite for achievement of continuity of care.[2,7] The philosophy of patient care, for example, in an organization that values family-centered care and interdisciplinary care is more likely to foster continuity. Well-defined standards of care may be used as a guide to achieve continuity of care.

It is important to consider the rationale behind the current emphasis on continuity. Beyond our acceptance of continuity as a desirable goal, positive outcomes have been identified as a result of patients receiving continuity of care. The most commonly cited outcomes include quality of care, patient satisfaction, nurse and physician satisfaction, and a decrease in complications or unnecessary hospital admissions.[4,5,8-11]

Standards of Oncology Nursing Practice indicates that achievement of any standard is contingent on continuity in the care provided. The standards emphasize the use of an interdisciplinary approach and identify patient needs to include issues such as comfort, coping, mobility, and elimination. To practice excellence in oncology nursing, therefore, is not to question the need for continuity of care but, rather, to question how cancer care can exist without continuity.

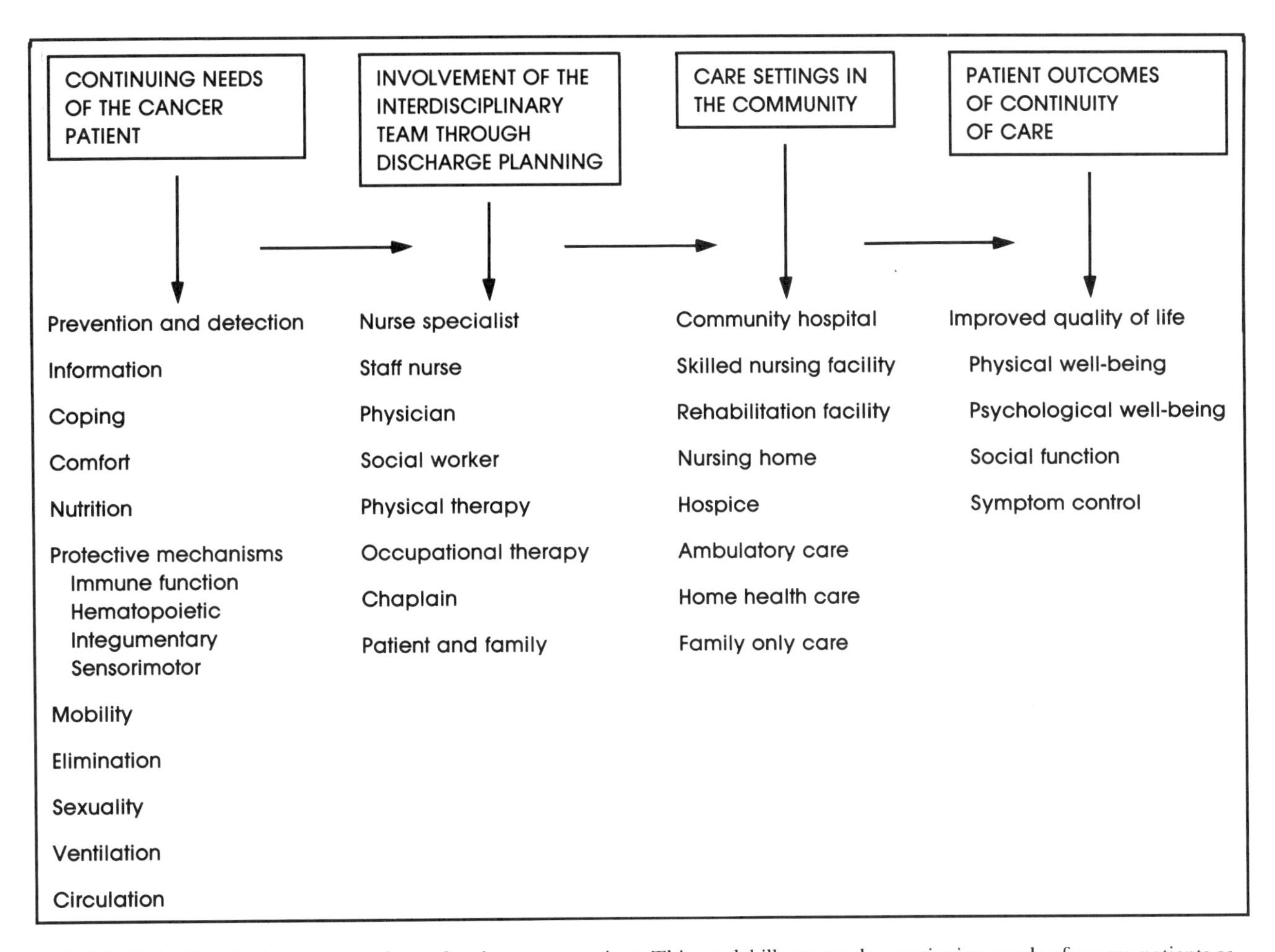

FIGURE 49-1 Model of continuity of care for the cancer patient. This model illustrates the continuing needs of cancer patients as derived from the Standards of Oncology Nursing Practice. Through involvement of an interdisciplinary team in discharge planning, care continues in community settings. The outcomes of effective continuity of care are dimensions of quality of life.

TABLE 49-1 Characteristics of Continuity of Care

C	Communication exists between settings
O	Organization exists in the form of policies, procedures, or standards of care
N	Nursing care is delivered at a level consistent with the patients' needs
T	The patient and family are informed and involved in care
I	Interdisciplinary care is provided
N	Nursing care is efficient
U	Unplanned and unavoidable events are minimal
I	Individual goals are established for each patient
T	There is adequate written documentation of care
Y	Your discharge-planning process begins prior to or at the time of admission

Specific Concerns Related to the Person with Cancer

Continuity of care is being emphasized by all areas of health care and among disciplines. The concept has particular significance for oncology. Although often perceived as a terminal diagnosis cancer is, in fact, a chronic disease. Patients with cancer are now living longer with this illness, and many achieve long-term survival and cure.

Patients with cancer can develop complex problems during the course of their disease. It is not uncommon for patients with cancer to experience disruption of several major body systems. Current technology and therapy can enable patients to overcome these disruptions; however, there may be residual effects to cope with.

Treatment of cancer involves various modalities: surgery, radiation, chemotherapy, immunotherapy, and multiple support therapies. The number of health care providers interacting with the cancer patient is reason alone for concern about continuity. An individual with newly diagnosed colon cancer, for example, may receive direct care provided by a medical oncologist, a radiation oncologist, the surgical oncology staff, an oncology nurse clinical specialist, staff nurses, an enterostomal therapist, and a dietitian. This is without mention of the additional encounters with the hospital chaplain, volunteer services, patient support groups, and other medical consultants.

Many characteristics of cancer patients' experiences place them at increased risk of compromised continuity of care. Coupled with complex physical needs is the intense psychologic impact of a diagnosis of cancer. Responses commonly cited in association with cancer include shock, fear, anxiety, depression, and hopelessness.[12] These psychologic responses can be barriers to the patients' participation in care.

Cancer patients are frequently elderly individuals with special needs for continuity of care.[13] Coupled with the burdens of a cancer diagnosis are the factors associated with aging, including decreased social supports, diminished financial resources, and multiple medical problems.

Continuity of care, therefore, is an essential element in achieving quality of care. The oncology nursing profession must evaluate current systems and devise strategies for enhancing continuity of care. This is best accomplished through careful evaluation of the specific settings used by cancer patients and planning of the transition from the acute care hospital to those settings.

CARE SETTING ALTERNATIVES AND ISSUES: FROM HOSPITAL TO COMMUNITY

Hospital to Hospital

Transition between hospitals is often necessary at the time of cancer diagnosis if the patient is referred from a community hospital to a more comprehensive cancer center. Other common transition points are at the completion of treatment when the patient resumes care closer to home or when a terminally ill patient prefers to be closer to home during the final stage of illness.

The most effective tool for continuity of care between hospitals is written communication. Most hospitals have discharge-planning tools that document the patient's status and anticipated needs after discharge. Written care instructions are essential between settings but are particularly important when the patient will continue to receive acute care and complex treatments.

Verbal communication between nurses is an effective avenue for exchanging pertinent information about the patient. Some cancer centers have established systems for nurses in community hospitals to telephone the patient's primary nurse from the cancer center to discuss care issues verbally.

Nursing Home or Skilled Nursing Facility

Since they have approximately three times as many beds as hospitals have in the United States, nursing homes represent a major segment of the health care system.[14] Contrary to popular beliefs, nursing homes care for a dynamic population of patients constantly in transition between settings, including home, hospitals, and other long-term care institutions.[14] Eighty percent of residents in nursing homes are admitted from acute care hospitals, 13% are admitted from home, and another 7% are transferred from other nursing homes.[14] Patients admitted to the nursing home are likely to be older, poorer, sicker, mentally impaired, and to have fewer family members or friends than those discharged to their own homes.[14] Discharges from the nursing home include 50% to the hospital, 40% to the patients' homes, and 10% to other nursing homes.[15]

With the increase in long-term survival of patients with cancer, the nursing home and the skilled nursing facility will likely be common settings for many patients with cancer. A major limitation to continuity of care in these settings is the reliance on a predominantly nonprofessional staff of nursing assistants and medication aides. Certain patients, such as those who require aggressive management of pain or continuous parenteral infusions, require highly skilled care, and the average nursing home, convalescent setting, or skilled nursing facility may not be appropriate. Patients at particular risk in this setting include those who have recently completed chemotherapy. Delayed complications of chemotherapy, such as myelosuppression or neurotoxicity, require careful assessment and early intervention by skilled professionals.

Oncology nurses from the acute care hospital can greatly enhance care in the nursing homes and skilled nursing facilities by offering education programs related to cancer care. Teaching basic principles of oncology nursing, such as nutrition needs, oral care, and pain management, can contribute to improved care and increased communication among staff.[16]

A major problem in care for nursing home or skilled nursing residents is inadequate documentation in the medical record. All too frequently, patients arrive from the hospital for admission to the nursing home or skilled nursing facility with little or no medical history. Patients in this setting are often not able to provide this information because of communication deficits, dementia, or poor memory. Miller et al.[17] documented that as many as 60% of primary diagnoses and 80% of secondary diagnoses were inaccurate in the nursing home record. Adverse drug reactions and inappropriate prescriptions have been associated with inaccurate diagnosis and poor medical records.[18]

In contrast, excellent care is available in some nursing homes. Many skilled nursing facilities can provide highly technical procedures for nursing, pharmacy, respiratory, and rehabilitation therapy. With the variable availability of technology and quality of care in nursing homes and skilled care facilities, there is no substitute for a thorough knowledge of individual facilities within the community.

As with all settings, basic patient information is important on transfer to and from the nursing home or the skilled nursing facility. Specific information, in addition to the nursing care plan, includes mental status information, for example, to determine the risk of falls. Other specific information needed on transfer to a nursing home would include the time of last medication administration, functional status, mental status, specific nutritional needs, and skin condition.[19]

Hospice

The transition from acute care to the hospice setting raises several important issues. The first issue is the psychologic impact on the patient and family of transfer to a hospice. While the hospice is usually considered a positive setting desired by patients and families, admission to a hospice can signify a transition from active treatment to terminal illness. Patients and families may be facing the reality of death for the first time as goals of care shift from cure to palliative care.[20] This transition requires careful attention to the psychologic needs of the patient and the family.

Another area of concern for continuity of care during a transfer to a hospice is the need for continuous symptom control. Primarily a home-based service, hospice care usually means that the family assumes responsibility for providing relief of symptoms. Studies have documented that symptom control is a chief concern of family members and that the ability to manage symptoms such as pain will influence the family's adjustment during bereavement.[21-23]

A national survey by Lauer et al.[24] examined home-based hospice services for terminally ill children. Major challenges reported were the need for hospice programs with pediatric expertise, the need for a cohesive working relationship between family and hospice staff, and the need for continued pain management.

Ambulatory Care

Ambulatory care has evolved as a major setting for oncology practice and is expected to grow in the future. Effective continuity of care provided in an ambulatory care setting can greatly reduce the need for hospitalization.

The major issues in the ambulatory setting are teaching patients and families self-care measures and preparing patients to detect an adverse reaction early enough to avoid serious sequelae or hospitalization. Outpatient radiation therapy is an example of a setting in which nurses can assure continuity of care. Patients may experience many acute and chronic symptoms related to radiation therapy, including skin alterations, gastrointestinal symptoms, fatigue, and potential disruption of major organ systems.[25] Intervention by the nurse is critical to prepare the patient for self-management of symptoms that may not occur until the conclusion of treatment or later. Dodd[9] has documented that patients who receive adequate education are more capable of self-care activities.

Tighe et al[26] conducted a comparative study of the roles of oncology nurses and non-oncology nurses in ambulatory care. Their findings indicate that oncology nurses have a greater role in interdisciplinary communication and in direct physical care of cancer patients.

Home Care

One of the primary areas for continuity of care in the home is symptom control. The author's research[27,28] indicates that management of cancer pain is not effectively provided in the home. Family members undermedicate patients for pain because of their fears of drug addiction and respiratory depression and their general misunderstanding of pain relief.

Continuity in the management of symptoms is strongly correlated with the patient's ability to function and his or her overall quality of life.[29] Few home health agencies specialize in cancer care, and therefore home care providers may not be skilled in the special needs of the cancer patient. One approach to provision of that expertise has been the integration of oncology services into home care agencies. The pain management team at Mercy Health Center in Oklahoma City has a pain team nurse provide consulting visits through the hospital home health agency to insure continuity and adequacy in pain management.[30]

Family members may be so overwhelmed by their own emotional response to having a loved one with cancer that they are less able to provide direct care. Yet social influences have encouraged families to provide care at home rather than to seek institutional care. Studies in geriatrics have indicated that, in fact, home care is often immensely burdensome on the family members.[31-33] The authors' research in the area of home care for the dying patient[23] indicates that while family members want to care for the dying patient at home, the experience may have deleterious effects on the physical and psychologic health of the surviving family members. Home care of children requires special consideration of family readiness, role confusion between home care nurses and family, flexibility, and availability of emergency back-up.[10]

Another issue of concern for continuity of care is the increase in "high-tech" home care for oncology patients, including such procedures as tube feedings, epidural catheters, intravenous infusions, or blood transfusions.[34,35] It is imperative that the family be involved throughout the hospitalization to learn the skills necessary to provide care when the patient goes home. Instructions given to families in the final hours before discharge are often not learned and can result in compromised care for the patient and feelings of inadequacy for the family. Home care has been cited as a valuable asset in the transition from care in a major hospital setting to eventual resumption of primary care by the community physician.[36]

Rehabilitation Facility

Many patients will be discharged from the hospital with continuing acute care needs that are more appropriately met through a skilled nursing facility or a rehabilitation setting. Both settings are designed as interim care facilities to help in the patient's transition from acute care to home or alternate care.

The diagnosis of cancer once carried the stigma of certain and immediate death. Patients may live for long periods after diagnosis, however, and will need time and skills to adjust to the deficits or changes they have incurred. Cancer is a chronic disease that necessitates rehabilitation measures as an integral part of therapy for some patients.[37] Rehabilitation is the action taken to return the patient to a maximum level of function and, as such, implies the need for continuity of care across settings. Mutual goal setting by the patient and the staff and interdisciplinary collaboration are particularly important for the achievement of continuity of care in cancer rehabilitation.[38,39]

Cancer rehabilitation includes not only the traditional areas of physical rehabilitation and mobility but also psychologic and social recovery.[40] Even today, patients with cancer may find it difficult to return to work or to social activities because of misconceptions and fears by employers or friends. A woman undergoing bilateral radical mastectomies could require both occupational therapy and vocational counseling to adjust to physical and social deficits. On discharge of the patient from the hospital setting to the rehabilitation setting, it is important to communicate information regarding the patient's psychologic status and social concerns.

The Patient with No Follow-Up Care

Alternative care settings have become such a common part of the health care system that it is often assumed that all patients will receive ongoing care after hospital discharge. This is not the case; moreover, the majority of cancer patients are discharged from hospital settings to self-care or family care only.[2] Financial constraints, geographic location, and resource limitations are the primary barriers to continuing services.

Oncology nurses are often uneasy about discharging the patient, realizing that while the DRG demands discharge, the patient may be inadequately prepared for or incapable of meeting the care demands. One innovative way to enhance care at home when families are the only care providers is to designate a primary care provider at home. This person can be targeted to receive instructions and can be involved in actual care during the hospitalization.

Patients and their families may elect discharge without community referral, assuming that they can meet the patient's needs. It is not until the reality of being alone in the home sets in that they are aware of the scope of care needed. For this reason, all families should be advised on how to obtain services at a later time if arrangements are not made before hospital discharge.

Because of financial constraints or third-party reimbursement limitations, many patients are ineligible for home or hospice care, even though they have definite needs for care. Nurses should be particularly alert to the patient and family who are resistant to being discharged. Requests for "just one more day" in the hospital usually indicate hesitancy and feelings of inadequacy to assume care. Additional support and teaching may be helpful.

The concerns regarding caregiver burden are crucial in the instances of care by family alone. The nursing staff can help the family to realistically address the responsibilities that await them and to plan for assumption of care at home. Volunteer groups may be able to offer some relief or assistance.

Preparation of families to assume care at home centers around family involvement during the hospitalization with ample opportunity to demonstrate procedures, such as dressing changes or tube feedings, before discharge. Responsibilities should be assumed gradually (for example, from first having the family care provider perform a single procedure to eventually assuming all the care during a shift). Another strategy is to plan the first 24 hours after discharge in great detail to assist with this critical time period. Family "care plans" and a "cardex" can be used. An example of such a plan is included in Figure 49-2.

SELECTING AND RECOMMENDING SETTINGS

Assessment of Patient and Family Needs

The importance of the patient's involvement in the process of discharge planning cannot be overstated. Continuity of care must be based on a comprehensive nursing assessment specific to the needs of the patient with cancer. There are model tools available that provide an excellent assessment base for oncology nursing.[2,35,41]

It is essential to first identify who is "family" for the patient. Family is broadly interpreted to include whoever is identified as such by the patient.[42] Assessment includes evaluation of the normal family routine, normal roles in the family, and the health status of the family members. Rose[43] has identified a number of excellent tools for the assessment of families with school-age children. Wright and Leahey[44] have identified effective interviewing methods to assess families as well as intervention strategies for enhancing family care. They present the use of interviewing skills to assess relationships within the family and interventions that maximize family strengths. Our clinical experiences have included arriving for a home visit to find the patient in better health than the family members.

The best approach to assessment of family and patient needs is one characterized by individuality. It is a tremendous challenge to balance both the patient's and the family members' best interests. Accurate assessment of patient and family needs is a prerequisite to effective intervention.

Collaborative Planning and Roles of the Health Care Team

The benefits of collaborative practice and their impact on improved outcomes have been documented.[45-47] Patients benefit from clear communication between health care providers and from consistent goals of care. Patients experience a sense of support and reduced conflict when care is based on collaborative planning.

NAME: ____________ PHYSICIAN: ____________ PHONE: ____________

PATIENT GOALS:
1. To be able to remain at home while I get my radiation therapy treatments.
2. To gain my strength back and gain some weight.

MEDICATIONS:
1. Metamucil—take one teaspoon two times a day.
2. Doxidan—take one capsule every day.
3. Tylenol #3—take one tablet every 4 hours if needed for pain. Contact your physician if your pain increases or if the medicine isn't working.

ACTIVITY RESTRICTIONS:
1. Take a short walk each day if weather permits.
2. Do not lift anything heavier than 1 pound for the next 4 weeks.

DIET:
1. Eat 3 meals a day and continue your Ensure®, one can two times a day.
2. Use the suggested foods list from the dietician.
3. Weigh yourself once a week. Report any weight loss to the home health nurse.

TREATMENTS:
Clean your suture site two times a day with peroxide for the next week. After that time, clean your suture site with warm water only during shower.

NOTES:
1. The American Cancer Society will provide your transportation for radiation therapy. Call them at ____________ to make arrangements.

2. The Hospital Home Health Care nurse will visit 3 times a week on Monday, Wednesday, and Friday. The first visit will be tomorrow. Their number is ____________.

3. Your Radiation Therapy will begin on 5-14-90 and is scheduled once a day for 2 weeks at 10:00 a.m. Call the Radiation Therapy Department with any questions at ____________.

4. You may also call the Hospital Oncology Patient Hot Line for any questions about your care. The number is ____.

FIGURE 49-2 Family care plan. A family care plan will enhance continuity of care at home. Note that the instructions are clearly written for family understanding on the basis of patient goals.

Multidisciplinary care is not necessarily interdisciplinary care.[48] While there may be many disciplines involved, it is critical that these multiple care providers are interacting to avoid conflict. Territorial struggles and political battles can greatly impede continuity of care for the patient and may result in either duplication and conflicting goals or the absence of planning as the patient falls through the system.

Discharge-planning teams exist in most acute care settings, either in a formal structure or often in an informal sense. Models of discharge planning include formal teams who develop coordinated plans of care through conferences, discharge planners functioning as consultants to staff, and staff nurses or social workers who assume discharge-planning functions within their normal roles.[2]

The nurse has the central role in the discharge-planning team.[2,49] As the provider with the greatest amount of interaction with the patient and the most comprehensive view of the total needs, the nurse is best suited to coordinate the team approach. The nurse member of the discharge-planning team can be an advanced practitioner, a clinical specialist, or the staff nurse. As the primary provider of inpatient care, the staff nurse generally is best informed of the patient's care and response. Rusch[49] has presented a model program in which staff nurses are educated about community resources and discharge-planning principles to enhance their role in discharge planning. This includes knowledge of the specific resources as well as procedures for making these resources available to a patient.

The social worker also has an important role in discharge planning.[48] Nurses and social workers collaborate to provide a comprehensive approach to discharge planning. This is facilitated by clear delineation of responsibilities.

Communication among the discharge team members greatly influences achievement of continuity of care. Written documentation is essential as discharge plans are made. Methods to promote communication include weekly discharge-planning conferences, walking rounds for discharge planning, or daily communication among team members.

Case management is a care-delivery method that is emerging and being refined.[50,51] Developed during the 1970s in the areas of psychiatric and geriatric care, case management is now being extended to other areas of health care. Zander et al.[51] have developed the concept to include a primary nurse/case manager who uses a production plan process to organize, direct, revise, and evaluate care. The case manager model emphasizes the need for interdisciplinary collaboration while maintaining the central role of the nurse as case manager.

Case management uses specific outcome criteria and predicted time frames to monitor the patient's hospital stay and discharge. Case management is a nursing delivery system that uses standards or critical paths to map out the patient's expected progress.[52] The nurse case manager is responsible for the total management of the patient and collaborates with other disciplines to achieve the outcomes. Schwab and Pierce[53] evaluated the case-management system in an ambulatory pediatric setting and reported that it was useful in achieving desirable patient outcomes.

This concept has potentially a great deal to offer oncology, particularly as a method to assure continuity of care. Since this is a new service-delivery method, research is warranted to evaluate the use of case management in other areas such as oncology.

Evaluation of Alternatives

Individual attention to the needs and goals of the patient is a critical part of the evaluation and selection of alternative care arrangements. Discharge from the hospital setting can become a routine with little attention given to careful identification of the most appropriate alternatives. It is not uncommon for a patient to be admitted to home health care when his or her needs would have more appropriately been met by hospice care.

Cost is a critical consideration in the evaluation of alternatives. If applicable, insurance coverage and benefits should be thoroughly checked for important information on alternative care choices. If insurance coverage is not available, the patient and the family should receive realistic estimates of potential expenses. Example: when a patient with leukemia was admitted to the home health agency, the nurse calculated the cost of necessary supplies for the management of a central line catheter. Both the patient and the nurse were distressed to learn that the costs of supplies exceeded the patient's total income. The hospital social worker had assumed that the cost of supplies in the home would be covered by insurance but, in fact, no coverage was available.

To make appropriate referrals, health care providers must be well informed of the services provided by the alternative care settings or agencies. For example, when one is referring a patient for home chemotherapy, it is necessary to know the qualifications of the home care nurse who will administer the chemotherapy and the availability of on-call services for help with potential problems. A patient discharged to nursing home care after administration of chemotherapy will require laboratory services for follow-up blood work. Since cancer patients may move among multiple settings, it is incumbent on the referring agency to carefully evaluate the services available in the potential setting.

To insure continuity, the referring nurse should be aware of the quantity of services needed and the ability of the alternative agency to provide those services. Knowing that the home health nurse will be available to visit only once a week will indicate the need for intense family teaching, since the family will assume responsibility for most of the patient's care.

Choices

When the assessment and evaluation of alternatives are completed, an informed choice can be made and the specific arrangements can begin. Patients should be advised that choices may be flexible and that alterations can be made at any time. A patient who finds that return trips to the hospital ambulatory care center are too exhausting may need reevaluation for possible change to a closer community clinic or to in-home chemotherapy.

In most instances there is a wide variety of services for the patient to select. The nurse, functioning in a patient-advocacy role, should encourage the patient and the family to be assertive consumers in their choices of care. A family selecting a nursing home setting should inquire specifically into the experience of that facility in caring for cancer patients. The family preparing for transfer of the patient to hospice care should be informed of the extent or limit of emergency on-call services so that an informed choice between home care and hospice can be made.

Assessment of the Care Setting

Continuity of care requires integration of the patient's past, present, and future in the planning and provision of care.[3] Nurses must remember that some of the patient's current needs could have existed before admission to a health care service. The nurse determines how the patient's needs were met before the current hospitalization in order to evaluate future plans. An effective approach for assessment of the proposed transfer setting includes a visit to the setting before the patient's hospital discharge. A visit to the patient's home by the home health nurse prior to discharge can provide valuable insight into specific needs for continued care. Another assessment strategy is to have the patient describe the environment and routines that existed before the present hospitalization.

If the patient is not going home, the family should be encouraged to visit the alternative care setting in advance of the discharge. If the patient is going to be transferred to a hospice, a visit from the hospice nurse may greatly allay the patient's and family's anxiety regarding discharge.

Hospital staff members may fall into a pattern of discharge planning that does not adequately assess individual needs. Settings that routinely refer cancer patients for home care may fail to recognize that some patients may best be served through a short stay in a skilled nursing facility. Some discharge-planning programs have home care nurses to assist in appropriate referrals.

TRANSITION

Coordination

Regardless of the amount of prior planning, transfer from one setting to another evokes anxiety for the patient, the family, and the health care staff. It is common to find that the patient who had been eagerly awaiting discharge is quite hesitant when the actual day arrives.

The stress of transition may be greatly reduced by active involvement of the staff nurse. The primary nurse is in the best position to assess the patient's status and to provide instruction to patient and family in a timely and coordinated manner. The staff nurse coordinates the involvement of specialists and support staff to help the patient during the transition. In addition, discharge instruction given over a period of time will most likely be more effective than teaching that occurs on the day of discharge when anxiety is at a peak.[54,55]

Communication Process and Tools

Since cancer patients are now receiving their care in multiple settings throughout the course of their disease, innovative strategies to improve and facilitate communication will be needed. Preuss et al[56] developed a model program that includes a statewide telecommunication system to facilitate communication between nurses at a tertiary referral center and a community hospital. The project, entitled CHILD (Continued Help in Lending Direction), has resulted in improved patient outcomes, increased patient satisfaction, and continuity of care.

A comprehensive patient-assessment tool is invaluable during the transition from the hospital to any community setting. Miaskowski and Nielson[41] developed a cancer nursing assessment tool that provides the new setting with a rich data base from which to plan care. Another tool, developed by O'Neil-Page for use in discharge planning based on self-care theory, is included in Figure 49-3.

Acceptance and Adjustment

The concept that discharge planning begins on admission to the hospital has changed from a desirable process to a required process. Family members and patients must understand the need for early discharge planning and must be involved from the time of admission. New models for better utilization of health care resources are beginning the discharge-planning process before the patient's admission to the hospital.

Experience has shown that gradual transition from the acute care setting to the community is best accomplished through transfer to a day hospital, respite care, or gradual assumption of care by the family during hospitalization. Unfortunately, it is often assumed that the transition is over and continuity of care has been achieved when the patient is discharged and all the appropriate forms have been completed. The characteristics for continuity of care (see Table 49-1) can be a useful checklist for evaluation of ongoing care.

The previous decade has witnessed a movement away from acute care settings. However, there is interest in the idea that the acute care setting should be the center of care for the patient amid the multiple alternative settings. Model programs, such as the Supportive Care Program at Memorial Sloan-Kettering Cancer Center,[8] have demonstrated the ongoing role of the hospital in coordinating continuity of care. This program emphasizes the central role of nursing in the extension of the acute care setting into the community. The Supportive Care Program provides expertise to insure that standards of care, particularly in the area of patient comfort, are met after hospital discharge.

EVALUATION AND FOLLOW-UP

Evaluation to determine the effectiveness of health care is based on patient outcomes. These outcomes are individualized and are derived from the patient assessment. For example, a priority in the care of a patient after radical surgery for a neck tumor is continued nutritional support. To determine the status of care at home, evaluation of outcomes would be based on measures of nutrition, such as intake, weight gain, and wound healing.

Hospitals have used follow-up questionnaires or surveys of the primary physician to obtain information regarding the patient's status after discharge. To fully appreciate the cancer patient's experience, one would need to evaluate every care setting and service encountered by that person. Further research is needed to determine the quality of transitions of cancer patients among settings and to evaluate such settings according to standards of care.

PATIENT NAME: ______________________ ADDRESS: ______________________

PHONE: ______________ PHYSICIAN: ______________________

DISCHARGE DATE: __________ TIME: __________ AMBULATORY CONDITION: ______________

DIAGNOSIS: ______________________

HOSPITAL COURSE: (a summary of the major events during the hospitalization)

TREATMENT: (chemotherapy, radiation, etc.)

MEDICATIONS: (list all medications, dose, schedule, PRNs, patients understanding of medications and allergies)

PATIENT'S SELF-CARE STATUS AT DISCHARGE:

Ability to maintain sufficient ventilation and circulation:
(Shortness of breath, cough, respiratory rate, pulse and BP, chest pain, edema, fatigue)

Ability to maintain sufficient fluid status:
(Oral intake, oral mucosa)

Ability to maintain food intake:
(Current weight, weight changes, nausea, food intake, diet restrictions, stomatitis, dentures)

Ability to maintain elimination:
(Bowel and bladder habits, medications for elimination, problems or changes in elimination)

Ability to balance activity and rest:
(Patterns of sleep and activity, changes in activity and rest, aids to sleep, prescribed activity)

Ability to prevent hazards and achieve safety:
(Mental status, gait, sensory status, fatigue)

Ability to maintain balance of social interaction:
(Family relationships, support systems, sexuality and changes in sexual activity, occupation)

Ability to maintain comfort:
(Pain description, location and amount; pain medications; non drug pain relief; other symptoms)

Ability to cope with illness and treatment:
(Anxiety, depression or other emotions; communication, self-esteem, role changes)

Patient Concerns at Discharge:

Referrals to community agencies or continuing care:

Nursing Diagnosis/Problem List:
(Include anticipated teaching needs)

FIGURE 49-3 Self-care nursing discharge tool. Careful assessment is critical to continuity of care after hospital discharge. This comprehensive assessment will enhance continuing care.

CONCLUSION

Evaluation of services is clearly a challenge amid the constraints of the health care system at present. Evaluation is essential to assuring the quality of services but is undoubtedly time-consuming. One innovative evaluation program, which has been reported by Siegel et al,[57] uses a computer-automated telephone outreach system to follow up chemotherapy outpatients.

One implication of continuity of care relates to the education of future health care providers. Students in nursing and other health disciplines need curricula that include knowledge of continuity of care.[3,11] Nursing students need to evaluate patients in a broad spectrum of care rather than only in their current care setting. Nursing education can incorporate knowledge and experience in continuity of care into student experiences by exposure of students to advanced practitioners, oncology clinical specialists, and nurse managers who are familiar with nursing roles in interdisciplinary discharge-planning teams. Such concepts as case management should be included in continuing education in oncology.

Continuity of care provides nurses with greater professional satisfaction.[58] Oncology nurses are characterized by concern and involvement with the cancer patient. The inpatient nurse can become frustrated without follow-up contact with the patient after discharge from the hospital. Communication channels made available through continuity-of-care systems can provide feedback to inpatient nurses. It is hoped that when a complete feedback loop exists for care providers to communicate and evaluate outcomes of continuity of care, cancer patients will achieve an improved quality of life.

REFERENCES

1. American Nurse's Association and Oncology Nursing Society: Standards of Oncology Nursing Practice. Kansas City, ANA, 1987.
2. O'Hare P, Terry M: Discharge Planning: Strategies for Assuring Continuity of Care. Rockville, Md, Aspen Publications, 1988.
3. Ruane T, Brody H: Understanding and teaching continuity of care. J Med Educ 62:969-973, 1987.
4. Wasson J, Sauvigne A, Mogielnicki P: Continuity of outpatient medical care in elderly men. JAMA 252:2413-2417, 1984.
5. Magill M, Senf J: A new method for measuring continuity of care in family practice residencies. J Fam Pract 24:165-168, 1987.
6. Rehr H: Discharge planning: An ongoing function of quality care. QRB 12(2):47-50, 1986.
7. Notkin MS: Collaboration and communication. Nurs Admin Q 7:1-7, 1983.
8. Coyle N: A model of continuity of care for cancer patients with chronic pain. Med Clin North Am 71:259-270, 1987.
9. Dodd M: Patterns of self-care in patients receiving radiation therapy. Oncol Nurs Forum 11(3):23-30, 1984.
10. Feetham S: Hospitals and home care: Inseparable in the 80s. Pediatr Nurs 12:383-386, 1986.
11. Klingbeil G, Fiedler I: Continuity of care: A teaching model. Am J Phys Med 67:77-81, 1988.
12. Welch-McCaffrey D: Cancer: Anxiety and quality of life. Cancer Nurs 8:151-158, 1985.
13. King F, Figge J, Harman P: The elderly coping at home: A study of continuity of nursing care. J Adv Nurs 11:41-46, 1986.
14. Kane RL, Matthias R: From hospital to nursing home: The long term care connection. Gerontologist 24:604-609, 1984.
15. Lewis MA, Shan C, Kane RL: The natural history of nursing home patients. Gerontologist 25:382-388, 1985.
16. Goldman L, Miller D, Moeller T: Hospital-nursing home collaboration. QRB 12(6):215-217, 1986.
17. Miller MB, Elliot F, Elliot DF: Errors and outcomes in diagnostic records on admission of patients to nursing homes. J Am Geriatr Soc 34:108-116, 1976.
18. Segal JL, Thompson JF, Floyd RA: Drug utilization and prescribing patterns in a skilled nursing facility: The need for a rational approach to therapeutics. J Am Geriatr Soc 27:117-122, 1979.
19. Wright H, Lancot A: From hospital to nursing home. QRB 6(8):7-10, 1980.
20. Martocchio B: Living While Dying. New York, Robert Brady Company, 1983.
21. Hine V: Dying at home: Can families cope? Omega 10:175-187, 1979.
22. Martinson I: Care for the dying child. Nurs Clin North Am 1:467-475, 1979.
23. Ferrell BR: Home versus hospital cancer deaths and bereavement outcomes. Am J Hospice, July-August:18-23, 1985.
24. Lauer M, Mulhern R, Hoffmann R, et al: Utilization of hospice/home care in pediatric oncology. Cancer Nurs 9:102-107, 1986.
25. Strohl R: The nursing role in radiation oncology: Symptom management of acute and chronic reactions. Oncol Nurs Forum 15:429-434, 1988.
26. Tighe M, Fisher S, Hastings C, et al: A study of the oncology nurse role in ambulatory care. Oncol Nurs Forum 12:23-27, 1985.
27. Ferrell BR, Schneider C: Experience and management of cancer pain at home. Cancer Nurs 11(2):84-90, 1988.
28. Ferrell BR, Patterson B: Pain at home. Caring 6(11):22-25, 1987.
29. Ferrell BR, Ferrell BA: Comfort, in Corr D, Corr C (eds): Nursing Care in an Aging Society. Springhouse, Pa, Springhouse Publishers (in press).
30. Ferrell BR, Wisdom C, Wenzl C: Evolution and evaluation of a pain management team. Oncol Nurs Forum 15(3):285-289, 1988.
31. Litman T: Health care and the family. Med Care 9:67-81, 1971.
32. Zarit S: Subjective burden of husbands and wives as caregivers: A longitudinal study. Gerontologist 26:(3) p 253-259, 1986.
33. Hinds C: The needs of families who care for patients with cancer at home: Are we meeting them. J Adv Nurs 10:575-581, 1985.
34. Birmingham J: Home Care Planning Based on DRGs. Philadelphia, JB Lippincott, 1986.
35. Bulau J: Clinical Policies and Procedures for Home Health Care. Rockville, Md, Aspen Publishers, 1986.

36. Mor G, Joseph A, Carel C, et al: Evaluation of the annual activity of a continuing medical and home care unit. Soc Sci Med 24:967-972, 1987.
37. Broadwell D: Rehabilitation needs of the patient with cancer. Cancer 60:563-568, 1987.
38. Dudas S, Carlson C: Cancer rehabilitation. Oncol Nurs Forum 15:183-188, 1988.
39. Gruca J: Oncology rehabilitation. Rehabil Nurs 9(3):27-30, 1984.
40. Dietz J: Adaptive rehabilitation in cancer. Cancer Rehabil 68:145-153, 1980.
41. Miaskowski C, Nielson B: A cancer nursing assessment tool. Oncol Nurs Forum 12:37-42, 1985.
42. Leahey M, Wright L: Families and Life Threatening Illness. Springhouse, Pa, Springhouse, 1987.
43. Rose D: Assessing families of school aged children with cancer, in Leahey M, Wright L (eds): Families and Life Threatening Illness. Springhouse, Pa, Springhouse, 1987.
44. Wright L, Leahey M: Families and Chronic Illness. Springhouse, Pa, Springhouse, 1987.
45. Crowley S, Wollner I: Collaborative practice: A tool for change. Oncol Nurs Forum 14:59-63, 1987.
46. Anderson DJ, Finn MC: Collaborative practice: Developing a structure that works. Nurs Admin Q 7:19-25, 1983.
47. Ryan LS, Edwards R, Rickles F: A joint practice approach to the care of persons with cancer. Oncol Nurs Forum 7:8-11, 1980.
48. Blumenfield S: Discharge planning: Changes for hospital social work in a new health care climate. QRB 12(2):51-54, 1986.
49. Rusch S: Continuity of care: From hospital unit into home. Nurs Management 17:38-41, 1986.
50. McIntosh L: Hospital based case management. Nurs Econ 5:232-236, 1987.
51. Zander K, Etheredge M, Bower, R: Nursing Case Management: Blueprints for Transformation. Massachusetts, Winslow, 1987.
52. Weisman E: Practical approaches for developing a case management program. QRB 13(1):380-382, 1987.
53. Schwab S, Pierce P: Assessment of clinical nursing practice in a rural decentralized case-management system. Public Health Nurs 3:111-119, 1986.
54. Knowles M. The Modern Practice of Adult Education. New York, Association Press, 1970.
55. Rankin S, Duffy K: Patient Education: Issues, Principles, and Guidelines. Philadelphia, JB Lippincott, 1983.
56. Preuss N, Perez N, Randall J, et al: Continued help in lending direction: A proposed nurse to nurse communication system. Issues in Comprehensive Pediatric Nursing 9:229-237, 1986.
57. Siegel K, Mesagno F, Chen J, et al: Computerized telephone assessment of the concrete needs of chemotherapy outpatients: A feasibility study. J Clin Oncol 6:1760-1767, 1988.
58. Rulin M, Hayashi T, Badway D: Continuity of ambulatory care in an obstetrics and gynecology residency program. Obstet Gynecol 71:787-790, 1988.

Chapter 50

Ambulatory Care

Dolores Esparza, RN, MS

AMBULATORY CARE: AN OVERVIEW

Ambulatory care, synonymous with outpatient care, is a system of services for the diagnosis, treatment, and care of patients who are not hospitalized.[1,2] Patients who do not stay more than 24 hours can obtain health care in an ambulatory facility.[1] Services obtainable in an ambulatory cancer care facility include diagnostic testing, screening, and detection, minor surgical procedures, chemotherapy, radiation therapy, and psychosocial intervention.[3]

The earliest account of ambulatory care dates back to the 1600s when outpatient care was traditionally reserved for the impoverished.[4,5] Ambulatory cancer care has gone through an evolutionary cycle directly affected by the economy, politics, and technologic improvements in the treatment of cancer. Today ambulatory care is available to persons of all socioeconomic levels in modern settings that compete to attract a market share that includes private-pay patients. The current trend in ambulatory care reflects a response to economic pressure for less expensive health care delivery systems, a high degree of competitiveness between institutions, and the need to provide improved and more accessible patient services.

As a result of the tremendous growth in outpatient care, alternative settings in addition to clinics and hospital-based centers have been developed. These settings include highly specialized outpatient facilities designed to offer consolidated cancer services under one roof.[6] The attractive feature of these settings is that the patient has the convenience of one-stop care. The advantages for the clinician are efficiency, expediency, and improved communication among team members. Other features include home care and physician group practices.

Patient Selection

Outpatient facilities should determine specific screening criteria for patient selection to ensure the safe administration of treatment in the ambulatory setting. By definition, ambulatory patients are able to intervene on their own behalf in health promotion, prevention, detection, and treatment.[7] For patients to qualify for ambulatory status, they should be able to care for themselves and have a strong support system. The requirements and expectations of outpatient care places great responsibility on the patients and their families to provide social support and physical assistance. As health care providers, we often expect the family and friends to learn complex facts and treatment and observation skills in a short period of time. The management of ambulatory cancer care is easier for those patients who have a solid base of support in the home. It is important to assess the family's ability and level of motivation to care for the patient.

Criteria for outpatient treatment should include the ability of the patient to withstand the prescribed therapy and the ability of the facility to care for the potential complications that could occur during therapy. For example, when a patient is scheduled to receive cisplatin on an outpatient basis, it will be critical to determine whether that patient is at risk for congestive heart failure or has inadequate respiratory or renal function to tolerate the extensive regimen required.[8] If these risk factors exist, the decision may be made to provide treatment in an inpatient setting until patient's tolerance of the regimen is evident. Other persons with questionable potential as outpatients are bedridden patients with inadequate support in the home, patients who are dehydrated as a result of nausea and vomiting, those who require heavy sedation and have no one to stay with them at home, and those who are not willing to cooperate with predetermined self-care activities of therapy. These as well as other clinical parameters must be evaluated before a patient is treated on an ambulatory basis.

However, the preceding description of a candidate for ambulatory cancer care does not always hold true today. Most ambulatory cancer programs provide the full scope of therapy aimed at cure, control, or palliation. As a result of the progress in cancer therapy and management of symptoms, many cancer patients with advanced disease can be treated and cared for as outpatients. It is not unusual for a patient to be transported by ambulance to an ambulatory center for cancer treatment. Often the patient with limited physical mobility or advanced disease will elect to receive care as an outpatient in order to retain some portion of the social integrity of the family unit. Clearly, the family plays the most critical role in the care of the patient who is receiving cancer therapy as an outpatient. The nurse provides education for the patient and the family and gives reassurance throughout the treatment course. Both the patient and the family need to be assessed frequently to determine their continued ability and motivation to sustain care for the outpatient.

Economic Considerations

Ambulatory care constitutes the largest volume of medical care in the United States.[9] Furthermore, today's economic climate favors the continuation of the prevailing trend for expansion of outpatient facilities.[10] Historical trends indicate that by the year 2000 national health expenditures will exceed a staggering $1.5 trillion, of which ambulatory care costs will be a significant part.[10]

Effective care of the person with cancer can take place in a myriad of settings. The outpatient setting has received widespread acceptance as the most economical and socially beneficial environment in which to treat cancer, a disease that can be financially devastating.[11-14] In outpatient care, the main financial saving is the per diem room fee assessed to hospitalized patients. Laboratory fees, patient-chargeable items, and pharmacy fees are usually similar for both inpatients and outpatients.

In addition to the economic savings in the direct cost of health care, ambulatory care can sometimes enable patients to receive cancer therapy with a minimal disruption of work schedules and family routines. Caring for a patient with cancer in the home often places inordinate stress on children and spouse.[6] Clinicians should weigh the toll on the family's integrity against the benefits of outpatient therapy.

Types of Ambulatory Care Programs

Ambulatory care is a rapidly expanding method for health care delivery. Diversification into ambulatory care can be attributed to a variety of factors, including technologic advances, consumer awareness, entrepreneurism, and a changing attitude toward health care.[2]

The 1971 National Cancer Act stimulated funding and development of regional comprehensive cancer centers. Their broad mission was interdisciplinary collaboration in basic and clinical research, detection, diagnosis, and treatment of cancer.[15] These comprehensive cancer centers were based at major medical institutions that were strategically located to promote their leadership role in cancer activities in their respective regions. The centers received federal funding for administration, construction, and research.[15] Ambulatory cancer care facilities are usually components of these federally funded comprehensive cancer centers. Many of the outpatient therapy protocols and patient-management methods used in ambulatory cancer care today were initially developed and studied by the regional comprehensive cancer centers. In addition to federal programs, the private sector is emerging as an important presence in provision of outpatient cancer care.

Reimbursement issues, economic constraints, and competition have forced hospitals to establish programs, services, and settings to attract patients.[16] Joint ventures between the private sector and the nonprofit sector yield ambulatory facilities that specialize in cancer treatment that offers an alternative to traditional hospital care and provides a competitive edge in the health care market. Joint ventures afford hospitals additional capital to construct and operate outpatient cancer centers that are accredited as hospital-based facilities.[17] Hospital-based ambulatory care centers can make significant financial and clinical contributions by expanding outpatient services.

Growth of independent for-profit ambulatory centers has introduced a new source for expansion of health care facilities unparalleled since the Hill Burton legislation of 1946.[18] Today's ambulatory cancer centers are also able to provide increasing numbers of patient services, such as nutrition counseling, psychosocial consultation, pain management, pharmacy services evaluation, diagnostic services, medical consultation, and treatment.[17] There are four basic models for outpatient cancer care: hospital-based ambulatory centers, free-standing outpatient facilities, office-based care, and home care.

Hospital-based programs

Of the four basic types of ambulatory cancer care facilities, hospital-based programs are the most common and offer the patient the most options for care. Hospital-based ambulatory cancer care facilities can offer patients a full range of clinical services, support staff, and specialists. Since cancer patients can fluctuate between hospitalization and ambulatory status during the course of the disease, many patients and families welcome the familiarity and continuity of a hospital-based ambulatory cancer program. Some hospital-sponsored ambulatory centers offer nursing and medical care during off-hours. This convenience means that patients do not have to seek out an emergency room to receive care for the complications that may arise from their cancer treatment.

Free-standing programs

Free-standing outpatient cancer facilities usually offer more limited patient services than hospital-based programs, since they are not able to supply the diverse clinical resources that a hospital-based outpatient facility offers. This is primarily because free-standing clinics may be physically removed from the main source of clinical services. However, free-standing ambulatory cancer care centers are often easily accessible and less confusing to the patient than those based in a large hospital.

Physician's office–based care

Care in the physician's office is expected to outpace overall future spending for health care since physician reimbursement is currently not subject to prospective payment schedules.[10] A payment-reform program is being developed for possible modifications of part B Medicare reimbursement. The Department of Health and Human Services is evaluating the benefits and effectiveness of chemotherapy in the physician's office.[19] The type and extent of cancer care offered in a physician's office are restricted only by facilities, staff, and support services. There are a few disadvantages of being treated in a physician's office.[6] The most restrictive variable is office hours. Once the office is closed, patients have to go to an emergency room if care is needed. On the other hand, an advantage of care in a physician's office is the close relationship developed between the patient, the office staff, and the physician.

Home care

Patients who are homebound but do not require hospitalization may receive some of their cancer care in the home. Nutritional support, antibiotics, blood products, and chemotherapy are being given if the therapy and the patient's status are appropriate for home administration. The chapters on "Home Care" and "Chemotherapy" offer a more in-depth review of home care for the cancer patient.

Characteristics of Ambulatory Cancer Care

Many ambulatory cancer care programs have been developed in recent years. The following should be considered in the development of an ambulatory cancer care program[20]:

- Outpatient care is a rapidly changing field that requires flexibility and ability to adapt to new technologies, treatments, and financial constraints.
- Cancer care is a research-oriented field that requires evaluation and exploration of new approaches.
- Cancer has a devastating effect on patients and their families. Both crisis care and ongoing support will be needed.
- Areas for privacy, counseling, and teaching need to be included in the design of the facility.
- Coordination of health services must be provided by primary facility or may be contracted.
- It should provide accessible services in terms of both location and times that are convenient to the patient.
- Development should respond to community needs.
- Services may be provided at hospitals, free-standing facilities, or private physician offices.

Environment

It would be safe to predict that ambulatory cancer care has not reached the pinnacle of its development. In the past, ambulatory facilities had a reputation as high-patient-volume clinics with crowded waiting rooms, multiple appointment bookings, and long waiting periods.[21] The focus of ambulatory cancer care is changing as competition increases and patients have more choices of where to receive their care. The current focus is on provision of an individualized, private environment where patients have definite appointments and waiting periods are kept to a minimum. Every effort is made to eradicate previous negative connotations of a clinic.

Patient and family education

Outpatients, by definition, must be able to care for themselves with support from their families. The reliance on the patient's self-care skills makes it essential that the nurse and ancillary staff prepare the family and the patient adequately for handling medications, treatments, and special procedures. If the patient is unable to follow instructions or to comply with the requirements of return visits or proper use of medication, a decision may have to be made to hospitalize the patient.

Family involvement

Family involvement is of paramount importance in such areas as assisting the patient with therapy, transporting the patient to and from appointments, and monitoring the patient's condition at home. The pressure on the family to assimilate extensive information regarding the patient's care, equipment (ie, infusion pump maintenance), and medications can tax the family unit significantly. An assessment by the nurse will determine whether the patient has adequate family support to be treated safely on an outpatient basis. The family situation must be closely monitored, since advancing disease and a deteriorating condition can have a dramatic impact on the amount of family involvement and their ability to meet the patient's needs on a daily basis. Additional supports or an alternative care setting may help a highly stressed family.

Rehabilitation

Rehabilitation of the patient is an important aspect of ambulatory care. As cancer patients are living longer, it is critical to assure the highest possible quality of life. Physical, occupational, psychologic, and social rehabilitation needs should be assessed frequently during ambulatory care. Body image and sexuality are major issues for some cancer patients. Innovative programs are including such supports as the services of make-up artists and hair designers.

Continuity of care

In an ambulatory cancer care program it is important to provide consistency and continuity for both the patients and the staff. Primary nursing, the case-management model, and primary physician-nurse teams are methods for providing continuity of care. With these models, there is a specific staff member for the patient to call with regard to problems or complications. The patient load can be shared with additional nurses if the practice size warrants it.

Ambulatory Care Clinical Services

A broad array of cancer care services can be offered through an ambulatory cancer care program. Some programs provide comprehensive services, while others are limited. Radiation therapy and administration of chemotherapy are the most common outpatient cancer care services. As the focus on outpatient care sharpens, more centers are developing core services for therapy and are also implementing additional services to become comprehensive outpatient cancer centers.

Diagnostic procedures

Ambulatory patients with cancer receive many diagnostic and therapeutic services during the course of their disease. Provision of cost-effective, quality diagnostic services is a focal point of competition between many health care facilities.[22] Most patients prefer to continue with therapy at the place where their cancer was diagnosed. For the cancer patient, the availability of both diagnostic and therapeutic services within one setting can mean less time spent seeking out services and less time traveling from one facility to another. The major diagnostic services for cancer patients include radiology, magnetic resonance imaging, nuclear medicine, surgical diagnostic procedures, and clinical laboratory.

In the diagnostic services, the staff will sometimes encounter a situation in which the patient comes to the realization that he or she could have cancer. Registered nurses and technicians should be prepared to help patients with this crisis. The patient may be alone, particularly if he came for a follow-up visit unsuspecting that the disease has recurred. Some patients may experience claustrophobic reactions from the closed rooms and ominous equipment. Adverse physical reactions to contrast media can occur with specific diagnostic procedures. This can be frightening to the patient and the family. The nurse is a provider not only of technical skill but also of support and education for the patient and the family.

Chemotherapy

A major type of therapy provided in ambulatory settings is chemotherapy. The principles of administration and management of side effects are the same as those for inpatients. There are two important contrasts with inpatient care; one is a financial advantage, and the other is the responsibility placed on the family for administering medications, observing response and reactions, performing treatments, transporting the patient for treatment, and reporting any changes in the patient's condition.[6] Implicit in the patient's and family's responsibility is the need for thorough, careful education by the nursing staff.

Chemotherapy administered on an outpatient basis is less expensive than when it is administered on an inpatient basis.[23] Chemotherapy in a physician's office is often even less expensive. This is probably due to the less stringent financial regulations for physician's offices. Prager[23] demonstrated that chemotherapy administered in a physician's office yielded a cost savings of 34%, as compared to inpatient costs. Chemotherapy administered in a hospital-sponsored ambulatory center is also significantly less costly than inpatient care. The savings of outpatient care are attributed to the lack of a per diem room charge.

Advances in technology and management approaches are among the factors that have enabled clinicians to treat patients with complex chemotherapy protocols in the outpatient setting. Examples include continuous infusions of chemotherapy through central venous catheters or arterial lines while the patient remains an outpatient.[24-28]

Safety in handling chemotherapy in the workplace has been a concern of many professionals, regulatory agencies, and institutions.[29] In addition, clinicians have been concerned with the safe handling and disposal of chemotherapeutic agents that are taken or administered at home. Patients and families should be instructed to dispose of agents separately and to place them into a closed container, such as a coffee can or a special impervious chemotherapy container, provided by the outpatient staff. If possible, the remains of the chemotherapy equipment and drug should be returned to the outpatient facility if the next visit occurs soon after the treatment. Every precaution should be taken to avoid disposing of these agents and the equipment through the domestic rubbish or common sewer system. This issue is one of environmental control and needs further investigation before alternatives can be safely used.

Radiation therapy

Radiation therapy services play a major role in ambulatory cancer care since more than 50% to 60% of persons with cancer will receive radiation therapy at some point in their course of treatment.[30-32] A total of 85% to 90% of this group receiving radiation will be treated as outpatients.[30-32] While nurses do not administer the radiation treatment, the nurse prepares the patient for treatment, manages side effects, and provides supportive care. The nurse assesses the patient before each treatment and develops a problem list and interventions to prevent or minimize complications of therapy. Grant et al[33] surveyed radiation oncology facilities to identify the most common responsibilities of the radiation oncology nurse. Highest-priority activities identified were patient education before treatment, explanation of radiation therapy, management of side effects, assistance with examinations, and assessment of the patient.

The acute and chronic side effects of radiation therapy are generally predictable. This predictability aids in the implementation of preventive care measures and makes teaching more manageable and organized. Side effects may be categorized for reference into the seven major systems shown in Table 50-1.[34] The nurse can anticipate potential problems and initiate measures to reduce or avoid these problems with nursing interventions and patient instructions delineated in Table 50-1. Nursing care of the radiation therapy patient is discussed in greater detail in Chapter 12. The expected outcome of treatment may be improved by intensive efforts to improve or maintain the patient's general condition at a high level.[35] Considerable time and effort are needed to care for patients treated with radiation therapy.

Radiation therapy facilities are usually designed to comfortably accommodate a large volume of outpatients and inpatients in wheelchairs and on stretchers. Inpatients may have an assortment of catheters, tubes, and pumps. The radiation therapy nurse needs to have the skills to identify a malfunction of the equipment and to intervene accordingly. The therapy staff should exercise appropriate safety precautions, such as the use of monitoring devices and film badges to measure occupational exposure.[36] Equipment is monitored and maintained according to the Radiation Therapy Safety Guidelines for the safety of the staff and the patient. Quality assurance is carefully monitored, and the criteria for equipment purchase, replacement, and maintenance are critical in all departments.

Radiation therapy can be administered on an outpatient basis to provide curative, adjuvant, and palliative treatment. It is an area of cancer care that requires extensive nursing interventions with the patient and the family.

Surgery

Lengths of hospitalization for surgery can be reduced with a subsequent reduction in cost to patients. Outpatient surgical procedures are being done safely in ambulatory settings with increasing frequency. It is predicted that 50%

TABLE 50-1 Major Acute and Chronic Side Effects of Radiation Therapy and Related Nursing Interventions

Site	Acute Effect	Chronic Effect	Nursing Intervention	Patient Instructions
Skin	Erythema (3000-4000 cGy), dry desquamation, moist desquamation (4500-6000 cGy) Epilation of brows and lashes (2000 cGy), first-degree erythema	Fibrosis, atrophy, telangiectasis, permanent darkening of skin	Avoid: trauma to skin, extremes of temperature, harsh chemicals, soaps	*During treatment:* Use tepid water for bathing, pat dry with soft towel, electric razors only, use cotton or silk garments next to skin, open-neck shirts with scarves, caution around nose with glasses, avoid drugs that increase sensitivity to radiation (check with doctor), avoid use of tape on treated area *After treatment care:* Gentle washing with warm water and mild soap, lanolin or moisturizing creams may be applied to areas where dry/dead skin is present Use sunscreen when outdoors or cover skin
Mucosa				
Oral cavity	Change or loss of taste, dryness, mucosity (3000-4000 cGy) Mucositis (3000-4000 cGy)	Permanent xerostomia (dependent on dose and patient age), permanent taste alterations, dental caries (if proper dental care is not initiated)	Monitor weight, use artificial saliva, viscous Xylocaine, preventive dental care with fluoride, nutritional counseling to maintain dietary status, gargling with salt/soda, instruct patient on high protein diet	Dental visit to detect and repair infected teeth, brush teeth before and after meals with soft toothbrush, use mouthwashes, high-protein diet
Esophagus	Pain, esophagitis, dysphagia	Fibrosis	Antacids, viscous Xylocaine, nutrition counseling	Soft easily swallowed diet, avoid ice or hot fluids; take analgesic solution before meals
Stomach	Nausea and vomiting (1000-3000 cGy)	Obstruction, ulceration, fibrosis	Antiemetics 1 hour prior to treatment and as needed	Nourishing diet of carbohydrates, protein, fats, high fluids
Intestines	Diarrhea (2000-5000 cGy), severe colic	Malabsorption, strictures, necrosis (6000-7000 cGy), avitaminosis, obstruction	Medication for diarrhea, dietary modifications, low-residue diet, teach good skin care and perineal hygiene	Avoid all high-roughage foods; take antidiarrheal and antispasmodic medications before therapy and as needed, increase fluid intake
Rectum	Tenesmus	Proctitis, fistula	Sitz baths PRN	Avoid all high-roughage foods
Chest	Cough, dyspnea (1500-3000 cGy)	Radiation pneumonitis, fibrosis	Pulmonary hygiene measures	Discontinue smoking, avoid areas of secondary smoke, increase room humidification to about 40%
Pelvis	Diarrhea, cystitis (5000 cGy), proctitis, rectal frequency		Dietary changes, monitor intake and output	Sitz baths, antidiarrheal and antispasmodics PRN

TABLE 50-1 Major Acute and Chronic Side Effects of Radiation Therapy and Related Nursing Interventions (continued)

Site	Acute Effect	Chronic Effect	Nursing Intervention	Patient Instructions
Intrathoracic cavity				
Respiratory system	Cough, pneumonitis (1500-3000 cGy)	Fibrosis, cough, breathlessness, pulmonary fibrosis	Pulmonary hygiene measures to alleviate cough and dyspnea, avoid smoke, increase humidity	Discontinue smoking; avoid secondary smoke; increase humidity Avoid places of high-risk infection (crowds, theaters); cough suppressant may be used
Cardiovascular system	Pericarditis, myocarditis, (doses greater than 4000 cGy)	Fibrosis, increased risk of coronary vessel disease	Recognize symptoms of deteriorating cardiac status	Follow up with regular evaluations by internist
Reproductive system				
Testes	Low sperm count after 90-120 days, temporary sterility (100-300 cGy)	Sterility (>1000 cGy)	Counsel patient re: effect of radiation on fertility, birth control measures	Sperm banking facilities available, birth control methods
Ovaries	Sterility (500-1000 cGy) depends on age	Menopause	Counsel patient re: effect of radiation on fertility, birth control measures	
Vagina	Vaginitis, discharge (doses greater than 5000 cGy)	Fibrosis, vaginal dryness	Peri-care. Counsel patient re: sexual activity, hygiene	Douching helps control risk of infection, topical estrogen, vaginal dilators
Renal system				
Kidney	Radiation nephritis (doses greater than 2000 cGy)	Radiation nephritis	Monitor blood pressure, look for signs of renal failure	Hypertensive medication, recognize signs of nephritis
Bladder	Cystitis (>3000 cGy), dysuria, frequency	Fibrosis, contracted bladder (6500-7000 cGy)	Increase fluid intake, may use prophylactic urinary antibiotics, diagnose and treat UTI	Fluids should be forced, antispasmodics as prescribed
Bone				
Bone	Pain, hypercalcemia	Growth disturbances if growth plate of bone is in field (2000-3000 cGy), spontaneous fracture	Increase fluid intake, adequate pain relief regimens, counseling re: growth disturbances if child	Analgesics to relieve pain, avoid weight bearing on long bones, support arm in sling
Bone marrow	Neutropenia, thrombocytopenia, anemia, granulocytopenia	Chronic anemia especially with combined modality treatment	Initiate bleeding precautions, measures to prevent infection as indicated, transfuse as needed, promote rest, nutritional counseling	Precautions regarding infection and bleeding, rest frequently

TABLE 50-1 Major Acute and Chronic Side Effects of Radiation Therapy and Related Nursing Interventions (continued)

Site	Acute Effect	Chronic Effect	Nursing Intervention	Patient Instructions
Central nervous system				
Brain and spinal cord	Edema and inflammation, increased intracranial pressure (1000-3000 cGy)	Infarction, occlusion, necrosis, gliosis, myelitis, endarteritis (doses greater than 5000 cGy)	Monitor sequelae of steroids, assess neurologic status, monitor for headaches, signs of increased intracranial pressure, edema	Keep head well powdered, report neurologic changes
Peripheral nerves	Paresthesia, hyperesthesia, changes in temperature discrimination Pain: Cervical: arm, hand, fingers Dorsal: girdle pain Lumbar: legs, back of thighs, front of legs	Paralysis, dysfunction (5000-6000 cGy)	Monitor neurologic status; maintain accurate documentation of response and changes	Adjust activities of daily living accordingly, analgesics for pain
Eye	Conjunctivitis, keratitis (2500-3000 cGy), inhibition of lacrimal gland secretion, iritis (3000 cGy)	Glaucoma, shrinkage of globe, corneal scarring, cataracts, epiphora	Avoid eye trauma or stress, emphasize need for eye protection and care	Avoid overwiping or rubbing eyes, dab eye with soft tissue and discard, avoid using handkerchief, irrigation of eye may soothe discomfort, sun glasses may serve as protection

Adapted from Strohl RA: The nursing role in radiation oncology: Symptom management of acute and chronic reactions. Oncol Nurs Forum 15:429-434, 1988.

of all surgery will be performed on an outpatient basis by 1990.[37]

In cancer treatment, biopsies, removal of superficial lesions, and placement of venous access devices will be done in the ambulatory setting. Procedures that require general anesthesia are usually limited to the operating room. However, short procedures that require less lengthy anesthesia time can be performed effectively on an outpatient basis. Typically the person is assessed as an outpatient and arrives at the ambulatory surgery facility just before the scheduled procedure. Once the procedure is completed and the patient has recovered satisfactorily, the patient is discharged to his or her home. Significant savings are realized in terms of room fees, lost work days, and numerous indirect costs.

A comparison of average charges for inpatients versus outpatients treated with the same surgery revealed that the outpatients' charges were considerably lower than inpatients' charges.[37] The difference is attributed in large part to the decreased use of hospital resources in the care of an outpatient. The family and the patient assume a greater role in medication and care, thus decreasing the use of hospital resources.

Patient counseling and support

Patient counseling and support services are important components of ambulatory cancer care, since the quality and availability of social support is believed to play a role in the patient's adaptation to illness. The fear and uncertainty experienced by cancer patients and their families pose many challenges for the health care team.[38] Some ambulatory cancer centers have a specialty staff that includes a psychosocial support team for the patients and their families. It may be necessary to contract or arrange for special services, such as those provided by relaxation experts or recreational staff.

A multiprofessional approach to patient support can be most effective. For example, the nurse provides information about therapy and management of side effects and determines the appropriate referrals needed, while the social worker assists in the coördination of resources and referrals to home care and community agencies. The nurse and the social worker also assess the needs for long- and short-term psychotherapeutic intervention. The nutritionist addresses significant changes in eating habits, while a psychologist evaluates the patient for behavior modification techniques, such as relaxation.

Ambulatory cancer care is not complete without access to support groups or programs for patients and families, relaxation sessions, peer support, and volunteer involvement. If this is not provided by the ambulatory center, many communities have organized support groups that are available.

Nutritional support

Ambulatory patients with cancer usually need nutritional intervention in a number of areas, such as decreased food intake, desire for weight gain, food-preparation problems, and questions about diet and cancer. Ambulatory patients are often receiving complex chemotherapy regimens, radiation therapy, or treatment for pain that may result in a compromised physical condition. For example, patients receiving some types of chemotherapy experience problems with reduced food intake attributable to anorexia, nausea and vomiting, and other side effects of the drugs.[39] If the problem goes untreated, the nutritional deficit could result in a loss of physical function and the patient may not be able to remain an outpatient for the rest of the treatment program.[39]

A specific problem for outpatients may be eating away from home or in restaurants. Nutrition counseling includes recognition of food groups and substitutions. The patient is encouraged to ask for special food preparation, a request with which most restaurants willingly comply.

Diet and its relationship to cancer is a controversy that nutritionists address frequently. Care should be taken to avoid making dietary recommendations for reducing cancer risk that are not based on prudent health habits.[40] At this time, most of the correlations between diet and cancer have not been scientifically validated and thus may be controversial.

COMMON PATIENT CARE PROBLEMS MANAGED IN AMBULATORY SETTINGS

Since outpatient cancer care includes aggressive therapy and palliative management, the range of patient care problems managed by the nurses is wide. Treatment toxicities, tumor effects, advanced disease, and anticipatory management are a few of the issues that require creative and effective nursing care. The common problems selected for discussion in this chapter are pain, progressive disease management, neutropenia, and equipment malfunction.

Pain

Pain management is a critical component of ambulatory cancer care since 30% to 40% of patients with intermediate-stage cancer and 55% to 90% of patients whose cancer is in an advanced stage experience moderate to severe pain.[41] The clinical assessment and management of pain in cancer patients often require the collective skills of a multidisciplinary group, which may include a nurse, a pharmacist, a social worker, an anesthesiologist, a psychologist, and a neurosurgeon. Some ambulatory cancer care facilities have a formal pain-management team. Ambulatory care programs that do not have the benefit of a formal pain team can also provide excellent pain management through interdisciplinary collaborative efforts.

The objective of pain management is to evaluate the patient's symptoms, reach a well-defined explanation for the pain complaint, and ultimately to provide the appropriate interventions based on etiologic factors. Sources of cancer pain are associated with direct tumor involvement, as in metastasis to vertebral bodies, tumor infiltration of the nerve or spinal cord, postmastectomy or phantom limb pain, and postradiation pain, as in radiation myelopathy.[42,43] Pain coupled with other variables (eg, age, sex, culture, environment, and psychologic as well as physiologic status) can produce a complex and demanding clinical situation.

Nurses are at the core of pain management, since they usually have more interaction with the patient. The nurse's responsibilities in outpatient pain management include coordinating the pain-control approach, facilitating the exchange of information among disciplines, implementing pain-reducing behaviors,[44] evaluating and modifying the approach, and providing the patients with the continuity of care from the beginning of the problem throughout its course.

The multidisciplinary approach to pain management offers the patient the benefit of the talents and skills of various experts. Psychosocial professionals evaluate the impact that pain has on all areas of the patient's life and provide nonpharmacologic interventions, such as cognitive-behavioral techniques, hypnosis, relaxation, and biofeedback training. These nonmedical treatment strategies have been shown to reduce pain and to increase the patient's level of comfort.[45] Social service workers intervene to tap economic and social sources that could benefit the patient and subsequently alter the treatment plan. Pharmacists profile the patient's problems and current medications, suggest appropriate medications, and monitor the drugs with respect to possible side effects and related adverse reactions. The benefits of a team approach to the patient's pain problem are numerous.

Communication of the pain-management plan, a stumbling block in many settings, can be facilitated by the use of standardized pain-assessment and pain-management forms.[46] For example, a preassessment form (Figure 50-1[47]) can be initiated by a nurse. A McGill pain questionnaire could be incorporated as part of the initial patient assessment to determine a description of the pain and its location. The preassessment form can become a permanent part of the medical record.

Another communication tool may be used to document the outcome of an interdisciplinary pain-control plan (Figure 50-2). This form calls for impressions of the problem, a plan of care, a psychologic note, and a postevaluation follow-up. A section of the form has been designed to

PAIN PREASSESSMENT

PREASSESSMENT DATE: ______________________ Signature of Assessor ______________________

1. Where is your pain? (mark "X" on diagram)
2. When did it start? ______________________
3. Is it getting:
   ____ better ____ same
   ____ worse ____ changes
4. What makes pain better? (check all that apply)
   ____ heat/warmth ____ rest
   ____ cold ____ position change
   ____ medication ____ other
   ____ massage
5. What makes pain worse?
   ____ position ____ cold
   ____ stress ____ fatigue
   ____ exertion ____ other
6. Current pain meds:

Name *Dose*	*Effectiveness*	
	none *somewhat*	*very*

7. Past pain meds and procedures:

Name *Dose*	*Effectiveness*	
	none *somewhat*	*very*

8. How does the pain limit your normal daily routine and activities? What can't you do that you could do before?
   ____ eat ____ sex
   ____ sleep ____ bend or change position
   ____ walk ____ other
   ____ be with friends
9. READ: "We have a team of pain specialists. Do you feel that a specialized consultation regarding your situation would be of interest to you?"
   ____ yes ____ not at this time
10. Have you ever received any formal relaxation training?
   ____ yes ____ no

   If so, do you practice it now?
   ____ yes ____ no
11. Are you on any regular exercise program?
   ____ yes ____ no
12. Comments: ______________________

FIGURE 50-1 Pain preassessment sample form for ambulatory patients referred for pain evaluation. (Adapted from McMillan SC, Williams FA, Chatfield R, et al: A validity and reliability study of two tools for assessing and managing cancer pain. Oncol Nurs Forum 15:735-740, 1988.)

include modification of the treatment plan. Additional notes are part of the progress notes in the chart.

The management of cancer pain offered by a multidisciplinary group approach could include cognitive strategies such as imagery and attention-diversion techniques,[48] behavioral manipulations such as hypnosis and biofeedback, and physical interventions such as surgery or drug therapy. Physical interventions include: traditional analgesic regimens, adjuvant analgesics (ie, anticonvulsant agents, antidepressants, and nerve blocks), and continuous-infusion methods.[46,49] Technologic advances in venous access ports and ambulatory pumps have enhanced the use of effective pharmacologic agents in the control of pain in outpatients.

Signs/Symptoms of Progressive Disease

Ambulatory cancer patients are evaluated, treated, and followed up in an outpatient setting. The nurse is responsible for assessment of the patient on each visit to the

PAIN TEAM INTERDISCIPLINARY NOTE

Date: ______________________

I. PRESUMPTIVE DIAGNOSIS AND PLAN BASED UPON PREASSESSMENT DATA:

____

____

____

Signatures: ______________________

Date: ______________________

II. EVALUATION

A. Pain Management Physician Impressions:

____

____

Plan (include follow-up dates, labs, meds, consults):

____

____

____

Signature: ______________________

Date: ______________________

B. Pain Management Psychologist Impressions:

____

____

Plan (include follow-up dates, tests):

____

____

____

Signature: ______________________

Date: ______________________

III. POST EVALUATION TEAM CONFERENCE AND FOLLOW-UPS (include any modification to treatment plan):

____

____

____

____

____

Signatures: ______________________

IV. DATES OF FOLLOW-UP TEAM CONFERENCES*:

____

____

____

*Refer to Progress Notes on date(s) listed.

FIGURE 50-2 Documentation form from pain planning conference team.

I. PATIENT STATUS: (Describe how patient arrived—in ambulance, per wheelchair, ambulatory; accompanied by whom, appearance, no acute distress)

II. INFORMANT:

III. CHIEF COMPLAINTS: (Duration, intensity, and precipitating factors)

IV. HISTORY OF PRESENT ILLNESS (short):

V. MEDICATIONS:

VI. ALLERGIES:

VII. SIGNIFICANT MEDICAL HISTORY:

VIII. VITAL SIGNS:

IX. NURSING ASSESSMENT: (Review of Systems [HEENT, Cardio/Resp., GI, GU, etc.])

X. NURSING DIAGNOSIS:

XI. INTERVENTION IN RELATION TO NURSING DIAGNOSIS

XII. PLAN

FIGURE 50-3 Assessment criteria for a new outpatient.

setting. The nurse is in a position to observe both the subtle and the obvious changes in the patient's status that may be indicative of progressive disease.

A baseline assessment is made on the first visit, or shortly thereafter, to enable the nurse to formulate a plan of care for the patient. The major areas for assessment include history of the present problem, family history, review of medications, nutritional screening, psychosocial screening, pain assessment, and review of systems (Figure 50-3). A nutrition-status screening tool (Figure 50-4) is a preliminary screen to identify high-risk patients who need nutrition counseling. These tools provide the essential elements for a database.

The intermittent and episodic nature of ambulatory cancer care challenges the nurse to perform discriminating patient assessments. A standard assessment tool can help the nurse identify early signs of complication or the spread of disease. The organs most frequently affected by metastatic cancer are the brain, lung, bone, and liver. The use of a standard assessment tool to monitor the patient is a time-saving method to assist the nurse and provide a consistent method for comparing patient progress from visit to visit.

Febrile Episodes from Neutropenia

Patients with cancer are susceptible to infection for a variety of reasons, that is, underlying disease process, poor nutritional status, or impaired immunologic system.[50] Some chemotherapeutic agents cause myelosuppression and consequently predispose the patient to infection.[51] Radiation to vulnerable areas and at certain dosages can also induce myelosuppression. Outpatients need to learn to recognize the signs and symptoms of infection, to take their temperature, and to avoid unnecessary risks of exposure to infections. During patient-teaching sessions and at each visit, the nurse emphasizes the importance of immediately reporting temperature elevations. Time is a critical factor in effective management of infections. Expediency is required in determining the source of an infection.

In an ambulatory care setting, standardized treatment protocols provide one way to expedite the patient's care. Standardized protocols, if permitted by the particular state's Nurse Practice Act,[52] delineate specific measures that nurses can independently exercise in patient assessment and initiation of treatment. Figure 50-5 serves as an example of a nursing protocol for neutropenic patients.[51]

Antibiotic treatment can be initiated in an ambulatory setting and administered at home with the use of a central venous catheter and an infusion pump.[53,54] The loading dose of the antibiotic is usually administered in the ambulatory setting, where the nursing staff can evaluate reactions. The patient is taught to administer the other doses at home. Patients are visited on a daily basis for follow-up assessment and for preparation of the medication for the

1. Height: _____ cm
2. Weight: _____ kg

	Y	N
3. Is the patient <18 or >70 years of age?	___	___
4. Is the patient currently experiencing changes in appetite?	___	___
5. Is the patient currently following any restrictive diet plan?	___	___
6. Is the patient diabetic?	___	___
7. Has the patient had a weight loss >10 lbs during the past month?	___	___
8. Has the patient had a weight loss >20 lbs during the past 4 months?	___	___
9. Is the patient going to receive more than two courses of:		
High-dose cisplatin?	___	___
High-dose methotrexate?	___	___
10. Is the patient going to receive more than 2000 rad (cGy) to one of the following areas:		
Head and neck?	___	___
Abdomen?	___	___
Pelvis?	___	___
11. Would the patient like to have a nutritional consult with the dietician?	___	___

FIGURE 50-4 A nutrition screening tool for initial assessment for patients in ambulatory cancer facility.

1.00 Standard of Care:
The professional nurse shall assume accountability and responsibility in the assessment and treatment of the febrile neutropenic patient.

2.00 Objective:
Patients with a temperature of 100 degrees or greater warrant immediate assessment and intervention.

3.00 Policy:
- 3.01 Responsible personnel: Registered Nurse and Physician.
- 3.02 Circumstances under which the standardized procedure for febrile neutropenic patients may be implemented:
  - a. Patient presents with a temperature of 100 degrees or greater and other stable vital signs, and
  - b. Patient is at nadir post chemotherapy.
- 3.03 The registered nurse may take the following standardized procedure actions after trying to contact the attending physician to obtain orders. If no immediate response, proceed as follows:
  - a. Collect data base:
    1. Take vital signs every 2 hours and p.r.n.
  - b. Examine thorax, lungs, buccal mucosa, abdomen, CVC exit site; c/o dysuria, perianal discomfort.
  - c. Laboratory:
    1. Draw and send a stat CBC and differential.
    2. If absolute neutrophile count is less than 1000, proceed to
    3. Send culture specimens to lab
       - a. Blood
       - b. Throat and urine
       - c. Other sites as indicated
         1. Sputum
         2. Central venous catheter exit site
         3. Draining wounds
- 3.04 Intravenous fluids:
  - a. Begin 1000 cc D5w at a KVO rate.
- 3.05 Contact physician with lab results and await further orders.

FIGURE 50-5 A standardized procedure for the febrile neutropenic patient.

next 24-hour doses. Patients and families will need time and support to learn to care for the equipment and medications. Home care nurses will provide professional assistance and reinforcement of techniques.

Equipment Malfunction

Cancer treatments involving chemotherapy, antibiotics, and nutritional components can be delivered by means of central venous access devices and pumps for ambulatory patients. Technologic advances in medical equipment have helped clinicians treat ambulatory patients with a variety of drug protocols. However, occasional problems arise with the use of this equipment.

Central venous access devices

Central venous access devices (VADs) have made life more comfortable for the patient during cancer treatment. A central venous access device allows ambulatory patients to receive chemotherapy, analgesics, nutritional supplements, antibiotics, and hydration at home and in the outpatient setting.

The rationale for using VADs is divided into two categories: clinical and financial. On the clinical side, VADs allow the patient to be treated in the home with chemotherapy, antibiotics, and hydration. Continuous-infusion pumps have added greatly to the ease with which this can be accomplished. Also, VAD administration decreases the risk of chemical phlebitis experienced with vesicant administration.[55] The patient's anxiety level is substantially decreased when the need to experience frequent venipuncture is removed. Cost savings are realized with the use of VADs since the patient can receive most intravenous therapy on an outpatient basis. Resource use is decreased and nursing time need not be spent in seeking new venipuncture sites each time the patient has to be treated.

There are primarily three types of venous access device: the silicone silastic atrial catheter, the small-gauge central venous catheter, and the subcutaneously implanted port.[55] The competitive medical equipment market offers an assortment of venous access devices; thus clinicians are able to choose the most appropriate model for a given patient.

Atrial catheters are used for chemotherapy, antibiotics, blood component therapy, and blood drawing. A major advantage of this catheter is the availability of a double lumen and the fact that the catheter can be inserted on an outpatient basis.

Peripheral central venous catheters or small-gauge silicone catheters have the same indications for use as the atrial catheters. They can be inserted at the bedside with the use of only a local anesthetic. A nurse who has received specialized training in the insertion of these catheters and has expanded professional privileges can place and maintain the VAD. Improved catheters can now remain in place for more than 6 months without complications.

Infusion ports have a wide range of uses. Bolus injections, vesicant infusions, blood products, and antibiotics can be administered through an implanted port. The port can also be used for drawing blood specimens. Nursing skill and practice are required to access the ports. Several variables, such as the size and anatomy of the patient, determine the ease with which blood can be drawn. A sterile technique is required to introduce the Huber needle into the self-sealing, multipuncturable port.

Infection and occlusion are two potential complications that have occurred with every type of venous access device.[50] Infection is of primary concern, since it can result in systemic complications.[50] Both the catheter-insertion site and the lumen itself serve as potential ports of entry for pathogens. Procedures that safeguard against infection need to be developed, particularly for cannulation or accessing of the device and for care of the catheter-insertion site. Simple procedures will be more consistently applied and adhered to by staff, patient, and home care providers.

It is important that the procedures taught to the patient and home care givers be the same as those used by staff members in the ambulatory care setting. Patient education for care of the venous access device includes procedures to prevent infection, methods to monitor for signs and symptoms of infection, and actions to take if complications develop. The patient and the family are taught to care for the catheter or port and to change the dressings. The most important principles are good handwashing and aseptic technique.

Catheter or port clotting and occlusion problems are managed in the outpatient setting. Nurses can implement standardized procedures for declotting or replacing the catheter by using a technique labeled "over the wire exchange."[52,56] This procedure should not be attempted unless the nurse has demonstrated proficiency in the procedure.

Ambulatory infusion pumps

Ambulatory pumps are commonly used to deliver chemotherapy in an outpatient setting. A variety of pumps, each with distinctive engineering features, are available. Pumps deliver chemotherapy by continuous or intermittent infusion. While in the continuous mode, most pumps have the capability for delivering bolus doses.

The pumps have locking mechanisms to prevent tampering or accidental alteration of the programmed dose to be delivered. Another type of locking device secures the cassette containing the medication, thus preventing removal of the drug from the cassette. The pump that best suits the patient's therapy requirements and level of self-care skill can be selected.

The most frequent source of equipment malfunction is an occlusion of the infusion tubing, which results in restriction of flow. This usually occurs because the clamps on the infusion line have inadvertently closed or the tubing is kinked or knotted. The presence of air in the tubing triggers an alarm, but this seldom occurs since the air should be completely removed during setup preparation. These and other problems can be easily resolved, usually during a telephone consultation between the nurse and the patient. Pumps are designed to shut off in the event of a malfunction in order to protect the patient from receiving an inappropriate dose of drug. Likewise, pumps automatically shut off when the infusion is completed. These safety features allow patients to receive chemotherapy infusions at home in a safe and cost-effective manner.

High-technology equipment affords the patient and the clinician a vast selection from which to choose. Treatments and problems can be managed in the outpatient setting without requiring hospitalization.

NURSING STAFF

Role of Nurses in Ambulatory Cancer Care

Nurses in an ambulatory cancer care setting deliver care and execute the plan designed by the health team. Nurses assess and evaluate the patient's status and progress from the initial visit through the end of the patient's experience. Clinical skills are important and should be accurate and up to date. Nurses provide services ranging from diagnosis and treatment of patients to management of the actual or potential health problems that can be encountered in an outpatient setting.[20] In addition to specialized cancer care activities, routine activities of the nurse include assessing patients, assisting physicians with procedures, documenting information, and specimen collection.[20]

The outpatient nurse communicates pertinent information to the patient and the family. Patients recall health care communications as a very important aspect of their cancer experience.[38] The patient and the family are expected to carry on a major part of the treatment; therefore the nurse must provide concise, clear, and timely instructions. The objective of patient education is to prepare the patient and his or her family to understand the course of the disease, its management, and the control of side effects in order to comply with specific instructions.[57] There are many tools and strategies for accomplishment of this goal.[58-61] An important principle to keep in mind is that the patient and the family must be ready to learn complex procedures. It is the nurse's responsibility to ascertain the competency and readiness of the patient and the family and to teach accordingly.

An integral component of the nurse's role in ambulatory care is provision of social support for the patient. Simply defined, social support is the provision of information and facts that lead individuals to believe that they are valued as members of a network of communication and that they have mutual responsibility.[62] The nurse provides support by demonstrating caring, empathy, and trust in patients' abilities to take care of themselves. Ambulatory care nurses also provide informational support by teaching patients what they will need to know for taking care of their health problems.

Follow-up assessment and follow-up evaluation are other aspects of care provided by the ambulatory care nurse. When patients return for follow-up visits, it is often the nurse who will conduct the assessment. Although assessments differ from one institution to another, the purpose of follow-up assessments is to determine whether there is any change in the patient's status. Information from this assessment is then communicated and channeled to the appropriate members of the multidisciplinary team. Written documentation and telephone communication are the most common methods used to relay pertinent information. To facilitate documentation, a telephone consultation form may be useful. These forms can be adhesive backed and become a permanent part of the medical record. Figure 50-6 illustrates an example of a communications tool that can be used by all members of the team.

Staff Education and Support

Nurses in an ambulatory cancer care program should have previous experience working with individuals with chronic illness. Ideally, previous work experience would be with cancer patients. The orientation and education of new staff should be based on competence in order to achieve measurable objectives and assure the quality of patient services.[63,64] Each employee should understand the philosophy of care and be apprised of the job expectations. A preceptor or instructor is an essential resource for new staff members.

Continuing education and professional development are priorities for individuals who care for cancer patients. Because the technology involved in cancer care is changing rapidly, conferences and professional communications are of the utmost importance. Staff members should be encouraged to read current literature and share information with each other.

Staff nurses caring for patients with cancer may experience more stress than staff members who care for other groups of patients.[65] Furthermore, oncology nurses report significantly more relational difficulties with cancer patients than other nurses.[65] Several stressors may account for this, among them the fact that many patients have terminal disease. Other factors to consider may be the shortage of nursing personnel and conditions of the work environment. The use of stress-management strategies will help to decrease potential conflict. It is hoped that support groups, improved working conditions, clarification of goals and roles, and improved communication with administrators will reinforce a caring attitude and relieve stress among the staff. Working in an ambulatory cancer care environment offers a multitude of opportunities for staff members to use skills in assessment, planning, intervention, and evaluation. For this reason, the continuous development of a qualified staff is the highest priority for the overall quality of ambulatory cancer care.

TELEPHONE CONSULT　Call Date: ______ Call Time: ______

Patient's Name: ______ Phone # ______ Med. Rec. # ______

Informant: ______ Physician: ______ Contacted: Yes ______ No ______

Problem: ______

Intervention: ______

Signature: ______ Date: ______ Time: ______

FIGURE 50-6 Telephone consult form for documentation of communication from ambulatory patients.

CONCLUSION

Ambulatory care is a safe and often preferred method of treating a patient for cancer. Many of the same procedures that are typically done on an inpatient basis can be achieved outside the hospital environment. Chemotherapy, blood component therapy, antibiotic administration, diagnostic studies, and special surgical procedures may be provided in an ambulatory care setting.

The safety of the procedures is dependent in part on appropriate selection of patients and professional competence in caring for the cancer patient in the ambulatory setting. With the support of modern technology, clinicians are able to maintain patients on treatment regimens that were formerly reserved for inpatient use. In the ambulatory setting nurses have a multidimensional role that involves assessing patients and teaching them to assume self-sustaining health care behaviors and duties.

There are many benefits of ambulatory care. The most important for the patient is the ability to be at home, close to family and friends. Another advantage is the financial benefit to both patients and insurers, who realize a significant cost savings. There are many indirect social and personal savings that should be considered.

The future holds many challenges, such as the need to classify acuity of illness for outpatients, consistent charging mechanisms and reimbursement policies, and the need for improved technology and equipment for the care of the cancer patient in an ambulatory setting. The field of ambulatory oncology practice will continue to develop and prosper as improvements in technology and quality come about.

• • •

The author gratefully acknowledges the support of Salick Health Care, Inc, Beverly Hills, CA, during the writing of this chapter.

REFERENCES

1. Title 42, Code of Federal Regulations, 405.1032 Washington, DC, 1983, pp 303-311.
2. Howard DM: Past experiences and future directions in ambulatory care, in Howard DM (ed): New Business Development in Ambulatory Care. Chicago, American Hospital Publishing Inc, 1988, pp 15-24.
3. Nathanson SN, Lerman D: Directions in cancer care, in Nathanson SN, Lerman D (eds): Outpatient Cancer Centers. Chicago, American Hospital Publishing Inc, 1988, pp 1-13.
4. Sand R: The Advances to Social Medicine, London, Staples Press, 1952.
5. Roemer M: Origins of organized ambulatory health care, in Ambulatory Health Care Services in America. Rockville, Md, Aspen, 1981, pp 15-27.
6. Esparza DM, Young N, Luongo JA: Effective planning for office and outpatient chemotherapy administration. Semin Oncol Nurs 5:8-14, 1989 (suppl).
7. Levin L: Patient education and self-care: How do they differ? Nurs Outlook 26:170, 1978.
8. Miller SA: Considerations in the outpatient and office administration of cisplatin. Semin Oncol Nurs 3:3-7, 1987 (suppl).
9. Robin DL, Spector KK, Bush PJ: Ambulatory care in the community. Public Health Rep 95:511-519, 1980.
10. National health expenditures. Health Care Financing Rev 8:1-36, 1987.
11. Wodinsky HB, DeAngelis C, Rusthoven JJ, et al: Reevaluating the cost of outpatient cancer chemotherapy. Can Med Assoc J 137:903-906, 1987.
12. Plasse T, Ohnuma T, Bruckner H, et al: Portable infusion pumps in ambulatory cancer chemotherapy care. Cancer 50:27-31, 1982.
13. Mor V, Stalker MZ, Gralla R, et al: Day hospital as an alternative to inpatient care for cancer patients: A random assignment trial. J Clin Epidemiol 41:771-785, 1988.
14. Berk AA, Phil M, Chalmers TC: Cost and efficacy of the substitution of ambulatory for inpatient care. N Engl J Med 304:393-397, 1981.
15. Carbone PP: Organization of clinical oncology in the USA: Role of cancer centers, cooperative groups and community hospitals. Eur J Cancer Clin Oncol 21:149-154, 1985.
16. Katz G, Zavodnick L, Markezin E: Strategic planning in a restrictive and competitive environment. Health Care Manage Rev 8:7-12, 1983.
17. Outpatient cancer centers begin to get attention. Hospitals 59:54, 1985.
18. Mannisto M: For-profit systems pursue growth in specialization and diversification. Hospitals 55:71-76, 1981.
19. HCFA seeks comments on payment for chemotherapy in physician offices. Cancer Economics Nov 18:1-2, 1988.
20. Lattal LA: Operational issues, in Nathanson SN, Lerman D (eds): Outpatient Cancer Centers. Chicago, American Hospital Publishing Inc, 1988.
21. Brown JK: Ambulatory services: The mainstay of cancer nursing care. Oncol Nurs Forum 12:57-59, 1985.
22. MacDonald AS: Strategic planning, in Howard DM (ed): New Business Development in Ambulatory Care, Chicago, American Hospital Publishing Inc, 1988, pp 27-28.
23. Prager D: Chemotherapy in the physician's office. Socioeconomics 87:50-52, 1984.
24. Benahmed M, Carde P, Laplanche A, et al: Chemotherapy by ambulatory continuous infusion using a portable pump: A feasibility trial. Bull Cancer 72:30-36, 1985.
25. Sullivan RD, Otis PT: Ambulatory arterial infusion cancer chemotherapy for liver cancer: Salient technique modifications. Proc Am Soc Clin Oncol 3:142, 1984 (abstr).
26. Lokich JJ, Perri J, Bothe A, et al: Cancer chemotherapy via ambulatory infusion pump. Am J Clin Oncol 6:355-363, 1983.
27. Plasse T, Ohnuma T, Bruckner H, et al: Portable infusion pumps in ambulatory cancer chemotherapy. Cancer 50:27-31, 1982.
28. Greidanus J, de Vries EG, Nieweg MB, et al: Evaluation of a totally implanted venous access port and portable pump in a continuous chemotherapy infusion schedule on an outpatient basis. Eur J Cancer Clin Oncol 23:1653-1657, 1987.
29. Frank RM: Safety in handling chemotherapy. J NYSNA 18:23-31, 1987.
30. Rubin P: The emergence of radiation oncology as a distinct medical specialty. Int J Radiat Oncol Biol Phys 11:1247-1270, 1985.
31. Radiation oncology in integrated cancer management. Report of the Inter-Society Council for Radiation Oncology, November, 1986.

32. Mulkerin LE: Practical Points in Radiation Oncology. Garden City, NY, Medical Examination Publishing Company, 1979.
33. Grant M, Dodd M, Hilderly L, et al: Radiation oncology nurses' role: A national survey. Oncol Nurs Forum 2:107, 1984 (suppl) (abstr).
34. Strohl RA: The nursing role in radiation oncology: Symptom management of acute and chronic reactions. Oncol Nurs Forum 15:429-434, 1988.
35. Oberst MT, Thomas SE, Gass KA, et al: Caregiving demands and appraisal of stress among family caregivers. Cancer Nurs 12:209-215, 1989.
36. Hassey K: Principles of radiation safety and protection. Semin Oncol Nurs 3:23-29, 1987.
37. Keithley J, Glandon GI, Llewellyn J, et al. The cost effectiveness of same day admission surgery. Nursing Economics 7:90-93, 1989.
38. Thorne SE: Hopeful and unhelpful communication in cancer care: The patient perspective. Oncol Nurs Forum 15:167-172, 1988.
39. Hartlapp JH: Nutrition of the ambulatory tumor patient, especially under chemotherapy. Proceedings of the International Symposium for Physicians, Nurses and Social Workers on Supportive Care in Cancer Patients, pp 23, 1987 (abstr).
40. Byers T: Food, additives, and cancer. Food Cancer 84:275-281, 1988.
41. Bonica JJ: Treatment of cancer pain: Current status and future needs. Pain 2:196, 1984 (suppl) (abstr).
42. Coyle N, Foley K: Pain in patients with cancer: Profile of patients and common pain syndromes. Semin Oncol Nurs 1:93-99, 1985.
43. Foley KM: Control of pain in cancer, in Calabresi P, Schein PS, Rosenberg SA (eds): Medical Oncology: Basic Principles and Clinical Management of Cancer. New York, Macmillan Publishing Company, 1985, pp 1385-1405.
44. Wilkie D, Lovejoy N, Dodd M, et al: Cancer pain control behaviors: Description and correlation with pain intensity. Oncol Nurs Forum 15:723-741, 1988.
45. Subramanian K, Rose SD: Social work and the treatment of chronic pain. Health Soc Work 13:49-60, 1988.
46. Ferrell BR, Wenzl C, Wisdom C: Evolution and evaluation of a pain management team. Oncol Nurs Forum 15:285-289, 1988.
47. McMillan SC, Williams FA, Chatfield R, et al: A validity and reliability study of two tools for assessing and managing cancer pain. Oncol Nurs Forum 15:735-740, 1988.
48. Fernandez E: A classification system of cognitive coping strategies for pain. Pain 26:141-151, 1986.
49. Portenoy RK, Moulin DE, Rogers AG, et al: Intravenous infusions of opioids in cancer related pain: Review of cases and guidelines for use. Adv Pain Res Ther 8:413-424, 1986.
50. Petrosino B, Becker H, Christian B: Infection rates in central venous catheter dressings. Oncol Nurs Forum 15:709-717, 1988.
51. Brandt B: A nursing protocol for the client with neutropenia. Oncol Nurs Forum 11:24-28, 1984.
52. Anderson RD: Legal Boundaries of California Nursing Practice. Sacramento, Calif, Anderson Publishing Co, 1981.
53. Rosen G, Lamnin M, Young R: Efficacy and cost-effectiveness of outpatient treatment with ceftriaxone and gentamicin in febrile, neutropenic patients. Rev Infect Dis (in press).
54. Poretz DM, Wooland D, et al: Outpatient use of ceftriaxone: A cost-benefit analysis. Am J Med 77:77-83, 1984.
55. Goodman MS, Wickham R: Venous access devices: An overview. Oncol Nurs Forum 11:16-23, 1984.
56. Snyder RH, Archer FJ, Endy T, et al: Catheter infection: A comparison of two catheter maintenance techniques. Ann Surg 208:651-653, 1988.
57. Villejo LA, Gilloth BE, Zerbe DA: Patient education services, in Nathanson SN: Outpatient Cancer Centers, Implementation and Management. Chicago, American Hosp Publishing Inc, 1988, pp 151-167.
58. Hennessy J, et al: Home instructions for post-chemotherapy care. Oncol Nurs Forum 15: 201, 1988.
59. Howser DM, Meade CD: Hickman Broviac care: Developing organized teaching strategies. Cancer Nurs 10:70-76, 1987.
60. Nieweg R, Greidanus J, de Vries EGE: A patient education program for a continuous infusion regimen on an outpatient basis. Cancer Nurs 10:177-182, 1987.
61. Goodman M: External venous catheters: Home management. Oncol Nurs Forum 15:357-360, 1988.
62. Cobb S: Social support is a moderator of life stress. Psychosom Med 38:300-314, 1976.
63. Alspach JG: Designing a competency-based orientation for critical care nurses. Heart Lung 13:655-662, 1984.
64. Scott B: A competency-based learning model for critical care nursing. Int J Nurs Stud 21:9-17, 1984.
65. Delvaux N, Razavi D, Farvacques C: Cancer care: A stress for health professionals. Soc Sci Med 27:159-166, 1988.

Chapter 51

Home Care

Joy Stair, RN, MS

Joan McNally, RN, MSN

INTRODUCTION

A variety of services and supplies are offered to assist persons with a diagnosis of cancer and their families and to enable them to remain in their home. The availability of services varies within different communities and tends to be more accessible in urban areas. Selection of the type of service and type of agency depends on the needs of the patient and family and their financial base for health care.

The delivery of home care to individuals with cancer who have a multiplicity of needs challenges even the most creative and energetic practitioners. The home becomes a high-technology setting[1,2] to accommodate the dramatic changes in technically complex patient care. In the home setting, nurses function in an independent role. Often they are the only health care professionals with whom the homebound individual has contact on a consistent basis. The home care nurse provides direct nursing care, coordinates services, teaches and initiates patient self-care behaviors, and acts as advocate for the individual and family.

HOME CARE: AN OVERVIEW

The family is the core unit for care in the home. The family is the focus of home nursing care inasmuch as the family unit is expected to pull itself together, mobilize resources, and assume the responsibility for care in the home setting.[3] Throughout this chapter the words *family*, *caregivers*, and *caretakers* are used interchangeably, defining family in a broad sense to include those persons who provide care and support for the individual with a diagnosis of cancer.

The nurse is the initial manager of care in the home and is responsible for coordinating all patient care activities, including referrals to various health care disciplines. To be most effective, home care programs provide 24-hour availability of staff members to patients and families.

The nurse who cares for individuals with cancer and their families at home has the following general goals:

1. To assist the patient and family develop strategies to achieve optimal independence and attain client-identified goals
2. To assist the patient to attain optimal physical and psychosocial status in collaboration with other members of the health care team
3. To assist the patient and family to develop support systems to facilitate a therapeutic environment
4. To assist the individual and family in planning for the future by providing adequate information and support

Patient and Family Needs: A Literature Review

As a result of the extended survival period of patients with cancer and their use of multiple treatment facilities, demands on community health services have increased dramatically. Consequently, increased attention has been focused on identifying the at-home needs of individuals with cancer and their families. The demands on spouse/caregivers of terminally ill adult patients with cancer were explored by Stetz,[4] who identified nine categories related to the types of interventions provided by caregivers: managing the physical care and treatment regimens; managing the household and finances; coping with unmet expectations from the health care system; coping with alterations in the spouse/caregiver's well being and patterns of living (eg, lack of sleep); exercising constant vigilance; standing by (observing the effects of the illness); anticipating the future; dealing with cancer itself; and adjusting to alterations in relationship with the patient. Rose[5] interviewed relatives who had cared for family members at home sometime during the 8 weeks preceding the patient's death. Most families reported that the person's physical needs were met by immediate relatives or close friends. Identified concerns were special equipment, teaching in areas that required judgment such as pain control or special foods, transportation to or from the clinic or hospital, lack of sleep, child care, and finances.

Parsons[6] has pinpointed the home care needs of individuals with advanced cancer. Physical needs included help in clarifying diet and medication instructions, realistic goal setting for activity levels, and ostomy management. Methods for controlling pain and assistance in investigating community resources for home care also were listed as needs.

Googe and Varricchio[7] interviewed 15 individuals with cancer and their families to determine home care needs. Study data indicated that daily living needs are met by family members, with some assistance from home health agency personnel. Assistance with pain, sleep, and elimination often was needed. Transportation to the physician's office was an area of universal need but one that generally was not met. The most helpful functions of the home care nurse were identified: making a list of medicines, giving baths and backrubs, checking blood pressure, and lessening the number of visits to the physician. Most caregivers, however, saw the provision of emotional support as most helpful. Data also indicated that the home care nurse was able to provide more and better information than either the physician or hospital nurse.

In another study of needs in the preterminal period,[8] family groups mentioned a greater need for medical monitoring in the home than did patients, and half the family groups believed a nurse rather than a physician could meet this need. Assistance with obtaining equipment, transportation, and personal care was considered necessary by approximately half the respondents, as was help with household chores and meals. Comparison of responses of 22 patients with those of corresponding caregivers revealed a 28% to 68% disparity in the identified need for all services and in the physical symptoms perceived. More patients than family members reported the need for better management of dyspnea and dietary counseling. Needs perceived by families more than by the patients were for family relief care, recreation and emotional support for the family, and hospital beds.

To improve the ability of the family to care for the individual with cancer at home, the contributions of a home health nurse or aide are usually most significant in two areas. First, the specific services provided, such as monitoring the health status of both patient and caretaker, changing a catheter, bathing the patient, assisting with exercises, or performing homemaking tasks, directly contribute to the maintenance of the patient, caretaker, and household. Second, the home visits serve a more diffuse but often equally crucial purpose—that of providing the caretaker with reassurance and practical and emotional support.[9]

Welch[3] conducted an exploratory study to identify components of family coping during the cancer experience. Difficult factors in the home setting included (1) fear of leaving the patient alone, (2) being a long distance from the medical center, (3) having to prepare different meals, (4) lack of help with the patient's emotional needs, (5) lack of knowledge about how to care for the patient, (6) child care, (7) trying to work while caring for the patient, and (8) lack of help with the patient's physical care.

Welch also asked family members, "What would be the *most* helpful action nurses could do to help you cope with your relative's illness?" Overwhelmingly, the most helpful nursing measure identified was for the nurse to give excellent, personalized patient care. This need was supported by Skorupka and Bohnet's study,[10] in which they interviewed 20 primary caregivers in a home hospice setting to determine which nursing behaviors were perceived as most helpful. Four of the five most helpful behaviors identified by the entire sample referred to the patient rather than the family member. They included (1) providing the patient with the necessary emergency measures if the need arises, (2) assuring the patient that nursing services will be available 24 hours a day, 7 days a week, (3) allowing the patient to do as much for himself/herself as possible, and (4) teaching family members how to keep the patient physically comfortable. The fifth most helpful behavior identified by family members was to have their questions answered honestly, openly, and willingly.

Giacquinta[11] has proposed a model for working with families facing cancer, which systematically describes the needs and coping strategies of family members during the patient's illness and after death has occurred. During the stage of living with cancer, family members often face feelings of despair, isolation, vulnerability, and helplessness. Nursing interventions that foster cohesion of the family unit and that strengthen interaction, communication, cooperation, and social and emotional involvement will combat isolation and enable the family to increase its autonomy and decrease its instability. The direction of nursing intervention toward daily problem solving minimizes the helplessness that families feel.

Patient Selection

Home care is not for everyone; its feasibility is determined by assessing the needs of the individual with a diagnosis of cancer and the patient and family's ability to meet those needs. The individual's diagnosis alone may not reflect the degree of illness, the complexity of care, or the number of support personnel required to assist the person at home.[12] Although the physical facilities may be adequate and the family willing, the emotional adjustments and 24-hour commitment to provide care may be more than the individual and family bargained for. On the other hand, caring for a loved one at home can be a positive experience that enables families to function in their natural environment.

The majority of candidates for home care have advanced disease that is metastatic and incurable but not imminently terminal.[13] Palliation of symptoms and pain control are major care issues. A second group of individuals for whom home care is indicated are those whose treatments result in self-care difficulties (either temporary or long-term) such as colostomy, laryngectomy, or total parenteral nutrition. A third group for whom home care is appropriate consists of those who are experiencing the effects of treatment (eg, the person with altered skin integrity as a result of radiotherapy). A fourth category includes those individuals who are homebound and require chemotherapy or blood products. Home care agencies are expanding services to meet the demands of this growing population.

An important factor in eligibility for insurance coverage of home care is determining whether the care required can be classified as "skilled" and therefore reimbursable under the person's health insurance. Skilled nursing care has been interpreted as consisting not only of technical procedures required by the individual but also patient assessment and evaluation, management of a prescribed medical regimen, and patient teaching.

Until recently, unless a person was fairly independent

in meeting self-care needs, the critical factor in determining whether a person was cared for at home was the degree of family/caregiver support and willingness to take on the task.[14] This criterion, which has been documented in the care of elderly persons[15,16] also is valid in the care of individuals with cancer. However, today's reimbursement environment and spiraling health care costs have impacted greatly in this area. In the past, if a caregiver was reluctant or unwilling to take the patient home, there was a good chance that the patient's stay at home would be brief and that the family would find reasons to return the patient to a health care facility. Today, financial considerations often eliminate an outside facility as an option for many families.

Transition to home care can be eased by assessing the wishes and concerns of individual and family, as well as beginning discharge planning early to prepare the patient and caregiver to manage at home. This is particularly relevant in those cases in which families are willing but afraid. In fact, the concept of prehospital admission discharge planning is being implemented by combining preadmission testing programs with discharge planning programs to begin patient/family education before hospitalization.[17]

A second factor in determining the potential for success in home care concerns the availability and type of home health services to assist in the supervision and management of the patient. A family usually can manage well if it knows that a home care nurse will be providing direction and assistance.

The degree of informal support has an impact on the family's ability to manage home care.[15] Informal support refers to support systems outside the home such as friends, neighbors, and church groups. Assistance from others may range from check-in telephone calls or running errands to providing relief to the caregivers by staying with the ill person.

The amount of care or the complexity of required technical procedures does not seem to correlate with the degree of success in home care. It might appear that increased care needs and technical skills would have a negative impact on the ability to maintain a person at home, but this is not the case. It is not unusual to observe one family managing total parenteral nutrition, colostomy care, or parenteral analgesics without apparent difficulty whereas a second family opts to transfer an individual to a health care facility when an indwelling Foley catheter becomes necessary.

How well a patient and family manage home care relates to the length of time a person requires higher levels of care from the in-home caregivers. Families often are able to manage well for short periods of time (weeks to several months). It is not unusual, however, for caregivers to "burn out" if a person stabilizes at a level in which intense or complete care is necessary and caregivers cannot see an end in sight.[18]

Finally, in spite of the family's willingness and the presence of both formal and informal support systems, some patients and families are unable to manage home care. Sometimes the patient is frightened and desires to be in a setting in which health professionals are in charge of care. As home care becomes increasingly complex, family caregivers may not be comfortable with the required level of knowledge and skills. The amount of physical and emotional stamina needed to manage the care of an individual with cancer at home should not be minimized. What may have appeared reasonable at the time of hospital discharge may become temporarily or permanently impossible at home. It is the responsibility of the nurse to assist and support patients and families in these difficult decisions regarding other settings for care.

Discharge/Referral Planning

Referrals for home care may be made by physicians and nurses in in-patient settings and in office practices, clinic nurses, families, or friends. The majority of referrals, however, are initiated when the patient is being discharged from a hospital; therefore *discharge planning* is the commonly accepted term for planning patient referrals for home care.

Discharge planning has been defined as a process that consists of activities to determine a patient's need for follow-up care and the arrangement for such care.[19] It is generally an interdisciplinary process. Full patient/family involvement in developing a plan for posthospital care is critical to the successful implementation of a discharge plan.[20]

The Medicare diagnosis-related group (DRG)–based prospective payment system has had a great impact on discharge planning activities in hospitals. One study investigated the influence of DRGs on discharge planning and concluded that patients with certain medical diagnoses, including cancer, were most affected because their hospitalization tended to exceed the DRG-allowed period and patients were not able to manage independent care.[21]

Because shortened hospital stays are now common, individuals are being discharged with highly complex treatment plans that must be managed in the home environment. The home setting, which reflects the person's uniqueness, life-style, and family interactions, must incorporate an unfamiliar set of routines and conditions that may be distasteful or misunderstood and may seem more appropriate procedures for the hospital than for the home.

The Joint Commission on Accreditation of Healthcare Organizations includes standards for nursing care that mandate patient discharge planning, discharge teaching, and documentation, which are identified as key factors in the accreditation decision process.[22] In 1986 the Health Care Financing Administration (HCFA) announced the new conditions of participation for hospitals for the Medicare and Medicaid programs. These include standards that mandate that the hospital have an ongoing plan, consistent with available community and hospital resources, to provide or make available social, psychological, and educational services to meet the medically related needs of its patients. The hospital also must have an effective ongoing discharge planning program that facilitates the provision of follow-up care.[23]

Excellent discharge planning is based on good communication between the referring professionals (eg, nurses in clinics or inpatient facilities) and the home care nurse, with recognition of the expertise of each. There can be serious discontinuity between inpatient treatment and the levels of care and compliance that occur after the person returns home.[24] One study compared differences in how discharge planning nurses and home health nurses view their patients.[25] Findings generally demonstrate that discharge planners focus on the specific details of facilitating patients' discharge whereas home health nurses view the patient more holistically. Ongoing communication between these two groups could provide home care nurses with a more complete patient and family picture before the first home visit.

A predischarge hospital visit and an assessment of the home situation by the home care nurse may be helpful. Some insurance companies will reimburse the home care agency for one assessment visit to the home before the patient's discharge, and some home care agencies will absorb the cost of this service to promote continuity of care in cases with multiple, complex care requirements.

Frequent communication between the hospital or clinic nurse and the home care staff promote continuity of care. Written reports about the patient's status and verbal updates facilitate high-quality care, particularly when patients move between settings.

Patient problems that require follow-up care include an inadequate support system or an absence of one, inadequate financial resources, poor environmental conditions, inability to provide the treatment and medication regimen, inability to carry out activities of daily living, poor socialization, and potential or anticipated problems resulting from one of these factors.[26]

To design a discharge/referral plan that is realistic and appropriate, the following questions are addressed:

1. What is the physical/functional status of the individual?
2. What physical care tasks will be performed by the individual and/or caregiver?
3. What is the individual's mental/emotional status? Is the person able to understand instructions?
4. What is the type and extent of the person's support system?
5. What equipment and supplies are needed?
6. What are the individual's financial resources (eg, health insurance)?
7. What services will be required to assist the individual and family with home care?
8. What is the physical setup of the home?

These areas will be discussed further from the perspective of the home care nurse, but they are essential components of a discharge/referral planning assessment. The answers to these questions provide a framework to prepare the individual and family for discharge to the home or to identify those persons unsuitable for home care.

Discharge planning ideally begins as soon as the patient is admitted to the hospital.[27,28] This is particularly important in this day of short hospital stays and early discharges. Hospital nurses no longer have the luxury of determining "readiness" of the patient and family to learn; rather they now are challenged to determine how best to teach self-care behaviors in the quickest and most efficient way possible and to assist the patient and family to understand why this is necessary. The caregivers need to learn the basic skills required to manage on a 24-hour basis and to be given time to modify the home environment and gather equipment and resources.

It is important to be realistic about what can be accomplished in the home. It is unlikely the patient who has been unable to get into the shower in the hospital will be able to do so at home. Setting simple, realistic goals will foster the confidence and satisfaction of the patient and family.

A concept currently gaining much attention as a result of the complexity of needs and the variety of services available is that of case management. This is the process of identifying the patient's needs and assisting the patient to use a variety of services and service systems in a coordinated manner. This process may be accomplished by a variety of methods, from the hospital nurse actually making home visits to facilitate care to functioning as the overseer of all care needs. Thus the patient may be followed up for long periods of time (months to years) by the case manager nurse.[29]

Types of Home Care Agencies

Home care services today are provided by a variety of agencies. Choosing a home care agency frequently is confusing to patients, families, and even health care providers who are not in the home care field.

Selection of the most appropriate type of home care agency is based primarily on patient and family needs, the financial arrangement or the patient's health care insurance coverage, and availability of family and community support, as well as the type of home care services available in the patient's community.

The three primary classifications of agencies that provide home care services are the official agency of the public health departments, the Medicare-certified home health agencies, and the private duty agencies.

Official public health agencies

Official agencies are organized and administered within city, county, or multicounty health departments. Historically the major focus of official health agencies has been preventive health care and infectious disease control. As such, home nursing care consists of biweekly or monthly home visits for patient teaching and supervision rather than provision of direct physical care. State and local tax revenues fund the health department's traditional health promotion and disease prevention programs.

A number of official health departments have expanded the scope of their services and have developed

Medicare-certified home health agencies. These operate as separate entities within their organizations.

Medicare-certified home health agencies

Home health agencies are structured and operated within the specific guidelines defined by the Health Care Financing Administration in their conditions of participation so that they may be certified to participate in the federal health insurance program (Medicare). When certified, the home health agency is reimbursed for services to Medicare patients when that service is provided within these guidelines.

Medicare certification also authorizes the home health agency to provide and be reimbursed for services to Medicaid patients when those services are provided within the guidelines defined by each state for home care for the indigent. Generally Medicare certification of a home health agency also is required by private insurance companies before reimbursement for home care services can be considered by those companies.

It is essential that home care nurses be aware of the type of insurance coverage for each patient in their case load and the guidelines defined by each reimbursement source in order to obtain the necessary approvals for care, to complete the required forms, and to provide services within the guidelines for reimbursement of home care services.

In terms of ownership and management there are many types of Medicare-certified home health agencies. Three types, however, are common: voluntary agencies, private agencies, and hospital-based agencies.

Voluntary home health agencies are managed by a board of directors composed of members of the local community. They generally are nonprofit organizations that are certified for Medicare reimbursement, as well as other insurances. In addition, they receive private funds and those that are not generated by taxes for services provided to patients who do not have health insurance.

The best known and oldest group of voluntary home health service providers are the Visiting Nurse Associations (or Services), known as the *VNAs* (or the *VNS*). Nationally they still comprise the majority of the voluntary organizations. Voluntary agencies were responsible for the initial development of health care delivery in the home.

Private home health agencies may be either nonprofit or for-profit organizations. Those that are both privately owned and operated for profit are called *proprietary* home health agencies. Proprietary agencies can be licensed and certified for Medicare purposes only in those states that have special laws allowing licensing of proprietary agencies. Private nonprofit home health agencies are those that are tax exempt under section 501 of the Internal Revenue Code.

Private agencies are financed on a fee-for-service basis. Most of their patients have Medicare, Medicaid, or private insurance, and reimbursement from third-party insurers accounts for nearly all their revenue. Nationwide corporations such as Homemakers-Upjohn operate Medicare-certified home health agencies in various communities across the country.

Hospital-based home care agencies have proliferated in recent years as a result of the emphasis on moving care into the community. Hospital-based home care agencies differ from the community-based agencies by their affiliation with a hospital. Most home care patients in hospital-based programs become agency clients directly on discharge from the hospital. For financial reasons, hospital-based agencies often set limitations on the persons they will serve. These limits usually define geographic residence and patient need for the kind of home care that these agencies provide. Some hospitals make their in-home care available only to those individuals who have used the hospital's facilities (either as inpatients or outpatients) or to those persons whose personal physicians are on staff. Although hospital-based agencies depend heavily on reimbursement from third-party insurers, other means of financing also are available, such as private donations, grants, or public tax monies.

Private duty agencies

Private duty agencies provide home nursing care by registered nurses, licensed practical nurses, home health aides, and companions. The services are contracted by the patient or family for a specific block of time (eg, 4, 8, 12, or 24 hours per day) and frequently are paid privately by the patient or family. These agencies are often large, national organizations that operate for profit.

Home Care Services

Although there is an increased emphasis on an interdisciplinary team approach to home health care, the various agencies offer different home health services. A general discussion of commonly provided home care services follows. The needs of the individual must be delineated so that a referral can be made to the agency that can best meet those needs.

Nursing

Nursing is the foundation of home health care. Historically, nursing was the first health service to be provided in the home and remains the one most frequently used. Federal legislation has reinforced the position of nursing in home health care by requiring that nursing services be available in all home health agencies certified to receive Medicare or Medicaid funds. The nurse is the coordinator of all care provided to the patient. Home care nursing responsibilities include assessment, direct physical care, evaluation of patient progress, patient and family teaching, supervision and coordination of patient care, and provision of psychosocial support.

Home health care nursing differs from private duty nursing in that care is provided on an intermittent basis (eg, per visit) rather than for an extended time period (eg, 8-hour shift). Previously, home nursing care was available only during daytime hours; however, this was changed as home care demands have increased, and 24-hour availability of home nursing care is now the rule.

Clinical nurse specialist involvement in home care agencies has become more prevalent for particular populations of patients with increasingly complex problems and needs. The role of the clinical nurse specialist is primarily one of consultant to staff members, with direct patient contact limited to more complex or acute cases. Because the home care nurse often is a generalist, nurse-to-nurse consultation in specialty areas such as oncology is becoming more common.

Homemaker–home health aide

The availability of homemaker–home health aide service often is the determining factor as to whether a patient and family can select home care. The National Council for Homemaker–Home Health Aide Services defines responsibilities of the home health aide to include assistance with personal hygiene and homemaking tasks. The home health aide must have successfully completed a home health aide certification course and is supervised by the home care nurse, who is responsible for developing a care plan for the aide to follow.

Under the direction of the nurse the home health aide may assist the patient and family to follow through on a treatment plan (eg, wound care, decubitus ulcer care, range-of-motion exercises, or ambulation exercises). The aide may perform personal care activities for the individual such as feeding, bathing, and grooming. Although housekeeping duties are not heavily emphasized, responsibilities of the home health aide may include preparing meals, marketing, laundry, and light housekeeping.

One of the most beneficial aspects of the placement of a home health aide is the relief or respite it provides the family. A home health aide can generally assist for 2- or 4-hour periods depending on individual need and reimbursement regulations. The primary caregiver in the home can use these blocks of time to accomplish other tasks, rest, or "regroup." A study was conducted at a large VNA in the Southwest to evaluate empirically the objective, quantity, and quality of services provided by home health aides, as well as to define their roles.[30] The data showed that 82.5% of the respondents expected that the home health aide would provide relief for the primary caregiver. Respondents also stated that the assistance of a home health aide reduced loneliness and isolation and prevented the necessity of placing the patient in a nursing home.

Medical care

Physician involvement in home care depends on patient needs, agency policy, and the individual physician's interest. All home health agencies require a physician's order before home care services can be initiated. This policy is reinforced by federal health insurance regulations, which require a physician to establish the plan of treatment for each insured patient.

Typically the physician orders home care services from an agency in the community and then works cooperatively with the agency staff to plan and provide care. Less commonly, a physician may be an employee of a home health agency who directs the medical care for agency clients; this method exists in some hospital-based agencies and most prepaid group health plans.

Because home care for the patient with cancer is primarily nursing care, it is important that the nurse communicate with the physician on a regular basis to report changes in patient status and to outline the plan of care, delineating what is needed to carry out the nursing care plan. The physician depends heavily on the nurse's input in planning and ordering of home care services and medical treatments inasmuch as the nurse has consistent contact with the patient and family.

Physical therapy

A major goal of home health care is to promote the individual's functioning at an optimal level. For patients with cancer to achieve this goal, physical therapy and occupational therapy services are integral to the multidisciplinary team.

Physical therapists provide maintenance, preventive, and restorative treatment for individuals at home. Maintenance physical therapy programs are directed toward maintaining the individual's current level of functioning. Preventive programs attempt to prevent patients from losing functional ability or to minimize such losses. In home care the most common physical therapy program is directed at restoring function. For example, physical therapy can be effective to restore function lost by brain tumor or pathologic bone fracture. This emphasis on restorative therapy is reinforced by the present interpretation of Medicare regulations, which basically restricts reimbursement to restorative physical therapy.

Occupational therapy

Occupational therapists assist individuals to achieve their highest functional level and to be as self-reliant as possible by developing and maintaining the ability to perform those tasks essential to daily living. The occupational therapist can teach the individual adaptive techniques and use of adaptive equipment that will allow continuation of household duties. Occupational therapists provide preprosthetic and prosthetic training. They also assist in the selection or construction of splints to correct or prevent a deformity.

Speech pathology

Speech pathologists provide therapy to individuals with communication difficulties caused by speech, language, or hearing problems and to those with swallowing disorders. A major treatment goal is to facilitate maximum speech and language recovery and to enable the person to use to the optimal level whatever speech ability is present. Individuals with head and neck malignancies often are referred to a speech pathologist for speech and language problems or to promote swallowing function.

Social work

Social workers in the home care setting traditionally have been considered referral agents with knowledge of and access to all available community resources, particularly those involving money. Although this is one aspect of their work, equally important in home health are their roles as counselor and patient advocate.

There has been much discussion over the difference between a medical social worker and a mental health clinical nurse specialist in the area of patient and family counseling. The two professions overlap, and there are similarities in practice. A major difference is that the clinical nurse specialist can incorporate knowledge of patient medications in the treatment plan for counseling services.

Nutrition services

The role of the nutritionist in home health care encompasses direct patient care through diet counseling and indirect care through staff consultation and education regarding dietary practices. In most instances direct care often is secondary to consultation and staff education because few third-party insurers will reimburse for direct patient counseling by the nutritionist at home.

Laboratory services

Laboratory services are available in most communities through the health care agency or independent laboratories. The availability of a laboratory that will send technicians into a person's home to draw blood is becoming an important component of home care for the person with cancer, particularly as in-home administration of chemotherapy and total parenteral nutrition become more frequent. As a rule, third-party insurers will reimburse the laboratory fees, but the individual is responsible for the fee charged by the laboratory staff member to come to the home. Because there is a fee for the house call, home care nurses can help their patients by using reliable laboratory services whose cost is minimal.

Infusion therapy

Infusion therapy is becoming a frequently used home care service. Infusion therapy includes chemotherapy administration, total parenteral nutrition, parenterally administered antibiotics, fluid replacement, and administration of blood components.[31-33] Drug and hospital supply companies are entering this market independently or jointly with home care agencies inasmuch as growth in this area is anticipated over the next few years. Issues related to home infusion services include patient selection, reimbursement considerations, qualifications of the agency and nurse, and patient/family education. Appropriate policies and guidelines for collaboration among agencies need to be developed for the population that requires home care.

Other services

As home health care becomes more comprehensive in its scope, additional services are being offered through home health agencies or community resources. Some of the services that have been useful to individuals with cancer are transportation for health-related purposes (such as for radiotherapy), furnishing medical supplies and equipment, and supplying home-delivered meals. Depending on the person's insurance program, transportation and medical supplies/equipment may be reimbursed if ordered by a physician.

Financing Home Health Care

In the current political atmosphere in which cost containment is a major factor, home care nurses struggle with issues such as who should have access to their care, what the quality of care should be, and who needs care at public expense.[34] Home care, because of its desirability and potential cost effectiveness, is taking a place at the negotiation table to create its own set of answers to these topics.

In today's environment, nurses need to be familiar with the reimbursement guidelines for home health care if comprehensive patient care is to be facilitated in a financially responsible manner. Knowledge of the services, equipment, and supplies covered by the individual's insurance is necessary.

Before 1966 most individuals personally paid for home health services, and donations subsidized the care of those who could afford only partial payment or none at all. In the years since the implementation of federally funded Medicare and Medicaid, these health insurance programs have become major funding sources for home care services. Additionally, private insurance companies have begun to expand coverage for coordinated home health care services.

In 1974 the Blue Cross Association developed a manual that described a model benefit program and related guidelines for home health care. The Blue Cross and Blue Shield approach to home care reimbursement identifies three levels of care.[35] The intensive category of care benefits usually requires professional coordination of health care services, central administration of those services, and active medical and nursing management of patient care. Intermediate home care includes a less concentrated array of health care services, usually concentrating on a single service or a combination of nursing and therapeutic services. The basic category of home care benefits usually consists of a minimum of services that are needed to maintain a person's health and well being.

The Blue Cross and Blue Shield model concentrates home health care benefits in the intensive and intermediate categories in an effort to contain health care costs and improve the quality of care that individuals receive. Because most insurers have adopted this model, various plans offer home care benefits that include nurse and home health aide visits, physical therapy, speech pathology, prescription services, prosthetic devices, outpatient services, ambulance services, and medical and surgical supplies as a part of their package. Relatively few insurance plans include homemaker services or nutritional guidance as part of their covered benefits.

Medicare has had the most profound impact on the delivery of care in the home. Eligibility and benefits for services under Medicare remain the same nationwide, whereas eligibility and benefits under other programs vary from state to state or from program to program. Because there are no other nationally accepted standards, Medicare regulations have been accepted de facto by many providers in the industry. Aspects of the Medicare guidelines are presented here to illustrate areas to consider in the planning and implementation of home care.

Home health services available to Medicare recipients include nursing, physical therapy, speech therapy, occupational therapy, home health aide care, social service, and medical supplies and appliances. Medicare regulations dictate that a person be "homebound" to be eligible for home health services. This does not mean that the person is unable to leave the house but that leaving home requires considerable effort. The regulations also state that the person requires home health care on a part-time or intermittent basis. "Part-time" has been interpreted to mean that nurses and home health aides combined are in the home for fewer than 8 hours per day or 35 hours per week. "Intermittent" has been interpreted to mean that services are required at least once every 60 days on the basis of a medically predictable recurring need.

A key in determining whether nursing care will be reimbursed is if the care is "skilled." Skilled nursing care consists not only of those technical procedures required for the patient's care but also patient assessment and evaluation, nursing intervention for a prescribed medical regimen, and patient teaching. Medicare regulations provide guidelines to indicate when skilled nursing services will be covered as a Medicare benefit. Those procedures that require the technical skill and knowledge of a nurse are covered when they are appropriate treatment techniques for the individual's illness. For example, nursing services would not be reimbursable under Medicare if the nurse administered an enema because the homebound person preferred it to self-treatment; however, if the patient recently had had rectal surgery, the nurse visit would be reimbursable by Medicare.

Home health aide services are covered by Medicare only when they are provided in conjunction with nursing services, speech therapy, or physical therapy. Therefore, when the need for these professional services no longer exists, reimbursement for the home health aide will cease even though aide service still may be needed by the patient and family.

Documentation in the patient record must reflect that the care and services were required in accordance with the designated regulations for appropriate reimbursement. The individual's homebound status needs to be established and documented. All skilled care falls within the realm of professional nursing; however, all professional nursing measures are not deemed skilled care. For example, counseling family members regarding breast self-examination for early detection is an appropriate nursing measure but does not meet the requirement for skilled care. A written nursing care plan and documentation of services include specific data about the individual's status, the need for ongoing assessment and evaluation, details of treatments being provided as ordered by the physician and the person's response, and patient and family teaching that facilitates self-care behaviors and their response to teaching. Other areas that the professional nurse manages in the home to provide comprehensive care for the individual and family also need to be documented to reflect the quality and quantity of care. Specific and measurable outcomes are identified, with documentation to reflect patient progress toward those outcomes.

SPECIAL CHARACTERISTICS OF THE HOME

The home presents a set of circumstances and conditions that are unlike those encountered in other health care settings. When the nurse enters a person's home, the protective environment of the clinic/hospital and the control it provides the professional person are absent.

Most important, the patient and family are in control of the way care will be provided at home. Not only are they in control of the manner in which the treatment plan is carried out but they also can decide when and how the plan of care will be implemented. It is desirable and necessary for the patient and family to assume responsibility for the care; this is the overall goal of home care. It is exciting to see an individual or family member state how things will be done, because it reflects a desire to maintain independence. The patient and family's wishes should be recognized and respected and the necessary adjustments incorporated into the plan of care.

Lewis[36] has examined the association of personal control and quality of life for individuals with late-stage cancer. It was hypothesized that greater control would be associated with a higher quality of life as measured by self-esteem, anxiety, and perceived meaningfulness. Results were as predicted: greater personal control over an individual's life was associated with higher levels of self-esteem, lower self-reported anxiety, and more purpose in life. These findings can be beneficially applied to the person who receives home care and to the family.

Working with the patient and family in the home demands that the nurse be flexible in the use of equipment and supplies. Financial limitations or lack of availability may preclude obtaining what might be considered the most up-to-date or desirable equipment or supplies. For instance, disposable irrigation syringes may not be used in the home because the cost is prohibitive for many individuals; the caregiver usually will be instructed by the nurse in the sterilization and proper handling of a reusable glass syringe.

The patient's or caregiver's personality may be different from what it seemed to be in the clinic or hospital.

The person who is rather docile and compliant in an institutional setting sometimes turns out to be a dominant figure in the home. The reverse may be true; the person who is comfortable exerting authority in the hospital may defer decisions to the caregiver in the home. In the home the nurse has the opportunity to observe the individual and family in a natural setting and formulate a realistic approach to care.

APPLYING THE NURSING PROCESS IN HOME CARE

Assessment Factors

In this section, areas of assessment specific to the individual with cancer and to the family in the home setting are discussed. General assessment factors and those specific to various tumor types can be found in other chapters of this text.

Excellent assessment skills are helpful because the nurse in the home setting has no peer close at hand on whom to rely for assistance in evaluating an individual or to validate observations. Accurate assessment can result in early detection of threats to health and avoidance of potentially costly and dangerous health problems.

Patient history

When a person is referred to the home care agency, basic information is needed; standardized information forms streamline this initial process. The home care nurse may not have access to the individual's medical records. Referral information primarily consists of pertinent data related to the individual's hospital course or any significant problems. If a person is referred for home care by a physician or family member, more general information is provided that allows the home care nurse to begin working with the patient and family.

In the planning of comprehensive care the following data are obtained for the patient history:

1. *Primary tumor site(s) and tumor histology.* This information often is difficult to obtain inasmuch as the medical record usually is not available to the nurse. Because of the complexity of cancer as a disease, many health care professionals and family members do not understand the difference between primary versus metastatic disease or the implications of tumor histology. A referral may be made for a person with "lung cancer," and the home care nurse's initial assessment will elicit that the individual had a mastectomy for breast cancer in the past and the lungs are now sites of metastasis. The natural history of the disease and the individual's anticipated clinical course will have nursing implications.

2. *Site(s) of metastasis.* To anticipate potential problems and to alleviate current problems, the extent and sites of disease are important factors.

3. *Past and present treatment(s).* This includes previous and planned surgeries (types and dates), chemotherapy agents and related side effects, radiotherapy (location, duration, and dates), and biotherapy (type and dates). The overall goal of the therapies should be identified. The use of unproved treatment methods is important information. The person at home has access to a myriad of "cancer cures" and may be living on distilled water and stewed tomatoes or ingesting a large number of calcium tablets per day that pose risks for multiple problems.

4. *Family cancer history.* It is not unusual to elicit a lengthy family history of cancer. The home care nurse needs to collect these data to plan preventive and comprehensive family care. Previous experiences with cancer may facilitate or confound current care.

5. *Other medical conditions.* Additional health problems, age-related factors, and responses to therapy need to be identified so that appropriate nursing care can be planned.

6. *Chief complaint.* It always is a surprise to enter a person's home where multiple complex problems exist only to have the individual identify the chief complaint as constipation. Although the nurse may wish to address the major problems first, the patient's concern takes priority. Because the patient and family are in charge in the home, the nurse first will work collaboratively with them to resolve the identified problem(s) so that other aspects of care can be addressed. For example, a person who complains of constipation may not be amenable to learning wound care unless the nurse provides assurance of assistance in resolving the chief complaint.

The individual's presenting health problem(s) or chief complaint(s) can be described in terms of the following components: (a) date and time of onset, (b) type of onset (gradual/abrupt), (c) course of the problem (continuous or intermittent, improving or getting worse), (d) duration (length of time of each episode, frequency of episodes), (e) character (description of quality and severity), (f) interference with usual activites, (g) location and any radiation pattern, (h) associated symptoms, (i) precipitating conditions, and (j) relieving factors.

Physical assessment

A physical assessment is performed on admission to the home care program. Complete baseline data should include the integumentary system; eyes, ear, nose, and throat; hematopoietic/lymphatic systems; respiratory system; breasts and cardiovascular system; gastrointestinal/abdominal areas; genitourinary system; nervous system; and musculoskeletal system. The complete data base allows for comprehensive problem identification and ongoing assessment.

Functional status

Individual need for home-based services is not defined in diagnostic terms but rather in functional terms.[37] Data indicate that chronic illness, diagnostically defined, is not necessarily concurrent with limitations in ability to perform activities essential for living at home.

If a major goal of home care is to promote or maintain the individual's optimal functional ability, then a baseline assessment is necessary to determine the person's status and directions for care. Most important, a functional assessment should define the type and amount of assistance required.

Performance scales are used by oncology health professionals to record the physical status of individuals before initial treatment (such as chemotherapy) and at each subsequent examination. Functional assessment tools of varying degrees of detail and complexity also are available (see the Karnofsky Performance Scale in Chapter 10).

Functional assessment may be performed by means of a variety of tools, depending on the nurse's or agency's preference. It is important to develop a tool that facilitates the assessment and documentation of the individual's performance status as a basis for planning the level of care and type and amount of services required.

Physical care tasks

A systematic approach is used to assess the specific physical tasks involved in the individual's care. Procedures such as wound care or administration of tube feedings are obvious physical care tasks, but is is imperative to anticipate all potential aspects of care so that it can proceed smoothly and problems can be prevented. A useful framework could integrate the functional assessment and common patient care areas identified in the *Standards of Oncology Nursing Practice.*[38] These standards include comfort, nutrition, protective mechanisms, mobility, elimination, sexuality, ventilation, and circulation.

Several questions must be answered by the home care nurse. First, what specific care tasks are to be performed to maintain the individual in the home setting? Second, who will perform the tasks, and what assistance will the person require to perform the identified care tasks? Third, what equipment, assistive devices, and/or supplies are required? And finally, are there associated factors that have an impact on the individual's ability to carry out identified care? Table 51-1 summarizes these points.

Caregiver assessment

The following assessment takes into account the complex nature of the caregiver's role and the stresses involved[39]:

1. Has the caregiver's age been considered, as well as the patient's?
2. Does the caregiver's mental and physical condition allow that person to assume this responsibility?
3. If the caregiver does not live in the patient's home, how accessible will that person be?
4. Is the caregiver aware of the patient's medical condition?
5. Is the caregiver aware of the expected course of treatment, as well as signs/symptoms to report?
6. Who can relieve or assist the caregiver?

Equipment and supplies

Most individuals will require special equipment, assistive devices, or supplies not normally found in the home. Equipment may range from a simple bedpan or urinal to more complex apparatus such as oxygen equipment or intravenous infusion pumps.

The number of medical equipment companies that sell or rent equipment and supplies to the consumer of home care has grown significantly in the last decade. Whatever equipment is required, it is imperative that the caregivers be thoroughly instructed in its use and have resources available should problems arise.

Assistive and safety devices often are necessary to facilitate the patient's functional status. Assistive devices may be as simple as a long-handled bath brush or raised toilet seat. The occupational therapist can be helpful in selecting appropriate equipment.

Supplies such as dressings or ostomy appliances may be available from the local cancer society or other organizations. Ideally, the patient will begin the home stay with sufficient supplies for a week or two so that the family has time to settle in, identify sources, and obtain additional supplies before they are needed. The patient's health insurance may cover a portion or all of the cost of equipment or supplies.

Psychosocial assessment

The individual with cancer learns somehow to integrate the cancer experience into everyday life. Contrary to clinic or hospital activity, which can be an excellent distractor, at home the individual is left to deal with feelings and fears.

Areas pertinent to the psychosocial assessment of the individual in the home setting are as follows:

1. Patient's mood or affective state
2. Causative factors and associated problems that affect the patient's mood state
3. Impact of mood on the person's functioning (role performance, sexual functioning, functional performance status, activities of daily living)
4. Coping mechanisms used by the individual
5. Social supports[40]
6. Diversional activities

Family assessment

Because it is accepted that the family is the unit of care in the home and that the caregivers are central to whether home care is successful, a detailed family assessment is important. The caregiver's role affects virtually all aspects of the caregiver's life to some degree, but the impact varies with the circumstances. Four variables appear to be especially important[9]: (1) the patient's level of disability and dependence, (2) the caregiver's own health and functional mobility, (3) the presence or absence of other assistance, and (4) the caregiver's other roles and responsibilities.

The milder the patient's disability and dependence, the

TABLE 51-1 Patient Assessment: Physical Care Tasks

Oncology Nursing Society Standard	Specific Care Tasks (Examples)	Assistance Required (Examples)	Equipment/ Supplies (Examples)	Associated Factors
Comfort	Medication administration (oral, suppositories, injections, IV); backrubs; positioning; odor control methods	To what degree is the person able to meet comfort needs? Self-medication vs. mild, moderate, or total assistance?	Hospital bed; medications; syringes; IV supplies	Anxiety; family conflict
Nutrition	Preparation of special diets; management of nausea/vomiting; preparation/administration of tube feedings; hyperalimentation administration; measures to deal with anorexia	To what degree is the person able to meet nutritional needs? Needs assistance with food purchase, preparation, feeding?	Blenders; food supplements, special foods; infusion pumps; gavage equipment; hyperalimentation supplies	Urine testing
Protective mechanisms	Personal hygiene needs; general measures to promote skin integrity; management of impaired skin/mucosal integrity (stomatitis, decubitus ulcers, wounds, radiation dermatitis); prevention/ management of infection (medication administration, cleansing/care of equipment)	To what degree is the person able to accomplish activities of daily living; independent in activities of daily living vs. moderate or total assistance? Degree of assistance required with measures to maintain skin integrity?	Shower equipment (bars, chairs); dressings; irrigating syringes	Individual's mobility status
Mobility	Active/passive range-of-motion exercises; transferring, turning, positioning, application of braces; management of edema	To what degree is the person able to ambulate, turn, move, or transfer independently? How many assistants are needed?	Wheelchair; walker; trapeze; Hoyer lift; splints; braces	Individual's pain; fatigue; fractures; bone metastases; edema/ ascites; altered respiratory status
Elimination	Foley catheter care; self-catheterization; suprapubic catheter care; stoma management; ostomy bag changes; irrigations; skin care; management of constipation/diarrhea; use of bedpans; administration of enemas	To what degree is the person able to manage elimination needs? How much and what type of assistance is required?	Bedpan; urinal; bedside commode; enema equipment; laxatives; ostomy supplies	Individual's nutritional status; hydration; use of narcotic analgesics
Sexuality	Measures to maintain vaginal integrity (e.g., dilator); douching; intermittent catheterization	To what degree is the person able to perform tasks related to sexuality needs?	Foley catheters; straight catheters; douche equipment	Urinary elimination needs
Ventilation	Oxygen use; suctioning; tracheostomy care; postural drainage; chest percussion and vibration; medication administration	To what degree is the person able to perform tasks related to respiratory care?	Oxygen; suction catheters/machine; humidifier; tracheostomy care sets	Modification of environmental temperature and humidity; removal of pollutants (smoke, chemicals, exhaust, dust)

better the caregiver's health, and the more available the assistance of others, the less arduous is the caregiver role and the less disruptive to his or her other roles or involvements. Conversely, the more physically and emotionally taxing the caregiver role, the greater the likelihood that other roles and activities will be sacrificed. The most frequently mentioned and severe effects for caregivers involve confinement within the home and restrictions on their outside activities. For the majority of caregivers, role fatigue is the most difficult problem.[9]

Googe and Varricchio[7] interviewed 15 patients with cancer and their families to investigate home health care needs. Study data indicate that family members who serve as primary caregivers often are themselves in a state of unsatisfactory health. Many have additional help during the daytime, but few have help at night.

Clinical research has delineated three types of family units: supportive, ambivalent and hostile.[41] The manner in which family members functioned in the past generally is the way that they will confront the cancer experience; it is unusual to learn new coping behaviors in the face of a crisis. This is evident in the home setting as people function within their own environment. It is commonly thought that when a family member is faced with the threat of a potentially fatal disease, people will forgive old behaviors, forget past misunderstandings, and band together for a common cause. Although this certainly is true for some families, it is not the case for many. Knowledge of a family's response to previous crises can provide insight into basic patterns of coping behavior already within the family's repertoire.[42]

The following are questions to be addressed in a family assessment:

1. What is the composition of the family? Who is living in the household, and how are the household activities distributed? If care is to be planned realistically, consider those family members in the home as well as those outside the home. This facilitates the delineation of roles. For example, if there are young children at home, consider the caretaker's role of parent and associated time and energy constraints. The nurse can be helpful in assisting the family to redefine roles and redistribute household tasks or responsibilities.

2. What are the strengths of the family and its individual members? The number and complexity of patient and family problems sometimes can be overwhelming to the point of immobilizing the family. Identifying positive characteristics of individuals and positive aspects in the environment may be a starting point.[43] It can be helpful to point out what the patient and family are able to do and accomplish rather than focusing on the negative aspects.

3. What is the pattern of authority in the home? Who makes the decisions? It is important to answer these questions early and make allies of those persons in authority so that care can proceed in the most efficient way.

4. What kinds of relationships exist among various family members? Which members work together? The nurse can use this information to coordinate and facilitate care. For example, two adult sisters who are competitive with each other may not be the ideal candidates to enlist in a task that requires cooperation. Their individual capabilities, however, can be put to good use.

5. What is the general pattern of family activities? Do family members do things together? If promoting the optimal functioning of the patient and family is a goal, determining family activities that are important will provide direction for care. For instance, if dinner taken together as a family is valued, nursing interventions are directed at facilitating this goal (eg, establishing a pain control regimen to enable the individual to get to the kitchen and sit through the meal, as well as obtaining necessary ambulation aids).

6. What is the level of family development that is being interrupted or affected? As with individuals, families have certain developmental tasks.[44] If successfully completed, a sense of accomplishment and growth is felt. For example, a young couple addresses the developmental tasks of establishing a household and planning for a family. A cancer diagnosis for either spouse disrupts the ability of the couple to achieve the identified tasks. Understanding and acknowledging the larger impact of a cancer diagnosis on the family can assist in the development of alternate acceptable goals for an intervening time period.

7. What is the health and functional status of the caretaker(s)? Because 24-hour care of a loved one is physically and emotionally taxing, attention to the health of the caregiver(s) is imperative. Assessment also includes the caretaker's physical ability to perform the necessary tasks or procedures (such as lifting, moving, or transferring).

8. Are there stressors aside from the individual's illness that may have an impact on the family? Additional burdens that the family may be carrying often are overlooked by health care professionals in the face of a potentially fatal illness of one family member. These outside stressors, however, may interfere with the delivery of care to the patient (eg, a drug-dependent child who is taking the patient's narcotics) or with the energy level and emotional ability of the family to cope with the cancer experience.

9. What outside support systems or assistance are available to the family? Patients and families are reluctant to ask for help when friends or relatives often are looking for something to do to alleviate their own sense of helplessness. Also, the family living with cancer may not be aware of the community support or resources available. The nurse can assist the family to identify and gather support in an attempt to prevent or diminish caretaker role fatigue.

10. What is the meaning of the cancer event to the family? The vulnerability of the family unit to a crisis event (such as cancer) is related to the ability of the family members to modify their respective roles, perform tasks essential for the continuity of family life, and redefine personal expectations and goals.[42] If a mother's cancer interferes with her adolescent daughter's autonomy and peer relationships because the teenager is depended upon to participate in care, the daughter may become a resentful or unwilling caregiver. Attention by the nurse to the perceived (or actual) threats resulting from a relative's cancer can assist family members to identify measures to alter the experience and cope more effectively.

11. What is the family's level of comprehension related to health practices? Because the family members provide the major portion of care, an assessment of their cognitive skills is necessary for the nurse to develop strategies to appropriately teach the caregivers the necessary patient care.

12. What are the family's values regarding health care? The caregiver who values health promotion is more likely to perform tasks to prevent problems than the individual whose orientation is that of illness or problem management.

Environmental assessment

An important area for assessment is environmental safety, both in general and as adaptations are made in the environment to facilitate care. In particular, those areas that impose threats for the patient with an actual or potential altered immune status include heat and ventilation, cleanliness, and sanitation.[45]

Consideration should be given to general safety such as fire protection and emergency exit routes. For example, an obese 16-year-old girl with osteogenic sarcoma underwent amputation of her right upper extremity and had become paraplegic as her disease advanced. She was placed in halo traction. Her bedroom was in the rear of a third-story flat. The girl had been brought home from the hospital by ambulance, and there was no way her mother could have managed to move her out of the apartment in case of a fire. The fire department was notified of the girl's status and location, and an emergency sticker was placed on her bedroom window that would have directed firemen to that location first in the event of a fire.

Attention should be given to the physical layout of the home, particularly if equipment is needed. Locations of bedrooms and bathrooms are important in determining if the person requires a bedside commode. The number of stairs into and within the house and the width of doorways are considerations if ambulatory aids are needed. For the individual with a wheelchair, the following factors should be assessed: the size of the bedroom and doors to manipulate the wheelchair, height of the bed, bathroom space to transfer from wheelchair to toilet, height of the tub, type of tub rim, and accessibility to kitchen appliances and sink.[46]

Environmental assessments include safety factors. Location of furniture, scatter rugs, and other small objects should be noted and these items removed if potentially dangerous. Safety factors in the bathroom are important if the person is weak or unsteady. Railings for the bathtub and toilet are helpful, as are adhesive-backed rubber strips in the tub or shower to prevent slipping.[47] The use of oxygen needs to be assessed on each home visit and safety guidelines posted for all to see.

Financial assessment

The cost of a chronic illness and the potential catastrophic effect on individuals and families have been well documented in the literature. More than half the families surveyed by Groebe, et al[8] expressed a need for financial assistance or counseling. In another home care study[6] additional expenses related to patient care were problems for 73% of families. An early study of the impact of cancer home care[5] indicated that 15% of families experienced great financial disruption, which included accepting welfare benefits, selling personal property, or accruing numerous unpaid bills and great debt.

The financial costs to the family of implementing the prescribed plan of home care should be estimated early. Supplies, medications, equipment, and laboratory tests usually are reimbursed by third-party payers while the person is hospitalized; however, the expense of these items can become the responsibility of the individual at home unless insurance benefits specifically include these areas:

The following are questions to be answered:

1. What services and supplies are covered by the individual's insurance? This information is needed to determine if recommended care will be covered. Insurers can be contacted directly to determine specific details of home care coverage. For example, some insurance plans will not cover the placement of a home health aide but will cover the placement of a private duty nurse (registered nurse or licensed practical nurse). In these cases it is to the benefit of the individual to employ a private duty nurse for a full day rather than a home health aide for 2 or 4 hours.
2. What is the income of the family? Do family members believe that their income is adequate to meet their needs; that is, are expenses greater, less than, or equal to income? This will provide a general idea about how much money is available for health care expenses. It cannot be assumed that because income is large there will be no financial problems; expenses and obligations may be greater.
3. How has the person's illness affected the financial status of the family? Health professionals should not make assumptions about the financial impact of illness. An individual with excellent long-term disability benefits may be affected minimally. On the other hand, the costs of a long-term illness can be devastating to the disposable income and financial security of many families.

Planning Home Care

Self-care and family equilibrium are general objectives of home care.[47] The initial nursing assessment provides the information necessary to identify and prioritize basic patient and family needs. The first visit includes teaching those aspects of care the patient and caregiver will be implementing before the next nursing visit (such as transfer techniques, tube feedings, use of the bedpan, turning and positioning, and medication administration). Appropriate supplies and equipment will make the tasks of care easier. Referrals to other health care providers (such as a home health aide, physical therapist, or social worker) are made as soon as the need is identified so that these services can begin early.

A vital point to keep in mind is that the patient and family's initial impressions regarding the transition to home care will influence their ongoing experience. If the transition is made easier with adequate support and assistance, they most likely will approach care comfortably and with confidence. A 1- or 2-week delay in obtaining a home health aide may seem minimal, but it may be critical to the caregiver who has been unable to leave the house during this time. The decision to "wait and see" if a hospital bed is required may be an unnecessary stressor to the patient and caregiver. Equipment and services always can be discontinued if the needs change.

Frequency of visits

Appropriate planning regarding the frequency of nursing visits is crucial. Home care can be divided into three stages: introduction/transition stage, working stage, and termination stage.

Patients and families need increased support during the initial transition to home care. Daily or frequent visits are appropriate during this stage to facilitate a smooth transition, inasmuch as the patient and caregiver's learning needs are great during this time. Nursing interventions during this stage include assessment and monitoring, direct patient care, and patient/family teaching.

As the patient and family settle into home care—the working stage—nursing visits may decrease to two to three visits per week. Nursing interventions will include assessment of the patient's status and evaluation of the patient's care, as well as the provision of direct care and ongoing patient and family education. The nurse provides support that is important to foster the patient and family's participation in the plan of care.

The third stage of home care is the termination stage. Depending on the patient's condition and family's ability to manage care, nursing visits may either increase or decrease in frequency. As the patient and family progress to independence in care and the patient's condition stabilizes, nursing visits may taper off and plans are made for termination of service. If the patient's status is deteriorating and/or the family is unable to manage care at home, the frequency of nursing visits may increase to provide needed support and care and to assist the family in making alternate plans. Frequent or daily nursing visits also are appropriate for the individual with end-stage disease whose condition is rapidly deteriorating and who chooses to die at home.

Planning for emergencies

Early recognition of problems often is the key to successful home care. Emergencies should be anticipated and caregivers educated regarding their management. For example, the obstruction of a Foley catheter always is a possibility, and measures to unplug or remove the catheter should be explained during the initial visit. Individuals with tracheostomies should have a suction machine available and know how to use it even though routine suctioning may not be required. The patient and family need to know what constitutes an emergency and when it might be necessary to go to the emergency room. Signs and symptoms that require immediate attention should be clearly identified (eg, impending spinal cord compression), as should those signs and symptoms that can be anticipated and dealt with at home (eg, mild or moderate hematuria). Caregivers may need assistance in differentiating between significant and minor problems. If the potential for a severe emergency exists (eg, seizures or hemorrhage), the family needs to be prepared. Although it is a threatening topic to discuss, it can be more terrifying if the emergency occurs and the family has not been forewarned and prepared either to respond to the emergency or to allow death to occur. A written emergency plan should be discussed with the patient and family, one that identifies the specific signs and symptoms to monitor, the most appropriate person or service to contact (ie, physician, nurse, or ambulance), and the relevant telephone number. The nursing care plan includes documentation of teaching related to management of emergencies and patient/family response.

Developing realistic patient/family outcomes

Evaluation of care is based on patient outcomes. Expected outcomes should be realistic and achievable so that the patient, caregiver(s), and health care providers are able to provide good care and to feel a sense of satisfaction and accomplishment. This is not to say that patient outcomes reflect minimal goals but rather that the goals are realistic.

Implementing Home Care

Division of labor

Implementation of home care is divided into two components: care provided by the nurse and other health care professionals and care provided by the family. The role of the nurse and other health care providers should be clearly defined so that the patient and family know what to expect. The importance of this factor cannot be overemphasized. Problems develop when the patient and caregivers have different expectations of the health professionals and anticipate services that may be unrealistic, inappropriate, or unavailable.

Some tasks may be shared by home care staff and family members. For example, wound care to be done three times a day may be accomplished in the morning by a home health aide, in the afternoon by the home care nurse, and in the evening by a family member. This frees the family caregivers from three dressing changes a day and facilitates ongoing assessment of the wound by the nurse. As the patient's condition stabilizes and family members become more comfortable with the dressing change procedure, they will assume increased responsibility for the wound care.

TABLE 51-2 Formulas for Common Solutions

Acetic Acid Solution (0.25%)
2 cups of water plus 2 Tbsp of 4% vinegar (white)
or
$2\frac{1}{2}$ cups of water plus 2 Tbsp of 5% vinegar (white)
Normal Saline
1 quart of water (4 cups) plus 2 Tbsp of salt

Source: From the *Field Guide,* Visiting Nurse Association of Metropolitan Detroit, 1980.

Minimizing costs

The cost of such items as supplies and medications often is a burden and worry for patients and families. Improvising and using creative approaches to care can facilitate good care in a less costly manner. For example, families can be taught to make their own irrigating solutions (Table 51-2) at a greatly reduced cost. Another cost-effective strategy to consider is the use of equipment that can be sterilized and reused rather than the use of disposable equipment (eg, glass irrigating syringe).

Infection prevention and control

Patients with cancer are at high risk of infection. Intrinsic factors that predispose individuals to infection include altered defense mechanisms, chronic disease, and age. Extrinsic factors can further predispose individuals to infection. Therapies such as chemotherapy, corticosteroids, and radiotherapy can be immunosuppressive. Also, antibiotics can alter normal host microbial flora, thereby enabling the growth of resistant organisms.[48]

Medical devices and procedures to treat diseases and prolong life also may predispose patients to infection by providing portals of entry and reservoirs for microbial growth. As the result of an early hospital discharge, a patient may go home with multiple devices or the need for procedures, or both, that previously would have been managed in the hospital (eg, venous access lines). For many medical devices and procedures, there may be insufficient data regarding the safety of necessary care methods. Therefore care methods for infection control often are based on knowledge of microbial growth and transmission.

The following principles of infection control underlie care in the home setting[48]:

1. Thorough handwashing before donning gloves and after contact with secreta, excreta, and contaminated fomites and after removing gloves is of paramount importance.
2. With the possible exception of intravascular and intra-abdominal devices, aseptic technique usually can be modified safely to clean technique in the home.
3. Mechanical cleansing with a mild soap and water followed by thorough rinsing will remove most contaminating organisms. For tenacious secretions, hydrogen peroxide in a 1:3 dilution is an effective adjunct to mechanical cleansing.
4. Disinfection can be accomplished by the use of household products. For devices that will have direct contact with mucous membranes, a 1:3 dilution of white vinegar to water is both safe and effective. Large pieces of equipment can be disinfected with a 1:3 dilution of a phenolic agent such as Lysol or Pinesol but should be carefully rinsed and thoroughly dried to decrease phenolic residue and should not be used on surfaces used for food preparation or food serving because of its toxic potential. Surfaces contaminated with blood should be disinfected with a 1:9 dilution of household chlorine bleach.
5. Thorough drying and storage in a clean, dry area help to prevent proliferation of gram-negative waterborne organisms.
6. To protect the care provider from potential contact with the human immunodeficiency virus, the universal precautions recommended by the Centers for Disease Control should be followed.[49]

Adapting Therapies to the Home

Chemotherapy administration

The demand for more cost-effective methods of treating patients with cancer has stimulated the development of outpatient facilities that provide comprehensive services, including administration of chemotherapy. For those patients whose physical conditions preclude travel to an outpatient setting, administration of chemotherapy in the home has become a viable option. Technologic advances have made it possible to produce sophisticated equipment for the administration of antineoplastic drugs, and clinical research has provided methods for the control of side effects, which enables safe administration at home. In addition to cost reduction, home chemotherapy reduces the risk of complications as a result of nosocomial infections, it is convenient for the patient and caregiver, and it provides psychologic benefits to the patients who desire the comfort of their homes.

Criteria for patient selection Specific criteria must be adhered to before administration of chemotherapy in the home:

1. The patient meets the requirements for admission to home care as determined by the agency's licensing or certification agency.
2. The patient is stable and free of symptoms that preclude the safe administration of antineoplastic drugs.
3. The patient desires chemotherapy and is willing to pay for that portion of drugs and services not covered by medical insurance.
4. The patient has received the initial course of chemotherapy with no untoward effects before administration in the home.

5. The patient and family are willing and able to assume related caregiving activities.
6. Resources are available in the community for medications, supplies, laboratory services, and additional nursing or caregiving services.

Insurance reimbursement for antineoplastic drugs, equipment, supplies and nursing services varies. Before referral for home chemotherapy, medical coverage should be determined inasmuch as the patient may not be able to assume the costs.

Policies for chemotherapy administration Home care agencies that offer chemotherapy as a service must develop specific policies and procedures,[50] including the following:

1. Specific patient eligibility requirements
2. Specific antineoplastic drugs to be administered at home
3. Acceptable criteria for laboratory tests and their frequency and timing
4. Procedures for each route of administration, which includes preparation, administration, and disposal of the drugs[51,52]
5. Specific criteria for withholding the antineoplastic drugs
6. Eligibility requirements for nurses who administer antineoplastic drugs

Consideration must be given to the antineoplastic agents that will be given at home. Some agencies limit approved drugs to nonvesicant[51] or noncaustic agents.[52] Many home health agencies will administer only those drugs that can be infused within 1 to 2 hours. Companies that provide home infusion therapy usually will administer those antineoplastic drug protocols that require hydration and infusion over several hours, such as cisplatin. Investigational drugs should be considered for home administration only if the side effects are known and documented, and written information describing action and side effects is provided to the agency. Although this information is readily available to the hospital or clinic nurse, it is more difficult for home care agencies to obtain.

The frequent use of venous access devices has made the administration of chemotherapy at home easier. However, not all patients who receive chemotherapy have an existing intravenous (IV) line. An agency must determine whether the nurses will be expected to perform venipunctures. Some agencies require that a patient have an existing line if chemotherapy is to be given at home. Others mandate the establishment of a free-flowing IV line through which chemotherapy is administered rather than direct IV push administration. This action ensures venous access and facilitates the flushing of the tubing.

Specific laboratory criteria must be designated for the minimal levels of white blood cell and platelet counts at which chemotherapy will be administered. A complete blood cell count and differential and platelet counts are obtained 36 to 48 hours before administration of each series of drug(s) and the physician contacted to confirm, adjust, or withhold the dose of the antineoplastic agent. The Michigan Cancer Foundation Home Care Program's policy states that chemotherapy will not be administered when the white blood cell count is below 3000/mm^3 or the platelet count is below 75,000/mm^3. In the home, serial laboratory testing that may indicate bone marrow recovery generally is not available.

Staff education As in any setting, the nurse who administers chemotherapy must have a theoretic knowledge base and technical skills necessary to ensure the safety of the patient. Many home care agencies have developed a chemotherapy certification course based on the *Cancer Chemotherapy Guidelines* developed by the Oncology Nursing Society.[53] To be eligible to administer chemotherapy at home, the nurse should demonstrate the following:

1. Knowledge of administration procedures and the purpose, action, and side effects of drugs, as well as measures to manage untoward effects
2. The ability to administer IV drugs via venous access ports, catheters, pumps, and peripheral lines
3. Knowledge of appropriate preparation, transportation, and disposal of antineoplastic agents. A comprehensive review of this information is included in Chapter 13.

Safety considerations Several studies have suggested that mutagenic changes may occur in persons who handle chemotherapy drugs.[54-56] Potential hazards associated with the administration of antineoplastic agents have prompted the Occupational Safety and Health Administration (OSHA) to set guidelines for compounding, transporting, administering, and disposing of toxic chemotherapy agents.[57]

Potential risks to persons who come into contact with chemotherapy drugs and associated safety. measures should be discussed with the patient and family before the initial home chemotherapy treatment.

Safety considerations include drug transport, preparation, spill control, patient care, and disposal.

Transport of drugs In the home care situation, the antineoplastic drugs often are obtained by the family or nurse. The drugs are labeled as cytotoxic, and they are capped securely and sealed and packaged in an impervious packing material for transport. The family is cautioned to protect the package from breakage and taught the necessary procedures should a spill occur.

Preparation of drugs An area of the patient's home that is apart from frequent family activity and food preparation is selected to prepare the drugs. Ceiling fans, if present, should be turned off. A work surface area that can be cleansed should be used (eg, a card table). All family members should remain outside the rooms in which the drugs are prepared and administered. If possible, the family should make arrangements for children to be cared for outside the home on the day of chemotherapy.

Supplies are assembled on a disposable, absorbent, plastic-backed pad that is taped over the work surface area. Only syringes, needles, and IV sets with Luer-lock fittings are used. A plastic or metal tray can be lined with sterile gauze squares to catch and collect excess solution. A closable, puncture-resistant, shatter-resistant container is necessary for the disposal of contaminated sharp or breakable materials. Appropriate containers may be purchased from medical supply companies, but empty coffee cans with reinforced lids have been used, with care taken to direct the "sharps" toward the bottom of the can. Sealable 4-mil thick polyethylene or 2-mil polypropylene plastic bags with wire ties and labeled "cytotoxic hazard" must be used for disposal of all supplies used in the preparation and administration of antineoplastic drugs.

Before donning a protective disposable gown, surgical latex gloves, and goggles, the nurse reminds the patient and caregiver of the need for protection from exposure to the drugs. During the preparation and administration of the drugs, care is taken to prevent aerosolization; for example, sterile gauze is wrapped around ampules before they are broken and around needle tips while air is expelled from syringes, IV lines are primed, or needles are inserted into vials or IV lines. During the administration of antineoplastic drugs the universal precautions for prevention of transmission of human immunodeficiency virus, hepatitis B virus, and other bloodborne pathogens must be followed.[49] The patient or caregiver who participates in administering the drug also should wear protective gloves.[50]

In many parts of the country the drugs may be prepared in an appropriate laminar-flow hood in a licensed pharmacy and then delivered to the home by the nurse. In the home these drugs (which usually require refrigeration) must be stored away from food, cosmetics, and frequently used household areas.[50]

Spills Spills and breakages must be cleaned up immediately by a person wearing a protective gown, gloves, and goggles. Liquids and solids are wiped up with absorbent pads or gauze and the area cleansed three times with detergent solution and rinsed with clean water. All contaminated materials are placed in the plastic bag labeled "cytotoxic hazard."

Patient care The blood, emesis, and excreta from patients who have received antineoplastic agents within a 48-hour period may be contaminated. The health care providers and caregivers must be informed of the need to wear protective garments if the potential exists to become contaminated, for example, when caring for the bedbound or incontinent patient. All contaminated linens are prewashed separately once and then laundered again with the family laundry. All disposable bed pads, tissues, gowns, and gloves must be sealed in a plastic bag for disposal. Children should be discouraged from visiting the patient during the 48-hour period after chemotherapy administration.

Disposal When administration is completed, all items that have been in contact with the drug are wrapped in an absorbent pad, including unused portions of the drug, unless it is to be used in the future, and placed into the plastic bag labeled "cytotoxic hazard." A reusable drug vial is cleaned with an alcohol pad, placed in a plastic bag with a zip lock, and stored according to package directions regarding environmental temperature. The patient and family are warned that all persons must avoid contact with the drug (especially children). The nurse will transport the bag of contaminated wastes to the home care agency for disposal. OSHA[57] recommends that all hazardous wastes be disposed of in a licensed sanitary landfill or by appropriate high-temperature incineration. Therefore home care agencies that administer antineoplastic drugs must have a contract for disposal of the wastes.

Patient and family responsibility The family that assumes responsibility for obtaining the drugs, solutions, and equipment will need a list of specific items required and information as to where they may be purchased. Some agencies require a caregiver to be present on the day(s) chemotherapy is administered to observe for problems and to assist the patient to manage side effects. Written information about the potential side effects is provided along with the symptoms to be reported immediately to the physician or nurse. It is helpful to include the telephone number of these health care providers on the written instructions.[58] Patient and family education regarding management of side effects is an obvious need.

Total parenteral nutrition

The administration of total parenteral nutrition (TPN) at home is a cost effective and beneficial therapy for the malnourished patient with cancer.[59] It is a rapidly developing option in home cancer care.[60,61] In 1968 the first person in the United States received TPN at home,[60] and by 1970 the University of Washington developed a system to permit home administration of TPN.[61]

Criteria for patient selection Certain criteria are recommended for acceptance of a patient into a home parenteral nutrition (HPN) program:

1. The patient's physical status is sufficiently stable to allow hospital discharge and safe home care for a reasonable period of time
2. To prevent problems related to parenteral nutrition, the patient has received parenteral nutrition for a minimum of 1 week before discharge from the acute care facility
3. The patient and/or family members are willing and able to learn and maintain the procedures necessary for HPN
4. The amount and types of care requirements, as well as the benefits, risks, and financial considerations, have been evaluated and explained to the patient and caregiver before discharge
5. Adequate resources are available in the community for obtaining medications and supplies, as well as troubleshooting support, on a 24-hour basis. Additionally, laboratory services and home nursing care are accessible. Most areas in the United States currently are serviced by home infusion therapy companies that provide the necessary supplies, medications, and equipment
6. The home environment is conducive to providing safe HPN, including running water, electricity, and a telephone

The patient and family assume primary responsibility for the administration of HPN. If the patient lives alone, a caregiver must be identified who will stay with the patient and administer the HPN until the patient is able to manage this care. Private duty nurses may be considered if a family member or willing caregiver is not available. Frequently the patient with cancer who requires HPN has additional complex care requirements, and the total amount of care required, especially at night, can impose a severe burden on the caregiver.[3] Therefore consideration is given to available supports to provide respite for the caregiver.

The financial costs of HPN vary according to locale and patient needs. In 1985 Konstantinides[60] estimated the cost to be approximately $55,000 to $70,000 per year, which included solutions and supplies, home nursing visits, and cost of clinical follow-up with laboratory tests. The patient's medical insurance must be reviewed by the discharge planner or home infusion company to determine if it covers HPN. Handy[32] reports that many third party payers have extended coverage to include IV administration of drugs and solutions in the home because of the substantial savings involved. Frequently the patient's insurance will cover 80% of the cost, as with Medicare Part B coverage, with the other 20% the patient's responsibility. The company that provides infusion therapy usually directly bills the patient's provider of medical insurance.

Initial home care assessment The initial visit by the home care nurse should occur soon after the patient's arrival at home and coincide with the delivery of the supplies, equipment, medication, and the home infusion therapy company personnel. This will allow time to review the medical orders for HPN with the patient and caregiver, test the infusion pump, review the schedule and procedures for ordering supplies, and define the specific responsibilities of the home care nurse and the infusion therapy company personnel. It is essential that agencies that participate in the administration of HPN provide 24-hour service. Because HPN usually is infused at night, most problems occur at this time.

The complete patient assessment may span several visits because of the many essential activities required during the initial home visit related to HPN. The initial assessment includes the following:

1. The type and status of the venous access device, such as the single, double, and triple lumen catheters, right atrial catheters, and implanted ports
2. The patient and family's knowledge of the management of HPN and other caregiving needs
3. Evaluation of the home environment for safety and cleanliness factors that are required for HPN (eg, running water, electricity, and working telephone)

Most acute care facilities have developed complete teaching programs that include catheter care, home monitoring techniques, solution preparation (if applicable), administration techniques, and emergency care.[61] Because the prospective payment system fosters earlier discharges, however, patients may be sent home before they are fully knowledgeable in HPN management.

Adequate refrigeration must be available in the home to store the 2- to 4-week supply of solutions. Most companies that supply infusion therapy will provide a small refrigerator if needed. An electric infusion pump is necessary for safe administration of HPN.[61,62] Most infusion pumps have a battery backup that can operate the pump for several hours during an electrical outage. Thick carpeting or steps in multilevel homes may impede the patient's mobility during the infusion inasmuch as the pumps are attached to IV poles.

Nursing management Initially, twice-a-day home nursing visits usually are required to start the infusion of HPN in the evening and discontinue it in the morning. The role of the nurse encompasses ongoing assessment and evaluation of the patient's status, direct patient care (eg, HPN administration), supervision of the patient/family management of HPN, and patient/family education.

Written instructions for HPN procedures usually are given to the patient at time of discharge. It is helpful to adjust the HPN infusion time to the family's routine. HPN often is administered over 10 to 16 hours, including the patient's sleeping time.[63] The infusion rate for the first and last hours is decreased to prevent hyperglycemia on initiation and rebound hypoglycemia on withdrawal of the HPN. A typical 10-hour schedule will start at 80 to 100 mL/hour, increase to 200 mL/hour over 8 hours, and then decrease to 80 to 100 mL for the last hour.

A flow sheet for recording the multiple monitoring needs and tasks can be helpful. The patient and family are instructed to record the date, time, and results of the following data:

- Time of initiation/completion of HPN infusion
- Daily temperature, pulse, respirations
- Weight
- Urine fractionals (glucose)
- Intake (HPN, additional IV fluids, oral fluids)
- Output
- Medications added to HPN; other medications given
- Catheter care (heparinization, cap change, dressing change)
- Blood drawings for laboratory testing

Although complications occur less frequently in the home than in the inpatient setting,[64] the patient and caregiver need oral and written instructions regarding symptoms that require notification of the nurse or physician. The caregiver(s) and nurse also should observe the patient for depression or anxiety, which can occur with long-term HPN.[65]

Blood transfusions

The expanded services offered by many home health agencies include home blood transfusion programs. Issues to be considered include referral and preparation, blood transport, and the blood transfusion process.[66] The Transfusion Practices Committee of the American Association of Blood Banks offers guidelines for home health agencies to establish protocols for out-of-hospital transfusions.[67] Their recommendations are grouped into three main areas.

Patient criteria In-home transfusions of blood components may be considered for a patient who has physical limitations that would make transportation to a hospital difficult; has a stable cardiorespiratory status; has not had an untoward reaction to the most recent transfusion; is cooperative and can respond to verbal commands; has a responsible adult available to stay with the nurse and patient during the transfusion; and has access to a usable telephone during the transfusion.

Nursing criteria The nurse who is eligible to be a member of the home transfusion team should be a registered nurse with experience in acute patient care and proven skills in venipuncture and IV therapy. It is suggested that the nurse (1) has been supervised in the administration of blood components before independent performance and (2) has successfully completed a basic education program in transfusion therapy.

Transfusion administration The basic areas of transfusion therapy are the same in any setting with regard to patient identification, patient education, administration procedure, and patient monitoring. Areas that require adaptation to home care are discussed next.

Method of obtaining physician orders Written orders are required, including the component to be transfused, the number of units, the rate of infusion, the date of transfusion, pretransfusion and post-transfusion tests to be performed, and any premedications. Any telephone requests must be followed with written prescriptions before the transfusion.

Transportation Blood products must be transported in a container with the coolant appropriate for the products. For example, wet ice is used to ensure an ambient temperature between 1° and 10°C during transport of blood. Platelets are maintained between 20° and 24°C (no wet ice is used).

Disposal of equipment All equipment is collected in a biohazard bag, including the containers and infusion devices, and returned to the blood bank in the transportation container for proper disposal. Blood-contaminated supplies and containers constitute a biohazard, and federal law requires proper disposal.

Patient consent form A home care agency obtains a consent form that includes patient acknowledgment of the risks and benefits of receiving an in-home transfusion.

Transfusion reaction A transfusion policy includes specific nursing actions to be taken in the event of an adverse reaction, and the nurse carries medications to be administered in an emergency.

Other considerations Additional recommendations regarding home transfusion policies include the following guidelines[66]:

- Transfusions are administered during customary physicians' office hours, Monday through Friday only.
- The primary physician must be readily available by telephone during the administration period.

Intravenous antibiotic therapy

Antibiotic therapy is the most commonly used IV therapy at home.[68,69] Home parenteral antibiotic therapy (HPAT) is a preferred method for delivering a course of therapy for many infectious diseases—those that require prolonged, repeated, or short-term antibiotics.[70]

Criteria for patient selection for HPAT include the following[69]:

1. Signs and symptoms of infection are under control.
2. Other aspects of the patient's treatment plan can be monitored or performed at home; hospitalization continues for IV therapy only.
3. The patient and family understand and agree with the plan for home therapy.
4. The patient and/or caregiver can perform the necessary procedures for in-home therapy. Some agencies require that the patient have a primary caregiver or support person who has agency-documented training in the specific therapy ordered.[71]
5. The patient has peripheral veins suited for repeated cannulizations or has a central venous catheter in place.
6. The patient has a suitable home environment for therapy (eg, refrigerator, freezer, telephone, and transportation).
7. The arrangement of payment for supplies, medication, skilled nursing visits, laboratory tests, and clinic appointments is agreeable to the patient and family.

Before the patient is discharged from the hospital, arrangements are made for the preparation and delivery of pharmaceutical supplies to the home. The patient usually is given enough supplies to last a week, with subsequent replenishment at least once a week. If antibiotics are prepared in batches by a hospital or a pharmacy that provides private home care and then sent to the patient for storage, frequent deliveries may be required, depending on the stability of the specific agent.[72]

During the active treatment phase, nursing visits may vary in frequency from three times a day to once a week. On each visit the nurse monitors the vital signs, laboratory test results, equipment operation, supplies, drug effects, and signs/symptoms of complications. Although the patient may prepare, store, and administer the HPAT, the home care nurse is responsible for ensuring that specific pharmaceutical guidelines are followed during the course of therapy (eg, storage and mixing of drugs).

By far the simplest and least costly drug delivery system is gravity infusion, which is easily adapted to the home. If particular antibiotics could cause phlebitis or if the flow rate is a critical factor in administration, it is preferable to use a mechanized infusion (eg, infusion pump).

Dosing intervals or adverse effects are important factors in the selection of a drug for home administration. If all other factors are equal, a drug that needs to be administered only once or twice daily is especially attractive in the home setting.

The stability of the medication and type of storage required must be considered. Recommended refrigeration temperature of 2° to 8° C (36° to 44° F) can be achieved in most home and commercial refrigerators.[72] To prevent unnecessary freezing or warmth however, the temperature should be tested before a supply of prepared parenteral bags is placed in the refrigerator. It is advisable to purchase a refrigerator thermometer to monitor the temperature during drug storage. Some antibiotics have a stability of 30 days or more and are available in commercially prepared frozen piggyback solutions, as well as piggybacks prepared and frozen by pharmacies. If antibiotics are frozen, it is necessary to use proper thawing techniques to prevent inactivation or degradation. With conventional thawing techniques, the antibiotic needs to be left at room temperature until it is completely thawed (approximately 1 to 3 hours and 4 to 6 hours for 50 mL and 100 mL bags, respectively).[72] Except for certain drugs a 24-hour supply of frozen small volume parenteral bags can be thawed in advance and then refrigerated for use the next day.

Patient education is the key to safe administration of antibiotics in the home. Teaching includes venous access site care, signs/symptoms of recurrent infection, proper drug admixture procedures, drug administration techniques, infusion pump operation (if applicable), and the identification and resolution of problems. The individuals responsible for HPAT should be assessed for psychomotor skills and dexterity, basic mathematical skills, reading ability, and the ability to comprehend and follow instructions.[73]

Sheehan and Gildea[74] present an interesting case study on teaching a complex regimen of IV antibiotic therapy to an elderly couple, thereby demonstrating that physical impairments need not prevent self-care IV therapy. Because various procedures were simplified (eg, prepriming IV tubings and needles), the couple was able to achieve a workable level of self-care.

The home care nurse monitors the overall effectiveness of the home IV therapy. A quality assurance instrument has been developed that identifies outcome criteria in six areas of at-home IV antibiotic care[69]: infusion-related complications, drug-related complications, home care management, psychosocial response of patient/caregiver, cost, and recovery (cure).

Pain management

Principles of pain management for the patient at home include the following guidelines:

1. An analgesic regimen should provide sufficient pain relief to allow optimal functioning of the patient. The regimen should be simple to administer.
2. Pain medications should be given around the clock, not PRN. Continuous pain requires continuous treatment.
3. Measures other than analgesics to decrease pain may be fully and effectively employed in the home setting (eg, relaxation techniques).
4. Interventions to prevent the potential side effects of a narcotic analgesic regimen should be initiated (eg, anticonstipation medications).
5. Comprehensive assessment of the patient's pain is an ongoing process. The source of pain should be identified whenever possible; it should not be assumed that the patient's pain is due to the malignant process.
6. Patient and family misconceptions about the use and abuse of narcotic analgesics should be addressed.

Oral analgesics or analgesic combinations should, when possible, be used in the management of chronic cancer pain. The oral route is preferable for long-term cancer pain management for a number of reasons: comfort, ease of administration, compliance, and freedom of movement; also, no equipment is required. Oral administration is equally effective as parenteral routes once serum equilibration has been achieved.[75] Oral medications with high potency and long duration of action permit longer dosing intervals, which is advantageous in the development of medication schedules to allow the patient to sleep through the night.

Chapter 20 provides an in-depth review of medications for mild, moderate, and severe pain. Morphine, however, is the prototypic agent for cancer pain and often is the analgesic of choice. It is easy to use, safe, versatile, effective, and well-tolerated.[75,76] Newer preparations, such as concentrated solution and sustained-release tablets, facilitate better pain control for the patient at home.

Intermittent or continuous infusion therapy can be administered in the home setting via a variety of routes: subcutaneous, intravenous, epidural, and subarachnoid.[77,78] For continuous infusions, ambulatory infusion pumps offer unimpeded mobility.[77]

The epidural or subarachnoid route is indicated for pain that is refractory to analgesics administered by conventional means or analgesics that have produced severe, intolerable side effects that cannot be managed by alterations in drug therapy.[78] Epidural analgesia permits control or alleviation of severe pain without the opioid-mediated side effects because a smaller dose of drug is given.[78,79] The analgesic most frequently administered is preservative-free morphine. The nurse is usually responsible for filling the analgesic pump in the home. Patients and families are taught preparation and administration procedures, dressing change procedures, and administration of naloxone (Narcan) for respiratory depression. Home catheter care is accomplished by means of clean rather than aseptic technique.[79]

Patient-controlled analgesia (PCA) is an intravenous drug delivery system that allows patients to administer predetermined doses of analgesic with the use of a programmed ambulatory pump. The ability to self-administer medication and manage the pain produces a sense of control for the patient that seems to decrease feelings of powerlessness and vulnerability.[80] Several studies have examined the efficacy of using PCA with patients with cancer. Keeri-Szanto[81] found that PCA provided effective pain relief and reduced total drug dose requirements. Citron et al[82] reported that PCA-administered morphine produced significant pain relief without undue sedation during severe cancer pain episodes. A research study that compared PCA with IV bolus hydromorphone administration in patients with advanced cancer demonstrated no significant difference in the amount of narcotic administered, pain response, sedation level, anxiety score, self-care, or activity between subjects who received PCA versus those who received IV bolus medication.[80]

PCA pumps that deliver both continuous and incremental dosing are particularly useful. Small, portable, computerized PCA pumps available for home use are lightweight and easy to use. Most pumps can deliver a continuous amount of medication along with an incremental dose that is self-administered for breakthrough pain. The caregiver and patient are taught to attach the pump to the indwelling venous catheter and to change the medication cassette as needed.

The logistics of obtaining narcotics for home use require planning. Prescriptions for intravenously administered narcotics cannot be telephoned to a pharmacy unless prior arrangements have been made by the physician. Therefore, the analgesic requirements must be anticipated and the obtaining of new prescriptions planned. Arrangements can be made with local pharmacies to obtain (or stock) certain narcotics for the patient with cancer.

Measures other than narcotic analgesics to decrease pain may be fully and effectively employed in the home setting. Behavioral coping strategies and noninvasive techniques can be quickly taught to patients and families, including distraction, relaxation,[83-85] and cutaneous stimulation. Diversions such as music, hobbies, visitors, and television may be useful distractors in the home setting. Ensuring a quiet environment for relaxation exercises often is more easily achieved at home than in an acute care setting. Cutaneous stimulation includes the use of cold packs, hot packs or heating pads, massage and backrubs, warm baths, and topical ointments or anesthetics. Patients and caregivers also can be taught comfort measures such as repositioning or range-of-motion exercises.

Other types of medications may be considered for adjunct therapy. The emotional and psychologic components of pain must be recognized. Tricyclic antidepressants are one group of drugs that can play a role in pain management.[86] Other categories of medications include anticonvulsants (especially carbamazepine) and steroids for nervous system involvement.[86] Over-the-counter medications such as hypnotics, antitussives, and antacids frequently are found in home medicine cabinets and may be helpful.

Critical assessment of pain is ongoing. A change in the location, severity, or type of pain may indicate an acute problem that requires additional intervention. Little clues that may signal a change can go unheeded if all pain is simply attributed to the malignant disease. For example, a patient with cancer of the prostate and diffuse bony metastases complained to the home care nurse that his pain was getting worse. The nurse conducted a detailed pain assessment and determined that the pain was now sharp versus dull, localized to the center of the back, and became excruciating when the patient attempted to sit. Previously the patient had described his pain as more diffuse regardless of position. No neurologic deficits were noted. After conferring with the physician, the patient was transported by ambulance to the hospital where radiologic studies confirmed the presence of three vertebral compression fractures.

Patients and caregivers often have a negative influence on the treatment of pain as a result of their fears regarding narcotics. In an attempt to prevent dependence or addiction, they may increase the dose interval, withhold doses, and avoid certain medications or routes. Physical dependence and development of tolerance are anticipated potential effects that are managed easily by adjusting the dose upward according to need or, conversely, slowly decreasing the dose over time before discontinuing the narcotic.[75] Twycross and Lack[87] note that patients who receive morphine and other opioid-like drugs usually require increased doses over time, which indicates the development of tolerance. Similar studies, however, have shown that the longer a patient receives morphine therapy: (1) the rate at which the dose rises is slower; (2) the intervals between dose increases are longer; and (3) the chance that the dose will be reduced is greater (especially when optimal pain control has been achieved through combination methods).[87] Addiction (psychologic craving for a drug's psychic effects) is a phenomenon so rarely seen in cancer pain management that concern is needless.[75] This information is helpful to share with patients and families as they struggle to manage cancer pain at home.

DISCHARGE FROM HOME CARE

Critics of home care often express concern that individuals will receive care for longer periods of time than necessary and therefore that the cost effectiveness of home care may not be achieved. This rarely is the case because the overall goal of home care is to facilitate the patient and family's independence in managing daily life within the constraints imposed by the malignant disease. Furthermore, guidelines for reimbursable services are specific and well-defined so that services are discontinued or modified when the level of care required by the person changes.

The obvious reason for discontinuing home care services occurs when the patient and family have achieved the identified outcomes developed by the nurse, patient, and family. For example, a person who is being followed for wound care may be discharged from home care when it is apparent that the individual and family are demonstrating safe wound care management and can identify signs/symptoms of potential problems. This set of circumstances does not necessarily mean that the wound is healed but rather that the patient can manage independently and safely. This is particularly true in the case of severely disrupted tissue integrity for which healing is not anticipated.

A person will be discharged from the home care program when the service needs change. For instance, if professional nursing is no longer required but assistance with household tasks still is necessary, the person can be referred to more appropriate agencies to meet these needs.

Another reason for discharge is the decline of the person's health status so that family members are physically, mentally, or emotionally unable to provide care at home. In an exploratory study conducted to determine primary caregivers' perceptions of nurse behaviors that best met their needs in the home care setting, male respondents identified that an important nurse behavior was to provide assurance that the person could be readmitted to an inpatient setting if necessary.[10] Patients and families need to be assisted and supported in their decision to discontinue home care and move the patient to another setting. With increased emphasis on the home as the ideal (and financially advantageous) setting for care, families often feel as if they have failed when they decide to place the person in an extended care facility or to return the patient to the hospital. Guilt occurs even when families have done an excellent job for long periods of time. Sometimes just knowing that there are options enables a family to maintain the person at home.

A person whose status changes so that physical and comfort needs can be more effectively met in a setting other than the home should be transferred to an appropriate inpatient setting, for instance, the person with severe ascites and nausea/vomiting who becomes dehydrated. The patient can be admitted to a hospital for IV hydration and paracentesis if these procedures cannot be accomplished at home. A person with a severely compromised respiratory status (eg, respiratory rate of 50 to 60/minute) is sometimes more comfortable in the hospital where close monitoring and intravenously administered medication ease respiratory distress. There is nothing as frightening to the patient and family at home as severe respiratory difficulty.

Discharge from the home care program is planned carefully. Components of a discharge assessment include the following points:

1. What is the patient's physical/functional status? Is the individual's status stable, or can changes be anticipated in the near future? If so, the patient and/or family need to be instructed to anticipate the change.
2. Have the identified outcomes been achieved?
3. Is the care provided in the home safe and reasonable? Have modifications been incorporated to make it as simple as possible?
4. Do the individual and family feel ready to be on their own? Are resources available for them to call with their questions? Do they know what to do in an emergency?
5. Can the patient and family identify problems that require the attention of the health care team (such as signs/symptoms of hypercalcemia)?
6. What are the patient and family's needs in terms of continuing services? Are they aware of community resources?

In the evaluation of the discharge process, important points for consideration and documentation are (1) the patient's status on discharge, (2) evidence of planning for discharge, and (3) timeliness of the decision.

EVALUATING HOME CARE

Quality Assurance Program

A comprehensive quality assurance program is essential in home health care in light of the recently enacted federal regulations to monitor the quality of care (Public Law 100-203, 1987), the increased risks associated with expanded, highly technologic services, and a growing industry's need to quantify credibility.[88] A quality assurance program begins with identification and adoption of standards for home health care. Such standards have been developed by the home health regulatory bodies (eg, Department of Public Health and the Health Care Financing Administration), professional organizations (eg, American Nurses' Association and Oncology Nursing Society), credentialing organizations (eg, National League for Nursing and the Joint Commission on Accreditation of Health Care Organizations), and national organizations for home care. Home health care agencies should incorporate these standards in the development and revision of their philosophy, purpose, goals, and objectives, as well as their policies and procedures for operations. Standards that are pertinent to home care for persons with cancer include American Nurses' Association and Oncology Nursing Society's *Standards of Oncology Nursing Practice*[38] and the American Nurses' Association's *Standards of Home Health Nursing Practice.*[89]

Donabedian's model[90] for evaluation of quality examines the home care agency's organizational structure, the process of service delivery, and the outcomes of care for the level of achievement of each identified standard of care. Evaluation of the home health agency's organizational structure includes review of the agency's philosophy, goals, objectives, organizational chart, financial resources, human resources, staff education, and the community served.

The process of service delivery is regularly evaluated by most home health agencies in quarterly utilization and review committees, periodic process audits, and routine clinical record review by supervisors.[91] There is, however, a move to measure quality on the basis of client-centered outcomes, including functional assessment of the patient[92] or achievement of expected outcomes.[93] The Visiting Nurse Association of Omaha developed a comprehensive quality assurance program that evaluates client-focused domains (environmental, psychosocial, physiologic, and health-related behaviors) and signs and symptoms addressed by nurses in the community health setting.[94] These domains represent the broad areas of community health practice. One study is defining and testing the following client-centered outcome criteria: general symptom distress, discharge status, caregiver strain, functional status, physiologic indicators, and knowledge of major diagnosis/ health problems.[95] Additional studies and measures of quality of care are discussed in Chapter 53.

Documentation

Documentation is the hinge on which an effective quality assurance program hangs. We all remember that old adage, "If it is not written, it was not done." This adage can be expanded, "If it is not written appropriately, it will have the following consequences:

- Impact negatively on the agency's fulfillment of state licensure and certification requirements
- Delay or prohibit third-party reimbursement
- Place the agency at risk in a legal suit
- Reflect a negative image of the agency and the quality of care provided"

CONCLUSION

The home is an appropriate health care setting for individuals with cancer and other chronic or long-term illnesses. The number and types of home care agencies and services have increased greatly as the rising costs of health care and cost-containment measures have shifted the focus of care to alternate delivery sources and away from inpatient facilities. Society's awareness of the scope of patient needs has increased, as evidenced by the hospice movement, and more families are willing to care for their members in the home. Finally, individuals are living longer with a cancer diagnosis because of earlier detection and more effective treatment methods. The major portion of the life of a person with a diagnosis of cancer is spent in the home setting.

Home health agencies continue to expand their services and move to coordinate support services. It is anticipated that varied charge structures for different levels of care and units of care will be developed for effective use of personnel and services.

The patient and family require a range of health and social services to help maintain optimal levels of physical, psychologic, and social functioning. The nurse in the home setting has the opportunity to use his or her education and skills to the maximum in providing and directing care.

On a very human level the nurse has the privilege of entering the homes of individuals and families living with cancer at extremely critical times. The home setting provides an opportunity for full understanding of the impact of the cancer experience on the lives of those involved and allows the nurse to interact with patients and families on a level that often is difficult to achieve in other settings.

REFERENCES

1. Knollmueller RN: The growth and development of homecare: From no-tech to high-tech. Caring 3:3-8, 1985.
2. Rose MA: Home care nursing practice: The new frontier. Holistic Nurs Pract 3(2):1-8, 1989.
3. Welch D: Planning nursing interventions for family members of adult cancer patients. Cancer Nurs 4:365-369, 1981.
4. Stetz KM: Caregiving demands during advanced cancer: The spouse's needs. Cancer Nurs 10:260-268, 1987.
5. Rose MA: Problems families face in home care. Am J Nurs 75:416-418, 1976.
6. Parsons JB: A descriptive study of intermediate state terminally ill cancer patients at home. Nurs Dig 5(3):1-26, 1977.
7. Googe M, Varricchio G: A pilot investigation of home health care needs of cancer patients and their families. Oncol Nurs Forum 8(4):24-29, 1981.
8. Groebe ME, Ahmann DL, Ilstrup DM: Needs assessment for advanced cancer patients and their families. Oncol Nurs Forum 9(4):26-30, 1982.
9. Goldstein V, Regnery G, Wellin E: Caretaker role fatigue. Nurs Outlook 29:24-30, 1981.
10. Skorupka P, Bohnet N: Primary caregivers' perceptions of nursing behaviors that best meet their needs in a home care hospice setting. Cancer Nurs 5:371-374, 1982.
11. Giacquinta B: Helping families face the crisis of cancer. Am J Nurs 77:1585-1588, 1977.
12. Tolkoff-Rubin NE: Coordinated home care, the Massachusetts General Hospital experience. Med Care 16:453-464, 1978.
13. Rosenbaum E, Rosenbaum I: Home care of patients with advanced cancer. Your Patient and Cancer 2(7):86-91, 1982.
14. Baird SB: Nursing roles in continuing care: Home care and hospice. Semin Oncol 7:28-38, 1980.
15. Hays A: Family care: The critical variable in community-based long-term care. Home Healthcare Nurse 6(1):26-31, 1988.
16. Haltiwanger JK: Home health services and nursing home care—Are they competing factions or unique entities? Nurs Homes 31(1):4-7, 1982.
17. Smeltzer CH, Flores SM: Preadmission discharge planning: Organization of a concept. JONA 16(5):18-24, 1986.
18. Thobaben M: Preventing caregiver depression. Home Healthcare Nurse 5(2):42-43, 1987.
19. McKeehan K: Continuing Care: A Multidisciplinary Approach to Discharge Planning. St Louis, CV Mosby, 1981.
20. Simmons WJ: Planning for discharge with the elderly. Quality Review Board 12(2):68-71, 1986.
21. Bull MJ: Influence of diagnosis-related groups on discharge planning, professional practice, and patient care. J Prof Nurs 4:415-421, 1988.
22. Joint Commission on Accreditation of Healthcare Organizations: Nursing services, in Accreditation Manual for Hospitals. Chicago, The Commission, 1988, pp 138-139.
23. Hartigan EG: Discharge planning: Identification of high-risk groups. Nurs Management 18(12):30-32, 1987.
24. Tulga G: Bridging the gap between hospital and home. Fam Community Health 4(3):57-60, 1981.

25. Drew LA, Biordi D, Gillies DA: How discharge planners and home health nurses view their patients. Nurs Management 19(4):66-70, 1988.
26. Slevin AP, Roberts AS: Discharge planning: A tool for decision making. Nurs Management 18(12):47-50, 1987.
27. Delaney M, Trachtenberg J: Discharge planning: A quality assurance program in a cancer research hospital. Cancer Nurs 3:138-144, 1980.
28. Esper PS: Discharge planning—A quality assurance approach. Nurs Management 19(10):66-68, 1988.
29. Peters DA: A concept of nursing discharge. Holistic Nurs Pract 3(2):18-25, 1989.
30. Fashimpar GA, Grinnell RM: Homemaker–home health aides. Health Soc Work 3(1):148-165, 1978.
31. Garvey EC: Current and future nursing issues in the home administration of chemotherapy. Semin Oncol Nurs 3(2):142-147, 1987.
32. Handy CM: Home care of patients with technically complex nursing needs. Nurs Clin North Am 23:315-328, 1988.
33. Miller P: Home blood component therapy: An alternative. National Intravenous Therapy Association 9(1):213-217, 1986.
34. Pera MK, Gould EJ: Home care nursing: Integration of politics and nursing. Holistic Nurs Pract 3(2):9-17, 1989.
35. Koncel JA: Home health care can be reimbursed. Hospitals 53(20):44-45, 1979.
36. Lewis FM: Experienced personal control and quality of life in late-stage cancer patients. Nurs Res 31(2):113-119, 1982.
37. Fortinsky R, Granger C, Seltzer G: The use of functional assessment in understanding home care needs. Med Care 19:489-497, 1981.
38. American Nurses' Association and Oncology Nursing Society: Standards of Oncology Nursing Practice. Kansas City, Mo, The Association, 1987.
39. Feuer LC: Discharge planning: Home caregivers need your support, too. Nurs Management 18(4):58-59, 1987.
40. Pierangeli LP, Spencer GA: Social network discharge planning tool. Home Healthcare Nurse 5(6):38-40, 1987.
41. Speese-Owens N: Psychological components of cancer nursing, in Bouchard-Kurtz R, Speese-Owens N (eds): Nursing Care of the Cancer Patient (ed 4). St Louis, CV Mosby, 1981, pp 45-57.
42. MacVicar MG, Archbold P: A framework for family assessment in chronic illness. Nurs Forum 15(2):180-194, 1976.
43. Popkess S: Diagnosing your patient's strengths. Nursing '81, 11(7):34-37, 1981.
44. Duvall EM: Family Development. Philadelphia, JB Lippincott, 1971.
45. Siegel H: Assessing an environment for safety first. J Gerontol Nurs 8:509-518, 1982.
46. Reinhardt A, Quinn M: Family-Centered Community Nursing—A Sociocultural Framework. St Louis, CV Mosby, 1980.
47. Rehr H: Discharge planning: An ongoing function of quality care. Quality Rev Bulletin 12:47-50, 1986.
48. Pfaff SJ, Terry BA: Discharge planning—Infection prevention and control in the home. Nurs Clin North Am 15:893-908, 1980.
49. Centers for Disease Control: Update: Universal precautions for prevention of transmission of human immuno-deficiency virus, hepatitis B virus and other bloodborne pathogens. Health Care Settings. MMWR 37(24):377-382, 1988.
50. Weinstein SM: Biohazards of working with antineoplastics. Home Healthcare Nurse 5(1):30-34, 1987.
51. Gullo SM: Safe handling of antineoplastic drugs: Translating the recommendations into practice. Oncol Nurs Forum 15:595-601, 1988.
52. Barry LK, Booher RN: Promoting the responsible handling of antineoplastic agents in the community. Oncol Nurs Forum 12(5):41-46, 1985.
53. Oncology Nursing Society: Cancer Chemotherapy Guidelines. Pittsburgh, The Society, 1988.
54. Gross J, Johnson BL, Bertino JR: Possible hazards of working with cytotoxic agents: A review of the literature. Oncol Nurs Forum 8(4):10-12, 1981.
55. Cloak M, Connor TH, Stevens KR, et al: Occupational exposure of nursing personnel to antineoplastic agents. Oncol Nurs Forum 12(5):33-39, 1985.
56. Rogers B, Emmett EA: Handling antineoplastic agents: Urine mutagenicity in nurses. Image: J Nurs Scholarship 19(3):108-113, 1987.
57. Occupational Safety and Health Administration: Work practice guidelines for personnel dealing with cytotoxic (antineoplastic) drugs. OSHA Instruction pub no. 8-11. Washington, DC, Office of Occupational Medicine, Jan 29, 1986.
58. Teich CJ, Raia K: Teaching strategies for an ambulatory chemotherapy program. Oncol Nurs Forum 11(5):24-28, 1984.
59. Blackburn G: Home TPN: State of the art. Am J Intravenous Therapy Clin Nutr 11:20-32, 1984.
60. Konstantinides NW: Home parenteral nutrition: A viable alternative. Oncol Nurs Forum 12(1):23-29, 1985.
61. Dudrick SJ, O'Connell JJ, Englert DM, et al: 100 patient years of ambulatory home total parenteral nutrition. Ann Surg 199:770-781, 1984.
62. Weiss SM, Worthington PH, Prioleau M, et al: Home total parenteral nutrition in cancer patients. Cancer 50:1210-1213, 1982.
63. Dudrick SJ, Englert DM, VanBuren C, et al: New concepts of ambulatory home hyperalimentation. J Parenter Enter Nutr 3:72-76, 1979.
64. Dudrick SJ: A clinical review of nutritional support of the patient. Am J Clin Nutr 34:1191-1198, 1981.
65. Gulledge AD, Gipsom WT, Steiger E, et al: Home parenteral nutrition for the short bowel syndrome: Psychological issues. Gen Hosp Psychiatry 2:271-281, 1980.
66. Pluth NM: A home care transfusion program. Oncol Nurs Forum 14(5):43-46, 1987.
67. American Association of Blood Banks: Blood transfusions outside the hospital. Am J Nurs 89:486-489, 1989.
68. Barfoot KR, Ross KL: Intravenous therapy at home: An overview. Home Healthcare Nurse 6(4):11-13, 1988.
69. Dolbee SF, Creason NS: Outcome criteria for the patient using intravenous antibiotic therapy at home. Home Healthcare Nurse 6(4):22-29, 1988.
70. Kasmer RJ, Hoisington LM, Yukniewicz S: Home parenteral antibiotic therapy. I. An overview of program design. Home Healthcare Nurse 5(1):12-18, 1987.
71. Bontempo T, Eggland ET: Nursing implications for home parenteral therapy. Home Healthcare Nurse 6(4):14-19, 1988.
72. Kasmer RJ, Hoisington LM, Yukniewicz S: Home parenteral antibiotic therapy. II. Drug preparation and administration considerations. Home Healthcare Nurse 5(1):19-29, 1987.
73. Gorski LA: Effective teaching of home IV therapy. Home Healthcare Nurse 5(5):10-17, 1987.
74. Sheehan K, Gildea J: Home antibiotic therapy—A less than ideal candidate. National Intravenous Therapy Association 8:157-159, 1985.
75. Tartaglia MJ: The management of chronic cancer pain, principles and practices. J Intravenous Nurs 11(2):79-87, 1988.
76. Stephany T: Oral medication for pain relief. Home Healthcare Nurse 7(2):44-45, 1989.

77. Dennis EMP: An ambulatory infusion pump for pain control: A nursing approach for home care. Cancer Nurs 8:309-313, 1984.
78. Patt RB: Interventional analgesia: Epidural and subarachnoid therapy. Am J Hospice Care (March/April):11-14, 1989.
79. Lonsway RA: Care of the patient with an epidural catheter: An infection control challenge. J Intravenous Nurs 11(1):52-55, 1988.
80. Panfilli R, Brunckhorse L, Dundon R: Nursing implications of patient-controlled analgesia. J Intravenous Nurs 11(2):75-77, 1988.
81. Keeri-Szanto M: Demand analgesia for the relief of pain problems in terminal illness. Anesth Rev 2:29-31, 1987.
82. Citron ML, Early AJ, Boyer M, et al: Patient controlled analgesia for severe cancer pain. Arch Intern Med 146:734-736, 1986.
83. Mast D, Meyers J, Urbanski A: Relaxation techniques: A self-learning module for nurses, Unit I. Cancer Nurs 10:141-147, 1987.
84. Mast D, Meyers J, Urbanski A: Relaxation techniques: A self-learning module for nurses, Unit II. Cancer Nurs 10:217-225, 1987.
85. Mast D, Meyers J, Urbanski A: Relaxation techniques: A self-learning module for nurses, Unit III. Cancer Nurs 10:279-285, 1987.
86. Enck RE: Adjuvant analgesic drugs. Am J Hospice Care (March/April):9-10, 1989.
87. Twycross R, Lack S: Oral Morphine in Advanced Cancer. Bucks, UK, Beaconsfield Publishers, 1984.
88. Daniels K: Planning for quality in the home care system, in Fishen K, Gardner R (eds): Quality and Home Care: Redefining the Tradition. Chicago, The Joint Commission on Accreditation of Healthcare Organizations, 1987.
89. American Nurses' Association: Standards of Home Health Nursing Practice. Kansas City, Mo, The Association, 1986.
90. Donabedian A: Explorations in Quality Assessment and Monitoring. The Definitions of Quality and Approaches to its Assessment. Ann Arbor, Mich, Health Administration Press, 1980.
91. Sorgen LM: The development of a home care quality assurance program in Alberta. Home Health Care Serv Q 7(2):13-28, 1986.
92. Wilson AA: Measurable patient outcomes: Putting theory into practice. Home Healthcare Nurs 6(6):15-18, 1988.
93. Buck JN: Measuring the success of home health care. Home Healthcare Nurse 6(3):17-23, 1988.
94. Martin KS, Scheet NJ: The Omaha system: Providing a framework for assuring quality of home care. Home Healthcare Nurse 6(3):24-28, 1988.
95. Lalonde B: Assuring the quality of home care via the assessment of client outcomes. (Overview of research being conducted in conjunction with the Home Care Association of Seattle, Wash). Unpublished paper.

Chapter 52

Hospice Care

Candace Carter Childs, RN, MS

Mary Taverna, RN

INTRODUCTION

Hospice programs have developed in the United States in response to the developing awareness of society that dying individuals and their families need specialized and personalized care. Inherent in the hospice philosophy is the belief that care for terminally ill individuals does not cease when curative therapy is no longer appropriate. Hospice care is designed to enhance the quality of remaining life for the dying patient and family members by responding to the many physical, psychosocial, spiritual, and practical needs that accompany a terminal illness.

This chapter describes the historical perspective of hospice development, discusses the philosophy and characteristics of hospice care, and considers several model approaches to delivery of care. The role of the hospice nurse is discussed in detail, including direct patient care, teaching, counseling, bereavement follow-up, and research. Hospice staffing issues also are discussed, including desirable staff qualities and ways to help avoid staff burnout.

HISTORICAL PERSPECTIVE

Researchers such as Quint,[1] Sudnow,[2] and Kübler-Ross[3] studied the type of care offered to dying individuals in the United States and the circumstances surrounding death. Care often was found to be impersonal, inappropriate, or inadequate to meet the many needs of terminally ill individuals and their families. The resulting explosion of interest in the care provided dying persons has led to many improvements and innovative approaches to sensitive and difficult problems. With increasing frequency, members of the health professions, as well as the lay public, agree with Stoddard,[4] who writes that "it is a modern and ignorant prejudice to consider death a failure."

Hospice care programs are designed specifically to offer unique care to terminally ill individuals and their families. Unburdened by the restrictions of acute care hospitals, hospice programs can fulfill what Craven and Wald[5] describe as the most important needs of the dying: "relief from the distressing symptoms of their disease, the security of a caring environment, sustained expert care, and the reassurance they and their families won't be abandoned." The goal of hospice care is to help each person live the remainder of his or her life to the fullest, surrounded by loved ones and free from pain.

Many individuals with a diagnosis of cancer choose to continue with every possible aggressive/curative treatment measure until the last few days of life. With increasing frequency, however, people are reconsidering the balance between quality of life and quantity of life. Choosing hospice care does not rule out palliative treatment to enhance comfort and improve the quality of the patient's life.

The hospice concept originated in the time of the Crusades or Holy Wars, when men, women, and children left home in large numbers on pilgrimages. In response to the illness and fatigue experienced by these travelers, way stations were established, often by religious groups. These medieval hospices served as both hotel and hospital, providing care for travelers, as well as for the sick, destitute, or dying.

The concept of hospice is deeply rooted in the Christian tradition of caring for one's neighbor as for oneself and the belief in the innate value of each human life. It is not surprising that religious orders are among the pioneers of hospice work and have continued this work to the present. Mother Mary Aikenhead founded the Irish Sisters of Charity in 1815 in Dublin. The Sisters combined nursing skills with concern for the spiritual care of every person, and Mother Mary's philosophy of care continues today at St. Joseph's Hospice in London.

In 1967, after working and training at St. Joseph's, Cicely Saunders established the now well-known English hospice, St. Christopher's in London.[6] Dr. Saunders, who is a physician, nurse, and social worker, serves as the medical director of this 62-bed facility. St. Christopher's is regarded as the prototype of excellence in care for the dying by providing total care that includes attention to any problem that causes a patient or family distress, whether physical, psychological, social, or spiritual. In a warm and loving atmosphere, patients are aided by a mutually supportive, interdisciplinary team to live fully and comfortably until death or discharge to the home care (domiciliary) program. Dr. Saunders and her staff pioneered and successfully demonstrated pain and symptom control techniques, developed philosophies for the care of patient and family units, including bereavement follow-up, and served as teachers for hundreds of visitors and students studying the hospice philosophy.

In the United States the hospice movement proliferated rapidly during the past decade. With a strong base of support from the principles identified in Great Britain, the numbers grew from only one hospice in 1974 to nearly 1600 hospices by the end of 1988.[7] Hospices now are located in every state and serve thousands of patients and families in rural, suburban, and urban settings. Primarily, hospice care in the United States is delivered at home. There are four types of hospice: hospital based, community based, home care agency based, or affiliated with a skilled nursing facility; all, however, subscribe to the basic principles of specific and continuous care to the dying, delivering similar services from different bases. Strong grassroots support for the hospice movement has translated into a greater involvement by volunteers in US hospices. Thus a social movement that started tentatively less than two decades ago now has become an essential part of the health care delivery system in the United States. Hospice has been welcomed for its principles, appropriateness, and cost effectiveness.

PHILOSOPHY AND PRACTICE OF HOSPICE CARE

In Europe, hospice generally refers to a place or facility such as St. Christopher's or St. Joseph's in London. Caregivers in the United States studied the European models and then adapted the basic hospice philosophy to the varied circumstances of their communities. Therefore, in the United States, hospice refers to a philosophy of care rather than to an institution or particular setting.

Hospice can be defined as a coordinated program of palliative and supportive services provided in both home and inpatient settings that offers physical, psychological, social, and spiritual care for dying persons and their families. Care is given by a medically directed interdisciplinary team of professionals and volunteers.[8] The team can be composed of the following primary and auxiliary members:

- *Primary members,* including attending and hospice physicians, nurse team coordinator, primary nurse, community/admissions nurse, bereavement services coordinator, counselor, social worker, chaplain and volunteer coordinator
- *Auxiliary members,* including per diem nurses, home health aides, homemakers, dietitians, physical therapists, occupational therapists, speech/language pathologists, and volunteers

Because no single person can meet the total needs of a patient or family, true teamwork of a nurse-coordinated interdisciplinary care team is essential. The nurse assumes responsibility for case management and assesses the patient/family needs. The nurse's initial assessment is aided by a similar assessment conducted by a mental health professional. Together the nurse and social worker determine the most appropriate care and services to be provided. The nurse is responsible for committing the plan to paper, obtaining additional input and guidance from the attending physician, implementing the plan, and ensuring that the care and services are delivered in a timely and effective manner. Most teams meet on a weekly basis to review the plan of care, consider new symptoms, and develop ongoing treatment plan goals.

Trained volunteers can offer valuable support to the family such as providing respite to family caregivers, helping with household chores, running errands, or simply befriending the person who is ill. Volunteers are particularly helpful to the family in offering them a break from the constancy of caregiving.

A primary goal of hospice care is symptom control, including attention to physical, emotional, and spiritual needs. Severe pain and physical symptoms can be controlled and comfort provided in nearly all cases by means of current medical and nursing knowledge and skills. In addition, many patients continue to receive active palliative treatment of the cancer until the very last stages of the disease. Emotional support for both the individual and family considerably reduces stress and anxiety, enhances comfort, and provides an atmosphere of honesty and security. Spiritual needs must never be forgotten. It is the responsibility of all team members to respect the individual's personal beliefs and to help with spiritual concerns as they arise. Each person's physical, emotional, and spiritual needs can constantly change, and the team should be attentive to subtleties and react appropriately.

Because concerns or crises can arise during the night or on weekends, as well as during weekdays, hospice services are available 24 hours a day and 7 days a week. Continual availability involves a tremendous obligation and coordinating effort by the nurse and staff members who are on call for the hospice. It is important to provide support and care whenever needed and to call in other team members if necessary.

A distinguishing characteristic of hospice care is follow-up care in the bereavement period. Staff involvement with the family does not stop with the patient's death but continues throughout the bereavement depending on family needs and resources. Because strong emotional reactions often are evidenced on birthdays, holidays, or the 1-year anniversary of the death, the availability of hospice team members may be critical.

Ongoing support for the hospice care team is critical and includes formal and informal methods for mutual support and evaluation. Hospice work can be as draining as it is rewarding. It is important to be aware of each staff member's emotional state and provide critical support as needed on a day-to-day basis. Development of a caring hospice community includes caring for each other as well as for the patients.

TYPES OF PROGRAMS

Several different types of hospice programs have developed in response to varying community resources and needs. The particular needs of each community should be assessed carefully and existing resources and programs explored before implementing a hospice program. Most hospice programs can be categorized into three general administrative types: community-based or free-standing, home health agency–based, and institution-based (mainly hospital based).

Institution-based hospices are owned and governed by acute care or skilled nursing facilities. Home health agency–based hospices are usually part of established home care agencies or departments that also provide traditional home health services. The community-based or free-standing hospices are independent, most often non-profit organizations governed by community boards.

The hospice concept can be organized effectively through other administrative forms, such as coalitions of providers working together; regional hospice networks of multiple organizations; small, predominantly volunteer programs located in more rural areas; hospices participating as affiliates or subsidiaries of larger health care networks or corporations; and a parent organization operating a chain of hospices. Most hospices currently operate on a not-for-profit basis, although there are a growing number of for-profit ventures.[9]

There has been a distinct trend away from hospitalization of the terminally ill, with an increasing demand for alternative care programs to support the dying person. Consequently, many hospice programs in this country began as home care programs rather than through inpatient facilities as they did in Europe. A survey by the Joint Commission on Accreditation of Healthcare Organizations (the Joint Commission) in 1982 stated that 40% (457) of 1145 established hospices were hospital-based and 60% (688) were community-based home care programs.[10] More recently the National Hospice Organization (NHO) reported that 31% of hospices are hospital-based, 21% are home health agency–based, 41% are independent, and the remainder are coalitions (personal conversation, Ira Bates, NHO, April 1989). It seems likely that the trend toward hospice care will continue in view of escalating health care cost-containment efforts.

Advantages of hospice home care for the patient are significant. First and most important, the individual and family are in control and can direct activities of daily life to achieve maximum comfort and satisfaction. They do not have to worry about schedules, tests, treatments, interruptions, and unfamiliar food. Second, the environment is familiar and contributes to both security and comfort. Sleep and pain control are easier to achieve with the familiar routines of sleeping in one's own bed, wearing one's own clothes, and perhaps having the family pet nearby. Third, family and friends are more available without limits to visiting hours except for those imposed by the patient or family. The person with cancer can be a part of the ongoing life at home. Many patients in hospice programs have their beds set up in family or living rooms where they can observe daily activities and possibly participate, even if only by listening.

Home care necessitates the active involvement of family members, thus increasing their awareness of their loved one's status and encouraging anticipatory grieving. Participation by family members may lead to feelings of extreme satisfaction and facilitate the grieving process as family members gain awareness and anticipate their feelings of loss. Active involvement may decrease family members' feelings of helplessness and focus attention on anticipatory problem solving. It also fosters an openness to assistance that may enable family members to accept support in their grief process. However, with home care the demands and responsibilities on the family are great. The hospice team's role is to mobilize and augment the resources available to the family. When home care is not feasible, the team helps evaluate the options for relocating the patient and continuing support and services as appropriate.

The cost advantage of home care is important. The financial savings of home care can be significant, even if part-time caregivers are employed to help with the nursing care. Many insurance carriers are offering more extensive coverage of home care, thus further reducing the financial burden of cancer care.

Additional experience, evaluation, and research are necessary to compile a more complete picture of which hospice approaches prove most successful, although the method of delivery of hospice care most likely always will be related to the unique needs and resources of each community. The type of hospice that provides the care is not as important as compliance with the basic philosophy of hospice care that seeks to support each patient and family as the person with cancer faces the ultimate experience—death.

STANDARDS OF HOSPICE CARE

The NHO, the largest hospice specialty organization in the United States, identified development of standards of care as one of its purposes. In the mid-1970s, as hospices were just beginning in the United States, leaders were already working on standards, and in 1978 the initial standards of care for hospice were adopted by NHO. These standards, designed to ensure the quality of hospice programs, were revised in 1983 and 1987. The NHO standards for a hospice program are listed in Table 52-1.[8]

There is concern regarding possible exploitation of the hospice concept through renaming hospital units, convalescent homes, or residential care centers "hospices" without incorporating the essential standards into a total care program. Great care must be taken to protect the basic hospice philosophy to ensure the public and health care payers of a legitimate service. In 1983 the Joint Commission, in close cooperation with hospice providers, focusing on quality and continuity of care, established standards and a voluntary accreditation procedure for hospice programs. Compliance with standards for every aspect of hospice care is being monitored by the Joint Commission, and standards are being refined as appropriate on the basis of data gathered during the accreditation process and the further development of programs. To date 380 hospice programs have secured accreditation (B. McCann, personal communication, The Joint Commission, April 1989).

The NHO was developed in 1978 as a national coordinating body and information clearinghouse. Annual meetings provide a forum for information sharing and a national voice in support of the hospice movement. The purposes of the NHO are as follows[11]:

1. To develop a clear understanding of the hospice concept among health care professionals as well as the public
2. To provide for a steady flow of information and communication among existing hospice groups and others that are evolving
3. To develop and maintain standards of care in program planning and implementation

4. To provide technical assistance to hospice organizations in their formative years and to evaluate their programs
5. To make available basic training materials to assist new groups and their boards, members, and volunteers
6. To monitor health care legislation and regulation at all government levels relevant to the hospice movement

FUNDING

Financial considerations and reimbursement matters are of great concern, both to the development and future of hospice programs. Before 1982, hospice services were generally nonreimbursable. Philanthropic support was key to

TABLE 52-1 Standards of a Hospice Program of Care: National Hospice Organization

1. The hospice program establishes and maintains appropriate reports, policies and procedures to assure that the hospice is accountable to the community for the services it provides.
2. The hospice program complies with applicable local, state, and federal laws and regulations governing the organization and delivery of health care to patients and families.
3. Access to hospice medical and nursing services is available to identified hospice patients on a 24-hour basis, 7 days a week. During hours covered by on-call staff, hospices provide for at least a minimum of medical and nursing coverage with visit capability should further assessment or treatment be needed. Provisions are made to assure that on-call staff are informed and updated regarding care plans and level of care. Reporting mechanisms are in place to assure continuity and coordination among members of the hospice interdisciplinary team.
4. The hospice program has admission criteria that reflect the patient/family's desire and need for hospice care; the extent and role of physician participation; and diagnosis and prognosis. To the maximum extent possible, the hospice program will admit patients regardless of their diagnosis or ability to pay for services.
5. The hospice program organizes its services to respond to patient/family needs whenever they arise. It provides both structure and staff to ensure continuation of the hospice care plan in all settings (home and inpatient).
6. Access to hospice inpatient care is available either directly by the hospice or through contract or arrangement with an inpatient facility. This hospice inpatient unit must comply with all applicable local, state and federal regulations including fire and safety code regulations.
7. At a minimum, the hospice inpatient unit provides for: medical direction and coverage for all patients either directly or through agreement with the patient's personal physician; staffing coverage by an interdisciplinary team available to meet the needs of the patient/family on a 24-hour basis as needed; and, specific policies and procedures, as well as personal comfort amenities and courtesies that support and encourage a non-institutional, "home-like" environment for the patient/family. All hospice inpatient personnel must be appropriately trained in the provision of hospice interdisciplinary team care.
8. The patient/family is the unit of care in hospice and support is provided to both the patient and the family. The hospice program encourages patient/family participation in the development of the interdisciplinary team plan of care and in the provision of hospice services.
9. The hospice program acknowledges that each patient/family has its own values and beliefs and is respectful of them.
10. The hospice program seeks to identify, teach, coordinate and supervise those persons acting as primary caregivers for the patient. If a primary care person is not available, the hospice program seeks to develop a substitute network. If the hospice program does not accept patients without primary caregivers, then it must provide adequate information about community resources available to them.
11. The goal of hospice care is to provide optimum relief of pain and control of symptoms through appropriate palliative therapies.
12. Symptom control includes assessing and responding to the physical, emotional, social and spiritual needs of the patient/family.
13. A hospice program offers volunteer support to each patient/family admitted to its program of care.
14. A hospice program has an organized training program and procedures for the selection, supervision and continuing evaluation of volunteers.
15. The hospice identifies and maintains an appropriately qualified interdisciplinary team of health professionals and lay persons.
16. Emotional support for staff/volunteers is provided as an integral part of a hospice program.
17. Inservice training and continuing education are offered on a regular basis to both paid and volunteer staff.

TABLE 52-1 Standards of a Hospice Program of Care: National Hospice Organization (continued)

18. The hospice program has a written, interdisciplinary team plan of care for each patient/family unit that includes assessments, identified problems, proposed interventions, level and frequency of services, and their outcomes.
19. The hospice program maintains accurate, current, integrated clinical records for all patient/family units and provides assurances for the confidentiality of these records.
20. These clinical records must include a signed informed consent form completed by the patient or a designated representative. The consent form must inform the patient/family of the palliative nature of hospice care; the avoidance, if at all possible, of injections, diagnostic testing and curative measures; and the non-use of heroic measures to prolong the dying process.
21. These clinical records must include specific, signed instructions regarding actions to be taken when life-threatening situations occur to the patient. These instructions should be prepared by the physician and the interdisciplinary team following consultation with the patient/family and must be consistent with the patient/family's wishes.
22. The hospice program provides bereavement services to the surviving family members for at least one year after the death of the patient.
23. The hospice program maintains a process of risk assessment for surviving family members that identifies those individuals at risk of pathological grief. For those individuals at high risk, appropriate referrals are made to mental health professionals in the community.
24. The hospice program has quality assurance and utilization review programs that include the following: statement of goals and objectives and established policies for conducting an ongoing assessment program that reflects the interdisciplinary nature of hospice services; designation of person(s) responsible for implementing policies and procedures; provisions for addressing specific problems identified in the quality assurance and utilization review process.
25. At a minimum, the hospice program conducts on a regular basis the following activities: evaluation of services provided by both professionals and volunteers, audit of patient charts for outcomes of interventions, organizational review of hospice program, interdisciplinary team care plan review, evaluations provided by patient/families of care received, and review of appropriate/inappropriate use of services, facilities and personnel.

From National Hospice Organization: Meeting the Challenge for a *Special* Kind of Caring: Standards of a Hospice Program of Care Recommended by the National Hospice Organization (position paper). Arlington, Va, The Organization, 1987.

covering the more limited profile of hospice services offered in the late 1970s and early 1980s.

In 1980 Congress commissioned the National Hospice Study to develop a knowledge base from which to make legislative decisions about hospice. The study was conducted by the Health Care Financing Administration (HCFA). Twenty-six hospices participated as demonstration sites and were funded for virtually all previously nonreimbursed hospice services, including home nursing care, outpatient drugs, and bereavement visits. These 26 funded hospices were compared with 14 nonfunded hospices and 14 traditional care settings in terms of psychosocial, physical, and financial progress of the patients enrolled in the programs. Even before publication of the final report, national hospice leaders were working with Congress to establish Medicare coverage for hospice care. This study contributed to enactment of the Hospice Medicare Benefit. The findings supported the cost savings associated with the delivery of hospice care.[12]

In 1982 Congress included in the Tax Equity and Fiscal Responsibility Act (TEFRA) benefits for Medicare-eligible individuals who were medically certified as terminally ill (6 months or less to live). Presently, about 41% of hospice programs in the United States are certified as providers of the Medicare hospice benefit (personal communication, Ira Bates, NHO, 1989). The key elements of the law are as follows:

1. The certified hospice program is responsible for all elements of care. Nursing, physician, medical, social, and counseling services must be provided directly by the hospice interdisciplinary team who are required to be employees of the hospice program. Supplemental services, for example, inpatient services (general and respite) related to the terminal illness, are also the financial and clinical responsibility of the hospice program. Bereavement care is required but is not reimbursed. Volunteers must be represented as part of the interdisciplinary team.

2. There is no limit to the days covered as long as the physician certifies that the patient has a limited life expectancy of 6 months or less. Days are broken up into four special benefit periods (two 90-day, one 30-day, and a new open-ended fourth period). If a patient chooses hospice care but then later decides not to use it, he or she can cancel it any time and resume standard hospital benefits under Medicare Part A. If cancellation is made before the end of a hospice period, any days left in that period are forfeited, but the patient still is eligible for any remaining hospice periods. For example, if a patient cancels at the end of 60 days in the first 90-day period, he or she loses the remaining 30 days. However, the patient is still eligible at a future time for the remaining periods. Cancellation within the fourth period would render the patient ineligible for any further hospice benefit.

3. Hospices are paid directly by Medicare for services provided. Patients who are eligible under Medicare for hospice benefits cannot be billed for any services, drugs, or equipment related to the terminal illness except as follows: Hospices are authorized to charge patients the minimal amount of 5% of the cost for (1) each outpatient prescription for pain relief and symptom management and (2) short-term inpatient respite care.

Today, hospice benefits have become the rule rather than the exception for the insurance industry. Most major and many smaller insurance companies provide hospice benefits. However, hospice care providers, in seeking reimbursement, experience inconsistent reimbursement policies by these companies, which often are unfamiliar with the hospice concept and services.[13]

Hospice coverage by private insurance companies can be difficult to evaluate because of the myriad plans offered by different companies. Although this patchwork quilt of coverage and exclusions may be confusing, the good news is that coverage may not necessarily be limited to what is explicitly stated in the benefit. In fact, many hospice care providers are able to maximize private insurance reimbursement by negotiating modifications or alternative approaches with payers. As long as the hospice can demonstrate that an alternative approach or customized coverage will prevent expensive hospitalizations, thereby reducing health care costs, payers can be flexible in considering and authorizing coverage and payment more in line with the hospice's actual costs and services.[13]

Hospice leaders encourage private insurance companies to convert from the per visit, fee-for-service reimbursement method to a per diem basis following the Medicare hospice benefit model. Those involved in hospice work believe that this method offers several advantages. First, patient/family needs can be responded to individually, enabling the hospice team to work in a flexible and authoritative manner as under the Medicare benefit. Second, a case management approach, which leads to quality of care and cost-effective methods, is encouraged. Third, the billing process is simplified for the provider, patient/family, and payer.

The preceding discussion of administrative information, although essential, serves only to establish the setting and methods by which hospice care can be delivered to those who seek this alternative. In delivering this care, the hospice nurse is key. Hospice nurses have provided not only bedside care but also have administered hospice programs and provided national leadership, and the major portion of this chapter will be devoted to the nurse's role.

ROLE OF THE HOSPICE NURSE

With an interdisciplinary team structure, care is provided at our hospice program (Hospice of Marin) by two nurse-managed teams, each composed of a nurse team leader, staff nurses, a counselor, home health aides, and a homemaker. The team's function is to provide comprehensive care to patients. The primary nurse performs the functions of case management and direct care. The team meets at the beginning and end of each work day to exchange information and to plan visits.

Weekly interdisciplinary team meetings include the hospice medical director, chaplain, volunteer coordinator, bereavement services coordinator, and patient services manager. The team meetings allow staff members to review case developments, revise the plan of care, develop new approaches to problem areas, and provide team input to each plan of care. Role divisions among physicians, nurses, counselors, home health aides, and homemakers tend to blur with the team approach, thus helping to diffuse patient responsibility to a team rather than placing it on one individual.

The critical responsibility for coordination of services between the home, hospital, or extended care facility rests with the hospice nurse. Hospice nursing is truly an opportunity to practice in an expanded role, caring for the entire family as well as responding to the holistic needs of the patients. Nurses and other members of the interdisciplinary team are offered an immense challenge: they use their human skills in conjunction with their technical skills to assist families in a time of crisis. It is particularly important for hospice caregivers to remember that the individual with a diagnosis of cancer is a member of a family or community in addition to being a patient. Family members will have questions, fears, and feelings of loss. They will need support, practical assistance, and emotional care as they provide care for the terminally ill individual. Every family member is affected by long-term illness; efforts must be made to support those who are experiencing the dying process of a loved one.

The key staff position in any hospice program regardless of size, type, or location is the hospice nurse. The hospice nurse is a case manager as well as a provider of care. Case management is a system of care that incorporates health assessment; planning, procurement, delivery, and coordination of services; and monitoring to ensure that the multiple service needs of the client are met.[14] Case management is a particularly useful approach to the complex care of hospice patients or chronically ill patients who receive care at home.

The goals of case management are "provision of quality health care along a continuum, decreased fragmentation of care across many settings, enhancement of client's quality of life, and cost containment."[14] Hospice patients are ill, often elderly or in crisis, with complex medical, social, spiritual, and psychological needs. Case management enhances the provision of care in the least restrictive environment—the patient's home—and can prevent unnecessary institutionalization. The hospice team can serve as the client's advocate across varied settings and multiple providers. The hospice philosophy and program are totally oriented toward quality of life for the patient.

Hospice nursing has many facets, all of which come into prominence at different times in the care of terminally ill individuals. Certain aspects of the role illustrate the wide scope of care hospice nursing encompasses. The nursing role includes (1) direct patient care, (2) teaching, (3) counseling, (4) bereavement follow-up, and (5) research/evaluation.

Direct Patient Care

Direct patient care includes symptom and pain control as well as physical care for the patient, both of which are priorities for the patient and family. In interviews conducted with 115 individuals being treated for cancer at a large university teaching hospital, researchers found that patients cited medical control of symptoms as most important in a list of 10 services available through a hospice program. The other important services identified were home nursing care and psychological counseling.[15]

Pain is often a problem for people with cancer, although not all individuals with cancer experience pain. For patients with chronic pain, every effort must be made to alleviate their discomfort and minimize other distressing symptoms. Hospice health care professionals have developed effective principles and methods of pain control, such as scheduled administration of narcotics rather than administration on a demand basis (see Chapter 11). Other discomforts associated with pain control measures or the cancer process, such as constipation, nausea, fatigue, anxiety, and sedation, are important priorities for the nurse to address in the individual's plan of care (Table 52-2[16]).

In addition to symptom and pain control, direct patient care includes physical care. Comfort care best describes the focus of physical care for the terminally ill. The family or employed caregivers usually prefer to give the physical care, but the hospice nurse occasionally is needed to change dressings, insert an indwelling catheter, give an enema, aid with a linen change, or otherwise provide the care needed to maintain comfort. The nurse also assesses the patient's need for medical equipment and makes arrangements for its delivery. Patience, gentleness, and respect for modesty are important in providing physical care. Hands-on care is a special part of nursing, and in the hospice setting it helps develop a trusting bond between the nurse and patient.

To recognize or prevent the development of serious physical problems, careful evaluation of the patient's physical status is essential. The frequency of home visits and communication with the primary physician increase as the patient's health declines. Consistently assessing appetite, bowel activity, comfort level, mobility, new symptoms, and emotional status helps the team evaluate the progress of each patient and suggest measures that might be offered to relieve any distress.

Nurses are the primary professionals responsible for assessing the problems, planning and implementing a care plan, evaluating the effect of interventions, and working with the hospice team to achieve maximum patient comfort.

Patient-Family Teaching

Patient and family involvement in care is one of the most beneficial aspects of a hospice home care program. Most individuals prefer to remain independent and care for themselves as long as possible. However, when the dying patient no longer can manage self-care, the family needs careful instruction and preparation, as well as constant support from nurses who are available whenever needed (24 hours a day) and who are skilled in the challenges of home care. Most families, given the necessary support, can cope with the demands of home care; 95% of the patients who have received care from the Hospice of Marin die at home.

Experience at our hospice indicates that initial assessment includes identification of the family members who will require concentrated teaching efforts in particular areas. Sometimes one family member will carry out the majority of the patient care while another member may prefer to keep the house running smoothly. Sometimes the primary caregiver is unable or unwilling to give physical care. If so, it is necessary to discuss alternatives such as employing caregivers. It is also important to discuss openly the decision to help alleviate that family member's guilt over not being able to provide the care. Each family member differs in the degree to which he or she wishes to be involved. Hospice nurses should respect these differences and support whatever level of involvement each family member chooses. Each person has unique talents to contribute, from that special massage to bringing home a colorful picture as a present.

Repetition, role modeling, and reinforcement are crucial in teaching patient care. First, a concept is explained in lay terms, possibly many times, depending on learner readiness; second, that concept is demonstrated to the family; and third, plenty of positive reinforcement is given to the caregivers when the task is accomplished. These elements keep recurring throughout the course of a person's illness as the nurse explains, demonstrates, and constantly reinforces the efforts of the caregivers. The family may not adhere to the suggested schedule of care or provide care as efficiently as nurses, but the benefits of having control over the daily routine and the warmth and personal concern of family caregivers seem to far outweigh any criticism of home nursing skills.

Good basic nursing care is timeless; the principles rarely change. For example, transferring from a bed to wheelchair or wheelchair to car often is a difficult problem because of the patient's pain or weakness. One patient explained to the hospice nurse that she could not go to see her doctor because of difficulty in getting into the car. A short lesson in transfer technique alleviated the problem, and she was on her way to her appointment.

TABLE 52-2 Nursing Care for Symptom Control Management

Problem	Nursing Diagnosis	Intervention
Elimination	• Alteration in bowel elimination (constipation) related to Medication reaction Poor fluid/dietary intake Immobility	Add bran or prunes to diet to add bulk. Increase fluid intake, particularly fruit juices. Stool softeners such as docusate (eg, Colace) and lactulose, and laxatives (Milk of Magnesia) help constipation. Stimulants such as bisacodyl (Dulcolax) tabs or suppositories and senna (Senokot) are useful. Prevention of constipation through a daily bowel regimen is preferable to enemas for impactions. Bulk laxatives are not recommended for constipation as they depend on large fluid intakes to be effective; they can cause impaction, especially in persons receiving opiates.
	• Alteration in bowel elimination (diarrhea) related to Impaction Disease process	For diarrhea, check first for fecal impaction, and remove. Metamucil may absorb excess fluid, causing watery stools. Kaolin/pectin (Kaopectate), diphenoxylate/atropine (Lomotil), or paregoric may be necessary for persistent diarrhea. Frequent skin care after incontinent stools is mandatory to prevent ulceration and pain; any good barrier such as Sween cream protects sensitive skin.
	• Alteration in bowel elimination related to Obstruction Incontinence as a result of Weakened state Semicomatose/comatose state	No laxatives are recommended in the case of obstruction. High-dose stool softeners in subacute instances; antispasmodics and antiemetics in intractable obstruction. Nasogastric tubes not needed.
Ventilation/respiration	• Ineffective airway clearance related to inability to eliminate secretions • Impaired gas exchange related to shortness of breath • Alteration in tissue perfusion related to respiratory distress syndrome • Ineffective breathing pattern related to Dysphagia Pain Rales/rhonchi Obstruction Semicomotose/comatose state	Positioning, head elevation, use of oxygen Suppression of chronic coughs with a narcotic such as codeine 15 to 60 mg q 4-6h Humidified air Routine use of suction machine is not necessary but may be of use in special circumstances. "Death rattles": explanation to family and use of transdermal scopolamine, which dries secretions, potentiates analgesia, and provides some sedation. The patch can be cut to tailor dose and can be left in place for 3 days. Hiccoughs: chlorpromazine (Thorazine) 25-50 mg q4-6h, or diazepam (Valium) 5-10 mg po q4-6h, or metoclopramide (Reglan) 10-20 mg q6-8h po. Drug therapy: opiates, aminophylline, diazepam, bronchodilators, diuretics.
Problems of the mouth	• Alteration in comfort related to stomatitis caused by Dehydration Continuous mouth breathing Local trauma	*For oral pain:* Several times a day before eating, have patient swish and swallow a mixture of magnesium hydroxide (Mylanta), diphenhydramine (Benadryl), and lidocaine (Xylocaine 2% viscous) and avoid alcohol and smoking. *For oral dryness:* Ice chips, hard candy, artificial saliva, and petroleum jelly (Vaseline) or mineral oil for dry lips. Can use syringe for delivery of small amounts of fluids.
	• Alteration in oral mucosa related to disease caused by Impaired immune system Decreased protein intake • Alteration in oral mucosa related to effects of treatment: Chemotherapy Radiation Administration of continuous oxygen	*For oral thrush infection:* Nystatin (Mycostatin) oral suspension or systemic ketoconazole (Nizoral) *For mouth care:* Toothettes instead of toothbrushes. May use simple solution of hydrogen peroxide and normal saline (1:4) for cleaning if no open sores are present. Full-strength baking soda or added to water is excellent for cleansing dried secretions from teeth and oral mucosa.

TABLE 52-2 Nursing Care for Symptom Control Management (continued)

Problem	Nursing Diagnosis	Intervention
Anorexia	• Alteration in nutritional intake (less than body requirement) related to	In debilitated persons the appetite is decreased, yet the need for caregivers to feed is great. The hospice team can help family members learn to accept a dying person's lessening interest in food and tailor their actions appropriately.
	Nausea and vomiting as a result of Chemotherapy Medication interactions Obstructions in gastrointestinal tract Anxiety	Control nausea/vomiting with regular administration of phenothiazines (oral or suppository) or metoclopramide (Reglan), or corticosteroids.
	Altered taste as a result of Dysphagia Weakness Depression	Capitalize on high nutritional intake (protein and calories) during patient's best meal. Serve several small meals daily instead of traditional three; serve small portions on small plates. Socialize with patient during meals amid pleasant surroundings. Replace bedside water with fruit nectar or milkshakes for increased calories. Replace distasteful foods (often meats) with other protein sources such as eggs, cheese, fish, or chicken. A small cocktail before mealtime may help stimulate the appetite.
Skin impairment	• Impairment of skin integrity related to immobility	Cushion bony prominences. Turn immobile patients q2h. Massage reddened areas to promote circulation.
	• Potential for impaired skin integrity related to symptoms of disease such as Urinary incontinence Sweating Cachexia	Keep bed clothes clean, dry, and smooth, changing incontinent patients frequently. Sheepskins, egg-crate, foam mattresses, water beds, and alternating-pressure mattresses assist in preventing skin breakdown.
	Fungating tumors	Fungating wounds such as in breast cancer require special attention because of noxious odors. Plain yogurt spread over the wound may change the flora and decrease odor. Some patients require systemic antibiotics such as cephalexin (Keflex) or tetracycline 250 mg, one tablet a day to eliminate odor. Radiation therapy, hormones, and chemotherapy also may palliate fungating lesions.
	• Potential for impairment of skin integrity related to complications of treatment Reactions to medications	Oral antihistamines may benefit intense itching. These include diphenhydramine (Benadryl) 25-50 mg po q6h; hydroxyzine (Atarax) 25-50 mg po q6-8h; or cyproheptadine (Periactin) 4 mg po q6-8h. Diazepam (Valium) may be indicated for some patients. Topical applications of lanolin, Alpha-Keri, or hydrocortisone ointment 1% may provide temporary relief.
	• Poor tissue perfusion related to Infrequent turning/repositioning Circulatory impairment • Alteration in comfort (pain/inflammation/edema) related to Immobility Poor turning/positioning Poor dressing technique	If infected, decubitus ulcers should be cleansed with povidone-iodine (Betadine) or other antiseptic, dried and covered with Op-site or Tegaderm. Betadine or peroxide are not recommended as general cleansers because they interfere with epithelialization. It is best to cleanse with clear water and then apply covering; leave the semipermeable membrane dressing in place as long as possible until it begins to come off by itself.
Fluid balance	• Potential or actual fluid volume deficit related to Low fluid intake as a result of weakness Fever Reduced extracellular fluid volume Dysphagia Gastrointestinal fluid losses Oliguria Polyuria	For dehydration, force oral fluids and/or decrease or eliminate medication that promotes diuresis.

TABLE 52-2 Nursing Care for Symptom Control Management (continued)

Problem	Nursing Diagnosis	Intervention
	• Alteration in fluid volume related to Altered cardiac output Effects of medication	Oral hyperglycemic medications may control corticosteroid-induced diabetic polyuria
	• Potential for skin integrity impairment related to edema	For edema, elevation of swollen extremities is important. Diuretics may help with edema and ascites. Paracentesis may alleviate discomfort from ascites. Nursing support and teaching to caregivers will help in the success of preventive measures such as fluid restrictions or fluid-forcing.
Rest and sleep	• Sleep pattern disturbance related to Fear of dying Uncertainty about future Pain Shortness of breath Metabolic effects of disease Drug interactions/untoward drug reactions Night sweats Restlessness Depression	Family or patient emotional support or counseling may help with anxiety or depression. A tricyclic antidepressant such as amitriptyline (Elavil) may help alleviate depression and promote sleep. Anxiety may be relieved by the use of diazepam (Valium) on a regular or as-needed schedule. Doxepin (Sinequan) or lorazepam (Ativan) 1-2 mg several times a day or at bedtime, also may help. If patient is receiving narcotics, flurazepam (Dalmane) is useful for sleep rather than a barbiturate that could interact with a narcotic. Back rubs, warm milk, and proper positioning promote relaxation. The hospice team can address financial or spiritual problems that may be contributing to insomnia. Restlessness may be controlled with chlorpromazine (Thorazine) given in small doses (10-15 mg po) during the day and larger doses (50-100 mg po) at night. Hallucinations that prevent sleep usually are eliminated by the administration of chlorpromazine (Thorazine) or haloperidol (Haldol). Pain control narcotics may need to be changed if they cause hallucinations.
Elimination of urine	• Alterations in urinary elimination patterns related to Reaction to medications Obstruction of the urinary tract Reduced fluid intake Nausea • Potential for urinary tract infection related to Reaction to medication Urinary retention	Conservative measures include warm compresses to the perineum, gentle compression of the bladder, and running water within earshot of the patient to trigger voiding.
	• Knowledge deficit related to Purpose of Foley catheter Intake and output Infection Catheterization equipment • Potential for injury related to Poor catheterization technique Poor handwashing technique Skin breakdown Poor irrigation technique • Ineffective individual/family coping related to Catheter discomfort Dependence on others for care • Actual/potential skin integrity related to Catheter leakage Poor personal hygiene Tape allergy Infection	Teach correct methods for care of catheter, bag, and urinary meatus. Leave handouts in the home for caregivers. Teach proper irrigation techniques and proper handwashing. Condom catheters for male patients may help with urinary frequency. Anticholinergic drugs also may be useful. Caregiver competency with Foley care tasks can prevent panic calls when problems occur at night or on weekends.

TABLE 52-2 Nursing Care for Symptom Control Management (continued)

Problem	Nursing Diagnosis	Intervention
Body movement	• Impaired physical mobility related to Weakness Contractures Pain Infection Semicomatose/comatose state Paralysis • Activity intolerance related to Depression Shortness of breath • Alteration in comfort level related to Pain Exhaustion • Potential for injury as a result of Metastases to bone Confusion Seizures	Proper equipment can help both with mobility and safety. An overhead trapeze is useful for helping patients turn themselves. Side rails are useful for turning, as well as for safety. A physical therapist is helpful in instructing the patient and family in the correct use of exercises, in ambulation devices such as canes, walkers, and wheelchairs, and with the use of lifting devices such as a Hoyer lift. Steroid administration may help combat feelings of malaise that hinder mobility.
Temperature regulation	• Alteration in comfort related to Medication reaction Fever/chills Decreased fluid intake Advance in condition	Chronic fevers may be palliated by lowering room temperature, lightening bed clothes, and increasing fluid intake. Persistent fevers may best respond to a regular schedule of aspirin or indomethacin (Indocin) or acetaminophen (Tylenol). Propantheline (Pro-Banthine) may help night sweats. Patients who feel too cold may respond to warm water bottles at the feet, careful use of heating pads, socks, flannel sheets, electric blankets, or down comforters. Caution always should be exercised in the use of heating devices around patients with sensory impairment or circulatory problems who are at high risk for burns. Chills may require the use of systemic antibiotic therapy for infection control or relaxants such as diazepam (Valium) or chlorpromazine (Thorazine).

Adapted from Amenta MO, Bohnet NL: Nursing Care of the Terminally Ill. Boston, Little, Brown & Co, 1986.

The hospice nurse is a resource person able to provide information in answer to many questions and help solve patient management problems. The hospice nurse identifies any lack of understanding about the disease process, current therapies, or treatment side effects. It is important for the nurse to transmit information clearly without becoming involved in value judgments concerning treatments or care. The nurse identifies and coordinates the many community resources that may be helpful, such as the American Cancer Society, county social services, and Meals on Wheels (see Yellow Pages of this text for a list of the oncology self-help organizations available to individuals with a diagnosis of cancer and their families).

Teaching is not limited to the patient and family. New staff members can observe and learn by working with experienced staff members. The community needs to be made aware of the services hospice programs offer. Staff members of local hospitals and convalescent homes should understand hospice philosophy and hospice pain control techniques to ensure the continuity of care when the individual moves from home to hospital or nursing facility. The Hospice of Marin has developed a community liaison/admissions nurse role to facilitate the information flow between settings. Development of cooperative professional relationships with staffs of local institutions takes time and patience, but the effort is richly rewarded.

Patient-Family Counseling and Support

A large part of the hospice nurse's role is listening to and talking with the patient and family. Much of the care hospices can offer depends on developing mutually trusting relationships over a period of time with each family.

Involvement of support systems

Identification and understanding of the support systems available to each family are important. The family's relationship with a church, the availability of close friends or neighbors who can help, and how well the family members cooperate will have an impact on the patient and family's progress through the course of terminal illness.

The aim of identifying support systems is to help families realize that they are not alone, that in fact many people are available to help in different ways. Often family members hesitate to ask for help until they realize that friends and neighbors want to help out but need direction to do so. Identifying and utilizing support systems available to each family help to prevent the development of crisis situations.

When a crisis does occur, the hospice nurse should respond immediately. Most crises seem to involve physical problems (eg, vomiting, breakthrough pain, and catheter problems). Sometimes, however, intrafamily conflict or a personal crisis precipitates a call to the nurse. Generally, a visit to the home, attention to physical problems, and recognition and discussion of the severe stress each family member is under greatly relieves the anxiety and helps the family mobilize. More time sometimes is spent with the family than with the patient, helping family members cope with stress so that they can then continue to care for the patient.

It is important to reaffirm that the caregivers are doing a good job and are giving the dying person the best gift of all—themselves. This reassurance often keeps families going when times are difficult and they are doubting their ability to provide necessary care. It is appropriate in some instances to suggest alternative care, but sincere reassurance generally relieves doubts. When situations arise that necessitate hospitalization, the hospice nurse can help alleviate the guilt the family may feel regarding hospitalization by discussing and supporting their decision. The nurses also can provide continuity of care between the home and the hospital. The primary nurse and physician will collaboratively outline the patient and family's problems at home and facilitate timely hospitalization. Communication between hospice nurse and hospital nurse ensures continuity of established routines for such needs as medication, diet, and physical care. The family can be reassured of their continued participation in patient care even in the hospital, and visits from hospice staff members will continue regardless of the setting.

Counseling of the individual and family is an extremely important part of the hospice nurse's role. Chapters 16 through 18 explore the counseling process in depth.

Facilitation of anticipatory mourning

Facilitation of anticipatory mourning is a sensitive and crucial part of the hospice nurse's care. Anticipatory mourning is considered a normal process associated with chronic disease, whereby a grieving person begins to work through part of his or her grief before the patient dies.

The hospice nurse can help the dying individual by being a consistent and concerned person with whom the patient feels free to talk. Dying individuals sometimes find it easier to talk with a trusted and empathic nurse than with a family member. This requires that the nurse be attentive, listen nonjudgmentally, and then, if appropriate, foster more open communication between the dying person and the family.

Open communication often occurs once family members realize that the "ice has been broken." For example, one woman was very close to her sister, with whom she had lived all her life. As the patient drew close to death, she and her sister experienced tremendous anxiety and fear. Each could talk to the nurse but not to each other. Very gently, the nurse suggested that the sister talk with the dying person, give her permission to let go, and assure her that she would be able to carry on alone. Both sisters felt enormous relief and comfort in sharing their most intimate feelings.

The nurse can help the patient redefine goals. Previous long-term goals pale compared with the immediate goals of comfort, enjoying music, seeing friends, or completing unfinished business. One person, realizing that her death was nearing, organized her family into helpers who assisted her in cataloging all her precious possessions. Then she carefully divided them among her daughters. She talked frequently of her death, which she saw as a release from this world, where she was incapacitated, to the beautiful new heavenly world where she would be whole.

The willingness of hospice nurses to face their patients' imminent death and to help other family members prepare for it is an important aspect of care that seems to occur more easily in a hospice milieu. Helping individuals and families prepare for the inevitable is a prime concern of nurses in every setting when patients are near death, but the acute care orientation can discourage the full engagement of such caring in many ways. It is hoped that as nurses and physicians become more aware of how much genuine help and support hospice care offers, especially to dying individuals, the facilitation and preparation for a patient's decline will be practiced more fully.

Preparation for the decline

When the patient is obviously nearing death, the hospice nurse can reduce family members' anxiety in several ways. Because this is a time of great stress, care is taken to relate to the family in a calm and concerned but unhurried and unafraid manner.

It is sometimes necessary, although not easy or always indicated, to check with the family regarding funeral arrangements. Discussing the wishes of various family members not only helps take care of a vital piece of business but also helps to facilitate and consolidate the family's mourning process. At this point some families may realize that they do not know the dying person's preferences. Sometimes the dying person has given a great deal of thought to this subject and may have carefully written out specific wishes. One dying woman was a devout Catholic, and her funeral plans focused on a religious service. Two days before she died, she was overjoyed when she was accepted into the Third Order of the Carmelite Sisters in a beautiful bedside service.

Religion may play an important role, especially as death draws near. Someone who previously had declined religious support may now desire a visit with a chaplain.

Some may want to talk about funeral arrangements, or sometimes a simple prayer with the nurse may be significant. Each nurse should be sensitive to the potential for some degree of religious reinvolvement.

The hospice nurse can help the family prepare for the patient's decline by explaining the probable signs and symptoms of impending death. Families invariably ask what to expect, and they want to be certain that the person will not be in great pain. Most families want to know if the person can still hear even when he or she cannot respond, and, of course, family members want to know what they can do to help. The nurse can help the family maintain a sense of control, as well as decrease anxiety, by sharing as much knowledge as possible in an attempt to "limit the uncertainty."[17] Many unrealistic fears can be eliminated by a frank but sensitive discussion of realistic probabilities.

Nearly all families realize that no one can know when a person will die. They usually are grateful, however, for any information that can help them understand what is happening. It is important to discuss signs and symptoms that are easy to determine. Failing circulation may cause extremities to become cool or slightly cyanotic. The pulse may become rapid or irregular and then gradually slow. A simple explanation of Cheyne-Stokes respirations may prevent anxiety if the patient's breathing becomes irregular. Rattling or gurgling respirations frequently occur. Elevation of the head and positioning the patient to one side may relieve labored respirations and reduce gurgling. Incontinence may be more frequent but can easily be handled with Chux and disposable diapers. Responsiveness to stimulation can decrease gradually or can suddenly reverse to complete awareness. In either event it is important to stress and demonstrate respect for the dying person by continuing communication and by maintaining physical contact.

Physical care becomes extremely important at this time. Frequent mouth care is necessary because of mouth breathing; dry skin requires a softening lotion; eyes need frequent cleansing; and attention is given to decreasing any objectionable odors. The hospice nurse can assist the family with physical care at this time when it might be most difficult for the family to carry on.

One of the most difficult human dilemmas is the question of when a person will die. Families desperately want to know so that they can be with the person, call other family members, or simply measure their strength to meet the person's demands over a period of time. Waiting for a death that everyone has come to expect but does not happen at the expected time must be one of the hardest tests of human endurance. It is particularly important that nursing support be increased during this period and that much attention be given to the caregivers. Acknowledgment that waiting is a difficult time helps families release some pent-up anxiety and express their tacit wish that it end soon.

Death itself usually comes quietly and without surprise. It is helpful and comforting to share with families that the moment of death frequently is more like a peaceful sigh than the violent struggle so often portrayed on television. Helping family members narrow their areas of uncertainty aids tremendously in reducing their understandable anxiety, thus preparing them to stand by the person when his or her needs are greatest.

Occasionally the progression of events is not smooth, or the bonding of family members does not occur. Nurses cannot and should not be all things to all people. They can offer their best efforts but should be constantly aware that they are working with independent persons who will make their own decision as to how they will live their lives. It seems that a person's manner of dying is a direct reflection of his or her manner of living. Under all circumstances, nurses must respect and value that manner.

Provision of support at the time of death

When death finally arrives, it is usually a time of quiet relief and grieving. If the hospice nurse is not present, the nurse may be called soon after the death. Some families are so well prepared that they request that the nurse not come. In most instances, however, the hospice nurse goes to the home to offer support.

If the family wishes, the nurse calls the physician for a pronouncement or notifies the mortuary after the person is pronounced dead. To avoid unnecessary involvement of law enforcement officials strict attention must be paid, both before and after death, to the county regulations regarding home deaths.

Assurance of dignified care of the patient's body includes helping with bathing, if necessary, and helping to select clothes to send to the funeral home. Other tasks include careful disposal of all unused narcotic medications (with a witness), removal of as much equipment as possible, and then general help in returning the room to its original state.

During the wait for the mortician to arrive, family members may want to spend time alone with the patient's body to say their good-bys. This is to be respected and encouraged. An explanation of general mortuary practices helps the family mentally prepare for the physical removal of their loved one. The family may desire to participate in the ritual of removal as a continuation of their total involvement. Often it is appropriate to ask that the person's head be left uncovered if the family wishes, again symbolizing the continuation of dignified care even after death.

After removal of the body, there generally is an opportunity for all to sit down and review the events. Some family members may want to be alone, whereas others need encouragement to talk about the events leading up to the death, to review the death itself, and to begin to make plans for the upcoming hectic time surrounding the funeral services and burial or scattering of ashes. One of the most important gifts the nurse can give family members is the confirmation that they did a good job and that the dying person received the best of care. Family members characteristically are proud of their roles in fulfilling the desires of the dying person, and this sense of achievement fosters the normal grieving process and provides support in the bereavement period.

Bereavement Follow-Up

Nursing support continues after the death, into the bereavement period. The degree of involvement with each family differs according to individual needs.

Attending the funeral or memorial service when appropriate can be important because it shows continuing concern for the family and provides an opportunity for the nurse to pay respects and say good-by to the deceased. Strong bonds of affection are formed when a nurse shares a family's struggle to allow a member to die at home with dignity and comfort. Attendance at the ritual of farewell for the person can be useful in helping the nurse also to experience closure.

A written note or personal visit by the primary nurse 2 to 3 weeks after the death is helpful. This is a time when public activity around the death is declining. Then the family is assured of ongoing involvement with the hospice staff if it desires.

A bereavement program can include monthly gatherings that may give survivors a reason to go out again, as well as a chance to learn more about the bereavement process. These informal, nonthreatening gatherings allow survivors to meet others who have experienced similar losses. Not only is personal sharing among survivors of great value, but new friendships are initiated, social activities are planned, and life is carried on with optimism. Grief support groups are another form of assistance offered. Individual counseling is available to those survivors who experience particular difficulty.

Research and Evaluation

Research and evaluation represent the cornerstones for the future of hospice nursing. Random clinical observation of techniques and approaches is not sufficient to ascertain which are most effective. Nurses must turn their energies toward systematic evaluation and careful, well-planned investigation of nursing actions. Organizations such as the American Nurses' Association, Oncology Nursing Society, and Association of Pediatric Oncology Nurses have published standards of nursing practice based on patient outcomes. Incorporating these standards into nursing care in the hospice setting will help guide interventions, direct research efforts, and assist in evaluation of nursing care in the hospice setting.

Hospice nursing provides many potential avenues for research. Among priorities for study are various pain and symptom control approaches and patient responses. Nurses must learn more about patient and family responses to severe stress, coping mechanisms, and the types of nursing interventions that help alleviate or prevent the occurrence of such stress. Research on bereavement could identify methods of coping with loss and how successful coping can be fostered in families. Study of the family as a unit will reveal whether hospice interventions support familial integrity. In the planning and conducting of any kind of research, however, particular concern and attention must be paid to the difficult circumstances and stressful situations that surround terminally ill individuals.

HOSPICE STAFF

Qualities of the Hospice Nurse

Hospice nursing is challenging and rewarding but also extremely demanding. Several basic characteristics are essential in nurses who are continuously under high levels of stress while providing care. Other providers of care for patients with cancer, such as staff members of oncology units and home health programs, also experience similarly stressful circumstances.

The first characteristic of a hospice nurse is maturity. Each nurse must carefully examine his or her motivations for choosing to enter this field. What are the nurse's goals and expectations? Is the nurse ready to give care under continuously stressful situations? What is the nurse's philosophy of death? The nurse's personal beliefs or expectations must not dominate his or her actions. Each nurse needs to be aware of personal weaknesses and strengths and be prepared to examine, learn, and grow through experience.

A second characteristic of the nurse is flexibility. The ability to work independently and assume great responsibility, yet be able to consult and work with a team, is crucial. Patience during long periods of waiting may be necessary when caring for terminally ill individuals, yet quick, decisive action may be needed during a person's sudden decline. The nurse must be sensitive in responding to each person's needs and be emotionally strong to endure continued encounters.

Finally, a hospice nurse needs to maintain a sense of perspective through other rewarding activities. Achieving a balance in life among work, play, and companionship serves to keep the nurse from becoming totally immersed in a difficult job.

Avoidance of Burnout

Caring for persons experiencing severe stress inevitably affects the nurse. It is easy to reach that stage of total physical and emotional exhaustion called *burnout*, particularly in the care of those with terminal illness. How can burnout be prevented and hospice nurses remain responsive to the needs of their patients and colleagues?

The entire staff may benefit from meeting weekly for a patient care conference. Reports of recent deaths are presented in summary, each active patient/family situation is discussed, and bereavement contacts are reviewed. Several goals are achieved by the conference, including (1) updating team members on current patient care status, (2) providing a mechanism for interdisciplinary input into the total care plan, (3) offering opportunities for staff teaching and learning through analyzing successful and unsuccessful approaches to patient care, and (4) providing a formal setting for mutual staff support. Individual achievements are recognized and group efforts are devoted to solving persistent dilemmas. Fostering the sense of shared responsibility for the total care of any person helps to diffuse the inevitable frustration and guilt that arise when working with persons who are terminally ill.

Daily morning and afternoon conferences also can be held for the patient care staff to share reports and information, discuss assignments, and further provide mutual peer support on a regular basis. Most important, each staff member can share reports with the team leader and other staff members at the end of the day, providing that vital chance to "unload" reactions and receive spontaneous feedback before taking problems home. A mechanism for day-to-day release and reward is crucial.

Peer support is prominent in both the patient care conference and the daily reports. However, it also occurs among individuals in a spontaneous, ongoing fashion. Development of such staff interactions is an elusive but important part of helping each staff member deal with day-to-day aggravations. How often do nurses take the extra 2 minutes to pass on to another nurse the report of glowing feedback received from a patient about that nurse's sensitive care? Recognizing that a coworker has had a particularly hard day or week may help unleash some pent-up frustration. Nurses must take an active role in consciously giving support to one another and in providing recognition for excellent care or innovative ideas. Sensitivity to how others feel is a valuable nursing attribute, and nurses should strive to make themselves available to colleagues who need someone with whom to share their victories and defeats. A support group for clinical staff members, led by an outside counselor, offers staff an opportunity to express feelings and reactions to work issues.

Finally, time away from the hospice setting aids tremendously in maintaining perspective. Regular vacations are essential. Weekend and night nursing coverage could be provided by staff members hired specifically for those hours. This staffing pattern allows the primary nurses to relax completely, knowing that another nurse is available to respond to any crisis.

Preventing burnout is a concern in hospice nursing. It can be prevented if careful attention is devoted to the problem by both the individual and the hospice organization.

CONCLUSION

Hospice nursing is both exceptionally fulfilling and extraordinarily demanding. Each team member supports other team members and strives to maintain a sense of balance and perspective to continue to be available emotionally for patients and family members.

Hospice philosophy is deeply rooted in history, flourishing during the Middle Ages, and again today as society becomes more conscious of the innate worth and dignity of each human life and death. Health care personnel in particular must examine and protect the manner in which individuals are treated as they approach death.

Hospice nursing is an opportunity to practice the full spectrum of nursing skills by providing direct patient care, teaching, counseling, bereavement follow-up, and research. As an independent caregiver and as a team member, the hospice nurse experiences fulfillment of a truly professional relationship with other staff members. The nursing care and philosophy of hospice programs are not new. Many home care organizations and religious groups have provided elements of hospice care for years. However, the need for comprehensive, specialized care programs for terminally ill individuals is growing rapidly. The development of hospice programs is a response to this unmet need in the medical care system.

As each community develops hospice services according to the unique resources and demands of the area, the philosophy of hospice care must continue to be paramount. Regardless of whether the setting is a free-standing hospice, home care program, or in-hospital unit, hospice care is a part of our health care system that will continue to flourish.

REFERENCES

1. Quint JC: Awareness of death and the nurse's composure. Nurs Res 15(1):49-55, 1966.
2. Sudnow D: Passing On. Englewood Cliffs, NJ, Prentice-Hall, 1978.
3. Kübler-Ross E: On Death and Dying. New York, Macmillan, 1969.
4. Stoddard S: The hospice movement. Briarcliff Manor, NY, Stein & Day, 1978, p xvii.
5. Craven J, Wald F: Hospice care for dying patients. Am J Nurs 70:1816-1821, 1975.
6. Liegner LM: St. Christopher's hospice, 1974. JAMA 234:1047-1048, 1975.
7. National Hospice Organization: The 1989 Guide to the Nation's Hospices. Arlington, Va, The Organization, 1989.
8. National Hospice Organization: Meeting the Challenge for a *Special* Kind of Caring: Standards of a Hospice Program of Care Recommended by the National Hospice Organization (position paper). Arlington, Va, The Organization, 1987.
9. National Hospice Organization: Hospice Operations Manual. Arlington, Va, The Organization, 1988.
10. Pryga E, Bachofer H: Hospice care under Medicare. Chicago, American Hospital Association, 1983.
11. National Hospice Organization: Hospice in America. Arlington, Va, The Organization, 1978.
12. National Hospice Study Final Report: Executive Summary. Providence, RI, Brown University, 1982.
13. Beresford L: Private insurance reimbursement. Calif Hospice Rep 6(4):1-12, 1988.
14. Task Force on Case Management in Nursing: Nursing Case Management (position paper). Kansas City, Mo, American Nurses' Association, 1988.
15. Rainey LC, Crane LA, Breslow DM, et al: Cancer patients' attitude toward hospice services. CA 34(4):191-201, 1984.
16. Amenta MO, Bohnet NL: Nursing Care of the Terminally Ill. Boston, Little, Brown & Co, 1986.
17. Martinson IM: Why don't we let them die at home? RN 39(1):59-65, 1976.

PART VIII

PROFESSIONAL ISSUES FOR THE CANCER NURSE

Chapter 53

Quality of Care

Diane Scott Dorsett, RN, PhD, FAAN

CONCEPTUAL FOUNDATIONS OF QUALITY CARE

Historical Context and Origins

Well over a century ago, Nightingale[1] said that the prime objective in nursing was "to put the patient(s) in the best condition for nature to act." Since then, both conceptually and operationally, care has become the essence of nursing. During the past 10 years, a science of caring has emerged as a discrete theme in the nursing literature,[2-6] but only recently has care been accorded the importance recognized by Nightingale so long ago.

The relevance of care to society's health is becoming increasingly evident as demographic trends, such as an expanding elderly population, accelerate the incidence of chronic disease and as an increasingly advanced treatment technology extends life. Cure, once an important concept in the history of illness, when disease was primarily acute and infectious, has been replaced by the notion of prolonged remission with maximal quality of life. As modern science ushers in a biologic wave of modalities influencing prevention, detection, and treatment, clinical health care providers will continue to face the reality of increasingly rigorous treatments and more critically acute, morbid episodes superimposed on the chronic illness itself. Thus, as Benner[2] eloquently states, "In health care, caring sets up the possibility for cure."

As physicians attempt to master the rapidly changing complexities of cancer treatment in an increasing number of sicker patients, nursing care becomes a central issue. Quality of care is challenged by a health care system that contracts hospital stay time and health care cost coverage and by a health care environment in which large segments of the most vulnerable members of society (nonwhite, poor, less educated), who have greater than average health care needs, also have less than equal access to health care. Furthermore, those disadvantaged who do gain access often receive health care of lower quality—especially when measured in terms of appropriateness, timeliness, comprehensiveness, and continuity.[7] Documented in a publication of the President's Commission for the Study of Ethical Problems in Medicine and Biomedical and Behavioral Research, *Securing Access to Health Care,*[8] cancers of white Americans are detected earlier than those of nonwhites and those of paying patients are found earlier than those of nonpaying ones.

Although the reasons for these trends are complexly interwoven into the social, political, and economic fabric of American society, the outcome places a heavy burden not only on the underserved population but on all other segments of the society as well. Given today's challenges of specialization, complex technology, patterns of chronic illness, and a restrictive health care environment, the quality care of cancer patients and their families demands an interdisciplinary team approach and the extension of the role of nursing in its total management.

By the end of 1988, the Oncology Nursing Society had revised and expanded its scope of practice statement on the basis of a philosophic recognition that persons with cancer and their families need to be fully informed and to participate actively in their care and treatment and, further, that competent, humane care demands a complementary team of specialty practitioners who communicate with one another and augment one another's efforts. Increasingly, the notion of the patient as the owner-manager of his or her total health, with the need for a head coach and a qualified, well-coordinated health care team, has been gaining acceptance.[9]

Recognizing the emerging health care system as possessing an ever-expanding place for the nurse as direct caregiver, educator, administrator, and researcher, the Oncology Nursing Society statement emphasized the importance of the oncology nurse as a *coordinator* of care, collaborating with other health care team members to make the best use of resources available to patients and families and, as their *advocate,* assessing and communicating the uniqueness of each patient's response to cancer, thereby promoting maximum independence and autonomy. In short, oncology nurses, by virtue of their knowledge, skills, and holistic (biopsychosocial) perspective of persons with cancer, are often viewed as the most qualified practitioners to assume the head coach role.

Care and caring

To care is to respond to another in need because of pain, illness, or distress. Caring involves a sense of commitment and responsibility and, when taken to higher levels, can be considered a body of knowledge and skill known tacitly, empirically, or scientifically to accomplish change for the good. Although caring behavior is central to most public and private human activity, when defined for nursing, caring becomes a set of meaning-laden actions.[2,10] To wit, early in the education of most nursing students, Virginia Henderson's classic definition of nursing is introduced:

> Nursing is primarily assisting individuals (sick or well) with those activities contributing to health, or its recovery (or to a peaceful death) that they perform unaided when they have the necessary strength, will or knowledge; nursing also helps individuals carry out prescribed therapy and be independent of assistance as soon as possible.[11]

The definition of nursing as a profession, discipline, and practice, through such theaters of relevance, becomes public domain through the Nurse Practice Act. Nurse practice acts are state determined but are remarkably similar in wording throughout the country. Most legislate nursing as the diagnosis and treatment of human responses in health and illness—a broad definition, further operationalized in the interest of public safety by a regulated and standardized system of education, registration, certification, standards of practice, and quality assurance.

After the broad, formative brushstrokes of Nightingale,[1] who recognized "the fundamental needs of the sick and principles of good care," a concise, comprehensive definition of nursing by Harmer and Henderson,[11] and the more recent revisions that modernized nurse practice acts in this country, nursing began the establishment of a taxonomy of nursing diagnoses.[12-14] Nursing diagnoses operationalize the nurse practice act terminology, "human responses to an actual or potential health problem."[15]

Diagnostic taxonomies generally allow for a clear definition of professional purpose and for faster communication among the practitioners of a discipline, and they become the basis for a profession's research and development activity. As Herberth and Gosnell[13] advise, the next step is the integration of standards of practice and nursing diagnoses (Table 53-1) to foster relevant research, promote therapeutic interventions, and, ultimately, advance the quality of care.

Caring actions cannot be separated from intent, however, if the outcome is to be effective. It is not enough to practice according to a guiding set of rules and regulations. To achieve even an acceptable level of quality of care, one must have commitment, creativity, and a willingness to innovate at reasonable risk. Knowing one's craft well is not enough. Caring requires knowing our patients and their beliefs, values, and cultural norms and tailoring care accordingly. Thus understanding and defining quality of care in terms of practices that enable health promotion

TABLE 53-1 Functional Health Pattern Categories and Nursing Diagnoses

Health perception–health management pattern

Health maintenance alteration
Health management deficit (total)
Health management deficit (specify)
Health seeking behavior
Noncompliance (specify)
Potential noncompliance (specify)
Potential for infection
Potential for physical injury
Potential for poisoning
Potential for suffocation

Nutritional-metabolic pattern

Alteration in nutrition: potential for more than body requirements or potential obesity
Alteration in nutrition: more than body requirements or exogenous obesity
Alteration in nutrition: less than body requirements or nutritional deficit (specify)
Ineffective breast feeding
Impaired swallowing
Potential for aspiration
Alterations in oral mucous membranes
Potential fluid volume deficit
Fluid volume deficit (actual) (1)
Fluid volume deficit (actual) (2)
Fluid volume excess
Potential or actual impairment of skin integrity or skin breakdown
Decubitus ulcer (specify stage)
Impaired skin or tissue integrity
Altered body temperature
Ineffective thermoregulation
Hyperthermia
Hypothermia

Elimination pattern

Alteration in bowel elimination: constipation or intermittent constipation pattern
Alteration in bowel elimination: diarrhea
Alteration in bowel elimination: incontinence or bowel incontinence
Altered urinary elimination pattern
Urinary incontinence: functional, stress, urge or total
Stress incontinence
Urinary retention

Activity-exercise pattern

Potential activity intolerance
Activity intolerance (specify level)
Fatigue
Impaired physical mobility (specify level)
Potential for disuse syndrome
Total self-care deficit (specify level)
Self-bathing–hygiene deficit (specify level)
Self-dressing–grooming deficit (specify level)
Self-feeding deficit (specify level)
Self-toileting deficit (specify level)
Self-care skills deficit
Diversional activity deficit
Impaired home maintenance management (mild, moderate, severe, potential, chronic)
Potential joint contractures
Ineffective airway clearance
Ineffective breathing pattern
Impaired gas exchange
Decreased cardiac output
Altered tissue perfusion
Dysreflexia
Altered growth and development

Sleep-rest pattern

Sleep-pattern disturbance

Cognitive-perceptual pattern

Pain
Chronic pain
Pain self-management deficit
Uncompensated sensory deficit (specify)
Sensory-perceptual alterations: input deficit or sensory deprivation
Sensory-perceptual alterations: input excess or sensory overload
Unilateral neglect
Knowledge deficit (specify)
Uncompensated short-term memory deficit
Potential cognitive impairment
Impairment thought processes
Decisional conflict (specify)

TABLE 53-1 Functional Health Pattern Categories and Nursing Diagnoses (continued)

Self-perception–self-concept pattern

Fear (specify focus)
Anticipatory anxiety (mild, moderate, severe)
Anxiety
Mild anxiety
Moderate anxiety
Severe anxiety (panic)
Reactive depression (situational)
Hopelessness
Powerlessness (severe, low, moderate)
Self-esteem disturbance
Body image disturbance
Personal identity confusion

Role-relationship pattern

Anticipatory grieving
Dysfunctional grieving
Disturbance in role performance
Unresolved independence-dependence conflict
Social isolation
Social isolation (rejection)
Impaired social interaction
Altered growth and development: social skills (specify)
Translocation syndrome
Altered family process
Weak mother-infant attachment or parent-infant attachment
Potential altered parenting
Altered parenting
Parental role conflict
Impaired verbal communication
Altered growth and development: communication skills
Potential for violence

Sexuality-reproductive pattern

Sexual dysfunction
Altered sexuality patterns
Rape trauma syndrome
Rape trauma syndrome: compound reaction
Rape trauma syndrome: silent reaction

Coping–stress tolerance pattern

Coping, ineffective (individual)
Avoidance coping
Defensive coping
Ineffective denial
Impaired adjustment
Post-trauma response
Family coping: potential for growth
Ineffective family coping: compromised
Ineffective family coping: disabling;

Value-belief pattern

Spiritual distress (distress of human spirit)

Source: Reproduced by permission from Gordon M: Manual of nursing diagnosis 1988-1989, St. Louis, The CV Mosby Co.

and recovery from illness requires that caring be intrinsic to the process. Leininger[5] defined caring as behavioral attributes characterized by empathy, support, compassion, protection, succor, and education, firmly grounded in a comprehension of the needs, problems, values, and goals of the person or group being assisted.

Quality

The nature of quality is multifaceted and difficult to define, especially in relation to nursing care. Yet quality has emerged as the most important issue in patient care services in the final two decades of the twentieth century. The 1980s witnessed an integration of quality management, control, and assurance in nursing practice. To some observers, this integration has changed practice habits and promoted the individuation of care in innovative ways. These new ways of practice have led to the development of standards of care as the basic unit of analysis in the evaluation of quality in practice.[16]

Quality has become the focus of all cancer service provider groups, including the Commission on Cancer of the American College of Surgeons, the National Cancer Institute, the American Cancer Society, the College of American Pathology, the American College of Radiology, and, in joint affiliation, the American Nurses' Association and the Oncology Nursing Society.[17] Quality was, as Beyers[16] stated, "the banner of the 1980s" and will be the established base for the next major advance in clinical nursing during the 1990s and beyond.

Quality, by definition, is a set of properties, attributes, and capacities that are essential and unique to the focus of evaluation, be it nursing or a work of art. In a generic sense, quality connotes a degree of excellence as measured by recognized standards. Standards are characterized by utility, durability, stability, flexibility, and aesthetics and, in the health care environment, require the definition of correlates related to both clinical and organizational qualities. Beyers[16] defines these correlates of quality as cost, productivity, and risk.

Historically, approaches to quality management in the United States have gone through several "eras," from inspection and statistical accounting measures (time and motion studies), to quality assurance processes and procedures (chart audit), to the newest era of "strategic quality management."[18] Strategic quality management is based on the realities of market share and fiscal viability since health care is big business and the driving force has become patient satisfaction. The "new" approach to quality recognizes four important factors: (1) recognition of consumer need and response, (2) integrated service teams, (3) standards of practice, organization, and professional performance, and (4) data management systems that document structure, process, and outcome elements.[16]

Beyers[16] views these factors as interactive and as having the potential for a positive effect. When patient needs are understood, recognized, and met by a well-coordinated team of clinicians who are guided by high standards, the associated documentation will allow clinical outcomes to be "known," ultimately modifying patient response for the better.

Thus quality embraces the dimensions of structure (patient and environment norms), process (strategies of quality management), and outcome (documentation of clinical outcomes and patient satisfaction). For many experts, quality is driven by the profit motive. For nursing, quality must be powered both by its value as a public service and by the caring ethic for maximal effect.

The concept of quality of care is grounded in the integration of a sound body of knowledge and skill, standards of practice and performance that promote excellence, a coordinated team approach, and a built-in capacity for innovation (research), with all components fired by a deep sense of caring.

Quality of Care Model

A model of quality of care (Figure 53-1) has been designed to represent the major goals in cancer care and treatment and those structural factors that ensure quality in terms of process and outcomes.

Structure

In the 1980s, several critical components were set in place that allowed for a guiding definition of quality in cancer care. These structural elements include overall *standards for oncology nursing practice and for the professional performance of the nurse* who cares for patients with cancer and their families. These standards are currently undergoing integration with the classification of nursing diagnoses and further categorization into Gordon's 11 functional health pattern categories.[14] Another major structure that promotes quality of care is clinical research and the development of nursing technology to test and improve interventions and maximize positive results. Nursing research in cancer care can be built into every patient care environment on some level. For some, this might mean keeping up with the nursing research literature or participating in a journal club, or it might involve undertaking a small study of one's own or participating in a larger multisite research project. Research allows for the development of nursing technology as well: Audiovisual patient teaching programs, drug dispensers that allow for safer self-administration of the many medications that cancer patients take at home, or measures that aid mobility, protect the skin and mucous membrane, or improve ventilation are examples of methods that achieve practical purposes toward the improvement or refinement of care. As these innovations are developed, they need to be tested and the results shared with others.

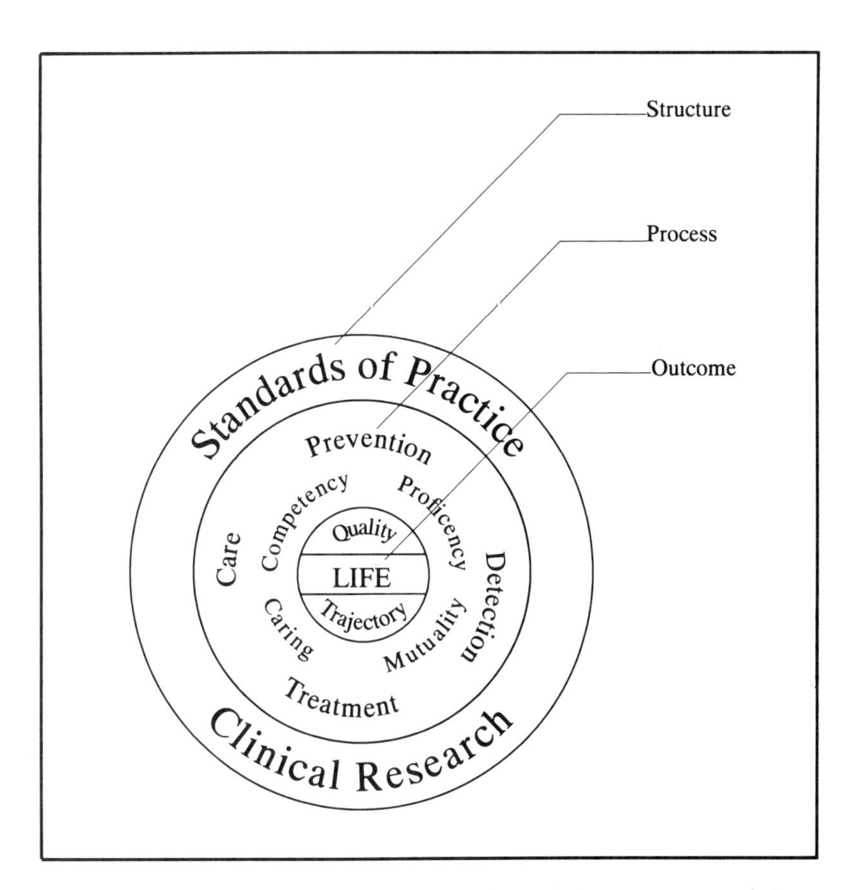

FIGURE 53-1 This model represents the major goals in cancer care and those structural factors that ensure quality of care in terms of process and outcome.

Process

The second dimension of the quality of care model is represented by the process variables of cancer prevention, detection, treatment, and nursing care. This dimension brings together the nursing care–medical treatment complex because the components of this complex are mutually dependent in achieving the desired outcome. More often than not, nursing care revolves around medical treatment but, in the best sense, extends itself beyond the immediate goals of interest to the physician. Cell kill and reduced tumor size are important, but without attention to management of side effects and promotion of functional recovery, the effect is diminished at best and ineffective at worst. In this sense, cure and care are not dichotomous. Care augments and enhances cure and in the process humanizes the total outcome.

Outcome

On a structural bed of sound standards and research innovation, the processes of prevention, detection, treatment, and care lead to patient outcome variables. The objectives of oncology care providers do not stop with the elimination of disease. Given the current status of cancer treatment today, with a documented 50% cure rate in all patients with a diagnosis of cancer,[19,20] Paul Marks, president of Memorial Sloan-Kettering Cancer Center, placed the current climate in perspective:

> The implication of this [sic, cancer biologic revolution] massive research effort is not that cancer will fade away in the next few years, or even decades. The discovery of oncogenes suggests that cancer may be an integral part of living, the result of interaction of our genes with the environment. Certainly, an understanding of the fundamental nature of carcinogenesis will transform the nature of clinical care. But it will not yield a magic bullet to cure the disease, nor a vaccine to prevent it. Cancer will not be eradicated like smallpox or polio. Rather, what seems likely to emerge are new approaches to early diagnosis of cancers and new techniques to treat them, providing steady gains in our ability to cure and, more important, to prevent cancer.[20]

The bottom-line results of 30 years of massive biomedical scientific effort has been an extension of life for many patients with a diagnosis of cancer. Paralleling the work on this frontier, the biopsychosocial scientific effort in nursing has promoted advances in the quality of the lives that medical science has extended. The amalgamation of life extension and quality of life makes clear the ultimate and optimal outcome of cancer care: maximal quality of life for cancer patients and their families.

Standards of Care

Nursing, as a science of caring, is based on a theoretical foundation for practice, continuously tested, refined, and verified by research, and a clearly articulated set of principles guiding that practice. Central to the concept of quality care is a set of standards that exists to guide practice by operationalizing its essence.

The publication of *Outcome Standards for Cancer Nursing Practice*[21] in 1979 and of its integration into the *Standards of Oncology Nursing Practice*[22] in 1987 were joint ventures of the Oncology Nursing Society (ONS) and the American Nurses' Association (ANA). Although the revision, *Standards of Oncology Nursing Practice*,[22] is rooted in the ANA published standards of nursing practice,[23] the former is a separate statement developed in recognition of cancer as a major health problem and of the importance of oncology nursing as a specialty practice devoted to the care of cancer patients and their families.

There are 11 Standards of Oncology Nursing Practice,[22] 6 that address professional practice and 5 that concern professional performance (Table 53-2). Practice standards focus on the process involved in patient care (theory, data collection, diagnosis, planning, intervention, and evaluation), with emphasis on 11 commonly occurring problem areas. Performance standards, in contrast, are criteria for professional development, interdisciplinary collaboration, quality assurance, ethics, and research in nursing as a discipline. To complement practice standards, ONS published *Outcome Standards for Cancer Nursing Education*,[24] *Cancer Patient Education*,[25] and *Public Cancer Education*.[26] A summation of the oncology nursing practice standards follows:

Standards of oncology nursing practice

I. The central core of oncology nursing is a logically articulated theoretical framework derived from the biologic, social, behavioral, and physical sciences. There are at least a dozen major nursing theories that have been constructed to guide practice, but two of the most frequently used in oncology nursing are Orem's self-care deficit theory[27] and the Johnson behavioral system model.[28] With a sound theoretical base, the nursing process is firmly grounded in established knowledge that can be constantly tested, evaluated, modified, and shared with colleagues.

II. Effective communication, assessment, and analytic skills are necessary to enable the oncology nurse to plan appropriate interventions for clients. The result is a sound database, available to the multidisciplinary team, that is maintained to reflect the most current and accurate clinical status of the patient.

III. The ability to make nursing diagnoses from the theoretical framework and the patient's database is essential to the plan of care. The diagnoses may emerge from actual or potential problems in 11 parameters: (1) prevention-detection, (2) information, (3) coping, (4) comfort, (5) nutrition, (6) protective mechanisms, (7) mobility, (8) elimination, (9) sexuality, (10) ventilation, and (11) circulation. Nursing diagnoses enable nurses to document problems and risks, planning, evaluation, and ultimately the research in care and collegial sharing that fosters continuity of care.

IV. Planning care is the first step in actively ensuring quality of care. During the planning process, goals are

TABLE 53-2 Standards of Oncology Nursing Practice

Standards of Professional Practice

I. *Theory:* The oncology nurse applies theoretical concepts as a basis for decisions in practice.

II. *Data collection:* The oncology nurse systematically and continually collects data regarding the health status of the client. The data are recorded, accessible, and communicated to appropriate members of the interdisciplinary team.

III. *Nursing diagnosis:* The oncology nurse analyzes assessment data to formulate nursing diagnoses.

IV. *Planning:* The oncology nurse develops an outcome-oriented care plan that is individualized and holistic. This plan is based on nursing diagnoses and incorporates preventive, therapeutic, rehabilitative, palliative, and comforting nursing actions.

V. *Intervention:* The oncology nurse implements the nursing care plan to achieve the identified outcomes for the client.

VI. *Evaluation:* The oncology nurse regularly and systematically evaluates the client's reponses to interventions in order to determine progress toward achievement of outcomes and to revise the data base, nursing diagnoses, and the plan of care.

Standards of Professional Performance

VII. *Professional development.* The oncology nurse assumes responsibility for professional development and continuing education and contributes to the professional growth of others.

VIII. *Multidisciplinary collaboration:* The oncology nurse collaborates with the multidisciplinary team in assessing, planning, implementing, and evaluating care.

IX. *Quality assurance:* The oncology nurse participates in peer review and interdisciplinary program evaluation to assure that high-quality nursing care is provided to clients.

X. *Ethics:* The oncology nurse uses the *Code for Nurses** and *A Patient's Bill of Rights*† to guide ethical decision making in practice.

XI. *Research:* The oncology nurse contributes to the scientific base of nursing practice and the field of oncology through the review and application of research.

*American Nurses' Association: Code for Nurses with Interpretive Statements. Kansas City, Mo, The Association, 1985.

†American Hospital Association: A Patient's Bill of Rights. Chicago, The Association, 1972.

Source: Reprinted with permission from Standards of Oncology Nursing Practice, © 1987, American Nurses' Association, Kansas City, Mo.

established and methods addressing the above 11 parameters are decided.

V. The implementation of the plan uses independently and interdependently determined actions to achieve its goals. In most cases, however, the nurse should function autonomously but collaboratively with others. Intervention should be flexible, documented, and provide measurable evidence of effect in light of the plan.

VI. Finally, the evaluation of the plan and its outcomes allows for continuous update, revision, improvement, and refinements in the database and diagnoses and for resulting modifications in intervention. This evaluation is done in collaboration with the patient and family and the health care team, is fully documented, and ultimately leads to scholarly, scientific analysis through research.

Standards of professional performance

VII. The first standard for professional performance makes clear (1) that the nurse is accountable for keeping abreast of advances in the field, maintaining current knowledge and skill, and incorporating them into practice and (2) that there is a commitment to the betterment of self, patients, colleagues, and the profession.

VIII. The complexity of cancer care today requires a multidisciplinary approach. Learning how to communicate effectively and to collaborate with team members is another indicator of professional development. There is considerable latitude in this standard in that the nurse may function effectively as participant, coordinator, and leader.

IX. Peer review and program evaluation have become mandated mechanisms in today's health care structure. Actively participating with an open, inquiring, and creative mind maximizes the possibility of quality improvement on individual, unit, and organizational levels.

X. The cancer care experience provides ample opportunity for ethical judgments. The rationale for the ethics standard spells out the profound ethical concerns in oncology nursing: right of self-determination, surrogate decision making, informed consent, treatment options, nontraditional treatment modalities, decisions about quality of life, confidentiality, distribution of resources, and matters of economics and value. Involvement with these issues can be demanding and challenging as well as stressful and exhausting. Continuing education and peer support are important vehicles for professional growth in this area.

XI. The 1970s and 1980s ushered in a new era of research-based practice in nursing. Oncology nursing practice must be kept therapeutically effective through research. The latitude in this performance standard is substantial. Minimally, the practitioner should keep abreast of research-based studies published in the most relevant specialty journals and incorporate findings into practice. Through expanded education, the nurse might ultimately become the principal investigator of his or her own study and might cultivate a scholarly interest in research that becomes a lifelong pursuit and vehicle for the enhancement of quality care.

The most recent 1987 revisions of the *Standards of Oncology Nursing Practice* incorporated the separately published *Outcome Standards for Cancer Nursing Practice* published in 1979. The original outcome standards reflected 10 high-incidence problem areas (Table 53-3) common to cancer as a major chronic disease with "intermittent acute episodes." When integrated with the 1987 revised practice standards concerned with data collection (II), nursing diagnoses (III), planning (IV), and evaluation (VI), the outcome assumes a patient-family-community focus, cuts across all phases of the cancer experience from prediagnosis to death, and recognizes the multiplicity of settings where patients are cared for today. These 10 high-incidence areas provide an essential link between the operating practice standard and quality assurance.

TABLE 53-3 High-Incidence Problems in Cancer Nursing Practice

I.	*Prevention and early detection:* Client and family possess adequate information about cancer prevention and detection.
II.	*Information:* Client and family possess knowledge about disease and therapy in order to attain self-management, participate in therapy, optimal living and peaceful death.
III.	*Coping:* Client and family manage stress optimally according to their individual capacity and in accord with their value system.
IV.	*Comfort:* Client and family manage factors that influence comfort.
V.	*Nutrition:* Client and family manage nutrition and hydration optimally.
VI.	*Protective mechanisms:* Client and family possess knowledge to prevent or manage alterations in protective mechanisms.
VII.	*Mobility:* Client and family maintain optimal mobility.
VIII.	*Elimination:* Client and family manage problems with elimination.
IX.	*Sexuality:* Client and partner can manage threats to sexual function and satisfaction and maintain their sexual identity.
X.	*Ventilation:* Client and family can anticipate factors that impair ventilatory function and maintain optimal ventilatory capacity.

Source: Adapted from Oncology Nursing Society. Outcome Standards for Cancer Nursing Practice. Pittsburgh, Pa, The Society, 1979.

RESEARCH AND EVALUATION IN QUALITY OF CARE

Background and Context

Research-based clinical practice and quality care are the hallmarks of professional nursing. These important processes are based on a theoretical body of knowledge, standards for practice, and valid and reliable measurements that allow for the evaluation of care and the expansion of the scientific foundation of practice.

The nursing literature of the 1970s saw a significant expansion in standardized approaches to measuring the quality of nursing care. As early as 1966, Donabedian[29] identified structure, process, and outcome variables in medicine as the three classic approaches to patient care evaluation.

One of the earliest studies of quality in nursing additionally tested the research tool "Patient Indicators of Nursing Care."[30] Seven physiologic indicators reflecting nursing care–related complications were assessed. This study was a prototype of today's research evaluating patient outcome standards and nursing diagnosis–specific interventions. Majesky et al[30] chose three broad functional categories from Dorothy Johnsons' theoretical framework—infection, immobility, and fluid imbalance—and operationalized them using 27 measurable indicators. The overall goal was to establish a reliable, valid, easy-to-use, clinically useful instrument to evaluate quality of nursing care.

Oncology nursing literature came of age with the beginning publication of two journals, *Cancer Nursing* and *Oncology Nursing Forum.* In a review[31] of research-based articles published in these journals through 1984, a total of 15 were found to evaluate nursing care programs. All interventions tested were educative or of a supportive, counseling nature, perhaps reflecting Herberth and Gosnell's finding[13] that over 40% of diagnoses involve knowledge deficit. Most of the studies did not allow for control group comparisons. Nine articles described tools designed to evaluate patient outcomes. Rarely was care measured directly, and most measures were constructed by the investigator because of the lack of sound instrumentation at that time. Few were tested for accuracy or consistency.

A distinct shift in the cancer nursing literature, noted from 1985 onward, seemed to coincide with the establishment of oncology nursing standards and their clinically useful format (patient outcome standards and functional health classification). Clearly, more authors attempted schema that integrated patients' clinical problems and deficits, nursing diagnoses, assessment parameters, causes, and interventions into plans for care that provided a useful guide for the practicing nurse and a methodical approach for quality assurance programs.

The following review of methods for measuring quality of cancer nursing care recognizes the seminal work of early researchers[32-36] but concentrates on studies published in the cancer nursing literature since 1985 that reflect more recent trends in the field (ie, standards, nursing diagnoses, quality assurance, and measurement methods).

Approaches to Measuring Quality of Care

There are three major approaches to measuring quality of care: (1) quality assurance programs, (2) clinical research that includes both program evaluation and experimental studies of interventions, and (3) measurement tool or instrument development that includes both the construction of quantitative scales, questionnaires, and inventories and qualitative measures that include the establishment of clinical indicators, predictors, and guidelines for assessment.

Quality assurance

The Joint Commission on Accreditation of Health Care Organizations publishes standards used in the accreditation of hospitals and five other types of health care organizations (long-term care, psychiatric care, ambulatory health care, hospice care, and home care organizations) in this country.[37] These standards are concerned with the structures, processes, and outcomes of patient care activities in all services provided by the organization, including nursing services. There are eight standards that address the provision, management, and monitoring of nursing services regardless of location or institutional type. Four of the eight standards are concerned directly with the quality of nursing care: NR3 requires maintenance of established standards of nursing practice; NR5 mandates the use of the nursing process; NR7 delineates written documentation that care reflects optimal standards of practice; and NR8 provides for the monitoring and evaluation of care and the identification and resolution of problems.

The Joint Commission on Accreditation of Health Care Organizations distinguishes between standards of care and standards of practice.[37] Whereas standards of care reflect expected patient outcomes of care activities, standards of practice are concerned with "the structure and process elements used by the nurse and nursing service to provide patient care."[38] Thus a standard of care focuses on the patient, and a standard of practice focuses on the nurse. Patterson[38] differentiates the two concepts further by explaining that a standard of care is what the patient outcome should be and what the patient can expect from nursing service, whereas standards of practice relate to what and how the nurse provides care to achieve the patient outcome. The outcomes of care are generally based on clinical criteria or well-defined indicators that are measurable and that reflect the quality and appropriateness of intervention. Quality, in this sense, depicts the degree of adherence between the standard of care and actual patient outcome, and appropriateness reflects the degree of congruence between what the patient needed to achieve in terms of a desired outcome and what the nurse provided.

Therefore, to operationalize a quality assurance program, the health care institution must maintain a sound system for documentation of nursing care activities and patient outcomes and must establish a system to review and assess regularly both quality and appropriateness. In addition to evaluation, there is need for a system to rectify or resolve problems or breeches of quality in all aspects of care: diagnostic, preventive, therapeutic, rehabilitative, supportive, and palliative.

Depending on the nature and specialization of the nursing care unit, there may be need for a more precise definition of both patient outcomes and nursing practices to achieve those outcomes, or what is known as clinical functions. Oncology nursing is a prime example of the need for care and practice standards to be tailored to the unique needs and problems of the cancer patient and for more precise operationalization of clinical functions such as assessment, evaluation of learning needs, provision of physical care, teaching, goal setting, nursing interventions based on nursing diagnosis, implementation of the medical plan of care and required medications and treatments, and the coordination of nursing goals and plans for care with those of other professional team members.[38]

In these specific cases, both health care institutions and accrediting organizations look to the professional specialty group to establish and promulgate those standards of nursing practice. Quality assurance structures look to organizations such as ONS for current, state-of-the-art research-based standards.[38] On the basis of these published specialty guides, the hospital or agency customizes the standards further to be in line with the nature and character of its own care-giving environment. For example, nursing practice standards at one of the nation's five major cancer centers might differ from those in a small community hospital, where there may or may not be a discrete oncology unit or where there may or may not be a department of nursing research that focuses on oncology care. However, no matter how specialized or how large or small the institution might be, mandated quality assurance accords the *right* to quality of care as defined by the ONS standards of nursing practice to every oncology patient.

The literature is sparse in studies evaluating the quality of cancer nursing care by using patient outcomes as evidence. However, several articles stand out in their effort to improve the quality assurance process. This small body of literature reflects the complexities involved in studying quality and the many dimensions in focus and approach. Five issues important to quality assurance (QA) were examined in nine studies reported in the period from 1985 to 1988: (1) QA audit results for specific areas of care, (2) oncology patient classification systems, (3) Occupational Safety and Health Administration (OSHA) guidelines, (4) clinical database development, and (5) methods to identify and measure oncology nursing competencies and practice proficiency.

Oleske et al[39] conducted a controlled study that measured the effects of both nurse specialist consultation and continuing education on the home care of cancer patients, using an audit measure documenting assessment, intervention, and evidence of outcomes for patients with breast and colon cancers. Findings revealed that improvement in nursing assessment and management performance occurred over time in all three intervention groups. However, only half the criteria for optimal nurse performance were achieved, with little increase in patient outcome scores. The greatest improvements were noted in patients' nutrition, and little improvement was noted overall in the management of pain and physiologic complications. The authors recommend replication and offer the complete set of audit forms on request.

Similarly, Stephany[40] tested the reliability and validity of the Hope Hospice Quality Assurance Tool (HQAT), which assesses physical concerns, patient and caregiver education, and emotional and spiritual support, using operationally defined critera. Test-retest stability and internal consistency of the tool were established. Content, criterion-related, and construct validities were tested and found to be high in the nurse group but only moderate for lay volunteers. The tool was modified, with subsequent improvement in reliability and validity scores. The report provides detailed descriptions of the QA program, standards, and criteria and of the assessment form. The rigor of the study produced an effective audit tool to measure the quality of hospice care.

Arenth[41] developed and validated an acuity classification of oncology patients based on the definition of four categories of emergent status. The system has served as the basis for calculating nursing hours per patient day, patient volumes, nursing utilization or productivity, and variable staffing in a large medical center.

Dudjak[42] described the Radiation Therapy Nursing Care Record, comprising six flowsheets designed to document the nursing care of patients undergoing radiation therapy. The record allows for baseline assessment of risk factors and problems and for nursing practices in assessment, teaching, and other interventions. The record has been used to justify staff needs and cost of nursing care and to establish standards of practice further.

Because safety is a cornerstone of quality assurance for both patients and health care providers, periodic updates such as Gullo's review[43] of safe handling of antineoplastic drugs are essential to the application of the OSHA guidelines to practice. Recommendations for avoiding exposure, for safe disposal, and for health evaluation and monitoring are given clearly according to a well-articulated knowledge framework. Gullo estimated that more than 60% of nurses were not using safe handling techniques, an important factor in quality assurance. Two articles by Williamson et al[44,45] reviewed the occupational risks of infection, musculoskeletal injury, exposure to antineoplastic agents, stress in the work environment, shift work, and reproductive health concerns of nurses. Their articles call for a greater intensity of clinically oriented research efforts in this area.

Two articles suggest methods of establishing a clinical database to provide a structured framework for the collection of critical data with which to formulate nursing diagnoses. Miaskowski and Nielsen[46] developed the Cancer Nursing Assessment Tool to evaluate the integrity of 15 functional systems at high risk because of cancer and its treatment. The assessment included teaching needs and discharge planning. Gray et al[47] published a clinical database that provides description and analysis of age, metastatic sites, diagnoses, and associated symptoms of hospitalized patients with advanced cancer. Their study of 1103 patients generated more than 400 variables and provided important information on problem areas related to cancer metastasis. Since symptom management is the "cornerstone of care" in this patient group, the database facilitated the identification of relevant nursing diagnoses and related nursing practices that improved the measurement of quality of care.

On another level, two separate studies by Moore et al[48] and McGee et al[49] sought to establish nurse competencies and to measure proficiency in cancer nursing practice. The Moore team constructed the Appraisal of Practice Behaviors Instrument, based on the five dimensions of the theoretical framework used by ONS to develop the Standards of Oncology Nursing Practice. Three classes enrolled in a master's level oncology nursing graduate program were tested before and after each of the 2 years of their educational program for both frequency and self-assessed proficiency in achieving the ONS outcome standards of oncology practice. The instrument consists of 92 items divided among six subscales. Findings revealed that frequency of practice and proficiency were positively related and that students significantly increased in self-assessed proficiency as their educational program progressed. The investigators suggest further evaluation of the instrument in both academic and clinical settings to expand the database.

In contrast, McGee et al[49] conducted a two-round Delphi survey to identify oncology clinical nurse specialist (OCNS) competencies. The initial pilot study amassed 363 competencies, which the investigators further divided into knowledge, skill, attitude, and human trait categories. Ranking by means for each category revealed that attitude and human traits were ranked highest in importance by the 47 respondents. Attitudes of greatest importance had to do with ethical practice, respect for humanity, responsibility for behavior, and commitment to continued learning. Identifying nursing diagnoses and commitment to cost-effective practices were ranked lowest in the category. The human traits most valued included accountability, common sense, caring, flexibility, and resourcefulness. Of lower importance were sympathy and abstract thinking. The highest number of competencies, 173, were amassed in the "skills" category, and knowledge ranked second in number of competencies, totaling 137. The investigators, in interpreting their results, concluded that attitudes and human traits concerned with caring, commitment, and professionalism were ranked as those most important to OCNS functioning. They considered their results to be consistent with Yasko's survey[50] of 185 OCNSs, who reported a decided "care orientation" described as "keeping the client comfortable, maintaining a therapeutic environment, providing emotional support, personalized care, friendliness, emotional acceptance and ensuring that clients understand their medical problems."

The information generated from these key studies helps to expand and facilitate attempts to improve quality of care. By integrating findings from these and future studies on acuity, audit assessment tools, safety guidelines, clinical databases, and nursing competencies and practice proficiency, quality assurance will move into the era of strategic quality management predicted by Garven[18] and Beyers.[16]

Clinical research

Research offers a means of improving and refining practice to ensure optimal outcomes. The desired result of practice is usually defined as a valuable change in the patient for the better. In most institutional settings, this means cost-effective patient outcomes and consumer satisfaction.

Clinical research, in the context of evaluating quality of care, includes two major categories: (1) experimental studies of nursing interventions and (2) evaluations of programs of care. The program of research in most disciplines is shaped by the intellectual and practical problems and challenges encountered in carrying out its objectives and by the diagnostic and functional categories that constitute its focus. For nursing, these areas for investigation can best be illustrated by the results of two Delphi surveys conducted during the past decade to examine research priorities in cancer nursing.

Oberst[51] polled a group of 575 oncology nurses throughout the United States, asking them what they thought was important to investigate systematically in order to improve their clinical practice. From those nurses giving the most direct care to cancer patients, Oberst's goal was to capture a heuristic force that would have an impact on patient welfare by using the research process as a catalyst. She asked nurses to identify the problems they confront every day in practice, the problems cancer patients have from the time of diagnosis, and how these problems arrange themselves in priority.

The results of Oberst's study determined 10 priorities for cancer nursing research: (1) chemotherapy- or radiation-induced nausea and vomiting, (2) pain, (3) discharge needs, (4) grief, (5) stomatitis, (6) venipuncture in long-term therapy, (7) comfort and dignity of the terminally ill patient, (8) effective analgesia, (9) assistance with providing effective pain management, and (10) understanding the nurses' own attitudes toward pain and how it affects their ability to provide effective pain management. In addition, the oncology nurses responding to Oberst's survey reported that patient- and nurse-related research needs parallel one another. Optimal patient outcomes were inextricably tied to the reduction of deficits in nurse knowledge and skill in the 10 patient-focused research priority areas.

Ten years later, a partial replication of Oberst's work was conducted with 143 practicing oncology nurses from the four western provinces of Canada.[52] Results were similar but were expressed by requests for studies of specific interventions. Of the top 15 research priorities, the following areas emerged as most important: relaxation, imagery, and biofeedback techniques in the reduction of anticipatory nausea and vomiting and other side effects of treatment and in the enhancement of quality of life; ways to increase effectiveness of patient teaching in areas of patient compliance, self-care, and coping; approaches to improve discharge planning programs; methods of communicating diagnosis and prognosis to patients and families; approaches to strengthen effectiveness in primary care; ways to improve preceptorship programs; and therapeutic approaches to the relief of treatment- and disease-related symptoms and side effects. The emphasis of the Canadian results was clearly on studying nursing practices that improve the patient's condition, rather than on the problem itself. This shift may reflect the result of descriptive nursing research efforts and a more sophisticated practice during the past 10 years after Oberst's survey.[51]

In a review of research-based articles appearing in the cancer nursing literature between 1976 and 1984, Scott[31] found 122 articles representing 25% of all articles published. More than 60% of the studies were published after 1981, most concerned with side effects of treatment (26%) or with oncology nurses themselves (24%). Approximately 15% examined the impact of cancer on the family, and another 16% described phenomena about cancer patients. Only 12% were intervention-management studies, and fewer (7%) offered assessment-measurement approaches to evaluate care.

In a developmental sense, the era before 1985 may be viewed as a descriptive phase when the rich database that exists today was established. Clinical research, comprising both program evaluation and experimental studies of interventions, began slowly between 1980 and 1985, marked by the seminal work of Satterwhite et al,[53] Edlund,[35] Dodd and Mood,[54,55] Johnson,[56] Miller and Nygren,[57] Marty et al,[58] Watson,[59] and Henrich and Schag.[60] Since 1985, there has been an expansion of the cancer research literature addressing the priorities in the two Delphi surveys and testing the therapeutic effect of larger-scale programs of care.

Fourteen experimental studies published since 1984[61-74] (Table 53-4) addressed 3 of the 10 (30%) outcome standards for cancer nursing practice, with more than half testing interventions to promote patient comfort and reduce treatment-related side effects. Five studies (36%) tested interventions to optimize protective mechanisms by preventing infection or reducing skin and mucous membrane integrity deficits. One study (7%) evaluated an educational program to promote early cancer detection practices. As a whole, these studies reflected a growing sophistication in research design and measurement. Most were randomized, controlled investigations of the effect of a clearly defined intervention on a small, homogeneous sample. The instruments employed to measure patient outcomes generally had been tested for reliability and validity or consisted of well-defined clinical indicators rated for construct validity by a panel of experts. All reports discussed study limitations, the generalizability of results, and implications for further research. Moreover, practically all made useful contributions to clinical knowledge.

In the period from 1984 to 1989, a total of 14 program evaluation reports[75-88] (Table 53-5) covering a wider range of outcome standards were published. The largest number (5, or 36%) evaluated programs designed to assist patients and families to cope with cancer. The next largest category (4, or 29%), comfort, described multidisciplinary pain

TABLE 53-4 Experimental Studies of Oncology Nursing Interventions and Patient Outcomes by Functional Pattern Category

Author	Problem	Method	Findings	Implications
I. Prevention and early detection				
Rudolf and Quinn[61]	Education to promote TSE	N = 64 college men; Health Beliefs Survey for Testicular Cancer and Testicular Self-Examination Survey (modified by authors); pretest and posttest; educational program with film and silicone practice model	Subjects lacked knowledge about testicular cancer and TSE Increased perception in benefits and decrease in barriers to TSE resulted Of "never performers," 63% did TSE at least once after program Perception of susceptibility and disease seriousness did not increase	Need for education and for research testing of a variety of educational approaches Nurses should take lead Replication with time between testing and more controlled methods Further testing of instrument
IV. Comfort				
Cotanch et al[62]	Self-hypnosis as antiemetic therapy	N = 20 children, aged 9-18 years, receiving chemotherapy Experimental and control groups Investigator-constructed visual analog scale, self-report, nurse's charting Experimental subjects trained in relaxation and self-hypnosis	Decrease in intensity and severity of nausea and vomiting in experimental group Increased oral intake in experimental group No difference in antiemetic administration between groups	Further research in other age groups
Frank[63]	Music and guided imagery as antiemetic therapy	N = 15 adults on variety of chemotherapy regimens 13 women, 2 men Single group Pretest and posttest STAI Nausea and Vomiting Questionnaire Intervention: musical tapes and poster images during and after chemotherapy	Decreased anxiety (STAI) Decreased intensity of vomiting No difference in perception of nausea, but duration showed nonsignificant downward trend	Test intervention in other stressful, threatening situations (ie, crisis and pain)
Scott et al[64]	Progressive Muscle Relaxation (PMR), guided imagery, and slow-stroke back massage vs drug regimen as antiemetic therapy	N = 17 women with gynecologic cancer receiving chemotherapy Relaxation and drug groups Drug group received high-dose metaclopramide Emetic Process Rating Scale (EPRS) Relaxation group received 1-hour educational program with slide tape and were coached by nurse in relaxation	Relaxation group had reduced total duration Drug group had reduced peak vomiting phase No difference in intensity or amount of emesis between groups Drug group experienced significantly increased diuresis unexplained by intake Content validity of EPRS established Verification of phase periodicity	Testing interventions combining both methods Replication in other populations Continued testing of EPRS Data on norm phase periodicity for other chemotherapy regimens

Cotanch and Strum[65]	PMR as antiemetic therapy	N = 60 Three-group design: experimental, placebo control (music), true control (no intervention) Dukes Descriptive Scale Diary of Food Intake STAI Upper skin-fold size Blood pressure Admission-discharge assessments	PMR most effective in reducing frequency and duration of vomiting, general anxiety, and physiologic arousal and in improving caloric intake in patients 48 hours after chemotherapy	Replication
Parker[66]	Scalp hypothermia to reduce alopecia	N = 12 subjects receiving cyclophosphamide randomly assigned to 2 groups: experimental and control SPENCO Hypothermia Cap Samples of hair loss for 7 days after treatment Scalp photographs	Control subjects have significantly more hair loss than experimental subjects	Clinical use
Dudjak[67]	Mouth care for mucositis therapy	N = 15 subjects receiving radiation therapy to head and neck area Random assignment of experimental and control groups Experimental subjects received hydrogen peroxide solution Control subjects received baking soda and water Oral examination guide Oral Comfort Guide Subjects evaluated 8 times: once before radiation therapy and then once weekly for 5 weeks, at completion, and 1 month after completion	Increase in perceived comfort in experimental group No difference in mouth condition between groups Hydrogen peroxide treatment judged more effective Both groups at lower incidence than published norms Rate of infection equal in both groups	Replication Test other interventions Clinical use

TABLE 53-4 Experimental Studies of Oncology Nursing Interventions and Patient Outcomes by Functional Pattern Category (continued)

Author	Problem	Method	Findings	Implications
Winningham and MacVicar[68]	Aerobic exercise as antiemetic therapy	N = 42 breast cancer patients Matched age and functional capacity Three-group design: experimental (stationary bike), placebo control (mild stretching), control (no treatment) Treatment: supervised 10-week 3-times-per-week aerobic training on cycle ergometer Symptom-Limited Graded Exercise Text (SLGXT) Symptom Checklist 90—Revised Somatization Subscale All tests given before and after treatment	Marked improvement in experimental compared with other groups in patient reports of nausea Increase in somatization scores in experimental groups	Studies of other types of exercise, emetic treatment protocols, and studies to determine difference between exercise and relaxation
Giaccone et al[69]	Scalp hypothermia to reduce alopecia	N = 39 patients receiving doxorubicin Randomly assigned to experimental (scalp hypothermia) or control (no treatment) group SPENCO Hypothermia Evaluations after 2 full chemotherapy cycles Hair loss evaluated by nurse and physician using an operationalized scale	Control subjects (100% alopecia) Experimental subjects, 37% prevention of hair loss No or slight hair loss in 7 of 19 No instances of scalp metastasis in either group	Clinical use
VI. Protective mechanisms				
Shell et al[70]	Dressings to treat radiation therapy skin reactions	N = 16 patients with moderate to severe radiodermatitis Comparison of moisture-permeable to conventional hydrous lanolin gauze Evaluation of healing time by use of 4 visual inspection parameters in number of days	Healing time for Mvp: 19 days vs 24 days for lanolin gauze	Warrants further study

Harwood and Bachur[71]	DMSO vs local cooling in extravasation therapy	Animal study using 4 pigs Posttest control experimental design Micro measurements by primary investigator Measured time to healing DMSO vs local cooling with ice vs no treatment control	Local cooling more highly effective in preventing tissue necrosis after extravasation No difference between DMSO and control groups Time to healing increased with DMSO DMSO not recommended for treatment	More studies to determine optimal schedule of cooling
Jones[72]	Catheter care procedures in central venous catheter infection	Evaluation of 2 catheter care procedures, one using fewer supplies and less time Assessment of observable evidence of infection, neutrophil count, and blood cultures	No difference Only common factor connected with likelihood of infection: low neutrophil count at time of positive blood culture	Conduct further studies to refine predictive risk factors
MacGeorge et al[73]	Mixing vs reinfusion methods in drawing blood from Hickman catheter	N = 18 bone marrow transplant patients Hematocrit (Coulter counter) Visual determination of hemolysis by expert laboratory technician	No statistical difference in accuracy of laboratory values between 2 methods Mixing has advantage of less infection	Replication in pediatric population with larger sample in variety of clinical settings
Petrosino et al[74]	Dressing to reduce central venous catheter infection	N = 52 patients with central venous catheters Random assignment to 4 dressing groups: Tegaderm transparent, Op-Site, gauze, no dressing Observation at 7 and 30 days for 5 indicators: skin culture, oral temperature, erythema, tenderness, drainage	No difference among groups No dressing option seems simpler and less costly	Further research on skin cleansing techniques

TSE, Testicular self-examination; *STAI*, State-Trait Anxiety Inventory; *PMR*, progressive muscle relaxation; *DMSO*, dimethyl sulfoxide.

TABLE 53-5 Care Program Evaluation Studies

Program	Author	Method	Results
I. Prevention and detection			
Family High Risk Program	Beck et al[75]	Health Family Tree Questionnaire Family health survey to assess satisfaction with program, health practices, health history, and behavior; includes retrospective data	Evaluation ongoing No results as of publication
II. Information			
Patient Education Program	Nieweg et al[76]	Comparison of patient self-care of chemotherapy port infection rates with literature-based norms Weekly clinical assessments No standardized evaluation methods used	Empirically judged effective Takes considerable time Required teaching materials Greater social support involvement Less need for hospitalization Greater patient freedom
III. Coping			
We Can Weekend	Lane and Davis[77]	Postprogram participant evaluation Staff feedback Director-evaluation of training sessions, staff, facilities, schedule, public relations, and supplies	Recommended use of preprogram questionnaires to enable advance custom planning Also use of postprogram questionnaire
Living With Cancer	Fredette and Beattie[78]	Precourse and postcourse knowledge test Precourse and postcourse personal needs assessment Postcourse interviews Written comments of specialist-observer End-of-class and end-of-program evaluations	Coping skills can be taught Profiles "good coper" as one who pursues information and seeks opportunities to learn Adaptive, resilient, optimistic, and assertive Need further exploration into program design for those who desire less or differently structured programs Teaching skills of coping was primary value of program
Cancer Caregivers Program	Cawley and Gerdts[79]	Committee-constructed evaluation tool: evaluates 8 dimensions of care in terms of time, instructor, handouts	Provides steps in establishment of program Evaluation tool developed and provided Ongoing evaluation No results
I Can Cope	Diekmann[80]	Postprogram mail questionnaire	Demographic characteristics Overall evaluation: valuable to help people learn about cancer More research to improve impact on coping
Bereavement Outreach Program	Mosely et al[81]	No formal means of evaluation	Excellent client response Need to tailor program to institution

management programs. The rest were divided among prevention-detection (1, or 7%), information (1, or 7%), nutrition (1, or 7%), and two economic feasibility studies (14%) of an adult day care hospital and a home transfusion program.

The therapeutic programs generally were well defined, as was the patient population. Most were service innovations based on the institution's database of patient needs and problems. In a majority of these studies, evaluation methods proved to be the weakest component. Although all programs were judged as valuable by the investigators, only half employed evaluation criteria developed before program initiation. Some measured quality by the number of clients seen or by unsolicited patient feedback. Others, however, made use of standardized surveys, questionnaires, interviews, and preprogram and postprogram

TABLE 53-5 Care Program Evaluation Studies (continued)

Program	Author	Method	Results
IV. Comfort			
Home Pain Management Program	Coyle et al[82]	Evaluated 123 patients with advanced disease for pain management at home	Nurse becomes primary liaison Successful pain management at home with use of analgesic and behavioral modes Team as expert information resource in community
Continuous SC Infusion Pain Management Program	Coyle et al[83]	Evaluated 15 patients for quality of pain management	Avoids repeated injection, need for intravenous access, analgesia delay, pain breakthrough
Pain Management Team	Ferrell et al[84]	No evaluation of effect of interventions on pain	Patient visits: 7500 (750 patients) over course of 5 years Community presentations: 300
Patient-controlled Analgesia (PCA) Service	Kane et al[85]	Patient questionnaire on discharge Nurse evaluation of two pumps re safety, ease of use, saving of time Bedside flow sheets to rate pain and sedation Daily patient evaluation by PCA team	Use of pump gives excellent control of pain in postsurgical patients, has few problems, and frees nurse to care for patient Further studies in chronic pain populations needed Choice of one pump over another
V. Nutrition			
Home Parenteral Nutrition Program	Konstantinides[86]	Patient teaching flow sheet No formal evaluation methods presented	Cost estimated between $55,000 and $70,000 for nutritional solutions, supplies, home visits, clinic follow-up, and laboratory costs Guides for patient teaching, discharge planning, laboratory monitoring, and follow-up given
VI. General Focus			
Day Hospital for Cancer Patients	Clark[87]	Economic feasibility measures	One-year pilot project Ongoing as of publication
Home Care Transfusion Program	Pluth[88]	Cost comparisons with patients receiving transfusions in different settings Client satisfaction Difficulties in implementation	Cost-effective and beneficial to patients' quality of life

comparisons of knowledge tests or needs assessments with baseline findings. Almost all investigative teams communicated willingness to share their programs with others but advised tailoring them to the unique needs of the institution and their patient populations. Most suggested the need for further study and program modifications or refinements.

Although the program evaluations reflected significant effort in planning and execution by hardworking teams, it must be remembered that program evaluation is a mature methodology, generally requiring an expert team of outside investigators to conduct the study. Two noteworthy examples include the Brown University evaluation of the Adult Day Care Hospital, Memorial Sloan-Kettering Cancer Center[89] and the as yet unpublished University of Washington study of the effect of the Planetree Unit, a primary-nursing, family-centered care facility at Pacific Presbyterian Medical Center, San Francisco.

The overall picture of 28 studies published over a 4-year period suggests the beginning establishment of a clinical scientific base for practice. Clearly, much more research is needed in all standards-of-practice domains. Research that replicates or builds on the work of others and that refines established interventions may be the most economic ventures. However, to address meaningfully the issue of quality of care, longitudinal studies expanding the clinical database and testing effects of nursing intervention over time are critically needed. The oncology nursing research program, to have an impact on quality of care, will need not only to continue building the growing knowledge base in symptom management and patient education but also to turn attention to the issues of quality of life, recovery, transition, and the effect of a host of new modalities on patients' lives and health.

Measurement tool development: Quantitative

As psychometric theory advances and the results of nursing research build over time, better methods for measuring quality of care will emerge. Hartshorn.[90] Duffy,[91] and Lynn[92] emphasize the importance of using reliable and valid instruments in clinical research. Duffy said that research-based practice should be precise enough to be replicable and to produce predictable patient outcomes. Hartshorn warned that results from studies employing poor instruments cannot be accepted or implemented. Indeed, many nursing studies that have required considerable time and effort conclude with a long list of limitations to the generalizability of their findings and with an underdeveloped interpretation of important data because of faulty design, inadequate sampling technique, and use of untested measurement tools.

The basic ingredients of sound quantitative measurement techniques include adequate reliability and validity of the instrument. Reliability tests both the stability (test-retest correlations) and the internal consistency (intercorrelations among items or alpha coefficient) of an instrument. Correlations of at least 0.8 in internal consistency and test-retest correlations ensure that the instrument is reliably measuring the construct it purports to measure and is stable in its ability to reproduce results in repeated testing of the sample. A third type of reliability, interrater reliability, is also important to ensure that all persons using a set of evaluation criteria have closely correlated results.[93]

Validity testing offers a way to assess the ability of the instrument to measure the construct of interest accurately and objectively. The three most important types of validity include construct, content, and criterion related (predictive or concurrent).[90,93] One of the most definitive signs of increasingly improved and sophisticated cancer nursing research is growing evidence that reliable and valid instruments were used.

Table 53-6 provides a partial list of cancer nursing measurement tools* grouped by functional category, including the construct measured and whether evidence of reliability and validity testing are given.[94-114] Note that most of these instruments quantify patient attributes. The aim is to establish further a normative database or to measure the qualitative outcomes of nursing practice, or both.

Measurement tool development: Qualitative

During the past few years, an increasing interest in qualitative methods of research has become evident in the nursing literature. Measuring quality of care quantitatively does not readily capture the contextual nature and natural richness of the situational and interpersonal data that compose the nursing care environment.

Nursing literature generally reflects attempts at establishing patient databases composed of qualitative sets of indicators, predictors, and assessment parameters that form the etiologic foundations of patient concerns and nursing practices. For example, if we review the available quantitative tools, most are based on the identification of indicators grouped to facilitate diagnostic reasoning. However, less precision is found in scoring instrument results. Few scoring systems are based on large amounts of normative data, particularly those established in healthy populations that allow clear comparisons and interpretation of new data.

The most recognized qualitative approaches include case study, grounded theory, phenomenology, and ethnography, among others (Ammon-Gaberson and Piantanida.)[115] Qualitative research begins with carefully conceptualized and clearly articulated research questions to guide data collection and later interpretation. The motive is to understand an aspect of human experience and to shape a representation of it from the data. The results of the qualitative method may include (1) operationalizing a single concept, (2) developing a conceptual framework, (3) establishing guidelines for practice, (4) creating portraits, paradigm cases, or typologies, and (5) forming theory.

Although reliability testing and validity testing in the conventional sense do not have a place in the qualitative process, there are sound principles and methods to guide study design, data gathering, data analysis and management, data interpretation, and paradigm construction. These processes are no less rigorous than those of the quantitative approach. In many areas of quality of care research, the qualitative paradigm or a combination of the qualitative and quantitative paradigms may be the best approach.

The qualitative cancer nursing research literature represents a mixed bag of clinically relevant information that, for the purposes of a quality-of-care discussion, may be categorized according to format and content considerations. The research articles have been grouped as either indicators, predictors, or guidelines for care.

Indicators are sets of variables that describe empirically an important clinical manifestation. These sets are derived generally from a review of published work on the subject or a descriptive exploratory or qualitative study, or both. For example, Saunders and Valente's article[116] on suicide in cancer patients brings together their wealth of empirical knowledge as well as general information about depression and suicide. One outcome is a useful "Brief Suicide Assessment Guide" for practitioners. In contrast, Thorne[117] reported the results of her phenomenologic study of the family cancer experience, providing important insights into family perceptions and coping strategies when a member has cancer. Therefore information in a wide variety of content areas produced sets of clues to facilitate better understanding of many common clinical issues.

Predictors are variables that have been tested to deter-

*For a current, inclusive discussion of clinical research tools in nursing, consult Frank-Stromborg's *Instruments for Clinical Nursing Research*.[94]

TABLE 53-6 Tools to Measure Patient Outcomes

Tool	Author	Construct	Findings	Implications
Quality of Life Index (QLI)	Ferrans and Powers[95]	Quality of life	Likert scales (2) to determine importance and satisfaction in 18 life areas: life goals, general satisfaction, stress, physical health; reliability established; validity established; versions for normal, healthy adults and for kidney transplant, heart transplant, kidney dialysis, and cancer patients	Establishing norms in different populations
Cancer Malaise Scale	Kobashi-Schoot et al[96]	Physical fatigue, mental fatigue, malaise, psychologic complaints in radiotherapy cancer patients; validity established	Malaise increased during course of treatment; physical symptoms increased late in course of treatment; malaise correlates with "feeling ill" or "not well"	Further correlation stratified by treatment level of radiation exposure
Quality of Life Index (QLI)	Padilla and Grant[97]	Linear analog: psychologic well-being, physical well-being, symptom control; 14 items; reliability established; validity established		Further testing in variety of subject populations; use to test intervention effectiveness
Information Preference Questionnaire (IPQ)	Hopkins[98]	Information seeking; 5-point scale measuring preference for treatment information	Information seeking negatively related to age and severity of disease; reliability established; validity established	Needs additional testing to establish criterion and construct validities
Emetic Process Rating Scale (EPRS)	Scott et al[64]	Analog scale: nausea, retching, vomiting, intake, output, vital signs, treatment; validity established	Evaluated antiemetic effect of clinical relaxation vs drug intervention; scale found clinically useful	Further reliability and validity testing
Sexual Adjustment Questionnaire (SAQ)	Waterhouse and Metcalf[99]	Desire, activity level, relationship, arousal, techniques, orgasm	Persons with cancer significantly reduced scores on activity level, relationships, and techniques	Continued refinement and larger sample testing
Derdiarian Informational Needs Assessment (DINA)	Derdiarian[100]	Informational needs related to disease: personal, family, and social parameters		Further instrument assessment and use in patient referral and follow-up
Patient Care Needs Survey	Fleming et al[101]	Comfort needs in advanced cancer patients: physiologic, spiritual, psychosocial, patients' rights, dignity, self-worth	Identified 7 themes of comfort; decreased with severity of illness; calls for social support approach, including multidisciplinary	Further development and testing
Human Needs Assessment Scale	Lilley[102]	Likert scale of 35 human needs based on work by Yura and Walsh; modified to a 4-point scale; reliability established; evaluates importance of need	Instrument easy to use; nurses perceived patients' human needs similarly to patients' own assessment	Suggest development of nursing diagnosis and evaluation of nursing care to be based on this Human Need Model
Quality of Life Questionnaire (QLQ)	Young-Graham and Longman[103]	Likert-type brief scale: social dependency, symptom distress, behavior-morale, direction of life change; reliability established	Pilot study of patients with melanoma to test model of major hypothesized factors in quality of life	Further use in other populations; internal consistency confirmed

TABLE 53-6 Tools to Measure Patient Outcomes (continued)

Tool	Author	Construct	Findings	Implications
Derogatis Sexual Functioning Inventory (DSFI) (modified)	Blackmore[104]	Affect, body image, symptoms, drive, satisfaction, activity	Reduction in sexual activity postoperatively in orchidectomy cancer group	More research on sexuality of cancer patients
McGill Pain Questionnaire	Camp[105]	Location, quality, pattern, increase, intensity, verbal-nonverbal symptoms; reliability established; validity established	Compared patient perceptions and nurse documentation; less than 50% of patients' pain perceptions were documented	Replication and assessment of pain management protocols
Hypercalcemia Knowledge Questionnaire (HKQ)	Coward[106]	Hypercalcemia risk factors and knowledge		Need for educational program to evaluate
Derdiarian Behavioral System Model	Derdiarian[107]	Achievement, affiliation, aggressive-protective, dependence, elimination, ingestion, restoration, sexuality; based on Johnson Behavioral Symptom Model; reliability established; validity established	Defines imbalance in behavioral subsystems caused by illness; predicts direction and quality of change; sensitive to age, site of cancer, and stage of cancer	Further studies in larger samples
Oral Assessment Guide	Eilers et al[108]	Stomatitis or oral mucositis and mucosal changes in radiotherapy and chemotherapy patients: voice, swallow, lips, tongue, saliva, mucous membranes, gingivae, teeth and dentures	Clinical guide to evaluate oral care protocols and toxic effects of treatment protocols and persons at risk	Further clinical use
Breast Self-examination (BSE) Belief and Attitude Questionnaire	Lauver[109]	Remembering, competence, comfort, interference, efficacy; reliability established	Positive relationship between frequency of BSE and competence, remembering, and comfort	Replication in larger, heterogeneous population with test-retest reliability; further testing for methods to promote competence and remembering
Pain Assessment Tool (PAT) and Pain Flow Sheet (PFS)	McMillan and Williams[110]	Ongoing assessment of pain and its management	Pain intensity and level of sedation documented in two-group study	Further research with both tools
Self-care and Symptom Report Interview	Rhodes et al[111]	Symptom distress, self-care activities, coping strategies regarding fatigue and weakness; based on Orem's self-care deficit theory	Lays foundation for tool to measure symptom occurrence and distress and to assess self-care efficacy	Ongoing development and testing
Linear Analogue Modification (LAM) of Profile of Mood States (POMS)	Sutherland et al[112]	Emotional distress: fatigue, anxiety, confusion, depression, energy, anger	Significant correlation between LAM and POMS in 29 subjects	To evaluate patients' ongoing emotional status as base for psychosocial interventions over time
Cancer Knowledge Test	Weinrich and Weinrich[113]	Belief in cancer myths, recall of American Cancer Society 7 warning signals, recognition of disease symptoms	Overall significant difference in cancer knowledge based on race, education, and income	Evaluation of health teaching on elderly, less educated, and low-income black persons
Champion's Instrument and Williams' Breast Inventory	Williams[114]	Likert scale of 5 constructs of Health Belief Model, health history, and personal knowledge	Health motivation represents 18% of variance; barriers, 8%; age differences	Further testing of variables

mine their ability to predict a future event with some degree of accuracy. Predictors are critical to nursing's role in health promotion and prevention. For example, Hays' article[118] on predictors of hospice utilization identified specific patient and family parameters that, when taken into consideration early enough in the nursing plan of care, have a good chance of strengthening the family unit so that the patient can be maintained at home under quality care conditions for longer periods. Another illustration of the establishment of predictors is the research that has identified clusters of variables predicting the occurrence of anticipatory nausea and vomiting.[119,120]

Guidelines for care are organized, integrated schemata for practice. These presentations are readily identifiable by title descriptors such as nursing care, nursing interventions, nursing implications, the nursing role, nursing assessments, nursing management, and nursing plans for a variety of patient problems, specialized treatments, or situations. In most cases, guidelines are in tabular format, resembling the traditional nursing care plan (problem, care, scientific rationale) with updated language such as nursing diagnoses, nursing etiology, nursing interventions, and nursing evaluations by outcome criteria.

Table 53-7 provides a list of indicators, predictors, and assessment guidelines used in recent studies addressing quality of care.[121-153] These articles report studies of cancer-related disease and treatment problems, psychosocial adjustment, risk factors, and family response and coping.

QUALITY IN PERFORMANCE: APPLICATIONS IN PRACTICE

No discussion of care is complete without a look at process—the performance of nursing care and its meaning for both patient and nurse. Although patient outcome has become the basis for care evaluation, the multiple forces impinging on a patient's condition often make this method

TABLE 53-7 Indicators, Predictors, and Guidelines for Quality of Care

Indicators

Fever patterns in neutropenic patients (Henschel[121])

Psychologic model of adjustment in gynecologic cancer patients (Krouse[122])

Family cancer experience (Thorne[117])

Sexual and reproductive issues for women with Hodgkin's disease (Cooley and Cobb[123,124])

Cancer-induced hypercalcemia (Coward[125])

Primary caregiver's perception of the dying trajectory (Holing[126])

Alterations in taste during cancer treatment (Huldij et al[127])

Family responses to cancer hospitalization (Lovejoy[128])

Characteristics of pain in hospitalized cancer patients (Donovan[129])

Sexual changes after gynecologic cancer treatment (Jenkins[130])

Cisplatin-related peripheral neuropathy (Ostchega et al[131])

Weakness, fatigue, and self-care abilities (Rhodes et al[111])

Suicide in cancer patients (Saunders and Valente[116])

Cancer pain control behavior (Wilkie et al[132])

Predictors

Patterns of lung cancer dyspnea (Brown et al[133])

Anticipatory nausea and vomiting associated with cancer chemotherapy (Duigon[119])

Patterns of hospice utilization (Hays[118])

Radiotherapy symptom profile (King et al[134])

Carotid artery rupture (Lesage[135])

Colorectal cancer (Messner et al[136])

Glucocorticosteroid-induced depression (Post-White[137])

Needs of family members of cancer patients (Tringali[138])

Anticipatory nausea and vomiting (Coons et al[120])

Patterns of nausea, vomiting, and distress with antineoplastic drug protocols (Rhodes et al[139])

Guidelines for Care

Prevention of chemotherapy-associated pneumonia in non-Hodgkin's lymphoma (Foote[140])

Primary, secondary, and tertiary interventions for lymphedema (Getz[141])

Management of disseminated intravascular coagulation (Rooney and Haviley[142])

Care of patients treated with intrapleural tetracycline for malignant pleural effusion (Rossetti[143])

The compromised host (Gurevich and Tafuro[144])

Management of venous access ports (Moore et al[145])

Morphine infusion for intractable cancer pain by implanted pump (Paice[146])

Care of head and neck cancer patients receiving myocutaneous flap reconstructive surgery (Rodzwic and Donnard[147])

Care of patients receiving radiation therapy for rectal cancer (Hassay[148])

Care of patients receiving third-generation cephalosporins (Link[149])

Assessment of gynecology patients (Moreland[150])

Needs of the spouse of the patient with advanced cancer (Stetz[151])

Care of the family with cancer (Lewandowski and Jones[152])

Skin care during radiotherapy (Strohl[153])

partially precise at best. Outcomes are relative and frequently are only partly related to the quality of nurse performance. More often, quality is deeply embedded in the rich mutual interpretations of care and caring that constitute the nurse-patient bond. Measuring quality of care by documented patient outcome is only one aspect of the multipronged approach demanded, an important indication that evaluation must go beyond the standard.

Determining the quality of a process is tricky and yet critical to the search for excellence. There are four important patterns to the process of giving and receiving care. The first is *mutuality*. Care behavior and the caring attitude forge a mutuality of response between two people that is characterized by reciprocity and complementarity. The experience is shared and cooperative, and the roles of caregiver and care receiver are complementary in that there is a degree of dissimilarity in the nature of the role relationship that works in a nondissonant way, allowing for harmony. However, the degree of dissimilarity is important in that the effect of care can be compromised if patient-nurse perceptions are either too much alike or radically different.

The nature of the mutual experience of caregiver and care receiver and their interacting perceptions are central to the quality of care. A growing literature focused on the congruity of nurse and patient perceptions reflects this phenomenon. In an early study by Jennings and Muhlenkamp,[154] caregivers' perceptions of their patients' affective states and the patients' self-reports of their anxiety, hostility, and depression were significantly different. Caregivers (eg, physicians, nurses, nursing assistants) assessed patients as feeling significantly worse than patients reported feeling. Findings were interpreted in light of "Wright's requirement-of-mourning hypothesis" that caregivers may perceive patients as having negative feelings so that the caregivers' own value systems, which place emphasis on health, will be supported."[155]

In 1987, Verron et al[156] hypothesized that attitudes of health care providers, grounded in their values, influence the quality of patient care. The authors cited work linking learning, experience, and consequent changes in attitude with positively modified behavior that endured for long periods.[157] Further, they attempted to identify and measure attitude themes pertinent to caring for oncology patients. The "Ideas About Oncology Patient Care Scale" (IAOPC) resulted, generating four attitude-related factors: therapy, future outlook, terminality, and drug use. Through repeated instrument testing, the attitudes were found to be multidimensional, another indication of the complexities of measuring human responses to caregiving and care receiving.

Larson[3,158,159] laid a foundation for unraveling the intricacies involved in giving and receiving care. She interviewed two separate samples of patients and nurses to determine what nurse behaviors were most and least important in making cancer patients feel "cared for." Her assumption was that the optimal expectation of nursing care is for patients to feel cared for as a result of nursing actions. Feeling cared for was defined as a sensation of well-being and safety linked to the behavior of the nurse. Nurses and patients were asked to rank, in order of importance, 50 nurse caring behaviors categorized by six action themes: anticipation, accessibility, explanation-facilitation, provision of comfort, establishment of trust, and monitoring with follow-through. Findings revealed that patients and nurses held very divergent opinions of what was most important. The highest-ranked behaviors reported by patients were those demonstrating competency, actions mostly concerned with monitoring and follow-through and with accessibility. Actions rated highest by nurses were more focused on meeting comfort and psychosocial needs such as listening and touch. In an examination of the top 10 responses of both groups, however, several mutual choices appeared: being quickly accessible, giving good physical care, putting the patient first, and listening. These choices indicated several important shared values.

Mayer[160] replicated Larson's study and found similar results. There was 100% agreement between samples of nurses in both studies regarding the most and least important caring behaviors. Comparisons of the two patient groups revealed 40% agreement for the most important behaviors and 80% for the least important. Across both studies and all samples, conventions of professional etiquette such as appearance, cheerfulness, and polite social behavior were viewed as least important. In Mayer's study, listening was again rated highest by nurses, and knowing how to give injections and intravenous infusions, and managing technical equipment remained most important to patients. Mayer concluded that patients seem to value the instrumental, technical caring skills and that nurses are more attuned to expressive caring behaviors.

These results might reflect understandable differences in perception between the two groups. Patients seemed to value those competencies and skills most concretely apparent and directly linked to their welfare. Nurses, on the other hand, may have perceived expressive and instrumental dimensions of care as inextricably connected, similar to the mutuality of care and cure. Who can deny the effect when patient preparation, technical skill, and gentleness are integrated during administration of an uncomfortable, intrusive procedure? To emphasize one aspect without the others decontextualizes care and strips it of its healing quality.

Several other comparison reports have documented discrepancies between patients' self-reports and their nurses' knowledge and understanding of patients' needs. Sodestrom and Martinson[161] found that 76% of a sample of nurses caring for hospitalized terminally ill patients considered spiritual needs low on the list of priorities because of the lack of time to incorporate spiritual assessment into care. Although the nurses correctly identified the meaning and purpose of their patient's relationship with God and the patient-nurse definitions of the term *spiritual* did not differ significantly, the nurses in this study did not view themselves as essential in meeting the spiritual needs of their terminally ill patients.

As the location of cancer care increasingly moves into the home, the concept of caregiver expands to include family members and others in charge of the patient's welfare. In light of this trend, congruence between caregiver and care recipient perceptions of quality of life was examined in 23 care dyads in a home hospice program (Curtis and Fernsler[162]). The overall trend, although not statistically significant, was for patients to report a higher quality of life for themselves in comparison with their caregivers' assessments. Patients reported better sleeping and pain control than did caregivers, but much less fun and sexual satisfaction. Thus nurse caregivers are not alone in their struggle to interpret the patient's situation accurately.

The needs of family members as they care for their loved ones with cancer are emerging as an important dimension in quality of care. Dyck and Wright[163] found that almost half of their sample of next-of-kin said that nurses did not do anything for them as family members, nor did they expect anything. Their expectation, however, seemed to be a function of limitations in their knowledge of the role of the nurse and what was thought to be the appropriate focus—the patient. If the patient was competently cared for and the nurse kept the family accurately informed, families said they could not expect more. Yet, a parallel analysis of their needs documented acceptance, support, and comfort as being very important to them. Furthermore, their rank-order of traits looked for in nurses differed depending on the stage of the patient's illness. Competence was number one in the early diagnostic stage, friendliness when the disease recurred, and compassion during the terminal stage. The authors concluded that appropriate emphasis of a trait is contextually determined and a significant way that nurses may express "caring for" patients.

The second major pattern in the caregiving and care-receiving process is *contextuality*. The contextual aspects of care have been highlighted repeatedly in these studies, with location of care and phase of illness emerging as two important determinants of the most appropriate clinical approach. Often, phenomenologic studies provide the best look at contextuality.

For example, Thorne,[117] in studying helpful and unhelpful communications in care, refers to cancer as "a modern metaphor for human confrontation with existential uncertainty." She found that communication is important in shaping the illness experience. Patients in Thorne's study were able to recall communication with health care providers during their illness and distinguish between styles that were more and less helpful. She found that the more uncertain a patient's situation, the greater was the vulnerability to communication characterized by lack of concern. On the other hand, the providers' feelings of failure, vulnerability, and hopelessness were part of the total picture as well. Nurses did not figure prominently into this compilation of opinions about helpful and unhelpful communicators, although study subjects reported that physicians communicated more about the disease and nurses provided advice about treatment and the illness. More often, a communication was perceived to be helpful if it was thought to be intentionally supportive. The most frequent unhelpful type was described as advice that was intentionally unhelpful, when the person withheld information or abused his power. Moreover, most important to the caring process was content, style, and a manner perceived by the patient as intentionally designed to be useful, encouraging, and supportive.

As a unit, these studies highlight the importance of mutuality and contextuality in determining the quality of nursing care performance. Yet, two other patterns have emerged as major influences on quality of performance; these patterns are so mutually dependent that they must be considered as one: *competence and proficiency*.

Benner[164,165] says that the practical knowledge embedded in expert nursing needs to be understood and yet has not been fully elucidated. Since clinical practice involves constant interpretation and prediction based on complex, contextual information, expertise increases as the nurse becomes intuitively able to read the situation as a whole as a result of past experience. The experience of the nurse is central to proficiency, which Benner views as having five levels: novice, advanced beginner, competent nurse, proficient nurse, and expert. Experience is the vehicle by which the nurse passes through these phases.

Progress in the movement from novice to expert is reflected by three gradual changes in performance. Initially, rather than relying solely on abstract principles and procedures to guide nursing practice, the nurse acquires a personal knowledge rich in "paradigms" of various care issues. The paradigms emerge from past experience that not only challenges previously held perceptions but is powerful enough to change and refine those preconceptions and understandings. Later, as the nurse gains experience, situations are viewed holistically, with the nurse focusing only on the most relevant elements and having a deep sense of confidence in intuitive interpretations. Finally, there is full involvement in the situation as a confident, effective performer.

The fourth major pattern of the care process is *intentionality of caring*. Intentionality of caring represents the connecting pattern or matrix holding together mutuality, contextuality, and competence with proficiency. Intentionality of caring requires awareness and a determined effort to provide quality care in any setting or to facilitate others as they provide care for cancer patients. Intentionality of caring serves to enhance quality in practice by the following:

- Recognizing that care is mutual—a cooperative venture between two human beings, based on a balanced complement of perceptions
- Considering the context of the care environment on the basis of an understanding of the shared meaning of the circumstances
- Encouraging pride in one's acquired competencies (knowledge, skills, attitudes, and traits) and having a desire to increase proficiency and become expert

Overall, intentionality of caring links the science and art of nursing knowledge and skill. Its most overt manifestation in practice is known as clinical judgment.

CONCLUSION

Every health care provider group today is struggling with the definition, provision, and evaluation of quality care. Nursing comes to the task from a long tradition of empirically established caring skills and a more recent scientific knowledge based on clinical research.

For two decades, experts in the quality assurance field have advocated a three-dimensional approach to the quality question based on structure, process, and outcome variables and their relatedness (see Figure 53-1). Structural elements are those grounding fundamentals that provide a sense of shared purpose and criteria against which effect can be measured. The structural elements include nursing's direction, definition, education, legislation, diagnostic taxonomy, standards of practice, research and technology, and programs of peer review and quality assurance.

Process is a much more elusive phenomenon in that it represents the individualized enactment of competencies characterized by knowledge, skills, human traits, and attitudes[49] under diverse and unique environmental conditions (contextuality) where the mutuality of caregiver and care receiver is central. Process is most manifest in the intentionality of caring of the care provider and in the proficiency with which competencies are revealed. Therefore process is much more difficult to evaluate in comparison with the components of structure and outcome.

Oncology nursing has come closest to evaluating the process dimension by defining standards of performance that recognize several critical determinants of quality: continuously working to perfect the art, science, and skill of practice; participating as a contributing, valued member of the health care team; utilizing the problem-solving process in the planning, organization, and execution of care and in its evaluation through the conduct or utilization of research; and providing a health care service to patients on the basis of a host of both independent and interdependent interventions conducted in an autonomous way. The measurement of process is based generally on written documentation and periodic peer evaluation. Some attempts have been made to categorize[164] and to measure[48] proficiency, and the literature on caring as a science is expanding rapidly.

Outcome criteria have been defined in terms of patient outcomes, quality of life, and, for nursing to some degree, maximum life extension. These criteria are best represented by patient outcome standards and by a burgeoning literature focused on the quality of life of the person with cancer and his or her family. As we gain knowledge about the quality of life, the purpose of nursing as a science of caring will more clearly be understood, and will further enable us to foster, nurture, and strengthen its quality.

REFERENCES

1. Nightingale F: Notes on Nursing. New York, Appleton-Century-Crofts, 1859.
2. Benner P: Nursing as a caring profession. Working paper for the Academy of Nursing Annual Meeting, October 16-18, 1988, Kansas City, Mo.
3. Larson P: Cancer nurses' perceptions of caring. Cancer Nurs 9(2):86-92, 1986.
4. Gaut DA: A philosophic orientation to caring, in Leininger MM (ed): Care: The Essence of Nursing and Health. Thorofare, NJ, Slack, 1984, pp 17-26.
5. Leininger MM: Care: The Essence of Nursing. Thorofare, NJ, Slack, 1984.
6. Watson J: Nursing: The Philosophy and Science of Caring. Boston, Little, Brown, 1979.
7. Dougherty CJ: American Health Care: Realities, Rights, and Reforms. New York, Oxford University Press, 1988.
8. President's Commission for the Study of Ethical Problems in Medicine and Biomedical and Behavioral Research: Securing Access to Health Care, vol I. Washington, DC, US Government Printing Office, 1983.
9. Oncology Nursing Society: Board approves revised scope of practice statement. ONS News 3(6):1-2, 1988.
10. Taylor C: Philosophic Papers, vols I and II. Cambridge, Cambridge University Press, 1985.
11. Harmer C, Henderson V: Principles and Practices of Nursing. New York, Macmillan, 1956.
12. Mundinger L: Nursing diagnoses for cancer patients. Cancer Nurs 1:221-226, 1978.
13. Herberth L, Gosnell DJ: Nursing diagnosis for oncology nursing practice. Cancer Nurs 10(1):41-51, 1987.
14. Gordon M: Nursing Diagnoses: Process and Application. New York, McGraw-Hill, 1982.
15. American Nurses' Association: Nursing: A Social Policy Statement. Kansas City, Mo, The Association, 1980.
16. Beyers M: Quality: The banner of the 1980s. Nurs Clin North Am 23:617-623, 1988.
17. Winchester DP: The assurance of quality for the cancer patient. Paper presented at the American Cancer Society Symposium on Advances in Cancer Management, Hilton Towers, Los Angeles, Calif, December 1988.
18. Garven DA: Managing Quality: The Strategic and Competitive Edge. New York, The Free Press, 1988.
19. National Cancer Institute: Five-year survival rates. SEER Program. Washington, DC, US Government Printing Office, 1983.
20. Henderson M: Introduction, in Roberts L (ed): Cancer Today: Origins, Prevention, and Treatment. Washington, DC, National Academy of Sciences Press, 1984.
21. Oncology Nursing Society: Outcome Standards for Cancer Nursing Practice. Pittsburgh, Pa, The Society, 1979.
22. Oncology Nursing Society and American Nurses' Association: Standards of Oncology Nursing Practice. Kansas City, Mo, The Association, 1987.
23. American Nurses' Association: A Plan for Implementation of Standards of Nursing Practice. Kansas City, Mo, The Association, 1979.
24. Oncology Nursing Society: Outcome Standards for Cancer Nursing Education. Pittsburgh, Pa, The Society, 1982.
25. Oncology Nursing Society: Cancer Patient Education. Pittsburgh, Pa, The Society, 1982.

26. Oncology Nursing Society: Public Cancer Education. Pittsburgh, Pa, The Society, 1983.
27. Orem DE: Nursing Concepts of Practice. New York, McGraw-Hill, 1987.
28. Johnson DE: The behavioral system model for nursing, in Riehl JP, Roy C (eds): Conceptual Model for Nursing Practice (2nd ed). New York, Appleton-Century-Crofts, 1980.
29. Donabedian A: Structure, process and outcome standards. Am J Public Health 59:1833, 1969.
30. Majesky SJ, Brester MH, Nishio KT: Development of a research tool: Patient indicators of nursing care. Nurs Res 27:365-371, 1978.
31. Scott DW: The Research Connection: Practice, Research, Theory. Keynote Address: American Cancer Society Nursing Research Conference, Honolulu, Hawaii, June 1985. Proceedings. Denver, American Cancer Society, 1986.
32. Brown MH, Kiss ME: Cancer audit. Cancer Nurs 2:1-6, 1979.
33. Legge JS, Reilly BJ: Assessing the outcomes of cancer patients in a home nursing program. Cancer Nurs 3:357, 1980.
34. Valencius JC, Packard R, Widiss T: The ONS-ANA Outcome Standards for Cancer Nursing Practice: Two models for implementation—Implementation of the Nutrition Standard at City of Hope National Medical Center. Oncol Nurs Forum, 7:137-140, 1980.
35. Edlund BJ: Patient education: Determining the effectiveness of an ostomy care guide in facilitating comprehensive patient care. Oncol Nurs Forum, 8(3):43-46, 1981.
36. Wood HA, Ellerhorst JM: Using site-specific nursing algorithms as an adjunct to oncology nursing guidelines. Oncol Nurs Forum 10(3):22-27, 1983.
37. Joint Commission on the Accreditation of Hospitals: Accreditation Manual for Hospitals (AMH/88). Chicago, The Commission, 1987.
38. Patterson CH: Standards of patient care: The Joint Commission focus on nursing quality assurance. Nurs Clin North Am 23:625-638, 1988.
39. Oleske DM, Otte DM, Heinze S: Development and evaluation of a system for monitoring the quality of oncology nursing care in the home setting. Cancer Nurs 10:190-198, 1987.
40. Stephany TM: Quality assurance for hospice programs. Oncol Nurs Forum, 12(3):33-40, 1985.
41. Arenth LM: The development and validation of an Oncology Patient Classification System. Oncol Nurs Forum, 12(6):17-27, 1985.
42. Dudjak LA: Radiation Therapy Nursing Care Record: A tool for documentation. Oncol Nurs Forum 15:763-777, 1988.
43. Gullo SM: Safe handling of antineoplastic drugs. Translating the recommendations into practice. Oncol Nurs Forum 15:595-601, 1988.
44. Williamson KM, Selleck CS, Turner JC, et al: Occupational health hazards for nurses: Infection. Image 20:48-53, 1988.
45. Williamson KM, Turner JG, Brown KC, et al: Occupational health hazards for nurses. Part II. Image 20:162-168, 1988.
46. Miaskowski CA, Nielsen B: A cancer nursing assessment tool. Oncol Nurs Forum 12(6):37-42, 1985.
47. Gray G, Adler D, Fleming C, et al: A clinical data base for advanced cancer patients: Implications for nursing. Cancer Nurs 11(2):77-83, 1988.
48. Moore IM, Piper B, Dodd MJ, et al: Measuring oncology nursing practice: Results from one graduate program. Oncol Nurs Forum 14(1):45-49, 1987.
49. McGee RF, Powell ML, Broadwell DC, et al: A Delphi survey of oncology nurse specialist competencies. Oncol Nurs Forum, 14(2):29-34, 1987.
50. Yasko JM: A survey of oncology clinical nursing specialists. Oncol Nurs Forum 10(1):25-30, 1983.
51. Oberst MT: Priorities in cancer nursing research. Cancer Nurs 1:281-290, 1978.
52. Western Consortium for Cancer Nursing Research: Priorities for cancer nursing research. Cancer Nurs 10:319-326, 1987.
53. Satterwhite BA, Pryor AS, Harris MB: Development and evaluation of chemotherapy fact sheets. Cancer Nurs 3:277-284, 1980.
54. Dodd MJ, Mood DW: Chemotherapy: Helping patients to know the drugs they are receiving and their possible side effects. Cancer Nurs 4:311-318, 1981.
55. Dodd MJ: Self-care for side effects in cancer chemotherapy: An assessment of nursing interventions. Part II. Cancer Nurs 6:63-67, 1983.
56. Johnson J: The effects of a patient education course on persons with a chronic illness. Cancer Nurs 5:117-123, 1982.
57. Miller MW, Nygren C: Living with cancer: Coping behaviors. Cancer Nurs 1:297-302, 1978.
58. Marty PJ, McDermott RJ, Gold RS: An assessment of three alternative formats for promoting breast self-examination. Cancer Nurs 6:207-211, 1983.
59. Watson PJ: The effects of short-term postoperative counseling on cancer/ostomy patients. Cancer Nurs 6:21-29, 1985.
60. Heinrich RL, Schag CC: A behavioral medicine approach to coping with cancer: A case report. Cancer Nurs 7:243-247, 1984.
61. Rudolf VM, Quinn KL McE: The practice of TSE among college men: Effectiveness of an educational program. Oncol Nurs Forum 15:45-48, 1988.
62. Cotanch P, Hockenberry M, Herman S: Self-hypnosis as antiemetic therapy in children receiving chemotherapy. Oncol Nurs Forum 12(4):41-46, 1985.
63. Frank JM: The effects of music therapy and guided visual imagery on chemotherapy-induced nausea and vomiting. Oncol Nurs Forum, 12(5):47-52, 1985.
64. Scott DW, Donahue DC, Mastrovito RC, et al: Comparative trial of clinical relaxation and an antiemetic drug regimen in reducing chemotherapy-related nausea and vomiting. Cancer Nurs 9:178-187, 1986.
65. Cotanch P, Strum S: Progressive muscle relaxation as antiemetic therapy for cancer patients. Oncol Nurs Forum 14(1):33-37, 1987.
66. Parker R: The effectiveness of scalp hypothermia in preventing cyclophosphamide-induced alopecia. Oncology Nurs Forum 14(6):49-53, 1987.
67. Dudjak LA: Mouth care for mucositis due to radiation therapy. Cancer Nurs 10:131-140, 1987.
68. Winningham ML, MacVicar MG: The effect of aerobic exercise on patient reports of nausea. Oncol Nurs Forum 15:447-450, 1988.
69. Giaccone G, DiGuilio F, Morandini MP, et al: Scalp hypothermia in the prevention of doxorubicin-induced hair loss. Cancer Nurs 11:170-173, 1988.
70. Shell JA, Stanutz F, Grimm J: Comparison of moisture vapor permeable (MVP) dressings to conventional dressings for management of radiation skin reactions. Oncol Nurs Forum 13(1):11-16, 1986.
71. Harwood KVS, Bachur N: Evaluation of dimethylsulfoxide and local cooling as antidotes for doxorubucin extravasation in a pig model. Oncol Nurs Forum 14(1):39-44, 1987.

72. Jones PM: Indwelling central venous catheter–related infections and two different procedures of catheter care. Cancer Nurs 10:123-130, 1987.
73. MacGeorge L, Steeves L, Steeves RH: Comparison of the mixing and reinfusion methods of drawing blood from a Hickman catheter. Oncol Nurs Forum 15:335-338, 1988.
74. Petrosino B, Becker H, Christian B: Infection rates in central venous catheter dressings. Oncol Nurs Forum 15:709-717, 1988.
75. Beck S, Breckenridge-Patter S, Wallace S, et al: The Family High-Risk Program: Targeted cancer prevention. Oncol Nurs Forum 15:301-306, 1988.
76. Nieweg R, Greidanus J, deVries EGE: A patient education program for a continuous infusion regimen on an outpatient basis. Cancer Nurs 10:177-182, 1987.
77. Lane CA, Davis AW: Implementation: We Can Weekend in the rural setting. Cancer Nurs 8:323-328, 1985.
78. Fredette S, La F, Beattie HM: Living with cancer: A patient education program. Cancer Nurs 9:308-316, 1986.
79. Cawley MM, Gerdts EK: Establishing a cancer caregiver's program: An interdisciplinary approach. Cancer Nurs 11:266-273, 1988.
80. Diekmann JM: An evaluation of selected "I Can Cope" programs by registered participants. Cancer Nurs 11:274-282, 1988.
81. Mosely JR, Logan SJ, Tolle SW, et al: Developing a bereavement program in a university hospital setting. Oncol Nurs Forum 15:151-155, 1988.
82. Coyle N, Monzillo E, Loscalzo M, et al: A model for continuity of care for cancer patients with pain and neuro-oncologic complications. Cancer Nurs 8:111-119, 1985.
83. Coyle N, Mauskop A, Maggard J, et al: Continuous SC infusions of opiates for cancer patients with pain. Oncol Nurs Forum, 13(4):53-57, 1986.
84. Ferrell BR, Wenzl C, Wisdom C: Evolution and evaluation of a pain management team. Oncol Nurs Forum 15:285-289, 1988.
85. Kane NE, Lehman ME, Drugger R, et al: Use of patient-controlled anesthesia in surgical oncology patients. Oncol Nurs Forum 15:29-32, 1988.
86. Konstantinides NI: Home parenteral nutrition: A viable alternative for patients with cancer. Oncol Nurs Forum 12(1):23-29, 1985.
87. Clark M: A day hospital for cancer patients: Clinical and economic feasibility. Oncol Nurs Forum 13(6):41-45, 1986.
88. Pluth NM: A home transfusion program. Oncol Nurs Forum 14(5):43-46, 1987.
89. Lewis PM: Implementing practice and organizational models. Cancer Nurs 8:75-78, 1985 (suppl 1).
90. Hartshorn JC: Research-based practice: The need for, use and reporting of instrument reliability and validity. Heart Lung 16:100-101, 1987.
91. Duffy ME: Research in practice: The time has come. Nurs Health Care 6:127, 1985.
92. Lynn MR: Reliability estimates: Use and disuse. Nurs Res 34:254-256, 1985.
93. Nunally JC: Psychometric Theory. New York: McGraw-Hill, 1978.
94. Frank-Stromborg M (ed): Instruments for Clinical Nursing Research. Norwalk, Conn, Appleton & Lange, 1988.
95. Ferrans C, Powers M: Quality of Life Index: Development and psychometric properties. Adv Nurs Sci 8(1):15, 1985.
96. Kobashi-Shoot JAM, Gerrit JFPH, Frits SAM et al: Assessment of malaise in cancer patients treated with radiotherapy. Cancer Nurs 8:306-313, 1985.
97. Padilla G, Grant M: Quality of life as a cancer nursing outcome variable. Adv Nurs Sci 8(1):45, 1985.
98. Hopkins MB: Information seeking and adaptational outcomes in women receiving chemotherapy for breast cancer. Cancer Nurs 9:256-262, 1986.
99. Waterhouse J, Metcalf MC: Development of the sexual adjustment questionnaire. Oncol Nurs Forum 13(3):53-59, 1986.
100. Derdiarian AK: Informational needs of recently diagnosed cancer patients. Cancer Nurs 10:156-163, 1987.
101. Fleming C, Scanlon C, D'Agostino NS: Patient care needs survey. Cancer Nurs 10:237-243, 1987.
102. Lilley LL: Human need fulfillment alteration in the client with uterine cancer: The registered nurse's perception versus the client's perception. Cancer Nurs 10:327-337, 1987.
103. Young-Graham K, Longman AJ: Quality of life and persons with melanoma: Preliminary model testing. Cancer Nurs 10:338-346, 1987.
104. Blackmore C: The impact of orchidectomy upon the sexuality of the man with testicular cancer. Cancer Nurs 11:33-40, 1988.
105. Camp LD: A comparison of nurses' recorded assessments of pain with perceptions of pain as described by cancer patients. Cancer Nurs 11:237-243, 1988.
106. Coward DD: Hypercalcemia knowledge assessment in patients at risk of developing cancer-induced hypercalcemia. Oncol Nurs Forum 15:471-476, 1988.
107. Derdiarian AK: Derdiarian Behavioral System Model (DBSM). Scholarly Inquiry for Nursing Practice, 2(2):103-121, 1988.
108. Eilers J, Berger AM, Petersen MC: Development, testing and application of the oral assessment guide. Oncol Nurs Forum 15:325-330, 1988.
109. Lauver D: Development of a questionnaire to measure beliefs and attitudes about breast self-examination. Cancer Nurs 11:51-57, 1988.
110. McMillan SC, Williams FA, Chatfield R, et al: A validity and reliability study of two tools for assessing and managing cancer pain. Oncol Nurs Forum 15:735-741, 1988.
111. Rhodes VA, Watson PM, Hanson BM: Patients' descriptions of the influence of tiredness and weakness on self-care abilities. Cancer Nurs 11:186-194, 1988.
112. Sutherland HJ, Walker P, Till JE: The development of a method for determining oncology patients' emotional distress using linear analogue scales. Cancer Nurs 11:303-308, 1988.
113. Weinrich SP, Weinrich MC: Cancer knowledge among elderly individuals. Cancer Nurs 9:301-307, 1987.
114. Williams RD: Factors affecting practice of BSE in older women. Oncol Nurs Forum 15:611-616, 1988.
115. Ammon-Gaberson KB, Piantanida M: Generating results from qualitative data. Image 20:159-161, 1988.
116. Saunders JM, Valente SM: Cancer and suicide. Oncol Nurs Forum 15:575-581, 1988.
117. Thorne SE: Helpful and unhelpful communications in cancer care: The patient perspective. Oncol Nurs Forum 15:167-172, 1988.
118. Hays JC: Patient symptoms and family coping. Cancer Nurs 9:317-325, 1986.
119. Duigon A: Anticipatory nausea and vomiting associated with cancer chemotherapy. Oncol Nurs Forum 13(1):35-40, 1986.
120. Coons HL, Leventhal H, Nerenz DR, et al: Anticipatory nausea and emotional distress in patients receiving cisplatin-based chemotherapy. Oncol Nurs Forum 14(3):31-35, 1987.

121. Henschel L: Fever patterns in the neutropenic patient. Cancer Nurs 8:301-305, 1985.
122. Krouse HJ: A psychological model of adjustment in gynecologic cancer patients. Oncol Nurs Forum 12(6):45-49, 1985.
123. Cooley ME, Cobb SC: Sexual and reproductive issues for women with Hodgkin's disease. I. Overview of issues. Cancer Nurs 9:188-193, 1986.
124. Cooley ME, Yeoman AC, Cobb SC: Sexual and reproductive issues for women with Hodgkin's disease: Application of PLISSIT Model. Cancer Nurs 9:248-255, 1986.
125. Coward DD: Cancer-induced hypercalcemia. Cancer Nurs 9:125-132, 1986.
126. Holing EV: The primary caregiver's perception of the dying trajectory: An exploratory study. Cancer Nurs 9:29-37, 1986.
127. Huldij A, Giesbers A, Poelhuis EHK, et al: Alterations in taste appreciation in cancer patients during treatment. Cancer Nurs 9:38-42, 1986.
128. Lovejoy N: Family responses to cancer hospitalization. Oncol Nurs Forum 13(2):33-37, 1986.
129. Donovan MI, Dillon P: Incidence and characteristics of pain in a sample of hospitalized cancer patients. Cancer Nurs 10:85-92, 1987.
130. Jenkins B: Patients' reports of sexual changes after treatment for gynecological cancer. Oncol Nurs Forum 15:349-354, 1988.
131. Ostchega Y, Donahue M, Fox N: High-dose cisplatin-related peripheral neuropathy. Cancer Nurs 11:23-32, 1988.
132. Wilkie D, Lovejoy N, Dodd M, et al: Cancer pain control behaviors: Description and correlation with pain intensity. Oncol Nurs Forum 15:723-731, 1988.
133. Brown ML, Carrieri V, Janson-Bjerklie S, et al: Lung cancer and dyspnea: The patient's perception. Oncol Nurs Forum 13(5):19-24, 1986.
134. King KB, Nail LM, Kreamer K, et al: Patients' descriptions of the experience of receiving radiotherapy. Oncol Nurs Forum 12(4):55-61, 1986.
135. Lesage C: Carotid artery rupture: Prediction, prevention, preparation. Cancer Nurs 9:1-7, 1986.
136. Messner RL, Gardner SS, Webb DD: Early detection: The priority in colorectal cancer. Cancer Nurs 9:8-14, 1986.
137. Post-White J: Glucocorticosteroid-induced depression in the patient with leukemia or lymphoma. Cancer Nurs 9:15-22, 1986.
138. Tringali CA: The needs of family members of cancer patients. Oncol Nurs Forum 13(4):65-70, 1986.
139. Rhodes VA, Watson PM, Johnson MH, et al: Patterns of nausea, vomiting and distress in patients receiving antineoplastic drug protocols. Oncol Nurs Forum 14(4):35-44, 1987.
140. Foote M: Nursing care of the patient with non-Hodgkin's lymphoma: Prevention of pneumonia associated with combination chemotherapy. Cancer Nurs 8:263-271, 1985.
141. Getz DH: The primary, secondary and tertiary nursing interventions of lymphedema. Cancer Nurs 8:177-184, 1985.
142. Rooney A, Haviley C: Nursing management of disseminated intravascular coagulation. Oncol Nurs Forum 121(1):15-22, 1985.
143. Rossetti AC: Nursing care of patients treated with intrapleural tetracycline for control of malignant pleural effusion. Cancer Nurs 8:103-109, 1985.
144. Gurevich I, Tafuro P: The compromised host: Deficit-specific infection in the spectrum of prevention. Cancer Nurs 9:263-275, 1986.
145. Moore CL, Erickson KA, Yanes LB, et al: Nursing care and management of venous access ports. Oncol Nurs Forum 13(3):35-39, 1986.
146. Paice JA: Intrathecal morphine infusion for intractable cancer pain: A new use for implanted pumps. Oncol Nurs Forum 13(3):41-47, 1986.
147. Rodzwic D, Donnard J: The use of myocutaneous flaps in reconstructive surgery for head and neck cancer: Guidelines for nursing care. Oncol Nurs Forum, 13(3):29, 1986.
148. Hassay KM: Radiation therapy for rectal cancer and the implications for nursing. Cancer Nurs 10:311-318, 1987.
149. Link DL: Antibiotic therapy in the cancer patient: Focus on third generation cephalosporins. Oncol Nurs Forum 14(5):35-41, 1987.
150. Moreland BJ: A nursing form for gynecology patient assessment. Oncol Nurs Forum 14(2):19-23, 1987.
151. Stetz KM: Caregiving demands during advanced cancer: The spouse's needs. Cancer Nurs 10:260-268, 1987.
152. Lewandowski W, Jones SL: The family with cancer: Nursing intervention throughout the course of living with cancer. Cancer Nurs 11:313-321, 1988.
153. Strohl RA: The nursing role in radiation oncology: Symptom management of acute and chronic reactions. Oncol Nurs Forum 15:429-434, 1988.
154. Jennings BM, Muhlenkamp AF: Systematic misperception: Oncology patients' self-reported affective states and their care-givers' perceptions. Cancer Nursing 4:485-489, 1981.
155. Wright BA: Physical Disability: A Psychological Approach. New York, Harper & Row, 1960.
156. Verron JA, Longman A, Clark M: Development of a scale to measure undergraduate students' attitudes about caring for patients with cancer. Oncol Nurs Forum 14(5):51-55, 1987.
157. Robb S: Attitudes and intentions of baccalaureate nursing students toward the elderly. Nurs Res 28(1):43-50, 1979.
158. Larson P: Important nurse caring behaviors perceived by patients with cancer. Oncol Nurs Forum 11(6):46-50, 1984.
159. Larson P: Comparison of cancer patients' and professional nurses' perceptions of important nurse caring behaviors. Heart Lung 16:187-192, 1987.
160. Mayer DK: Oncology nurses' versus cancer patients' perceptions of nursing care behaviors: A replication study. Oncol Nurs Forum 14(3):48-52, 1987.
161. Sodestrom KE, Martinson IM: Patients' spiritual coping strategies: A study of nurse and patient perspectives. Oncol Nurs Forum 14(2):41-46, 1987.
162. Curtis AE, Fernsler JI: Quality of life of oncology hospice patients: A comparison of patient and primary caregiver reports. Oncol Nurs Forum 16:49-53, 1989.
163. Dyck S, Wright K: Family perceptions: The role of the nurse throughout an adults' cancer experience. Oncol Nurs Forum 12(5):53-56, 1985.
164. Benner P: From Novice to Expert: Excellence and Power in Clinical Nursing Practice. Menlo Park, Calif, Addison-Wesley, 1984.
165. Benner P, Wrubel J: The Primacy of Caring: Stress and Coping in Health and Illness. Menlo Park, Calif, Addison-Wesley, 1989.

Chapter 54

Economics of Cancer

Arlene E. Fleck, RN, MNEd

INTRODUCTION

In the past, the ability to apply clinical expertise to solve patient care problems was the major concern of the cancer nurse specialist. However, in today's health care arena the challenge is to integrate this clinical expertise and apply it in a cost-effective manner. A cost-effective approach is one that emphasizes balancing cost requirements and standards of excellence.

Cancer care is changing rapidly because of new technology, innovative therapy, and current economic and health care policy issues. Nurses specializing in oncology must be prepared to adapt to this constant change. This chapter will explore the economic environment, which is a major influencing factor in the practice of oncology nursing. The discussion begins with a review of basic economic theory and the historical and current issues that have an impact on health care economics. The remainder of this chapter will emphasize how these economic changes are affecting cancer care.

SCOPE OF THE PROBLEM

Since the early 1980s, revolutionary changes have occurred in the health care economics of this country. Before that time, the word "economics" did not have the strong association with health care that it does today. In today's health care environment, nurses are exposed to new phrases: "cost justification," "more does not mean better," "quality versus cost," and "lack of resources," to name just a few. These phrases represent dramatic changes that were introduced when expenditures for health care reached 9.4% of the US gross national product (GNP), or $147 billion, in 1982; this figure was a sharp contrast to the 1960 statistics, in which health care expenditures were only 4.5% of the GNP. It has been estimated that by the turn of the century, health care will account for 15% of the GNP. These rising figures have waved red flags in front of government officials who continually are trying to trim the federal budget. The rise in health care costs is being scrutinized not only by politicians but by business leaders and consumers as well. Pressure by these groups has been applied to constrain the use of health care resources. To accomplish this task, nurses and other health care professionals must continue to deliver patient care in sufficient quantities and of acceptable quality to meet public demands—in other words, to do more with less.

ECONOMICS THEORY

Historically, economics has not been a popular elective course among student nurses, nor has there been a demand for the ability to apply economic principles to the health care field. However, with the current major emphasis on the high costs of health care and national health policy changes, an introduction to economics could become not only interesting but also beneficial. An ability to analyze economic issues can provide important insights into the operation of health care systems and the evaluation of health care policies.

Economics is the science that deals with the production, distribution, and consumption of wealth, or resources. The economy is the management of the production, allocation, and consumption of resources in this country. In simple words, it is the study of supply and demand. Figure 54-1 illustrates a normal, or balanced, economic environment.[1] Two parties are involved in the exchange of money. One party is the supplier, who provides the goods or services to the other party, the consumer. The consumer is responsible for the demand of the goods or services. Pricing is established to balance the supply and demand of goods and services. This pricing establishes an important equilibrium:

Supply = Demand
and
Demand = Supply

The ability of price to act as a balance point between the supply and demand of a good or service is referred to as the concept of *price elasticity* or *price sensitivity*. This concept is illustrated in Figure 54-2. It can be predicted that when the price of a good or service falls, the quantity demanded will rise. The significance of this concept is readily apparent in health care provided during the late 1960s and early 1970s. For most Americans, health care had no price; it was essentially free. Health insurance coverage was a standard part of virtually every employee benefit package. Most Americans believed health care services

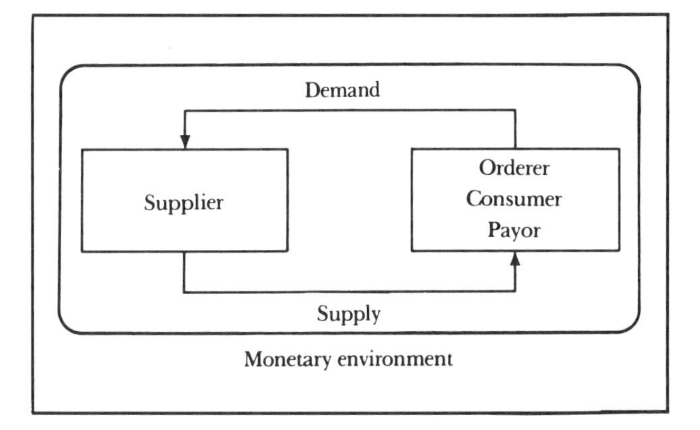

FIGURE 54-1 Normal economic environment. In a normal economic environment, there are essentially two parties—supplier and consumer (also referred to as payor and orderer). The former supplies goods and services, and the latter demands goods and services. Money, or the promise of it, is exchanged between the two parties, thus establishing a market price for the goods and services. (Source: Ward WJ Jr: An Introduction to Health Care Financial Management. Owings Mills, Md, Rynd Communication, 1988, p 5.)

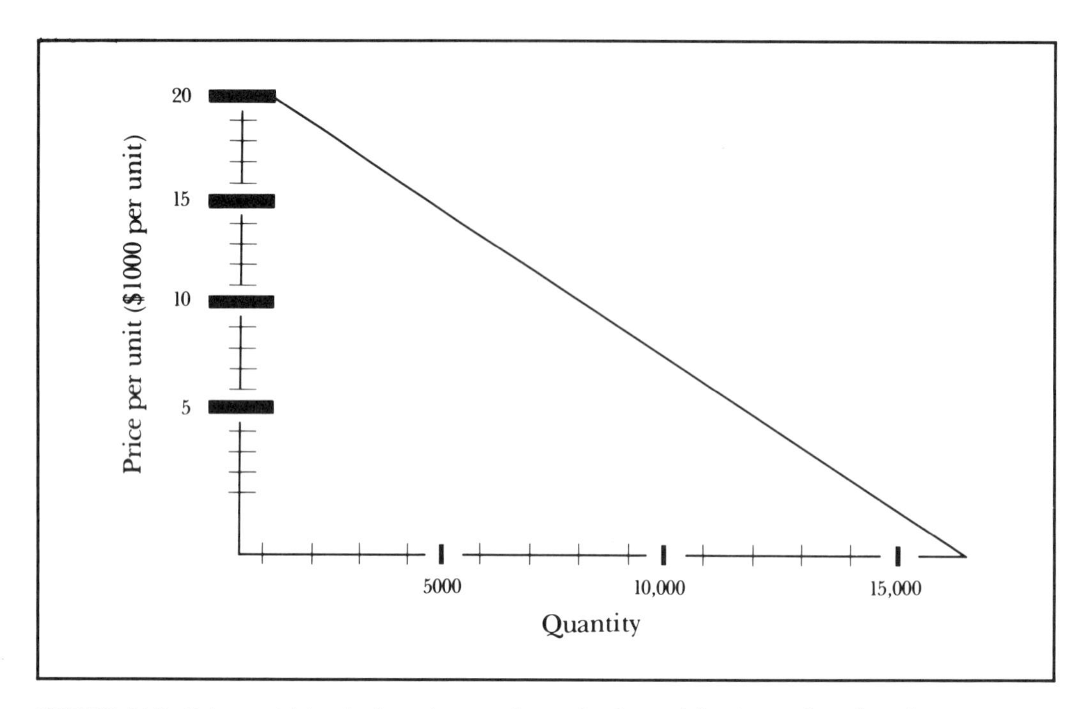

FIGURE 54-2 Price sensitivity. As the price goes down, the demand for the goods and services goes up.

to be their "right"—not a privilege. The cost of any health care was never an issue because only insurance companies, rarely the consumer, saw the bill or charges. The ready access to health care coverage as an employee benefit often encouraged indiscriminate use of high-cost services. The prevailing attitude was that of obtaining the best and most sophisticated care regardless of cost. This health care behavior caused costs to spiral.

Persons who were unemployed or retired, and who did not have health care insurance coverage provided by an employer, were often eligible for federal health insurance programs (ie, Medicare or Medicaid). The method of federal payment for services was retrospective and cost based. Hospitals were reimbursed by the government for their incurred costs of treating patients after the treatment and care had been delivered. The incentive for hospitals (where 70% of all Medicare dollars were spent[2]) was to spend as much money as possible on the care of each patient. The more money a hospital spent, the more the government paid. This system of payment for services provided resulted in overutilization of resources, extended hospitalization, duplication of equipment, and more treatments and diagnostic tests than were actually necessary.

The health care economic environment of the late 1960s and early 1970s is depicted in Figure 54-3.[1] This diagram illustrates why problems arose in the US health care economic system.[1] Because neither the consumer, physician, or health care professional was concerned with the price of the goods or services, the demands became unlimited. Consumers came to expect a health care system that provided everything possible. Physicians, nurses, and other health care professionals continued to use all available technology and resources to care for the patient, often in excess of what was required. The increased number of

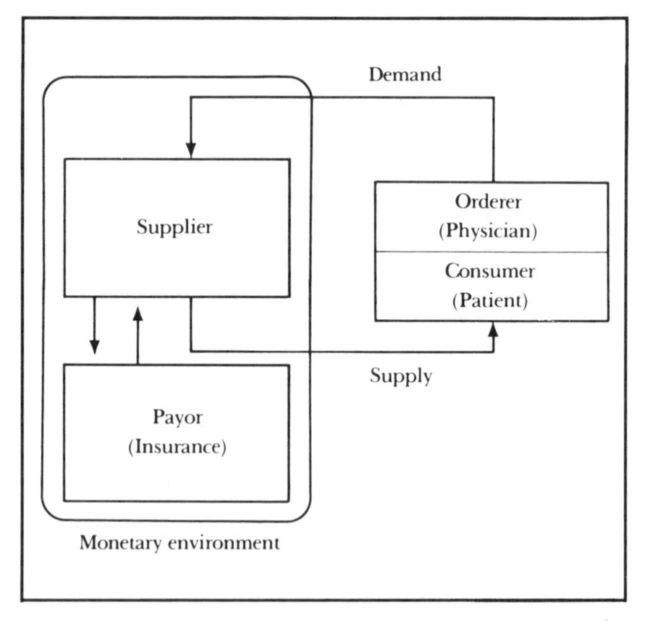

FIGURE 54-3 Health care economic environment. The economic environment as applied to health care is significantly different. Note that there are now four parties instead of two and that the supply of and demand for health care services no longer include the payor for those services. Because the monetary environment does not include the orderer, or consumer, price is unable to establish a balance between supply and demand. (Source: Ward WJ Jr: An Introduction to Health Care Financial Management. Owings Mills, Md, Rynd Communication, 1988, p 8.)

malpractice lawsuits caused physicians to practice defensive medicine, ordering more tests than usual and thereby driving costs upward. Moreover, costs rose because people were living longer and thus contributing to the increasing number of elderly citizens, many of whom have chronic health care needs. Thus, in the 1980s, there was a resultant demand for more available health care resources than could be satisfied. To address and sustain these increasing demands, the Ninety-seventh Congress passed the Tax Equity and Fiscal Responsibility Act (TEFRA) in August 1982. This payment system changed the method of providing inpatient services for Medicare and Medicaid beneficiaries from a retrospective, cost-based payment system to a prospective payment system.

PROSPECTIVE PAYMENT SYSTEM

History

The prospective payment system (PPS) was signed into Public Law 98-21 as part of the Social Security Amendment of 1983. This system reimburses hospitals with a fixed payment that is based on the complexity of the problems that precipitated during the patient's hospitalization. The exact amount is determined by using one or more of the 477* diagnosis related groups (DRGs). Each DRG is assigned a specific, fixed rate of payment for which the hospital is reimbursed regardless of the actual cost of the patient's care. The individual DRGs originally were developed by a group of researchers at Yale University as a hospital management tool; they were adapted for use as a federal payment system, after being field-tested in New Jersey. In the pilot study, the major factor observed was the number of days that a patient stayed in the hospital.[3] It was believed that if the number of days a patient stayed in the hospital could be decreased, the overall hospital bill would also be decreased. By 1982, all acute care hospitals in New Jersey were reimbursed according to the PPS; a 6% reduction in comparison with national hospital costs was observed.[4]

To help standardize hospital costs throughout the country, researchers assigned a specific weight to each DRG. This weighting factor reflects the estimated relative costs of hospital resources used (ie, laboratory tests, medications, medical and surgical supplies, room, ancillary services) per patient discharge. The principal sources of data to compile the cost weights originally were based on the Medicare cost reports for 1981 and on a national representative sample of inpatient Medicare claims.

The Health Care Financing Administration (HCFA) agency of the federal government now assigns the appropriate weighting factor for each DRG. An average standardized cost for each of the original 468 DRGs was developed from the cost data received; the statistical method of regression was used to establish a variance for each DRG. It can be estimated statistically that 95% of the patients assigned to a specific DRG actually will incur the cost allocated within the parameter of the DRG.[5]

This system was integrated gradually over the first five years of its inception (1983-1987); hospitals were reimbursed at a prospective payment rate for each discharge that was a blend of national and regional data and the respective hospital's historic cost per case. Effective Aug. 21, 1988, the method to determine payment rates was adjusted and was based only on national/regional standardized information. The individual hospital's costs were no longer recognized as a factor.

*In 1982, when DRGs were first used in the hospitals, there were 470 of them. As the need for other DRGs was established, the number increased. In 1989 there were 477 DRGs.

Calculation

An example of a 1989 prospective payment calculation is shown in Figure 54-4. An understanding of how a payment is calculated for a hospital is important for nurses because it provides a basis for understanding many of the current and future trends of health care economics. For a more extensive history on the DRGs or calculation details, see references 6, 7, 8, 9, and 10.

Exemptions

All hospitals that participate in the Medicare system are reimbursed by the PPS with the exception of the following:

1. Long-term hospitals: average length of inpatient stay more than 25 days.
2. Psychiatric hospitals and units: primarily engage in treatment of mentally ill persons.
3. Rehabilitation hospitals and units: meet federally established criteria for a rehabilitation center.
4. Children's hospitals.
5. Hospitals located in states with state-regulated PPS plans (Maryland, New Jersey).
6. Veterans Administration hospitals.
7. Cancer hospitals: those recognized by the National Cancer Institute (NCI) as comprehensive cancer centers or as clinical cancer research centers. The entire facility must be organized primarily for the treatment of, and research on, cancer. As of 1989, the hospitals recognized under this exemption included MD Anderson Cancer Center, Houston, Tex; Fox Chase Cancer Center, Philadelphia, Pa; Kenneth Norris, Jr., Cancer Center, University of Southern California, Los Angeles, Calif; City of Hope National Medical Center, Duarte, Calif; Fred Hutchinson Cancer Center, Seattle, Wash; Memorial Sloan-Kettering Cancer Center, New York, NY; Roswell Park Memorial Institute, Buffalo, NY; and Dana-Farber Cancer Institute, Boston, Mass.

DRGs were developed with a primary orientation toward the short-term, acute care hospitals. Their applicability in specialty (exempt) hospitals is limited.

Baseline Data

1. Fiscal Year 1989
2. 300-bed acute care hospital (urban)
3. Census Region 2
4. Principal diagnosis example: DRG 82, Respiratory Neoplasms

Formula

$$\left[\begin{array}{c}\text{Adjusted labor component} = \\ \text{Labor component} \times \text{Wage index} \\ \$2{,}374.22 \times 1.0206 = \\ \$2{,}423.13\end{array}\right]^{1} + \begin{array}{c}\text{Nonlabor component}^{2} \\ \$840.95\end{array} \times \begin{array}{c}\text{DRG weight}^{3} \\ 1.2367\end{array} = \$4{,}036.69$$

Payment rate to hospital = $4,036.69
Hospital costs for patient "A" = 3,200.00
Profit for hospital $ 836.69

[1] *Adjusted labor component* is determined by the mean urban or rural cost per discharge and is then adjusted to reflect regional differences in hospital wages. This figure is derived from regional and national aggregate data of cost reports submitted by hospitals and reflects labor-intensive costs (ie, wages, salaries, employee benefits, professional fees).

[2] *Nonlabor component* is adjusted to the appropriate regional or national standardized figure. The geographic location and the urban or rural designation of the hospital is also considered. This figure accounts for all other resource consumption for patient care.

[3] *DRG weights* are based on a nationwide random sample study. The variables reviewed in hospitals to arrive at a cost-reimbursement figure per case includes length of stay, per diem cost in routine and special care, estimated cost of ancillary services (eg, laboratory work, radiography, drugs, medical supplies). From these reports, each DRG is assigned a relative weight that reflects the resources needed to care for a patient with a specific diagnosis. PROPAC annually recommends to the secretary of the US Department of Health and Human Services the appropriate annual percentage change in payment for hospital inpatient discharges. This report is due by March 1 of each year.

FIGURE 54-4 Prospective payment calculation. Specific details for calculating a prospective payment reimbursement are outlined. Although there is no need to memorize this calculation, it is important to understand which components are used to compute the reimbursement. This knowledge will help the student to understand many of the dilemmas encountered by the prospective payment system.

Hospital Cost-Per-Case Comparisons

To establish a set price per DRG for every acute care hospital in the United States is virtually impossible. A variety of variables can cause fluctuations in the federal payment amount. The variables that are used to compare one hospital's cost per case to another's include the case mix (a classification by diagnosis of a hospital's caseload or patient population), labor costs, urban or rural location, and teaching intensity. These adjustment factors, which were incorporated into the PPS system, explain an estimated 65% of the variation in the average cost per case.[11] The teaching-intensity variable was originally a "pass-through" reimbursement (the costs of education were reimbursed). However, in the past several years the system has been adjusted in such a manner that only a percentage of teaching costs are reimbursed.

The current PPS assumes that variations in cost per case that are not accounted for by the above-described adjustment factors are due to differences in hospital efficiency. As hospitals become more efficient (ie, produce targeted health care outcomes with the least costly input), these additional variations in costs will be significantly reduced.[12]

Monitoring Activities

The PPS legislation requires close monitoring of costs. Each hospital is required to contract with a peer review organization (PRO) established by the US Department of Health and Human Services. The purpose of the PROs is to conduct required medical reviews to ensure that quality patient care is provided and maintained and that the duration of hospital stay is appropriate to the level of required care. The Health Care Financing Administration (HCFA) also will review periodically the records of each hospital for compliance with the PPS regulations and will deny payment if the regulations are not followed.

To update and maintain the new Medicare payment system, Congress established the Prospective Payment Assessment Commission (PROPAC).* A 15-member commission of experts was appointed by the Office of Technology Assessment (OTA)† in 1983.[13] The PPS law mandates that PROPAC make recommendations annually to the secretary of the US Department of Health and Human Services and to Congress in two primary areas[14]: the annual percentage increase in Medicare expenditures on a per-case basis (the update factor) and the DRG patient classification categories and weights. In recent years, PROPAC has been reviewing several other areas: the hospital market-basket structure (a figure used to estimate inflation rates in the price of patient-utilized goods and services purchased by hospitals); improvements in the case-mix measurement (measurement of a hospital's inpatient population and its severity of illness or resource needs); capital expenditure policy (outlay made by a hospital to the purchase of a fixed asset such as a piece of equipment for a period greater than a year[1]); and the effects of PPS on rural hospitals.

Impact of PPS

The change in hospital reimbursement from costs incurred to fixed rates has caused drastic restructuring of health care incentives. If the actual cost of a patient's care is less than the fixed or assigned DRG rate, the hospital retains the excess amount. These DRGs are known as "winners." If the hospital's costs exceed the fixed payment scale, the hospital must absorb the excess costs. These DRGs are known as "losers." Hospitals are striving to reduce costs to an efficient and effective level. Adaptation to prospective reimbursement has caused changes in the health care environment. The following section will discuss several key trends that have resulted from the implementation of PPS; the decrease in the length of stay in the hospital, the restraint of technologic advancement, and the limitation of access to health care. Each trend will be discussed in terms of its history or development, its relation to current issues, and its impact on nursing.

Decrease in length of stay

History The original studies at Yale University that provided the methodology for the DRGs used length of stay (LOS) as the dependent variable. This variable was chosen because the initial purpose of developing DRGs was to improve utilization review activities, which consisted of reviewing the appropriateness of patient care services by a single-diagnosis method.[3] Before the Yale study, a single-diagnosis patient classification system (the International Classification of Diseases, Adapted, Eighth Revision [ICDA-8]) was used for the review of patient care. This scheme was limited to classifying patients only by similar ailments. Yale researchers adjusted the classification system by adding the LOS variable. After the Yale researchers reviewed the results of their work, they concluded that the LOS variable was not entirely appropriate, because variations were too wide. They therefore found it necessary to consider several other classification factors in addition to ICDA-8 codes and LOS. The revisions included classifying diseases on the basis of 23 major diagnostic categories (MDCs) based on human anatomy. These 23 MDCs are divided further by factors that have an impact on the patient's LOS: the patient's age, the presence of comorbidities (ie, the presence of diseases or conditions concurrently with the patient's principal condition), disease complications, and the use of surgical procedures (Figure 54-5). These additional factors still are not an inclusive list for determining a patient's LOS. The assumed homogeneity* of each particular DRG needs to be examined critically because many other factors can contribute to variations in a patient's LOS. Some of these factors are listed below:

1. The severity index reflects the stage of the patient's illness within each DRG, which significantly influences the extent of resource consumption. As an example, a patient with cancer who has just been informed of disease progression is undergoing 5 days of inpatient chemotherapy. The patient has a vascular access device that is malfunctioning. Chemotherapy based on DRG 410 is used. This classification gives no consideration to special services such as patient teaching for chemotherapy side effects, adjustment of procedures because of a malfunctioning vascular access device, or increased psychologic support needed because of disease metastasis.
2. The socioeconomic status of the patient is a concern, because the disadvantaged patient may require more resources (such as nursing care, education, discharge planning, and social service) than others with similar diagnoses.
3. Hospitals that care for patients with severe and complex cases will likely be underpaid relative to hospitals who have less complex cases.
4. A physician's or surgeon's practice that is unique may affect the patient resource consumption. As an example, reconstructive surgery after mastectomy may require an extra 5 days in the hospital.

Current trends A great emphasis in hospital care management is to decrease the number of hospital days, which strongly affects the utilization of resources. Consequently, there is a powerful incentive to discharge patients earlier

*A person interested in keeping abreast of PROPAC's latest recommendations, as reported to the secretary of the US Department of Health and Human Services, can be added to the mailing list to receive these reports by calling the PROPAC office at (202)453-3986.

†The OTA was created in 1972 as an analytic arm of Congress. OTA's basic function is to help legislative policy makers anticipate and plan for the consequences of technologic changes. OTA provides Congress with independent and timely information about the potential effects of the changes. The board is composed of the OTA director and members of the US House of Representatives and US Senate.

*Homogeneity is defined as the expectation that the variances in cases classified under the same DRG are equal.

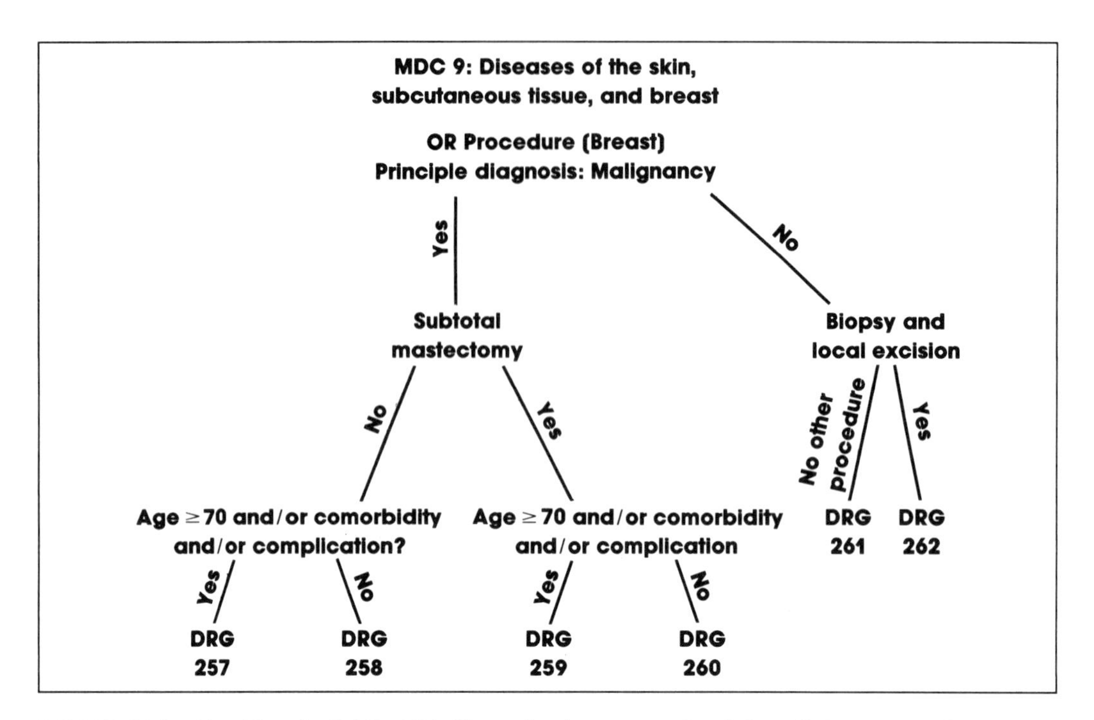

FIGURE 54-5 Algorithm for DRGs. This illustration is an example of the splitting process for a major diagnostic category, MDC 9. This decision tree, or algorithm, helps the medical records department to classify a patient's discharge status under a particular DRG category. The criteria or splitting process used to select the appropriate DRGs includes the use of an operating room (OR procedure), the principal diagnosis, the type of OR procedure, the age of the patient, and the type or severity of complication or comorbidity.

than before. During the past several years, Medicare's reimbursed LOS has progressively decreased. Since 1984 the average decrease for each year has been 2.1%; in 1989 the average LOS was 8.8 days.[15] Of greatest concern is the pressure for inappropriately shortening the LOS, especially for the elderly patient. The job of the PROs is to monitor this factor carefully.

Greater responsibility has been given to the hospital's medical records department for providing data for current and retrospective patient care studies. These studies can be used to document the complex care required by patients with cancer.

Nursing implications Nurses have a greater need than ever before to increase patients' self-care knowledge and skills. Teaching self-care is not a specific intervention but, rather, is an attempt to provide a model of care. The emphasis is on managed care throughout a lifetime.[16]

Coordinating discharge planning is a vital role for the nurse. Continuity of care between the hospital and home must be ensured. Because patients are leaving the hospital setting sooner, home care agencies have grown, increasing the need for home care nurses, especially those with acute care experience.

Nursing case management models have been developed to maximize resources and expertise needed in the care of hospitalized patients who have similar diagnoses. An example of a case management model is that of the New England Medical Center Department of Nursing. A strategy was initiated that formally joins a specific group of nurses together into a group practice. This group nursing practice is then linked to a specific physician. Together the nurses and physicians care for patients throughout the continuum of hospitalization. Case management assignments may be aligned with caseloads in a variety of ways; for example, a nurse may be assigned to a physician and all his or her patients, assigned to manage cases within a geographic unit, or assigned to cases on the basis of diagnosis. Collectively, the nurses and physicians are responsible for developing standards, management tools, and designs for delivery of care.[17] This plan can be very effective because nurses and physicians together are responsible for more than 80% of all the resources expended during each hospitalization.[15] A case management plan at the New England Medical Center is used to discuss possible cause-and-effect relationships in commonly encountered patient problems. The plan also results in the development of intermediate patient goals that outline appropriate nursing and physician interventions needed to achieve the specific desired clinical outcomes. The entire plan is designed to function within the DRG LOS framework.[18] Through these strategies, this center was able to reduce the LOS for patients undergoing induction therapy for leukemia from 48 to 32 days.[18] Case management requires the nurse to be prepared at a bachelor's or master's degree level of education, because nurses in this role must define and facilitate clinical and financial outcomes.[15]

Restraint of technologic advancement

History With the birth of the PPS, new terminology has evolved in health care agencies. Words such as cost-effectiveness, cost efficiency, cost saving, competition, and feasibility echo in the administrative offices. When a request is made for an item that uses new technology, administrators want documentation or a feasibility report before approving the purchase. Items using new technology include drugs, devices, diagnostic equipment, and any equipment needed for medical and surgical procedures that prevent, diagnose, and treat disease. It is estimated that 20% to 50% of the growth in health care costs can be attributed to new technology.[12] Initially, under the PPS, capital expenditures were reimbursed on the basis of the actual costs, a "pass-through." The initial cost of the purchase was not the major concern; rather, the indirect costs of operation, maintenance, and salary for trained personnel were the issues. These indirect costs are accounted for in the DRG calculation under the labor and nonlabor components. If a hospital's indirect figures are not in line with the standard DRG calculation, the hospital loses money for the specific DRG.

Not only are the indirect costs a concern, but Congress continues to mandate percentage reductions in hospital capital payments. In fiscal year 1989, hospitals received only 85% of Medicare's share of allowable capital-related costs.[12]

The government uses different avenues to influence the development and utilization of technology. The following are some of these avenues[12]:

- National Institutes of Health: supplies financial support for both basic and applied research related to the development of new medical technologies.
- Food and Drug Administration (FDA): reviews the safety and efficacy of new medical technologies, drugs, and medical devices.
- State government: regulates, in many states, the purchase of new equipment through a certificate of need (CON) program.
- Medicare and Medicaid: influence indirectly the availability of new technology through decisions regarding reimbursement.
- Office of Health Technology Assessment (OHTA): evaluates safety and efficacy of new technology and recommends for or against Medicaid coverage.
- Patent laws: provide manufacturers with a monopoly for a period of several years.

Current trends In addition to the federal government's historic involvement, third-party payers (insurance companies) have developed techniques to control costs. This involvement is in response to the soaring health care costs, high insurance premiums, and the introduction of the PPS. Some of the techniques are as follows[12]:

- Technologic assessment. Many third-party payers have established formal processes for evaluating the clinical and economic effects of new technology.
- Utilization review. Insurers are constantly reviewing the course of treatment provided and establishing protocols for appropriate treatment. If their protocols are not followed, payment is not given.
- Case management. Insurers are using case management techniques to direct patients to efficient providers.
- Selective contracting and price discounting. Some health care systems have developed contracting mechanisms with suppliers of drugs, medical supplies, and equipment. These mechanisms provide patient care at a fixed, discounted price.

Several major concerns regarding the PPS have been raised in regard to technologic advancement. Some of the concerns that have been discussed in the literature include the incentives provided to hospitals for restricting the adoption of new technology; the access to purchasing new technology, which may be given only to those hospitals that have proven cost reductions in the DRG categories utilizing the technology; the possibility that new technologies that increase costs of treatment within specified DRGs may not be readily adopted, even if they can effect an improvement in patient care; the restrictions in state-of-the-art medical care for hospitalized Medicare recipients; and the possible reduction of expenditures by manufacturers of technologic equipment for research and development, as a response to cost-cutting policies. Although there are no data to confirm the occurrence of these phenomena, the concerns are realistic.

In 1989, consideration was given to a proposal that would give the US Department of Health and Human Services the authority to evaluate new medical technology and to judge its cost-effectiveness for patient care.[19] Moreover, several years ago, Project Hope, under contract to PROPAC, began studies to investigate which technologies would significantly increase inpatient operating costs and which would decrease costs. Some examples from Project Hope of cost-increasing technologies estimated for fiscal year 1990 were implantable infusion pumps, magnetic resonance imaging, and monoclonal antibodies used as diagnostic agents.[20] Among those technologies estimated to be cost decreasing were endoscopic lasers, gallstone lithotripsy, and peripheral vascular angioplasty.[20]

Updating the current reimbursement system is an omnibus job, but it must be done on a routine, consistent, scientific basis. Many of the technologic advancement issues relate directly to the care of patients with cancer. These issues will be explored in a later section of this chapter.

Nursing implications No longer is it appropriate for nurses to base decisions regarding patient care on the assumption that resources are unlimited. In any economy or organization, resources are scarce relative to demands.

There will always be more demands on available resources than can be satisfied. As a result of these demands, output must be rationed. The objective of rationing is to use available resources to maximize social welfare or institutional well-being.[21] As health care expenditures continue to take a large share of our society's total resources, pressure will continue to increase on the industry to justify outcomes relative to their costs.

Nurses must be able to justify the resources that are needed for improving patient care. This goal can be accomplished through the use of financial management tools or techniques. Some examples of these techniques include feasibility studies and cost analysis studies.

A feasibility study is a documentation process to determine whether a new program should be developed and implemented in a health care agency.[22] These studies provide a comprehensive economic and financial forecast for a new idea or program.

The basic steps of a feasibility study include the following:

- Define objectives: List the goals that the study is to achieve.
- List assumptions: Discuss the existing conditions that the reader of the feasibility study would otherwise not be familiar with if he or she had not read it. This section allows the reader to understand the writer's global perspective of the situation or problem.
- Describe the current situation: Answer the question, Why is this project possible? Then present relevant background data on the project, list who or what is in competition, and discuss the macroenvironment (eg, government, legal issues).
- Develop a plan of action: List what will be done, assign a person or persons to act, provide a time line or framework, and document the cost.
- Record the projected profit and loss: Discuss the expected financial gains or losses of the project.
- Enlist the assistance of the institution's finance department for the coordination of this section.
- Describe controls: Present a plan for monitoring the study.
- Prepare an executive summary: Write an abbreviated overview of the proposed plan. This section of the proposal is usually the one that most decision makers on the management team will review. It should therefore be as brief and concise as possible—usually one page. The executive summary is the first section of the feasibility study.

Cost-analysis techniques generally are classified as one of two types: cost-benefit analysis (CBA) or cost-effective analysis (CEA). Larson and Peters[23] define each of these techniques: "Cost-benefit analysis assigns monetary value to all costs and benefits of a potential program, practice or product, resulting in a cost-benefit ratio" (eg, a decision needs to be made on whether an outpatient oncology unit will be designed or on whether an outpatient department will be expanded). Cost-effective analysis is defined as follows: "All the costs measured in dollars necessary to achieve a certain effect (benefit) are calculated and expressed as cost/unit of effectiveness."[23] This technique is used to compare relative costs of several alternatives. All the alternatives are designed to have the same outcomes (eg, inserting an indwelling catheter for a chemotherapy regimen versus administering individual doses via venipuncture). Steps used in conducting either analysis also have been delineated by the Office of Technology Assessment (OTA). Larson and Peters[23] reviewed the OTA analysis steps as follows:

1. Define the problem.
2. State objective of the proposed program, practice change, or product.
3. Identify alternatives.
4. Define the perspective of the analysis. (For example, does it represent costs and benefits to the patient or to employees? If it represents more than one viewpoint, each should be analyzed separately.)
5. Analyze costs (include both direct and indirect costs).
6. Evaluate benefits (in dollars for CBA, in effects for CEA).
7. Determine the present value of any future costs and benefits by calculating a discount. This is called discounting. Formula: Present value = Future value (1 + Interest rate) interval in years
8. Analyze uncertainties. Substitute different values from within the range of possible values for costs and benefits calculated to determine whether changes in the values will alter the conclusions of the analysis. (This is called a sensitivity analysis.)
9. Address ethical issues (ie, the appropriate distribution of limited resources in the population, the accessibility of programs and resources, the extent to which the analysis can be influenced by bias).
10. Interpret results.

Another important contribution that nurses can make in an evaluation of new technology is to organize a product evaluation committee (PEC) or to serve as a member of the committee. The PEC is responsible for controlling which product or service will be used in a health care agency. Larson and Maciorowski[24] describe a four-step process to be utilized by a PEC:

- Step 1: All requests for new products or changes in the use of existing products are directed to the PEC.
- Step 2: Product options are explored in depth by potential users and by the PEC.
- Step 3: Product options are carefully evaluated on the basis of a review of the literature (historical and research perspectives), consultation with other experts, and field testing of products. Methods of field testing should be consistent for everyone involved. The PEC should use objective criteria (eg, quality of product compared with that of others, safety, serviceability, cost, standardization, prevention of duplication of products).

- Step 4: Summarize findings in a comparison chart.

When nurses increase their understanding and utilization of these processes, cost-effectiveness will no longer be a "buzz word" but, rather, a significant approach for the justification of resources needed to care for patients and their families.

Limitation of access to health care

History "Access to care" refers to a person's ability to pay for the health care services provided. Before the early 1980s, few patients had financial burdens from medical expenses; their health care insurance carrier paid any bills, and the burden of health care expenses was therefore on the third-party payer. With the implementation of the PPS, the issue of access to care has gained prominence.

A brief history of health care coverage in the United States is helpful in gaining a perspective on this issue[25]:

- Before the 1930s: Ninety percent of the money spent on medical bills came directly from the patient's own pocket.
- During the great depression, beginning in 1929: The cost of medical care rose sharply, and people had less money to spend on medical bills. Doctors were collecting only 40% of the fees they charged.
- 1935: The American Hospital Association, which represented hospitals throughout the United States, promoted Blue Cross insurance to pay for hospital stays.
- During World War II, beginning in 1941: Although the federal government halted price and wage increases, health insurance was not counted as a wage. This enabled labor unions to negotiate for better health care coverage.
- 1950: The high cost of national health care was beginning to gain attention by the politicians. The cost per person was $80.
- 1965: Medicare and Medicaid federal health insurance programs started. Medicare is a program for people 65 years of age or older and for certain disabled people; Medicaid is a program for people with very low income (federal regulations mandate that each state be responsible for administering the program and establishing income levels for cash assistance). Health insurance coverage became a common employee benefit. Federal and state governments paid about 26% of all monies spent for health care in the United States. National health care costs rose to $141 per person.
- 1970: Medical costs went up faster than the general rate of inflation. In this era of explosive growth for medical technologies and services, intensive care units became very popular. The cost of national health care continued to climb, until it reached $340 per person.
- 1980: The early 1980s were regarded as a time of economic recession. The government's share of the national medical bill rose to 43%, and national health care costs rose to $1054 per person. Health care costs consumed one fourth of the corporate profits left after paying taxes. As a result government and industry (the employers) started paying closer attention to the health benefit package.
- 1983: TEFRA was passed. Prospective reimbursement was implemented for the national Medicare program; however, each state had the responsibility for establishing its own reimbursement process for the Medicaid program.

Throughout the 50-year period from the 1930s to the 1980s, many uninsured, indigent Americans were not eligible for employee or government-assistance benefits. Hospitals provided charity care to these patients by shifting costs. Cost shifting is the practice of charging higher rates to those patients whose care is paid through an insurance plan and then using the extra income to compensate for the cost of care for those patients who are unable to pay their bills. As a result of this cost-shifting practice, insurance premiums rose. For example, in some states the cost of insuring a family of four rose about 400% between 1980 and 1989.[26] With these enormous increases, corporations reduced their health care benefits. Today it is becoming more difficult, with cutbacks by both the government and big business, for hospitals to afford to provide uncompensated care to the 37 million uninsured Americans.[12] To do so would require an increase in a hospital's gross revenue, which is not the focus of cost-containment efforts.[27]

Current trends The demand for charity care is steadily increasing at a time when many hospitals have negative operating margins. (A 1988 American Hospital Association report indicated that about half of all hospitals had lost money and were concerned about their financial failure[28]; about 200 hospitals have closed since the PPS began in 1983.[7]) A significant reason for the increased need for charity care is the number of persons who are in the active work force but who do not receive health insurance as an employee benefit. Approximately 90% of uninsured persons are employed in companies or businesses that do not offer employee health insurance.[12] These small companies cannot afford to offer health coverage benefits. As our nation continues the transition from a manufacturing to a service economy, this category of uninsured persons will increase. Service companies are usually small and nonunionized, and both of these characteristics are associated with limited employer-sponsored insurance plans. Almost half of uninsured persons are under 25 years of age, and one third of this group are children or other dependents.[12]

Many employers are changing their traditional health insurance benefits, in which the worker chooses his own physician and receives reimbursement for all or part of the incurred expenses. Instead, they are adopting programs that restrict both the extent of coverage and physician selection. As recently as 1984, a total of 96% of insured workers were covered by the traditional plan, compared with the current 28% of workers enjoying such plans in 1989.[26] Newly organized care delivery systems have been introduced.

Alternative care delivery systems An array of acronyms such as HMO, IPA, and PPO (see below) have emerged in the literature. They represent models of health care coverage in which companies offer employee health benefits and at the same time monitor and evaluate the "appropriateness" of medical care prescribed by physicians. A term that may be used to summarize this activity is "managed care."

One of the most popular alternatives is the *health maintenance organization* (HMO). HMOs are membership organizations that provide health care ranging from prevention to treatment for a prenegotiated price during a fixed period. Members may solicit care from only those doctors and hospitals designated by the HMO. This type of alternative care delivery system is the oldest alternative to the traditional health insurance plan. Prepaid group practices, as they were first called, started in farming communities in the 1800s.[25] In the 1940s, Henry Kaiser, an industrialist, founded the HMO known as Kaiser-Permanente. He believed in the "preventive" approach to medicine, rather than the "curing the sick" approach.[29] He encouraged persons to visit a physician before illness developed—preventive health maintenance. These visits were paid for by the HMO and was a distinctly different approach from traditional health care benefits (eg, Medicare, Blue Shield), which would only pay if the patient had a problem that needed treatment. Today, Kaiser-Permanente represents one of the biggest corporation-backed HMO chains in the United States. HMOs first gained national prominence in the 1970s under President Nixon's Administration. During that time, Congress passed the Health Maintenance Organization Act, which created a national policy designed to control escalating health care costs. Federal loans and other incentives were provided to increase HMO growth. HMOs provide corporations with the financial advantage of fixed rates of reimbursement, rather than steadily increasing health insurance premiums. Under this plan, physicians are salaried employees of the HMO.

The *individual practice association* (IPA) is a type of HMO in which the participating physician accepts patients who are HMO members and those who are "fee for service" patients. The physician is reimbursed for care provided to the HMO patients according to a set fee schedule. This fee includes the cost of diagnostic tests and the fee for a referral to a specialist if needed. The physician who does not spend all the allotted money received from the set fee schedule may keep some portion or all of the balance. However, if costs exceed the predetermined rates, the physician must pay the difference.

A *preferred provider organization* (PPO) is another alternative plan for health care coverage. This is a negotiated business arrangement between an industry or business (the buyer) and a hospital or physician (the seller). A limited number of physicians and hospitals join a network and offer a discounted fee for service. In PPO plans, members pay a reduced fee or nothing at all when they are seen by a PPO physician. The physicians and hospitals in the PPO are able to discount their fees in return for a guaranteed volume of patients. The PPO offers the employer cost-controlling mechanisms through a claims review process. This process provides for prospective review of recommended diagnostic tests, surgery, and hospitalizations. Any care that is considered unnecessary is not approved. The PPOs usually offer a wider selection of physicians and hospitals than HMOs offer.

It is estimated that before the year 2000, up to 80% of the insured population will be enrolled in HMOs or PPOs.[26] The greatest controversy surrounding these alternative health care systems is in the implications of the strong incentive to reduce overall spending. Some persons believe that these delivery systems result in fewer tests and procedures or in delays in their being prescribed, to the detriment of the patient's health. Moreover, strong ethical concerns are raised when physicians have the authority to approve or disapprove patient referrals to specialists and at the same time are permitted to keep a percentage of the money they save by not referring patients to specialists. One questions whether such a system can produce unbiased judgment. There are few data available to confirm or deny this phenomenon.

In defense of the alternative care delivery system, the results of two studies showed that there were no statistical differences between the HMO population and the fee-for-service population in the care provided for the diagnosis and treatment of patients with breast cancer or colorectal cancer.[30,31] Variables analyzed for these studies included the mean age of diagnosis, the duration of symptoms before diagnosis, the number of physician visits for symptoms due to cancer before diagnosis, the stage of disease at which diagnosis was made, the methods of diagnosis and treatment, the length of hospital stay, the severity and type of complications, and survival rates. Further research is needed to explore the pros and cons of managed care and validate data and conclusions.

National health care Many Americans have been "spoiled" by the fact that they have been able to receive immediate access to almost any kind of medical treatment. However, health care is not a constitutional right, a fact that has become more apparent as the impact of the PPS continues to be felt. The news media have covered numerous stories about the state and federal funding cutbacks that are causing important public health programs, clinics, and county hospitals to close. Even television entertainment has portrayed persons going to an emergency department and being denied care because they do not have health insurance. A county in the San Francisco Bay area even hired bioethics consultants to help them decide priorities for emergency care.[32] Oregon was one of the first states to ration health care for the poor. In June 1987 the Oregon legislature voted to stop using Medicaid funds to pay for heart, liver, bone marrow, and pancreas transplants.[33] In December 1987 a 7-year-old leukemia patient from Portland, Oregon, whose mother was on welfare, died after the state refused to pay for a bone marrow transplant.

In addition to poor persons, elderly persons, who generate 29% of this nation's health care expenses, are suffering.[33] Physicians who care for frail elderly persons are penalized for having patients who require longer hospitalization. Proposed legislation such as the Catastrophic Health Care Act were attempts to assist the elderly, but at the current time little has been accomplished to help this struggling segment of the population.

Another startling fact that has an impact on the care of elderly persons is that $50 billion a year is spent on patients during the last 6 months of life.[33] This fact has raised questions about the rationing of medical care for persons with a limited life expectancy (ie, elderly persons). For example, should an elderly person with a diagnosis of incurable adenocarcinoma of the lung be given chemotherapy, and if so, for how long?

A growing number of persons in this country are arguing that the American health care system has failed and that the nation needs some kind of nationalized health insurance system. A 1989 poll showed that 89% of Americans believed that fundamental changes are needed.[34] In the past, physicians have strongly opposed the idea of a nationalized health insurance system; however, proposals are being developed, such as the one outlined by Hummelstein and Woolhandler,[35] in which the government would fund all health care but would leave the existing private delivery structure intact; hospitals would not be owned, nor would physicians be employed, by the government.

The United States is one of the few remaining industrial nations that does not have some kind of national health financing program. In the United States, the per capita health care cost is 41% higher than in Canada, 61% higher than in Sweden, 85% higher than in France, 131% higher than in Japan, and an astounding 171% higher than in Great Britain.[36]

An organization that compares the health care of 24 wealthy countries is the Organization for Economic Cooperation and Development (OECD). The OECD reveals that medical practice is similar everywhere and that physicians are quick to learn about the medical advances in other countries; however, the biggest difference between wealthy countries and poorer ones is in the organization and financing of health care in the former.[37] The OECD has also addressed the phenomenon that although countries have much different health care systems, their problems are the same: how to financially restrict the practices of hospitals and physicians, how to secure adequate treatment for poor and elderly persons, and how to control an apparently infinite demand for health care.[37]

The next logical question that comes to mind is, Is the quality of care in the United States better than in other countries? When quality indicators such as life expectancy and infant mortality rates are considered, the United States ranks low. However, in the United States, rationing of medical care through waiting lists (as in countries with nationalized health care systems) is not yet the norm. In Great Britain, waiting lists for elective procedures such as hip replacements or cataract surgery can stretch up to 2 years.[29] Moreover, kidney dialysis ordinarily is not provided for anyone more than 55 years of age,[33] whereas in the United States, this procedure is available to anyone. The fact that the United States does have the highest health care costs but produces the most sophisticated care is an outcome that must not be dismissed.

Our country is pondering the idea of a nationalized health care plan. The time for radical reform is fast approaching as the health care budget continues to soar. Corporate business leaders believe that many Americans are demanding more health care than is needed.[36] However, concern regarding the assessment and definition of quality care is an even bigger issue for many Americans. Reports such as "Quality of Medical Care: Information for Consumers"* have been prepared by the OTA for Congressional review. Paul M. Elwood, Jr, MD, founder of InterStudy, a Minnesota-based health-care-policy think tank, is generally credited with coining the term "health maintenance organization." He is investigating a new theory known as outcome management, in which a collection of objective criteria would help providers, payers, and purchasers to define the relationship between medical interventions and health outcomes.[38] For collection of these data, a quality-of-life scale has been designed and tested. It is based on a 5-minute test, self-administered by patients, that measures their ability to function.[38] This tool is now in the testing stage.

In the 1990s, cost-effective quality care will be a dominant theme. Keeping abreast of the latest information and research is imperative for health care professionals.

Nursing implications There has not been a more important period than the present for nurses to become proactively involved in helping to formulate our nation's health care policies in relation to access to care. A variety of directions can be taken:

- Initiate an educational program to increase the knowledge and skills of the public in regard to decision-making ability, balancing quality with cost. According to competitive theory, the cost and quality of care will be guided by the consumers who weigh price and quality levels in the selection of health insurance and medical care providers.[12]
- Develop clinical nursing research methods that investigate strategies to reduce health care costs without compromising care. According to Fuch,[39] "10% of delivered care may be considered harmful and another 10% is delivered with marginal benefits. If funding cuts were concentrated on this 20% the overall negative effect on health care would be minimal." The results from nursing research can be presented to legislators to assist them in making decisions about cutbacks. Nursing research can answer questions about which cutbacks have serious health implications versus those that will not have any adverse clinical affects.
- Engage in political activities. As drastic changes continue to appear on the horizon, nurses must take a proactive stance in health care decisions, rather than being reactive and merely trying to justify or rectify

*A copy of this report can be purchased through the Superintendent of Documents, US Government Printing Office, Washington, DC (GPO stock no. 052-003-01114).

the current changes. There is a political movement in this country for organizing grass-roots health care organizations. To date, 10 states have organized groups of concerned citizens who tell their legislators how they want their tax dollars spent on health care issues such as rationing and biomedical ethics. (See the Yellow Pages for information regarding this organization.)

- Nurses are advocates of patient care and should assist consumers in the decision-making process of selecting the alternative care system that is the best for their needs. Millensen[25] identified several questions to help people who are considering health care provided by an HMO or PPO:

  1. What do comments from friends or acquaintances indicate about the reputation of the physicians and hospitals that belong to the HMO?
  2. How are the HMO physicians paid? Is there a financial incentive to withhold certain kinds of services or specialist referrals?
  3. What happens if a person becomes sick away from home or outside his HMO service area? Does the HMO pay for care provided elsewhere?
  4. Can consumers choose their primary physician, or are they assigned?
  5. Are all the physicians who are listed as members of the HMO actually available? (Sometimes a popular physician is unable to accept referrals for new patients.)
  6. What are the benefits of the particular HMO? For example, are home prescription drugs and home care visits available?

  For those consumers considering a PPO, it is appropriate to consider the following questions:

  1. Do the participating physicians and hospitals meet the consumer's specific needs for medical care? For example, are specialized services for certain illnesses or treatments, pediatric facilities, maternal care, prescriptions, and home care available?
  2. How much will the PPO pay toward the care provided by a physician who is not participating in the discounted fee arrangement?
  3. Are financial incentives given to physicians that might motivate them to increase the number of office visits and prescribed tests to make up for discounted fees?
  4. Will the PPO pay for a second opinion if it is sought before consumers undergo any tests or treatments that might not be warranted?

- Develop mechanisms to document, in financial terms, the nursing care needed to care for indigent patients. Reports show that the acuity level of the indigent patient is higher.[40,41] This information should be directed to members of PROPAC and Congress—the persons who are responsible for recommending reimbursement figures for indigent care.
- Read *In Search of Excellence,* by Peters and Waterman.[42] This book provides insight into how companies have arrived at strategies for cost savings, cost-effectiveness, and quality services and thus offers the nurse an added perspective on how to influence such changes in the future. A major theme of the book, which can serve as a caution for the hospital industry, is that low-cost providers are not winners over the long term.
- Keep abreast of agenda of the Joint Commission on Accreditation of Healthcare Organizations (the agency responsible for accrediting health care organizations) for the study of change. This study is a major research and development project that is intended to improve the Joint Commission's ability to evaluate health care organizations and generate greater attention to the quality of patient care. Clinical indicators will be used to evaluate specific areas of patient care (eg, obstetrics, oncology). The Association of Community Cancer Centers (ACCC) is developing a multistep method for validating clinical indicators in cancer care. Organizations such as the American College of Surgeons, the ACCC, the American Society of Clinical Oncology, and the Oncology Nursing Society usually provide updated reports on the status of this study.

SPECIFIC ECONOMIC ISSUES IN CANCER CARE

Economics has a major effect on the outcome and delivery of today's patient care. Unfortunately, the specialty of oncology did not escape the PPS regulations. During the 1970s and early 1980s, cancer care has had a "sacred cow" reputation with an "ask and you shall receive" attitude. However, this honeymoon phase is coming to an end in the eyes of today's insurance providers and federal officials. The specialty must now begin to justify all its resource costs. For some hospitals and administrators, cancer is not seen as a "winner" from a cost perspective; consequently, resources such as specialized personnel and state-of-the-art technology are scarce. In this section of the chapter, current issues imposing threats to the specialty of oncology will be addressed.

Oncology as a specialty embodies several unfavorable economic conditions: trend of increasing patient volume; hospital intensive, high acuity care needs; chronicity; a need for intensive monitoring throughout treatment; and the abundant need for psychologic interventions. The specific details of the problems change frequently, but the overall picture of cancer care is that it is expensive, in need of budgetary cuts and under the scrutiny of the legislators.

Cancer-Specific DRGs

The ACCC has been the leader in reporting information specific to cancer DRGs. In the past several years, this organization has gathered information from 90 of its affiliated hospitals. Information of interest from the compilation and analysis of these data includes the following[43]:

- There are 76 cancer or cancer-related DRGs. Forty-four DRGs, or 9.2% of all DRGs are designated as "pure" cancer DRGs for their title includes the presence of the word cancer. These are indicated in Table 54-1 by a "P."
- The 15 DRGs with the highest total gross reimbursement or relative income for each cancer DRG have been identified by calculating the total gross reimbursement, or overall income, for each of the specified cancer or cancer-related DRGs in the 90 institutions surveyed by the ACCC[44] (Table 54-2). Please note that these high-gross-reimbursement DRGs do not necessarily constitute "winning DRGs" for hospitals. In fact, many of the DRGs that have the highest gross reimbursement are "losers"—unprofitable for hospitals. For example, the type of cancer with the highest incidence in this country is lung cancer; thus the highest number of cancer patients are categorized under DRG

TABLE 54-1 Cancer and Cancer-related DRGs

DRG No.	DRG Title
"P" 10	Nervous System Neoplasms, Age ≥70 and/or Complications
"P" 11	Nervous System Neoplasms, Age <70 W/O Complications
46	Other Disorders of the Eye, Age ≥18 W/Complications
47	Other Disorders of the Eye, Age ≥18 W/O Complications
48	Other Disorders of the Eye, Age to 17
"P" 64	Ear, Nose, and Throat Malignancy
73	Other Ear, Nose, and Throat Diagnoses, Age ≥18
"P" 82	Respiratory Neoplasms
145	Other Circulatory Diagnoses W/O Complications
164	Appendectomy W/Complicated Principal Diagnosis, W/Complications
165	Appendectomy W/Complicated Principal Diagnosis, W/O Complications
"P" 172	Digestive Malignancy, Age ≥70 and/or Complications
"P" 173	Digestive Malignancy, Age <70 W/O Complications
185	Dental and Oral Disease Excluding Extraction and Restoration, Age ≥18
187	Dental Extractions and Restorations
188	Other Digestive System Diagnoses, Age ≥70 and/or Complications
189	Other Digestive Diagnoses, Age 18 to 69 W/O Complications
190	Other Digestive System Diagnoses, Age to 17
"P" 199	Hepatobiliary Diagnostic Procedure for Malignancy
"P" 203	Malignancy of Hepatobiliary System or Pancreas
"P" 239	Pathologic Fractures and Musculoskeletal and Connective Tissue Malignancy
256	Other Diagnoses of Musculoskeletal System and Connective Tissue
"P" 257	Total Mastectomy for Malignancy, Age ≥70 and/or Complications
"P" 258	Total Mastectomy for Malignancy, Age 70 W/O Complications
"P" 259	Subtotal Mastectomy for Malignancy, Age >70 and/or Complications
"P" 260	Subtotal Mastectomy for Malignancy, Age <70
261	Breast Procedure for Nonmalignancy Except Biopsy and Local Excision
262	Breast Biopsy and Local Excision for Nonmalignancy
272	Major Skin Disorders, Age ≥70 and/or Complications
273	Major Skin Disorders, Age <70 W/O Complications
"P" 274	Malignant Breast Disorders, Age >70 and/or Complications
"P" 275	Malignant Breast Disorders, Age <70 W/O Complications
276	Nonmalignant Breast Disorders
284	Minor Skin Disorders, Age <70 W/O Complications
300	Endocrine Disorders, Age ≥70 and/or Complications
301	Endocrine Disorders, Age <70 W/O Complications
"P" 303	Kidney, Ureter, and Major Bladder Procedure for Neoplasm

TABLE 54-1 Cancer and Cancer-related DRGs (continued)

DRG No.	DRG Title	DEG No.	DRG Title
"P" 318	Kidney, Urinary Tract Neoplasms, Age ≥70 and/or Complications	399	Reticuloendothelial and Immunity Disorders, Age <70 W/O Complications
"P" 319	Kidney and Urinary Tract Neoplasm, Age <70 W/O Complications	"P" 400	Lymphoma or Leukemia W/Major OR Procedure
334	Major Male Pelvic Procedures W/O Complications	"P" 401	Lymphoma or Leukemia W/Minor OR Procedure, Age ≥70 and/or Complications
"P" 336	Transurethral Prostatectomy, Age ≥70 and/or Complications	"P" 402	Lymphoma or Leukemia W/Minor OR Procedure, Age <70 W/O Complications
"P" 338	Testes Procedure for Malignancy	"P" 403	Lymphoma or Leukemia, Age ≥70 and/or Complications
"P" 344	Other Male Reproductive System OR Procedure for Malignancy	"P" 404	Lymphoma or Leukemia, Age 15 to 69 W/O Complications
345	Other Male Reproductive System OR Procedure Except for Malignancy	"P" 405	Lymphoma or Leukemia, Age to 17
"P" 346	Malignancy, Male Reproductive System, Age ≥70 and/or Complications	"P" 406	Myeloproliferative Disorder or Poorly Differentiated Neoplasm W/Major OR Procedure and Complications
"P" 347	Malignancy, Male Reproductive System, Age <70 W/O Complications	"P" 407	Myeloproliferative Disorder or Poorly Differentiated Neoplasm W/Major OR Procedure W/O Complications
352	Other Male Reproductive System Diagnoses	"P" 408	Myeloproliferative Disorder or Poorly Differentiated Neoplasm W/Minor OR Procedure
"P" 353	Pelvic Evisceration, Radical Hysterectomy and Radical Vulvectomy	"P" 409	Radiotherapy
"P" 357	Uterus and Adenexal Procedures for Malignancy and/or Complications	"P" 410	Chemotherapy
"P" 363	Conization and Radioimplant for Malignancy	"P" 411	History of Malignancy W/O Endoscopy
"P" 366	Malignancy, Female Reproductive System, Age ≥70 and/or Complications	"P" 412	History of Malignancy W/Endoscopy
"P" 367	Malignancy, Female Reproductive System, Age <70 W/O Complications	"P" 413	Other Myeloproliferative Disorder or Poorly Differentiated Neoplasm, Age ≥70 and/or Complications
368	Infections, Female Reproductive System	"P" 414	Other Myeloproliferative Disorder or Poorly Differentiated Neoplasm, Age <70 W/O Complications
369	Menstrual and Other Female Reproductive System Disorders	"P" 465	Aftercare W/History of Malignancy as Secondary Diagnosis
395	Red Blood Cell Disorders, Age ≥18	467	Other Factors Influencing Health Status
396	Red Blood Cell Disorders, Age to 17	"P" 473	Acute Leukemia W/O Major OR Procedure, Age >17
398	Reticuloendothelial and Immunity, Disorders, Age ≥70 and/or Complications		

OR, Operating room; *"P"*, "pure" cancer DRGs; *W/*, with; *W/O*, without.

82 (respiratory neoplasms). Hospital care for these patients is usually more expensive than the allowed DRG reimbursement. If a hospital's largest number of cancer patients are in the DRG 82 category, its highest gross reimbursement will be from this DRG. However, each time a hospital seeks reimbursement through Medicare for patients with lung cancer, they lose money, making this DRG unprofitable for the hospital.

- Variations in cancer DRG profits and losses are also related to regional location. Patterns of care vary

TABLE 54-2 Fifteen Cancer or Cancer-Related DRGs with the Highest Total Gross Reimbursement

	DRG Title		DRG Title
DRG 188	Other Digestive System Diagnoses, Age ≥70 and/or Complications	DRG 172	Digestive Malignancy, Age ≥70 and/or Complications
DRG 400	Lymphoma or Leukemia W/Major OR Procedure	DRG 257	Total Mastectomy for Malignancy, Age >70 and/or Complications
DRG 401	Lymphoma or Leukemia W/Minor OR Procedure, Age ≥70 and/or Complications	DRG 82	Respiratory Neoplasms
DRG 303	Kidney, Ureter, and Major Bladder Procedure for Neoplasm	DRG 203	Malignancy of Hepatobiliary System or Pancreas
DRG 10	Nervous System Neoplasms, Age ≥70 and/or Complications	DRG 395	Red Blood Cell Disorders Age ≥18
DRG 403	Lymphoma or Leukemia, Age ≥70 and/or Complications	DRG 239	Pathologic Fractures and Musculoskeletal and Connective Tissue Malignancy
DRG 408	Myeloproliferative Disorder or Poorly Differentiated Neoplasm W/Minor OR Procedure	DRG 409	Radiotherapy
		DRG 410	Chemotherapy

OR, Operating room; *W/*, with
Source: Adapted from Mortenson LE, Young JL Jr, Ney MS: Variations in cancer DRG profit and loss by hospital size and region of the nation. Oncol Issues 3(4):19, 1988.

throughout the United States and include recommended types of treatment and average length of stay in a hospital setting. In a 1988 ACCC study, 4 of the 15 cancer DRGs with the highest total gross reimbursement in Table 54-2 were selected for review (Table 54-3). Twelve hospitals from the Northeast and Mid-Atlantic areas, 9 hospitals in the Southeast, 14 hospitals in the Midwest, 3 hospitals in the Southwest, and 9 hospitals in the West participated in the study. If a hospital is located in a high-cost region for the DRG chemotherapy category, such as in the Midwest (see Table 54-3), the hospital will probably lose money on this DRG.[44] On the other hand, hospitals located in the southeastern region of the United States will probably make money on this DRG. (Note that the financial figures for the northeastern region in the chemotherapy category listed in Table 54-3 are also a good example of high gross reimbursement for a DRG but a "loser" for hospitals.) Examples of other DRG variations by regional location can also be seen in Table 54-3.[44]

A copy of similar reports may be requested from a hospital's finance department. An oncology clinical nursing specialist (OCNS) should examine this institutional list to identify which DRGs are "winners" and which are "losers." Individual hospitals can compare their data with those of national studies such as the one completed by the ACCC. If there is a negative difference between a hospital's financial DRG data compared with the regional data, measures to improve this status should be investigated. (For example, can length of stay be decreased? Are procedures such as intravenous chemotherapy administration, dressing changes, mouth care protocols, and antibiotic protocols too costly?) If there is a significant difference between the hospital's DRG data and the regional data, this information should be shared with other OCNSs.

When an institution's profit-loss DRG list is reviewed, the variability of volume must be considered. It is important to ensure that those DRGs with the highest volume are monitored to produce "winning" DRGs for the hospital. If a DRG is a "loser," the hospital, with the assistance of an OCNS, must find ways to improve profit margins with such strategies as reducing the length of inpatient stay; by reviewing the necessity and appropriateness of tests, procedures, and drugs that are prescribed; and by determining other variable costs that might be financially draining factors.

In an analysis of the profit-and-loss nature of a cancer program, it is important to avoid two major pitfalls. First, the patient with cancer should not be used as the unit of analysis. This practice ignores the importance of multiple admissions for patients with cancer. Instead, the unit of analysis should be the cancer admissions. A report from the ACCC data revealed that half of all cancer patients' admissions are generated by one fourth of the cancer patients.[45] Second, a limit should not be set on the number of DRGs analyzed for the entire oncology product line. For example, if one is interested in assessing the hospital's profitability in the treatment of lung cancer, data from numerous DRGs (eg, numbers 82, 75, and 76, or a total of 26 others) should be used to analyze profitability, rather than limiting the data to only DRG 82 (Respiratory Neo-

TABLE 54-3 National Regional Variations in DRG Profits and Losses

Region	No. of Discharges	Average Profit/Loss	Average Reimbursement	Average Cost	Total Reimbursement
DRG 82: Respiratory neoplasm					
NE	812	$(517)	$4536	$5054	$3,683,491
SE	633	284	3665	3950	2,820,120
MW	939	645	4505	3860	4,230,550
SW	176	339	5042	4703	887,413
WEST	431	(287)	4531	4818	1,953,049
DRG 257: Total mastectomy for malignancy, age ≥70 and/or complications					
NE	257	$ 403	$3725	$3322	$ 845,559
SE	248	(109)	3277	3387	812,754
MW	290	547	4102	3556	1,189,650
SW	82	443	3603	3159	295,434
WEST	262	810	4110	3300	1,076,926
DRG 409: Radiation therapy					
NE	275	$(1416)	$4978	$6394	$1,368,964
SE	45	1101	3318	2216	149,293
MW	76	(481)	3733	4214	283,718
SW	10	235	3554	3319	35,537
WEST	55	(28)	3501	3529	192,551
DRG 410: Chemotherapy					
NE	1831	$ (53)	$1486	$1539	$2,720,180
SE	854	93	1346	1252	1,149,567
MW	851	(302)	1714	2016	1,458,328
SW	388	(76)	1472	1548	571,101
WEST	1057	(73)	1654	1727	1,748,484

NE, Northeast and Mid-Atlantic; *SE,* Southeast; *MW,* Midwest; *SW,* Southwest.

Source: Adapted from Mortenson LE, Young JL Jr, Ney MS: Variations in cancer DRG profit and loss by hospital size and region of the nation. Oncol Issues 3(4):17-18, 1988.

plasms). The combined DRG list best reflects the true profit or loss figure. If these two mistakes are made, a significant portion (up to 40%) of the cancer program revenues are likely to be missed.[45]

Clinical Trials

The future of clinical trials has been a major concern since the inception of DRGs. In 1983 a study was done to illustrate that the cost of conducting clinical research was too great. The results of this New Jersey–based study concluded that the average loss for each patient in a clinical trial was $1057, or 30 times greater than the loss for patients not in a clinical trial.[46] Additional costs for clinical trials occur because of the increased use of laboratory and radiology tests, the need for an environment conducive to safe, high-quality care (eg, a special unit, an educated interdisciplinary team, higher staff/patient ratios, nutritional support) and data management. The HCFA's response to this inflated figure was that "the Medicare program has always been prohibited from paying the research costs and for items or services that are either experimental in nature or that are paid for by another government entity."[47] The HCFA also commented "that there is substantial federal support through NCI's programs."[47]

This issue became most problematic as a result of work done by researchers at Yale University in assigning weights to the cancer-related DRGs. Patients in clinical trials were not differentiated from others. Thus, when hospitals conducting research (eg, in community clinical oncology programs [CCOPs]) were reimbursed under the PPS, they lost money. Ironically, before the PPS, Medicare did pay for the costs of research, such as the patient's care on specialized oncology units, services provided by the interdisciplinary team, and laboratory and radiology services.[10]

One potential solution to this problem was the suggestion by the ACCC to create "DRG 471" for patients in clinical trials. This strategy was initially rejected by the HCFA. In the spring of 1983, an amendment was passed to provide exemption or adjustment for hospitals involved in providing cancer treatments or engaged in cancer research. Congress limited the amendment by including only three comprehensive cancer centers: MD Anderson Cancer Hospital, Fox Chase Cancer Center, and City of Hope National Medical Center. Since then, five more hospitals were added (refer to DRG cancer hospital exemptions on page 1181). This amendment, however, still did not solve all the problems. Thus many patients who were eligible to receive investigational drugs through clinical trials (eg, patients whose cancer is refractory to all known forms of standard therapy) would not be covered because they were receiving care in a hospital that was not exempt. Thus the cost of receiving investigational drugs was prohibitive for such patients.

To intensify the problem, many insurance companies are following the HCFA's policy. An NCI report to the U S Senate, "Remedies and Cost of Difficulties Hampering Clinical Research," noted that Medicare policy excludes coverage for investigational therapy because treatment with agents not yet approved by the FDA does not satisfy the "reasonable and necessary" criteria included in the legislative language relating to Medicare.[48] In addition, this same report pointed out that many third-party insurance contracts are excluding payments for patient care costs associated with investigational drugs. Although this exclusion has been a part of most insurance contracts for many years, it was not enforced until recently because of the growing emphasis on cost containment. Thus some insurance companies are denying claims whenever an investigational agent is clearly a part of the therapy. Claims that are denied may include the entire cost of hospitalization regardless of what the cost would be without the investigational treatment.[48] The NCI and other health-related organizations are attempting to convince third-party carriers that the treatment received by patients in clinical trials represents the best approach medically that can be offered.[48]

To draw the attention of Congress to the need for change in this reimbursement trend, factual data documenting the scope of the problem must be presented. The National Center for Health Services Research and the NCI are conducting a retrospective research study entitled the Hospital Cost and Clinical Research Project (HCCRP). The principal objectives of the study are (1) to determine whether there are cost differences between protocol and nonprotocol patients and (2) to estimate the extent to which incentives for hospitals to participate in clinical trials may have changed after the implementation of the PPS.[49]

The most frightening concern expressed occasionally by third-party payers is that living longer can waste resources because new technology does not prevent or cure disease but, rather, prolongs the course of illness, especially for patients who are near death. This disturbing concept surfaces at times when budget problems in health care are being discussed. Treating cancer patients with stage III or stage IV disease is viewed by some as a financially ineffective use of national resources. Reese[50] discussed the cost-effectiveness of cancer treatment in the United Kingdom, which has a national health program, and reported that patients with cancer are being denied the best treatment available because of the spending limits imposed by the National Health Service. For example, treatment to reduce pain and improve the quality of life were not always available, and some hospitals could not afford to give chemotherapy because of the costs. Costs were determined by dividing a measure of the effectiveness of intervention in avoiding death or long-term disability into the cost of treatment for one patient.[50] A maximum of 17,000 francs (approximately $25,000) was documented as the amount available to save a life or avoid severe disability (a high-dose methotrexate chemotherapy regimen would exceed this figure). Fortunately, these cost-assessment procedures are not the primary sources for decision making about care to be provided. The thought of calculating the worth of a person's life by a formula is astounding. Yet Reese[50] concludes that the rationing of resources for cancer patients is inevitable and that cost assessment is a means of enabling hospitals and physicians to make optimal use of resources.

Changes in reimbursement policies occur on an almost daily basis. Medicare, Medicaid, and private insurers presently handle reimbursement on a case-by-case basis and usually require a written narrative (a preauthorization) of the patient's diagnosis, prognosis, treatment plan, effectiveness of prior treatment, and supporting data on the efficacy of the drugs to be used.[51] Policies and regulations vary from one state to another.

Funds are available for clinical trials from the NCI. However, the designated budget is not adequate to support the current explosion in scientific discovery and biotechnology. For example, President Bush's budget request in 1989 for the NCI was $1.6 billion; an additional $90 million was needed to sustain the existing level of services.[48]

Pharmaceutical companies often assist in funding clinical trials because the trials provide a means of testing their products. Companies usually pay an agreed-on dollar figure per accrued patient, with funding for laboratory tests, clinical coordination, data management, and physician fees, but rarely does the budget allocate money for the cost of routine patient care and clinical management, including the cost of hospitalization.[51]

To add further confusion to the reimbursement scenario, new institutions or corporations are being developed outside the auspices of the NCI to deliver advanced technologic care to patients whose cancer is refractory to standard therapy. An example of such an institution was the Biologic Therapy Institute, Biotherapeutics, Inc, of Franklin, Tennessee where patients paid their own medical expenses to receive experimental therapy. Unfortunately, financial difficulties caused Biotherapeutics, Inc, to close. Such delivery systems are called patient sponsored and promulgate the notion that care is available for those who can pay. In addition, we live in the era of the "baby boom" generation, when consumers are willing to pay extra for high-quality services.[52] The future for patient-sponsored research is not well defined, but already the National Academy of Sciences Institute of Medicine is proposing guidelines for responsible behavior in research.[53]

Through self-education, patients, legislators, and nurses can have an impact on the issue of reimbursement for clinical trials. Barbara Hoffman, JD, vice-president of the National Coalition for Cancer Survivorship, summarizes the predicament of clinical trials[54]:

The current lack of adequate health insurance coverage for experimental clinical trials and newly developed treatment bodes poorly for improving cure rates in the near future. The costs that society is paying now for cancer treatments is slight when compared with the cost of productive lives lost to oncology care that is dictated by M.B.A.s rather than M.D.s.

Unlabeled Use of FDA-Approved Chemotherapy Drugs

The government and insurance companies began in the late 1980s to deny reimbursement for drugs used for indications that do not fall within the package-insert guidelines approved by the FDA (unlabeled drugs). Some insurers (in northern California and Michigan) are denying reimbursement for unlabeled indications of chemotherapy, calling the use of such drugs experimental.[55]

The ACCC conducted an audit of 3500 patients' records from 1986 in 165 oncologists' offices. The audit concluded that of the eight most frequently used chemotherapy drugs, 46% were being used for unlabeled indications[56] (Table 54-4). The impact of this conclusion for the third-party payers who can deny payment is an annual savings of $150 to $200 million; for patients with cancer, it means that 372,000 were denied treatment with vincristine, 218,000 were denied treatment with cyclophosphamide, 88,000 were denied treatment with cisplatin, and 121,000 were denied treatment with methotrexate.[55] All these treatments are considered standard medical practice. In addition, approximately 90% of chemotherapy is given in standard combination regimens, and none of these combinations have ever had FDA approval.[55]

Insurers are asking drug manufacturers to obtain FDA approval for indications not listed on the label. Pharmaceutical representatives say that this process of supplemental application is a very time-consuming and costly endeavor, ranging from $500,000 to $5 million.[57] In addition, the burden on the FDA would be astronomic! However, "under Section 502 of the Federal Drug and Cosmetic Act, the FDA must support the policy that an approved drug must be labeled, promoted and administered only for uses for which its safety and efficacy have been established."[57] This guideline has not always been followed, however. In the past, the package inserts were mainly used only as a guide for physicians.

As the reader can surmise, we are just beginning to see cost-cutting warfare. Nurses must keep abreast of the most current information for creating profitable strategies for oncology programs. Keeping well informed will also enable nurses to react quickly as advocates for patients who are being denied payment for their health care.

TABLE 54-4 Eight Chemotherapy Agents with High Frequencies of Unlabeled Uses

Agent	Unlabeled Diagnoses
Adriamycin	GI/digestive cancers Other malignancies
Cytoxan	GI/digestive cancers Lung cancers Other malignancies
Fluorouracil	Lung cancers Metastatic adenocarcinoma Metastatic prostate cancer
Methotrexate	GI/digestive cancers Ovarian cancers Other malignancies
Mutamycin	Rectal cancers Lung cancers Breast cancers Ovarian cancers Other malignancies
Oncovin	GI/digestive cancers Breast cancers Lung cancers Other malignancies
Platinol	GI/digestive cancers Lung cancers Metastatic thyroid cancer Malignant melanoma Metastatic uterine cancer Other malignancies
Vepesid	GI/digestive cancers Ovarian cancers Brain cancer Hematologic malignancies

Source: Mortenson LE: Audit indicated half of current chemotherapy uses lack FDA approval. Oncol Issues 3(1):22, 1988.

Outpatient Oncology Care

Implementation of the PPS caused a major shift in the treatment environment, from inpatient to outpatient care. Patients who were receiving treatment for cancer, especially chemotherapy, felt the impact most heavily. The DRG limit for reimbursement, pressure for early patient discharge, and patient preference have been strong incentives for the accelerated growth of outpatient cancer care facilities. The delivery of quality outpatient care has quickly become possible through advanced technologic support (eg, vascular access devices, ambulatory infusion pumps), the results of pharmacology research (eg, oral chemotherapeutic agents), and the specialized knowledge and skills of oncology nurses and physicians. Management of toxic effects has become possible on an outpatient basis by increasing the education and responsibility of patients and their families. Moreover, triage by telephone has become an important monitoring modality in outpatient cancer care (see Chapter 50, Ambulatory Care).

Shifting chemotherapy to the outpatient setting has not sheltered it from the scrutiny of insurance coverage, however. The HCFA received an allocation of $70,000 in 1988 to study the reasonableness of current Medicare payment levels for outpatient chemotherapy.[58] Recommendations based on the study will be made to Congress.

To ensure payment from an insurance company, the health care provider should contact the company to determine whether it will pay for outpatient treatment, which billing codes should be used, and which limitations are applicable to a particular patient. In 1989 a group practice of oncologists working in a hospital outreach clinic was ordered to return $75,000 in chemotherapy supervision fees charged during the prior 2½ years.[59] The ruling was based on a long-standing Medicare regulation whereby only the entity that owns or leases the space in which outpatient chemotherapy is delivered and that pays the employees can charge for the office visit, drug charges, and administration and supervision for chemotherapy.[59]

Preventive Cancer Care

The concept of wellness has been part of nursing and medicine for years and is reflected in the axiom "An ounce of prevention is worth a pound of cure." However, not until the medical world convinced the industrial world, through profitable financial data reports, did industry understand that this concept was both medically and economically sound. A report from the National Cancer Health Statistics indicates that $10.3 million was spent for medical care for cancer in 1985.[60] Care for male patients with lung cancer accounted for $1 million of this figure (48% of these patients were younger than 62 years of age, and 52% were 65 and older); $0.9 million was spent on female lung cancer patients (74% were less than 65 years of age and 26% were 65 and older). The investment in smoking cessation programs has the potential to effect great savings for industry. Another federal study demonstrated that hospital care expenditures account for roughly 60% to 75% of the total direct cost of cancer, compared with about 35% to 50% spent on hospital care for all other diseases.[61] The American Cancer Society estimates the average cost of treating a malignancy to be $60,000.[62] At the time of publication, more current information had not been compiled. One study at the University of Pennsylvania's Wharton School, Institute of Health Economics, found that companies can save more than 40% in hospitalization costs by implementing wellness programs for employees.[26] Wellness programs are increasingly popular; two of every three firms with 50 employees or more now offer some health promotion activity.[26] Worried about the skyrocketing costs of caring for employees with cancer, industry has also started cancer screening programs. Lately, more insurance providers are investigating mammography screening. However, a discouraging report in *Newsweek* noted that the expense to insurers would be about $5 billion if a third of the nation's women had screening mammograms annually, rather than $2 billion per year to treat cancer.[29] Such calculations can have only a negative impact on reimbursement. On the positive side, legislators are taking actions to ensure that mammograms will be covered for Medicare beneficiaries. Also, close to half of the states in the nation have laws requiring that third-party insurers pay for screening mammography. For changes in the future of cancer prevention and screening to be positive, many cost-benefit studies must be initiated and must produce evidence of overall cost savings.

THE FUTURE OF NURSING IN THE ECONOMICS OF HEALTH CARE

Changes in health care policy and economics are not new. In each decade there has been a different reason—the 1960s access to care, the 1970s technologic advancements, the 1980s cost containment, and the 1990s cost containment with quality care. The birth of the prospective payment system has offered nursing the chance to turn from a reactionary, follow-the-textbook, nostalgic approach and to become a proactive, creative, open-minded, economically aware profession. It is important to retain the successes and values that nursing has obtained throughout the years while also being ready to advance to a new era of influence and power.[2]

An initial impact of the PPS on nursing was to uncouple nursing services from hospital per diem charges along with charges for housekeeping, dietary, and laundry services. The effort to make this change began in 1977 when the New Jersey Health Department initiated the development of a nursing allocation-of-resources model that was DRG specific; the model was called relative intensity measures (RIMs) of nursing.[10] The RIMs have been criticized for methodologic failure; the necessary time for planning care, obtaining the resources needed for patient care, and evaluating the care was not allocated.[10,63] These daily nursing activities are often more time-consuming than nursing assessments or interventions. However, in the RIMs study, emphasis was given to these components of assessment and intervention. Also criticized was the assumption that care delivered equals care required.[64]

Various other schemes have been used to determine the cost of nursing services or to estimate nursing resource utilization. In 1985 a report from the American Nurse's Association Center for Research,[65] entitled "DRGs and Nursing Care," was submitted to the HCFA. The project was funded through an HCFA grant. The pilot study examined the relationship between DRGs and both nursing resource utilization and nursing costs. This report noted that the DRGs were developed without explicit attention to nursing resource use or nursing costs in hospitals, which is a significant component of overall hospital activities and costs. Data from the study consisted of approximately 1600 patient records from two hospitals in Wisconsin. Twenty-one DRGs, selected in relationship to high frequency with which they were encountered among the hospitalized Medicare beneficiaries, were examined for this study. The principal findings outlined in the study were as follows:

- DRG relative cost weights generally appear to reflect differences in nursing resource requirements among the DRGs in the study.
- Some DRGs in the study are interpretable groupings of patients, both in terms of total hours of nursing care by DRG and in terms of the daily pattern of nursing resource consumption during the course of hospitalization.
- Even though nursing care was not given explicit attention when the prospective pricing was developed, nursing costs as defined in the study have been shown to account for between 20% and 28% of hospital costs for two thirds of the DRGs in the study.
- Sufficient variations in nursing resources utilization patterns and in nursing costs were found to suggest further study in the refinement of prospective pricing. This study clearly defines the need for nursing to be identified in prospective pricing. However, to date, the Prospective Payment Assessment Commission has not acknowledged this fact. The only concern related to nursing that the Commission discussed in its June 1989 report to Congress was the shortage of registered nurses.[66]

Although there has been great interest and concern about determining nursing care costs for separate billing in the past several years, rapid movement in that direction has been limited because of the lack of financial and hospital administration support. Unfortunately, some of the nursing literature even suggests that such cost assessments may not be helpful and may not be effective unless the professional nursing staff is salaried.[63] Even with these restraints, success has been achieved in many hospitals toward the goal of billing patients directly for nursing costs. Hospitals in Arizona, Connecticut, New York, and Miami have been noted for their achievement in this area.[2]

CONCLUSION

The PPS will not be static: changes will occur over time and will further restrict health care payments. A significant opportunity for nurses will be to conduct or participate in the clinical research needed to determine which nursing interventions are most beneficial from a cost-benefit perspective. Although nurses have traditionally developed a variety of interventions to manage patient care problems, there has been minimal research to determine which approaches produce the best results. It is important to determine not only which approaches are the best but also which are the best at the lowest possible cost. When nurses collaborate in this type of research, they will have an impact on the cost of health care and consequently will gain recognition by health care and policy leaders. Seldom are nurses appointed to advisory committees that are involved in research studies with a direct influence on changing our nation's health policy. The nursing profession must strive for this recognition.

Perhaps the greatest impact of the DRGs on nursing is in delivery systems for nursing care, which often have not kept pace with the rapid and complex changes in health care.[16] A current popular nursing delivery system is primary nursing. This delivery system is being monitored by nursing executives not only for its quality but for its patient care costs. However, newer changes in nursing care delivery systems are on the horizon. O'Malley et al[16] note that these delivery systems will have to be redesigned to (1) integrate with hospital business plans, (2) be consumer driven, outcome focused, and flexible, and (3) define more clearly the practice of professional nursing, which requires an advanced level of clinical and management skills at the bedside. One example of a redesigned system that was discussed earlier in this chapter is case management.

In the decade of the 1990s, the profession of nursing should continue to pursue recognition by health care leaders as the most vital link in successfully managing quality patient care at low cost. By unifying the large number of nurses in this country through professional nursing organizations, nurses can become a strong and powerful voice in the health care arena.

The role of the clinical nurse specialist (CNS) will be a pivotal position in the nursing organization structure. Yasko and Fleck[10] state:

> The CNS, with emphasis on the word nursing as the focus of their practice, will be needed to ensure the implementation of sophisticated patient care, which includes: the development, implementation, and evaluation of standards of care; systematic early discharge programs; methods to document accurately the delivery of nursing care; systems to determine the cost/benefit [ratio] of new supplies and equipment; methods to more effectively and efficiently teach patients and significant others self care; and systems to determine the cost of planning, implementing and evaluating nursing care.

REFERENCES

1. Ward W: An Introduction to Health Care Financial Management. Owings Mills, Md, National Health Publishing, 1988.
2. Davis CK: Health care economic issues: Projection for oncology nurses. Oncol Nurs Forum 12(4):17-22, 1985.
3. Diagnosis Related Groups: Their Evolution. Current Applications and Future Implications. (Executive Series No. J58341.) Cleveland, Ernst and Whinney, 1980.
4. Bird S, Mailhot C: DRGs: A new way to reimburse hospital costs. AORN J 38:773-777, 1983.
5. Joel L: DRGs: The state of the art of reimbursement for nursing services. Nurs Health Care 4:560-563, 1983.
6. Medicare program: Proposed rules. Federal Registry 54(87):19663, May 1989.
7. Hunt K: DRG: What it is, how it works and why it will hurt. Med Econ Sept 5, 1983, pp 262-272.
8. Shaffer F: DRGs: History and overview. Nurs Health Care 4:389-396, 1983.

9. Vladek BC: Medicare hospital payment by diagnosis related groups. Ann Intern Med 100:576-591, 1984.
10. Yasko JM, Fleck AE: Prospective payment (DRGs): What will be the impact on cancer care? Oncol Nurs Forum 11(3):63-72, 1984.
11. US Department of Health and Human Services: Report to Congress: DRG refinement: Outliers, severity of illness and intensity of care. Washington, DC, The Department, 1987.
12. National Committee for Quality Health Care: An American health strategy: Ensuring the availability of quality health care. Washington, DC, The Committee, 1988.
13. Young D: Prospective Payment Assessment Commission: Mandate, structure and relationships. Nurs Econ 2:309-311, 1984.
14. Young D: PROPAC: Future directions. Nurs Econ 4:12-15, 1986.
15. Tokarski C: Hospital inflation: A recurring problem. Mod Healthc 18(45):38-43, 1988.
16. O'Malley J, Loveridge C, Cummings S: The new nursing organization. Nurs Manage 20(2):29-33, 1989.
17. Definition. The Center for Nursing Case Management, New England Medical Center 3:1-3, 1988.
18. Definition. The Center for Nursing Care Management, New England Medical Center 2:1-4, 1987.
19. Tokarski C: Group hit government plan to access technology coverage. Mod Healthc 19(14):21, 1989.
20. Prospective Payment Commission: Report and recommendations to the Secretary, US Department of Health and Human Services. Washington, DC, The Commission, March 1989.
21. Hicks L: Using benefit cost and cost-effectiveness analysis in health care resource allocation. Nurs Econ 3(2):78-84, 1985.
22. Hochhauser M: A format for health care feasibility studies. Health Mark Q 4(2):35-41, 1986.
23. Larson E, Peters D: Integrating cost analysis in quality assurance. J Nurs Quality Assurance 1(1):1-7, 1986.
24. Larson E, Maciorowski L: Rational product evaluation. J Nurs Adm 16(7,8):31-36, 1986.
25. Millenson M: New options in health insurance, in Zeleny RO (ed): The World Book Health and Medical Annual. Chicago, World Book, 1988, pp 99-107.
26. Miller A, Bradburn E, Hager M, et al: Can you afford to get sick? Newsweek 113(5):45-51, 1989.
27. Murphy E: Health care: Right or privilege? Nurs Econ 4(2):66-68, 1986.
28. Wagner L, Toakrski C: Speculation begins. Mod Healthc 19(3):24-31, 1989.
29. Easterbrook G: The revolution in medicine. Newsweek 109(4):40-74, 1987.
30. Hughes J, Heckel V, Vernon S, et al: HMO versus FFS practice: A four-year retrospective analysis of colorectal cancer diagnosis and treatment—is there a difference in quality of care? Quality versus reimbursement and other conundrums. Proceedings of the 15th National Association of Community Cancer Care, 1989 (abstr).
31. Kulkarni PR, Vernon SW, Jackson GL, et al: Stage at diagnosis of breast cancer, comparison in a fee-for-service and health maintenance organization practice. Med Care 27:608-621, 1989.
32. Hilton B: Time for hard choices in health care. Pittsburgh Press, section 1B, p 3, March 15, 1989.
33. Robinson D: Who should receive medical aid. Parade Magazine, pp 4-5, May 28, 1989.
34. News at deadline. Hospitals 63(5):14, 1989.
35. Hummelstein DU, Woolhandler S: A national health program for the United States: A physician's proposal. N Engl J Med 320(2):102-108, 1989.
36. Iacocca L: Not ready for national health insurance but . . . Houston Chronicle, April 16, 1989, Sec H, p 1.
37. Sick health service. The Economist, July 16, 1988, pp 19-22.
38. Ellwood explains his theory, terminology and outcomes method of managing care. Mod Healthc 19(2):30, 1989.
39. Fuch VR: The ratio of medical care. N Engl J Med 311:1572-1573, 1984.
40. Studnick J: Differences in length of stay of Medicaid and Blue Cross patients and the effect of intensity of services. Public Health Rep 94(5):43845, 1979.
41. Presgrove M: Indigent patients: More nursing or less revenue. Nurs Manage 16(1):47-51, 1985.
42. Peters TJ, Waterman RH: In Search of Excellence. New York, Harper & Row, 1982.
43. Young JL, Mortenson LE, New MS: Hospital reimbursement, charges, and profit and loss for cancer and cancer-related DRGs. Oncol Issues 3(4):9-15, 1988.
44. Mortenson LE, Young JL, Ney MS: Variations in cancer DRG profit and loss by hospital size and region of the nation. Oncol Issues 3(4):16-20, 1988.
45. Katterhagen JG, Clarke RT, Mortenson LE: Understanding the economics of outpatient care. Oncol Issues 4(1):11-14, 1989.
46. Mortenson LE, Winn R: The potential negative impact of prospective reimbursement on cancer treatment and clinical research progress. Cancer Prog Bull 9(3):7-9, 1983.
47. Medicare regulations: final report. Federal Register 49(1):234, January 3, 1989.
48. The Cancer Letter 15(11):1-6, March 17, 1989.
49. Coffey R, Wallen J: Hospital cost and clinical research project. Washington, DC, National Center for Health Services Research, National Cancer Institute, 1985.
50. Reese GJ: Cost-effectiveness in oncology. Lancet 2:1405-1407, 1985.
51. Yasko J: Biological response modifier treatment: Reimbursement—present status and future strategies, Oncol Nurs Forum Suppl 15(6):28-34, 1988.
52. Jensen J: Consumers consider quality in deciding on a hospital, but measurements differ. Mod Healthc 19(10):88, 1989.
53. Report on the responsible conduct of research in the health sciences. Cope Magazine 3(6):12, 13, 1989.
54. Oncology Forum: Is the current system of reimbursement for experimental cancer treatment appropriate for the patient and/or oncologist? Cope Magazine 3(6):17-18, 1989.
55. Mortenson LE: Insurers target chemotherapy payments. Wall Street Journal 83(92):A16, May 11, 1989.
56. Mortenson LE: Audit indicates half of current chemotherapy uses lack of FDA approval. Oncol Issues 3(1):21-25, 1988.
57. FDA review of new indications is lengthy, costly process. Oncol Issues 3(1):19, 1988.
58. HCFA studies outpatient chemotherapy payment levels. Oncol Issues 3:7, 1988.
59. Medicare demands supervision fee refunds in Indiana. Oncol Issues 4:5, 1989.
60. US Department of Health and Human Services: Cancer rates and risks (3rd ed). Washington, DC, National Institutes of Health, 1985, pp 33-35.
61. Baird S: Changing economics of cancer care, challenges, opportunities. Proceedings of the Fifth National Conference on Cancer Nursing. New York, American Cancer Society, 1987, pp 1-16.

62. O'Grady E: Health investment: Firms back worker wellness. Houston Post (Business Section), June 12, 1989, p 1.
63. Kramer M, Schmalenberg C: Magnet hospitals talk about the impact of DRGs on nursing care. Nurs Manage 18(10):33-40, 1987.
64. Mowry, Mychelle, Korpman: Do DRGs reimbursement rates reflect nursing costs? J Nurs Adm 15(7,8):29-35, 1985.
65. American Nurses' Association Center for Research: DRGs and Nursing Care. (HCFA Grant No. 15-C-98421/7-02.) Kansas City, Mo, The Association, 1985.
66. Prospective Payment Commission: Medicare prospective payment and the American health care system. Report to the Congress. Washington, DC, The Commission, 1989.

Chapter 55

Ethics in Cancer Nursing Practice

Constance T. Donovan, RN, MSN, FAAN

INTRODUCTION

The tremendous advances in health-related science and technology of the second half of the twentieth century have resulted in an increased ability to exert control over the lives of human beings. This phenomenon has created an urgent need for a new emphasis on the ethical dimensions of decision making in health-related matters.[1] In fact, an entire field called bioethics (health care ethics, medical ethics, biomedical ethics) has emerged.

Gorovitz,[2] in 1978, defined this field as follows: "Bioethics is the critical examination of the moral dimensions of decision-making in health related contexts and in contexts involving the biological sciences." Questions about what is right or what should be done are raised, and the issues are organized in a way that allows for rational deliberation. Complexities are revealed about such situations as allowing a person with refractory leukemia to die or performing clinical phase I cancer studies. In the process of deliberation, conflict between ethical principles comes to light as alternative choices are considered. While no one "right" ethical answer or set of rules is produced, the potential of wrong action toward persons is minimized. In addition, choices based simply on current practices, universalization of personal convictions (frequently and emotionally expressed as "I feel"), or scientific knowledge can be avoided. In essence, more morally responsible choices in health-related matters can emerge.

Within nursing, considerable attention has been given to the question of whether nursing ethics is a subcategory of or separate from medical ethics. In general, there is a growing concern to develop nursing ethics as a unique field. Scholars in nursing ethics have been engaged in a continuing discourse regarding the moral foundation of nursing[3-6] and the extent to which nursing should borrow from the ethical theory approach or the moral development approach to ethics.[7] Although it is uncertain as to the degree to which the current lack of clarity about nursing ethics has created confusion within the nursing community and impeded integration of ethics into nursing curricula, Thompson and Thompson[8] concluded that formal preparation for ethical decision making lags behind our recognition of the need.

With increasing responsibility and expanding areas of professional decision making, cancer nurses are among those who have become increasingly aware of the importance of being prepared to participate in making ethical choices. They recognize that simple answers based on general statements about patients' rights are inadequate, do not identify the role of nursing in the ethical decision-making process, and certainly do not convince professional colleagues. These colleagues may view a particular situation as requiring only a clinical-scientific decision, rather than a decision that includes an ethical dimension. On the other hand, attempts to resolve ethical dilemmas by focusing strictly on the legal aspects often lead to frustration, because what is legal may not be congruent with what should be done ethically.

This chapter explores the influence of the nurse-patient relationship on bioethical decision making and examines issues that are most relevant to cancer nursing. To provide background for these discussions, the initial section focuses on information about ethical dilemmas and models of ethical reflection.

BACKGROUND INFORMATION

Ethical Dilemmas

Recognition of the fact that every health care decision has a value component is fundamental to the ethical practice of nursing. Although clinical-scientific data contribute to judgments, final decisions involve either the implicit or explicit consideration of values. Alternative actions reflect these values.

Actions are not always preceded by extensive ethical analysis. Veatch[9] notes that numerous health decisions are either so ordinary or have such obvious moral choices that immediate actions are possible. Veatch[9] points out, however, that it is only because some general guidelines have emerged as a result of our previous experiences that we are able to act without being immobilized by ethical considerations. Other situations do present serious dilemmas that require ethical deliberation before action is taken. The alternative choices of action within the situation represent conflicting moral claims for which no best choice is easily identified. Davis and Aroskar[1] define a dilemma as a choice between equally unsatisfactory alternatives and indicate that such questions as the following are asked: What should I do? What is the right thing to do? What harm and benefit result from this decision or action?

An example from the recent past where the alternatives were equally unsatisfactory involved pain management. Before approaches were developed to control the pain of persons with terminal cancer without endangering life, a choice often had to be made between preserving life and relieving suffering. Should a high dose of pain medication be administered or withheld? The best choice was not always easily decided nor mutually agreed on by patient, physician, and nurse.

Ethical problems are not limited, however, to specific patient situations. At times, choices must be defended on the policy-making level, as in the use of human subjects in experimentation and in the allocation of limited health care resources.

Choosing the best or right action requires careful deliberation. The data must be carefully collected. Davis and Aroskar[1] note that "the process of reflective thinking provides data by asking questions related to identifying the actors in the situation, the required action(s), possible and probable consequences of the proposed action(s), the intention or purpose of the action(s), the range of alternatives or choices, and the context of the action(s)." Once the data have been collected, the formulation of the problem is reviewed to be sure that it has been identified accurately and to clarify the values or moral principles that are in conflict.

Models for Ethical Reflection

What is a morally right act? To provide for careful analysis of choices and to move toward deciding the best choice of action, one must have knowledge of the various models of ethical reflection. Veatch[9] describes normative ethics as that area of ethics that determines whether there are general principles or norms related to a situation that make actions right or wrong. Beauchamp[10] describes normative ethics as divided into two fields: applied and general. In applied ethics, general ethical principles such as utility, truth telling, and keeping promises are used to resolve problems. In general ethics, the general ethical principles are organized into a system that is referred to as an ethical theory or position. The two dominant positions in the West are utilitarianism and formalism.

Taylor[11] describes *utilitarianism* as a teleologic ethical system (from the Greek word *telos*, meaning end or purpose) in which an action is morally right if it brings about good consequences. Therefore, in a utilitarian system, it is the goodness or badness of the consequences of actions that make them right or wrong. Taylor[11] describes *formalism* as a deontologic system (from the Greek word *deon*, meaning duty) in which an action is right if it accords with a moral rule and wrong if it violates such a rule, regardless of the end or purpose of the action. In formalism, there exists a set of conditions that are necessary and sufficient for any rule of moral obligation to apply to an action.

In using the utilitarian position to determine which alternative action in a situation of choice will provide the greatest general happiness, one can employ either of two approaches, the act-utilitarian or the rule-utilitarian approach.

The following case study may be used to consider each of these approaches:

> Mrs. H. has had a diagnosis of advanced cancer of the esophagus. Her children report that Mrs. H.'s husband has recently died. They insist that they do not wish their mother to be told about her diagnosis because they believe that she will "give up." They request that she be told that she has a narrowing in her esophagus. One day Mrs. H. says to her primary nurse, "I know I'm very sick; I can't eat very much." The next day she asks the same nurse to tell her what is wrong. Should Mrs. H. be told her diagnosis?

According to the act-utilitarian approach, an attempt would be made to predict the possible consequences for the alternative choices of action: (1) withholding information about the diagnosis of esophageal cancer and (2) explaining to Mrs. H. that she has cancer of the esophagus. The consequences would be listed as empiric statements based on experience or knowledge. Some argue that a possible consequence for the first action is that Mrs. H. will maintain hope and for the second action is that Mrs. H. will become anxious and depressed. After all the possible consequences for each action are outlined, each consequence would be assigned a happiness value, and the alternative with the greatest general happiness value for the greatest number involved would be selected.

In the rule-utilitarian approach, the alternative actions would be compared with an established rule that would have predetermined, by a listing of consequences, the actions that would produce the greatest general happiness for the greatest number of persons involved. An example of such a rule might be that depression and fear should be prevented. The alternative that is consistent with the rule would then be considered the right choice.

Finally, according to the deontologic approach, the method would be simply to compare alternative actions with rules or ethical principles such as keeping promises and telling the truth. These principles are seen as independent of consequences or of the good to be achieved. The alternative that is consistent with all appropriate principles would be viewed as the right action. For example, in the case study, telling the patient about her diagnosis might be seen as the right action because it is consistent with the principles of telling the truth and allowing self-determination.

Each of these approaches seems to have practical limitations. For example, in the utilitarian approach, consequences may be hard to predict or validate, and estimates of happiness values may be difficult to determine. In the deontologic approach, if both alternatives are consistent with some principles and conflict with others, choosing the right action might be difficult.

The adequacy of each theory can also be questioned. For the utilitarian approach, achieving the greatest happiness for the greatest number of persons could mean infringing on the rights of some. As an example, consider a clinical study in which cancer cells are to be injected into persons who do not have cancer and who have not consented to the procedure. It could be argued that the happiness of the majority resulting from the knowledge obtained would definitely outweigh the unhappiness of the research subjects. Therefore it could be decided that undertaking such a study is a right act. Some argue, however, that respect for the rights of individuals is of more fundamental moral value than the greatest happiness for the greatest number.[12] Thus, at times, using the concept of greatest happiness as a central focus for ethical decisions may be inappropriate.

For the deontologist, a difficulty unfolds when duties and obligations conflict. Davis and Aroskar[1] explain: "It does not resolve the dilemma for the nurse who decides to follow the rule that one should always tell the truth but realizes that the truth will undoubtedly hurt a particular patient in a given situation where the principle of telling the truth conflicts with the principle of doing no harm."

To avoid the limitations of each of these models, some authors[13,14] have arrived at a pluralistic model in which consideration is given to both consequences and inherent characteristics. Thus, in the situation of telling the truth, one relevant factor considered would be the duty to tell the truth, but the significance of consequences also would be recognized.

Although these and other models do not provide answers and, indeed, should not be used as "recipes," disciplined ethical reasoning is used to try to arrive at decisions about morally right actions.

NURSE-PATIENT RELATIONSHIPS IN CANCER CARE

It can be argued that attention to what constitutes an ethical dilemma, patterns of ethical reasoning, and analysis of ethical issues, although essential to ethical deliberation, is not sufficient; that is, the relational aspect inherent in the clinical situation must also be taken into consideration. In fact, several authors[15-17] have suggested that the key to creating an ethical climate lies in the relationship between the health professional and the patient; they note that the type of relationship will affect directly who makes the decision and how and what kinds of decisions are made.

Several models of the nurse-patient relationship were identified by Gadow[18] in 1977: nurse as healer, parent surrogate, physician surrogate, health educator, patient advocate, and contracted clinician. Gadow[18] noted, however, that each type of relationship raised some ethical questions, such as the following:

> Does the nurse, if acting as parent surrogate, have the right to act paternalistically when the patient does not make "health" decisions? Does the nurse, if acting in contractual partnership with the patient, have the right to withdraw care when the patient refuses to assume responsibility for his or her health? Does the nurse, if acting as healer, analogous to the physician, have the right to cultivate the placebo effect that is thought to accompany all the actions of a healer, even to the point of patient deception? Or does the nurse, if acting as patient advocate, have an obligation to protect the patient from every erosion of human dignity and value, including deceptions in the name of health?

Faced with these alternative conceptions and their related ethical difficulties, what has been nursing's choice? American nursing, in general, seems to have rejected most of these models, including the "nurse as parent surrogate" conception, in which the nurse decides what is best for the patient. Rather, the numerous articles and books that have been written promoting the role of the nurse as patient advocate[19-25] suggest that nursing has adopted the "nurse as patient advocate" conception of the nurse-patient relationship.

However, there is a need to clarify the meaning of advocacy in nursing.[26,27] For example, advocacy at times seems to mean assuring the quality of care for groups of patients, whereas at other times, it seems to mean being a spokesperson for the patient or information provider and "watchdog" as the patient representative model and the patient's rights model, respectively, suggest. In addition, there are those times when advocacy seems to mean promoting and enhancing patient autonomy (self-determination).

Ultimately, it may be decided that the concept of advocacy in nursing should encompass a variety of meanings. However, careful analysis would be required for clarification of each meaning and to avoid including morally incompatible meanings. Consider, as an example, the various meanings identified above in which the nurse's involvement could range from political action or negotiation for change, to protection of particular patients' human rights or best interests, to interactions with patients that promote their autonomy. It is not entirely clear whether all these meanings represent a commitment to the same moral position. For example, if protection of a patient's best interests could be interpreted to mean that, in general, the nurse could act without the competent patient's permission or could decide what was in the competent patient's best interest, then such a paternalistic position clearly would be incompatible with the moral position of the promotion of patient autonomy.

Gadow[28-31] offers one of the most instructive analyses of the meaning of advocacy in the patient-nurse relationship. She characterizes advocacy as based on the primacy of the human right of freedom of self-determination,[28] and describes it as

> the effort to help persons become clear about what they want to do, by helping them discern and clarify their values in the situation, and on the basis of that self-determination, to reach decisions which express their reaffirmed, perhaps recreated, complex of values. Only in this way, when the valuing self is engaged and expressed in its entirety, can a person's decision be actually self-determined instead of being a decision which is not determined by others.[29]

Thus, in Gadow's view, advocacy involves "nurse-patient interactions that enhance the patient's autonomy."[31] In some instances, this may mean that the nurse must respect a patient's truly autonomous choice not to know particular information. Gadow contrasts this view of advocacy with both paternalism, in which decisions are made by the nurse without ascertaining or respecting the patient's wishes, and consumerism, in which the patient is supplied with the facts and then left unassisted to reach a decision.[31]

It could easily be argued that patients with cancer are in particular need of the type of advocacy that enhances autonomy. Not only is their autonomy diminished by disease, treatment, and, all too frequently, the health care system, but they are also confronted with many difficult choices.

Clinical observation suggests that cancer care nurses are very much aware of the vulnerability of the patients they care for. Accordingly, they inform patients about decisions that they need to make and assist them in their understanding of treatment options. To the extent that they also assist patients to identify and clarify their beliefs, values, and goals in relation to the available options, they would, in Gadow's view of advocacy,[31] be truly involved in a patient-nurse relationship that enhances patient autonomy.

Cancer care nurses are also concerned about those patients who are unable to communicate their values. (Gadow uses the term silent patients "because all that can be known with certainty about them is that communication—not necessarily competence—is lacking."[32]) Gadow notes that although the values of some silent patients can be known through advance directives or proxy instructions from someone who knows the patient's values well enough to decide as he or she would, access to the values of other silent patients has not seemed possible.[32] For these other silent patients, it is tempting for nurses to abandon the moral position of advocacy for self-determination and to adopt another moral approach, such as utilitarianism or beneficence (promoting the individual patient's best interest as defined by the professional).[32]

Gadow notes the moral chaos for the nurse that results from changing moral positions from patient to patient. She proposes that if the nurse considers himself or herself to be a full-fledged advocate for patient self-determination, the nurse must set aside the notion that the only access to patients' values is through standard communication and consider ways of illuminating the subjective world of silent patients.[32]

MAJOR BIOETHICAL ISSUES

Telling the Truth

Cancer care nurses' commitment to patient self-determination is implicit in a document entitled *Standards of Oncology Nursing Practice,* which was developed jointly by members of the American Nurses' Association (ANA) Council on Medical-Surgical Nursing Practice and the Oncology Nursing Society (ONS).[33] Of particular interest is the section on planning care, in which the outcome criteria for Information reads as follows:

> The client—1) Describes the state of the disease and therapy at a level consistent with his or her educational and emotional status. 2) Participates in the decision-making process pertaining to the plan of care and life activities. 3) Identifies appropriate community and personal resources that provide information and services. 4) Describes appropriate actions for highly predictable problems, oncological emergencies, and major side effect of the disease or therapy.[33]

This content, as well as some content in other sections, suggests that two major assumptions underlie this document: individuals generally desire to exercise their moral right to obtain information; and cancer care nurses should have the competence, collaboration with colleagues, and rapport with patients necessary to fulfill their moral obligation (duty, responsibility) to provide the information or to see that it is provided.

The implementation of the ANA/ONS standards in relation to information giving remains a challenge. Two central questions emerge: (1) Exactly what information should individuals with a diagnosis of cancer be given concerning such matters as the seriousness of their illness or the specifics of various treatment options? (2) Should the nurse be the one to tell the patient?

Traditional and recent views of truth telling

The issue of truth telling historically has received little attention in the medical profession's codes and oaths.[34] This avoidance of the issue of veracity, which Beauchamp and Childress[35] describe as including the obligations to disclose information, not to lie, and not to deceive, seems to have been related to the desire to be free to choose, in each particular situation, the types of information that would result in the greatest good for the particular person and prevent harm, including suffering, fear, and anxiety. Veatch[36] refers to this approach to moral reasoning as individualistic, situational, and a special sort of utilitarianism. From this position, each individual situation is viewed as unique, the greatest good is considered only in relation to potential benefit or harm, with a special emphasis on eliminating harm. Because truthful information was often viewed as harmful (as an example, the effect of telling the patient of a terminal diagnosis), one can see why concealment, evasion, and withholding of information were not prohibited and, in fact, were often justified.

In recent years, professional views regarding truth-telling have undergone a gradual shift.[36] In a 1953 study about disclosure of a cancer diagnosis, Fitts and Ravdin[37] found that 3% of physicians who responded always told their patients and 28% usually did, but 57% usually did not tell and 12% never told. By the early 1970s, studies about physicians' stated policies of disclosure revealed the following information: 25% always told their patients of any diagnosis of a malignancy and only 9% never told[38]; 13% always and 80% usually told the patient with a critical illness the nature of his disease[39]; and 53% always or frequently told terminal patients of their prognosis.[40] However, by 1979, Novack and colleagues,[41] who asked questions almost identical to those asked by Oken in 1961,[42] found that 98% of physicians reported that their usual policy was to tell patients their cancer diagnosis; in contrast, Oken[42] had found that only 12% of physicians usually told their patients.

The reason for this shift in physicians' stated policies of disclosure is not entirely clear. (The issue of actual practices of disclosure will be considered in the section on the Realities of Daily Practice.) Gadow[43] notes that professionals' empirical beliefs regarding truth telling have changed; in the past, professionals emphasized the potential dangers of truth telling, whereas now, other beliefs regarding the potential therapeutic value of truth telling and the potential negative consequences of not telling the truth seem to prevail. Thus, in the weighing of benefit versus harm, it becomes clear why it is more likely that the contemporary professional will decide to tell the truth in the majority of cases. However, such an approach to decision making is paternalistic; that is, the criterion of benefit versus harm is used and the professional decides. In essence, the professional is deciding whether and how much truth will benefit the patient. And, as Gadow notes: "Candor is no less paternalistic a response than deception."[43]

Novack and colleagues[41] offer several other possible reasons for the shift in disclosure practices. One reason is the availability of more treatment options for cancer, including research therapies. Such availability of options clearly has influenced the information given to individuals with cancer, because professionals are now required to disclose information necessary for consent to, or refusal of, further medical treatment. This necessary information includes two major types: information about diagnosis and prognosis and information about diagnostic and therapeutic procedures and alternatives, including their risks and benefits.[44]

Disclosure of information

In general, there are two major contexts in which the disclosure question arises: that in which consent to, or refusal of, treatment is not at issue and that involving consent to, or refusal of, standard or research therapies or procedures.

For patients with a diagnosis of terminal cancer, when no cancer treatment options are available, there is an ethical obligation of veracity that requires disclosure of information regarding diagnosis and prognosis and any other information that affects the patient's understanding and decision making. However, it is important to note that, first, there is no legal obligation of veracity in these situations that do not involve consent; that is, the law requires only disclosure of information about procedures to which patients consent.[35] Second, some argue that limited disclosure and deception can sometimes be justified even though violations of the rules of veracity are viewed as prima facie wrong.

Bok[34] states that the three major arguments for not being truthful with patients are (1) that truthfulness is impossible, (2) that patients do not want bad news, and (3) that truthful information harms them. After careful analysis of each argument, Bok concludes that the three arguments that defend lies to patients do not serve as a counterweight to the right to be informed.

Beauchamp and Childress,[35] in an analysis of the same three arguments, came to a similar conclusion. They point out that some health professionals justify not telling the truth on the basis of their assessment that some patients, particularly the very sick and dying, indicate by various signals that they do not want to know the truth about their condition, despite the conclusions of opinion surveys that they do want to know.[35] Beauchamp and Childress[35] caution that such claims set dangerous precedents for paternalistic actions under the guise of respect for autonomy. They and other authors[44,45] suggest that the best policy is to ask the patient at various points during the illness about the extent to which he or she wants information or autonomy in decision making.

When standard or experimental treatment or procedures are proposed for patients with cancer, professionals have both an ethical and a legal obligation to disclose information necessary for consent or refusal. This information is of two major types: information about diagnosis and prognosis and information about diagnostic and therapeutic procedures and alternatives, including their risks and benefits.[44]

For situations involving research treatments or procedures, the US Department of Health and Human Services (DHHS)[46] presents the kind of information that must be included to constitute "informed consent." These basic elements of informed consent are listed below:

1. A statement that the study involves research, an explanation of the purposes of the research and of the expected duration of the subject's participation, a description of the procedures to be followed, and identification of any procedures that are experimental
2. A description of any reasonably forseeable risks or discomforts to the subject
3. A description of any benefit to the subject or to others that may reasonably be expected from the research
4. A disclosure of appropriate alternative procedures or courses of treatment, if any, that might be advantageous to the subject
5. A statement describing the extent, if any, to which confidentiality of records identifying the subject will be maintained
6. For research involving more than minimal risk, an explanation as to whether any compensation and medical treatments are available if injury occurs and, if so, what they consist of or where further information may be obtained
7. An explanation of who to contact for answers to pertinent questions about the research and about the research subject's rights, and who to contact in the event of research-related injury to the subject
8. A statement that participation is voluntary, refusal to participate will involve no penalty or loss of benefits to which the subject is otherwise entitled, and the subject may discontinue participation at any time without penalty or loss of benefits to which the subject is otherwise entitled.

The following additional elements should be included when appropriate:

1. A statement that the particular treatment or procedure may involve risks to the subject (or to the embryo or fetus, if the subject is or may become pregnant) that currently are unforeseeable
2. Anticipated circumstances under which the subject's participation may be terminated by the investigator without regard to the subject's consent
3. Any additional costs to the subject that may result from participation in the research
4. The consequences of a subject's decision to withdraw from the research and the procedures for orderly termination of participation by the subject
5. A statement that significant new findings developed during the course of the research that may relate to the subject's willingness to continue participation will be provided to the subject
6. The approximate number of subjects involved in the study

Although some of the elements listed apply only to research consent, many are appropriate for consent to standard therapy. However, since these elements identify only the kind of information that must be disclosed, it is still necessary to make judgments about exactly what information to disclose to the patient in each of these categories. Clearly, some standard for making judgments is necessary. From court cases, two standards of disclosure have emerged: the professional practice standard and the reasonable person standard. In addition, some have proposed a third: the subjective standard.

In the professional practice standard, adequate disclosure is determined by inquiring into the customs of the other practitioners in the community.[35] Thus the customary practices of physicians establish the amount and kind of information that patients should be told. A major objection to this standard, therefore, is that it can affect the patient's right of autonomous choice[35] in that some patients may want more information than is uniformly disclosed.

In the reasonable person standard, the information that must be disclosed is that which a reasonable person, in the patient's position, would want to know to decide whether to undergo the treatment or procedure. From court cases, this has come to mean that physicians must include in their disclosure the diagnosis, the nature and purpose of the proposed treatment, the risks and consequences of the proposed treatment, the probability that the proposed treatment will be successful, feasible treatment alternatives, and the prognosis if the proposed treatment is not given.[47]

A major difficulty with this standard is that the informational needs of an "objective, reasonable person" may not be the same as the informational needs of an individual patient. Thus some have proposed a third standard: the subjective standard. According to this standard, professionals must disclose what a reasonable person would want to know, modified by what the practitioner knows or ought to know about the unique needs and desires of the patient.[48]

In addition to a consideration of disclosure standards that address adequacy of information, problems that involve the question of when less than complete disclosure is justified must also be considered.

Legally, exceptions to the disclosure necessary for consent have been allowed in emergency situations and in situations involving competency, waiver, and the like. Exceptions also have been permitted when, in the judgment of the physician, the information would potentially be harmful to an emotionally unstable individual.[35] This latter exception, termed the therapeutic privilege, is not only controversial but is also not uniformly defined across legal jurisdictions. After careful analysis, Beauchamp and Childress[35] conclude that there are difficult and rare nonresearch situations in which a physician's judgment of the patient's welfare takes precedence over the patient's right to information.

Other questions regarding less than complete disclosure have arisen in the context of randomized clinical trials. Included is the question of whether patients should be told about the fact that therapy will be selected by chance and not by clinical judgment. It has been concluded that, in general, there is no ethical justification for not providing complete disclosure in randomized clinical trials, including information about the method of assignment.[35]

In summary, although withholding of information may be justified in a few situations, in general, competent patients, unless they specifically ask not to be informed, should be given complete information. It appears that the subjective standard is most in concert with advocacy for patient autonomy.

Realities of daily practice

A great deal of intellectual and emotional turmoil is involved in deciding exactly what information to give to patients with a diagnosis of cancer. Despite the fact that physician self-reports indicate that they usually favor disclosure, the majority of physicians, according to the study by Novack et al,[41] also report making exceptions to their usual policy of disclosing information, which are manifested in the timing, pattern, and completeness of disclosures. Blumenfield and colleagues[49] found that, although 90% of medical residents held that patients have a right to be told, only 47% thought that the patient should be informed as soon as possible. Other researchers have found evidence that physicians are distinguishing between telling the truth and telling the "complete truth" and between the right to know for patients who ask and for those who do not ask.[50]

Clinical observations seem to agree with these findings. For example, information about the extent of the disease may be withheld; some medically acceptable alternative treatments or the availability of clinical trials may not be discussed; and information about a plan to reduce drug doses to decrease toxic effects and about the disease implications of such a plan may be withheld. Thus, despite a tendency toward more full disclosure, the information necessary for patients to reach a truly autonomous choice may not, in some instances, be provided.

The following case study is an example of the complexity of the current intellectual and emotional pressures. It combines the issues of providing adequate disclosure about the nature, benefits, and risks of treatment and of the withholding of information about the extent of disease.

> A 72-year-old competent woman with a left mastectomy was hospitalized for symptoms resembling a stroke. She was aware that she had breast cancer and that she was receiving chemotherapy for metastatic disease. During this hospital admission, she was informed by her physician that she had a brain lesion that was a metastasis from the breast cancer. After receiving information about the nature, benefits, and risks of the proposed treatment and the effects of no treatment, she consented to treatment. The physician and family decided, however, to withhold information that she had multiple brain lesions. This decision was based on the fact that her brother had died of a primary brain tumor, and it was predicted that disclosure of information about the multiple lesions would be too upsetting for her. The woman did not request any further information about the brain metastasis. However, she did ask the nurse, one day, whether her liver scan was positive or negative. At that point, the physician entered the room and asked the nurse to step outside. He informed her that he,

with the concurrence of the family, had decided not to tell the woman that her liver scan was positive. They believed that if the woman knew about the liver involvement, she would not only recognize that her time was limited and consequently become very depressed but also refuse current treatment for her brain metastasis as well as any future cancer therapy.

This situation raises at least two major concerns. First, should family members be given information about a competent patient without the competent patient's consent? (This question will be considered in the section on Confidentiality.) Second, does the nurse have any responsibility in this situation of limited disclosure and apparent invalid consent? (The patient's consent to the current therapy for brain metastasis and to any future cancer therapy is not valid because the patient was not fully informed about the extent of disease and thus about the degree of potential benefit.)

The almost total focus in the literature on the physician's role and responsibility in informed consent suggests that it is totally the prerogative of the physician to decide whether information should be given to a particular patient and to disclose such information. Furthermore, feedback to nurses in many instances in daily practice seems to support this traditional position. However, careful reflection leads to the suggestion that nurses do have a moral responsibility in matters of disclosure.

Role of the nurse

In a consideration of the role of the nurse in disclosure of information, the key issue seems to be as follows: Is the question of whether information should be given to a particular patient with a diagnosis of cancer essentially a medical-scientific one or a moral one? Yarling,[51] in his discussion about whether persons with terminal cancer should be informed about their condition, clearly argues that such questions are essentially moral ones. He notes that although telling the patient requires medical-scientific knowledge, the decision to inform is a moral decision because it recognizes the patient's moral right to such information. Accordingly, Yarling[51] concludes that no one professional group has a special position in making judgments about whether to inform persons with terminal cancer of their condition. Medical expertise cannot be generalized to other areas; therefore nurses and physicians stand as moral equals.

It follows, therefore, that questions regarding disclosure of information in the context of consent to medical treatment or procedures are also essentially moral ones that require morally responsible judgments on the part of nurses as well as physicians. In fact, Pellegrino[52] argues that, although physicians are legally responsible for obtaining a valid consent, all team members are morally responsible for the quality of the consent. Clearly, disclosure of information, an element of informed consent, is an important factor influencing the quality of the consent.

Given that nurses have moral responsibility in disclosure matters and that physicians and nurses may disagree as to the kind and amount of information to provide, it is important that nurses be prepared to articulate their ethical position clearly. Ordinarily, these disagreements involve a physician's decision to limit disclosure rather than to provide complete and full information. The physician may justify, on the basis of acting in the patient's best interests, plans to withhold such information as the extent of disease, a terminal diagnosis, a medically acceptable alternative treatment, or the amount of expected benefit from treatment. Furthermore, the physician may "order" the nurse to avoid disclosing such information. If, however, the nurse, after careful thought, thinks that plans to interfere with the person's right to self-determination are not justified, what course of action should the nurse take?

Initially, the nurse makes an effort to engage the physician in a thoughtful and respectful dialogue. Concurrently, the nurse could also, if the patient wishes, assist the patient to identify the information that he or she might want to know to reach a decision about treatment or care. Through such efforts, the disagreement might be resolved. For example, the nurse might be persuaded by either the physician's arguments or the patient's explicit requests not to be told certain information to change her or his position, or the physician might be persuaded by either the nurse's arguments or the patient's specific requests for information to change her or his position, or the physician and nurse might agree to a mutually acceptable compromise position, such as a plan to assist the patient to ask questions regarding diagnosis, care, and treatment and to provide the information (which was previously to be withheld) within the context of these specific questions.

If, however, the disagreement is not resolved, the nurse will consider the following question: Does the nurse's moral obligation regarding disclosure extend to informing the patient about such matters as diagnosis and medical treatment? There are two distinct contexts in which this question can be asked: (1) the patient is not asking the nurse for information or has directly and specifically requested not to be told, and (2) the patient directly and clearly asks the nurse for information.

In the first context, which through therapeutic interaction is always subject to change, the patient is not exercising his or her moral right to information, and therefore the corresponding moral responsibility for the nurse to disclose the information does not exist.[51] The patient does not have a moral obligation to know. However, it is important to note that if procedures or treatments are being proposed, any consent would be without legal effect.

The second context, however, is more common. Yarling[51] argues as follows regarding disclosure of a terminal diagnosis: Given that the nurse has the medical knowledge and psychosocial skills necessary to make a competent disclosure, collaborates and communicates with the physician before responding to facilitate quality care, and has the requisite rapport with the patient, as evidenced by the patient's asking the nurse, the nurse can be seen as having the moral obligation to disclose the information. The same argument could be applied to situations involving procedures and treatments.

Legally, the situation of the nurse who discloses information that the physician has withheld and perhaps has "ordered" the nurse not to disclose is ambiguous. Would the nurse be seen as interfering with the patient-physician relationship? There seems to be room for precedent-setting action by nurses. Besch[53] takes the following position:

> If one profession has not adequately met the patient's needs or has neglected to tell the patient facts he might consider relevant in making a decision, it is the responsibility of another profession to meet these needs. One does not need permission to foster patient autonomy. The only permission necessary is the patient's. If there is some question that a doctor-patient relationship has been interfered with, it seems reasonable that the patient is capable of deciding this for himself.

This position seems to suggest that prior communication with the physician about plans for disclosure is not necessary. However, communicating with the physician differs from requesting the physician's permission, and communication with the physician before responding to the patient is desirable because it provides the possibility of facilitating quality care. Furthermore, such communication offers the opportunity for further ethical deliberation, which could help to prevent such situations from arising in the future.

Informed Consent

A review of the history of informed consent in the twentieth century reveals that it emerged from two different ethical concerns.[54] In the early years, the primary concern was the protection of the patient from harm and the promotion of the patient's welfare, which, in the research situation meant reduction of risk and avoidance of unfairness and exploitation. During the last two decades, the protection of autonomy has emerged as the primary concern and, indeed, the primary justification for the requirements of informed consent. Thus the primary goal of informed consent in medical care and in research is now considered to be that of enabling individuals to make autonomous decisions about whether to authorize medical and research interventions.[35] This more recent ethical perspective is consistent with twentieth-century American case law, which typically appeals to the right of self-determination as the justifying principle for the requirement of informed consent.[54]

Not surprisingly, the focus of the professional's obligation in informed consent has been influenced by this more recent ethical perspective and case law. In the past, the emphasis was on disclosure of information; now, the focus increasingly is on the *quality* of a patient's or subject's understanding and consent.[35] This shift in emphasis suggests that informed consent increasingly is being viewed as an active ongoing process rather than an isolated event.

The standard elements of informed consent, which can be viewed as imposing conditions for valid consent, have been listed as follows by Beauchamp and Childress[35]: I. Threshold Element: Competence; II. Information Elements: Disclosure of information, Understanding of information; III. Consent Elements: Voluntariness, Authorization. The following is a discussion, based on the work of Beauchamp and Childress,[35] of each of these conditions.

Competence

To determine whether one ought to solicit a decision from a particular patient, one must determine whether the individual is capable of adequate decision making. Incompetent patients would be unable to give a valid consent or valid refusal of consent to medical procedures. In the following considerations, the term "competence" will not be used in the legal sense but rather will refer to decision-making capacity.

Unfortunately, there is no established standard of competence. Thus determining whether a person is capable of adequate decision making requires judgments about (1) what capacities are needed (capacities range from ability to evidence a choice to ability to reach a reasoned decision), (2) the threshold required for each of the selected capacities, and (3) how these thresholds will be determined.[35]

Decisions by professionals will vary in relation to how the professional balances concerns about benefit and harm with concerns about autonomy; that is, if the professional's primary concern is protection of autonomy, then a less stringent level of capacity and testing will be decided on, but if the primary concern is that patients receive the best medical care, then a more stringent level of capacity and testing will be required.[35] (The reader is referred to Drane's model[55] of competency as an instructive example of how concerns about benefit and harm might be balanced with the importance of autonomy.

Another instructive example of the process of determining competence is offered by Brody,[56] who suggests that there are five capacities that constitute the patient's competency to participate in health care decision making: (1) the ability to receive information, (2) the capacity to remember the information received, (3) the ability to make a decision and give a reason for it, (4) the ability to use the relevant information in making the decision, and (5) the ability to assess the relevant information appropriately.

Brody[56] notes, in his discussion, that it is relatively easy to test, through mental-status examinations, the first two components—that is, to test whether a patient can receive information and the status of the patient's short-term memory—whereas the latter three components are more difficult to define and assess. For example, is the patient not coming to a decision because he is being careful or because, continually vacillating, he cannot make a decision? Is the patient not using the relevant information because he cannot understand it or is denying it or because he finds the information not relevant from the perspective of his values? Does the patient come to a decision that differs from the professional's because the patient is more or less optimistic than the professional or because he truly cannot appropriately estimate outcomes?

The process of determining competence is complex, and the judgments involved are often difficult. However, the importance to patients of a careful evaluation is enormous in that it protects competent patients from being declared incompetent simply because they refuse treatment that professionals judge to be essential to health and protects incompetent patients from being considered competent simply because they agree with the professionals' treatment plan.

Finally, even if a patient is determined, by careful evaluation, to have adequate decision-making capacity, professionals must take the law into account. In general, persons less than 18 years of age are not seen as legally competent to consent, although exceptions may apply, depending on the nature of the decision. However, whether young persons have legal authority to consent should not influence their involvement in the decision-making process. Their role in this process should be consistent with their decisional capacity.

Disclosure of information

The reader is referred to the previous discussion in the section on Telling the Truth.

Understanding of information

Studies suggest that attaining the comprehension necessary for valid consent may be difficult. On the day after signing consent forms for cancer treatment, only 60% of the 200 patients studied by Cassileth et al[57] understood the purpose and nature of the treatment, and only 55% were able to identify one major risk. Similarly, Muss et al[58] found that only 29% of the patients they studied could recognize the purpose of their treatment even though they had signed the consent form. Parenthetically, even if patients in these studies were able to recall the material, this would not necessarily be evidence of comprehension and certainly would not indicate whether patients believed what was disclosed.

Many of the environmental, patient, and communication barriers to achieving comprehension are well known. Thus the focus here will be on those that are less frequently discussed: the framing of information about risk and acceptance of information.

A recent study by McNeil and colleagues[59] reveals that presenting risk information as a gain or a loss influences choices. Three groups of people—outpatients with chronic medical problems, radiologists, and graduate students in business—were asked to make a hypothetical choice between two alternatives for lung cancer: radiation therapy and surgery. In all three groups, preferences were affected by how the information was framed. When the information about surgery was framed in terms of probability of dying, 42% preferred radiation. However, when the information about surgery was framed in terms of probability of survival, only 25% chose radiation over surgery.[59] The implication of this important study is clear: patient comprehension is affected by how risk information is framed.

Distinguishing between patient comprehension of information and patient acceptance of information is important. Some patients may understand the information disclosed and yet may not believe it. For example, a patient may be given all appropriate information about the diagnosis and the proposed radiation therapy treatment and may demonstrate an understanding of the material, and yet he may refuse treatment because he does not believe that he has cancer. As another example, a patient may demonstrate full understanding about a phase 1 clinical trial, but his agreement to participate is based on the false belief that he will be cured; that is, he does not believe the information about the purpose of the study.

Some might argue that false beliefs are evidence of lack of understanding and that it is not possible to judge a patient as comprehending if he evidences false beliefs. There seems to be a difference, however, between objective understanding of disclosed information and subjective integration of that information. If so, then it is possible to judge a patient who has false beliefs as having comprehension of the disclosed information. Interventions to assist these individuals include more than providing information or simply correcting a false belief that is based on misinformation. Thus the reason for suggesting that comprehension and acceptance not be conflated becomes clearer.

Voluntariness

The key question in determining whether the patient is free to act is as follows: Is the patient free from controlling influences? In general, influences can be divided into three major categories: coercion, manipulation, and persuasion.[35]

Beauchamp and Childress[35] view coercion as the intentional use of "a credible and severe threat of harm or force to control another." An example of coercion is a threat by a professional to abandon a patient unless the patient complies with treatment. In contrast, persuasion occurs when a person is convinced by logical reasoning to believe in something. Manipulation consists of getting people to do what the manipulator wants by means other than coercion or persuasion, such as lying, withholding of information, or distortion of the facts.

Influences that are coercive or manipulative are controlling influences; influences that are persuasive are not controlling in that they appeal to reason. However, professionals must be aware that some attempts to persuade may bypass reasoning or irrationally influence the patient and thus become controlling; for example, distressing information may overwhelm a patient with fear and panic and thus bypass reasoning; patients who are weak and dependent may not be able to resist influences that they ordinarily would and thus even attempts at rational persuasion may irrationally influence them.[35]

Authorization

Simply electing a medical intervention is not sufficient. The patient must give approval or consent.

Summary

For the consent of a patient or subject to be considered valid, the consent must be competent (legally), voluntary, informed, and comprehending. *Since all members of the health care team are morally responsible for the quality of the consent,*[52] *nurses should be prepared to participate in disclosure of information, evaluation of decision-making capacity, facilitation of understanding, and mitigation of patients' vulnerabilities. In addition, they should ensure that consent has actually been given before proceeding with treatment.*

Research Involving Human Subjects

Cancer care nurses continually are involved in research involving human subjects. This involvement may be as investigator, member of a research team or institutional review board, clinician, or user of results. Therefore an understanding of the ethical considerations of the conduct of clinical research is essential.

Six general ethical norms emerge from the various codes and regulations on research involving human subjects.[60] There should be (1) good research design, (2) competent investigators, (3) a favorable balance of harm and benefit, (4) informed consent, (5) equitable selection of subjects, and (6) compensation for research-related injury.

The reader is referred to the American Nurses' Association's *Human Rights Guidelines for Nurses in Clinical and Other Research.*[61] The following discussion will address some of the ethical concerns in clinical research from two broad perspectives: the design of the research and the involvement of human subjects.

Research design

Good research design is one of the conditions necessary for justifying research on human subjects. Evidence of this requirement can be found in the Nuremberg Code[62] and the Declaration of Helsinki[63]:

> The experiment should be so designed and based on the results of animal experimentation and a knowledge of the natural history of the disease or other problems under study that the anticipated results will justify the performance of the experiment. [Nuremberg Code 3]
>
> Biomedical research involving human subjects must conform to generally accepted scientific principles and should be based on adequately performed laboratory and animal experimentation and on a thorough knowledge of the scientific literature. [Helsinki 1.1]

In addition, the US Department of Health and Human Services (DHHS) regulations[46] (Section 26.111a) charge the institutional review board (IRB) to make a determination of the "importance of the knowledge that may reasonably be expected to result." Levine[60] suggests that this statement may be construed as a charge to the IRB to make determinations as to the adequacy of research design.

Generally, a review of research design involves attention to scientific validity, benefit-risk ratio for the human subject, investigator bias, and methods of analysis. Consider the situation of the controlled clinical trial with a randomization procedure. Such a design could certainly minimize investigator bias, but the benefit-risk ratio for the human subjects also must be explored. Rutstein's commentary[64] on a proposal to perform internal mammary artery operations for angina pectoris (which uncontrolled evidence had suggested might be helpful) on one group of patients and sham operations on the control group is instructive for two reasons: It demonstrates the ethical importance of benefit-risk ratio considerations, and it serves to highlight the tremendous need for stronger research guidelines. Rutstein[64] states:

> Although scientifically sound, I do not believe that it is ethical to perform sham operations on human subjects because of the operative risk and the lack of potential benefit to the patient. Instead, controlled studies could have been performed with randomly allocated control patients being given the best medical treatment of the time together with a period of bed rest similar to that of the surgical convalescent.

Current DHHS regulations clearly mandate a favorable balance between the projected benefits and the projected harms[46]: "Risks to the subjects (must be) reasonable in relation to anticipated benefits, if any, to subjects, and the importance of the knowledge that may reasonably be expected to result" (DHHS, Section 46.111a).

Identifying a design that is both scientifically valid and meets the benefit-risk requirements calls for careful deliberation. Sutnick and colleagues[65] demonstrate such deliberations in their discussion regarding studies to test the effectiveness of screening methods. First, a controlled clinical trial could be designed in which an identified population at high risk for cancer could be randomly divided into two subgroups, one receiving the screening techniques and the other serving as the control subjects; no change in care would be offered to the control group. Sutnick and colleagues[65] point out that such a design raises serious ethical questions. For example, the control group, known to be at high risk for cancer, will most likely not receive any benefits and might indeed be harmed. This potential harm could arise from the possibility that the control group "for whom more extensive screening procedures are not recommended will have the false security of feeling that they are not required."[65]

The authors[65] therefore consider the possibility of telling the control group about their increased risk and advising them to have periodic examinations. They decide, however, that such an action would probably minimize the difference between the subgroups and render the information obtained from the study less conclusive. Finally, they conclude that an alternative design is needed. They suggest an adaptive design in which the study group is selected from a large population that is already under medical surveillance for other reasons: "In this way, a representative sample could be selected for the institution of screening procedures and appropriate follow-up, while prospective or even retrospective examination of the records of the remainder of the population, or of a similarly selected or evenly matched sample population, could serve as the control observations."[65]

Decisions about benefits and risks are not limited, however, to the preimplementation period:

> During the course of the experiment the scientist in charge must be prepared to terminate the experiment at any stage, if he has probable cause to believe . . . that a continuation . . . is likely to result in injury, disability or death to the experimental subject. [Nuremberg Code 10[62]]
>
> The investigator . . . should discontinue the research if in his/her . . . judgment it may, if continued, be harmful to the individual. [Declaration of Helsinki 111.3[63]]
>
> Where appropriate, the research plan makes adequate provision for monitoring the data collected to insure safety of the subjects. [DHHS, Section 46.111a[46]]
>
> An IRB shall have authority to suspend or terminate approval of research . . . that has been associated with unexpected serious harm to subjects. [DHHS, Section 46.113[46]]

Clearly, to make such decisions in situations involving controlled clinical trials with randomization procedures, the method of data analysis must be valid.

Research subjects

Usually, concerns regarding the ethical involvement of human subjects focus on such considerations as whether there is good and ethical research design, including a favorable balancing of harms and benefits along with measures to maximize benefits and reduce harms; adequate provisions for the protection of privacy and maintenance of confidentiality of data; and valid consent. Although these considerations are both essential and important, explicit attention must also be given to the equitable distribution of the harms and benefits of research. This concern raises questions regarding subject selection. The following discussion highlights considerations and recommendations on subject selection by Levine.[60]

Selection of subjects based exclusively on informed consent may result in inequitable distribution of the harms and benefits of research. Although truly autonomous persons are capable of adequately negotiating informed consent, those with diminished autonomy may not be able to look after their own best interests; that is, they may accept an unfair share of the burdens of research participation. Levine[60] defines those persons who are incapable of protecting their own interests as vulnerable and includes uneducated subjects; seriously ill persons who are desperate and willing to take any risk for a possibility of relief; those with dependent relationships who fear that they will place their relationships in jeopardy if they refuse to cooperate with the investigator; members of minority groups who are impoverished, seriously ill, or dependent; and elderly persons with reduced capacities.

Involving vulnerable persons in research is not forbidden by codes and regulations, but it must be justified. Justification becomes more difficult, however, as the degree of risk and the degree of vulnerability increase. Therefore, efforts must be made to reduce the ethical problems associated with selecting vulnerable persons as research subjects. In general, these efforts are directed toward improving the quality of the consent. This may include clarifying the fact that individuals have a right to refuse to participate in research or to withdraw at any time without prejudicing their care or relationships. If, however, patients' capacity for consent cannot adequately be increased, then they should be excluded from the study and less vulnerable persons from the populations being studied should be selected.[60]

In the field of cancer medical research, one area of intense concern regarding patient vulnerability is the situation of phase 1 clinical studies.[66] In these studies, patients with advanced cancer whose disease is not amenable to known effective treatment constitute the population from which subjects are selected. In addition, these studies ordinarily offer only a remote possibility of any medical therapeutic benefit for enrolled patients[67]; the potential benefit is for future patients with cancer.

Some might suggest that members of this population be considered as a vulnerable group. This does not seem appropriate, because they are not homogeneous in regard to such factors as degree of desperateness or willingness to take any risk, perceptions of imminent death, and concerns about prejudicing their relationships with professionals. To consider these persons as vulnerable would suggest, among other things, that all patients with advanced cancer whose disease is not amenable to therapy are incapable of looking after their own best interests.

However, the capacity of some does not mean that many other individuals within this population are not vulnerable. Thus it is appropriate to consider each patient as potentially vulnerable and to take measures to improve the quality of consent in the event that it is needed. Such measures may include defining more clearly the fact that the expected benefits are for future patients; assuring patients that their relationships and care will not be prejudiced if they refuse to participate; and outlining the kind of care (eg, support, symptom control, and monitoring for unexpected events) that can be provided if the patient does not participate. In some instances, it may be necessary for the investigator to decide or for other health professionals to recommend that a patient not be selected for study.

Confidentiality

Basic to an understanding of the issues of confidentiality is an appreciation of the fact that privacy and confidentiality are two distinct concepts even though the concepts partially overlap and the terms are often used interchangeably. Privacy can be defined as "the freedom of the individual to pick and choose for himself the time and circumstances under which, and most importantly, the extent to which, his attitudes, beliefs, behavior and opinions are to be shared with or withheld from others."[68] Respect for privacy requires that professionals not invade patients' privacy (through such activities as taking a personal history; touching, listening to, or observing the body; or conducting tests) without their permission.

In the situation of a patient's voluntary admission to a

hospital, there is both explicit and implicit consent to limited losses of privacy. However, the patient's voluntary admission to the hospital does not grant unlimited access.[35] The right to restrict some access is reflected in the American Hospital Association's *Statement on a Patient's Bill of Rights*,[69] which states that persons not directly involved in a patient's care must have the permission of the patient to be present.

In contemporary society, the most poignant example of a privacy issue is the screening and testing of individuals to determine whether they have antibodies to the human immunodeficiency virus (HIV). Some proposed policies would infringe on privacy in that they would not involve permission or consent; that is, screening or testing would be mandatory. Whether such infringements are justified and, if so, under what conditions remain matters of continuing debate. The point is that this particular aspect of the acquired immunodeficiency syndrome (AIDS) debate is about whether intrusions into individuals' privacy are justified, not about what to do with the private information (that persons have detectable antibodies or AIDS) once it is generated; the question of what to do with, or how to manage, private information is a confidentiality issue.

In general, respect for confidentiality requires that private information that is shared by a patient, whether through words or an examination, not be disclosed to others without the patient's authorization. Although most professionals accept this ideal, there are informational needs in the contemporary health care setting that have altered the meaning of confidentiality.[35] The large and diversified health care team needs relevant information to provide care for the patient; therefore, in most cancer care settings today, information shared by the patient with one health professional is usually disclosed to other health professionals involved in the patient's care, except for information that is judged to be "confidential." In addition there are numerous other persons with legitimate needs and responsibilities to examine the patient's chart.

The difficulty is that many patients do not know about these practices. In addition, judgments about what information is too "confidential" to disclose, either verbally with other members of the health care team or in the chart, are made by the health professional. Patients should be informed about these contemporary practices so that they, not the health care professional, can decide what is too "confidential" to be disclosed.

Bok[70] points out, however, that there are justifiable limits to the obligation of confidentiality. Walters,[71] in an earlier work, identified three possible grounds for violating the principle of confidentiality. First, the principle may come into conflict with the rights of the patient himself. As an example, a temporarily but seriously depressed patient with cancer may tell the nurse "in confidence" that he plans to commit suicide. In such a life-threatening situation, the nurse's duty to act in the patient's best interest might require temporarily interfering with the patient's self-determination by disclosing, without the patient's consent but with the patient's knowledge, the information to a third party.

Second, the principle of confidentiality may be violated when it conflicts with the rights of an innocent third party.[71] As a contemporary example, a patient, on being told that HIV antibodies have been detected in his serum, not only refuses to tell his wife but insists that the health care professional maintain absolute confidentiality. If the professional is unable to persuade the patient either to disclose the information or to give permission for the disclosure, then a strong ethical argument can be made that the professional should disclose the portion of the information that is necessary to protect the wife from harm.[35] (The reader is referred to a report by the American Medical Association's Council on Ethical and Judicial Affairs[72] for the medical profession's position on and procedures for warning third parties.)

Finally, the principle of confidentiality may be violated when there exists a serious conflict between the principle and the rights or interests of society in general.[71] One type of situation involves persons with communicable diseases. For many years, it was agreed that the mandatory reporting of persons with communicable diseases by health care professionals to public health officials was justified; that is, the public health objectives underlying the reporting requirements were substantial enough to justify the violation of confidentiality. However, in the specific situation of a new disease, AIDS, new and complex questions have been raised. Currently the focus is not, for the most part, on mandatory reporting of AIDS. (All states require the reporting of AIDS, as defined by the Centers for Disease Control, to public health officials.[73]) Rather, the focus is on proposals that would require the mandatory reporting of HIV-positive test results with identifiers. Some would argue that the public health objectives are not substantial enough at this time to justify either a violation of confidentiality or the possibility of serious harm from wrongful and damaging public disclosure of the information.

With the three broad categories of justified exceptions to the obligation for confidentiality in mind, it seems that disclosures of information to family members without the competent patient's consent cannot, in general, be ethically justified. One approach to this not uncommon problem would be to assist patients to clarify and explicitly to communicate what information they want shared and with whom. In this way, disclosures to family members without patient consent would require strong explicit justification by any health team member proposing such action.

CONCLUSION

This chapter focuses on bioethical decision making in the context of cancer nursing practice. Special emphasis is placed on relationships in cancer care and the challenge of protecting and promoting patient self-determination. The issues of telling the truth, informed consent, research on human subjects, and confidentiality are used to illustrate ethical deliberation and explore advocacy nursing.

FUTURE TRENDS

To promote continued growth and development in ethical decision making, cancer nurses may wish to develop a forum for deliberation within their practice settings.[74] These discussions initially could be among nurse colleagues and then expand to include other health care professionals. The outcome of such discussions could be the prevention of some recurring ethical dilemmas; the clarification of professional responsibilities, particularly in relation to persons who have detectable HIV antibodies; the development of research studies; and the identification of areas for action on the public policy level.

One of the most urgent issues in the latter category is the "fair" allocation of limited health care resources; that is, who should receive what kind of care. Cancer nurses must become active in considering these and other questions involving distributive justice.

REFERENCES

1. Davis AJ, Aroskar MA: Ethical Dilemmas and Nursing Practice (ed 2). Norwalk, Conn, Appleton-Century-Crofts, 1983.
2. Gorovitz S: Bioethics and social responsibility, in Beauchamp TL, Walters L (eds): Contemporary Issues in Bioethics. Encino, Calif, Dickenson, 1978, pp 52-60.
3. Yarling RR, McElmurry BJ: The moral foundation of nursing. Adv Nurs Sci 8:63-73, 1986.
4. Bishop AH, Scudder JR: Nursing ethics in an age of controversy. Adv Nurs Sci 9:34-43, 1987.
5. Cooper MC: Covenantal relationships: grounding for the nursing ethic. Adv Nurs Sci 10:48-59, 1988.
6. Packard JS, Ferrara M: In search of the moral foundation of nursing. Adv Nurs Sci 10:60-71, 1988.
7. Yeo M: Integration of nursing theory and nursing ethics. Adv Nurs Sci 11:33-42, 1989.
8. Thompson JE, Thompson HO: Teaching ethics to nursing students. Nurs Outlook 37:84-88, 1989.
9. Veatch RM: Case Studies in Medical Ethics. Cambridge, Mass, Harvard University Press, 1977.
10. Beauchamp TI: Ethical theory, in Beauchamp TL, Walters L (eds): Contemporary Issues in Bioethics. Encino, Calif, Dickenson, 1978, pp 1-5.
11. Taylor P: Utilitarianism, in Beauchamp TL, Walters L (eds): Contemporary Issues in Bioethics. Encino, Calif, Dickenson, 1978, pp 12-22.
12. Campbell AV: Moral Dilemmas in Medicine. New York, Churchill Livingstone, 1975.
13. Veatch RM: Death, Dying, and the Biological Revolution: Our Last Quest for Responsibility (ed 1). New Haven, Conn, Yale University Press, 1976.
14. Childress J: Ethical issues in the experimentation with human subjects. Conn Med 43:26-31, 1979.
15. Pellegrino ED: Protection of patients' rights and the doctor-patient relationship. Prev Med 4:398-403, 1975.
16. Curtin LL: The nurse as advocate: A philosophical foundation for nursing. Adv Nurs Sci 3:1-10, 1979.
17. Bandman EL: The rights of nurses and patients: A case for advocacy, in Bandman EL, Bandman B (eds): Bioethics and Human Rights. Boston, Little, Brown, 1978, pp 332-338.
18. Gadow S: Humanistic issues at the interface of nursing and the community. Conn Med 41:357-361, 1977.
19. Donahue MP: The nurse: A patient advocate? Nurs Forum 17:143-151, 1978.
20. Kohnke M: The nurse as advocate. Am J Nurs 80:2038-2040, 1980.
21. Laszewski M: Patient advocacy in primary nursing. Nurs Adm Q 5:28-30, 1981.
22. Brower HT: Advocacy: what it is. J Gerontol Nurs 8:141-143, 1982.
23. Fay P: In support of patient advocacy as a nursing role. Nurs Outlook 26:252-353, 1978 (editorial).
24. Namerow MJ: Integrating advocacy into the gerontological nursing major. J Gerontol Nurs 8:149-151, 1982.
25. Ash CR: Are you an advocate? Cancer Nursing: An International Journal for Cancer Care 7:447, 1984 (editorial).
26. Winslow GR: From loyalty to advocacy: a new metaphor for nursing. Hastings Cent Rep 14:32-40, 1984.
27. Nelson ML: Advocacy in nursing. Nurs Outlook 36:136-141, 1988.
28. Gadow S: Advocacy nursing and new meanings of aging. Nurs Clin North Am 14:81-91, 1979.
29. Gadow S: Existential advocacy, in Spicker SF, Gadow S (eds): Nursing: Images and Ideals. New York, Springer, 1980, pp 79-101.
30. Gadow S: A model for ethical decision-making. Oncol Nurs Forum 7:44-47, 1980.
31. Gadow S: An ethical case for patient self-determination. Semin Oncol Nurs 5:99-101, 1989.
32. Gadow S: Clinical subjectivity: advocacy with silent patients. Nurs Clin North Am 24:535-541, 1989.
33. American Nurses' Association, Oncology Nursing Society: Standards of Oncology Nursing Practice. Kansas City, Mo, American Nurses' Association, 1987.
34. Bok S: Lying: Moral Choices in Public and Private Life. New York, Pantheon Books, 1978.
35. Beauchamp TL, Childress JF: Principles of Biomedical Ethics (ed 3). New York, Oxford University Press, 1989.
36. Veatch RM: Death, Dying, and the Biologic Revolution: Our Last Quest for Responsibility (ed 2). New Haven, Conn, Yale University Press, 1989.
37. Fitts WL Jr, Ravdin IS: What Philadelphia physicians tell patients. JAMA 153:901-904, 1953.
38. Friedman HJ: Physician management of dying patients. Psychiatry Med 1:295-305, 1970.
39. Mount BM, Jones A, Patterson A: Death and dying: Attitudes in a teaching hospital. Urology 4:741-747, 1974.
40. Travis TA, Noyes R Jr, Brightwell DR: The attitude of physicians toward prolonging life. Int J Psychiatry Med 5:17-26, 1974.
41. Novack DH, Plumer R, Smith RI, et al: Changes in physicians' attitudes toward telling the cancer patient. JAMA 241:897-900, 1979.
42. Oken D: What to tell cancer patients: A study of medical attitudes. JAMA 173:1120-1128, 1961.
43. Gadow S: Advocacy and paternalism in cancer nursing, in McCorkle R, Hongladarom G (eds): Issues and Topics in Cancer Nursing. Norwalk, Conn, Appleton-Century-Crofts, 1986, pp 19-28.
44. Schoene-Seifert B, Childress JF: How much should the cancer patient know and decide? CA 36:85-94, 1986.
45. Angell M: Respecting the autonomy of competent patients. N Engl J Med 310:1115-1116, 1984.
46. US Department of Health and Human Services: Final reg-

ulations amending basic HHS policy for the protection of human research subjects: final rules: 45 CFR 46. Federal Register: Rules and Regulations 46:8366-8392, 1981.
47. Rosoff AJ: Informed Consent. Rockville, Md, Aspen, 1981.
48. Veatch RM, Fry ST: Case Studies in Nursing Ethics. Philadelphia, JB Lippincott, 1987.
49. Blumenfield M, Levy N, Kaufman D: The wish to be informed of a fatal illness. Omega 9:323-326, 1978–1979.
50. Hatfield CB, Hatfield RE, Geggie PHS, et al: Attitudes about death, dying, and terminal care: differences among groups at a university teaching hospital. Omega 14:51-63, 1983–1984.
51. Yarling RR: Ethical analysis of a nursing problem: the scope of nursing practice in disclosing the truth to terminal patients—an inquiry directed to the National Joint Practice Commission of the AMA and the ANA. Part I and Part II. Supervisor Nurse 9:28-34, 40-50, 1978.
52. Pellegrino ED: The moral foundations for valid consent. Proceedings of the American Cancer Society Third National Conference on Human Values and Cancer. New York, American Cancer Society, Inc, 1981, pp 171-177.
53. Besch LB: Informed consent: a patient's right. Nurs Outlook 27:32-35, 1979.
54. Faden RR, Beauchamp TL (in collaboration with King NNP): A History and Theory of Informed Consent. New York, Oxford, 1986.
55. Drane JF: The many faces of competency. Hastings Cent Rep 15:17-21, 1985.
56. Brody B: Life and Death Decision Making. New York, Oxford, 1988.
57. Cassileth BR, Zupkis RV, Stuton-Smith K, et al: Informed consent—why are its goals imperfectly realized? N Engl J Med 302:896-900, 1980.
58. Muss HB, White DR, Michielutte R, et al: Written informed consent in patients with breast cancer. Cancer 43:1545-1550, 1979.
59. McNeil BJ, Pauker SG, Sox HC, et al: On the elicitation of preferences for alternative therapies. N Engl J Med 306:1259-1262, 1982.
60. Levine RJ: Ethics and Regulation of Clinical Research (ed 2). New Haven, Conn, Yale University Press, 1988.
61. American Nurses' Association: Human Rights Guidelines for Nurses in Clinical and Other Research. Kansas City, Mo, American Nurses' Association, 1985.
62. Nuremberg Code, 1964, in Reich WT (ed): Encyclopedia of Bioethics, vol 4. New York, The Free Press, 1978, pp 1764-1765.
63. World Medical Association Declaration of Helsinki as Revised by the 29th World Medical Assembly, October, 1975, in Beauchamp TL, Walters L (eds): Contemporary Issues in Bioethics. Encino, Calif, Dickenson, 1975, pp 405-407.
64. Rutstein D: The ethical design of human experiments, in Beauchamp TL, Walters L (eds): Contemporary Issues in Bioethics. Encino, Calif, Dickenson, 1975, pp 421-426.
65. Sutnick A, et al: Ethical issues in investigation of screening strategies. Med Pediatr Oncol 3:133-136, 1977.
66. Lipsett MB: On the nature and ethics of phase 1 clinical trials of cancer chemotherapies. JAMA 248:941-942, 1982.
67. Lipsett MB: Ethics of phase 1 clinical trials. JAMA 249:883, 1983.
68. Kelman HC: Privacy and research with human beings. J Soc Issues 33:169-195, 1977.
69. American Hospital Association. Statement on a patient's bill of rights. Hospitals 4:41, 1973.
70. Bok S: The limits of confidentiality. Hastings Cent Rep 13:24-31, 1983.
71. Walters L: Ethical aspects of medical confidentiality, in Beauchamp TL, Walters L (eds): Contemporary Issues in Bioethics. Encino, Calif, Dickenson, 1975, pp 169-175.
72. Council on Ethical and Judicial Affairs. Ethical issues involved in the growing AIDS crisis. JAMA 259:1360-1361, 1988.
73. Gostin LO: Public health strategies for confronting AIDS: legislative and regulatory policy in the United States. JAMA 261:1621-1630, 1989.
74. Donovan CT: Toward a nursing ethics program in an acute care setting. Top Clin Nurs 5:55-62, 1983.

Chapter 56

Unproven Methods of Cancer Treatment

Connie Henke Yarbro, RN, BSN

INTRODUCTION

Defined as "methods that have not been shown to be active in tumor animal models or in acceptable clinical trials and yet are promoted as effective methods for the cure, palliation, and control of cancer," unproven methods are a major concern for health care professionals in the United States.[1] Unproven, unorthodox, and alternative treatments have existed for decades and continue to be a problem today, with the public spending four billion dollars a year on unproven cancer cures.[2,3] Questionable nutritional supplements alone are a two-billion-dollar-a-year business in the United States.[4] According to Cassileth and colleagues,[5-8] more than half of all cancer patients eventually try an unproven method either in conjunction with conventional treatment or as a substitute for treatment.

In a discussion of unproven methods, it is important to remember that for thousands of years, individuals in need of medical care have turned to those who were offering what they felt or hoped would meet their needs. Only in relatively recent times has the scientific method, in conjunction with organized medicine and government, been able to provide a measure of confidence in a given treatment's safety and efficacy.

HISTORICAL PERSPECTIVES

Before the Food and Drug Act of 1906, thousands of unproven treatments were promoted to the American public. Often the treatments were not harmful in themselves, but as an anonymous physician of the era noted in a letter to the *National Quarterly Review,* "Quackery kills a larger number annually than the disease it pretends to cure."[9]

Advertisements frequently guaranteed the effectiveness of a particular treatment. For example, promotions for "Dr. Chamlee's Cancer Specific," which appeared in the 1930s, informed readers that "any lump in [a] woman's breast is cancer" and "any tumor, lump, or sore on the lip, face, or anywhere six months is, nearly always, cancer."[9] Dr. Chamlee's treatment involved "no knife or pain, no x-ray or other swindle." The promoter of this treatment was so confident that he required no payment until the person was cured. He further promised to pay $1000 to any individual he failed to cure of cancer. With sufficient information to evaluate these treatments, fewer qualified medical experts to consult with, and human nature being what it is, it is not difficult to understand how such a promoter could make a fortune.

Even well-intentioned and educated individuals were duped. In 1748 the Virginia General Assembly, whose members included George Washington and James Madison, appointed a committee to investigate the efficacy of Mary Johnson's recipe for curing cancer. The cure included sorrel, bark celandine, and springwater. Witnesses' statements that they had been cured of various cancers were read into the Assembly's record, and in good time the legislators voted that Mrs. Johnson's recipe was indeed effective in treating cancer and consequently awarded her 100 pounds for her achievement.[10]

The promotion of unproven methods was not significantly affected even by the passage of the Food and Drug Act in 1906. Janssen[11] reported that in 1910 a crucial test of the new law found the US Supreme Court ruling that the law involved only the truthful labeling of ingredients used in drugs, not the false therapeutic claims on the drug label. Justice Oliver Wendell Holmes, Jr, concluded that individuals could not be prosecuted for what he termed "mistaken praise" of their treatments even though the claims were false.

Noting the dangers of permitting unsafe and ineffective drugs on the market, President Taft exhorted the Congress, in 1911, to pass tougher legislation:

> There are none so credulous as sufferers from disease. The need is urgent for legislation which will prevent the raising of false hopes of speedy cures of serious ailment by misstatements of facts as to the worthless mixtures on which the sick will rely while their disease progresses unchecked.[12]

In 1912 Congress passed the Sherley Amendment, which stated that it was a crime to make false or fraudulent claims regarding the therapeutic efficacy of a drug. The problem encountered with this legislation was that it was necessary to prove that the promoter intended to defraud the public. Mistaken claims could still be made, and patients could continue to be defrauded. In 1938 Congress eliminated this difficulty by passing legislation that required scientific proof of safety before a drug could be marketed. This law was the direct result of a disaster in which over 200 individuals lost their lives. A drug promoter had marketed a sulfanilamide with a diluting agent consisting of automobile antifreeze.

In 1962 Congress clarified some of the language of the previous legislation and further added that drugs must demonstrate efficacy in addition to safety before they can be marketed. Thus a process was created by which a substance can become approved for prescription use. First, a sponsoring group submits data, generally first from animal studies that demonstrate some measure of safety and probable efficacy. The sponsor then files an Investigational New Drug (IND) application with the Food and Drug Administration (FDA). If approved, clinical testing with human volunteers is permitted. Following the completion of clinical testing, the company may make the drug available if it can be determined reliably that the drug is indeed safe and effective.

The Food and Drug Commissioner[13] noted that the Food and Drug Act of 1962 means that the "the absolute freedom to choose an ineffective drug was properly surrendered in exchange for the freedom from danger to each person's health and well-being from the sale and use of worthless drugs." This is, in fact, the same decision made by those in government who have decided over the years that only persons certified by experts may practice medicine and are qualified to help the patients who would choose to seek their assistance.[13] Although the Food and Drug Act of 1962 frequently has been challenged over the years by those who promote unproven methods, the act was upheld by a decision of the US Supreme Court in 1973.

MOTIVATIONS FOR THE USE OF UNPROVEN METHODS

People in the twentieth century seek unproven methods in conjunction with or in lieu of standard medical procedures for many of the same reasons their ancestors did. Following are some of the more common reasons:

- "I have nothing to lose."
- "If it won't hurt me, why not?"
- "I want to feel that I tried everything."
- "They wouldn't put that in the papers if it wasn't true."
- "The doctor told me there is nothing more that can be done."
- "I heard of a person who was terminal, took it, and was cured."

Cancer creates many fears, such as fear of death, an uncertain future, pain, mutilation, loss of family, dependency, alienation, and costly medical care. Given these fears, it is not difficult to understand that many individuals with cancer are in great need of hope and are likely to seek out those individuals who seem most capable of providing this desired commodity. Unfettered by standard methods, ethics, and regulations, a purveyor of unproven methods has a distinct advantage over individuals within the established medical system. The current norm is for a person to be informed of treatment alternatives, all of which necessarily have risks that are inextricably linked with a potentially positive outcome. Emotionally, an individual may regret having ever gone to the physician who diagnosed cancer. Cancer patients want a treatment without risks and pain and with a good probability of cure. Yet they are confused and frustrated by some reports claiming that cancer is a curable disease with a cure rate approaching 50% and others claiming that no major advances have been made in treatment of the major types of cancer.[7,8] Turning to some dietary or enzyme therapy that promises no side effects or uses "the body's natural defenses" may coincide with patients' fantasies about being cured. That is, by utilizing unconventional therapy, the patient hopes for an unconventional cure.[14]

The use of an unproven method may provide an individual with a greater sense of control. This desire for control may partially be a response to fear but may also be a reaction to the feeling of being merely a passive recipient of treatments designated by the health care team rather than being a partner in the fight against the disease. Better educated and highly motivated patients fighting their disease are more likely to turn to unproven methods because the promoters of such methods falsely promise that "you can control your disease."[5,15,16] The age-old cry of the quack, placing the blame of failure on the patient, remains: "It is the patient's fault if it fails. You came to us too late."[17] Inasmuch as the provider of unproven methods is often supplying an illegal or unapproved therapy requested by the patient with cancer, a bond may easily be formed between them. This relationship may assist the person with cancer in rebelling against his or her fate and the medical system that provided the fearful diagnosis of cancer. The promoter of unproven methods often appears to be an underdog battling the medical system to make some new risk-free treatment available to neglected people with cancer. Those individuals within the conventional medical system may be seen as profiting from the plight of the poor and sick. The purveyors of unproven methods frequently suggest that the government and organized medicine are in a conspiracy against curing cancer. It is easy for the cancer patient to identify with the isolation projected by the marketer of unproven methods. Patients with cancer frequently resent those who do not have it. It is perfectly acceptable for an individual to feel this way, but it is also important for the health care professional to ensure that this anger does not interfere with communication. The patient with cancer who is made to feel persecuted might seek out someone who "understands," even if—or especially if—the new care provider is also at odds with established medicine.

Other influences for using unproven methods can come from pressures exerted by family or friends.[18] The family often plays the most important role in providing emotional support. Family members, who have many of the same fears as the patient with cancer, are susceptible to the same influences. They often share responsibility for deciding the patient's treatment, and this responsibility itself can be overwhelming and frightening. "We want to feel that we tried everything" is commonly heard from concerned family members. The health care provider also may hear an unspoken wish to avoid guilt if the patient with cancer does not recover. Not being in a position to understand completely what treatments can and cannot do, the family may feel that the best course is to try everything with the hope that something will work. In turn, the patient with cancer may feel obligated to meet the family's expectation to submit to these treatments or may be afraid of alienating his or her support system at this crucial time by doing otherwise. In contrast, others might want to try everything. In such instances the family might feel pressured to unearth "cancer cures," and friends may bring in newspaper articles or stories that tell of someone who was cured by some method or another. Although the friend's intentions are admirable, such information might foster feelings of guilt in the patient with cancer or in the family members if these avenues are not explored.

Even with the best intentions of all parties concerned, the course of the disease can be torturous for everyone. How difficult this time will be greatly depends on the types of personalities and relationships that existed before the cancer was diagnosed, the quality of communication that takes place, the availability of accurate information on treatment options and outcomes, and the effects of disease and therapy.

UNPROVEN METHODS: 1940s TO 1970s

Unproven approaches to cancer treatment have existed for centuries, and a specific alternative seems to develop and thrive during each decade. Examples of unorthodox approaches, listed according to their eras of popularity, are identified in Table 56-1. We have gone from the nineteenth-century "holistic," or "natural," movement to the so-called-drug approach of the early and mid 1900s, and back to the holistic, natural, or diet-oriented regimens of today.[7] According to Cassileth et al,[5-8] among all unproven therapies today, the most commonly used are, in order of frequency, metabolic therapy, diet therapy, megavitamin therapy, mental imagery, faith or spiritual healing, and "immune" therapy. The following discussion will review the alternative approaches from the era of the 1940s through the 1980s.

Koch Antitoxin Therapy: 1940s to 1950s

First mentioned in 1919,[19] the Koch antitoxin therapy was a popular unproven cancer treatment during the 1940s and 1950s. The treatment consisted of extremely pure distilled water mixed with one part per trillion of a chemical called glyoxylide. Glyoxylide is merely glyoxylic acid with water removed. Glyoxylic acid is a normal body constituent, but it would take nearly a trillion of the 2 mL ampules that Koch distributed to equal the quantity the body produces normally in a single day.[13] Koch proposed that cancer was caused by a microorganism that was susceptible to the differential poison in his antitoxins. Associated therapies included enemas and a special diet. Over 3000 health practitioners in the United States employed this regimen, paying $25 per ampule for it and charging patients as much as $300 for a single injection.[11] The Koch Cancer Foundation promoted the treatment through lectures, pamphlets, and magazines. In 1942 the Food and Drug Administration held hearings across the United States in an effort to gather information regarding the promotion and use of the Koch antitoxins. In 1943, Dr. Koch was indicted. Although 43 expert witnesses testified that the Koch method was a worthless cancer therapy, the defense produced 104 witnesses who alleged that the treatment was useful in the management of some 69 diseases, including herpes zoster, appendicitis, allergies, and cancer. A mistrial was declared after the jury could not come to a unanimous decision.

TABLE 56-1 EXAMPLES OF MAJOR UNORTHODOX APPROACHES 1800–PRESENT

Era Popular In US	Unorthodox Approach
1800–1850	Thompsonianism Belief: All disease results from one general cause (cold), and can be cured by one general remedy (heat). Opposed "mineral" drugs and the "tyranny" of doctors. Remedy: Emetics and hot baths.
1850–1900	Homeopathy Belief: Like cures like ("Law of Similia"); disease results from suppressed itch ("psora"). Remedy: More than 3000 different drugs, each a highly distilled organic or inorganic substance.
1890–	Naturopathy Belief: Disease results not from external bacteria but from violation of natural laws of living; drugs are harmful; "natural" products and activities cure. Remedy: Diets, massages, colonic irrigation.
1890–	Early Osteopathy and Chiropractic Belief: Mechanistic view of the body; disease caused by dislocation of bones in spine. Rejected drugs and germ theory. Remedy: Spinal manipulation.
1900s	Tablet and Ointment Cancer Cures Bye, Buchanan, Chamlee, Curry, Leach (Cancerol), Mixer, Griffith (Radio-sulpho), Warner, Wells (Radol).
1920s	"Energy" Cancer Cures Abrams (Radio Wave cure), Brown (Radio Therapy), Kay (cosmic energy "vrilium"), Ghadiali (Spectro-Chrome Light Therapy); Cayce's psychic diagnoses and treatments
1940s	Koch's Glyoxylide
1950s	Hoxsey's Cancer Treatment
1960s	Ivy's Krebiozen
1970s	Laetrile
1980s	Metabolic Therapies Diet, High Colonics, Vitamins, and Minerals

Source: Reprinted with permission from Cassileth B: Unorthodox cancer medicine. Cancer Invest 4:591-598, 1988. By courtesy of Marcel Dekker, Inc.

In 1943 the Canadian Cancer Foundation issued a report on a clinical trial using the Koch method. None of the patients in the study benefited from the treatment.[20] In 1948 Koch closed his laboratory and moved to Brazil. Three years later the Federal Trade Commission issued a court order forbidding the promotion of Koch antitoxins because of their lack of therapeutic value. Although Koch's antitoxins are illegal in the United States, they can be obtained through the underground medical community or in Mexico.

Hoxsey Method: 1950s

Promoted since the early 1920s, the Hoxsey method aimed to restore the body to physiologic "normalcy."[21] Hoxsey maintained that cancer was a result of a chemical imbalance that caused the body's healthy cells to mutate and become cancerous. The aim of the therapy was to restore the chemical environment and kill the cancerous cells. Hoxsey's Herbal Tonic consisted of several different formulas: the "black medicine" was composed of cascara (a laxative) in an extract of licorice root, alfalfa, burdock root, red clover blossoms, buckthorn bark, barberry root, pokeweed, and prickly ash bark; the "pink medicine" contained potassium iodide and lactated pepsin.[21] Hoxsey claimed that a horse his grandfather owned had been cured of a leg cancer after eating a mixture of these plants, and this chance event led to his using this form of therapy for cancer in humans. Except for potassium iodide and the laxative, which are effective drugs but have no value in treating cancer, all the other ingredients have been discarded as medically ineffective.[11]

Hoxsey began promoting his treatment in the early 1920s, at which time it was called "Hoxide." After having been convicted of practicing medicine without a license in Illinois and Iowa, Hoxsey opened a small clinic in Dallas, Texas, and a second clinic in Portage, Pennsylvania, where Hoxsey's medicines were given in tablet form. The Hoxsey therapy was available at the clinic until 1960, when a federal court injunction, after 10 years of litigation, declared the sales of the treatment illegal.[11]

During the 10 years of litigation, a University of British Columbia panel investigated the Hoxsey method and found "that the methods of diagnosis are inadequate, that the treatments for internal cancer do not affect the progress of the disease, that no serious attempt is made to follow up treated cases in order to evaluate results, and that no significant research has been done."[22]

The Food and Drug Administration (FDA) investigated nearly 400 cases of persons who claimed to be cured of cancer through the use of the Hoxsey method. No case of a bona fide cure was discovered. Janssen[11] notes that one group of persons had never been diagnosed as having cancer, a second had received conventional therapy in addition to the Hoxsey treatment, and the final group still had cancer or had died from it. At the time the Hoxsey Clinic was closed, more than 10,000 individuals were enrolled as current patients. The FDA estimated that more than $50 million had been spent for the Hoxsey drugs.[23]

As of 1985, Hoxsey's medicines were thriving at the Bio-Medical Center in Tijuana, Mexico. The cost of therapy ranged from $150 to $450 for the blood test and examination to $2000 for the herbal remedies and physician consultation. A down payment of 30% was required.[24]

Krebiozen: 1960s

Krebiozen was allegedly first produced by a Yugoslavian physician named Steven Durovic. Durovic claimed that the first 200,000 doses (2 g in all) were obtained from blood extracted from some 2000 Argentinian horses. The horses were said to have been previously inoculated with a special mold before the blood sample was obtained.

Dr. Andrew C. Ivy, professor emeritus of the University of Illinois, endorsed the substance as an effective cancer therapy in the mid-1950s. Thousands of physicians across the country used Krebiozen as an investigational drug and charged nine dollars per ampul.[11] In 1961 the National Cancer Institute (NCI) obtained a sample of Krebiozen, and the substance was identified as creatine monohydrate, an amino acid found in all animal tissue.[25] Subsequent investigation of samples of Krebiozen actually distributed to physicians found that pre-1960 samples contained mineral oil and a small amount of amyl alcohol and methylhydantoin.[26]

The Krebiozen Research Foundation submitted 504 case records to the NCI in an effort to demonstrate therapeutic efficacy and help justify a clinical trial. A team of 24 scientists reviewed these records and unanimously concluded that Krebiozen is an ineffective drug.[27] Although no clear scientific evidence of efficacy has been brought forward, the treatment was available until 1977.[11]

Laetrile: 1970s

Laetrile is a term applied to various cyanogenic glucosides, derived from a variety of food products (eg, apricot pits, peaches, cherries, and almonds). It is also known as amygdalin and "vitamin B_{17}." It has been known as a killer of people since the Pharoahs' priests in ancient Egypt used it in the form of a water extract of peach kernels as the official means of execution of their enemies. Laetrile has been a quack remedy since 1840, 10 years after its isolation in pure form by two French chemists.[28] Ernst T. Krebs, Sr, a physician, claimed to be the first individual to use a cyanogenic glucoside as an anticancer agent. In the 1940s, Dr. Krebs used amygdalin, derived from apricot kernels, and found it to be too toxic for use in humans despite what he claimed were encouraging results. In 1952 his son, Ernst Krebs, Jr, reported that he had made an empiric apricot formula that was safe for parenteral administration.

Kreb's patent on laetrile was for a chemical different from amygdalin, and yet amygdalin is what is typically distributed as laetrile.[13] Laetrile's purported mechanism of action has changed over the years. Perhaps the most common hypothesis is that an enzyme called β-glucosidase is present in cancer cells in larger quantities than in healthy tissue. In turn, normal tissue is alleged to have greater quantities of the enzyme rhodanese, which supposedly is not present in cancerous tissue. The theory notes that the β-glucosidase in the cancerous tissues causes the laetrile to be broken down into glucose and mandelonitrile, which breaks down further into hydrogen cyanide (a toxic substance) and benzaldehyde (a mild anesthetic). The cyanide kills the cancer cells while the healthy tissue is protected by rhodanese, which converts cyanide into nontoxic sodium thiocynate. Manner et al[29] expand this theory and suggest, for example, that benzaldehyde may interfere with respiration in cancer cells. They also claim to have demonstrated a differentiation in quantities of rhodanese and β-glucosidase in the directions predicted by theory. However, this result is inconsistent with the findings of other investigators.[30-32] Greenberg[32] theorized that the majority of the parenterally injected laetrile is probably excreted intact in the urine.

Claims have been made that laetrile is a nontoxic form of "vitamin B_{17}," and that taking this vitamin can prevent cancer. Because no disease state exists in the absence of laetrile, however, it does not fulfill the requirements of a vitamin.[33] Evidence suggests that laetrile has toxic effects. The gastric lumen is thought to have enzymes capable of breaking laetrile down into hydrogen cyanide and mandelonitrile.[34] Numerous reports have associated cyanide toxicity with the ingestion of fruits or seeds containing cyanogenic glucosides, including amygdalin.[35-39] Ingestion of laetrile with certain other foods, such as sweet almonds, lettuce, certain fresh fruits, or mushrooms, can potentiate the toxic reaction. In addition, a number of deaths attributed to cyanide poisoning from oral laetrile have been reported,[28,40,41] and laetrile by enema is so poisonous.[42,43]

Another area of potential risk for the laetrile user is that the FDA has no control over the manufacture, importation, and distribution of laetrile. Laetrile that is used in the United States is either imported illegally or brought in under court order (exempting the substance from FDA supervision). There have been reports of fungal contamination of parenterally formulated laetrile, variations in dosage, and mislabeling of contents of laetrile imported from Mexican manufacturers.[44] For the cancer patient, whose immune system may already be compromised, an infection resulting from contamination could be fatal.

With regard to tests of efficacy, it is worth noting that laetrile has been the most extensively tested unproven method of all time. Numerous animal studies[45-49] and two retrospective studies have showed no therapeutic benefit.[50,51] Throughout the 1970s the FDA took legal action against many of the proponents of laetrile, there was a movement to legalize laetrile in many states, and approximately 75,000 US cancer patients were seeking laetrile therapy; many of these patients were discontinuing effective conventional therapy.[52] Laetrile was a billion-dollar-a-year industry in 1979.[28] Thus, in 1980, the FDA gave approval to the NCI for the first prospective clinical trial of laetrile and once again demonstrated laetrile to be ineffective against cancer.[53]

Today, many of the proponents of laetrile have changed their strategy of using it as a single agent and are combining it with vitamins, enzymes, or so-called metabolic therapy. For example, the Centro Medico Del Mar, in Tijuana, which is known for its laetrile treatments, has provided a therapy program consisting of laetrile, enzymes, diet, detoxification with enemas, "vaccines," vitamin A, and extracts of thymus tissue. The treatments last approximately 3 weeks and cost about $4000.[24]

MOST POPULAR UNPROVEN METHODS OF TODAY

Metabolic Therapy

Developed by German physician Dr. Max Gerson in the 1920s, metabolic cancer therapy proposes that constipation, or inadequate elimination of wastes from the body, interferes with metabolism and healing. Cure can be achieved through manipulation of diet and "detoxification," or purging the body of so-called toxins. There are many adaptations of Dr. Gerson's original program, but all have a consistent approach, which includes (1) avoidance of exposure to carcinogens, (2) positive mental outlook, and (3) eliminating wastes from the body. The diet is high in potassium, low in sodium, low in fats and oils, and includes reduced amounts of animal proteins. Individuals are encouraged to drink raw vegetable and fruit juices, take coffee enemas, and ingest supplemental vitamins, minerals, and enzymes.[54]

Cassileth et al[5] reported that 45% of the patients in their study used metabolic therapy with or without conventional therapy. Metabolic therapies are available from individual practitioners and clinics in the United States, Europe, and Canada, with the majority of such therapy given at the Gerson Therapy Hospital, in Tijuana, Mexico.[7,16,24] Treatment in the Mexican clinic costs approximately $3000 to $4000 and lasts from 3 to 6 weeks.[55] There is a long waiting list of US patients to receive a 1-week treatment, for $1700, of 13 glasses of carrot juice per day and coffee enemas.[24] Repeated enemas and purgatives are more likely to lead to metabolic imbalance than to correct it, and coffee enemas have killed people.[56,57] There are no objective data showing that the Gerson method has any benefit in the treatment of cancer.[58]

Harold Manner, PhD, is another proponent of metabolic cancer therapy. He is founder and president of the Metabolic Research Foundation, in Glenview, Illinois. He supervises his Tijuana Clinic, in Mexico, and has 168 Manner Metabolic Clinics in the United States, Canada, Japan, and Scotland. He claims that "metabolic therapy" enhances the body's immune system, causing tumors to disappear. The "Manner cocktail" consists of an intravenous solution of 10mL dimethyl sulfoxide, 25 g vitamin C, 9 g laetrile, and 5% dextrose given over a 2-week period at a cost of approximately $6000.[24] There are various protocols for this metabolic therapy, which may also include coffee enemas, megavitamins, and enzymes.[59] More important, there is no objective evidence that Harold Manner's metabolic therapy has any benefit in the treatment of cancer.[59]

Macrobiotic Diets

Over the years, a variety of diet therapies have been purported to be useful in the treatment of cancer. The macrobiotic diet is probably the most common today and is promoted both as a cure for cancer and a preventive measure. This diet has its origin in Zen mysticism, which proposes two antagonistic and complementary forces, yin and yang, governing everything in the universe. Each food can be classified as yin or yang, whereas each tumor can be classified as being caused by an imbalance of either yin or yang. The diet is matched to the tumor to restore the balance between yin and yang, resulting in a cure or prevention, as the case may be.[16] In addition to diet, balance is also achieved through cooking techniques and a correct attitude toward life.[60]

The original version of the diet, developed by George Ohsawa (1893–1966), involved 10 macrobiotic diets ranging from diet −3 to diet 7. As an individual progresses from diet −3 toward diet 7, more and more foods are forfeited, until in diet 7 the diet exclusively consists of cereal grains. In the 1970s, Michio Kushi,[61] recommended a more "standard macrobiotic diet" that was less restrictive than diet 7. This standard approach consists of 50% to 60% whole cereal grains, 20% to 25% vegetables, 5% to 10% soups, 5% to 10% beans and sea vegetables, occasional fish and fruits, and liquids used sparingly. The foods that are not allowed because they are excessively "yin" or "yang" include meat, animal fat, poultry, eggs, dairy products, bananas, citrus fruits, potatoes, tomatoes, spinach, coffee, sugar, and vitamin supplements.[61] Thus the macrobiotic diet uses only plant proteins and is high in bulk and low in fat. It is necessary to consume a large quantity of macrobiotic foods to meet the daily recommended energy allowance. For example, a healthy man who requires 2700 kilocalories would need 17 cups of food in volume.[62] Kushi[61] also recommends that modern medicine be avoided except for emergency lifesaving treatment.

Macrobiotic therapy may result in malnutrition and may cause a variety of serious health problems.[63] With adequate planning, vegetarian diets may be nutritionally sound, but the diet recommended by Kushi is unsound. The American Cancer Society[64] (ACS) recently reviewed the literature and available information and found no objective evidence that macrobiotic diets are of benefit in the treatment of cancer. There are also no valid data on the efficacy of the macrobiotic diet in the prevention of cancer.[63]

Megavitamins

The use of supplemental vitamins is another approach that has been exploited and promoted as an unproven method for the treatment of cancer. Megadoses of vitamin C, vitamin A, and pangamic acid ("vitamin B_{15}") have been alleged to have antitumor properties. However, excessive vitamin intake can be useless and, more important, very toxic.

Vitamin C

Vitamin C, consumed in megadoses, is probably the most popular self-administered vitamin supplement. Vitamin C has been promoted as a remedy for conditions ranging from the common cold to arthritis. It gained popularity as a therapy for cancer when Cameron and Pauling[65] published a study claiming that patients with terminal cancer who received massive doses of vitamin C survived much longer. However, their study was not valid because they selected the patients who received vitamin C and the control subjects were selected from files; thus the groups were not comparable.[66] Objective studies have shown such therapy to be worthless.[28,67,68] In fact, megadoses of vitamin C may cause severe kidney damage,[69] release cyanide from laetrile,[70] and cause death if administered intravenously.[67,71,72]

Vitamin A

Megadoses of vitamin A have also become popular, used either alone or in combination with other agents, for the treatment of cancer. Doses of vitamin A supplements as low as five times the recommended dietary allowance (RDA) may be toxic; moreover, vitamin A has no clear value in the treatment of cancer.[73]

Pangamic acid (vitamin B_{15})

Pangamic acid is a vitamin in name only, has no standard identity, and does not exist except as a label.[16] In the United States, it is illegal to sell this agent as either a drug or a food supplement.[74-76] There is evidence that the two most widely used chemicals in products labeled "B_{15}" or "pangamate" are diisopropylamine dichloroacetate (DIPA-DCA) and dimethylglycine hydrochloride (DMG), which actually may promote the development of cancer.[77,78]

Mental Imagery: Simonton Method

The Cancer Counseling and Research Center (CCRC), in Fort Worth, Texas, was established by O. Carl Simonton, a board-certified radiologist, and Stephanie Matthews-Simonton, a motivational counselor. The Simontons hypothesized that attitude and stress could be crucial factors in both causation and potential cure of cancer. It is their belief that a positive mental attitude can improve an individual's physiologic responses, resulting in improved response to standard therapies. Patients with cancer and their partners are taught to use mental imagery and relaxation techniques to visualize cancer cells as weak and sick and to imagine body defenses as a strong army that attacks and eliminates cancer cells.[79] The Simontons strongly advocate that individuals who participate in their counseling sessions continue to receive conventional medical treatment.

Although the scientific and medical communities support the notion that a positive mental attitude may increase patient comfort and promote a sense of control and well-being, the following problems remain concerning the Simonton method:

1. There are no carefully controlled clinical studies that show an objective benefit of the Simonton method for the treatment of cancer.

2. Patients may be made to feel guilty by leading them to believe that they are responsible for the development of cancer because they have a particular personality type.
3. If individuals become overly reliant on the Simonton method, they may be encouraged to abandon standard medical therapy.

Until such time as the efficacy of the Simonton method is documented by carefully controlled clinical studies, the American Cancer Society has determined that the Simonton method should be listed as an unproven method.[80]

The CCRC enrolls many patients and families in each session, and many people derive benefit from the sessions (ie, improved confidence, sense of well-being, and improved quality of life). In counseling patients about available options, nurses can point out potential benefits of the Simonton program while stressing that the method has no scientific documentation of effectiveness.

Spiritual, Faith, or Mind Healing

Many people find empowerment and comfort through various aspects of spiritual or faith healing. Cassileth and Brown[7] noted that in their study of 378 patients, 71 were attracted to this method of therapy, which involved use of prayer, "laying on of hands," incantation, or other ways of obtaining divine intervention to rid themselves of the disease. Many patients resort to commercialized faith healers who defraud people of their money by claiming that they can cure cancer. Other healers, such as Louise Hay, espouse self-love as a way to improve health and a possible cure.[81] Holland[18] notes that some methods that require patients to accept the idea that emotions contributed to their cancer may render patients even more vulnerable to guilt and depression. More important, these methods may be more hazardous to the patients' well-being than is usually recognized.

Immunoaugmentive Therapy

Dr. Lawrence Burton (doctor of zoology) is the originator of immunoaugmentive therapy (IAT) for cancer; treatment is given at his Immunology Research Center, located in the Bahamas. IAT is based on the theory that stimulation of the immune system will enable the body's normal defenses to destroy tumor cells. Although the therapeutic approach is based on reasonable scientific theory, scientific documentation of results of this therapy is lacking.[82] Evidence reported in 1985 suggested that his therapy not only is worthless but in fact may spread hepatitis and acquired immunodeficiency syndrome (AIDS).[83]

The ACS maintains a file of unproven methods and is therefore a good resource for information concerning them. Table 56-2 lists a variety of unproven methods that have been used for cancer diagnosis, prevention, or treatment.[84]

PROMOTERS OF UNPROVEN METHODS

Promoters of unproven cancer treatment methods survive, thrive, and grow rich. They invest time, effort, and money in public relations and media presentations that use legitimate scientific words or phrases in a misleading and deceptive manner while retaining their emotional impact. The promoters and purveyors omit the facts that their remedies have never been objectively tested and found valid. They omit citing the lack of benefit resulting from their regimen. Instead, they rely on testimonials and anecdotes that do not separate fact from fiction or from coincidence resulting from the natural history of the disease.[16]

In the last decade, the strategies used by the promoters of unproven treatment methods have become more sophisticated. Several points should be made about these new strategies: (1) the public's reasonable interest in nutrition, good mental attitude, and physical fitness is being exploited for personal profit; (2) the prevention of cancer is represented by purveyors of unproven methods as achievable with their remedies at a time when health professionals and the government also are emphasizing prevention; (3) there has been a movement to combine many questionable methods to make objective evaluation difficult; and (4) a rising distrust of health professionals is being exploited.[16,17] Highly motivated and better-educated individuals are more likely to turn to unquestionable methods because of the promise that "you can control your disease."[5,15]

The Subcommittee on Unorthodox Therapies of the American Society of Clinical Oncology[85] lists 10 questions to ask in making a decision as to whether a treatment should be suspected of being questionable (Table 56-3). Although these questions were developed as a guide for the layperson, they are also an excellent resource for the health professional.

INTERVENTIONS

The health care professional who discusses unproven methods of treating cancer with a patient or a family member must first assess the underlying motivations of the individual's desire to use these therapies. What information has the patient heard regarding the method in question? Where was the information obtained? What does the individual perceive as the benefits of pursuing this therapy? If a family member is asking about such a method, has the individual discussed this therapy with the patient?

Individuals who raise questions regarding unproven methods are usually aware that such techniques are not likely to be approved by the health care professional. For the professional, these questions provide an opportunity to discover unmet needs of the patient and family and to assess their understanding of the therapies that have been

TABLE 56-2 Unproven Methods for Diagnosis or Treatment of Cancer

Unproven Methods
Alkylating punch
Almonds
Aloe vera plant
American International Hospital's program
Anti-cancer factor in clams
Anticacergen Z-50 and Zuccala lytic test
Antineol
Arthur morphologic immunostatus differentials
Asparagus oil
Bacteria enema
Bamfolin
H. H. Beard methods
Bio-medical detoxification therapy
Bonifacio anticancer goat serum
Cancer lipid concentrate and the malignancy index
Carcin and neo-carcin
Carrot/celery juice
Carzodelan
Cath$_2$O$_2$LIC therapy
Cedar cones
CH-23
Chamonils
Chaparral tea
Chase dietary method
Chelation
Cinical El Buen Samaritano
C.N.T.
Coffee enemas
Coley's mixed toxins or mixed bacterial toxins (MBT)
Collodaurum and bichloracetic acid Kahlenbury
Compound X
Contreras methods
Cresson method
Crofton immunization method
Cytec system
Diamond carbon compound
DMSO
Dotto electronic reactor
Drown radio-therapeutic instrument
Esterlit
Ferguson plant products
Fonti methods
Francis diet
Fresh cell therapy
Frost method
Ganner petroleum or "Petroleum pal"
Germanium
Gerson method
Gibson method
Glover method
Goat's milk
Grape cure
Greek cure
H. 11
Hadley vaccine and blood and skin test
Haematoxylon dissolved in DMSO
Heat therapy or hyperthermia
Hemacytology index (HCI)
Hendricks natural immunity therapy
Helt "cancer serum" and Gruner blood smear test
Hoxsey method or Hoxsey chemotherapy
Hubbard E. Meter
Hypnosis
Immuno-augmentation cancer therapy program
Iscador
Issels combination therapy
Kallzyne
Kanfer neuromuscular or handwriting test
KC-555
Kelley malignancy index and ecology therapy
Koch antitoxins
Laetrile
Lewis method
Livingston vaccine
M-P virus
Makari intradermal cancer test
Manner's metabolic cancer prevention program
Marijuana
Megadose vitamin therapy
Mexican clinics and hospitals
Millet bread
Millrue
Miniburg system
Mucorhicin
Multiple enzyme therapy
Naessens serum or anablast
Nichols escharotic method
Nieper
Olive oil
OM-12
Oncone juice
Orgone energy devices
Oscilloclast
Pap-Chek, Female laboratory testing
Polonine
Psychic methods
Rand coupled fortified antigen (RCFA) and Delayed double diffusion (3-D) test
Revici cancer control
Samuels causal or "endogenous endocrinotherapy"
Sander's treatment
Simonton method
Snake meat
Snake oil capsules
Spears hygienic system
Staphylococcus phage lysate or Lincoln bacteriophage lysate
Sunflower seeds
Ultraviolet blood irradiation intravenous treatment
Wigmore program
Zen macrobiotic diet

Source: Reprinted with permission from Miller NJ, Howard-Ruben J. Unproven methods of cancer management: Part I. Background and historical perspective. Oncol Nurs Forum 10(4):46, 1983.

administered. If the patient receives a strong negative response concerning the unproven method, the communication channel between the health care professional and the patient will likely be impaired. A nonjudgmental attitude facilitates the caregiver's assessment of the patient's and family's motivations for wanting to try an unproven method. In turn, the patient and family will likely be more receptive to the information provided by a nonjudgmental health care professional.

Anything that can be done to make the patient feel a part of the therapeutic effort may help prevent the use of unproven methods by the patient. Information on exercise or nutrition provided in a positive context will help the patient feel less isolated. Keeping the patient and family well informed by answering questions concerning the type of therapy being received will also combat feelings of isolation. Pamphlets available from the ACS or NCI may increase communication because they provide background material that can put the health care team's information into perspective. The goal of communication is to have the patient feel that he or she is being treated humanely. The person who feels like an adversary of the health care team is not likely to see the hospital staff as human beings. Many individuals will say that health care professionals could cure cancer if they wanted to but that there is no profit in doing so. Those who make such statements forget

TABLE 56-3 Ten Questions to Ask in Deciding Whether a Treatment is Questionable

1. Is the treatment based on an unproven theory?
2. Is there a purported need for special nutritional support?
3. Is there a claim for painless, nontoxic treatment?
4. Are claims published only in the mass media and not in reputable peer-reviewed scientific journals?
5. Are claims for benefit merely compatible with a placebo effect?
6. Are the major proponents recognized experts in cancer treatment?
7. Do proponents claim benefit for use with proven methods of treatment? For prolongation of life? For use as a cancer preventive?
8. Is there a claim that only specially trained physicians can produce results with the drug, or is the preparation secret?
9. Is there an attack on the medical and scientific establishment?
10. Is there a demand by promoters for "freedom of choice" regarding drugs?

Source: Subcommittee on Unorthodox Therapies, American Society of Clinical Oncology: Ineffective cancer therapy: A guide for the layperson. J Clin Oncol 1:154-163, 1983.

that health care professionals are human and that their loved ones also die of cancer.

In evaluating communication patterns, the health care professional also needs to examine communications between the patient and family. The family may become preoccupied with seeking various therapies as a means of coping with stress. Such a situation may be sufficiently intense to cause the family to engage in a conspiracy to exclude the patient from the decision-making process. The patient then becomes alienated from the family's communication system and from the psychologic and physical support that is so important. The family must be made aware of the impact of their actions on the patient. A social worker, chaplain, or patient-family support group might facilitate more effective intrafamily communication.

Frequently, discussion will focus on the use of unproven methods for individuals who are terminally ill. For many such patients, standard therapy will be able to extend life. Should "terminal" be used to describe a state in which no therapeutic modalities can be effective? Palliative care may still be able to extend the person's life, whereas an unproven method may shorten it. When a patient is interested in experimental research, the options should be explored by the physician. In all instances the issue of quality of life versus quantity of life should be discussed. The advantages and disadvantages for each individual should be examined. For many, a second opinion concerning therapeutic options may prove helpful. Second opinions can provide two positive outcomes:

1. They can make the patient aware of additional therapeutic alternatives.
2. They reassure both patient and family that the therapeutic assessment that has been made is likely a sound one.

The health care professional must be informed both regarding technical information on the most frequently encountered unproven methods and regarding the particular aims of a given individual's therapy. The health care professional should be able to explain the risks of unproven methods, such as toxic effects and, in instances where the unproven method is being used as the sole form of therapy, the risk of further progression of disease. For individuals who are using an unproven method in combination with standard therapy, it is still important to be aware of possible side effects. A drug analysis may prove valuable for any substances that the patient has been given from an unproven methods clinic. For example, one Mexican clinic provided a "vitamin" that was actually a potent chemotherapeutic agent. The patient was at the same time taking standard chemotherapy at a university medical center. Fortunately, the physicians discovered the true identity of the "vitamin" after noting an unusually low white blood cell count.[14] The risks of adverse effects can be increased when drugs are mixed with unorthodox substances, and the patient must be informed that all risks may not even be known.

Finally, health care professionals who are caring for patients with cancer must be kept informed regarding hospital, state, and federal policies regarding any drug—experimental, standard, or unproven. The term "unproven," as originally noted, suggests that the substance is being promoted even though it has not been proven effective. However, the fact that a promoted therapy has not been proven effective does not necessarily mean that it has no therapeutic value. It must be tested to determine its safety and efficacy. The present system permits the scientific method to play a strong role in determining what therapies will be on the market, and improvements are continually being made in methods of evaluation. In this way the health care consumer is protected from unsafe and fraudulent therapies.

REFERENCES

1. Olson KB: Drugs, cancer and charlatans, in Horton J, Hill GJ (eds). Clincal Oncology. Philadelphia, WB Saunders, 1977, pp 182-191.
2. House Subcommittee on Aging: Quackery: A 10-Billion-Dollar Scandal—Report. Committee publication No. 98-435. Washington, DC, Government Printing Office, 1984, pp 1-250.

3. House Subcommittee on Aging: Quackery: A 10-Billion-Dollar Scandal—Hearing. Committee publication No. 98-463. Washington, DC, Government Printing Office, 1984.
4. Herbert V, Barnett S: Vitamins and "Health" Foods: The Great American Hustle. Philadelphia, George F Stickley, 1981.
5. Cassileth B, Lusk E, Strouse T, et al: Contemporary unorthodox treatments in cancer medicine. Ann Intern Med 101:105-112, 1984.
6. Cassileth B: Unorthodox cancer medicine. Cancer Invest 4:591-598, 1986.
7. Cassileth B, Brown H: Unorthodox cancer medicine. CA 38:176-186, 1988.
8. Cassileth BR, Berlyne B: Counseling the cancer patient who wants to try unorthodox or questionable therapies. Oncology 3:29-33, 1989.
9. Janssen WF: The cancer "cures": A challenge to rational therapeutics. Anal Chem 50:197A-202A, 1978.
10. Grant RN, Bartlett I: Unproven cancer remedies: A primer, in Unproven Methods of Cancer Management. New York, American Cancer Society, 1971.
11. Janssen WF: Cancer quackery: the past in the present. Semin Oncol 6:526-536, 1979.
12. Message from President Taft. Congressional Record 62 Cong., 1 Sess. 2380 (June 21, 1911).
13. Kennedy D: Commissioner decision on status. Federal Register 42:39806-39967, 1977.
14. Luurs KJ: Unproven methods of treatment, in Groenwald SL (ed): Cancer Nursing Principles and Practice. Boston, Jones & Bartlett, 1987, pp 405-413.
15. Hiratzka S: Knowledge and attitudes of persons with cancer toward use of unproven treatment methods. Oncol Nurs Forum 12:36-41, 1985.
16. Herbert V, Yarbro CH: Nutrition quackery. Semin Oncol Nurs 2:63-69, 1986.
17. King M: Falling victim twice. Cancer News 39:8-11, 1985.
18. Holland JC: Why patients seek unproven cancer remedies: A psychological perspective. CA 32:10-14, 1982.
19. Koch WF: A new and successful treatment and diagnosis of cancer. Detroit Med J, 1919.
20. Letter to the Editor: Senator Langer abuses franking privilege by circulation of propaganda for Koch's cancer quackery. JAMA 137:1333, 1948.
21. Hoxsey HM: You Don't Have to Die: The Amazing Story of the Hoxsey Cancer Treatment. New York, Milestone Books, 1956.
22. Mather JM: Report of a committee of faculty members of the University of British Columbia concerning the Hoxsey treatment for cancer. Unpublished report, December 19, 1957.
23. Press Release HEW-020: US Department Health, Education, and Welfare, Food and Drug Administration. Washington, DC, Steptember 21, 1960.
24. Kreiger L: Unorthodox clinics flourishing in Tijuana. Am Med News 3:25-27, 1985.
25. Holland JF: The Krebiozen story: Is cancer quackery dead? JAMA 200:213-218, 1967.
26. American Cancer Society: Unproven methods of cancer management. New York, American Cancer Society, 1971.
27. Report of Director, National Cancer Institute, to Secretary of Department of Health, Education, and Welfare concerning decision of the Institute not to undertake clinical testing of Krebiozen. Washington, DC, FDA Records 539.1.PX, October 16, 1963.
28. Herbert V: Nutrition Cultism: Facts and Fictions (ed 3). Philadelphia, George F. Stickley, 1981.
29. Manner HW, DiSanti SJ, Michalsen TL: The Death of Cancer. Evanston, Ill, Advanced Century Publishing, 1978.
30. Conchie J, Findlay L, Levvy GA: Mammalian glycosidases: Distribution in the body. Biochem J 71:318-325, 1959.
31. Gal EM, Fung FH, Greenberg DM: Studies on the biological action of malonitriles. II. Distribution of rhodanese (transulfurase) in the tissues of normal and tumor-bearing animals and the effect of malononitrile thereon. Cancer Res 169:449-450, 1952.
32. Greenberg DM: The vitamin fraud in cancer quackery. West J Med 122:345-348, 1975.
33. Greenstein JP: Quantitative nutritional studies with water-soluble chemically defined diets. I. Growth, reproduction and lactation in rats. Arch Biochem Biophys 72:396-416, 1957.
34. Everly RC: Laetrile: Focus on the facts. CA 26:50-54, 1976.
35. Grabois B: Exposure to hydrogen cyanide in processing of apricot kernels. Monthly Review: New York Department of Labor 33:33-36, 1954.
36. Sayre JW, Kaymakcalan S: Cyanide poisoning from apricot seeds among children in central Turkey. N Engl J Med 270:1113-1115, 1964.
37. Gunders AE, Abrahamov A, Weisenberg E: Cyanide poisoning following the ingestion of apricot *(Prunus armeniaca)* kernel. J Israel Med Assoc 76:536-538, 1969.
38. Humbert JR, Tress JH, Braico KT: Fatal cyanide poisoning: Accidental ingestion of amygdalin. JAMA 238:482, 1977 (letter).
39. Sadoff L, Fuchs K, Hollander J: Rapid death associated with laetrile ingestion. JAMA 239:1532, 1978.
40. Herbert V: Laetrile: The cult of cyanide—Promoting poison for profit. Am J Clin Nutr 32:1121-1158, 1979.
41. Vogel SN, Sultan TR: Cyanide poisoning. Clin Toxicol Exp Ther 18:367-383, 1981.
42. Ortega JA, Creek J: Acute cyanide poisoning following administration of laetrile enemas. J Pediatr 93:1059, 1978.
43. Eisele JW, Reay DT: Deaths related to coffee enemas. JAMA 244:1608-1609, 1980.
44. Food and Drug Administration: Toxicity of laetrile. FDA Drug Bull 7:25-32, 1977.
45. Wodinsky I, Swiniarsky JK: Antitumor activity of amygdalin as a single agent and with beta-glucosidase on a spectrum of transplantable rodent tumors. Cancer Chem Rep 59:939-950, 1975.
46. Hill GJ, Shine TE, Hill HZ, et al: Failure of amygdalin to arrest B16 melanoma and BW5147 AKR leukemia. Cancer Res 36:2102-2107, 1976.
47. Stock CC, Tarnowski GS, Schmid FA, et al: Antitumor tests of amygdalin in transplantable animal tumor systems. J Surg Oncol 10:81-88, 1978.
48. Stock CC, Martin DS, Suguira K, et al: Antitumor tests of amygdalin in spontaneous animal tumor systems. J Surg Oncol 10:89-123, 1978.
49. Ovejira AA, Houchens DP, Barker AD, et al: Inactivity of DL-amygdalin against human breast and colon tumor xenografts in athymic (nude) mice. Cancer Treat Rep 62:576-578, 1978.
50. California Medical Association, Cancer Commission: The treatment of cancer with "Laetriles." Calif Med 78:320-326, 1953.
51. Ellison NM, Byar DP, Newell GR: Special report on laetrile: the NCI laetrile review. N Engl J Med 299:549-552, 1978.
52. Henney JE: Unproven methods of cancer treatment, in DeVita VT, Hellman S, Rosenberg SA (eds): Cancer Principles and Practice of Oncology (ed 2). Philadelphia, JB Lippincott, 1985, pp 2333-2342.
53. Moertel CG, Fleming TR, Tubin J, et al: A clinical trial of

amygdalin (laetrile) in the treatment of human cancer. N Engl J Med 306:201-207, 1982.
54. Gerson M: The cure of advanced cancer by diet therapy: A summary of 30 years of clinical experimentation. Physiol Chem Phys 10:449-464, 1978.
55. Donsbach KW, Walker M: Metabolic Cancer Therapies. Huntington Beach, Calif International Institute of National Health Sciences, 1981.
56. Istre GR, Kreiss K, Hopkins RS, et al: An outbreak of amebiasis spread by colonic irrigation at a chiropractic clinic. N Engl J Med 307:339-342, 1982.
57. Markman M: Medical complications of "alternative" cancer therapy (letter). N Engl J Med 312:1640-1641, 1985.
58. American Cancer Society: Unproven methods of cancer management: Gerson method of treatment for cancer. CA 23:314-317, 1973.
59. American Cancer Society: Unproven methods of cancer management: The metabolic cancer therapy of Harold W. Manner, Ph.D. CA 36:185-189, 1986.
60. Ohsawa G: Cancer and the Philosophy of the Far East. Binghamton, NY, Swan House Publishing, 1971.
61. Kushi M: Macrobiotic Approach to Cancer. Wayne, NJ, Avery Publishing Group, 1982.
62. Arnold C: The macrobiotic diet: A question of nutrition. Oncol Nurs Forum 11:50-53, 1984.
63. Bowman BB, Kushner RF, Dawson SC, et al: Macrobiotic diets for cancer treatment and prevention. J Clin Oncol 2:702-711, 1984.
64. American Cancer Society: Unproven methods of cancer management: Macrobiotic diets for the treatment of cancer. CA 39:248-251, 1989.
65. Cameron E, Pauling L: Supplemental ascorbate in the supportive treatment of cancer, prolongation of survival time in terminal human cancer. Proc Natl Acad Sci USA 73:3685-3689, 1976.
66. Sampson WI: When the big C is a vitamin. Coping 2:35, 1988.
67. Marshall CW: Vitamins and Minerals: Help or Harm? Philadelphia, George F Stickley, 1983.
68. Creagan ET, Moertel CG, O'Fallon JR, et al: Failure of high-dose vitamin C to benefit patients with advanced cancer. N Engl J Med 301:687-690, 1979.
69. Swartz RD, Wesley JR, Somermeyer MG, et al: Hyperoxaluria and renal insufficiency due to ascorbic acid administration during total parental nutrition. Ann Intern Med 100:530-531, 1984.
70. Backer RC, Herbert V: Cyanide production from laetrile in the presence of megadoses of ascorbic acid. JAMA 241:1891-1892, 1979.
71. Herbert V: The rationale of massive-dose vitamin therapy: Megavitamin therapy—hot fiction vs cold facts, in Whilte PL, Selvey N (eds): Proceedings of the Fourth Western Hemisphere Nutrition Congress. Acton, Mass, Publishing Sciences Group, 1975, pp 84-91.
72. Hodges RE: Nutrition in Medical Practice. Philadelphia, WB Saunders, 1980.
73. Herbert V: Toxicity of 25,000 IU vitamin A supplements in "health" food users. Am J Clin Nutr 36:185-186, 1982.
74. Herbert V: Pangamic acid (vitamin B_{15}). Am J Clin Nutr 32:1534-1540, 1979.
75. Herbert V, Herbert R: Pangamate (vitamin B_{15}) in Ellenbogen L (ed): Controversies in Nutrition. New York, Churchill Livingstone, 1981, pp 159-170.
76. McPherrin EW, Herbert V, Herbert R: "Vitamin B_{15}": Anatomy of a Health Fraud. New York, American Council on Science and Health, 1981.
77. Colman N, Herbert V, Gardner A, et al: Mutagenicity of dimethylglycine when mixed with nitrite: Possible significance in human use of pangamates. Proc Soc Exp Biol Med 164:9-12, 1980.
78. Gelernt MD, Herbert V: Mutagenicity of diisopropylamine dichloroacetate, the "active constituent" of vitamin B_{15} (pangamic acid). Nutr Cancer 3:129-133, 1982.
79. Simonton OC, Matthews-Simonton S, Creighton J: Getting Well Again: A Step-by-Step, Self-Help Guide to Overcoming Cancer for Patients and Their Families. Los Angeles, Jeremy P. Tarcher, 1978.
80. American Cancer Society: Unproven methods of cancer management: O. Carl Simonton, MD. CA 32:58-61, 1982.
81. Irish AC: Maintaining health in persons with HIV infection. Semin Oncol Nurs 5:302-307, 1989.
82. Easy cures for cancer still find support. JAMA 246:714-716, 1981.
83. OT briefs. Oncol Times 7:26, 1985.
84. Miller NJ, Howard-Ruben J: Unproven methods of cancer management. Background and historical perspectives. Oncol Nurs Forum 10:46-52, 1983.
85. Subcommittee on Unorthodox Therapies, American Society of Clinical Oncology: Ineffective cancer therapy: A guide for the layperson. J Clin Oncol 1:154-163, 1983.

Chapter 57

Teaching Strategies: The Public

Marion E. Morra, MA

INTRODUCTION

Communicating to and educating the public in the area of health has been a responsibility of nurses for many years. Health care professionals in the cancer field view themselves as role models, not only to the patients they serve but also to the public at large.

DEFINITION OF TERMS

There are many definitions of health education. Some relate to the field of education as a whole; others are based in the areas of communications, behavior, and marketing.

The President's Committee on Health Education views health education as a process that bridges the gap between health information and health practices. Health education motivates the person to take information and do something with it—to keep healthier by avoiding actions that are harmful and by forming habits that are beneficial.[1] The World Health Organization (WHO) defines health education as any combination of planned activities leading to a situation where people want to be healthy, know how to obtain health, do what they can individually and collectively, and seek help when needed.[2] Green et al[3] have a broader definition: Health education is any combination of learning experience designed to facilitate voluntary adoption of behavior conducive to health. This increases the scope as well as the purpose of health education, allowing for a wide variety of programs, activities, and methods to enrich the field.

THEORIES AND MODELS

Health education embodies theories in the fields of education, psychology, and communications. Following are several theories relating to health education.

The Health Belief Model

The Health Belief Model, often considered the basis for health behavioral research, was developed in the 1950s[4] and established a framework for explaining and predicting why people engage in specific preventive behaviors. The Health Belief Model provides insight into how an individual makes such a decision. Based on the tenet that the beliefs and values acquired over a lifetime affect a person's decisions, it combines variables such as the person's perception of being susceptible to that condition, the perceived seriousness of the problem, and the availability of specific actions that prevent or treat the condition. This model is discussed in detail in Chapter 6.

PRECEDE

The PRECEDE model of health education[3] provides an organizing framework within which more detailed theories might be integrated. The PRECEDE (an acronym for predisposing, reinforcing, and enabling causes in educational diagnosis and evaluation) framework is highly focused on intervention, be it with people whose health is in question or with those who control resources or rewards, such as community leaders, parents, peers, teachers, or health care professionals. PRECEDE has seven phases: (1) assessment of social problems of concern, (2) identification of specific health-related problems, (3) identification of specific health-related behaviors linked to the health problems, (4) categorization of factors that have direct impact on these behaviors (predisposing, enabling, or reinforcing factors), (5) assessment of relative importance of factors and resources available to influence them, (6) development and implementation of programs, and (7) evaluation.

PAR

The PAR (population attributable risk) theory[1] is based on the incidence of a disease with a fraction of a population due to exposure to a specific risk factor. It then focuses on those priority health behaviors that must influence the health of the target communities.

Communications Theory

In communication theory,[5] six basic elements are described as essential to any process of communications: (1) a source (that constructs a message), (2) an encoder (that produces it), (3) the message itself, (4) a channel (that carries it), (5) a decoder (that translates it), and (6) a receiver (that gets the message). Within the source and the receiver, four factors impinge on the success of communications: communications skills, attitudes, knowledge level, and social or cultural systems.

Social Marketing Theory

Social marketing is a theory that introduces the principles and practices of marketing to social issues, causes, and ideas.[6] It takes the attitudes and needs of the target audience into account in planning programs and campaigns. A social marketer uses research as a basis for segmenting audiences, positioning the offering, and identifying audience needs, wants, expectations, satisfactions, and dissatisfactions. In addition to the offering, social marketing contains other essential elements, such as price strategies, channel strategies, and communications. It embraces classic health promotion models and other behavioral theories and disciplines. Social marketers believe in designing related products and services, making them available when and where consumers are, and using effective channels to promote the wares.

Since health behavior is caused and determined by

many factors, education must incorporate different methods and channels to effect changes in behaviors.

BARRIERS TO EDUCATING THE PUBLIC

The National Cancer Institute (NCI) has defined several barriers to the publics' acceptance of health messages[7]:

1. Health risk is an intangible concept. Many people underestimate their risk of common health problems, such as cancer, stroke, and diabetes. People believe a serious illness will not happen to them, regardless of their actual risk.
2. The public responds to easy solutions. People are more likely to respond to simple actions (such as getting a blood test for cholesterol checking) than to a more complicated one (such as quitting smoking).
3. People want absolute answers. In the cancer field, there are not many firm answers from scientists.
4. The public may react unfavorably to fear. Frightening information may result in denial, hysteria, anxiety, and helplessness, which may be compounded if there are not immediate actions to take.
5. The public doubts the verity of science. People may not believe a scientist's prediction.
6. The public has other priorities. Many times daily problems are more important than intangible health information.
7. The public holds contradictory beliefs. Even though an individual believes "it can't happen to me", he or she can still believe "everything causes cancer" and can find no need to alter behavior. Only 38% of the population believes that life-style is related to cancer.[8]
8. The public lacks a future orientation. Many Americans, especially lower socioeconomic groups, have trouble relating to the concept of changing their behaviors for something that may not happen to them.

It is important to take such barriers into consideration during the various phases of program development. It may be possible to turn barriers into opportunities, thus creating better programs.

DEVELOPMENT OF PROGRAMS

The extent of the planning process for a health education program will depend on many factors. For example, a nationwide program will entail a more extensive planning process than will a program carried out in one community. However, several planning steps should be considered for every program and a decision made on their applicability to each situation.

The Office of Cancer Communications of the NCI outlines six stages in developing health communications programs[7]:

Stage 1: Planning and Strategy Selection

Careful assessment is made of the problem to determine whether it can be addressed by communication strategies. During this phase, information is gathered and available data are reviewed to identify existing activities and any gaps that must be addressed. Goals and objectives are written to establish what the program will accomplish. Target audiences are defined and described. The direction the program will take and the strategy for reaching the target audiences are planned. Major obstacles and barriers are identified. Resources needed to carry out the strategies are identified. Finally, a program plan and timetable are produced.

Stage 2: Selecting Channels and Materials

In this stage, the decisions made in the planning process are used to select the kinds of materials needed to reach the target audience. An assessment is made on whether existing materials can be used or adapted or whether new materials must be produced. Decisions about how the target audience will be reached (channel to be used) are also made during this stage—whether it will be a face-to-face campaign, one delivered in a classroom or a worksite, one using mass media or community groups, or a combination of more than one channel.

Stage 3: Developing Materials and Pretesting

If new materials are to be developed, this state is essential. Pretesting is used to determine whether materials produced by you or by someone else will be suitable for use with a specific target audience. This phase assures that all messages in the materials reinforce each other, are based on the strategies determined in Stage 2, and are presented in a way that is understandable to the target audience. Both the written material and the illustrations are pretested to be sure they convey the proper response. For example, when the NCI tested the phrase "cancer prevention" with an apple substituted for the "o" in prevention, it found respondents failed to link apples to either good health or prevention and thus did not use it.[7]

Stage 4: Implementing the Program

During this stage, the program is introduced to the target audience. The promotion and distribution of the materials is begun. Before starting this stage, it is essential to assure that all materials are ready in sufficient quantities, that promotion plans are in place, and that methods of tracking progress (process evaluation) have been developed. The written program plan for this phase will also contain a strategy for informing and working with other organizations involved, information on when resources are needed, when specific events are planned, and ways to identify potential problems. Specific periodic assessments are planned to determine whether the target audiences and time schedule are being reached, whether some strategies are more successful than others, how the program is operating, whether the target audience is responding, and whether the resources are being used as planned. Written progress reports and modification of program components are important aspects of this phase.

Stage 5: Assessing Effectiveness

Assessment of the effectiveness of the program is based on the goals and objectives planned in Stage 1 and used throughout the life of the program. This stage determines the outcome or results of the program, that is, whether the target audience learned, acted, or made a change. Outcome evaluation usually consists of a comparison of target audience awareness, attitudes, or behavior before and after the program.

Stage 6: Feedback

Using the information gathered at each stage—about the audience, the messages, the channels of communication, and the program's intended effect—this phase prepares to improve an ongoing program, revise it, or plan a new cycle of program development. It is also a time for sharing what has been learned about others, such as writing an article, sending materials to a related clearinghouse or agency, or presenting a poster or an abstract at a professional meeting.

OPPORTUNITIES AND CHALLENGES

The NCI, in establishing its Year 2000 goal to achieve a 50% reduction in the 1985 cancer death rate, has set a challenge for concentrated efforts by health organizations, voluntary and professional associations, government agencies, industry, and the media. The Year 2000 goal offers a framework for action and has been further enhanced by the setting of cancer-control objectives[9] based on the goal (Table 57-1). The prevention objectives center on the reduction of smoking—responsible for some 30% of all cancer deaths—and on diet, which is associated with several cancers, including colorectal cancer, the leading cause of cancer deaths after lung cancer.[9] The screening objective relate to detecting cervical and breast cancers in asymptomatic women. There are effective screening tech-

TABLE 57-1 Cancer Control Objectives to Meet Year 2000 Goal

Action	Target	Rationale	Year 2000 Objectives
Prevention	Smoking	The causal relationship between smoking and cancer has been scientifically established.	Reduce the percentage of adults who smoke from 34% to 15% or less.
			Reduce the percentage of youths who smoke by age 20 from 36% to 15% or less.
	Diet	Research indicates that high-fat and low-fiber consumption may increase the risk for various cancers.	Reduce average consumption of fat from 37% or 30% to 30% or less of total calories.
			Increase average consumption of fiber from 8 to 12 g to 20 to 30 g per day.
Screening	Breast	The effectiveness of breast screening in reducing mortality has been scientifically established.	Increase the percentage of women ages 50 to 70 who have an annual physical breast examination coupled with mammography from 45% for physical examination alone and 15% for mammography to 80%.
	Cervix	The effectiveness of cervical screening in reducing mortality has been scientifically established.	Increase the percentage of women who have a Pap smear every 3 years from 79% (ages 20 to 39) to 90% and from 57% (ages 40 to 70) to 80%.
Treatment	Transfer of research results to practice	Review by NCI of clinical trial and NCI's SEER Program data indicates that, for certain cancer sites, mortality as shown by SEER data is greater than that experienced in clinical trials.	Increase adoption of state-of-the-art treatment.

Source: National Cancer Institute: Cancer Control Objectives for the Nation: 1985-2000. NCI monograph no. 2, Appendix B. Bethesda, Md, Division of Cancer Prevention and Control, The Institute, October 1986.

niques available for both types of cancers, and women who are diagnosed early have excellent prognoses. These objectives form a strong basis for program planning and offer widespread opportunities. These opportunities also offer many challenges to health education. A few will be discussed further: segmenting audiences, reaching the disadvantaged, and using the media as a gatekeeper.

Segmenting Target Audiences

A major challenge in public education is to identify the main audience for the program. The most basic way to segment audiences is by age into adult and child learners. Factors other than age, however, must be taken into account, including sex, education, income levels, race and ethnic origin, attitudes, and beliefs. Audience segmentation has become so complex that it encompasses an entire new field of study called psychographics.

Psychographics

Psychographics, sometimes referred to as attitudinal or life-style research, segments the country into neighborhood types, personality types, media users, product and brand buyers, and benefit seekers. Its roots come from sociology, political science, and developmental psychology. Psychographics goes beyond demographics in identifying smaller, more targeted clusters in the population. One branch of psychographics is called *geodemographics.* Based on the theory that people in similar neighborhoods have similar life-styles, geodemographics divides the country into neighborhoods with specific characteristics. Using these techniques in the cancer field can give direction into who is the targeted learner—who is at highest risk and who is most needy of learning about the particular issue—as well as what kind of message to deliver.

The NCI reinforces the need for segmenting audiences to increase the likelihood that the targeted learner is reached by the educational program. Several studies on the national level have detailed cancer prevention opportunities as well as the knowledge, attitude, and behavior of specific target groups. The NCI outlines several opportunities for health education in cancer prevention[8]:

1. The lung cancer rate for women is rising much faster than that for men and has surpassed the death rate for breast cancer. The American Cancer Society (ACS) has found that 20% more women are heavy smokers (a pack or more a day) than in the 1960s.[10]
2. Cigarette smoking among adolescent girls (ages 17 to 19) is now greater than among boys in the same age group. Young women are starting to smoke at an earlier age (50% before 10th grade). The ACS estimates that female smokers are starting to smoke an average of 9 years earlier than they did in the 1960s.[10]
3. Women older than 50 who have annual physical breast examinations and mammograms can reduce their risk of breast cancer death by as much as 30%, but only 15% of women age 50 and over have an annual mammogram and only 45% have a physical breast examination.
4. Since many cancers (breast, prostate, colorectal) occur more often in people age 50 or over, this age group is a prime target for early detection tests.[11]

Primary and secondary targets

In segmenting audiences, it may be useful to identify both primary and secondary audiences. A "primary" target audience is one that will be affected in some way by the messages given. A "secondary" target audience is one that has some influence on the primary audience or who must do something to help cause the change in the primary target audience. For instance, women over age 50 may be the primary audience for a mammography education program. Physicians serving this population can be a secondary target audience to be reminded to refer these women for the screening test.

One of the steps to developing a successful education program is to get to know as much as possible about the target audience and to write as detailed a description as can be defined. Items that should be delineated include[7]:

- Age, sex, ethnic background, area of residence or work
- Knowledge, attitudes, and behavior as related to the patterns to be changed
- Available health-related services and patterns of use
- Media preference and habits
- Information sources considered credible by the potential target group.

Obtaining information about audiences

There are many ways to obtain information about potential target audiences. Census data, reports from Chambers of Commerce, health departments, economic development agencies, and local hospitals can all offer demographic information. Advertising agencies, television and radio stations, newspapers, and media guides can provide data on the use of the media and the composition of the media's audiences. Knowledge and attitudes of various groups are available from polling companies, voluntary health agencies, health professional organizations, and universities. Library searches may yield useful data for audience segmentation.

New data may be needed to pinpoint specific information about the target audience. Focus group interviews is one method often used to provide insight into the beliefs, perceptions, and feelings about topics among a particular group of people. Usually consisting of 12 to 14 persons, a focus group is good for stimulating discussion of issues and for gathering opinions in a short time. However, it is not a representative sample of target populations, usually has too few participants for concensus or decision making, and depends greatly on a skilled moderator. Focus groups can be especially useful for testing materials before production in the areas of appropriate language, the appeal of a message, or the appeal of a particular spokesman to a specified target population. For instance, the NCI, in planning a major national survey on public knowledge attitudes of breast cancer, conducted separate focus groups with white, black, and Hispanic men and women to help develop the wording for specific questions. Focus groups can also be used to (1) clarify the results of survey research (especially if the results are different from those expected), (2) to generate hypotheses, or (3) to give depth to feelings about health-related issues.

Personal interviews, either by mail, telephone, or at home, are another method to gather vital data but are more expensive to conduct. If the questions that need answering are few, it may be possible to add them to an ongoing survey (such as polls that are conducted by newspapers or other enterprises to determine consumer attitudes). Mailed questionnaires are a relatively inexpensive way to reach large numbers of people. However, response rates may be low, respondents may not be representative of the whole sample, and minimum information may result. Telephone interviews generally give a higher response rate but may limit the questionnaire length. Interviews in the home, although they may give the most information, also cost the most.

Whatever the method used, it is worth the time to identify the people who are most important to reach so that pertinent messages can be developed and communication channels established. In this process, decisions can be made about audiences that will not be targeted, assuring that the available resources will be used in the most cost-effective manner.

Reaching the Disadvantaged

In 1987 and 1988, the NCI's National Advisory Board sponsored public hearings in Los Angeles, Atlanta, Miami, Dallas and Philadelphia. As a result of these hearings, the Board recommended intensified efforts to provide cancer information, prevention, and early detection programs to special population groups for whom a combination of economic disadvantage and indigenous cultural factors impede access to the health care system.[12] Groups to be included are the poor, older Americans, blacks, Hispanics, Asian-Americans, and native Americans.

Several studies[13-17] have defined serious cancer problems in the disadvantaged populations. For instance, from 1978 to 1981, blacks experienced annual cancer mortality substantially higher than did whites for several cancer sites (cervix, uterus, esophagus, larynx, lung, pancreas, prostate, and stomach).[13] Blacks delay for 3 to 12 months before seeking diagnosis and treatment for cancer.[8] There is also evidence of a relationship between low socioeconomic levels and cancer incidence. Several racial and ethnic groups have severe problems in this area (Table 57-2). For example, women of lower socioeconomic status are less likely to have regular examinations, such as Papanicolaou (Pap) tests for cervical cancer.[17] Hispanic

TABLE 57-2 Sociodemographic Characteristics of United States Population Subgroups

	Ethnic/Racial Background				
Characteristics	White	Black	Hispanic	Asian Pacific	Native American
Percentage of total US population	79.6	11.5	6.4	1.6	0.9
Median age	31.6	24.9	23.2	28.7	22.4
Percentage high school graduates	88	79	58	75	31
Median annual income in dollars	23,270±	13,270±	16,228±	22,713*	15,900*
Percentage below poverty level	11‡	34‡	30§	13.1*	29*
Percentage unemployed	8.6§	18.9§	13.8§	4.7*	13§
Average fertility rate per family	1.7†	2.3†	2.3†	—	4.0†
Percentage of households headed by women	10.9	37.7	23	11	24

*1979
†1980
‡1981
§1982
Source: Reprinted with permission from Ramirez AG, MacKellar DA, Gallion K: Reaching minority audiences: A major challenge in cancer reduction. Cancer Bull 40:334-343, 1988. Copyright Medical Arts Publishing Foundation, Houston, Texas.

women have twice the incidence of cervical cancer as do non-Hispanic white women.[14]

Other issues related to ethnic minorities create special requirements for cancer prevention information. On the average, blacks are less aware of cancer signs, available treatment options, and early detection techniques and their importance.[13] Both blacks and Hispanics underestimate the prevalence of cancer and have a fatalistic attitude about the disease.[17] There are also voids in almost every area of research in the minority population. For instance, the literature on the black population and cancer prevention research, cancer intervention studies, and clinical trials studies is particularly scant,[18] signalling a major opportunity for nurses.

There are several strategies for implementing health education programs in communities where the socioeconomically disadvantaged live and work. It is useful, especially in the early planning stages, to make a list of leaders who can provide information and access into the community. The list includes those persons who are respected and have personal contacts with the specific audience to be reached. The influentials can include any of the following categories[8]: church leaders, leaders in the school system, merchants and other members of the business community, members of the media, health care providers, government and civic leaders, officers of fraternal orders, and leaders in teenage communities. The influential leaders can help identify the needs of the community and assist with education programs where people live, work, and play.

Social service and health organizations are an important point of entry into these communities. A program's success can be increased by coordinating with these trusted and respected organizations and working through their existing programs. Creating special health events that address the concerns of the audience and adding them to established neighborhood-based efforts can also help ensure success.

Health education programs must take into consideration the many socioeconomic and cultural characteristics among minorities. The following considerations must be addressed during the development stage to assure successful programs for reaching the socioeconomically disadvantaged audiences.

1. *The family.* The family is a dominant influence on many minority populations and can be a credible source of health-related information. On the other hand, depending on factors, such as the disease being discussed or the type of program being planned, the family can also be a major barrier. For instance, in the Native American population, tribal elders may need to be used as role models to assure the program's success.

2. *The community.* Many minority groups, especially those who have recently come to this country, strongly identify with neighborhood and community groups. In rural areas and in some neighborhoods, the community may act as an extension of the family and become the focus of social interaction. There may be a distinct microculture, such as a religious society, within a community. Knowing the community structure is essential. It can open up different locations for presenting health education messages—such as in churches and barber shops, libraries and malls, and gyms and bodegas (stores in Hispanic neighborhoods).

3. *The language.* Language can be a significant barrier, especially in those areas where new settlers to the country are located. It is crucial, when producing materials in different languages, to involve persons who understand the nuances of the language. In some communities, language can be a major obstacle to conducting successful health education programming, and extra time and planning will be needed to ensure success.

4. *Folk beliefs and traditions.* Some minorities have strong beliefs and traditions in folk medicines, depending on cultural mores. Programming may need to incorporate these beliefs and traditions to enhance messages or at least to determine their potential impact.

5. *The influence of poverty.* Some people who live in poverty develop a sense of powerlessness, a loss of control over the outcomes of day-to-day living. Self-esteem may be lost, along with the hope for a better life. In addition, some may have a short-term perspective in living. The day-to-day stresses of crime and drugs, of foraging for meals and an existence, make issues like cancer risk seem unimportant. These influences create serious obstacles to programming for health education on issues such as cancer prevention and behavioral changes.

Reaching the Elderly

As people grow older, there seems to be a greater need to reach them, especially with messages concerning cancer screening. Approximately 50% of all cancers occur in persons over 65, with certain ones (stomach, prostate, colon and rectum in men, breast in women) accounting for over 50% of invasive cancers in persons over 60.[10] Stromborg-Frank[11] notes that the elderly are being divided into three categories: young-old (65 to 74 years), older-old (75 to 85 years) and old-old (85 years and over), a practice that helps in delivering public education messages, since cancer incidence of specific sites varies significantly with age.

The elderly population provides different challenges and obstacles to anyone presenting health education messages. These individuals have beliefs and attitudes acquired over a lifetime that may significantly influence their health practices.

A study conducted at Fox Chase Cancer Center[17] showed that most older people did not realize they are at increased risk for cancer. In addition, more than 50% of the older people surveyed believed cancer treatments are worse than the disease and had negative attitudes about physicians (80% thought that physicians cause patients to worry because they do not explain everything). In general, older persons are usually not as aware of their risk of developing cancer, are less likely to participate in screening programs, and are less likely to practice self-examination. The elderly also are more apt to underreport significant symptoms and thus present to the health care system with more advanced disease. This may be due to the fact that aches and pains are seen as more normal occurrences among the elderly and taken for granted rather than viewed as a potential symptom of disease.[19]

Dellefield[19] defines several topics that must be addressed in educating older persons: (1) the increased risk of developing cancer with advancing age, (2) the seven warning signals of cancer, (3) normal vs abnormal changes of aging, (4) the health maintenance practices recommended by the ACS, (5) the benefits of early detection in relation to reduced morbidity and mortality, (6) the acceptability and management of cancer treatments, (7) the skills and coping strategies needed to make the elderly more successful as patients in the contemporary health care system, and (8) the community resources available to provide early detection services and assistance in developing better self-care skills.

On average, the elderly do not learn as quickly and as easily as do younger persons. They may not see and hear as well. They may have had many negative lifetime experiences with cancer and cancer treatment. In preparing materials and in presenting programs to this target group, special attention must be paid to specific strategies to overcome these barriers.

Socializing and social atmospheres are attractive to this target population. Taking advantage of already existing meetings, such as senior citizens groups, may add to a program's success. Using positive, wellness-related tactics is another strategy. A gastroenterologist in Connecticut found that entitling his program "The Care and Feeding of Your Digestive Tract" rather than "Cancer of the Colon" increased his audiences twofold. Older Americans are an important group to target. They present special problems and have distinct barriers that must be overcome if programming is to be successful. Table 57-3 summarizes the strategies for reaching special audiences.

TABLE 57-3 Reaching Special Audiences

Production of Materials	Strategies for Older Learners	Strategies for Lower Socioeconomic Groups
Use language appropriate to different cultural groups (one word may have different meanings to different groups).	Keep learning sessions brief (10 to 15 minutes) and pace instruction.	Work through existing programs and agencies.
Understand values and customs for each cultural group.	Avoid rushing the learner.	Work through people already trusted in the community.
Identify channels that will be credible and most capable of reaching minority audiences.	Proceed from the simple to the complex.	Try to create programs incorporating your needs into already ongoing programs.
Use current information to choose the best channels and message strategies.	Focus and maintain attention on a single well-defined piece of information.	Use concern for family as a motivator.
Develop separate message appeals for each minority group, since perceived needs, values, and beliefs may differ.	Use concrete examples, short sentences, slow speech, and much repetition.	Stress payoffs for changing attitudes or beliefs.
Use simply written print materials, reinforced with graphics and pretested.	Use redundant or multiple cuing; say it, draw it, write it.	Create simple, concrete messages.
Pretest both print and graphics. People perceive graphics and illustrations in different ways, just as words have different meanings.	Allow the initial learning tasks to proceed slowly.	Use visual materials—people learn more by seeing than by any other method.
Use bilingual materials to ensure that intermediaries and family members who are most comfortable with English can help readers understand content.	Do not present new information until earlier concepts have been mastered.	Use both visual and written materials to reinforce messages.
Do not simply translate print materials from the English; rewrite the material, since concepts and appeals may differ by culture just as the words do.	Allow ample time for learning tasks involving psychomotor skills.	Repeat the same message and same themes.
Consider audiovisual materials or interpersonal communication that may be more successful for some messages and audiences.	Deemphasize tasks involving abstract reasoning.	Use television as a primary channel.
	Minimize the number of alternative responses available.	Use personalized, direct mail messages.
	Compensate for sensory changes by using nonglare lighting, large print, mid- to low-pitched speaking voice, and a quiet environment.	
	Use social support to reinforce learning.	
	Provide positive feedback to make learner aware of progress.	
	Express warmth and respect.	

Source: Adapted from National Cancer Institute: Making Health Communications Programs Work: A Planner's Guide. Bethesda, MD, Office of Cancer Communications, The Institute, NIH pub. no. 89-1493, 1989; and Dellefield ME: Informational needs and approaches for early cancer detection in the elderly. Semin Oncol Nurs 7:156-168, 1988.

Making Written Materials Easier to Read

One of the major problems facing those producing printed health communications materials is how to make them easy to read. About 20% of the adult American population reads at or below the fifth-grade level. An additional 35% reads at the fifth- to tenth-grade level.[20] Yet cancer materials being used for general information and education are written at higher levels. For instance, the NCI pamphlet "Goods News for Blacks About Cancer" is written at a seventh-grade level. The ACS pamphlet "Fry Now, Pay Later," about skin cancer, is written at an 11th-grade level. A Readers Digest article, "Why Can't We Get the Medicine We Need," tests at a 14th-grade level.

In the area of patient information, there is also a wide gap between the readability level of commonly used health-teaching materials and patients' reading comprehensive skills. Much of the material is written at a 10th-grade level, although the average patients have word-recognition skills at about the seventh-grade level; they state, however, that they are high school graduates.[20]

Both the NCI and the ACS are working to produce more materials in easy-to-read language and format. A series of simple, one-page cards on each of the major cancer sites has been produced by the ACS (Figure 57-1) with the message in English on one side and Spanish on the other. These have a fifth-grade readability level.

Performing readability tests

Readability testing measures the approximate level of education needed to understand printed materials. Most of the formulas used to test how readable an item is take into account the difficulty of the words being used and length of sentences. Short sentences and words of two syllables or less make materials easier to read. The Office of Cancer Communications of the NCI reviewed twelve readability formulas and chose the SMOG grading system for testing its own materials because it is easy to use and accurate.[7]

A basic description of how the SMOG system is used follows:

1. Pick 10 consecutive sentences near the beginning, in the middle, and at the end of the material (30 sentences total).
2. Count the words that have three or more syllables, including repeats of those words.
3. Using the conversion numbers listed below, find the approximate grade level that a person must have reached to understand fully the text being examined (the grade will be plus or minus 1.5 grades).

Word count	*Grade level*
0-2	4
3-6	5
7-12	6
13-20	7
21-30	8
31-42	9
43-56	10
57-72	11
73-90	12
91-110	13
111-132	14
133-156	15
157-182	16
183-210	17
211-240	18

Guidelines for producing simpler material

To produce materials that will be understandable to the general audience, use the following guidelines:

- Pick short words—two syllables or less.
- Create short sentences. It makes you write more simply.
- Use short paragraphs—limit each one to one idea.
- Pick simple language.
- Write to one person, using action verbs and a conversational style.
- Use the same words to describe an item. Do not say "cancer" one time and "tumor" the next.
- Use examples to illustrate important points.
- Do not use abbreviations.
- Repeat the same information in several ways. Write it. Show a picture or sketch of it. Make a chart out of it.
- Use subheads to tell the reader what is coming.
- Break up the text with graphics at key points, using bold face type, bullets, underlining, or boxed text.
- Summarize at the end of major points.
- Do a readability test; if the level is too high, go back and try again.

THE MEDIA AS GATEKEEPER

The media is an essential part of many programs for communicating with and educating the public. The mass media, which includes radio, television, wire service, newspapers, and magazines, can also involve other channels such as direct mail, billboards, and transit cards. Mass media transmits information quickly to a broad audience and is probably the public's main source of information. The media plays an important role for some target au-

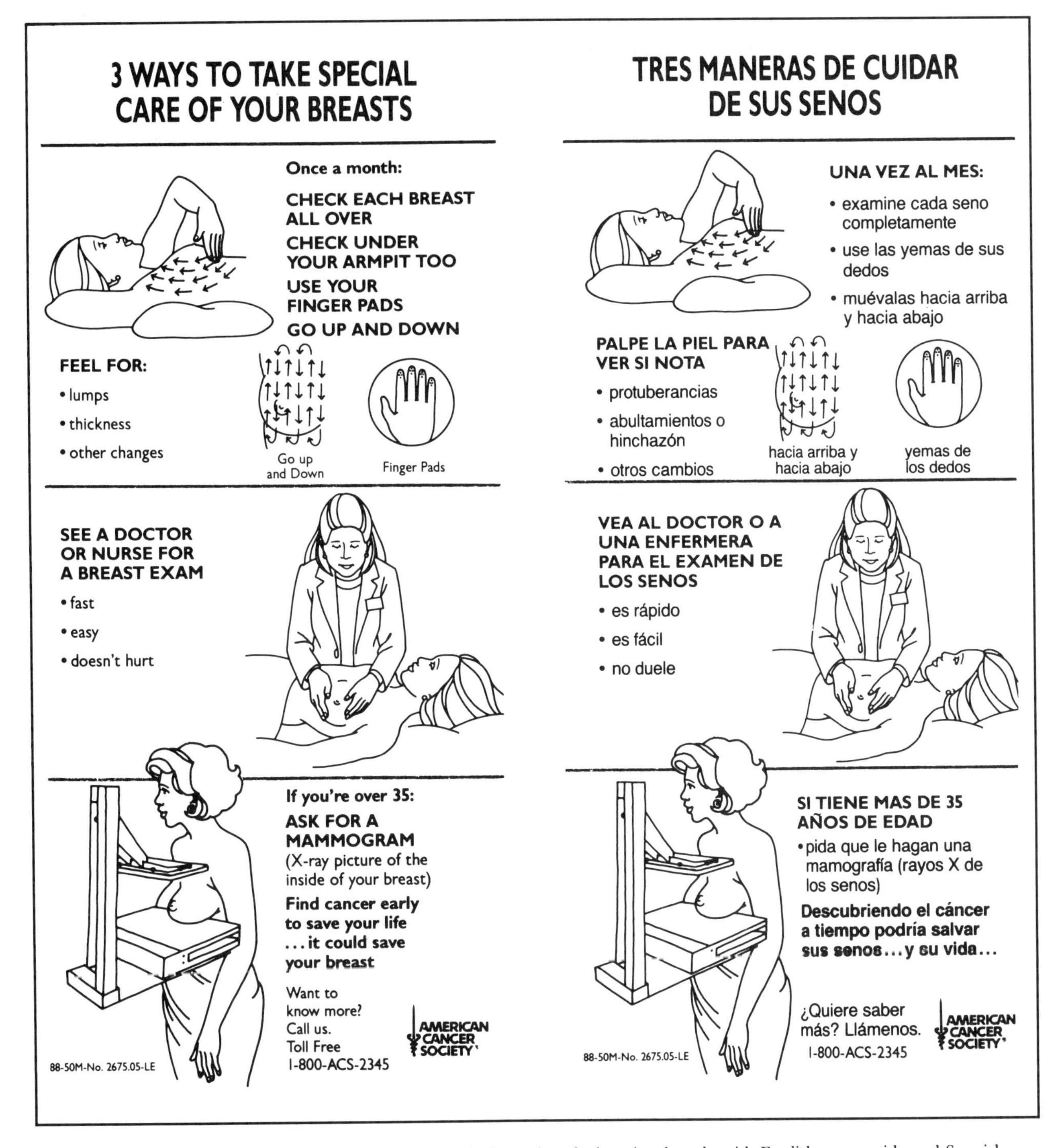

FIGURE 57-1 The American Cancer Society has published a series of educational cards, with English on one side and Spanish on the other, written at a fifth-grade level. (Source: American Cancer Society: Three Ways to Take Special Care of Your Breasts. Atlanta, Ga, The Society, pub no. 88-2675.05-LE, 1988.)

diences, since the average American has a television set turned on for almost 7 hours a day and individual family members watch television approximately 3 hours each. In addition, most Americans read a newspaper daily.

Drawbacks of Mass Media

Mass media has several drawbacks when used for public education about cancer: (1) its main purpose is to inform and entertain rather than to educate, (2) it is difficult to use for transmitting complex messages, (3) it has major constraints on space and time, and (4) it carries a high risk of miscommunication, particularly if the material is controversial (Table 57-4).

Public service announcements (PSAs), which the mass media will carry for free for nonprofit organizations, are often thought of as the major use of the mass media for public education purposes. Since deregulation, however, television and radio stations are no longer required to

TABLE 57-4 Characteristics of Mass Media Channels

	Television	Radio	Magazines	Newspapers
Audiences	Potentially largest/wide range of audiences, but not always at times when public service announcements (PSAs) are most likely to be broadcast.	Various formats offer potential for more audience targeting than television (eg, teenagers through rock stations). May reach fewer people than television.	Can more specifically target to segments of public (young women, people with an interest in health)	Can reach broad audiences rapidly.
	Can reach low-income and other audiences not as likely to turn to health sources for help.	Can reach audiences who do not use the health care system.	Audience has chance to clip, reread, contemplate material.	Easy audience access to in-depth issue coverage is possible.
Availability of public service announcements	Deregulation ended government oversight of station broadcast of PSAs, public affairs	Deregulation ended government oversight of stations' broadcast of PSAs, public affairs programming.	No requirement for PSA use; PSAs more difficult to place.	PSAs are virtually nonexistent.
Special opportunities	Opportunity to include health messages through broadcasts, public affairs/interview shows, dramatic programming.	Opportunity for direct audience involvement through call-in shows.	Can explain more complex health issues, behaviors.	Can convey health news/breakthroughs more thoroughly than television or radio and faster than magazines. Feature placement possible.
Visual and audio appeals	Visual as well as audio make emotional appeals possible. Easier to demonstrate a behavior.	Audio alone may make messages less intrusive.	Visual effects can be intensified	Print may lend itself to more factual, detailed, rational message delivery.
Convenience	Passive consumption by viewer; viewers must be present when message aired; less than full attention likely. Message may be obscured by commercial "clutter."	Generally passive consumption; exchange with audience possible, but target audience must be there when aired.	Permits active consultation; may pass on; read at reader's convenience.	Short life of newspaper limits rereading, sharing with others.
Flexibility	PSAs can be expensive to produce and distribute. Feature placement requires contacts and may be time-consuming.	Live copy is very flexible and inexpensive; PSAs must fit station format. Feature placement requires contacts and may be time-consuming.	Public service advertisements are inexpensive to produce; ad or article placement may be time-consuming.	Small papers may take public service ads; coverage demands a newsworthy item.

Source: National Cancer Institute: Making Health Communications Programs Work: A Planner's Guide. Bethesda, Md, Office of Cancer Communications, National Cancer Institute, NIH pub no. 89-1493, 1989.

donate a specific amount of time to public service programming, and the number of PSAs being carried has diminished. Although well-planned and well-produced PSAs can be effective, many other opportunities exist in the mass media, such as news programs, public affairs programs, interview and talk shows, local television panel discussions, call-in programs, editorials, letters to the editors, and health and political columns.

There are professionals ("media gatekeepers") in the media who decide what material will be used and when it will be used. It is their responsibility to understand what the public wants. If the health information messages or programming do not fit into the gatekeepers' needs, they will not be used or they will be used at odd hours or, in the case of print media, will be placed in nonprominent positions. It is a challenge to produce materials that are appealing to media formats and relevant to media needs as well as to target audiences.

Beliefs Among Gatekeepers

Stuyck and Chilton [21] conducted a study to examine the role of mass media gatekeepers in disseminating cancer information. The study gathered information on the beliefs among gatekeepers of the major health problems, the perception of their roles, and their opinions on materials they received for cancer information. The following are observations and recommendations based on the information gained from the study:

1. Disease mortality and morbidity in themselves do not guarantee media interest. Cancer and acquired immune deficiency syndrome (AIDS) ranked highest as important health care issues. Cardiovascular disease was ranked by less than half to be among the three major health concerns (although heart disease annually kills more than twice as many Americans as does cancer). There was little correlation between the prevalence or impact of disease and related problems and their relative rank among health issues.

2. Health professionals should be armed with information before approaching the media. Most gatekeepers feel a responsibility to educate the public but consider themselves trained to report and write, and they expect health educators to be informed about the issues and about the needs of the media.

3. Health communicators should be aggressive if they wish to achieve results. In the Stuyck and Chilton survey,[21] there was a correlation between how often the gatekeepers were contacted by persons in the cancer field and how often they covered cancer news. Since the gatekeepers did not consider reporting cancer news as a top priority for their media, health communicators must be knowledgeable and active advocates for their causes.

4. The media are more likely to pay attention to information from sources they perceive to be credible. Among seven factors with the potential for influencing news coverage, the credibility of the news source was ranked highest, significantly above others such as management interests and audience or readership surveys. Gatekeepers also said they were most likely to cover a news story from an institution with a reputation in cancer.

5. Media gatekeepers want information they consider useful to their audiences. Gatekeepers showed great interest in helping their audiences become informed consumers in the area of cancer, especially in advances in cancer treatment and risk reduction (tobacco and nutrition).

6. Media gatekeepers want information that is clearly written and is brief. The main reason for not using materials sent to them by health professionals were inappropriate format (43%), lack of space or time (28%), and uninteresting material (18%). Complicated terminology and inability of physicians and scientists to discuss findings in simple language were also cited. Ways in which the information could be improved include tailoring the information to local audiences (29%), making information more concise (18%) or simple and clear (13%), and sending information on a regular basis (8%). Gatekeepers from all types of media were interested in receiving materials they perceived as relevant to their audiences and of help in doing their jobs.

This study emphasizes the importance of looking at material being produced and disseminated through the eyes of the people who control its use, be they news directors or public service directors at radio and television stations or medical reporters, science writers, life-style editors, or journalists in the print media.

EXAMPLES OF PUBLIC EDUCATION ACTIVITIES

If one were to consider all the activities that educate and inform the public about health in the media and in community sites of various descriptions, around the country, they would number in the thousands per month. In the government arena alone, some 20 agencies directly offer information related to cancer prevention and detection (Table 57-5). The activities range from a simple talk before a woman's group to complex curricula proposed for school systems in entire states, from an 8-second mention on a local television news program to the organization of a national 1-day event such as the Great American Smokeout. The evaluation of these programs also varies widely—from none at all to highly sophisticated. Two major activities have been selected and will be considered in this section—smoking-related programs and the Cancer Information Service.

Helping People to Stop Smoking

There have been programs in the United States to help people to stop smoking since the 1950s. Although more than 40 million Americans have stopped smoking since the first Surgeon General's report on smoking and health in 1964, over 50 million Americans continue to smoke.[10] There are more heavy smokers today than ever before.[10] To help these people quit and to make the Surgeon General's goal of a smoke-free society by the year 2000 will require a major effort by all the health groups in this country. It will also require knowledge of the most effective intervention strategies and widespread implementation of these strategies.

The NCI commissioned a comprehensive review and evaluation of smoking cessation methods in the United States and Canada for the years 1978 to 1985, as an update to a review carried out under the auspices of the Centers for Disease Control (CDC) for the years 1969 to 1977 (an earlier review of smoking control methods was supported by the National Clearinghouse for Smoking and Health

TABLE 57-5 Government Agencies as Resources for Cancer Education

Agency	Major Programs	Special Features
CENTER FOR HEALTH PROMOTION AND EDUCATION CENTERS FOR DISEASE CONTROL Building 1 South, Room SSB249 1600 Clifton Road, NE Atlanta, GA 30333 (404) 329-3492	Provides technical assistance to state and local health departments Coordinates Behavior Risk Factor Surveillance System (BRFS). Implements School Health Education Program (SHED). Maintains Health Education Database (HED).	Tracks risk factors in population with BRSF-telephone survey on smoking, alcohol, nutrition. SHFD evaluates impact of program on students' health related behaviors. HED gives on line, computer summary of health education efforts.
CLEARINGHOUSE FOR OCCUPATIONAL SAFETY AND HEALTH INFORMATION NATIONAL INSTITUTE FOR OCCUPATIONAL SAFETY AND HEALTH Technical Information Branch 4676 Columbia Parkway Cincinnati, OH 45226 (513) 684-8326	Provides technical information to Institute's research programs. Gives information to others on request.	
CLEARINGHOUSE ON HEALTH INDEXES NATIONAL CENTER FOR HEALTH STATISTICS Division of Epidemiology and Health Promotion 3700 East-West Highway, Room 2-27 Hyattsville, MD 20782	Provides informational assistance in development of health measures for researchers, administrators and planners.	
CONSUMER INFORMATION CENTER GENERAL SERVICES ADMINISTRATION Pueblo, CO 81009 (303) 948-3334	Distributes consumer publications on many topics, such as food and nutrition, health, and exercise.	Provides *Consumer Information Catalog* from which to order publications.
CONSUMER PRODUCT SAFETY COMMISSION Washington, DC 20207 (301) 492-6800 (800) 638-2772 (Hotline)	Sets standards and conducts information programs on potentially hazardous products, such as carcinogens.	Independent Federal regulatory agency. Has jurisdiction over consumer products in and around home.
FOOD AND NUTRITION INFORMATION CENTER U.S. DEPARTMENT OF AGRICULTURE National Agricultural Library Building-Room 304 Beltsville, MD 20705 (301) 344-3719	Serves information needs of professionals interested in nutrition education, food services and food technology.	Acquires and lends books, journal articles and audiovisual materials.
NATIONAL AUDIOVISUAL CENTER NATIONAL ARCHIVES 8700 Edgeworth Drive Capitol Heights, MD 20743-3701 (301) 763-1896 (301) 763-4385 (TDD)	Distributes more than 8000 programs on over 600 topics, including cancer and environment, cancer detection, smoking, specific cancer sites.	Central source for federally sponsored audiovisuals. Charges for audiovisuals and accompanying materials.
DIVISION OF CANCER PREVENTION AND CONTROL NATIONAL CANCER INSTITUTE National Institutes of Health Bethesda, MD 20892-4200 (301) 496-6616	Plans and conducts basic and applied research programs aimed at reducing cancer incidence, morbidity and mortality. Plans, directs and coordinates the support of basic and applied research on cancer prevention and control at cancer centers and community hospitals. Coordinates programs activities with Federal and state agencies. Establishes liaison with professional and voluntary health agencies, labor organizations, cancer organizations and trade associations.	Activities carried out across five phases of research: hypothesis development, methods testing, controlled intervention, trials, defined population studies and demonstrations relevant to the prevention and management of cancer.

TABLE 57-5 Government Agencies as Resources for Cancer Education (continued)

Agency	Major Programs	Special Features
OFFICE OF CANCER COMMUNICATIONS NATIONAL CANCER INSTITUTE National Institute of Health Bethesda, MD 20892 (301) 496-6631	Provides information on all aspects of the cancer problem to physicians, scientists, educators, Congress, the Executive Branch, the media and the public. Fosters and coordinates a national cancer communications programs designed to provide the public and health professionals with information they need to take more responsible health actions.	The Cancer Information Service (1-800-4-CANCER) is located with this office, with a network of locations across the country.
OFFICE OF PREVENTION, EDUCATION, AND CONTROL NATIONAL HEART, LUNG, AND BLOOD INSTITUTE (NHLBI) National Institute of Health 9000 Rockville Pike Bethesda, MD 20892 (301) 496-5437	Initiates educational activities for NHLBI which fosters informational and educational activities designed to reduce preventable heart, lung, and blood disease morbidity and mortality.	
NATIONAL CLEARINGHOUSE FOR ALCOHOL INFORMATION NATIONAL INSTITUTE ON ALCOHOL ABUSE AND ALCOHOLISM P.O. Box 2345 Rockville, MD 20852 (301) 468-2600	Gathers and disseminates current information on alcohol-related subjects. Provides literature searches, referrals, a library and reading room and summaries of current alcohol-related information.	Responds to requests from the public, health professionals, scientists, and other professionals.
NATIONAL LIBRARY OF MEDICINE NATIONAL INSTITUTES OF HEALTH 8600 Rockville Pike Bethesda, MD 20892 (301) 496-6308 Public Information Office (301) 496-6095 Reference Station	Collects, organizes and disseminates both printed and audiovisual materials, technical and scientific in nature, primarily for medical professionals. Offers extensive computerized literature retrieval service.	Listing of bibliographies, catalogs and indexes with specific ordering instructions is available from the Public Information Office.
NATIONAL MATERNAL AND CHILD HEALTH CLEARINGHOUSE 38th and R Street, NW Washington, DC 20057 (202) 625-8410	Provides information and publications on maternal and child health and genetics, including topics such as smoking and pregnancy and nutrition and pregnancy.	Provides materials to consumers and health professionals.
NATIONAL TOXICOLOGY PROGRAM NATIONAL INSTITUTE OF ENVIRONMENTAL HEALTH SCIENCES M.D. B2-04, Box 12233 Research Triangle Park, NC 27709 (919) 541-3991	Develops and disseminates scientific information regarding potentially hazardous chemicals, including those which can cause cancer. Coordinates research conducted by four agencies of the Department of Health and Human Services.	Information in the form of technical reports is available free of charge to scientists and other health professionals.
OFFICE OF CONSUMER AFFAIRS FOOD AND DRUG ADMINISTRATION 5600 Fishers Lane Rockville, MD 20857 (301) 443-3170	Responds to consumer inquiries. Serves as clearinghouse for consumer publications on a variety of topics including pregnancy, food and nutrition, cosmetics, proper use of drugs and health fraud.	Over 250 publications available free of charge.

TABLE 57-5 Government Agencies as Resources for Cancer Education (continued)

Agency	Major Programs	Special Features
NATIONAL HEALTH INFORMATION CLEARINGHOUSE OFFICE OF DISEASE PREVENTION AND HEALTH PROMOTION P.O. Box 1133 Washington, DC 20013-1133 800-336-4797 (202) 429-9091	Central source of information and referral for health questions from the public and health professionals. Maintains computer database of government agencies, support groups, professional societies and other organizations that can answer questions on specific health topics. Offers library containing medical and health reference books, directories, information files and periodicals; database development on organizations that provide health information; and a number of publications including resource guides and bibliographies.	Among publications prepared are *Prevention Abstracts,* which summarizes prevention-oriented findings in the scientific literature; *Prevention Activities Calendar,* which highlights major prevention events for the month; *Healthfinder Series* which provides resource lists on specific health topics such as exercise for older Americans, health risk appraisals, health statistics and many other issues; *Staying Healthy: A Bibliography of Health Promotion Materials,* which serves as a guide to current information on health promotion and disease prevention topics.
OFFICE ON SMOKING AND HEALTH U.S. DEPARTMENT OF HEALTH AND HUMAN SERVICES Technical Information Center Park Building-Room 1-10 5600 Fishers Lane Rockville, MD 20857 (301) 443-1690	Produces and distributes a number of informational and educational materials. Offers bibliographic and reference services to researchers and others. Produces pamphlets, posters and public service announcements which contain various health messages.	Materials and services are available free of charge.
PUBLIC INFORMATION CENTER ENVIRONMENTAL PROTECTION AGENCY 820 Quincy Street, NW Washington, DC 20210 (202) 829-3535	Provides information on programs and activities of the Environmental Protection Agency including topics such as hazardous wastes, the school asbestos project, air and water pollution, pesticides and drinking water.	
PUBLICATION DISTRIBUTION OFFICE OCCUPATIONAL SAFETY AND HEALTH ADMINISTRATION U.S. Department of Labor 200 Constitution Ave., NW–Room s4203 Washington, DC 20210 (202) 523-9667	Responds to inquiries about a limited number of job-related carcinogens and toxic substances.	Single copies of materials available free to general public, health professionals, industry, educational institutions and other sources.
INFORMATION OFFICE NATIONAL INSTITUTE ON AGING Federal Building, 6th Floor 9000 Rockville Pike Bethesda, MD 20892 (301) 496-1752	Distributes information for older Americans on many topics, including cancer and smoking.	
OFFICE OF MINORITY HEALTH RESOURCE CENTER P.O. Box 37337 Washington, DC 20013-7337 1-800-444-MHRC(6472)	Provides minority health information and referrals. Maintains computerized database of materials, organizations and programs. Provides network of professionals active in the field.	Provides bilingually staffed toll-free number.

Source: National Cancer Institute: Cancer Prevention Resource Directory, Bethesda, Md, Office of Cancer Communications, The Institute, NIH pub no. 86-2827, 1986.

and published in 1969). The conclusions of this review are as follows[22]:

1. Smokers prefer to quit on their own with the help of instructions, medicines, and guides. Less complex quit guides achieve higher success rates. Of people who select to quit on their own, 16% to 20% are not smoking 1 year later. These data are supported by national studies that show that of those who try to quit, 20% report that they succeed. Self-quitting seems to involve cumulative learning over repeated efforts.
2. Many people who quit act on the advice or warning of a health professional. Physician advice and counseling encourage many individuals to attempt to break their cigarette habit. Where the physician adds a stronger message, gives tips on how to quit, or provides follow-up support, the results improve.
3. The nurse is an ideal person to counsel smokers, since the nurse is viewed as a credible health worker. The nurse involves the patient's family in the counseling process so that family members can provide support and encouragement.
4. The roles of other health professionals such as dentists, dental hygienists, physician's assistants, nurse practitioners, inhalation therapists, paramedics, pharmacists, and others have not been studied adequately in terms of their effects on influencing patients to quit smoking.
5. Nicotine chewing gum (Nicorette) can be an effective tool for persons who are motivated to quit. Longer use (6 months to 1 year) appears to improve quit rates. Other methods (counseling, support) should be used to supplement the gum.
6. Hypnosis and acupuncture are popular treatments, but evaluation has been inadequate. In general, counseling and support also are needed.
7. The media reaches a wide number of smokers with instructions on how to quit smoking. Long-term quit rates are low, but these programs could be more effective if combined with group or individual instructions. Use of the telephone to promote maintenance support is noteworthy.
8. Community studies have mixed results but suggest that a combination of mass media and intensive instruction is more successful than media alone.
9. Behavioral techniques reveal a wide range of success. Adversive therapy (electric shock, breath holding, unpleasant taste, etc.) showed poor results. Rapid smoking appears to be effective in the short term. Covert sensitization (use of subject's imagination) has failed to produce long-term results but, like rapid smoking, may be useful combined with other procedures.
10. The worksite offers an excellent opportunity for implementing strategies that lead to cessation of smoking. There is a growing movement to restrict smoking in employee work areas. Some companies offer smoking cessation programs, such as educational programs, distribution of self-help kits, and physician advice during physical examinations and groups.
11. Maintenance support is the critical ingredient in the long-term success of smoking cessation. Successful quitters score higher than recidivists in personal security, ease of quitting on last attempt, expectation of success in giving up smoking, and social support. They had smoked fewer cigarettes a day before quitting and had lower levels of anxiety.
12. Leading causes of relapse are anxiety, stress, anger, frustration, social pressures, weight gain, and lack of inner resources. Being around other smokers, eating, and drinking alcohol or coffee also contribute to relapse.
13. The highest median quit rates for trials with 1-year follow-up were scored by physician intervention programs for patients with cardiac disease (these patients are highly motivated due to life-threatening illness). High quit rates were also scored by physician intervention with patients with pulmonary disorders, risk factor studies, and rapid smoking and satiation when each was combined with other procedures. Support groups and nicotine chewing gum, combined with behavioral treatment or therapy, came next.
14. A significant trend is the increased negative attitude toward cigarette smoking, as exemplified by the numerous regulations for nonsmoking sections in schools, restaurants, worksites, military areas, and other public places.

The smoking, tobacco and cancer program In 1982, the NCI launched an intervention research effort, the Smoking, Tobacco and Cancer Program, which is today supporting 60 intervention trials. These trials are evaluating the use of specific channels (schools, health care providers, mass media and self-help strategies) among target populations (youth, women, ethnic minorities, heavy smokers, and smokeless tobacco users). About half these trials have been completed, with the remaining to be completed in 1992.

These target groups were selected based on the latest smoking statistics. In 1987, 33% of men and 28% of women smoked (down from 53% and 34%, respectively, in 1964). However, because of an increase in total population, there are now 1 million more smokers than existed 10 years ago—over 50 million regular smokers.[10]

There are also many signs of problems among population groups. The proportion of teens, ages 12 through 17, who smoke increased from 12% in 1979 to over 15% in 1985. Smoking quit rates among adults have slowed, with more adults hard-core addicted smokers and more heavy smokers (25 or more cigarettes a day). Black men are more likely to smoke, are more likely to use cigarettes with a higher tar and nicotine content, and are 50% more likely to develop lung cancer than are white men. In addition, the use of smokeless tobacco products has increased, particularly among adolescent males and young men. It is estimated that at least 12 million people used smokeless tobacco in 1985.[10]

The ASSIST/2000 program The ASSIST/2000 program, a new initiative launched by the NCI in the early

1990s, supports large-scale demonstrations in states and large metropolitan areas. It includes a broad range of organizations and community groups capable of working together to coordinate the area's tobacco control resources and to implement intervention trials. The program has two phases: an 18- to 24-month planning phase, and a 5-year implementation phase.

Activities include the training of health care professionals to deliver cessation counseling, the provision of targeted cessation interventions in worksites and other locations, the implementation of tobacco-use prevention curricula in schools, and the use of print and electronic media to cover the smoking issue. The target groups are minorities, women, heavy smokers, low-income smokers, and youth. The lead organizations on the local levels are the state (or local) health departments and the ACS. The interventions will be based on the trials presently underway. An independent evaluation will be conducted using baseline and follow-up surveys of smoking and tobacco use in each geographic area funded. It is estimated that some 20 areas will be funded to begin phase II work in 1992.

The investigators involved in the Smoking, Tobacco and Cancer Program are testing the strategies to be used in ASSIST/2000 and by 1988 had already produced 166 articles in journals and scientific reports on these studies.[23] This scientific base will be used to plan the intervention by the organizations involved. ASSIST/2000 is a massive effort that will provide many challenges and opportunities for nurses.

The Cancer Information Service

As public educator

The Cancer Information Service (CIS), a program of the NCI, is a toll-free telephone service that answers questions about cancer prevention and control, diagnosis, treatment, and rehabilitation. Begun in 1976, the CIS has a network of offices throughout the country based in comprehensive cancer centers, community cancer centers, and hospitals. Using a common number (1-800-4-CANCER), calls are routed automatically to CIS offices in local areas. Since 1976, when the CIS received 47,000 calls, the calls have grown steadily to nearly 400,000 a year in the late 1980s.

CIS counselors, after completing a standardized training program, provide accurate, up-to-date information tailored to the needs of individual callers. The NCI's computerized database, PDQ (Physician's Data Query), which contains state-of-the-art treatment information and NCI-aproved clinical trials, is a major resource for treatment information.

Between 1983 and 1986, almost 50% of inquiries to the CIS were from the general public, that is, people without symptoms. The callers are predominately white (86%), female (70%), over age 30 (74%), and with at least a high school education (89%). A national user survey, carried out in 1983, of a random sample of over 7600 CIS callers, showed that the respondents found the information helpful (94%) and clear and easy to understand (96%). The CIS staff was seen as knowledgeable (95%), courteous (97%), and friendly (97%). Nearly 98% said they would call the service again if they had questions, and more than 50% had already recommended the use of CIS to others. About 93% of the callers reported taking some kind of action, with 58% sharing the information with at least one other person (information from 4091 initial inquiries reached 11,386 people). In addition, 91% indicated the CIS was important in their decisions to take action following the call.[24] As one of the oldest continuously funded programs of the NCI and as its major outreach arm, the CIS has grown in size, in quality, and in the services it offers.

As change agent

The CIS, in addition to its roles in public and patient information and in education, is increasingly acting as a change agent in the area of cancer prevention and risk reduction. In CIS offices across the country, telephone counselors have been trained in techniques to help smokers who wish to quit, based on a research project conducted at the Roswell Park CIS[24] and on basic strategies for behavior change (using a protocol concentrating on steps including precomtemplation, contemplation, action, and maintenance). The counselors assess the individual's needs, identify roadblocks and facilitators to altering personal behavior, and give the appropriate advice, referrals, and written materials to help the caller make the change. A similar training program has been conducted to enable counseling about clinical trials.

A study, currently being conducted at the University of California at Los Angeles and the University of Southern California, uses the CIS as an instrument to increase breast screening among female callers. This project attempts to change the CIS from a passive system, which depends on a specific request from the caller, to an active one, which targets particular subgroups of high-risk callers for specific cancer control messages. All female CIS callers 40 years and older who are not currently being treated for cancer will be randomized within these groups: group I (information about mammography will only be given in response to a specific request by the caller); group II (information about breast screening and age-specific behavioral recommendations will be given, following a strict intervention protocol, to all callers regardless of their initial reason for calling the CIS; and group III (will receive the same intervention as group II but will be contacted 2 weeks after the initial call to reinforce adherence to the behavioral recommendations).

The intervention protocol is grounded in communications and persuasion theory. Assessment of the outcome (self-reported adherence to the mammography recommendations made by the CIS) will be by telephone interview 6 months after the initial call, along with measures of attitudes, barriers, beliefs, and intentions related to mammography.[24]

This new thrust of the CIS into the role of change agent has the potential for major impact. It uses an existing system with a proven track record for satisfying the needs of people who wish cancer information in a new and different way. These studies, showing that a telephone system can be used to reinforce positive health messages and stimulate encouraging behavioral change, could provide a new catalyst to altering knowledge and health practices.

CHALLENGES FOR THE FUTURE

There have been many changes in public information and education during the 1980s. The cancer field, led by the NCI and the ACS, has kept pace, using sophisticated marketing techniques. New opportunities will continue, and health professionals must join with colleagues in other areas to meet them.

As health professionals work toward reaching the NCI's Year 2000 goals, a number of challenges present themselves: how to develop interventions most effectively to reduce the cancer risk, how to implement those interventions to reach the greatest number of people at risk, how to plan public education programs that will use resources, both nationally and locally, to their greatest benefits, and how to plan and implement programs that will be sensitive to the needs of minority and other target audiences. These challenges demand new ways of thinking, new interrelationships, and new methods of operation. Nurses can assume a leadership role in providing innovative, research-based educational opportunities that will help meet these challenges.

REFERENCES

1. Gochman DS: Health Behavior: Emerging Research Perspectives. New York, Plenum Press, 1988.
2. Kolbe LJ: The application of health behavior and research: Health education and health information, in Gochman DS (ed): Health Behavior: Emerging Research Perspectives. New York, Plenum Press, 1988, pp 381-396.
3. Green LW, Kreuter MW, Deeds SG, et al: Health Education Planning: A Diagnostic Approach. Palo Alto, Calif, Mayfield Publishing Co, 1980.
4. Rosenstock IM: Historical Origins of the Health Belief Model. Health Ed monographs 2:328-35, 1974.
5. Berlo DK: The Process of Communication: An Introduction to Theory and Practice. New York, Holt, Rinehart & Winston, 1960.
6. Kotler P, Andreasen AR: Strategic Marketing for Nonprofit Organizations (ed 3). Englewood Cliffs, NJ, Prentice-Hall, 1987.
7. National Cancer Institute: Making Health Communications Programs Work: A Planner's Guide. Bethesda, Md, Office of Cancer Communications, The Institute, NIH pub no. 89-1493, 1989.
8. National Cancer Institute: Making The Right Connection. Bethesda, Md, Office of Cancer Communication, The Institute, 1989.
9. National Career Institute: Cancer Control Objectives for the Nation: 1985-2000. NCI monograph no. 2, Appendix B. Bethesda, Md, Division of Cancer Prevention and Control, The Institute, October 1986.
10. American Cancer Society: Cancer Facts and Figures—1989. Atlanta, Ga, The Society, 1989.
11. Stromborg-Frank M: The role of the nurse in early detection of cancer: Population sixty-six years and older. Oncol Nurs Forum 13(3):66-74, 1986.
12. National Cancer Institute: Fighting Cancer in America: Findings and Recommendations of the 1987-88 Public Participation Hearings of the National Cancer Advisory Board on Cancer Prevention and Early Detection. Bethesda, Md, Office of Cancer Communications, The Institute, 1989.
13. US Department of Health and Human Resources: Report of the Secretary's Task Force on Black and Minority Health (Vol III), Cancer, 1986. Washington, DC, US Government Printing Office, 1986.
14. US Department of Health and Human Resources: Report of the Secretary's Task Force on Black and Minority Health (Vol VIII), Hispanic Health Issues. Washington, DC, US Government Printing Office, 1986.
15. Porter/Novelli: Cancer Prevention and Control Needs of Disadvantaged Americans: An Exploratory Study. Atlanta, Ga, The American Cancer Society, 1988.
16. Ramirez AG, MacKellar DA, Gallion K: Reaching minority audiences: A major challenge in cancer reduction. Cancer Bull 40:334-343, 1988.
17. Wilson CM, Rimer BK, Bennett DJ, et al: Educating the older cancer patient: Obstacles and opportunities. Health Ed Q 10:76-87, 1984.
18. National Cancer Institute: Annotated Bibliography of Cancer-Related Literature on Black Populations. Bethesda, Md, The Institute, Division of Cancer Prevention and Control, NIH pub no. 89-3024, 1989.
19. Dellefield ME: Informational needs and approaches for early cancer detection in the elderly. Semin Oncol Nurs 7:156-168, 1988.
20. Doak CC, Doak LG, Root JH: Teaching Patients with Low Literary Skills. Philadelphia, JB Lippincott, 1985.
21. Stuyck SC, Chilton JA: Examining the role of mass media gatekeepers in disseminating cancer information. Cancer Bull 40:334-343, 1988.
22. Schwartz JL: Review and Evaluation of Smoking Cessation Methods: The United States and Canada, 1978-1985. Bethesda, MD, National Cancer Institute, Division of Cancer Prevention and Control, NIH pub no. 87-2940, 1987.
23. National Cancer Institute: Assist/2000: American Stop Smoking Intervention Study. Presentation to Board of Scientific Counselors. Bethesda, Md, The Institute, Division of Cancer Prevention and Control, October, 1988.
24. Ward JD, Duffy K, Sciandra R, et al: What the public wants to know about cancer: The Cancer Information Service. Cancer Bull 40:384-389, 1988.
25. National Cancer Institute: Cancer Prevention Resource Directory. Bethesda, Md, Office of Cancer Communications, The Institute, NIH pub no. 86-2827, 1986.
26. American Cancer Society: Three Ways To Take Special Care of Your Breasts. Atlanta, GA, The Society, pub no. 88-2675.05-LE, 1988.

Chapter 58

Teaching Strategies: The Patient

Barbara D. Blumberg, ScM

Judith (Judi) L. Bond Johnson, RN, PhD

INTRODUCTION

Approximately 75 million, about 30%, of Americans now living are expected to get cancer.[1] Given the complexity of the disease, along with the wide range of physiologic and economic accompaniments, one would expect the education of patients and their family members to be of prime concern. Within the broader context of cancer education itself, the education of those who are ill has been overshadowed by public and preventive efforts.[2]

HISTORICAL PERSPECTIVE

Patient education itself is not a new concept in health care. For years doctors and nurses, in the course of regular contact with patients, have explained illness and its consequences. As a rule, however, these efforts have been sporadic and lacking in consistency.[3]

Literary references to patient education first appeared in the 1950s. A prime factor responsible for increased attention to the field was the development of prepaid health care plans. A basic tenet of these plans was that informed self-care could reduce the costs of long-range patient care.[4] Patient education was viewed by some as a factor that facilitated such self-care.

At a 1964 conference on health education, the American Hospital Association took the position that it should act as the nationwide agency for stimulating the development of patient education programs. Their advocacy served as a milestone in the recognition of patient education within the health care system. Patient education was recommended as an integral part of patient care. This conference served as the impetus for *A Patient's Bill of Rights*,[5] which was approved by the Association's House of Delegates in 1973.

Both the National Cancer Institute's document entitled *Adult Patient Education in Cancer*[6] and the Oncology Nursing Society's *Outcome Standards in Cancer Patient Education*[7] identify a number of tasks for patient education. These include helping patients and family members adjust to the disease, participate in treatment, carry out treatment regimens, manage stress, recognize and control side effects, prevent social isolation and strengthen relationships with significant others, mobilize and manage resources, and adapt to a life of uncertainty.

In addition to these efforts are several other factors that contribute both to the historical development of patient education and to its role in the future.

1. As the population of older Americans increases, so will the number of individuals who have chronic diseases and disabilities. The emergence of chronic illness as a major health problem has provided much stimulus for the development of patient education services.[8]
2. The consumer rights movement has resulted in more patients asking for greater amounts of information and in *A Patient's Bill of Rights*. This document outlines the patient's right to know. It states that "the patient has the right to obtain . . . complete current information concerning his diagnosis, treatment, and prognosis in terms that he can be reasonably expected to understand . . ." and that "the patient has the right to refuse treatment to the extent permitted by law and to be informed of the medical consequences of his action . . . ."[5] In addition, legislation passed in Massachusetts, California, Minnesota, and Wisconsin mandates that patients be given information on treatment options for breast cancer (Massachusetts and California) or alternate modes of treatment for any disease (Minnesota and Wisconsin).
3. As a result of increasing health care costs and changing medical reimbursement policies, cost effectiveness of patient education has become a matter of concern.
4. Accountability by the health care provider has become more of a necessity and, as a result, issues related to informed consent are of greater concern. In addition, auditing of medical and nursing records, an attempt to document accountability, has become more of a routine practice.

Recent Literature

A review of articles on cancer patient education published between 1970 and 1985[9] cited growing evidence that cancer patient education can improve knowledge, attitudes, behavior, and health status. Specifically, Dodd's work with chemotherapy patients[10-13] provided evidence that planned patient education is capable of increasing self-care practices. In a study by Beck,[14] which looked at the effect of an oral care protocol on stomatitis after chemotherapy, patient education was credited with reducing infection and thus lowering financial as well as physiologic and psychologic costs of cancer. Other patient education programs have resulted in decreased anxiety and/or increased knowledge,[15-18] as well as improved self-concept and self-esteem.

On the basis of their review, Rimer and colleagues[9] suggest concise considerations for patient education programming that include the following:

- Use of a combination of education methods[11-14,17,19)]
- Enhancement of educational methods by combining them with behavioral modalities such as relaxation, guided imagery, and/or hypnosis[20-23]
- Use of repetition to improve the generally compromised recall facilities of those with cancer[24]
- Preparation of informed consent forms at a reading level and in a format conducive to their use as educational vehicles
- Development of programs with the objective of teaching self-care as part of treatment regimens[10,11,25]

- Development of programs targeted at the special needs of the older patient as well as other high-risk patient audiences

An additional review of articles on cancer patient education based on a search of the Cancerlit data base, yielded more than 200 articles and abstracts published from 1979 to 1989. Subject areas receiving the greatest attention in terms of the number of publications during this time period were AIDS, patient information needs, self-care, and chemotherapy. The cancer that received the most attention in terms of patient education publications was breast cancer.

Program Priorities

Activities of the National Cancer Institute's (NCI) Patient Education Program[26] help shed light on extant national priorities in this area:

- A needs assessment conducted with hospital-based patient educators was conducted to determine what services their institutions provide, sources of educational materials used, and continuing education needs. Responses to the needs assessment will be used to provide direction for new Patient Education Program activities directed toward health professionals.
- A directory of patient education program contacts at clinical and comprehensive cancer centers nationwide has been prepared and distributed to encourage interaction and networking.
- A specific program area targeted to the special needs of older patients has been undertaken. A state-of-the-art paper describing the needs of this audience and services available for them has been developed. In addition, a working group of experts on cancer and aging has convened to help determine program priorities. Exhibits at meetings whose members are either representative of this audience or serve their needs are ongoing, as are the preparation of print advertisements for journals that cater to these two audiences.
- Collaboration with the National Coalition for Cancer Survivorship has been undertaken to create an information and education kit for cancer survivors.
- A project has been undertaken, in conjunction with NCI's Division of Cancer Treatment, with the hope of doubling patient participation in NCI-sponsored clinical trials by 1992. Called "Patients Helping Progress: Cancer Clinical Trials," activities include presentations and seminars at Oncology Nursing Society Congress meetings, development of a training program for Cancer Information Service telephone counselors, videotapes for patient and lay audiences, and a series of "updates" on clinical trials initiatives.
- NCI's International Cancer Information Center and the Office of Cancer Communications (OCC) have joined together to revise the current patient information file (PIF) component of the Physician Data Query (PDQ) cancer treatment data base. The PIF contains information about prognosis and treatment for different types and sites of cancer. Written in lay language, it is intended for use by patients and their families.

As more people live longer, and as more of those who have cancer experience long-term control or cure, the needs of two specific audiences—the elderly and cancer survivors—take on greater importance. Specific needs of older audiences must be considered, including their peculiar beliefs, myths, and misconceptions about the disease, information style preference,[27] and concomitant medications and diseases. Although these variables are necessary considerations in the education of any audience, older persons have needs and predispositions that are unique to them and should be considered in any effort to reach them.

Fitzhugh Mullan,[28] a physician and cancer survivor, brought new light to the definition of the terms *patient* and *survivor*. He maintains that the lives of all those living with cancer are similar in concept, if not always in form, and views their needs and concerns in a continuum that he has referred to as "seasons of survival."

There are specific implications for patient education in this updated definition of "patient" as one who should be considered a "survivor" from diagnosis onward. Educational needs of the "survivor," however, change according to the specific point in the continuum that the patient inhabits at a particular point in time.

The first season—the medical or acute stage—commences with diagnosis and is focused on efforts, both diagnostic and therapeutic, to contain the illness. Educational effort at this time should focus on the medical and psychosocial needs for information and self-care. The emphasis should be on maintenance of as good a quality of life as possible by fostering a "surviving" rather than a "getting by" attitude.

The next season begins when the patient has gone into remission or has completed the primary course of treatment. This period, aptly termed "watchful waiting," has as its governing force the fear of recurrence. During this phase, the person with cancer reintegrates into the community; medical personnel do not play the major role that they did during the previous phase. Educational efforts should address both the need for continuing medical surveillance and ways to live as normal a life as possible. Teaching strategies incorporate health-promotion behaviors and a wellness concept.

The final "season" is "permanent survival" or cure. Besides "victory over the disease," those who have entered this phase of the continuum have a very special comradeship with those in the previous "seasons of survival." This phase is characterized by concerns about employability, insurability, and long-term effects of treatment (see Chapter 19, Psychosocial Dimensions: Issues in Survivorship). Educational concerns are similar to those previously mentioned. Teaching people to be their own advocates is a means of empowering them to speak for their rights.

In recognition of the ever-growing network of cancer survivors, the American Cancer Society prepared a *Cancer Survivors' Bill of Rights* to call public attention to the 5 million Americans alive today who have a history of cancer.[1] The purpose of this document is to call attention to the specific needs of the cancer survivor in areas that include continued excellence in acute cancer care, as well as ongoing lifelong medical care, health insurance, job opportunities, and interpersonal happiness. In addition, 1986 saw the birth of the National Coalition for Cancer Survivorship, an organization dedicated to the needs of the survivor.

In summary, this new emphasis on the patient as a survivor should be a major theme in patient education programming. Considering all who are diagnosed with cancer as survivors, with needs peculiar to the specific "season" they inhabit, appears to be more timely than using the more traditional medical model to delineate patient needs in the educational arena.

DEFINITIONS

In an earlier article,[29] a composite definition of patient education was developed. Patient education is a series of structured or nonstructured experiences designed to help patients cope voluntarily with the immediate crisis response to their diagnosis, with long-term adjustments, and with symptoms; gain needed information about sources of prevention, diagnosis, and care; and develop needed skills, knowledge, and attitudes to maintain or regain health status.

Patient education is able to accomplish all of this by enabling patients and their families to plan strategies for change; interpret and integrate needed information for achieving the desired attitudes or behaviors; and meet patients' specific learning needs, interests, and capabilities.[30] Patient education through a combination of learning experiences derived from joint planning by patients, significant others, and health care professionals is considered part of total health care.[31]

RATIONALE FOR PATIENT EDUCATION

Teaching is integral to healing. It is a facet of cancer rehabilitation programs. Providing structured patient education courses and classes gives people an option for coping with their cancer diagnosis. The adaptation process is enhanced by patient education efforts.[32]

First, a structured patient education program ensures that important medical and psychosocial information is made available in a consistent manner. The key word is *consistency*. When procedures or treatments are being explained as part of routine care, interruptions are certain to occur that lead to disruption in teaching time and inadvertent deletion of pieces of information. Distractions and lack of privacy inherent in the hospital environment also create a less than ideal learning environment. This can be remedied by providing a planned and scheduled time for patient education. This is not to say that the informal bedside exchange of information is not valuable. This approach should continue to be viewed as an integral part of patient care. Both approaches to providing patient education are incorporated into an overall plan. They work in concert, with each reinforcing information exchange.

Second, patient education addresses one of the major difficulties experienced by people with cancer—the loss of control over their disease and over their lives. In addition to providing information, patient education offers options, choices, and ways to engage self-care. It sets forth an expectation that people can be involved in their treatment decisions and obtain what they want and need from their health care providers. It promotes a proactive stance.

Patient education classes bring together people who have a common purpose or problem, providing opportunity for the exchange of ideas, problems, and solutions. Patients can learn from each other because of their similar situations. The educational setting is different from that of the neighborhood gathering or the doctor's waiting room. It provides a forum for exchange and a constructive guided direction for interaction between participants.

Finally, patient education broadens the opportunity for patient and provider to interact. Their roles in this setting are that of trainee and teacher. Patients gain a different perspective of their health care provider—that of facilitator and patient advocate. The relationship between patients and their health care providers can be strengthened by a broadening of the concept of partnership in health care.

DEVELOPING PATIENT EDUCATION MATERIALS AND PROGRAMS

Integral to the success of any patient education material or program is the extent to which the needs of the intended audience are met. Also called "social marketing," this perspective incorporates assessment of audience needs at particular points in the program/material development and implementation process.

Developing patient education materials and programs is viewed as a process whereby time and available resources are allocated in quantities sufficient to include concept, message, and actual resource development, along with attendant evaluations. This process is conceptualized in a six-part wheel (Figure 58-1)[33] whereby each section of the wheel represents a stage in a circular process in which the last stage feeds back to the first one in a continuous loop of replanning and improvement.

The key to the development process is pretesting, a qualitative research method executed during the development of materials and programs. The purpose of pre-

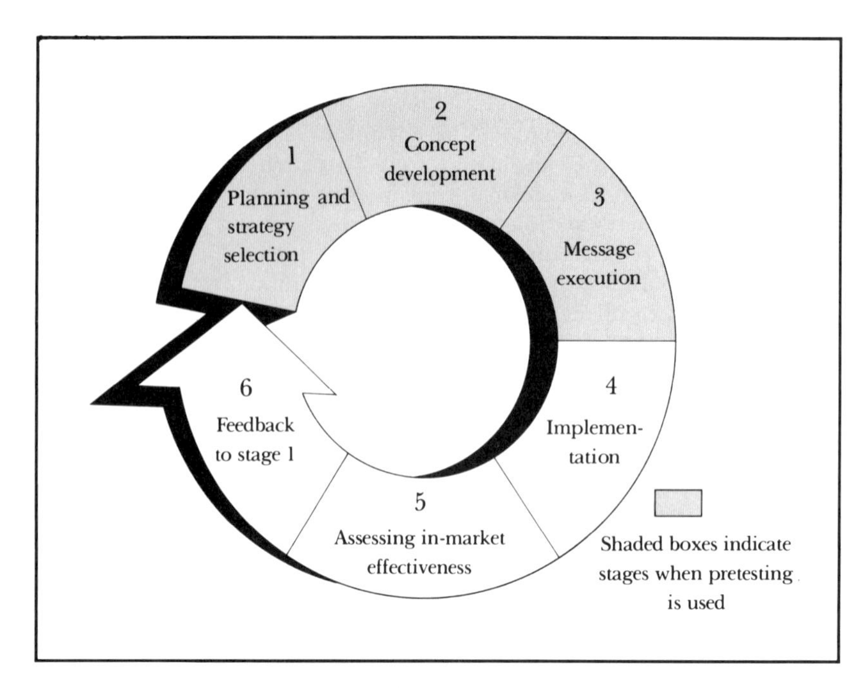

FIGURE 58-1 Stages in the development of patient education materials and resources. (Source: United States Department of Health and Human Services. Pretesting in Health Communications [NIH pub no. 84-1493]. Washington DC, US Government Printing Office, 1984.)

testing is to systematically gather target audience reactions to draft concepts and materials before final production and implementation. Pretesting is useful in determining which version of a concept, message, or material is most likely to meet stated objectives. In addition, pretesting is useful in identifying strengths and weaknesses of draft materials. Variables particularly amenable to pretesting are awareness and interest, comprehension, audience relevance, believability, acceptability, and gain in short-term knowledge.

Pretesting provides important diagnostic information that can lead to improvements in draft materials and programs before they are made widely available. It is important to recognize, however, that pretesting is a qualitative method and, as such, does not yield findings that are reportable in terms of their statistical significance. Results of pretesting are not absolutely predictive of potential success or failure of items in terms of variables pretested. Rather, pretesting provides direction on the basis of perception of needs of representative members of the target audience.

Pretesting Techniques

A host of research techniques can be usefully employed in pretesting. The particular method chosen depends on the target audience, the message or concepts being tested, objectives of the pretest, the best mode of access to the target audience, and time and resources available. In general, the techniques most conducive to pretesting of patient education materials and programs are the following: readability testing, focus group interviews, individual in-depth interviews, self-administered questionnaires, and gatekeeper review.

Readability testing is an easily employed technique that is used to predict the level of reading comprehension necessary to understand a particular written piece. After extensive review of 12 selected formulas,[33] the Office of Cancer Communication of the National Cancer Institute chose the SMOG grading formula for readability testing of its public and patient education materials.[34] SMOG was chosen because of the ease of its use and its accuracy in determining readability. This formula considers the number of words of at least three syllables in determining the grade level needed for comprehension. Table 58-1[33] describes how to apply this formula.

Focus group interviews are guided group discussions with a group of 8 to 10 individuals who share specific target audience characteristics. Interviews are led by a facilitator who uses a list of open-ended questions to guide the discussion. This technique is particularly appropriate during the concept-development stage and provides insight into audience beliefs and perceptions. Adapted from group therapy, focus group discussion encourages participants to converse about specific topics. Frequently, direct or paraphrased dialogue from focus groups can be incorporated into educational materials, making them more realistic and readable. Reactions to artwork and logos can also be gathered through use of this pretesting technique.

Individual in-depth interviews or one-on-one discussions are carried out by an interviewer who uses a prepared questionnaire that consists of both open-ended and closed-end items. This technique is appropriate when

TABLE 58-1 The SMOG Readability Formula

To calculate the SMOG reading grade level, begin with the entire written work that is being assessed, and follow these four steps:

1. Count off 10 consecutive sentences near the beginning, in the middle, and near the end of the text.

2. From this sample of 30 sentences, circle all of the words containing three or more syllables (polysyllabic), including repetitions of the same word, and total the number of words circled.

3. Estimate the square root of the total number of polysyllabic words counted. This is done by finding the nearest perfect square, and taking its square root.

4. Finally, add a constant of three to the square root. This number gives the SMOG grade, or the reading grade level that a person must have reached if he or she is to fully understand the text being assessed.

A few additional guidelines will help to clarify these directions:

- A sentence is defined as a string of words punctuated with a period (.), an exclamation point (!) or a question mark (?).
- Hyphenated words are considered as one word.
- Numbers which are written out should also be considered, and if in numeric form in the text, they should be pronounced to determine if they are polysyllabic.
- Proper nouns, if polysyllabic, should be counted, too.
- Abbreviations should be read as unabbreviated to determine if they are polysyllabic.

Not all pamphlets, fact sheets, or other printed materials contain 30 sentences. To test a text that has fewer than 30 sentences:

1. Count all of the polysyllabic words in the text.

2. Count the number of sentences.

3. Find the average number of polysyllabic words per sentence as follows:

$$\text{Average} = \frac{\text{Total \# of polysyllabic words}}{\text{Total \# of sentences}}$$

4. Multiply that average by the number of sentences *short of 30.*

5. Add that figure on to the total number of polysyllabic words.

6. Find the square root and add the constant of 3.

Perhaps the quickest way to administer the SMOG grading test is by using the SMOG conversion table. Simply count the number of polysyllabic words in your chain of 30 sentences and look up the approximate grade level on the chart.

SMOG Conversion Table*

Total Polysyllabic Word Counts	Approximate Grade Level (+ 1.5 Grades)
0-2	4
3-6	5
7-12	6
13-20	7
21-30	8
31-42	9
43-56	10
57-72	11
73-90	12
91-110	13
111-132	14
133-156	15
157-182	16
183-210	17
211-240	18

*Developed by Harold C. McGraw, Office of Educational Research, Baltimore County Schools, Towson, Maryland.

Source: United States Department of Health and Human Services: Pretesting in Health Communications (NIH pub no. 84-1493). Washington DC, US Government Printing Office, 1984.

the subjects addressed are sensitive or require in-depth probing.

Self-administered questionnaires that can be completed by the subject without the assistance of an interviewer are more widely used in gathering reactions to draft materials. Use of short, closed-end questions and a data-collection technique that ensures return of completed questionnaires is advised when this technique is employed. Hand delivering and retrieving questionnaires, offering a small incentive for return of completed questionnaires, and/or including a postage-paid return envelope are techniques that have yielded higher return rates.

Since many health education materials and programs reach their audiences by way of a health professional, it is prudent to seek review and comment from such persons during the development of programs and materials. Because of their role in determining whether a particular material or program reaches its intended audience, such health professionals are referred to as "gatekeepers." Review of draft materials by gatekeepers can be carried out through short self-administered questionnaires and can occur at the same time as the target audience review. If a discrepancy occurs between target audience needs and gatekeeper perception of these needs, deference should be made to the needs of the target audience. A memo announcing the availability of the program or material can summarize the extensive process and note that information ultimately included reflects the viewpoints of a number of persons.

The Development Process

Planning and strategy selection are the first activities in development of patient education materials and programs. During this period, a concise definition of what the material or program will address, objectives, and target audience identification are addressed. Planning and selection of educational strategies can be facilitated by conducting a needs assessment. Perusal of literature in the field and identification of other analogous materials and programs are undertaken. In addition, it may be useful to conduct a more formal assessment to determine education needs and strategies that have the greatest potential for meeting objectives.

Before development of the National Cancer Institute publication *What Are Clinical Trials All About?* a small-scale needs assessment survey was conducted, with patients, family members, and health professionals participating in clinical trials. This survey helped the staff determine that a booklet addressing specific topics would be most useful to the target audience, patient, and family members given the option of clinical trial participation.[35] Useful pretesting techniques during this stage are in-depth interviews, focus group interviews, and small-scale surveys.

During the concept-development stage, draft educational resources are developed on the basis of concepts that appear to have the greatest potential for educating the target audience. Drafts can take a variety of forms, ranging from short manuscripts with rough artwork, to slides or storyboards with accompanying dialogue, to draft posters. During the message-execution stage, draft educational resources are pretested before final production. Gatekeeper review takes place as part of pretesting to assure that those responsible for disseminating the education to the target audience are familiar with it and have had a chance to submit comments. Self-administered questionnaires are the most unobtrusive method of pretesting to employ during this stage. Pretesting comments can then be incorporated before final production.

During the next stage—implementation—the educational material or program is used with the target audience, with initial reaction monitored closely. With both informal comments and observations, along with more formal methods, initial use and usefulness of materials and programs can be assessed. Number of copies distributed, how often the program is carried out, and the value of short evaluation forms accompanying a material or program are all to be considered during this period of process evaluation.[36]

During the next stage—assessment of in-market effectiveness—the effectiveness of materials and programs in terms of meeting stated objectives is assessed. Self-administered questionnaires completed before and after exposure to the material or programs and assessment of behavioral change targeted by the material or program are sample means of outcome assessment.

The final stage in the development of educational materials and programs involves critical assessment of information gathered during pretesting, process, and outcome evaluations for the purpose of replanning. Problems incurred in use of the material or program, strengths of the material or program, and other feedback are assessed in terms of changes necessitated by actual implementation.

CLIMATE FOR LEARNING

Considerable time, energy, and money can be committed to providing quality patient education programs. However, unless peoples' health beliefs, attitudes, cultural backgrounds, and personal values are considered, patient education efforts may be less than successful.

Chaisson[37] reports on past patient education efforts from which the following mistakes were discovered by default:

1. Telling people what they should know rather than what they are ready and willing to learn.
2. Failure to individualize patient teaching content to accommodate the person's personal background, attitude, and motivation.
3. Failure to assess a person's knowledge before beginning the teaching process.
4. Lack of coordination of patient teaching efforts across the continuum of care.
5. Expecting people to be effective teachers when they are not knowledgeable about educational principles, methods, and evaluation.
6. Use of an incidental, informal approach as a basis for a patient education program.

In summary, studies of the clinical practice of health care show that more emphasis needs to be placed on the "how" of patient teaching.

Techniques of teaching are nearly as varied as people. Each person should be viewed as a special learner! There are a host of factors to be considered if a climate for learning is to be created.

*H*uman
- Interpersonal relations
- Individual needs and wants

*O*rganization
- Policy
- Structure

*P*hysical
- Environmental factors

*E*ducational options
- Methods
- Materials

The first aspect is the human factor. There has to be interest and involvement on the part of both teacher and learner. The learners should be offered ways to participate actively throughout the entire educational process. To maximize readiness to learn, it is necessary to ascertain the concerns people have at that particular moment. Unless these concerns are addressed first, additional health teaching will not be heard.

A person's age will directly affect his or her ability to understand and master information and skills. Ability to learn depends on maturation. Growth and development of children is a crucial element of the teaching-learning process. Intellectual development moves from concrete to abstract. As children mature, they move toward a clearer distinction between what is internal and what is external to themselves.

Knowles[38] provides some valuable insights into the adult as a learner. He coined the word *andragogy,* the science of teaching adults, to distinguish the adult learner from the child. He proposes four assumptions about the adult learner. As people mature, (1) their self-concept moves from dependency to self-direction, (2) they accumulate life experiences that are an increasing resource for learning, (3) their readiness to learn is increasingly oriented to developmental tasks and social roles, and (4) time perspective changes and orientation to learning shifts to immediate application of knowledge and learning that is problem-centered rather than subject-centered.

Adult learners are motivated to learn when they recognize a gap between what they know and what they want to know. They accept a share of the responsibility for planning and carrying out a learning experience and therefore have a feeling of commitment toward it. The learning process capitalizes on their past experiences.[39]

Changes brought on by aging need to be acknowledged when the learner is an older adult. Intellectual ability does not necessarily diminish with age; rather, it changes. The speed of learning declines, not the ability! Thus, factors other than age are more likely to be barriers to learning for the older adult.[40] Alford[41] identifies the following changes:

1. Slowed processing time requires that older persons have more time to think through and absorb new information.
2. Stimulus persistence means that older persons must be given time to explore each concept in its entirety and to ask questions.
3. Decreased short-term memory causes older persons to have difficulty in remembering new information. Learning can easily become frustrating if learning requires recent recall. Ways can be devised to reinforce learning, such as linking it with past experiences or providing written data to supplement the verbal information.
4. Test anxiety occurs because older persons sense they cannot remember as well. Taking tests would prove this fact. If tests are necessary, verbal ones should be considered. Elderly learners need to be given a sense of confidence in their ability to maintain independence.

Material for older adults is printed in 10- or 11-point type on paper with a dull finish, and two-tone beige or green-tone colors are avoided. The print size used in written materials, the volume and speed of visual presentations, and the amount of information given at any one time are paced. Teaching is limited to 3 to 5 points. Older persons are accustomed to being in control, and teaching addresses this need whenever possible.

In addition to age, differences in culture, language, level of literacy, and physical impairment (for example, hearing and/or sight deficiencies) must be considered in providing the appropriate educational climate for each particular patient. Cultural differences significantly influence communication and subsequent education. Recognizing the importance of the person's family and even the immediate community as a support system is essential. Acknowledging culture-specific medical and religious beliefs and practices and attempting to incorporate them into educational opportunities is also advisable. Communicating in a language or dialect that is not the one most frequently used by a person can change both the expression of symptoms and the level of comprehension. When educating a patient with a different cultural background, it is wise to consider the use of a variety of methods to both convey and understand messages. For example, the use of pictures to illustrate instructions, and/or materials that have been translated into the person's primary language is helpful.[42]

In addition to cultural differences, level of literacy is an important consideration in the education of any patient. Although concise communication can enhance the education of any patient, those with poor reading or comprehension skills require special consideration concerning their educational needs. A major caveat in working with this audience is to simplify the language used. In addition, Chatham and Knapp[43] suggest the following: Speak and write in short sentences, conveying no more than one concept per sentence; use words of no more than two syllables as often as possible; use nontechnical language that the patient understands in offering explanations of medical terms; speak or write in the active voice. An excellent reference by Doak, Doak, and Root[44] entitled *Teaching Patients With Low Literacy Skills* provides a variety of additional suggestions.

A second aspect to consider when establishing a climate for learning is the need for support from the organization or institution. Squyres[45] proposes a foundation for health education services. It requires integration of a person's personal philosophy and goals with that of the organizations, along with the position statements of professional, legal, and accrediting bodies. Often patient education is given only lip service by an institution. Strategies for gaining support and recognition include knowing the state-of-the-art literature, supporting claims of effectiveness with research data, and presenting a cost-effective plan for implementing a program that addresses quality patient care. Patient education addresses accreditation standards, requirements for informed consent, self-care interests of consumers, and trends for earlier discharge with home care collaboration. Quality patient education is nurtured by a supportive administrative and medical staff. The physical component also must be considered in creation of a climate conducive to learning. The environment can be used to focus peoples' attention on what is to be learned. A learning resource center facilitates self-initiated learning. Visual aids, such as anatomic charts or a human torso, heighten peoples' interest in their own body parts. A positive learning environment offers mutual respect, acceptance of differences, and freedom of expression. If patient education is valued as an integral part of patient care, then time and space should be allocated for carrying it out. It is less than ideal to teach when there are frequent interruptions, a lack of privacy, and interference by hospital routines. For group classes, chairs and tables should be arranged in advance; lighting and microphones adequate for group size and the availability of group leaders who are knowledgeable about audiovisual equipment are important factors. Otherwise, distractions will interfere with class interaction and the group process.

A final factor to consider when establishing a climate conducive to learning is the choice of educational methods and materials. Consideration must be given to ways to best present the content to be taught. People learn better when more than one of their senses is involved in the learning process.[46] Hearing alone is a passive activity. Thus the use of only a lecture method to present information does not promote optimal learning. For each sense that is included, the more involved the learner and the more likely learning will occur.

Audiovisual materials are the tools of patient education programs. However, their use alone is not considered an adequate means for providing patient education.[47] Education is a process that requires human interaction. Appropriate materials enhance the teaching-learning process and are selected with that purpose in mind.

CONCLUSION

The rapid changes in health care technology as well as the complexities of the health care system present a challenge to both the health care professionals and the consumers within the health care system. People enter the system, become patients, and find themselves faced with a life-threatening illness that requires multiple changes. They need assistance in the form of guidance and information. Facilitating adaptation to these changes comes in the form of patient education. The process begins before an illness is diagnosed and continues long after the acute phase of an illness is over. Patient education has as its ultimate goal the restoration of a person to his or her highest state of wellness and reentry into society.

REFERENCES

1. American Cancer Society: Cancer Facts and Figures. Atlanta, American Cancer Society, Inc, 1988, p 3.
2. Green LW: The future of cancer patient education. Health Educ Q 10:102-110, 1984 (special suppl).
3. Brechon D: Highlights in the evolution of hospital-based patient education program. J Allied Health 3:35, 1976.
4. Shapiro I: The patient and control of quality in medical care. Proceedings Tenth Annual Group Health Association of America. Chicago, 1960.
5. American Hospital Association: A Patient's Bill of Rights. AHS Catalog No. 2415, Chicago, The Association, 1975.
6. National Cancer Institute: Adult Patient Education in Cancer. NIH pub no. 83-2601. Washington, DC, The Institute, 1983.
7. Oncology Nursing Society: Outcome Standards for Cancer Patient Education. Pittsburgh, Oncology Nursing Society, 1982.
8. Simonds S: Current Issues in Patient Education. New York, American Group Practice Association and Core Communications in Health, 1974.
9. Rimer B, Keintz MK, Glassman B: Cancer patient education: Reality and potential. Prev Med 14:801-818, 1985.
10. Dodd M: Assessing patient self-care for side effects of cancer chemotherapy. Part I. Cancer Nurs 5:263-268, 1982.
11. Dodd M: Cancer patients' knowledge of chemotherapy: Assessment and informational interventions. Oncol Nurs Forum 9:39-44, 1982.
12. Dodd M: Self-care for side effects in cancer chemotherapy: An assessment of nursing interventions. Part II. Cancer Nurs 6:63-67, 1983.
13. Dodd M, Mood D: Chemotherapy: Helping patients to know the drugs they are receiving and their possible side effects. Cancer Nurs 4:311-318, 1981.
14. Beck S: Impact of a systematic oral care protocol on stomatitis after chemotherapy. Cancer Nurs 2:185-199, 1979.
15. Cassileth BR, Heiberger RM, March V, et al: Effects of audiovisual cancer programs on patients and families. J Med Educ 57:54-59, 1982.
16. Jacobs C, Ross R, Walker IM, et al: Behavior of cancer patients: A randomized study of the effects of education and peer support groups. Am J Clin Oncol 6:347-350, 1983.
17. Johnson J: The effects of a patient education course on persons with a chronic disease. Cancer Nurs 5:117-123, 1982.
18. Watson PG: The effects of short-term postoperative counseling on cancer/ostomy patients. Cancer Nurs 6:21-29, 1983.
19. Green LW, Kreuter MW, Deeds SG, et al: Health Education Planning. Palo Alto, Calif, Mayfield, 1980.
20. Burish T, Lyles J: Effectiveness of relaxation training in reducing the aversiveness of chemotherapy in the treatment of cancer. Behav Ther Exp Psychiatry 10:357-361, 1979.
21. Burish T, Lyles J: Effectiveness of relaxation training in reducing adverse reaction to cancer chemotherapy. J Behav Med 14:65-78, 1981.
22. Redd W, Andresen G, Minagwa R: Hypnotic control of anticipatory emesis in patients receiving cancer chemotherapy. J Consult Clin Psychol 50:114-119, 1982.
23. Redd W, Hendler C: Learned aversions to chemotherapy treatment. Health Educ Q 10:57-64, 1984 (special suppl).
24. Ley P: Towards better doctor-patient communications, in Bennett AE (ed): Communication Between Doctors and Patients. London, Oxford University Press, 1976, pp 75-98.
25. Thomas NP, Cloak M, Crossan K, et al: Preparing cancer patients to administer medication. Patient Couns Health Educ 3:137-143, 1982.
26. National Cancer Institute, Office of Cancer Communication Patient Education Program: Overview of Current Activities, September 1988 (unpublished).
27. Wilson CM, Rimer B, Kane-Williams E, et al: Educating the older cancer patient: Obstacles and opportunities. Health Educ Q 10:76-87, 1984 (special suppl).
28. Mullan F: Seasons of survival: Reflections of a physician with cancer. N Engl J Med 313:270-273, 1985.
29. Johnson JL, Blumberg BD: A commentary on cancer patient education. Health Educ Q 10:7-18, 1984 (special suppl).
30. DeJoseph J: Writing and evaluating educational protocols, in Squyres W (ed): Patient Education: An Inquiry Into the State of the Art. New York, Springer, 1960.

31. Ulrich M, Kelley K: Patient care includes teaching. Hospitals 46:59-65, 1972.
32. Johnson J, Flaherty M: The nurse and cancer patient education. Semin Oncol 7 (March):63-70, 1980.
33. National Cancer Institute: Pretesting in Health Communications. NIH pub no. 84-1493, Washington, DC, The Institute, 1984.
34. Rader LA: The SMOG Grading Readability Formula. Michigan State University, 1980 (unpublished).
35. Blumberg B, Nealon E: Educational needs of the patient considering clinical trials. Paper presented at the Oncology Nursing Society Congress, Toronto, Canada, 1984.
36. Blumberg BD: Evaluating patient education programs. Oncol Nurs Forum 8(2):29-31, 1981.
37. Chaisson GM: Patient education: Whose responsibility is it and who should be doing it. Nurs Admin Q 4(2):1-11, 1980.
38. Knowles M: The Modern Practice of Adult Education, New York, Associated Press, 1975.
39. Woldum K, Ryan-Morrell V, Towson M, et al: Patient Education Foundations of Practice, Rockville, Md, Aspen, 1985.
40. Casserly D, Strock E: Educating the older patient. Caring 7(11):60-67, 1988.
41. Alford PM: Tips for Teaching Older Adults. Nurs Life 2:60-64, 1982.
42. American Hospital Association, Center for Health Promotion: Culture Bound and Sensory Barriers to Communication With Patient: Strategies and Resources for Health Education. Chicago, The Association, May 1982.
43. Chatham MAH, Knapp BL: Teaching patient with low literacy skills, in Patient Education Handbook. Bowie, Md, Robert J Brady, 1982, pp 145-150.
44. Doak CC, Doak LG, Root JH: Teaching Patients With Low Literacy Skills. Philadelphia, JB Lippincott, 1985.
45. Squyres W: Patient Education and Health Promotion in Medical Care. Palo Alto, Calif, Mayfield, 1985.
46. Bille DA: Practical Approaches to Patient Teaching. Boston, Little Brown, 1981.
47. Monaco RM, Salfen L, Spratt J: The patient as an education participant in health care. J Mo Med Assoc, 69(12):932-937, 1972.

Chapter 59

Cancer Nursing Education

Alice J. Longman, RN, EdD

INTRODUCTION

Cancer nursing as a specialized area of professional nursing practice has an important role in the decades ahead. The practice of cancer nursing has been influenced by "(1) national and international recognition of cancer as a major chronic health problem; (2) scientific and technological developments; (3) changes in professional and public perceptions of cancer, and (4) changes within the nursing profession."[1] These changes occurred as a result of a shift within nursing toward more extended and expanded roles. As these roles emerged, there was more emphasis on professionalism. The extension and expansion of cancer nursing practice have been related to organizational developments, educational developments, and research developments.[2]

The management of the care of individuals with cancer or at risk for the development of cancer is one of collaboration and coordination among various health professions. Changes in undergraduate nursing education have been marked by the gradual shift from hospital-based education to college-based education. More nurses practice nursing in a variety of settings, and practice is based increasingly on the use of findings from research.

CHARACTERISTICS OF CANCER NURSING PRACTICE

The Social Policy Statement issued by the American Nurses' Association in 1980 defined four characteristics of nursing: phenomena, theory application, nursing action, and evaluation of effects in relation to phenomena.[3]

Phenomena and Theory Application

The phenomena of concern in cancer nursing are multiple. Cancer no longer is regarded as one disease but rather "a group of diseases with clinically distinct presentations, and differing biologic behavior and clinical manifestations."[4] The impact of cancer on individuals has implications for numerous biologic, social, behavioral, and physical interventions. Furthermore, cancer can be described as a group of chronic diseases for which treatment is possible. Theoretic concepts for cancer nursing are drawn from biologic and social theories, as well as from systems, developmental, and change theories.

Improved observations that relate to levels of health and illness need to be stressed by nursing personnel. Individuals, families, and communities thus can be assisted in the early identification of potential or real problems. Of importance to the practice of cancer nursing are the facts that prevention and early detection of cancer are within the purview of nursing and that most cancers can be treated successfully at early stages.

Nursing Action

Actions in cancer nursing are based on a sound knowledge base to provide care for those individuals or groups at risk for the development of cancer or those who are being treated for cancer and its sequelae. A sound knowledge base is acquired in basic nursing education programs, continually updated through continuing education and expanded in graduate nursing education programs. Toward this end the major purpose of the Education Committee of the Oncology Nursing Society is to promote high-quality cancer education for nurses.[5] The Education Committee oversees and promotes the quality of all educational activities generated by the Oncology Nursing Society.

The complexity of care for individuals with cancer necessitated the development of a systematic process for nursing actions. The nursing process, including the formulation of nursing diagnoses, serves as an organizing framework for cancer nursing practice. In 1979 the American Nurses' Association and the Oncology Nursing Society published *Outcome Standards for Cancer Nursing Practice*.[6] Ten high-incidence problems were identified for individuals in primary, acute, or long-term care settings. The 10 areas were prevention and early detection, information, coping, comfort, nutrition, protective mechanisms, mobility, elimination, sexuality, and ventilation. Criteria for evaluation of nursing actions were provided.

Standards of Oncology Nursing Practice, published in 1987, presents professional practice standards and professional performance standards. The practice standards address theory, data collection, diagnosis, planning, intervention, and evaluation. Eleven high-incidence problem areas common to individuals with cancer are addressed. These are prevention and early detection, information, coping, comfort, nutrition, protective mechanisms, mobility, elimination, sexuality, ventilation, and circulation. The professional performance standards examine professional development, interdisciplinary collaboration, quality assurance, ethics, and research. Examples of nursing diagnoses in relation to the high-incidence problem areas are included in the document.

Care for individuals with cancer and their families is provided through the services of many health professions. These include but are not limited to diagnostic radiologists, nuclear medicine specialists, radiotherapists, surgeons, medical oncologists, hematologists, dietitians, social workers, physical therapists, and nurses. For individuals with the suspected or confirmed diagnosis of cancer and their families, the vast array of health care professionals may be overwhelming. Collaboration among health professionals is essential to assist individuals to achieve optimum health. Such collaboration provides consistency in the ongoing plan of treatment. Nurses often assume the role of coordinator in such collaboration.

Evaluation of Effects of Action

Evaluation of the effects of nursing actions suggests whether the actions have improved or resolved the conditions toward which they were directed. The knowledge base is continually examined and updated. The results of cancer nursing research provide evidence of the efficacy of nursing actions.

DEVELOPMENT OF CANCER NURSING PRACTICE

Recognition of cancer as a major health problem led to the development of the specialty of cancer nursing. A comprehensive approach to cancer care has contributed to the expansion of the boundaries of cancer nursing practice. Cancer nursing is practiced by nursing generalists and nursing specialists. Nursing generalists have conceptual knowledge and skills acquired through basic nursing education, clinical experience, and professional development. Nursing generalists meet the concerns of individuals with cancer and provide care in a variety of health care settings. Continuing education is a mechanism to update their knowledge of and skills in cancer care. Nursing specialists have substantial theoretic knowledge gained through preparation for the master's degree. Nursing specialists meet diversified concerns of individuals with cancer and their families and function in a discrete area of practice. The scope of cancer nursing practice includes clinical practice, education, administration, and research.

Oncology Nursing Society

In 1975 the Oncology Nursing Society was established to promote communication among cancer nurses, to generate new knowledge about cancer nursing, to promote cancer research in general, and to enhance the level of care being given to patients and families.[4] Activities of the Society include an annual congress to provide a forum for nurses to present and exchange information, major standing committees to foster the professional development of cancer nurses, a professional journal to disseminate scientific and clinical information, and a newsletter that reports on the activities of the Society. Formal and informal communication among and between individual nurses involved in cancer nursing has contributed to the impact of professional collaboration on cancer nursing. Yarbro[7] summarized the major accomplishments on the Oncology Nursing Society from 1975 to 1983.

Association of Pediatric Oncology Nurses

The Association of Pediatric Oncology Nurses was established in 1975 and became a nonprofit corporation in 1976.[8] A significant contribution of the Association has been the development of expanded nursing roles in pediatric cancer nursing. The organization has striven to provide a forum for mutual support, the exchange of ideas, and the comparison of practice models through annual conferences and a professional journal. Close relationships are maintained with other specialty nursing organizations, in particular the Oncology Nursing Society.

National Cancer Institute

The National Cancer Act of 1971 has had a major impact on cancer and cancer control programs. The Act authorized a broad intensive program to reduce the incidence, morbidity, and mortality of cancer in human beings. The National Cancer Institute is a unique structure that systematically attacks the complex cancer problem.[9] Its mission is to support a network that provides information, distributes funding for research, and establishes research and treatment centers. Comprehensive cancer centers have been developed, and specialized clinical and research centers are in operation. Nursing generalists and nursing specialists are involved in the planning and development of specialized cancer units in general hospitals. The development of the Comprehensive Cancer Centers Outreach programs, community-based programs, and the Clinical Hospital Oncology programs also have involved nursing generalists and nursing specialists.

Individual predoctoral and postdoctoral research fellowships for cancer nurses are available from the National Cancer Institute. Nurses have had representation on the National Cancer Institute Cancer Control Grant Review Committee since the 1970s. In addition, with the assistance of a grant from the National Cancer Institute, the Oncology Nursing Society has offered a cancer nursing research short course at the Society's Congress for the past several years. A national forum for exchange between students and faculty is provided for those selected to participate in the research experience.[9]

American Cancer Society

The American Cancer Society appointed the first nursing consultant in 1948. The first Nursing Advisory Committee of the American Cancer Society was established in 1951, and its purpose was to offer advice on educational programs and materials.[10] Nurses were eligible to become members of all professional education and service committees at the divisional and local levels of the American Cancer Society. Since 1980 support for graduate students enrolled in master's degree programs that offer specialization in cancer nursing has been available. The scholarship program was expanded in 1986, and assistance also is available for those nurses engaged in doctoral studies. Through the efforts of the American Cancer Society a program was established for professorships in cancer nursing. By 1988 nine nurse educators were named professors in cancer nursing. These professors are actively involved in the education of graduate students and practicing nurses and in the activities of the Society.

PERSPECTIVES OF CANCER NURSING EDUCATION

The development of cancer nursing education reflects the changes in nursing practice, changes in nursing education, and rapid changes in cancer therapy and cancer care settings. In particular, two specific trends in cancer nursing education were noted by Tiffany[2]: the acceptance of the World Health Organization's definition of health as a state of complete physical, mental, and social well-being and not merely the absence of disease and infirmity and the recognition that patients and families should be active participants in their treatment and recovery process. The proliferation of roles that require definition and differentiation in cancer nursing also has influenced cancer nursing education. These roles have included the nurse specialist, the nurse clinician, the nurse oncologist, the oncology nurse practitioner, the oncology coordinator, and the clinical nurse specialist.[11-13]

General Cancer Nursing Education

Continuing education has been the most widely used method to increase the knowledge and skills of those engaged in cancer nursing. Because of the nature of educational preparation at the generalist level, that is, baccalaureate, associate degree, and diploma, nurses who required expertise in cancer nursing were unprepared. Thus continuing education programs were necessary to provide nurses with the opportunity to gain the knowledge essential for the practice of cancer nursing. Programs in cancer nursing in the early 1940s and 1950s, which were sponsored by the American Cancer Society in cooperation with professional nursing organizations, usually consisted of 1-day seminars.[10]

Many cancer nursing education programs were provided by cancer hospitals. Memorial Sloan-Kettering Cancer Center was a pioneer in offering educational programs in cancer nursing. The Center's activities included continuing education programs, in-service education, clinical practice for undergraduate and graduate students, and the development of teaching materials in cancer nursing.[14] Other cancer hospitals in the country, such as Roswell Park Memorial Hospital, Ellis Fischel State Cancer Center, City of Hope National Medical Center, and MD Anderson Hospital and Tumor Institute, also have provided continuing education for nurses through the years.[14]

The need for special training for nurses in cancer care was stressed in a report of the Division of Cancer Control Program.[15] In 1950 a 3-week institute on cancer nursing was conducted for 30 nurse instructors under the auspices of the National Cancer Institute.[14] After the completion of the institute, a Cancer Production Committee was formed and an outline developed to demonstrate how cancer nursing could be incorporated into basic nursing programs.[16]

Through the years the Nursing Advisory Committee of the American Cancer Society has been concerned with the preparation and publication of educational resources for nurses. The first *Cancer Source Book for Nurses* was published in 1950; subsequent revisions have been published through the years.

The incorporation of cancer content in baccalaureate nursing programs was addressed in the early 1950s. The National Cancer Institute awarded grants to four baccalaureate nursing programs to integrate cancer nursing content into the nursing courses.[15] Tools were developed to measure knowledge about cancer among students within existing baccalaureate nursing programs.[17,18] The tools served to interest other faculty members in cancer content. Instruments for use by nursing instructors then were designed to evaluate cancer nursing education.[19] Courses for public health nurses, institutional nurses, and nursing faculty also were in progress in various states.[20]

In 1971 the National Cancer Institute contributed seed funding for a 10-week work-study program for students enrolled in baccalaureate nursing programs. Students were provided the opportunity to increase their knowledge and skills in caring for individuals with cancer in the areas of prevention, detection, diagnosis, treatment, and rehabilitation.[21] The program was successful in recruiting nurses for cancer nursing practice.

Currently, the National Cancer Institute offers a Cancer Nurse Training Program, which is a 9-month clinical traineeship for new baccalaureate nursing graduates.[22] The program offers a comprehensive review of current cancer practice and its implications for nursing. A monthly stipend is given to participants in the program.

Another project funded by the National Cancer Institute in recent years was the evaluation of the current essential cancer content in an undergraduate nursing program.[23] Five activities were included in the project: measurement of students' attitudes toward cancer patients and cancer knowledge of students, research experiences for selected students, research symposia related to cancer nursing, an update on cancer treatment for nursing faculty, and the development and implementation of an interdisciplinary elective course. As a result the content was integrated more logically into the program. Two instruments, Ideas About Oncology Patient Care and a Knowledge Inventory, were developed and tested.

Graduate Cancer Nursing Education

Teachers College of Columbia University offered the first academic courses in cancer nursing at the graduate level.[10,14] Two eight-credit courses were offered over two semesters. The theoretic content included the nature of cancer as a biologic phenomenon, the theoretic basis for specific nursing care measures, and the community health aspects of cancer for individuals and their families. The course included a clinical practicum, which was conducted at Memorial Sloan-Kettering Cancer Center. Through the efforts of the director of nursing at the hospital, a grant of $30,000 was received from the American Cancer Society, New York Division, for support of the program.[14]

When funding was discontinued, the courses were dropped.

The earliest reported survey of graduate programs to determine those that offered cancer nursing was conducted in 1958 by the American Cancer Society. Representatives of 30 graduate programs were contacted; 22 responded and only two programs indicated that cancer nursing was included in their programs.[10] Nursing guidelines, entitled "Assessing Graduate Education in Oncology Nursing,"[24] were published by the Education Committee of the Oncology Nursing Society to assist those nurses interested in graduate education with a specialty in cancer nursing. By 1988 more than 45 graduate programs offered specialization in cancer nursing. An annual listing of such programs is prepared by the Education Committee of the Oncology Nursing Society and published in the *Oncology Nursing Forum.* Additional information about graduate education content is available from the Oncology Nursing Society in the publication, *The Master's Degree with a Specialty in Oncology Nursing: Role Definition and Curriculum Guide.*[25]

Two programs that prepare graduates of master's programs as teachers of cancer nursing were supported by the National Cancer Institute for 5 years (1979-1984). The dissemination of the model curriculum and evaluation results were important parts of the project.[26]

Support for graduate students enrolled in master's degree programs specializing in cancer nursing has been available since 1980 through the efforts of the American Cancer Society.[27] Graduate scholarships for those pursuing additional preparation also are awarded by the Oncology Nursing Foundation. Five doctoral programs offer specialization in cancer nursing. Support also is available from the American Cancer Society for those engaged in doctoral studies. One program offers a postdoctoral fellowship in cancer nursing.

Certificate programs are available for those who specialize in cancer nursing. Preparation in the management of care for selected individuals with cancer and their families is provided. Advanced practitioner skills related to taking health histories, performing physical examinations, and monitoring laboratory results are included.

Educational Needs of Nurses

The educational needs of cancer nurses have been studied. An early study identified the need for further education in assisting patients to meet their psychosocial needs.[28] Grant and Padilla[29] reviewed the status of cancer nursing research and categorized the studies into two groups, those on cancer nursing knowledge and those on oncology nurses. The studies on cancer nurses concerned nurses' attitudes toward cancer patients, death, cancer nursing care, and cancer care. The Western Consortium for Cancer Nursing Research, a regional collaborative research group in Canada, conducted a Delphi study to establish priorities for cancer nursing research.[30] The top-ranked topic with respect to nursing practice was to determine strategies to promote morale and prevent burnout among oncology nurses.

The Education Committee of the Oncology Nursing Society developed educational standards to provide guidelines for cancer nursing education.[31-33] *Outcome Standards for Cancer Nursing Education: Fundamental Level*[31] delineated the knowledge needed to provide cancer nursing care consistent with *Outcome Standards for Cancer Nursing Practice.*[6] The latter was developed to delineate the knowledge needed by those with cancer.[32] *Outcome Standards for Public Cancer Education*[33] was developed to provide information on prevention, early detection, rehabilitation, and living with cancer. To address the implementation of the education standards, examples were published in the *Oncology Nursing Forum.* The first example described the development of a clinical elective for senior nursing students using the education standards[34] whereas the second example was the development of a program for nurses to integrate into clinical practice current knowledge and research results related to antineoplastic drug treatment of cancer.[35] The determination of readiness for learning in cancer care was addressed in the third example.[36] A model for cancer patient education was proposed in terms of the cancer patient education standards. The final example described an approach to provide the public with information on cancer prevention, detection, and treatment.[37] A Cancer Information Day was planned and proved to be a valuable and worthwhile enterprise. The public cancer education standards were used to guide the program.

EDUCATION FOR CANCER NURSING PRACTICE

Because of the high incidence of cancer, most practicing nurses become involved in the care of individuals with cancer and their families. As a result of the basic education in nursing, however, the knowledge and skills nurses have about cancer nursing vary. It is incumbent on nurses who care for individuals with cancer to become knowledgeable about current cancer care practices so that they can provide optimal nursing care to these patients and their families.

To determine the status of cancer nursing education in the United States, a descriptive study was conducted by the Oncology Nursing Society.[38] The impetus of the study, which was supported by the American Cancer Society, was the concern that the basic education of nurses in cancer care may be inadequate.

Questionnaires were sent to 982 professional schools in the United States that were accredited by the National League for Nursing. The total number of returned questionnaires was 672 (68%). The results indicated that some content areas received considerable attention, whereas others did not. Content areas inadequately covered were prevention and detection; acute problems; late effects of treatment; unorthodox treatments; attitudes toward cancer; home care; social and political issues; resources for patients, families, and nurses; and legal implications in cancer nursing practice. The most frequent amount of time designated for cancer nursing content was 14½ hours.

The results of the survey indicated the need to maximize the time designated for cancer nursing content in basic nursing programs. There was a need for educational resources that are current and readily available. Suggestions were made to improve the knowledge necessary for cancer nursing practice.

The Education Committee of the Oncology Nursing Society proposed an organizing framework and approach for the education of nurses in cancer nursing practice.[39] Two levels were proposed: fundamental and advanced education. Education at the fundamental level provides the basic knowledge, skill, and attitudes for cancer nursing practice whereas the advanced level provides in-depth knowledge, skills, and attitudes. To reflect the changes within the profession, as well as the changes within cancer nursing, the terms *generalist* and *specialist* currently are used.

Conceptual Framework

A conceptual framework for cancer nursing education was developed that was consistent with those in *Outcome Standards for Cancer Nursing Practice*.[6] Four concepts were included in the framework: individual-family, health-illness continuum, health care system, and community-environment.[31] The four concepts interact with one another as they apply to caring for individuals with cancer and their families. The individual-family concept is the central focus of cancer nursing practice. The health-illness concept is defined as adaptation of the individual and family along a continuum. The health care system concept is the setting for the practice of cancer nursing, and the community-environment concept refers to the resources and support necessary for those with cancer. The nursing process and the research process are the methods used for the organization of knowledge for cancer nursing practice.

Generalist Level

The generalist level of cancer nursing education encompasses basic education for nurses, continuing education to improve current nursing practice, and professional development. With the use of the concepts of individual-family, health-illness continuum, health care system, and community-environment, an outline of content for cancer nursing education is presented in Table 59-1.

Individual-family

Individuals are viewed as having biologic, psychologic, spiritual, cultural, developmental, and economic dimensions. These dimensions should be considered in assessing the impact of the diagnosis of cancer on individuals and their families. The strengths and limitations of each individual can be determined, and they provide direction for nursing actions.

Three strategies are important in managing the care of individuals and families dealing with the impact of cancer. Communication strategies employed by individuals and families should be assessed and used in planning nursing care. Basic communication strategies are obtained in preservice preparation and then are expanded in nursing curricula. The sophistication of the strategies depends on the organization of the nursing program, but most faculty

TABLE 59-1 Outline of Content for Cancer Nursing Education

Individual and Family	Health-Illness Continuum	Health Care System	Community-Environment
Impact of cancer: biologic, psychologic, spiritual, cultural, developmental, economic	Cancer epidemiology terminology	Organizational design: primary care, acute care, ambulatory care, long-term care	Cancer-related resources: local, regional, national
Communication strategies	Incidence: trends, patterns of occurrence, cancer risk factors	Accessibility/availability of health care services	Community: economic, legal, political, employability/insurability
Decision-making strategies	Prevention and early detection	Continuity of health care services	Environment: occupational, physical
Stress management strategies	Diagnosis and staging	Utilization of health care services	
Individual and family resources	Pathophysiology of cancer	Accountability (standards for practice)	
	Treatment: surgery, radiation therapy, chemotherapy		
	Other modalities: immunotherapy, hyperthermia, biologic response modifiers		
	Rehabilitation: economic, physical, psychosocial, life cycle		

members would agree that graduates of basic nursing programs need to have acquired a variety of communication strategies. Decision-making strategies employed by individuals and their families are important in planning interventions to meet identified short- and long-term needs. Content related to these strategies usually is offered in preservice courses and further expanded in successive nursing courses. Various stressors are brought about by the nature of cancer and its treatment. Stress management strategies are numerous and are provided in both preservice courses and nursing courses.

The resources that individuals and families use to assist them in their life activities need to be identified because they often can be mobilized to assist them during the course of the disease. Accurate information about cancer, treatment options, consequences of treatment, potential problems, and alternative care settings is necessary for individuals and their families. The need for adequate preparation based on sound knowledge and experience is evident.

Health-illness continuum

The health-illness continuum is defined as the adaptation individuals and families undergo during the cancer experience. Because cancer is a major and prevalent disease, information about the epidemiology of cancer is provided and includes national, regional, and local incidence rates. Trends in the incidence of cancer in certain populations, as well as the patterns of occurrence, are addressed. Cancer risk factors and prevention and early detection of cancer are discussed at several levels in nursing programs. In addition, the causes of cancer, as well as the cellular biology of cancer, are addressed. The epidemiology of cancer and cell growth processes often are provided in science courses in most nursing programs. Additional information then is given as major cancers are described. Although information on the characteristics of major cancers may vary from program to program, content related to lung cancer, breast cancer, colon cancer, genitourinary cancer, gynecologic cancer, and the leukemias is included. Other cancers related to specific populations may or may not be added, depending on the region of the country. Content related to common diagnostic tests is included in nursing courses. The importance of diagnostic and staging procedures is best discussed in relation to the characteristics of major cancers.

The rationale for and principles of the major treatment modalities should be included, along with the specific skills appropriate to the treatment modalities. Management of comfort, nutrition, mobility, elimination, sexuality, ventilation, and circulation is necessary to assist individuals in dealing with their treatment regimens. The final consideration in the health-illness continuum is rehabilitation, which includes economic, physical, and psychosocial needs of individuals and their families. Life cycle considerations and the level of functioning each person had achieved or is capable of achieving are of utmost importance.

Health care system

Cancer nursing is practiced in multiple settings. Primary care settings provide a range of services required by individuals and their families during initial diagnostic examinations. Acute care settings also provide multiple services necessary for individuals with cancer. The organizational design of community hospitals, major medical centers, and major cancer centers should be well understood by those who practice in them. The roles of the members of the health care team need to be defined and understood by the other members so that assistance can be rendered most appropriately to the patients served by the institution. Ambulatory care settings are becoming increasingly important in the care of patients with cancer. The resources needed by individuals and their families are important for satisfactory delivery of care in these settings. Long-term care settings such as hospice also provide services required by individuals with cancer.

Mutual understanding of each of the systems should be well known by those who practice cancer nursing. Individuals with cancer and their families need to be assisted to search for the appropriate components of the health care system available to them. Accountability for nursing actions is an integral part of this concept.

Community-environment

Cancer-related resources at the local, regional, and national levels are available. Students are apprised of the services offered by the American Cancer Society at each level. Home care services and bereavement services in each community are included in the content of courses.

Content related to the economic impact of cancer often is included in preservice preparation and expanded in the nursing courses. Political factors that influence cancer care, legal implications of cancer nursing practice, issues of employability and insurability, the identification of environmental carcinogens, and knowledge of safety measures related to hazards of cancer treatment are necessary components of curricula that prepare individuals for cancer nursing practice.

The fostering of the development of empathy in those who will care for individuals with cancer and their families is important in basic nursing education programs. It is recommended that the promotion of empathy be incorporated at the beginning of nursing programs.[40] Attitudes and feelings of students toward caring for patients with cancer need to be assessed. A clinically useful instrument to evaluate nursing students' attitudes toward caring for patients with cancer has been designed and tested.[41] This instrument, Ideas About Oncology Patient Care, measures the multidimensional nature of attitudes toward caring for cancer patients.

Strategies for increasing undergraduate nursing students' knowledge about cancer have been proposed. These include the development of a clinical elective for students[34]; the use of an independent study option for selected students[42]; the use of alternate methods of obtaining information beyond assigned textbook readings[43]; and an annual nursing student cancer workshop.[44] These strategies were developed in response to the amount of information necessary to practice cancer nursing.

Clinical experience

The relationship of theory to practice is crucial to cancer nursing. Students are given the opportunity to practice their skills in multiple care settings. Through the use of the nursing process, including nursing diagnosis, acquired clinical skills can be used in meeting individual and family needs. Physical and psychosocial assessment is necessary in the provision of direct care. Technical skills need to be carefully and meticulously integrated into each student's program.

In the past several years numerous resources have become available to educators. These have included journals devoted exclusively to cancer nursing, audiovisual resources that detail specific aspects of cancer prevention and detection, diagnosis, and treatment, and textbooks that include content on cancer nursing care.

For students enrolled in baccalaureate nursing programs the Cancer Work-Study Program sponsored by the National Institutes of Health is another option. Students must have completed their junior year toward a baccalaureate degree in nursing. Twenty students are selected, paid a stipend, and complete a 10-week program. Opportunity is provided for enhancement of knowledge and skills in caring for individuals with cancer in the areas of prevention, detection, diagnosis, treatment, and rehabilitation.

The "Position Statement on Nursing Roles—Scope and Preparation"[45] addressed the necessity to improve the quality of nursing education programs and described the range of nursing practice roles. *Standards for Professional Nursing Education*[46] was designed to help the nursing profession meet the changing needs of society. Both documents stated that professional nursing practice requires the minimum of a baccalaureate degree with a major in nursing, and technical nursing practice requires an associate degree or a diploma in nursing.

Continuing education

For nurses who are consistently involved in cancer nursing practice and have been prepared at the baccalaureate level, associate degree level, or diploma level, continuing education becomes a practical necessity. Educational opportunities are provided by universities, nursing organizations, hospitals, and health departments and may be offered either on a short- or on a long-term basis. The Oncology Nursing Society was granted accreditation as an approver and provider of continuing education for nurses by the American Nurses' Association in 1988. As an approver of continuing education the Oncology Nursing Society reviews applications for educational programs, offerings, and independent studies. Contact hours are awarded to registered nurses who attend programs. As a provider of continuing education the Oncology Nursing Society is committed to planning and implementing continuing education according to the standards of the American Nurses' Association.

Standards of Oncology Nursing Practice[1] provides guidelines for continuing education programs. That practicing nurses are eager to acquire further knowledge and skill is evident in the attendance at conferences throughout the country. Since 1973 the American Cancer Society has sponsored a national conference on cancer nursing every 4 years. At the first conference in 1973, more than 2500 nurses participated in the activities, and successive conferences have been equally well attended.

The Department of Nursing Education at Memorial Sloan-Kettering Cancer Center presents an Overview of Cancer Nursing four times annually. Content includes information related to the major modalities of cancer treatment, content on the major cancers, and implications for nursing care in terms of individual needs. Observational experiences are available throughout the program. The University of Texas System Cancer Center, MD Anderson Hospital and Tumor Institute, sponsors cancer prevention and detection programs for nurses. The offerings vary from 1 day to 3 weeks in length. Scripps Memorial Hospital Cancer Center sponsors an annual cancer symposium for nurses. The conference is 3 days in length and attracts participants from all across the country.

The Institute of Continuing Education for Nurses at the University of Southern California sponsors an annual cancer nursing seminar. Workshops during the seminar are planned to suit individual learning needs. The opportunity to meet other cancer nurses from across the country is an important outcome of the conference.

To assist nurses with the development of continuing education programs in cancer nursing, the Education Committee of the Oncology Nursing Society presented an instructional session at the 11th Annual Congress.[47] The session was based on the assumption that consumers of continuing education programs in cancer nursing are adult learners. How to conduct a learning needs assessment with examples was presented in the first paper.[48] Formulating educational objectives was the focus of the second paper.[49] Examples of objectives for continuing education programs were given. In the third paper the need for congruency between content and methodology and program objectives was discussed.[50] Examples were given to illustrate the material. The benefits of specific methods were described. Finally, program evaluation was addressed, with a discussion of the process, as well as the components, of the programs.[51]

The efficacy of the benefits of short-term programs has been a subject of interest to educators. The advantages of the acquisition of knowledge in a short period of time are debatable. For many practicing nurses, however, short-term programs offer information that they might not otherwise obtain. To determine the effects of an intensive 3-day cancer nursing workshop on nurses' attitudes toward patients and cancer nurses, 36 participants were evaluated before and 6 weeks after the completion of the course.[52] The Activity Vector Analysis, an adjective checklist of 81 nonderogatory adjectives to describe human behavior, was used. The results suggested that perhaps no one type of nurse is attracted to cancer nursing and that nurses in the specialty of cancer nursing need to develop realistic expectations about their roles.

Long-term continuing education programs have been offered to provide a broad overview of cancer nursing and specific knowledge in the different types of cancer. Most of these courses include advanced physical assessment skills, supervised clinical practice, and the awarding of a certificate at the completion of the program. *Standards of Oncology Nursing Practice* presents useful guidelines for the implementation of these programs. Because of the length of these programs, a more comprehensive offering is possible. An annual listing of long-term continuing education programs is prepared by the Education Committee of the Oncology Nursing Society and published in the *Oncology Nursing Forum.*

Meeting the needs of individuals with cancer and their families continues to be a challenge for those engaged in cancer nursing. By organizing the necessary knowledge, practicing nurses can continue to increase their expertise in cancer nursing.

To assist in the planning and evaluation of generalist level education, *Standards of Oncology Nursing Education: Generalist and Advanced Practice Levels*[53] is useful. Designed to guide the achievement of quality education for nurses, these standards reflect structure, process, and outcomes of educational offerings. Another publication, *Standards of Oncology Education: Patient/Family and Public,*[54] is available to assist in the planning and evaluation of formal and informal patient and family teaching and public education programs. Descriptive statements guide the achievement of quality education for these populations. Additionally, materials related to patient, family, and public education are available from the American Cancer Society, the Leukemia Society of America, and the National Cancer Institute.

Specialist Level

The specialist level of cancer nursing education encompasses graduate education for nurses to develop a broader scope of practice, as well as the development of resources and an increased emphasis on coordination, continuity, and evaluation of care.[39] Specialists require substantial theoretic knowledge in cancer nursing and proficient use of this knowledge in providing expert care to individuals with cancer and their families.[1]

A cancer nursing workshop, Curriculum Construction and Role Definition, was convened by the American Cancer Society in 1978. The purpose was to reach a consensus about the educational preparation for nursing specialists in cancer nursing.[14] Content for preparation as a clinical nurse specialist was outlined and has proved beneficial inasmuch as programs have continued to offer specialization in cancer nursing at the master's level. The publication, *Master's Degree with a Specialty in Oncology Nursing: Role Definition and Curriculum Guide,*[25] is useful for nurse educators in planning graduate cancer nursing education. Its content, which is based on the current body of knowledge in advanced cancer nursing practice, is organized by role components, that is, clinical practice, education, consultation, administration, research and professionalism, and steps of the nursing process.

Individual-family

The dimensions ascribed to individuals at the generalist level are considered in the delineation of content at the graduate level. Courses should be available that address the recurrent phenomena related to cancer such as depression, pain, anxiety, body image, and coping. Courses often are available in other departments of a university or may be available in the graduate program in nursing.

Communication strategies are included and specifically related to individuals with cancer and their families. These may include self-help groups, support groups, or group work that addresses counseling needs of individuals and their families. Decision-making strategies are most effectively taught as they relate to role preparation in graduate education. Ethical implications of cancer is an area that is included in many graduate programs; thus the decisions made by individuals and their families related to cancer treatment and its consequences can be supported. Stress management theories are incorporated into the major courses of the program. These theories can be related to stressors that individuals encounter as they adapt to living with cancer. Nurses prepared at the specialist level are in a position to act as advocates for individuals with cancer and their families. Those who assume this role must of course be trained to do so. Specialists in cancer nursing have the ability to integrate and evaluate the factors that have an impact on coping with the disease.[13]

The identification of resources available to individuals and their families is crucial to their care. Content related to health care agencies and community resources should be included to assist students in early and rapid identification of available assistance. Specialists need to be knowledgeable in the identification of high-risk individuals in terms of complications resulting inside and outside of the health care system. The problems of long-term survival also need to be addressed.

Health-illness continuum

Determination of the individual's position on the health-illness continuum is a major emphasis in graduate programs. Building on the basic sciences of undergraduate programs, graduate education broadens this foundation. Courses in advanced physiology and pathophysiology are recommended for students interested in cancer. Special attention is given to the acquisition of knowledge related to cellular biology, cellular kinetics, radiation biology, and immunology. Courses often are offered in other departments of the universities, and every effort should be made to have students participate in these courses.

Analysis of the cancer problem in terms of the application of epidemiologic techniques is an important component of the curriculum. Indications for prevention and early detection, identification of high-risk populations, and diagnostic techniques are crucial for understanding the continuum. Emphasis in graduate programs often is placed on the pathophysiology of malignant processes. The goals and general principles of therapy, including cure, control, and palliation, are discussed. Surgery, radiotherapy, chemotherapy, and other treatment modalities then are discussed in relation to the physiologic aberrations that have occurred. Unproved methods and their implications are described. The relationship of medical management to nursing management then is analyzed. Research that has been conducted or is being conducted is an integral part of the content.

Not all graduate programs have as their major focus the management of the acute manifestations of cancer. Some may be concerned with the management of advanced disease or the rehabilitative aspects of care. Nonetheless, medical management and nursing management are necessary for cancer nursing practice at the specialist level. Indications for supportive management such as nutritional support, pain control, infection control, and blood component therapy also are studied. Other content areas include acute problems related to cancer, such as cardiac tamponade, disseminated intravascular coagulation, hypercalcemia, inappropriate antidiuretic hormone syndrome, sepsis, spinal cord compression, superior vena cava syndrome, and tumor lysis syndrome.

Health care system

Role preparation is an integral component of graduate education at the master's degree level and includes clinical specialist, practitioner, educator, and administrator.[55,56] Because most students enrolled in graduate programs have practiced in the health care system before returning for further education, their experiences should be considered. The organization of each of the major health care systems is discussed in relation to the functional area in which the student is or will be practicing. Ideally, students may be able to practice in ambulatory care settings, home care settings, or hospice settings during their graduate program. Although this may not always be possible, it certainly is desirable. Continuity of health care service can thus be described and implementation ensured. Utilization of health care services can be clearly explained in relation to continuity of health care services. Professional, legal, and ethical issues in the management of the care of individuals with cancer and their families are inherent in practice accountability. Content related to informed consent, human investigation, legal aspects of cancer nursing practice, cancer economics, and employability and insurability is presented.

Community-environment

Resources that are available for individuals and their families should be investigated and understood by cancer nurses. The expertise of the members of the cancer health team provides assistance with problem solving. The political implications of cancer care is one other area that should be addressed in graduate education. In the future the politics of cancer care will play an increasing role in cancer nursing.

Clinical experience

The application of theory to practice is crucial to graduate preparation in cancer nursing. Clinical experience for graduate students is directed by the overall program objectives. The objectives generally specify performance in clinical specialization, functional roles, and research.[57,58]

By means of organized approaches to nursing care problems, the objectives of the clinical components of the program can be met. The approaches most widely used involve the nursing process, including nursing diagnosis, and the research process. Both approaches enable students to accomplish the objectives of the program.

Physical and psychosocial assessment skills are necessary for the provision of direct care and are acquired before admission to the program or concurrent with attendance. Technical skills are reinforced during the course of the program. The rationale for the use of technical skills is explained, and students need to investigate the basis for the use of technical skills. The need to acquire teaching skills is important in graduate education because graduates are involved in the teaching of other nurses, patients and their families, and community personnel.

Three different groups of personnel interact with graduate students as they engage in clinical practice during their program. These groups—faculty members, practicing clinical nurse specialists, and nursing service administrators in health care settings—all influence the students as they progress in the program.[59,60] Ample time should be allowed for students to integrate the expectations of these professionals.

The role of the clinical nurse specialist in cancer nursing has received considerable attention in the last few years. Consistency in preparation has been alluded to, but to date few studies have been conducted to verify the role of the clinical nurse specialist in practice. A national invitational conference entitled "The Oncology Clinical Nurse Specialist-Role Analysis and Future Projections" was held in 1984. The conference, sponsored by the Cancer Nursing Service at the Clinical Center, National Institutes of Health, was held for the purpose of providing guidelines for currently practicing cancer clinical nurse specialists to optimize current practice and to provide goals for future development. Most would agree that the role of the clinical nurse specialist encompasses direct patient care, teaching nursing personnel, role modeling for other nursing personnel, consultation, and research.[11,13,58,61]

The characteristics of the clinical nurse specialist in cancer nursing are summarized in Table 59-2. Achieving this role in nursing practice remains a challenge, and problems have been cited in relation to role implementation.[62,63] A survey conducted by Yasko[64] described the characteristics and perceptions of nurses with a master's degree in

TABLE 59-2 Characteristics of Clinical Nurse Specialist in Cancer Nursing

Clinical competence
Direct nursing care
Coordinate patient care services
Patient/family advocate
Teaching
Patient/family
In-service education
Basic, continuing, and graduate education
Public education
Research
Conduct of research
Clinical trials
Research protocols
Experimental regimens
Consultation
Resource for nursing personnel
Intraprofessional resource
Evaluation of health programs
Evaluation of health delivery

nursing, who were currently employed as clinical nurse specialists in cancer nursing; 185 nurses with master's degrees participated in the study. Variations in master's level curricula were apparent, as well as variations in the implementation of the role. A modified Delphi survey with 47 participants, conducted by McGee et al,[65] identified 363 competencies required of cancer clinical nursing specialists. Attitudes and human traits received the highest mean ratings of the competency categories identified. Findings indicated a consistent ranking of knowledge and skill categories. Moore et al[66] reported on a longitudinal evaluation of students' abilities to apply new knowledge to clinical behaviors. The Appraisal of Practice Behaviors Instrument was developed to measure cancer nursing practice and tested on 38 enrollees in a master's program.

Trends that affect the future role of the clinical nurse specialist have been examined and include those related to societal changes, new developments in health care, and professional directions. It will be up to the clinical nurse specialist to describe the changes in practice, to identify new arenas for practice, and to continue to evaluate the impact of the role.

Continuing education

For those nurses prepared at the master's degree level and consistently involved in cancer nursing, continuing education is a practical consideration. The direction this education takes depends on the position and the setting in which nursing specialists practice. Often clinical nurse specialists are engaged in numerous teaching activities. These may include but are not limited to patient/family education, in-service education, public education, and education at the generalist or specialist level. Further preparation in teaching strategies and methods may be sought and is available through university programs and professional organizations.

Standards of Oncology Nursing Practice,[1] *Standards of Oncology Nursing Education: Generalist and Advanced Practice Levels*[53] and *Standards of Oncology Education: Patient/Family and Public*[54] provide useful guidelines for promoting continuing education for practicing nursing specialists. Conferences often are arranged around such themes as symptom management, management of pain, and strategies used by individuals with cancer. Interdisciplinary conferences also are available for cancer nursing specialists.

The International Union Against Cancer was established in 1934 to provide leadership and an international forum for the exchange of information in the fight against cancer.[67] Meetings are held every 4 years in various parts of the world and offer an opportunity for nurses to participate in the sessions or to present papers. A permanent activity of the UICC is the Nurses' Cancer Education Project. The first International Conference on Cancer Nursing, sponsored by the Royal Marsden Hospital, London, was held in 1978, and the second took place in 1980. A commitment was then made to conduct an international conference every 2 years beginning in 1984. These conferences offer an opportunity for nurses to present clinical findings at international conferences.

ISSUES IN CANCER NURSING EDUCATION

Education of Ancillary Health Workers

As more individuals with cancer are cared for at home, the preparation of family members and other health workers will assume greater importance. Cancer nurses are in a position to offer assistance and education for both family members and ancillary health workers. Continuing education has a role to play in the offering of programs to meet community needs.

Certification and Recertification

For the past few decades many nursing specialty organizations have developed certification programs. Soon after World War II, the American Association of Nursing Anesthetists developed its certification program. The American Nurses' Association established its certification program in 1973 to provide recognition of professional achievement in a defined clinical or functional area of nursing. The American Nurses' Association's definition of certification is that it is the process by which the Association's Committee of Examiners validates, on the basis of predetermined standards, an individual nurse's qualifications, knowledge, and practice in a defined functional or clinical area in nursing.[68] The American Nurses' Association offers more than 17 programs in nursing administration certification. Most nursing specialty organizations offer certification.

The definition of certification most widely used is that stated in the report entitled *The Study of Credentialing in Nursing: A New Approach:*[69]

> Certification is a process by which a non-governmental agency or association certifies that an individual licensed to practice a profession has met certain predetermined standards specified by that profession for specialty practice. Its purpose is to assure various publics that an individual has mastered a body of knowledge and acquired skills in a particular specialty.

The principal advantage of certification is that it provides an additional measure of quality nursing care for the consumer. More important, certification assists the entire nursing profession in upgrading its performance and provides individual nurses with tangible acknowledgment of professional achievement in nursing. Through a system of peer review, recognition of expertise in both current knowledge and in clinical practice is provided.

A survey of the Oncology Nursing Society members indicated a strong interest in certification for cancer nursing.[70] In 1981 the Board of Directors of the Oncology Nursing Society voted to explore the possibility of a certification program. A Task Force on Certification in Oncology Nursing was established to explore the methodology for a certification program and to determine the cost of such a program.[71] A survey of the members of the Oncology Nursing Society was undertaken in 1982 to determine the commitment to certification in cancer nursing. The questionnaire was sent to 4365 nurses; 693 returns, or 15.9%, were used as the study base of the survey.[72]

The response indicated support of a certification program, as well as a sense of commitment to the process. The results of the survey were presented to the members at the 1983 Oncology Nursing Society Congress through an instructional session and an open forum.[72] The task force recommended that a certification program be considered for members and be directed first at the generalist level. Plans for subspecialization and specialist level were to be considered in the future.

The Core Curriculum Task Force of the Oncology Nursing Society prepared a core curriculum and a bibliography for the development of the certification examination, a study guide for those preparing for the examination, and a format for workshops.[73] The Oncology Nursing Certification Corporation (ONCC) was established for the development, administration, and evaluation of the certification program. The ONCC contracted with the Educational Testing Services for the development of the certification examination. Members of the Test Specification Committee developed test items for inclusion in the examination. Before the test administration, rigorous procedures were used to determine the examination's cut score.[74] The cut score represents the lowest score qualifying a candidate for certification. The test development was supported by the Oncology Nursing Society and in part by a grant from the American Cancer Society.

Nurses with an RN license, 3 years' experience as a registered nurse within the last 5 years, and a minimum of 1000 hours of cancer nursing practice within the last 3 years are eligible for certification. Nursing experience may be in the areas of nursing administration, education, clinical practice, or research. The first examination was offered in 1986, and subsequent examinations have been offered twice yearly since. Successful candidates receive a certificate from ONCC and use the designation of Oncology Certified Nurse (OCN). Certification for cancer nursing is valid for 4 years. The total number of OCNs in 1989 was 5116, and a task force was formed to address recertification issues.[75] Recommendations were that the renewal of certification should be a voluntary credentialing process similar to the initial process. Candidates must meet the same criteria as before, and an examination will constitute the requirements for recertification. OCNs certified in 1986 are eligible for recertification in 1990.

A bulletin is prepared each year for candidates. The bulletin includes information regarding the examination process, core curriculum for the certification examination, selected references, and sample questions.[76] Additionally, a textbook has been developed for use by those preparing for certification.[77] A role delineation study is under way to identify critical indicators to help determine the content of future examinations of cancer nursing. Issues being considered by the ONCC are identifying the focus of educational efforts and providing a body of knowledge for the development of a specialist core curriculum and a baseline to describe specialist practice.

Research

The research process is an integral component of cancer nursing education. Nursing education at the generalist level, particularly in baccalaureate programs, fosters a beginning knowledge of the research process. Students are encouraged to use research findings, both in the theoretic portion of the program and in their practice. For practicing nurses the identification of nursing practice problems is an ongoing process. Assistance should be sought from those qualified to engage in the investigation of these problems.

For those engaged in graduate education the research process is applied in most courses of the program. Nursing practice problems are identified and analyzed on the basis of systematic use of the process. A thesis or research project often is required for completion of the program. For those engaged in doctoral education the conduct of research is required and the application to nursing practice mandated.

Using the criteria of *Outcome Standards for Cancer Nursing Education: Fundamental Level,*[31] Grant and Padilla[29] undertook a review of the current status of cancer nursing research. More than 300 studies were reviewed and categorized. Suggestions for the future development of clinical nursing research were made. Fernsler et al[78] conducted a study of cancer nursing research from 1975 to 1982. The findings described the quantity and nature of cancer nursing research and affirmed that patient needs were the focus of most of these studies. The Oncology Nursing Society has conducted two surveys of research priorities.[79,80] Both these studies used the educational standards as the framework for the categorization of the studies. Research priorities were symptom management, including pain control, patient education, coping and stress management, and prevention and early detection. The results of the 1988 survey were submitted to the National Center for Nursing Research as the organization's top research priorities. To guide the development of cancer nursing research in western Canada, five priority topics were identified by a regional collaborative group.[30] Collaborative approaches hold promise for generating solutions to researchable problems.

Funds are required for the conduct of research, and qualifying for funds will be a challenge in the decade ahead. Sound research proposals that address cancer morbidity and mortality will have to be developed.

CONCLUSION

Nursing as a professional discipline has a unique place in society. Cancer nursing as a component of this professional discipline must meet the challenges of society, and its practice must continue to be based on a sound theoretic and clinical base.

REFERENCES

1. American Nurses' Association and Oncology Nursing Society: Standards of Oncology Nursing Practice. Kansas City, Mo, American Nurses' Association, 1987.
2. Tiffany R: The development of cancer nursing as a specialty. Int Nurs Rev 34:35-39, 1987.
3. Nursing: A Social Policy Statement. Kansas City, Mo, American Nurses' Association, 1980.
4. Marino LB: Cancer Nursing. St Louis, CV Mosby, 1981.
5. Oncology nursing society education committee. Oncol Nurs Forum 6:20-21, 1979.
6. American Nurses' Association and Oncology Nursing Society: Outcome Standards for Cancer Nursing Practice. Kansas City, Mo, American Nurses' Association, 1979.
7. Yarbro CH: The early days: Four smiles and a post office box. Oncol Nurs Forum 11:79-85, 1984.
8. Greene PE: The association of pediatric oncology nurses: The first ten years. Oncol Nurs Forum 10:59-63, 1983.
9. ONS salutes NCI on its 50th anniversary. Oncol Nurs Forum 14:14-16, 1987.
10. Hilkemeyer R: A historical perspective in cancer nursing. Oncol Nurs Forum 9:47-55, 1982.
11. Siehl S: The clinical nurse specialist in oncology. Nurs Clin North Am 17:753-761, 1982.
12. Spross J: An overview of the oncology clinical nurse specialist role. Oncol Nurs Forum 10:54-58, 1983.
13. Welch-McCaffrey D: Role performance issues for oncology clinical nurse specialists. Cancer Nurs 9:287-294, 1986.
14. Craytor JK: Highlights in education for cancer nursing. Oncol Nurs Forum 9:51-59, 1982.
15. Peterson R: Federal grants for education in cancer nursing. Nurs Outlook 4:103-105, 1956.
16. Peterson R, Soller G: Cancer nursing in the basic professional nursing curriculum. Washington, DC, US Government Printing Office, 1951.
17. Peterson R, Heil L: Tools for the evaluation of cancer nursing for nursing instructors. Washington, DC, US Government Printing Office, 1957.
18. Diller D: An Investigation of Cancer Learning in Ninety-One Selected Schools of Nursing. Saratoga Springs, NY, Skidmore College, 1955.
19. Diller D: An Investigation of Cancer Learning in Ninety Selected Schools of Nursing. Third Report. Saratoga Springs, NY, Skidmore College, 1957.
20. Hilkemeyer R, Kinney H: Teaching cancer nursing. Nurs Outlook 4:177-180, 1956.
21. Barckley V: Work study program in cancer nursing. Nurs Outlook 19:447-452, 1971.
22. National Cancer Institute: Cancer Nurse Training Program. Washington, DC, National Institutes of Health, 1987.
23. Longman AJ, Verran JA, Clark M: Improving oncology nursing content in an undergraduate program. J Nurs Ed 27:42-44, 1988.
24. Education Committee, Oncology Nursing Society: Assessing graduate education in oncology nursing. Oncol Nurs Forum 7:37-38, 1980.
25. The Master's Degree with a Specialty in Oncology Nursing: Role Definition and Curriculum Guide. Pittsburgh, Pa, Oncology Nursing Society, 1988.
26. Seigele D: Longitudinal evaluation of a model post-master's program in oncology nursing. Oncol Nurs Forum 11:61-71, 1984.
27. Frerichs M, Yasko JM: The American Cancer Society's scholarship program. Oncol Nurs Forum 12:62-64, 1985.
28. Craytor JK, Brown JK, Morrow GR: Assessing learning needs of nurses who care for persons with cancer. Cancer Nurs 1:211-220, 1978.
29. Grant M, Padilla G: An overview of cancer nursing research. Oncol Nurs Forum 10:58-69, 1983.
30. Priorities for cancer nursing research: A Canadian replication. Cancer Nurs 10:319-326, 1987.
31. Oncology Nursing Society: Outcome Standards for Cancer Nursing Education: Fundamental Level. Pittsburgh, Pa, The Society, 1982.
32. Oncology Nursing Society: Outcome Standards for Cancer Patient Education. Pittsburgh, Pa, The Society, 1982.
33. Oncology Nursing Society: Outcome Standards for Public Cancer Education. Pittsburgh, Pa, Oncology Nursing Society, 1983.
34. Nevidjon B, Deatrich J: An oncology clinical elective. Oncol Nurs Forum 12:57-59, 1985.
35. Kimball DD, Heft PL: The development of an antineoplastic drug education program. Oncol Nurs Forum 12:59-62, 1985.
36. Welch-McCaffrey D: Evolving patient education needs in cancer. Oncol Nurs Forum 12:62-66, 1985.
37. Vega T: Outcome standards for public cancer education: The foundation for community education programs. Oncol Nurs Forum 12:66-67, 1985.
38. Brown J, Johnson J, Groenwald S: Survey of cancer nursing education in US schools of nursing. Oncol Nurs Forum 10:82-83, 1983.
39. Given B: Education of the oncology nurse: The key to excellent patient care. Semin Oncol 7:71-79, 1980.

40. Welch-McCaffrey D: Promoting the empathetic development of nursing students in the care of the patient with cancer. J Nurs Ed 23:73-75, 1984.
41. Verran JA, Longman A, Clark M: Development of a scale to measure undergraduate students' attitudes about caring for patients with cancer. Oncol Nurs Forum 14(5):51-55, 1987.
42. Mooney M, Dudas S: Undergraduate independent study in cancer nursing. Oncol Nurs Forum 14(1):51-53, 1987.
43. Daly JM, Erdmann WS: Oncology search: An innovative teaching method. Nurs Ed 13:28-30, 1988.
44. Quinn-Casper P, Holmgren C: Enhancing nursing concepts in undergraduate curricula. Cancer Nurs 10:274-278, 1987.
45. Position statement on nursing roles—scope and preparation. Nurs & Health Care 3:212-213, 1982.
46. Standards for professional nursing education. Kansas City, Mo, American Nurses' Association, 1984.
47. Fernsler J: An overview. Oncol Nurs Forum 14:59-60, 1987.
48. Volker DL: Learning needs assessment. Oncol Nurs Forum 14:60-62, 1987.
49. Itano J: Developing educational objectives. Oncol Nurs Forum 14:62-65, 1987.
50. Belcher AE: Defining content and methods. Oncol Nurs Forum 14:65-67, 1987.
51. McMillan SC: Program evaluation. Oncol Nurs Forum 14:67-70, 1987.
52. Johnson J, Mosier MA, Johnson C: Registered nurses: Perceptions of patients, cancer nurses and themselves. Oncol Nurs Forum 9:27-31, 1982.
53. Oncology Nursing Society: Standards of Oncology Nursing Education: Generalist and Advanced Practice Levels. Pittsburgh, Pa, The Society, 1989.
54. Oncology Nursing Society: Standards of Oncology Education: Patient/Family and Public. Pittsburgh, Pa, The Society, 1989.
55. Holzemer WL: Quality in graduate nursing education. Nurs & Health Care 3:536-542, 1982.
56. Piemme JA: Oncology clinical nurse specialist education. Oncol Nurs Forum 12:45-48, 1985.
57. Hodges LC, Poteet GW, Edlund BJ: Teaching clinical nurse specialists to lead and to succeed. Nurs & Health Care 6:192-196, 1985.
58. Paulen A: Practice issues for the oncology clinical nurse specialist. Oncol Nurs Forum 12:37-39, 1985.
59. Cason CL, Beck CM: Clinical nurse specialist role development. Nurs & Health Care 3:25-38, 1982.
60. Wyers MEA, Grove SK, Pastorino C: Clinical nurse specialist: In search of the right role. Nurs and Health Care 6:202-207, 1985.
61. Kwong M, Manning MP, Koetters TL: The role of the oncology nurse specialist: Three personal views. Cancer Nurs 5:427-434, 1982.
62. Starck P: Factors influencing the role of the oncology clinical nurse specialist. Oncol Nurs Forum 10:54-58, 1983.
63. Spross J, Donoghue M: The future of the oncology clinical nurse specialist. Oncol Nurs Forum 11:74-78, 1984.
64. Yasko JM: A survey of oncology clinical nursing specialists. Oncol Nurs Forum 10:25-30, 1983.
65. McGee RF, Powell ML, Broadwell DC, et al: A Delphi survey of oncology clinical nurse specialist competencies. Oncol Nurs Forum 14:29-34, 1987.
66. Moore IM, Piper B, Dodd MJ, et al: Measuring oncology nursing practice: Results from one graduate program. Oncol Nurs Forum 14:45-49, 1987.
67. Ash CR: Cancer nursing: An international perspective. Cancer Nurs 9:172-177, 1986.
68. American Nurses' Association 1988 Certification Catalog. Kansas City, Mo, American Nurses' Association, 1988.
69. The study of credentialing in nursing: A new approach, vol 1: The Report of the Committee. Kansas City, Mo, American Nurses' Association, 1979.
70. Cobb ME, Maier P: Informational needs of the oncology nursing society membership. Oncol Nurs Forum 8:58-61, 1981.
71. Moore P, Hogan C, Longman A, et al: Report of the task force on certification in oncology nursing. Oncol Nurs Forum 9:75-80, 1982.
72. Longman A, Hogan C, McNally J, et al: Report of the task force on certification in oncology nursing. Oncol Nurs Forum 10:84-88, 1983.
73. Certification committee. Oncol Nurs Forum 11:77-79, 1984.
74. Ewing T: Determining examination cut scores. Oncol Nurs Forum 14:88, 1987.
75. Piper BF, Longman A, Protho P, et al: Certification renewal task force and recommendations. Oncol Nurs Forum 13:97-98, 103-105, 1986.
76. Oncology Nursing Certification Corporation Bulletin and Application 1989. Pittsburgh, Pa, Oncology Nursing Certification Corporation, 1989.
77. Ziegfeld CR: Core curriculum for oncology nursing. Philadelphia, Pa, WB Saunders, 1987.
78. Fernsler J, Holcombe J, Pulliam L: A survey of cancer nursing research January 1975-June 1982. Oncol Nurs Forum 11:46-52, 1984.
79. McGuire D, Frank M, Varricchio C: 1984 ONS research committee survey of membership's research interests and involvement. Oncol Nurs Forum 12:99-103, 1985.
80. Funkhouser SW, Grant MM: 1988 ONS survey of research priorities. Oncol Nurs Forum 16:413-416, 1989.

Chapter 60

Cancer Nursing Research

Marcia M. Grant, RN, DNSc, OCN

Geraldine V. Padilla, PhD

INTRODUCTION

Research has provided critical knowledge concerning the care of cancer patients. Basic science, medical science, and nursing science all form the foundation important in the prevention, detection, treatment, and management of cancer. The focus of this chapter is the role of the cancer nurse in the implementation of medical research and in the development, implementation, dissemination, and application of cancer nursing research. An examination of the role of the nurse in each of these activities provides a basis for understanding the rapid development of nursing research in the provision of care for today's cancer patient.

RESEARCH DEFINED

Research involves a structured approach to answering questions or discovering new knowledge.[1] It is conducted for the broad purpose of increasing scientific knowledge. Research can be considered valid only when it is replicated. The process of research involves an orderly and standardized series of steps. These steps can be compared to the steps in the nursing process; that is, both processes are specialized forms of problem solving.[2] Differences between the two processes involve amount of detail and accuracy of measurement. In addition, research focuses on a group of patients and includes the obligation to disseminate the results for critique by others. A comparison of the research and nursing processes is found in Table 60-1.

TABLE 60-1 Comparison of Clinical Nursing and Research Processes

Steps Involved	Clinical Nursing	Nursing Research
Defining the problem	Individual patient assessment	Identify area of concern
	Nursing diagnosis	Review literature and select a conceptual or theoretical framework Conduct preliminary studies Define methods Select population Define designs Define samples Operationally define variables Describe procedures Identify data analysis
Carrying out the action	Intervention implementation	Implement study Accrue consenting subjects Administer standardized tools Check reliability of data collection
Evaluating the results	Outcome evaluation	Code and analyze data Interpret findings Publish results

DEVELOPMENT OF MEDICAL RESEARCH IN CANCER

The focus of medical research and nursing research differs. In the development of cancer treatment, medical research is used to describe the natural history of the diseases, to test new treatment approaches and evaluate the value of singular and multimodal approaches to cancer treatment. Through these endeavors have developed surgical, chemotherapeutic, radiation, and biologic response-modifier approaches to the treatment of cancer, as well as supportive care measures.

Until the 1950s surgery was the primary approach to the treatment of cancer.[3] After World War II, radiation therapy began to develop as an offshoot of diagnostic radiation activities.[4] As radiation therapy improved and doses and schedules were adapted to specific cancers such as those of the skin, oral cavity, larynx, and breast, it became available as both a singular treatment for some diseases (eg, Hodgkin's disease) and in combination with surgery for other diseases (eg, breast and cervical cancer).

The development of chemotherapy for cancers (eg, leukemia) that were not amenable or responsive to either surgery or radiation gave the nurse a primary role in implementation of medical research.[5] The chemotherapeutic agents were administered intravenously over a course of therapy given on a regular (daily, weekly, etc) basis.

The Chemotherapy Research Nurse

The chemotherapy nurse assumed one of the first specialty roles in the development of cancer nursing practice. These nurses were responsible for the administration and monitoring of chemotherapy. They accrued patients for medical protocols, administered medications, counseled patients on management of side effects, collected data, and kept the physician informed of the patient's condition. Because of the complex nature of the medications and the potentially lethal side effects, chemotherapy nurses sought out and developed an extensive knowledge base about chemotherapeutic principles. Their involvement with accruing, monitoring, and teaching chemotherapy patients increased their familiarity with the research process as used in clinical chemotherapy research. These nurses were among the first nurses to participate as collaborators in cancer research. With their research skills as background, many of them sought further education and developed into primary researchers interested in either medical or nursing aspects of cancer care.

The first survey of research skills of Oncology Nursing Society (ONS) members conducted by the ONS Research Committee revealed that a large proportion of oncology nurses had participated in a variety of steps in the research process.[6] The continued participation of oncology nurses in the implementation of medical research is considered in further detail in our discussion of the members of the clinical research team and their roles.

The Clinical Trials Approach

The medical research approach to clinical investigation of cancer treatment methods has resulted in a specialized approach to clinical research called the clinical trials approach.[7] Developed and encouraged under the influence of studies funded by the National Cancer Institute (NCI), this approach involves several phases of study, each designed to answer specific clinical questions at a different time in the development of applied scientific knowledge. Each study or research protocol includes a well written and detailed guide which serves as the procedure for implementation of the study.

Clinical trials are divided into phase 1, 2, and 3 studies.[7] Each has a different purpose and design. After testing of medical treatment approaches (surgical, chemotherapeutic, or radiation) with appropriate animal or cell models, phase 1 studies are implemented as the first clinical tests of new treatments on human patients. The purpose of a phase 1 study is the determination of dose schedules and toxicities. Because new drugs and treatments are used, the population eligible to participate in phase 1 clinical trials includes patients for whom standard therapy has failed. Since the determination of how to use a drug or treatment in a phase 1 clinical trial has not yet been made, patients for whom standard treatments can be issued are *not* eligible or enrolled in phase 1 studies.

Data in phase 1 clinical trials include determination of the maximum tolerated dose (MTD), drug toxicities, and the response of tumors. Pharmacokinetic data on the medication being tested may be conducted as well. Thus the collection of timed specimens is common and requires precision by the nursing staff implementing the protocol. An example of a current phase 1 trial is the use of new investigational drugs for patients in whom standard chemotherapy has failed and who are not eligible for other treatments, such as radiation therapy. A phase 1 clinical trial requires accrual of the smallest number of patients to determine at what dose or schedule of treatments toxicities occur. Frequently the only benefit to a phase 1 patient is the satisfaction of having contributed to scientific knowledge for treatment of other cancer patients. However, patients often view participation in a phase 1 study from a hopeful perspective—prolongation of life for themselves or for other patients.

In phase 2 trials, the focus shifts to specific tumor types for which the treatment appears promising.[7] To be eligible for phase 2 trials, patients must either be not able to participate in standard therapy or have failed standard therapy. Specific tumors are selected that have shown some positive responses in preclinical or phase 1 trials. An example of a current phase 2 trial is the use of LAK and IL2 for patients with colorectal cancer and renal cell carcinoma. Toxicities during phase 2 trials are frequently profound, and close monitoring of patients is necessary to provide data for evaluation of patient response and early detection of toxicities.

The focus shifts again for phase 3 studies.[7] These studies determine (1) the effects of a treatment relative to the natural history of the disease, (2) whether a new treatment is more effective than a standard therapy, and (3) whether a new treatment is as effective as a standard therapy but is associated with less morbidity. In phase 3 trials, the focus is on comparison of a new treatment with the standard treatment. These studies involve randomization of patients to the experimental or the standard treatment.

Phase 1 clinical trials are implemented only at NCI-designated cancer centers (see Yellow Pages for list of these centers). This specification is done to assure the full spectrum of clinical support needed in studies in which toxicities are not predictable and close monitoring of patients is critical. Depending on the nature of the treatment being tested, phase 2 trials may also be conducted in NCI-designated cancer centers. Phase 3 trials, which require the greatest number of subjects to answer the research question, are conducted in large medical centers, university hospitals, and community centers with qualified cancer researchers and needed clinical support resources. Participation of cancer patients in all three kinds of clinical trial has been the critical element in the rapid development of current cancer treatment options. Through clinical trials we have developed options for primary breast cancer treatment involving either radiation therapy or surgery and options for Hodgkin's disease involving either chemotherapy or radiation. An interesting corollary to this approach to medical research is the increased participation and involvement of the patient in the selection of medical treatment. Today an informed citizen may read about a new cancer treatment in the newspaper and seek out a physician who is able to provide that approach to treatment.

The Medical Research Team

Implementation of clinical trials for cancer is carried out by a research team composed of a variety of multidisciplinary members: principal investigator, coinvestigator, research or protocol nurse, data manager, investigational pharmacist, statistician, and clinical nursing staff. Clinical nurses are important members of this team. The principal investigator is generally a physician and is responsible for the scientific integrity of the study. Responsibilities include development of the protocol, presentation of the study to the Institutional Review Board for review of appropriate informed consent procedures, and implementation of the study. Coinvestigators may include other physicians whose patients may be eligible for the study and other scientists (eg, molecular biologists or psychologists) interested in other aspects of cancer patients' responses.

The research nurse is responsible for patient accrual, implementing the physician's orders as described in the protocol, and observing patient responses and toxicities. In implementing the role, the nurse is involved in informed consent issues, astute clinical care, and education of supporting nursing staff.

While the principal investigator is legally responsible for obtaining informed consent from the patient, all members of the research team share this responsibility.[5] The research nurse ensures that patients understand what has been defined as the treatment, what the risks and benefits are, what alternative treatment approaches are available, and what the probability is that the patient will receive personal benefit from the treatment. This is especially important if the patient is participating in phase 1 or phase 2 clinical trials, wherein personal benefit to the individual patient is infrequent or nonexistent. Since many patients are reluctant to ask questions of the physician, the nurse is frequently in a position to answer patients' questions, explain further, define more clearly, and generally help the patient understand the research. Identification of patients who obviously do not understand the treatment approach being administered or the implications of the research in relation to personal benefits requires that the principal investigator be notified, so that before any treatment is administered further clarification of the patient's concerns is provided and any possibility of coercion is eliminated.

The nurse also carries out astute clinical care in implementing the study for the research patient. Since many of the patients involved in phase 1 and phase 2 trials may have profound toxicities, the observation and reporting of these toxic effects are critical for safe patient care. The nurse is in a key position to monitor the patient's symptoms and report toxicities that are a threat to the patient's comfort. For some studies, toxicities are unknown, and life-threatening complications are a possibility. Both anticipated and nonanticipated toxicities occur and make it essential for the nurse to observe patients frequently and thoroughly.

The observation and evaluation of toxic responses to the research protocol are important priorities in clinical research trials. When the research or protocol nurse is not present, responsibilities must be delegated to someone else. Thus a major responsibility of the protocol nurse is the education of the patient's caregiver. Education may involve the clinical nursing staff, the patient, and/or the family or significant other. Depending on the protocol, observations for specific reactions may be necessary. For example, the occurrence of nausea and vomiting may be an expected toxic response but needs to be monitored and treated so that nutritional depletion does not occur. The patient and the caregiver need to know when to notify the physician or the research nurse of side effects. The use of one-to-one teaching followed by discussion of standard educational materials is a common and effective way to provide the patient with the information needed to recognize and report significant toxic effects.

The role of the data manager is to collect the information on toxicities from the chart and to enter these data into the computer for statistical analysis. Various forms in the chart are used. Laboratory responses, pathology reports, and physician's progress notes are frequent sources of data. The toxicity data are usually collected from standardized forms, which include a grading system for rating various symptoms. The data manager does not have to be a nurse, and thus the job description does not generally include any clinical observations for which clinical nursing skills are needed.

The investigational pharmacist is a part of the team when the focus of the clinical trial is chemotherapy. Many phase 1 and 2 trials involve investigational drugs, which are not available for public use, and for which specific records need to be kept. The investigational pharmacist is responsible for dispensing these medications, making sure that the records on the drugs are in order. This person also is usually the first to learn about changes in drug administration, dosage changes, problems reported by other research institutions, and reclassification of the medications. Once a drug moves from an investigational drug to a medication available for general use (usually with a physician's prescription), the drug is no longer available free of charge. This change may have a major impact on the patient's ability to continue the protocol.

The statistician is responsible for a variety of activities in relation to a clinical trial. These include determination of initial sample size, study design and protocol review, data evaluation and analysis, interpretation of findings, and preparation of manuscripts. Frequently data managers report to the statistician, and protocol tracking, randomization, data entry, and statistical analysis are carried out in the department of biostatistics. This support is vital to maintenance of the integrity of the study design.

Members of the clinical nursing staff make up the remainder of the research team. While most of the patients in medical research protocols are hospitalized, other settings may be involved as well. Thus, staff includes nurses in hospital units, ambulatory care settings, physicians' offices, and home care agencies. The protocol nurse is frequently involved in the education of clinical nursing staff, ensuring that patient assessments are relevant and charted. Introduction and explanation of toxicity rating forms are frequently needed. The clinical nursing staff has a major contribution to make in terms of patients' responses to the research therapy.

SETTINGS FOR MEDICAL RESEARCH

Medical research related to cancer treatment may be conducted in a number of settings. Four types of cancer centers are defined by the NCI. While all four types are required to have a broad foundation of peer-reviewed research activities, they differ from each other in the type of research that is conducted. Basic science centers conduct laboratory research (for example, research on the biology of cancer). Clinical cancer centers conduct a combination of basic and clinical research. Comprehensive cancer centers include the same research as clinical cancer centers, plus cancer-control research. Consortium centers involve clinical and cancer control research, plus cancer-control activities. Cancer-control research focuses on the reduction in incidence of cancer by primary and secondary disease-prevention activities. Medical research related to cancer treatment may be conducted at any of these settings. Oncology nurses have been involved in all aspects, ranging from extravasation studies that use animal models, to clinical trials of experimental therapies, to research and activities on cancer prevention and early detection.

The conduct of phase 1 clinical trials is restricted to NCI-designated cancer centers. However, because of the low number of all cancer patients proportionately treated at cancer centers, programs have been developed to allow patients at community agencies to participate in cancer treatment research. Phase 2 and 3 clinical trials are thus conducted at institutions with cooperative arrangements with NCI-designated cancer centers. This not only provides for a larger number of patients available for research accrual; it also provides patients with options that are not available in the practices of their own private physicians. As increased numbers of patients are accrued into phase 2 and 3 trials, results will accumulate more rapidly and new, successful treatments may be demonstrated earlier and made available to a wider spectrum of patients.

Studies on cancer treatment are also conducted by principal investigators who are not located at NCI-designated centers. Thus nurses from a variety of settings may be involved in medical research and learn a variety of research skills useful in nursing studies as well.

DEVELOPMENT OF NURSING RESEARCH IN CANCER

The focus of nursing research differs from that of medical research. Nursing research is defined as the systematic investigation of the responses of patients to actual or potential health problems.[8] Nursing research focuses on the patient rather than on the disease and may encompass biologic, psychologic, and social aspects.

Because of the profound effect of cancer and cancer treatment on the patient, cancer nursing care has provided a rich source of questions and problems for nursing research investigators. The inclusion of a large proportion of data-based articles in the primary cancer nursing journals (ie, *Oncology Nursing Forum* and *Cancer Nursing*) attests to the flourishing amount of nursing research relevant to cancer care. In the first edition of this book, it was possible to catalog cancer nursing research and identify areas of diverse activity, beginning investigations, and areas of no activity.[9] Since then, expansion in the number of cancer nursing studies makes such a review unrealistic. This discussion will examine the development of cancer nursing research by focusing on the role of the nurse in clinical research, emphasizing the increasing participation in research, the resources available for cancer nurses, and the priorities for research questions as identified by cancer nurses. A summary of cancer nursing research is used to exemplify recent activity.

The Role of the Nurse in Clinical Research

Currently the nurse has several roles in the implementation of research for cancer patients. For a protocol nurse or a clinical staff nurse, the role is that of a member of the research team conducting medical research. Another role is that of initiator of a study conducted along with a medical protocol. This arrangement has been useful in the testing of a variety of nursing approaches. Advantages include the participation of patients already being accrued to another study and the provision of many of the basic demographic and treatment variables needed for study analysis. Cotanch's work on relaxation for chemotherapy-related nausea and vomiting provides a good example of such a study.[10]

The nurse may also act as a principal investigator, initiating the study, writing up the protocol, selecting the subjects, and evaluating the results. The shift to increased numbers of nurses participating as principal investigators is evident from the latest Research Committee survey.[11] The advantage of this shift is that study results can expand the knowledge basic to the development of nursing science. Several recent developments have made the expansion of cancer nursing research possible. Resources for nursing research have increased and include financial as well as knowledge-dissemination opportunities.

Resources for Oncology Nursing Research

Financial support for oncology nursing research has expanded in the last few years and is a major resource for the growth of cancer nursing research activities. While some research can be carried out with a minimum of expense, most research requires financial support for literature searches, proposal development time, supplies, space, data management, secretarial assistance, statistical analysis, and manuscript preparation. Support is available in both educational and clinical settings.

One source that is increasingly available to nurses is internal support at one's own institution. This is an especially valuable resource for the investigator with limited or no grant-writing experience. In educational institutions, seed money is frequently available through the school or college of nursing, as well as the general institution budget. These funds are specifically focused toward increasing research productivity in faculty. Senior faculty or faculty members with other financial resources for research are frequently not eligible for these seed funds, unless a major change in research focus is being attempted. Funds may also be available from an alumni association.[12]

Biomedical support grants from the federal government are available for both educational and clinical institutions that have already achieved a specific level of research support from the government. These biomedical support funds are used to fund beginning or pilot studies that are expected to develop into large-scale projects submitted for outside funding. Each institution establishes criteria by which these funds are distributed. The application process is usually relatively simple, involving a one- to three-page proposal.

External funds are available for individual investigators and can be divided into those available from the government and those available from private foundations. For cancer nursing research, two major sources for federal funds are the National Center for Nursing Research and the National Cancer Institute. Federal funds for research support are by far the biggest resource, and are distributed through a well-defined application and review process. One of the most valuable resources for cancer nurses looking for federal funds is the publication entitled *NIH Guide for Grants and Contracts*. Published by the National Institutes of Health, this document is mailed at regular intervals and lists grant programs and deadline dates for grants and contracts administered by the National Institutes of Health. This free publication can be ordered from NIH Guide, Distribution Center, National Institutes of Health, Room B4B-N-08, Building 31, Bethesda, MD 20892. This publication provides program descriptions and calls for research proposals in specific problem areas.

Private funds for cancer nursing research have expanded and are found in both oncology nursing organizations and outside groups. The Oncology Nursing Foundation funds a variety of research projects yearly. Sigma Theta Tau, both the national organization and local chapters, funds many research projects. Multidisciplinary private groups that fund oncology nursing research include the American Cancer Society and the Robert Wood Johnson Foundation. Addresses for some of these resources are found in Table 60-2. This financial support has increased through the last few years as the educational background and experience of cancer nurses has increased and the demand for research support has risen.

Changing characteristics of oncology nurses can be viewed as an additional resource. According to J. Kinzler (personal communication, June 13, 1989), the number of nurses has increased tremendously, as illustrated by an increase in membership of the Oncology Nursing Society to 15,198 members in 1989. This membership represents an increase of 2578 members from 1988 to 1989. Two surveys of this membership illustrate the changes in research focus that have occurred in the membership. Grant and Stromborg[6] reported findings of a survey conducted by the ONS Research Committee. This mailed survey was sent to the total 1980 membership of ONS (N = 2205) and was returned by 988 members, a response rate of 45%. The respondents reported a high degree of interest in participating in research, with 42% giving research a large or highest priority, 41% giving it a moderate priority, and 17% giving it a lower or no priority. A majority of the respondents (52%) had participated in research as part of their education experiences; 40% reported participation in one to three projects after completion of their last educational experience. Participation involved a variety of tasks associated with research implementation. Data collection was by far the most common activity, with 75% of the respondents reporting this as part of their nursing role. Implementation of clinical protocol was done by 42%, data analysis by 37%, writing up project results by 36%, and development of a research protocol by 35%. A reported 10% of the respondents had published research results.

Education preparation is likely to influence participation in various research activities, and respondents also illustrated a level of education that paralleled their reported research activities. A comparison of the educational

TABLE 60-2 Contacts for Cancer Nursing Research Support

Service	Contact Person/Address
American Cancer Society	Trish Greene, RN, MS Vice-President for Cancer Nursing American Cancer Society 1599 Clifton Rd., NE Atlanta, GA 30029
American Nurses' Foundation	Pauline Brimmier, RN, PhD Director, Center for Nursing Research America Nurses' Foundation 2420 Pershing Rd. Kansas City, MO 64100
National Cancer Institute	Ann Bavier, RN, MN Program Director Community Oncology and Rehabilitation Program Division of Cancer Prevention & Control Blair Bldg. Room 7A-05 National Cancer Institute Bethesda, MD 20892
National Center for Nursing Research	Ada Sue Hinshaw, RN, PhD Director, National Center for Nursing Research Building 31, Rm. B1-C02 National Institutes of Health Bethesda, MD 20892
National Institute of Aging	National Institute of Aging Building 31, Rm. 5C05 National Institutes of Health Bethesda, MD 20892
Oncology Nursing Foundation	Pearl Moore, RN, MS Executive Director Oncology Nursing Foundation 1016 Greentree Rd. Pittsburgh, PA 15220
Sigma Theta Tau	Sigma Theta Tau International Honor Society of Nursing 1200 Waterway Blvd. Indianapolis, IN 46202

preparation of the members of the American Nurses' Association with that of members of the Oncology Nursing Society revealed that ONS members had a higher percentage of nurses with baccalaureate preparation (39% versus 25%) and with master's preparation (24% versus 16%).[6]

A second survey revealed changes in the characteristics of oncology nurses relevant to today's increased productivity in research activities. Participants in this second survey responded to a questionnaire published in the *Oncology Nursing Forum.*[13] The 350 respondents represented 46 states. The typical respondent (1) had either a baccalaureate or a master's degree, (2) had been in nursing under 10 years and in oncology nursing less than 6 years, (3) worked in a hospital setting or a school of nursing, and (4) was employed as either a clinical specialist or an educator. A major difference reported in this survey was the increase in the number and variety of research roles in which participation was reported. Findings that contrast with the 1981 survey revealed that between 1981 and 1985 the primary role changed from that of data collector to a variety of more independent research roles, including proposal development, individual investigation, and statistical analysis, as well as data collection. These expanding roles in research reflect a growing sophistication in ability to conduct oncology nursing research.

A third resource for development in cancer nursing research is support from nursing administration in both educational and clinical settings. In educational settings, more and more faculty members are prepared at the doctoral level and are expected to conduct research on a regular basis and within a program of research interests. Students frequently work with faculty in their programs of research. As doctoral programs for nurses have increased, dissertation research involving cancer patients' clinical problems has increased. Because of these research expectations, educational settings have developed additional resources for researchers. Computer facilities are common; statistical consultation is generally available and at reasonable rates for students; data coding and management assistance are provided.

In clinical settings, the expectations for conducting research are less frequent. An initial institutional commitment to research is exemplified by a statement in the clinical nurse specialist job description that specifies that research is a job expectation.[14] Such commitment may be found in institutions that have no specific individual or department with a designated nursing research focus. For clinical nurses in these settings to conduct research, success is related to the enthusiasm and tenacity of the individual nurse. A trend that has become evident recently is the increased frequency of establishment of a specific position or department for nursing research.[15] This position or department may be a separate department, or it may be combined with either education and/or quality-assurance departments. The kind of research carried out by investigators in clinical settings differs from that carried out by investigators in educational settings. In the clinical setting a larger percentage of investigators plan and conduct evaluation research specific to the institution and its problems.[16] Such research may emerge from quality-assurance studies. For example, vascular access devices show an increased occurrence of infection. A study comparing currently used but different dressing techniques for these devices may be launched in response to the quality-assurance findings.

Resources for oncology nursing research have changed over the last few years, and these changes have been positive. Increased financial support has become available. The education and experience of oncology nurses reflect increased academic preparation for research and increased involvement in a variety of research activities. These resources will continue to expand the knowledge base of cancer nursing care as studies become more sophisticated and are replicated.

Priorities for Cancer Nursing Research

One method that has proved useful in the development of depth in the scientific foundation for nursing practice has been a systematic targeting of researchers and resources to areas of needed knowledge. The identification of priorities for studies has provided information useful in the development of a program for nursing research that leads to well-tested areas of study. With such an approach, the accurate information needed for development of clinical nursing practice is possible. The National Center for Nursing Research has been involved in identification of clinical nursing research priorities through the development of a national nursing agenda.[17] One aspect of this endeavor has been to seek out research priorities identified by various nursing groups.

Cancer nursing research priorities have been identified and revised over the years. One of the first reports was published by Oberst.[18] This list of priorities was developed through a Delphi survey technique in which 254 oncology nurses participated. The following five top priority areas were identified:

1. Relieving nausea/vomiting induced by chemotherapy/radiation
2. Pain management
3. Discharge planning and follow-up
4. Grief and death
5. Stomatitis

This study was followed by several other studies conducted through the Oncology Nursing Society, the Canadian Consortium, and the National Cancer Institute.[6,13,19,20] The most recent survey is that by Funkhouser and Grant.[11] This survey was sent to 700 ONS members who had previously identified research as their major focus, members who had participated as research faculty in ONS short courses, and/or members who had functioned in leadership positions in ONS. A total of 213 respondents returned the survey. Respondents had practiced nursing for an average of 15 years and had specialized in oncologic nursing for an average of 9 years. Distribution of highest educational degrees was as follows: doctoral degree, 30%; master's de-

TABLE 60-3 1988 Cancer Nursing Research Priorities

1 Prevention and early detection	23 Hospice care
2 Symptom management	24 Oncologic emergencies
3 Pain control and management	25 Characteristics of oncology nurses
4 Patient or health education	26 Role of specialist
5 Coping and stress management	27 Bereavement
6 Home care	28 Comfort
7 Economic influences on oncology	29 Physiologic aspects
8 Cancer rehabilitation	30 Epidemiology
9 AIDS	31 Quality of life
10 Compliance with treatment	32 Pediatric oncology
11 Self-care	33 Body image
12 Early detection activities	34 Protective mechanisms
13 Nurse burn-out	35 Labor costs
14 Cancer in the elderly	36 Cancer survival
15 Cost containment	37 Stomatitis
16 Spiritual aspects/religiosity	38 Family issues
17 Counseling	39 Primary nursing
18 Nutrition	40 Acuity/staffing
19 Sexuality	41 Health care delivery systems
20 Implementation of ONS standards	42 Outcome measures for interventions
21 Quality assurance	43 Occupational hazards
22 Smoke cessation	44 Mobility
	45 Elimination
	46 Ethnic/cultural issues

gree in nursing, 24%; bachelor's degree in nursing, 30%. Of the 213 respondents, 150 reported that their current position included research expectations. Table 60-3 contains a listing of the research topics rank-ordered between 1 and 5 by respondents.

Why changes in priorities have occurred over the years is not clear. One interpretation is that some research activity has been completed and findings are being implemented in the management of patient care. One area in which considerable medical and nursing research activity has occurred is that of nausea and vomiting associated with chemotherapy or radiation therapy. It is interesting to note that symptom management and pain persist in the top-priorty positions and that prevention and early detection is No. 1. This listing may be of assistance to nurses who are interested in developing a focus for a research program or even a specific research project. The breadth of topics reflects the extent of nursing care problems and researchers' interests.

Examples of Recent Cancer Nursing Research Publications

To provide examples of the progress in cancer nursing research, Padilla[11] analyzed the 1986 issues of *Cancer, Nursing, Oncology Nursing Forum, Nursing Research, Research in Nursing and Health, Western Journal of Nursing Research,* and *Advances in Nursing Science.* The three research journals published 120 scientific articles, excluding features, editorials, and the like. Of these 120 articles, 8 (6.6%) were considered to concern cancer nursing research since they dealt with oncology patients, oncology nursing problems, or hospice care. The two cancer journals published 79 articles, excluding features, editorials, etc. Of these, 40 (50.6%) were identified as scientific investigations.

The 48 cancer nursing research articles published in the five journals included 4 instruments-development studies; 3 descriptive program-evaluation studies; 27 one-group descriptive studies and 9 two- or three-group comparison descriptive studies with infrequent use of a random selection procedure; and 5 experimental or quasi-experimental studies. Data collection covered periods of 6 months or less. Units of analysis were patients (27 studies), families or care givers (4 studies), nurses (15 studies), healthy subjects (5), and agencies (2). Some studies included more than one type of unit of analysis. Number of subjects ranged from one agency[22] whose "day hospital for cancer patients" was being evaluated, to 823 nurses[23] who returned a mailed survey questionnaire on prevalence and quit rates of smoking-related behaviors. Diagnoses of patients participating in these research studies were not always stated. Mail-out/mail-return surveys were conducted as part of five studies. The return rate for these surveys was quite good, ranging from 46%[24] to 88%,[25] with the mean at 63%.

The nursing research studies were classified, according to Padilla and Grant,[9] into five categories. The categories were population descriptors,[23-35] impact of the diagnosis,[36-46] impact of cancer treatment,[47-58] impact of cancer prognosis,[22,59-63] and education regarding cancer and death.[64-66]

FUTURE DIRECTIONS FOR CANCER NURSING RESEARCH

By comparing the results of the review of cancer nursing research[21] with the recommendations made by Grant and Padilla in the first edition of this book, areas of continued concern can be identified. These areas can be viewed as the authors' personal observations of where studies will occur and are still needed. (1) Descriptive studies of patient care questions continue to form the bulk of cancer nursing efforts and are likely to continue. (2) Recommended population descriptor studies on nurse needs and incidence of patient care problems have been published. (3) Recommended studies on the impact of the cancer diagnosis in relation to pain control and adjustment have been published. However, studies on blame and guilt are still needed, as are studies on nutrition, weight loss, and physical activity. (4) Recommended investigations related to the impact of treatment have included hospitalization and cognitive, physical, and emotional side effects of therapy and standards of care. Lacking are studies on disruptions in sleep and sexual activity and neglect of cancer patients. (5) Recommended studies on the impact of cancer prognosis in relation to needs of dying patients and alternative care systems for these patients have been published. There continues to be a paucity of information on physiologic aspects of the dying process, related care, and quality of life. (6) Only three studies relating to education about cancer and death were identified in the 1986 cancer nursing research publications.

There continues to be a need for investigations of the cost of oncology nurse and patient education programs in relation to cancer prevention, hospitalization, self-care, and adaptation to illness. Also needed are studies that investigate the impact of patient and nurse education programs on desired patient and nurse behavioral outcomes.

CONCLUSION

Research continues to be an important aspect of the cancer nursing specialty. Both medical and nursing research activities are important in improving the care, treatment, and quality of life for patients with cancer. A review of the nature of medical research in cancer care and of nursing research activities provides ample evidence of the essential role that nurses play in this aspect of care. Recent review of cancer nursing research publications reveals a rapidly growing collection of valuable studies. Nurses have made and will continue to make important contributions through research endeavors.

• • •

Partial support was provided by NIH Cancer Support Grant CA 33572.

REFERENCES

1. Polit D, Hungler B: Nursing Research: Principles and Methods. Philadelphia, JB Lippincott, 1987.
2. Padilla GV: Incorporating research in a service setting. J Nurse Admin 9:44-49, 1979.
3. Eilber FR: Principles of cancer surgery, in Haskell CM (ed): Cancer Treatment (ed 2). Philadelphia, WB Saunders, 1985, pp 7-13.
4. Rubin P: The emergence of radiation oncology as a distinct medical specialty. Int J Radiat Oncol Biol Phys 2:1247-1270, 1985.
5. Hubbard SM: Cancer treatment research: The role of the nurse clinical trials of cancer therapy. Nurs Clin North Am 17:763-783, 1982.
6. Grant M, Stromborg M: Promoting research collaboration: ONS research committee survey. Oncol Nurs Forum 8(2):48-53, 1981.
7. Fisher B: Clinical trials for the evaluation of cancer therapy. Cancer 54:2609-2617, 1984.
8. American Nurses' Association: Nursing—A social policy statement. Kansas City, Mo, American Nurses' Association, 1980.
9. Padilla GV, Grant MM: Cancer nursing research, in Groenwald SL (ed): Cancer Nursing: Principles and Practice. Boston, Jones & Bartlett, 1987, pp 827-853.
10. Cotanch PH: Relaxation training for control of nausea and vomiting in patients receiving chemotherapy. Cancer Nurs 6:277-283, 1983.
11. Funkhouser SW, Grant MM: 1988 ONS survey of research priorities. Oncol Nurs Forum 16:413-416, 1989.
12. Schmitt MH, Chapman MK: Alumni involvement in nursing research development. Nurs Outlook 28:572-574, 1980.
13. McGuire D, Frank-Stromborg M, Varricchio C: 1984 ONS research committee survey of membership's research interest and involvement. Oncol Nurs Forum 12:99-103, 1985.
14. Varricchio C, Mikos D: Research: Determining feasibility in clinical setting. Oncol Nurs Forum 14(1):89-90, 1987.
15. Pranulis M, Gortner S: Researchmanship: Characteristics of productive research environments in nursing. West J Nurs Res 7:127-131, 1985.
16. McArt E: Research facilitation in academic and practice settings. J Prof Nurs 3(2):84-91, 1987.
17. Hinshaw AS, Heinrich J, Bloch D: Evolving clinical nursing research priorities: A national endeavor. J Prof Nurs 4:398, 458-459, 1988.
18. Oberst M: Priorities in cancer nursing research. Cancer Nurs 1:281-290, 1978.
19. Degner L, Arcand R, Chekryn J, et al: Priorities for cancer nursing research. Cancer Nurs 10:319-326, 1987.
20. Dodd M: Problem approaches and priorities in oncology nursing research. AARN Newsletter 43(2):13-14, 1987.
21. Padilla GV: Progress in cancer nursing research, in Grant MM, Padilla GV (eds): Cancer Nursing Research: A Practical Approach. New York, Appleton-Lange, 1990, pp 14-18.
22. Clark M: A day hospital for cancer patients: Clinical and economic feasibility. Oncol Nurs Forum 13(6):41-45, 1986.
23. Feldman BM, Richard E: Prevalence of nurse smokers and variables identified with successful and unsuccessful smoking cessation. Res Nurs Health 9:131-138, 1986.
24. Dalton JA, Swenson I: Nurses and smoking: Role modeling and counseling behaviors. Oncol Nurs Forum 13(2):45-48, 1986.
25. Gritz ER, Kanim L: Do fewer oncology nurses smoke? Oncol Nurs Forum 13(3):61-64, 1986.
26. Kesselring A, Lindsey AM, Dodd MJ, et al: Social network and support perceived by Swiss cancer patients. Cancer Nurs 9:156-163, 1986.
27. Blesch KS: Health beliefs about testicular cancer self-examination among professional men. Oncol Nurs Forum 13(1):29-33, 1986.
28. Massey V: Perceived susceptibility to breast cancer and practice of breast self-examination. Nurs Res 35:183-185, 1986.
29. Weinrich SP, Weinrich MC: Cancer knowledge among elderly individuals. Cancer Nurs 9:301-307, 1986.
30. Karani D, Wiltshaw E: How well informed? Cancer Nurs 9:238-242, 1986.
31. Martin BA, Belcher JV: Influence of cultural background on nurses' attitudes and care of the oncology patient. Cancer Nurs 9:230-237, 1986.
32. Larson PJ: Cancer nurses' perceptions of caring. Cancer Nurs 9:86-91, 1986.
33. Trygstad L: Professional friends: The inclusion of the personal into the professional. Cancer Nurs 9:326-332, 1986.
34. Jenkins JF, Ostchega Y: Evaluation of burnout in oncology nurses. Cancer Nurs 9:108-116, 1986.

35. Williams HA, Wilson ME, Hongladarom, et al: Nurses attitudes toward sexuality in cancer patients. Oncol Nurs Forum 13(2):39-43, 1986.
36. Solodky M, Mikos K, Bordieri J, et al: Nurses' prognosis for oncology and coronary heart disease patients. Cancer Nurs 9:243-247, 1986.
37. Derdiarian AK: Informational needs of recently diagnosed cancer patients. Nurs Res 35:276-281, 1986.
38. Tringali CA: The needs of family members of cancer patients. Oncol Nurs Forum 13(4):65-70, 1986.
39. Kesselring A, Dodd MJ, Lindsey AM, et al: Attitudes of patients living in Switzerland about cancer and its treatment. Cancer Nurs 9:77-85, 1986.
40. Waterhouse J, Metcalfe MC: Development of the sexual adjustment questionnaire. Oncol Nurs Forum 13(3):53-59, 1986.
41. Longman AJ, Graham KY: Living with melanoma: Content analysis of interviews. Oncol Nurs Forum 13(4):58-64, 1986.
42. Brown ML, Carrieri V, Janson-Bjerklie S, et al: Lung cancer and dyspnea: The patient's perception. Oncol Nurs Forum 13(5):19-24, 1986.
43. Bressler LR, Hange PA, McGuire DB: Characterization of the pain experience in a sample of cancer outpatients. Oncol Nurs Forum 13(6):51-55, 1986.
44. Austin C, Eyres PJ, Hefferin EA, et al: Hospice home care pain management: Four critical variables. Cancer Nurs 9:58-65, 1986.
45. Barbour LA, McGuire DB, Kirchhoff KT: Nonanalgesic methods of pain control used by cancer outpatients. Oncol Nurs Forum 13(6):56-60, 1986.
46. Coyle N, Mauskip A, Maggard J, et al: Continuous subcutaneous infusions of opiates in cancer patients with pain. Oncol Nurs Forum 13(4):53-57, 1986.
47. Lovejoy NC: Family responses to cancer hospitalization. Oncol Nurs Forum 13(2):33-37, 1986.
48. Fernsler J: A comparison of patient and nurse perceptions of patients self-care deficits associated with cancer chemotherapy. Cancer Nurs 9:50-57, 1986.
49. Hopkins MB: Information-seeking and adaptational outcomes in women receiving chemotherapy for breast cancer. Cancer Nurs 9:256-262, 1986.
50. Moore IM, Kramer J, Ablin A: Late effects of central nervous system prophylactic leukemia therapy on cognitive functioning. Oncol Nurs Forum 13(4):45-51, 1986.
51. Post-White J: Glucocorticosteroid-induced depression in the patient with leukemia or lymphoma. Cancer Nurs 9:15-22, 1986.
52. Scott DW, Donahue DC, Mastrovito RC, et al: Comparative trial of clinical relaxation and an antiemetic drug regimen in reducing chemotherapy-related nausea and vomiting. Cancer Nurs 9:178-187, 1986.
54. Stajich GV, Barnett CW, Turner SV, et al: Protective measures used by oncologic office nurses handling parenteral antineoplastic agents. Oncol Nurs Forum 13(6):47-49, 1986.
55. Strauman JJ: Symptom distress in patients receiving phase I chemotherapy with taxol. Oncol Nurs Forum 13(5):40-43, 1986.
56. Huldij A, Giesbers A, Poelhuis EHK, et al: Alterations in taste appreciation in cancer patients during treatment. Cancer Nurs 9:38-52, 1986.
57. Shell JA, Stanutz F, Grimm J: Comparison of moisture vapor permeable (MVP) dressings to conventional dressings for managment of radiation skin reactions. Oncol Nurs Forum 13(1):11-16, 1986.
58. La Monica EL, Oberst MT, Madea AR, et al: Development of a patient satisfaction scale. Res Nurs Health 9:43-50, 1986.
59. Sawyer PF: Breast self-examination: Hospital-based nurses aren't assessing their clients. Oncol Nurs Forum 13(5):44-48, 1986.
60. Holing EV: The primary caregiver's perception of the dying trajectory: An exploratory study. Cancer Nurs 9:29-37, 1986.
61. Francis MR: Concerns of terminally ill adult Hindu cancer patients. Cancer Nurs 9:164-171, 1986.
62. Reed PG: Religiousness among terminally ill and healthy adults. Res Nurs Health 9:35-41, 1986.
63. Lauer ME, Mulhern RK, Hoffmann RG, et al: Utilization of hospice/home care in pediatric oncology. Cancer Nurs 9:102-107, 1986.
64. Martinson IM, Moldow DG, Armstrong GD, et al: Home care for children dying of cancer. Res Nurs Health 9:11-16, 1986.
65. Hauck SL: Pain: Problem for the person with cancer. Cancer Nurs 9:66-76, 1986.
66. Fredette SL, Beattie HM: Living with cancer: A patient education program. Cancer Nurs 9:308-316, 1986.
67. Brailey LJ: Effects of health teaching in the workplace on women's knowledge, beliefs, and practices regarding breast self-examination. Res Nurs Health 9:233-231, 1986.

PART IX

YELLOW PAGES FOR THE CANCER NURSE

Marilyn Frank-Stromborg, RN, EdD, NP, FAAN

Beth Savela, RN, BSN

AUDIOVISUAL

Audiovisual Sources

The past few years have witnessed a dramatic growth in the use of video technology in all areas of professional health care education. Many institutions such as schools and hospitals are finding audiovisual material to be a highly efficient information and training medium. The number of available audiovisual programs (software) continues to increase substantially each year. Several directories or catalogs that index software may be rented or purchased. These indexes list the following for each entry: physical description (including format, width, and mode of videotape and length of program), indication of additional materials, audience level, costs to rent or purchase, year of production, producer/distributor, subject headings, and a brief summary of the contents of the program.

1. American Cancer Society
   Tower Place
   3340 Peachtree Road NE
   Atlanta, GA 30026
   (404) 320-3333

   The American Cancer Society (ACS) has films, videos, filmstrips, slides, and audiotapes available for free loan. Contact the national office or your local ACS unit for a catalog on the available audiovisual materials.
2. American Hospital Association
   Catalog of Publications and Audiovisual Products
   840 North Lake Shore Drive
   Chicago, IL 60611
   (312) 645-9400

   Free Catalog
3. National Audiovisual Center
   Information Services SF
   Washington, DC 20409
   (301) 763-1896/763-4385 (TDD)

   This center distributes over 13,000 US government–sponsored productions at low prices. Contact the center for your specific area of interest and request free catalogs. Example of listings in the catalog are as follows: *Diet and Cancer Prevention,* 1986, 58 min., videocassette, Dr. Peter Greenwald, Director, Division of Cancer Prevention and Control, NCI explores the effects of fat on breast and colon cancer.
4. NLN Directory of Educational Software for Nursing
   Christine Bolwell
   National League for Nursing
   350 Hudson Street
   New York, NY 10014
   (800) 669-1656
   Pub no. 41-2215

   This directory provides information for anyone interested in using the microcomputer to teach nursing. Each program listed in this directory was reviewed and described along with ratings of the software and the educators' comments that accompany each computer-assisted instruction. There are complete descriptions and purchasing information for over 300 programs, program ratings by a pool of more than 730 health care professionals, and sections on how to evaluate computer-assisted instruction. There are several oncology-related programs listed in this directory.
5. Media Review Digest
   Lesley Orlin (ed)
   The Pierian Press
   Ann Arbor, MI 48104

   This reference book is an annual index to and digest of reviews, evaluations, and descriptions of all forms of nonbook media. This text reviews films, videotapes, filmstrips, records, and tapes.
6. Many universities and medical centers produce audiovisual material that can be purchased. Contact your local university to see if they produce audiovisuals that can be loaned or if the film library contains cancer-related audiovisuals that you could borrow. Several examples are listed below:

   The University of Michigan Media Library
   Department of Postgraduate Medicine and Health Professionals' Education
   R4440 Kresge
   Box 0518
   Ann Arbor, MI 48109-0518
   (313) 763-2074

   You can request a free catalog of medical and nursing audiovisuals.

   Carle Medical Communications
   510 West Main
   Urbana, IL 61801
   (217) 384-4838

   This company produces several cancer-related films/videotapes. One example is *Controlling the Behavioral Side Effects of Chemotherapy.*

Cancer Communications Pretesting

The NCI's Office of Cancer Communications has been experimenting with various pretesting techniques and has gained experience with a number of approaches among a variety of individuals. It has published three booklets that provide information and guidance about measuring the effectiveness of the health message. All three booklets are provided free of charge and can be obtained by calling the **1-800-4-CANCER** telephone number.

1. Making Health Communication Programs Work: A Planner's Guide
   NIH pub no. 89-1493, 1989

   Originally published in 1984 and revised in 1988, *Making Health Communication Programs Work: A Planner's Guide* discusses the purpose of pretesting, planning the health message, conducting pretesting research, conducting the pretest, and measuring the readability of the health message. It also provides an extensive bibliography about pretesting as well as suggestions on how to write the message and determine its readability.
2. Pretesting Television PSAs
   NIH pub no. 85-2670, 1985

   Pretesting Television PSAs is a guidebook developed to assist in designing, implementing, analyzing, and interpreting television public service announcements. The booklet provides specific step-by-step directions for the pretesting process and provides examples of how to handle communication with the pretesting audience. There is also a discussion of what the pretest results should mean to the individual planning the public service announcement.

3. Making PSAs Work—TV and Radio. A Handbook for Health Communication Professionals
NIH pub no. 83-2485, 1983

Making PSAs Work—TV and Radio. A Handbook for Health Communication Professionals is the third booklet designed to provide assistance in planning health messages. The booklet offers guidelines for producing effective messages and for planning, pretesting, implementing, and evaluating a PSA campaign. There is a discussion of how to define the campaign objectives, who the target audience is, selecting an appropriate medium format and length, and what is involved in the technical aspects of filming and recording the PSA. This booklet, like the other two, also provides the user with a helpful bibliography and appropriate appendixes.

ACADEMIC PROGRAMS AND CONTINUING EDUCATION OPPORTUNITIES

Master's Degree Oncology Nursing Programs

Several nursing schools offer graduate education in oncology, and the potential student can choose from several types of programs. Some programs offer separate, distinct, oncology clinical specialist master's curricula, whereas others offer the oncology component within the graduate program in medical-surgical nursing. Because curricula and programs change, the reader is advised to contact local universities to determine if the school of nursing offers a master's program in oncology nursing. In addition, the Oncology Nursing Society publication, "The Master's Degree With a Specialty in Oncology Nursing: Role Definition and Curriculum Guide" (1988), serves a dual purpose as a guide for (1) nursing educators in establishing new oncology programs or evaluating current ones and for (2) prospective students in selecting a program. Another excellent source is the article "Survey of Graduate Programs in Cancer Nursing" in *Oncology Nursing Forum* 15:825-831, 1988. This article details specific information about each program (clinical focus, program length, application deadline, NLN accreditation, etc).

Graduate Oncology Nursing Programs

Alabama

University of Alabama
School of Nursing
Judy Holcombe, RN, DSN
Associate Professor
University of Alabama at Birmingham
University Station
Birmingham, AL 35294

Arizona

University of Arizona
Alice J. Longman, RN, EdD
Associate Professor
College of Nursing
Tucson, AZ 85721

California

University of California, Los Angeles
School of Nursing
Ada Lindsey
Dean
Los Angeles, CA 90024

University of California, San Francisco
Co-Program Directors
Marylin Dodd, RN, PhD
Patricia Larson, RN, DNSc
School of Nursing
Department of Physiological Nursing
San Francisco, CA 94143

Connecticut

Yale University
School of Nursing
Dorothy Sexton, RN, EdD
Associate Professor and Chairperson
Medical-Surgical Nursing Program
New Haven, CT 06520

Delaware

University of Delaware
Jayne Fernsler, RN, DSN
Assistant Professor
College of Nursing
University of Delaware
Newark, DE 19716

District of Columbia

Catholic University of America
Janice Hallal, RN, DNSc
Coordinator—Graduate Oncology Nursing
School of Nursing
Washington, DC 20064

Florida

University of Miami
School of Nursing
Beverly Nielsen, RN, EdD
Oncology Nursing
Miami, FL 33124

University of South Florida
College of Nursing
Susan McMillan, RN, PhD
Chairperson, Oncology Nursing
Tampa, FL 33612

Georgia

Emory University
Rose F. McGee, RN, PhD
Professor
Oncology Nursing
Atlanta, GA 30322

Illinois

Loyola University of Chicago
Niehoff School of Nursing
Claudette Varricchio, RN, DSN
Associate Professor
Medical-Surgical Nursing
Chicago, IL 60626

Northern Illinois University
School of Nursing
Marilyn Stromborg, RN, EdD
Professor, Adult Oncology
DeKalb, IL 60115

Northwestern University
Center for Nursing
Janet A. Deatrick, RN, PhD
Associate Director, Graduate Program in Nursing
750 North Lake Shore Drive
Chicago, IL 60611

Rush University
College of Nursing
Judith Paice, RN, MS
Acting Coordinator, Graduate Program in Oncology Nursing
Chicago, IL 60612

University of Illinois at Chicago
College of Nursing
Susan Dudas, RN, MSN
Associate Professor
Chicago, IL 60612

Indiana

Indiana University
Judy Lambert, RN, MSN
Assistant Professor
School of Nursing
Indianapolis, IN 46223

Massachusetts

Massachusetts General Hospital Institute of Health Professions
Sylvia Drake Page, RN, DNSc
Coordinator, Oncology
Boston, MA 02108-9990

Missouri

St. Louis University
School of Nursing
Ramona M. Wessler, RN, PhD
St. Louis, MO 63104

University of Missouri, Columbia
Ann Rosenow, RN, PhD
Associate Dean for Research
Director, Graduate Studies
Columbia, MO 65211

New York

Columbia University
School of Nursing
Anne Hubbard, MS, MPH
Director, Master's Program in Oncology Nursing
New York, NY 10032

Russell Sage College
Marjory Keenan, EdD
Professor of Nursing
Troy, NY 12180

State University of New York, Buffalo
Yvonne Sherer, RN, EdD
School of Nursing
Department of Graduate Education
Faculty of Health Sciences
Buffalo, NY 14214

University of Rochester
School of Nursing
Jean Johnson, RN, PhD
Cancer Center Nursing
Rochester, NY 14642

North Carolina

Duke University
School of Nursing
Dorothy Brundage, RN, PhD
Interim Dean
Durham, NC 27710

University of North Carolina at Chapel Hill
Inge Corless, PhD, FAAN
Chairman, Secondary Care Nursing
School of Nursing
Chapel Hill, NC 27514

Ohio

Frances Payne Bolton
School of Nursing
Case Western Reserve University
Ellen Rudy, RN, PhD
Chairperson
Cleveland, OH 44106

Medical College of Ohio
School of Nursing
Sharon Utz, RN, PhD
Associate Professor
Medical-Surgical Nursing
Toledo, OH 43699

University of Cincinnati
M. Linda Workman, RN, PhD
Assistant Professor
College of Nursing and Health
Cincinnati, OH 45221

Pennsylvania

Gwynedd-Mercy College
Patricia Bennett, RN, MA
Oncological Nursing
Graduate Nursing Division
Gwynedd Valley, PA 19437

University of Pennsylvania
Ruth McCorkle, RN, PhD, FAAN
Nursing Education Building
School of Nursing
Philadelphia, PA 19104

University of Pittsburgh
School of Nursing
Catherine Bender, RN, MN
Assistant Professor
Graduate Program Oncology Nursing
Pittsburgh, PA 15261

Widener University
Jean Fergusson, RN, MSN (Pediatrics)
Susan Cobb, RN, MSN, CS, OCN (Adult)
Graduate Program
School of Nursing
Chester, PA 19013

South Carolina

University of South Carolina
College of Nursing
Janet F. Nussbaum, RN, EdD
Oncology Nursing
Columbia, SC 29208

Tennessee

University of Tennessee
College of Nursing
Dianne Greenhill, RN, EdD
Associate Dean
Memphis, TN 38163

Vanderbilt University
James Pace, RN, DSN

Dana Rutledge, RN, PhD
Oncology Specialty Coordinators
Nashville, TN 37240

Texas

University of Texas
Health Science Center
Patricia Bohannan, RN, PhD
Program Coordinator
School of Nursing
Houston, TX 77030

Utah

Brigham Young University
Camilla Wood, RN, PhD
Professor and Oncology Nursing Program Coordinator
College of Nursing
Provo, UT 84602

Virginia

George Mason University
Graceann Ehlke, RN, DNSc
Coordinator, Advanced Clinical Nursing
Fairfax, VA 22030

Virginia Commonwealth University
Medical College of Virginia
Ethelyn Exley, RN, EdD
Assistant Dean of Academic Affairs
Richmond, VA 23298

Washington

University of Washington
Betty Gallucci, RN, PhD
Professor, Department of Physiological Nursing
Seattle, WA 98195

University of Washington
Marion Rose, RN, PhD
Professor, Department of Parent and Child Nursing SC-74
Seattle, WA 98195

Wisconsin

University of Wisconsin
Marilyn Oberst, RN, EdD
School of Nursing
Clinical Science Center
Madison, WI 53792

Enterostomal Therapy Programs

Enterostomal therapy (ET) is an allied healthcare field specializing in the care of patients with all types of abdominal stomas as well as the management of patients with a wide variety of draining sinus tracts and fistulas. This nurse specialist is called an enterostomal therapist. Currently, an applicant must be an RN with a baccalaureate degree in nursing with 1 year of recent (within 5 years) clinical experience in medical-surgical nursing. Tuition varies among programs. Scholarships are available through the International Association for Enterostomal Therapy, Inc. (IAET), ACS, United Ostomy Association, and many of the individual ET nurse programs.

It is best to first obtain a list of IAET-approved professional education programs from:

IAET
2081 Business Center Drive
Suite 290
Irvine, CA 92715
(714) 476-0268

IAET-accredited ET Nurse Education Programs are listed below:

Abbott Northwestern ET Nursing Education Program
800 East 28th Street at Chicago Avenue
Minneapolis, MN 55407
(612) 863-4601

Emory University ET Nursing Education Program
1365 Clifton Road, NE, Room 360, Emory Clinic
Atlanta, GA 30322
(404) 321-0111 ext. 3321

Harrisburg Hospital School of Enterostomal Therapy
South Front Street
Harrisburg, PA 17101
(717) 782-5565

M. D. Anderson Hospital and Tumor Institute
Department of Nursing
6723 Bertner
Houston, TX 77030
(713) 792-7132

Northwest Community Hospital
ET Education Program of the Department of Continuing Education
800 West Central Road
Arlington Heights, IL 60005
(312) 259-1000 ext. 5161

R. B. Turnbull Jr. School of ET
Cleveland Clinic Foundation
9500 Euclid Avenue 3L20
Cleveland, OH 44106
(216) 444-5966

Tucson Medical Center
c/o Restorative Services
ET Nurse Education Program
5301 East Grant Road
Box 42195
Tucson, AZ 85733
(602) 327-5461 ext. 5400

University of Southern California
c/o MSN Program
Leavey Hall
320 West 15th Street
Los Angeles, CA 90015
(213) 743-2362

PRINT SOURCES

Library Retrieval Services

For those readers who are not familiar with the benefits of mechanized literature search or the "how-to's," the following articles will supply this information. In addition, you are advised to consult your local librarian or the closest college or university library near you. Most higher education libraries now have public access terminals for students and the public to conduct their own computer search.

1. Treece E, Treece J: The library and computer-based literature searches, in *Elements of Research in Nursing* (ed 4). St Louis, CV Mosby, 1986, pp 91-112. This chapter discusses how to use the MEDLARS retrieval service.

2. Nieswiadomy R: Review of the literature, *Foundations of Nursing Research.* Norwalk, Conn, Appleton-Lange, 1987, pp 73-89. This chapter details the multiple computer-assisted literature searches that are available to the nurse desiring to do a literature review.
3. Polit D, Hungler B: Locating and summarizing existing information on a problem, *Nursing Research. Principles and Methods* (ed 2). Philadelphia, JB Lippincott, 1987, pp 62-78. This chapter provides a guide to selected abstracts and indexes for nursing and related subjects and relationship to computer searches and databases.
4. Woodbury M: Computerized retrieval services, *A Guide to Sources of Educational Information.* Washington, DC, Information Resources Press, 1982. This chapter gives an in-depth description of computerized retrieval services—location, information stored, cost, and availability.

In addition, the following catalog contains extensive information on data banks and computerized retrieval services.

1. *Dialog Database Catalog 1988,* Dialog Information Services, Inc., a subsidiary of Lockheed Corporation, contains a description of all available databases, including years the database covers, number of records in the database, when the database is routinely updated, who provides the database, and costs to access the database.

A partial list of computerized retrieval services follows, with an emphasis on medically oriented systems.

1. MEDLARS: MEDLARS is a computer-based bibliographic processing system operated by the National Library of Medicine (NLM) at Bethesda, MD. It has been designed to achieve rapid bibliographic access to over 3000 international journals published in the United States and 70 other countries. Included is all the material in *Index Medicus, International Nursing Index,* and *Index to Dental Literature* from 1966 to the present. MEDLARS is identical to MEDLINE (MEDLARS ON-LINE), but MEDLINE makes it possible for the researcher to obtain the bibliographic retrieval faster. Over 40% of records added since 1975 contain author abstracts taken directly from the published articles. Over 250,000 records are needed each year, of which over 70% are English language. Cost as of 1989 is $36 each hour of computer connect time, $0.20 for a full record printed offline, and $0.05 for a full record typed or displayed online.
2. AVLINE: AVLINE (audiovisuals-on-line) is a computer information service available through the MEDLARS system of the NLM. The AVLINE database is searchable through any MEDLARS terminal by using the classification established in the medical subject headings of the *Index Medicus.* AVLINE is a clearinghouse of nontextbook educational materials to assist the health science community. All audiovisual material is catalogued, indexed, abstracted, and described according to physical characteristics and rated (highly recommended, recommended, or not recommended). It is updated weekly, with approximately 100 records added per month.
3. CHEMLINE: A chemical dictionary, it is used primarily to aid in searching other databases. It is produced by *Chemical Abstracts* and the NLM.
4. TOXLINE: All aspects of toxicology are on this computer tape, including material from *Chemical Abstracts, Toxicity Bibliography, Bio Research Index, Health Effects of Environmental Pollutants,* etc. The database covers from 1930 to the present. It is part of the NLM database.
5. HEALTH (Health planning and administration): Bibliographic citations covering nonclinical aspects of health care delivery. Subject areas emphasized include the administration and planning of health facilities, services and personnel, health insurance, health policy, aspects of financial management, etc. Citations are prepared by the NLM, the American Hospital Association (AHA), and the National Health Planning Information Center.
6. CATLINE: This database is available through the NLM (as are MEDLINE, HEALTH, TOXLINE, CHEMLINE, CANCERLINE, and AVLINE). It contains a listing of over 600,000 books and serials acquired since 1965 by the NLM. The cost of doing a MEDLINE search is based on the actual cost of searching the database. For example, a 5-minute search on MEDLINE may cost $3 (based on the average cost of $36 an hour). You can print citations on your printer or have them printed elsewhere and sent to you ("offline").
7. Smoking and Health: Smoking and Health contains bibliographic citations and abstracts to journal articles, reports, and other literature that discuss the effects of smoking on health. The files contain information from 1960 to the present and are updated every 2 months. Presently Smoking and Health contains over 37,000 records. This database corresponds to the printed government publication "Smoking and Health Bulletin." It is operated by the NIH, Office of Smoking and Health, Rockville, MD. Cost is $45 for each hour of computer connect time and $0.20 for a full-record printed offline.
8. CANCERLINE: A computer-based system for on-line retrieval of abstracts derived from published results of cancer research. Includes material from *Carcinogenesis Abstracts* and *Cancer Therapy* (1963 to present). CANCERLINE is available at all terminals linked to the computer system at the NLM in Bethesda, MD. This service is available to scientists, physicians, nurses, and other health care professionals and educators. Terminals for the NLM are located at more than 700 medical library locations throughout the United States and in 12 foreign countries. The CANCERLINE system is composed of three separate computer databases:
   a. CANCERLIT (CANCERLITerature): This database contains more than 617,812 records and is updated monthly. CANCERLIT contains abstracts that appeared in *Carcinogenesis Abstracts* from 1963 to 1969 and in *Cancer Therapy Abstracts* from 1967 to 1979. In 1977 the database was enlarged to include cancer-related articles from a variety of sources.
   b. CLINPROT (CLINICAL PROTOCOLS): CLINPROT, sponsored by the NCI, has been designed to disseminate information to clinical oncologists engaged in the development and testing of clinical protocols. It is also useful to other clinicians who wish to learn about new cancer treatment methods currently being evaluated in controlled clinical trials. It provides descriptions of the clinical trials, including patient entry criteria, the therapy regimen, and special study parameters.
   c. PDQ (PHYSICIAN DATA QUERY): The PDQ database has three major files: (1) a file that summarizes the most current approaches to cancer treatment, (2) a file of research treatment protocols that are open to patient entry, and (3) a directory of physicians that provide cancer treatment and health care organizations that have programs of cancer care. At any time, the PDQ protocol file contains approximately 1000 treatment protocols, 20% of which have been voluntarily submitted. Each protocol is indexed according to disease and stage-specific eligibility criteria,

as well as details of treatment, to allow users to narrow down geographically classified information on participating investigators.

PDQ, CANCERLIT, and CLINPROT are available through the NLM's MEDLARS computer system at U.S. medical libraries and health care organizations. For more information contact:

MEDLARS Management Section
National Library of Medicine
Building 38, Room 4 N 421
8600 Rockville Pike
Bethesda, MD 20894
301-496-6193
800-638-8480 (toll free)

The staff of NCI's Cancer Information Service network (toll free 1-800-4-CANCER) will also provide information on PDQ.

9. Nursing and Allied Health: This database provides access to more than 300 English-language nursing journals, publications of the American Nurses' Association and the National League for Nursing. It also includes citations from approximately 3200 biomedical journals in *Index Medicus* and from the psychological, management, and popular literature. It contains over 72,764 records and is updated bimonthly. Beginning with 1986 issues, abstracts from approximately 45 nursing journals were added to the database. The cost is $54 per computer connect hour and $0.25 for a full-record printed offline.
10. Education Resources Information Center (ERIC): The ERIC system is a network of clearinghouses, each devoted to collecting, evaluating, storing, abstracting, and disseminating resource material in its own area of specialization. Materials included are research projects, theses, speeches, books, proceedings, and project reports. ERIC corresponds to two printed indexes: *Resources in Education,* which is concerned with identifying the most significant and timely education research reports, and *Current Index to Journals in Education,* an index of more than 700 periodicals of interest to every segment of the education profession. Consult the university library, state department of education, or state library system nearest you for the availability of this service and the specific procedures to be followed at that institution, or write:

    ERIC Processing and Reference Facility
    4350 East-West Highway
    Suite 1100
    Bethesda, MD 20814-4475
11. EMBASE (formerly EXCERPTA MEDICA): EMBASE is one of the leading sources for searching the biomedical literature. It consists of abstracts and citations of articles from over 4000 biomedical journals published throughout the world. Updated every 2 weeks, EMBASE contains over 3,021,722 records on file that correspond to the 43-specialty abstract journals and 2 literature indexes that make up the printed EXCERPTA MEDICA. More information can be obtained from:

    EMBASE
    Elsevier Science Publishing Co., Inc.
    North American Data Base Department
    52 Vanderbilt Avenue
    New York, NY 10017
12. Dissertation Abstracts Online: Dissertation Abstracts Online is a definitive subject, title, and author guide to every American dissertation accepted at an accredited institution since 1861. This is a computerized bibliographic file of abstracts of doctoral theses originally listed in *Dissertation Abstracts* and *Dissertation Abstracts International.* Abstracts are included for a large majority of the degrees granted after January 1980. It is updated every month and contains over 955,147 records. The database also contains citations to master's theses appearing in the quarterly "Masters Abstracts" published by University Microfilms International since 1962. For more information contact:

    University Microfilms International
    A Bell and Howell Information Company
    300 North Zeeb Road
    Ann Arbor, MI 48106
13. Psyc INFO: Worldwide literature in psychology and the related disciplines of psychiatry, sociology, anthropology, education, linguistics, and pharmacology are covered in this database. This database corresponds to the printed *Psychological Abstracts* and covers 1967 to the present. Write to the following for information on costs and location of terminals:

    American Psychological Association
    1400 N. Uhle Street
    Arlington, VA 22201
14. Clinical Abstracts: Clinical Abstracts is designed to meet the needs of the practicing clinician. The database provides access to more than 300 leading English-language medical journals. Major subject areas include pediatrics, family practice, internal medicine, general surgery, and cardiovascular surgery. Material from 1981 to the present is included, and the database is updated monthly. Contact:

    Medical Information Systems
    Reference and Index Services
    Indianapolis, IN 46223
15. SCISEARCH: SCISEARCH is a multidisciplinary index to the literature of science and technology prepared by the Institute for Scientific Information (ISI). It contains all the records published in *Science Citation Index.* The ISI staff indexes all significant items from about 2600 major scientific and technical journals. This database contains over 8,000,000 records and is updated biweekly.

Oncology Periodicals

An excellent resource for a discussion of cancer journals and serials is *Cancer Journals and Serials. An Analytical Guide,* compiled by Pauline Vaillancourt (New York, Greenwood Press, 1988). The content of each journal is discussed along with costs, where published, price, frequency of the journal, and number of cancer-related articles usually found in each issue.

Acta Haematologica
Acta Oncologica
Advances in Cancer Research
American Journal of Clinical Oncology
American Journal of Hematology
Anticancer Research
Australian Cancer Society
Breast Cancer and Research Treatment
Breast/Diseases of the Breast
British Journal of Cancer
British Journal of Haematology
British Journal of Preventive and Society Medicine
Ca—A Cancer Journal for Clinicians
Canadian Cancer Society
Cancer Cells
Cancer: A Journal of the American Cancer Society
Cancer Chemotherapy Reports
Cancer Detection and Prevention: International Study Group for Detection and Prevention of Cancer

Cancer Federation, Inc.
Cancer Forum
Cancer Genetics and Cytogenetics
Cancergram (abstracts of selected cancer-related articles): Breast Cancer, Cancer Detection and Management, Cancer Research: Techniques and Applications, Cell Biology, Dietary Aspects of Carcinogenesis, Environmental and Occupational Carcinogenesis, Metastasis, Molecular Biology, Organ Site Carcinogenesis (Liver), Organ Site Carcinogenesis (Skin), Pediatric Oncology
Cancer Immunology and Immunotherapy
Cancer Letters
Cancer Metastasis Review
Cancer Nursing: An International Journal for Cancer Care
Cancer Review
Cancer Treatment Reports
Cancer Treatment Reviews
Cancer Update
Carcinogenesis
Clinical Cancer Letter
Clinical Oncology: The Journal of the British Association of Surgical Oncology
Clinics in Oncology
Current Problems in Cancer
Cancer Victors Association
European Journal of Cancer
European Journal of Gynaecological Oncology
European Journal of Nuclear Medicine
Fox Chase Cancer Center
Gynecologic Oncology: An International Journal
Important Advances in Oncology
Indian Cancer Society
International Journal of Cancer
International Journal of Radiation Oncology, Biology, Physics
International Union Against Cancer
Journal of Cancer Education
Journal of the British Association of Surgical Oncology
Journal of Clinical Hematology and Oncology
Journal of Clinical Oncology
Journal of the National Cancer Institute
Journal of Psychosocial Oncology
Journal of Surgical Oncology
Journal of Tumor Marker Oncology
Lancet
Leukemia Research
Medical and Pediatric Oncology
National Cancer Institute Monographs
Neoplasma
Oncology
Oncology: International Journal of Cancer Research and Treatment
Oncology: Journal of Clinical and Experimental Cancer Research
Oncology Nursing Forum
Preventive Medicine: An International Journal Devoted to Practice and Theory
Proceedings of the American Association for Cancer Research
Progress in Clinical Research
Radiotherapy and Oncology
Recent Results in Cancer Research
Seminars in Oncology
Seminars in Oncology Nursing
Yearbooks in Cancer
UCLA Cancer Center

Oncology Patient Education Material

Many of the self-help organizations offer literature that emphasizes their organization, and the reader is advised to contact these groups for special-interest material. There are many excellent sources for patient education material, and a partial list follows:

1. American Academy of Dermatology
   PO Box 3116
   Evanston, IL 60204-3116

   The American Academy of Dermatology offers brochures, audiovisuals, and posters. Information is available to the public by writing the above address and enclosing a self-addressed stamped envelope; it is free of charge unless requested in quantities. The Academy gives referrals to physicians in the patient's area.
   Brochures:
   The Sun and Your Skin
   Melanoma/Skin Cancer
   Posters:
   Be Sun Smart
   Ban the Burn
   Lighten Up—Cover Up
2. American Cancer Society
   Tower Place
   3340 Peachtree Road, NE
   Atlanta, GA 30026
   (404) 320-3333

   The reader is urged first to contact the American Cancer Society in his or her area. The Society has an extensive collection of material for both the public and the professional. The material covers all aspects of cancer and is available as books, films, reprints, posters, audiotapes, programs, and proceedings.
   Patient education rehabilitation pamphlets (partial listing):
   Care of Your Sigmoid Colostomy
   First Aid for Laryngectomees
   Helping Words (for Laryngectomees)
   Reach to Recovery—After Mastectomy: A Patient Guide
   Sex and the Male Ostomate; Sex and the Female Ostomate; Sex, Courtship and the Single Ostomate
   What is Reach to Recovery
   Your New Voice
   Breast Reconstruction—After Mastectomy
   Emergency Info for Tracheo-Esophageal Fistula Users
   Help for the Patient Going Home
   Another Spring: The Diary of a Radiation Patient
   Patient education site pamphlets (partial listing):
   Cancer of the Breast
   Cancer of the Colon
   Cancer of the Larynx
   Cancer of the Lung
   Cancer of the Mouth
   Cancer of the Prostate
   Cancer of the Skin
   Cancer of the Stomach
   Cancer of the Uterus
   Childhood Cancers
   Hodgkin's Disease
   Testicular Cancer
   Patient education pamphlets (partial listing):
   Finding a Lump in Your Breast
   The Last Day in April (the story of a child with leukemia, written by her mother)

Cancer Facts for Men
Cancer Facts for Women
Parents' Handbook on Leukemia
Sexuality and Cancer for the Woman who has Cancer and Her Partner
Sexuality and Cancer for the Man who has Cancer and His Partner
Facts on Cancer Treatment

3. American Lung Association
1740 Broadway
New York, NY 10019
(212) 315-8700

The reader is encouraged to contact his or her local American Lung Association for a free catalog of public education materials. *The following is a partial list of available materials:*
Asbestos: Lung Hazards on the Job
Lung Hazards in the Workplace
Occupational Lung Cancer
Lung Cancer—You Need to Know the Facts
Your Lung Facts
Carcinogens and Synonyms
About Smoking and Cancer

4. *Candelighters Childhood Cancer Foundation Youth Newsletter*
Candelighters Childhood Cancer Foundation
Suite 1001
1901 Pennsylvania Avenue
Washington, DC 20006
(202) 659-5136

Candelighters Childhood Cancer Foundation Youth Newsletter is written by and for adolescent cancer patients and teenage siblings.

5. *Coping*
Pulse Publications, Inc.
377 Riverside Drive
PO Box 1677
Franklin, TN 37065-1677
(615) 791-5900

The magazine *Coping* is published quarterly for cancer patients and their families. It includes such categories as education, support, life-style, treatment, research, and progress reports. Cost is $14 for 1 year (outside the United States it is $22) and $24 for 2 years.

6. Ellis Fischel State Cancer Hospital
Business 70 and Garth Avenue
Columbia, MO 65201
(314) 875-2100

Several pamphlets are available designed specifically to answer the questions of cancer patients undergoing chemotherapy, radiation, and surgery.
Pamphlets (partial list):
Chemotherapy
Radiotherapy Information and Hints for You
Radium Implant Booklet

7. Office of Cancer Communications
National Cancer Institute
Building 31, Room 10A24
Bethesda, MD 20892
1-800-4-CANCER

A variety of pamphlets and booklets are available that discuss symptoms, diagnosis, and treatment of different cancer sites as well as research. In addition, there are pamphlets designed to help the parents of children with cancer.
Partial list of materials available (these are frequently updated):
Breast Exams: What You Should Know
Diet, Nutrition and Cancer Prevention: The Good News
Help Yourself: Tips for Teenagers with Cancer
Progress Against Cancer of the Skin
Progress Against Cancer of the Larynx
Questions and Answers About Breast Lumps
Research Report Series (includes many sites such as kidney, bladder, pancreas, stomach, uterus, etc)
Services Available to Cancer Patients
What You Need to Know About Cancer Series (includes many sites such as brain, breast, lung, etc)
Booklets:
Chemotherapy and You
Eating Hints
Questions and Answers About DES Exposure During Pregnancy and Before Birth
Radiation Therapy and You
What are Clinical Trials All About?
Young People with Cancer

8. National Alliance of Breast Cancer Organizations
1180 Avenue of the Americas
2nd Floor
New York, NY 10036
(212) 719-0154

NABCO is a central resource of information on breast cancer. The Breast Cancer Resource List compiled by NABCO in 1988 is shown on p. 1290. The list includes resources available from the NCI and other sources.

9. Patient Education Center
The North Carolina Memorial Hospital
Manning Drive
Chapel Hill, NC 27514
(919) 966-4131

Series of patient education booklets are available that cover a variety of topics. For example, the *Series of Home Health Care Procedures* includes booklets on wound drainage, tracheostomy care, intracavity radiation therapy, biliary catheter care, and turning and positioning a patient. Each booklet is illustrated, uses simple language, and has questions throughout to test the patient's understanding of the material. The catalog is currently being revised, but a list of series and booklets is available. Each booklet costs $2.

10. The Skin Cancer Foundation
245 Fifth Avenue, Suite 2402
New York, NY 10016
(212) 725-5176

On request, the Skin Cancer Foundation will provide samples and an ordering form for brochures, leaflets, booklets, and posters. A contribution of $25 or more entitles the contributor to a 1-year subscription of *Sun and Skin News* and *The Melanoma Letter,* four issues each.
The following is a limited list of materials available:
It's Never Too Early to Stop Skin Cancer . . . Or Too Late
Skin Cancer Booklet
Types and Descriptions of Skin Cancers
The ABCD's of Moles and Melanomas
The Many Faces of Malignant Melanoma
For Every Child Under the Sun, A Guide to Sensible Sun Protection
Basal Cell Carcinoma, The Most Common Cancer
Simple Guidelines on Sun Protection
Malignant Melanoma—Guidelines and Early Warning System
Dysplastic Nevi and Malignant Melanoma

Breast Cancer Resources
Overview Information and Treatment Choices

Title	Author	Source	Catalogue Number or Publisher	Number of Pages	Charge
What You Need To Know About Breast Cancer		NCI	88-1556	33	None
Breast Cancer: We're Making Progress Every Day		NCI	86-2409	12	None
The Breast Cancer Digest: A Guide To Medical Care, Emotional Support, Educational Programs and Resources		NCI	84-1691	212	None
Alternatives	R. Kushner	Bookstores	Warner Books, 1986	438	$5.95
If You've Thought About Breast Cancer (1987 edition)	R. Kushner	Women's Breast Cancer Advisory Center, PO Box 224, Kensington, MD 20895			$3.00
Every Woman's Guide To Breast Cancer	V.L. Seltzer, MD	Bookstores	Viking Books, 1987	209	$17.95
A Real Choice	R. Moss	Bookstores	St. Martin's Press, 1984	249	$13.95
Breast Biopsy: What You Should Know		NCI	87-657	12	Free
Breast Cancer: Understanding Treatment Options		NCI	87-2675	19	Free
Mastectomy: A Treatment For Breast Cancer		NCI	87-658	24	Free
Radiation Therapy: A Treatment For Early Stage Breast Cancer		NCI	87-659	20	Free
Radiation Therapy and You: A Guide To Self-Help During Treatment		NCI	88-2227	39	Free
Breast Reconstruction: A Matter Of Choice		NCI	88-2151	19	Free
Breast Reconstruction After Mastectomy		ACS	4630-PS	20	Free
An Informed Decision: Understanding Breast Reconstruction	M. Snyder	Bookstores	Little, Brown, 1989	201	$10.95

The following books are excellent resources for cancer patients and their families. There is a great deal of useful information that can help with care and decision making. Further resources also may be found within these books addressing many aspects of diagnosis, treatment, and care.

Benjamin H, Trubo R: *From Victim to Victor.* New York, Dell, 1987.

Bergman T: *One Day at a Time: Children Living with Cancer.* Milwaukee, Gareth Stevens, 1989.

Bloch A, Bloch R: *Cancer . . . There's Hope.* Kansas City, Mo, Cancer Connection, 1987.

Bloch A, Bloch R: *Fighting Cancer.* Kansas City, Mo, Cancer Connection, 1988.

Borysenko J: *Minding the Body, Mending the Mind.* New York, Bantam, 1988.

Bruning N: *Coping with Chemotherapy.* New York, Ballantine, 1985.

Cousins N: *Anatomy of an Illness.* New York, Bantam, 1983.

Doan Nayes D, Mellody P: *Beauty & Cancer: A Woman's Guide to Looking Great while Experiencing the Side Effects of Cancer Therapy.* Los Angeles, AC Press, 1988.

Gaes J: *My Book for Kids with Cansur.* Aberdeen, SD, Melius Peterson, 1988.

Grollman E: *Talking about Death: A Dialogue between Parent and Child.* Boston, Beacon Press, 1976.

Harwell A: *When Your Friend Gets Cancer.* Wheaton, Ill, Harold Shaw, 1987.

Holleb A (ed): *The American Cancer Society Cancer Book.* New York, Doubleday, 1986.
Le Shan L: *Cancer as a Turning Point: A Handbook for People with Cancer, their Families, and Health Professionals.* New York, Dutton, 1989.
Matthews-Simonton S: *The Healing Family.* New York, Bantam, 1984.
Morra M, Potts E: *Choices: Realistic Alternatives in Cancer Treatment.* New York, Avon, 1987.
Muraa A, Stewart B: *Man to Man: When the Woman You Love Has Breast Cancer.* New York, St. Martin's Press, 1989.
O'Toole D: *Aarvy Aardvark Finds Hope.* Burnsville, NC, The Rainbow Connection, 1988.
Patterson JT: *The Dread Disease: Cancer and Modern American Culture.* Cambridge, Mass, Harvard University Press, 1987.
Rosenfeld I: *Second Opinion: Your Guide to Alternative Treatment.* New York, Bantam, 1988.
Sattilaro A: *Recalled by Life.* New York, Avon, 1984.
Shook RL: *Survivors: Living with Cancer.* New York, Harper & Row, 1983.
Siegel B: *Love, Medicine & Miracles.* New York, Harper & Row, 1988.
Simonton C, Matthews-Simonton S, Creighton J: *Getting Well Again.* New York, Bantam, 1988.

ORGANIZATIONS: PROFESSIONAL AND CLIENT SELF-HELP

Nonsmokers Organizations

Between 1964 and 1975, a dramatic change occurred in adult smoking behavior; more than 29 million Americans quit smoking during this period. A growing concern for the rights and health of nonsmokers has resulted in social and legislative pressures on smokers, and new antismoking education and information materials and programs have been introduced in local communities around the country. The following is a list of some national organizations for the rights of nonsmokers. This list was obtained from The Action on Smoking and Health (ASH) Organization.

1. Action on Smoking and Health (ASH)
   2013 H Street, NW
   Washington, DC 20006
   (202) 659-4310

   ASH is a national nonprofit legal-action organization fighting for the rights of nonsmokers everywhere and helping nonsmoking passengers to protect their rights. ASH is the organization primarily responsible for the airline nonsmoking rules and their enforcement. ASH also publishes a bimonthly newsletter on smoking and nonsmokers' rights, has available a variety of other educational materials, and sells signs, buttons, stickers, etc. to help nonsmokers speak out. ASH has compiled a list of nonsmoking organizations (updated January 1989) in every state that can be requested. A partial listing is given below.
2. Group Against Smokers' Pollution (GASP)
   PO Box 632
   College Park, MD 20740
   (301) 577-6427

   Provides information about activities in support of nonsmokers' rights. GASP chapters are found throughout the United States.
3. Non-smokers Travel Club
   8929 Bradmoor Drive
   Bethesda, MD 20034
   (301) 530-1664

   Arranges smoke-free tours—both domestic and international.
4. Citizens Against Tobacco Smoke (CATS)
   PO Box 2232
   Rockville, MD 20852
   (301) 369-1473

   A national organization with chapters throughout the United States.
5. Stop Teenage Addiction to Tobacco (STAT)
   PO Box 60658
   Longmeadow, MA 01116
   (413) 567-7587

   Chapters of STAT are found throughout the United States.

Smoking Cessation Information

I have frequently urged people to stop smoking but have difficulty really substantiating why they should stop. Where can I obtain scientific information on the hazards of smoking? Also, what types of programs are available for the person who desires to stop smoking? Many different approaches to smoking cessation are being offered around the country. These approaches include group therapy, individual counseling, physician messages, and self-help guides. Methods of therapy include the use of drugs, electric shock, hypnosis, and acupuncture. The following is a discussion of the various types of smoking cessation methods, educational materials that can be obtained, health organizations, and professional material that discusses all aspects of smoking (psychological, economic, social, and physiologic).

1. The Health Consequences of Smoking (1988)
   DHHS pub no. (CDC) 88-8406

   May be ordered from the Superintendent of Documents, US Government Printing Office, Washington, DC 20402. Updated annually, presenting new topics each year (ie, addiction of nicotine).
2. The Health Consequences of Involuntary Smoking (1986)
   DHHS pub. no. (CDC) 87-8398

   May be ordered from the Superintendent of Documents, US Government Printing Office, Washington, DC 20402. Definitive presentation of the hazards of smoking to nonsmokers.
3. Smoking and Health Bulletin
   US Department of Health and Human Services
   Public Health Service
   Centers for Disease Control
   Center for Health Promotion and Education
   Office on Smoking and Health

   The Smoking and Health Bulletin is a bimonthly publication from the Technical Information Center of the Office on Smoking and Health. The Bulletin presents abstracts from the medical, nursing, sociology, public health, political, biological, and psychological literature on smoking, tobacco, and tobacco use. The yearly cumulation of the Smoking and Health Bulletin is titled *Bibliography on Smoking and Health.*
4. National Cancer Institute
   Office of Cancer Communications
   Building 31, Room 10A30
   Bethesda, MD 20892

Materials for health care professionals.
"Quit for Good" kit—a complete packet of materials designed specifically for health care professionals to assist their smoking patients to quit. Each kit contains enough materials for 50 patients. There is a similar kit for pharmacists, and the pharmacist kits contain enough material for 25 patients.

"Smoking Programs for Youth" (81-2156)—this paperback book (92 pages) is a comprehensive state-of-the-art report covering demographics of youth smoking in the United States, smoking regulations in schools and examples of how specific school systems are dealing with the problem, past approaches to smoking education and how these approaches have changed, factors likely to influence smoking among young people, and descriptions of innovative smoking solutions for youth today.
Public information:
Quit for Good
Why Do You Smoke?
Clearing the Air. A Guide to Quitting Smoking
Life as a Nonsmoker
How to Quit Smoking
Chew or Snuff is Real Bad Stuff

5. American Cancer Society

Some examples of available pamphlets, booklets, posters, buttons, and films are listed below. Contact your local ACS for more information.
Pamphlets:
Quit Cigarettes—Live Longer (in Spanish)
Quit Smoking—Live Longer (for black Americans)
Danger
The Smoke Around You: Risk of Involuntary Smoking
Decision Maker's Guide (workplace smoking booklet)
Why Start Life Under a Cloud?
Can They Stop Smoking (for black women)
How to Quit Cigarettes
The Decision is Yours
Don't Bite Off More Than You Can Chew
The Dangers of Smoking—Benefits of Quitting
Smokeless Tobacco: Cause for Concern?
Just a Pinch Between Your Cheek and Gum (Ohio Division)
Everything You Wanted to Know About Chewing and Dipping—But Were Afraid to Ask (Texas Division)
Regular Films and Video Tapes:
Women and Smoking (film and videotape)
Let's Call it Quits
Breaking Free (film and videotape)
The Feminine Mistake (film and videotape)—powerful film showing the effects of smoking. Although the film is geared to women, it is effective for men.
Taking Control (slide/tape and video)—provides an introduction to a healthy, enjoyable lifestyle that may prevent cancer. The program gives an overview of five "protective factors" against cancer and five preventable "risk factors."
Smokeless Tobacco (slide/tape and video)—presents all the health hazards related to smokeless tobacco.
Breaking Free—a film designed to promote smoking cessation especially among students who concentrate on vocational/career classes (film and video)
Posters and Buttons:
Smoking is Very Glamorous (poster)
Sean Marsee Poster
Best Tip Yet, Don't Start (poster)
Quite Smoking, Lives You Could Save (poster)
Thank You for Not Smoking
Kiss a Non-smoker, Taste the Difference (poster)
Smoking Stinks (buttons)
Are You a Draggin' Lady? (poster)
Archie, Smoke-Free Young America (poster)
His Spittin' Image (poster)

6. American Lung Association

Some of the smoking literature, posters, buttons, and smoking cessation materials are listed below. Contact your local American Lung Association.
Pamphlets:
How Not To Love Your Kids (English and Spanish)
Emphysema—The Facts About Your Lungs
Cigarette Smoking—The Facts About Your Lungs
Marijuana: A Second Look at Health Hazards
Is There a Safe Tobacco?
Facts About Second-Hand Smoke
A Guide to Smokeless Tobacco
A No-Smoking Coloring Book (coloring booklet for children)
Help a Friend Stop Smoking
Nonsmokers' Rights, What You Can Do
Me Quit Smoking? How?
Posters:
This Is a Smoke-Free Workspace
Thanks For Not Smoking
Almost 35 Million Americans Quit Smoking
Brooke Shields: Smoking Spoils Your Looks
Be Kind to Nonsmokers
Films:
Breathing Easy Film—film for 5th and 8th graders.
As We See It—made for pre-teens.
Everything You Always Wanted to Know About How to Stop Smokers But Were Afraid to Try—interviews with nonsmokers, filled with humor and imagination.
Anti-smoking programs:
Freedom From Smoking Booklets—Freedom From Smoking in 20 Days—self-help book shows you how to quit smoking in 20 days
Freedom From Smoking Home Video Program "In Control"
Freedom From Smoking T-Shirt Iron-Ons
Freedom From Smoking The Workplace Booklets
Freedom From Smoking buttons and posters and tent cards
Puzzles:
Have Fun!! Figure Out the Smoking Puzzle

7. Narcotics Education, Inc.
6830 Laurel Street, NW
Washington, DC 20012-9979
(1-800-548-8700)

This organization has multiple pamphlets, booklets, films, videos, posters, and teaching aids that stress smoking cessation as well as advocating not starting to smoke. Request a free catalog of their materials. A sample of a few items are given below:
Pamphlets:
How to Stop Smoking and Breathe Free ($8.95 per 25)
Your Health: What Smoking May Do
One Strike Against You
Booklets:
I Love Not Smoking—coloring book (grades 1 to 3) ($12.50 per 25)
To Smoke Or Not (grade 7 to adult) ($0.95 each)
Audiovisuals:
Death in the West. (Grade 7 to adult)—can be purchased or rented. A British television documentary showing six real-life cowboys who are dying of disease caused by their smoking (in contrast to the Marlboro man).

Smokeless Tobacco—It Can Snuff You Out (grade 7 to adult)—can be purchased or rented. Young people tell their own experiences, including their difficulties in quitting, and one young man's death emphasizes the hazards of smokeless tobacco.

Teaching aids:

Real Human Lung Sections (grade 5 to adult) ($128.75 per item)

Mr. Gross Mouth (grade 1 to adult) ($65.00 for model that accurately shows the oral effects of chewing and dipping tobacco, including cancers)

8. American Cancer Society
Local Units

Assists hospitals and organizations in establishing Fresh Start or I Quit Clinics where participants attempt to learn why they smoke, identify ways to quit, and are motivated and encouraged by the leader, usually an ex-smoker, and other group members. The ACS provides all materials for the sessions, including films and books, free of charge, but the institutions usually charge for the clinic itself.

9. Narcotics Education Division
6840 Eastern Avenue, NW
Washington, DC 20012

They offer a smoking cessation program called "The Breathe-Free Plan to Stop Smoking." A Director's Kit can be purchased at a cost of $59.95. This kit includes (1) The Director's Manual—How-to explanation of the entire program includes a planning and advertising guide for attracting people to the program, (2) Program Scripts—These scripts are so complete that when the traditional physician-minister team is not available, other health care professionals, counselors, and experienced laypersons may competently conduct the plan, and (3) Handout Masters—one-time activity sheets. Buttons, diplomas, personal plan booklet, and matchless pens/lighter plugs can be purchased for the program, as can pamphlets, posters, advertising materials and films, and videos and slide-tape programs.

10. Schick Laboratories
Los Angeles, CA
(213) 553-9771 or 1-800-CRAVING

Schick Laboratories operates 13 smoking cessation centers in the western part of the United States, which conduct individual therapy sessions for 1 hour on 5 consecutive days. The centers' goal is behavior modification, and aversion therapy is stressed. Methods include a rapid smoking (quick puff) and an "electrostimulus" applied to the participant's arm. Schick charges participants $625 for the 5-day program. There is also a 6-week support phase following the 5-day program, with weekly telephone calls from a counselor and one "booster" session in the second week. For more information see Smith J: Long term outcomes of clients treated in a commercial stop smoking program. *Journal of Substance Abuse Treatment* 5:33-36, 1988.

11. Office on Smoking and Health
Department of Health and Human Services
Public Health Service
Rockville, MD 20857
(301) 443-1575

The following materials can be obtained from this government office:

Public Information:

Two Reasons to Quit (English and Spanish poster and brochure)

If Your Kids Think Everyone Smokes

No More Butts

Adult Self Test

A Self Test for Teenagers

Why People Smoke Cigarettes

A Decision Maker's Guide to Reducing Smoking at the Worksite

Passive Pamphlet

Technical Information:

Review and Evaluation of Smoking Cessation Methods

Smokeless Tobacco Report

Smoking and Health—A National Status Report

Smoking and Health Bulletin

Surgeon General's Report:

1985—Cancer and Chronic Lung Disease in the Workplace

1986—Involuntary Smoking

1988—Nicotine Addiction (GPO Stock #017-001-00468-5)

1989—25 Years of Progress (Summary)

Self-Help Organizations

1. American Cancer Society: CanSurmount

This program is composed of the patient, family member, trained volunteer (also a cancer patient), and health care professional. The program is designed to have volunteers visit cancer patients in the hospital and home and to provide patient and family education, information, and emotional support.

2. American Cancer Society: I Can Cope

I Can Cope is a formal educational program designed to provide information (treatment, side effects, nutrition, resources, etc.) and support to people with cancer and their families. Contact your local ACS for details about this program in your area.

3. American Cancer Society: Loan Closets and Transportation Services

Many ACS units have loan closets that supply sickroom equipment for home cancer patients. Equipment may include wheelchairs, walkers, surgical dressings, bedpans, hospital beds, shower chairs, etc. This equipment can be borrowed for as long as needed. Contact your local unit for this free service. In some communities the ACS offers patient transportation to physicians' offices, hospitals, or clinics for diagnosis and treatment. This service is run by ACS volunteers.

4. American Cancer Society: Reach to Recovery

This is one of the best-known self-help groups. It was founded in 1952 by Terese Lasser and has been part of the ACS since 1969. Reach to Recovery works through its volunteer visitors, who have adjusted successfully to their own mastectomies. Once the patient's physician has given permission, the volunteer makes a hospital visit a few days after surgery. She brings a kit containing a manual of information about rehabilitation exercises and exercise equipment and a temporary breast form. Volunteers have up-to-date lists of prostheses and bathing suits available locally, which may be given to patients along with lists of national manufacturers. Volunteers who have had reconstructive surgery are available to visit women who are deciding about this type of surgery. Some units have women volunteers who have had chemotherapy or radiation meet with women before surgery. Reach to Recovery services are free and can be secured by contacting your local ACS unit.

5. Association of Brain Tumor Research
3735 North Talman Avenue
Chicago, IL 60618
(312) 286-5571

This organization works to raise funds for brain tumor research and patient education materials. The purposes are to raise funds for brain tumor research, raise the level of public awareness about the prevalence of brain tumors, and to help the victims of the disease and their families by making them aware that they are not alone and by disseminating information to them. ABTR furnishes on request a list of experimental treatment centers and brain tumor study groups. Twelve publications, in lay language, are available free of charge to patient and family members. Organizations may purchase these pamphlets:
Chemotherapy of Brain Tumors
A Primer of Brain Tumors
Radiation Therapy of Brain Tumors Part 1: A Basic Guide
Radiation Therapy of Brain Tumors Part 2: Background and Research Guide
Living With a Brain Tumor
Coping With a Brain Tumor
When Your Child is Ready to Return to School
Shunts
Tumor Specific
About Glioblastoma Multiforme and Malignant Astrocytoma
About Medulloblastoma
About Meningioma
About Oligodendroglioma

6. Cancer Care
1180 Avenue of the Americas
New York, NY 10036
(212) 221-3300

Founded approximately 44 years ago, this organization offers services to cancer patients and their families and friends at all stages of the disease to help them cope with the emotional, psychological, and financial impact of cancer. This social service agency directly provides professional counseling and offers referrals for nursing care, homemakers, home health aides, and housekeepers to patients with cancer and their supportive others. They also distribute cancer education materials. Although they primarily serve New York City and its tristate, metropolitan region, they answer letters and telephone calls from all over the United States, providing information and referrals to these inquiries whenever possible. The pamphlet "Listen to the Children" (a study of the impact on children's mental health when a parent has a catastrophic illness) is available from Cancer Care.

7. Cancer Information Service
1-800-4-CANCER
Hawaii: Oahu 524-1234 (call collect from neighbor islands)
Alaska: 1-800-638-6070
National Office: 1-800-638-6694

The Cancer Information Service is a program of the NCI. It is a network of regional offices with trained staff and volunteers that provide accurate and confidential telephone information to questions concerning cancer (rehabilitation, research, causes, prevention and detection, diagnosis, treatment, support services, etc) from patients and their supportive others, health care professionals, and the public.

8. Candelighters Childhood Cancer Foundation
Suite 1001
1901 Pennsylvania Avenue
Washington, DC 20006
(202) 659-5136

Candelighters began in April 1970 as a group of parents of young cancer patients at local hospitals and clinics in the Washington, DC, area. The group's focus is children, adolescents, and teens. There are presently 250 chapters in the United States. Candelighters have two primary goals: to obtain consistent and adequate federal support for cancer research and to help parents and other family members who share the particularly difficult experience of living with a child with cancer. A national newsletter is published quarterly, which serves as a communication link among parents and parents' groups and concerned professionals. A quarterly youth newsletter is also published to provide information to young cancer patients. The free newsletters include information about research in childhood cancer, bibliography materials, and group activities. Local groups usually have their own newsletter. Candelighters also publishes a resource list of childhood cancer education materials. All the above information is available free on request.

9. Children's Hospice International
1101 Kings Street, Suite 131
Alexandria, VA 22314
(800) 24-CHILD
(703) 684-0330

The purpose of Children's Hospice International is to "create a world of hospice support for children, providing medical and technical assistance, research and education for these special children, families and health care professionals." Membership (individual is $35) includes a quarterly newsletter titled, *CHI*, 10% discount on publications and other purchases, national conference discount, and update information mailings. Also available are two teddy bears (one with a tape player and special tapes that can be purchased) and dolls, one of which, Zaadi, is an overstuffed soft cloth doll with embroidered insides (heart, ribs, lungs, etc) that is useful in teaching children.
A partial list of publications is as follows:
Home Care for Children: A Manual for Parents
Palliative Pain and Symptom Management for Children and Adolescents
My Life, Melinda's Story

10. Concern for the Dying
250 West 57th Street
New York, NY 10107
(212) 246-6962

A nonprofit organization, founded in 1967, Concern for the Dying is an educational council that advocates an individual's right to participate in the decisions regarding her or his treatment, particularly those decisions when a person is near death. Concern for the Dying developed the Living Will, a document that specifies one's wishes concerning life-sustaining measures. This organization offers the Living Will, up-to-date information on the current laws of each state, and registration of the will in the Living Will Registry. Other services provided include assistance to terminally ill patients whose wishes are not being honored, a quarterly newsletter for annual contributors of $5 or more, a staff attorney and legal advisors committee for assistance with patients' rights issues, conferences on death and dying (professional and lay), audiovisual materials (purchase or rent), publications, an extensive library, and a multidisciplinary forum for health care professionals in educational settings to address issues related to the terminally ill.

11. Corporate Angel Network, Inc.
Westchester County Airport
Building One

White Plains, NY 10604
(914) 328-1313

CAN is a nonprofit organization that arranges free air transportation for cancer patients going to or from recognized treatments, consultations, or checkups. The program uses available seats on corporate aircraft. A person must be in stable condition, able to board unassisted, and have backup reservations on commercial airlines, since travel is not guaranteed. This service is available regardless of financial need.

12. Encore
National Board, YWCA
726 Broadway
New York, NY 10003
(212) 614-2827

Encore is a national program offered by the YWCA and sponsored by local YWCAs. It provides floor and pool exercises as well as discussion and support groups for women recovering from breast cancer surgery. The reader is encouraged to contact the local YWCA for details of program availability and cost.

13. International Association of Laryngectomees
c/o American Cancer Society
Tower Place
3340 Peachtree Road, NE
Atlanta, GA 30026
(404) 320-3333

The International Association of Laryngectomees was founded in 1952 and affiliated with the ACS and consists of 257 domestic and 14 foreign clubs whose members are laryngectomees. For the location of the "Lost Chord," "New Voice", or "Anamile" club nearest you, write the IAL or contact your local ACS. The goal of these lost chord clubs is to assist newly laryngectomized persons to make early adjustments to loss of voice and to overcome psychosocial problems. They accomplish this by serving as hosts for newly laryngectomized persons at club meetings and by collaborating with surgeons in preoperative and postoperative speech orientations. Members of the Lost Chord Club visit new laryngectomee patients in the hospital (at the invitation of the physician). The Lost Chord Club member discusses with both the spouse and the patient early home adjustment, speech therapy, the need for early return to normal work and recreation, required changes in the activities of daily living, and benefits of joining a Lost Chord Club. Meetings enable patients and their spouses to discuss common problems of caring for a laryngectomee and to offer moral support and encouragement and social confidence after similar surgery. Manuals and newsletters are available to members. A laryngectomy kit is available and contains stoma covers, an emergency identification card, booklets (first aid, stoma care, tracheostomy care, speech, etc), and an erasable writing board with a pen.
Other resources for laryngectomy patients:
Bruce Medical Supply
411 Waverly Oaks Road
P.O. Box 9166
Waltham, MA 02254
(800) 225-8446
This company has a catalog of tracheostomy supplies.

Communitrach
Implant Technologies, Inc.
7900 West 78th Street
Minneapolis, MN 55435
(800) 328-0925
A trach tube is available, which allows the intubated patient to speak laryngeally.

Medic-Alert Foundation International
P.O. Box 1009
Turlock, CA 95381
(800) 344-3226
(209) 668-3333 (California)
Contact the Foundation for medic-alert bracelets.

Vocaid (Texas Instruments) and Spelling Ace (Franklin Computers) are electronic voice communication aids.

14. Leukemia Society of America
733 Third Avenue
New York, NY 10017
(212) 573-8484

This is a national voluntary health agency dedicated solely to seeking the control and eventual eradication of leukemia and allied diseases. The Society supports a three-pronged program: research, patient aid, and public and professional education. The patient-aid program provides up to $750 per year on an outpatient basis: drugs for the care, treatment or control of leukemia; laboratory service charges for blood processing, cross-matching, typing, and transfusing; up to $300 per individual for radiotherapy in the first stages of Hodgkin's disease; also, up to $300 for prophylactic radiation for children with acute leukemia. The patient-aid program is conducted through the Society's local chapters, which also give counsel and referrals to other community resources to all leukemia patients and their families regardless of financial circumstances. Some local chapters also offer family support programs for patients and family members or friends. There are 56 chapters in 31 states and the District of Columbia.

15. Make A Wish Foundation of America
2600 North Central Avenue
Suite 936
Phoenix, AZ 85004
1-800-722-9474
(602) 240-6600

This foundation grants wishes for individuals under 18 years of age who are suffering from life-threatening illnesses. The wish includes the immediate family and expenses. The local Make a Wish chapter assigns a wish team for each wish. Common wishes include trips to Disneyland, meeting celebrities, visiting relatives, and requests for material things such as videorecorders and entertainment centers. The Foundation is a nonprofit organization composed of volunteers. There are 68 chapters serving 44 states in the United States and 5 international affiliates.

16. Make Today Count
101½ South Union Street
Alexandria, VA 22314
(703) 548-9674

Make Today Count is a mutual support group for persons with life-threatening illnesses. The purpose is to allow these people to discuss their personal concerns so that they may deal with them in a positive way. By sharing and exchanging experiences of living with a life-threatening illness, it is hoped that patients and their families will live their lives as fully and meaningfully as possible. Make Today Count chapter activities include formal programs, group discussions, chapter newsletters, social activities, workshops and seminars, community projects, educational activities, and monthly meetings. It was founded by Orville Kelly, a cancer patient, in January 1974 in Burlington, IA. There are over 200 chapters in the United States, Canada, and Europe. A national newsletter and the book *Make Today Count* may be purchased through the above address. Information about local chapters or establishing a chapter in your area can be obtained from the same address.

17. Meals on Wheels Program

This service provides at least one hot meal a day and in some cases an additional cold meal. The program varies from state to state, but the cost for the meals is usually minimal, and they are delivered Monday through Friday. Some programs require a referral from a physician. Programs may be run by local health departments, church groups, or community volunteer organizations. Local hospitals can provide information on this program through their social service departments.

18. National Coalition for Cancer Survivorship
323 Eighth Street, SW
Albuquerque, NM 87102
(505) 764-9956

"The mission of NCCS is to communicate that there can be vibrant, productive life following the diagnosis of cancer." The NCCS is a relatively new organization founded in 1986. It is composed of independent groups and individuals interested in issues of cancer survivorship and support of cancer survivors and their significant others. It provides a national communication network between persons and organizations involved with survivorship, advocates issues, research and interests of cancer survivors, and collects and distributes information. NCCS is a proponent of National Cancer Survivors' Day.

19. National Hospice Organization
1901 North Moore Street
Suite 901
Arlington, VA 22209
(703) 243-5900

Established in 1978, NHO is a nonprofit organization, promoting quality care to the terminally ill and their significant others. NHO has worked over the past decade to establish hospice as a part of the health care delivery system in the United States. As a result of its efforts, hospice is now included as a Medicare/Medicaid benefit and as an employee benefit for 66% of American workers. The number of hospices has also increased from one in 1974 to over 1725 in 1990. Most hospices are members of NHO and receives NHO's technical assistance, education programs and events, publications, and advocacy and referral services. Membership has several categories and includes *The Hospice Journal* among numerous other publications and workshops.

20. Nurses' Clubs: Loan Closets

Many communities have local nurses' clubs that provide free-of-charge hospital equipment to cancer patients for use in their homes. Equipment varies with clubs but ranges from bedpans to crutches.

21. Ronald McDonald Houses
Kathy Charlton, Coordinator
500 North Michigan Avenue
Chicago, IL 60611
(312) 836-7100

The first Ronald McDonald House opened in 1974 in Philadelphia. Currently there are over 100 such houses in the United States (and in some foreign countries). The purpose of the house is to provide temporary lodging for families of children who are undergoing treatment at a nearby hospital for cancer, leukemia, and other serious illnesses. Rooms are usually available on a first-come basis. Families are asked to donate financially toward their stay if they are able (ranging from $5 to $15 per day); if unable, their lodging is free. They are also asked to keep their room clean and to do their own cooking, laundry, and grocery shopping. Each house is a partnership consisting of volunteers, community organizations, local hospital(s), and area McDonald's restaurants.

22. Society for the Right to Die
250 West 57th Street
New York, NY 10107
(212) 246-6973

The Society for the Right to Die is a national nonprofit organization in the United States that pursues a program on several fronts: legal services, legislation, and promotion for citizens' rights. It supports legislation enabling persons, while of sound mind, to execute a legally binding document directing that in the event of a terminal condition, medical procedures that prolong the dying process be withheld or withdrawn. Services include a newsletter, bibliographies, handbooks, and material related to the right to refuse treatment, journal articles, and several legislative handbooks. A physician in residence is on staff and available for consultation. A copy of a living will for each of 40 states will be sent free of charge on request. A declaration in general language is provided for those states that still lack living will legislation.

23. TOUCH
513 Tinsley Harrison Tower
University Station
Birmingham, AL 35294
(205) 934-3814

TOUCH is an acronym for Today Our Understanding of Cancer is Hope and is cosponsored by ACS Alabama Division, Inc. and Comprehensive Cancer Center, Birmingham, AL. It started in 1976 and grew from a small group to several hundred members in a number of different cities in Alabama. The program offers emotional and psychological support to cancer patients who are undergoing or have completed cancer treatment and their significant others. TOUCH's goal is to enable patients to cope with psychosocial difficulties caused by their disease such as side effects of treatment, employment, lack of adequate information, communication barriers with family or friends, and fear. Trained peer counselors offer group and individual counseling. TOUCH also seeks to combat unproved cancer treatment methods.

24. United Cancer Council
Parc Place Office Center
4010 West 86th Street, Suite H
Indianapolis, IN 46268-1704
(317) 844-6627

Founded in 1963, the purpose of the UCC is to serve cancer patients through service programs, public and professional education, and research. It is composed of 39 member agencies. Free patient services, provided by the member agencies, include counseling, financial assistance for treatment and medications, loan closets, transportation, and detection clinics. UCC offers public and professional educational services such as cancer prevention seminars, smoking clinics, screening programs, mastectomy group counseling, breast-self-

examination clinics, and pamphlets. Research is funded by UCC in the form of grants to institutions.
Pamphlets available:
Reduce Your Risk of Getting Cancer: Tips for people over 50
Cancer Prevention: Fact & Fiction
Facts on Cancer Risk Factors
"How Do You Talk with Someone who Has Cancer?"
Protect Your Skin
Breast Self-Examination Guide
MEN

25. United Ostomy Association
36 Executive Park
Suite 120
Irvine, CA 92714
(714) 660-8624

Local chapters are composed primarily of ostomates who provide aid, moral support, and education to those who have a colostomy, ileostomy, or urostomy surgery. The chapter supplements the work of the surgeon by offering rehabilitation through follow-up by people who have learned to live with an ostomy. Trained members make visits to homes and hospitals, on request, with the prior consent of the patient's physician. Chapters have medical advisory boards consisting of non-surgeon physicians, surgeons, and enterostomal therapists trained in ostomy care and the use of equipment. At regular monthly meetings, open to anyone who is interested, members can exchange practical, personal experiences about their ostomies, see ostomy equipment displayed, and hear speakers who are knowledgeable about ostomy. All local chapters are volunteer organizations. A list of the chapters is available on request from the UOA. Annual chapter dues vary from no fee to $30. Each member of the UOA receives the *Ostomy Quarterly* magazine and is eligible to participate in the UOA insurance programs. The UOA has both publications and slide programs, which cover every aspect of ostomies. The following is a list of some of these booklets and programs:
Sex, Courtship and the Single Ostomate, $1.50
Sex and the Female Ostomate, $1.50
My Child Has An Ostomy, $0.25
The Ostomy Handbook, $4.50
Ileostomy: A Guide, $5
Urinary Ostomies: A Guidebook for Patients
Colostomies—A Guide, $4 (In English, Spanish, French, and Chinese)

26. We Can Do
1800 Augusta, Suite 150
Houston, TX 77057
(713) 780-1057

This program offers psychological and educational support for cancer patients and their significant others addressing long-term needs. Support groups and referral to local resources are available in California, Washington, DC, and Texas.

27. Wellness Centers/Groups

The basic philosophy of these organizations is to provide psychosocial support for people with life-threatening illnesses. Some of the centers are specifically for people with cancer and their significant others, some cater to children and adults, others include the bereaved, and a few include people without any serious illness who want to improve the quality of their lives. Other services may include information such as books or pamphlets, free second opinions, workshops, mind-body exercises, coping skills, support groups, matching people with the same diagnosis, joke fests, hotlines (some staffed with cancer survivors), relaxation and guided imagery sessions, and social events. The reader is encouraged to contact a local Wellness Center or Group for details. The CIS (1-800-4-CANCER) provides location and telephone numbers of the nearest center or group.

Cancer Support Center
5300 Rockhill Road
Kansas City, MO 64111
(816) 932-8453 (Hotline 9 AM to 4:30 PM)

Cancer Wellness Center
9701 North Kenton, #18
Skokie, IL 60076
(312) 982-9689

Center for Hope
374 Middlesex Road
Darien, CT 06820
(203) 655-4693

Exceptional Cancer Patients
1302 Chapel Street
New Haven, CT 06511
(203) 865-8392

The Wellness Community
1235 Fifth Street
Santa Monica, CA 90401
(213) 393-1415

28. Y-ME
18220 Hardwood Avenue
Homewood, IL 60430
(312) 799-8228 Open 24 hours
(800) 221-2141 Weekdays 9 to 5

Founded in 1978 by Ann Marcou and Mimi Kaplan, two mastectomy patients, Y-ME has become the largest breast cancer support program in the USA. It provides hotlines staffed by volunteers who have personally experienced breast cancer, presurgery counseling, open door meetings, early detection workshops, speakers bureau, resource library, wigs and prosthesis bank, and inservice workshops for health care professionals. Volunteers are professionally supervised, and the information provided to patients is monitored by a medical advisory board. Contributing members receive a quarterly newsletter and an invitation to attend the Y-ME national conference at discounted rates.

Miscellaneous Consumer Groups

1. American Health Decision
Dept P 1200 Larimer
Campus Box 133
Denver, CO 80204

American Health Decisions are groups of concerned citizens in various states that tell their legislators how they want their tax dollars spent related to health care issues such as rationing of resources and other biomedical ethical questions.

2. National Alliance of Breast Cancer Organizations (NABCO)
1180 Avenue of the Americas
2nd Floor
New York, NY 10036
(212) 719-0154
(NABCO prefers written inquiries)

NABCO is a central resource of information on breast cancer. NABCO publishes a breast cancer resource list.

3. National Coalition for Cancer Survivorship
323 Eighth Street, SW
Albuquerque, NM 87102
(505) 764-9956

NCCS serves as a resource to network individuals and groups concerned with cancer survivorship issues by providing access to information, referrals, resources, educational opportunities, and professional and peer support.

AIDS-Related Organizations

1. AIDS Action Council
729 Eighth Street, SE
Suite 200
Washington, DC 20003
(202) 293-2886

The purpose of this organization is lobbying for AIDS education, research, and policy.

2. American Foundation for AIDS Research
1515 Broadway, Suite 3601
New York, NY 10036-8901
(212) 719-0033

The American Foundation for AIDS Research is a nonprofit fundraising organization for AIDS research. Funds are raised in forms of scientific and educational grants for individual researchers.

3. American Society of Psychiatric Oncology/AIDS
Mary Jane Massie, MD
Psychiatry Service
1275 York Avenue
New York, NY 10021

ASPOA established itself in November of 1988 as a national organization of psychiatrists working with patients with AIDS and cancer. It seeks to encourage research and education, enhance clinical care, and foster communication and disseminate information among its members. ASPOA will have semiannual meetings, a newsletter, and a directory. Associate membership is open to non-physicians.

4. Gay Men's Health Crisis
129 West 20th Street
New York, NY 10011
(212) 807-6655 (Hotline)
(212) 645-7470 (TTY)

GMHC is the world's first AIDS organization, founded by members of the gay community. Staffing includes 120 paid members and 1700 to 2000 volunteers. GMHC locally serves the New York City area. Its purposes are to maintain and improve the quality of life for persons with AIDS, ARC, and their care partners, to advocate for fair and effective public policies and practices concerning HIV infection, and through education and AIDS prevention programs, to increase awareness and understanding of HIV infection. Services include the buddy system (volunteers assigned to AIDS patients to help with daily chores), crisis intervention, meals, tickets to theaters, outings, exercise machines (at the facility), legal assistance, complaint department, AIDS profesional education program, and a speakers bureau. GMHC lobbys in New York City and Washington on AIDS issues. A newsletter on treatment issues and experimental drug therapies is published 10 times per year.

5. Health Education AIDS Liaison
PO Box 1103
Old Chelsea Station
New York, NY 10103
(212) 674-HOPE (Counseling)
(212) 243-3612 (Information packet—leave name and address)

Formed in 1982 to challenge the idea that AIDS is fatal, HEAL is a nonprofit organization providing holistic and alternative treatment approaches to people with AIDS. Their services include weekly information and support groups, monthly intensive healing workshops, forums, and a clearinghouse.

6. National AIDS Hotline
(800) 342-2437 (Open 24 hours, 7 days a week)
(800) 344-7432 (Spanish, live operator from 8 AM–2 PM)
(800) 243-7889 (TTY/TDD, Monday–Friday, 10 AM–10 PM)

The hotline is staffed by volunteers and paid workers with information from the CDC, Federal Government, etc. The hotline offers counseling, referrals to other agencies, hotlines and local AIDS testing sites, printed materials, and a wealth of additional information.
Sampling of pamphlets:
What About AIDS Testing
How You Won't Get AIDS
If Your AIDS Test is Positive
Surgeon General's Report on AIDS
Facts About AIDS
Understanding AIDS
Guidelines for Effective School Health Education to Prevent the Spread of AIDS
Information for Teachers and School Officials: AIDS and Children
Information for Parents: AIDS and Children
Pamphlets available in Spanish, Laotian, and Braille:
AIDS and the Safety of the Nation's Blood Supply
Caring for the AIDS Patient at Home

7. National AIDS Information Clearinghouse
PO Box 6003
Rockville, MD 20850
(800) 458-5231 (Publications)
(301) 762-5111 (Database)

This is a clearinghouse for free publications from the CDC and other organizations. A catalog is available on request. The database access provides additional information for speakers and other AIDS-related resources.
Partial list of publications:
Understanding AIDS (English, Spanish, Chinese, Braille, Portugese)
MMWR *(Morbidity and Mortality Weekly Report)*
Universal Precautions for Health Care Workers (Reprint)
Monthly Report CDC HIV/AIDS Surveillance
AIDS and Deafness Resource Directory
AIDS Education: A Business Guide (AIDS in the Workplace)

8. National AIDS Network
2033 M Street, NW
Suite 800
Washington, DC 20036
(202) 293-2437

NAN is a resource center and national voice for community-based volunteer organizations that provide AIDS services and education. Currently, 700 volunteer organizations and 200 health departments belong to the network. NAN offers

many services including technical assistance in areas such as volunteer management and buddy programs, a clearinghouse for current resources, directories, and publications.
Publications:
Network News (monthly newsletter)
NAN Multi-Cultural Notes (monthly newsletter)
NAN Monitor (quarterly newsletter)
NAN Directory of AIDS Education and Service Organizations
NAN Video Directory
NAN Directory of AIDS-Related Periodicals
AIDS Into the 90s: Strategies for an Integrated Response to the AIDS Epidemic
The CORO Report
Americans Who Care
Heads, Hearts, & Hands

9. National Association of People with AIDS
2025 Eye Street, NW
Suite 415
Washington, DC 20006
(202) 429-2856

NAPWA's members are people living with AIDS, ARC, and HIV helping themselves and others. Local chapters serve their own communities, offering housing, meals, peer support groups, information pamphlets, alternative therapies and holistic healing, forums on AIDS for health care professionals, and other programs. The national office service include the newsletter *NAPWA NEWS*, scholarships and traveling expenses to national meetings and conferences, technical assistance to local chapters in areas such as fundraising and grantwriting, and administering two funds that support education of and advocacy by people with AIDS.

10. National Minority AIDS Council
714 G Street, SE
Washington, DC 20003
(202) 544-1076

Composed of nearly 160 education and service or community-based minority AIDS organizations, NMAC is dedicated to "creating a greater, more coordinated response among People of Color to the devastating and disproportionate effect of AIDS on minority communities." It provides technical assistance to its member organizations and emerging organizations, promotes AIDS education among the minorities, influences policymakers on a community and national level, creates resources for AIDS programs and education, and acts as a national advocate for the minority response to the AIDS epidemic.

11. Project Inform
347 Dolores Street, Suite 301
San Francisco, CA 94110
(800) 822-7422 (national 10 AM to 2 PM PST)
(800) 334-7422 (California)
(415) 558-9051 (local)

This nonprofit volunteer organization gives current available information on drug treatment protocols for HIV, ARC, and AIDS. The information is available nationally and internationally free of charge with donations accepted. Project Inform publishes a quarterly newsletter, *P.I. Perspectives.*"

12. San Francisco AIDS Foundation
PO Box 6182
San Francisco, CA 94101
(415) 863-2437
(800) FOR AIDS (Northern California Hotline)
(415) 864-6606 (TTY)

Locally, the foundation offers an emergency housing and food bank, case management, and support groups to persons with ARC and AIDS. It also has two special programs: (1) a bilingual multicultural program with support groups and events in Spanish and other languages and (2) a program of women's services. Another aspect of the foundation is disseminating publications and information, which is available free to local San Francisco nonprofit agencies but with some restrictions to nonprofit agencies and individuals outside the San Francisco area.
Brochures:
AIDS and Healthcare Workers
Women and AIDS
Alcohol, Drugs and AIDS
Your Child and AIDS
Risky Business (comic book for teenagers)
When a Friend has AIDS

13. The Women AIDS Network
c/o San Francisco AIDS Foundation
PO Box 6182
San Francisco, CA 94101
(415) 863-2437

The Women's AIDS Network is a coalition of women providers to individuals with AIDS. Their monthly meeting is in San Francisco. Membership is $20 for individual and $30 for institution. Benefits of membership include monthly mailings encompassing new information about women and AIDS, legislation, conferences, and education.

Organizations Devoted to Pain

1. American Academy of Pain Medicine
43 East Ohio, Suite 914
Chicago, IL 60611
(312) 645-0083

Founded in 1983, the AAPM is comprised of physicians and surgeons whose practices involve a large number of patients with chronic intractable pain. Its mission is "to enhance the practice of pain medicine in the United States." Primary goals include quality and comprehensive treatment of patients with intractable chronic pain through education and research, and promoting "a socioeconomic and political climate which will be conducive to the practice of pain medicine in an effective and efficient manner." One of the objectives of the AAPM is to be the official organization representing physicians who specialize in the field of pain medicine in the USA.

2. American Chronic Pain Association
257 Old Haymaker Road
Monroeville, PA 15146
(412) 856-9676

ACPA, founded in Pittsburgh in 1980, is now a national organization with 174 chapters. Its purpose is to provide support groups for persons with chronic pain. The focus is on coping and living with chronic pain, moving from the role of the patient back to being a person. The groups are open to chronic pain sufferers, should not be affiliated with a hospital or other institution or meet in a hospital, and the facilitator is a person with chronic pain. Professionals are not allowed to practice therapy at group meetings. Members are chronic pain sufferers. Membership entitles one to the ACPA Member's Manual and relaxation tapes at reduced rates.

3. American Pain Society
1200 17th Street NW
Suite 400
Washington, DC 20036
(202) 296-9200

The APS, a national chapter of the International Association for the Study of Pain, is a professional multidisciplinary educational society promoting acute and chronic pain control. Membership includes the quarterly APS Newsletter, *Principles of Analgesic Use in the Treatment of Acute Pain and Chronic Cancer Pain,* meetings and special events information and discount rates at the annual meeting.

4. American Society of Clinical Hypnosis
2250 East Devon, Suite 336
Des Plaines, IL 60018
(312) 297-3317

The American Society of Clinical Hypnosis is comprised of 3500 doctorally prepared professionals (physicians, dentists, psychologists) who use hypnosis in their clinical practice. Of interest is the use of hypnosis in the treatment of pain and side effects of chemotherapy. The society publishes a quarterly journal, *American Journal of Clinical Hypnosis.* It also has a speakers bureau and a referral service.

5. Association for Applied Psychophysiology and Applied Biofeedback
10200 West 44th Avenue
Wheatridge, CO 80037
(303) 422-8436

The reader may contact this organization for resource people working with biofeedback in a particular specialty or region of the United States.

6. Commission on Accreditation of Rehabilitation Facilities
101 North Wilmot Road, Suite 500
Tucson, AZ 85711
(602) 748-1212

CARF provides national accreditation and standards on a variety of programs including chronic pain management. Many states recognize the value of CARF accreditation and require it for licensure. On request, CARF will send a list of accredited chronic pain management clinics.

7. The Committee on the Treatment of Intractable Pain
PO Box 9553
Friendship Station
Washington, DC 20016
(202) 965-6717

The major purpose of the committee is to promote education and research on more effective management and alleviation of intractable pain, particularly pain that is beyond the control of available drugs and conventional techniques. One activity of the committee is to seek the transfer of heroin from Schedule I of the Controlled Substance Act, which designates it of no medical use, to Schedule II, which places it in the same restricted category as morphine.

8. InControl: Cancer Pain Care Association
2320 Tracy Place NW
Washington, DC 20008
(202) 483-6108

Educational and consulting services are provided for a fee to physicians, nurses, patients, and significant others on pain and pain management. Telephone consultation is available without charge.

9. International Association for the Study of Pain
909 NE 43rd Street, Suite 306
Seattle, WA 98105
(206) 547-6409

The purposes of IASP are multifold and include promoting professional and public education, encouraging research, disseminating new information, developing a national and international data bank, formatting national associations for the study and treatment of pain, sponsoring world congresses, and encouraging the adoption of a uniform classification system of pain. Presently, there are 20 national chapters. Regular membership fees are salary based and include a subscription to the monthly journal *PAIN*, the IASP newsletter, and a members' directory.

10. National Chronic Pain Outreach Association, Inc.
4922 Hampden Lane
Bethesda, MD 20814
(301) 652-4948

Established in 1980, NCPOA is a nonprofit organization that receives its funds from the public. Its purpose is to reduce chronic pain suffering. Services provided include a clearinghouse for pain information and management, the quarterly newsletter *Lifeline,* seminars and lectures, local support groups for chronic pain sufferers and their families, and professional education. Membership has several categories and includes *Lifeline* and reduced rates for publications, pamphlets, and audio tapes.

Publications:
Recommended Reading List
Pain Management Strategies
Flare-up Coping Tips
Choosing a Pain Clinic or Specialist
The Mind-Body Dilemma
10 Hints for Helping Your Patients with Chronic Pain
Support Group Discussion Topics
Arthritis and Bradykinins
Neuropathy Pain

Audio cassette tapes:
Chronic Pain and Hypnosis
Progressive Relaxation Exercise

11. National Pain Association
Department of Family Health Care Nursing
Pain Study Office, N411Y
University of California, San Francisco
San Francisco, CA 94134
(415) 476-4400

Founded in the bay area relatively recently, the NPA seeks to encourage education, research, and high standards of nursing care in treating patients with acute and chronic pain. The NPA also fosters communication and dissemination of information among members and with other nursing colleagues. Membership requires one to be an RN and pay annual dues of $10.

12. Society for Behavioral Medicine
PO Box 8530
University Station
Knoxville, TN 37996
(615) 974-5164

The Society is a scientific multidisciplinary organization whose purpose is to communicate the relationship between behavior and health among researchers, academicians, and clinicians. One of its areas of research and clinical practice is chronic pain treatment. Membership has several categories and includes two quarterly journals, *Behavioral Medicine Abstracts* and *Annals of Behavioral Medicine,* as well as reduced rates on publications and the annual meeting.

13. Wisconsin Pain Initiative
3675 Medical Sciences Center
University of Wisconsin Medical School

1300 University Avenue
Madison, WI 53706

The Initiative started in 1986 as a statewide comprehensive effort to improve the management of cancer pain. The Initiative focuses on educating the patient, family, public, and professional, establishing patient care advocates to improve clinical cancer pain management, overcoming regulatory, legislative, and system barriers such as inadequate stocking of narcotics secondary to fear of theft, and determining through research and evaluation the success and future direction of the Initiative. The World Health Organization (WHO) designated Wisconsin as a demonstration state in the effort of worldwide cancer pain relief. *Handbook of Cancer Pain Management* can be purchased for $3 at the above address. A bimonthly newsletter, *Cancer Pain Update*, listing meetings and statewide activities can be obtained by contacting *Cancer Pain Update*, Jeanne Dosch (ed), 3717 Ross Street, Madison, WI 53705. A patient education booklet, *Cancer Pain Can Be Relieved*, is available through the ACS—Wisconsin Division, 615 North Sherman Avenue, Madison, WI 53704.

14. World Health Organization
Publications Center, USA
49 Sheridan Avenue
Albany, NY 12210

WHO sponsors the Cancer Pain Relief Program, which essentially proposes cancer pain relief as a worldwide priority. One can contact WHO to receive a booklet titled *Cancer Pain Relief*. The booklet discusses the prevalence of cancer pain, the need for education and training in pain management, legislative factors, pharmacologic guidelines, etc.

Oncology Nursing Organizations and Related Oncology Professional Organizations

1. American Association for Cancer Education
Samuel Brown, EdD
Secretary, AACE
Educational Research and Development
University of Alabama at Birmingham
401 CHSD University Street
Birmingham, AL 35294

The purpose of the AACE has been "to provide a forum for those concerned with education of groups who attempt to advance the cause of early cancer detection, promote individualized multimodality therapy, or develop programs of rehabilitation for cancer patients." This multidisciplinary organization brings together basic scientists, surgeons, internists, oncology nursing educators, pediatricians, pathologists, gynecologists, dentists, and radiation oncologists. They hold an annual fall meeting, and members receive the *Journal of Cancer Education* and other publications on cancer education.

2. American Association for Cancer Research
Margaret Foti, Executive Director
530 Walnut Street, Tenth Floor
Philadelphia, PA 19106
(215) 440-9300

AACR provides an organization of research workers for presentation and discussion of new and significant observations and problems in cancer.

3. American Cancer Society
Trish Greene, RN, MSN, Vice President, Cancer Nursing
Tower Place
3340 Peachtree Road, NE
Atlanta, GA 30026
(404) 320-3333

4. American Society of Clinical Oncology
435 North Michigan Avenue
Chicago, IL 60611-4067
(312) 644-0828

ASCO is a professional organization of physicians board-certified in neoplastic diseases and other health care professionals of the doctorate level whose interests involve biology, diagnosis, prevention, or treatment of human cancer. Affiliate membership is granted to oncology nurses, physician assistants, and other paramedical personnel involved with the care of oncology patients. Membership includes attendance at the annual meeting.

5. Association of Community Cancer Centers
Lee Mortenson, Executive Director
11600 Bevel Street, Suite 201
Rockville, MD 20852
(301) 984-9496

The ACCC acts as the national voice of community cancer care professionals. It serves as a forum on national issues and a source of information on clinical research organizations, new technology, and research results. Annual dues are $100 (1989). Members include institutions and individuals. Membership benefits include a copy of ACCC's quarterly publication, *Oncology Issues*, and an annual publication, *Community Cancer Programs in the United States*.

6. Association of Freestanding Radiation Oncology Centers
3960 Park Boulevard, Suite E
San Diego, CA 92103
(610) 692-1598

AFROC is a nonprofit organization composed of physicists, physicians, administrators, technicians, and clinical personnel working in freestanding, fully equipped radiation centers. It acts as a forum for addressing concerns and as an advocate for reimbursement and legislative policies affecting the centers. Full membership is $400, and benefits include a quarterly newsletter, *Source*, legislative information, reduced rates at the annual meeting, and current information on reimbursement, economic issues, practice development/marketing ideas, financial management, quality assurance, and more.

7. Association of Pediatric Oncology Nurses
11508 Allecingie Parkway, Suite C
Richmond, VA 23235
(804) 379-9150

APON has been in existence since 1973. Membership in the organization is open to all registered nurses who are either interested in or engaged in pediatrics or pediatric oncology. Annual dues are $55 (1989), which entitles the member to receive a copy of the quarterly journal, *J.A.P.O.N.*, *A.P.O.N. Newsletter*, and other pertinent publications, attend all business meetings and programs at a reduced rate, and vote on all issues concerning the organization. The objectives of the organization are to promote excellence in the specialty of pediatric oncology nursing, provide opportunities for communication among all nurses who work with children who have cancer through quarterly newsletters and an annual seminar, encourage dissemination of information among nurses about the medical and nursing care of pediatric oncology patients that is used in various areas of the country, encourage members to update professional and lay literature with regard to the care of children with cancer, and encourage and support research in nursing care of children with cancer.

8. Food and Drug Administration
Office for Consumer Affairs
HFE-88
5600 Fishers Lane
Rockville, MD 20857
(301) 443-3170

The FDA serves as a source for information regarding FDA regulations, cosmetics, foods, drugs, health fraud, and medical devices.

9. International Society of Nurses in Cancer Care
Carol Reed Ash, EdD, RN, FAAN
Secretary/Treasurer
Adelphi University School of Nursing
Box 516
Garden City, NY 11530
(516) 663-1001

Established in 1984, this society's goal is "to enable cancer nurses to share their knowledge and problems on a worldwide basis." Individual membership is $35 per year and entitles one to the bimonthly journal, *Cancer Nursing: An International Journal for Cancer Care,* and attendance at the biennial international meetings.

10. International Union Against Cancer
(Union Internationale Contre Le Cancer - UICC)
Rue de Conseil - General 3
1205 Geneva, Switzerland
Telephone: (41-22) 20 18 11

UICC is composed of multidisciplinary cancer organizations. Its purpose is to encourage the fight against cancer worldwide, promoting communication internationally in cancer research, treatment, and prevention. It is also a certifying government of legitimate cancer-fighting organizations. Membership dues are based on an organization's ability to pay. Congresses are held biennially.

11. National Institute for Occupational Safety and Health
US Department of Health and Human Services
Room 714B
200 Independence Avenue, SW
Washington, DC 20201
(202) 472-7134
(800) 35 NIOSH (Clearinghouse)

NIOSH is a federal research agency. Of interest is its research in the area of handling cytotoxic drugs and laminar airflow hoods. It also has developed guidelines for health care workers in preventing the transmission of hepatitis B virus and HIV. For information on printed materials, contact the clearinghouse.

12. National Tumor Registrars Association
11600 Nebel Street, Suite 201
Rockville, MD 20852
(301) 984-1748

The purpose of the NTRA is to provide support and promote tumor registry and its use. Both certified and noncertified tumor registrars may be members in this organization. The NTRA will assist certified members in maintaining their credentials. Information gathered from tumor registry is used for statistics, research, epidemiology, quality assurance, screening, etc, but its main focus is the patient and quality care.

13. Oncology Nursing Society
1016 Greentree Road
Pittsburgh, PA 15220-3125
(412) 921-7373

ONS was founded in 1975 to promote the highest professional standards of oncology nursing; study, research, and exchange information, experiences, and ideas leading to improved oncology nursing; encourage nurses to specialize in the practice of oncology nursing; identify resources within the group; and establish guidelines of nursing care for patients with cancer. Annual dues are $53 (1989), which entitles a member to the society's referred journal, *Oncology Nursing Forum,* and a newsletter, *ONS News,* which are published six times per year. Members are also entitled to reduced rates for the annual Congress, an opportunity to serve on society committees, and research and travel awards. ONS publishes guidelines and standards for various aspects of oncology nursing and makes these publications available through its national office. In 1989 there were more than 100 chapters of ONS across the country.

Partial list of publications:
Cancer Related Resources in U.S.
Graduate Programs in Cancer Nursing
Patient Classification Systems: An Annotated Bibliography (1987)
Membership Directory (1988-89)
Standards
Standards of Oncology Nursing Practice (1987)
Cancer Patient Education (1982)
Public Cancer Education (1982)
Modules—Cancer Chemotherapy Guidelines
Course Content and Clinical Practicum (1988)
Acute Care Setting (1988)
Outpatient Setting (1988)
Home Care Setting (1988)
Management of Extravasation and Anaphylaxis (1988)
Monographs
Oncology Nursing Reflections (1985)
The Role of the Oncology Nurse in the Office Setting
Oncology Nursing Forum
Oncology Nursing Forum Index
Oncology Nursing Forum Back Issues
Annual Congress Supplement
Audio/visual
Those Were Hard Days
History of ONS

14. Occupational Safety and Health Administration
US Department of Labor
200 Constitution Avenue, NW
Washington, DC 20210
(202) 523-8151

OSHA is a federal enforcement agency. It has published guidelines for handling antineoplastic drugs (currently being updated) and other information related to health care worker safety.

GOVERNMENT AGENCIES/PROGRAMS*

Resources for Cancer Education

1. Center for Health Promotion and Education
Centers for Disease Control
Building 1 South, Room SSB249
1600 Clifton Road, NE
Atlanta, GA 30333
(404) 329-3492

   The Center has a number of programs that emphasize prevention: providing technical assistance to state and local health departments on tracking risk factor conditions in the population; coordinating the Behavioral Risk Factor Surveillance System, a telephone-based survey on major risk factors such as smoking, alcohol, nutrition, hypertension, weight, and seat belt use; implementing School Health Education Evaluation project, an extensive evaluation of the impact of school health education programs on students' health-related behaviors; and maintaining a Health Education Database, a computer online summary of national health education efforts.
2. Clearinghouse for Occupational Safety and Health Information
National Institute for Occupational Safety and Health
Technical Information Branch
4676 Columbia Parkway
Cincinnati, OH 45226
(513) 684-8326

   Provides technical information to the National Institute for Occupational Safety and Health research programs and supplies information to others on request.
3. Clearinghouse on Health Indexes
National Center for Health Statistics
Division of Epidemiology and Health Promotion
3700 East-West Highway, Room 2-27
Hyattsville, MD 20782
(301) 436-7035

   Provides informational assistance in the development of health measures for health researchers, administrators, and planners.
4. Consumer Information Center
General Services Administration
Pueblo, CO 81009
(303) 948-3334

   The Consumer Information Center, a mail order operation, distributes consumer publications on topics such as children, food and nutrition, health, exercise and weight control. The *Consumer Information Catalog* is available free from the Center and must be used to identify publications being requested.
5. Consumer Product Safety Commission
Washington, DC 20207
(301) 492-6800
(800) 638-2772 (Hotline)

   An independent Federal regulatory agency with jurisdiction over consumer products used in and around the home, the Commission sets standards and conducts information programs on potentially hazardous products, among them carcinogens and other chronic hazards. Single copies of printed materials are available free of charge.
6. Food and Nutrition Information Center
US Department of Agriculture
National Agricultural Library Building - Room 304
Beltsville, MD 20705
(301) 344-3719

   Serving the informational needs of professionals interested in nutrition education, food service management, and food technology, the Center acquires and lends books, journal articles, and audiovisual materials.
7. National Audiovisual Center
National Archives
8700 Edgeworth Drive
Capitol Heights, MD 20743-3701
(301) 763-1896
(301) 763-4385 (TDD)

   The National Audiovisual Center, a nonprofit public service, is the central source for federally sponsored audiovisuals. The Center distributes more than 8000 programs on over 600 topics, including cancer and the environment, breast cancer, cancer detection and smoking. Costs for these audiovisuals and accompanying printed materials range from $50 to $350.
8. Division of Cancer Prevention and Control
National Cancer Institute
National Institutes of Health
Bethesda, MD 20892-4200
(301) 496-6616

   The Division of Cancer Prevention and Control (DCPC) plans and conducts basic and applied research programs aimed at reducing cancer incidence, morbidity and mortality. Activities are carried out across five phases of research: hypothesis development, methods testing, controlled intervention trials, defined population studies, and demonstrations relevant to the prevention and management of cancer. DCPC plans, directs and coordinates the support of basic and applied research on cancer prevention and control at cancer centers and community hospitals. It also coordinates program activities with Federal and state agencies and establishes liaisons with professional and voluntary health agencies, labor organizations, cancer organizations, and trade associations.
9. Office of Cancer Communications
National Cancer Institute
National Institutes of Health
Bethesda, MD 20892
(301) 496-6631

   The Office of Cancer Communications provides information on all aspects of the cancer problem to physicians, scientists, educators, Congress, the Executive Branch, the media, and the public and fosters and coordinates a national cancer communications program designed to provide the public and health care professionals with information they need to take more responsible health actions. The CIS (1-800-4-CANCER) is located within this office, with a network of locations across the country.
10. Office of Prevention, Education, and Control
National Heart, Lung, and Blood Institute
National Institutes of Health
9000 Rockville Pike
Bethesda, MD 20892
(301) 496-5437

*Adapted from Cancer Prevention Resource Directory, National Cancer Institute, NIH pub no. 86-2827. Bethesda, Md, US Government Printing Office, 1986.

The National Heart, Lung, and Blood Institute is congressionally mandated to develop and foster informational and educational activities designed to reduce preventable heart, lung, and blood disease morbidity and mortality. This office is responsible for initiating educational activities.

11. National Clearinghouse for Alcohol Information
National Institute on Alcohol Abuse and Alcoholism
PO Box 2345
Rockville, MD 20852
(301) 468-2600

The National Clearinghouse for Alcohol Information, a service of the National Institute on Alcohol Abuse and Alcoholism, gathers and disseminates current information on alcohol-related subjects. It responds to requests from the public, health care professionals, scientists, educators, and other professionals. The Clearinghouse provides literature searches, referrals, a library and reading room, and summaries of current alcohol-related information.

12. National Library of Medicine
National Institutes of Health
8600 Rockville Pike
Bethesda, MD 20892
(301) 496-6308 Public Information Office
(301) 496-6095 Reference Section

The National Library of Medicine collects, organizes, and disseminates both printed and audiovisual materials. The collection, technical and scientific in nature, is primarily for medical professionals. The Library offers an extensive computerized literature retrieval service. A list of bibliographies, catalogs, and indexes with specific ordering instructions is available from the Public Information Office.

13. National Maternal and Child Health Clearinghouse
38th and R Street, NW
Washington, DC 20057
(202) 625-8410

The National Maternal and Child Health Clearinghouse provides information and publications on maternal and child health and genetics to consumers and health professionals. Materials cover such topics as smoking and pregnancy and nutrition and pregnancy.

14. National Toxicology Program
National Institute of Environmental Health Sciences
M.D. B2-04, Box 12233
Research Triangle Park, NC 27709
(919) 541-3991

The National Toxicology Program develops and disseminates scientific information regarding potentially hazardous chemicals, including those that can cause cancer. The program also coordinates research conducted by four agencies of the Department of Health and Human Services. Information in the form of technical reports is available free of charge to scientists and the general public.

15. Office of Consumer Affairs
Food and Drug Administration
5600 Fishers Lane
Rockville, MD 20857
(301) 443-3170

The Office of Consumer Affairs, Food and Drug Administration, responds to consumer inquiries and serves as a clearinghouse for consumer publications on a variety of topics including pregnancy, food and nutrition, cosmetics, proper use of drugs, and health fraud. Over 250 publications are available free of charge.

16. National Health Information and Clearinghouse
Office of Disease Prevention and Health Promotion
PO Box 1133
Washington, DC 20013-1133
800-336-4797
(202) 429-9091 (in Washington, DC)

The National Health Information Clearinghouse, a service of the Office of Disease Prevention and Health Promotion, is a central source of information and referral for health questions from the public and health care professionals. It maintains a computer database of government agencies, support groups, professional societies, and other organizations that can answer questions on specific health care topics. In addition, the Clearinghouse offers a library containing medical and health reference books, directories, information files, and periodicals; database development on organizations that provide health information; and a number of publications including resource guides and bibliographies. Some publications prepared by this office are the Department of Health and Human Services (DHHS) *Prevention Abstracts,* which summarizes prevention-oriented findings in the scientific literature; the DHHS *Prevention Activities Calendar,* which highlights major prevention events for the month; the *Healthfinder Series,* which provides resource lists on specific health topics such as exercise for older Americans, health risk appraisals, health statistics and many other issues; and *Staying Healthy: A Bibliography of Health Promotion Materials,* which serves as a guide to current information on health-promotion and disease-prevention topics.

17. Office on Smoking and Health
US Department of Health and Human Services
Technical Information Center
Park Building - Room 1-10
5600 Fishers Lane
Rockville, MD 20857
(301) 443-1690

The Office on Smoking and Health produces and distributes a number of informational and educational materials. It also offers bibliographic and reference services to researchers and others. The materials and services are available free of charge. In addition, the Office produces pamphlets, posters, and public service announcements that contain various health messages.

18. Public Information Center
Environmental Protection Agency
820 Quincy Street, NW
Washington, DC 20011
(202) 829-3535

Materials on such topics as hazardous wastes, the school asbestos project, air and water pollution, pesticides, and drinking water are available from the Environmental Protection Agency's Public Information Center. The Center provides information on other Environmental Protection Agency programs and activities.

19. Publication Distribution Office
Occupational Safety and Health Administration
US Department of Labor
200 Constitution Ave, NW - Room s4203
Washington, DC 20210
(202) 523-9667

The Publication Distribution Office responds to inquiries from the general public, health care professionals, industry, educational institutions, and other sources about a limited number of job-related carcinogens and toxic substances. Single copies of materials are available free of charge.

20. Information Office
National Institute on Aging
Federal Building, 6th Floor
9000 Rockville Pike
Bethesda, MD 20892
(301) 496-1752

Distributes information for older Americans on many topics, including cancer and smoking.

21. Office of Minority Health Resource Center
PO Box 37337
Washington, DC 20013-7337
1-800-444-MHRC (6472)

An office of the Department of Health and Human Services, its activities include bilingually staffed toll-free number providing minority health information and referrals, a computerized database of materials, organizations, and programs, and a resource persons network of professionals active in the field.

Other Government Offices Related to Oncology

1. International Cancer Information Center
National Cancer Institute
Bethesda, MD 20205
(301) 496-7403

This agency provides information on the computerized databases, ie, CANCERLINE, that have been detailed previously.

2. Clinical Center of the National Institutes of Health
Bethesda, MD
(301) 496-4891—Patient Referral Service

Patients who are referred to the Clinical Center by their physician and who meet the criteria for the research studies being conducted at the Clinical Center receive free nursing and medical care. A limited number of patients are accepted.

Regional Cancer Centers

The National Cancer Act of 1971 authorized the development of new comprehensive research and demonstration centers known as comprehensive cancer centers and specialized cancer centers. Through community outreach activities, comprehensive cancer centers are to provide coordination and leadership within their geographic regions to ensure the availability of complete care for patients with cancer.

At present, there are 23 comprehensive cancer centers and 21 clinical cancer centers designated by the NCI. To receive this designation by the NCI, a treatment center must meet rigorous criteria set by the NCI, including the ability to perform advanced diagnostic and treatment methods, support a strong research program, and participate in an integrated nationwide system in prevention, diagnosis, and treatment.

The following is a list of the comprehensive* and clinical† cancer centers supported by NCI as of June 1989.

Alabama

University of Alabama Comprehensive Cancer Center*
1918 University Boulevard
Basic Health Sciences Building, Room 108
Birmingham, AL 35294
(205) 934-6612

Arizona

University of Arizona Cancer Center†
1501 North Campbell Avenue
Tucson, AZ 85724
(602) 626-6372

California

The Kenneth Norris Jr. Comprehensive Cancer Center* and The Kenneth Norris Jr. Hospital and Research Institute
University of Southern California
1441 Eastlake Avenue
Los Angeles, CA 90033-0804
(213) 226-2370

Jonsson Comprehensive Cancer Center (UCLA)*
10-247 Factor Building
10833 Le Conte Avenue
Los Angeles, CA 90024-1781
(213) 825-8727

City of Hope National Medical Center†
Beckman Research Institute
1500 East Duarte Rd.
Duarte, CA 91010
(818) 359-8111, ext 2292

University of California at San Diego Cancer Center†
225 Dickinson Street
San Diego, CA 92103
(619) 543-6178

Charles R. Drew University of Medicine and Science (consortium)
12714 South Avalon Boulevard, Suite 301
Los Angeles, CA 90061
(213) 603-3120

Northern California Cancer Center (consortium)
1301 Shoreway Road
Belmont, CA 94002
(415) 591-4484

Colorado

University of Colorado Cancer Center†
4200 East 9th Avenue, Box B190
Denver, CO 80262
(203) 270-3019

Connecticut

Yale University Comprehensive Cancer Center*
333 Cedar Street
New Haven, CT 06510
(203) 785-6338

District of Columbia

Howard University Cancer Research Center*
2041 Georgia Avenue, NW
Washington, DC 20060
(202) 636-7610 or 636-5665

Vincent T. Lombardi Cancer Research Center*
Georgetown University Medical Center
3800 Reservoir Road, NW
Washington, DC 20007
(202) 687-2110

Florida

Sylvester Comprehensive Cancer Center*
University of Miami Medical School
1475 Northwest 12th Avenue
Miami, FL 33136
(305) 548-4850

Illinois—Illinois Cancer Council* (includes institutions listed and several other organizations)

Illinois Cancer Council
36 South Wabash Avenue
Chicago, IL 60603
(312) 226-2371

University of Chicago Cancer Research Center
5841 South Maryland Avenue
Chicago, IL 60637
(312) 702-9200

Kentucky

Lucille Parker Markey Cancer Center†
University of Kentucky Medical Center
800 Rose Street
Lexington, KY 40536-0093
(606) 257-4447

Maryland

The Johns Hopkins Oncology Center*
600 North Wolfe Street
Baltimore, MD 21205
(301) 955-8638

Massachusetts

Dana-Farber Cancer Institute*
44 Binney Street
Boston, MA 02115
(617) 732-3214

Michigan

Meyer L. Prentis Comprehensive Cancer Center of Metropolitan Detroit*
110 East Warren Avenue
Detroit, MI 48201
(313) 745-5429

University of Michigan Cancer Center†
101 Simpson Drive
Ann Arbor, MI 48109-0752
(313) 936-2516

Minnesota

Mayo Comprehensive Cancer Center*
200 First Street Southwest
Rochester, MN 55905
(507) 284-3413

New Hampshire

Norris Cotton Cancer Center†
Dartmouth-Hitchcock Medical Center
2 Maynard Street
Hanover, NH 03756
(603) 646-5505

New York

Memorial Sloan-Kettering Cancer Center*
1275 York Avenue
New York, NY 10021
1-800-525-2225

Columbia University Cancer Center*
College of Physicians and Surgeons
630 West 168th Street
New York, NY 10032
(212) 305-6730

Roswell Park Memorial Institute*
Elm and Carlton Streets
Buffalo, NY 14263
(716) 845-4400

Mt. Sinai School of Medicine†
One Gustave L. Levy Place
New York, NY 10029
(212) 241-8617

Albert Einstein College of Medicine†
1300 Morris Park Avenue
Bronx, NY 10461
(212) 920-4826

New York University Cancer Center†
462 First Avenue
New York, NY 10016-9103
(212) 340-6485

University of Rochester Cancer Center†
601 Elmwood Avenue, Box 704
Rochester, NY 14642
(716) 275-4911

North Carolina

Duke University Comprehensive Cancer Center*
PO Box 3843
Durham, NC 27710
(919) 286-5515

Lineberger Cancer Research Center†
University of North Carolina School of Medicine
Chapel Hill, NC 27599
(919) 966-4431

Bowman Gray School of Medicine†
Wake Forest University
300 South Hawthorne Road
Winston-Salem, NC 27103
(919) 748-4354

Ohio

Ohio State University Comprehensive Cancer Center*
410 West 12th Avenue
Columbus, OH 43210
(614) 293-8619

Case Western Reserve University†
University Hospitals of Cleveland
Ireland Cancer Center
2074 Abington Road
Cleveland, OH 44106
(216) 844-8453

Pennsylvania

Fox Chase Cancer Center*
7701 Burholme Avenue
Philadelphia, PA 19111
(215) 728-2570

University of Pennsylvania Cancer Center*
3400 Spruce Street
Philadelphia, PA 19104
(215) 662-6364

Pittsburgh Cancer Institute†
200 Meyran Avenue
Pittsburgh, PA 15213-2592
1-800-537-4063

Rhode Island

Roger Williams General Hospital†
825 Chalkstone Avenue

Providence, RI 02908
(401) 456-2070

Tennessee

St. Jude Children's Research Hospital†
332 North Lauderdale Street
Memphis, TN 38101
(901) 522-0694

Texas

The University of Texas M.D. Anderson Cancer Center*
1515 Holcombe Boulevard
Houston, TX 77030
(713) 792-6161 (Physicians)
(713) 792-3245 (Patients)

Utah

Utah Regional Cancer Center†
University of Utah Medical Center
50 North Medical Drive, Room 2C10
Salt Lake City, UT 84132
(801) 581-4048

Vermont

Vermont Regional Cancer Center†
University of Vermont
1 South Prospect Street
Burlington, VT 05401
(802) 656-4580

Virginia

Massey Cancer Center†
Medical College of Virginia
Virginia Commonwealth University
1200 East Broad Street
Richmond, VA 23298
(804) 786-9641

University of Virginia Medical Center†
Box 334
Primary Care Center, Room 4520
Lee Street
Charlottesville, VA 22908
(804) 924-2562

Washington

Fred Hutchinson Cancer Research Center*
1124 Columbia Street
Seattle, WA 98104
(206) 467-4675

Wisconsin

Wisconsin Clinical Cancer Center*
University of Wisconsin
600 Highland Avenue
Madison, WI 53792
(608) 263-6872

COOPERATIVE CLINICAL TRIAL GROUPS IN THE UNITED STATES

Below are the United States Clinical Trials Cooperative Groups and telephone numbers from which information can be obtained on clinical trials being conducted, eligibility criteria, treatment plan on the clinical trial and how to refer a patient to one of these trials. Currently in the United States fewer than 10% of eligible adult patients are entered on clinical trials. The result of this low percentage of patients is a delay in answering important therapeutic and scientific questions and in disseminating therapeutic advances to the general oncology community. There are multiple clinical trials conducted within each of the Cooperative Groups.

1. BTCG
   Brain Tumor Cooperative Group
   For patient entry information:
   Lauren Rich, Data Manager, or
   Marie Topor, Project Manager
   Information Mgmt Services, Inc.
   1400 Spring Street, Suite 500
   Silver Springs, MD 20910
   (301) 495-0440
2. CALGB
   Cancer and Leukemia Group B
   Emil Frei III MD, Chairman
   Dana-Farber Cancer Institute
   For patient entry information:
   Daniel Paterson,
   Clinical Research Manager
   CALGB Headquarters
   303 Boylston Street
   Brookline, MA 02146
   (617) 732-3676
3. CCSG
   Children's Cancer Study Group
   Denman Hammond, MD, Chairman
   University of Southern California
   For patient entry information:
   John M. Weiner, Dr. PH
   Administrative Director
   University of Southern California
   199 North Lake Avenue, 3rd Floor
   Pasadena, CA 91101-1859
   (213) 681-3032
4. ECOG
   Eastern Cooperative Oncology Group
   Paul P. Carbone, MD, Chairman
   Wisconsin Clinical Cancer Center
   University of Wisconsin
   For patient entry information:
   Barbara Miller, Coordinator
   Medical Science Center, Room 4765
   420 North Charter Street
   Madison, WI 53706
   (608) 263-6650
5. GOG
   Gynecologic Oncology Group
   For patient entry information:
   George Lewis Jr., MD, Chairman
   GOG Headquarters
   1234 Market Street, 19th Floor
   Philadelphia, PA 19107
   (215) 854-0770
6. Intergroup Rhabdomyosarcoma Study
   For patient entry information:
   Harold M. Maurer, MD, Chairman
   Professor and Chairman
   Department of Pediatrics
   Virginia Commonwealth University
   Medical College of Virginia
   MCV Box 646
   Richmond, VA 23298
   (804) 786-9602

7. LCSG
Lung Cancer Study Group
E. Carmack Holmes, MD, Chairman
UCLA School of Medicine
For patient entry information:
Sherrill Long
Administrative Coordinator
IMS, Inc.
6110 Executive Boulevard, Ste 310
Rockville, MD 20852
(301) 984-3445

8. NSABP
National Surgical Adjuvant Project for Breast and Bowel Cancers
Bernard Fisher, MD
Project Chairman
University of Pittsburgh
For patient entry information:
Mary Ketner, RN, Assistant Director for Clinical Affairs
University of Pittsburgh
914 Scaife Hall, 3550 Terrace Street
Pittsburgh, PA 15261
(412) 648-9720

9. NWTSG
National Wilms' Tumor Study Group
Guilio D'Angio, MD, Chairman
Children's Cancer Research Center
Children's Hospital of Philadelphia
For patient entry information:
Juanita Guagenti, Administrator
Children's Cancer Research Center
Children's Hospital of Philadelphia
3400 Civic Center Boulevard
Ninth Floor
Philadelphia, PA 19104
(215) 387-5518

10. NCCTG
North Central Cancer Treatment Group
Charles G. Moertel, MD, Chairman
Mayo Clinic
For patient entry information:
Mrs. Rose Smith, Supervisor
Mayo Clinic
200 First Street, SW
Rochester, MN 55905
(507) 284-8384

11. POG
Pediatric Oncology Group
Teresa J. Vietti, MD, Chairman
The Edward Mallinckrodt
Department of Pediatrics
Washington University School of Medicine
For patient entry information:
Patricia Gensel, Administrator
4949 West Pine Street, Suite 2A
St. Louis, MO 63108
(314) 367-3446

12. RTOG
Radiation Therapy Oncology Group
James Cox, MD, Chairman
M.D. Anderson Cancer Center
For patient entry information, contact:
Sharon Hartson, Coordinator
RTOG Headquarters
American College of Radiology
1101 Market Street, 14th Floor
Philadelphia, PA 19107
(215) 574-3205

13. SWOG
Southwest Oncology Group
Charles A. Coltman, MD, Chairman
Cancer Therapy & Research Center
San Antonio, TX
For patient entry information:
Ms. Marj Godfrey, Coordinator
5430 Fredericksburg Road
San Antonio, TX 78229-3533
(512) 366-9300

INDEX